MAYO CLINIC
INTERNAL MEDICINE
BOARD REVIEW
2004-2005

MAYO CLINIC INTERNAL MEDICINE BOARD REVIEW 2004-2005

Thomas M. Habermann, M.D.

Editor-in-Chief

Associate Editors

S. Vincent Rajkumar, M.D.

Randall S. Edson, M.D.

Scott C. Litin, M.D.

Amit K. Ghosh, M.D.

Dennis K. McCallum, Pharm.D.

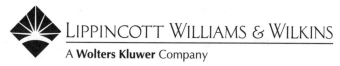
LIPPINCOTT WILLIAMS & WILKINS

A **Wolters Kluwer** Company

Philadelphia · Baltimore · New York · London
Buenos Aires · Hong Kong · Sydney · Tokyo

Acquisitions Editor: Danette Somers
Development Editor: Mary Choi
Production Editor: Robert Pancotti
Manufacturing Manager: Benjamin Rivera
Indexer: Mary Kidd
Cover Designer: Jeffrey A. Satre
Printer: Courier Westford

9 8 7 6 5 4 3 2 1

Printed in the USA

ISBN: 0-7817-5773-8

Care has been taken to confirm the accuracy of the information presented and
to describe generally accepted practices. However, the authors, editors, and
publisher are not responsible for errors or omissions or for any consequences
from application of the information in this book and make no warranty, express
or implied, with respect to the contents of the publication. This book should
not be relied on apart from the advice of a qualified health care provider.

The authors, editors, and publisher have exerted efforts to ensure that drug
selection and dosage set forth in this text are in accordance with current recommendations and practice at the time of publication. However, in view of
ongoing research, changes in government regulations, and the constant flow
of information relating to drug therapy and drug reactions, the reader is urged
to check the package insert for each drug for any change in indications and
dosage and for added warnings and precautions. This is particularly important
when the recommended agent is a new or infrequently employed drug.

Some drugs and medical devices presented in this publication have Food
and Drug Administration (FDA) clearance for limited use in restricted research
settings. It is the responsibility of the health care providers to ascertain the FDA
status of each drug or device planned for use in their clinical practice.

DEDICATED TO

All students of medicine,
whatever their level of experience
and whatever their needs

FOREWORD

The sixth edition of *Mayo Clinic Internal Medicine Board Review 2004-2005* reflects the continued commitment by the faculty of the Department of Internal Medicine to its mission of scholarship. One of the key traditions in medicine is the passing of knowledge from physician to physician. In 1928, William J. Mayo, M.D., wrote, "The glory of medicine is that it is constantly moving forward, that there is always more to learn. The ills of today do not cloud the horizon of tomorrow, but act as a spur to greater effort."* This edition is a response to these themes. My hope is that this book will aid in the study of medicine and in the care of patients.

Nicholas F. LaRusso, M.D.
Chair, Department of Internal Medicine
Mayo Clinic, Rochester, Minnesota

*Mayo WJ: The aims and ideals of the American Medical Association. Proceedings of the 66th Annual Meeting of the National Education Association of the United States, 1928, pp 158-163.

PREFACE

The pace of change in medicine is remarkable. These changes require physicians to remain abreast of the latest developments not only in their areas of expertise but also in areas beyond their sphere of expertise. To assist physicians in this endeavor, the Department of Internal Medicine at Mayo Clinic remains committed to providing continuing medical education to physicians in a timely manner. *Mayo Clinic Internal Medicine Board Review 2004-2005* is designed to meet the needs of physicians-in-training and practicing clinicians by updating their knowledge of internal medicine and also by helping them prepare for the certifying and recertifying examinations in internal medicine.

The success of the earlier editions of *Mayo Clinic Internal Medicine Board Review* is exemplified by the number of books published. The positive reaction to and the success enjoyed by the earlier editions prompted the Department of Internal Medicine to proceed with the publication of this, the sixth, edition.

The overall approach in learning medicine may perhaps be summed up in two questions. What is it? What do you do for it? Ongoing efforts have been made to improve the book and its answers to these questions. Each section is updated each year. Over time, algorithms and diagrams have been added and changed. The goal is to have an update that is readable and easy to study.

The book is divided into subspecialty topics, each chapter written by an author(s) with clinical expertise in the designated topic. Appropriate images and tables continue to be enhanced. Each chapter has bulleted items that highlight key points. These may be summary points from previous paragraphs or new points. Bulleted items also address typical clinical scenarios. These scenarios emphasize classic clinical presentations. Pharmacy tables are included with many of the chapters. The scenarios and pharmacy tables highlight two key issues. First, the general internist and the subspecialist diagnose diseases in internal medicine. Second, the predominant type of patient management is pharmacologic. Knowledge of the indications, toxic effects, and drug interactions is of paramount importance. Multiple-choice questions with a single answer follow each chapter. As many clinical cases as possible are included in the questions. This edition has approximately 300 multiple-choice questions. The answers with explanatory notes follow the questions. Material in the questions and answers is not included in the index.

Some points from the earlier editions are worth repeating. This book is not a comprehensive textbook of internal medicine. It should be used only as a guide containing selected topics considered important for physicians reviewing internal medicine or preparing for either the certifying or the recertifying examination offered by the American Board of Internal Medicine or other examining institutions. This book is prepared with the assumption that readers have studied one of the standard textbooks of internal medicine and have supplemented their study of this review with additional readings of the literature.

I thank everyone who offered important ideas for improvement during the development of this book. I am grateful to the authors of the previous editions for providing input into this edition and for permitting the use of some of their materials. I am indebted to all authors for their contributions. I thank the staffs of the Section of Scientific Publications, Department of Medicine, and Media Support Services at Mayo Clinic for their contributions to this edition. The support and cooperation of the publisher, Lippincott Williams & Wilkins, are gratefully acknowledged.

I trust that the sixth edition of *Mayo Clinic Internal Medicine Board Review* will serve to update and advance the reader's knowledge of internal medicine, as previous editions have done.

I hope that you have enjoyed this review as much as I have.

Thomas M. Habermann, M.D.
Editor-in-Chief

ACKNOWLEDGMENTS

I thank the Mayo Clinic production staff for their efforts and commitment to this book: O. E. Millhouse, Ph.D., LeAnn Stee, Roberta Schwartz, Virginia Dunt, and Renée Van Vleet, Scientific Publications; Jeff Satre, Media Support Services; and Cindy Cunningham, Internal Medicine.

CONTRIBUTORS

Timothy R. Aksamit, M.D.
Consultant, Division of Pulmonary and Critical Care Medicine and Internal Medicine,* Assistant Professor of Medicine†

Robert C. Albright, Jr., D.O.
Consultant, Division of Nephrology, Hypertension, and Internal Medicine,* Assistant Professor of Medicine†

Thomas Behrenbeck, M.D., Ph.D.
Consultant, Division of Cardiovascular Diseases and Internal Medicine,* Associate Professor of Medicine†

Eduardo E. Benarroch, M.D.
Consultant, Department of Neurology,* Professor of Neurology†

Peter A. Brady, M.D.
Senior Associate Consultant, Division of Cardiovascular Diseases and Internal Medicine,* Assistant Professor of Medicine†

Robert D. Brown, Jr., M.D.
Consultant, Department of Neurology,* Associate Professor of Neurology†

Darryl S. Chutka, M.D.
Consultant, Division of Preventive and Occupational Medicine and Internal Medicine,* Associate Professor of Medicine†

William F. Dunn, M.D.
Consultant, Division of Pulmonary and Critical Care Medicine and Internal Medicine,* Assistant Professor of Medicine†

Stephen B. Erickson, M.D.
Consultant, Division of Nephrology, Hypertension, and Internal Medicine,* Assistant Professor of Medicine†

Lynn L. Estes, Pharm.D.
Infectious Disease Pharmacist Specialist,* Assistant Professor of Pharmacy†

Fernando C. Fervenza, M.D., Ph.D.
Consultant, Division of Nephrology, Hypertension, and Internal Medicine,* Assistant Professor of Medicine†

Paul A. Friedman, M.D.
Consultant, Division of Cardiovascular Diseases and Internal Medicine,* Associate Professor of Medicine†

William W. Ginsburg, M.D.
Consultant, Division of Rheumatology and Internal Medicine,‡ Associate Professor of Medicine†

Thomas M. Habermann, M.D.
Consultant, Division of Hematology and Internal Medicine,* Professor of Medicine†

Gregory D. Hart, M.D.
Senior Associate Consultant, Division of Infectious Diseases and Internal Medicine,* Instructor in Medicine†

C. Christopher Hook, M.D.
Consultant, Division of Hematology and Internal Medicine,* Assistant Professor of Medicine†

Barry L. Karon, M.D.
Consultant, Division of Cardiovascular Diseases and Internal Medicine,* Assistant Professor of Medicine†

Kyle W. Klarich, M.D.
Consultant, Division of Cardiovascular Diseases and Internal Medicine,* Assistant Professor of Medicine†

*Mayo Clinic, Rochester, Minnesota.
†Mayo Clinic College of Medicine, Rochester, Minnesota.
‡Mayo Clinic, Jacksonville, Florida.

Lois E. Krahn, M.D.
Consultant, Department of Psychiatry and Psychology,* Associate Professor of Psychiatry†

Scott C. Litin, M.D.
Consultant, Division of Area General Internal Medicine,* Professor of Medicine†

William F. Marshall, M.D.
Consultant, Division of Infectious Diseases and Internal Medicine,* Assistant Professor of Medicine†

Marian T. McEvoy, M.D.
Chair, Division of Clinical Dermatology,* Associate Professor of Dermatology†

Virginia V. Michels, M.D.
Consultant, Department of Medical Genetics,* Professor of Medical Genetics†

Clement J. Michet, Jr., M.D.
Consultant, Division of Rheumatology and Internal Medicine,* Associate Professor of Medicine†

Kevin G. Moder, M.D.
Consultant, Division of Rheumatology and Internal Medicine,* Assistant Professor of Medicine†

Neena Natt, M.D.
Consultant, Division of Endocrinology, Diabetes, Metabolism, Nutrition and Internal Medicine,* Assistant Professor of Medicine†

Rick A. Nishimura, M.D.
Consultant, Division of Cardiovascular Diseases and Internal Medicine,* Professor of Medicine†

Scott H. Okuno, M.D.
Consultant, Division of Medical Oncology,* Assistant Professor of Oncology†

Steve R. Ommen, M.D.
Consultant, Division of Cardiovascular Diseases and Internal Medicine,* Assistant Professor of Medicine†

John G. Park, M.D.
Senior Associate Consultant, Division of Pulmonary and Critical Care Medicine and Internal Medicine,* Instructor in Medicine†

Steve G. Peters, M.D.
Consultant, Division of Pulmonary and Critical Care Medicine and Internal Medicine,* Professor of Medicine†

John J. Poterucha, M.D.
Consultant, Division of Gastroenterology and Hepatology and Internal Medicine,* Associate Professor of Medicine†

Frank A. Rubino, M.D.
Consultant, Department of Neurology,‡ Professor of Neurology†

Thomas R. Schwab, M.D.
Consultant, Division of Nephrology, Hypertension, and Internal Medicine,* Associate Professor of Medicine†

Gary L. Schwartz, M.D.
Consultant, Division of Nephrology, Hypertension, and Internal Medicine,* Associate Professor of Medicine†

Robert E. Sedlack, M.D.
Senior Associate Consultant, Division of Gastroenterology and Hepatology and Internal Medicine,* Assistant Professor of Medicine†

Marcia J. Slattery, M.D.
Consultant, Section of Adult Psychiatry,* Assistant Professor of Psychiatry†

Peter C. Spittell, M.D.
Consultant, Division of Cardiovascular Diseases and Internal Medicine,* Assistant Professor of Medicine†

Karen L. Swanson, D.O.
Senior Associate Consultant, Division of Pulmonary and Critical Care Medicine and Internal Medicine,* Assistant Professor of Medicine†

*Mayo Clinic, Rochester, Minnesota.
†Mayo Clinic College of Medicine, Rochester, Minnesota.
‡Mayo Clinic, Jacksonville, Florida.

Zelalem Temesgen, M.D.
Consultant, Division of Infectious Diseases and Internal Medicine,* Assistant Professor of Medicine†

Charles F. Thomas, Jr., M.D.
Consultant, Division of Pulmonary and Critical Care Medicine and Internal Medicine,* Assistant Professor of Medicine†

Sally J. Trippel, M.D., M.P.H.
Consultant, Division of Preventive and Occupational Medicine and Internal Medicine,* Instructor in Preventive Medicine†

Adrian Vella, M.D.
Senior Associate Consultant, Division of Endocrinology, Diabetes, Metabolism, Nutrition and Internal Medicine,* Assistant Professor of Medicine†

*Mayo Clinic, Rochester, Minnesota.
†Mayo Clinic College of Medicine, Rochester, Minnesota.
‡Mayo Clinic, Jacksonville, Florida.

Thomas R. Viggiano, M.D.
Consultant, Division of Gastroenterology and Hepatology and Internal Medicine,* Professor of Medicine†

Abinash Virk, M.D.
Consultant, Division of Infectious Diseases and Internal Medicine,* Assistant Professor of Medicine†

Gerald W. Volcheck, M.D.
Consultant, Division of Allergic Diseases and Internal Medicine,* Assistant Professor of Medicine†

Amy W. Williams, M.D.
Consultant, Division of Nephrology, Hypertension, and Internal Medicine,* Assistant Professor of Medicine†

John W. Wilson, M.D.
Consultant, Division of Infectious Diseases and Internal Medicine,* Assistant Professor of Medicine†

CONTRIBUTORS FOR PHARMACY REVIEW

Alma N. Adrover, R.Ph., M.S.
Jeffrey J. Armon, Pharm.D.
Kari L. Beierman, Pharm.D.
Sansana D. Boontaveekul, Pharm.D.
Lisa K. Buss, Pharm.D.
Julie L. Cunningham, Pharm.D.
Lynn L. Estes, Pharm.D.
Jamie M. Gardner, Pharm.D.
Darryl C. Grendahl, R.Ph.
Thomas M. Habermann, M.D.
Lisa G. Hall, Pharm.D.
Robert W. Hoel, R.Ph.
Todd M. Johnson, Pharm.D.
Carrie A. Krieger, Pharm.D.

Philip J. Kuper, Pharm.D.
Susan V. McCluskey, R.Ph.
Robert B. McMahan, Pharm.D., M.B.A.
Kevin W. Odell, Pharm.D.
Laura J. Odell, Pharm.D.
John G. O'Meara, Pharm.D.
Narith N. Ou, Pharm.D.
Lance J. Oyen, Pharm.D.
Michael A. Schwarz, Pharm.D.
Virginia H. Thompson, R.Ph.
Christopher M. Wittich, Pharm.D., M.D.
Kelly K. Wix, Pharm.D.
Robert C. Wolf, Pharm.D.

TABLE OF CONTENTS

1. **THE BOARD EXAMINATION** 1
   Darryl S. Chutka, M.D.

2. **ALLERGY** 11
   Gerald W. Volcheck, M.D.

3. **CARDIOLOGY** 39
   Thomas Behrenbeck, M.D., Ph.D.
   Kyle W. Klarich, M.D.
   Peter A. Brady, M.D.
   Paul A. Friedman, M.D.
   Steve R. Ommen, M.D.
   Rick A. Nishimura, M.D.
   Barry L. Karon, M.D.

4. **CRITICAL CARE MEDICINE** 147
   Steve G. Peters, M.D.
   William F. Dunn, M.D.

5. **DERMATOLOGY** 169
   Marian T. McEvoy, M.D.

6. **ENDOCRINOLOGY** 197
   Adrian Vella, M.D.
   Neena Natt, M.D.

7. **GASTROENTEROLOGY AND HEPATOLOGY** 253
   Thomas R. Viggiano, M.D.
   Robert E. Sedlack, M.D.
   John J. Poterucha, M.D.

8. **GENERAL INTERNAL MEDICINE** 331
   Scott C. Litin, M.D.

9. **GENETICS** 361
   Virginia V. Michels, M.D.

10. **GERIATRICS** 383
    Darryl S. Chutka, M.D.

11. **HEMATOLOGY** 411
    Thomas M. Habermann, M.D.

12. **HIV INFECTION** 479
    Zelalem Temesgen, M.D.

13. **HYPERTENSION** 511
    Gary L. Schwartz, M.D.

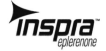

14. INFECTIOUS DISEASES **549**
    William F. Marshall, M.D.
    Abinash Virk, M.D.
    Gregory D. Hart, M.D.
    John W. Wilson, M.D.
    Lynn L. Estes, Pharm.D.

15. MEDICAL ETHICS **649**
    C. Christopher Hook, M.D.

16. NEPHROLOGY **665**
    Fernando C. Fervenza, M.D., Ph.D.
    Thomas R. Schwab, M.D.
    Amy W. Williams, M.D.
    Robert C. Albright, Jr., D.O.
    Stephen B. Erickson, M.D.

17. NEUROLOGY **721**
    Eduardo E. Benarroch, M.D.
    Robert D. Brown, Jr., M.D.
    Frank A. Rubino, M.D.

18. ONCOLOGY **775**
    Scott H. Okuno, M.D.

19. PREVENTIVE MEDICINE **807**
    Sally J. Trippel, M.D., M.P.H.

20. PSYCHIATRY **823**
    Marcia J. Slattery, M.D.
    Lois E. Krahn, M.D.

21. PULMONARY DISEASES **847**
    John G. Park, M.D.
    Timothy R. Aksamit, M.D.
    Karen L. Swanson, D.O.
    Charles F. Thomas, Jr., M.D.

22. RHEUMATOLOGY **943**
    Clement J. Michet, Jr., M.D.
    Kevin G. Moder, M.D.
    William W. Ginsburg, M.D.

23. VASCULAR DISEASES **1013**
    Peter C. Spittell, M.D.

Index **1035**

CHAPTER 1

THE BOARD EXAMINATION

Darryl S. Chutka, M.D.

Many physicians take the American Board of Internal Medicine (ABIM) certifying examination in internal medicine (IM) annually. The total number of candidates who took the ABIM certifying examination for the first time in 2002 was 7,074. Of these, 87% passed the examination. Currently, greater importance is being placed on achieving board certification. Many managed-care organizations now require board certification before employment. This chapter is aimed primarily at candidates preparing for the ABIM's certifying or recertifying examination in IM. However, candidates preparing for non-ABIM examinations also may benefit from the information, which covers various aspects of preparation for an examination, strategies to answer the questions effectively, and avoidance of pitfalls.

AIM OF THE EXAMINATION

The ABIM has stated that the certifying examination tests the breadth and depth of a candidate's knowledge in IM to ensure that the candidate has attained the necessary proficiency required for the practice of IM. According to the ABIM, the examination has two goals: the first is to ensure competence in the diagnosis and treatment of common disorders that have important consequences for patients, and the second is to ensure excellence in the broad domain of IM.

EXAMINATION FORMAT

The examination for ABIM certification in IM requires 2 days to complete and is divided into four sections of 3 hours each. Details regarding the examination, training requirements, eligibility requirements, application forms, and other related information can be obtained from the American Board of Internal Medicine, 510 Walnut Street, Suite 1700, Philadelphia, PA 19106-3699 (telephone numbers: 215-446-3500 or 800-441-2246; fax number: 215-446-3470). The Internet address of the ABIM is http://www.abim.org.

Almost all of the questions are clinical and based on a correct diagnosis and management. Because there is no penalty for guessing the answers, candidates should *answer every question*. Marking multiple answers for a single question is not allowed and will cause the question to be scored as incorrect. Most questions are based on the presentations of patients. Among these, 75% are in the setting of outpatient or emergency room encounters, and the remaining 25% are in the inpatient setting, including the critical care unit and nursing home. The ability to answer these questions requires integration of information provided from several sources (such as history, physical examination, laboratory test results, and consultations), prioritization of alternatives, or use of clinical judgment. Candidates should know that approximately 15% of questions are known as field questions, or pretest questions, and are included for experimental purposes only and test the question quality. Although field questions are not scored, they cannot be identified during the examination. The overall ability to manage the patient in a cost-effective, evidence-based fashion is stressed. Questions that require simple recall of medical facts have essentially been eliminated. The examination is reviewed by practicing internists to ensure the questions are relevant to a general internal medicine practice.

- Candidates should answer every question; there is no penalty for guessing.
- Most questions are based on presentations of patients.
- Questions that require simple recall of medical facts are in the minority.

A list of normal laboratory values and illustrative materials (electrocardiograms, blood smears, Gram stains, urine sediments, chest radiographs, and photomicrographs) necessary to answer questions are provided. Candidates should interpret the abnormal values on the basis of the normal values provided and not on the basis of the normal values to which they are accustomed in their practice or training. Candidates for the certifying examination receive an information booklet several weeks before the examination. The booklet provides a detailed description of the examination, including the types of questions used.

Although much of the information contained in this chapter is borrowed from the previous information booklets, candidates for ABIM examinations should read the booklet that is sent to them because the ABIM may change various components of the format of the examination.

- A list of normal laboratory values and illustrative materials necessary to answer questions are provided.
- The information booklet is sent several weeks before the examination by the ABIM and should be read by candidates.

SCORING

The passing scores reflect predetermined standards set by the ABIM. Passing scores are determined before the examination and therefore are not dependent on the performance of any group of candidates taking the examination.

- Passing scores are set before the examination.

THE CONTENT

The questions in the examination cover a broad area of IM, as listed below. They are divided into "primary" and "cross-content" groups. The subspecialties in the primary content areas have included cardiovascular diseases, gastroenterology, pulmonary diseases, infectious diseases, rheumatology/orthopedics, endocrinology/metabolism, oncology, hematology, nephrology/urology, neurology, psychiatry, allergy/immunology, dermatology, obstetrics/gynecology, ophthalmology, otolaryngology, and miscellaneous. The specialties in the cross-content group have included adolescent medicine, critical care medicine, clinical epidemiology, ethics, geriatrics, nutrition, palliative/end-of-life care, occupational/environmental medicine, preventive medicine, women's health, and substance abuse. Approximately 75% of the questions test knowledge in the following major specialties in IM: cardiology, endocrinology, gastroenterology, hematology, infectious diseases, nephrology, oncology, pulmonary diseases, and rheumatology. The remaining 25% of questions cover allergy/immunology, dermatology, gynecology, neurology, urology, ophthalmology, and psychiatry. Independent of primary content, about 40% of the questions encompass the cross-content topics. Table 1-1 shows the distribution of the contents for a recent ABIM certifying examination in IM.

- About 75% of the questions test knowledge in the major specialties.
- About 25% of the questions cover allergy/immunology, dermatology, gynecology, neurology, urology, ophthalmology, and psychiatry.

- About 40% of all questions encompass the cross-content topics: adolescent medicine, critical care medicine, clinical epidemiology, medical ethics, geriatrics, nutrition, occupational medicine, preventive medicine, and substance abuse.

QUESTION FORMAT

Each session contains 90 multiple-choice, single-best–answer questions. This format reflects a change that began with the 1995 examination. True-or-false, double-negative, and matching questions have been eliminated. The question may include

Table 1-1 Contents of the Certification Examination of the American Board of Internal Medicine

Area	% of test
Primary content	
Cardiovascular disease	14
Gastroenterology	10
Pulmonary disease	10
Infectious disease	9
Rheumatology/orthopedics	8
Endocrinology/metabolism	7
Medical oncology	7
Hematology	6
Nephrology/urology	6
Allergy/immunology	5
Psychiatry	4
Neurology	4
Dermatology	3
Obstetrics/gynecology	2
Ophthalmology	2
Miscellaneous	3
	100
Cross-content	
Critical care medicine	10
Geriatric medicine	10
Preventive medicine	6
Women's health	6
Medical ethics	3
Clinical epidemiology	3
Nutrition	3
Palliative/end-of-life care	3
Adolescent medicine	2
Occupational/environmental medicine	2
Substance abuse	2

From ABIM News Update: 1999 Internal Medicine Certification Examination. American Board of Internal Medicine, Philadelphia, Spring 1999. By permission.

a case history, a brief statement, a radiograph, a graph, or a picture (such as a blood smear or Gram stain). Each question has five possible answers, and the candidates should identify the *single-best* answer. More than one answer may appear correct or partially correct for a question. Also, the traditionally correct answer may not be listed as an option. In that situation, the one answer that is better than the others should be selected. As noted above, most questions are based on encounters with patients. Some questions are progressive; that is, more than one question is based on information about the same patient. The examples in this chapter, the questions at the end of each chapter in this book, and the examples included in the ABIM's information booklet should help candidates become familiar with the question format. Furthermore, the national in-training examination taken by most second-year residents in IM provides ample opportunity to become familiar with the question format.

- All questions are of the single-best–answer type.
- Various study guides should be used to become familiar with the question format.

EXAMPLES

Select the *one best answer* for each of the following questions.

1. A 56-year-old woman is referred to you for an evaluation of dyspnea and chest pain of 6 weeks in duration. The chest pain is nonpleuritic, nonexertional, and located along the lower right lateral chest cage. She has no fever, cough, or chills. During the past few weeks, she has been experiencing constant low back pain. The patient underwent right mastectomy 4 years ago because of carcinoma of the breast with metastatic involvement of the right axillary lymph nodes. She received radiotherapy followed by chemotherapy for 24 months. Examination now shows diminished breath sounds in the right lower lung field. The remainder of the examination is unremarkable. A chest radiograph suggests a moderate right pleural effusion. Which one of the following is most likely to be helpful in confirming the suspected diagnosis?
   a. Bone scan with technetium 99m diphosphonate
   b. Bone marrow aspirate and biopsy
   c. Scalene fat pad biopsy
   d. Thoracentesis
   e. Mammography

2. A 20-year-old male military recruit returns home from several weeks of summer training in boot camp. He appears in your office the following day with a 12-day history of fever (38°C), coryza, pharyngitis, and cough. Physical examination discloses a bullous lesion over the right tympanic membrane and scattered crackles in both lung fields. Blood cell count shows mild thrombocytopenia. A chest radiograph shows patchy alveolar-interstitial infiltrates in both lungs. Which one of the following is the best treatment for this patient?
   a. Erythromycin
   b. Penicillin
   c. Trimethoprim
   d. Clindamycin
   e. Ceftazidime

3. A 49-year-old male executive comes to your office with a 6-month history of cough, shortness of breath, and chest tightness soon after substantial exertion. He notices these symptoms soon after he finishes a game of racquetball. He is a nonsmoker and has no risk factors for coronary artery disease. Results of physical examination in your office are normal. His weight is normal for his height. The chest radiograph is normal. A treadmill test for ischemic heart disease is negative. Which one of the following diagnostic tests is indicated?
   a. CT of the chest
   b. Arterial blood gas studies at rest and after exercise
   c. Spirometry before and after exercise
   d. Ventilation-perfusion lung scanning
   e. Cardiopulmonary exercise testing

4. A 43-year-old asymptomatic man has chronic hepatitis C. Therapy for 12 months with a combination of interferon and ribavirin failed to clear the virus. Laboratory results are notable for an alanine aminotransferase value of 65 U/L and normal values for bilirubin, albumin, and prothrombin time. A liver biopsy shows a mild lymphocytic portal infiltrate but no fibrosis. Which one of the following statements about this patient is true?
   a. He should be given lamivudine
   b. He should have screening for hepatocellular carcinoma and undergo ultrasonography and α-fetoprotein testing every 6 months
   c. He should have endoscopy to look for esophageal varices
   d. He should be referred for liver transplantation
   e. He should receive the hepatitis A and B vaccines if he is not already immune

5. A hospitalized patient with acquired immunodeficiency syndrome (AIDS) dies of disseminated infection caused by *Mycobacterium avium* complex. Cough develops in the 28-year-old resident physician who cared for this patient. A chest radiograph shows a nodular infiltrate in the right upper lobe. Tuberculin skin test (purified protein

derivative) is positive (12 mm). Which one of the following is the most appropriate next step?
a. Begin antituberculous therapy with at least four drugs because *M. avium* is resistant to two-drug therapy
b. Obtain sputum and gastric washings for stain and culture of tubercle bacilli
c. Order human immunodeficiency virus (HIV) serologic testing now and in 6 months
d. Begin prophylactic isoniazid therapy 300 mg/day for 12 months
e. Treat with isoniazid 300 mg/day and rifampin 600 mg/day for 9 months

6. A 37-year-old woman was treated previously with prednisone and cyclophosphamide for biopsy-proven lupus nephritis. Two years ago the dosage of these medications was tapered and she did well. During the past several weeks she has noted increasing malaise, a low-grade fever, and polyarthralgias. Which one of the following tests might be helpful for deciding whether she has active systemic lupus erythematosus?
a. Antinuclear antibody
b. Anti-Sm
c. Anti-SSA
d. Anti-nDNA
e. Anti-RNP

7. An HIV-positive patient with low CD4 counts is receiving multidrug treatment. He complains of colicky flank pain, and many crystals are subsequently noted on urinalysis. Which one of the following drugs is most likely causative?
a. Ribavirin
b. Sulfamethoxazole/trimethoprim
c. Indinavir
d. Acyclovir
e. Ganciclovir

8. A 68-year-old woman, nonsmoker, presents with an 8-week history of low-grade fever, malaise, myalgias, sore throat, hoarseness, and cough. She also complains of headaches, cramps in the jaws, and intermittent visual blurring. The leukocyte count is normal, and the erythrocyte sedimentation rate is 86 mm in 1 hour. A chest radiograph is normal. Which one of the following treatments is likely to resolve these symptoms?
a. Cranial radiation and chemotherapy
b. Itraconazole
c. Corticosteroid
d. Amantadine
e. Antiplatelet (aspirin)

9. A 34-year-old woman comes to your office with a 4-week history of hemoptysis, intermittent wheeze, and generalized weakness. On examination her blood pressure is 186/112 mm Hg. She appears cushingoid and has noted these changes taking place during the past 12 weeks. Auscultation discloses localized wheezing in the left mid-lung area. The chest radiograph indicates partial atelectasis of the left upper lobe. She is referred to you for further evaluations. Which one of the following is least likely to provide useful information for diagnosis and treatment?
a. Serum adrenocorticotropic hormone level
b. 24-Hour urine test for 5-hydroxyindoleacetic acid level
c. Bronchoscopy
d. CT of the chest
e. Serum potassium level

10. A 62-year-old woman presents with the onset of eye discomfort and diplopia. She has not noted any other new neurologic symptoms. Neurologic examination shows a normal mental status and neurovascular findings. Reflexes are slightly decreased in the lower extremities. Gait and coordination are normal. Cranial nerves show an inability to adduct, elevate, and depress the eye. Pupillary reaction is normal. Motor strength testing is negative. Sensation is normal except there is decreased vibratory and joint position sensation in the feet. What abnormality would be expected?
a. Saccular aneurysm of the cavernous sinus on CT
b. Brain stem neoplasm on MRI
c. Left temporal sharp waves on electroencephalography
d. Increased fasting blood sugar
e. Increased erythrocyte sedimentation rate

11. A 42-year-old man who is an office worker presents to the emergency department with acute dyspnea. He has smoked 1 1/2 packs per day for 25 years and had been relatively asymptomatic except for a smoker's cough and mild dyspnea on exertion. Physical examination findings are not remarkable except for slightly diminished intensity of breath sounds over the right lung and some prolonged expiratory slowing, consistent with obstructive lung disease. The chest radiograph shows extensive infiltrates in the upper two-thirds of the lung fields. Which one of the following conditions is most likely responsible for this patient's symptoms?
a. Pulmonary alveolar proteinosis
b. Silicosis
c. Pulmonary eosinophilic granuloma (histiocytosis X)
d. Idiopathic pulmonary fibrosis
e. Sarcoidosis

12. In a 34-year-old man with acute myelomonocytic leukemia, fever and progressive respiratory distress develop, and the chest radiograph shows diffuse alveolar infiltrates. The patient completed intensive chemotherapy 6 weeks earlier. The total leukocyte count has remained less than 0.5 $\times 10^9$/L for more than 3 weeks. He is currently (for at least 10 days) receiving a cephalosporin (ceftazidime). Which one of the following is the most appropriate therapy for this patient?
   a. Clindamycin
   b. Blood transfusion to increase the number of circulating leukocytes
   c. Antituberculous (triple-drug) therapy
   d. Amphotericin intravenously
   e. Pentamidine aerosol

The answers to the questions are as follows: 1, d (metastatic pleural effusion); 2, a (*Mycoplasma* infection); 3, c (exercise-induced asthma); 4, e; 5, d; 6, e (hereditary angioneurotic edema); 7, c; 8, c (giant cell arteritis); 9, b (bronchial carcinoid); 10, d; 11, c (histiocytosis X or pulmonary eosinophilic granuloma with spontaneous pneumothorax); 12, d (disseminated aspergillosis in a leukopenic patient).

Questions 1 through 3 are examples of questions that are aimed at evaluating knowledge and judgment about problems that are encountered frequently in practice and for which physician intervention makes a considerable difference. These questions judge the candidate's minimal level of clinical competence. These questions include descriptions of typical clinical features of metastatic breast carcinoma, *Mycoplasma* pneumonia, and exercise-induced asthma, respectively. Therefore, the decision making is relatively easy and straightforward. Questions 4 through 12 are more difficult to answer because they are structured to reflect excellence in clinical competence rather than just minimal competence. In other words, they require more extensive knowledge (i.e., knowledge beyond that required for minimal competence) in IM and its subspecialties. Although most of the questions on the examination are based on encounters with patients, some require recall of well-known medical facts.

PREPARATION FOR THE TEST

Training during medical school forms the foundation on which advanced clinical knowledge is accumulated during residency training. However, the serious preparation for the examination actually starts at the beginning of the residency training in IM. Most candidates will require a minimum of 6 to 8 months of intense preparation for the examination. Cramming just before the examination is counterproductive and is unlikely to be successful. Some of the methods of preparation for the board examination are described below. Additionally, each candidate may develop her or his own system.

● Preparation for the ABIM examination should start at the beginning of the residency training in IM.

Each candidate should use a standard textbook of IM. Any of those available should provide a good basic knowledge base in all areas of IM. Ideally, the candidate should use one good textbook and not jump from one to another, except for reading certain chapters that are outstanding in a particular textbook. The most effective way to use the textbook is with patient-centered reading; this should occur throughout the residency program. This book and similar board review syllabi are excellent tools for brushing up on important board-relevant information several weeks to months before the examination. They, however, cannot take the place of comprehensive textbooks of internal medicine. This book is designed as a study guide rather than a comprehensive textbook of medicine. Therefore, it should not be used as the sole source of medical information for the examination.

● Candidates should thoroughly study a standard textbook of IM.
● This book is designed as a study guide and should not be used as the sole source of information for preparation for the examination.

The Medical Knowledge Self-Assessment Program (MKSAP) prepared by the American College of Physicians is extremely valuable for obtaining practice in answering multiple-choice questions. The questions and answers from the MKSAP are very useful to learn the type of questions asked and the depth of knowledge expected for various subjects. The text contents, however, are uneven in the coverage of topics. By design, the MKSAP is prepared for the continuing medical education of practicing (presumably ABIM-certified) internists rather than for those preparing for initial certification by the ABIM. For recertification examination purposes, the MKSAP textbook is an excellent aid.

Some find it helpful to prepare for the examination in study groups. Formation of two to five candidates per group permits study of different textbooks and review articles in journals. The group should meet regularly as each candidate is assigned reading materials. Selected review articles on common and important topics in IM should be included in the study materials. Indiscriminate reading of articles from many journals should be avoided. In any case, most candidates who begin preparation 6 to 8 months before the examination will not find time for extensive study of journal materials. The newer information in the recent (within 6 to 9 months of the examination) medical journals is unlikely to be included in the examination. Notes and other materials the candidates have gathered during their residency training are also good sources of information. These clinical "pearls" gathered from mentors will be of help in remembering certain important points.

- Study groups may help cover large amounts of information.
- Indiscriminate reading of articles from many journals should be avoided.
- Information in the recent (within 6 to 9 months of the examination) medical journals is unlikely to be included in the examination.

Candidates should try to remember some of the uncommon manifestations of the most common diseases (such as polycythemia in common obstructive pulmonary disease) and common manifestations of uncommon diseases (such as pneumothorax in eosinophilic granuloma). The large majority of the questions on the examination involve conditions most commonly encountered in clinical practice. Several formulas and points should be memorized (such as the alveolar gas equation). The clinical training obtained and the regular study habits formed during residency training are the most important aspects of preparation for the examination.

In general, the examination rarely has questions about specific drug dosages or specific chemotherapy regimens used in oncology. Rather, questions are geared toward concepts regarding the treatment of patients. Questions regarding adverse effects of medications are common on the examination, especially when the adverse effect occurs frequently or is potentially serious. The candidate is also expected to recognize when a clinical condition is a drug-related event.

- Study as much as possible about board-eligible topics.
- Learn about the uncommon manifestations of common diseases and the common manifestations of uncommon diseases.

DAY OF THE EXAMINATION

Adequate time is allowed to read and answer all the questions; therefore, there is no need to rush or become anxious. You should watch the time to ensure that you are at least halfway through the examination when half of the time has elapsed. Start by answering the first question and continue sequentially. Almost all of the questions follow a case presentation format. At times, subsequent questions will give you information that may help you answer a previous question. Do not be alarmed by lengthy questions; look for the question's salient points. When faced with a confusing question, do not become distracted by that question. Mark it so you can find it later, then go to the next question and come back to the unanswered ones at the end. Extremely lengthy stem statements or case presentations are apparently intended to test the candidate's ability to separate the essential from the unnecessary or unimportant information. You may want to underline important information presented in the question in order to review this information after reading the entire question and the answer options. You are not allowed to bring a highlighter to the examination.

- Look for the salient points in each question.
- If a question is confusing, mark it to find it and come back to the unanswered questions at the end.

Some candidates may fail the examination despite the possession of an immense amount of knowledge and the clinical competence necessary to pass the examination. Their failure to pass the examination may be caused by the lack of ability to understand or interpret the questions properly. The ability to understand the nuances of the question format is sometimes referred to as "boardsmanship." Intelligent interpretation of the questions is very important for candidates who are not well versed in the format of multiple-choice questions. Tips on "boardsmanship" include the following:

- All questions whose answers are known should be answered first.
- Spend adequate time on questions for which you are certain of the answers to ensure that they are answered correctly. It is easy to become overconfident with such questions and thus you may fail to read the questions or the answer options carefully. Make sure you never make mistakes on easy questions.
- Read the final sentence (that appears just before the multiple answers) several times to understand how an answer should be selected. Recheck the question format before selecting the correct answer. Read each answer option thoroughly through to the end. Occasionally a response may be only partially correct. At times, the traditionally correct answer is not listed. In these situations, select the best alternative listed. Watch for qualifiers such as "next," "immediately," or "initially."
- Avoid answers that contain absolute or very restrictive words such as "always," "never," or "must." Answer options that contain absolutes are likely incorrect.
- Try to think of the correct answer to the question before looking at the list of potential answers. Assume you have been given all the necessary information to answer the question. If the answer you had formulated is not among the list of answers provided, you may have interpreted the question incorrectly. When a patient's case is presented,

think of the diagnosis before looking at the list of answers. It will be reassuring to realize (particularly if your diagnosis is supported by the answers) that you are on the "right track."

- Abnormalities on, for example, the photographs, radiographs, and electrocardiograms will be obvious.
- If you do not know the answer to a question, very often you are able to rule out one or several answer options and improve your odds at guessing.
- Occasionally you can use information presented in one question to help you answer other difficult questions.

Candidates are well advised to use the basic fund of knowledge accumulated from clinical experience and reading to solve the questions. Approaching the questions as "real-life" encounters with patients is far better than trying to second-guess the examiners or trying to analyze whether the question is "tricky." As indicated above, the questions are never "tricky," and there is no reason for the ABIM to trick the candidates into choosing wrong answers.

It is better not to discuss the questions or answers (after the examination) with other candidates. Such discussions usually cause more consternation, although some candidates may derive a false sense of having performed well in the examination. In any case, the candidates are bound by their oath to the ABIM not to discuss or disseminate the questions. Do not study between examination sessions, particularly the night between the two examination days.

- Approach questions as "real-life" encounters with a patient.
- There are no "trick" questions.

CONNECTIONS

Associations, causes, complications, and other relationships between a phenomenon or disease and clinical features are important to remember and recognize. For example, Table 1-2 lists some of the "connections" in infectious and occupational entities in pulmonary medicine. Each subspecialty has many similar connections, and candidates for the ABIM and other examinations may want to prepare lists like this for different areas.

RECERTIFICATION

The diplomate certificates issued to successful candidates who have passed the ABIM examination in IM in 1986 and thereafter are valid for 10 years. The ABIM recently announced changes in the physician recertification process. This new process is called Continuous Professional Development and

consists of a three-step program. These three steps include verification of professional credentials, a self-evaluation component of five self-evaluation modules, and a proctored written secure examination. The self-evaluation modules evaluate performance in clinical skills, preventive services, practice performance, fund of medical knowledge, and feedback from patients and colleagues. Successfully completed self-evaluation modules are valid for 10 years. Candidates may apply to begin the recertification process any time after initial certification or recertification. The ABIM recommends that completion of the self-evaluation modules be spread out over time. It is anticipated that the candidate will complete one self-assessment module every 1 to 2 years.

- Candidates who passed the ABIM certification examination in IM in 1986 and thereafter have certificates that are valid for 10 years.
- The new recertification process is called Continuous Professional Development and consists of a three-step process.

Medical Knowledge Self-Evaluation Module

This is an open-book examination containing 60 single-best–answer multiple-choice questions regarding recent clinical advances in IM. This module tests the candidate's knowledge of IM and clinical judgment. The questions are written by board members and ABIM diplomates. Candidates may choose a module in internal medicine or a subspecialty (focused content). The module is available on paper or CD-ROM or on the Internet. Candidates must achieve a predetermined passing score to establish credit for the module. The module may be repeated as often as necessary to achieve a passing score.

Clinical Skills Self-Evaluation Module

This is an open-book examination containing audio and visual information pertaining to physical examination and physical diagnosis and physician-patient communication skills. The module contains 60 single-best answer multiple-choice questions. It is available on a CD-ROM format and eventually will be available on the Internet. Candidates must achieve a predetermined passing score to establish credit for the module. The module may be repeated as often as necessary to achieve a passing score.

Patient and Peer Feedback Module

Confidential and anonymous feedback regarding the candidate's professionalism, physician-patient communication skills, and overall patient care skills is obtained from colleagues and patients of the candidate by an automated telephone survey. The candidate selects 20 colleagues and 40 patients who

Table 1-2 Example of "Connections" Between Etiologic Factors and Diseases

Etiologic factor	Agent, disease
Cattle, swine, horses, wool, hide	Anthrax
Abattoir worker, veterinarian	Brucellosis
Travel to Southeast Asia, South America	Melioidosis
Squirrels, chipmunks, rabbits, rats	Plague
Rabbits, squirrels, infected flies, or ticks	Tularemia
Birds	Psittacosis, histoplasmosis
Rats, dogs, cats, cattle, swine	Leptospirosis
Goats, cattle, swine	Q fever
Soil, water-cooling tower	Legionellosis
Military camps	Mycoplasmosis
Chicken coops, starling roosts, caves	Histoplasmosis
Soil	Blastomycosis
Travel in southwestern United States	Coccidioidomycosis
Ohio and Mississippi river valleys	Histoplasmosis
Decaying wood	Histoplasmosis
Gardeners, florists, straw, plants	Sporotrichosis
Progressive, massive fibrosis	Silicosis, coal, hematite, kaolin, graphite, asbestosis
Autoimmune mechanism	Silicosis, asbestosis, berylliosis
Monday morning sickness	Byssinosis, bagassosis, metal fume fever
Metals and fumes producing asthma	Baker's asthma, meat wrapper's asthma, printer's asthma, nickel, platinum, toluene diisocyanate (TDI), cigarette cutter's asthma
Increased incidence of tuberculosis	Silicosis, hematite lung
Increased incidence of carcinoma	Asbestos, hematite, arsenic, nickel, uranium, chromate
Welding	Siderosis, pulmonary edema, bronchitis, emphysema
Centrilobar emphysema	Coal, hematite
Generalized emphysema	Cadmium, bauxite
Silo filler's lung	Nitrogen dioxide
Farmer's lung	*Thermoactinomyces, Micropolyspora*
Asbestos exposure	Mesothelioma, bronchogenic carcinoma, gastrointestinal cancer
Eggshell calcification	Silicosis, sarcoid
Sarcoid-like disease	Berylliosis
Diaphragmatic calcification	Asbestosis (also ankylosing spondylitis)
Nonfibrogenic pneumoconioses	Tin, emery, antimony, titanium, barium
Minimal pathology in lungs	Siderosis, baritosis, stannosis
Bullous emphysema	Bauxite lung

are asked to complete a brief, anonymous telephone survey. The candidate receives a summary of the survey findings.

Practice Improvement Module

This module is a computer-based instrument to help candidates assess the care they provide to patients and to help them develop a plan for improvement. Areas of the practice that have potential for quality improvement are identified. Completion of this module involves review of patient charts. This module requires data entry over at least 3 weeks. This module is available in CD-ROM format only at this time.

Secure Examination

A comprehensive, secure, computer-based examination is offered two times yearly, currently in May and November. The examination consists of three modules of 60 single-best–answer multiple-choice questions. Two of the three modules must be in internal medicine, and the third may be internal medicine, a medical subspecialty, or an area of added qualifications. Successful completion of the self-evaluation modules is not required before taking this examination. Questions are based on well-established information and assess clinical judgment more than pure recall of medical information. The examination contains clinically relevant questions. To pass the final examination, the candidate must achieve a predetermined passing score. The examination may be repeated as often as it takes to achieve a passing score. The examination is expected to be computer-based within the next year or so.

Details of the recertification program can be obtained by writing to the ABIM offices at the American Board of Internal Medicine, 510 Walnut Street, Suite 1700, Philadelphia, PA 19106-3699 (telephone numbers: 215-446-3500 or 800-441-2246; fax number: 215-446-3470). The Internet address of the ABIM is http://www.abim.org.

CHAPTER 2

ALLERGY

Gerald W. Volcheck, M.D.

ALLERGY TESTING

Standard allergy testing relies on identifying the IgE antibody specific for the allergen in question. Two classic methods of doing this are the immediate wheal-and-flare skin test (a small amount of antigen is introduced into the skin and evaluated at 15 minutes for the presence of an immediate wheal-and-flare reaction) and in vitro testing.

Allergy testing that does not have a clear scientific basis includes cytotoxic testing, provocation-neutralization testing or treatment, and "yeast allergy" testing.

Patch Tests and Prick (Cutaneous) Tests

Many seem confused about the concept of patch testing of skin as opposed to immediate wheal-and-flare skin testing. Patch testing is used to investigate contact dermatitis, a type IV hypersensitivity reaction. Patch tests require about 96 hours for complete evaluation (similar to tuberculin skin reactivity that requires 72 hours). Patch testing is useful only for investigating type IV hypersensitivity reactions that lead to contact dermatitis. Most substances that cause contact dermatitis are small organic molecules that can penetrate various barriers inherent in the skin surface. The mechanisms of hypersensitivity postulated to explain these reactions usually involve the formation of haptens of endogenous dermal proteins.

Inhalant allergens, in comparison, generally are sizable intact proteins in which each molecule can be multivalent with respect to IgE binding. These molecules penetrate the skin poorly and are seldom involved in cutaneous type IV hypersensitivity reactions. They cause respiratory symptoms and are identified by prick skin testing.

- Patch testing is used to investigate contact dermatitis.
- Prick (immediate) skin testing is used to investigate respiratory allergy to pollens and molds.

Prick, scratch, and intradermal testing involve introducing allergen to the skin layers below the external keratin layer. Each of these techniques becomes increasingly sensitive (but less specific) because with the deeper, intradermal tests, allergen is introduced more closely to responding cells and at higher doses. Allergen skin tests performed by the prick technique adequately identify patients who have important clinical sensitivities without identifying a large number of those who have minimal levels of IgE antibody and no clinical sensitivity. Intradermal testing is used in selected cases, including evaluating allergy to stinging insect venoms and to penicillin. Drugs with antihistamine properties, such as H_1 receptor antagonists, and many anticholinergic and tricyclic antidepressant drugs can suppress immediate allergy skin tests. The H_2 receptor antagonists have a small suppressive effect. Corticosteroids can suppress the delayed-type hypersensitivity response but not the immediate response.

- Intradermal skin tests are more sensitive but less specific than prick skin tests.
- Intradermal skin testing is used to investigate allergy to insect venoms and penicillin.

In Vitro Allergy Testing

In vitro allergy testing initially involves chemically coupling allergen protein molecules to a solid-phase substance. The test is then conducted by incubating serum (from the patient) that may contain IgE antibody specific for the allergen that has been immobilized to the membrane for a standard time. The solid phase is then washed free of nonbinding materials from the serum and incubated in a second solution containing a reagent (e.g., radiolabeled anti-IgE antibody). The various wells are counted, and the radioactivity is correlated directly with the preparation of a standard curve in which known amounts of allergen-specific IgE antibody were incubated with a set of standard preparations of a solid phase. In vitro allergy testing uses the principles of radioimmunoassay or chromogen activation.

It is important to understand that this test only identifies the presence of allergen-specific IgE antibody in the same way that the allergen skin test does. Generally, in vitro allergy testing is not as sensitive as any form of skin testing and has some limitations because of the potential for chemical modification of the allergen protein while it is being coupled to the solid phase by means of covalent reaction. Generally, it is more expensive than allergen skin tests and has no advantage in routine clinical work. In vitro allergy testing may be useful clinically for patients who have been taking antihistamines and in whom no positive histamine responsiveness can be induced in the skin or for patients who have primary cutaneous diseases that make allergen skin testing impractical or inaccurate (e.g., severe atopic eczema with most of the skin involved in a flare).

● Skin testing is more sensitive and less expensive than in vitro allergy testing.

ASTHMA

Pathology

The pathologic features of asthma have been studied chiefly in fatal cases; some bronchoscopic data are available about mild and moderate asthma. The histologic hallmarks of asthma are listed in Table 2-1.

● The histologic hallmarks of asthma include mucus gland hypertrophy, mucus hypersecretion, epithelial desquamation, widening of the basement membrane, and infiltration by eosinophils.

Pathophysiology

Bronchial hyperresponsiveness is common to all forms of asthma. It is measured by assessing pulmonary function before and after exposure to methacholine, histamine, cold air, or exercise. Prolonged aerosol corticosteroid therapy reduces bronchial hyperresponsiveness. Prolonged therapy with certain other

Table 2-1 Histologic Hallmarks of Asthma

Mucus gland hypertrophy
Mucus hypersecretion
Alteration of tinctorial and viscoelastic properties of mucus
Widening of basement membrane zone of bronchial epithelial
  membrane
Increased number of intraepithelial leukocytes and mast cells
Round cell infiltration of bronchial submucosa
Intense eosinophilic infiltration of submucosa
Widespread damage to bronchial epithelium
    Large areas of complete desquamation of epithelium into
      airway lumen
    Mucus plugs filled with eosinophils and their products

---

anti-inflammatory drugs, for example, cromolyn sodium or nedocromil, also reduces bronchial hyperresponsiveness. Note that although cromolyn and nedocromil both were originally touted as "antiallergic" (they inhibit mast cell activation), they affect most cells involved in inflammation; also, the effects on these cells occur at lower doses than those that inhibit mast cell activation.

● Bronchial hyperresponsiveness generally is present in all forms of asthma.
● Prolonged aerosol corticosteroid therapy reduces bronchial hyperresponsiveness.

Persons who have allergic asthma generate mast cell and basophil mediators that have important roles in the development of endobronchial inflammation and smooth muscle changes that occur after acute exposure to allergen. Mast cells and basophils are prominent during the immediate-phase reaction.

● In the immediate-phase reaction, mast cells and basophils are important.

In the so-called late-phase reaction to allergen exposure, the bronchi display histologic features of chronic inflammation and eosinophils become prominent in the reaction.

● In the late-phase reaction, eosinophils become prominent.

Patients who have chronic asthma and negative results on allergy skin tests seem to have an inflammatory infiltrate in the bronchi and histologic findings dominated by eosinophils when asthma is active. Patients with sudden asphyxic asthma may have a neutrophilic rather than an eosinophilic infiltration of the airway.

Various hypotheses explain the development of nonallergic asthma. One proposal is that the initial inflammation represents an autoimmune reaction arising from a viral or other microbial infection in the lung and, for reasons unknown, inflammation becomes chronic and characterized by a lymphocyte cytokine profile in which interleukin (IL)-5 is prominent. The intense eosinophilic inflammation is thought to come from the IL-5 influence of T cells in the chronic inflammatory infiltrate. Airway macrophages and platelets have low-affinity IgE receptors on their membranes and are activated by cross-linking of these receptors by allergen, suggesting that some phases of lung inflammation in allergy may involve the macrophage as a primary responder cell.

● IL-5 stimulates eosinophils.
● Airway macrophages and platelets have low-affinity IgE receptors.

The two types of helper T cells are TH1 and TH2. In general, TH1 cells produce interferon-γ (IFN-γ) and IL-2, and TH2 cells produce IL-4 and IL-5. IL-4 stimulates IgE synthesis. Hence, many clinical scientists believe that atopic asthma is caused by a preferential activation of TH2 lymphocytes.

- IL-4 stimulates IgE synthesis.
- TH2 lymphocytes produce IL-4 and IL-5.

Important characteristics of cytokines are summarized in Table 2-2.

Genetics of Asthma

The genetics of asthma is complex and confounded by environmental factors. No "asthma gene" has been discovered.

The gene encoding the beta subunit of the high-affinity IgE receptor is located on chromosome 11q13 and is linked to total IgE, atopy, and bronchial hyperreactivity. Polymorphic variants of the β_2-adrenergic receptor are linked to bronchial hyperreactivity. The gene for IL-4 is located on chromosome 5q31 and is linked to total IgE.

Occupational Asthma

Every patient interviewed about a history of allergy or asthma must be asked to provide a detailed occupational history. A large fraction of occupational asthma escapes diagnosis because physicians obtain an inadequate occupational history. An enormous range of possible industrial circumstances may lead to exposure and resultant disease. The most widely recognized types of occupational asthma are listed in Table 2-3.

Table 2-2 Characteristics of Cytokines

Cytokine	Major actions	Primary sources
IL-1	Lymphocyte activation	Macrophages
	Fibroblast activation	Endothelial cells
	Fever	Lymphocytes
IL-2	T- and B-cell activation	T cells (TH1)
IL-3	Mast cell proliferation	T cells
	Neutrophil, macrophage maturation	Mast cells
IL-4	IgE synthesis	T cells (TH2)
IL-5	Eosinophil proliferation and differentiation	T cells (TH2)
IL-6	IgG synthesis	Fibroblasts
	Lymphocyte activation	T cells
IL-8	Neutrophil chemotaxis	Fibroblasts
		Endothelial cells
		Monocytes
IL-10	Inhibits IFN-γ, IL-1 production	T cells
		Macrophages
IL-13	Promotes IgE synthesis	T cells
IFN-α	Antiviral activity	Leukocytes
IFN-γ	Activates macrophages	T cells (TH1)
	Stimulates MHC expression	
	Inhibits TH2 activity	
TNF-γ	Antitumor cell activity	Lymphocytes
		Macrophages
TNF-β	Antitumor cell activity	T cells
GM-CSF	Stimulates mast cells, granulocytes, macrophages	Lymphocytes
		Mast cells
		Macrophages

GM-CSF, granulocyte-macrophage colony-stimulating factor; IFN, interferon; IL, interleukin; MHC, major histocompatibility complex; TH, helper T cell; TNF, tumor necrosis factor.

● Inquiry into a possible occupational cause of asthma is important for all patients with asthma.

As new industrial processes and products evolve, occupational asthma may become more common. An example of this is latex-induced asthma among medical workers, associated with the widespread use of latex gloves. The incidence of occupational asthma is estimated to be 6% to 15% of all cases of adult-onset asthma.

● Allergy to latex is an important cause of occupational asthma.

Table 2-3 Industrial Agents That Can Cause Asthma

Metals
    Salts of platinum, nickel, chrome
Wood dusts
    Mahogany
    Oak
    Redwood
    Western red cedar (plicatic acid)
Vegetable dusts
    Castor bean
    Cotton
    Cottonseed
    Flour
    Grain (mite, weevil antigens)
    Green coffee
    Gums
Industrial chemicals and plastics
    Ethylenediamine
    Phthalic and trimellitic anhydrides
    Polyvinyl chloride
    Toluene diisocyanate
Pharmaceutical agents
    Phenylglycine acid chloride
    Penicillins
    Spiramycin
Food industry agents
    Egg protein
    Polyvinyl chloride
Biologic enzymes
    Bacillus subtilis (laundry detergent workers)
    Pancreatic enzymes
Animal emanations
    Canine or feline saliva
    Horse dander (racing workers)
    Rodent urine (laboratory animal workers)

Gastroesophageal Reflux and Asthma

The role of gastroesophageal reflux in asthma is not known. Two mechanistic hypotheses are 1) reflex bronchospasm from acid in the distal esophagus and 2) recurrent aspiration of gastric contents. Although a well-documented reflex in dogs links acid in the distal esophagus to vagally mediated bronchospasm, this reflex had not been demonstrated consistently in humans. The other hypothesis is that gastric contents reach the tracheobronchial tree by ascending to the hypopharynx.

Asthma-Provoking Drugs

It is important to recognize the potentially severe adverse response that patients with asthma may show to β-blocking drugs, β_1 and β_2 blockers, including β_1 selective β-blocking agents. Patients with asthma who have glaucoma treated with ophthalmic preparations of timolol and betaxolol (betaxolol is less likely to cause problems) may experience bronchospasm.

● β-Blocking drugs, including eyedrops, can cause severe adverse responses.
● Note that so-called β_1 selective β-blocking agents such as atenolol may also provoke asthma.

Persons taking angiotensin-converting enzyme inhibitor (ACEI) drugs may develop a chronic cough that can mimic asthma. This cough may not be accompanied by additional bronchospasm.

● ACEIs can cause coughing.

Aspirin ingestion can cause acute, severe, and fatal asthma in a small subset of patients with asthma. The cause of the reaction is unknown but probably involves the generation of leukotrienes. Most of the patients affected have nasal polyposis and hyperplastic pansinus mucosal disease and are steroid-dependent for control of asthma. However, not all asthma patients with this reaction to aspirin fit the profile. Many nonsteroidal anti-inflammatory drugs (NSAIDs) can trigger the reaction to aspirin; the likelihood of a drug causing the reaction correlates with its potency for inhibiting cyclooxygenase enzyme. Structural aspects of the drug seem unrelated to its tendency to provoke the reaction. Only nonacetylated salicylates such as choline salicylate (a weak cyclooxygenase inhibitor) seem not to provoke the reaction. Leukotriene-modifying drugs may be particularly helpful in aspirin-sensitive asthma.

● Aspirin and other NSAIDs can cause acute, severe asthma.
● Asthma, nasal polyposis, and aspirin sensitivity form the "aspirin allergy triad."
● Leukotriene modifiers may be helpful in aspirin-sensitive asthma.

Traditionally, asthma patients have been warned not to take antihistamines because the anticholinergic activity of some antihistamines was thought to cause drying of lower respiratory tract secretions, further worsening the asthma. However, antihistamines do not worsen asthma, and, in fact, some studies have shown a beneficial effect. Thus, occasionally an antihistamine is specifically prescribed for asthma because it may have some beneficial effect on asthmatic inflammation.

- Antihistamines are not contraindicated in asthma.

Cigarette Smoking and Asthma

A combination of asthma and cigarette smoking leads to accelerated chronic obstructive pulmonary disease. Because of accelerated decline in irreversible obstruction, all asthma patients who smoke should be told to stop smoking.

Environmental tobacco smoke is an important asthma trigger. In particular, children with asthma who are exposed to environmental smoke have more respiratory infections and asthma attacks.

Medical History

A medical history for asthma includes careful inquiry about symptoms, provoking factors, alleviating factors, and severity. Patients with marked respiratory allergy have symptoms when exposed to aeroallergens and often have seasonal variation of symptoms. If the allergy skin test results are negative, it is reasonably certain that person does not have allergic asthma.

- In allergic asthma, symptoms are sporadic and consistently related to exposure or are seasonal.

Respiratory infections (particularly viral), cold dry air, exercise, and respiratory irritants can trigger allergic and nonallergic asthma.

- Patients with allergic asthma are likely to respond to many nonimmunologic triggers.
- Cold dry air and exercise can trigger asthma.

Assessment of Severity

Asthma is mild intermittent if 1) the symptoms are intermittent (two times a week or less), 2) continuous treatment is not needed, and 3) the flow-volume curve during formal pulmonary function testing is normal between episodes of symptoms. Even for patients who meet these criteria, inflammation (albeit patchy) is present in the airways and corticosteroid inhaled regularly diminishes bronchial hyperresponsiveness.

- Corticosteroid inhaled regularly diminishes bronchial hyperresponsiveness.

Asthma is mild persistent or moderate when 1) the symptoms occur with some regularity (more than two times a week) or daily, 2) there is some nocturnal occurrence of symptoms, or 3) asthma exacerbations are troublesome. For many of these patients, the flow-volume curve is rarely normal and complete pulmonary function testing may show evidence of hyperinflation, as indicated by increased residual volume or an increase above expected levels for the diffusing capacity of the lung for carbon dioxide. Patients with mild, moderate, or severe persistent asthma should receive treatment daily with anti-inflammatory medications, usually inhaled corticosteroids.

Asthma is severe when symptoms are present almost continuously and the upper end of the dose range of the usual medications is needed to control the disease. Most patients with severe asthma require either large doses of inhaled corticosteroid or oral prednisone daily for adequate control. Most of them have been hospitalized more than once for asthma. The severity of asthma can change over time. Note that one of the first signs that asthma is not well-controlled is the emergence of nocturnal symptoms.

- Nocturnal symptoms suggest that asthma is worsening.

Methacholine Bronchial Challenge

A patient with a history suggestive of episodic asthma but who on the day of the examination has normal results on pulmonary function tests is a reasonable candidate for methacholine bronchial challenge. The methacholine bronchial challenge is also useful in evaluating patients for cough in whom baseline pulmonary function appears normal. Positive results indicate that bronchial hyperresponsiveness is present (Table 2-4). Some consider isocapneic hyperventilation with subfreezing dry air (by either exercise or breathing carbon dioxide/air mixture) or exercise testing as alternatives to methacholine challenge.

Do not perform a methacholine challenge in patients who have severe airway obstruction or a clear diagnosis of asthma.

Table 2-4 Medical Conditions Associated With Positive Findings on Methacholine Challenge

Current asthma
Past history of asthma
Chronic obstructive pulmonary disease
Smoking
Recent respiratory infection
Chronic cough
Allergic rhinitis

Usually, a 20% decrease in forced expiratory volume in 1 second (FEV_1) is considered a positive result.

● Patients with suspected asthma and normal results on pulmonary function tests are candidates for methacholine testing.

Differential Diagnosis

The differential diagnosis of wheezing is given in Table 2-5.

Medications for Asthma

Medications for asthma are listed in Table 2-6. Currently, the only anticholinergic drug available in the United States for treating asthma is ipratropium bromide, although it is approved only for treating chronic obstructive pulmonary disease. Several short-acting β-adrenergic compounds are available, but albuterol or pirbuterol is probably prescribed most. More side effects occur when these medications are given orally rather than by inhalation. Nebulized β-agonists are rarely used long-term in adult asthma, although they may be life-saving in acute attacks. For home use, the metered-dose inhaler or dry powdered inhalation is the preferred delivery system. Salmeterol and formoterol are two long-acting inhaled β-agonists. Both should be used in combination with inhaled corticosteroids. Theophylline is effective for asthma but has a narrow therapeutic index. Note that drug interactions (cimetidine, erythromycin, and quinolone antibiotics) can increase the serum level of theophylline.

● Theophylline has a narrow therapeutic index.
● β-Agonists are best delivered by the inhaler route.

Cromolyn and nedocromil are inhaled anti-inflammatory medications that are appropriate for treatment of mild or moderate asthma. The 5-lipoxygenase inhibitor zileuton and the leukotriene receptor antagonists zafirlukast and montelukast are approved for treatment in mild persistent asthma. These agents work by decreasing the inflammatory effects of leukotrienes. Zileuton can cause increased liver function tests. Cases of Churg-Strauss vasculitis have also been linked to zafirlukast, although a clear cause-and-effect relationship has not been established.

Corticosteroid Therapy

Many experts recommend inhaled glucocorticoids for mild persistent asthma because of the potential long-term benefits of reduced bronchial hyperresponsiveness and reduced airway remodeling (fibrosis). Long-term use of β-agonist bronchodilators may adversely affect asthma; this also argues for earlier use of inhaled glucocorticoids. Asthma mortality has

Table 2-5 Differential Diagnosis of Wheezing

Pulmonary embolism
Cardiac failure
Foreign body
Central airway tumors
Aspiration
Carcinoid syndrome
Chondromalacia/polychondritis
Löffler syndrome
Bronchiectasis
Tropical eosinophilia
Hyperventilation syndrome
Laryngeal edema
Vascular ring affecting trachea
Factitious (including psychophysiologic vocal cord
    adduction)
α_1-Antiprotease deficiency
Immotile cilia syndrome
Bronchopulmonary dysplasia
Bronchiolitis (including bronchiolitis obliterans), croup
Cystic fibrosis

Table 2-6 Medications for Asthma

Bronchodilator compounds
    Anticholinergic drugs (ipratropium bromide)
    β_2-Agonist drugs
        Short-acting (albuterol, pirbuterol)
        Long-acting (salmeterol, formoterol)
    Methylxanthines (theophylline)
"Anti-allergic" compounds
    Cromolyn
    Nedocromil
Glucocorticoids
    Systemic
        Prednisone
        Methylprednisolone
    Topical
        Triamcinolone acetonide
        Beclomethasone
        Flunisolide, budesonide
Antileukotrienes
    Leukotriene receptor antagonists (zafirlukast, montelukast)
    Lipoxygenase inhibitors (zileuton)

been linked to the heavy use of β-agonist inhalers. This association may simply reflect that patients with more severe asthma (who are more likely to die of an asthma attack) use more β-agonist inhalers. However, prolonged and heavy use of inhaled β-agonists may have a direct, deleterious effect on asthma, although this has not been proved. Certainly, asthma patients with regularly recurring symptoms should have inhaled corticosteroids (or cromolyn or nedocromil) as part of the treatment.

● Prescribe inhaled glucocorticoids for mild, moderate, and severe persistent asthma.
● Long-term use of β-agonist bronchodilators may worsen asthma.

The inflammatory infiltrate in the bronchial submucosa of asthma patients likely depends on lymphokine secretory patterns. Corticosteroids may interfere at several levels in the lymphokine cascade.

Bronchoalveolar lavage and biopsy studies show that corticosteroids inhibit IL-4, IL-5, and granulocyte-macrophage colony-stimulating factor (GM-CSF) in asthma.

Monocytes or platelets may be important in the asthmatic process. Corticosteroids modify activation pathways for monocytes and platelets. Furthermore, corticosteroids have vasoconstrictive properties, which reduce vascular congestive changes in the mucosa, and they tend to decrease mucus gland secretion.

● Corticosteroids reduce airway inflammation by modulating cytokines.
● Corticosteroids can inhibit the inflammatory properties of monocytes and platelets.
● Corticosteroids have vasoconstrictive properties.
● Corticosteroids decrease mucus gland secretion.

The most common adverse effects of inhaled corticosteroids are dysphonia and thrush. These unwanted effects occur in about 10% of patients and can be reduced by using a spacer device and rinsing the mouth after administration. Usually, oral thrush can be treated successfully with oral antifungal agents. Dysphonia, when persistent, may be treated by decreasing or discontinuing the use of inhaled corticosteroids.

Detailed study of the systemic effects of inhaled corticosteroids shows that these agents are much safer than oral corticosteroids. Nevertheless, there is evidence that high-dose inhaled corticosteroids can affect the hypothalamic-pituitary-adrenal axis and bone metabolism. Also, high-dose inhaled corticosteroids may increase the risk of future development of glaucoma, cataracts, and osteoporosis. Inhaled corticosteroids can decrease growth velocity in children and adolescents. The effect of inhaled corticosteroids on adult height is not known, but it appears to be minimal.

Poor inhaler technique and poor compliance can result in poor control of asthma. Therefore, all patients using a metered-dose inhaler or dry powder inhaler should be taught the proper technique of using these devices. Most patients using metered-dose inhaled corticosteroids should be using a spacer device with the inhaler.

● The most common cause of poor results is poor inhaler technique.
● Patients should use a spacer device with metered-dose inhaled corticosteroids.

Goals of Asthma Management
The goals of asthma management are listed in Table 2-7.

Management of Chronic Asthma
Baseline spirometry is recommended for all patients with asthma, and home peak flow monitoring is recommended for those with moderate or severe asthma (Fig. 2-1).

● Spirometry is recommended for all asthma patients.
● Home peak flow monitoring is recommended for those with moderate or severe asthma.

Environmental triggers should be discussed with all asthma patients, and allergy testing should be offered to those with suspected allergic asthma or with asthma that is not well controlled. Although allergy immunotherapy is effective, it is recommended only for patients with allergic asthma who have had a complete evaluation by an allergist.

Management of Acute Asthma
Inhaled β-agonists, measurements of lung function at presentation and during therapy, and systemic corticosteroids (for most patients) are the cornerstones of managing acute asthma (Fig. 2-2). Generally, nebulized albuterol, administered repeatedly if necessary, is the first line of treatment. Delivery of β-agonist by metered-dose inhaler can be substituted in less severe asthma attacks. Inhaled β-agonist delivered by continuous nebulization may be appropriate for more severe disease.

Table 2-7 Goals of Asthma Management

No asthma symptoms
No asthma attacks
Normal activity level
Normal lung function
Use of safest and least amount of medication necessary
Establish therapeutic relationship between patient and provider

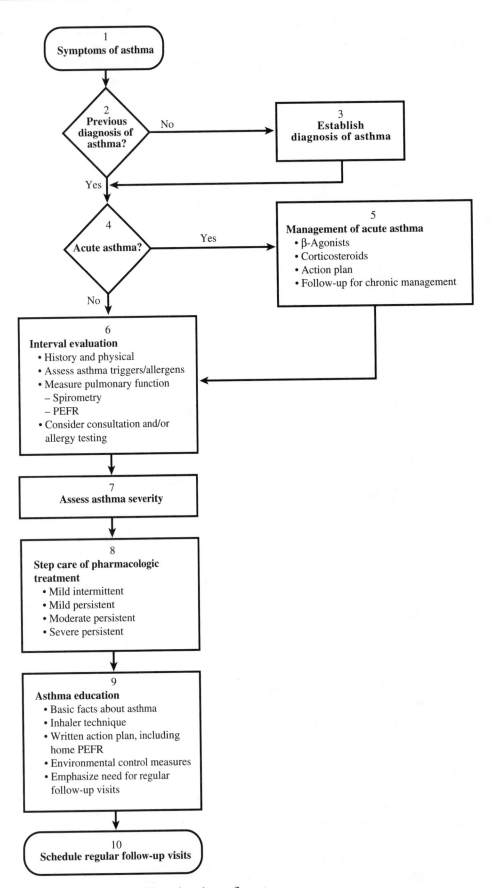

Fig. 2-1. Diagnosis and management of asthma. PEFR, peak expiratory flow rate.

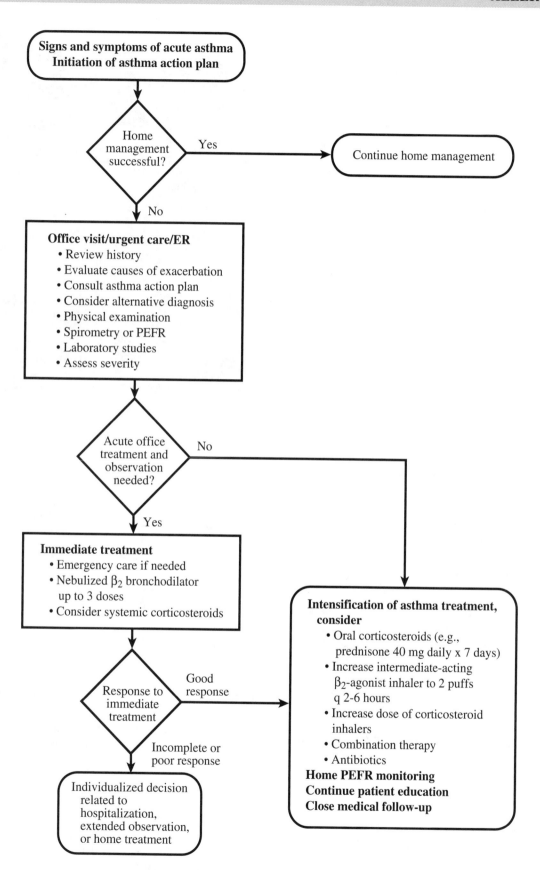

Fig. 2-2. Management of acute asthma in adults. ER, emergency room; PEFR, peak expiratory flow rate. (By permission of Institute of Clinical Systems Integration.)

● Inhaled β-agonist can be delivered by intermittent nebulization, continuous nebulization, or metered-dose inhaler.

It is important to measure lung function (usually peak expiratory flow rate [PEFR] but also FEV_1 whenever possible) at presentation and after administration of bronchodilators. These measurements provide invaluable information that allows the physician to assess the severity of the asthma attack and the response (if any) to treatment.

Patients who do not have a prompt and full response to inhaled β-agonists should receive a course of systemic corticosteroids. Patients with the most severe and poorly responsive disease should be treated on a hospital ward or in an intensive care unit.

● Measure pulmonary function at presentation and after giving bronchodilators.
● Most patients with acute asthma need a course of systemic corticosteroids.

ALLERGIC BRONCHOPULMONARY ASPERGILLOSIS

Allergic bronchopulmonary aspergillosis is an obstructive lung disease caused by an allergic reaction to *Aspergillus* in the lower airway. The typical patient presents with severe steroid-dependent asthma. Most patients with this condition have coexisting asthma or cystic fibrosis.

● Allergic bronchopulmonary aspergillosis develops in patients with asthma or cystic fibrosis.

The diagnostic features of allergic bronchopulmonary aspergillosis are summarized in Table 2-8. Fungi other than *Aspergillus fumigatus* can cause an allergic bronchopulmonary mycosis similar to allergic bronchopulmonary aspergillosis.

Chest radiography can show transient or permanent infiltrates and central bronchiectasis, usually affecting the upper lobes (Fig. 2-3). Advanced cases show extensive pulmonary fibrosis.

Table 2-8 Diagnostic Features of Allergic Bronchopulmonary Aspergillosis

Clinical asthma
Bronchiectasis (usually proximal)
Increased total serum IgE
IgE antibody to *Aspergillus* (by skin test or in vitro assay)
Precipitins or IgG antibody to *Aspergillus*
Radiographic infiltrates (often upper lobes)
Peripheral blood eosinophilia

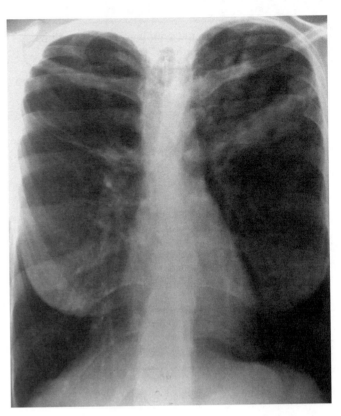

Fig. 2-3. Chest radiograph in allergic bronchopulmonary aspergillosis shows cylindrical infiltrates involving the upper lobes.

Allergic bronchopulmonary aspergillosis is treated with systemic corticosteroids. Total serum IgE may be helpful in following the course of the disease. Antifungal therapy has not been effective.

CHRONIC RHINITIS

Medical History

Vasomotor rhinitis is defined as nasal symptoms occurring in response to nonspecific, nonallergic irritants. Common triggers of vasomotor rhinitis are strong odors, respiratory irritants such as dust or smoke, changes in temperature, changes in body position, and ingestants such as spicy food or alcohol. This is considered a nonallergic rhinitis.

● Vasomotor rhinitis is defined as nasal symptoms in response to nonspecific stimuli.

Historical factors favoring a diagnosis of *allergic* rhinitis include a history of nasal symptoms that have a recurrent seasonal pattern (e.g., every August and September) or symptoms provoked by being near animals. Factors favoring *vasomotor* rhinitis include symptoms provoked by strong odors and humidity and temperature changes.

- Allergic rhinitis has a recurrent seasonal pattern and may be provoked by being near animals.
- Triggers of vasomotor rhinitis include strong odors and humidity and temperature changes.

Factors common to allergic rhinitis and vasomotor rhinitis (thus, without differential diagnostic value) include perennial symptoms, intolerance of cigarette smoke, and history of "dust" sensitivity. Factors that suggest fixed nasal obstruction (which should prompt physicians to consider other diagnoses) include unilateral nasal obstruction, unilateral facial pain, unilateral nasal purulence, nasal voice but no nasal symptoms, disturbances of olfaction without any nasal symptoms, and unilateral nasal bleeding (Table 2-9).

- Perennial symptoms, intolerance of cigarette smoke, and history of "dust" sensitivity are common to allergic and vasomotor rhinitis.
- Dust mite sensitivity is a common cause of perennial allergic rhinitis.

Allergy Skin Tests in Allergic Rhinitis

The interpretation of allergy skin test results must be tailored to the unique features of each patient.

1. For patients with perennial symptoms and negative results on allergy skin tests, the diagnosis is vasomotor rhinitis.
2. For patients with seasonal symptoms and appropriately positive allergy skin tests, the diagnosis is seasonal allergic rhinitis.
3. For patients with perennial symptoms, allergy skin tests positive for house dust mite suggest house dust mite allergic rhinitis. In this case, dust mite allergen avoidance should be recommended. Have patients encase their bedding with allergy-proof encasements, remove carpeting from the bedroom, and lower the relative humidity in the house to 40% to 50% or less.

Table 2-9 Differential Diagnosis of Chronic Rhinitis

Allergic rhinitis
Vasomotor rhinitis
Rhinitis medicamentosus
Sinusitis
Nasal polyposis
Nasal septal deviation
Foreign body
Tumor

Corticosteroid Therapy for Rhinitis

The need for systemic corticosteroid treatment for rhinitis is limited. Occasionally, patients with severe symptoms of hay fever may benefit greatly from a short course of prednisone (10 mg 4 times daily by mouth for 5 days). This may induce sufficient improvement so that topical corticosteroids can penetrate the nose and satisfactory levels of antihistamine can be established in the blood. Severe nasal polyposis may warrant a longer course of oral corticosteroids. Sometimes, recurrence of nasal polyps can be prevented by continued use of topical corticosteroids. Polypectomy may be required if nasal polyps fail to respond to treatment with systemic and intranasal corticosteroids.

- Treatment of nasal polyposis can include oral prednisone, followed by topical corticosteroids.

In contrast to systemic corticosteroid therapy, topical corticosteroid agents for the nose are easy to use and have few adverse systemic effects. Intranasal corticosteroids may decrease growth velocity in children.

- Intranasal corticosteroids may decrease growth velocity in children.

Most people are aware that long-term treatment with decongestant nasal sprays is a bad idea because of the "addictive" potential (a vicious cycle of rebound congestion called "rhinitis medicamentosa" caused by topical vasoconstrictors is common knowledge). Reassure patients that an inhaled corticosteroid does not induce any dependence.

- Unlike decongestant nasal sprays, intranasal corticosteroid does not induce tachyphylaxis and rebound congestion.

A substantial number of patients with vasomotor rhinitis also have a good response to intranasal (topical aerosol) corticosteroid therapy, especially if they have the nasal eosinophilia or nasal polyposis form of vasomotor rhinitis.

- Many patients with vasomotor rhinitis have a good response to topical aerosol corticosteroid therapy.

If a patient with hay fever does not receive adequate relief with topical corticosteroid plus antihistamine therapy, it may indicate the need for systemic corticosteroid treatment and the initiation of immunotherapy.

- If pharmacologic management fails, allergy immunotherapy should be considered for patients with allergic rhinitis.

An unusual side effect of intranasal corticosteroids is nasal septal perforation. Dry powder spray cannisters deliver a powerful jet of particulates, and a few patients have misdirected the jet to the nasal septum.

- Rarely, nasal topical corticosteroid sprays can cause perforation of the nasal septum.

Antihistamines and Decongestants

Antihistamines antagonize the interaction of histamine with its receptors. Histamine may be more causative than other mast cell mediators of nasal itch and sneezing. These are symptoms most often responsive to antihistamine therapy.

Pseudoephedrine is the most common agent in nonprescription drugs for treating cold symptoms and rhinitis and usually is the active agent in widely used proprietary prescription agents. Phenylpropanolamine has been removed from the market because of its association with hemorrhagic stroke in women. A large number of prescription and nonprescription combination agents combine an antihistamine and decongestant. Decongestant preparations are often the only therapeutic option for patients with vasomotor rhinitis unresponsive to topical glucocorticoids.

- Pseudoephedrine is the most common decongestant in nonprescription preparations.

Note that middle-aged and older men may have urinary retention caused by antihistamines (principally the older drugs that have anticholinergic effects) and decongestants; these patients should be alerted to this. Although there has been concern for years that decongestants may exacerbate hypertension because they are α-adrenergic agonists, no clinically significant hypertensive response has been seen in patients with hypertension that is controlled medically.

- Antihistamines and decongestants may cause urinary retention in men.

For antihistamines with anticholinergic activity, patients, especially older ones, should be warned about possible dizziness, dry mouth, blurred vision, and drowsiness.

- The elderly are more sensitive to the anticholinergic effects of antihistamines.

Immunotherapy for Allergic Rhinitis

Until topical nasal glucocorticoid sprays were introduced, allergen immunotherapy was considered first-line therapy for allergic rhinitis when the relevant allergen was seasonal pollen of grass, trees, or weeds. Immunotherapy became second-line therapy after topical corticosteroids were introduced because immunotherapy 1) requires more time commitment during the build-up phase and 2) carries a small risk of anaphylaxis to the immunotherapy injection itself. However, immunotherapy for allergic rhinitis can be appropriate first-line therapy in selected patients and is highly effective.

Immunotherapy is usually reserved for patients who have no satisfactory relief from intranasal corticosteroids or who cannot tolerate antihistamines. Controlled trials have shown a benefit for pollen, dust mite, and cat allergy and a variable benefit for mold allergy. Immunotherapy is not given for food allergy or nonallergic rhinitis. The practice is less uniform with respect to mold allergens, with endorsement divided in the subspecialty.

- Immunotherapy usually is reserved for patients who receive no relief from intranasal glucocorticoids or who cannot tolerate antihistamines.
- Controlled trials have shown that immunotherapy is effective for allergic rhinitis.
- Anaphylaxis is a risk of immunotherapy.
- Immunotherapy for allergic rhinitis can be first-line therapy in selected patients.

Environmental Modification

House Dust Mites

House dust mites are so small they cannot maintain their own internal water unless ambient conditions are high humidity. They eat all kinds of organic matter but seem to favor mold and epidermal scale shed by humans. They occur in all human habitations, although the population size varies with local conditions. The only geographic areas free of house dust mites are those at great elevations with extreme dryness.

- House dust mites require high humidity to survive.
- They are found in nearly all human habitations.

Areas in the home harboring the most substantial mite populations are bedding and fabric-upholstered furniture (heavily used) and any area where carpeting is on concrete (when concrete is in contact with grade). Although carpeting is often cited as an important mite-related problem, carpet on wooden floors in a dry, well-ventilated house usually harbors only a small number of dust mites. Aerosol dispersion of allergen from this source is not great compared with that from bedding and furniture. To prevent egress of allergen when the mattress and pillows are compressed by occupancy of the bed, encase the bedding (and sometimes, when practical, furniture cushions) in plastic dust-proof encasements. To some degree, this also prevents infusion of water vapor into the bedding matrix. These two factors combine to markedly decrease the amount of airborne allergen. Measures for controlling dust mites are listed in Table 2-10.

- Dust mite is an important respiratory allergen.
- The most substantial mite population is in bedding and fabric-upholstered furniture.
- Plastic encasements prevent egress of allergen.
- Recently, chemical sprays (acaricides) capable of either killing mites or denaturing the protein allergens from them have been marketed. However, neither agent is substantially helpful when applied in the home.

Pollen

Air conditioning, which enables the warm-season home to remain tightly closed, is the principal defense against pollinosis. Most masks purchased at local pharmacies are not capable of excluding pollen particles and are not worth the expense. Some masks can protect the wearer from allergen exposure. These include industrial-quality respirators designed specifically to pass rigorous testing by the Occupational Safety and Health Administration (OSHA) and the National Institute for Occupational Safety and Health (NIOSH) to certify them capable of excluding a wide spectrum of particulates, including pollen and mold. These masks allow persons to mow the lawn and do yard work otherwise intolerable because of exposure to pollen allergen.

- Only industrial-quality masks are capable of excluding pollen particles.

Animal Dander

No measure can compare with getting the animal completely out of the house. No air filtration scheme that is feasible for average homeowners to install can eliminate allergen from an actively elaborating animal. If complete removal is not tenable, some partial measure must be considered.

If the house is heated or cooled by a forced-air system with ductwork, confining the pet to a single room in the house is only partially effective in reducing overall exposure, because air from every room is collected through the air-return ductwork and redistributed through a central plenum. If air-return ducts are sealed in the room where the animal is kept and air can escape from the room only by infiltration, exposure may be reduced. The room selected for this measure should be as far as possible from the bedroom of the person with the allergy. Naturally, the person should avoid close contact with the animal and should consider using a mask if animal handling or entry into the room where the animal is kept is necessary. Most animal danders have little or nothing to do with animal hair, so its shedding status is irrelevant. Bathing cats about once every other week may reduce the allergen load in the environment.

- Complete avoidance is the only entirely effective way to manage allergy to household pets.

Sinusitis

Sinusitis is closely associated with edematous obstruction of the sinus ostia (the osteomeatal complex). Poor drainage of the sinus cavities predisposes to infection, particularly by microorganisms that thrive in low oxygen environments (e.g., anaerobes). In adults, *Streptococcus pneumoniae*, *Haemophilus influenzae*, anaerobes, and viruses are common pathogens. In addition, *Branhamella catarrhalis* is an important pathogen in children.

Important clinical features of acute sinusitis are purulent nasal discharge, tooth pain, cough, and poor response to decongestants. Findings on paranasal sinus transillumination may be abnormal.

- Purulent nasal discharge, tooth pain, and abnormal findings on transillumination are important clinical features of sinusitis.

Physicians should be aware of the complications of sinusitis, which can be life-threatening (Table 2-11). Mucormycosis can cause recurrent or persistent sinusitis refractory to antibiotics.

Table 2-10 Dust Mite Control

Encase bedding and pillows in airtight encasements
Remove carpeting in bedroom
Remove upholstered furniture from bedroom
Remove all carpeting laid on concrete
Discontinue use of humidifier
Wash bedding in hot water
Run dehumidifier

Table 2-11 Complications of Sinusitis

Osteomyelitis
Meningitis
Subdural abscess
Extradural abscess
Orbital infection
Cellulitis
Cavernous sinus thrombosis

Allergic fungal sinusitis is characterized by persistent sinusitis, eosinophilia, increased total IgE, antifungal (usually *Aspergillus*) IgE antibodies, and fungal colonization of the sinuses. Wegener granulomatosis, ciliary dyskinesia, and hypogammaglobulinemia are medical conditions that can cause refractory sinusitis (Table 2-12).

Untreated sinusitis may lead to osteomyelitis, orbital and periorbital cellulitis, meningitis, and brain abscess. Cavernous sinus thrombosis, an especially serious complication, can lead to retrobulbar pain, extraocular muscle paralysis, and blindness.

Persistent, refractory, and complicated sinusitis should be evaluated by a specialist. Sinus computed tomography (CT) is the preferred imaging study for these patients (Fig. 2-4).

Amoxicillin, 500 mg three times daily, or trimethoprim-sulfamethoxazole (one double-strength capsule twice daily) for 10 to14 days is the treatment of choice for uncomplicated maxillary sinusitis.

The sensitivity of plain radiography of the sinuses is not as good as that of CT (using coronal sectioning technique). Good-quality coronal CT scans show greater detail about sinus mucosal surfaces, but CT usually is not necessary in acute uncomplicated sinusitis. However, CT is indicated for patients being considered for a sinus operation and for those in whom standard treatment for sinusitis fails. Be aware that patients with extensive dental restorations that contain metal may generate too much artifact for CT to be useful. For these patients, magnetic resonance imaging (MRI) techniques are better.

- Sinus imaging is indicated for recurrent sinusitis.
- Sinus CT is preferred to sinus radiography for complicated sinusitis.

URICARIA AND ANGIOEDEMA

The distinction between acute and chronic urticaria is arbitrary and based on the duration of the urticaria. If it has been present for 6 weeks or longer, it is called "chronic urticaria."

Table 2-12 Causes of Persistent or Recurrent Sinusitis

Nasal polyposis
Mucormycosis
Allergic fungal sinusitis
Ciliary dyskinesia
Wegener granulomatosis
Hypogammaglobulinemia
Tumor

Secondary Urticaria

Most patients simply have urticaria as a skin disease (chronic idiopathic urticaria), but occasionally it is the presenting sign of more serious internal disease. It can be a sign of lupus erythematosus and other connective tissue diseases, particularly of the more difficult to categorize "overlap" syndromes. Malignancy, mainly of the gastrointestinal tract, and lymphoproliferative diseases are associated with urticaria, as occult infection may be, particularly of the gallbladder and dentition. Immune-complex disease has been associated with urticaria, usually with urticarial vasculitis, and hepatitis B virus has been identified as an antigen in cases of urticaria and immune-complex disease.

- Urticaria can be associated with lupus erythematosus and other connective tissue diseases, malignancy, infection, and immune-complex disease.

A common cause of acute urticaria and angioedema (other than the idiopathic variety) is drug or food allergy. However, drug or food allergy usually does not cause chronic urticaria.

- Chronic urticaria and angioedema are often idiopathic.
- A common secondary cause of acute urticaria and angioedema is drug or food allergy.

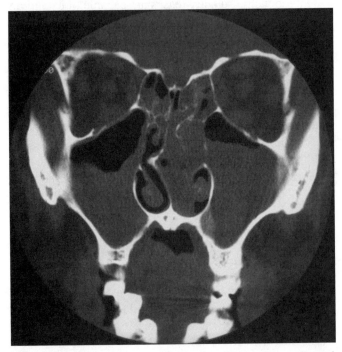

Fig. 2-4. Sinus computed tomogram showing opacification of the osteomeatal complex on the left, subtotal opacification of the right maxillary sinus, and an air-fluid level in the left maxillary antrum.

Relation Between Urticaria and Angioedema

In common idiopathic urticaria, the lesions itch intensely because histamine is one of the causes of wheal formation.

- Typical urticarial lesions last 2-18 hours and are pruritic.

The pathophysiologic mechanism is similar for urticaria and angioedema. The critical factor is the type of tissue in which the capillary leak and mediator release occur. Urticaria occurs when the capillary events are in the tightly welded tissue wall of the skin—the epidermis. Angioedema occurs when capillary events affect vessels in loose connective tissue of the deeper layers—the dermis. Virtually all patients with the common idiopathic type of urticaria also have angioedema from time to time. When urticaria is caused by allergic reactions, angioedema may also occur. The only exception is with the hereditary angioneurotic edema (HANE) type of disease, which is not related to mast cell mediator release but is a complement disorder. Patients with this form of angioedema rarely have urticaria.

C1 Esterase Inhibitor Deficiency

If HANE is strongly suspected, the diagnosis can be proved by the appropriate measurement of complement factors (C1 esterase inhibitor [quantitative and functional] and C4 [also C2, if seen during an episode of swelling]).

- C1 esterase inhibitor levels and C4 are decreased in hereditary angioedema.

The duration of individual swellings varies. Many patients with HANE have had at least one hospitalization for what appeared to be intestinal obstruction. If they avoid laparotomy on these occasions, the obstruction usually resolves in 3 to 5 days. Cramps and diarrhea may occur.

Lesions in HANE do not itch. The response to epinephrine is a useful differential point: HANE lesions do not respond well to epinephrine, but common angioedema usually resolves in 15 minutes or less. Laryngeal edema almost never occurs in the common idiopathic type of disease (although it may occur in allergic reactions, most often in insect-sting anaphylaxis cases); however, it is relatively common in HANE (earlier papers quoted a 30% mortality rate in HANE, with all deaths due to laryngeal edema). HANE episodes may be related to local tissue trauma in a high percentage of cases, with dental work often regarded as the classic precipitating factor.

- Most patients with HANE have been hospitalized for "intestinal obstruction."
- HANE lesions do not respond well to epinephrine.
- In HANE, laryngeal edema is relatively common.
- Dental work is the classic precipitating factor for HANE.

The common idiopathic form of urticaria and angioedema is usually unrelated to antecedent trauma except in special cases of delayed-pressure urticaria, in which hives and angioedema follow minor trauma of or pressure on (e.g., to the hands while playing golf) soft tissues. The response to pressure distinguishes this special form of physical urticaria from HANE.

It is reasonable to perform C4 and C1 esterase inhibitor assays (functional and quantitative) for all patients with unexplained recurrent angioedema, especially if urticaria is not present.

The three major types of HANE-like disorders are as follows:

1. Classic HANE is a genetic dysregulation of gene function for C1 inhibitor that is inherited in an autosomal dominant pattern. Therapy with androgens (testosterone, stanozolol, danazol) reverses the dysregulation and allows expression of the otherwise normal gene, resulting in half-normal plasma levels of C1, which are sufficient to eliminate the clinical manifestations of the disease.

- Classic HANE is a genetic dysregulation (autosomal dominant).
- Testosterone, stanozolol, and danazol reverse the dysregulation.

2. In some cases of HANE, the gene for the C1 inhibitor mutates, rendering the molecule functionally ineffective but quantifiable in the blood. Thus, plasma levels of the C1 inhibitor molecule may be normal in these patients. This is the basis for requesting immunochemical and functional measures of serum C1 inhibitor (with immunochemical measures only, the diagnosis is missed in cases of normal levels of an inactive molecule). Both classic HANE (low levels of C1 esterase inhibitor) and classic HANE with the mutated gene for C1 inhibitor (nonfunctional C1 esterase inhibitor) are inherited forms of the disease. However, the proband may start the mutational line in both forms of HANE, so the family history is not positive in all cases.

- Hereditary angioedema with normal levels of C1 esterase inhibitor but nonfunctional (by esterase assay) indicates a gene mutation.

3. C1 esterase inhibitor deficiency may be an acquired disorder with malignancy or lymphoproliferative disease. Plasma levels for C1, C4, and C1 esterase inhibitor are low in acquired C1 esterase inhibitor deficiency. The hypothesis for the pathogenesis of this form of angioedema is that the tumor has or releases determinants that fix complement, and with constant consumption of complement components, a point is reached at which the biosynthesis of C1 inhibitor cannot keep up with

the consumption rate, and the relative deficiency of C1 inhibitor allows episodes of swelling.

- C1 esterase inhibitor deficiency can be an acquired disorder in malignancy or lymphoproliferative disease.
- C1 levels are low in acquired C1 esterase inhibitor deficiency.

Physical Urticaria

Heat, light, cold, vibration, and trauma or pressure have been reported to cause hives in susceptible persons. Obtaining the history is the only way to suspect the diagnosis, which can be confirmed by applying each of the stimuli to the patient's skin in the laboratory. Heat can be applied by placing coins (soaked in hot water for a few minutes) on the patient's forearm. Cold can be applied with coins kept in a freezer or with ice cubes. For vibration, a laboratory vortex mixer or any common vibrator can be used. A pair of sandbags connected by a strap can be draped over the patient to create enough pressure to cause symptoms in those with delayed pressure urticaria. Unlike most cases of common idiopathic urticaria in which the lesions affect essentially all skin surfaces, many cases of physical urticarias seem to involve only certain areas of skin. Thus, challenges will be positive only in the areas usually involved and negative in other areas. Directing challenges to the appropriate area depends on the history.

- For physical urticaria, the history is the only way to suspect the diagnosis, which can be confirmed by applying stimuli to the patient's skin.

Food Allergy in Chronic Urticaria

Food allergy almost never causes chronic urticaria. However, urticaria can be an acute manifestation of true food allergy.

- Food allergy almost never causes chronic urticaria.
- Food allergy may cause acute urticaria, angioedema, or anaphylaxis.

Histopathology of Chronic Urticaria

Chronic urticaria is characterized by mononuclear cell perivascular cuffing around dermal capillaries, particularly involving the capillary loops that interdigitate with the rete pegs of the epidermis. This mononuclear cell cuff consists mostly of helper T cells, with some monocytes, macrophages, B cells, and mast cells. This is the usual histologic location for most skin mast cells. It appears there is about a tenfold increase in the number of mast cells in the cuff compared with the normal value. However, the number of mast cells is still small compared with that of other round cells in the cuff. This histologic picture is consistent throughout the skin, regardless

of recent active urtication. Most pathologists consider "vasculitis" to indicate actual necrosis of the structural elements of blood vessels; thus, the typical features of chronic urticaria do not meet the criteria for vasculitis. Immunofluorescence studies on chronic urticaria biopsy samples for fibrin, complement, and immunoglobulin deposition in blood vessels are negative.

Urticarial vasculitis shows the usual histologic features of leukocytoclastic vasculitis.

- The characteristic histopathologic feature of chronic urticaria is a mononuclear cell perivascular cuff around capillaries.

Management of Urticaria

The history is of utmost importance if the 2% to 4% of cases of chronic urticaria actually due to allergic causes are to be discovered. A complete physical examination is needed, with particular attention to the skin (including some test for dermatographism) to evaluate for the vasculitic nature of the lesions and to the liver, lymph nodes, and mucous membranes. Laboratory testing need not be exhaustive: chest radiography, a complete blood count with differential count to discover eosinophilia, liver enzymes, erythrocyte sedimentation rate, serum protein electrophoresis, total hemolytic complement, antinuclear antibody, urinalysis, and stool examination for parasites. Only if the patient has strong allergic tendencies and some element in the history suggests an allergic cause is allergy skin testing indicated. However, patients with idiopathic urticaria often have fixed ideas about an allergy causing their problem, and skin testing often helps to dissuade them of this idea.

- The history is of utmost importance in diagnosing allergic urticaria.
- Laboratory testing may include chest radiography, eosinophil count, liver enzymes, erythrocyte sedimentation rate, serum protein electrophoresis, total hemolytic complement, and stool examination for parasites.

Management of urticaria and angioedema consists of blocking histamine, beginning usually with H_1 antagonists. The addition of H_2 antagonists may be helpful. Tricyclic antidepressants, such as doxepin, have potent antihistamine effects and are useful. Systemic corticosteroids can be administered for acute urticaria and angioedema or for very severe chronic idiopathic urticaria and angioedema.

- Urticaria and angioedema: management is usually with H_1 antagonists.
- Urticaria and angioedema: systemic corticosteroids are used for severe cases.

FOOD ALLERGY

Clinical History

The clinical syndrome of food allergy should prompt patients to provide a history containing some or all the following: for very sensitive persons, some tingling, itching, and a metallic taste in the mouth occur while the food is still in the mouth. Within 15 minutes after the food is swallowed, some epigastric distress may occur. There may be nausea and rarely vomiting. Abdominal cramping is felt chiefly in the periumbilical area (small-bowel phase), and lower abdominal cramping and watery diarrhea may occur. Urticaria or angioedema may occur in any distribution or there may be only itching of the palms and soles. With increasing clinical sensitivity to the offending allergen, anaphylactic symptoms may emerge, including tachycardia, hypotension, generalized flushing, and alterations of consciousness.

In extremely sensitive persons, generalized flushing, hypotension, and tachycardia may occur before the other symptoms. Most patients with a food allergy can identify the offending foods. The diagnosis should be confirmed by skin testing or in vitro measurement of allergen-specific IgE antibody.

- Allergic reactions to food usually include pruritus, urticaria, or angioedema.

Common Causes of Food Allergy

Items considered the most common allergens are listed in Table 2-13.

Food-Related Anaphylaxis

Food-induced anaphylaxis is the same process involved in acute urticaria or angioedema to food allergens, except the severity of the reaction is greater in anaphylaxis. Relatively few foods are involved in food-induced anaphylaxis; the main ones are peanuts, shellfish, and nuts. Patients with latex allergy can develop food allergy to banana, avocado, kiwifruit, and other fruits.

- Anaphylaxis to food can be life-threatening.
- There is cross-sensitivity between latex and banana, avocado, and kiwifruit.

Table 2-13 Common Causes of Food Allergy

Eggs	Shellfish
Milk	Soybean
Nuts	Wheat
Peanuts	

Allergy Skin Testing in Food Allergy

Patients presenting with food-related symptoms may have food allergy, food intolerance, irritable bowel syndrome, nonspecific dyspepsia, or one of a large number of nonallergic conditions. A careful and detailed history on the nature of the "reaction," the reproducibility of the association of food and symptoms, and the timing of symptoms in relation to the ingestion of food can help the clinician form a clinical impression.

In many cases, allergy skin tests to foods can be helpful. If the allergy skin tests are negative (and the clinical suspicion for food allergy is low), the patient can be reassured that food allergy is not the cause of the symptoms. If the allergy skin tests are positive (and the clinical suspicion for food allergy is high), the patient should be counseled about the management of the food allergy. For highly sensitive persons, this includes strict and rigorous avoidance of the offending foods. These patients should also be given epinephrine for self-administration in case of emergency.

If the diagnosis of food allergy is uncertain or if the symptoms are mild and nonspecific, sometimes oral food challenges can be helpful. An open challenge is usually performed first. If negative, the diagnosis of food allergy is excluded. If positive, a blinded placebo-controlled challenge can be performed.

- Positive results on skin tests and double-blind food challenges can confirm the diagnosis of food allergy.
- If results of food skin tests are negative, food allergy is unlikely.
- Patients with anaphylaxis to food should strictly avoid the offending food and carry an epinephrine kit.

STINGING INSECT ALLERGY

In patients clinically sensitive to Hymenoptera, reactions to a sting can be either large local reactions or the systemic, anaphylactic reactions. With the large local sting reaction, swelling at the sting site may be dramatic but there are no symptoms distant from that site. Stings of the head, neck, and dorsum of the hands are particularly prone to large local reactions.

Anaphylaxis caused by allergy to stinging insects is similar to all other forms of anaphylaxis. Thus, the onset of anaphylaxis may be very rapid, often within 1 or 2 minutes. Pruritus of the palms and soles is the most common initial manifestation and frequently is followed by generalized flushing, urticaria, angioedema, or hypotension (or a combination of these). The reason for attaching importance to whether a stinging insect reaction is a large local or a generalized one is that allergy skin testing and allergen immunotherapy are recommended only for generalized reactions. Patients who experience a large local reaction are not at increased risk for future anaphylaxis.

- Two varieties of reaction to sting: large local and anaphylactic.

Bee and Vespid Allergy

Yellow jackets, wasps, and hornets are vespids, and their venoms cross-react to a substantial degree. The venom of honeybees (family Apidae) does *not* cross-react with that of vespids. Unless the patient actually captures the insect delivering the sting, uncertainty will likely attend many cases of insect-stinging anaphylaxis. Thus, we usually conduct skin testing to honeybee and each of the vespids. To interpret skin tests accurately, it is helpful to know which insect caused the sting producing the generalized reaction. Often, the circumstances of the sting can help determine the type of insect responsible. Multiple stings received while mowing the grass or doing other landscape jobs that may disturb yellow-jacket burrows in the ground are likely causes of yellow-jacket stings. A single sting received while near picnic tables or refuse containers at picnic areas is likely from a yellow jacket or possibly a hornet. Stings received while working around the house exterior (painting, cleaning eaves and gutters, attic work) are most likely from wasps.

- Yellow jackets, wasps, and hornets are vespids and their venoms cross-react.
- The venom of bees does not cross-react with that of vespids.
- It is helpful to know which insect caused the sting.

Allergy Testing

Patients who have had a generalized reaction warrant allergen skin testing. Patients who have had a large local reaction to one of the Hymenoptera stings do *not* warrant allergen skin testing because they are not at increased risk for future anaphylaxis.

- Generalized reaction warrants allergen skin testing.
- Large local reaction does not warrant allergen skin testing.

In many cases, skin testing should be delayed for at least 1 month after a sting-induced general reaction because tests conducted closer to the time of the sting have a substantial risk of being falsely negative. Positive results on skin testing that correlate with the clinical history are sufficient evidence for considering Hymenoptera venom immunotherapy.

- Skin testing should be delayed for at least 1 month after a sting-induced general reaction.
- Patients with clinical anaphylaxis and positive results on venom skin tests may benefit from venom immunotherapy.

Venom Immunotherapy

The decision to undertake venom immunotherapy can be reached only after a discussion between the patient and physician. General indications for venom immunotherapy are listed in Table 2-14. Patients must understand that once initiated the immunotherapy injection schedule has to be maintained and that there is a small risk of the immunotherapy inducing anaphylaxis. It is important that patients understand that despite receiving allergy immunotherapy, they must carry epinephrine when outdoors because of the 2% to 10% possibility that immunotherapy will not provide suitable protection. Most, but not all, patients can safely discontinue venom immunotherapy after 3 to 5 years of treatment.

- There is a small risk that venom immunotherapy will induce anaphylaxis.
- There is a 2%-10% chance that venom immunotherapy will not provide adequate protection.

Avoidance

The warnings that every patient with stinging-insect hypersensitivity should receive are listed in Table 2-15. The circumstances of each patient may provide additional entries to this list. Also, patients need to know how to use self-injectable epinephrine in its several forms. Many patients wear an anaphylaxis identification bracelet.

- All patients with stinging-insect sensitivity should carry an epinephrine kit.

Anaphylaxis

Anaphylaxis is a generalized reaction characterized by flushing, hypotension, and tachycardia. Urticaria and angioedema may occur in many cases, and in patients with moderate-to-severe asthma or rhinitis as a preexisting condition, the asthma and rhinitis can be made worse. This definition of anaphylaxis is based on clinical manifestations. A

Table 2-14   Indications for Venom Immunotherapy

History of anaphylaxis to a sting

Positive results on skin tests to venom implicated historically in the anaphylactic reaction

Patient's level of anxiety disrupts usual habits and activities in warm months

Occupational—higher than usual risk of sting

   House painters

   Outdoor construction workers

   Forestry workers

Table 2-15 Do's and Don'ts for Patients With Hypersensitivity to Insect Stings

---

Avoid looking or smelling like a flower

    Avoid flowered prints for clothes

    Avoid cosmetics and fragrances, especially ones derived from flowering plants

Never drink from a soft-drink can out-of-doors during the warm months—a yellow jacket can land *on* or *in* the can while you are not watching and go inside the can and sting the inside of your mouth (one of the most dangerous places for a sensitive patient to be stung) when you take a drink

Avoid doing outdoor maintenance and yard work

Never reach into a mailbox without first looking inside it

Never go barefoot

Always look at the underside of picnic table benches and park benches before sitting down

Never attempt physically to eject a stinging insect from the interior of an automobile, but pull over, get out, and let someone else remove the insect

---

cellular and molecular definition of anaphylaxis is "a generalized allergic reaction in which large quantities of both preformed and newly synthesized mediators are released from activated basophils and mast cells." The dominant mediators of acute anaphylaxis are histamine and prostaglandin D_2. The serum levels of tryptase may be increased for a few hours after clinical anaphylaxis. Physiologically, the hypotension of anaphylaxis is caused by peripheral vasodilatation and not by impaired cardiac contractility. Anaphylaxis is characterized by a hyperdynamic state. For these reasons, anaphylaxis can be fatal in patients with preexisting fixed vascular obstructive disease in whom a decrease in perfusion pressure leads to a critical reduction in flow (stroke) or in patients in whom laryngeal edema develops and completely occludes the airway.

- The clinical hallmarks of anaphylaxis are flushing, hypotension, and tachycardia.
- Urticaria and angioedema may be present.
- Histamine and prostaglandin D_2 are the dominant mediators of acute anaphylaxis.
- Peripheral vasodilatation causes hypotension of anaphylaxis.

Latex allergy is an important cause of intraoperative anaphylaxis. Patients with intraoperative anaphylaxis should be evaluated for possible latex allergy, usually by a skin test or in vitro assay. When persons with known latex allergy undergo invasive procedures, a latex-free environment is necessary.

Patients with spina bifida or those with dermatitis, rhinitis, or asthma caused by latex allergy are at increased risk for anaphylaxis to latex.

- Latex allergy is an important cause of intraoperative anaphylaxis.

DRUG ALLERGY

Classes of Drug Allergy Not Involving IgE or Immediate-Type Reactions

Stevens-Johnson Syndrome

Stevens-Johnson syndrome is a bullous skin and mucosal reaction; very large blisters appear over much of the skin surface, in the mouth, and along the gastrointestinal tract. Because of the propensity of the blisters to break down and become infected, the reaction often is life-threatening. Treatment consists of stopping the drug that causes the reaction, giving corticosteroids systemically, and providing supportive care. The patients are often treated in burn units. Penicillin, sulfonamides, barbiturates, diphenylhydantoin, warfarin, and phenothiazines are well-known causes. A drug-induced Stevens-Johnson reaction is an absolute contraindication to giving a causative drug to the patient.

- Stevens-Johnson syndrome is life-threatening and is an absolute contraindication for rechallenge with the drug.

Toxic Epidermal Necrolysis Syndrome

Clinically, toxic epidermal necrolysis syndrome is almost indistinguishable from Stevens-Johnson syndrome. Histologically, the cleavage plane for the blisters is deeper than in Stevens-Johnson syndrome. The cleavage plane is at the basement membrane of the epidermis, so even the basal cell layer is lost. This makes toxic epidermal necrolysis syndrome even more devastating than Stevens-Johnson syndrome because healing occurs with much scarring. Often, healing cannot be accomplished without skin grafting, so the mortality rate is even higher than for Stevens-Johnson syndrome. Patients with toxic epidermal necrolysis are always cared for in a burn unit because of full-thickness burns over 80% to 90% of the skin. The mortality rate is very high, as in burn patients with damage of this extent.

- Toxic epidermal necrolysis syndrome is a life-threatening exfoliative dermatitis.

Macular "Drug Red" Syndrome

Macular "drug red" syndrome is a generalized skin rash that is fairly characteristic because it is intensely bright red. It is nonpruritic, flat (macular), and usually causes no major discomfort. It cannot be predicted, and because it is potentially related to the serious syndromes above, most physicians regard this type of rash as a strong contraindication to giving the drug anytime in the future.

- Macular "drug red" rash is intensely bright red, nonpruritic, and flat (macular).

Ampicillin-Mononucleosis Rash

Ampicillin-mononucleosis rash is a unique drug rash that occurs when ampicillin is given to an acutely ill febrile patient who has mononucleosis. The rash is papular, nonpruritic, rose-colored, and usually on the abdomen and has a granular feel when the fingers brush lightly over the surface of the involved skin. It is not known why the rash is specific for ampicillin and mononucleosis. This rash does not predispose to allergy to penicillin.

- Ampicillin-mononucleosis rash is papular, nonpruritic, rose-colored, and on the abdomen.
- This rash does not predispose to penicillin allergy.

Fixed Drug Eruptions

Fixed drug eruptions are red to red-brown macules that appear on a certain area of the patient's skin; any part of the body can be affected. The macules do not itch or have other signs of inflammation, although fever is associated with their appearance in a few patients. The unique aspect of this allergic phenomenon is that if a patient is given the drug of cause in the future, exactly the same skin areas have the rash. Resolution of the macules often includes postinflammatory hyperpigmentation. Except for cosmetic problems due to skin discolorations, the phenomenon does not seem serious. Antibiotics and sulfonamides are the most frequently recognized causes.

- In fixed drug eruptions, the same area of skin is always affected.

Erythema Nodosum

Erythema nodosum is a characteristic rash of red nodules about the size of a quarter, usually nonpruritic and appearing only over the anterior aspects of the lower legs. Histopathologically, the nodules are plaques of infiltrating mononuclear cells. Erythema nodosum is associated with several connective tissue diseases, viral infections, and drug allergy.

- Erythema nodosum rash is usually nonpruritic, appearing only over the anterior aspect of the lower legs.
- It is associated with several connective tissue diseases, viral infections, and drug allergy.

Contact Dermatitis

Contact dermatitis can occur with various drugs. Commonly, it is a form of drug allergy that is an occupational disease in medical or health care workers. In some patients receiving topical drugs, allergy develops to the drug or various elements in its pharmaceutical formulation, for example, fillers, stabilizers, antibacterials, and emulsifiers. Contact dermatitis is a manifestation of type IV hypersensitivity and clinically appears as an area of reddening on the skin which progresses to a granular weeping eczematous eruption of the skin, with some dermal thickening and a plaque-like quality of the surrounding skin. Histopathologically, the affected area is infiltrated by mononuclear cells. When patients receiving treatment for some kind of dermatitis develop contact hypersensitivity to corticosteroids or other drugs used in treatment, a particularly difficult diagnostic problem arises unless the physician is alert to this possibility. When contact hypersensitivity to a drug occurs, it does not increase the probability of acute type I hypersensitivity and is not associated with serious exfoliative syndromes. However, patients can develop exquisite cutaneous sensitivity of this type so that almost no avoidance technique in the workplace completely eliminates dermatitis; even protective gloves are only partly helpful. Thus, it can be occupationally disabling.

- Contact dermatitis is a form of drug allergy.
- It is a manifestation of type IV hypersensitivity.

Drug Allergy Involving IgE or Immediate-type Reactions

Penicillin Allergy

Penicillin can cause anaphylaxis in sensitive persons. It is an IgE-mediated process that can be evaluated by skin testing to penicillin major and minor determinants. Patients with positive results on skin testing and a clinical history of penicillin allergy can be desensitized to penicillin, but the procedure may be hazardous.

- Penicillin can cause anaphylaxis.
- It is an IgE-mediated process diagnosed by penicillin skin testing.
- Patients can be desensitized, but the procedure may be hazardous.

Penicillin skin tests can be helpful in determining whether it is safe to administer penicillin to a patient with suspected penicillin allergy. About 85% of patients who give a history of penicillin allergy have negative skin tests to the major and minor determinants of penicillin. These patients generally are not at increased risk for anaphylaxis, and most can receive penicillin safely. If penicillin skin tests are positive, there is a

40% to 60% chance that an allergic reaction will develop if the patient is challenged with penicillin. Most of these patients should avoid penicillin and related drugs. However, if there is a strong indication for penicillin treatment, desensitization can be considered. The desensitization procedure involves the administration of progressively increasing doses of penicillin. Desensitization can be accomplished by the oral or intravenous route and is usually performed in a hospital setting.

Ampicillin, amoxicillin, nafcillin, and other β-lactam antibiotics cross-react strongly with penicillin. Early studies suggested that up to 20% to 30% of patients with penicillin allergy were also allergic to cephalosporins. More recent studies have suggested that the cross-sensitivity of penicillin with cephalosporins is much less, about 5%. Most studies have suggested that aztreonam does not cross-react with penicillin.

Radiographic Contrast Media Reactions

Radiographic contrast media can cause reactions that have the clinical appearance of anaphylaxis. Estimates of the frequency of these reactions are 2% to 6% of procedures involving intravenous contrast media. The incidence of intra-arterial contrast-induced reactions is lower. The anaphylactoid reactions *do not* involve IgE antibody (thus, the reason for the term "anaphylact*oid*" reactions). Radiocontrast media appear to induce mediator release on the basis of some other property intrinsic to the contrast agent. The tonicity or ionic strength of the media seems particularly related to anaphylactoid reactions. With availability of low ionic strength media, the incidence of reactions has been lower.

- The frequency of contrast media reactions is 2%-6% of procedures.
- The reaction does not involve IgE antibody.
- Nonionic or low osmolar contrast media cause fewer anaphylactoid reactions than standard contrast media.

The frequency of radiocontrast media reactions can be decreased with the use of low ionic strength media in patients with a history of asthma or atopy. Patients with a history of reaction to radiocontrast media who subsequently need radiographic contrast media procedures can be pretreated with a protocol of 50 mg oral prednisone every 6 hours for three doses, with the last dose 1 hour before the procedure. At the time of the last dose, also give 50 mg of diphenhydramine or equivalent H_1 antagonist. Some studies show that the addition of oral ephedrine can be beneficial. However, most studies show that the addition of an H_2 antagonist is unnecessary.

- Patients with a history of systemic reactions to radiocontrast media should be pretreated with systemic corticosteroids and an H_1 antagonist and should be offered nonionic contrast agents.

Mastocytosis

Systemic mastocytosis is a disorder of abnormal proliferation of mast cells. The skin, bone marrow, liver, spleen, lymph nodes, and gastrointestinal tract can be affected. The clinical manifestations vary but can include flushing, pruritus, urticaria, unexplained syncope, fatigue, and dyspepsia. Bone marrow biopsy with special stains for mast cells (toluidine blue, Giemsa, chloral acetate esterase, and immunochemical stains for tryptase) is the most direct diagnostic study. Serum levels of tryptase and urinary concentrations of histamine and histamine metabolites may be increased.

Treatment initially consists of antihistamines. Cromolyn given orally can be beneficial, especially in patients with gastrointestinal symptoms. Corticosteroids should be considered in severe cases, and interferon is a promising investigational treatment.

Eosinophilia

The differential diagnosis of eosinophilia is given in Table 2-16. The eosinophil myalgia syndrome is a systemic illness associated with a contaminant in specific batches of L-tryptophan preparations (these contaminated products are no longer available).

Table 2-16 Common Causes of Eosinophilia

Atopic
  Allergic rhinitis
  Allergic bronchopulmonary aspergillosis
  Asthma
  Atopic dermatitis
  Drug hypersensitivity
Pulmonary
  Eosinophilic pneumonia
  Löffler syndrome
Proliferative/neoplastic
  Idiopathic hypereosinophilic syndrome
  Eosinophilic leukemia
Vasculitis/connective tissue
  Churg-Strauss vasculitis
  Eosinophilic fasciitis
Eosinophilic gastroenteritis
Infectious
  Visceral larva migrans
  Helminth
Toxic
  Eosinophil myalgia syndrome
  Toxic oil syndrome

The clinical manifestations include weight loss, muscle weakness, and cutaneous induration. The laboratory hallmark is peripheral and tissue eosinophilia. Follow-up studies show that many affected patients continue to have marked disability months and years after the acute illness. Although corticosteroids are used in the treatment of this disorder, there is no evidence that corticosteroid therapy alters long-term disability or mortality.

Hypereosinophilia syndrome is an idiopathic disorder characterized by a total eosinophil count more than 1,500/µL (1.5 × 10^9/L) for 6 months or longer, signs or symptoms of organ involvement, and no other known cause of eosinophilia. The syndrome typically affects persons in the third through sixth decades of life; women are affected more often than men. It usually is a multisystem disorder that affects the heart, lungs, nervous system, or skin. Symptoms include fatigue, cough, shortness of breath, or rash. Cardiac involvement in hypereosinophilia syndrome is especially important: endomyocardial fibrosis, mural thrombi, and mitral and tricuspid incompetence can occur. The clinical syndrome is one of a restrictive cardiomyopathy with congestive heart failure. Echocardiography and endomyocardial biopsy are important diagnostic tests.

Treatment of hypereosinophilia syndrome usually includes systemic corticosteroids. Hydroxyurea or vincristine can be useful in cases of refractory disease.

Common Variable Immunodeficiency

Common variable immunodeficiency can affect persons of all ages, both males and females. It is not a hereditary disorder. Patients have recurrent infections and hypogammaglobulinemia. Recurrent pyogenic infections include chronic otitis media, chronic or recurrent sinusitis, pneumonia, and bronchiectasis.

Patients with common variable immunodeficiency often have autoimmune or gastrointestinal disturbances. About one-half of patients have chronic diarrhea and malabsorption. There may be steatorrhea, protein-losing enteropathy, ulcerative colitis, or Crohn disease. Other gastrointestinal problems associated with the disease are atrophic gastritis, pernicious anemia, giardiasis, and chronic active hepatitis. Pathologic changes in the gastrointestinal tract mucosa include loss of villi, nodular lymphoid hyperplasia, and diffuse lymphoid infiltration.

Autoimmune anemia, thrombocytopenia, or neutropenia is present in 10% to 50% of patients. Inflammatory arthritis and lymphoid interstitial pneumonia are other associated conditions. Also, patients have an increased risk of developing malignancy, particularly a lymphoid malignancy such as non-Hodgkin lymphoma.

The diagnosis of common variable immunodeficiency should be considered in patients with recurrent pyogenic infections and hypogammaglobulinemia. Associated gastrointestinal or autoimmune disease and the exclusion of hereditary primary immunodeficiencies support the diagnosis. Treatment is with intravenous gamma globulin.

Terminal Complement Component Deficiencies

Patients with deficiency of the terminal complement component C5, C6, C7, or C8 have increased susceptibility to meningococcal infections. The terminal complement components form the membrane attack complex that causes cell lysis; hence, deficiency of one of these components results in defective microbial killing. The terminal component C9 participates in membrane pore formation but is not essential for complement-mediated cell lysis. Thus, the rare patients with a C9 deficiency have limited increased susceptibility to infections.

Terminal complement component deficiency should be suspected in patients with recurrent meningococcal disease, a family history of meningococcal disease, systemic meningococcal infection, or those infected with an unusual serotype of meningococcus. Diagnosis is confirmed with assay of total hemolytic complement and measurement of individual complement components.

Allergy Pharmacy Review
Sansana D. Bontaveekul, PharmD, Todd M. Johnson, PharmD

Drug (trade name)	Toxic/adverse effects	Drug interactions	Comments
Bronchodilators	Palpitations, tachycardia, hypertension, arrhythmia, tremor, nervousness, headache, insomnia, GERD or pharyngitis	β-Blockers may inhibit bronchodilator effect in patients with asthma	Bronchodilators must be used cautiously for those with DM, cardiovascular disorders, hyperthyroidism, or seizure
Albuterol (Proventil, Ventolin, Volmax)			
Bitolterol (Tornalate)		Tricyclic antidepressants and sympathomimetics may cause hypertension	
Epinephrine (AsthmaHaler, Primatene Mist)			β-Blockers may precipitate asthma in asthmatics
Ipratropium (Atrovent)	Ipratropium may cause blurred vision & dry mouth		
Ipratropium & albuterol (Combivent)			
Isoetharine (Bronkosol)			
Isoproterenol (Isuprel, Medihaler-Iso)		Isoproterenol or epinephrine may sensitize myocardium to effects of general anesthetics	
Levalbuterol (Xopenex)			
Metaproterenol (Alupent)			
Pirbuterol (Maxair)			
Salmeterol (Serevent)			
Terbutaline (Bricanyl)			
Leukotriene receptor antagonists	Rarely may cause systemic eosinophilia with vasculitis consistent with Churg-Strauss syndrome		
Montelukast (Singulair)			
Zafirlukast (Accolate)		Zafirlukast & zileuton can increase warfarin effects	
Zileuton (Zyflo)		Zileuton can double theophylline concentrations	
Anti-inflammatory inhalant products			Corticosteroids, cromolyn, & nedocromil effective for relieving acute bronchospasm
Beclomethasone (Beclovent, Vanceril, Qvar)			When withdrawing systemic corticosteroids, inhaled corticosteroids do not provide systemic effects needed to prevent symptoms of adrenal insufficiency
Budesonide (Pulmicort)			
Cromolyn (Intal)			
Flunisolide (Aerobid)			
Fluticasone (Flovent)			
Fluticasone & salmeterol (Advair Diskus)			
Nedocromil (Tilade)			
Triamcinolone (Azmacort)			

Allergy Pharmacy Review (continued)

Drug (trade name)	Toxic/adverse effects	Drug interactions	Comments
First-generation antihistamines[*][†]			
Brompheniramine maleate (Dimetapp elixir, Dimetane Extentabs) Chlorpheniramine maleate (Chlor-Trimeton) Clemastine fumarate (Tavist) Cyproheptadine (Periactin) Dexchlorpheniramine maleate (Polaramine) Diphenhydramine HCl (Benadryl) Hydroxyzine HCl (Atarax) Hydroxyzine pamoate (Vistaril) Promethazine HCl (Phenergan) Tripelennamine (PBZ, PBZ-SR)	CNS depression (most frequent, sedation) Some patients, especially children, may have paradoxical excitement (restlessness, insomnia, tremors, nervousness, palpitation) Sensitivity reaction & photo-sensitivity Cardiovascular effects are uncommon & usually limited to overdosage Promethazine may lower seizure threshold Adverse anticholinergic effects: dryness of mouth, nose, throat; dysuria; urinary retention; blurred vision; thickening of bronchial secretions	Alcohol may potentiate CNS effects & should be avoided while taking antihistamines Additive CNS suppressant effects may occur in patients taking other CNS suppressants (sedatives, tranquilizers)	Histamine H_1 receptor antagonists block H_1 receptor sites, preventing action of histamine on cells; they do not chemically inactivate or prevent histamine release Antihistamines exert various degrees of anti-histaminic, anticholin-ergic, antimuscarinic activities & are useful as sedatives, antiemetics, anti–motion sickness, antitussive, & anti-parkinsonism agents Unlabeled use: increased appetite, weight gain (cyproheptadine) Caution for patients with angle-closure glaucoma, prostatic hypertrophy, stenosing peptic ulcer, pyloroduodenal obstruc-tion, bladder neck obstruction
Second-generation antihistamines[*][‡]			
Cetirizine HCl (Zyrtec)	Nausea, dyspepsia, dry mouth, headache, drowsiness	No clinically important drug interactions have been reported in patients taking cetirizine concomitantly with azithromycin, erythromycin, or ketoconazole	Cetirizine is a carboxylic acid metabolite of hydroxyzine The increase in polarity of cetirizine may decrease its distribution in CNS, thus reduced potential for CNS adverse effects compared with 1st-gener-ation antihistamines; incidence of certain adverse CNS effects (somnolence) is higher in patients taking cetiri-zine than in those taking other 2nd-generation antihistamines

Allergy Pharmacy Review (continued)

Drug (trade name)	Toxic/adverse effects	Drug interactions	Comments
Desloratadine (Clarinex)		Although AUC of desloratadine increases with concomitant use with erythromycin or ketoconazole, no clinically important changes measured by ECG, laboratory evaluations, vital signs, adverse events	Desloratadine, fexofenadine, & loratadine are selective for peripheral H_1 receptors & less sedating than 1st-generation antihistamines Desloratadine is a major metabolite of loratadine Dosage adjustment is recommended in patients with renal and/or hepatic impairment (cetirizine, desloratadine, loratadine, and fexofenadine—renal impairment only)
Fexofenadine HCl (Allegra)		Fexofenadine is active metabolite of terfenadine, but does not have cardiotoxic & drug interaction potentials of terfenadine; no clinically important adverse effects or changes in QT_c interval reported with concomitant use of erythromycin or ketoconazole despite increases in AUC and peak plasma concentration of fexofenadine	
Loratadine (Claritin, Claritin Reditabs, Tavist ND, Alavert)		Although AUC of loratadine increases with concomitant use of erythromycin or ketoconazole, no clinically important changes measured by ECG, laboratory evaluation, vital signs, adverse effects	
Nasal solution products Azelastine HCl (Astelin) Cromolyn sodium (Nasalcrom)	Bitter/bad taste, nasal burning/ stinging/irritation, pharyngitis, sneezing Somnolence & headache can occur	No clinically important drug interactions known	Histamine H_1 receptor antagonists Mast cell stabilizer; begin therapy before & continue at regular intervals during allergenic exposure

Allergy Pharmacy Review (continued)

Drug (trade name)	Toxic/adverse effects	Drug interactions	Comments
Histamine H$_1$ receptor antagonist ophthalmic products[§]			
Emedastine difumarate (Emadine) 0.05% ophthalmic solution	Transient eye burning/stinging, blurred vision, dry eyes, foreign body sensation, headache, bitter taste	Benzalkonium (preservative) may be absorbed by soft contact lens; wait at least 10 min after applying drug before inserting contact lenses	Shake bottle well before use (levocabastine)
Levocabastine HCl (Livostin) 0.05% ophthalmic suspension			
Mast-cell stabilizer ophthalmic products[§]			
Cromolyn sodium (Crolom) 4% ophthalmic solution	Same as above	Same as above	
Lodoxamide tromethamine (Alomide) 0.1% ophthalmic solution			
Pemirolast potassium (Alamast) 0.1% ophthalmic solution	Preservative in pemirolast is lauralkonium Cl; wait at least 10 min after applying drug before inserting contact lenses		
Nedocromil sodium (Alocril) 2% ophthalmic solution	Same as above	Same as above	
Histamine H$_1$ receptor antagonists and mast-cell stabilizer ophthalmic products[§]			
Azelastine HCl (Optivar) 0.5 mg/mL ophthalmic solution			
Ketotifen fumarate (Zaditor) 0.025% ophthalmic solution			
Olopatadine HCl (Patanol) 0.1% ophthalmic solution			

AUC, area under curve; CNS, central nervous system; DM, diabetes mellitus; ECG, electrocardiography; GERD, gastroesophageal reflux disease.

[*]Histamine H$_1$ receptor antagonists.

[†]Oral or parenteral products.

[‡]Available in oral products only.

[§]To prevent contamination of products, care should be taken not to touch eyelids or surrounding areas with dropper tip of bottle.

QUESTIONS

Multiple Choice (choose the one best answer)

1. A 24-year-old man developed sudden swelling of the lips, a few scattered hives, wheezing, and a feeling of a lump in his throat a few minutes after eating a shrimp salad. He has had a similar episode in the past after eating seafood. He states that he does not have a history of seasonal allergic rhinitis or asthma. Which of the following is the most appropriate initial treatment?
   a. Administer parenteral or oral H_1 receptor antagonist
   b. Administer subcutaneous or intramuscular epinephrine
   c. Delay treatment and observe
   d. Administer parenteral corticosteroid
   e. Obtain a chest radiograph and peak flow rate

2. A 50-year-old man reports three episodes of pruritus, weakness, and near syncope over the last 6 months, without associated wheezing or abdominal symptoms. There were no obvious environmental factors. Examination of the skin documented several reddish-brown papules. A biopsy specimen of the skin lesions shows mast cell infiltration. Which of the following tests is the most useful to determine if he has organ involvement consistent with mastocytosis?
   a. Serum tryptase level
   b. Upper gastrointestinal tract study
   c. Whole-body bone scan
   d. 24-Hour urine histamine level
   e. Bone marrow aspirate and biopsy

3. A 67-year-old woman presents with intermittent swelling of the hands and lips and abdominal cramping over the last year. This has not been accompanied by a skin rash or hives. She cannot attribute her problem to any medications, either prescribed or over-the-counter agents. She has never taken an angiotensin-converting enzyme inhibitor. In the last 6 months, she has also had night sweats and a 10-lb weight loss. What are the most likely laboratory findings?
   a. Normal C1 esterase inhibitor, decreased C1q
   b. Increased tryptase
   c. Decreased C1 esterase inhibitor, decreased C1q
   d. Decreased C1 esterase inhibitor, normal C1q
   e. Decreased C3 and C4

4. A 35-year-old woman presents with a progressive rash that has developed over the last 3 days. The patient was in good health until 10 days earlier when she was prescribed amoxicillin clavulanic acid for sinusitis. The current rash consists of "bulls-eye" type skin lesions that are erythematous. She has no hives or mucous membrane involvement. She does not have any other specific complaints except for the skin rash. At this time, management should consist of:
   a. Finish the 14-day course of the antibiotic with close observation
   b. Perform skin prick and intradermal testing to penicillin to check for allergy
   c. Discontinue the antibiotic and recommend she never use it again
   d. Discontinue the antibiotic and recommend that if it is needed again, a desensitization procedure could be done to administer the antibiotic
   e. Continue the antibiotic and treat with an H_1 receptor antagonist

5. A 32-year-old man presents for an asthma evaluation. He feels that he generally is doing well. He reports using his albuterol inhaler, on average, once a day for 4 days a week with good results. He has nighttime symptoms approximately twice a month and has required prednisone once in the past 2 years. The results of a current lung examination are within normal limits, and the forced expiratory flow volume is 3.9 L, which is 92% of predicted. How should his inhaler regimen be managed?
   a. Continue as he is doing with the as-needed use of albuterol
   b. Start scheduled albuterol 2 puffs every 6 hours
   c. Start treatment with a long-acting β-agonist, salmeterol, on a daily scheduled basis and use albuterol as needed
   d. Start treatment with an anti-inflammatory medication, low-dose inhaled corticosteroid on a daily basis, and use the albuterol as needed
   e. Start treatment with an H_1 antagonist in addition to the albuterol

6. A 20-year-old man has a history of acute difficulty breathing when he plays basketball. His symptoms include rapid breathing, throat tightness, and inspiratory wheezing. Pretreatment with an albuterol metered-dose inhaler does not help prevent the symptoms. The symptoms tend to begin and resolve abruptly. What is the most likely finding on pulmonary function testing performed when the patient is asymptomatic?
   a. Concavity of the expiratory flow loop
   b. Flattening of the expiratory flow loop
   c. Normal spirometry results
   d. Flattening of the inspiratory flow loop
   e. Flattening of the expiratory flow loop

7. A 62-year-old man reports three episodes of pneumonia and one episode of sinusitis in the last 18 months. Before that time, he did not have any history of respiratory difficulties. He is a nonsmoker. The infections responded to antibiotic treatment. His immunizations are current. The baseline chest radiograph is normal, but a CT scan of the chest shows a small area of bronchiectasis. Further evaluation would likely show a decreased:

a. IgG level
b. IgM level
c. IgA level
d. Leukocyte count
e. Neutrophil chemotaxis

ANSWERS

1. Answer b.

The patient is having an anaphylactic reaction. A delay in treatment could be fatal. Epinephrine is the first line of treatment and should be given immediately. The use of H_1 blockers and corticosteroids is also indicated as adjunctive treatment. Obtaining a chest radiograph and peak flow rate is not indicated initially.

2. Answer e.

The patient's episodes indicate possible systemic proliferation of mast cells beyond the urticaria pigmentosa seen in the skin. Bone marrow is the most common extracutaneous site of mast cell infiltration and would be most likely to confirm the diagnosis. The tryptase level and 24-hour urine histamine, even if elevated, could not confirm the presence of mastocytosis. An upper gastrointestinal tract study and bone scan should be performed only if there are symptoms referable to those organ systems.

3. Answer c.

The clinical scenario is suggestive of acquired C1 esterase inhibitor deficiency. This is commonly associated with a hematologic malignancy. As opposed to hereditary C1 esterase inhibitor deficiency, C1q is depressed in the acquired form. In both types, the C1 esterase inhibitor and C4 are decreased. The tryptase level is normal in this condition.

4. Answer c.

The type of reaction that has occurred is consistent with an erythema multiforme reaction. This is non-IgE mediated; thus, skin testing is of no value in the evaluation. The main concern is that erythema multiforme could lead to Stevens-Johnson syndrome. Therefore, the antibiotic should be discontinued and the patient advised to avoid it in the future. Desensitization is done mainly in patients with an IgE-mediated allergic reaction to a medication.

5. Answer d.

The patient's disease would be classified as "mild persistent asthma" because of the use of albuterol more than 2 days a week. Mild persistent asthma should be treated with a daily anti-inflammatory medication. The use of a long-acting β-agonist as a controller medication is associated with higher morbidity and mortality in asthma unless coupled with an anti-inflammatory medication.

6. Answer c.

The patient has vocal cord dysfunction. When asymptomatic, the results of spirometry will be normal, which is part of the difficulty in making the diagnosis. When symptomatic, there is a flattening of the inspiratory flow loop, which is typical for a variable extrathoracic obstruction. Flattening of both the inspiratory and expiratory flow loops is found in a fixed obstruction.

7. Answer a.

The repeated sinopulmonary infections and finding of bronchiectasis are suggestive of a humoral immunodeficiency. In the patient's age group, the most common cause is common variable immunodeficiency, in which the IgG level is decreased. The IgM and IgA levels may also be decreased, but this is not required for making the diagnosis. The leukocyte count typically is normal. Neutrophil defects are more common in the young population and typically associated with skin and lung abscesses.

CHAPTER 3
CARDIOLOGY

Thomas Behrenbeck, M.D., Ph.D.
Kyle W. Klarich, M.D.
Peter A. Brady, M.D.
Paul A. Friedman, M.D.
Steve R. Ommen, M.D.
Rick A. Nishimura, M.D.
Barry L. Karon, M.D.

PART I
Thomas Behrenbeck, M.D., Ph.D.
Kyle W. Klarich, M.D.

PHYSICAL EXAMINATION

Jugular Venous Pressure

This pressure is normally 6 to 8 cm H_2O and is best evaluated with the patient at 45°. When the pressure is increased, consider not only biventricular failure but also constrictive pericarditis, pericardial tamponade, cor pulmonale (especially pulmonary embolus), and superior vena cava syndrome. The normal waves are *a*, which reflects atrial contraction; *c*, closure of tricuspid valve followed by the *x* descent; and *v*, ventricular filling followed by *y* descent.

- Normal jugular venous pressure is 6 to 8 cm H_2O.
- Normal waves are *a*, atrial contraction; *c*, closure of tricuspid valve; and *v*, ventricular filling.
- *x* descent, downward motion of right ventricle.
- *y* descent, early right ventricular filling phase.

Abnormalities of the waves indicate various conditions, as follows:
1) large "a" wave: tricuspid stenosis, right ventricular hypertrophy, pulmonary hypertension (that is, increased right ventricular end-diastolic pressure)
2) cannon "a" wave: atria contracting intermittently against a closed atrioventricular valve (atrioventricular dissociation)
3) large, fused cv wave: tricuspid regurgitation
4) rapid x + y descent: constrictive pericarditis

5) Kussmaul sign: venous filling with inspiration, pericardial tamponade, or constriction

- Abnormalities of waves:
    large "a" wave: tricuspid stenosis, right ventricular hypertrophy, pulmonary hypertension.
    cannon "a" wave: atria contracting against a closed atrioventricular valve (atrioventricular dissociation).
    rapid x + y descent: constrictive pericarditis.

Arterial Pulse

Palpation of the radial pulse is useful only for rate; check the brachial or carotid pulse for contour. "Tardus" describes the timing and rate of rise of upstroke, and "parvus" describes the volume. In hypertension, radiofemoral delay (check radial and femoral pulses simultaneously) may reveal accompanying aortic coarctation.

Abnormalities of the arterial pulse and their indicated conditions are as follows:
1) parvus and tardus: aortic stenosis
2) parvus only: low output, cardiomyopathy
3) bounding: aortic regurgitation or atrioventricular fistulas
4) bifid: hypertrophic obstructive cardiomyopathy (from midsystolic obstruction)
5) bisferiens: aortic stenosis and regurgitation
6) dicrotic: left ventricular failure with hypotension, low output, and increased peripheral resistance

● Abnormalities of arterial pulse:
  parvus and tardus: aortic stenosis.
  parvus only: low output, cardiomyopathy.
  bisferiens: aortic stenosis and regurgitation.

Apical Impulse

This is normally a discrete area of localized contraction. It is usually maximal at the fifth intercostal space, midclavicular line.

Abnormalities of the apical impulse and their indicated conditions are as follows:

1) apex displaced (laterally or downward or both), impulse poor and diffuse: cardiomyopathy
2) sustained, but not necessarily displaced: left ventricular hypertrophy, aortic stenosis, often with large "a" wave
3) trifid (or multifid): hypertrophic cardiomyopathy
4) hyperdynamic, descended, and diffuse with rapid filling wave: mitral regurgitation, aortic regurgitation
5) tapping quality, localized: mitral stenosis

● Abnormalities of apical impulse:
  apex displaced, impulse poor and diffuse: cardiomyopathy.
  trifid: hypertrophic cardiomyopathy.
  tapping quality, localized: mitral stenosis.

Additional Cardiac Palpation

A palpable aortic (A_2) component at the right upper sternum suggests a dilated aorta (aneurysm, dissection, severe aortic regurgitation, poststenotic dilatation in aortic stenosis, hypertension).

Severe tricuspid regurgitation may result in a pulsatile liver palpable in the right epigastrium. Look for accompanying hepatojugular reflux, that is, distention of the external jugular vein 3 to 4 beats after compression of the liver. In patients with severe emphysema, the apical impulse rotates medially and may be appreciated in the epigastrium.

Right ventricular hypertrophy results in sustained lift, best appreciated in the fourth intercostal space 2 to 3 cm left parasternally. Diastolic overload (atrial septal defect, anomalous pulmonary venous return) results in a vigorous outward and upward motion but may not be sustained. In significant pulmonary hypertension, the pulmonic (P_2) component may be palpable (this may be physiologic in slender people with small anteroposterior diameter).

● Pressure overload usually results in sustained, lateralized impulses (left > right ventricle).
● Volume overload (regurgitant lesions, atrial septal defect) usually is appreciated as dynamic and forceful but not sustained impulses.
● Palpable A_2/P_2 components are pathologic in adults with average body habitus.

Thrills

These indicate turbulent flow (such as aortic stenosis, ventricular septal defect).

Heart Sounds

First

This consists of audible mitral valve closure followed shortly by tricuspid valve closure and normally silent aortic and pulmonic opening. A *loud* first heart sound occurs with a short PR interval and mitral stenosis because the mitral valve is wide open when the left ventricle begins to contract and then slaps shut (assumes some preserved pliability of the mitral valve leaflets). The first heart sound is also augmented in hypercontractile states (fever, exercise, thyrotoxicosis, pheochromocytomas, anemia). The intensity of the first sound is *decreased* if the mitral valve is heavily calcified and immobile (severe mitral stenosis) and also if the PR interval is long (occurs classically with acute rheumatic fever).

● Loud first heart sound: short PR interval, mitral stenosis, hypercontractile states.
● Decreased intensity of first heart sound: mitral valve heavily calcified, long PR interval.

Second

This consists of aortic closure followed by pulmonary closure. Intensity of both is increased by hypertension (loud P_2 with pulmonary hypertension, P_2 then audible at apex). Intensity is decreased with heavily calcified valves (severe aortic stenosis). Normally, the second sound widens on inspiration.

● The intensity of the second heart sound is increased by hypertension.
● The intensity is decreased with heavily calcified valves.

Abnormalities of splitting of the second heart sound and their indicated conditions are as follows:

1) fixed split, particularly during expiration: atrial septal defect, widest split occurs with a combination of atrial septal defect and pulmonary stenosis
2) paradoxic split (caused by delay in aortic closure so it closes after pulmonary valve): left bundle branch block, left ventricular hypertrophy

● Abnormalities of splitting of second heart sound:
  fixed split: atrial septal defect.
  paradoxic split: left bundle branch block, left ventricular hypertrophy.

- Mnemonic for S_1-S_2 (right ventricular-left ventricular sequence): many things are possible (MTAP; S_1=mitral> tricuspid; S_2=aortic>pulmonic).

Third

This is probably caused by tensing of the chordae as the blood distends the left ventricle during diastole. It is heard in young people (younger than 30 years—a normal variant due to excellent ventricular distensibility) and in older adults. In older adults, it is associated with volume load on the left ventricle, such as aortic regurgitation, mitral regurgitation, and cardiomyopathy.

- Third heart sound is a normal variant in young adults.
- Third heart sound in older adults is associated with volume load on the left ventricle (aortic regurgitation, mitral regurgitation, cardiomyopathy).

Fourth

This occurs with the atrial kick as blood is forced into the left ventricle by atrial contraction when the left ventricle is stiff and noncompliant but usually not failing, such as in aortic stenosis, systemic hypertension, hypertrophic cardiomyopathy, and ischemia.

- Fourth heart sound occurs in aortic stenosis, systemic hypertension, hypertrophic cardiomyopathy, and ischemia.

Opening Snap

This is virtually always caused by mitral stenosis, and the interval from the second heart sound to the opening snap helps determine the severity. With severe mitral stenosis, the left atrial pressure is very high and thus the valve opens earlier, and the interval is less than 60 m/s.

- Opening snap is virtually always caused by mitral stenosis.

Murmurs

The specific murmurs are discussed with the individual valvular lesions described later in this chapter, but some broad guidelines follow here.

A systolic ejection murmur begins after the first heart sound and ends before the second sound. It may have a diamond-shaped quality with crescendo and decrescendo components, but in general the more severe the obstruction (the narrower the orifice), the louder the murmur and the later the peak of the murmur. It may be preceded by an ejection click, if the pliability of the valve is preserved.

- Systolic ejection murmur: the more severe the obstruction, the louder the murmur and the later the peak.

A holosystolic murmur occurs when blood goes from a high-pressure to a low-pressure system (mitral regurgitation, ventricular septal defect). It engulfs the first and second heart sounds.

- A holosystolic murmur occurs with mitral regurgitation and ventricular septal defect.

MANEUVERS THAT ALTER CARDIAC MURMURS

- *Inspiration* increases venous return and thus increases right-sided murmurs, pulmonary stenosis, and pulmonary regurgitation.
- *Valsalva* increases intrathoracic pressure, inhibiting venous return to the right side of the heart.
- Most cardiac murmurs and sounds diminish in intensity during Valsalva maneuver because of decreased ventricular filling and decreased cardiac output (except hypertrophic obstructive cardiomyopathy and mitral valve prolapse).
- *Handgrip* increases cardiac output and systemic arterial pressure.
- A change in *posture* from supine to upright causes a decrease in venous return; therefore, stroke volume decreases, and this decrease causes a reflex increase in heart rate and peripheral resistance.
- *Squatting* and the *Valsalva maneuver* have opposite hemodynamic effects. Squatting increases peripheral resistance and increases venous return.

The effects of maneuvers are shown in Table 3-1.

VALVULAR HEART DISEASE

Aortic Stenosis

Supravalvular

The two major types of supravalvular aortic stenosis are diaphragmatic and localized hourglass-shaped narrowing immediately above the aortic sinuses, often associated with hypoplasia of the ascending aorta.

Supravalvular aortic stenosis is associated with Williams syndrome, which is characterized by so-called elfin facies, mental retardation, and hypercalcemia. Systemic hypertension is a common association. An important feature is large, dilated, thick-walled coronary arteries because the coronary ostia are proximal to the obstruction, causing premature atherosclerosis.

Table 3-1 Effects of Physical Maneuvers and Other Factors on Valvular Diseases

		Effect on murmur			
Maneuver	Result	Mitral regurgitation	MVP	Aortic stenosis	HOCM
Amyl nitrite	↓ afterload	↓	↑/0	↑	↑
Valsalva	↓ preload	↓	↑	↓	↑
Handgrip	↑ afterload	↑	↓/0	↓	↓
Post-PVC	↑ contractility ↓ afterload	=	↓	↑	↑*

HOCM, hypertrophic obstructive cardiomyopathy; MVP, mitral valve prolapse; PVC, premature ventricular complex.
*Although the murmur increases, the peripheral pulse decreases because of the increase in outflow obstruction.

Physical Examination

Findings include a prominent left ventricle, a thrill in the suprasternal notch and over the carotid artery (the thrill is often more marked in the right carotid artery and the pulse upstroke is often brisker on the right side than the left side), systolic murmur without click, and a loud A_2, because the valve is intact and the stenosis is downstream.

- Features of supravalvular aortic stenosis: thrill in the suprasternal notch and over the carotid artery, systolic murmur without click, and a loud A_2.

Subvalvular

The types of subvalvular stenosis are discrete ("membranous") and fibromuscular (fixed or dynamic). These two types can coexist.

Physical Examination

Findings include a prominent left ventricle, reduced pulse pressure, no click, and an arterial thrill when the stenosis is severe. Subvalvular aortic stenosis is commonly associated with aortic regurgitation because there is a jet lesion on the aortic valve cusps.

- Features of subvalvular aortic stenosis: prominent left ventricle, reduced pulse pressure, no click, arterial thrill when the stenosis is severe.
- Subvalvular aortic stenosis is commonly associated with aortic regurgitation.

Diagnosis

The diagnosis can usually be made with two-dimensional and Doppler echocardiography, often without the need for cardiac catheterization. Two-dimensional echocardiography can determine the severity of the stenosis and the site and presence or absence of additional valvular abnormality. In addition, it can assess the presence or absence of left ventricular hypertrophy. If cardiac catheterization is performed, when the catheter is pulled back from the left ventricle toward the aorta there is a low subvalvular left ventricular pressure tracing before the aortic valve is crossed.

- The diagnosis of subvalvular aortic stenosis is made with two-dimensional and Doppler echocardiography.
- Echocardiography can assess the presence or absence of left ventricular hypertrophy.

Valvular

Types

The *congenital bicuspid* type occurs in 1% of the population. It may be associated with obstruction in infancy through early adulthood. It is the most common cause of aortic stenosis in adults younger than 55 years. Frequently, the valve is still pliable and auscultation is thus different from that of degenerative aortic valve disease. An ejection click often precedes the systolic murmur. The earlier the click (i.e., the closer to the first sound), the more severe the stenosis. A_2 is delayed with progressive stenosis, and when severe there may be paradoxic splitting of the second sound. The lesion may be associated with coarctation of the aorta (10%). The diagnosis can usually be made successfully with two-dimensional and Doppler echocardiography without the need for cardiac catheterization in young people.

- Congenital bicuspid valvular aortic stenosis occurs in 1% of the population.
- It is the most common cause of aortic stenosis in adults younger than 55 years.
- An ejection click often precedes the systolic murmur.
- The earlier the click (closer to first heart sound), the more severe the stenosis.

- A_2 is delayed with progressive stenosis; when severe, there may be paradoxic splitting of the second sound.

Degenerative aortic valve disease is the most common cause of aortic stenosis in adults older than 55 years. The valve is tricuspid and calcified. When calcification is extensive, A_2 becomes inaudible.

- Degenerative aortic valve disease is the most common cause of aortic stenosis in adults older than 55 years.
- With extensive calcification, A_2 becomes inaudible.

The *rheumatic* type of aortic valve disease is less common. It is associated with thickening and fusion of the aortic cusps at the commissures. It always occurs with a rheumatic mitral valve, although significant mitral stenosis or regurgitation may not always be evident. It usually occurs in adulthood (age 40-60 years), usually 15±5 years after acute rheumatic fever.

- The rheumatic type of aortic valve disease is a less common cause of valvular aortic stenosis.
- It usually occurs at 40 to 60 years of age.

Symptoms

The classic symptoms of the valvular type of aortic stenosis include exertional dyspnea, syncope, angina, and sudden cardiac death. Most patients are symptom-free; the onset of symptoms is an ominous sign. The presence of angina does not necessarily indicate coexisting coronary disease.

- Symptoms of the valvular type of aortic stenosis: exertional dyspnea, syncope, angina, and sudden cardiac death.
- Angina does not necessarily indicate coexisting coronary disease.

Physical Examination

The pulse is parvus and tardus in hemodynamically significant aortic stenosis. The left ventricular impulse is localized, lateralized, and sustained. Arterial thrills may be palpable at the carotid, suprasternal notch, second intercostal space, or left and right sternal borders. A fourth heart sound may be present, both palpable and audible. A_2 is diminished or absent with decreasing pliability of the aortic cusps. The ejection systolic murmur becomes louder and peaks later with increasing severity, radiating to the carotid arteries and the apex.

- The pulse is parvus and tardus in hemodynamically significant aortic stenosis.
- The ejection systolic murmur becomes louder with increasing severity.
- A_2 is diminished or absent with progressive aortic stenosis.

Diagnosis

Electrocardiography may show left ventricular hypertrophy (not a sensitive index; echocardiography is better), but the results often are normal in young patients. Left bundle branch block is common, and in later stages of the condition conduction abnormalities may develop (e.g., complete heart block) if the calcium impinges on the conducting system. On chest radiography, the heart size is normal, until left ventricular remodeling occurs in the late stages, even when the stenosis is severe. The aortic root may show poststenotic dilatation. In degenerative aortic valve disease, calcium in the valve leaflets may be seen, especially on a penetrated lateral view.

- Electrocardiography is often normal in young patients.
- Left bundle branch block is common on electrocardiography.
- The aortic root may show post-stenotic dilatation on chest radiography.

Differential diagnoses include 1) hypertrophic cardiomyopathy (note different carotid upstroke and change in murmur with maneuvers) and 2) mitral regurgitation (murmur may radiate anteriorly and upward, particularly if there is rupture of a posterior mitral valve leaflet; there is no radiation to the carotid arteries).

Aortic stenosis can be diagnosed with bedside physical examination. The most important physical finding is the parvus and tardus pulse. However, the degree of aortic stenosis can be difficult to determine, particularly in older patients. Doppler echocardiography is useful for assessing gradients and correlates well with cardiac catheterization. Severe aortic stenosis is present when the mean Doppler gradient is more than 50 mm Hg and the valve area is less than 0.75 cm^2. Patients being considered for operation should also have coronary angiography if they are older than 50 years.

- Aortic stenosis can be diagnosed with bedside physical examination.
- The most important physical finding is the parvus and tardus pulse.
- Doppler echocardiography is useful for diagnosis.
- Severe aortic stenosis: gradient is >50 mm Hg and valve area is <0.75 cm^2.

Aortic Regurgitation

Etiology

Valvular

Causes of valvular aortic regurgitation include 1) congenital bicuspid valve, 2) rheumatic fever, 3) endocarditis,

4) degenerative aortic valve disease, 5) seronegative arthritis, 6) ankylosing spondylitis, and 7) rheumatoid arthritis.

Aortic Root Dilatation

Various conditions have been associated with aortic root dilatation. Marfan syndrome can be associated with progressive dilatation of the aortic root and sinuses (so-called cystic medial necrosis). Prophylactic β-adrenergic blocker therapy is effective for slowing the rate of aortic dilatation and reducing the development of aortic complications in some patients with Marfan syndrome. When the aortic root reaches 5.5 cm or more in diameter, it should be replaced. Syphilis is an uncommon cause of aortic regurgitation and usually causes aortic root dilatation above the sinuses (syphilis spares the sinuses). Remember that syphilis is associated with calcium in the aortic root on chest radiography. Age is also a related factor. With advancing age, the aorta dilates; hypertension also tends to accelerate this process. Acute aortic regurgitation may be associated with an aortic dissection.

- Marfan syndrome can be associated with aortic root dilatation.
- Hypertension is a common cause of (usually mild) aortic regurgitation.
- Syphilis is an uncommon cause of aortic regurgitation.

Symptoms

The symptoms of aortic regurgitation include fatigue, dyspnea, palpitations, and exertional angina.

Physical Examination

A bounding, collapsing Corrigan pulse resulting from wide pulse pressure is found. Other findings are de Musset head nodding, Durozier sign (systolic and diastolic ["to-and-fro"] murmur of gentle compression with stethoscope or tactilely) over the femoral artery, and Quincke sign (pulsatile capillary nail bed). The left ventricular impulse is diffuse and hyperdynamic, and the apex beat is often displaced downward. A diastolic decrescendo murmur is heard at either the left or the right sternal border, and the second heart sound may be paradoxically split because of increased left ventricular volume.

The duration of the murmur is related to the rate of pressure equilibration between the aorta and the left ventricle. Mild aortic regurgitation with physiologic diastolic pressures results in a holosystolic murmur. The shorter the murmur, the faster the pressure equilibration, the more severe the aortic regurgitation, or the higher the left ventricular end-diastolic pressure. The loudness of the murmur does not correlate with the severity of aortic regurgitation, particularly in acute aortic regurgitation (such as with dissection). A systolic flow murmur is common, because of the increased "shuttle" volume. It does not necessarily indicate coexistent structural aortic stenosis, and so the pulse upstroke should be checked.

- Findings indicative of aortic regurgitation: bounding, collapsing Corrigan pulse, diastolic decrescendo murmur, and a second heart sound that may be paradoxically split.
- The duration (shorter), but not the loudness, of the murmur, is related to the severity of the aortic regurgitation (more severe).

Diagnosis

On electrocardiography, features of left ventricular hypertrophy may be found. Ruptured sinus of Valsalva should be considered in the differential diagnosis. The diagnosis can be made at bedside clinical examination, but it can be missed if a patient with acute aortic regurgitation presents with little or no murmur. Doppler echocardiography is useful and also helps evaluate left ventricular size and function. If dissection is suspected, transthoracic echocardiography may be insufficient, and electron beam computed tomography, transesophageal echocardiography, magnetic resonance imaging, or even aortography may be needed.

- Electrocardiography may show left ventricular hypertrophy.
- Differential diagnosis: ruptured sinus of Valsalva.
- Doppler echocardiography is useful.

Timing of Surgery

The timing of surgical management is still controversial. Despite a large volume load on the left ventricle and compensatory left ventricular enlargement, patients with aortic regurgitation may remain asymptomatic for several years. The development of symptoms, however, usually reflects left ventricular dysfunction, and survival is limited unless surgical intervention is prompt. Once left ventricular dysfunction is established, patients are less likely to have a return of normal function after aortic valve replacement. There is still debate, however, regarding the timing of operation for patients who are asymptomatic or who have very mild symptoms. Other factors that have been used include echocardiographic data: a systolic dimension more than 55 mm or a diastolic dimension more than 80 mm. Asymptomatic patients with dilated left ventricles need to be followed carefully; if there is evidence of resting left ventricular systolic dysfunction, progressive diastolic dysfunction, or rapidly progressive left ventricular dilatation, operation should be performed. Angiotensin-converting enzyme inhibitors help slow ventricular dilatation in patients with severe aortic regurgitation and may help to delay operation. Chances for valve preservation (repair vs. replacement) may favor earlier operation before left ventricular dilatation has occurred.

- Patients with aortic regurgitation can be asymptomatic for several years.
- If symptoms develop, survival is limited unless surgical intervention is prompt.
- If ejection fraction decreases below normal, operation is needed.

When the cause of aortic regurgitation is acute infective endocarditis, antibiotics should always be the first line of therapy. Operation is indicated for uncontrolled infection, development of left ventricular dysfunction, or pulmonary congestion. Conduction abnormalities suggest an aortic root abscess and are an urgent indication for operation.

- If the cause of aortic regurgitation is acute infective endocarditis, antibiotic therapy should be given first.
- Indications for operation: uncontrolled infection, left ventricular dysfunction, or pulmonary congestion.
- Conduction abnormalities suggest aortic root abscess.

Mitral Stenosis

Mitral stenosis is almost always due to rheumatic heart disease causing leaflet thickening with fusion of the commissures and later calcification. Symptoms do not usually develop for several years after mitral stenosis is apparent on physical examination. These symptoms are usually dyspnea and later orthopnea with paroxysmal nocturnal dyspnea. Atrial fibrillation usually causes considerable deterioration of symptoms. Hemoptysis and pulmonary hypertension with signs of right-sided failure (that is, ascites and peripheral edema) are late manifestations. Systemic emboli also may result from atrial fibrillation (about 20% without anticoagulation).

- Mitral stenosis is almost always due to rheumatic heart disease.
- Symptoms do not develop for several years after mitral stenosis is found on physical examination.
- Symptoms: dyspnea, orthopnea with paroxysmal nocturnal dyspnea.
- Atrial fibrillation causes considerable deterioration of symptoms.

Physical Examination

The first heart sound is loud. The shorter the interval from the second heart sound (A_2) to the opening snap, the more severe the mitral stenosis. An opening snap occurs only with a pliable valve, and it disappears when the valve calcifies. The stenosis is mild if this interval is more than 90 ms, moderate if it is 80 ms, and severe if it is less than 60 ms. The diastolic murmur is a low-pitched apical rumble, and the longer it is, the more severe the stenosis. The murmur has presystolic

accentuation if sinus rhythm is present. Right ventricular lift and increased P_2 are associated with pulmonary hypertension.

- Physical examination in mitral stenosis:
   loud first heart sound.
   the shorter the interval from A_2 to the opening snap, the more severe the stenosis.
   diastolic murmur is a low-pitched apical rumble.
   the longer the murmur, the more severe the stenosis.

Diagnosis

Electrocardiography shows P mitrale and later right ventricular hypertrophy. Chest radiography (Fig. 3-1) shows straightening of the left heart border with a large left atrial shadow and dilated upper lobe pulmonary veins. With pulmonary hypertension, the central pulmonary arteries become prominent. In severe stenosis, Kerley B lines may be present, indicating a pulmonary wedge pressure of more than 20 mm Hg.

- Electrocardiography shows P mitrale and later right ventricular hypertrophy.
- Chest radiography shows straightening of the left heart border, a large left atrial shadow, and dilated upper lobe pulmonary veins.
- In severe stenosis, Kerley B lines may be present.

Two-dimensional and Doppler echocardiography is the tool of choice to diagnose mitral stenosis and determine its severity. Information is gained about valve gradient and valve area (Table 3-2), and pulmonary artery pressures can be noninvasively assessed. Cardiac catheterization is usually

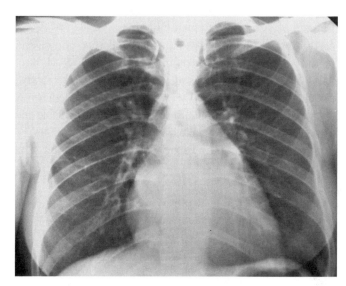

Fig. 3-1. Chest radiograph from a patient with severe mitral stenosis, showing a typical straight left heart border, prominent pulmonary artery, large left atrium, right ventricular contour, and pulmonary venous hypertension.

Table 3-2 Severity of Mitral Stenosis, by Valve Area

Severity	Valve area, cm^2	Mean gradient, mm Hg	Systolic PAP, mm Hg
Mild	1.5-2	<6	Normal
Moderate	1-1.5	6-11	≤50
Severe	<1	≥12	>50

PAP, pulmonary artery pressure.

unnecessary unless the coronary arteries need to be studied or the echocardiographic findings do not concur with the clinical situation. Severe stenosis usually correlates with a mean gradient of 12 or more mm Hg.

- Two-dimensional and Doppler echocardiography is used to diagnose mitral stenosis and determine its severity.
- For diagnosis of mitral stenosis, cardiac catheterization is usually unnecessary.
- Severe stenosis correlates with a mean gradient of ≥12 mm Hg.

Indications for Surgery

Because there is no concern about left ventricular dysfunction (left ventricle is small and underfilled) in mitral stenosis, operation is not needed until there are symptoms of exertional dyspnea, pulmonary edema, or pulmonary hypertension with the risk of irreversible pulmonary vascular changes. Atrial fibrillation does not necessarily indicate the need for operation because it often can be controlled medically. Because atrial fibrillation is frequent and intermittent in the early stages, anticoagulation should be considered early. With a pliable valve that is noncalcified and has no regurgitation, a commissurotomy can be performed without valve replacement, and this may preclude the need for valve replacement for at least 10 years. Another consideration is a percutaneous balloon valvuloplasty if the valve is pliable and there is no regurgitation. This is probably the procedure of choice; results compare favorably with those of surgical commissurotomy.

- Operation for mitral stenosis is indicated with exertional dyspnea, pulmonary edema, or serious pulmonary hypertension.
- Atrial fibrillation does not necessarily indicate the need for operation (if it can be controlled medically). Consider anticoagulation early.
- Percutaneous balloon valvuloplasty is probably the procedure of choice if the valve leaflets are pliable.

Mitral Regurgitation

Etiology

Causes of mitral regurgitation include the following: 1) rheumatic; 2) mitral valve prolapse (with or without ruptured chordae); 3) infective endocarditis; 4) papillary muscle dysfunction—as a result of ischemia, fibrosis, or rupture (note that the posteromedial papillary muscle with its single blood supply from the right coronary artery becomes infarcted more frequently than the anterior papillary muscle); 5) dilated left ventricle; 6) hypertrophic cardiomyopathy; 7) cleft mitral valve associated with primum atrial septal defect; 8) trauma; and 9) systemic lupus erythematosus. Mitral annular calcification, when severe, also can cause mitral regurgitation. This may be accelerated by systemic hypertension, diabetes, and hypercalcemic states (such as resulting from chronic renal failure and dialysis).

- In mitral regurgitation, the posteromedial papillary muscle becomes infarcted more often than the anterior papillary muscle.
- Mitral annular calcification may be accelerated by systemic hypertension, diabetes, and hypercalcemic states.

Symptoms

Fatigue, dyspnea (due to increased left atrial pressure), and pulmonary edema can be present. Symptoms worsen with atrial fibrillation.

Physical Examination

The findings include a diffuse and hyperdynamic left ventricular impulse, which may be visible, and a palpable rapid filling wave. The first heart sound is usually obliterated, and there is a holosystolic murmur. The second heart sound is widely split (early A$_2$), and there is a third heart sound. A low-pitched early diastolic rumble indicates severe regurgitation; it represents a volume murmur and usually not coexisting mitral stenosis.

In acute mitral regurgitation, the murmur may be short because of increased left atrial pressure. In severe mitral regurgitation, the carotid upstroke may appear parvus, because of the low forward stroke volume, but not tardus. The left atrium may be palpable with systole, and the left ventricle, with diastole; there may be both third and fourth heart sounds. If the cause is ruptured chordae, an anterior leaflet murmur radiates to the axilla and back, and a posterior leaflet murmur radiates to the base and carotid arteries. Consider acute mitral regurgitation with a normal-sized heart, pulmonary edema, and acute onset of symptoms.

- Physical examination in mitral regurgitation: first heart sound is usually obliterated.

holosystolic murmur is present.

second heart sound is widely split (early A_2).

low-pitched early diastolic rumble indicates severe regurgitation.

Diagnosis

Chest radiography may first show a dilated left atrium and then, as mitral regurgitation increases, dilatation of the left ventricle.

Pathophysiology

Mitral regurgitation "offloads" the left ventricle, so filling volume must increase to maintain adequate forward output. This results in a hyperdynamic ventricle, and thus many patients with significant mitral regurgitation remain asymptomatic for many years. A low or low-normal ejection fraction therefore suggests significant ventricular dysfunction.

- Many patients with mitral regurgitation remain asymptomatic for many years.
- A low or low-normal ejection fraction suggests significant ventricular dysfunction.

Timing of Surgery

Asymptomatic patients with a normal or hyperdynamic ejection fraction can continue to undergo regular observation. Operation should be considered for symptomatic patients (note that ventricular function considerably influences the postoperative outcome), and because "afterload is removed" when the mitral valve is replaced, left ventricular function may actually deteriorate temporarily. Mildly symptomatic patients may be considered for operation, particularly if serial examinations reveal progressive cardiac enlargement. Earlier operation may be indicated in those who are suitable for mitral valve repair rather than replacement.

- Symptomatic patients with mitral regurgitation should be considered for operation.
- Mildly symptomatic patients, particularly with progressive cardiac enlargement, may be considered for operation to increase the chance for repair rather than replacement.

Tricuspid Stenosis

The cause of tricuspid stenosis is almost always rheumatic, and it is never an isolated lesion. Carcinoid syndrome may cause tricuspid stenosis, and in rare cases atrial tumors may be the cause.

- The cause of tricuspid stenosis is almost always rheumatic; rarely, carcinoid syndrome and atrial tumors may be the cause.

Tricuspid Regurgitation

This is usually caused by dilatation of the right ventricle. When there is right ventricular hypertension, tricuspid regurgitation is also common. It often accompanies mitral valve disease, but it may be related to 1) biventricular infarction, 2) primary pulmonary hypertension, 3) congenital heart disease (such as Ebstein anomaly), or 4) carcinoid syndrome—more commonly associated with tricuspid regurgitation than tricuspid stenosis.

- Tricuspid regurgitation is usually caused by dilatation of the right ventricle.
- It often accompanies mitral valve disease.

Tricuspid Valve Prolapse

This may occur as an isolated entity or in association with other connective tissue abnormalities. The tricuspid valve may prolapse or become flail as a result of trauma or endocarditis (commonly fungal or staphylococcal in drug addicts).

Physical Examination

Findings on physical examination include jugular venous distention with a prominent v wave, a prominent right ventricular impulse, a pansystolic murmur at the left sternal edge, possibly a right-sided third heart sound, and peripheral edema, ascites, and hepatomegaly.

Surgical Therapy

Tricuspid annuloplasty may be helpful if regurgitation is a result of right ventricular dilatation. However, if there is significant pulmonary hypertension, tricuspid valve replacement is usually required with either a biologic or a mechanical valve. Biologic prostheses in the tricuspid position do not degenerate as quickly as prostheses in the left side of the heart. In patients with endocarditis, the tricuspid valve can be removed completely, and patients may tolerate this well for several years.

CONGENITAL HEART DISEASE

Atrial Septal Defect

Secundum Atrial Septal Defect

Patients with secundum atrial septal defect often survive to adulthood and may be asymptomatic. The condition is often detected on routine examination with the finding of a systolic flow murmur and "fixed" split second heart sound. If the defect has gone undetected, atrial fibrillation frequently develops by the fifth decade along with onset of symptoms, usually dyspnea with subsequent tricuspid regurgitation and right-sided heart failure. Stroke may occur as a result of paradoxical embolism.

- Patients with secundum atrial septal defect often survive to adulthood and may be asymptomatic.
- The condition is found on routine examination with the finding of a systolic flow murmur and "fixed" split second heart sound.
- Atrial fibrillation often develops in patients in their 50s with onset of symptoms.
- Stroke may occur as a result of parodoxical embolism.

Physical Examination

Findings include a normal or slightly prominent jugular venous pressure, a right ventricular heave or lift, an ejection systolic murmur in the pulmonary artery due to increased flow (usually less than grade 3/6), a fixed splitting of the second sound, and a tricuspid diastolic flow rumble if the shunt is large.

- Physical findings of secundum atrial septal defect:
    ejection systolic murmur in the pulmonary artery (never more than grade 3/6).
    fixed splitting of the second sound.
    tricuspid diastolic flow rumble with large shunts.

Diagnosis

Electrocardiography characteristically shows right bundle branch block and right axis deviation. Chest radiography shows pulmonary plethora, a prominent pulmonary artery, and right ventricular enlargement (Fig. 3-2). Young patients (younger than 40 years) with secundum atrial septal defect and sinus rhythm do not have left atrial enlargement. If the chest radiograph shows left atrial enlargement, consider another lesion, particularly primum atrial septal defect with mitral regurgitation.

- If the chest radiograph shows left atrial enlargement, consider primum atrial septal defect with mitral regurgitation.

Two-dimensional and color Doppler echocardiography usually can show the defect and right ventricular enlargement with volume overload. If visualization is poor, transesophageal echocardiography can be performed. Cardiac catheterization is usually unnecessary, unless coexisting coronary artery disease is suspected.

Sinus Venosus Atrial Septal Defect

An uncommon condition, this occurs in the superior portion of the atrial septum. It is often associated with anomalous pulmonary veins, usually the right upper. If echocardiography shows right ventricular volume overload and no secundum defect (because surface echocardiography can miss the sinus venosus area), consider sinus venosus atrial septal defect or anomalous pulmonary veins.

Primum Atrial Septal Defect (Partial Atrioventricular Canal)

This is a defect in the lower portion of the septum. The mitral valve is usually cleft and produces various degrees of regurgitation.

Diagnosis

On electrocardiography, findings are different from those of secundum type; left axis deviation and right bundle branch block are evident. More than 75% of patients have first-degree atrioventricular block. The chest radiographic findings are the same as those for secundum atrial septal defect, although there may be left atrial enlargement because of mitral regurgitation. Atrioventricular defects are the most common cardiac anomaly associated with Down syndrome.

- Electrocardiography shows left axis deviation with right bundle branch block and, commonly, first-degree atrioventricular block.
- Atrioventricular defects are the most common cardiac anomaly of Down syndrome.
- Typical clinical scenario: Middle-aged persons present with a gradual decrease in exercise tolerance and new-onset palpitations. Examination shows "fixed" split of the second heart sound and a systolic ejection murmur. Atrial fibrillation is found on electrocardiography, which also suggests right ventricular hypertrophy. Chest radiography shows filling in of the retrosternal clear space.

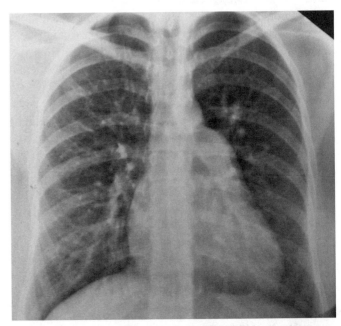

Fig. 3-2. Chest radiograph from a patient with a large left-to-right shunt due to a secundum atrial septal defect. Note cardiac enlargement with right ventricular contour, very prominent pulmonary artery, and pulmonary plethora.

Ventricular Septal Defect

Ventricular septal defect occurs in different parts of the ventricular septum, most commonly classified as either in the membranous septum or in the muscular septum. Small defects produce a loud noise, and patients are often asymptomatic. The size of the hole determines the degree of left-to-right shunting. Small defects may have a long holosystolic murmur, often with a thrill at the left sternal edge, usually around the fourth interspace. Large defects may produce a mitral diastolic flow rumble at the apex, especially when the shunt is more than 2.5:1.

- Ventricular septal defects are most common in the membranous septum or the muscular septum.
- Small defects produce a loud noise.
- The size of the hole determines the degree of left-to-right shunting.
- Typical clinical scenario: In adults, ventricular septal defect generally presents as a murmur in an asymptomatic patient. Large defects cause considerable symptoms early. It is critical to recommend prophylaxis for subacute bacterial endocarditis. Sometimes patients present with symptoms of this infection.

Patent Ductus Arteriosus

This condition is associated with maternal rubella. It produces essentially an "arteriovenous fistula." A small ductus is compatible with a normal lifespan. The ductus may calcify in adult life. A continuous "machinery" murmur envelops the second heart sound around the second interspace beneath the left clavicle. A large patent ductus arteriosus may produce ventricular failure. Surgical ligation is curative. Patients then do not need prophylaxis for endocarditis.

All of the above-described shunt lesions, when large, may produce increased pulmonary pressures and subsequently pulmonary vascular disease and pulmonary hypertension.

- Patent ductus arteriosus is associated with maternal rubella.
- A small ductus is compatible with a normal lifespan.
- A continuous "machinery" murmur is present.
- Surgical ligation is curative, and prophylaxis for endocarditis then is not needed.
- All of the above-described shunt lesions, when large, may produce increased pulmonary pressures and subsequently pulmonary vascular disease.
- Typical clinical scenario: A patient in an ambulatory clinic is an asymptomatic adult with a loud continuous "machinery" murmur. It is crucial to recommend prophylaxis for subacute bacterial endocarditis.

Eisenmenger Syndrome

This syndrome develops in the first few years of life when a large shunt (usually a ventricular septal defect or patent ductus arteriosus, less often atrial septal defect) produces pulmonary hypertension and irreversible pulmonary vascular disease. This condition causes the shunt to reverse so that blood flows from the right to the left, and subsequent cyanosis occurs. The condition is then inoperable. Death commonly occurs in the third or fourth decade of life as a result of exercise-induced syncope, arrhythmia, hemoptysis, and stroke. The cyanosis produces marked erythrocytosis, often with hemoglobin values in the teens or 20s. There is no need for phlebotomy in patients with a hemoglobin value less than 20 g/dL or a hematocrit value less than 65%. Also, repeated phlebotomies frequently lead to iron deficiency, and iron-deficient erythrocytes are more rigid than ordinary ones, and the risk of stroke is thereby increased. Phlebotomy may be necessary in symptomatic patients with a hemoglobin value more than 20 g/dL. Always remember to replace fluid concomitantly in patients with Eisenmenger syndrome because hypotension and syncope may be fatal as a result of exacerbation of right-to-left shunting and hypoxia.

- Eisenmenger syndrome develops in the first few years of life.
- The syndrome produces pulmonary hypertension and irreversible pulmonary vascular disease.
- Death is common in the third or fourth decade of life.
- Associated conditions: exercise-induced syncope, arrhythmia, hemoptysis, and stroke.
- Cyanosis produces marked erythrocytosis.
- Typical clinical scenario: Patients will have a long medical history because of the huge right-to-left shunts. A patient presents with syncope and erythrocytosis. Phlebotomy should not be used unless the patient has neurologic symptoms and a hemoglobin value >20 g/dL.

Pulmonary Stenosis

This may occur as an isolated lesion or in association with a ventricular septal defect. Valvular pulmonary stenosis often causes few or no symptoms. The valve is frequently pliable, and it may be bicuspid. Thickened dysplastic valves, often stenotic, occur in association with the Noonan syndrome.

- Thickened dysplastic valves, often stenotic, occur with the Noonan syndrome.

Physical Examination

Findings include a prominent "a" wave in the jugular venous pulse; right ventricular heave; ejection click—the earlier the click, the more severe the stenosis (the click indicates that the valve is pliable and noncalcified); ejection systolic murmur—the longer the murmur and the later peaking, the more severe the stenosis; and soft and late P_2 (with severe stenosis P_2 becomes inaudible). The click is the only right-sided sound that gets softer with inspiration. Later in life, the valve may become so thick, calcified, and immobile that the ejection click disappears.

- Findings of pulmonary stenosis:
    prominent "a" wave in the jugular venous pulse.
    ejection click (the earlier the click, the more severe the stenosis).
    pulmonary ejection click is the only right-sided sound that gets softer with inspiration.
    soft and late P_2.

Diagnosis

Electrocardiography shows right ventricular hypertrophy. On chest radiography, poststenotic pulmonary dilatation, especially of the left pulmonary artery (Fig. 3-3), is the hallmark.

The diagnosis can be reliably made with two-dimensional echocardiography, and Doppler reliably predicts the gradient and estimates right ventricular pressure. In asymptomatic patients, treatment is indicated when the right ventricular systolic pressure approaches two-thirds or more that of the systemic blood pressure. The treatment of choice for a pliable noncalcified valve is percutaneous balloon valvuloplasty, which has essentially replaced surgical valvotomy.

- The diagnosis of pulmonary stenosis is made with two-dimensional and Doppler echocardiography.
- The treatment for a pliable valve is percutaneous balloon valvuloplasty when the right ventricular systolic pressure is two-thirds or more that of the systemic pressure.
- Typical clinical scenario: A younger patient presents with dyspnea on exertion or exertional syncope. On examination, there is a murmur that is late-peaking and louder with inspiration. A systolic click is also heard, but it is softer with inspiration. A prominent "a" wave is seen on jugular venous profile. On echocardiography, the condition is diagnosed with a gradient >50 mm Hg across the pulmonary valve. If the valve is still pliable (usually to middle age), balloon valvuloplasty is the procedure of choice.

Coarctation of the Aorta

This is usually either a discrete or a long segment of narrowing adjacent to the left subclavian artery. It is more common in males and frequently is associated with a bicuspid aortic valve. Most cases of coarctation are diagnosed in childhood; only about 20% are diagnosed in adulthood. This is the most common cardiac anomaly associated with Turner syndrome. Other associations include aneurysms of the circle of Willis and aortic dissection or rupture. There is an increased incidence of aortic dissection or rupture in Turner syndrome, even in the absence of coarctation. As a result of the coarctation, systemic collateral vessels develop from the subclavian and axillary arteries through the internal mammary, scapular, and intercostal arteries.

- Coarctation of the aorta is more common in males.
- The condition is frequently associated with a bicuspid aortic valve.
- Only 20% of cases are diagnosed in adulthood.
- It is the most common cardiac anomaly associated with Turner syndrome.
- The incidence of aortic dissection or rupture is increased in Turner syndrome, even in the absence of coarctation.

There are five major complications of coarctation of the aorta: 1) cardiac failure, 2) aortic valve disease, 3) aortic rupture or dissection, 4) endarteritis, and 5) rupture of an aneurysm of the circle of Willis—this is exacerbated by the presence of hypertension, which occurs in the upper limbs. Systemic hypertension may be the presenting feature in adults. Some patients complain of pain and fatigue in the legs on exercise, reminiscent of claudication.

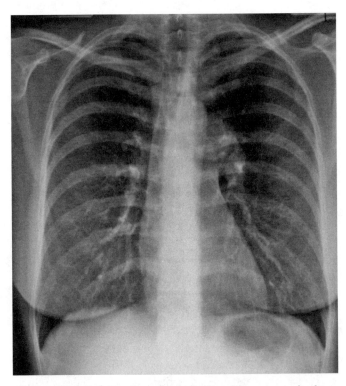

Fig. 3-3. Typical chest radiograph of valvular pulmonary stenosis, showing normal cardiac size and marked prominence of main and left pulmonary arteries, representing poststenotic dilatation. This does not occur with infundibular pulmonary stenosis. Lung fields appear mildly oligemic.

Physical Examination

Findings include an easily palpable brachial pulse; the femoral pulse is weak and delayed. There are differences in systolic pressure between the upper and the lower extremities. Exercise may exaggerate the systemic hypertension. An ejection click is present when there is an associated bicuspid valve. A_2 may be loud as a result of hypertension. A fourth heart sound may be present with associated left ventricular hypertrophy and hypertension. Murmurs may originate from 1) the coarctation, which can produce a systolic murmur over the left sternal edge and over the spine in the mid-thoracic region, and it sometimes extends into diastole in the form of a continuous murmur; 2) arterial collateral vessels, which are spread widely over the thorax; and 3) the bicuspid aortic valve, which may generate a systolic murmur.

- Physical findings of coarctation of the aorta: easily palpable brachial pulse, weak and delayed femoral pulse, differences in systolic pressure between the upper and the lower extremities.
- Coarctation can produce a systolic murmur over the left sternal edge and over the spine in the mid-thoracic region.
- Arterial collateral vessels are spread widely over the thorax.

Diagnosis

Electrocardiography may be normal. The more severe the coarctation stenosis and hypertension, the more likely is the finding of left ventricular hypertrophy with or without repolarization changes. Chest radiography may show rib notching from the dilated and pulsatile intercostal arteries and a "3" configuration of the aortic knob, which represents the coarctation site with proximal and distal dilatation.

- Chest radiographic findings in coarctation of the aorta are rib notching and a "3" configuration of the aortic knob.

The condition may be shown on echocardiography and Doppler, although imaging may be difficult in this area, and additional visualization may be necessary with digital subtraction angiography, magnetic resonance imaging, computed tomography, or angiography.

Treatment

Balloon angioplasty has been performed in some patients, although it has been associated with aneurysm formation and re-coarctation. Surgical treatment has been an accepted approach since 1945. However, there is a significant rate of hypertension after coarctation repair. As many as 75% of patients are hypertensive at 30-year follow-up. Surgically treated patients still often die prematurely of coronary artery disease, heart failure, stroke, or ruptured or dissected aorta.

Age at operation is important. The 20-year survival rate is 91% in patients who have operation when they are younger than 14 years and 79% in patients who have operation when they are older than 14 years.

- Surgical repair is the accepted treatment of coarctation of the aorta.
- Even after successful operation, there is a high rate of cardiovascular complications.
- Surgically treated patients often die prematurely of coronary artery disease, heart failure, stroke, or ruptured or dissected aorta.
- Typical clinical scenario: Coarctation should be considered in patients with hypertension who are younger than 50 years. There may be coexistent claudication of the lower extremities. Examination reveals differentiated blood pressure, upper extremity hypertension, and lower extremity hypotension. Simultaneous palpation of radial and femoral pulses reveals a delay, smaller in the femoral arteries. Patients may present with symptoms of aortic rupture, dissection, congestive heart failure, or associated conditions of Turner syndrome, circle of Willis aneurysm, or bicuspid valve.

Ebstein Anomaly

This is a congenital lesion of the right heart that has a variable clinical spectrum. It involves an inferior displacement of the tricuspid valve ring into the right ventricular cavity, causing a sail-like elongated anterior cusp or tricuspid valve on echocardiography. The degree of displacement is variable, as is the degree of abnormality of the tricuspid valve. The inferior displacement of the tricuspid valve results in "atrialization" of the right ventricle. Maternal lithium ingestion during pregnancy has been associated with this anomaly.

- Ebstein anomaly is thought to be associated with maternal lithium ingestion during pregnancy.
- The anomaly involves inferior displacement of the tricuspid valve ring into the right ventricular cavity, causing a sail-like tricuspid valve on echocardiography.

Physical Examination

The extremities are usually cool, often with peripheral cyanosis (a reflection of low cardiac output). A prominent "a" wave and, if tricuspid regurgitation is present, a v wave will be present in the jugular venous pressure (although this is variable because the large right atrium may accommodate a large tricuspid regurgitant volume). A right ventricular lift is noted. The first heart sound has a loud tricuspid (T_1) component. A holosystolic murmur increases on inspiration at the left sternal edge from tricuspid regurgitation. One or more systolic clicks are noted (often may be multiple). Common associated conditions are secundum atrial septal defect, pre-excitation syndrome, and bundle of Kent (atrioventricular accessory pathway in 13% of patients in a Mayo Clinic series). Patients with secundum atrial septal defects are often very cyanotic because of the increased right-to-left shunting, and they may present with neurologic events due to paradoxical embolism.

- Findings of Ebstein anomaly include cool extremities, often with peripheral cyanosis.
- A holosystolic murmur increases on inspiration.
- One or more systolic clicks are noted.
- Associated conditions: secundum atrial septal defect, pre-excitation syndrome, and bundle of Kent.
- Patients with secundum atrial septal defects are often very cyanotic.

Diagnosis

Chest radiography shows a narrow pedicle with an enlarged globular silhouette and right atrial enlargement. The lung fields are normal or oligemic. On electrocardiography, a tall P wave ("Himalayan" P waves) and right bundle branch block are found.

Two-dimensional and Doppler echocardiography delineates the anatomy precisely, and cardiac catheterization is unnecessary. Electrophysiologic study may be necessary to delineate the bypass tract, if present.

- Typical clinical scenario: Although findings are highly variable, most patients present with cyanosis and dyspnea with or without atrial arrhythmias. The cyanosis is due to right-to-left shunting at the atrial level.

PREGNANCY AND CARDIAC DISEASE

Physiologic Changes of Pregnancy

Plasma volume starts to increase in the first trimester and continues to increase through the third trimester to almost 50% more than normal. An increase in red cell mass also begins early and peaks in the second trimester, but not to the same degree as the plasma volume; thus, there is a relative anemia. The cardiac output increases by 30% to 50%, and peripheral resistance decreases. Heart rate also increases throughout pregnancy. Increased venous pressure in the lower extremities leads to pedal edema in 80% of healthy pregnant women.

- Physiologic changes of pregnancy include marked increased plasma volume and a moderate increase in red cell mass, causing a relative anemia.
- Peripheral resistance decreases.
- Cardiac output increases.

Because of these changes, the physical examination may suggest cardiac abnormalities to the unwary. Normal results of physical examination in a healthy pregnant woman include increased jugular venous pressure, bounding carotid pulses, and an ejection systolic murmur in the pulmonary area (should not be more than grade 3/6). The second heart sound is loud, and there is often a third heart sound or diastolic filling sound. A fourth heart sound occasionally may be heard.

- Ejection systolic murmur in the pulmonary area (not more than grade 3/6) is a normal finding in pregnancy.
- A third or fourth heart sound is common.

Although a third heart sound or diastolic filling sound is common, a long rumble should raise the possibility of mitral stenosis. Because of the decrease in peripheral resistance and increased output changes, stenotic lesions are less well tolerated than regurgitant ones; for example, a patient with aortic stenosis has exaggeration of the aortic valve gradient, whereas a patient with mitral regurgitation experiences "afterload reduction" with peripheral vasodilatation and so tolerates pregnancy better. Functional class of the patient is a consideration in terms of whether pregnancy is possible. Patients who are in New York Heart Association functional class III or IV have a maternal mortality rate approaching 7%.

- A third heart sound or diastolic filling sound is common in pregnancy, but a long rumble should raise the possibility of mitral stenosis.
- For patients in functional class III or IV, the maternal mortality rate approaches 7%.

Pregnancy is *absolutely contraindicated* in patients with the following conditions: 1) Marfan syndrome with a dilated aortic root—there is an increased risk of dissection and rupture because hormonal changes soften the connective tissue (there is unpredictable risk of dissection and rupture in Marfan syndrome and pregnancy even when the aortic root has normal size), 2) Eisenmenger syndrome (maternal mortality rate is 50%), 3) primary pulmonary hypertension, 4) symptomatic severe aortic stenosis, 5) symptomatic severe mitral stenosis, and 6) symptomatic dilated cardiomyopathy.

Although not absolute contraindications, the following conditions are also of concern in pregnancy: 1) atrial septal defect (deep venous thrombosis may lead to paradoxical embolus) and 2) coarctation (increased risk of dissection and rupture).

Patients at risk during pregnancy should minimize activity (decreases cardiac output), reduce sodium in the diet, and minimize anemia with iron and vitamin supplements.

If symptoms deteriorate and congestive heart failure supervenes, bed rest may need to be instituted. Arrhythmias such as atrial fibrillation need to be treated promptly in these situations. If necessary, cardioversion can be performed with apparently low risk to the fetus. Fetal cardiac monitoring should be performed at the same time. Occasionally patients need operative intervention. Operation during the first trimester is associated with a significantly increased rate of fetal loss. Percutaneous aortic, mitral, and pulmonary balloon valvuloplasty have been performed during pregnancy and may obviate cardiopulmonary bypass. Careful lead shielding of the fetus is needed during these procedures.

Drugs

Many cardiac drugs cross the placenta into the fetus but yet can be used safely when necessary and are not absolutely contraindicated in pregnancy. These include digoxin, quinidine, procainamide, β-adrenergic blockers, and verapamil. The β-adrenergic blockers can be associated with growth retardation of the fetus, neonatal bradycardia, and hypoglycemia. They may need to be used, however, in large doses in patients with hypertrophic cardiomyopathy, and fetal growth must be monitored.

Drugs that should be avoided are angiotensin-converting enzyme inhibitors (i.e., captopril), which cause fetal renal dysgenesis; phenytoin, which causes hydantoin syndrome and teratogenicity; and warfarin, which causes teratogenicity and abortion (should be especially avoided in the first and third trimesters). One noncardiac drug to avoid is tetracycline, which stains fetal teeth.

- Drugs to avoid in pregnancy: angiotensin-converting enzyme inhibitors (i.e., captopril), phenytoin, warfarin, and tetracycline.

Delivery

Delivery is a time of rapid hemodynamic swings. With each uterine contraction, about 500 mL of blood is released into the circulation. Cardiac output goes up with advancing labor. Oxygen consumption increases threefold. High-risk patients need careful monitoring with Swan-Ganz catheterization to maintain preload at an optimal level, maternal and fetal electrocardiographic monitoring, careful analgesia and anesthesia to avoid hypotension, delivery in the left lateral position so the fetus is not lying on the inferior vena cava (this position maintains venous return), and a short second stage of labor (delivery may need to be facilitated if labor progresses slowly).

Vaginal delivery is safer for most women because the average blood loss is less than 500 mL; with cesarean section it is 800 mL. Usually, cesarean section is performed only for obstetric indications. The new guidelines of the American Heart Association state there is no need for antibiotic prophylaxis in an uncomplicated vaginal delivery.

- With each uterine contraction, 500 mL of blood is released into the circulation.
- There is no need for antibiotic prophylaxis in uncomplicated vaginal delivery.

Prosthetic Valves and Pregnancy

Most women of childbearing age who need a valve replacement will receive a biologic valve, and if they are in sinus rhythm they will usually not be receiving anticoagulants. Women with mechanical valves will be taking warfarin, and this poses a problem with teratogenicity and increased risk of abortion. In general, diagnose pregnancy as soon as possible and switch the therapy to subcutaneous heparin (low-molecular-weight heparin has not yet been approved for this indication), monitoring the activated partial thromboplastin time, and continue this approach throughout pregnancy. This agent is also associated with increased fetal loss and an increased risk of maternal valve thrombosis.

- In pregnant patients with mechanical valves, switch therapy from warfarin to subcutaneous heparin.
- Heparin is associated with increased fetal loss.
- Warfarin is contraindicated in the first and third trimesters.

Hypertension and Pregnancy

High blood pressure during pregnancy is defined as an increment in systolic blood pressure of 30 mm Hg, an increment in diastolic blood pressure of 15 mm Hg or more, or an absolute diastolic blood pressure of 90 mm Hg or more. Hypertension during pregnancy may be 1) chronic hypertension (blood pressure ≥140/80 mm Hg before pregnant state), 2) transient hypertension (develops during pregnancy), 3) preeclampsia (starts ≥20 weeks of pregnancy), or 4) a combination of these.

For the medical management of hypertension, methyldopa is most extensively studied and is safe. β-Adrenergic blockers are safe and efficacious but may lead to growth retardation and fetal bradycardia. Angiotensin-converting enzyme inhibitors are contraindicated because they cause fetal renal failure. Hydralazine is used when additional drug treatment is needed, but it may be associated with fetal thrombocytopenia. Calcium channel blockers are not extensively studied. Diuretics are effective because the hypertension of pregnancy is "salt-sensitive." Although there is not total agreement, the Working Group on Hypertension in Pregnancy allows continuation of the use of diuretics if they had been prescribed before gestation.

PERICARDIAL DISEASE

The pericardium has an inner layer, the visceral pericardium, and an outer layer, the parietal pericardium. The space between the two layers contains 15 to 25 mL of clear fluid. The pericardium has three main functions: prevent cardiac distention, limit cardiac displacement because of its attachment to neighboring structures, and protect the heart from nearby inflammation.

Acute or Subacute Inflammatory Pericarditis

Presenting Symptoms

The chest pain of pericarditis is often aggravated by movement of the trunk, by inspiration, and by coughing. The pain is often relieved by sitting up. Low-grade fever and malaise are other findings.

Diagnosis

Pericardial friction rub may be variable. Chest radiography is usually normal. It may show globular enlargement if pericardial effusion is significant (at least 250 mL). Occasionally, pulmonary infiltrate or small pleural effusion is noted. Left pleural effusion predominates, and the cause is unknown. Electrocardiography shows acute concave ST elevation in all ventricular leads. The PR segment is also depressed in the early stages. Echocardiography allows easy diagnosis of pericardial effusion and determination of whether the pericardial effusion is hemodynamically significant.

- Chest pain is the presenting symptom of pericarditis.
- Electrocardiography shows concave ST elevation and a depressed PR segment.

Causes

The causes of pericarditis include viral pericarditis, idiopathic pericarditis, autoimmune and collagen diseases (systemic lupus erythematosus, rheumatoid arthritis, scleroderma), and postmyocardial infarction. The postcardiotomy syndrome follows open heart procedures. It presents with pyrexia, increased sedimentation rate, and pleural or pericardial chest pain. It occurs weeks to months after operation. Its incidence decreases with age, and it usually responds to anti-inflammatory agents. Pericarditis is also associated with radiation and neoplasm, namely, Hodgkin disease, leukemia, and lymphoma. Breast, thyroid, and lung tumors can metastasize to the pericardium and cause pericarditis or pericardial effusion. Melanoma also metastasizes to the heart. Uremia and tuberculosis also can cause pericarditis. If no cause can be documented, idiopathic viral pericarditis is the most likely diagnosis, and treatment with nonsteroidal anti-inflammatory agents or high-dose aspirin usually resolves the condition.

- Causes of pericarditis: autoimmune and collagen diseases; postmyocardial infarction; radiation; neoplasm; breast, thyroid, and lung tumors; uremia; tuberculosis.

Pericardial Effusion

The response of the pericardium to inflammation is to exude fluid, fibrin, and blood cells, causing a pericardial effusion. The condition is not seen on chest radiography until the amount of effusion is 250 mL. If fluid accumulates slowly, the pericardial sac distends slowly with no cardiac compression. If fluid accumulates rapidly, such as with bleeding, tamponade can occur with relatively small amounts of fluid. Tamponade restricts the blood entering the ventricles and causes a decrease in ventricular volume. The raised intrapericardial pressure increases the ventricular end-diastolic pressure and mean atrial pressure, and the increased atrial pressure increases the venous pressure. The decreased ventricular volume and filling diminish cardiac output. Any of the previously listed causes of pericarditis can cause tamponade, but other acute causes of hemopericardium should be considered, such as ruptured myocardium after infarction, aortic dissection, ruptured aortic aneurysm, and sequelae of cardiac operation.

- Pericardial effusion is not seen on chest radiography until the amount is 250 mL.
- Tamponade can occur with small amounts of fluid.
- Tamponade restricts the blood entering the ventricles and decreases ventricular volume.

Clinical Features

Tamponade produces a continuum of features, depending on its severity. The blood pressure is low, the heart is small and quiet, tachycardia may be present, jugular venous pressure is increased, and pulsus paradoxus develops (increased flow of blood into the right heart during inspiration, decreased flow into the left heart). An increase in inspiratory distention of the neck veins (Kussmaul sign) is infrequent unless there is underlying constriction.

Treatment

Emergency pericardiocentesis is performed with echocardiography-directed guidance.

Constrictive Pericarditis

Diastolic filling of both ventricles is prevented by the pericardium. The smaller the ventricular volume, the higher the end-diastolic pressure. The most common causes are recurrent viral pericarditis, irradiation, previous open heart operation, tuberculosis, and neoplastic disease.

Symptoms

Dominantly right-sided failure, peripheral edema, ascites, and often dyspnea and fatigue are present.

- Symptoms of constrictive pericarditis: peripheral edema, ascites, dyspnea, and fatigue.

Physical Examination

The jugular venous pressure is increased (remember to look at the patient when he or she is sitting or standing), and inspiratory distention of neck veins (Kussmaul sign) is present. The jugular venous pressure may show rapid descents, and pericardial knock is present in fewer than 50% of cases (sound is probably due to sudden cessation of ventricular filling). Ascites and peripheral edema may be present. Chest radiography may show pericardial calcification, but no specific changes are found on electrocardiography.

- Signs of constrictive pericarditis: increased jugular venous pressure, inspiratory distention of neck veins, rapid descents of jugular venous pressure, and pericardial knock (fewer than 50% of cases).
- Chest radiography may show pericardial calcification.
- No specific changes are found on electrocardiography.

Diagnosis

Echocardiography and Doppler may be helpful, particularly Doppler, which shows respiratory changes in mitral and tricuspid inflow velocities. Other methods such as computed tomography and magnetic resonance imaging help to delineate the thickness of the pericardium. The major confounding diagnosis is restrictive cardiomyopathy, and the distinction can be very difficult. Diastolic expansion of both ventricles is affected equally; therefore, diastolic pressure is increased and equal in all four chambers. Ventricular pressure curve shows characteristic " $\sqrt{}$ " from rapid ventricular filling and equalization of pressures (also may be seen in restrictive cardiomyopathy). The "a" and v waves are usually equal and x and y descents are rapid. If pulmonary artery systolic pressure is more than 50 mm Hg, myocardial disease is likely. If the end-diastolic pulmonary artery pressure is more than 30% of systolic pressure, myocardial disease is likely. Both of these findings are nonspecific, however. The treatment of choice for constrictive pericarditis is exploratory operation to remove the pericardium.

- Constrictive pericarditis is diagnosed from respiratory changes in mitral and tricuspid inflow velocities.
- The major confounding diagnosis is restrictive cardiomyopathy.
- Diastolic pressure is increased and equal in all four chambers.

THE HEART AND SYSTEMIC DISEASE

Many systemic diseases may have manifestations in the heart. This section describes those that are most likely to be included on the examination.

Hyperthyroidism

Effects

The cardiovascular manifestations of hyperthyroidism include an increase in heart rate, stroke volume, and cardiac output. Peripheral vascular resistance is decreased, and thus there is a widened pulse pressure. All of these lead to an increase in myocardial oxygen consumption and therefore may precipitate angina. Other potential symptoms include palpitations, tachycardia, presyncope or syncope, and shortness of breath on exertion.

- The effects of hyperthyroidism lead to increased myocardial work and oxygen consumption and therefore may precipitate angina and arrhythmias.

Physical Examination

Common physical findings are tachycardia and a bounding pulse with a wide pulse present with forceful apical pulse and a systolic ejection murmur due to increased flows. Cardiac arrhythmias are common, particularly supraventricular tachycardia and atrial fibrillation. Atrial fibrillation occurs in 10% to 20% of patients with hyperthyroidism. Therefore, always suspect thyrotoxicosis in patients with atrial fibrillation and check the thyroid function studies.

- Findings of hyperthyroidism: tachycardia, bounding pulse, forceful apical impulse, widened pulse pressure, and systolic ejection murmur.
- Cardiac arrhythmias are common, especially atrial fibrillation.
- Suspect thyrotoxicosis in patients with atrial fibrillation.
- Typical clinical scenario: An elderly woman (hyperthyroidism is 4-8 times as common in women as in men) presents with weight loss, weakness, and tachycardia and may or may not have angina or atrial fibrillation (15%). Examination shows tremor of fingers and tongue; may or may not include goiter.

Hypothyroidism

Effects

Hypothyroidism leads to cardiac enlargement and decreased function due to infiltration of the myocardium with mucoproteins. This disorder decreases the metabolic rate and circulatory demand and causes bradycardia, decreased myocardial contractility and stroke volume, and an increase in peripheral resistance. In one-third of patients, a pericardial effusion is present. The cardiomyopathy of hypothyroidism is reversible if detected early. The hypothyroid state can increase cholesterol levels and accelerate atherosclerosis.

● Hypothyroidism may lead to dilated cardiomyopathy.

Physical Examination

There may be cardiac enlargement due to the myocardial disease or to a commonly found pericardial effusion. The volume of pulses is decreased because of a decrease in myocardial contractility.

● Physical findings in hypothyroidism: cardiac enlargement, reduced myocardial contractility, and pericardial effusion (this occurs in a third of patients).
● Heart failure is less common, but it is reversible if found early.
● Atherosclerosis is accelerated.
● Typical clinical scenario: An elderly patient presents with depression, lethargy, and slowed mentation. Examination reveals scalp and eyebrow hair loss and macroglossia. Sinus bradycardia is usually present. Chest radiography shows increased cardiac size. Electrocardiography shows low voltage of QRS with prolonged intervals of QRS, PR, and QT.

Diabetes Mellitus

This condition frequently is associated with premature development of atherosclerosis. It is two times more prevalent in diabetic men and three times more prevalent in diabetic women than in a nondiabetic population. Patients with diabetes have an increased prevalence of hypertension and hyperlipidemia. Angina and myocardial infarction may often manifest as either atypical symptoms or silent ischemia. In fact, congestive heart failure may be the first manifestation of coronary artery disease among the diabetic population. There is also some evidence that cardiomyopathy unassociated with epicardial coronary atherosclerosis exists. This is speculated to be on the basis of small-vessel disease.

The BARI (Bypass and Angioplasty Revascularization Investigation) trial found that coronary artery bypass grafting reduced the death rate more than percutaneous transluminal coronary angioplasty in patients with diabetes mellitus and multivessel coronary artery disease. However, stents and glycoprotein IIb/IIIa inhibitors were not routinely used in that trial. It appears that patients with diabetes have a higher complication rate than nondiabetics regardless of the interventional strategy chosen. If percutaneous intervention is chosen, glycoprotein IIb/IIIa inhibition and stent placement have better long-term control.

Preventive strategy is important. Trials have shown that aggressive management of traditional risk factors for coronary artery disease lowers mortality. Diabetic-specific risk factors for coronary artery disease include glycemic control and urinary protein excretion.

Randomized control trials have found that the use of antihypertensives for aggressive lowering of blood pressure (diastolic pressure ≤80 mm Hg) reduces mortality. Statins and fibrates are effective for primary and secondary prevention of coronary artery disease in patients with both diabetes and hyperlipidemia. Aspirin is also effective for primary and secondary prevention. Angiotensin-converting enzyme inhibitors as a class reduce cardiovascular events and mortality in patients with diabetes who are older than 55 years and have additional risk factors (HOPE trial).

● Fatal myocardial infarction is more common in diabetics than in nondiabetics.
● Lipid lowering and glycemic control are important in the prevention of coronary artery disease.
● The prevalence of hypertension is increased in diabetes, but aggressive control lowers mortality.
● The incidence of silent myocardial ischemia is high.
● Angiotensin inhibition should be considered for primary and secondary prevention in diabetics with known vascular disease or with one or more traditional risk factors.
● Aspirin is beneficial for primary and secondary prevention in diabetes.

Amyloidosis

Amyloidosis is the result of multiple diseases leading to the extracellular deposition of insoluble proteins in organs. Organs involved typically are the liver, kidney, heart, gastrointestinal tract, and nervous tissue. In primary amyloidosis, nearly 90% of patients have clinical manifestations of cardiac dysfunction. The heart is enlarged, most often a result of thickened ventricular myocardium from the protein infiltration. Abnormalities of diastolic function, conduction, and ultimately systolic dysfunction can occur. Amyloid deposition in the cardiac valves leads to atrioventricular valvular regurgitation, which is usually not severe. Secondary amyloidosis occurs in association with chronic disease such as rheumatoid arthritis, tuberculosis, chronic infection, neoplasia (especially multiple myeloma), and chronic renal failure. Cardiac involvement occurs in secondary amyloidosis, but it is usually not a prominent feature. The entity of senile amyloidosis does exist, and the heart is the organ most commonly involved. The prevalence of this disorder increases after age 60 years. Familial amyloidosis is autosomal dominant. The characteristic amyloid protein is pre-albumin, and it can involve the heart.

Clinical Features

The following can occur in cardiac amyloid involvement: congestive heart failure, arrhythmias, sudden death, angina, chest pain, pericardial effusion (usually not hemodynamically significant), and murmurs. The natural history of the disease is usually intractable because of ventricular cardiac failure. Diastolic abnormalities are early common manifestations and are classic for "restrictive cardiomyopathy." The restrictive classification indicates a poor prognosis.

Diagnosis

The diagnosis of cardiac involvement is made on the basis of electrocardiography, which shows a classic low-voltage QRS complex, which is nonspecific. In addition, echocardiography is particularly useful. Classically, echocardiography shows an increase in left ventricular wall thickness, in contradistinction to the small (or normal) voltage on electrocardiography. Tissue characteristics on echocardiography are often described as granular. The atria are generally dilated. The cardiac valves may show some thickening and regurgitation. There may be a small pericardial effusion. Diastolic function is generally abnormal; in the early stages of the disease it shows a prolongation of the relaxation, and in the later stages it shows restrictive filling (consistent with high left ventricular filling pressures).

- In primary amyloidosis, 90% of patients have cardiac dysfunction.
- Echocardiographic features: thickened ventricular walls, granular myocardial appearance, dilated atria.
- Abnormal diastolic function: consistent with delay and relaxation in the early stages and with restrictive (increased ventricular filling pressure) patterns in the later stages.
- Hallmark: normal to reduced voltage on electrocardiography, in the face of "thick" walls on echocardiography.
- Typical clinical scenario: The diagnosis of amyloidosis should be given particular consideration when a patient (usually 40-70 years) presents with dyspnea and progressive lower extremity edema. Ancillary conditions such as vocal hoarseness, carpal tunnel syndrome, or peripheral neuropathy may be present and point to the systemic nature of the disease. The patient has often been treated with digoxin and a diuretic but has had little improvement. The key finding is a low-voltage QRS complex with or without other conduction abnormalities (such as increased PR interval or bundle branch block) coupled with echocardiographic findings of thick walls and usually preserved ventricular function.

Hemochromatosis

Hemochromatosis is an iron-storage disease. There is a primary or a secondary form related to exogenous iron (usually from repeated blood transfusions) deposits within the cardiac cells. Cardiac hemochromatosis generally does not occur alone and is accompanied by involvement of other organ systems, primarily the tetrad of diabetes, liver disease, brown

skin pigmentation, and congestive heart failure. The condition may present with cardiomegaly, congestive heart failure, and arrhythmias. This disease has features of poor systolic and diastolic function. Once clinical cardiac symptoms appear, the prognosis is very poor unless treatment is initiated with a combination of phlebotomy and iron chelation.

- Hemochromatosis is related to iron deposits within cardiac cells.
- Cardiac involvement in hemochromatosis does not occur alone; other organs are involved.
- The key to diagnosis is the tetrad of diabetes, liver disease, skin hyperpigmentation, and congestive heart failure.
- Typical clinical scenario: Patients are middle-aged and present with symptoms and signs of heart failure. Clues to hemochromatosis are a well-tanned patient with diabetes or, at minimum, increased blood sugar value, arthralgias, and loss of libido. The diagnosis is made on the basis of increased transferrin saturation and increased serum ferritin value.

Carcinoid Heart Disease

Carcinoid tumor is a malignant tumor. The primary site, usually gastrointestinal (terminal ileum), can produce a classic syndrome (in about 4% of patients) when metastatic to the liver or lungs. Malignant carcinoid tumors produce serotonin-like substances that cause cutaneous flushing, wheezing, and diarrhea, which is the carcinoid syndrome. These circulating substances are also toxic to valvular tissues. They are metabolized in the liver and lungs. Cardiac involvement occurs in approximately 50% of patients after hepatic or pulmonary metastasis. Therefore, toxic effects generally affect right-sided cardiac valves unless there is a shunt (generally a patent foramen ovale) that allows right-to-left movement of blood substances. Carcinoid lesions are fibrous plaques that form on valvular endocardium. The valve leaflets become thickened, relatively immobile, and retracted. The result is regurgitation with an element of stenosis of both the tricuspid and the pulmonary valves. Surgical therapies include tricuspid valve replacement and pulmonary valve resection.

- Carcinoid tumors produce serotonin-like substances that cause flushing, wheezing, and diarrhea.
- Changes occur in the tricuspid and pulmonary valves. Dominant lesions are tricuspid regurgitation, pulmonary regurgitation, and stenosis.
- Acquired tricuspid and pulmonary stenosis with or without regurgitation is rare and should always raise the possibility of carcinoid heart disease.
- Typical clinical scenario: A 50- to 70-year-old patient presents with weight loss, fatigue, watery diarrhea (>10 stools

daily), dyspnea on exertion, and audible wheezes. The patient has a red complexion and notes feeling hot flashes intermittently. Examination typically reveals a prominent v wave in an increased jugular venous pressure profile, a pulsatile liver that may be enlarged, ascites, and usually considerable peripheral edema. Electrocardiography typically shows right ventricular hypertrophy and right bundle branch block. Diagnosis is made by identification of a thickened tricuspid valve and pulmonary valve (left-sided valves only if a shunt is present) and the finding of liver metastasis on computed tomography, confirmed by a 24-hour urine study for 5-hydroxyindoleacetic acid.

Hypereosinophilic Syndrome

Effects

This syndrome affects young patients, generally male, who have a persistent eosinophil concentration of more than 1.5×10^9/L. The causes are several, including idiopathic hypereosinophilia, Löffler endocarditis, reactive or allergic eosinophilia, leukemic or neoplastic eosinophilia, or Churg-Strauss syndrome. All of these may have cardiac manifestations.

Clinical Features

Patients present with weight loss, fatigue, dyspnea, syncope, and systemic embolization. Cardiac manifestations include arrhythmias, myocarditis, conduction abnormalities, and thrombosis. Eosinophilic deposition occurs in the heart, where a clot forms in the apices of the ventricles and in the inflow portions under the mitral and tricuspid valves. This ultimately leads to matting down of the atrioventricular valve and causes considerable regurgitation. The clot ultimately scars, leading to endomyocardial fibrosis and restrictive cardiomyopathy.

- Hypereosinophilic syndrome may be present in patients with a persistent eosinophil value of more than 1.5×10^9/L.
- Hypereosinophilic syndrome presents with restrictive cardiomyopathy, atrioventricular valve regurgitation, and systemic embolization.
- Unexpected thromboembolism in the presence of normal left ventricular function should raise suspicion of this syndrome.
- Churg-Strauss syndrome should be considered if pulmonary involvement is present.
- Typical clinical scenario: A young patient has fatigue, weight loss, and dyspnea of relatively recent onset (months) and presents to the emergency department because of new right-sided weakness. Echocardiography shows a normal to small left ventricle, mitral valve abnormalities, and apical ventricular thrombus. The diagnosis is confirmed on the basis of a complete blood count with differential count.

Systemic Lupus Erythematosus

Effects

Systemic lupus erythematosus may involve any of the cardiac structures. Special features of involvement include the antiphospholipid syndrome, Libman-Sacks endocarditis, and congenital heart block in the offspring of mothers with lupus.

Offspring of mothers with anti-La and anti-Ro antibodies are at risk for development of neonatal lupus, characterized by myocarditis and inflammation and fibrosis of the conduction system, which may lead to congenital heart block.

Cardiac involvement in patients with systemic lupus erythematosus may include pericarditis, which is characterized by a positive antinuclear antibody in the pericardial fluid, myocarditis (more common in patients with anti-Ro antibody), a valvulopathy, coronary arteritis, and Libman-Sacks endocarditis.

Libman-Sacks endocarditis is a noninfective vegetation that may be present in up to 50% of patients with systemic lupus erythematosus. It does not generally embolize or interfere with valvular function.

- The offspring of mothers with anti-La and anti-Ro antibodies are at risk for congenital heart block.
- Approximately a third of patients with systemic lupus erythematosus may have clinical evidence of cardiac involvement, including pericarditis, endocarditis, myocarditis, and coronary arteritis.
- Typical clinical scenario: A mother with a history of multiple spontaneous abortions carries a baby to term, and the baby is born with complete heart block.

Scleroderma

Effects

Scleroderma affects the skin with sclerotic changes, the esophagus with dysphagia, and small vessels with manifestations such as Raynaud phenomenon. Cardiac involvement is manifested by intramural coronary involvement and immune-mediated endothelial injury, which is often associated with the Raynaud phenomenon clinically. Cardiac involvement is the third most common cause of mortality in patients with scleroderma. Conduction defects occur in up to 20% of patients, and a pericardial effusion is found in a third of patients, but it is often asymptomatic. Indirect cardiac involvement due to pulmonary hypertension and cor pulmonale is frequent.

- Cardiac involvement is the third most common cause of mortality in patients with scleroderma.
- Coronary vasculitis is associated with clinical Raynaud phenomenon.
- Conduction defects may occur in up to 20% of patients.

Rheumatoid Arthritis

Effects

Rheumatoid arthritis may be associated with involvement of nearly all cardiac components, including pericardium, myocardium, valves, coronary arteries, and aorta. Rheumatoid arthritis may cause both granulomatous and nongranulomatous inflammation of valve leaflets, which rarely leads to severe valvular incompetence. Pericarditis of rheumatoid arthritis is usually associated with a low glucose level and complement depletion in the pericardial fluid. Rheumatoid nodules may be deposited in the conduction system, leading to degrees of heart block. Aortitis and pulmonary hypertension due to pulmonary vasculitis are very rare complications of rheumatoid arthritis.

- Pericardial fluid in patients with rheumatoid pericarditis will be low in glucose and complement and is associated with nodular rheumatoid arthritis.
- Granulomatous involvement in the conduction system may lead to heart block.
- Nongranulomatous and granulomatous involvement of valvular tissue may lead to incompetence of cardiac valve structures.

Ankylosing Spondylitis

Aortic dilatation and aortic regurgitation may be present in approximately 10% of patients. Aortic valve cusps become distorted and retracted, leading to considerable aortic regurgitation. The conduction system may become involved as a result of both fibrosis and inflammation.

Marfan Syndrome

Marfan syndrome is an autosomal dominant condition associated with degenerative elastic tissues, leading to arachnodactyly, tall stature, pectus excavatum, kyphoscoliosis, and lenticular dislocation.

Common cardiac manifestations include mitral valve prolapse, aortic dilatation, and increased risks of aortic dissection. Long-term β-adrenergic blockade has been shown to decrease the rate of aortic dilatation and potential for dissection. Dissection occurs rarely in an aorta less than 55 mm. When dissection occurs, it tends to start in the ascending aorta and extend along the entire aorta.

Friedreich Ataxia

This is an autosomal recessive neurologic disorder that involves the heart in up to 90% of cases. It usually manifests as a symmetric hypertrophy and less commonly as a dilated cardiomyopathy.

Osteogenesis Imperfecta

Brittle bones, blue sclera, and deafness are the hallmarks of this condition, which leads to a lack of collagen-supporting matrix. Ultimately, there is a degeneration of elastic tissues, including aortic root dilatation, aortic regurgitation, annular dilatation, and chordal stretch leading to significant atrioventricular regurgitation.

Lyme Disease

Lyme disease is a spirochete infection by *Borrelia burgdorferi* organisms. Up to 10% of cases have clinical cardiac involvement. Cardiac manifestations include atrioventricular block and Lyme carditis. The diagnosis is generally made by biopsy of the right ventricular myocardium or gallium scanning.

Acquired Immunodeficiency Syndrome (AIDS)

Clinically apparent cardiac involvement may occur in up to 10% of patients with AIDS. Cardiac involvement has been reported as a myocarditis in up to 50% of patients at autopsy. This may be associated with ventricular arrhythmias, dilated cardiomyopathy, pericarditis, or infectious or malignant invasion of the cardiac structures.

Cardiac Trauma

Contusion, in the acute stage, may lead to arrhythmia, increased cardiac enzyme values, transient regional wall motion abnormalities, and pericardial effusion or tamponade. It also has been reported to cause disruption of the aorta or valves (tricuspid valve most often) or right ventricular rupture.

Commotio cordis is sudden cardiac death due to trauma, characteristically mild trauma to the chest wall, which is generally a nonpenetrating blow such as that delivered by a baseball or softball. This can occur in the absence of underlying cardiac disease and leads to instantaneous cardiac arrest. Research indicates that the trauma must be delivered during the vulnerable phase of the cardiac cycle, which is described as 15 to 30 ms before and after the T wave.

- Typical clinical scenario: An 11-year-old boy playing baseball is pitched a ball errantly and takes a blow to the chest. He falls to the ground pulseless.

PROSTHETIC VALVES

Bioprostheses

These are made of animal or human tissue, which may be unmounted or mounted in a frame. Different types include 1) homograft (human tissue), either aortic or pulmonary; 2) heterograft (porcine valve), for example, Hancock or Carpentier-Edwards; and 3) pericardial (bovine valve), for example, Ionescu-Shiley. Tissue valves have the advantage that they are not as thrombogenic as mechanical valves; thus, most patients in sinus rhythm do not require anticoagulation. There is a risk of systemic embolism, however, with biologic prostheses in patients with atrial fibrillation, particularly with a mitral prosthesis. The disadvantage is that tissue valves degenerate and calcify and thus patients will need reoperation. Approximately 50% of patients will need valve replacement at 10 years. In young patients (20 years or younger), these valves may calcify very rapidly. Tissue valves last a little longer in the tricuspid position than in positions on the left side of the heart. Aortic valves have a slightly better durability than mitral valves. Prosthesis failure can be detected by clinical evaluation and two-dimensional and Doppler echocardiography.

- Tissue valves are not as thrombogenic as mechanical valves.
- Most patients with tissue valves who are in sinus rhythm do not require anticoagulation.
- There is a risk of systemic embolism with biologic prostheses in patients with atrial fibrillation, particularly with a mitral prosthesis.
- Tissue valves degenerate and calcify.
- About 50% of patients will need valve replacement.

Mechanical Valves

An example of a *ball valve* is the Starr-Edwards. It has excellent longevity and is a so-called high-profile valve. A small valve may be associated with a higher transvalvular pressure gradient. Types of *tilting disc valves* are the Björk-Shiley and St. Jude. All mechanical valves have a risk of thromboembolism. Reported rates vary. Hemolysis often occurs with mechanical prostheses, especially in association with perivalvular leak. Anticoagulation also can be associated with hemorrhage and thrombosis. The rate of minor hemorrhages is 2% to 4% per year, and that of major hemorrhages is 1% to 2% per year.

- All mechanical valves have a risk of thromboembolism.
- Hemolysis often occurs with mechanical prostheses, especially in association with perivalvular leak.
- Anticoagulation can be associated with hemorrhage and thrombosis.

TUMORS OF THE HEART

Most cardiac tumors are metastatic. The most common primary cardiac tumor is myxoma.

Cardiac Myxoma

Most cardiac myxomas are sporadic, but there have been some reports of familial occurrence. A syndrome of cardiac myxomas with lentiginosis (spotty pigmentation) and recurrent myxomas has been recognized. About 75% are in the left atrium, 18% are in the right atrium, and the rest are in the ventricles. Most of the atrial tumors arise from the atrial septum, usually adjacent to the fossa ovalis. About 95% are single. Most myxomas have a short stalk, are gelatinous and friable, and tend to embolize. They occasionally calcify, so they may be visible on a chest radiograph.

The main clinical features are obstruction to blood flow, embolization, and systemic effects. Left atrial tumors prolapse into the mitral valve orifice and produce mitral stenosis. They mimic mitral valvular stenosis, with symptoms of dyspnea, orthopnea, cough, pulmonary edema, and hemoptysis. Classically, symptoms occur with a change in body position. Physical findings suggest mitral stenosis. Pulmonary hypertension also may occur. An early diastolic sound, the tumor "plop," may be heard. This has a lower frequency than an opening snap.

- Most cardiac tumors are metastatic.
- The most common primary cardiac tumor is myxoma.
- About 75% of cardiac myxomas are in the left atrium and 18% are in the right atrium; the rest are in the ventricles.
- Clinical features are obstruction to blood flow, embolization, and systemic effects.
- Symptoms occur with a change in body position.
- An early diastolic sound, tumor "plop," may be heard.

Embolization

Systemic emboli may occur in 30% to 60% of patients with left-sided myxoma, frequently to the brain and lower extremities. Histologic examination of embolized material is important. Coronary embolization is rare, but it should be considered in a young patient with no known previous cardiac disease. Systemic effects are fatigue, fever, weight loss, and arthralgia. Systemic effects may be associated with an increased sedimentation rate, leukocytosis, hypergammaglobulinemia, and anemia. Increased immunoglobulins are usually of IgG class.

Echocardiography is the preferred approach to diagnosis. Transesophageal echocardiography helps delineate the precise site of origin and accurately assesses tumor size and degree of mobility. Operation is indicated when the diagnosis is made.

- Systemic emboli occur in 30% to 60% of cases of left-sided myxoma, frequently to the brain and lower extremities.
- Coronary embolization is rare.
- Systemic effects: fatigue, fever, weight loss, and arthralgia.
- Systemic effects may be associated with an increased sedimentation rate, leukocytosis, hypergammaglobulinemia, and anemia.
- Increased immunoglobulins are usually of IgG class.

- Echocardiography is the preferred approach to diagnosis.
- Operation is indicated.

Primary Cardiac Neoplasm

Rhabdomyoma is most common in women and children. It can produce obstruction of cardiac valves, simulating other abnormalities, and can cause cardiac arrhythmias. Other tumors, such as Kaposi sarcoma associated with AIDS, do not usually cause cardiac symptoms.

Secondary tumors most often originate from bone, breast, lymphoma, leukemia, and thyroid. More than half of patients with malignant melanoma have metastases to the heart.

- Rhabdomyoma is most common in women and children.
- More than half of patients with malignant melanoma have metastases to the heart.

IMAGING IN CARDIOLOGY

An important part of cardiology is the appropriate choice of an imaging method to aid in the diagnosis, quantification, and prognosis of various diseases. The most commonly ordered test is assessment of left ventricular function. Various techniques are available, as outlined in Table 3-3. It is important for the clinician to have a focused question and subsequently choose the most appropriate technique to answer the clinical question.

Contrast Angiography

This imaging method was the first to visualize the cardiac chambers and directly assess left ventricular size and function with x-rays by injecting radiopaque material (iodine dye) into the cardiac chamber. Intracardiac access is usually required, and thus it is an invasive procedure, although new techniques (intravenous digital subtraction angiography) may allow a more noninvasive approach. With use of a 30° right ventricular oblique and an orthogonal (60°) left anterior oblique view (sometimes with a 20°-30° cranial tilt to avoid foreshortening of the left ventricle), biplane views are obtained over several cycles to assess left ventricular volumes and regional wall motion abnormalities. Several algorithms have been developed to extrapolate the information of these two views to the entire heart. This requires certain assumptions about the ventricular shape (regularity) and contraction pattern (concentric), which may not hold true in ischemia with resting wall motion abnormalities and previous myocardial infarction. Other concerns include the need for ionizing radiation, possible allergies to iodine, and impairment of renal function. These are usually managed with appropriate preparation (steroids, antihistamine, acetylcysteine) and by minimizing the amount of contrast agent used. Because coronary angiography, that is, the selective visualization of the coronary arteries, is the reference technique to assess the location (not necessarily the hemodynamic significance) of coronary artery stenosis, assessment of left ventricular function by contrast ventriculography should be performed only during accompanying coronary angiography. If the dye load needs to be minimized (renal failure), an alternative technique should be considered to save approximately 20 to 50 mL of contrast agent.

Echocardiography

Echocardiography uses a high-frequency (2-10 MHz) ultrasonic beam produced by a piezoelectric crystal from a transducer to generate images and acquire and process the various acoustic echoes. Currently, three methods are readily available: M-mode, two-dimensional, and Doppler-color Doppler.

Table 3-3 Cardiac Imaging Methods

Method	LVEF	RV function	LV mass	RWMA	Cost effective[*]
Contrast angiography	Yes	No	No	Yes	++++[†]
Two-dimensional echocardiography	Yes	Yes	Yes	Yes	++
First-pass RNA	Yes	Yes, quantitative[‡]	No	No	+
Blood pool RNA	Yes	No	No	Yes	+
Magnetic resonance imaging	Yes	Yes, quantitative[‡]	Yes	Yes	+++/+
Electron beam computed tomography	Yes	Yes, quantitative[‡]	Yes	Yes	+++

LV, left ventricular; LVEF, left ventricular ejection fraction; RNA, radionuclide angiography; RV, right ventricular; RWMA, regional wall motion abnormalities.
[*]+, Least expensive; ++++, most expensive.
[†]If performed without coronary angiography.
[‡]Quantitative, absolute measurements of global ventricular volumes possible to facilitate measure of RV ejection fraction.

M-Mode Echocardiography

A single cursor (beam) traverses the object of interest and traces its motion through time. Identification of characteristic borders (endocardium, epicardium, aorta, atria, valve leaflets) allows measurements of function (motion). M-mode echocardiography, because of its ease of application, is still the most commonly used method to assess function despite several shortcomings.

M-mode echocardiography provides only limited information about the structure of interest. Because of its dependence on the transducer position, appropriate placement of the M-mode cursor may not be possible. Because it represents a single-dimensional measurement (centimeters), extrapolations (cubing the measurements) need to be made, which can compound measurement errors.

Two-Dimensional Echocardiography

Two-dimensional imaging provides a beat-to-beat tomogram of the heart. Outlining the endocardial and epicardial borders allows determination of left ventricular volumes in end-diastole and end-systole and subsequently stroke volume, ejection fraction, and muscle mass. The algorithms used are similar to those used in contrast ventriculography, requiring certain assumptions about ventricular shape and contraction. The technique is, however, completely noninvasive and thus lends itself to serial image acquisition. Its easy availability (mobile equipment, "uncomplicated" technology, additional information) has made it the most widely used imaging technology in cardiology. With assessment of endocardial motion and wall thickening from various transducer positions, regional wall motion abnormalities also can be assessed. The morphologic features of valves (pliability, degree of calcification, morphologic abnormalities, i.e., flail segments) and intracardiac and pericardial structures also can be analyzed. With exercise or pharmacologic (usually dobutamine) stress, regional wall motion can be assessed both at rest and at stress for the diagnosis of coronary artery disease. Regional wall motion analysis requires a highly skilled interpreter, particularly in the presence of preexisting regional wall motion abnormalities.

Doppler-Color Doppler Echocardiography

Doppler-color Doppler echocardiography allows direct measurements of blood velocities across valves and along conduits (left ventricular outflow tract, vessels), which permit calculation of stroke volume, cardiac output, valve gradients, and severity of regurgitant lesions and semiquantitation of intracardiac and extracardiac shunts.

The crucial element for optimal echocardiographic image acquisition is the availability of appropriate acoustic "windows" to allow proper directing of the ultrasound beam to the structure of interest. Obese patients, very cachectic patients, and patients with extensive lung disease (smokers, chronic obstructive pulmonary disease, restrictive lung disease) may pose insurmountable problems for transthoracic echocardiography (10%-20% of cases). Transesophageal echocardiography may overcome this problem, but it is an invasive approach. Echocardiography also requires the most operator experience and is more dependent on the operator for both image acquisition and interpretation.

Contrast Echocardiography

Contrast echocardiography is a new technology, enhancing the echocardiographic signal with injection of an enhancing agent (such as albumin or agitated saline). Applications in the clinical arena are starting to emerge, including better visualization of the endocardium, particularly in patients with a body habitus (caused by obesity, emphysema, chest deformities) that is not conducive to sonographic access. Work is also progressing to use echocardiographic contrast agents as "flow" agents to assess myocardial perfusion, an additional, independent factor complementing regional wall motion analysis and cardiac function. Standardization of testing algorithms is in progress.

Radionuclide Imaging

Radionuclide imaging principally uses two techniques: labeling erythrocytes with an isotope to assess endocardial motion or using perfusion tracers (thallium, sestamibi) to assess differences between resting and stress blood flow.

Radionuclide Angiography

Erythrocytes are labeled with technetium, which can be imaged by a gamma camera, which usually is placed in the anteroposterior, left anterior oblique, and lateral positions. Sufficient photon capture is ensured by acquiring images over multiple cardiac cycles. This procedure requires electrocardiographic gating, which opens the aperture of the camera for fractions during the cardiac cycle. Patients with atrial fibrillation and markedly variable RR intervals are not suited for this approach. Quantification of left ventricular function is based on the number of photons in the ventricle at end-diastole and end-systole. This count-based method obviates any geometric assumptions and thus provides a very accurate assessment of left ventricular function, especially in patients with poor function. Because radionuclide angiography is dependent on the number of photons available at end-diastole and end-systole, there is a very good signal with little noise in large, poorly contractile ventricles, allowing excellent discrimination between low ejection fractions, particularly during serial assessment. In contrast, echocardiography relies on the endocardial inward motion, which is poor in severely dysfunctional ventricles, introducing a higher signal-to-noise ratio that makes discrimination between low ejection fractions difficult.

First-Pass Radionuclide Angiography

Recently, techniques have been developed to follow the passage of a radioisotope bolus through the right and left cardiac system, allowing assessment of left ventricular function. Subsequently, the tracer distributes according to coronary blood flow, and perfusion images are obtained. This technique, based on dye-dilution and videodensitometric principles, allows easy, economical assessment of both right and left ventricular function. Drawbacks are difficulties in administering the bolus (poor intravenous access), which lead to early diffusion of the bolus with poor discrimination of the dextro and levo phases. Similar to radionuclide angiography, first-pass radionuclide angiography is extremely sensitive to arrhythmias, particularly when they occur during the calculation phase of the first-pass acquisition.

Myocardial Perfusion Imaging

The two most commonly applied isotopes are thallium and sestamibi, which distribute to the myocardium according to blood flow. They are avidly taken up by the myocytes. These isotopes can subsequently be imaged at rest and after exercise (Fig. 3-4). Images are acquired by a planar technique in which the camera is positioned similar to that in radionuclide angiography in three positions. More accurate is a single photon emission computed tomography (SPECT) approach in which a camera rotates around the patient and takes images at certain narrow-angle intervals to compose a complete three-dimensional image of the entire heart without superpositrons. The views are then commonly displayed as short-axis tomograms spanning the entire heart (Fig. 3-4, upper left at stress; upper right at rest). The images are then compared with each other. During stress (exercise or pharmacologic), there is usually reduced uptake in the affected myocardium. Subsequently, at rest, there is redistribution of the isotope (thallium) where a preferential washout of the previously normal myocardium and a preferential uptake of the previously hypoperfused myocardium take place. With sestamibi, the isotope is taken up essentially irreversibly into the myocardium, and a repeat resting injection is mandatory to reflect the resting flow conditions. The extent and the severity of the perfusion defect provide additional important information in regard to the prognosis of the disease which goes beyond the mere diagnosis of the presence or absence of coronary artery disease. It is also helpful to assess residual

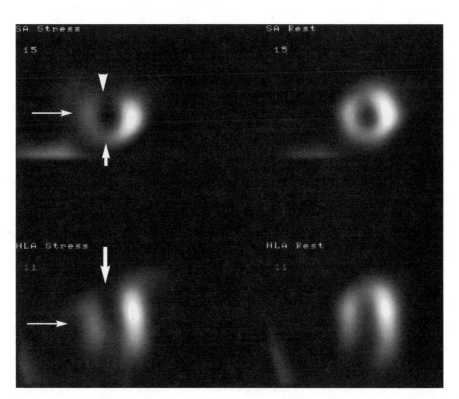

Fig. 3-4. Patient with exertional angina (class III) of recent onset. Low-level exercise with 1-mm ST-segment depression at 2 minutes into exercise. The left column depicts the stress images with a representative short-axis tomogram (upper left panel) and the horizontal long axis (lower left panel). In the right column are the rest images, with corresponding short-axis tomogram in the right upper panel and the corresponding horizontal long-axis tomogram in the right lower panel. Note the severely reduced uptake in the apical (*thick arrow*), septal (*thin arrows*), anterior (*arrowhead*), and inferior (*short arrow*) segments. At rest there is nearly complete normalization in all segments. Subsequent angiography indicated complete occlusion of the right coronary artery and 80% stenosis in the proximal left anterior descending coronary artery. The circumflex coronary artery did not show a critical lesion.

ischemia in patients with previous myocardial infarction and to assess therapeutic efficacy in patients treated medically or by intervention. The result of the imaging studies should always be viewed in conjunction with the data available from the exercise or stress electrocardiogram.

Gated Sestamibi Imaging

Improved imaging techniques and shortened image acquisition time due to dual- or triple-camera configurations have made gated imaging available, a technique similar to radionuclide angiography. Unlike multiple-gated acquisition scanning, in which the isotope remains in the left ventricular cavity (a "lumenogram"), with gated SPECT imaging the motion of myocardium is imaged throughout the cardiac cycle. This allows regional wall motion analysis similar to that of echocardiography. Because of technical circumstances, post-stress images are acquired with a considerable time delay and thus reflect mostly resting contractility.

Magnetic Resonance Imaging

Magnetic resonance imaging (MRI) is a noninvasive, three-dimensional imaging technique that allows noninvasive assessment of left ventricular size, function, and muscle mass. The technique is extremely precise. Recent technical advances have considerably shortened the acquisition time. Clinical applications are emerging aside from study of left ventricular function and anatomical structure. MRI may play a role in the detection of early atherosclerosis. It has the potential to differentiate plaque composition and thus may be able to identify vulnerable plaques. Currently, this technique is still in its developmental phase. Additional work indicates its usefulness in assessing myocardial perfusion.

Electron Beam Computed Tomography

Electron beam computed tomography (EBCT) uses a scanner without any movable parts in which an electron beam is deflected via magnetic fields rapidly on several rings around the patient, allowing high-fidelity, high-resolution, three-dimensional images of the entire heart in rapid succession. Like all complex imaging techniques it is dependent on electrocardiographic gating; however, it requires only one beat to complete a cycle. Because the entire heart is encompassed in the scan, no geometric assumptions need to be made. It is ideally suited for serial studies in left ventricular remodeling because of its high precision and accuracy. Drawbacks are the requirements for a contrast agent to be administered into a peripheral vein and for ionizing radiation.

EBCT has raised considerable interest in the early detection of coronary atherosclerosis because it opens the possibility for early, effective, and targeted intervention (primary prevention). It is currently the most widely used technique in this field because of its ease of application (rapid acquisition time, no contrast agent) and standardized imaging and analysis algorithms. It detects coronary calcium, an essential component of coronary plaque. Databases are being generated to assess the degree of calcification in relation to age, sex, and ethnic background. This information has been correlated with future risk for cardiac events, surpassing any currently available algorithm containing the conventional risk factor array (such as lipid profile, smoking history, family history, hypertension, and diabetes). Interest in the early detection of atherosclerosis has resulted in other scanning technology. It is not yet clear whether these other scanners are equivalent in their predictive accuracy.

Positron Emission Tomography

Positron emission tomography depends on the detection of a simultaneous pair of photons radiating into exact opposite directions. This principle, not unlike radionuclide angiography, allows high-spatial and temporal resolution imaging. Positron emission tomography currently is the reference standard for the assessment of myocardial viability. However, the complexity of the technology and the cost currently limit its use to tertiary academic centers.

PART II
Peter A. Brady, M.D.

MECHANISMS OF ARRHYTHMIAS

Three major mechanisms underlie abnormal cardiac rhythms: reentry, triggered activity, and abnormal automaticity (including parasystole).

Reentry

Reentry is the most common mechanism responsible for cardiac arrhythmias. Reentrant rhythms may be micro-reentrant or macro-reentrant. Examples of micro-reentrant circuits include the sinus node, atrioventricular (AV) node, or injured myocardium bordering a myocardial infarction (myocardial scar). Macro-reentrant circuits include reentry within the atrium (as in atrial flutter), AV conduction system, ventricle, or an accessory pathway (as in Wolff-Parkinson-White syndrome).

For reentry to occur, three conditions must be met (Fig. 3-5 and 3-6): 1) two or more anatomically or functionally distinct pathways (connected proximally and distally to form a closed circuit) must be present (e.g., slow and fast pathways in patients with supraventricular tachycardia due to AV nodal reentry), 2) unidirectional block must occur in one pathway, and 3) slowed conduction must occur in the second pathway to an extent that conduction in the first pathway has recovered by the time the impulse reaches its distal connection.

- Reentry is the most common mechanism for cardiac arrhythmias.

Triggered Activity

This mechanism is so-named because each abnormal complex is generated (triggered) by the preceding beat (complex).

During normal depolarization of the cardiac myocyte, partial (abnormal) depolarization also may occur which "triggers" complete depolarization of the cell, initiating an (early) abnormal complex. Two types of triggered activity exist depending on whether they arise before the end of the normal action potential (*early afterdepolarization*) or after the normal action potential during the rest phase (*delayed afterdepolarization*). Delayed afterdepolarizations arising during the resting phase of the action potential (phase 4) may be the mechanism for digitalis-induced arrhythmias. In contrast, *early afterdepolarizations* arise during the plateau (phase 2) or repolarization (phase 3) of the action potential and may be responsible for the polymorphic ventricular tachycardia (torsades de pointes) caused by antiarrhythmic drugs such as quinidine.

Automaticity

All cells in the heart possess the ability to discharge spontaneously in isolation of one another. This is normal and is termed "physiologic automaticity." Cells in the region of the sinus node discharge with the highest frequency and therefore act as the dominant pacemaker of the heart. The sinus node shows normal physiologic automaticity. Occasionally, cells outside the region of the sinus node discharge abnormally, and

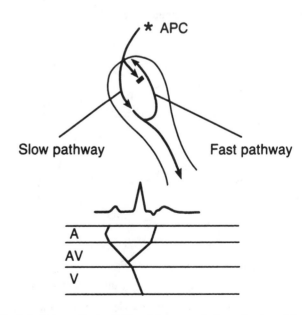

Fig. 3-6. Atrioventricular (AV) nodal reentrant tachycardia. An atrial premature complex (APC) blocks in fast pathway but conducts over slow pathway to ventricle. Impulse then returns to atria over recovered fast pathway and can reenter slow pathway and initiate tachycardia. A, atrium; V, ventricle.

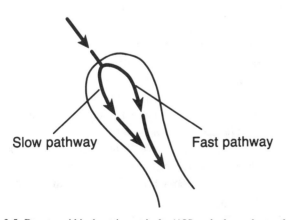

Fig. 3-5. Reentry within the atrioventricular (AV) node shows the two limbs of reentrant circuit. Recent evidence suggests that a portion of the reentrant pathway is separate from the AV node.

arrhythmias due to this mechanism are said to be due to "abnormal automaticity" and to accelerated phase 4 depolarization. Changes in the slope of spontaneous depolarization determine the rate of impulse formation (Fig. 3-7). Factors that enhance automaticity are listed in Table 3-4.

Abnormal automaticity may be the mechanism responsible for ectopic atrial tachycardia or multifocal atrial tachycardia in some patients with decompensated lung disease or ventricular ectopy early after myocardial infarction. Automaticity is enhanced by increased sympathetic tone, hypoxia, acid-base and electrolyte disturbances, and atrial or ventricular stretch. Accelerated idioventricular rhythm also may be due to abnormal automaticity.

● Automaticity is enhanced by increased sympathetic tone, hypoxia, acid-base and electrolyte disturbances, and atrial or ventricular stretch.

Parasystole

Parasystole is a special type of abnormal automaticity and occurs when an ectopic focus in the atrium or ventricle is isolated from the dominant rhythm because of conduction block into the focus. Cells within the focus are protected from the influence of surrounding cells and are not constantly "reset" by the sinus node or other focus. Thus, these cells are able to capture the regional myocardium unless it is refractory from a previously conducted beat resulting in a rhythm that is independent of the dominant rhythm. This mechanism accounts for approximately 3% of premature ventricular complexes (PVCs) noted during routine monitoring and is, in general, benign.

Table 3-4 Factors That Enhance Automaticity

Autonomic changes
    Increased sympathetic tone
    Decreased parasympathetic tone
Metabolic or ischemic changes
    Increased carbon dioxide
    Decreased oxygen
    Increased acidity
Mechanical factors
    Increased stretch
Drugs
    Isoproterenol
Electrolyte alterations
    Decreased potassium
    Increased calcium

● Due to an independently discharging ectopic focus in the atrium or ventricle.
● Causes 3% of PVCs during routine monitoring.
● Generally benign.

INVESTIGATIONS COMMONLY USED IN THE EVALUATION AND MANAGEMENT OF PATIENTS WITH SUSPECTED RHYTHM DISORDERS

Electrocardiography

Electrocardiography (ECG) remains a valuable tool in the evaluation of heart rhythm disorders. In many cases, ECG performed during symptoms of tachycardia is diagnostic of the tachycardia mechanism and is all that is needed to plan management. In other cases, ECG may provide clues to the probable diagnosis of symptoms. Whenever possible, a current ECG should be compared with previous recordings.

Ambulatory Electrocardiographic Monitoring and Transtelephonic Event Recording

Ambulatory (Holter) monitoring is useful for the evaluation of both symptomatic and asymptomatic rhythm disturbances and their relationship to daily activity (e.g., exercise). Symptoms, if present, must, however, occur frequently enough to be recorded during the 24- or 48-hour recording period. A diary in which patients record their activity and specific symptoms and precise duration of both allows correlation with heart rhythm recordings.

Ambulatory monitoring is also useful for assessing the impact of treatment on arrhythmias (e.g., determining the adequacy of ventricular rate control during drug therapy for atrial

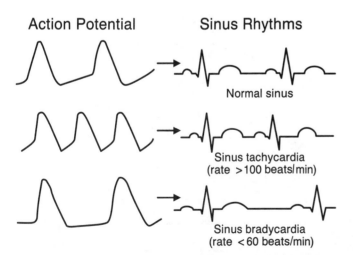

Fig. 3-7. Action potential corresponding to electrocardiographic manifestation of sinus node activity. Under physiologic conditions, sinus rate is a function of the slope of spontaneous depolarization during phase 4 of the action potential. A steep slope of the spontaneous depolarization corresponds to a faster sinus rate (sinus tachycardia). A flat slope of phase 4 depolarization corresponds to a slower sinus rate (sinus bradycardia).

fibrillation because control at rest may not reflect response during exercise or daily activity). In addition, ambulatory monitoring also can help assess pacemaker function (although newer devices can do this without the need for external monitoring) and confirm episodes of myocardial ischemia, most of which are not usually associated with the typical symptoms of angina.

- Ambulatory monitoring allows correlation of (frequent) symptoms with heart rhythm and helps assess response to treatment and pacemaker function.

Transtelephonic event recording is similar to ambulatory recording but is more useful for documenting heart rate and rhythm when symptoms are less frequent (less than one episode per 24-48 hours). Typically, patients either wear the recording device continuously for several days or weeks or briefly attach it to themselves during symptoms. The ECG is permanently stored in memory when the device is activated during symptoms by the patient. In most cases, continuous loop recorders record the ECG obtained 30 seconds to 4 minutes before the activation button is depressed. This feature is useful in patients whose symptoms are brief or of sudden onset. The ECG then can be transmitted when convenient over the telephone for evaluation. In most cases, depending on the specific population of patients in which the device is used, about 20% of transmissions document abnormal heart rhythm. However, even when completely normal, transmissions can be helpful for patient management when a normal rhythm is identified. Implantable loop event recorders also may be used when symptoms are more infrequent or are of such sudden onset that activation is not possible. These devices, which are implanted subcutaneously in the pectoral region, can be programmed to provide information regarding rhythm disturbances over several months.

- Transtelephonic event recording documents heart rate during symptoms that occur infrequently.
- About 20% of transmissions document abnormal heart rhythm.
- Transtelephonic event recording is often helpful for patient management even if a normal rhythm is identified.

Exercise Testing

Treadmill exercise testing is useful when symptoms occur during exercise because it allows evaluation of cardiac rhythm in a controlled setting with ECG monitoring. Exercise testing is also useful to determine whether the beneficial effect of a drug at rest is reversed with exercise. For example, patients with atrial fibrillation may have adequate control of heart rate at rest but poor control with moderate exercise. Similarly,

patients with ventricular tachycardia or complex ventricular ectopy may have adequate suppression of the arrhythmia at rest in response to medical therapy only to have ventricular tachycardia with exercise. Not infrequently, proarrhythmic effects of antiarrhythmic drugs may be provoked by exercise testing. This is particularly the case for class IC drugs (flecainide and propafenone) because of use-dependence (i.e., the pharmacologic effect of a drug is affected by heart rate) and their long unbinding times from the sodium channel.

- Exercise testing allows evaluation of cardiac rhythm disturbance during exercise.
- Useful for assessing whether the effect of a drug is reversed with exercise.

PVCs occur during exercise testing in 10% of patients without and 60% of those with coronary artery disease. The response of PVCs *during* exercise does not predict the severity of coronary artery disease. Elimination of PVCs with exercise is not an indication that coronary artery disease is less severe. Recent data suggest that appearance of frequent PVCs (defined as seven or more per minute, ventricular bigeminy or trigeminy, ventricular couplets or triplets, ventricular tachycardia or flutter, torsades de pointes, or ventricular fibrillation) during the recovery phase of treadmill exercise testing may be a better predictor of outcome than PVCs occurring during exercise.

- PVCs occur during exercise in 10% of patients without and in 60% of those with coronary artery disease.
- The response of PVCs during exercise does not predict the severity of coronary artery disease.
- Elimination of PVCs with exercise does not indicate less severe coronary artery disease.

Exercise testing is useful for assessing sinus node function, to diagnose chronotropic incompetence in a patient who complains of dyspnea on exertion or fatigue, and for assessing AV block. Exercise testing is most useful for assessing second-degree AV block in which the site of block is unknown (i.e., within the AV node vs. His-Purkinje system). This distinction is important because AV block occurring within the AV node (Wenckebach [Mobitz I]) is usually benign and does not require pacing. Characteristically, block within the AV node improves with exercise because increased catecholamines enhance AV node conduction. In contrast, AV block due to failure of conduction in the His-Purkinje system (Mobitz II) has a worse prognosis and a high incidence of progression to complete heart block and thus is an indication for permanent pacing. In contrast to block within the AV node, Mobitz II block typically worsens during exercise because enhanced AV node conduction increases the frequency of activation of the diseased His-Purkinje system, thus putting greater strain on the already diseased conducting system.

- Exercise testing is useful for assessing sinus node function.
- Mobitz I block usually improves with exercise.
- Mobitz II block usually worsens with exercise.
- Mobitz II block frequently progresses to complete AV block and therefore requires permanent pacing.

Signal-Averaged ECG

Signal-averaged ECG is a noninvasive test used to detect low-level signals, termed "late potentials," that result from delayed conduction through diseased myocardium. These signals usually arise in the border zone adjacent to a myocardial infarction, where conducting myocardial cells are mixed in among scar tissue. Disruption of myocardial architecture results in delayed conduction and is the substrate for myocardial reentry. Signal-averaged ECG amplifies this low-level signal by several thousandfold and averages multiple QRS complexes to eliminate random noise. The low-level activity is then measured to determine whether a late potential is present. Late potentials have independent prognostic value for identifying patients at risk for ventricular tachycardia after myocardial infarction and inducible ventricular tachycardia at the time of electrophysiologic testing. Signal-averaged ECG has a positive predictive accuracy of 25% to 50% and a negative predictive accuracy of 90% to 95% for identifying patients at risk for ventricular tachycardia. The test is used primarily to stratify patients at risk for ventricular tachycardia or ventricular fibrillation. It is not useful in the setting of bundle branch block or in patients without coronary artery disease.

- Signal-averaged ECG is noninvasive.
- Signal-averaged ECG identifies patients at risk for ventricular tachycardia.

Heart Rate Variability

Recently, attention has focused on how changes in the normal variability of the heart rate may be a predictor of future arrhythmic events. Specifically, heart rate variability decreases when there is relatively more sympathetic versus parasympathetic tone; the converse is also true. Decreased heart rate variability after myocardial infarction identifies a population of patients who are at increased risk of ventricular arrhythmias. However, at this time, determination of heart rate variability is not used routinely in clinical practice and should be considered a research tool.

Electrophysiologic Study

Electrophysiologic study involves the placement of electrode catheters in the heart to record and to stimulate heart rhythm. In most cases, pacing and recording electrodes (catheters) are positioned in the high right atrium, across the tricuspid valve in the region of the AV node in the region of the His bundle, in the right ventricular apex (Fig. 3-8). In select patients, additional catheters are placed (most commonly within the coronary sinus) to record from the left atrium and ventricle. Electrophysiologic testing is indicated in patients with cardiogenic syncope of undetermined origin, for determining the mechanism of supraventricular tachycardia, for assessing symptomatic patients with Wolff-Parkinson-White syndrome, and for evaluating patients with sustained ventricular tachycardia and survivors of out-of-hospital cardiac arrest. In the evaluation of patients with syncope, electrophysiologic study (including measurement of sinus and AV nodal function and ventricular stimulation to exclude ventricular arrhythmias as a cause for symptoms), when normal, also can be used in combination with tilt-table testing. Complications resulting from electrophysiologic study are usually minor and occur in 0.5% to 1.0% of cases. The most common complications include vascular injury and hematoma at the puncture site.

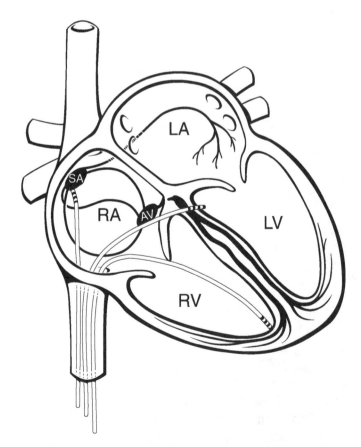

Fig. 3-8. Locations of intracardiac catheters for pacing and during cardiac electrophysiologic study.

- Electrophysiologic testing is invasive.
- It is indicated with a history suggestive of cardiogenic syncope or to determine the mechanism of a clinically documented or suspected heart rhythm disorder.
- Complications are uncommon and usually minor.

THERAPY FOR HEART RHYTHM DISORDERS

Several therapeutic options are available for heart rhythm disorders. These include drug therapy, radiofrequency ablation, surgical resection of abnormal tissue, and device therapy (pacing for bradyarrhythmias and implantable cardioverter-defibrillators for tachyarrhythmias).

Antiarrhythmic Drugs

Therapeutic range, half-life, and routes of metabolism of antiarrhythmic drugs are listed in Table 3-5. The relative effectiveness of these drugs for treating PVCs, ventricular tachycardia, paroxysmal tachycardia that uses the AV node as part of the reentrant circuit, and atrial fibrillation are listed in Table 3-6. The predominant target of the antiarrhythmic drugs is shown in Figure 3-9.

Half-life is an important concept in the use of antiarrhythmic drugs. It is the time required for 50% of the drug within the body to be eliminated. It takes 5 half-lives for a drug to reach steady state or to be eliminated completely. If a drug has a half-life of 90 minutes (e.g., lidocaine), a steady state will be reached in 6 hours; therefore, a loading dose is given to achieve a therapeutic level more promptly.

- Half-life is an important concept in the use of antiarrhythmic drugs.
- Half-life is the time required for 50% of the drug within the body to be eliminated.
- It takes 5 half-lives for a drug to reach steady state or to be eliminated completely.

Proarrhythmic effect (Table 3-7), a common problem of all antiarrhythmic drugs, occurs when the drug creates an adverse rhythm disturbance (Fig. 3-10), including sinus node suppression and sinus bradycardia, AV block, or increased frequency of or new-onset atrial or ventricular arrhythmias. It was first described in association with quinidine and causes quinidine syncope, which occurs in an estimated 3% of patients who take this drug. In such patients, a rapid polymorphic ventricular tachycardia, termed "torsades de pointes," develops. The frequency of proarrhythmia is higher in patients with decreased ventricular function and a history of sustained ventricular tachycardia or ventricular fibrillation. Unfortunately, it is these patients who most often require antiarrhythmic drugs. Also, proarrhythmia can occur in structurally normal hearts.

- Proarrhythmic effect occurs when a drug creates a rhythm disturbance.
- It is common to all antiarrhythmic drugs.
- Quinidine syncope due to polymorphic ventricular tachycardia (torsades de pointes) is an example of a proarrhythmic effect.

Table 3-5 Properties of Antiarrhythmic Drugs

Drug	Therapeutic range, µg/mL	Half-life, h	Route of metabolism Hepatic, %	Renal, %
Class IA				
Quinidine	2-5	6-8	80	20
Procainamide	4-10	3-6	50	50
Disopyramide	2-5	4-8	50	50
Class IB				
Lidocaine	1.5-5	1-4	100	...
Mexiletine	1-2	8-16	100	...
Phenytoin	10-20	24	~100	...
Class IC				
Flecainide	0.2-1	12-27	75	25
Propafenone	Not helpful*	2-10	100	...
Class III				
Amiodarone	1-2.5	25-110 days	80	...
Sotalol	~2.5	7-18	...	100
Ibutilide	Not established	2-12	...	80
Dofetilide	1-3.5	10	...	80

*Therapeutic effects for propafenone are generally associated with a QRS width increase of 10% above baseline.
Modified from MKSAP IX: Part C, Book 1, 1992. American College of Physicians. By permission.

Table 3-6 Relative Effectiveness of Antiarrhythmic Drugs

Drug	Effectiveness*			
	PVCs	VT	PSVT	AF
Quinidine	2+	2+	2+	2+
Procainamide	2+	2+	2+	2+
Disopyramide	2+	2+	2+	2+
Lidocaine	2+	2+	0	0
Mexiletine	2+	2+	0	0
Ibutilide[†]	-	-	-	2+
Flecainide	4+	2+	3+	2+
Propafenone	4+	2+	3+	2+
Dofetilide[‡]	2+	2+	-	2+
Amiodarone	4+	3+	3+	3+
Sotalol	3+	2-3+	3+	2+

AF, atrial fibrillation (prevention of paroxysmal AF); PSVT, paroxysmal
   tachycardia that uses atrioventricular node as part of reentrant circuit;
   PVCs, premature ventricular complexes; VT, ventricular tachycardia.
*0, not effective; 1+, least effective; 4+, most effective.
[†]Only intravenous form available; approved for acute cardioversion.
[‡]An option to maintain sinus rhythm in patients with atrial fibrillation and
   underlying heart disease.

The results of recent pharmacologic trials for the prevention of sudden cardiac death are summarized in Table 3-8.

Class I Antiarrhythmic Drugs

The Cardiac Arrhythmia Suppression Trial (CAST) was a landmark study that evaluated the use of flecainide, encainide, and moricizine to suppress asymptomatic or mildly symptomatic ventricular ectopy after myocardial infarction. The hypothesis tested was that patients in whom spontaneous ventricular ectopy could be suppressed would have improved outcome. In fact, patients who received class I agents showed a decrease in survival rates despite the adequate suppression of ventricular ectopy when compared with placebo. At the time, this was a totally unexpected and alarming finding. Similar results have been reported with class IA drugs (quinidine, procainamide, and disopyramide) and the class IB drug mexiletine.

- CAST reported decreased survival rate with drug therapy in patients with asymptomatic ventricular ectopy after infarction.

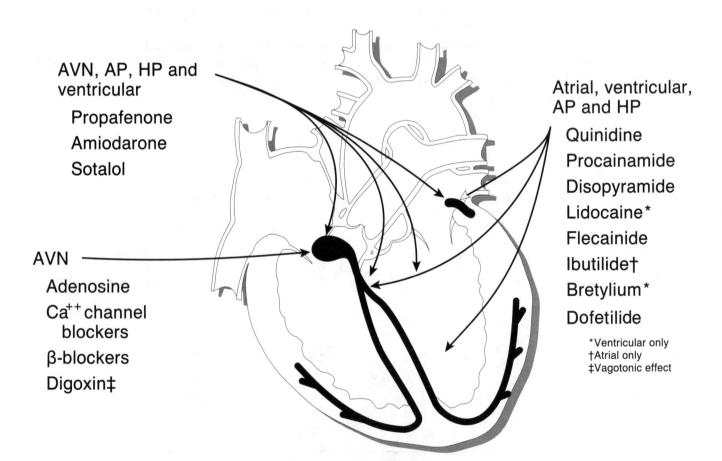

AVN, AP, HP and ventricular
   Propafenone
   Amiodarone
   Sotalol

AVN
   Adenosine
   Ca++ channel blockers
   β-blockers
   Digoxin‡

Atrial, ventricular, AP and HP
   Quinidine
   Procainamide
   Disopyramide
   Lidocaine*
   Flecainide
   Ibutilide†
   Bretylium*
   Dofetilide

*Ventricular only
†Atrial only
‡Vagotonic effect

Fig. 3-9. The predominant target of frequently used antiarrhythmic agents. AP, accessory pathway; AVN, atrioventricular node; HP, His-Purkinje system.

Table 3-7 Toxicity and Side Effects of Antiarrhythmic Drugs

Drug	Frequency of side effects, %	Organ toxicity	% proarrhythmia during treatment for VT	Risk of congestive heart failure*		Side effects
				EF >30%	EF ≤30%	
Quinidine	30	Moderate	3	0	0	Nausea, abdominal pain, diarrhea, thrombocytopenia, hypotension, ↓ warfarin clearance
Procainamide	30	High	2	0	1+	Lupus-like syndrome, rash, fever, headache, nausea, hallucinations, diarrhea
Disopyramide	30	Low	2	1+	4+	Dry mouth, urinary hesitancy, blurred vision, constipation, urinary retention
Lidocaine	40	Moderate	2	0	0	L-H, seizure, tremor, confusion, memory loss, nausea
Mexiletine	40	Low	2	0	0	L-H, tremor, ataxia, confusion, memory loss, altered liver function
Ibutilide†	25	Low	4	0	0	Nausea, headache
Flecainide	30	Low	5	1+	3+	L-H, visual disturbance, headache, nausea
Propafenone	30	Low	5	0-1+	2+	L-H, headache, nausea, constipation, metallic taste, ↓ warfarin clearance
Dofetilide	20	Low	4	0	0	Headache, chest pain, dizziness
Amiodarone	65	High	4	0	1+	Corneal deposits, photosensitivity, sleep disturbance, nausea, anorexia, tremor, ataxia, neuropathy, pulmonary fibrosis, thyroid disorders, hepatotoxicity, ↓ warfarin clearance
Sotalol	30	Low	5	1+	3+	L-H, fatigue, dyspnea, nausea

EF, ejection fraction; L-H, light-headedness; PVC, premature ventricular complex; VT, sustained ventricular tachycardia.
*Congestive heart failure risk: 0, no risk; 4+, high risk.
†Intravenous therapy for acute cardioversion in patients with atrial fibrillation.
Modified from MKSAP IX: Part C, Book 1, 1992. American College of Physicians. By permission.

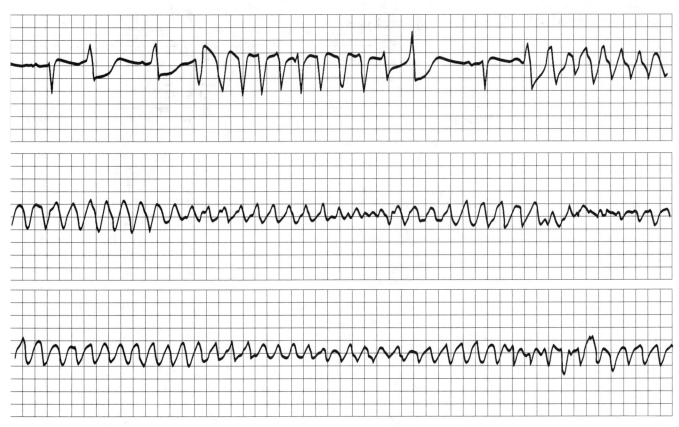

Fig. 3-10. Proarrhythmic response to quinidine. Quinidine resulted in prolongation of QT interval, and late-coupled premature ventricular complex initiated polymorphic ventricular tachycardia, termed "torsades de pointes."

Table 3-8   Results of Trials on Pharmacologic Prevention of Primary Sudden Cardiac Death

| Trial | Patients | No. | Drug | Follow-up, mo | Total mortality, % | | Significance |
					Placebo	Drug	
Julian et al., 1982	MI <2 wk	1,456	*d-, l*-Sotalol	12	8.9	7.3	No
CAST, 1989	MI, EF <55%, >6 PVCs/h	1,455	Flecainide Encainide	10	3.0	7.7	Yes
CAST II, 1992	MI, EF ≤40%, >6 PVCs/h	1,155	Moricizine	18	12.4	15.0	No
SWORT, 1996	MI, EF ≤40%	3,121	*d*-Sotalol	5	3.1	5.0	Yes
Diamond-MI, 1997	MI	1,510	Dofetilide	≥12	32.0	31.0	No
GESICA, 1994	CHF	516	Amiodarone	24	41.4	33.5	Yes
STAT-CHF, 1995	CHF, EF <40%	674	Amiodarone	45	29.2 (2 y)	30.6 (2 y)	No
CAMIAT, 1997	MI, ≥10 PVCs/h or ± NSVT	1,202	Amiodarone	22	11.4	9.4	No
EMIAT, 1997	MI, EF ≤40%	1,486	Amiodarone	21	13.7	13.9	No

CHF, congestive heart failure; EF, ejection fraction; MI, myocardial infarction; NSVT, nonsustained ventricular tachycardia ; PVCs, premature ventricular complexes.

Amiodarone

Results from two randomized trials of amiodarone after myocardial infarction (European Myocardial Infarction Amiodarone Trial [EMIAT] and Canadian Amiodarone Myocardial Infarction Arrhythmia Trial [CAMIAT]) suggested that amiodarone may decrease arrhythmia-related death. However, overall mortality was not improved. Results from amiodarone trials among patients with congestive heart failure are also mixed. The Survival Trial of Antiarrhythmic Therapy in patients with Congestive Heart Failure arrhythmia (STAT-CHF) study showed that overall mortality was not significantly different between patients treated with amiodarone and those receiving placebo. In contrast, the Gruppo de Estudio de la Sobrevida en la Insuficiencia Cardiaca en Argentina (GESICA) study (randomized trial of low-dose amiodarone in severe congestive heart failure) showed that low-dose amiodarone therapy reduced total mortality in comparison with placebo therapy in patients with congestive heart failure. The differences in outcome may be explained by differences in patient population. In the STAT-CHF study, approximately 70% of the study population had coronary artery disease, compared with 30% in the GESICA study. Currently, the routine use of amiodarone after myocardial infarction or in unselected patients with congestive heart failure is not recommended. However, if patients have frequent and complex PVCs associated with documented symptoms in the setting of compromised left ventricular dysfunction, it is not unreasonable to consider a trial of amiodarone therapy.

- The routine use of amiodarone after myocardial infarction or in unselected patients with congestive heart failure for PVC suppression or primary prevention of sudden cardiac death is not recommended.

Adenosine

Adenosine slows conduction in the AV node and is eliminated by uptake in endothelial cells and erythrocytes. Its half-life is 10 seconds. Adenosine is indicated in supraventricular reentrant tachycardia that uses the AV node as part of the reentrant circuit (i.e., AV nodal reentry or reentry using an accessory pathway). The drug does not terminate atrial fibrillation, flutter, or tachycardia, and it slows the ventricular rate for only a few seconds because of its short half-life. Both adenosine and verapamil have equal efficacy at the highest recommended doses (adenosine, 12 mg; verapamil, 10 mg). Because of the short half-life of adenosine, approximately 10% of patients have recurrent supraventricular tachycardia after its administration, whereas recurrent supraventricular tachycardia is rare after termination by verapamil. In patients who present with wide QRS tachycardia (ventricular tachycardia) or atrial fibrillation and associated Wolff-Parkinson-White syndrome, hemodynamic collapse is common when they are given verapamil. This hemodynamic collapse is not associated with adenosine. The cost of adenosine is approximately twice that of verapamil.

- Adenosine slows conduction in the AV node.
- Adenosine can terminate supraventricular reentrant tachycardia that relies on conduction through the AV node.
- Adenosine does not terminate atrial fibrillation, flutter, or atrial tachycardia (exceptions exist, so adenosine should not be used to "diagnose" atrial tachycardia by exclusion).
- The efficacy of 12 mg of adenosine is equal to that of 10 mg of verapamil.
- The cost of adenosine is twice that of verapamil.

Electrophysiology-Guided Serial Drug Testing

In the era before more widespread availability and use of implantable cardioverter-defibrillators, serial drug testing frequently was used to help identify an effective drug for patients with life-threatening ventricular arrhythmias in whom outpatient management was unsafe. The technique involved induction of arrhythmia at baseline state followed by administration of an antiarrhythmic drug until therapeutic levels had been achieved, followed by repeat electrophysiologic study. A drug that prevented subsequent induction of tachycardia was deemed effective.

Among patients presenting with ventricular tachycardia due to coronary disease, the chance of inducing clinical tachycardia in the laboratory is 95% but decreases to 75% in patients with dilated cardiomyopathy or valvular heart disease. Among patients who present with out-of-hospital cardiac arrest or ventricular fibrillation, the chance of life-threatening ventricular arrhythmia being induced at testing decreases to 70%. Serial drug testing primarily has been abandoned due in large part to the poor long-term efficacy of antiarrhythmic drug therapy in patients with life-threatening ventricular arrhythmias compared with the proven effectiveness of implantable cardioverter-defibrillators. In current practice, serial drug testing is largely limited to determining the efficacy of drug therapy for ventricular arrhythmias in patients who already have an implanted cardioverter-defibrillator and have frequent shocks due to recurrent ventricular arrhythmias.

- Electrophysiology-guided serial drug testing, performed before hospital dismissal, attempts to identify an effective drug for patients with life-threatening arrhythmias.
- With out-of-hospital cardiac arrest and ventricular fibrillation, the chance of inducing life-threatening arrhythmia during testing is 70%.
- Serial drug testing identifies an effective drug in only 40% of patients with ventricular tachycardia.

Transcatheter Radiofrequency Ablation

Transcatheter ablation therapy using a radiofrequency energy source to heat tissue (RFA) has revolutionized the treatment of almost all heart rhythm disorders. With currently available technology, supraventricular tachycardias such as AV nodal reentrant tachycardia or tachycardia due to an accessory pathway (such as Wolff-Parkinson-White syndrome) are completely curable with RFA in more than 95% of cases. Ectopic atrial tachycardias are curable in more than 90% of cases. Table 3-9 lists heart rhythm disorders amenable to catheter ablation therapy. In addition, considerable progress has been made in recent years in the treatment of atrial fibrillation (especially paroxysmal atrial fibrillation) and ventricular tachycardia due to reentry around a scar after myocardial infarction.

The technique of RFA is similar to that described for electrophysiologic testing and, in most cases, is performed during the same procedure if an abnormal rhythm is found or has been documented clinically. When an area of tissue critical for initiating or sustaining the abnormal rhythm has been identified (mapped), a specially designed electrode catheter capable of delivering radiofrequency energy is maneuvered in proximity and radiofrequency energy is delivered, thus preventing further conduction of electrical impulses and preventing the abnormal rhythm from occurring.

- Supraventricular tachycardia due to AV nodal reentrant tachycardia, accessory pathway in Wolff-Parkinson-White syndrome, automatic atrial focus, atrial flutter, and some cases of atrial fibrillation and ventricular tachycardia can be cured with RFA.
- RFA is performed with radiofrequency energy passed through a catheter.

Table 3-9 Heart Rhythms Amenable to Catheter Ablation

Rhythm	Curable	Treatable
SVT	AVNRT	AF
	AVRT (bypass tract)	
	EAT	
	AFL (without fibrillation)	
Ventricular	RV outflow tract tachycardia	VT due to coronary disease and scar after MI
	Idiopathic LV tachycardia	

AF, atrial fibrillation; AFL, atrial flutter; AVNRT, atrioventricular node reentry tachycardia; AVRT, atrioventricular reentry tachycardia; EAT, ectopic atrial tachycardia; LV, left ventricular; MI, myocardial infarction; RV, right ventricular; VT, ventricular tachycardia.

About 1% to 2% of patients experience complications, including vascular injury at the site of catheter insertion, cardiac perforation, and infection. In addition, if the site of the critical area, such as an accessory pathway, is close to the normal conduction system, or if AV nodal reentrant tachycardia is ablated, there is a 5% risk of creating complete heart block that requires permanent pacing. When compared with previous surgical approaches for the treatment of similar tachycardias, the technique has reduced the hospital stay from 7 days to 1 to 2 days and the time to return to work or school from 6 to 8 weeks to 3 to 5 days. The cost is approximately 40% of the surgical cost.

- Catheter ablation is successful in 95% of cases of accessory pathway or reentrant tachycardia in the AV node.
- The complication rate is 1%-2%.
- Catheter ablation reduces hospital stay to 1-2 days.
- The cost is 40% of the surgical cost.

Catheter ablation also may be used to achieve complete heart block in some cases of supraventricular tachycardias (usually atrial fibrillation or atrial flutter) that are refractory to medications and associated with rapid ventricular rates. With either direct-current ablation or RFA, complete heart block can be achieved in more than 95% of patients. In such cases, permanent pacing is required. In select patients, this approach results in substantial improvement in symptoms (because of regularization of the heart rate) and in exercise capacity with use of rate-responsive pacing. However, one disadvantage is that patients are pacemaker-dependent and require long-term follow-up.

- Catheter ablation achieves complete heart block in supraventricular tachycardias that are refractory to medication and associated with rapid ventricular rate.
- Catheter ablation results in heart block in >95% of patients; permanent pacing then is required.
- Symptoms improve substantially.

Antitachycardia Surgery

Endocardial resection is a standard technique for treating ventricular tachycardia associated with aneurysm. The border zone adjacent to a myocardial scar (including aneurysm) is generally the location for the reentrant circuit. This border zone is located with mapping systems at the time of operation and is then removed with a technique called subendocardial resection. The operative mortality rate is approximately 10%; arrhythmia is cured in 85% of survivors.

- Endocardial resection is an option for treating ventricular tachycardia associated with aneurysm.

- Operative mortality rate is 10%.
- Arrhythmia is cured in 85% of survivors.

In the past, endocardial resection was used to treat refractory arrhythmias due to accessory pathways or AV nodal reentry; it has now largely been replaced by RFA.

Current therapeutic interventions available to patients with symptoms due to tachycardia are summarized in Table 3-10.

Device Therapy

Device therapy is available for abnormal heart rhythms due to bradycardias (permanent cardiac pacemaker implantation) and tachycardias (implantable cardioverter-defibrillators [ICDs]).

Permanent Cardiac Pacemaker Implantation

An internationally recognized four-letter system is used to classify different types of implantable pacemakers and ICDs (Table 3-11). The initial letter is used to denote the chamber paced, the second letter the chamber sensed, and the third letter the programmed mode of response of the pacemaker (inhibited, triggered, or both). Recently, a fourth letter was added to denote whether rate-responsiveness is possible. In a pacemaker with rate-responsiveness, the programmed rate automatically increases in response to sensor-detected activity. Usually, the sensor is located within the pulse-generator or is part of the implanted lead system. Common pacing modes include VVI (ventricular paced, ventricular sensed, inhibited in response to a ventricular event), VVIR (same as previous entry but also has rate responsiveness), DDD (atrial and ventricular pacing and sensing with triggered and inhibited response to a sensed atrial or ventricular event), and DDDR (same as previous entry but also has rate responsiveness).

Table 3-10 Summary of Tachyarrhythmia Therapy

Supraventricular tachycardia	Drug	Ablation	ICD	Surgery
AVNRT	+	++	-	-
AVRT	+	++	-	-*
EAT	+	+	-	-*
IAST	++	o	-	-
Typical A flutter	+	++	-	-*
AFib	++	+	o	+

Symbols: +, effective; ++, preferred; o, investigational; -, no indication; -*, few indications, can be effective.
A, atrial; AFib, atrial fibrillation; AVNRT, atrioventricular nodal reciprocating tachycardia; AVRT, atrioventricular reciprocating tachycardia; EAT, ectopic atrial tachycardia; IAST, inappropriate sinus tachycardia; ICD, implantable cardioverter-defibrillator.

The precise choice of pacemaker used depends in large part on clinical circumstances.

Physiologic pacing (with a DDD pacemaker) attempts to maintain heart rate with normal AV synchrony and to increase heart rate in response to physical activity. In patients with normal sinus node activity, DDD pacemakers can "track" atrial activation. This has the advantage that as sinus node activity increases (e.g., in response to exercise or some other stress), the pacemaker rate increases accordingly so that the ventricle is paced at the appropriate rate but with normal AV conduction delay (PR interval). In patients with chronic atrial fibrillation, rate-modulated pacing (the "R" in VVIR) is used to increase heart rate in response to physical demand. In such cases, a sensor that responds to body motion, respiratory rate, blood temperature, or some other variable is used to drive the pacemaker so that the rate at which pacing occurs is appropriate to metabolic demands. Patients fitted with this type of pacemaker have increased exercise endurance during treadmill testing. Patients with both sinus node dysfunction and AV conduction system disease benefit most from DDDR pacing.

- Physiologic pacing maintains heart rate with normal AV synchrony and increases the rate during physical activity.
- Rate-modulated pacing increases exercise endurance during treadmill testing.

Complications of Permanent Pacing

Complications of device therapy (pacing and ICD) may be classified as early (usually within 30 days of implant) or late. Early complications are most commonly related to vascular injury, hematoma, pneumothorax, dislodgment of the lead, and extracardiac stimulation (e.g., diaphragmatic stimulation). In most cases, repositioning of the lead or reprogramming of the device remediates the problem. Late complications include lead fracture or insulation defect, infection, pacemaker syndrome, and pacemaker-mediated tachycardia.

Pacemaker syndrome may develop during dominant ventricular pacing in a minority of patients with intact retrograde conduction between the ventricle and the atrium (Fig. 3-11). When the ventricle is paced, the impulse conducts retrogradely to the atrium and simultaneous atrial and ventricular contraction results. Because the atria are contracting against closed tricuspid and mitral valves, the atrial contribution to ventricular filling is prevented and the atria are distended. The increased atrial pressure distends the neck veins, leading to a sensation of "fullness in the neck" and symptoms due to decreased forward cardiac output such as light-headedness and fatigue. Symptoms and signs due to pacemaker syndrome can be eliminated with dual-chamber pacing.

Table 3-11 Code of Permanent Pacing

Chamber(s) paced	Chamber(s) sensed	Mode(s) of response	Programmable capabilities
V = Ventricle	V = Ventricle	T = Triggered	R = Rate modulated
A = Atrium	A = Atrium	I = Inhibited	
D = Dual (atrium and ventricle)	D = Dual (atrium and ventricle)	D = Dual (triggered and inhibited)	
	O = None	O = None	

- In pacemaker syndrome, atria contract against closed tricuspid and mitral valves, resulting in backward blood flow and decreased forward blood flow (cardiac output).
- Symptoms are typically "fullness in the neck," light-headedness, and fatigue.
- Dual-chamber pacing eliminates symptoms.

Pacemaker-mediated tachycardia is a well-recognized complication of dual-chamber pacemakers (DDD pacing) and occurs when retrograde conduction between the ventricle and atrium is intact. In this type of tachycardia, the pacemaker generator acts as one limb of the reentrant circuit. Typically, a spontaneous PVC occurs which conducts retrogradely to the atrium. This early retrograde atrial activity is sensed by the pacemaker, which awaits the normal AV delay and then paces the ventricle. The "early" ventricular activity generated by

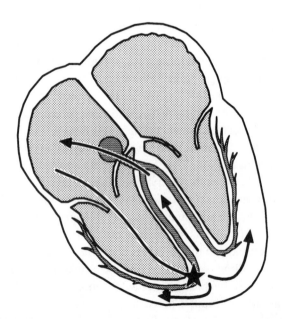

Fig. 3-11. Pacemaker syndrome with retrograde atrial activation during ventricular pacing (*star*), resulting in simultaneous atrial and ventricular contractions.

the pacemaker then conducts retrogradely to the atrium, and the reentrant circuit is completed. Typically, the tachycardia rate is close to the upper rate limit of the device. Most pacemaker devices possess algorithms that recognize and attempt to abort pacemaker-mediated tachycardia. Alternatively, the device can be programmed to reduce or eliminate it.

- Pacemaker-mediated tachycardia occurs with DDD pacing when there is intact retrograde conduction between the ventricle and atrium.
- The abnormality is corrected by programming changes of the pacemaker generator.

Indications for Permanent Pacemaker Implantation

Guidelines for permanent pacemaker implantation are well established. Indications for specific conduction system disease are discussed in Table 3-12. Indications are generally grouped according to the following classification: class I indication—conditions for which there is general agreement that permanent pacemakers should be implanted; class II—conditions for which permanent pacemakers are frequently used but opinions differ about the necessity of implantation; and class III—conditions for which there is general agreement that pacemakers are not necessary. Clinical symptoms such as syncope, presyncope, or exercise intolerance that can be correlated with and attributed to a bradycardia disorder usually constitute a class I indication for permanent pacemaker implantation. If symptoms cannot be correlated with bradycardia, it is less certain that permanent pacemaker implantation is indicated.

Implantable Cardioverter-Defibrillators

Because serial drug testing identifies only 40% of patients with life-threatening ventricular arrhythmias, an alternative therapy has been developed to treat recurrences of tachycardia. The most effective therapy has been the implantable cardioverter-defibrillator (ICD). This device continuously monitors heart rhythm and can detect and treat abnormal ventricular arrhythmia with overdrive pacing (antitachycardia pacing), low-energy cardioversion, or up to 30- to 40-J shocks. In most cases, an ICD can be implanted in the pectoral region in a fashion similar to that of permanent pacemakers. Moreover, with improvements in ICD technology, earlier problems with limited battery life, larger pulse generators, and frequent inappropriate shocks (often due to atrial fibrillation with rapid ventricular response being confused with a rapid ventricular tachycardia) are rapidly being resolved.

In terms of benefit, ICDs have clearly been shown to improve mortality among patients who survive a sudden cardiac death episode when compared with historical controls. Historically, such patients had a 70% survival rate at 1 year without treatment or with empiric antiarrhythmic drug therapy. Use of the ICD has improved the overall 1-year survival rate to 90%; recurrent sudden cardiac death occurs in 2% of patients at 1 year and in 4% of patients at 4 years. The Antiarrhythmic Versus Implantable Defibrillator (AVID) trial reported that an ICD is superior for reducing overall mortality in comparison with empiric amiodarone therapy in patients with a history of out-of-hospital cardiac arrest or symptomatic sustained ventricular tachycardia (secondary sudden cardiac death prevention).

Several trials have reported on the role of the ICD among patients at high risk of sudden cardiac death (i.e., primary prevention). One of the first was the Multicenter Automatic Defibrillator Implantation Trial (MADIT), which found that patients with prior myocardial infarction, ejection fraction less than 35%, and nonsustained ventricular tachycardia with electrophysiologically inducible sustained monomorphic ventricular tachycardia not suppressible with procainamide had improved survival with ICD when compared with the best medical (including antiarrhythmic) therapy. Similar observations were confirmed in the Multicenter Unsustained Tachycardia Trial (MUSTT). Recently, MADIT II addressed prophylactic implantation of an ICD in a group of patients with prior myocardial infarction and reduced ejection fraction (<30%), without additional risk stratification; survival improved compared with no ICD therapy. Currently, defibrillator implantation can be considered in select patients at high risk for primary sudden cardiac death.

Table 3-12 Indications for Pacemaker Implantation

Sinus node dysfunction
Class I
Documented symptomatic bradycardia
Class II
HR <40 beats/min, symptoms present but not clearly correlated with bradycardia
Class III
Asymptomatic bradycardia (<40 beats/min)
AV block
Class I
Symptomatic 2° or 3° AV block, permanent or intermittent
Congenital 3° AV block with wide QRS
Advanced AV block 14 d after cardiac surgery
Class II
Asymptomatic type II 2° or 3° AV block with ventricular rate >40 beats/min
Class III
Asymptomatic 1° and type I 2° AV block
Myocardial infarction
Class I
Recurrent type II 2° AV block and 3° AV block with wide QRS
Transient advanced AV block in presence of BBB
Class II
Persistent advanced AV block with narrow QRS
Acquired BBB in absence of AV block
Class III
Transient AV block in absence of BBB

AV, atrioventricular; BBB, bundle branch block.

- Implantation of a defibrillator is indicated for secondary sudden cardiac death prevention. Exceptions are cardiac arrest due to a correctable or transient substrate such as a metabolic disturbance or within hours of acute myocardial infarction.
- For prevention of primary sudden cardiac death, implantation of a defibrillator is indicated in selected high-risk patients, such as those with prior myocardial infarction, compromised ejection fraction, and inducible sustained ventricular tachycardia during electrophysiologic study.

PART III
Paul A. Friedman, M.D.

SPECIFIC ARRHYTHMIA PROBLEMS

Sinus Node Dysfunction

Sinus node dysfunction, also called "sick sinus syndrome," includes sinus bradycardia, sinus pauses, tachycardia-bradycardia syndrome (Fig. 3-12), and sinus arrest. It usually is associated with conduction system disease and lack of an appropriate junctional escape focus during sinus pause or sinus bradycardia. The diagnosis is made from the medical history and results of electrocardiographic (ECG) and Holter monitoring, which are the most useful diagnostic tests. Electrophysiologic testing is used to evaluate patients with a history consistent with sinus node disease in whom ECG or Holter monitoring has not shown the mechanism because of infrequent spells. Electrophysiologic testing has low sensitivity because patients may be in an increased adrenergic state in the laboratory and catecholamines prevent the sinus bradycardia or sinus pauses from being apparent. Prolonged monitoring with an event recorder is also useful for diagnosis.

- Sinus node dysfunction includes sinus bradycardia, sinus pauses, tachycardia-bradycardia syndrome, and sinus arrest.
- Sinus node dysfunction is associated with conduction system disease.
- The diagnosis is made from the history and the results of ECG and Holter monitoring.
- Electrophysiologic testing is used for patients in whom the mechanism of dysfunction is not shown by ECG or Holter monitoring.

Asymptomatic patients with sinus node dysfunction are followed without specific therapy. Symptomatic patients are usually treated with pacemakers. Often, patients with tachycardia-bradycardia have atrial fibrillation that at times presents with rapid ventricular rates and at other times with inappropriate, symptomatic bradycardia. Pacemakers are used to prevent the bradycardia, and drugs are used to slow conduction through the atrioventricular (AV) node and to prevent episodes of rapid ventricular rate.

- Asymptomatic patients with sinus node dysfunction: followed without specific therapy.
- Symptomatic patients with sinus node dysfunction: treated with pacemakers.

Conduction System Disorders

First-degree AV block results in a prolonged PR interval and is usually due to conduction delay within the AV node. In patients with associated bundle branch block, the conduction delay may be distal to the AV node in the His-Purkinje system. Patients with second-degree AV block of the Mobitz I (Wenckebach) variety have a gradual prolongation of the PR interval before the nonconducted P wave. The subsequent PR interval is shorter than the PR interval before the nonconducted P wave (Fig. 3-13 and 3-14). Also, the RR interval that encompasses the nonconducted P wave is shorter than two RR intervals between conducted beats. Wenckebach conduction often accompanies an inferior myocardial infarction, which results in ischemia of the AV node. This problem generally does not require pacing unless documented hemodynamic problems are associated with the slow heart rate.

- First-degree AV block results in a prolonged PR interval.
- Second-degree AV block of Mobitz I type results in gradual prolongation of the PR interval before the nonconducted P wave.

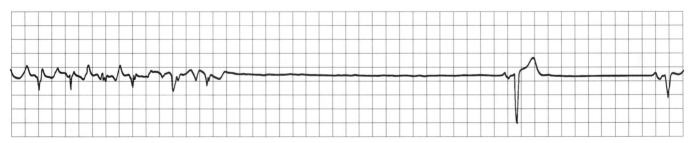

Fig. 3-12. Tachycardia-bradycardia with episode of atrial fibrillation terminating spontaneously; these are followed by a 4.5-second pause until the sinus node recovers. (From MKSAP IX: Part C, Book 1, 1992. American College of Physicians. By permission.)

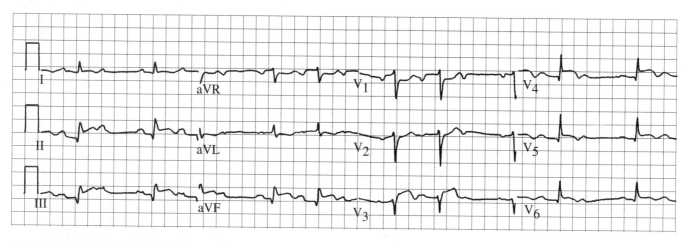

Fig. 3-13. 3:2 Mobitz I (or Wenckebach) second-degree atrioventricular block in a patient with acute inferior myocardial infarction.

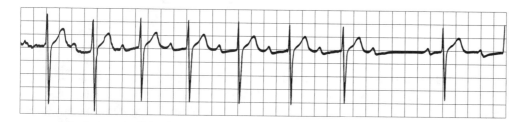

Fig. 3-14. Mobitz I second-degree atrioventricular block; note gradual PR prolongation. The PR interval after a nonconducted P wave is shorter than the PR interval preceding the nonconducted P wave.

- Wenckebach conduction may accompany inferior myocardial infarction.
- Wenckebach conduction does not require pacing unless hemodynamic problems are associated with slow heart rate.

Second-degree AV block due to the Mobitz II mechanism generally is caused by conduction disease in the His-Purkinje system and is associated with bundle branch block (Fig. 3-15). This conduction abnormality is shown on the ECG as a sudden failure of a P wave to conduct to the ventricle, with no change in the PR interval either before or after the nonconducted P wave. This problem often heralds complete heart block, and strong consideration should be given to permanent pacing. "Complete heart block" is diagnosed when there is no relation between the atrial rhythm and the ventricular rhythm and *the atrial rhythm is faster than the ventricular escape rhythm* (Fig. 3-16). The ventricular escape rhythm is either a junctional escape focus, with a conduction pattern similar to that seen during normal rhythm, or a ventricular escape focus, with a wide QRS conduction pattern. In most cases, complete heart block is treated with permanent pacing.

- Second-degree AV block of Mobitz II type is usually due to conduction disease in the His-Purkinje system.

- It often heralds complete heart block; consider permanent pacing.
- Complete heart block: no relation between atrial rhythm and ventricular rhythm, and atrial rhythm is faster than ventricular escape rhythm. Treatment: pacing.

"Bifascicular block" refers to left bundle branch block, right bundle branch block with left anterior fascicular block (marked left-axis deviation), or right bundle branch block with left posterior fascicular block (right-axis deviation). Bifascicular block usually is associated with underlying structural heart disease and has a 1% chance of progressing to complete heart block in asymptomatic persons. Patients presenting with syncope and bifascicular block may have intermittent complete heart block caused by conduction system disease or ventricular tachycardia caused by the underlying myocardial disease. Permanent pacing can be used to treat syncope due to complete heart block, but syncope due to ventricular tachycardia typically is treated with an implantable defibrillator, although antiarrhythmic medications or surgery may be prescribed, depending on the clinical situation. Patients with syncope and bifascicular block should have electrophysiologic testing (especially if the ejection fraction is decreased) to determine whether they have ventricular

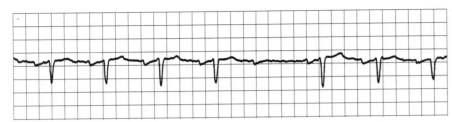

Fig. 3-15. Mobitz II second-degree atrioventricular block with no change in the PR interval before or after a nonconducted P wave.

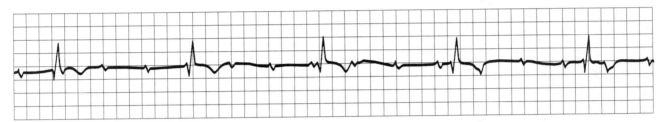

Fig. 3-16. Complete heart block with an atrial rate at 70 beats/min and a ventricular escape rhythm at 30 beats/min.

tachycardia, because this rhythm occurs in 40% of these patients. Although treatment with permanent pacing only does not decrease the risk of sudden death in these patients, it improves their syncope.

- Bifascicular block usually is associated with structural heart disease.
- Bifascicular block progresses to complete heart block in 1% of asymptomatic persons.
- Permanent pacing is used to treat syncope in complete heart block.
- Syncope due to ventricular tachycardia typically is treated with an implantable defibrillator, although antiarrhythmic drugs or surgery may be prescribed in some cases.
- Patients with syncope, bifascicular block, and ventricular tachycardia who receive only permanent pacing have improvement in syncope but no decrease in risk of sudden death.

High-degree AV block is diagnosed when there is a 2:1 or higher AV conduction block (Fig. 3-17). It might be caused by a Wenckebach or a Mobitz II mechanism. A Wenckebach mechanism is more likely if the QRS conduction is normal, and a Mobitz II-type mechanism is more likely if the QRS complex demonstrates additional conduction disease, such as bundle branch block.

Carotid Sinus Syndrome

Carotid sinus massage is performed to identify carotid sinus hypersensitivity (Fig. 3-18). Approximately 40% of patients older than 65 have a hyperactive carotid sinus reflex (3-second pause or a decrease in systolic blood pressure of 50 mm Hg), although most of these patients do not have spontaneous syncope. Carotid sinus massage should be performed over the carotid bifurcation at the angle of the jaw in patients without evidence of carotid bruit on carotid auscultation or a history of cerebrovascular disease. Carotid sinus massage is performed with moderate pressure over the carotid bifurcation for 5 seconds while monitoring heart rate and blood pressure. Approximately 35% of patients with a hyperactive carotid sinus reflex have a pure cardioinhibitory component manifested only by a pause in ventricular activity exceeding 3 seconds. Fifteen percent of patients have a pure vasodepressor component, with a normal heart rate maintained but a decrease in systolic blood pressure of more than 50 mm Hg. Sixty percent of patients have a combined response, with both cardioinhibitory and vasodepressor components. In such patients, permanent pacing may prevent the cardioinhibitory response, but the vasodepressor response continues to produce symptoms.

- Carotid sinus massage is used to identify carotid sinus hypersensitivity.
- About 40% of patients >65 years have a hyperactive carotid sinus reflex (3-second pause or decrease in systolic blood pressure of 50 mm Hg).

Occasionally, associated neck abnormalities, including lymph node enlargement, previous neck surgery, and regional tumor, result in carotid sinus syndrome. Surgical techniques to treat this condition are usually unsuccessful, and the primary form of therapy is AV sequential pacing for the cardioinhibitory

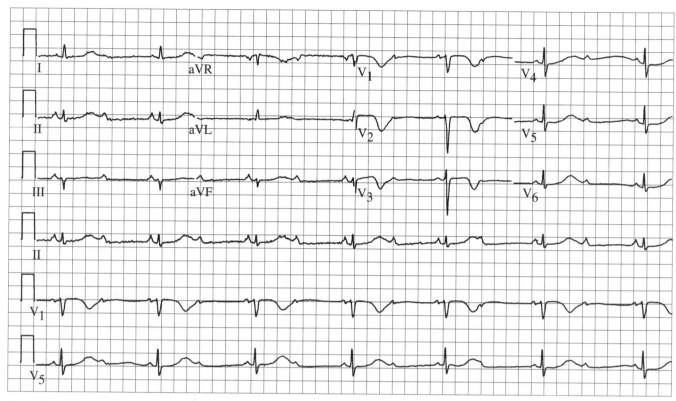

Fig. 3-17. High-grade 2:1 atrioventricular conduction block.

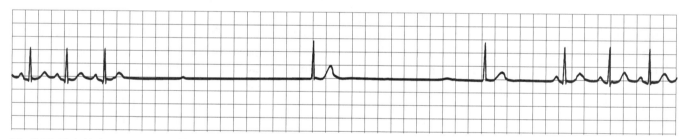

Fig. 3-18. Carotid sinus massage resulting in sinus pause with junctional escape beats before sinus rhythm returns.

component and elastic stockings for the vasodepressor component. Occasionally, the condition responds to anticholinergic medications.

Summary of Indications for Pacemakers

To summarize, pacemakers generally are indicated for symptomatic bradycardias. Commonly, these are AV block (second-degree Mobitz II, high-grade, or third-degree), sinus node dysfunction, and carotid sinus hypersensitivity. They usually are best documented by correlating the symptoms with an ECG recording. In asymptomatic patients, pacing should be considered in complete heart block (particularly with escape <40 beats/min or pauses >3 seconds), Mobitz II block (especially associated with bifascicular or trifascicular block), and postoperative AV block.

- Pacing is indicated for symptomatic bradycardias due to second- or third-degree heart block, sinus node dysfunction, and carotid sinus hypersensitivity.
- Asymptomatic patients with complete heart block, Mobitz II AV block, or postoperative AV block should also be considered for pacing.

Atrial Flutter

Atrial flutter is identified by the characteristic sawtooth pattern of atrial activity at a rate of 240 to 320 beats/min. Patients with normal conduction systems maintain 2:1 AV conduction; thus, the ventricular rate is often close to 150 beats/min. Higher degrees of AV block (3:1 or higher) in the absence of drugs to slow AV node conduction (digoxin, β-adrenergic blocker, calcium antagonist) imply AV conduction disease (Fig. 3-19). In patients with 2:1 AV conduction and a heart rate of 150 beats/min, one of the flutter waves is often buried in the QRS complex. Carotid sinus massage results in increased AV block, revealing the flutter waves and establishing the diagnosis.

- Atrial flutter: atrial activity at 240-320 beats/min.
- The ventricular rate is close to 150 beats/min.

Pharmacologic therapy for atrial flutter is used to slow AV node conduction and to control the ventricular rate or to control the flutter itself. The same medications used to treat atrial fibrillation (discussed below) are used to treat atrial flutter. Success rates for the control of atrial flutter are 30% to 50%.

Nonpharmacologic therapy for typical atrial flutter has been well established. Unlike atrial fibrillation, which is composed of multiple reentrant wavelets that travel through the atria, typical atrial flutter consists of a single reentrant circuit that follows the tricuspid valve annulus (Fig. 3-20). This fixed reentrant pathway results in a surface ECG with very stable flutter waves (see Fig. 3-19) and provides a target for ablation. Radiofrequency catheter ablation of this single circuit has a success rate higher than 90%. This procedure must not be confused with AV node ablation for atrial fibrillation. In atrial flutter ablation, a lesion is placed in the atrium to interrupt the flutter circuit; AV node conduction is not impaired and normal sinus rhythm (with no need for pacing) ensues. In AV node ablation for atrial fibrillation, the AV node (or His bundle) is ablated, preventing atrial impulses from reaching the ventricles, thus controlling ventricular rate; the atria, however, continue to fibrillate, and because of the presence of AV block, a pacemaker is required.

The ablation lesions for atrial flutter are placed between the tricuspid annulus and the inferior vena cava.

- Typical atrial flutter ablation has a success rate >90%.
- Atrial flutter can be associated with thromboembolism and probably should be treated similarly to atrial fibrillation with regard to anticoagulation.

Atrial Fibrillation

Atrial fibrillation is the most common arrhythmia encountered in clinical practice. Its frequency increases with age. Atrial fibrillation is characterized by continuous and irregular activity of the ECG baseline caused by swarming electrical currents in the atria. According to population-based studies, its prevalence is 5% among persons 65 and older. Common causes and associated conditions include hypertension, cardiomyopathy, valvular heart disease (particularly mitral stenosis), sick sinus syndrome, Wolff-Parkinson-White syndrome (especially in young patients), alcohol use ("holiday heart"), and thyrotoxicosis. The presence of these conditions should be sought in the history and physical examination of patients with atrial fibrillation. It has been discovered recently that atrial fibrillation can have a discrete focal source or trigger. These triggers are often from the muscle in the proximal portions of the pulmonary veins.

- Common causes of atrial fibrillation include hypertension, cardiomyopathy, valvular heart disease, sick sinus syndrome, Wolff-Parkinson-White syndrome, thyrotoxicosis, and alcohol use.
- Atrial fibrillation must be distinguished from atrial flutter (uniform flutter waves) and multifocal atrial tachycardia

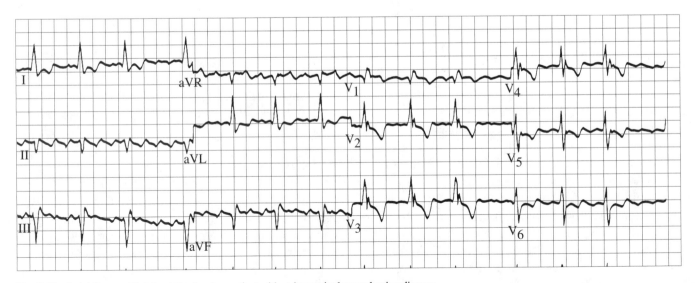

Fig. 3-19. Atrial flutter with 3:1 conduction in a patient with atrioventricular conduction disease.

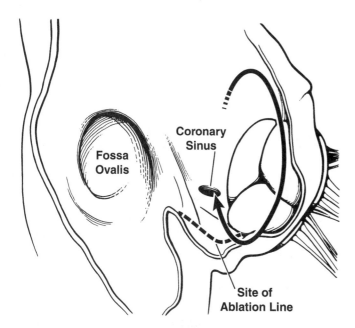

Fig. 3-20. View of the right atrium, with the tricuspid valve on the right. The atrial flutter circuit is confined to the path depicted by the circular arrow adjacent to the valve. An ablation lesion along the dashed line ("Site of Ablation Line") interrupts the circuit, eliminating atrial flutter. In contrast to atrial flutter, atrial fibrillation has wandering wavefronts throughout the atria which will not respond to the flutter ablation line.

(isoelectric interval between premature atrial contractions that have three or more different morphologies).

Therapy for Atrial Fibrillation

Therapy for atrial fibrillation can be divided into two broad categories: ventricular rate control (by slow conduction through the AV node) with stroke prophylaxis (for ongoing atrial fibrillation) and maintenance of sinus rhythm (rhythm control). The choice of the approach depends partly on the degree of the patient's symptoms, age, and preference and the coexisting conditions. Currently, it is not known whether one approach is superior; this issue is being evaluated by a multicenter trial.

- It is important to know which agents are useful for rate control and which for rhythm control (Table 3-13).

Rate Control and Anticoagulation

The three main categories of drugs used to blunt the AV node response in atrial fibrillation are digitalis glycosides, β-adrenergic blocking agents, and calcium channel blockers. These are summarized in Table 3-13. None of these agents has been shown to be effective in the prevention of recurrent atrial fibrillation. There is one exception: continuation of β-blockers after cardiac surgery may prevent recurrent atrial fibrillation.

Digoxin has primarily an indirect effect by increasing vagal tone and, thus, slowing AV node conduction. Because of its mechanism of action, digoxin is less effective than β-blockers or calcium channel blockers, particularly with exercise, when an increase in sympathetic tone results in more rapid AV node conduction. Thus, the optimal role for digoxin in atrial fibrillation is therapy for patients with left ventricular dysfunction (because of the drug's positive inotropy) or adjunctive therapy for patients receiving β-blockers or calcium channel blockers.

- Digoxin alone is no better than placebo for terminating atrial fibrillation.
- Digoxin is less effective than β-blockers or calcium channel blockers in controlling ventricular rate and is best used as an adjunctive agent or for treating impaired ventricular function.

Table 3-13 Pharmacologic Therapy for Atrial Fibrillation

Agents	Comments
Control of ventricular rate	
β-Blockers (e.g., atenolol, metoprolol, propranolol, carvedilol)	Ideal postoperatively and in hyperthyroidism, acute MI, and chronic CHF (especially carvedilol)
Calcium channel blockers (verapamil, diltiazem)	Nifedipine, amlodipine, and felodipine are not useful for slowing AV conduction
Digoxin	Less effective than β-blockers and calcium channel blockers, especially with exercise. Useful in heart failure
Maintenance of sinus rhythm	
Class IA: quinidine, disopyramide, procainamide	Enhance AV conduction—rate must be controlled before use. Monitor QTc
Class IC: propafenone, flecainide	Slow AV conduction. Often first choice for patients with normal heart. Monitor QRS duration
Class III: sotalol, amiodarone	Amiodarone is agent of choice for ventricular dysfunction and after MI

AV, atrioventricular; CHF, congestive heart failure; MI, myocardial infarction.

β-Blockers such as propranolol, metoprolol, and atenolol are effective in slowing AV node conduction and may be particularly useful when atrial fibrillation complicates hyperthyroidism or myocardial infarction (in which case they reduce the risk of death from myocardial infarction). β-Blockers also decrease the risk of postoperative myocardial infarction, making them well suited for postoperative atrial fibrillation. Carvedilol decreases mortality of patients with chronic heart failure and may be a good choice in that setting. Esmolol, because of its intravenous formulation and short half-life, is particularly useful for acute management of atrial fibrillation.

- β-Blockers are effective in slowing ventricular rate in atrial fibrillation, but they do not terminate atrial fibrillation (although they may prevent it postoperatively).
- β-Blockers are particularly useful postoperatively and in hyperthyroidism, acute myocardial infarction, and chronic heart failure.

Calcium channel blockers are divided broadly into two groups: dihydropyridines (nifedipine, amlodipine, felodipine) and nondihydropyridines (diltiazem, verapamil). Dihydropyridine agents have little or no effect on AV node conduction and no role in the management of atrial fibrillation. Verapamil and diltiazem are both available as intravenous and oral preparations and are well suited for acute and chronic rate control. Also, both agents have negative inotropic effects and should be used cautiously in congestive heart failure.

- Diltiazem and verapamil are both effective for rate control in atrial fibrillation; nifedipine, amlodipine, and felodipine are not and have no role in the management of atrial fibrillation.

Adenosine is very effective at slowing AV node conduction; however, because of its short half-life, it has no role in the treatment of atrial fibrillation. It can be useful diagnostically by slowing ventricular rate transiently, permitting visualization of atrial activity if the diagnosis is in question.

Nonpharmacologic AV Node Rate Control

If the rate cannot be controlled pharmacologically or rhythm control medications (discussed below) are either ineffective or not well tolerated, catheter ablation of the AV junction is an alternative. For patients with chronic atrial fibrillation, a VVIR pacemaker is implanted, and for those with paroxysmal atrial fibrillation, dual-chamber pacemakers with mode switching functions are used. These permit the tracking of P waves during sinus rhythm and revert to VVIR (or DDIR) pacing when atrial fibrillation recurs. With this approach, the risk of thromboembolism is unchanged because the fibrillation itself persists in the atria; thus, appropriate stroke prophylaxis must be prescribed.

A new approach to ablation to cure atrial fibrillation is based on the discovery of discrete triggers in the pulmonary vein. In this procedure, the source for the fibrillation is ablated in the pulmonary vein. The chance of a successful cure is about 40%. This procedure has rapidly become popular because AV node conduction is not impaired and permanent pacing is not required.

Rhythm Control

Rhythm control (maintenance of sinus rhythm) can control symptoms effectively. However, maintaining sinus rhythm has not been shown to decrease the likelihood of thromboembolism, nor has it been shown to prolong survival. In fact, some drugs used to prevent recurrences may cause new arrhythmias (proarrhythmias).

- Class IA agents (quinidine, procainamide, and disopyramide) can be associated with torsades de pointes, particularly at the time of reversion of atrial fibrillation to normal sinus rhythm, and treatment should be initiated in a monitored setting.
- Class IA agents also enhance AV node conduction, so before these agents are used, rate control agents should be administered.
- Class IB agents (lidocaine, mexiletine, tocainide) have no marked effect in treating atrial fibrillation and should not be used for that purpose.
- For patients with a normal heart, class IC agents (propafenone, flecainide) are often a good first choice and often can be given safely in an outpatient setting (with ECG and treadmill testing at 3 days to exclude proarrhythmia).
- Amiodarone has been proven safe for patients who have had myocardial infarction and those with systolic dysfunction and is preferable in these situations.

Stroke Prevention

Acute Cardioversion to Normal Sinus Rhythm—Electrical cardioversion from atrial fibrillation is commonly used to control atrial fibrillation. According to current guidelines, patients with atrial fibrillation lasting more than 2 days should receive anticoagulation before cardioversion. It has been demonstrated that several weeks of warfarin therapy before cardioversion can decrease the incidence of cardioversion-associated thromboembolism to 0% to 1.6% (compared with up to 7% in the absence of anticoagulation). Also, anticoagulation should be continued for 4 weeks after cardioversion because of the increased risk of thromboembolism in the weeks following cardioversion. Although few data are available about cardioversion in the absence of anticoagulation for atrial fibrillation of recent onset (<48 hours), current guidelines do not mandate anticoagulation in this setting.

Historically, atrial flutter was thought to confer a very low risk, but more recent data have contested this observation, suggesting that guidelines similar to those for atrial fibrillation should be followed.

- Patients with more than 2 days of atrial fibrillation must receive anticoagulation for 3 weeks before cardioversion and for 4 weeks afterward.
- An alternative approach for patients with more than 2 days of atrial fibrillation is transesophageal echocardiography with cardioversion (if no thrombus is found) and then 3-4 weeks of anticoagulation.

Chronic Stroke Prevention—Patients with atrial fibrillation due to rheumatic valvular disease have a markedly increased risk of stroke and should receive warfarin therapy. Most patients encountered in clinical practice have nonrheumatic atrial fibrillation. A series of landmark studies has demonstrated that warfarin decreases the incidence of thromboembolism by 68% to 84% in this population. The risk of thromboembolism can be determined by clinical and echocardiographic risk factors, which should be used to guide treatment (Tables 3-14). The risk factors are advanced age, previous transient ischemic attack or stroke, history of hypertension, diabetes mellitus, and congestive heart failure. Echocardiographic risk factors include depressed left ventricular function and left atrial enlargement. Patients who are younger than 60 years and have no clinical heart disease or hypertension are at extremely low risk and require no treatment, although some physicians recommend aspirin. Thus, a strategy based on age and risk factors has emerged and is summarized in Table 3-15. Patients younger than 65 (60 in some reports) with no risk factors can be given no therapy or aspirin. Patients older than 75 or those with risk factors should be given warfarin. For patients given warfarin, the international normalized ratio (INR) should be maintained in the range of 2.0 to 3.0 (although 2.0-2.5 may be preferable for those older than 75). INR values are preferable to prothrombin times for management because prothrombin time assays vary among laboratories.

- The clinical risk factors for stroke in nonrheumatic atrial fibrillation are age >75 years, previous transient ischemic attack or stroke, history of hypertension, diabetes mellitus, and congestive heart failure (know these for the board examination).
- The echocardiographic risk factors are depressed ventricular function and left atrial enlargement.
- Patients <60 years with structurally normal hearts and no hypertension are at low risk for thromboembolism and require no specific therapy.

Table 3-14 Risk Factors for Thromboembolism in Non-rheumatic Atrial Fibrillation

Clinical risk factors	Echocardiographic risk factors
Advanced age (>65 y)	Left ventricular dysfunction
Previous TIA or stroke	
Hypertension	
Diabetes (in pooled analysis)	
Congestive heart failure	
Other high-risk clinical settings	
Prosthetic heart valves	
Thyrotoxicosis	

TIA, transient ischemic attack.

Table 3-15 Recommended Management of Patients With Nonrheumatic Atrial Fibrillation

Age, y	Risk factors	Recommendations
<65	Present	Warfarin INR 2-3
	No risk factors	Aspirin or nothing
65-75	Present	Warfarin INR 2-3
	No risk factors	Warfarin or aspirin (based on discussion with patient of relatively low risk of stroke, decrease in risk with warfarin, monitoring needs, etc.)
>75		Warfarin INR 2-3 (but should be kept closer to 2.0-2.5 because of increased risk of hemorrhage in this age group)

INR, international normalized ratio.

- Warfarin should be used to maintain an INR of 2.0-3.0 (although 2.0-2.5 is preferable in the elderly).
- Studies have shown no difference between paroxysmal and chronic atrial fibrillation in stroke rate risk.

Supraventricular Tachycardia

"Paroxysmal supraventricular tachycardia" (PSVT) refers to cardiac arrhythmias of supraventricular origin using a reentrant mechanism with an abrupt onset and termination, a regular RR interval, and a narrow QRS complex, unless there is a rate-related or preexisting bundle branch block (Fig. 3-21). In patients with a normal QRS during sinus rhythm (lack of preexcitation), PSVT is due to reentry within the AV node in 60%, reentry using a concealed accessory pathway in 30%, and reentry in the sinus node or atrium in

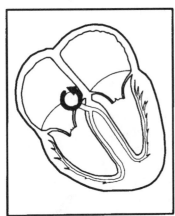

Fig. 3-21. Paroxysmal supraventricular tachycardia.

the other 10% (Fig. 3-22). Episodes usually respond to vagal maneuvers; if these fail, intravenously administered adenosine or verapamil terminates the arrhythmia in 90% of patients.

- PSVT is an arrhythmia with an abrupt onset and termination.
- Acutely, PSVT usually responds to vagal maneuvers; if not, adenosine or verapamil terminates the arrhythmia in 90% of patients.

PSVT generally is not a life-threatening arrhythmia and only occasionally is associated with near-syncope or syncope. The rhythm is more serious when it is associated with severe heart disease and cardiac decompensation results, with the sudden increase in heart rate. This can occur in patients with congenital heart disease, cardiomyopathy, or ischemic heart disease. Patients with AV nodal reentrant tachycardia usually have simultaneous activation of the atrium and ventricle, in which case the atria contract against closed tricuspid and mitral valves (similar to pacemaker syndrome) and produce symptoms associated with atrial distention, including a fullness in the neck, hypotension, and polyuria. Hypotension and polyuria are due partly to the release of atrial natriuretic peptide.

- PSVT generally is not a life-threatening arrhythmia; it is often seen in an otherwise normal heart.
- PSVT is more serious when associated with heart disease.

Chronically, PSVT responds to most antiarrhythmic drugs, including drugs that suppress AV node conduction (digoxin, β-adrenergic blockers, and calcium antagonists), assuming that part of the reentrant circuit uses the AV node, and to drugs that slow conduction within the reentrant circuit, including class IA (quinidine, procainamide, disopyramide), IC (propafenone, flecainide), and III (amiodarone, sotalol) antiarrhythmic drugs.

Most forms of PSVT can be "cured" permanently with catheter ablation, with success rates greater than 90%. For young patients in whom β-blocker or calcium channel blocker therapy fails or who choose not to take these agents, catheter ablation is usually preferred over class I or class III antiarrhythmic drugs. For patients with PSVT and hypertension that require treatment, the best treatment is β-blockers or calcium channel blockers, which might treat both conditions.

- PSVT responds to most antiarrhythmic drugs chronically.
- PSVT usually can be "cured" permanently with catheter ablation.

"Multifocal atrial tachycardia" is an automatic atrial rhythm diagnosed when three or more distinct atrial foci (P waves of different morphology) are present and the rate exceeds 100 beats/min (Fig. 3-23). The rhythm occurs primarily in patients who have decompensated lung disease with associated hypoxia, increased catecholamines (exogenous and endogenous), atrial stretch, and local tissue acid-base and electrolyte disturbances. This rhythm is made worse by digoxin, which shortens atrial refractoriness, but it does respond to improved oxygenation and slow channel blockade with verapamil or diltiazem.

AV node

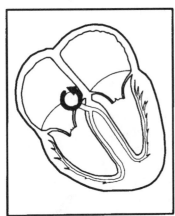

Accessory pathway

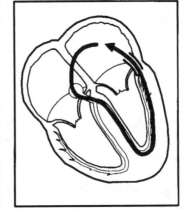

Sinus node, atrium

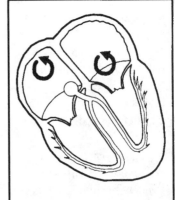

Fig. 3-22. Mechanisms of paroxysmal supraventricular tachycardia in patients with a normal ECG during sinus rhythm. AV, atrioventricular.

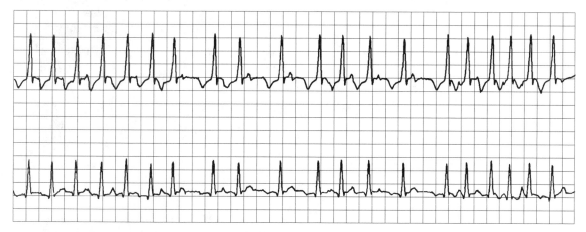

Fig. 3-23. Simultaneous recordings from a patient with multifocal atrial tachycardia showing three or more P waves of different morphology. (*Lower tracing*, From MKSAP IX: Part C Book, 1, 1992. American College of Physicians. By permission.)

- Digoxin worsens multifocal atrial tachycardia.
- Multifocal atrial tachycardia is best treated with calcium channel blockers and correction of the underlying medical illnesses.

Differentiating Supraventricular Tachycardia With Aberrancy From Ventricular Tachycardia

A wide QRS tachycardia may be due to supraventricular tachycardia with aberrancy or to ventricular tachycardia. Useful findings to identify ventricular tachycardia are listed in Table 3-16.

Approximately 85% of wide QRS tachycardias are ventricular in origin and are often well tolerated. The absence of hemodynamic compromise during tachycardia is not a clue that the tachycardia is supraventricular in origin. In patients with a wide QRS tachycardia and a history of ischemic heart disease (angina, myocardial infarction, Q wave on ECG), the tachycardia is ventricular in origin in 90% to 95%. Therefore, most wide QRS complex tachycardias are ventricular tachycardia (Fig. 3-24).

Table 3-16   Findings That Identify Ventricular Tachycardia

Evidence of AV dissociation with P waves "marching through" the QRS complexes
A QRS width >0.14 s if the tachycardia has a right bundle branch block pattern and >0.16 s if the tachycardia has a left bundle branch block pattern
Northwest axis (axis between -90° and -180°)
A different QRS morphology in patients with a preexisting bundle branch block
A history of structural heart disease

AV, atrioventricular.

- About 85% of wide QRS tachycardias are ventricular in origin.
- In patients with wide QRS tachycardia and ischemic heart disease, tachycardia is ventricular in origin in 90%-95%.

Avoid intravenous administration of verapamil in patients with a wide QRS tachycardia unless the tachycardia is supraventricular in origin. Most patients with a wide QRS tachycardia have ventricular tachycardia, and verapamil causes hemodynamic deterioration that requires cardioversion in more than half of the patients. The use of verapamil results in peripheral vasodilatation, further increase in catecholamines, and decreased cardiac contractility—all of which contribute to adverse hemodynamics.

- Avoid intravenously administered verapamil for wide QRS tachycardia.
- Verapamil causes hemodynamic deterioration requiring cardioversion in ventricular tachycardia.

Wolff-Parkinson-White Syndrome

This abnormality is defined as 1) symptomatic tachycardia, 2) short PR interval (<0.12 second), 3) a delta wave, and 4) prolonged QRS interval (>0.12 second).

In Wolff-Parkinson-White syndrome, normal activation of the ventricle is a fusion complex. Part of the activation is due to conduction over the accessory pathway, and the remaining activation is due to conduction through the normal His-Purkinje conduction system. Not all patients with preexcitation have a short PR interval. Normal PR conduction may occur if the accessory pathway is far removed from the AV node. In patients with a far left lateral accessory pathway, the heart is activated through the AV node before atrial activation reaches the accessory pathway. Thus, the PR interval may be normal before the onset of the delta wave.

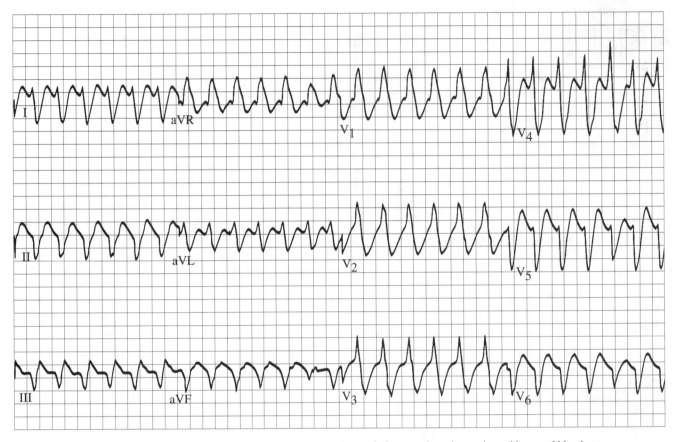

Fig. 3-24. Ventricular tachycardia with a wide QRS complex, northwest axis, and fusion complexes in a patient with normal blood pressure.

Ventricular activation is abnormal in patients with Wolff-Parkinson-White syndrome. Infarction, ventricular hypertrophy, and ST-T wave changes should not be interpreted after the diagnosis is established, because these changes are usually due to the abnormal pattern of ventricular activation.

- In Wolff-Parkinson-White syndrome, the PR interval may be normal before the onset of the delta wave.
- Ventricular activation is abnormal in Wolff-Parkinson-White syndrome.

Preexcitation occurs in about 2 of 1,000 patients; tachycardia subsequently develops in 70%. Of patients with tachycardia, 70% have PSVT and 30% have atrial fibrillation. The atrial fibrillation often occurs after a short episode of PSVT. Elimination of PSVT after surgery or catheter ablation generally eliminates problems with atrial fibrillation. The most serious rhythm disturbance is the onset of atrial fibrillation with rapid ventricular conduction over the accessory pathway resulting in ventricular fibrillation (Fig. 3-25). Most asymptomatic patients do not benefit from risk stratification with electrophysiologic testing, including induction of atrial fibrillation, unless they have a high-risk

occupation. Patients who are asymptomatic have a negligible chance of sudden death, and for patients who are symptomatic, the incidence of sudden death is 0.0025 per patient-year.

- Preexcitation occurs in 2/1,000 patients; tachycardia develops in 70%.
- Of patients with tachycardia, 70% have PSVT and 30% have atrial fibrillation.
- Asymptomatic patients have a negligible chance of sudden death.
- For symptomatic patients, the incidence of sudden death is 0.0025 per person-year.

Patients with Wolff-Parkinson-White syndrome may have either 1) a manifest accessory pathway resulting in preexcitation on the ECG (Fig. 3-26) due to anterograde conduction over the accessory pathway or 2) a concealed accessory pathway that is capable of conducting only in the retrograde direction; thus, the surface ECG in sinus rhythm is normal. Both manifest and concealed accessory pathways have the same mechanism of reentrant tachycardia, in which anterograde conduction over the normal conduction system results in a

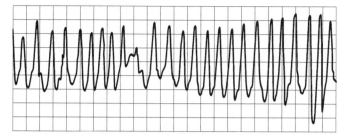

Fig. 3-25. Atrial fibrillation in a patient with Wolff-Parkinson-White syndrome shows a wide QRS complex and irregular RR intervals.

normal QRS complex (unless there is rate-related bundle branch block) and conduction continues through the ventricle, returns retrogradely over the accessory pathway, and continues through the atrium to complete the reentrant circuit, termed "orthodromic AV reentry" (Fig. 3-27). Five percent of patients may have reentrant tachycardia that goes in the reverse direction ("antidromic AV reentry"), in which ventricular activation over the accessory pathway activates the ventricle from an ectopic location; the result is a wide QRS complex tachycardia that is often confused with ventricular tachycardia (Fig. 3-28).

Electrophysiologic testing should be performed in patients with *symptomatic* Wolff-Parkinson-White syndrome. This testing identifies the pathway location, confirms that the pathway is an integral part of the reentrant circuit and not an innocent bystander (i.e., the arrhythmia is AV node reentry), and evaluates for a second accessory pathway that occurs in approximately 15% of patients.

Atrial Fibrillation in Wolff-Parkinson-White Syndrome

Atrial fibrillation in Wolff-Parkinson-White syndrome is of special interest because it can be life-threatening and requires therapy that is different from the usual treatment for atrial fibrillation. Patients with Wolff-Parkinson-White syndrome have an accessory pathway that can conduct electrical activity from the atrium to the ventricle, bypassing the AV node. Because the accessory pathway does not slow conduction in the same manner as the AV node, the ventricular response to atrial fibrillation can be extraordinarily and dangerously rapid. Also, wide, irregular, and rapid ventricular complexes are seen because activation down the accessory pathway does not use the normal His-Purkinje system (see Fig. 3-25). The use of agents such as calcium channel blockers, β-blockers, or digoxin can result in an even more rapid ventricular response due to blocking of conduction down the AV node (which can limit concealed conduction into the pathway). Therefore, the agent of first choice is procainamide, which slows accessory pathway and intra-atrial conduction. Should a patient with Wolff-Parkinson-White syndrome and atrial fibrillation become hypotensive, cardioversion should be performed.

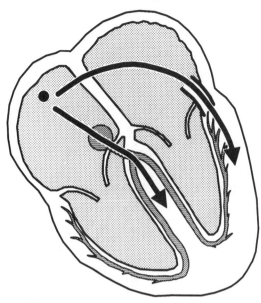

Fig. 3-26. Conduction of sinus impulses in Wolff-Parkinson-White syndrome. The ventricles are activated over the normal atrioventricular node–His-Purkinje system and accessory pathway; the result is a fusion complex (QRS and delta wave).

- Atrial fibrillation in Wolff-Parkinson-White syndrome should not be treated with digoxin, adenosine, β-blockers, or calcium channel blockers.
- In atrial fibrillation in Wolff-Parkinson-White syndrome, procainamide can be given to slow the ventricular rate (by slowing atrial and accessory pathway conduction) and to restore sinus rhythm.
- If the heart rate is rapid and there is hemodynamic compromise, perform cardioversion.

PSVT in patients with an accessory pathway often ends with vagal maneuvers or intravenously administered adenosine or verapamil. Additional episodes can be prevented with a β-adrenergic blocker, a calcium antagonist, and class IA (quinidine, procainamide, disopyramide), class IC (propafenone, flecainide), and class III (amiodarone, sotalol) antiarrhythmic drugs. Radiofrequency ablation is used to ablate the accessory pathway and to cure the tachycardia, thus eliminating the need for medical therapy.

- Additional PSVT is prevented with a β-adrenergic blocker, a calcium antagonist, and class IA, IC, and III antiarrhythmic drugs.
- Radiofrequency ablation is used to cure tachycardia and should be strongly considered for symptomatic patients.

Tachycardia-Mediated Cardiomyopathy

Supraventricular tachycardia, atrial fibrillation with a rapid ventricular rate, and ventricular tachycardia have been associated

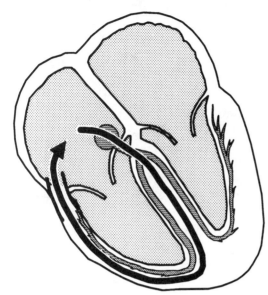

Fig. 3-27. Typical mechanism of supraventricular tachycardia in patients with Wolff-Parkinson-White syndrome (orthodromic atrioventricular re-entry): the result is a narrow QRS complex because ventricular activation is over the normal conduction system.

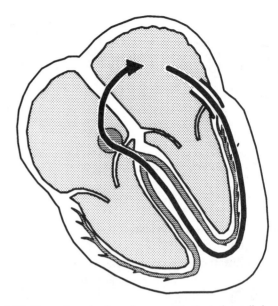

Fig. 3-28. Unusual mechanism of supraventricular tachycardia in patients with Wolff-Parkinson-White syndrome; the result is a wide QRS complex because ventricular activation is over an accessory pathway. This arrhythmia is difficult to distinguish from ventricular tachycardia.

with cardiomyopathy. Treatment of the tachycardia has allowed cardiac performance to return to near normal. When patients present with heart failure and tachycardia is identified, determine whether the heart failure is causing the tachycardia or the tachycardia has caused the heart failure. Control of ventricular rate often improves ventricular function. In a patient with heart failure who has a rhythm with an abnormal P-wave axis, tachycardia-mediated cardiomyopathy should be suspected.

Ventricular Ectopy and Nonsustained Ventricular Tachycardia

Management of frequent ventricular ectopy and nonsustained ventricular tachycardia is predicated upon the underlying cardiac lesion. For patients with structurally normal hearts, the long-term prognosis is excellent and no specific therapy is warranted in the absence of symptoms. If symptoms are present, management includes reassurance, β-blockers or calcium channel blockers for disturbing symptoms, and, in rare cases of frequent monomorphic symptomatic ventricular ectopy, catheter ablation.

In patients with previous myocardial infarction, depressed ventricular function (ejection fraction ≤35%), and nonsustained ventricular tachycardia, electrophysiologic study can risk stratify, even in the absence of symptoms. If, in this population, tachycardia is inducible, the mortality rate is decreased with implantation of a defibrillator. The management of patients with dilated cardiomyopathy is not well defined, although amiodarone may be appropriate in some settings (it has been shown to decrease mortality in this population).

- Patients with a structurally normal heart and complex ectopy or nonsustained ventricular tachycardia have an excellent prognosis; management includes reassurance or, if bothersome symptoms persist, calcium channel blockers or β-blockers.
- Patients with depressed ventricular function and nonsustained ventricular tachycardia are at increased risk for sudden cardiac death; patients with previous myocardial infarction can be risk stratified with electrophysiologic study.

Ventricular Tachycardia and Fibrillation

Patients who present with ventricular tachycardia or fibrillation or who survive sudden cardiac death (out-of-hospital cardiac arrest who were successfully resuscitated) have lethal ventricular arrhythmias and a substantial risk of recurrence. Survivors of sudden cardiac death have a risk of death approaching 30% in the first year after hospital dismissal. They should receive electrophysiologic-guided therapy, which improves outcome. For about 40% of patients, an antiarrhythmic drug is identified that prevents induction of ventricular tachycardia or fibrillation, and these patients have approximately a 5% chance of death at 1 year if discharged with that medication. Patients in whom the baseline electrophysiologic study is negative or an antiarrhythmic drug cannot be identified to prevent tachycardia continue to have an increased risk of sudden death and should be considered for antitachycardia surgery or an implantable cardioverter-defibrillator. This device has reduced the recurrence rate of sudden death to 2% at 1 year and to 4% at 4 years; the overall mortality rate is 10% at 1 year and 20% at 4 years.

- Patients with ventricular tachycardia or fibrillation who survive sudden cardiac death have a substantial risk of recurrence.
- Survivors of sudden cardiac death have a risk of death of 30% at 1 year after hospital discharge.
- Electrophysiologic-guided therapy improves outcome.
- For 40% of patients, an effective antiarrhythmic drug can be identified.

Torsades de Pointes

This is a form of ventricular tachycardia with a characteristic polymorphic morphology described as a "twisting of the points" (torsades de pointes) (see Fig. 3-10). The QT interval is prolonged, and the tachycardia is initiated by a late-coupled premature ventricular contraction. The arrhythmia usually is due to a medication (quinidine, procainamide, disopyramide, sotalol, tricyclic antidepressants), an electrolyte disturbance (hypokalemia), or bradycardia (especially after myocardial infarction). After the tachycardia has been converted to sinus rhythm (electrically or spontaneously), treatment should be aimed at shortening the QT interval until the offending drug can be metabolized or the electrolyte disturbance or bradycardia corrected. Treatment options include temporary overdrive pacing, isoproterenol infusion, or magnesium. Patients with a prolonged QT interval in the absence of medications, electrolytes, or bradycardia have a congenital form of this problem and are usually treated with a β-adrenergic blocker.

- Torsades de pointes is a form of ventricular tachycardia involving a prolonged QT interval.
- Torsades de pointes usually is due to a medication, an electrolyte disturbance, or bradycardia.
- Treatment includes temporary overdrive pacing, isoproterenol, or magnesium.

Ventricular Arrhythmias During Acute Myocardial Infarction

Prevention of myocardial ischemia and the use of β-adrenergic blockers are essential during and after acute myocardial infarction to decrease the frequency of life-threatening ventricular arrhythmias. Asymptomatic complex ventricular ectopy, including nonsustained ventricular tachycardia, should not be treated empirically in the acute phase of myocardial infarction because the risk of proarrhythmia outweighs the potential benefit of therapy for reducing the incidence of sudden cardiac death after hospital dismissal.

The results from amiodarone trials are mentioned above. The routine use of lidocaine or amiodarone in suppressing ventricular arrhythmias in the acute phase of myocardial infarction is not recommended.

Ventricular tachycardia and fibrillation occurring within 24 hours after myocardial infarction are independent risk factors for in-hospital mortality at the time of the acute myocardial infarction but are not risk factors for subsequent total mortality or mortality due to an arrhythmic event after hospital dismissal and do not require antiarrhythmic therapy.

Ventricular tachycardia and fibrillation occurring 24 hours or longer after an acute myocardial infarction in the absence of reinfarction are independent risk factors for increased total mortality and death due to an arrhythmic event after hospital dismissal. Patients should be assessed with electrophysiologic testing, and the treatment option is usually an implantable cardioverter-defibrillator.

Episodes of refractory ventricular tachycardia and fibrillation during acute myocardial infarction should be treated with intravenously administered lidocaine, procainamide, bretylium, or amiodarone, and patients should have adequate oxygenation and normal electrolyte values. Recent data suggest that amiodarone may be a reasonable choice if lidocaine fails to control the arrhythmia. If these drugs are ineffective, alternative therapies to prevent recurrences of tachycardia include overdrive pacing if the tachycardia follows a bradycardia event, intra-aortic balloon pump, and coronary revascularization.

- Refractory ventricular tachycardia and fibrillation during acute myocardial infarction should be treated with intravenously administered lidocaine, procainamide, bretylium, or amiodarone.
- Alternative therapies are overdrive pacing and coronary revascularization.

Role of Pacing in Acute Myocardial Infarction

Among patients with an acute inferior myocardial infarction, 5% to 10% have Mobitz I second-degree or third-degree block in the absence of bundle branch block, and the site commonly is in the AV node. This usually is transient, tends not to recur, and requires pacing only if there are symptoms as a result of bradycardia.

Bundle branch block occurs in 10% to 20% of patients with an acute myocardial infarction; in half of these patients, it is detected at the initial presentation, often representing preexisting conduction system disease. The appearance of a new bundle branch block is an indication for prophylactic temporary pacing.

Death of patients with myocardial infarction and bundle branch block usually is due to advanced heart failure and ventricular arrhythmias rather than to the development of complete heart block. Patients in whom transient complete heart block develops in association with a bundle branch block are at risk for recurrent complete heart block and should undergo permanent pacing. A new bundle branch block that never progresses to complete heart block is not an indication for permanent pacing.

- Death of patients with myocardial infarction and bundle branch block usually is due to advanced heart failure.
- New bundle branch block that never progresses to complete heart block is not an indication for permanent pacing.
- Second-degree (Mobitz II) block with bilateral bundle branch block and third-degree AV block warrants pacing.

SYNCOPE

"Syncope" is a transient loss of consciousness with spontaneous recovery. It is a frequent clinical syndrome that requires medical evaluation. Its causes can be categorized as cardiovascular, noncardiovascular, and unexplained syncope, as summarized in Table 3-17. It is estimated that 30% of cases of syncope have a cardiogenic cause (an arrhythmia), 35% have a vasovagal cause, and 10% to 25% are related to a miscellaneous disorder such as orthostatic or situational syncope or seizures or are drug-related episodes. In 10% to 25% of cases, the cause is—and often remains—unknown.

The most important aspect of evaluation for syncope is the clinical history and physical examination. The initial history and physical examination provide the key information in 40% to 75% of the patients for whom a diagnosis is eventually established. The factors associated with increased cardiogenic causes for syncope are listed in Table 3-18. In patients with increased risk of cardiogenic syncope, electrophysiologic testing should be considered. If an arrhythmogenic cause (bradycardia or tachycardia) for syncope has been established by noninvasive tests such as ECG, Holter monitoring, or transtelephonic monitoring, electrophysiologic testing is not indicated unless other arrhythmias are suspected. In patients at low risk for cardiogenic syncope, a noninvasive approach should be considered.

Tilt table testing is effective in eliciting a vasovagal response. For diagnostic purposes, tilt table testing is indicated for patients with recurrent syncope without evidence of structural cardiac disease or for those with structural heart disease but after other causes of syncope have been excluded by appropriate testing. Tilt table testing generally is not indicated for patients with a single episode of syncope without

Table 3-17 Major Causes of Syncope

Cardiovascular	Noncardiovascular
Cardiogenic syncope	Neurologic
Structural heart disease	Metabolic
Coronary artery disease	Psychiatric
Rhythm disturbances	
Reflex syncope	
Vasovagal	
Carotid sinus hypersensitivity	
Situational	
Micturition	
Deglutition	
Defecation	
Glossopharyngeal neuralgia	
Postprandial	
Tussive	
Valsalva maneuver	
Oculovagal	
Sneeze	
Instrumentation	
Diving	
After exercise	
Orthostatic hypotension	

From Shen W-K, Gersh BJ: Syncope: mechanisms, approach, and management. *In* Clinical Autonomic Disorders: Evaluation and Management. Edited by PA Low. Boston, Little, Brown and Company, 1993, pp 605-640. By permission of Mayo Foundation.

injury or in a high-risk setting with clear-cut vasovagal clinical features.

After the diagnosis of syncope has been established, the treatment usually is straightforward. Pacemaker therapy is appropriate for sinus node dysfunction and AV conduction disease. Various treatment options for tachyarrhythmias are discussed above. Pharmacologic therapy can be effective in selected patients with marked symptomatic vasovagal syncope. These therapeutic options include β-blockers, anticholinergic drugs, vasoconstrictors, increased intravascular volume, and maneuvers to prevent venous pooling. Recent reports suggest that serotonin reuptake blockers may be effective in a subgroup of patients. Pacemaker therapy can be effective in preventing syncope in patients with a predominant cardioinhibitory subtype of vasovagal syncope and may be effective in patients with very frequent recurrent vasovagal syncope.

Table 3-18 Risk Stratification in Patients With Unexplained Syncope

High-risk factors	Low-risk factors
Coronary artery disease, previous myocardial infarction	Isolated syncope without underlying cardiovascular disease
Structural heart disease	Younger age
Left ventricular dysfunction	Symptoms consistent with a vasovagal cause
Congestive heart failure	Normal ECG
Older age	
Abrupt onset	
Serious injuries	
Abnormal ECG (presence of Q wave, bundle branch block, or atrial fibrillation)	

ECG, electrocardiogram.

From Shen W-K, Gersh BJ: Syncope: mechanisms, approach, and management. *In* Clinical Autonomic Disorders: Evaluation and Management. Edited by PA Low. Boston, Little, Brown and Company, 1993, pp 605-640. By permission of Mayo Foundation.

PART IV

Steve R. Ommen, M.D.
Rick A. Nishimura, M.D.

Coronary heart disease, principally myocardial infarction, accounts for approximately one of three deaths in the United States, or nearly 600,000 deaths annually. The substantial decrease in the death rate from acute myocardial infarction that has occurred in the last 4 decades (Fig. 3-29) is attributed to efforts in primary prevention and new interventions in the treatment of myocardial infarction. The variable presentation of patients with coronary heart disease includes patients who are asymptomatic (with or without silent ischemia), patients who have stable or unstable angina or myocardial infarction, and patients with sudden death.

- About 1/3 of the deaths annually in the United States are due to myocardial infarction.
- The substantial decrease in the last 4 decades in death from acute myocardial infarction is due to primary prevention and new treatments of myocardial infarction.

PREVENTION OF CORONARY HEART DISEASE

Risk factors for coronary artery disease, which intervention has been proven to reduce cardiac events, include tobacco abuse, serum low-density lipoprotein (LDL) cholesterol level, and hypertension. Factors that clearly increase the risk of coronary artery disease, which intervention likely decreases, include diabetes mellitus, physical inactivity, obesity, serum high-density lipoprotein (HDL) level, and serum triglyceride levels.

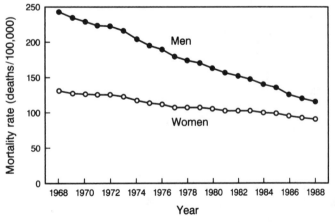

Fig. 3-29. Annual mortality rates from acute myocardial infarction among men and women in the United States, 1968-1988. (From Manson JE, Tosteson H, Ridker PM, et al: The primary prevention of myocardial infarction. N Engl J Med 1992;326:1406-1416. By permission of the Massachusetts Medical Society.)

Factors for which intervention may improve subsequent risk include psychosocial factors (anxiety and depression), homocysteine level, and alcohol intake. The nonmodifiable risk factors for coronary artery disease are age, sex, and family history. Primary prevention includes modification of the following risk factors (J Am Coll Cardiol 2003;41:159-168):

- Smoking more than doubles the incidence of coronary heart disease and increases mortality by 50%.
- The relative risk of smokers who have quit smoking decreases rapidly, approaching the levels of nonsmokers within 2-3 years.
- Plasma levels of total cholesterol and LDL cholesterol are important risk factors for coronary heart disease. This relationship is strongest at high levels of cholesterol.
- A 1% decrease in total serum cholesterol yields a 2%-3% decrease in the risk of coronary heart disease.
- Lowering increased plasma levels of LDL cholesterol slows progression and promotes regression of coronary atherosclerosis.
- Lowering increased plasma levels of LDL cholesterol prevents coronary events, presumably because of stabilization of lipid-laden plaques.
- The estimated decreased risk of myocardial infarction is 2%-3% for each 1-mm Hg decrease in diastolic blood pressure.
- The estimated decrease in the risk of myocardial infarction with the maintenance of an active compared with a sedentary lifestyle is 35%-55%.
- The adjusted mortality rates for coronary heart disease are two to three times higher in men with diabetes mellitus and three to seven times higher in women with diabetes mellitus.
- There are no definitive data to suggest that estrogen replacement therapy in women prevents cardiovascular disease.
- Although heavy alcohol use increases the risk of cardiovascular disease, moderate consumption decreases the risk of heart disease.

Secondary prevention refers to efforts to prevent recurrent ischemic events in patients with known coronary artery disease. The role of antiplatelet agents, β-blockers, and angiotensin-converting enzyme inhibitors (ACEIs) is discussed below. Aggressive treatment of cholesterol levels is of value. The statin drugs reduce events after myocardial infarction to a greater degree than would be expected from their effect on atherosclerosis progression alone. This may be related to stabilization of lipid-rich plaques, which are prone to rupture. In patients who have had a myocardial infarction and have increased levels of cholesterol (>220 mg/dL), treatment with a statin drug decreases overall mortality by 30% and disease mortality from coronary events by 42%. In patients who have had a myocardial infarction and have "average" levels of cholesterol (cholesterol, <240 mg/dL; LDL, >125 mg/dL), treatment with a statin drug reduces the chance of fatal heart disease or recurrent myocardial infarction by 24%.

Current indications for instituting cholesterol-lowering therapy are as follows:

- Known coronary artery disease (or diabetes mellitus): LDL >100 mg/dL.
- Risk factors for coronary artery disease: LDL >130 mg/dL.
- Others: LDL >160 mg/dL.

Newer "risk factors" have been proposed for the diagnosis and management of patients with coronary heart disease. Abnormal levels of Lp(a), homocysteine, and fibrinogen may be markers for coronary artery disease in patients who may not have the conventional risk factors. In patients with known coronary artery disease, inflammatory or infectious markers have been associated with adverse outcomes. These include inflammatory markers such as C-reactive protein, tumor necrosis factor-alpha, interleukin 1 and 6, and infectious agents such as *Chlamydia*, cytomegalovirus, and *Helicobacter*. New data suggest that increased levels of C-reactive protein is associated with a two- to threefold increase in the rate of myocardial infarction. There is the suggestion that some drugs (i.e., statins) may be beneficial in patients with inflammatory markers, although the data are preliminary.

MECHANISM OF ATHEROSCLEROSIS

The "response to injury" hypothesis is the most prevalent explanation of atherosclerosis (N Engl J Med 1992;326:242-250). According to this hypothesis, chronic minimal injury to the arterial endothelium is caused mainly by a disturbance in the pattern of blood flow (type I injury), potentiated by high cholesterol levels, inflammation, infections, and tobacco smoke. Type I injury leads to the accumulation of lipids and macrophages. The release of toxic products by macrophages produces type II injury, which is characterized by the adhesion of platelets. Macrophages and platelets with endothelial-release growth factors cause migration and proliferation of smooth muscle cells, which form a fibrointimal lesion or lipid lesion. Disruption of a lipid lesion that has a thin capsule causes type III damage, with thrombus formation. The thrombus may organize and contribute to the growth of the atherosclerotic lesion or become totally occluded, culminating in unstable angina or myocardial infarction (Fig. 3-30).

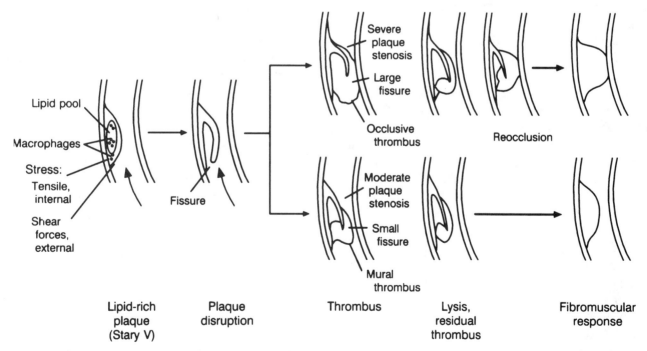

Fig. 3-30. Typical dynamic evolution of a complicated disrupted plaque. Curved arrows indicate direction of blood flow. (From Fuster V, Badimon L, Badimon JJ, et al: The pathogenesis of coronary artery disease and the acute coronary syndromes [first of two parts]. N Engl J Med 1992;326:242-250. By permission of the Massachusetts Medical Society.)

- The most prevalent explanation for atherosclerosis is the "response to injury" hypothesis.
- Type II injury is characterized by the adhesion of platelets.
- Type III damage is disruption of a lipid lesion leading to thrombus formation.
- Lipid-laden coronary artery lesions with less severe angiographic stenosis are more prone to rapid progression because of atherosclerotic plaque disruption.
- In up to two-thirds of cases of unstable angina or myocardial infarction, the lesion is a vessel with <50% stenosis.

CHRONIC STABLE ANGINA

Pathophysiology

In chronic stable angina, myocardial ischemia is caused by a mismatch between myocardial oxygen demand and myocardial oxygen supply. Less important factors are perfusion pressure (aortic–to–right atrial gradient), autoregulation (maintenance of coronary blood flow through a physiologic range of perfusion pressures), autonomic tone, and compressive effect (high left ventricular end-diastolic pressure decreases subendocardial flow). Normally, coronary blood flow can increase up to five times to meet effort-related increases in myocardial oxygen demands. Ischemia occurs when flow reserve is inadequate, usually the result of fixed coronary artery disease. Restriction of resting blood flow to levels sufficient to cause ischemia at rest does not occur unless vessel stenosis is greater than 95%. However, a decrease in overall flow reserve begins to occur with about 60% stenosis, at which point symptoms of exercise-induced ischemia may begin.

The four factors that determine myocardial oxygen consumption (demand) are heart rate, afterload, contractility, and wall tension [wall tension = (left ventricular radius) × (left ventricular pressure)]. With a dilated, poorly contractile left ventricle, the contribution of wall tension to myocardial oxygen consumption outweighs the other factors. The temporal sequence of events includes metabolic ischemia → diastolic dysfunction → perfusion abnormalities → regional wall motion abnormalities → electrocardiographic (ECG) changes → pain.

- In chronic stable angina, myocardial ischemia is caused by increased myocardial oxygen demand.
- Normally, coronary blood flow can increase up to five times to meet myocardial oxygen demand.
- Resting blood flow does not cause ischemia unless stenosis is >95%.
- The four factors of myocardial oxygen consumption: heart rate, afterload, contractility, and wall tension.
- The temporal sequence of events: ischemia → diastolic

dysfunction → perfusion abnormalities → regional wall motion abnormalities → ECG changes → pain.

Symptomatic Chronic Coronary Artery Disease

Many patients have symptoms of angina pectoris during physical activity. The pain is described variously as "pressure," "burning," "stabbing," "ache," "hurt," or "shortness of breath." It can be substernal or epigastric and radiate to the neck, jaw, shoulder, elbow, or wrist. In chronic stable angina, the pain lasts 2 to 30 minutes and is usually relieved by rest. It generally is precipitated by any activity that increases myocardial oxygen consumption. Physical signs that occur with the pain include the onset of a fourth heart sound and mitral regurgitant murmur due to papillary muscle dysfunction. ST-segment depression may be found on the ECG, indicating subendocardial ischemia. The double product [(heart rate) × (systolic blood pressure)] is useful for defining myocardial oxygen demand. Nocturnal angina can be caused by unstable angina and also by increased wall tension with left ventricular dysfunction.

- The pain of angina pectoris during physical exercise is described in various ways.
- Physical signs occurring with the pain are a fourth heart sound and mitral regurgitant murmur due to papillary muscle dysfunction.
- The double product [(heart rate) × (systolic blood pressure)] is useful for defining myocardial oxygen demand.

Silent Ischemia

Silent ischemia is common in patients with symptomatic stable coronary artery disease or unstable angina or after myocardial infarction. It is diagnosed by the presence of ST-segment depression in the absence of symptoms. The treatment is similar to that for chronic stable angina: risk factor modification, aspirin, and β-blockers are effective. Whether percutaneous transluminal coronary angioplasty or coronary artery bypass grafting should be performed for silent ischemia alone is debated unless there are other markers of exceptionally high risk. The prognosis for this condition is the same as for symptomatic ischemia.

- Silent ischemia is common in patients with symptomatic stable coronary artery disease or unstable angina or after myocardial infarction.
- Silent ischemia is diagnosed by the presence of ST-segment depression in the absence of symptoms.
- Treatment is similar to that for chronic stable angina.
- β-Blockers are effective therapeutic agents in silent ischemia.
- Whether coronary angioplasty or bypass grafting should be performed for silent ischemia is debated.

- The prognosis is the same for silent ischemia and symptomatic ischemia.

Ancillary Testing

Ancillary tests for coronary artery disease include measurement of left ventricular function, stress testing, and coronary angiography. Left ventricular function is the most important predictor of prognosis and should be measured in all patients by two-dimensional echocardiography, radionuclide angiography, or left ventricular angiography. Exercise testing is performed with the treadmill or bicycle exertion test in conjunction with ECG monitoring, thallium or technetium-sestamibi scanning (perfusion of the myocardium), radionuclide angiography (left ventricular function), or echocardiography (left ventricular function) to assess for ischemia. During a standard treadmill test (i.e., exercise with stepped increases in workload every 2-3 minutes), heart rate, blood pressure, and the onset of subjective symptoms are monitored. The cardiac rhythm and the 12-lead ECG are monitored continuously. The ECG is positive for ischemia if there is a flat or downsloping ST-segment depression of 1 mm or greater. The ECG response is uninterpretable when there is more than 1 mm of resting ST-segment depression, left bundle branch block, left ventricular hypertrophy, paced rhythm, digoxin therapy, or preexcitation (Wolff-Parkinson-White syndrome). For interpreting the results of any test, Bayes theorem is important. According to this theorem, the predictive value of a test depends on the prevalence of the disease in the population studied.

- The most important predictor of prognosis is left ventricular function.
- The ECG is positive for ischemia if there is a flat ST-segment depression of ≥1 mm.
- Complete left bundle branch block, resting ST-segment depression >1 mm, left ventricular hypertrophy, paced rhythm, digoxin therapy, or preexcitation will render the exercise ECG uninterpretable.
- Bayes theorem: the predictive value of a test depends on the prevalence of the disease in the population studied.

The sensitivity and specificity of ECG treadmill exertion testing are about 70% and 75%, respectively. Thus, a young patient with atypical chest pain and no risk factors (A in Fig. 3-31) has a low pretest probability (5%) of coronary artery disease. If the test results are negative, the probability decreases to 3%. However, if the results are positive, the probability is less than 15%. In comparison, an older man (B in Fig. 3-31) with typical chest pain and multiple risk factors has a high pretest probability (90%) of coronary artery disease, and even with negative test results, the probability is higher than 70%. The treadmill exertion test should not be used to make the *diagnosis* of coronary artery disease.

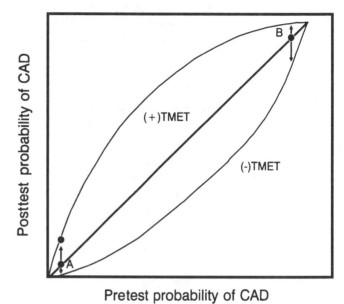

Fig. 3-31. The effect of Bayes theorem on the ability of treadmill exertion testing (TMET) to diagnose coronary artery disease (CAD). Representative patients A and B are described in the text.

Several different types of cardiac imaging modalities add to the sensitivity and specificity of ECG treadmill exertion testing. In thallium imaging, thallium 201 injected at peak exercise labels areas of perfusion; "cold spots" are nonperfused regions. Scanning is repeated 3 to 24 hours later. Persistent cold spots indicate previous infarction, and reperfused areas indicate ischemia. Single photon emission computed tomography thallium scanning (use of multiple tomographic planes) is more accurate than planar thallium scanning. In patients with left bundle branch block and severe left ventricular hypertrophy, thallium scanning gives false-positive results during exercise stress.

Sestamibi scanning uses an isotope with a half-life different from that of thallium. Also, because this isotope is more powerful than thallium, it is routinely used in women and obese patients to avoid artifact. However, the results are interpreted in the same way as those of thallium scanning, with "cold" spots indicating lack of perfusion.

In radionuclide angiography (multiple-gated acquisition scanning [MUGA]), erythrocytes are labeled with technetium 99m and the left ventricular cavity is imaged during the cardiac cycle to measure (at rest and at peak exercise) left ventricular volume, ejection fraction, and regional wall motion abnormalities. MUGA is positive if the ejection fraction decreases or new regional wall motion abnormalities appear. Because multiple cycles are gated, MUGA cannot be used with irregular rhythms.

In exercise echocardiography, two-dimensional echocardiography is performed at rest and at peak exercise. Digital acquisition allows side-by-side comparisons of images from the same view. The test is positive for ischemia if global systolic function decreases or new regional wall motion abnormalities appear.

- The sensitivity and specificity of ECG treadmill exertion testing are about 70% and 75%, respectively.
- The treadmill exertion test should not be used to make the diagnosis of coronary artery disease.
- Thallium or sestamibi scanning gives false-positive results during exercise in patients with left bundle branch block and severe left ventricular hypertrophy.
- MUGA is positive if the ejection fraction decreases or new regional wall motion abnormalities appear.
- Two-dimensional echocardiography is positive for ischemia if global systolic function decreases or new regional wall motion abnormalities appear.

All these imaging modalities are more expensive than the ECG treadmill exertion test. Because Bayes theorem applies, imaging modalities should not be used instead of ECG treadmill testing to diagnose coronary artery disease except in cases of an uninterpretable ECG or false-positive ECG results or for localizing specific regions of ischemia (for future revascularization procedures).

Pharmacologic stress tests that provoke ischemia have been developed for patients who cannot exercise. These tests include the use of dipyridamole thallium, which redistributes flow away from ischemic myocardium. Adenosine thallium works in the same way as dipyridamole. In dobutamine echocardiography, the myocardial oxygen demand is increased. Pacing echocardiography increases heart rate.

Treadmill exertion testing identifies high-risk patients. If the following are obtained on testing, the patient is high risk: less than stage I of the Bruce protocol, heart rate less than 120 beats/min, ST-segment depression greater than 2 mm, ST-segment depression greater than 6 minutes' duration after stopping, decreased blood pressure, multiple perfusion defects, and a decrease in ejection fraction greater than 20%. In patients with poor prognostic factors, it is reasonable to proceed with coronary angiography to define the anatomy of the coronary arteries and the need for intervention. However, in patients who achieve a good workload without significant ST-segment depression and have appropriate blood pressure and heart rate responses, medical management may be indicated because of the excellent prognosis.

- The major usefulness of stress testing is to identify high-risk patients, not to diagnose coronary artery disease.
- The treadmill exertion test should not be performed on patients with either unstable angina or severe aortic stenosis.

Coronary Angiography

Although coronary angiography has many limitations, it is the standard method for defining the severity and extent of coronary artery disease. Subjective visual estimation of the percentage of stenosis may grossly underestimate the severity of the disease, especially if it is diffuse, because angiography outlines only the vessel lumen. The risk of serious complications of coronary angiography is less than 1%. These complications include myocardial infarction (0.4%), stroke (0.4%), and death (0.1%). The risk is greater for older patients or for those with severe left ventricular dysfunction, left main coronary artery disease, or other coexistent diseases. Other complications include vascular complications (1.0%) and renal failure.

- Coronary angiography is the standard method for defining the severity of coronary artery disease.
- Visual estimation of the percentage of stenosis may grossly underestimate disease severity.
- The risk of serious complications in coronary angiography is <1%.

Medical Therapy

Medical treatment for chronic stable angina should be given in a stepwise manner according to symptoms. Sublingual nitroglycerin should be given as needed. A first-line drug should be increased to the optimal dosage before a second or third drug is added. β-Blockers are the most effective drugs for patients with coronary artery disease and should be the first-line drug of choice. β-Blockers relieve angina mainly by decreasing heart rate, reducing contractility, and decreasing afterload (blood pressure). They are the most effective drugs for reducing the double product (heart rate × blood pressure) with exercise. Also, these drugs may improve survival for some patients with known coronary artery disease, particularly those who have had a myocardial infarction and those with depressed left ventricular systolic function. β-Blockers should not be prescribed if the paient has marked bronchospastic disease, severely symptomatic congestive heart failure, or bradycardia. However, β-blockers can and would be given to patients with left ventricular systolic dysfunction in the absence of overt heart failure. β-Blockers should be given at a dosage that keeps the resting heart rate less than 70 beats/min.

Long-acting nitrates should be added sequentially if symptoms continue. Nitrates relieve angina mainly by producing venodilatation, which decreases wall tension. Nitrate tolerance can occur with continuous exposure (use a nitrate-free interval with dosing three times daily). Isosorbide dinitrate, at least 20 to 30 mg three times daily, needs to be given.

Calcium channel blockers are effective in relieving angina by decreasing afterload, heart rate, and contractility; they may be used as a third-line drug. However, short-acting calcium channel blockers, specifically the dihydropyridines, may increase mortality of patients with ischemic heart disease. This detrimental effect probably does not occur with the longer acting calcium channel blockers in patients with normal systolic function, but the use of these agents should be avoided if the patient has left ventricular systolic dysfunction. If a calcium channel blocker is required for patients with left ventricular systolic dysfunction, amlodipine should be given.

Always look for treatable underlying factors that contribute to ischemia (anemia, thyroid abnormalities, and hypoxia). For patients with left ventricular dysfunction and nocturnal angina, diuretics and ACEIs may be helpful in decreasing wall tension. Data suggest that ACEIs may be beneficial in preventing future cardiovascular events in high-risk patients with known coronary artery disease regardless of the level of systolic function.

- The initial therapy for chronic stable angina is β-blockade with sublingual nitroglycerin as needed.
- Add long-acting nitrates sequentially if symptoms continue.
- Nitrates relieve angina by producing venodilatation, which decreases wall tension.
- β-Blockers relieve angina by decreasing heart rate, reducing contractility, and decreasing afterload (blood pressure).
- β-Blockers are the most effective drugs for reducing the double product.
- Nitrate tolerance can occur with continuous exposure.
- Do not prescribe β-blockers if the patient has marked bronchospastic disease, severely symptomatic congestive heart failure, or bradycardia.
- β-Blockers should be given at a dosage to keep the resting heart rate <70 beats/min.
- Look for treatable underlying factors contributing to ischemia.
- Diuretics and ACEIs may be helpful for patients with left ventricular dysfunction and nocturnal angina.
- Short-acting calcium channel blockers should be avoided if the patient has coronary artery disease.
- For patients with left ventricular dysfunction, all calcium channel blockers except amlodipine should be avoided.

Antiplatelet agents may be helpful in patients with chronic stable angina pectoris. A low dose of aspirin probably does not prevent progression of atherosclerosis, but it may prevent acute myocardial infarction in patients with known coronary artery disease. In two large primary prevention trials, aspirin produced a 33% decrease in the risk for first, nonfatal myocardial infarction in men. The data are conflicting about the potential for a sex difference in the antithrombotic effects of aspirin; however, there is clear benefit for both men and women when aspirin is used in a secondary prevention strategy. The role of aspirin in primary prevention of stroke or overall cardiovascular mortality is uncertain.

- A low dose of aspirin probably does not prevent progression of atherosclerosis, but it prevents acute myocardial infarction in patients with known coronary artery disease.
- The role of aspirin in primary prevention of stroke or overall cardiovascular mortality is uncertain.

Catheter-Based Treatment

Percutaneous coronary intervention (PCI), a treatment for coronary artery disease, is performed at the time of coronary angiography. During percutaneous transluminal coronary angioplasty (PTCA), which is PCI with only a balloon, a small balloon is placed across a coronary stenosis and inflated to increase the area of the lumen at the site of stenosis. The mechanism of PTCA is a combination of "splitting" the atheroma and stretching the noninvolved segment of artery. In experienced laboratories, the success rate now is greater than 95%. The potential complications include myocardial infarction (<5%), vascular complications (<5%), emergency coronary artery bypass grafting (<1%), and mortality (1%). The risks of the procedure are increased in long, tubular eccentric lesions, which are calcified, and the risk is also increased in older women. Overall, more than 500,000 catheter-based therapies are performed annually in North America. The major problem with PTCA is restenosis, which occurs in 30% to 40% of patients within 6 months. Treatment with antiplatelet agents before PTCA may decrease the rate of acute closure but does not prevent restenosis. Glycoprotein IIb/IIIa inhibitors may decrease acute complications in high-risk patients but probably do not prevent restenosis. Other catheter-based therapies such as atherectomy, rotoblator, and laser have been used but they (and other therapies) have a high restenosis rate, similar to that of PTCA.

Placement of an intracoronary stent at the time of PCI is the only procedure that has been shown to decrease restenosis. The restenosis rate after successful stent implantation is 20% to 30%. Stents also are effective in treating the acute complications of PTCA such as acute dissection and have decreased the need for emergency bypass operation. However, for patients who have restenosis within a stent, the restenosis rate is high (>60%) if another procedure is performed. Although gamma and beta radiotherapy may decrease this high rate of restenosis, the long-term outcome of the procedure is not known and the risk of acute thrombosis is slightly increased. Radiation at the time of initial stent implantation has been associated with higher rates of subacute stent thrombosis. Stents that are coated with and elute drugs have been shown in randomized trials to significantly decrease the rate of restenosis. These stents were approved in April 2003 by the U.S. Food and Drug Administration for clinical use.

It is important to emphasize that for the treatment of chronic stable angina, catheter-based strategies clearly relieve symptoms, but they have not been shown to have an effect on subsequent myocardial infarction or death.

- PTCA is a combination of splitting the atheroma and stretching the uninvolved segment of artery.
- Currently, the initial success rate is >95%.
- Restenosis is a major problem of PTCA. Stents can decrease the rate of restenosis in selected patients.
- Antiplatelet agents reduce the problem of acute events but do not prevent restenosis.

Surgical Treatment

The surgical treatment for severely symptomatic patients with chronic stable angina is coronary artery bypass grafting (CABG) with either saphenous vein or internal mammary artery grafts. CABG provides excellent relief from symptoms (partial relief in >90% of patients and complete relief in >70%). In-hospital mortality after CABG varies widely from less than 1% to 30%. Mortality increases with age, poor ventricular function, female sex, left main coronary artery disease, unstable angina, and diabetes mellitus. Complications of CABG include sternal wound infection (especially in patients with diabetes mellitus), severe left ventricular dysfunction (from perioperative myocardial infarction or inadequate cardioprotection), and late constrictive pericarditis. The procedure is not without latent problems. Closure rates of saphenous vein grafts are 20% at 1 year and 50% at 5 years. The patency rate is higher for internal mammary arteries, possibly up to 90% patency at 5 years. A minithoracotomy with a left internal mammary artery–left anterior descending artery anastomosis may shorten hospitalization, but long-term follow-up is needed.

- CABG provides excellent relief from symptoms.
- CABG gives partial relief in >90% of patients and complete relief in >70%.
- In-hospital mortality after CABG varies widely from <1% to 30%.
- Mortality increases with age, poor ventricular function, female sex, left main coronary artery disease, unstable angina, and diabetes mellitus.
- Closure rates of saphenous vein grafts are 20% at 1 year and 50% at 5 years.

Several randomized trials have compared CABG with medical therapy, and the intermediate-term follow-up results are as follows:

- CABG does not prevent myocardial infarction.
- CABG does not uniformly improve left ventricular function.

- CABG does not decrease ventricular arrhythmias.
- CABG only improves survival for patients with 1) left main coronary artery disease, 2) three-vessel disease and moderately depressed left ventricular function, 3) three-vessel disease and severe symptoms of ischemia at a low workload, and 4) multivessel disease with involvement of the proximal left anterior descending artery. For all other subsets of patients, CABG should not be performed to improve survival.
- The indications for CABG instead of medical therapy are 1) relieving symptoms in patients who have limiting symptoms unresponsive to medical management and 2) prolonging the life of the subsets of patients listed above.
- These recommendations were based on the randomized trials of CABG vs. medical therapy, which all had a small number of patients and limited use of internal mammary artery grafts. In larger meta-analyses, there was a survival benefit for CABG vs. medical therapy for all patients with three-vessel disease.

Medical Versus Catheter-Based Versus Surgical Therapy

The decision about which therapy to use for a patient with chronic, stable angina is an individual one and must be based on the patient's age, lifestyle, and personal preference. However, randomized trials have compared the medical, catheter-based, and surgical therapies, and the results help in guiding decisions about which therapy to use for a selected subset of patients. The following summarizes the results of these trials.

1. Medical therapy versus PTCA (one-vessel disease):

- PTCA has a similar or higher incidence of myocardial infarction and emergency CABG.
- PTCA does not decrease the future risk of myocardial infarction.
- PTCA does not improve resting left ventricular function.
- PTCA does not increase survival.

2. PTCA versus surgical therapy (multivessel disease—excluding left main coronary artery disease and totally occluded vessels):

- The rates of procedure-related mortality are similar (1%-2%).
- There are more procedure-related Q-wave infarctions with CABG than with PTCA (4.6% vs. 2.1%), but events are well tolerated.
- The duration of initial hospitalization is longer for CABG than for PTCA.
- The overall incidences of death or myocardial infarction are similar at 5-year follow-up (85%-90% free of death and 80% free of myocardial infarction).

• Patients who have CABG have less angina, require less antianginal medication, and are less likely to need a repeat revascularization procedure than those who have PTCA (8% vs. 54% at 5-year follow-up).

• For patients with diabetes mellitus, 5-year survival is higher with CABG than with PTCA (80% vs. 65%). Increased survival is associated with a patent left internal mammary artery–left anterior descending artery graft.

Postcardiotomy Syndrome

Postcardiotomy syndrome occurs 2 weeks to 2 years postoperatively and consists of fever, pericarditis, and increased erythrocyte sedimentation rate. Rarely, it can present as pericardial tamponade. It probably is an autoimmune process (associated with antimyocardial antibodies); treatment is with aspirin and nonsteroidal anti-inflammatory drugs. Postperfusion syndrome is also characterized by fever and pericarditis, but it is associated with increased liver function tests and atypical lymphocytes, presumably due to cytomegalovirus syndrome. If a patient has fever and pleuritic chest pain postoperatively, measure the erythrocyte sedimentation rate and perform a special blood smear to check for postperfusion or postcardiotomy syndrome.

• Postcardiotomy syndrome occurs 2 weeks-2 years postoperatively.

• It consists of fever, pericarditis, and increased erythrocyte sedimentation rate.

• It probably is an autoimmune process (associated with antimyocardial antibodies).

• Treatment: aspirin and nonsteroidal anti-inflammatory drugs.

• Postperfusion syndrome: fever, pericarditis, increased liver function tests, and atypical lymphocytes.

• If the patient has fever and pleuritic chest pain postoperatively, measure the erythrocyte sedimentation rate and perform a special blood smear to check for postcardiotomy or postperfusion syndrome.

CORONARY ARTERY SPASM

The vasomotor tone of coronary arteries is important in the pathogenesis of coronary artery disease. Coronary artery vasoconstriction can be seen as a response to arterial injury. The endothelium affects vascular tone by releasing relaxing factors, for example, prostacyclin and endothelium-derived relaxing factor, which prevent vasoconstriction and platelet deposition. With dysfunctional endothelium, these factors are absent and the coronary arteries may be more prone to spasm. Most clinical episodes of coronary artery spasm are superimposed on atherosclerotic plaques. However, patients may have primary coronary artery spasm and angiographically normal coronary arteries.

• Endothelium affects vascular tone by releasing relaxing factors, e.g., prostacyclin and endothelium-derived relaxing factor.

• With dysfunctional endothelium, coronary arteries may be more prone to spasm.

• Most episodes of spasm are superimposed on atherosclerotic plaques.

• Patients may have primary coronary artery spasm and angiographically normal coronary arteries.

The typical presentation of coronary artery spasm consists of recurrent episodes of rest pain in association with ST-segment elevation, which reverses with administration of nitrates. Coronary angiography with ergonovine or methylergonovine challenge has been used to diagnose coronary artery spasm, but the sensitivity and specificity are not known. The use of acetylcholine to provoke spasm may be helpful because it directly examines the status of the endothelium. ST-segment elevation on the resting 12-lead ECG during an episode of rest pain is the standard criterion for diagnosing coronary artery spasm. Coronary artery spasm is treated with long-acting nitrates or calcium channel blockers (or both).

• The typical presentation of coronary artery spasm is recurrent episodes of rest pain and ST-segment elevation that is reversed with nitrates.

• The standard criterion for diagnosis: spontaneous ST-segment elevation on resting 12-lead ECG during an episode of rest pain.

ACUTE CORONARY SYNDROMES

The term "acute coronary syndrome" refers to any constellation of clinical symptoms that are compatible with acute myocardial ischemia (Fig. 3-32). Acute coronary syndromes encompass acute myocardial infarction (ST-segment elevation and depression, Q wave, and non–Q wave) as well as unstable angina.

The resting ECG is essential in the evaluation of a patient presenting with an acute coronary syndrome. Patients without ST-segment elevation and myocardial ischemia may have unstable angina or they may develop non–Q-wave myocardial infarction. Unstable angina and non–Q-wave myocardial infarction have a similar pathogenesis. Patients with ST-segment elevation most likely have complete occlusion of an epicardial coronary artery that causes transmural injury. If untreated, a Q-wave myocardial infarction eventually develops. A small proportion of patients with non–ST-segment elevation

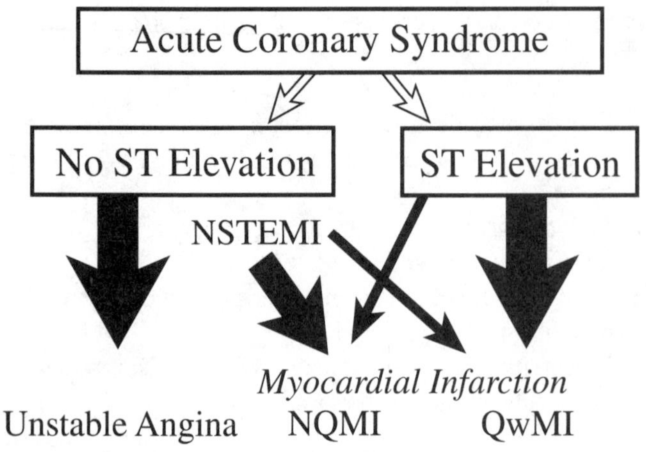

Fig. 3-32. Nomenclature of acute coronary syndromes. Patients with ischemic discomfort may present with or without ST-segment elevation on the ECG. The majority of patients with ST-segment elevation (large arrows) ultimately develop a Q-wave anterior myocardial infarction (QwMI), whereas a small proportion (small arrow) develop a non–Q-wave anterior myocardial infarction (NQMI). Patients who present without ST-segment elevation are experiencing either unstable angina or non–ST-segment elevation myocardial infarction (NSTEMI). The distinction between these two diagnoses is ultimately made on the basis of the presence or absence of a cardiac marker detected in the blood. Most patients with NSTEMI do not develop a Q wave on the 12-lead ECG and are subsequently referred to as having "sustained a non–Q-wave myocardial infarction" (NQMI); only a small proportion of NSTEMI patients develop a Q wave and are later diagnosed as having Q-wave myocardial infarction. Not shown is Prinzmetal angina, which presents with transient chest pain and ST-segment elevation but rarely with myocardial infarction. The spectrum of clinical conditions that range from unstable angina to NQMI and QwMI is referred to as "acute coronary syndromes." (From the Committee on the Management of Patients With Unstable Angina: ACC/AHA Guidelines for the management of patients with unstable angina and non-ST-segment elevation myocardial infarction. A report of the American College of Cardiology/American Heart Association Task Force on Practice Guidelines. J Am Coll Cardiol 2000;36:970-1062. By permission of American College of Cardiology.)

myocardial infarction develop Q-wave myocardial infarction. Patients who have ST-segment elevation and receive thrombolytic therapy may develop non–Q-wave myocardial infarction. Acute coronary syndromes should be considered a continuous spectrum of diseases in patients who present with myocardial ischemia.

When patients present with a suspected acute coronary syndrome, they should be evaluated immediately in the emergency department, and those who have ST-segment elevation should be treated immediately (see below, ST-Segment Elevation Myocardial Infarction). For patients who do not have ST-segment elevation, chest pain units have been developed in emergency departments that allow dismissal of low-risk patients, observation of intermediate-risk patients, and admission of high-risk patients.

- "Acute coronary syndrome" refers to clinical symptoms compatible with acute myocardial ischemia.

Unstable Angina and Non–ST-Segment Elevation Myocardial Infarction

These conditions are characterized by an imbalance between myocardial oxygen supply and demand. They may be caused by an increased myocardial oxygen demand in the presence of a fixed myocardial oxygen supply. They also may be caused by a decrease in myocardial oxygen supply, which usually results from narrowing of the coronary artery due to a noninclusive thrombus that developed on a disrupted atherosclerotic plaque. Superimposed spasm may also cause this syndrome.

All patients with the tentative diagnosis of an acute coronary syndrome should have continuous ECG monitoring and treatment to improve the myocardial oxygen demand-supply mismatch. Sedation should be used to decrease anxiety and catecholaminergic stimulation of the heart. β-Blocker therapy is the treatment of choice for decreasing myocardial oxygen demand. Antiplatelet agents, such as aspirin, should be given immediately because they are effective in decreasing the incidence of progression to myocardial infarction. Heparin also decreases the incidence of progression to myocardial infarction and should be given to all patients who do not have contraindications to this treatment. Continuous intravenous administration of unfractionated heparin or subcutaneous injections of low-molecular-weight heparin can be given. Glycoprotein IIb/IIIa inhibitors should be prescribed for patients who are at high risk (ongoing chest pain, transient ST-segment depression with angina at rest, marked increase in troponin levels), particularly if PCI is likely.

Unstable angina and non–ST-segment elevation myocardial infarction are differentiated on the basis of cardiac enzymes. Previously, creatine kinase-MB was the principal serum marker used in the evaluation of acute coronary syndromes. However, monoclonal antibody-based immunoassays have been developed to detect cardiac-specific troponin T and cardiac-specific troponin I. An increase in the level of these enzymes in patients with an acute coronary syndrome indicates myocardial necrosis and identifies patients who are at high risk for future events.

There are two accepted therapeutic pathways for patients who present with unstable angina or non–ST-segment elevation myocardial infarction. The first is a conservative approach in which aggressive medical management is used to stabilize the patient's condition. If additional ischemic episodes occur despite optimal medical therapy or if left ventricular function is reduced, coronary angiography is indicated. The second accepted therapeutic pathway is an early invasive approach in which all patients who present with an acute coronary syndrome have coronary angiography and high-grade coronary lesions are treated. If the conservative pathway is taken, patients should undergo stress testing before dismissal. Although there may be subgroups that will benefit more from one strategy, the optimal general approach is still debated.

- Unstable angina differs from non–ST-segment elevation myocardial infarction in that cardiac-specific enzymes are increased in the latter.

ST-Segment Elevation Myocardial Infarction

The underlying pathogenesis of a patient presenting with ST-segment elevation myocardial infarction is usually rupture of an intracoronary plaque. This leads to platelet adhesion, aggregation, thrombus formation, and sudden, complete occlusion of an epicardial coronary artery. Without collateral circulation, 90% of the myocardium that is supplied by the occluded coronary artery is infarcted within 3 hours. If untreated, transmural myocardial infarction develops. Patients with ST-segment elevation myocardial infarction require urgent diagnosis and therapy to preserve the myocardium. It is for this group of patients that aggressive reperfusion therapy has improved survival.

- ST-segment elevation myocardial infarction usually implies acute occlusion of an epicardial coronary artery.
- If untreated, a transmural myocardial infarction will develop within 3 hours.

Myocardial infarction accounts for a large percentage of morbidity and mortality in the United States. More than 500,000 patients are admitted annually to a hospital because of myocardial infarction. More than 50% of patients who have a myocardial infarction die before reaching the hospital. With the advent of coronary care units 4 decades ago, mortality from myocardial infarction has decreased from 30% to 15%, primarily because of treatment of ventricular arrhythmias. β-Blockade has further decreased in-hospital and posthospital mortality by 30% to 40%. In the 1980s, reperfusion therapy became the standard of care and has been shown to further improve survival. Currently, the overall in-hospital mortality for a patient with ST-segment elevation myocardial infarction is 5% to 10%.

Several new concepts about myocardial infarction have arisen in the past 2 decades: stunned myocardium, ischemia at a distance, and infarct remodeling. "Stunned myocardium" occurs when a coronary artery is completely occluded and then opened. If reperfusion occurs early enough, systolic contraction of the affected myocardium may be decreased after the event, but the myocardium is viable. Systolic contraction returns hours to days later. Currently, no clinical test differentiates stunned myocardium from infarcted, dead myocardium. "Ischemia at a distance" refers to infarction occurring in the distribution of one coronary vessel and

ischemia and subsequent hypokinesis developing in the distribution of a second vessel that has a high-grade stenosis. When this is seen on echocardiography, the prognosis is poor because of recurrent myocardial infarction and increased mortality. "Infarct remodeling" occurs mainly after a large anteroapical myocardial infarction. An area of infarction may undergo thinning, dilatation, and dyskinesis. This remodeling is associated with a high incidence of congestive heart failure and posthospital mortality. ACEIs may help prevent infarct remodeling.

- Stunned myocardium: a coronary artery is completely occluded and then opened, and transient akinesis of the myocardium occurs.
- Ischemia at a distance: infarction occurs in the distribution of one coronary artery and ischemia and subsequent hypokinesis develop in the distribution of a second vessel that has a high-grade stenosis.
- Infarct remodeling: occurs after a large anteroapical myocardial infarction.
- ACEIs may help prevent infarct remodeling.

Presentation and Diagnosis

The usual presentation of ST-segment elevation myocardial infarction is angina-like pain that lasts longer than 30 to 45 minutes and is associated with typical ECG changes and increased levels of creatine kinase-MB fraction or troponin. However, more than 25% to 30% of myocardial infarctions are silent and present later as new ECG abnormalities or regional wall motion abnormalities. Silent myocardial infarctions occur especially in patients with diabetes mellitus and in the elderly. The increased incidence of myocardial infarction in the early morning is perhaps related to increased platelet aggregation. The pain of myocardial infarction mimics that of other diseases, for example, gastrointestinal tract or pericardial disease or musculoskeletal pain.

- More than 25%-30% of myocardial infarctions are silent.
- Silent myocardial infarctions occur especially in patients with diabetes mellitus and in the elderly.
- The increased incidence of myocardial infarction in the early morning is perhaps related to increased platelet aggregation.
- The pain of myocardial infarction mimics that of other diseases.

Basic and Drug Treatments

Bed rest and sedation are essential and beneficial in the acute stage of myocardial infarction for decreasing myocardial oxygen demand. Analgesics, particularly morphine, are beneficial for recurrent pain. Currently, prolonged bed rest is not recommended, and the effort to shorten hospitalization is increasing. Many physicians recommend a gradual increase in activity level over 3 to 6 days for an uncomplicated myocardial infarction. During the acute 3- to 4-day period, ECG monitoring is recommended for both tachyarrhythmias and bradyarrhythmias. Oxygen can be given at the initial presentation but has little benefit after 2 or 3 hours unless hypoxia is present. However, modest hypoxemia is not uncommon, even with uncomplicated myocardial infarction, and is due to ventilation-perfusion lung mismatch.

- Prolonged bed rest is not recommended.
- Oxygen has little benefit beyond 3 hours after the initial presentation unless hypoxia is present.

Heparin is important in treating acute myocardial infarction. It prevents recurrent infarction (especially after thrombolytic therapy), deep venous thrombosis, and intracardiac thrombus formation. Historically, intracardiac thrombus formation occurs in 40% of patients with anterior myocardial infarction, and almost 50% of these patients have a systemic embolic event. Thus, intravenous unfractionated heparin therapy is especially indicated for these higher risk patients. Low-molecular-weight heparin given subcutaneously may be more effective. Aspirin decreases recurrent infarction by 50% in patients not receiving thrombolytic therapy. It also reduces mortality when given in addition to thrombolytic therapy.

- Heparin is important in treating acute myocardial infarction.
- Heparin prevents recurrent infarction, deep venous thrombosis, and intracardiac thrombus formation.
- Intracardiac thrombus formation occurs in 40% of patients with anterior myocardial infarction.
- Aspirin decreases recurrent infarction by 50% in patients not receiving thrombolytic therapy.

Nitroglycerin is useful for subsets of patients with myocardial infarction—for those with heart failure (by decreasing wall tension) and for those with continued pain. To prevent acute decreases in blood pressure in the early stages of myocardial infarction, intravenous nitroglycerin should be given instead of long-acting oral nitrates. Intravenous nitroglycerin may reduce infarct size by decreasing wall tension and affecting "remodeling." Also, it may decrease susceptibility to ventricular fibrillation. If the mean blood pressure is greater than 80 mm Hg, intravenous nitroglycerin may reduce mortality by 10% to 25%, specifically among patients with anterior myocardial infarction and poor left ventricular function. However, for patients with low blood pressure and those with inferior and right ventricular infarctions, nitroglycerin may decrease blood pressure too much, increasing mortality. The dosage of intravenous nitroglycerin is a 15-μg

bolus and an initial infusion of 10 μg/min. This infusion should be increased every 5 to 10 minutes, up to a maximum of 150 to 200 μg/min, until blood pressure decreases 10% to 15%. Mean blood pressure should be kept higher than 80 mm Hg. Nitrate intolerance develops with infusions that last longer than 24 hours. Do not give intravenous nitroglycerin to patients with low blood pressure or right ventricular infarction. Intravenous nitroglycerin may improve mortality for patients with large anterior myocardial infarctions and congestive heart failure.

- Nitroglycerin is useful for patients with myocardial infarction who have heart failure and for those with continued pain.
- Intravenous nitroglycerin may reduce infarct size by decreasing wall tension and affecting remodeling.
- Nitroglycerin may decrease susceptibility to ventricular fibrillation.
- Nitrate intolerance occurs with infusions that last longer than 24 hours.
- Do not give intravenous nitroglycerin to patients with low blood pressure or right ventricular infarction.
- Intravenous nitroglycerin may improve mortality for patients with a large anterior myocardial infarction and congestive heart failure.

β-Blockers are useful for both acute myocardial infarction and postmyocardial infarction. If given early, they decrease infarction size and in-hospital mortality. If given after myocardial infarction has been completed, β-blockers can reduce posthospital reinfarction and mortality. In an acute setting, the typical dosage of metoprolol is 5 mg given intravenously three times, 5 minutes apart, followed by 100 mg given orally twice daily. β-Blockers decrease pain and the incidence of ventricular fibrillation. The beneficial effects are probably multifactorial but include decreased myocardial oxygen demand, increased threshold for ventricular fibrillation, decreased platelet aggregability, and decreased sympathetic effects on the myocardium. β-Blockers are most beneficial for patients with a large infarction, that is, those at higher risk for complications. Acute intravenous β-blockers are also beneficial for patients receiving thrombolytic therapy. β-Blockers are especially useful for patients with hyperdynamic circulation and continued postinfarction pain and should be given to patients presenting with less than 12 hours of pain who do not have contraindications, especially those with anterior myocardial infarction.

- Acute intravenous β-blockers decrease infarction size and in-hospital mortality.
- Acute intravenous β-blockers decrease the incidence of ventricular fibrillation.

- Contraindications to β-blockers are bradycardia, atrioventricular block, hypotension, severe heart failure, and inferior myocardial infarction with high vagal tone.

Calcium channel blockers have been used to treat myocardial infarction, but their routine use has no proven benefit. Routine use of verapamil and nifedipine has no benefit and may increase mortality. However, by producing coronary vasodilatation and decreasing myocardial oxygen demand, calcium channel blockers may be beneficial in treating postinfarction angina if β-blockade is ineffective or cannot be used.

- Routine use of calcium channel blockers for myocardial infarction has no proven benefit.
- Routine use of verapamil and nifedipine to treat myocardial infarction may increase mortality.

In most patients, magnesium does not appear to have a therapeutic role after myocardial infarction. Although initial studies suggested that it may decrease infarct size, subsequent studies have not borne this out. Magnesium should be given only if a patient has documented hypomagnesemia (from diuretics) or for the treatment of torsades de pointes.

ACEIs have been studied extensively in patients with ST-segment elevation myocardial infarction. These inhibitors appear to prevent the infarct remodeling that occurs after a large anteroapical myocardial infarction. Although these drugs should not be given acutely intravenously, data support the initiation of ACEI therapy within the first 24 hours after anterior myocardial infarction as long as blood pressure is stable. It is debated whether ACEIs should be given to all patients with myocardial infarction.

Other medications are being studied for treating ST-segment elevation myocardial infarction. Although glycoprotein IIb/IIIa inhibitors are given to high-risk patients with non–ST-segment elevation myocardial infarction, there are conflicting data regarding their use either alone or in combination with other treatments during an ST-segment elevation myocardial infarction. Hirudin, a direct thrombin inhibitor, also has been studied in patients with acute ST-segment elevation myocardial infarction. However, hirudin has an increased bleeding risk and is not more effective than heparin therapy. Therefore, it should be prescribed only for patients who have heparin-induced thrombocytopenia and require anticoagulation.

Reperfusion Therapy

Early reperfusion therapy has had a tremendous effect on the treatment of acute myocardial infarction. Overall, mortality is decreased 27%±3% when reperfusion is given early. For more than 50,000 patients in the ISIS-3 and GISSI-2 studies, the 35-day in-hospital mortality was only 10% with thrombolytic

therapy. Time is of the essence when giving reperfusion therapy. The sooner the reperfusion, the better the extent of myocardial salvage and the better the effect on mortality. Without collaterals, 90% of the myocardium at risk is infarcted within 3 hours after occlusion. Very early reperfusion has a major effect on direct myocardial salvage. In a study in which thrombolysis was given less than 90 minutes after the onset of pain, mortality was 1%. In most U.S. studies, the average time from pain onset to artery opening is 3.7 hours. The delay is in patient presentation (22%), transport (21%), in-hospital institution of the drug (35%), and reperfusion drug time (19%). Reperfusion at 2 to 6 hours salvages the peri-infarction zone, depending on the degree of collateral circulation. Thus, there is a lesser effect on myocardial salvage but an important effect on survival. The "open artery concept" describes a benefit in improvement in posthospital mortality in the presence of an open artery after thrombolytic therapy that is not reflected in improved ventricular function. The reason for this is unclear, but it may be related to improved electrical stability or prevention of ventricular remodeling.

- Overall, mortality is decreased 27%±3% when reperfusion is given early.
- For more than 50,000 patients, the 35-day in-hospital mortality was 10% with thrombolytic therapy.
- The sooner the reperfusion, the better the extent of myocardial salvage.
- Without collaterals, 90% of the myocardium at risk is infarcted within 3 hours after occlusion.

Controversy exists about the effectiveness of intravenous thrombolytic therapy versus emergency PTCA for patients with acute myocardial infarction. After administration of thrombolytic therapy, emergency PTCA is not indicated in the absence of ongoing pain because of a higher incidence of complications than in patients not undergoing emergency PTCA (usually with a stent). The controversy is about whether intravenous thrombolytic therapy should be given instead of direct PTCA. Intravenous thrombolysis may not be as effective (65%-70%) in opening arteries as PTCA (90%), and there is a higher incidence of TIMI grade 3 flow after direct PTCA. However, this is counterbalanced by faster administration of intravenous thrombolysis and wider availability of the intravenous drug. Fewer than 10% of all hospitals have the capability of performing emergency PTCA, and these centers must be able to provide rapid treatment, with balloon opening within 90 minutes. Late patency (>24 hours) is 70% to 80% for both methods. Thus, with the lack of available resources, intravenous thrombolytic therapy is the treatment of choice at most medical centers for patients with acute myocardial infarction. Emergency PTCA may be used for patients with 1) contraindication for intravenous thrombolysis, 2) cardiogenic shock, 3) continued ischemia after thrombolytic therapy, or 4) immediate access to a high-volume catheterization laboratory.

- The effectiveness of intravenous thrombolytic therapy vs. emergency primary PTCA in patients with acute myocardial infarction is debated.
- After thrombolytic therapy has been administered, emergency PTCA is not indicated in the absence of ongoing pain.
- Intravenous thrombolysis may not be as effective (65%-70%) in opening arteries as PTCA (90%).
- Fewer than 10% of hospitals have the capability of performing emergency PTCA.
- Intravenous thrombolytic therapy is the treatment of choice at most medical centers for patients with acute myocardial infarction who have no contraindications and a stable condition.

Thrombolytic therapy definitely is indicated for patients younger than 75 who have ST-segment elevation myocardial infarction and no contraindications and who present within 12 hours after the onset of pain. It also should be given to patients who present within 6 hours after the onset of pain and have left bundle branch block. Thrombolytic therapy is not indicated for patients who have pain and other ECG abnormalities (ST-segment depression) or for those who after 12 hours are without pain.

- Thrombolytic therapy definitely is indicated for patients who have ST-segment elevation and no contraindications and who present within 12 hours after the onset of pain.
- Thrombolytic therapy is not indicated for patients with pain and other ECG abnormalities (ST-segment depression).
- Thrombolytic therapy is not indicated for patients who after 12 hours are without evidence of continued ischemia.

Contraindications to thrombolytic therapy include a history of bleeding, severe hypertension, recent stroke, diabetic hemorrhagic retinopathy, recent cardiopulmonary resuscitation, previous allergy to streptokinase, recent surgical procedure, suspected aortic dissection or pericarditis, and pregnancy. Major complications of intravenous thrombolysis include major bleeding (5%-6% of patients), intracranial bleeding (0.5%), major allergic reaction (0.1%-1.7%), and hypotension (2%-10%). A higher incidence of myocardial rupture may occur in patients who are given thrombolytic therapy late (>12 hours after pain onset).

- Major complications of intravenous thrombolysis are major bleeding (5%-6% of patients), intracranial bleeding (0.5%),

major allergic reaction (0.1%-1.7%), and hypotension (2%-10%).
- A higher incidence of myocardial rupture may occur in patients given thrombolytic therapy late (>12 hours after pain onset).

Several agents are available for intravenous thrombolysis. Streptokinase, a nonselective thrombolytic agent, combines with circulating plasminogen to split circulating and thrombus-bound plasminogen into plasmin, which splits fibrin. It lyses circulating fibrinogen and thus has systemic effects. The dosage is a 250,000-U bolus and 1.5×10^6 U in 1 hour. Tissue plasminogen activator (TPA) binds preferentially to preformed fibrin and lyses it without activating plasminogen in the general circulation. Thus, it has less effect on circulating fibrinogen and is "fibrin-specific." It has the fastest onset of action. The dosage is 100 mg over 90 minutes. Anisoylated plasminogen streptokinase activator complex (APSAC) is composed of anisoylated plasminogen and streptokinase bound together and inactivated by plasminogen. It requires spontaneous deacylation, which occurs in the plasma before the active plasminogen–streptokinase complex is generated, splitting plasminogen to plasmin. Thus, anistreplase is a more stable agent and may be given as a single intravenous bolus. The dosage is 30 U over 5 minutes. Several new thrombolytic agents with properties of better selectivity for active thrombus and easier application are being investigated. These include r-TPA, n-TPA, and TNK-TPA.

The large European trials did not demonstrate any benefit of one thrombolytic therapy over the others. In the GUSTO trial, the mortality rate was lower when an accelerated dose of TPA was given with intravenous heparin than when given with streptokinase. Compared with streptokinase, TPA is more expensive and has a slightly increased risk of cerebral hemorrhage, especially in the elderly. It is reasonable to give TPA preferentially to younger patients who present very early with a large myocardial infarction.

After intravenous thrombolysis, a high-grade residual lesion is usually present. Reocclusion or ischemia occurs in 15% to 20% of patients and reinfarction occurs in 2% to 3%. In the United States, both heparin and aspirin are given after intravenous thrombolysis with the specific tissue plasminogen activators to prevent reinfarction. After TPA, heparin is given as a bolus injection, followed by a continuous infusion to keep the activated partial thromboplastin time at 50 to 70 seconds. The indication for coronary angiography or PTCA after intravenous thrombolysis is continued pain or ischemia documented on functional testing. No benefit results from routine intervention in all patients.

- After intravenous thrombolysis, reocclusion or ischemia occurs in 15%-20% of patients and reinfarction occurs in 2%-3%.

- Both aspirin and heparin are given after intravenous thrombolysis to prevent reinfarction.
- The benefit is clear with aspirin but not with heparin.
- Streptokinase is the least expensive thrombolytic therapy.
- TPA is the most clot-specific thrombolytic therapy.
- The least amount of antigenicity is with TPA.

Acute Mechanical Complications of Myocardial Infarction

Cardiogenic shock after myocardial infarction has a high rate of mortality, but with newer interventions, the mortality has decreased from 90% to 60%. However, it is important to determine the cause of cardiogenic shock. Although most cases are due to extensive left ventricular dysfunction, there are other causes, for example, right ventricular infarction and mechanical complications of myocardial infarction. Pulmonary artery catheterization and two-dimensional echocardiography may help in determining the cause (Table 3-19).

- Cardiogenic shock after myocardial infarction approaches 90% mortality.
- Most cases of cardiogenic shock are due to extensive left ventricular dysfunction.
- Pulmonary artery catheterization and two-dimensional echocardiography may help determine other causes of cardiogenic shock.

Right ventricular infarction occurs in up to 40% of patients with inferior myocardial infarction and is diagnosed by increased jugular venous pressure in the presence of clear lung fields. It can present anywhere from hours to several days after the onset of infarction. ST-segment elevation in a V_{4R} lead is diagnostic of a large right ventricular infarction and portends a high mortality rate. In extreme circumstances, right ventricular infarction can cause cardiogenic shock because the right ventricle is not able to effectively pump enough blood to fill the left ventricle. Treatment includes large amounts of fluids given intravenously and infusion of dobutamine. If right ventricular infarction is recognized early, reperfusion therapy is indicated.

- Right ventricular infarction occurs in up to 40% of patients with inferior myocardial infarction and presents with increased jugular venous pressure with clear lung fields.

Myocardial free wall rupture may occur and cause abrupt decompensation. Free wall rupture occurs in 85% of all ruptures. It occurs suddenly, usually 2 to 14 days after transmural myocardial infarction, most commonly in elderly hypertensive women, and usually presents as electromechanical dissociation or death. If rupture is contained in the pericardium, tamponade may occur. If the diagnosis can be made by emergency echocardiography, surgery should be performed. If the rupture is sealed off, a pseudoaneurysm may occur; surgical treatment is required because of the high incidence of further rupture.

- Free wall rupture occurs in 85% of all ruptures.
- It occurs suddenly, usually 2-14 days after transmural myocardial infarction.

Papillary muscle rupture occurs in 5% of all ruptures and usually 2 to 10 days after myocardial infarction. It is associated with inferior myocardial infarction because of the single blood supply to the posteromedial papillary muscle. Rupture of papillary muscle is heralded by the sudden onset of dyspnea and hypotension. Although a murmur may be present, it may not be audible because of equalization of left atrial and left ventricular pressures. The diagnosis is made with echocardiography or pulmonary artery catheterization, which demonstrates a large "V" wave on pulmonary artery wedge pressure. The treatment is intra-aortic balloon pump and an emergency operation.

- Papillary muscle rupture occurs in 5% of all ruptures.
- It usually occurs 2-10 days after myocardial infarction.

Table 3-19 Diagnosis of Cause of Cardiogenic Shock

Cause	Pulmonary artery catheterization			Catheterization findings	2-Dimensional echocardiography
	RA	PAWP	CO		
Left ventricular dysfunction	↑	↑↑	↓↓		Poor left ventricle
Right ventricular infarction	↑↑	↓	↓↓		Dilated right ventricle
Tamponade	↑↑	↑↑	↓↓	End-equalization	Pericardial tamponade
Papillary muscle rupture	↑	↑↑	↓↓	Large "V"	Severe mitral regurgitation
Ventricular septal defect	↑	↑↑	↑	Step-up	Defect seen
Pulmonary emboli	↑↑	=	↓	PADP > PAWP	Dilated right ventricle

CO, cardiac output; PADP, pulmonary artery diastolic pressure; PAWP, pulmonary artery wedge pressure; RA, right atrial pressure.

- It is associated with inferior myocardial infarction.
- It is heralded by sudden dyspnea and hypotension.
- It is diagnosed with echocardiography and pulmonary artery catheterization.

Ventricular septal defects occur in 10% of all ruptures, usually 1 to 20 days after myocardial infarction, and are equally frequent in inferior and anterior myocardial infarctions. Ventricular septal defects associated with inferior myocardial infarctions have a poorer prognosis because of the serpiginous nature of the rupture and associated ventricular infarction. They are indicated by the sudden onset of dyspnea and hypotension. A loud murmur and systolic thrill are always present. The diagnosis is made with echocardiography or pulmonary artery catheterization, which demonstrates a step-up in oxygen saturation from the right atrium to the pulmonary artery. Treatment is intra-aortic balloon pump and an emergency operation.

- Ventricular septal defects occur in 10% of all ruptures.
- They are equally frequent in inferior and anterior myocardial infarctions.
- They are indicated by the sudden onset of dyspnea and hypotension.
- A ventricular septal defect almost always has a thrill and loud murmur.

Prehospital Dismissal Evaluation

To properly evaluate a patient with myocardial infarction before dismissal from the hospital, determine the predictors of mortality. These include status of the left ventricle, ventricular arrhythmias, and presence of continued myocardial ischemia.

After myocardial infarction, most patients should have rehabilitation treadmill exertion testing to detect continued ischemia, particularly patients who did not have thrombolytic therapy. A submaximal treadmill test can be performed before dismissal, within 4 to 6 days after myocardial infarction. Alternatively, a symptom-limited treadmill test can be performed safely 10 to 21 days after myocardial infarction. If a submaximal treadmill test is performed before dismissal, a late symptom-limited treadmill test should be performed at follow-up evaluation 3 to 6 weeks after myocardial infarction. High-risk patients identified by treadmill exertion testing have an ST-segment depression greater than 1 mm, a decrease in blood pressure, or an inability to achieve 4 metabolic equivalents on the exercise test. Imaging exercise tests may identify additional high-risk patients by demonstrating multiple areas of ischemia. Pharmacologic stress tests (dobutamine echocardiography, dipyridamole thallium scanning, or adenosine thallium scanning) may be useful for patients unable to exercise. The role of stress testing for patients after thrombolytic therapy is less clear because most of them do well without intervention. However, stress testing is of value in providing an exercise prescription to patients.

- After myocardial infarction, most patients should undergo rehabilitation treadmill testing.
- It is a low-risk test for properly selected patients.

To prevent infarct remodeling and expansion, ACEIs should be given to all patients who have large anterior myocardial infarctions. In patients with an ejection fraction less than 40%, ACEI therapy prevents future congestive heart failure and improves mortality. Data suggest that ACEIs may be beneficial in preventing recurrent myocardial infarction and cerebrovascular accidents in all high-risk patients who have coronary artery disease. Whether or not ACEIs should be given to all patients after myocardial infarction is still debated.

Coronary angiography is indicated after myocardial infarction if the results of a rehabilitation treadmill exertion test are highly positive or postinfarction angina occurs. These patients usually have substantial regions of myocardium at risk, and the coronary anatomy should be defined to determine whether they should undergo either catheter-based therapy or CABG. Other indications for coronary angiography include patients who have had hemodynamic instability. Patients who have had heart failure during hospitalization are at high risk and should be considered for coronary angiography. Because CABG improves mortality for patients with three-vessel disease and depressed systolic function, it has been suggested that coronary angiography be performed in all patients who have a depressed ejection fraction to look for severe three-vessel or left main coronary artery disease.

- Coronary angiography is indicated if the results of a rehabilitation treadmill exertion test are positive or postinfarction angina occurs.

No randomized trials have examined the benefit of PTCA or bypass grafting after myocardial infarction. However, in high-risk patients (i.e., those with continued ischemia or positive results on a treadmill exertion test), it is reasonable to proceed with intervention. PTCA can be undertaken if there is a single-vessel high-grade lesion amenable to the procedure. CABG should be performed if there is left main coronary artery or proximal three-vessel disease or two- or three-vessel disease that supplies a large portion of the myocardium, especially when associated with moderate depression in left ventricular function.

Aggressive modification of risk factors is essential in the treatment of patients who have had a myocardial infarction. An exercise program, weight loss, and diet are mandatory for all patients following myocardial infarction. Many physicians determine the cholesterol level upon admission to the hospital. The goal of treatment is to decrease LDL cholesterol to less than 100 mg/dL. If LDL cholesterol is greater than 100 mg/dL, the trend is to start treatment with a statin drug before dismissal, even before instituting diet and weight loss.

The following apply to patients who survive acute myocardial infarction:

- Aspirin decreases recurrent myocardial infarction by 31% and late mortality by 15%, more so in cases of non–ST-segment elevation myocardial infarction.
- Warfarin may cause a similar decrease in mortality and reinfarction, but it is not used routinely in the United States.
- Statin drugs reduce recurrent events and mortality in patients with increased cholesterol levels (total cholesterol >200 mg/dL).

- Statin drugs reduce recurrent events in patients with "average" cholesterol levels (LDL >125 mg/dL).
- β-Blockers improve survival after myocardial infarction.
- β-Blockers are most effective in high-risk patients (i.e., decreased left ventricular function and ventricular arrhythmias) and may not be required for low-risk patients.
- β-Blockers are also effective after thrombolytic therapy.
- Because antiarrhythmic agents are associated with increased mortality, they should not be used to suppress ventricular ectopy.
- ACEIs decrease mortality after anterior myocardial infarction and depressed left ventricular function, presumably by inhibiting infarct remodeling.
- A rehabilitation program is essential for the patient's well-being and cardiovascular fitness.

PART V
Barry L. Karon, M.D.
Rick A. Nishimura, M.D.

HEART FAILURE

Heart failure is a clinical syndrome characterized by the inability of the heart to meet the metabolic demands of the body while maintaining normal ventricular filling pressures. Although the most common cause is left ventricular systolic dysfunction (as in dilated cardiomyopathy), other causes must be considered. For correct treatment of heart failure, the cause and precipitating factors must be identified. "Backward heart failure" is caused by increased filling pressure, which affects the pulmonary venous circulation and causes shortness of breath and paroxysmal nocturnal dyspnea. Increased filling pressure also can affect the systemic venous circulation and cause edema and ascites. "Forward heart failure" is caused by low cardiac output, which produces symptoms of fatigue and lethargy. Most patients have a combination of the symptoms of backward and forward heart failure.

Myocardial dysfunction causing heart failure may manifest as impaired contractile function (systolic dysfunction), resulting in low stroke volume. Abnormal diastolic filling also is usually present and is as important as systolic dysfunction in causing the signs and symptoms of heart failure. However, a number of patients who present with heart failure have normal systolic function; diastolic dysfunction is predominantly the cause of their heart failure.

- Heart failure is the inability of the heart to meet the metabolic demands of the body while maintaining normal filling pressures.

- The most common cause of heart failure is left ventricular myocardial contractile dysfunction (systolic dysfunction).
- High ventricular filling pressures cause dyspnea and edema (backward heart failure).
- Reduced cardiac output (forward heart failure) causes fatigue and lethargy.
- Diastolic dysfunction is as important as systolic dysfunction in causing signs and symptoms of heart failure.
- A number of patients with diastolic dysfunction and heart failure have normal systolic function.

Ventricular diastolic function is a complex process. Three of its major components are relaxation, passive filling, and atrial contraction. Relaxation is an active, energy-requiring process in which calcium is removed from the actin-myosin filaments, causing contracted muscle to return to its original length. After relaxation, filling of the ventricle continues along the pressure gradient from the left atrium to the left ventricle (passive filling). The amount of filling during this phase is determined by left atrial pressure and left ventricular compliance; compliance is the increase in ventricular volume per unit of driving pressure. Thus, abnormally low compliance impairs filling and produces high end-diastolic pressure. The contribution from atrial contraction further increases ventricular volume by as much as 15% to 20% in normal subjects and 45% to 50% in those with abnormal ventricular relaxation and passive filling (Table 3-20).

Table 3-20   Abnormal Diastolic Function in Myocardial Disease

Phase	Influencing factors	Treatment
Relaxation	Ischemia, hypertrophy	Treat ischemia, hypertension
Passive filling	Myocardial compliance, heart rate	Slow heart rate
Atrial contraction	Atrial contraction, atrioventricular synchrony	Maintain sinus rhythm

- Three major components of ventricular diastolic function are relaxation, passive filling, and atrial contraction.
- Relaxation is impaired in myopathic ventricles.
- Impaired ventricular compliance means higher pressures are needed to produce volume changes.
- Atrial contraction takes on greater importance in patients with reduced ventricular relaxation or compliance.

Etiology

The mechanism and cause of heart failure must be defined to select proper therapy. A simple categorical framework is given in Table 3-21.

Clinically, the most common cause of heart failure is left ventricular myocardial contractile dysfunction. Because the treatment and prognosis are different for other causes of heart failure, accurate diagnosis is essential and is made on the basis of physical examination and noninvasive testing, such as echocardiography or radionuclide angiography.

Precipitating Factors

The appearance or worsening of heart failure symptoms may merely represent natural disease progression. Often, however, one or more precipitating factors are responsible for symptomatic deterioration (Table 3-22). If these factors are not identified and corrected, symptoms of heart failure frequently return after initial therapy. The most common precipitants are dietary indiscretion (sodium, fluid, alcohol) and medication noncompliance (cost, regimen complexity, patient understanding). The evaluation of each patient with heart failure follows these steps: 1) a medical history (include sodium and fluid intake, medication use and compliance, and sleep history from bedroom partners), 2) chest radiography to look for pneumonitis, 3) electrocardiography and creatine kinase-MB or troponin blood tests to document the rhythm and identify ischemia or myocardial injury, and 4) culture specimens of blood, urine, and sputum as appropriate. Other tests should include determination of complete blood cell count and thyroid-stimulating hormone, creatinine, and arterial blood gas values (if pulmonary embolus is a clinical concern).

- For different causes of heart failure, treatment and prognosis are different.

Table 3-21   Causes of Heart Failure and Treatment

Cause	Treatment
Myocardial	
Dilated cardiomyopathy (including ischemic)	Angiotensin-converting enzyme inhibitors, nitrates, digoxin, diuretics, nitrates and hydralazine in combination, transplantation, coronary revascularization, left ventricular aneurysmectomy, β-adrenergic blockers (carvedilol, metoprolol, bisoprolol), amlodipine
Hypertrophic cardiomyopathy	β-Adrenergic blockers, verapamil, disopyramide, surgical myectomy, dual-chamber pacing
Restrictive cardiomyopathy	Diuretics, heart transplant, treatment of underlying systemic disease
Pericardial	
Tamponade	Pericardiocentesis
Constrictive pericarditis	Pericardiectomy
Valvular	Valve repair or replacement
Hypertension	Antihypertensive treatment
Pulmonary hypertension	Heart-lung transplant, calcium channel blockers, prostacyclin infusion
High output	Correction of underlying cause
Hyperthyroidism, Paget disease	
Arteriovenous fistula	

Table 3-22   Precipitating Factors in Heart Failure

Diet (excessive sodium or fluid intake, alcohol)
Noncompliance with medication or inadequate dosing
Sodium-retaining medications (NSAIDs)
Infection (bacterial or viral)
Myocardial ischemia or infarction
Arrhythmia (atrial fibrillation, bradycardia)
Breathing disorders of sleep
Anemia
Metabolic (hyperthyroidism, hypothyroidism, chronic renal
  failure)
Pulmonary embolus

NSAIDs, nonsteroidal anti-inflammatory drugs.

- For every patient with heart failure, precipitating factors must be sought and treated.

Acute Heart Failure Syndromes

Acute heart failure syndromes usually present as pulmonary edema with or without shock. The most common cause is ischemic heart disease; less common causes include uncontrolled hypertension, progressive valvular disease, or infective endocarditis. Evaluation and treatment often proceed simultaneously. Testing includes hematologic studies; determination of electrolyte, cardiac enzyme, creatinine, and arterial blood gas values; chest radiography; electrocardiography; and echocardiography (if the mechanism of heart failure is clinically indeterminate). Initial treatment includes oxygen, intravenous loop diuretic, and morphine sulfate. Angiography should be considered for active ischemia or an evolving infarction.

CARDIOMYOPATHIES

According to the 1995 World Health Organization Task Force, a cardiomyopathy is a disease of myocardium associated with cardiac dysfunction. Major categories are dilated, hypertrophic, restrictive, arrhythmogenic right ventricular, and unclassified cardiomyopathies. The task force also defined several specific cardiomyopathies, but pathophysiologically all of these behave as dilated, hypertrophic, or restrictive cardiomyopathies. The different anatomical and pathophysiologic processes for each cardiomyopathy are listed in Table 3-23.

Dilated Cardiomyopathy

Etiology

The major abnormality in dilated cardiomyopathy is decreased systolic function (low ejection fraction) with enlargement of the left ventricular cavity and often increased left ventricular end-diastolic pressure due to coexistent diastolic dysfunction. The increased filling pressures and low cardiac output produce symptoms of shortness of breath and fatigue.

A true dilated cardiomyopathy is indicated by left ventricular dysfunction without any known cause. Many of these are genetic; an affected family member can be identified in up to 30% of cases. Other causes of severe left ventricular dysfunction include severe coronary artery disease ("hibernating myocardium"), multiple areas of previous infarction, uncontrolled hypertension, ethanol abuse, hyperthyroidism or hypothyroidism, postpartum cardiomyopathy, toxins and drugs, tachycardia-induced cardiomyopathy, infiltrative cardiomyopathy (i.e., hemochromatosis, sarcoidosis, or amyloidosis, but in amyloidosis, restrictive cardiomyopathy is more common), acquired immunodeficiency syndrome (AIDS), and pheochromocytoma.

- In dilated cardiomyopathy, the major abnormality is decreased systolic function (low ejection fraction).
- There is a genetic link in dilated cardiomyopathy (up to 30% of cases).
- Other causes of severe left ventricular dysfunction: severe coronary artery disease ("hibernating myocardium"),

Table 3-23   Anatomical and Pathophysiologic Processes for Each Cardiomyopathy

Type	Left ventricular cavity size	Left ventricular wall thickness	Systolic function	Diastolic function	Other
Dilated cardiomyopathy	↑	N/↑	↓	↓/N	
Hypertrophic cardiomyopathy	↓/N	↑	↑	↓	Left ventricular outflow obstruction
Restrictive cardiomyopathy	N/↑	N	N	↓	

↓, decreased; N, normal; ↑, increased.

multiple areas of previous infarction, uncontrolled hypertension, ethanol abuse, hyperthyroidism or hypothyroidism, postpartum cardiomyopathy, toxins and drugs, tachycardia-induced cardiomyopathy, infiltrative cardiomyopathy (i.e., hemochromatosis, sarcoidosis, or amyloidosis), AIDS, and pheochromocytoma.

Clinical Presentation

The presentation of dilated cardiomyopathy is highly variable. The patient may be asymptomatic, in which case the diagnosis is made on the basis of examination, chest radiography, electrocardiography (ECG), or echocardiography. Patients may have symptoms of mild to severe heart failure (New York Heart Association [NYHA] functional class II-IV). Other patients may present with the sudden onset of a systemic embolus. Atrial and ventricular arrhythmias are common in dilated cardiomyopathy. The following may be found on physical examination: jugular venous pressure is increased (if there is right heart involvement), low-volume upstroke of the carotid artery, displaced and sustained left ventricular impulse (possibly with a rapid filling wave), audible third or fourth heart sounds, and an apical systolic murmur of mitral regurgitation. Pulmonary examination is often normal but may reveal crackles or evidence of pleural effusion.

- Presentation of dilated cardiomyopathy is highly variable.
- Carotid volume is low, third heart sound is often present, and the apex is displaced and sustained.

ECG frequently shows left ventricular hypertrophy, intraventricular conduction delay, or left bundle branch block. Rhythm abnormalities may include premature atrial contractions, atrial fibrillation, premature ventricular contractions, or short bursts of ventricular tachycardia. The chest radiograph often shows left ventricular enlargement and pulmonary venous congestion. The diagnosis is made on the basis of reduced ejection fraction measured by echocardiography, radionuclide angiography, or left ventriculography.

- ECG may show left ventricular hypertrophy, intraventricular conduction delay, or left bundle branch block.
- Atrial and ventricular rhythm disturbances are common.
- The chest radiograph often shows left ventricular enlargement and pulmonary venous congestion.
- The diagnosis requires demonstration of reduced ejection fraction.

Evaluation

After impaired left ventricular contractile function is diagnosed, treatable secondary causes of left ventricular dysfunction should be excluded. Sensitive thyroid-stimulating hormone level should be determined to exclude hyperthyroidism or hypothyroidism. Iron and iron-binding capacities should be measured to screen for hemochromatosis. The serum angiotensin-converting enzyme level should be measured if sarcoidosis is a possibility. The metanephrine level should be measured if there is a history of severe labile hypertension or unusual spells. A history of ethanol or drug abuse must be sought.

In severe coronary artery disease, reversible left ventricular dysfunction can be caused by hibernating myocardium. In this situation, long-standing diffuse ischemia depletes adenosine triphosphate stores in myocardial cells, which are thus functionally inactive. However, with revascularization, left ventricular function may gradually improve. Identifying affected patients is difficult. Currently, the reference standard is positron emission tomography (PET), which can demonstrate metabolic activity. Viability protocols used in stress echocardiography and radionuclide perfusion imaging are more widely available than PET and are also useful in identifying hibernating myocardium.

Tachycardia-induced cardiomyopathy can occur in patients with prolonged periods of tachycardia (usually atrial fibrillation, flutter, or incessant atrial tachycardia). This is an important cause to establish because systolic dysfunction can be completely reversed after the tachycardia is treated.

- After depressed left ventricular function is diagnosed, seek treatable causes of reversible left ventricular dysfunction.
- Perform blood tests for thyroid dysfunction, sarcoid, and hemochromatosis, which are reversible causes of cardiomyopathy.
- Hibernating myocardium is a reversible cause of left ventricular dysfunction.
- Tachycardia-induced cardiomyopathy is reversible.

Some patients have left ventricular dysfunction caused by acute myocarditis. The natural history of these patients is unknown. Many patients have development of permanent left ventricular dysfunction, whereas others experience improvement with time. Thus, it is necessary to remeasure left ventricular function 3 to 6 months after making the diagnosis and initiating treatment. Although endomyocardial biopsy may help diagnose myocarditis, immunosuppressive therapy has not been demonstrated to improve outcome and should be reserved for patients with concomitant skeletal myositis or clinical deterioration despite standard pharmacologic therapy.

Pathophysiology

For understanding the treatment of heart failure associated with dilated cardiomyopathy, the hemodynamic, pathophysiologic, and biologic aspects of heart failure must be appreciated.

Preload can be thought of as the ventricular end-diastolic volume. The relationship of stroke volume to preload is shown on the Starling curve in Figure 3-33. *Afterload* is the tension, force, or stress acting on the fibers of the ventricular wall after the onset of shortening. Left ventricular afterload is increased by aortic stenosis and systemic hypertension but is decreased by mitral regurgitation. Importantly, afterload is increased by ventricular enlargement and therefore the compensatory preload adjustment to contractile dysfunction has a putative effect on stroke volume via its effects on afterload.

Figure 3-34 illustrates the neurohumoral response to decreased myocardial contractility. Decreased cardiac output activates baroreceptors and the sympathetic nervous system. Sympathetic nervous system stimulation causes an increased heart rate and contractility. Alpha-stimulation of the arterioles causes an increase in afterload. The renin-angiotensin system is activated by sympathetic stimulation, decreased renal blood flow, and decreased renal sodium. This system in turn activates aldosterone, causing increased renal retention of sodium and, thus, more pulmonary congestion. A low rate of renal blood flow results in renal retention of sodium. An increased level of angiotensin II causes vasoconstriction and an increase in afterload. In congestive heart failure, the compensatory mechanisms that increase preload eventually cause a malcompensatory increase in afterload, in turn causing further decrease in stroke volume.

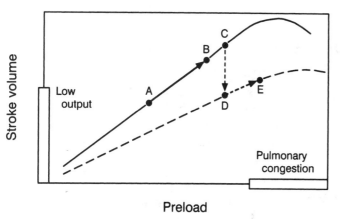

Fig. 3-33. Starling curve. Solid line is patient with normal contractility, and dotted line is one with depressed systolic function. Normally, stroke volume depends on preload of the heart. Increasing preload increases stroke volume (*A* to *B*). Myocardial dysfunction causes a shift of the curve downward and to the right (*C* to *D*), causing a severe decrease in stroke volume, which leads to symptoms of fatigue and lethargy. The compensatory response to decrease in stroke volume is an increase in preload (*D* to *E*). Because the diastolic pressure-volume relationship is curvilinear, increased left ventricular volume produces increased left ventricular end-diastolic pressure, causing symptoms of pulmonary congestion. Note flat portion of the curve at its upper end; here, there is little increase in stroke volume for increase in preload.

Finally, neurohormonal (adrenergic, angiotensin II) and other signaling pathways (endothelin, tissue necrosis factor-α, stretch, and wall stress) lead to altered myocyte gene expression (and thus impaired myocyte function) and progressive myocyte loss. These contribute to the progressive myocardial dysfunction and remodeling, which are the natural history of untreated myocardial dysfunction.

- An increase in preload causes an increase in stroke volume.
- An increase in afterload causes a decrease in stroke volume.
- Either an increase in afterload or a decrease in myocardial contractility can shift the Starling curve downward and to the right.
- Initial compensatory neurohormonal mechanisms lead to long-term malcompensatory increase in afterload, with a further decrease in stroke volume.
- The biologic aspects of myocyte dysfunction help explain the benefits of angiotensin-converting enzyme inhibitor and β-adrenergic blocker therapy.

Treatment

For treatment of dilated cardiomyopathy, it is important to identify and remove precipitating factors. Treatment of congestive heart failure in patients with dilated cardiomyopathy should be based on the pathophysiologic mechanisms described above (Fig. 3-35).

Nonpharmacologic treatment is crucial to patient management. It includes sodium and fluid restriction, avoidance of alcohol, daily patient monitoring of weight (with a definition of, and plan for responding to, excessive gain), and regular aerobic exercise. Ongoing patient and family education and regular outpatient follow-up (often with nurse specialists) reduce heart failure exacerbations, emergency room visits, and hospitalizations.

The mainstays of therapy are angiotensin-converting enzyme (ACE) inhibitors. By blocking conversion of angiotensin I to angiotensin II, ACE inhibitors decrease afterload by inhibition of angiotensin II and decrease sodium retention by inhibition of aldosterone. ACE inhibitors also directly affect myocyte gene expression, growth, and remodeling. Overall, ACE inhibitors provide symptomatic improvement in patients with NYHA functional class II-IV failure and improve mortality in patients with moderate and severe heart failure. In asymptomatic patients, ACE inhibitors prevent onset of heart failure and reduce the need for hospitalization.

- ACE inhibitors decrease afterload, decrease sodium retention, and directly reduce adverse biologic effects on myocytes.
- ACE inhibitor use decreases mortality in patients with moderate and severe heart failure.
- ACE inhibitors provide symptomatic improvement in patients with NYHA class II-IV heart failure symptoms.

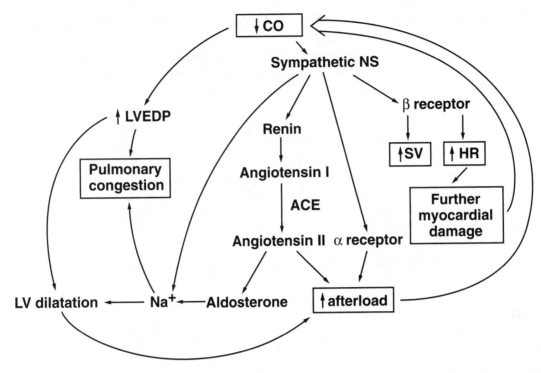

Fig. 3-34. Neurohormonal response to decreased myocardial contractility. ACE, angiotensin-converting enzyme; CO, cardiac output; HR, heart rate; LV, left ventricle; LVEDP, left ventricular end-diastolic pressure; NS, nervous system; SV, stroke volume.

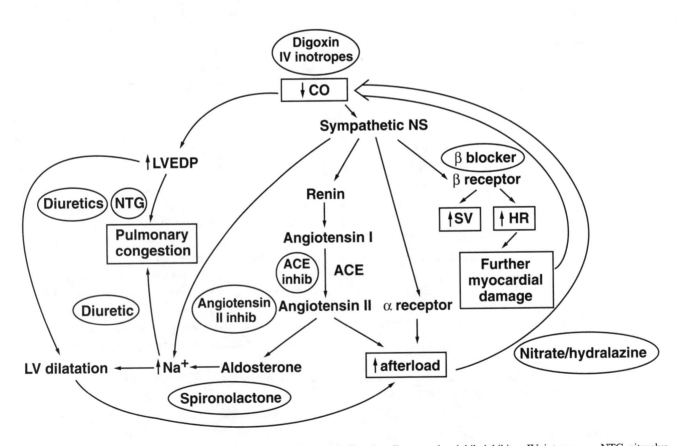

Fig. 3-35. The effect of various drugs used to treat heart failure in patients with dilated cardiomyopathy. inhib, inhibitor; IV, intravenous; NTG, nitroglycerin. Other abbreviations as in Figure 3-34.

• In asymptomatic patients, ACE inhibitors reduce the incidence of heart failure and reduce the need for hospitalization.

ACE inhibitors are given initially in small doses because of possible hypotensive effects. Dosage should be titrated up as tolerated on the basis of symptoms, blood pressure, and potassium and creatinine measurements. Even if a patient is clinically compensated on a low or intermediate ACE inhibitor dose, upward dose adjustment as tolerated is beneficial. For optimal ACE inhibitor doses to be achieved, the diuretic dose may need to be reduced. Common side effects of ACE inhibitors include hypotension, hyperkalemia, azotemia, cough, angioedema (mild or severe), and dysgeusia.

• ACE inhibitor doses are initially low but should be titrated upward; concomitant diuretic dose may need reduction.
• ACE inhibitor side effects: hypotension, hyperkalemia, azotemia, cough, angioedema, and dysgeusia.

Although less well studied than ACE inhibitors, direct angiotensin II receptor blockers provide similar hemodynamic benefits to patients with dilated cardiomyopathy. They cause less cough and angioedema than ACE inhibitors and should be tried in patients who cannot tolerate ACE inhibitors because of these bradykinin-mediated side effects.

Drugs that directly affect contractility include digoxin and phosphodiesterase inhibitors (milrinone and amrinone). Digoxin provides symptomatic relief when the ejection fraction is less than 40%, but it does not improve survival. Because digoxin is excreted by the kidneys, its dosage needs to be decreased with increased levels of creatinine and in older patients. The typical dosage is 0.25 mg/day but should be decreased to 0.125 mg/day if creatinine clearance is less than 70 mL/min • m^2 body surface area. In patients with chronic renal failure, the digoxin dose is adjusted on the basis of trough digoxin levels. Because of drug-drug interactions, digoxin dosage should be decreased with concomitant administration of quinidine, verapamil, and amiodarone. Although short-term parenteral inotropic agents (milrinone and amrinone) may improve symptoms, long-term use increases mortality and therefore these drugs should be used transiently and only in severe cases of congestive heart failure.

• Digoxin and phosphodiesterase inhibitors (milrinone and amrinone) directly affect contractility.
• Digoxin dosage needs to be decreased in azotemic and older patients.
• Digoxin dosage should be decreased with concomitant administration of quinidine, verapamil, and amiodarone.

Diuretics should be used only in patients with symptoms of pulmonary congestion or physical or radiographic evidence of fluid overload. Regular diuretic use causes neurohormonal activation and electrolyte imbalances. Mild fluid overload is initially treated with thiazide diuretics if renal function is normal. Loop diuretics are needed if there is significant fluid overload, renal dysfunction, or fluid overload resistant to thiazides. Occasionally, a combination of thiazides and loop diuretics is needed for severe fluid retention. The addition of spironolactone can help in patients with hypokalemia and may provide additional benefit by blocking aldosterone-mediated sodium retention. It has demonstrated survival benefit when added to standard therapy in patients with dilated cardiomyopathy and severe congestive heart failure; however, potassium must be carefully monitored.

Nitrates reduce preload and afterload through venodilatation. They also are anti-ischemic agents, may improve endothelial function, and combat ventricular remodeling. They should be given with a nitrate-free interval to prevent nitrate tolerance. Hydralazine may potentiate nitrate therapy by reducing nitrate tolerance when they are used in combination.

The combination of high-dose nitrates and hydralazine provides symptomatic improvement and improved mortality in patients with heart failure. However, the rate of intolerance to the necessary doses of medications is high, and their demonstrated mortality benefit is less than that achieved with ACE inhibitors.

• Diuretics and nitrates reduce pulmonary congestion.
• Nitrates reduce preload and afterload.
• Nitrate tolerance is best avoided by providing a nitrate-free interval.
• The combination of nitrates and hydralazine improves symptoms and mortality.

β-Adrenergic blockers have now been shown to be beneficial (symptoms, ejection fraction, mortality) as an adjunct to standard therapy with ACE inhibitors, digoxin, and diuretics in the treatment of patients with dilated cardiomyopathy. Although acutely they may have unwanted hemodynamic effects (negative inotropes, attenuation of heart rate response that may be maintaining cardiac output in the setting of reduced stroke volume), they provide long-term (may take up to 6 months) benefit by modifying the unfavorable biologic effects of enhanced adrenergic tone. These drugs should not be given to patients with decompensated heart failure and are most useful for patients with NYHA class II or III symptoms. Their role in asymptomatic left ventricular dysfunction is uncertain. Initial dosing should be low, clinical follow-up should be close, and upward titration of the β-blocker dose should be slow and cautious. Well-studied β-blockers in patients with heart failure include metoprolol, carvedilol, and bisoprolol (although only carvedilol currently has the approval of the U.S. Food and Drug Administration for the treatment of heart failure).

- β-Blockers have been shown to be effective as adjunctive therapy to ACE inhibitors, digoxin, and diuretics in patients with dilated cardiomyopathy.
- β-Blockers have a long-term beneficial effect on ventricular function and slow or reverse pathologic remodeling in dilated cardiomyopathy.
- β-Blockers need to be given carefully to avoid left ventricular decompensation.

A 48-hour infusion of dobutamine may give symptomatic relief, but the effect is often temporary and mortality may be increased. The infusion should be given with continuous ECG monitoring to look for arrhythmia. The usual dosage is 10 to 25 µg/kg per minute to get the resting heart rate 15 to 20 beats per minute above baseline. Dobutamine may replenish low catecholamine stores. Milrinone may also be used in this fashion and is preferred over dobutamine in patients who are chronically receiving β-blockers. Those therapies are reserved for severely symptomatic patients who are unresponsive to other therapies; they may receive continuous outpatient infusions.

- A 48-hour infusion of dobutamine or milrinone may give temporary symptomatic relief.
- Dobutamine and milrinone may cause increased mortality.

Amlodipine and felodipine are safe in patients with dilated cardiomyopathy but do not provide any survival benefit. First-generation calcium channel blockers (verapamil, diltiazem, nifedipine), however, are relatively contraindicated because of their negative inotropic effects.

Anticoagulation with warfarin is recommended for patients in atrial fibrillation and those with intracardiac thrombus or a history of systemic or pulmonary thromboembolism. Aspirin may diminish the benefits of ACE inhibitors by blocking prostaglandin-induced vasodilatation. Accordingly, most advise aspirin use in small doses only in patients with coronary artery disease.

- Anticoagulation with warfarin is recommended in patients with atrial fibrillation, intracardiac thrombus, or a history of thromboembolism.
- Aspirin therapy should be reserved for patients with coronary artery disease.

The prognosis for patients with dilated cardiomyopathy varies with functional class. Even with standard therapy, patients who have mild to moderate heart failure have a 40% mortality at 4 years, whereas patients with severe heart failure have a 1-year mortality of up to 35%. Patients with asymptomatic left ventricular systolic dysfunction do well initially but have a 40% mortality at 7 years, a finding emphasizing the need to treat these patients aggressively with ACE inhibitors. The long-term prognosis in patients treated with β-blockers in addition to "standard" therapy has not been defined. Heart transplantation is the procedure of choice for patients with severe dilated cardiomyopathy and severe symptoms. With successful transplantation, the 1-year survival is 90%. The major contraindication for transplantation in an otherwise healthy patient is a high pulmonary arteriolar resistance. In the United States, donor availability is the major limiting factor. Long-term complications after heart transplantation include rejection, infection, hypertension, hyperlipidemia, malignancy, and accelerated coronary vasculopathy.

- The 1-year mortality is 35% for patients with severely symptomatic dilated cardiomyopathy receiving standard medical therapy.
- Patients with asymptomatic dilated cardiomyopathy have increased mortality.
- The procedure of choice for patients with severely symptomatic dilated cardiomyopathy is heart transplantation. With successful transplantation, 1-year survival is 90%.

Recapitulation of Drug Therapy for Heart Failure
- ACE inhibitors improve symptoms and decrease mortality in patients with symptomatic dilated cardiomyopathy.
- ACE inhibitors prevent deterioration and subsequent hospitalizations in patients with asymptomatic dilated cardiomyopathy.
- The combination of high-dose nitrates and hydralazine improves symptoms and survival (although the survival benefit is less than with ACE inhibitors), but intolerance to the high doses limits their usefulness.
- Nitrates should be used with a nitrate-free interval to prevent nitrate tolerance.
- Digoxin is useful for symptomatic treatment of patients with dilated cardiomyopathy but provides no survival benefit.
- Phosphodiesterase inhibitors and prolonged infusion of dobutamine directly increase contractility and may improve symptoms transiently, but they probably increase mortality.
- β-Blockers are beneficial when given (in addition to ACE inhibitors, digoxin, and diuretics) to patients with NYHA class II-III heart failure.

Hypertrophic Cardiomyopathy

Etiology
Hypertrophic cardiomyopathy is a genetically and phenotypically heterogeneous family of disorders characterized by

defects involving myocyte proteins with hypertrophy as a compensatory response. There is usually dynamic left ventricular outflow tract obstruction, but 20% to 40% of patients have no obstruction. The diagnosis is currently based on the echocardiographic finding of severe hypertrophy of the myocardium in the absence of a secondary cause, such as hypertension, aortic stenosis, chronic renal failure, or infiltrative disease (although in the future it will increasingly become a diagnosis made with genetic testing). Because hypertrophic cardiomyopathy is a hereditary disease, all patients should have their first-degree relatives screened, and genetic counseling is advised for potential parents.

- Hypertrophic cardiomyopathy is a heterogeneous family of disorders of myocyte proteins with compensatory myocardial hypertrophy.
- Dynamic left ventricular outflow tract obstruction occurs in 60%-80% of patients.
- Diagnosis is based on the echocardiographic finding of severe myocardial hypertrophy in the absence of a secondary cause.
- Family screening and genetic counseling are advised.

Symptoms

Hypertrophic cardiomyopathy has several different manifestations. There appears to be a bimodal age distribution of presentation. Young males (usually in the teens or early 20s) have a high propensity for syncope and sudden death. Older patients (in their 50s and 60s) present with symptoms of shortness of breath and angina and may have a better prognosis than young patients. The classic presentation of the younger group is a young athlete undergoing a physical examination to participate in sports who is found to have a heart murmur or left ventricular hypertrophy on ECG. The classic presentation of the older group is an older woman in whom pulmonary edema develops after noncardiac surgery and whose condition worsens with diuresis, afterload reduction, and inotropic support (all of which worsen dynamic left ventricular outflow tract obstruction). The classic symptom triad is syncope, angina, and dyspnea (symptoms similar to those of valvular aortic stenosis). Some hypertensive patients have a small hyperdynamic left ventricle with hypertrophy and dynamic left ventricular outflow tract obstruction—"hypertensive-hypertrophic cardiomyopathy." Although the pathophysiology is the same as in hypertrophic cardiomyopathy, these patients are not at increased risk for sudden death and ventricular fibrillation.

There is a 1.5% per year frequency of evolution from hypertrophic to dilated cardiomyopathy. This may reflect either the natural history or a superimposed secondary process such as ischemia. The treatment of a "burnt-out hypertroph" is then the same as that for other dilated cardiomyopathies.

- The classic presentation of hypertrophic cardiomyopathy is the triad of angina, syncope, and dyspnea.
- There is a bimodal distribution of presentation: young males with high incidence of sudden death and older patients with dyspnea and angina.
- The prognosis for older patients may be better than that for younger patients.
- Patients with hypertension may have hypertrophy and dynamic left ventricular outflow tract obstruction similar to those of patients with hypertrophic cardiomyopathy.

Pathophysiology

Signs and symptoms of hypertrophic cardiomyopathy are caused by four major abnormalities: diastolic dysfunction, left ventricular outflow tract obstruction, mitral regurgitation, and ventricular arrhythmias.

Diastolic dysfunction is caused by many mechanisms. Severe hypertrophy and increased muscle mass produce decreased compliance so that there is increased pressure per unit volume entering the left ventricle during diastole. Marked abnormality in calcium metabolism causes abnormal ventricular relaxation. High afterload due to left ventricular tract obstruction also delays ventricular relaxation. All these events cause increased left ventricular diastolic pressure, which leads to angina and dyspnea.

In many patients, dynamic left ventricular tract obstruction is caused by the hypertrophied septum encroaching into the left ventricular outflow tract. This subsequently "sucks in" the anterior leaflet of the mitral valve (systolic anterior motion), creating left ventricular outflow tract obstruction. Because of this pathophysiologic process, dynamic outflow tract obstruction increases dramatically with decreased preload, decreased afterload, or increased contractility.

Systolic anterior motion of the mitral valve distorts the mitral valve apparatus during systole and may cause significant mitral regurgitation. The degree of mitral regurgitation is also dynamically influenced by the degree of left ventricular outflow tract obstruction. Patients with severe mitral regurgitation usually have severe symptoms of dyspnea.

Because of cellular disarray in patients with hypertrophic cardiomyopathy, the electrical conduction system is dispersed, leading to a high propensity for ventricular arrhythmias. The frequent occurrence of ventricular arrhythmias may cause sudden death or syncope.

- A major pathophysiologic abnormality in patients with hypertrophic cardiomyopathy is diastolic dysfunction.
- Left ventricular outflow tract obstruction and mitral regurgitation are caused by distortion of the mitral valve apparatus (systolic anterior motion), and they are dynamically influenced by preload, afterload, and contractility.

● The propensity for ventricular arrhythmias causing syncope and sudden death is high.

Examination

Hypertrophic cardiomyopathy is suspected on the basis of abnormal carotid artery upstroke and left ventricular impulse. The carotid artery upstroke is rapid compared with that of patients with aortic stenosis. If left ventricular outflow tract obstruction is extensive, the carotid artery upstroke has a bifid quality. The left ventricular impulse is sustained, indicating considerable left ventricular hypertrophy. It frequently has a palpable "a" wave. Patients with excessive left ventricular outflow tract obstruction may have a triple apical impulse. The first heart sound is normal, and the second heart sound is paradoxically split. A loud systolic ejection murmur indicates left ventricular outflow tract obstruction. The murmur changes in intensity with changes in loading conditions (Table 3-24). A holosystolic murmur of mitral regurgitation may be present; it increases in intensity with increases in the dynamic left ventricular outflow tract obstruction. Maneuvers affect the mitral regurgitant murmur of hypertrophic obstructive cardiomyopathy differently than other mitral regurgitant murmurs. When mitral regurgitation is not due to hypertrophic obstructive cardiomyopathy, it increases with increasing afterload and varies little with changes in

Table 3-24 Dynamic Left Ventricular Outflow Tract Obstruction

Increased obstruction
Decreased afterload
Amyl nitrite
Vasodilators
Increased contractility
Postpremature ventricular contraction beat
Digoxin
Dopamine
Decreased preload
Squat-to-stand
Nitrates
Diuretics
Valsalva maneuver (strain phase)
Decreased obstruction
Increased afterload
Handgrip
Stand-to-squat
Decreased contractility
β-Blockers
Verapamil
Disopyramide
Increased preload
Fluids

contractility and preload. When mitral regurgitation is due to hypertrophic cardiomyopathy, however, increased afterload decreases the dynamic left ventricular outflow obstruction and thus the amount of secondary mitral regurgitation.

In patients with hypertrophic obstructive cardiomyopathy, the ejection murmur increases in intensity, whereas the arterial pulse volume decreases on the beat following a premature ventricular contraction. This is called the Brockenbrough sign, and it is due to post-ectopic increased contractility and decreased afterload, resulting in more dynamic obstruction. In contradistinction, in patients with fixed left ventricular outflow tract obstruction (e.g., aortic stenosis), both the murmur intensity and the pulse volume increase with the beat following a premature contraction.

● The diagnosis of hypertrophic cardiomyopathy is suspected by palpating a sustained left ventricular impulse and rapid upstroke of the carotid artery.
● The outflow murmur intensity and carotid upstroke change with changes in loading conditions of the heart.
● In hypertrophic obstructive cardiomyopathy, the secondary mitral regurgitation murmur changes in the same direction as that of the left ventricular outflow obstruction murmur under different loading conditions. This differs from the auscultatory findings when mitral regurgitation is due to other conditions.

Diagnostic Testing

Patients with hypertrophic cardiomyopathy usually have an abnormal ECG, which shows considerable left ventricular hypertrophy (Fig. 3-36). Because ECG abnormalities may precede echocardiographically detected phenotypic expression, surveillance echocardiography is appropriate in patients with suspicious ECG results. Apical hypertrophic cardiomyopathy is a variant of hypertrophic cardiomyopathy in which the hypertrophy is localized at the apex of the left ventricle. Although patients with apical hypertrophic cardiomyopathy do not have outflow tract obstruction (no murmur or secondary mitral regurgitation), they do have diastolic dysfunction and a predisposition to ventricular arrhythmias. The ECG in these patients typically has large, diffuse, symmetric T-wave inversions across the precordium (Fig. 3-37).

Hypertrophic cardiomyopathy is diagnosed with echocardiography, which shows severe hypertrophy of the myocardium (left ventricular wall thickness >16 mm in diastole) without any known cause. Formerly, asymmetric septal hypertrophy was required for the diagnosis, but it is now recognized that hypertrophy can be in any part of the myocardium. Doppler echocardiography can be used to diagnose left ventricular outflow tract obstruction, measure its severity, and detect mitral regurgitation. Cardiac catheterization is no longer necessary

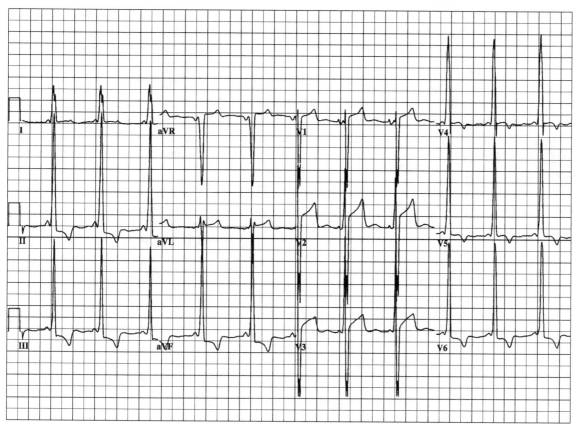

Fig. 3-36. Electrocardiogram in hypertrophic cardiomyopathy, showing marked left ventricular hypertrophy.

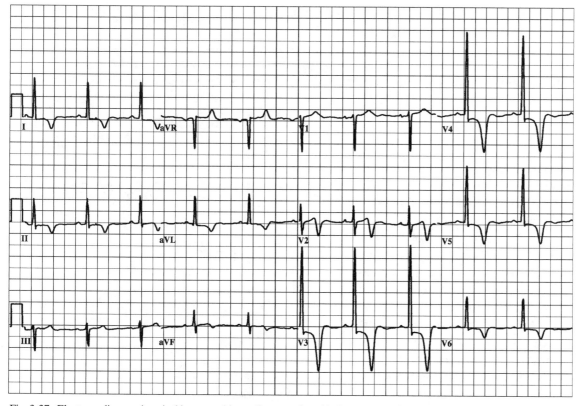

Fig. 3-37. Electrocardiogram in apical hypertrophic cardiomyopathy with deep symmetric T-wave inversions in precordial leads.

for diagnosing dynamic left ventricular outflow tract obstruction because all diagnostic data can be obtained by two-dimensional and Doppler echocardiography.

Sudden death is a problem in patients with hypertrophic cardiomyopathy. Because of a strong association between ventricular arrhythmias and sudden death, 48- to 72-hour Holter monitoring is recommended for all patients with hypertrophic cardiomyopathy. Predictors of sudden death include a personal or family history of sudden death, left ventricular hypertrophy, ventricular tachycardia at electrophysiologic study, young male, history of syncope, and non-sustained ventricular tachycardia. Genetic markers may identify patients with a strong propensity for sudden death. In some patients, carefully supervised stress testing also is indicated to search for ventricular tachycardia, to objectify symptom threshold, and to evaluate the variables contributing to symptoms.

- ECG usually shows evidence of left ventricular hypertrophy in cases of hypertrophic cardiomyopathy.
- Apical hypertrophy is suspected in the presence of large symmetric inverted T-waves in precordial leads on ECG.
- The diagnosis of hypertrophic cardiomyopathy is made with echocardiography, which shows hypertrophy in the absence of any known cause.
- Predictors of sudden death: personal or family history of sudden death, young male, history of syncope, nonsustained ventricular tachycardia, massive left ventricular hypertrophy, and sustained ventricular tachycardia at electrophysiologic study.
- 48- to 72-Hour Holter monitoring recommended for all patients with hypertrophic cardiomyopathy.

Treatment

Symptomatic Patients

For symptomatic patients with hypertrophic cardiomyopathy, initial treatment is with drugs that decrease contractility in an attempt to decrease left ventricular outflow tract obstruction (Fig. 3-38). The most effective medication is a high dose of β-adrenergic blockers (>240 mg equivalent of propranolol/day). Although verapamil may be used if β-adrenergic blockade fails, it may cause sudden hemodynamic deterioration in patients with high resting left ventricular outflow tract gradients because of its vasodilating properties. Disopyramide may improve symptoms by decreasing left ventricular outflow tract obstruction, but anticholinergic side effects limit its use. All drugs that reduce afterload or preload and those that increase contractility must be avoided in patients with hypertrophic cardiomyopathy. Cautious diuretic use for volume-overloaded states is permitted.

Surgical myectomy is reserved for patients who are severely symptomatic despite optimal medical therapy and produces dramatic symptomatic relief. Mortality associated with this procedure is less than 5% overall in experienced centers and less than 1% in patients younger than 40 years. Its complications are rare but include complete heart block, aortic regurgitation, and ventricular septal defect. Myectomy is a highly operator-dependent procedure and should be performed only at medical centers that specialize in this procedure. Catheter ablation of the septum by alcohol infusion is an as yet experimental surrogate for the operative procedure.

Dual-chamber pacing is an accepted alternative to myectomy for patients with hypertrophic cardiomyopathy and severe left ventricular outflow tract obstruction. Dual-chamber pacing can produce a reduction in gradient and symptomatic improvement in some patients, but this approach is not recommended for all patients with symptomatic hypertrophic obstructive cardiomyopathy.

Asymptomatic Patients

Whether to treat asymptomatic patients with nonsustained ventricular tachycardia is a controversial subject (Fig. 3-39). No antiarrhythmic agent is uniformly effective, and any may make the arrhythmia worse. In selected patients with multiple risk factors for sudden death, empiric amiodarone or an automatic implantable cardiac defibrillator might be chosen. In patients who have already had an out-of-hospital arrest, the treatment of choice is an automatic implantable cardiac defibrillator.

- β-Adrenergic blockade is the treatment of choice for patients with symptomatic hypertrophic cardiomyopathy.
- Verapamil may cause sudden hemodynamic deterioration in patients with high resting left ventricular outflow tract obstruction because of its vasodilating properties.

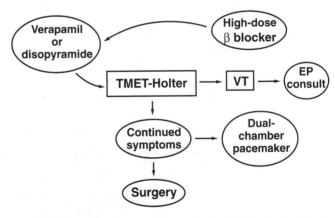

Fig. 3-38. Treatment of symptomatic patients. EP, electrophysiologic; TMET, treadmill exercise test; VT, ventricular tachycardia.

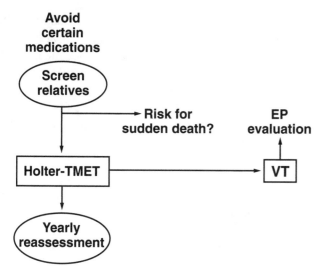

Fig. 3-39. Treatment of asymptomatic patients. Abbreviations as in Figure 3-38.

- Surgical myectomy is reserved for severely symptomatic patients unresponsive to medical therapy.
- Dual-chamber pacing is an accepted treatment strategy, but its role relative to medical management or surgical myectomy is not known.
- No antiarrhythmic agent is uniformly effective, and any may worsen the arrhythmia.
- Automatic implantable cardiac defibrillator is the treatment of choice for patients with out-of-hospital arrest.

Restrictive Cardiomyopathy

Definition

The primary abnormality in restrictive cardiomyopathy is diastolic dysfunction. Diastolic dysfunction causes abnormal left ventricular filling such that a greater than usual increase in filling pressure is required to fill the ventricle. This is reflected back to the pulmonary and systemic circulations, causing symptoms of shortness of breath and edema. In addition, the ventricle cannot fill adequately to meet its preload requirements, thus resulting in low cardiac output (Starling mechanism), fatigue, and lethargy. Normal myocardial contractile function is maintained in most patients with restrictive cardiomyopathy. However, at the end stage of the disease, there can be loss of contractile function as well.

- In restrictive cardiomyopathy, the primary abnormality is diastolic dysfunction.
- Diastolic dysfunction means a greater pressure per unit volume is required to fill the ventricle, causing dyspnea and edema.
- The left ventricle cannot fill to meet its preload requirements, causing low output, fatigue, and lethargy.

The cause of primary restrictive cardiomyopathy is unknown. There are two major categories: idiopathic restrictive cardiomyopathy and endomyocardial fibrosis. In idiopathic restrictive cardiomyopathy, there is progressive fibrosis of the myocardium. Familial cases, often with peripheral myopathy as well, have been reported. Endomyocardial fibrosis is probably an end stage of eosinophilic syndromes in which there is intracavitary thrombus filling of the left ventricle. This restricts filling and causes increased diastolic pressures. This fibrosis also may involve the mitral valve, causing severe mitral regurgitation. There may be two different forms of endomyocardial fibrosis: active inflammatory eosinophilic myocarditis in temperate zones and chronic endomyocardial fibrosis in tropical zones.

Diseases that cause infiltration of the myocardium (such as amyloidosis) have a presentation and pathophysiology similar to those of primary restrictive cardiomyopathy. Signs and symptoms similar to those of restrictive cardiomyopathy also may develop after radiation therapy, anthracycline chemotherapy, and heart transplantation. Although other infiltrative diseases (sarcoidosis, hemochromatosis) initially may mimic restrictive cardiomyopathy, they usually have progressed to a dilated cardiomyopathy by the time they cause cardiac symptoms.

- Restrictive cardiomyopathy may be idiopathic or due to infiltrative diseases (amyloidosis).
- Endomyocardial fibrosis is probably an end stage of eosinophilic syndromes.
- Secondary fibrosis may involve the mitral valve, causing severe mitral regurgitation.

Signs and Symptoms

Patients with restrictive cardiomyopathy usually present with edema, dyspnea, ascites, and low output symptoms. Atrial arrhythmias due to passive atrial enlargement are frequently present, and the patient may present with atrial fibrillation. Jugular venous pressure is almost always increased, with rapid X and Y descents. The precordium is quiet, and heart sounds are soft. There may be an apical systolic murmur of mitral regurgitation and a left sternal border murmur of tricuspid regurgitation. A third heart sound may be present. Dullness at the bases of the lungs is consistent with bilateral pleural effusions. ECG is usually low or normal voltage with atrial arrhythmias. Chest radiography shows pleural effusions with normal cardiac silhouette or atrial enlargement.

- Restrictive cardiomyopathy: biventricular failure, dyspnea, edema, and low output symptoms.
- Atrial arrhythmias are frequently present.
- Jugular venous pressure is increased, with rapid X and Y descents.

Diagnosis

Restrictive cardiomyopathy is diagnosed with echocardiography. Typical findings are normal left ventricular cavity size and function and marked enlargement of both atria. If there is right heart failure, the inferior vena cava is enlarged. Echocardiography is usually nonspecific about the cause except in two instances. First, in amyloid heart disease, echocardiography demonstrates thickened myocardium with a scintillating appearance as well as pericardial effusion and thickened regurgitant valves. Second, in endomyocardial fibrosis, there is an apical thrombus (without underlying apical akinesis) or thickening of the endocardium under the mitral valve, which often tethers the valve, causing mitral regurgitation. Cardiac catheterization shows elevation and end-equalization of all end-diastolic pressures. A typical "square-root sign" or "dip-and-plateau" pattern consistent with early rapid filling is present. Endomyocardial biopsy usually is not helpful unless there is a systemic disease that has caused infiltration of the myocardium (i.e., amyloidosis).

- Restrictive cardiomyopathy is diagnosed with echocardiography.
- Typical findings: normal left ventricular cavity size and function and marked enlargement of both atria.
- Amyloid heart disease: thickened myocardium with scintillating appearance, pericardial effusion, valvular regurgitation.
- Endomyocardial fibrosis: thrombus in left ventricular apex (without apical akinesis) or posterior mitral leaflet tethering causing mitral regurgitation.

Treatment

There is no medical treatment for idiopathic restrictive cardiomyopathy. Diuretics decrease filling pressures and give symptomatic relief, but this may be at the expense of further decreasing cardiac output. Digoxin usually is not helpful, because systolic contractility is maintained. Heart transplantation is the only proven therapy for patients with severe restrictive cardiomyopathy. Corticosteroids and cytotoxic drugs are appropriate during the early stages of eosinophilic endocarditis. Endomyocardial fibrosis can be surgically resected and the mitral valve can be replaced, although mortality is significant.

- There is no medical treatment for idiopathic restrictive cardiomyopathy.
- Diuretics decrease filling pressures.
- Digoxin usually is not helpful.
- Heart transplantation is the only proven therapy for severe restrictive cardiomyopathy.
- Medical therapy is used for early stages of eosinophilic endocarditis, and operation is used for endomyocardial fibrosis in selected cases.

It is important to differentiate restrictive cardiomyopathy from constrictive pericarditis. Both have similar presentations and findings on clinical examination and diagnostic studies. However, in constrictive pericarditis, pericardiectomy produces symptomatic improvement and, frequently, survival. Therefore, exploratory thoracotomy may be indicated in patients with normal left ventricular systolic function, large atria, and severe elevation of diastolic filling pressures if doubt remains after anatomical (fast computed tomography) and other tests (echocardiography, cardiac catheterization).

- It is important to differentiate restrictive cardiomyopathy from constrictive pericarditis.
- In constrictive pericarditis, pericardiectomy produces symptomatic improvement and may prolong survival.

Cardiology Pharmacy Review
Jeffrey J. Armon, PharmD, Narith N. Ou, PharmD, Lance J. Oyen, PharmD

Drugs Commonly Used for Cardiac Resuscitation

Drug	Primary use	Toxic/adverse effects	Comments: precautions (P) and contraindications (C)
Adenosine	Narrow complex PSVT	Chest pain, ischemia, bronchoconstriction, increased ICP, VF (infants)	Wide complex tachycardia (P) Drug/poison-induced arrest (C)
Amiodarone	Pulseless VT/VF, stable VT of unknown origin, AF	AV block, hypotension, proarrhythmias	Dose-related hypotension (P) Renal failure (P) Concomitant use of QT-prolonging drugs (e.g., procainamide) (P)
Atropine	Sinus bradycardia, type IIa AVB, asystole	Tachyarrhythmias, ischemia	Hypothermic bradycardia (C) Avoid in advanced infranodal (type II) AVB or new 3rd-degree AVB with wide QRS (C)
β-Blockers (atenolol, metoprolol, esmolol)	Myocardial infarction, supraventricular tachycardia	Bronchospasm, hypotension, bradycardia, exacerbation of heart failure	Bradycardia (<60 bpm) or 2nd- or 3rd-degree heart block (C) Poison/drug-induced arrest (C) Concomitant calcium channel blocker (P) Severe reactive airway disease (P) Wolff-Parkinson-White syndrome (P)
Calcium channel antagonists (diltiazem, verapamil)	Supraventricular tachycardia	AV block, hypotension, bradycardia, exacerbation of heart failure	Wolff-Parkinson-White syndrome (C) Ventricular arrhythmia (P) Concomitant use of β-blocker (P)
Catecholamines (dobutamine, dopamine, epinephrine, norepinephrine)	Bradycardia, hypotension (except dobutamine), asystole (epinephrine)	Hypertension, tachycardia, ischemia, arrhythmia, hypotension (dobutamine)	Evolving myocardial infarction (P) Peripheral administration may cause severe extravasation (P) Use only after volume resuscitation (P) SBP <100 mm Hg and signs of shock (dobutamine) (P)

Cardiology Pharmacy Review (continued)

Drugs Commonly Used for Cardiac Resuscitation (continued)

Drug	Primary use	Toxic/adverse effects	Comments: precautions (P) and contraindications (C)
Digoxin	Supraventricular tachycardia	Proarrhythmia	Hypokalemia, hypercalcemia, or hypomagnesemia (C) Concomitant defibrillation (P) Wolff-Parkinson-White syndrome (P) AV block (P)
Lidocaine	Ventricular tachyarrhythmias	Proarrhythmia, seizures, exacerbation of heart failure	Prophylaxis post-MI (C) Liver dysfunction or CHF (P) Evolving myocardial ischemia = more proarrhythmic (P)
Procainamide	Ventricular & supraventricular tachyarrhythmias	Proarrhythmias (torsades de pointes), hypotension, exacerbation of heart failure	Low magnesium or potassium (P) Evolving myocardial ischemia = more proarrhythmic (P) Hypotension: slow infusion important (P) Polymorphic VT (C)
Vasopressin	Pulseless VT/VF, vasodilatory shock	Bradycardia, ?ischemia	Coronary artery disease (P)

AF, atrial fibrillation; AV, atrioventricular; AVB, atrioventricular block; bpm, beats/minute; CHF, congestive heart failure; ICP, intracranial pressure; MI, myocardial infarction; PSVT, paroxysmal supraventricular tachycardia; SBP, systolic blood pressure; VF, ventricular fibrillation; VT, ventricular tachycardia.

Cardiology Pharmacy Review (continued)

Drugs Commonly Used in Cardiology

Drug	Toxic/adverse effects
Aldosterone antagonists (spironolactone, eplerenone)	Serious hyperkalemia if renally impaired, gynecomastia (less with eplerenone)
Angiotensin II receptor antagonists	Rarely angioedema (30% cross-reaction if h/o ACE inhibitor angioedema), hepatitis, headache, dizziness, fatigue
ACE inhibitors	Angioedema, renal failure, hypotension, hyperkalemia, hepatitis, neutropenia, cough, skin rashes, taste disturbance
β-Blockers	Bronchospasm, hypotension, bradycardia, decompensated heart failure, CNS effects (lipophilic agents > nonlipophilic: depression, psychosis, dizziness, weakness, fatigue, vivid dreams, insomnia), GI effects, reduced peripheral vascular perfusion, impotence, hypo-/hyperglycemia
Calcium channel antagonists	Hypotension, bradycardia (verapamil, diltiazem), worsen heart failure symptoms (verapamil, diltiazem), dizziness, flushing, peripheral edema, constipation, postural hypotension, taste disturbances
Centrally acting agents (clonidine, methyldopa)	Withdrawal hypertension, hypotension, hepatitis (methyldopa), bradycardia (clonidine), frequent CNS effects (depression, sedation), GI effects, sexual dysfunction, xerostomia (clonidine)
Digoxin	Cardiovascular effects (heart block, ectopic arrhythmias, ventricular extra beats, ventricular tachycardia, paroxysmal supraventricular tachycardia), GI effects (anorexia, nausea, vomiting, diarrhea), CNS effects (drowsiness, dizziness, confusion, vision abnormalities, photophobia)
Direct thrombin inhibitors (lepirudin, argatroban, bivalirudin)	Bleeding (no available antidote for reversal), allergic reaction to reexposure and antibody formation (lepirudin)
Hydralazine	Hypotension, hepatitis, neuropathy, flushing, GI effects, LLS
Loop diuretics	Dehydration, hypokalemia, hyponatremia, pancreatitis, jaundice, deafness (high dose), thrombocytopenia, serious skin disorders, dizziness, postural hypotension, gout
Nesiritide (Natrecor)	Dose-related hypotension, headache
Organic nitrates	Syncope, TIAs, headache, flushing, palpitations, peripheral edema
Potassium-sparing diuretics	Hyperkalemia, dehydration, GI effects (nausea, vomiting, diarrhea), CNS effects (headache, weakness), rashes, gynecomastia in men and breast enlargement/soreness in women (spironolactone)
Thiazide diuretics	Dehydration, rarely thrombocytopenia, cholestatic jaundice, pancreatitis, hepatic encephalopathy (in patients with cirrhosis), dizziness, gout, hyperglycemia, orthostasis, hypokalemia, hypermagnesemia, hypercalcemia, GI effects
Warfarin	Abnormal bleeding, rarely necrosis and/or gangrene of skin and other tissues, purple toe syndrome (cholesterol microembolization), osteoporosis

ACE, angiotensin-converting enzyme; CNS, central nervous system; GI, gastrointestinal tract; h/o, history of; LLS, lupus-like syndrome; TIA, transient ischemic attack.

Cardiology Pharmacy Review (continued)

Selected Important Cardiac Drug Interactions

Drug	Drug	Net effect and suggested actions
Amiodarone	Digoxin	Amiodarone increases serum digoxin levels
		Reduce digoxin dose by 25%-50% (monitor digoxin levels)
	Cyclosporine	Amiodarone increases serum cyclosporine
		Monitor cyclosporine levels
	Dofetilide	Amiodarone must be withdrawn for at least 3 mo or amiodarone level <0.3 mg/mL before initiating dofetilide therapy
	Fosphenytoin or phenytoin	Phenytoin level can increase × 2-3, amiodarone levels may decrease by >30%
		Monitor amiodarone effectiveness & phenytoin levels
	Procainamide	Amiodarone increases procainamide level; 20% reduction of procainamide dose is suggested
		Monitor procainamide levels; combination is rarely used
	Quinidine	Amiodarone increases quinidine levels; 50% reduction of quinidine dose is suggested
		Monitor quinidine levels; rarely used together
	Simvastatin	Amiodarone increases risk of myopathy or rhabdomyolysis with simvastatin. If >20 mg per day of simvastatin required, different agent is recommended
	Warfarin	Amiodarone increases warfarin effect
		Decrease warfarin dose by 25%-50%; monitor INR
Digoxin	Amiodarone	Amiodarone increases serum digoxin levels
		Reduce dose of digoxin by 25%-50% (monitor digoxin levels)
	Propafenone	Propafenone increases digoxin levels
		Empirically reduce digoxin dose; monitor levels and signs of increased digoxin
	Quinidine	Quinidine may increase digoxin levels
		Monitor ECG and digoxin levels
	Verapamil	Verapamil increases serum digoxin levels
		Reduction of digoxin dose may be required; monitor digoxin levels & signs of elevated digoxin
Dofetilide	Amiodarone	Torsades de pointes risk
		Amiodarone must be withdrawn for at least 3 mo or amiodarone level <0.3 mg/mL before initiating dofetilide therapy
	Class I & III antiarrhythmic agents	Torsades de pointes risk
		Washout period of at least 3 half-lives of other antiarrhythmics before starting dofetilide
	Cimetidine	Cimetidine is contraindicated because increased serum level of dofetilide = torsades de pointes effect
	Hydrochlorothiazide	Hydrochlorothiazide is contraindicated because increased serum level of dofetilide and decreased potassium = risk of torsades de pointes
	Ketoconazole	Ketoconazole is contraindicated because increased serum level of dofetilide = torsades de pointes effect

Cardiology Pharmacy Review (continued)

Selected Important Cardiac Drug Interactions (continued)

Drug	Drug	Net effect and suggested actions
Dofetilide (continued)	Megestrol	Megestrol is contraindicated because increased serum level of dofetilide = torsades de pointes effect
	Prochlorperazine	Prochlorperazine is contraindicated because increased serum level of dofetilide = torsades de pointes effect
	Trimethoprim-sulfamethoxazole	Trimethoprim-sulfamethoxazole is contraindicated because increased serum level of dofetilide = torsades de pointes risk
	Trimethoprim	Trimethoprim is contraindicated because increased serum level of dofetilide = torsades de pointes risk
	Verapamil	Verapamil is contraindicated because increased serum level of dofetilide = torsades de pointes risk
	Ziprasidone	Ziprasidone is contraindicated because increased serum level of dofetilide = risk of torsades de pointes
Propafenone	Digoxin	Propafenone increases digoxin levels
		Empirically reduce digoxin dose; monitor levels & signs of elevated digoxin
	Metoprolol	Propafenone increases metoprolol level 1.5-5 times
		Monitor cardiac function (especially blood pressure)
	Warfarin	Propafenone increases warfarin effect by 25%
		Monitor INR when adding/withdrawing propafenone
Warfarin	Amiodarone	Amiodarone increases warfarin effect
		Decrease warfarin dose by 25%-50% & monitor INR
	Cholestyramine	Cholestyramine decreases effectiveness of warfarin
		Use colestipol as alternative
	Cyclooxygenase-2 inhibitors (celecoxib [Celebrex], rofecoxib [Vioxx])	These inhibitors increase INR (monitor INR closely)
	Propafenone	Propafenone increases warfarin effect by 25%
		Monitor INR when adding/withdrawing propafenone
	Glycoprotein IIb/IIIa inhibitors (abciximab [ReoPro], eptifibatide [Integrilin], tirofiban [Aggrastat])	These inhibitors increase hemorrhagic risk (use with caution) Abciximab contraindicated if PT>1.2 × control
	Thrombolytics	Thrombolytics increase hemorrhagic risk (use with caution) Alteplase contraindicated if PT>15 s

ECG, electrocardiogram; INR, international normalized ratio; PT, prothrombin time.

QUESTIONS

Multiple Choice (choose the one best answer)

1. A 45-year-old slender man presents to your office for evaluation of chest pain. His pain does not seem to be related to exercise or physical exertion. He is a non-smoker and is not limited by dyspnea. On examination, you notice a 2/6 apical murmur radiating into the axilla. With the Valsalva maneuver, the murmur becomes more pronounced. Which additional finding is *most consistent* with your diagnosis?
   a. The murmur becomes louder with a postectopic beat
   b. Midsystolic clicks are more audible with the Valsalva maneuver
   c. A pronounced S_1 is noted
   d. A diffuse, lateralized left ventricular apical impulse is noted
   e. A postectopic beat increases the intensity of the murmur

2. To confirm the diagnosis of and to quantify the degree of mitral regurgitation in the patient described in question 1, you perform echocardiography. In addition to confirming the diagnosis, it shows that the left ventricle and left atrium are normal in size with hyperdynamic left ventricular function (ejection fraction, 72%). The degree of mitral regurgitation is deemed mild; the mitral valve leaflets show mild thickening and myxomatous degeneration. The patient is active, without specific complaints other than nonspecific chest pain, as noted in question 1. What is the most appropriate next step in the evaluation or management of this patient?
   a. Consider a treadmill exercise test to rule out underlying coronary artery disease
   b. Consider early operation to prevent unfavorable left ventricular dilatation
   c. Recommend prophylaxis for subacute bacterial endocarditis
   d. Advise that prophylaxis for subacute bacterial endocarditis is unnecessary because the mitral regurgitation is mild
   e. Recommend abstinence from physical exertion and aerobic exercise

3. A 20-year-old college student is sent to your office for an examination before joining the school's wrestling team. He is entirely asymptomatic, except for occasional headaches, particularly after exertion. On examination, you note a 3/6 early peaking systolic murmur over the left ventricular outflow tract with minimal radiation to the carotid arteries. The A_2 component of S_2 is preserved.

What is the most appropriate next step in the evaluation or management of this patient?
   a. Perform coronary angiography
   b. Refer the patient to a neurologist to evaluate his headaches
   c. Arrange for a treadmill exercise test
   d. Measure blood pressure in the upper and lower extremities
   e. Reassure the patient that his condition is benign and allow him to participate in wrestling

4. A 65-year-old man is referred to you after an exertional syncopal spell. This is his first episode of syncope. He denies any history of exertional chest pain or dyspnea before or since the syncopal spell. You notice a loud 3/6 murmur over the left ventricular outflow tract; the murmur is late peaking and the A_2 component appears slightly reduced. Which of the following findings would be *most consistent* with your suspected diagnosis?
   a. The left ventricular impulse is nondisplaced and crisp
   b. The carotid upstroke is full without bruits
   c. The murmur decreases in intensity and its peak occurs earlier with amyl nitrite
   d. With hand grip, the murmur increases in intensity
   e. After premature ventricular contraction, the murmur decreases in intensity

5. You are evaluating a 45-year-old immigrant woman for a complaint of insidious-onset exertional dyspnea of several months' duration. She is not aware of any childhood diseases, nor is she aware of any immunizations. On examination, you notice a loud S_1, a right ventricular lift, and an augmented P_2 component of the S_2. She is in regular rhythm with a rate of 86 beats per minute. Which of the following statements is true?
   a. This patient will not benefit from a β-adrenergic blocker
   b. Hoarseness is not a complication in this patient if untreated
   c. The patient requires anticoagulation
   d. The disappearance of an opening snap with time is a good sign
   e. The longer the diastolic murmur, the less significant the mitral stenosis

6. Unfortunately, in the patient described in question 5, atrial fibrillation and considerable worsening of her symptoms develop. She does not tolerate verapamil because of constipation, and other medications fail to control her heart rate. You are considering other alternatives. What is the most appropriate recommendation for this patient?
   a. Mitral valve replacement with a bioprosthesis to obviate anticoagulation

b. Surgical mitral commissurotomy

c. Mitral valve replacement with a mechanical prosthesis, because it is more durable

d. Atrioventricular node ablation to ensure a slower heart rate

e. Balloon valvuloplasty, given that the valve is not too calcified (Abascal score ≤7)

7. You are called urgently to the emergency department to help assess a 27-year-old woman who is severely orthopneic. She was in her usual state of good health and was working out strenuously at her athletic club when acute shortness of breath developed. On arrival in the emergency department, you find the patient sitting upright and gasping for breath. She is clearly ill. A chest radiograph shows essentially a whiteout pattern of her lungs. However, the size of the left ventricle appears normal. Her jugular veins are distended, and you notice that the ventricular impulse is not displaced, but an S_3 is present. On auscultation, only a brief systolic murmur is heard over the apex, decrescendo in nature. Which one of the following statements is true?

a. The patient has had an acute myocardial infarction with rupture of her mitral papillary muscle

b. A cardiovascular surgeon should be consulted immediately to attempt mitral valve repair

c. Oxygen should not be administered

d. Intravenous therapy with furosemide and digitalis is contraindicated

e. The patient should undergo emergency coronary angiography

8. A 67-year-old man presents to your office with chest pain that has occurred over the past 3 weeks which is not clearly associated with exertion. Cardiovascular history does not indicate any risk factors. On physical examination, a loud murmur is detected. It is best heard over the fourth intercostal space radiating into the carotid arteries. No heart failure is present. Echocardiography also is performed to confirm the diagnosis. Which of the physical findings listed below most likely will accompany the examination?

a. A loud S_3

b. An apical impulse that is lateralized, but not diffuse

c. A normal carotid upstroke

d. A loud S_2

e. An increased jugular venous pulse

9. The patient is visiting you again after 6 months, because he initially was reluctant to undergo surgery. Which of the following changes in the cardiovascular history and

examination would most likely motivate you to recommend surgery at the present time?

a. The murmur is peaking later in systole

b. A diastolic murmur is now present

c. You can no longer detect the aortic component of S_2

d. A syncopal event has occurred

e. An S_4 is now present

10. The patient is convinced by your arguments and wants to proceed with surgery. What is the best approach?

a. Go directly to surgery for aortic valve repair

b. Go directly to surgery for aortic valve replacement

c. Perform carotid ultrasonography

d. Perform echocardiography

e. Perform coronary catheterization

11. A 46-year-old mother of two children presents with a long history of hypertension. She recalls that as a teenager she had trouble competing in athletics and keeping up with her peers because of fatigability, described as heaviness in her legs. She had marked hypertension during both pregnancies. Recently, she has noted marked exertional pain in her buttocks and lower extremities and progressive fatigability with dyspnea. Her medications include atenolol, 100 mg orally twice daily, diltiazem extended release, 180 mg orally daily, and Dyazide (a combination of triamterene and hydrochlorothiazide), 1 capsule orally daily. A treadmill exercise test was terminated after 3 minutes because of severe hypertensive blood pressure response and 2 mm of ST depression on electrocardiography. Physical examination findings include blood pressure, 150/100 mm Hg in both arms in the seated position; pulse rate, 80 beats/min; carotid pulsation, normal; jugular venous pressure, normal; and lungs, clear. Cardiac examination showed a 1+ left ventricular lift with a normal S_1, a normal S_2, and a palpable S_4 at the apex. A grade 2/6 ejection murmur was heard along the left sternal border, audible in the posterior intrascapular area. Lower extremity blood pressure was 90/40 mm Hg. Femoral, popliteal, dorsal pedis, and posterior tibial pulses were palpable but diminished. The results of laboratory studies were essentially normal, except for a creatinine value of 1.6 mg/dL. An electrocardiogram showed sinus rhythm with voltage criteria for left ventricular hypertrophy. Laboratory tests were essentially normal. The chest radiograph is shown for review (Figure). Which of the following tests is most likely to yield the correct diagnosis?

a. Renal arteriography

b. Magnetic resonance angiography of the thoracic aorta

c. Serum catecholamine determination

d. Ultrasonography of the abdomen

e. CT of the abdomen

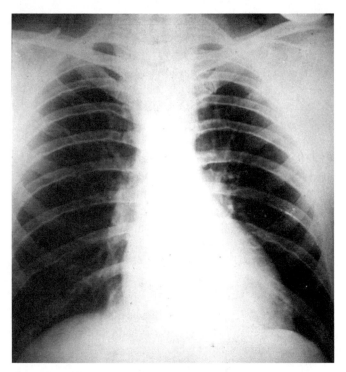

Question 11

12. An 18-year-old male, college long-distance runner seeks an opinion for approval for track team eligibility. He was told that as a child he had a heart murmur, but when he had pre-competition physical examinations throughout high school, this problem was never brought to his attention. Currently, he is asymptomatic. On physical examination, resting pulse rate is 45 beats/min and irregular, blood pressure is 90/40 mm Hg, jugular venous pressure is not increased, and the carotid pulse is normal. Chest examination shows a slight pectus deformity and a normal apical impulse. S_1 and S_2 are normal, with physiologic splitting. There is a soft early systolic click, and a grade 2/6 ejection murmur is heard best at the left intercostal space, with a soft grade 2/6 decrescendo murmur heard along the left sternal border and appreciated best with the patient leaning forward with a held expiration. A soft early diastolic filling sound (S_3) is heard at the apex with the patient in the left lateral decubitus position. There is no S_4. The systolic murmur decreases with a Valsalva maneuver. Peripheral pulses are all normal. An electrocardiogram shows sinus bradycardia with sinus arrhythmia and pauses up to 1 second in duration with normal QRS morphology. What would be the next most appropriate step for the evaluation of this athlete?
   a. Multigated image acquisition analysis (MUGA) for ejection fraction
   b. Echocardiography

   c. 24-Hour Holter electrocardiography
   d. Stress echocardiography
   e. Chest radiography

13. In addition to further diagnostic testing for the patient in question 12, what other management recommendation can be made at this time?
   a. Cardiac surgery consultation
   b. Electrophysiology/pacemaker consultation for consideration of pacemaker placement
   c. Institution of endocarditis prophylaxis
   d. Reassurance and no further follow-up because this is likely a benign flow murmur
   e. Discontinue all participation in competitive athletics

14. A 26-year-old woman consults you about her ability to become pregnant. She explains that she has a heart murmur and many years ago one of her doctors told her that she should check with a physician before becoming pregnant. Pregnancy should be *discouraged* in which one of the following situations?
   a. Mitral valve prolapse with moderate mitral regurgitation
   b. Bicuspid aortic valve with normal valve hemodynamics
   c. Patent foramen ovale
   d. Pulmonary hypertension due to ventricular septal defect with Eisenmenger physiology
   e. Systemic hypertension more than 150/85 mm Hg

15. A 35-year-old woman is evaluated for gradually increasing dyspnea with exertion. There are no risk factors for coronary artery disease and, in fact, the cholesterol level recently was determined to be 165 mg/dL. On physical examination, a normal, regular pulse of 80 beats/min and a blood pressure of 110/66 mm Hg are found. The lungs are clear, jugular venous pressure is 10 cm H_2O, and the carotid upstrokes are brisk and equal bilaterally. Cardiac examination shows a subtle sternal lift, and the left ventricular apical impulse was thought to be in the sixth intercostal space. S_1 is normal, and S_2 is split widely and persistently. A grade 2/6 systolic crescendo/decrescendo mid peaking murmur is heard in the second to third left interspace and increases with inspiration. Electrocardiography shows sinus rhythm with an incomplete right bundle branch block and right-axis deviation. The chest radiograph is shown (Figure). Echocardiographic results are consistent with a secundum atrial septal defect and dilated right atrium and right ventricle. What would be the next most appropriate step for treating this patient?
   a. No therapy
   b. Recommendations for endocarditis prophylaxis

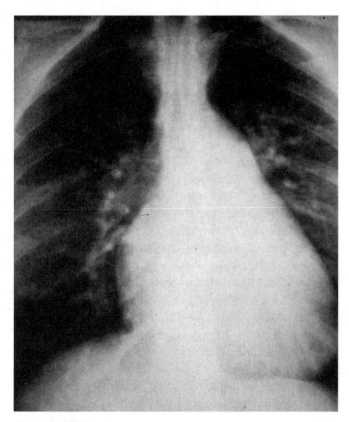

Question 15

c. Cardiac catheterization

d. Corrective cardiac surgery

e. Delay corrective surgery until the development of atrial fibrillation, paradoxical emboli, or right ventricular failure

16. A 35-year-old man with a history of hypertension and obesity presents with the chief complaints of fatigue and dyspnea. During the past 6 to 12 months, he has noticed a gradual decrease in his exertional tolerance, which he experiences if he walks for more than a block. He denies chest pain, nausea, vomiting, palpitations, syncope, or presyncope, but he has had frequent episodes of spontaneous diaphoresis. He has noted a 20-kg weight loss over the past year. Otherwise, his past history is unremarkable. He denies smoking, drinking, use of illegal drugs, hypercholesterolemia, or family history of premature heart disease. Physical examination findings include blood pressure, 146/80 mm Hg; pulse rate, 120 beats/min and irregular; weight, 121 kg; and height, 170 cm. He is somewhat anxious, has a fine tremor, and is very diaphoretic. Thyroid gland is enlarged. Bibasilar crackles are found on chest examination. Heart examination shows a displaced apex into the seventh intercostal space, mid-axillary

line, and an S_4. No murmur is heard. There is abdominal obesity, but the liver edge is palpable 2 cm below the rib margin. Extremities have 2+ pitting edema of the pretibial region bilaterally. Pulses are intact and equal bilaterally. Chest radiography shows cardiomegaly and evidence of pulmonary venous congestion. Electrocardiography shows atrial fibrillation with a rapid ventricular response and a heart rate of 128 beats/min. There is no evidence of Q waves on electrocardiography. You request echocardiography because you believe the patient has left ventricular dysfunction. Which one of the following groups of tests also should be done at this time?

a. Coronary angiography, ventilation-perfusion scanning, and complete blood count

b. Ventilation-perfusion scanning and sensitive thyroid-stimulating hormone test

c. Exercise echocardiography, ventilation-perfusion scanning, and sensitive thyroid-stimulating hormone test

d. Exercise thallium test, echocardiography, and fasting serum glucose test

e. 24-Hour Holter monitoring, echocardiography, and sensitive thyroid-stimulating hormone test

17. A 22-year-old woman reports to an ambulatory clinic with symptoms of upper respiratory tract infection. She is in the second trimester of her pregnancy. Her blood pressure is 140/50 mm Hg and pulse rate is 80 beats/min. Jugular venous pressure is 6 cm H_2O, and the carotid upstrokes are brisk and equal. The oral mucosa appears normal, but the nasal mucosa is swollen and red. The lungs are clear. A murmur is detected and described as a systolic ejection murmur, mid peaking, with a soft S_3 audible at the apex. The rest of the examintion findings are normal. Which one of the following would you recommend?

a. Diuretics to decrease pulmonary congestion

b. Antibiotics for subacute bacterial endocarditis prophylaxis in the setting of a murmur and acute infection

c. Referral to an infectious disease specialist

d. Reassurance, because a systolic ejection murmur and S_3 are normal at this stage of pregnancy

e. Referral to a high-risk pregnancy specialist

18. A 48-year-old woman comes to your office for a health maintenance visit. Her only complaint is worsening palpitations. She describes these as fluttering sensations in the chest, lasting only a few seconds but occurring on a daily basis. She has not had syncope or symptoms of presyncope. Her past medical history is unremarkable. There is no family history for any cardiovascular diseases. Physical examination, complete blood count, chest radiograph, and a 12-lead electrocardiogram are normal.

Which one of the following tests is most appropriate in the evaluation of this patient?

a. Echocardiography
b. Treadmill exercise test
c. 24-Hour Holter monitoring
d. Loop event recording
e. Coronary angiography

19. You are evaluating a 72-year-old man because of two episodes of syncope in the past week. Both episodes occurred abruptly while the patient was in the sitting position. Each episode lasted no more than 1 minute. The patient's spouse witnessed one of the two episodes. She reports that the patient's eyes rolled back and he did not respond to her verbal commands. The past medical history is significant for a myocardial infarction 3 years ago. Last year, the ejection fraction was 35% on echocardiography. Currently, the patient denies any serious ischemic symptoms and is taking atenolol 50 mg and aspirin 325 mg once daily. Cardiovascular examination is unremarkable except for a 1/6 holosystolic murmur at the apex radiating to the axilla and trace edema in both ankles. Complete blood count is unremarkable. The 12-lead electrocardiogram is shown in the Figure. Which

of the following tests would be most appropriate to document the suspected diagnosis?

a. Coronary angiography
b. Implantable loop recording
c. Exercise thallium scanning
d. Electrophysiologic testing
e. 24-Hour Holter monitoring

20. A 62-year-old man is being evaluated for palpitations that previously had been correlated with documented nonsustained ventricular tachycardia. He has been aware of occasional palpitations for 1 year, but he has no other cardiovascular symptoms. During a routine examination 2 years ago, he was told he had borderline hypertension and has been following a low-salt diet. The family history is unremarkable for cardiovascular diseases. The physical examination is unremarkable except for borderline hypertension of 150/90 mm Hg. Blood chemistry studies and complete blood counts are unremarkable. A 12-lead electrocardiogram shows normal sinus rhythm with borderline left ventricular hypertrophy. Results of 24-hour Holter monitoring show a total of 210 premature ventricular contractions with three episodes of nonsustained ventricular tachycardia. The longest run of nonsustained ventricular

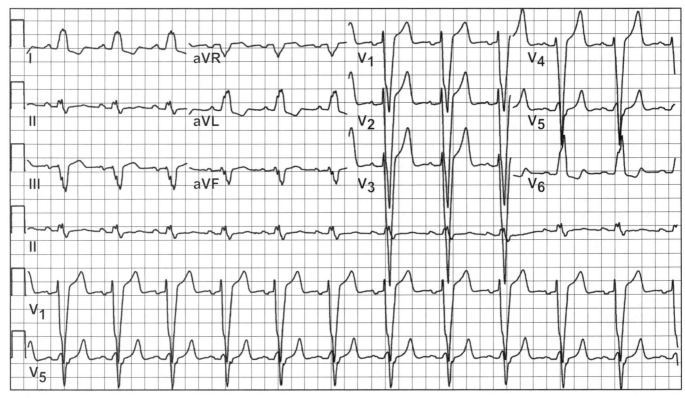

Question 19

tachycardia is 5 beats in duration. The maximal rate is 167 beats per minute. Which of the following is the most appropriate next step in the evaluation of this patient?

a. Order coronary angiography
b. Order exercise echocardiography
c. Order electrophysiologic testing
d. Initiate β-blocker therapy
e. Initiate amiodarone therapy

21. A 24-year-old woman comes to the emergency department because of sudden onset of palpitations. She reports symptoms of light-headedness without syncope. On physical examination, pulses are barely palpable and blood pressure in 90/60 mm Hg. The 12-lead electrocardiogram is shown in the Figure. Which one of the following is the most appropriate therapy for this patient?

a. Cardioversion
b. Digoxin 0.25 mg intravenously
c. Adenosine 6 mg intravenously
d. Verapamil 10 mg intravenously
e. Procainamide 4 mg/min intravenously

22. A 68-year-old man comes to your office because of fatigue. His past health has been excellent. Several years ago,

digoxin therapy was initiated after one episode of palpitations, and he has been taking digoxin 0.125 mg once a day since then. Physical examination is unremarkable except for a heart rate of 55 beats per minute. Total blood count and chemistry group results are within normal limits. The 12-lead electrocardiogram is shown in the Figure. Which one of the following is the most appropriate next step in the evaluation or management of this patient?

a. Refer the patient to a cardiologist for pacemaker implantation
b. Discontinue digoxin therapy
c. Order 24-hour Holter monitoring
d. Perform a treadmill exercise test
e. Order echocardiography

23. A 60-year-old woman was brought to the emergency department because of acute chest pain. A 12-lead electrocardiogram (Figure) showed changes consistent with acute anteroseptal infarction. Streptokinase thrombolytic therapy was initiated and was associated with immediate resolution of symptoms. Electrocardiographic changes gradually normalized during the next 24 hours. On day 2 after thrombolytic therapy and while the patient was being monitored in the coronary care unit, the patient

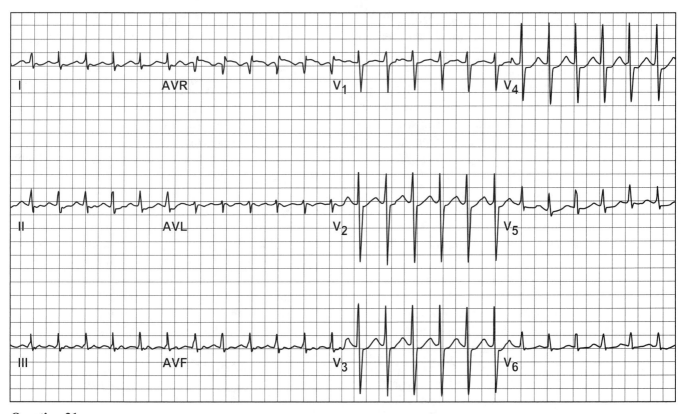

Question 21

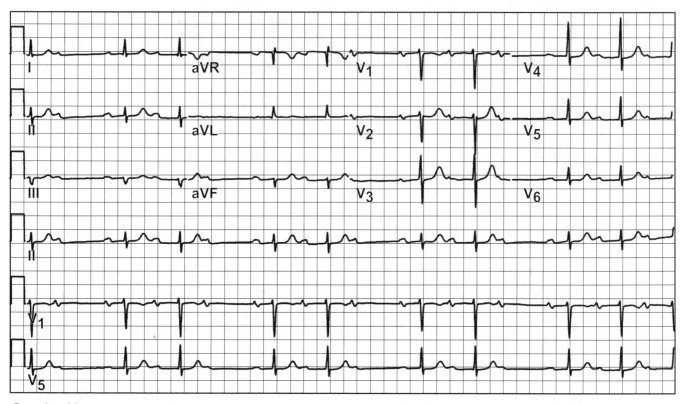

Question 22

had several episodes of ventricular tachycardia. One of the episodes was sustained and required cardioversion. The total blood count showed a hemoglobin value of 11.8 g/dL with normal leukocyte count. Serum potassium value was 4.2 mEq/L, sodium 141 mEq/L, and magnesium 2.2 mEq/L. Lidocaine boluses were given, and an infusion was started. What is the most appropriate next step in the evaluation or management of this patient?

a. Refer the patient to an electrophysiologist for implantation of a cardioverter-defibrillator
b. Implant a temporary pacemaker
c. Add esmolol drip
d. Refer the patient to a cardiologist for coronary angiography
e. Induce general anesthesia and intubate immediately

24. An 18-year-old woman comes to your office for a pre-college physical examination. She is healthy and has no significant past medical history. She denies any cardiovascular symptoms and does not smoke, drink alcohol, or use recreational drugs. Cardiovascular examination is unremarkable except for a midsystolic click. Total blood count and chemistry group values are within normal limits. The 12-lead electrocardiogram is shown in the Figure. Which of the following is the most appropriate next step in the evaluation or management of this patient?

a. Continue observation
b. Order a treadmill exercise test
c. Order echocardiography
d. Order coronary angiography
e. Refer the patient to an electrophysiologist for radiofrequency ablation

25. A 55-year-old man who had an anterior wall myocardial infarction 6 months previously is admitted after a sudden syncopal event, which occurred on a warm day when he was working in his yard. He has only a vague memory of the episode but now feels well and wants to go home. What is the most appropriate *next* step?

a. Home with instructions to maintain adequate salt and fluid intake while working outside on warm days
b. Home with a 24-hour Holter monitor
c. Echocardiography
d. Immediate referral for an implantable cardioverter-defibrillator
e. Determine serum cardiac enzyme values

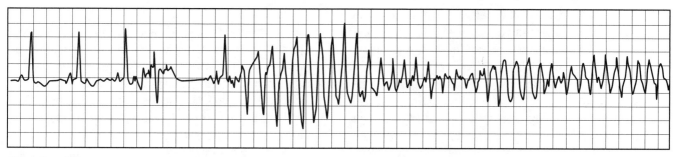

Question 23

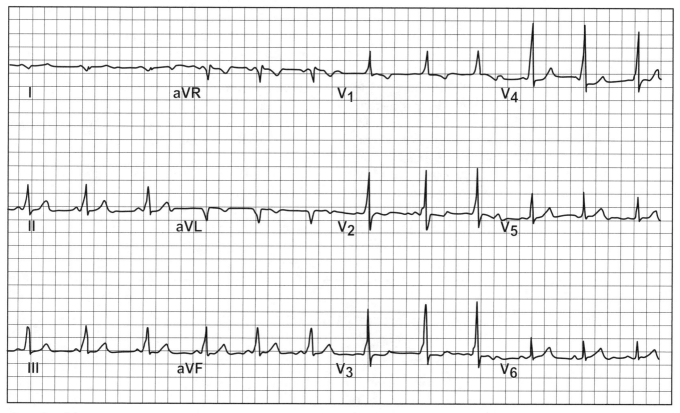

Question 24

26. A male student nurse comes to you having experienced a syncopal spell while observing a dressing change. He remembers feeling hot and clammy at the time and having a sensation of "not being there" before losing consciousness. He was informed by his fellow students that he "came around" quickly but looked pale. He felt "washed out" and somewhat embarrassed. Results of examination are unremarkable. Blood pressure, peripheral pulses and neurologic evaluation, and an electrocardiogram are normal. What is your next step?

   a. Electrophysiologic testing to rule out an arrhythmic cause for the symptoms

   b. Signal-averaged electrocardiography

   c. Tilt-table testing

   d. Reassurance

   e. Echocardiography

27. A 64-year-old woman with a history of hypertension was evaluated for irregular palpitations that were associated with shortness of breath. Electrocardiography was performed (Figure). In the emergency department, the patient received an intravenous infusion of diltiazem and her shortness of breath rapidly resolved. Physical examination showed no evidence of mitral stenosis, and the ventricular rate was 80

beats/min and irregular. She has no previous history of transient ischemic attack or stroke. She reported that the irregular palpitations had been present for the last 12 hours. Further evaluation revealed no evidence of coronary artery disease, and echocardiography showed preserved ventricular function. After additional diltiazem, oral digoxin, and flecainide, the heart rhythm became regular. Which one of the following is *least likely* in this setting?

a. Development of complete atrioventricular (AV) block and junctional escape rhythm
b. Development of atrial flutter
c. Restoration of sinus rhythm
d. Digitalis toxicity
e. Development of a left atrial thrombus

28. A 62-year-old executive presents for a physical examination. He is completely asymptomatic. He is overweight and has a relatively sedentary lifestyle. His past medical history is notable for mild hypertension and hyperlipidemia. His father had early-onset coronary artery disease. His current medications include triamterene and hydrochlorothiazide. On physical examination, his blood pressure is 150/90 mm Hg and the pulse rate is 82 beats/min. Jugular venous pressure is normal. Carotid upstrokes are normal without bruits. The lungs are clear to auscultation. The heart rate is regular. The first and second heart sounds are normal. A fourth heart sound is present. No murmurs are appreciated. The apical impulse is in the normal location and is of normal quality. The abdomen is soft and has no masses or bruits. The extremities have no clubbing, cyanosis, or edema, and the peripheral pulses are normal. Chest radiographic findings are unremarkable. The resting electrocardiogram shows normal sinus rhythm and no ST- or T-wave changes. A complete blood count, serum electrolytes, and chemistry panel are all normal. His total cholesterol value is 252 mg/dL, low-density lipoprotein cholesterol 142 mg/dL, and high-density lipoprotein 38 mg/dL. His triglyceride value is 160 mg/dL. What is the most appropriate next step in the evaluation or management of this patient?

a. Order coronary angiography
b. Order a treadmill exercise test to diagnose the presence of coronary artery disease
c. Increase therapy for blood pressure control, initiate cholesterol-lowering therapy, and begin aspirin therapy
d. Perform an imaging stress test to define the presence of coronary artery disease
e. Obtain a resting echocardiogram to define left ventricular systolic function

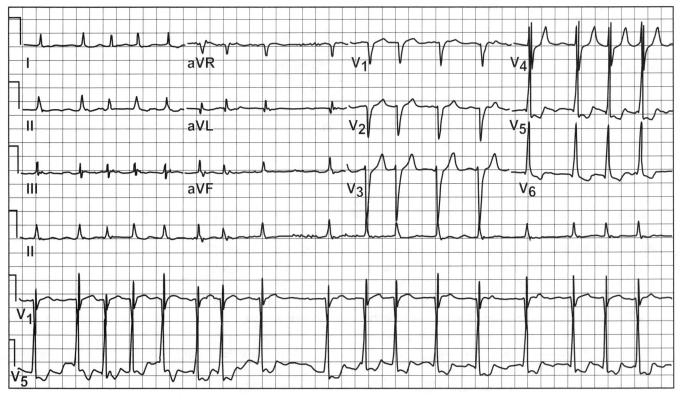

Question 27

29. During the next 12 months, the patient described in question 28 notes the onset of classic anginal symptoms with exertion. These are noted when he climbs 3 flights of stairs to his office daily. The symptoms are relieved with 1 minute of rest at the top of the stairs. He is currently taking atenolol 50 mg daily, aspirin 325 mg daily, and pravastatin 20 mg daily. Results of his physical examination are unchanged. Which one of the following interventions is *least* likely to lessen his risk for subsequent death or myocardial infarction?
    a. Percutaneous revascularization
    b. Lowering the low-density lipoprotein <100 mg/dL if the current value is >130 mg/dL
    c. Lowering the low-density lipoprotein to <100 mg/dL if the current value is between 100 and 129 mg/dL
    d. Exercise training program
    e. Further intensification of antihypertensive therapy

30. A 67-year-old farmer presents with a 3-day history of intermittent chest pressure and dyspnea with minimal exertion. He had one episode of nocturnal dyspnea 3 days ago. He is currently asymptomatic. He has a history of hypertension and hyperlipidemia. He currently takes metoprolol 25 mg twice daily and aspirin 325 mg once daily. On physical examination, his blood pressure is 140/85 mm Hg and his pulse rate is 76 beats/min and regular. His jugular venous pressure is normal. His carotid upstrokes are normal and without bruits. His lungs are clear to auscultation. His heart rate is normal and the rhythm is regular. The apical impulse is in the normal location and is of normal quality. The first and second heart sounds are normal. No murmurs or gallops are appreciated. The abdomen is soft and has no masses or bruits. The extremities have no clubbing, cyanosis, or edema, and the peripheral pulses are normal. The electrocardiogram shows nonspecific ST- and T-wave changes. Chest radiographic findings are normal. A complete blood count, electrolytes, and cardiac biomarkers are all normal. What is the most appropriate next step in the evaluation or management of this patient?
    a. Treadmill exercise stress testing
    b. Diagnostic coronary angiography with possible percutaneous revascularization
    c. Pharmacologic stress testing
    d. Start therapy with tirofiban 0.1 µg/kg per minute and reassess in 24 hours
    e. Administer alteplase 0.75 mg/kg over 30 minutes, then 0.5 mg/kg over 60 minutes

31. After appropriate diagnostic work-up and medical therapy are commenced, the patient described in question 30

is found to have a 95% stenosis in the middle left anterior descending coronary artery. This was successfully treated with an intracoronary stent. What is the most appropriate next step in the evaluation or management of this patient?
    a. Therapy with aspirin 325 mg and clopidogrel 75 mg daily should be commenced
    b. Noninvasive stress testing is required at 3 to 6 months after the percutaneous procedure regardless of the patient's symptom status
    c. Add long-acting nitrates to the medical therapy
    d. Surveillance coronary angiography to detect in-stent restenosis at 6 months
    e. Therapy with aspirin 81 mg plus warfarin adjusted to an international normalized ratio of 2.0-2.5 should be initiated

32. One year later, the patient described in questions 30 and 31 is in need of cholecystectomy. He remains asymptomatic. The surgeon had ordered a treadmill exercise test, and the results are available for your review. The patient exercised to an equivalent of 9.0 metabolic equivalents (METs) and had a normal heart rate and blood pressure response. The electrocardiogram was interpreted as positive at peak exercise and resolved by 3 minutes into recovery. What is the most appropriate next step in the evaluation or management of this patient?
    a. Repeat coronary angiography and possibly coronary revascularization to improve the patient's operative outcome
    b. Proceed with cholecystectomy and continue therapy with β-blockade perioperatively
    c. Postpone the operation until an imaging stress test can be performed
    d. Recommend intravenous β-blocker and intravenous nitroglycerin therapy with pulmonary artery catheter monitoring and proceed with the cholecystectomy
    e. Add clopidogrel 75 mg orally daily and proceed with cholecystectomy

33. A 72-year-old man underwent coronary angiography because of a history of chest pain. He had a 75% stenosis of the middle right coronary artery, a 40% stenosis of the middle left anterior descending coronary artery, and three 30% lesions in the left circumflex system. What is the most appropriate next step in the evaluation or management of this patient?
    a. Pharmacologic therapy with β-blockade and aspirin therapy and treatment of modifiable risk factors.
    b. Coronary artery bypass grafting to prevent subsequent myocardial infarction

c. A high-sensitivity C-reactive protein level test to assess overall risk

d. Percutaneous revascularization of the right coronary artery to prevent myocardial infarction

e. Exercise nuclear perfusion imaging stress test to assess the functional significance of the stenoses

34. A nondiabetic 68-year-old man has known stable coronary artery disease, ejection fraction of 40%, and class III angina pectoris despite aggressive pharmacologic therapy. Which of the following is the best therapy to improve survival and decrease the need for subsequent revascularization?

a. Percutaneous revascularization with intracoronary stenting

b. Coronary artery bypass grafting regardless of the number of diseased vessels

c. Coronary artery bypass grafting and percutaneous revascularization can be used interchangeably

d. Coronary artery bypass grafting if the patient has three-vessel disease

e. Percutaneous revascularization with intracoronary stenting and intravenous glycoprotein IIb/IIIa inhibition

35. A 63-year-old woman is hospitalized because of congestive heart failure. Her past medical history includes a mechanical aortic valve prosthesis, recent normal coronary angiography, hypertension, and chronic atrial fibrillation. Exertional dyspnea has progressed over 4 months to orthopnea and paroxysmal nocturnal dyspnea. Medications are verapamil, furosemide, and warfarin. On examination, blood pressure is 160/90 mm Hg and heart rate is 80 beats per minute. Obesity precludes accurate assessment of jugular venous pressure or carotid contours. There are bibasilar crackles. There is a grade 2/6 high-pitched systolic ejection murmur radiating from the apex to the base. No diastolic murmur or S_3 is heard. There is slight lower extremity pitting edema. Chest radiography shows cardiac enlargement and pulmonary venous congestion. Electrocardiography shows atrial fibrillation and left ventricular hypertrophy. Laboratory values include potassium 2.9 mEq/L, creatinine 1.9 mg/dL, and international normalized ratio 1.3. Aggressive potassium chloride supplementation and intravenous heparin therapy are begun. Which of the following is the most useful diagnostic test at this point?

a. Coronary angiography and left ventriculography

b. Echocardiography

c. Dipyridamole thallium perfusion imaging

d. Cine CT of the chest to assess pericardial thickness

e. Holter monitoring

36. A 79-year-old man being evaluated in the office notes progressive exertional dyspnea. He has a past history of coronary artery bypass grafting, and he has rare angina with extreme exertion. His medications are aspirin, diltiazem, and furosemide. On examination, blood pressure is 130/80 mm Hg, and heart rate is 84 beats per minute. Jugular venous distention is present, carotid upstrokes are reduced, and the lungs are clear. The cardiac apex is enlarged and displaced with an apical S_3 and a grade 3/6 holosystolic murmur radiating to the axilla. There is no hepatosplenomegaly or lower extremity edema. Chest radiography shows cardiomegaly. Echocardiography shows left ventricular enlargement, ejection fraction 20%, and structurally normal mitral valve but severe mitral regurgitation. A complete blood count and electrolyte values are normal. An exercise perfusion study shows moderately impaired exercise tolerance and large fixed perfusion defects without ischemia. Which initial medical treatment strategy is most appropriate?

a. Add long-acting nitrates and an angiotensin-converting enzyme inhibitor to the therapy

b. Add long-acting nitrates, increase the diltiazem dose, and add digoxin to the therapy

c. Begin use of an angiotensin-receptor blocker and spironolactone

d. Discontinue use of diltiazem and add digoxin and a long-acting nitrate to the therapy

e. Discontinue use of diltiazem and add a β-adrenergic blocker and angiotensin-converting enzyme inhibitor

37. A 55-year-old woman has exertional dyspnea and orthopnea. Angiographic findings within the past 8 months are an ejection fraction of 30% and single-vessel occlusion with good collateral vessels. Lisinopril and carvedilol were prescribed and the doses were upwardly adjusted. Initially, episodes of worsening dyspnea responded to diuretics. She was stable at target doses for months before contracting a mild upper respiratory viral illness. For the past 2 months, exertional dyspnea and orthopnea have returned. Hospitalization for aggressive diuresis has twice resulted in azotemia without weight loss or symptom improvement. Her blood pressure is 110/75 mm Hg, and pulse is 52 beats per minute. She has normal jugular venous pressure, clear lungs, distant heart sounds, and mild ankle edema. Complete blood count and electrolyte and creatinine values are normal. Chest radiography shows mild cardiomegaly and no pulmonary congestion or pleural effusions. On echocardiography, ejection fraction is 44%. What is the most appropriate recommendation?

a. Refer the patient for pulmonary evaluation

b. Add digoxin to the regimen

c. Use an angiotensin-receptor blocker instead of the angiotensin-converting enzyme inhibitor

d. Order transesophageal echocardiography

e. Order chest radiography, decubitus position, to look for subpleural effusions

38. A 57-year-old man is seen in the office because of exertional dyspnea, orthopnea, and paroxysmal nocturnal dyspnea. He denies both chest discomfort and rhythm awareness. Pulse is irregular at 140 beats per minute, and blood pressure is 110/85 mm Hg. There are bibasilar lung crackles, mildly increased jugular venous pressure, and an S_3. Electrocardiographic findings are atrial fibrillation with a rapid ventricular response but no abnormalities of the QRS complex or repolarization. Chest radiography shows cardiomegaly and small bilateral pleural effusions, and left ventricular enlargement and an ejection fraction of 25% without valvular abnormalities are found on echocardiography. What is the most appropriate next step?

a. Blood tests for thyroid function testing

b. Right ventricular endomyocardial biopsy

c. Electrophysiologic study followed by atrioventricular node ablation and pacemaker implantation

d. Gated radionuclide angiography (multiple gated acquisition)

e. Electrical cardioversion

39. A 62-year-old man seen in the office has hypertrophic obstructive cardiomyopathy and is treated with a β-adrenergic blocker. He denies any cardiopulmonary symptoms. His examnation is notable only for a 2/6 midpeaking systolic ejection murmur that increases in intensity with the performance of a Valsalva maneuver. Chest radiography is normal, and electrocardiography shows left ventricular hypertrophy with repolarization changes. On echocardiography, the ejection fraction is 70% and asymmetric septal hypertrophy with dynamic outflow tract obstruction is found. The gradient at rest is 15 mm Hg and it increases to 25 mm Hg with inhalation of amyl nitrite. On a treadmill he is able to walk 92% of his predicted time and his peak heart rate is 115 beats per minute. Which of the following is the most appropriate treatment?

a. Surgical septal myectomy

b. Dual-chamber permanent pacing

c. Addition of disopyramide to the regimen

d. Continuation of the β-blockade with no other changes

e. Alcohol septal ablation

40. A 47-year-old woman is discovered to have an idiopathic dilated cardiomyopathy after presenting with nonspecific fatigue. On physical examination, her blood pressure is 130/85 mm Hg and pulse is 84 beats per minute. Jugular venous pressure is normal. The lung fields are clear to examination. Precordial examination shows a slightly displaced and sustained apical impulse with a soft S_3. There is no peripheral edema. Mild cardiomegaly is found on chest radiography. No coronary artery lesions are found on coronary angiography. Laboratory studies do not suggest amyloidosis, hemochromatosis, or a thyroid disorder. Which of the following has been shown to forestall the development of symptomatic congestive heart failure in this type of patient?

a. Digoxin

b. Angiotensin-receptor blockers

c. Nesiritide (intravenous BNP)

d. Spironolactone

e. Angiotensin-converting enzyme inhibitors

ANSWERS

1. Answer b.

Patients with mitral valve prolapse often present with non-specific symptoms. The maneuver described on physical examination (Valsalva) leads to reduced ventricular filling. This augments the valve/left ventricular mismatch (remember the mitral valve leaflets are redundant in mitral valve prolapse) and subsequently the "flopping" of the leaflets during closure, which is believed to be responsible for the midsystolic clicks. A postectopic beat will lead to increased ventricular filling, reducing the murmur. In severe mitral regurgitation, an S_3 is sometimes identified, presumably due to the premature tensing of the mitral valve chord caused by the enhanced inflow (shuttle volume). S_1 is pronounced in mitral stenosis, and the left ventricular apical impulse should be hyperdynamic with considerable mitral regurgitation.

2. Answer c.

In a patient with structural (myxomatous thickening) changes of the mitral valve apparatus and regurgitation, endocarditis prophylaxis is recommended. Coronary artery disease is not more frequently associated with mitral valve prolapse. Early operation does have the advantage of a better chance at mitral valve repair, rather than valve replacement, but no adaptive changes have been noted yet. Thus, observation and serial follow-up would be the preferred therapeutic option. Physical activity and exercise are not contraindications.

3. Answer d.

This young patient has congenital bicuspid aortic stenosis. Given the clinical scenario, there is a suspicion for coarctation, which accompanies bicuspid aortic stenosis in about 10% of patients. Initially, the best way to assess for the presence of hemodynamically significant coarctation is to measure the blood pressure in both the upper and the lower extremities. The most comprehensive way to assess this patient's condition is with echocardiography, which allows quantification of the aortic valve disease and evaluation of the distal arch and proximal descending aorta. A treadmill exercise test might be helpful to document the hemodynamic response to physical activity in this patient.

4. Answer d.

The valvular disease suspected in this case is aortic stenosis. This disease can progress silently for many years, and syncope is often the first clinical manifestation. Answers "a" and "b" are classic clinical findings. Generally, any maneuver that enhances the transvalvular gradient, be it increased filling (after premature ventricular contraction, reverse Valsalva) or reduced peripheral resistance (after premature ventricular contraction,

amyl nitrite), will increase the intensity of the murmur. Handgrip, which increases the afterload (increase in peripheral resistance), would decrease the intensity of the murmur (as would the Valsalva maneuver).

5. Answer c.

Mitral stenosis is most commonly caused by rheumatic fever. Once thought nearly eradicated, it is now increasing in frequency, especially in immigrants from underdeveloped countries. Once symptomatic, there is a high incidence (approximately 50%) for occurrence of atrial fibrillation necessitating chronic anticoagulation because of the high risk of systemic emboli (about 20% a year without anticoagulation). Thus, despite the presence of sinus rhythm, and in view of secondary pulmonary hypertension, anticoagulation should be given. The disappearance of the opening snap indicates a loss of mitral valve pliability, that is, progression of the disease. A long diastolic murmur would indicate a persistent left atrial-to-left ventricular pressure gradient, supporting the finding of more severe mitral stenosis. Natural progression can lead to severe left atrial enlargement with impingement of the recurrent laryngeal nerve, leading to hoarseness. Initial medical therapy aims to allow as much time as possible for pressure equilibration. This may be achieved with a β-blocker or calcium-channel blocker, such as verapamil.

6. Answer e.

This patient has become symptomatic, and rate control poses a therapeutic challenge. Valvuloplasty in a patient whose valve is not markedly calcified and deformed can be very beneficial and can delay the need for valve replacement by as much as 10 years. Replacing the valve in the presence of a significant, symptomatic mitral stenosis is an option. The prosthesis used in this young patient should probably be a mechanical one, because she is beyond childbearing age and mechanical prostheses are more durable. Surgical commissurotomy is a successful procedure and is still performed often in developing countries (e.g., India), because it does not require the use of a cardiac bypass pump during operation. Atrioventricular node ablation is not a therapy of choice. In this patient, the underlying problem is hemodynamic and not primarily arrhythmogenic.

7. Answer b.

This patient has myxomatous mitral valve disease, possibly with prolapse. Rupture of chordae tendineae is not uncommon. With strenuous isometric exercise (weight lifting), a group of weakened chordae can rupture, resulting in severe acute mitral regurgitation. Because adaptive processes cannot occur in such a short time, acute cardiac shock results. Therapy is rapid surgical intervention. Other measures are merely temporizing, including the intravenous therapy with digitalis and furosemide to ameliorate her heart failure and acute pulmonary edema. Oxygen also can be helpful to lower the pulmonary pressures. This patient does not have coronary artery disease and preoperative angiography is unnecessary.

8. Answer b.

This patient presents with aortic stenosis. His leading symptom is chest pain, not heart failure. Thus, an S_3 is unlikely and most likely would be associated with systolic heart failure. Aortic stenosis should be accompanied by parvus and tardus carotid pulse. The S_2 in aortic stenosis is usually diminished. The apical impulse, particularly in chronic significant asymptomatic aortic stenosis, results in left ventricular hypertrophy, shifting the apical impulse to the left. Unless marked secondary pulmonary hypertension has occurred, the jugular venous examination should be normal.

9. Answer d.

Answers a, b, c, and e indeed represent progression in the degree of aortic stenosis. The diastolic murmur suggests that the aortic cusps have become frozen with an added component of aortic regurgitation (loss of residual pliability). However, the clinical presentation is the most pressing determinant for the timing of surgery.

10. Answer e.

There is a good chance (>50%) that this patient will have accompanying coronary artery disease necessitating concurrent bypass grafts. Carotid ultrasonography may be helpful for the anesthesiologist to guide the hemodynamics during surgery (avoid hypotension), but even the presence of significant carotid artery disease would not result in reversal of surgical procedures (carotid endarterectomy preceding aortic valve/coronary artery bypass grafting). The risk of stroke is lower than the risk of lethal perioperative myocardial infarction. The echocardiogram would not change the treatment because significant aortic stenosis with no clinical symptoms had been established before this visit.

11. Answer b.

The vignette contains important clues that indicate the patient has a secondary cause for hypertension. She is a young adult who has had a long history of hypertension requiring multiple medications to control blood pressure. Clues that coarctation of the aorta is present include claudication, diminished or absent femoral pulses, and difficult-to-control blood pressure. Supporting evidence would include a marked decrease in blood pressure between the arms and the legs; such a decrease was documented in the patient and was 90 mm Hg systolic and 40 mm Hg diastolic. Also, the finding of left ventricular hypertrophy on the electrocardiogram is consistent with the patient's history of long-standing hypertension and evidence that her medical management has not been adequate to avoid end-organ changes. The diagnosis of coarctation of the aorta may be made with a computed tomographic study of the chest, magnetic resonance angiography of the thoracic aorta, transesophageal or transthoracic echocardiography, spiral computed tomography of the thorax, or aortography or angiography of the thoracic aorta. If one study does not provide positive evidence of coarctation but it is strongly suspected clinically, a study should be performed with another imaging method. This can be a difficult area of the body to visualize. Teaching point: in all young persons with hypertension, it is important to palpitate *simultaneously* the *radial and femoral* pulses and observe for potential *radial-femoral delay*, which if present strongly suggests coarctation clinically. Coarctation of the aorta is managed by surgical repair and involves resection of the affected part of the aorta, with end-to-end anastomosis of the aorta. Occasionally, the procedure requires bypass of the coarcted segment of the aorta with an artificial woven graft from the aortic arch to the descending thoracic aorta. The patient's features at presentation, medical history, and physical examination findings are not indicative of renal artery stenosis or pheochromocytoma. Therefore, renal arteriography and serum catecholamine measurement or CT or ultrasonography of the abdomen would not be recommended.

Reference: Hougen TJ, Sell JE: Recent advances in the diagnosis and treatment of coarctation of the aorta. Curr Opin Cardiol 1995;10:524-529.

12. Answer b.

The physical examination findings indicate the patient has a bicuspid aortic valve with aortic regurgitation. The key physical examination clue is the early systolic click or "ejection click." Although the systolic murmur decreases with the Valsalva maneuver (suggesting that this is not a case of hypertrophic cardiomyopathy), it does not disappear, as would a benign flow murmur. A diastolic murmur always indicates abnormality and requires further investigation in any patient. In an athlete, a grade 2 systolic murmur that does not disappear with maneuvers should be investigated further to rule out aortic stenosis, hypertrophic cardiomyopathy, pulmonic stenosis, and atrial septal defect. Nuclear imaging has no role in the evaluation of murmurs. Although chest radiography may be indicated, it is not the definitive study. The sinus bradycardia with sinus arrhythmia is common in athletes because of hypervagotonia. The isolated finding of a systolic murmur may or may not indicate pronounced aortic obstruction because many young athletes have an increase in stroke volume in both the left and the right ventricular outflow tracts, creating turbulence. Stress echocardiography is helpful to rule out coronary artery ischemia, which is unlikely in this young patient, with no apparent risk factors. It also might give you ancillary information about exercise tolerance and chronotropic incompetence. Yet, these are not suspected clinically. A 24-hour Holter monitoring provides mostly rhythm information and one should recognize that younger athletes normally have considerable resting bradycardia and sinus arrhythmia. Although chest radiography is probably indicated, it is unlikely to give definitive information for making further recommendations. MUGA gives isolated, relatively inexpensive information for left ventricular function, which is not really the issue here.

Reference: Maron BJ, Isner JM, McKenna WJ: 26th Bethesda Conference: recommendations for determining eligibility for competition in athletes with cardiovascular abnormalities. Task Force 3: hypertrophic cardiomyopathy, myocarditis and other myopericardial diseases and mitral valve prolapse. J Am Coll Cardiol 1994;24:880-885.

13. Answer c.

The patient has a diastolic murmur, which is always abnormal and indicates valvular abnormality. Once a valvular lesion has been identified, the risk of bacterial endocarditis increases and patients need to receive prophylaxis. The issue of competition will be better defined after echocardiography has been performed. If severe aortic regurgitation or stenosis is found, this patient should not compete.

Reference: Seto TB, Kwiat D, Taira DA, et al: Physicians' recommendations to patients for use of antibiotic prophylaxis to prevent endocarditis. JAMA 2000;284:68-71.

14. Answer d.

Contraindications to pregnancy include severe pulmonary hypertension, especially in patients with Eisenmenger physiology (equalization of right ventricular and left ventricular pressures) due to long-standing left-to-right shunting, severe obstructive lesions (including aortic stenosis, mitral stenosis, coarctation of the aorta, or hypertrophic obstructive cardiomyopathy), severe left ventricular dysfunction, and Marfan syndrome with an enlarged aortic root. Regurgitant lesions are generally better tolerated if the patient does not have heart failure.

15. Answer d.

This patient has secundum atrial septal defect. Even large atrial septal defects are likely to be asymptomatic until patients reach the third or fourth decade, and then they are often detected on a general examination. At this time, patients also may begin to identify symptoms such as shortness of breath and possibly some atrial arrhythmia (usually atrial fibrillation) due to volume overload of the right ventricle and right atrium. In this vignette, the diagnosis is supported by the physical examination findings of right ventricular volume overload (sternal lift on physical examination), which is due to left-to-right shunting through the atrial septal defect. The electrocardiogram also shows right ventricular strain with incomplete right bundle branch block, which is characteristic. Chest radiography confirms a hemodynamically significant shunt by an increased cardiac silhouette and prominence of pulmonary artery shadows. The murmur heard on physical examination is a flow murmur through the pulmonary valve, represented as increased blood volume through the shunt. In addition, a fixed split of S_2 is pathognomonic. Consultation for corrective cardiac surgery is recommended to relieve the patient's symptoms and potentially to avoid the long-term complications of arrhythmia and pulmonary hypertension. The question of whether to close an atrial septal defect is based primarily on the hemodynamic significance, which is assessed by observing 1) right ventricular and atrial enlargement and 2) whether the pulmonary-to-systemic shunt (flow ratio) is greater than 1.5 to 1. In patients younger than 50 years, operative mortality is low (1%-2%) and 5- to 10-year survival is excellent. If corrective surgery is delayed, outcome is more likely to be unfavorable (atrial fibrillation, paradoxical emboli, pulmonary artery hypertension, right ventricular failure). Nonsurgical closing with a "clamshell" device is now possible, having recently been approved by the FDA.

Reference: Perloff JK: The Clinical Recognition of Congenital Heart Disease. Third edition. Philadelphia, Saunders, 1987.

16. Answer e.

The patient presents with obvious left ventricular dysfunction and congestive heart failure, complicated by atrial fibrillation (irregular pulse). At the bedside, you are trying to determine the cause and, thus, need to obtain laboratory data to rule out some of the reversible causes of dilated cardiomyopathy. The screening laboratory evaluation would include ruling out thyroid disease, hemochromatosis, alcoholic cardiomyopathy, and tachycardia-induced cardiomyopathy. Electrocardiography provides clues that the patient may have rapid rates with minimal provocation because his resting heart rate, both on resting electrocardiography and in the office, was increased. Persistent tachycardia, usually due to unrecognized atrial fibrillation, can lead to left ventricular dysfunction. In view of this patient's atrial fibrillation, 24-hour Holter monitoring will give a better idea of his average heart rate and certainly could be a major cause of left ventricular dysfunction in this particular patient. Measuring the ferritin level would help determine whether the patient has hemochromatosis. Although coronary angiography may be warranted in the future, in a young patient who does not have a history of smoking or chest pain, coronary artery disease would be low on the list of differential diagnoses. Similarly, ventilation-perfusion scanning and stress thallium study may be in the work-up but are not warranted before noninvasive studies. Tachycardia-induced cardiomyopathies are a commonly unrecognized cause of left ventricular dysfunction. In this patient, atrial fibrillation may be related to lone atrial fibrillation, due to thyrotoxicosis, or even pickwickian syndrome. The key is that these patients generally are unaware of their atrial fibrillation; that is, they do not feel palpitations or experience syncope or presyncope. Many patients with atrial fibrillation are highly symptomatic and generally present before left ventricular dysfunction develops. It is important to identify these patients because tachycardia-induced left ventricular dysfunction is a reversible cause of dilated cardiomyopathy. Also, it probably is the most likely cause of this patient's left ventricular dysfunction in the setting of thyrotoxicosis. Treating thyrotoxicosis would be important before attempting cardioversion.

Reference: Grogan M, Smith HC, Gersh BJ, et al: Left ventricular dysfunction due to atrial fibrillation in patients initially believed to have idiopathic dilated cardiomyopathy. Am J Cardiol 1992;69:1570-1573.

17. Answer d.

During pregnancy, plasma volume begins to increase as early as 6 weeks after conception and approaches its maximum in the second trimester but increases overall by 50% in the third trimester, when it reaches a plateau. Cardiac output increases overall early in pregnancy, primarily in relation to an increase in stroke volume, which is accompanied by a decrease in systemic vascular resistance. In addition, it is not uncommon for a murmur to develop during these high-flow states. The murmur disappears after delivery and normalization of hemodynamics. These hemodynamic changes are normal and generally well tolerated. Marked hypertension and increased jugular venous pressure should prompt further evaluation.

Reference: Longo LD: Maternal blood volume and cardiac output during pregnancy: a hypothesis of endocrinologic control. Am J Physiol 1983;245:R720-R729.

18. Answer c.

The patient's symptoms are consistent with extrasystoles in isolated forms or in short runs. In the absence of any serious cardiovascular diseases or malignant symptoms, such as syncope or presyncope, a noninvasive approach that documents the rhythm disturbances and correlates them with

symptoms is most appropriate. Because the symptoms are occurring on a daily basis, 24-hour Holter monitoring would be most effective.

19. Answer d.

The patient most likely has cardiogenic syncope. Both episodes occurred without any warning and in the sitting position. The patient has a history of significant cardiovascular disease with a compromised ejection fraction. The 12-lead electrocardiogram shows left bundle branch block, suggestive of conduction system disease. The presence of these risk factors puts the patient in a high-risk group for cardiogenic syncope. The causes usually include ventricular arrhythmias or intermittent bradycardia. An electrophysiologic study is most appropriate to establish the diagnosis.

20. Answer b.

The patient has newly documented nonsustained ventricular tachycardia on Holter monitoring which correlates with his symptoms of palpitations. He has modest risk factors for coronary artery disease, including age, sex, and mild hypertension. The prognostic importance of nonsustained ventricular tachycardia is dependent on the presence or absence of underlying structural or coronary artery disease. Exercise echocardiography would be most appropriate at this point to exclude any significant ischemia or structural heart disease. If ischemia or structural heart disease is not present, a trial of β-blocker therapy could be considered to also treat the documented mild hypertension. Additional diagnostic procedures may be necessary if any significant ischemia or structural disease is present. Empirical drug therapy for premature ventricular contractions or nonsustained ventricular tachycardia suppression is not recommended.

21. Answer c.

The 12-lead electrocardiogram shows paroxysmal supraventricular tachycardia. Adenosine is the treatment of choice; its success rate is more than 90%.

22. Answer b.

The patient's symptoms are likely related to relative bradycardia, although other causes have not been excluded. The 12-lead electrocardiogram shows a Wenckebach pattern with normal QRS complex morphology. The site of Wenckebach atrioventricular block is most likely at the atrioventricular node, which could be related to digoxin therapy. Because the precise indication for digoxin therapy is not clear, the most appropriate action is stopping digoxin therapy. There is no urgent indication for pacemaker implantation unless symptomatic bradycardia persists after the use of digoxin has been discontinued.

23. Answer d.

The single-lead monitoring strip demonstrates polymorphic ventricular tachycardia ("torsades"). This is highly suggestive of an ischemic nature for the arrhythmia. The serum electrolyte values are within normal limits. The most appropriate step at this time would be immediate coronary angiography to identify coronary anatomy and possible intervention.

24. Answer a.

The 12-lead electrocardiogram is consistent with preexcitation and Wolff-Parkinson-White syndrome. The low-grade outflow tract murmur is most likely physiologic in this young adult. In asymptomatic patients with Wolff-Parkinson-White syndrome, no additional evaluation is required. Should documented paroxysmal supraventricular tachycardia or symptoms develop, such as syncope, an electrophysiologic evaluation for consideration of radiofrequency ablation would be appropriate.

25. Answer c.

Although this patient's symptoms could well have been due to orthostasis exacerbated by dehydration, in view of his previous history any syncopal event requires thorough evaluation. A Holter monitor would be useful only if he had a subsequent event while wearing the device and, as could be the case in this patient, the next event could be fatal. For this reason, echocardiography should be performed to evaluate the ejection fraction. If the ejection fraction is reduced (<40%), the patient should be referred to an electrophysiologist for further evaluation and possible implantation of a cardioverter-defibrillator.

26. Answer d.

The clinical scenario is typical for vasovagal syncope. No further action is required. If there is a recurrence, however, tilt-table testing would be appropriate to document hemodynamic changes during episodes and to guide therapy.

27. Answer e.

If sudden normalization of the heart rhythm and regularization of the RR intervals are noted during atrial fibrillation, several possibilities need to be considered. This does not always signify restoration of sinus rhythm. The usual criteria for diagnosing complete AV block are irregular PP intervals, irregular RR intervals, and varying PR relationship. With atrial fibrillation, there is no discernible P activity, and one cannot comment on the regular PP or varying PR intervals. As a result, the only feature that can be found is an irregular RR interval in spite of continuing atrial fibrillation. This regularization results from a junctional escape rhythm, which can be a manifestation of digitalis toxicity. With the use of a class IC antiarrhythmic

agent, atrial fibrillation may convert to atrial flutter. If a constant ratio of conduction between atrium and ventricle occurs during the flutter, the ventricular rates will become regular. The development of left atrial thrombi has no relation to the ventricular response rates during atrial fibrillation.

28. Answer c.

This patient has multiple risk factors for coronary artery disease. The most important step to take for managing his subsequent cardiovascular risk is to treat his modifiable risk factors. These are principally hypertension and hyperlipidemia. Coronary angiography would not be indicated as an initial step for this asymptomatic patient. Exercise testing to *diagnose* coronary artery disease is not particularly useful for someone in this age group who already has a high pretest probability of having the disease. The more appropriate use of functional testing for this type of patient would be for *prognostic* information.

29. Answer a.

Once chronic stable angina develops, all the therapies listed decrease subsequent death and nonfatal myocardial infarction rates except percutaneous revascularization. This treatment relieves symptoms but does not improve survival for patients with stable coronary artery disease.

30. Answer b.

By definition, this patient has an unstable angina syndrome. Generally, noninvasive stress testing without intensification of anti-ischemic therapy is contraindicated in unstable syndromes. The patient does not have markers of increased risk (such as positive biomarkers, evidence of congestive heart failure, ongoing or prolonged chest pain, or electrocardiographic changes). Therefore, the administration of glycoprotein IIb/IIIa inhibitors is not indicated. Multiple studies have suggested that both conservative strategies (increased pharmacologic therapy and follow-up stress testing) and early invasive strategies can be used with similar outcomes for patients such as the one described. There is a tendency to prefer invasive strategies for patients in the higher risk categories. Thrombolytic therapy is contraindicated in non–ST-segment elevation acute coronary syndromes.

31. Answer a.

Intracoronary stents have a 15% to 20% restenosis rate in the first 6 months. The rates of subsequent death, myocardial infarction, and ischemic stroke are dramatically reduced with the combination of aspirin and clopidogrel (or aspirin and ticlopidine). Warfarin is not part of standard care after intracoronary stenting and should be used only if there is another indication. Follow-up testing is not mandated after percutaneous revascularization and is generally performed only when indicated from the clinical symptoms. Nitrates are useful for the relief of anginal symptoms; however, this patient may not have angina after successful revascularization, and nitrates do not have an effect on cardiac event rates.

32. Answer b.

Patients who have undergone coronary revascularization within the past 5 years and remain active and asymptomatic do not need preoperative cardiac stress testing. In this case, the patient did undergo treadmill exercise testing, which demonstrated good exercise capacity (9 METs), confirming his relatively good prognosis. Pulmonary artery catheterization is not supported by trial data (albeit scant). Patients at very high risk (such as evidence of congestive heart failure) undergoing high-risk procedures (major vascular) may be an exception.

33. Answer a.

More myocardial infarctions occur from the rupture of stenoses with less than 50% luminal diameter obstruction than from those with more than 50% obstruction. This reflects that most patients generally have far more mild-moderate stenoses in the coronary arterial tree. It is the stability of the plaque, rather than the size of the plaque, that is crucial. Currently, no method can determine the stability of a plaque. Appropriate pharmacologic therapy will treat overall myocardial oxygen demand and, if statins are indicated, may help to stabilize the plaques. Revascularization techniques have not been shown to prevent myocardial infarction. The high-sensitivity C-reactive protein and stress tests would not change the overall management of this patient.

34. Answer d.

Percutaneous revascularization has been shown to relieve symptoms. In patients with stable coronary artery disease (as opposed to acute coronary syndromes), no percutaneous revascularization strategy has been shown to improve mortality or prevent infarction. Overall, coronary artery bypass grafting and percutaneous techniques have similar subsequent death and myocardial infarction rates, but patients undergoing percutaneous techniques generally have more subsequent revascularization procedures. Patients with diabetes seem to have improved survival with coronary artery bypass grafting (compared with medical therapy), including those with left main coronary artery disease and those with three-vessel disease and left ventricular dysfunction or severe symptoms.

35. Answer b.

The mechanism of the patient's congestive heart failure is unclear. Physical examination cannot clearly discriminate whether the problems are confined to the left or right heart or whether it is a biventricular process. There is a mechanical valve with inadequate anticoagulation of indeterminate duration. Echocardiography would provide the most information about ventricular and prosthetic valve function. Coronary angiography would not be a first step, and the ability to perform left ventriculography is limited by the mechanical aortic prosthesis. The presentation is not sufficiently suggestive of an ischemic syndrome to make perfusion imaging the most helpful test, especially with a recent normal coronary angiogram. Although the patient could have constrictive pericarditis, there are not strongly suggestive findings to make cine CT the first test. The patient has a history of chronic atrial fibrillation, and her current electrocardiographic results fit with that and there are no historical features to suggest a primary rhythm component to her decompensation; thus, Holter monitoring is unlikely to be helpful.

36. Answer e.

This patient has an ischemic cardiomyopathy without serious angina or evidence of viable ischemic myocardium, which would make coronary angiography with an eye to revascularization appropriate. The foundations of treating ventricular dysfunction are to use an angiotensin-converting enzyme inhibitor and a β-blocker. Diltiazem is relatively strongly contraindicated because of its negative inotropic properties. Digoxin, nitrates, and spironolactone also could be used in addition to the angiotensin-converting enzyme inhibitor and β-blocker, as indicated by findings at follow-up.

37. Answer a.

This patient had dilated cardiomyopathy treated with appropriate medications. Ventricular function improved. In the past her spells of heart failure responded readily to furosemide, but more recently they have not responded symptomatically and the diuretic-induced azotemia and the current physical examination suggest the possibility that she is not fluid-overloaded. Because she is being treated with a nonselective β-blocker, her symptoms worsened after a respiratory infection, and her symptoms are behaving differently than they did in the past, the question of noncardiac disease must be considered. Adding digoxin would be appropriate if this was definite heart failure. There is no suggestion of a reaction to the angiotensin-converting enzyme inhibitor to warrant a switch to an alternative agent. There are no findings to suggest the patient has a disease process that would be better assessed with transesophageal echocardiography or findings of pleural effusions that would justify decubitus chest radiography.

38. Answer a.

The patient has a tachydysrhythmia of indeterminate duration. Identifying treatable causes of atrial fibrillation is appropriate and should include thyroid function testing. Right ventricular biopsy might be appropriate after further diagnostic testing, but not as the next step. Electrophysiologic study of atrial fibrillation generally is not indicated and an "ablate and pace" strategy is reserved for patients whose rhythm cannot otherwise be controlled. Gated radionuclide angiography is compromised in irregular heart rhythms and would serve only to provide an alternative measure of left ventricular function. Cardioversion in a patient with new atrial fibrillation of indeterminate duration is inappropriate without addressing potential atrial thrombus issues.

39. Answer d.

The patient has hypertrophic cardiomyopathy with a mild obstruction. He has no symptoms with β-blocker therapy, and objective testing confirms near normal exercise tolerance. The goal of adding disopyramide is unclear because diminishing the gradient has no proven benefit in the absence of symptoms. The other measures are designed to reduce the degree of obstruction and similarly have no proven use in an asymptomatic patient.

40. Answer e.

All of the choices have a beneficial role to play in patients with symptomatic dilated cardiomyopathy. However, only therapy with an angiotensin-converting enzyme inhibitor has been shown to delay the onset of symptomatic congestive heart failure in patients with asymptomatic left ventricular dysfunction. Although angiotensin-receptors or β-blockers may share that benefit, this has not yet been proved.

CHAPTER 4

CRITICAL CARE MEDICINE

Steve G. Peters, M.D.
William F. Dunn, M.D.

Critical care medicine encompasses multidisciplinary aspects of the management of severely ill patients. All areas of medicine may have relevance for critically ill patients, but this review focuses on aspects of cardiopulmonary monitoring and life support, technologic interventions, and disease states typically managed in the intensive care unit (ICU).

RESPIRATORY FAILURE

Effective functioning of the respiratory system requires normal central nervous system control, neuromuscular transmission and bellows function, and gas exchange at the alveolar-capillary level. Respiratory failure may result from disease at any of these levels.

Physiologic Definitions and Relationships

Lung Volumes

"Total lung capacity" (TLC) is the total volume of gas in the chest at the end of a maximal inspiration. "Vital capacity" (VC) is the volume of a maximal breath (expired or inspired). "Tidal volume" (VT) is the volume of a normal breath. "Functional residual capacity" (FRC) is the lung volume at the end of a normal expiration. It reflects the relaxation point of the respiratory system or the point at which outward recoil of the chest wall is balanced by inward recoil of the lungs.

Compliance and Resistance

"Compliance" (C) of the lungs or respiratory system is defined by the change in volume (ΔV) for a given change in pressure (ΔP):

$$C_{STATIC} = \frac{\Delta V}{\Delta P}$$

where ΔV is measured in liters (L) and ΔP in centimeters of water (cm H_2O). Emphysema causes the loss of recoil and, thus, increased compliance. Most other disease states, particularly interstitial diseases, fibrosis, pulmonary edema, and

acute respiratory distress syndrome (ARDS), cause decreased compliance (i.e., "stiff" lungs, or increased transpulmonary pressure for a given volume change).

- Normal compliance is approximately 0.2 L/cm H_2O.
- Emphysema causes the loss of recoil and increased compliance.
- Interstitial diseases, fibrosis, pulmonary edema, and ARDS cause decreased compliance.

Resistance (R) to airflow is defined by the change in pressure (ΔP) for a given change in flow ($\Delta \dot{V}$):

$$R = \frac{\Delta P}{\Delta \dot{V}}$$

where ΔP is measured in cm H_2O and $\Delta \dot{V}$ in L/s. Common causes of increased airway resistance include bronchospasm and airway secretions.

- Common causes of increased airway resistance are bronchospasm and airway secretions.

The total pressure required to inflate the respiratory system (spontaneously or with a mechanical ventilator) is the pressure required to overcome elastic recoil (due primarily to lungs and chest wall) plus the pressure to overcome flow resistance (due primarily to airways and endotracheal tube):

$$P \text{ inflation } = \frac{\Delta V}{C_{ST}} + R \times \Delta \dot{V}$$

(Elastic Load)   (Resistive Load)

Evaluation of Hypoxia

Gas exchange requires alveolar ventilation for the elimination of carbon dioxide, oxygen uptake across the alveolar-capillary membrane, and the delivery of oxygen to tissues. Hypoxemia may result from 1) a decrease in the inspired partial pressure of oxygen (e.g., high altitude, including air travel), 2) hypoventilation, 3) ventilation-perfusion ($\dot{V}/Q$) mismatch, 4) shunting, or 5) diffusion barrier. Estimation of the alveolar-arterial gradient (A-a) for oxygen is essential in analyzing the cause of hypoxemia. Important relationships include the following:

The partial pressure of carbon dioxide ($Paco_2$) in the blood is directly proportional to the amount of carbon dioxide produced ($\dot{V}co_2$) and inversely proportional to alveolar ventilation ($\dot{V}A$):

$$Paco_2 = k \, \frac{\dot{V}co_2}{\dot{V}A}$$

Alveolar ventilation is equal to total ventilation ($\dot{V}E$) minus dead space ventilation ($\dot{V}D$). Thus, physiologic dead space is defined by the portion of a breath that does not participate in gas exchange. Dead space volume (VD) may be anatomical (conducting airways) or alveolar (areas of ventilation that receive no perfusion):

$$\dot{V}A = \dot{V}E - (VD \times f)$$

where f = breaths/min.

Calculation of Dead Space Ventilation

$$\frac{VD}{VT} + \frac{Paco_2 - P_Eco_2}{Paco_2}$$
$$\text{(Bohr Equation)}$$

$$\frac{VD}{VT} \text{ normally is } <0.25 \text{ to } 0.30$$

where P_Eco_2 is the partial pressure of expired carbon dioxide. The dead space–to–tidal volume ratio is calculated by measuring the partial pressure of carbon dioxide in an arterial blood gas sample ($Paco_2$) and an expired gas sample (P_Eco_2). The greater the dead space, the greater the difference between $Paco_2$ and P_Eco_2.

- Physiologic dead space is defined by the portion of breath not participating in gas exchange.
- Increased dead space leads to decreased elimination of carbon dioxide at any given level of total minute ventilation.

Calculation of PAO_2

Alveolar gas consists of inspired gases saturated with water vapor. The alveolus also contains carbon dioxide delivered from the blood. The sum of the partial pressures of all gases present equals the ambient barometric pressure. The alveolar air equation defines this relationship:

$$PAO_2 = FIO_2 (PB - PH_2O) - \frac{Paco_2}{R}$$

where PA is alveolar partial pressure, PB is barometric pressure (about 760 mm Hg at sea level), PH_2O is water vapor pressure (47 mm Hg), and R is the respiratory quotient ($\dot{V}co_2/\dot{V}o_2$, normally about 0.8). The simplified equation is

$$PAO_2 = FIO_2 (PB - 47) - \frac{Paco_2}{0.8}$$

Breathing room air ($FIO_2 = 0.21$) at sea level:

$$PAO_2 = 150 - \frac{40}{0.8}$$

or normal PAO_2 is approximately equal to 100 mm Hg.

The A-a Gradient

The A-a oxygen difference is defined by PAO_2 minus Pao_2, which is normally less than 10 to 20 mm Hg when breathing room air. The A-a gradient normally increases to approximately 50 to 100 mm Hg as the FIO_2 increases from 0.21 to 1.0, and it also increases slightly with age. Hypoxemia due to hypoventilation is characterized by increased $Paco_2$ and decreased Pao_2 but by a relatively normal A-a gradient. Hypoxemia due to ventilation-perfusion mismatch shows an increased A-a gradient.

- Hypoxemia due to hypoventilation: increased $Paco_2$, decreased Pao_2, normal A-a gradient.

Shunt Fraction and the Fick Equation

A shunt is defined by perfusion in the absence of ventilation (i.e., $\dot{V}/Q = 0$). With a pure shunt, Pao_2 does not increase even though FIO_2 is increased to 100%. Normal shunt fraction is less than 3% to 5% of total cardiac output. The shunt fraction is measured with the person breathing 100% oxygen and is expressed as follows:

$$\frac{Qs}{Qt} = \frac{Cc'o_2 - Cao_2}{Cc'o_2 - C\overline{v}o_2} = \frac{P(A\text{-}a)o_2 \times 0.003}{P(A\text{-}a)o_2 \times 0.003 + (Ca - C\overline{v})o_2}$$

The content of oxygen in the blood is the total amount of oxygen bound to hemoglobin (Hgb) plus the amount dissolved.

$$O_2 \text{ content: } CxO_2 = 1.34 \times Hgb \times S_xO_2 + 0.003 \times P_xO_2$$
$$\text{(Bound)} \qquad\qquad \text{(Dissolved)}$$

where x may equal arterial, venous, or capillary.

Under steady state conditions, the amount of oxygen used by the tissues equals the amount taken up by the lungs. The oxygen uptake, $\dot{V}O_2$, can be defined by the amount of oxygen leaving the lungs in pulmonary venous blood minus the amount of oxygen coming into the lungs in the pulmonary arteries. This should be familiar as the Fick equation:

$$\dot{V}O_2 = CO\,(CaO_2 - C\bar{v}O_2)$$

where CO is cardiac output.

- A shunt is defined by perfusion in the absence of ventilation, i.e., $\dfrac{\text{Ventilation}}{\text{Perfusion}} = 0$.
- The normal shunt fraction is <3%-5% of total cardiac output.
- A shunt leads to hypoxemia that shows little improvement after supplemental oxygen.

Mixed Venous Oxygen Saturation

Many applications of the Fick equation are important in managing critically ill patients. One application involves continuous monitoring of mixed venous oxygen saturation by a specialized type of pulmonary artery catheter. Expressing oxygen content in terms of saturation and rearranging the Fick equation to solve for $S\bar{v}O_2$ yields the following:

$$S\bar{v}O_2 = SaO_2 - \frac{\dot{V}O_2}{CO \times Hgb \times 1.34}$$

where CO is cardiac output and Hgb is hemoglobin.

Note that decreased mixed venous oxygen saturation may be due to decreased arterial saturation, increased oxygen consumption, decreased cardiac output, or decreased hemoglobin. Certain disease states, particularly early sepsis, may be characterized by normal or increased mixed venous oxygen saturation because cardiac output initially increases along with impaired oxygen uptake by the tissues. Later in sepsis, mixed venous $S\bar{v}O_2$ typically decreases because of decreased oxygen delivery.

- Decreased mixed venous oxygen may be due to decreased arterial saturation, increased oxygen consumption, decreased cardiac output, or decreased hemoglobin.
- Early sepsis: normal or increased mixed venous oxygen saturation.

Oxygen Delivery

Under normal circumstances, oxygen demand by the tissues is met by the supply. Oxygen delivery is defined by cardiac output (CO) times arterial oxygen content:

$$O_2 \text{ delivery} = CO \times CaO_2$$

Although cardiac output may decrease, $\dot{V}O_2$ of the tissues may be maintained by increased oxygen extraction.

Oxygen delivery = cardiac output × arterial oxygen content.

ACID-BASE BALANCE AND ARTERIAL BLOOD GASES

The production of acid byproducts is the normal result of cellular metabolism. An acid is defined as a hydrogen ion, $[H^+]$, or proton donor. A base accepts protons. The dissociation constant (K) for an acid (HA) may be defined as

$$K = \frac{[H^+][A^-]}{[HA]}$$

Buffer systems minimize the changes in pH associated with the addition of acid or base. For carbonic acid:

$$H_2O + CO_2 \longleftrightarrow H_2CO_3 \overset{K}{\longleftrightarrow} H^+ + HCO_3^-$$

$$\text{and } K = \frac{[H^+][HCO_3^-]}{[H_2CO_3]}$$

This relationship gives the Henderson-Hasselbalch equation:

$$pH = pK + \log \frac{[HCO_3^-]}{[H_2CO_3]}$$

where $pH = -\log[H^+]$ and $pK = -\log K$. The pK for carbonic acid is 6.1. $[H_2CO_3]$ is often measured by taking $0.03 \times PaCO_2$ (i.e., dissolved carbon dioxide). So the Henderson-Hasselbalch equation can be rewritten as

$$pH = 6.1 + \log \frac{[HCO_3^-]}{0.03 \times PaCO_2}$$

Hydrogen ions are buffered by several mechanisms in different body fluid compartments. In plasma and interstitial fluid, bicarbonate is the major buffer, with proteins and phosphate compounds contributing to a lesser extent. In erythrocytes, hemoglobin is the major buffer, but bicarbonate contributes approximately 30% and phosphate 10% of the buffering capacity. The kidney eliminates organic acid and also contributes by 1) reabsorption of bicarbonate from tubular fluids, 2) formation of titratable acid, and 3) elimination of $[H^+]$ as ammonium ions.

- Bicarbonate is the major buffer in plasma and interstitial fluid.
- In erythrocytes, hemoglobin is the major buffer.
- The kidney eliminates organic acid and reabsorbs bicarbonate from tubular fluids.

Given the importance of the carbonic acid-bicarbonate system, many acid-base problems involve some method for solving variables of the Henderson-Hasselbalch equation. Because pK is constant, if only two of the three values for pH, P_{CO_2}, and HCO_3^- are known, the missing variable can be calculated. Graphic displays are commonly used; two of the variables are plotted at constant values for the third variable (e.g., the Davenport diagram).

Patterns of Acid-Base Disorders

Common acid-base disorders and associated clinical scenarios are listed in Table 4-1.

Respiratory Acidosis

Acute respiratory acidosis is defined by the rapid development of carbon dioxide retention ($P_{aCO_2} >45$ mm Hg) with a concomitant decrease in pH (<7.35). Common causes include respiratory depression by drugs such as narcotics, central nervous system injury, acute diaphragm or neuromuscular weakness,

Table 4-1   Common Acid-Base Disorders and Associated Clinical Scenarios

Acid-base disorder	Typical clinical scenario
Respiratory acidosis	Severe COPD
Respiratory alkalosis	Pulmonary embolism, anxiety
Normal anion gap metabolic acidosis	Diarrhea, renal tubular acidosis
Increased anion gap metabolic acidosis	Diabetic ketoacidosis, lactic acidosis, uremia
Metabolic alkalosis	Vomiting
Respiratory and metabolic acidosis	Severe shock
Respiratory acidosis and metabolic alkalosis	COPD being treated with diuretics or corticosteroids
Metabolic acidosis and respiratory alkalosis	Sepsis, salicylate overdose
Metabolic alkalosis and respiratory alkalosis	Mechanical ventilation in a patient with metabolic alkalosis

COPD, chronic obstructive pulmonary disease.

severe parenchymal respiratory failure, and cardiac failure. Because carbon dioxide diffuses quickly into cells and the cerebrospinal fluid, the physiologic effects of the acidosis may occur rapidly. Confusion, obtundation, and signs of cerebral edema are commonly observed. Chronic respiratory acidosis is typically seen in patients with severe chronic obstructive pulmonary disease (particularly chronic bronchitis or bronchiectasis) and in other states associated with chronic alveolar hypoventilation. Chronic respiratory acidosis may be compensated partly by renal mechanisms, that is, increased reabsorption of bicarbonate and excretion of acid in the urine.

- Acute respiratory acidosis: rapid onset of carbon dioxide retention with concomitant decrease in pH.
- Chronic respiratory acidosis is typically seen in patients with severe chronic obstructive lung disease or in other states associated with chronic alveolar hypoventilation.

Respiratory Alkalosis

Acute respiratory alkalosis is the result of a rapid decrease in P_{aCO_2} due to hyperventilation. Hyperventilation usually is associated with anxiety or pain. Important causes also include early shock states, pulmonary embolism, other causes of hypoxemia, hyperthermia, salicylate intoxication, liver failure, and disorders of the central nervous system. Patients with unexplained hypocapnia should be evaluated for these disorders. In mechanically ventilated patients, respiratory alkalosis may result from inadvertent overventilation, that is, excessive tidal volume or respiratory rate (or both), especially in a volume preset assist-control ventilator mode.

- Respiratory alkalosis is the result of alveolar hyperventilation.
- Common causes include anxiety, pain, shock, pulmonary embolism, hypoxemia, fever, salicylate overdose, liver failure, and mechanical overventilation.

Metabolic Acidosis

Metabolic acidosis results from the accumulation of organic acids such as lactate, pyruvate, or keto acids. Acidosis may develop by increased acid production or decreased renal excretion of acid. Conditions causing metabolic acidosis are further characterized by the anion gap, that is,

$$[Na^+] - ([Cl^-] + [HCO_3^-])$$

with a normal value of 8 to 14 mEq/L.

A normal anion gap or non-anion gap acidosis is characterized by an increase in chloride balancing the loss of bicarbonate. Causes include gastrointestinal losses of bicarbonate (diarrhea), urinary diversion procedures, and intestinal fistulas. Renal losses of bicarbonate (renal tubular acidosis) are also associated with a normal anion gap. Causes of acidosis associated with other anions—increased anion gap disorders—are diabetic ketoacidosis, lactic acidosis, uremia, and toxins (e.g., ethylene glycol, methanol, paraldehyde, and salicylate).

The "delta gap" is a useful calculation that assists in defining the presence of a complicated anion gap metabolic acidosis. It is defined as follows:

Delta gap = (deviation of anion gap from normal) −
(deviation of HCO_3^- from normal)

In uncomplicated anion gap metabolic acidosis, the expected delta gap is 0 (±6).

A positive delta gap would be due to the presence of a concomitant metabolic alkalosis or (chronic) respiratory acidosis. A negative delta gap would be due to a concomitant non-anion gap metabolic acidosis or (chronic) respiratory alkalosis.

- Metabolic acidosis: result of accumulation of organic acids, e.g., lactate, pyruvate, keto acids.
- Normal anion gap or non-anion gap acidosis is characterized by an increase in chloride balancing the loss of bicarbonate (diarrhea, renal tubular acidosis).
- Increased anion gap disorders: diabetic ketoacidosis, lactic acidosis, uremia, toxins (e.g., ethylene glycol, methanol, paraldehyde, and salicylate).
- An abnormal "delta gap" reveals the presence of a complicated anion gap metabolic acidosis.

Metabolic Alkalosis

Primary metabolic alkalosis is characterized by increased bicarbonate and pH. Hypokalemia and hypochloremia are commonly associated and further perpetuate the alkalosis. Common causes are volume contraction states, particularly those associated with the loss of chloride and hydrogen ion (e.g., vomiting and nasogastric suctioning). Diuretic therapy and mineralocorticoids are also common contributing factors. Although respiratory compensation (hypoventilation) for metabolic alkalosis might seem counterproductive, it can occur and may contribute to hypoxemia. As with other acid-base disorders, therapy is directed at the underlying cause, but support with volume and potassium and chloride replacement are important.

- Primary metabolic alkalosis is characterized by increased bicarbonate and pH.
- Hypokalemia and hypochloremia are commonly associated and further perpetuate alkalosis.
- Common causes are volume contraction states, particularly those associated with further loss of chloride and hydrogen ion (e.g., vomiting and nasogastric suctioning).

Mixed Acid-Base Disorders

Mixed disorders are characterized by a combination of the primary abnormalities described above or by a primary disorder and compensatory changes in $Paco_2$ or bicarbonate. For example, combined respiratory and metabolic acidosis may occur in patients with depressed respiration and tissue hypoperfusion, as would occur with severe shock, after cardiorespiratory arrest, or with status epilepticus. In these situations, pH is severely depressed and immediate therapy is necessary. Treatment includes assisted ventilation plus measures to improve cardiac output and organ perfusion. Sodium bicarbonate might be given for severe acidemia (pH <7.0-7.1), but treatment must be directed at the underlying cause of the primary disorder.

- Combined respiratory and metabolic acidosis leads to severe acidemia.
- Treatment should be directed at the underlying disorder.

Respiratory acidosis and metabolic alkalosis typically occur in patients with chronic obstructive pulmonary disease (COPD) or chronic alveolar hypoventilation. Secondary bicarbonate retention may be augmented by concomitant corticosteroid therapy or diuretics. Because a given blood gas measurement showing increased $Paco_2$ and increased bicarbonate (with pH near 7.4) could occur by many mechanisms, the clinical history is essential for determining the most likely pathophysiologic mechanism. If patients with chronic hypercarbia are mechanically ventilated, there is a risk of severe alkalemia if the ventilator settings are adjusted to "normalize" the $Paco_2$ at approximately 40 mm Hg without recognizing the chronic compensatory nature of the increase in bicarbonate.

- Respiratory acidosis plus metabolic alkalosis is seen most commonly in patients who have chronic respiratory insufficiency plus bicarbonate retention.

Metabolic acidosis and respiratory alkalosis may occur in patients who have tissue hypoperfusion and respiratory stimulation, as is commonly seen with early shock states, sepsis, and liver or renal failure. This pattern is also typical of salicylate intoxication.

- The combination of metabolic acidosis and respiratory alkalosis is commonly seen in shock states, sepsis, or salicylate overdose.

Metabolic alkalosis and respiratory alkalosis rarely occur in spontaneously breathing patients but can develop quickly with mechanical ventilation. This usually is the result of a disorder that causes respiratory alkalosis, as described above, combined with a metabolic alkalosis induced by volume contraction, gastric suctioning, hypokalemia, diuretics, or corticosteroids. Seizures or cardiac arrhythmias or both may result from severe alkalemia. Treatment usually requires replacement of volume, potassium, and chloride.

CLINICAL APPROACH TO ARTERIAL BLOOD GASES

Problems of acid-base balance and gas exchange can be assessed in several ways. When interpreting arterial blood gases, the following approach is useful:

1. Consider the pH. Are conditions normal (pH 7.35-7.45), acidemic (<7.35), or alkalemic (>7.45)?
2. Assess $Paco_2$. Does the $Paco_2$ change (from 40 mm Hg) account for the pH change (from 7.40)? The evaluation of this relation requires calculation, graphic display, or a rule of thumb such as the following: an acute change in $Paco_2$ of 10 mm Hg should be associated with a pH change in the opposite direction of approximately 0.08 unit. If an abnormal pH can thus be accounted for by the change in $Paco_2$, a simple acute respiratory disturbance is present. If not, a mixed acid-base disorder is present.
3. The change in bicarbonate will confirm whether a metabolic disturbance is present. That is, base deficit or excess should confirm the conditions already defined by pH and $Paco_2$. Is the anion gap increased? If an anion gap is present, is the delta gap appropriate?
4. Consider Pao_2. If hypoxemia is present, estimate the A-a gradient. If this is normal and $Paco_2$ is increased, hypoventilation alone should account for the hypoxemia. The A-a gradient should be increased in conditions of ventilation-perfusion mismatching, shunting, or diffusion barrier.
5. Compare the Pao_2 and the arterial saturation, Sao_2. The Sao_2 should correspond to the expected values for a normal oxygen-hemoglobin dissociation curve. If saturation is lower than expected, consider the presence of other hemoglobin forms, for example, carboxyhemoglobin or methemoglobin. As examples, use the above approach to match the following arterial blood gases with the clinical scenarios listed below.

	pH	$Paco_2$	HCO_3^-	Pao_2 (room air)	Sao_2
A.	7.35	60	32	50	85%
B.	7.50	46	34	85	94%
C.	7.18	70	26	55	89%
D.	7.28	31	15	110	99%
E.	7.38	30	18	105	75%

1. 20-year-old woman with diabetic ketoacidosis
2. 20-year-old man with acute narcotic overdose
3. 60-year-old man 1 week after an abdominal operation, with continuous nasogastric suction and diuretic therapy
4. 60-year-old woman with severe emphysema
5. 60-year-old man with carbon monoxide intoxication
(Answers: 1. D, 2. C, 3. B, 4. A, 5. E)

- Consider the pH.
- Assess $Paco_2$.
- The change in bicarbonate should confirm the conditions already defined by pH and $Paco_2$.
- Consider Pao_2 and the A-a gradient.

Airway Management

Endotracheal intubation allows control of the airway, enables the delivery of specific inspired oxygen and positive pressure ventilation, and provides protection from aspiration. Indications for intubation include airway protection in cases of obstruction or loss of normal gag and cough reflexes, central nervous system injury or sedation with loss of normal control of ventilation, and any cause of respiratory failure requiring positive pressure-assisted ventilation. Oral-tracheal intubation is usually achieved through direct visualization with a laryngoscope. In experienced hands, this procedure should be relatively quick and safe. Complications may include vomiting and aspiration, hypoxemia during the procedure, and inadvertent intubation of the esophagus. The major contraindication for laryngoscopic intubation is an unstable cervical spine (due to trauma or degenerative conditions such as rheumatoid arthritis). In such cases, fiberoptic intubation (passing a tube over a bronchoscope) or tracheostomy may be necessary. In semiconscious and spontaneously breathing patients, nasotracheal intubation may be accomplished "blindly" and may be more comfortable for patients. Complications include bleeding, obstruction of sinus drainage with sinusitis, and damage to nasal structures.

- Endotracheal intubation allows control of the airway.
- Contraindication: unstable cervical spine (trauma or rheumatoid arthritis).
- In semiconscious, spontaneously breathing patients, nasotracheal intubation may be an alternative.

In emergency situations in which airway control is required, cricothyrotomy may be lifesaving. This procedure involves identifying and puncturing the cricothyroid membrane. For patients who require prolonged mechanical ventilation or airway support, the timing of tracheostomy is controversial. The use of high-volume, low-pressure endotracheal tube cuffs has decreased the frequency of tracheal injury and stenosis caused by prolonged intubation. Tracheostomy has the advantages of decreased laryngeal injury, increased patient comfort, ease of suctioning, and, in certain patients, allowance for oral ingestion and speech. Complications may include tracheal injury and stenosis, bleeding, tracheoesophageal fistula, and possibly increased bronchial or pulmonary infections. Tracheostomy is commonly considered for patients who have needed or are expected to need intubation and mechanical ventilation for more than 2 to 4 weeks.

- In emergency situations, cricothyrotomy may be lifesaving.
- High-volume, low-pressure endotracheal tube cuffs have decreased the frequency of tracheal injury and stenosis.
- Tracheostomy is considered for patients who have needed or are expected to need intubation and mechanical ventilation for >2 to 4 weeks.

Mechanical Ventilation

Mechanical ventilation may be valuable in various conditions of respiratory failure, including loss of respiratory control, neuromuscular or respiratory pump failure, and disorders of gas exchange. Many specific variables that have been suggested as criteria (or general guidelines) for ventilator support are listed in Table 4-2.

Complications of Mechanical Ventilation

Complications of mechanical ventilation may be related to airway access, physiologic responses to positive pressure, and complications related to other organ systems. Examples are given in Table 4-3.

Other complications, such as pulmonary embolism or malnutrition, may also reflect the underlying disease state. Management of these complications requires ongoing surveillance and recognition. Pneumonia may be difficult to diagnose in patients who are receiving mechanical ventilation because pulmonary infiltrates are frequently present, tracheal secretions may be colonized by bacteria, and signs such as fever and leukocytosis are frequently blunted. In this setting, quantitative cultures of secretions obtained from bronchoalveolar lavage or protected-specimen brush may aid in the diagnosis of ventilator-associated pneumonia. Prophylaxis is commonly given to

Table 4-2 Criteria for Ventilator Support

Respiratory rate >30/min
Minute ventilation >10 L/min
Maximal inspiratory pressure < −20 cm H_2O
Vital capacity <10 mL/kg
PaO_2 <60 mm Hg with FiO_2 >0.60
PaO_2/FiO_2 <100-150
$P(A-a)O_2$ >300 mm Hg with FiO_2 1.0
VD/VT >0.60
$PaCO_2$ >50 mm Hg

Table 4-3 Complications of Mechanical Ventilation

Airway injury, bleeding, infection
Ventilator malfunction—leaks, power loss, incorrect settings, or alarm failures
Barotrauma; pneumothorax; interstitial, subcutaneous, or mediastinal air
Decreased right ventricular filling, increased right ventricular afterload, decreased cardiac output, hypotension
Gastrointestinal tract bleeding, stress gastritis, ulceration
Decreased urine output
Alteration in intracranial pressure

reduce stress-related gastritis and ulceration. H_2-Blockers may increase colonization of the respiratory tract by gram-negative bacteria. Sucralfate or frequent use of antacids is an alternative. The hemodynamic complications of increased intrathoracic pressure may be overcome with the administration of fluid; however, there is often a coexisting condition of capillary leak and pulmonary edema that may worsen.

- Pneumonia may be difficult to diagnose in patients receiving mechanical ventilation.
- Prophylaxis is commonly given to reduce stress-related gastritis and ulceration.
- H_2-Blockers may increase colonization of the respiratory tract by gram-negative bacteria; sucralfate or frequent use of antacids is an alternative.

An important and occasionally subtle complication of positive pressure ventilation is called "intrinsic positive end-expiratory pressure (PEEP)," "auto-PEEP," "breath-stacking," or "dynamic hyperinflation." This refers to a phenomenon of inadequate time during the expiratory phase of the respiratory cycle so that a mechanically assisted breath is delivered before passive expiration of the lungs is complete. Thus, a new machine breath is delivered before the previous breath is completely exhaled. This may worsen hyperinflation, increase intrathoracic pressure, reduce venous return, and worsen the associated complications (e.g., barotrauma), especially in patients with airway obstruction. Intrinsic PEEP may exist in spontaneously breathing patients with obstructive airway disease, but the effect is most important in mechanically ventilated patients. Treatment typically involves optimizing bronchodilator therapy and altering the ventilator cycle to allow maximal expiratory time.

Pulmonary oxygen toxicity appears to be the result of direct exposure to high tensions of inspired oxygen or alveolar oxygen. For adults, oxygen toxicity is not believed to be a major clinical concern below an FiO_2 of 0.40 to 0.50. Higher levels of inspired oxygen may be associated with acute tracheo-bronchitis (most likely an irritant effect). After several days of exposure, a syndrome of diffuse alveolar damage and lung injury may develop. The pathologic features may resemble those of ARDS.

- Pulmonary oxygen toxicity is the result of direct exposure to high tensions of inspired oxygen or alveolar oxygen.
- The syndrome of diffuse alveolar damage and lung injury may develop.

Modes of Mechanical Ventilation

"Modes of mechanical ventilation" refers to the pattern of cycling of the machine breath and its relation to the spontaneous breaths of the patient, for example, assist/control mode, intermittent mandatory ventilation, and pressure support ventilation. "Volume preset assist/control mode" is defined by a machine-assisted breath for every inspiratory effort by the patient. If no spontaneous breaths occur during a preset time interval, a controlled breath of predetermined tidal volume is delivered by the ventilator. The backup rate should determine the minimum minute ventilation the patient will receive. The advantage of assist/control mode ventilation is that it should allow maximal rest for the patient and maximal control of ventilation. The disadvantage is that hyperventilation or air trapping (or both) can occur in patients making rapid inspiratory efforts.

"Volume preset intermittent mandatory ventilation (IMV)" allows a preset number of machine-assisted breaths of a given tidal volume. Between machine breaths, patients may breathe spontaneously. The IMV mode was developed as a mode for weaning patients from the ventilator so that the number of mechanical breaths could be decreased gradually, allowing for increasing spontaneous ventilation. However, recent trials have shown that this mode of weaning is inferior to weaning via T-piece trials or pressure support ventilation.

- Assist/control mode ventilation: machine-assisted breath for every inspiratory effort by the patient (a mandatory minimal frequency is set).
- Assist/control mode advantage: allows maximal rest for the patient and maximal control of ventilation.
- Assist/control mode disadvantage: hyperventilation or air trapping or both occur in patients making rapid inspiratory efforts.
- IMV: allows a preset number of machine-assisted breaths of a given tidal volume.
- Between machine breaths, patients may breathe spontaneously.
- IMV is not superior to other weaning techniques (T-piece trials or pressure support).

"Pressure support ventilation" may be used to assist spontaneously breathing patients, with or without IMV breaths. In this technique, for each inspiratory effort by the patient, the ventilator delivers a high rate of flow of inspired gas, up to a preset pressure limit. This pressure support occurs only during the spontaneous inspiratory effort, so that the rate and pattern of respiration are determined by the patient.

- With pressure support ventilation, for each inspiratory effort of the patient, the ventilator delivers a high flow of inspired gas, up to a preset pressure limit.

Use of PEEP in Mechanical Ventilation

PEEP is intended to increase functional residual capacity, recruit partially collapsed alveoli, improve lung compliance, and improve ventilation-perfusion matching. An adverse effect of PEEP is an excessive increase in intrathoracic pressure with decreased cardiac output. Overdistention of lung units may also worsen gas exchange because of ventilator-induced lung injury. At levels of PEEP greater than 10 to 15 cm H_2O, barotrauma is of particular concern. The optimal, or best, PEEP may be defined as the lowest level of PEEP needed to achieve satisfactory oxygen delivery at a nontoxic FIO_2.

- PEEP: to increase functional residual capacity, recruit partially collapsed alveoli, improve lung compliance, and improve ventilation-perfusion matching.
- Adverse effect of PEEP: excessive increase in intrathoracic pressure with decreased cardiac output.
- Overdistention of lung units may also worsen ventilation-perfusion matching and gas exchange.
- Optimal, or best, PEEP: lowest level of PEEP needed to achieve satisfactory oxygenation at a nontoxic FIO_2.

ACUTE RESPIRATORY DISTRESS SYNDROME

Diffuse lung injury with acute hypoxic respiratory failure may result from various injuries. Acute lung injury is a frequent primary cause of critical illness and may occur as a complication or a coexisting feature of multisystem disease. "Acute respiratory distress syndrome" (ARDS) is commonly defined as diffuse acute lung injury with the following major features: diffuse pulmonary infiltrates, severe hypoxemia due to shunting and ventilation-perfusion mismatch, and normal or low pulmonary capillary wedge pressure (i.e., noncardiogenic pulmonary edema). Criteria for the diagnosis of ARDS are listed in Table 4-4. Mortality from all causes averages about 50%. For nearly 30 years after this syndrome was described, no single therapy was shown to alter outcome, although gradual improvement in overall mortality was attributed to multidisciplinary ICU management. Recently,

Table 4-4 Criteria for Diagnosis of Acute Respiratory Distress Syndrome

---

Appropriate setting
  Pulmonary injury, shock, trauma
  Acute event
  Clinical respiratory distress, tachypnea
Diffuse pulmonary infiltrates on chest radiography
  Interstitial and/or alveolar pattern
Hypoxemia
  PaO_2/FIO_2 ratio <150
Exclude
  Chronic pulmonary disease accounting for the clinical
    features
  Left ventricular failure (most series require pulmonary
    artery wedge pressure measurement <18 mm Hg)

---

prospective, controlled trials have found that a strategy of mechanical ventilation with reduced tidal volumes is associated with improved survival (discussed below).

- Diffuse lung injury with hypoxic respiratory failure may result from various injuries.
- Mortality from all causes averages approximately 50%.

ARDS Etiology, Pathophysiology, and Prognosis

ARDS was described initially as a post-traumatic or shock-induced injury, but it occurs with various states, as outlined in Table 4-5.

The relative risks of developing ARDS have been estimated from studies of predisposed groups. The greatest frequency is among patients with sepsis (approximately 40%), gastric aspiration (30%), multiple transfusions (25%), pulmonary contusion (20%), disseminated intravascular coagulation (20%), pneumonia requiring ICU management (12%), and trauma with long-bone or pelvic fractures (5%).

The pathophysiologic mechanism of ARDS depends on damage to the alveolar-capillary unit. The earliest histologic changes are endothelial swelling, followed by edema and inflammation. Mononuclear inflammation, loss of alveolar type I cells, and protein deposition in the form of hyaline membranes may occur within 2 or 3 days. Fibrosis may develop after days or weeks of the process. Damage to type II alveolar cells leads to loss of surfactant. The surfactant that is produced may be inactivated by proteins present in the airways. Alveolar filling and collapse cause intrapulmonary shunting and ventilation-perfusion mismatch with hypoxemia.

Death from ARDS is not usually caused by isolated hypoxemic respiratory failure. The most frequent causes of mortality are complications of infection, sepsis syndrome, and failure

of other organ systems. In addition to the clinical risk factors listed above, specific variables associated with mortality include fewer than 10% band forms on a peripheral blood smear, persistent acidemia, bicarbonate less than 20 mEq/L, and blood urea nitrogen greater than 65 mg/dL. Therefore, the systemic effects associated with ARDS may be important to outcome.

- Death from ARDS is not usually caused by isolated hypoxemic respiratory failure.
- Infection, sepsis syndrome, and failure of other organ systems are the usual causes of mortality.
- Variables associated with mortality: <10% band forms on a peripheral blood smear, persistent acidemia, bicarbonate <20 mEq/L, blood urea nitrogen >65 mg/dL.

Therapy for ARDS

The traditional therapy for ARDS involves optimization of physiologic variables and supportive management of associated complications. Measures include optimization of gas exchange and hemodynamics, nutrition, ambulation, and control of infections. Hypoxemia typically is corrected with positive pressure ventilation with supplemental oxygen and PEEP. PEEP provides potential benefits of increased lung volume and lung compliance and improvement in ventilation-perfusion relationships. Maintaining PEEP at a level adequate to prevent repetitive opening and closing of gravitationally dependent lung units (i.e., above "closing volume") may be helpful in limiting tissue sheer forces that can potentiate capillary injury and worsen the degree of diffuse alveolar damage.

Table 4-5 Disorders Associated With Acute Respiratory Distress Syndrome

Shock	Any cause
Sepsis	Lung infections, other bacteremic or endotoxic states
Trauma	Head injury, lung contusion, fat embolism
Aspiration	Gastric, near-drowning, tube feedings
Hematologic	Transfusions, leukoagglutinin, intravascular coagulation, thrombotic thrombocytopenic purpura
Metabolic	Pancreatitis, uremia
Drugs	Narcotics, barbiturates, aspirin
Toxic	Inhaled—O_2, smoke
	Irritant gases—NO_2, Cl_2, SO_2, NH_3
	Chemicals—paraquat
Miscellaneous	Radiation, air embolism, altitude

Beyond an optimal level of PEEP, an increase in intrathoracic pressure may be associated with decreased venous return, increased pulmonary vascular resistance, decreased left ventricular filling, and a corresponding decrease in cardiac output.

Limiting the degree of alveolar distention during peak inflation may limit the potential for alveolar disruption and subsequent barotrauma, often referred to as "ventilator-induced lung injury." This is achieved by delivering tidal volumes of limited size, either by a volume preset or a pressure-targeted mode of ventilation. The use of PEEP levels chosen to prevent alveolar closure and tidal volumes chosen to prevent alveolar overdistention is termed the "protective ventilatory strategy" in the management of ARDS. A recent randomized study found improved survival in ARDS patients receiving a tidal volume of 6 mL/kg ideal body weight compared with a control group receiving a tidal volume of 12 mL/kg body weight. This represents the first specific therapy for ARDS that has been shown to improve survival. In many patients supported with these ventilator guidelines, the level of alveolar ventilation achieved results in an increase in arterial PCO_2. This phenomenon, termed "permissive hypercapnia," does not appear to be harmful. Indeed, recent evidence indicates that mild hypercapnia and respiratory acidosis may decrease the degree of ventilator-induced lung injury.

Supportive management of associated complications includes screening for underlying infections and early antibiotic therapy. Selective bowel decontamination by oral or nasogastric administration of a combination of nonabsorbable antibiotics may decrease the colonization of the airway by gram-negative organisms (reported to decrease the incidence of pneumonia in patients receiving mechanical ventilation).

- Hypoxemia typically is corrected with positive pressure ventilation with supplemental oxygen and PEEP.
- A "protective ventilatory strategy" in ARDS is designed to limit ventilator-induced lung injury.
- A tidal volume of 6 mL/kg is the first specific intervention shown to improve survival in ARDS.

Because increased capillary permeability allows greater intravascular fluid leak at any given hydrostatic pressure, intravascular volume is usually limited to that necessary for systemic perfusion. However, associated shock states may demand volume expansion or increased inotropic support. Crystalloids can provide adequate filling pressures in patients with shock states, but large volumes may be required. Specific applications for colloids in ARDS include blood products (e.g., for coagulopathies or anemia). Supplemental nutrition typically is provided throughout the course of critical illness. Many patients with ARDS have associated multiorgan injury and may have ileus or gastrointestinal tract dysfunction that precludes enteral feeding. Enteral feeding is recommended if tolerated. The consequences of malnutrition may include impairment of respiratory muscle function, depressed ventilatory drive, and limitation of host defenses. Mobilization, ambulation, and ventilator weaning are carried out as early as practical.

- Crystalloids can provide adequate filling pressures in patients with shock states.
- Many patients with ARDS have associated multiorgan injury.

Pharmacologic therapies have been directed against proposed biochemical and cellular mechanisms of ARDS. The explanation for the presumed pathogenesis of acute lung injury is centered on the role of polymorphonuclear leukocytes. Activation of complement by many stimuli associated with lung injury may lead to recruitment and activation of neutrophils, which may injure endothelium by releasing proteolytic enzymes and liberating toxic oxygen species (e.g., hydrogen peroxide, hydroxyl radical, singlet oxygen, and superoxide). Bronchoalveolar lavage fluid from patients with established ARDS and from high-risk patients may show an increased number of cells, predominantly neutrophils. (Normal lavage fluid contains about 93% alveolar macrophages, with 5% to 7% lymphocytes and few neutrophils.) The percentage of neutrophils is correlated with the abnormalities of gas exchange and alveolar protein content. However, experimental lung injury may occur in the absence of neutrophils, and typical ARDS is seen in severely neutropenic patients, so that other mechanisms also have a role.

Arachidonic acid metabolites are implicated in many biochemical events associated with acute lung injury. Arachidonic acid is released from cell membranes by phospholipases. Arachidonate may then be metabolized via the lipoxygenase pathway to leukotriene compounds or via the cyclooxygenase pathway to prostaglandins or thromboxane. These compounds are potentially crucial in the pathogenesis of acute lung injury. Thromboxane A_2, a potent vasoconstrictor, induces platelet aggregation. Prostacyclin, or prostaglandin (PG) I_2, has the opposite effects on smooth muscle and platelet aggregation and is a potential therapeutic agent for ARDS. PGE_1, a prostaglandin, relaxes vascular and bronchial smooth muscle and inhibits neutrophil chemotaxis.

- Acute lung injury: the pathogenesis centers on polymorphonuclear leukocytes.
- Neutrophils may injure endothelium by releasing proteolytic enzymes and liberating toxic oxygen species.
- Experimental lung injury may still occur in the absence of neutrophils.

- Arachidonic acid metabolites are implicated in many biochemical events associated with acute lung injury.
- Thromboxane A_2 is a potent vasoconstrictor that induces platelet aggregation.
- PGE_1: relaxes vascular and bronchial smooth muscle and inhibits neutrophil chemotaxis.

Potential therapeutic and prophylactic agents have been directed against steps in the arachidonate pathways. Corticosteroids decrease cell membrane disruption and have other anti-inflammatory properties. Specifically, no differences in mortality have been observed in prospective, randomized studies of ARDS patients receiving methylprednisolone or placebo. However, limited trials have suggested that corticosteroid therapy may be of benefit in the fibroproliferative phase of ARDS, and in some instances, corticosteroids are added if no improvement has occurred after 1 to 2 weeks of conventional therapy. Trials of high-dose corticosteroids in sepsis have also shown no difference in overall mortality. High-dose corticosteroid therapy may delay the resolution of secondary infections. An increased risk of death related to secondary infection after high-dose corticosteroid therapy has been observed.

- Corticosteroids decrease cell membrane disruption and have other anti-inflammatory properties.
- However, in early-phase ARDS, corticosteroids are potentially harmful and have no proven benefit.
- Corticosteroids may decrease the time to resolution of fibroproliferative (late-phase) ARDS.
- In sepsis, no difference has been shown in overall mortality with corticosteroids.

Nonsteroidal anti-inflammatory drugs (NSAIDs), for example, ibuprofen and indomethacin, block cyclooxygenase and thromboxane formation. In animal models of acute lung injury and septic shock, NSAIDs have beneficial effects if used prophylactically. However, no benefit is known for established ARDS. Other mediators, particularly those associated with sepsis, may be important factors in the pathogenesis of acute lung injury. Endotoxin, a complex lipopolysaccharide, may activate complement; it has been associated with neutrophilic alveolitis. Monoclonal antiendotoxin antibodies reportedly have beneficial effects in some patients with sepsis, but controlled trials have failed to show improved overall survival.

Recently, pulmonary vasodilators, of which nitric oxide has been studied most widely, have been used as adjuncts to traditional therapy. Inhaled nitric oxide, delivered by a mechanical ventilator, naturally distributes to relatively well-ventilated regions of each lung. Nitric oxide acts as a dilator of the alveolar capillary and is rapidly inactivated in the bloodstream, thereby potentially improving perfusion to ventilated areas without systemic vasodilation.

Several studies of inhaled nitric oxide have shown dramatic short-term improvement in oxygenation and pulmonary artery pressures in patients with ARDS. However, outcome studies have not shown improved survival. In a large-scale European trial, 67% of ARDS patients were identified as responders to inhaled nitric oxide, showing improvement in oxygenation and a decrease in pulmonary artery pressure. However, there was no difference in the time to reverse lung injury or in 30-day mortality. Other vasodilating agents, including prostacyclin and PGE_1, have also been tried. Currently, anti-inflammatory agents and pulmonary vasodilators should be considered investigational for the treatment of ARDS, with no documented effect on survival. The prognosis for recovery of lung function in patients who survive ARDS is good. Studies of survivors have shown nearly normal lung volumes and airflow 6 to 12 months after the illness, with mild impairment in gas exchange—decreased diffusing capacity, desaturation with exercise, or widened A-a gradient. Therefore, the incentive is strong to continue aggressive measures in patients with otherwise reversible organ dysfunction.

- The prognosis for the recovery of lung function in patients surviving ARDS is good.
- Mild decreases in lung volumes, oxygenation, and diffusing capacity are typically observed after 6 to 12 months.

CARDIOPULMONARY RESUSCITATION

General clinical algorithms for standardized responses to cardiac arrhythmias or arrest should be reviewed. Ideally, in ICUs, cardiorespiratory problems should be prevented or anticipated and recognized quickly.

Airway Control

Relieve obstruction. Remove any foreign bodies. If not dislodged or obstructing, dentures may improve the seal of a face mask. However, dentures are usually removed before endotracheal intubation.

Suction (saliva, emesis, blood). A rigid suction catheter is most useful. Use head-tilt, chin-lift, or forward thrust of the jaw to open the posterior pharynx. The oropharyngeal or nasopharyngeal airway may help maintain patency and facilitate suctioning and mask ventilation.

Supply a high rate of flow of supplemental oxygen. Ventilation is usually begun with a bag-valve-mask technique. Because a combined respiratory and metabolic acidosis is common, hyperventilation should be carried out to the extent possible.

Endotracheal intubation provides better control of the airway for ventilation, oxygenation, and suctioning and should be performed as soon as practical during the resuscitation effort. However, the best possible ventilation and oxygenation should be provided before any attempt at intubation, and efforts should be limited to 15 to 30 seconds before mask ventilation is resumed.

For chest compressions, a 15:2 compression-to-ventilation ratio is currently recommended for one-person and two-person resuscitation. Check the femoral pulse for effectiveness of compressions. Monitoring of expired carbon dioxide (capnometry) by various devices is used to assess the adequacy of ventilation and to confirm endotracheal (versus esophageal) intubation. Under conditions of controlled ventilation and cardiac resuscitation, expired carbon dioxide may be an indicator of effective chest compressions, because carbon dioxide delivery to the lungs depends on adequate cardiac output.

- Relieve obstruction.
- Oropharyngeal or nasopharyngeal airway may help maintain patency.
- Supply a high rate of flow of supplemental oxygen.
- Endotracheal intubation: better control of the airway for ventilation.

Electrical Therapy

Ventricular fibrillation is the most common rhythm in sudden cardiac arrest. The time to defibrillation is the most important factor determining successful resuscitation. In monitored patients in ICUs, defibrillation typically should be the first treatment, with other life support efforts initiated only after immediate attempts at electrical conversion. Electrical pacing may be useful in some cases of bradycardia and heart block.

- Ventricular fibrillation is the common rhythm in sudden cardiac arrest.
- Time to defibrillation is the most important factor determining successful resuscitation.
- In monitored patients in ICUs, defibrillation typically should be the first treatment.

Drug therapy for arrhythmias is discussed elsewhere in this text.

VASCULAR ACCESS AND HEMODYNAMIC MONITORING

Central Venous Catheterization

The first choice for access in stable patients requiring intravenous therapy is the peripheral veins. However, in ICUs, central venous catheterization is often necessary for the following indications: lack of adequate peripheral veins, need for hypertonic or phlebitic medications or solutions, need for long-term access, measurement of central pressures, and access for procedures (hemodialysis, cardiac pacing). Relative contraindications include inexperience of the practitioner, coagulopathy, inability to identify landmarks, infection or burn at the entry site, and thrombosis of the proposed central venous site. Central venous catheters are usually placed over a guidewire (modified Seldinger technique). Complications of central venous catheterization include infections, cardiac arrhythmias, pneumothorax, air embolism, catheter or guidewire embolism, catheter knotting, bleeding, and other potential complications of needle or catheter misplacement.

- Central venous catheterization is often necessary.
- Contraindications: inexperienced practitioner, coagulopathy, inability to identify landmarks, infection or burn at the entry site, thrombosis of proposed central venous site.
- Complications: infections, cardiac arrhythmias, pneumothorax, air embolism, catheter or guidewire embolism, catheter knotting, bleeding.

Catheter-related infections are usually attributed to the migration of bacteria from the skin along the catheter tract. Catheter-related infection is usually defined by more than 15 colony-forming units (CFU/mL) on semiquantitative culture of the catheter tip. Catheter-related bacteremia is defined by similar growth and blood cultures positive for the same organism. Risk factors include infected catheter site or cutaneous breakdown, multiple manipulations, the number of catheter lumens, and the duration of use of the same site (particularly after 3 or 4 days). Treatment should include catheter removal and replacement at another site if necessary.

- Catheter-related infections usually are attributed to migration of bacteria from the skin along the catheter tract.
- Risk factors: infected catheter site or cutaneous breakdown, multiple manipulations, number of catheter lumens, duration of use of same site.

Pulmonary Artery Catheterization

Although common use (or overuse) of pulmonary artery catheterization has been criticized, data from pulmonary artery catheterization may aid diagnosis and therapy in many disorders encountered in ICUs. The physiologic data that may be obtained are listed in Table 4-6.

Clinical conditions for which hemodynamic data may be useful include shock states, pulmonary edema, oliguric renal failure, indeterminate pulmonary hypertension, and myocardial and valvular disorders. Intravascular volume may be assessed more accurately, and the effects of therapeutic interventions (volume, vasodilator therapy, or inotropes) may be evaluated.

Table 4-6 Hemodynamic Data Obtained With Pulmonary Artery Catheterization

Variable	Normal value
Right atrial pressure (RAP)	2-8 mm Hg
Pulmonary arterial pressure (PAP)	16-24/5-12 mm Hg
Pulmonary capillary wedge pressure (PCWP)	5-12 mm Hg
Cardiac output (CO)	4-6 L/min
Cardiac index (CI = CO/body surface area)	2.5-3 L/min per m^2
Stroke volume (SV = CO/heart rate)	50-100 mL/beat
Stroke volume index (SVI = SV/body surface area)	35-50 mL/m^2
Systemic vascular resistance	10-15 mm Hg/L per min
[SVR = (blood pressure − RAP)/CO]	(×80 to convert to 800-1,200 dynes • s/cm^{-5})
Pulmonary vascular resistance	1.5-2.5 mm Hg/L per min
[PVR = (PAP − PCWP)/CO]	(100-200 dynes • s/cm^{-5})

Mixed venous oxygen saturation may also be measured, as indicated above. This may be particularly useful in assessing the effects of PEEP on oxygen delivery (i.e., improving arterial saturation but potentially decreasing cardiac output).

Complications of pulmonary artery catheterization include arrhythmias, right bundle branch block, complete heart block in patients with preexisting left bundle branch block, vascular or right ventricular perforation, thrombosis and embolism, catheter knotting, infection, and pulmonary infarction or rupture due to persistent wedging or overdistention of the balloon.

Case-control studies have found that the use of a pulmonary artery catheter was associated with higher mortality than no catheter in patients who had a similar severity of illness. However, the basis of this observation is uncertain, and catheter use is still common clinical practice. A recent prospective trial of pulmonary artery catheterization in high-risk surgical patients showed no differences in outcome (i.e., no clear evidence of benefit or harm) between those who had catheterization and control groups.

- Complications of pulmonary artery catheterization: arrhythmias, right bundle branch block, complete heart block in patients with preexisting left bundle branch block, vascular or right ventricular perforation, thrombosis and embolism, catheter knotting, infection, pulmonary infarction or rupture due to persistent wedging or overdistention of the balloon.

The use of pulmonary capillary wedge pressure (PCWP) as an indicator of left ventricular end-diastolic pressure assumes a continuous hydrostatic column extending from the pulmonary capillary to the left atrium. Although digital displays of PCWP are usually available, the pressure wave should be examined for potential artifacts and for the degree of respiratory variation. Because varying intrathoracic pressure may be sensed by the pulmonary artery catheter, recorded PCWP should be obtained at end-expiration. Even with these measures, PCWP may be influenced by airway pressure and, thus, not accurately reflect ventricular filling pressure, especially with high levels of PEEP.

- PCWP is an indicator of left ventricular end-diastolic pressure.
- PCWP may be influenced by airway pressure, especially with high levels of PEEP.

SHOCK STATES

"Shock" is defined by evidence of end-organ hypoperfusion, usually (but not necessarily) associated with hypotension. A common classification is cardiogenic (decreased cardiac output), hypovolemic (decreased blood volume), and septic (variable cardiac output, decreased systemic vascular resistance). All forms of shock may be characterized by hypotension, tachycardia, tachypnea, altered mental status, decreased urine output, and lactic acidosis. The clinical history often helps determine the diagnosis, for example, blood loss, trauma, myocardial infarction, or systemic infection. Compared with other causes, septic shock is often characterized by relatively warm extremities and normal or increased cardiac output.

- Shock is defined by evidence of end-organ hypoperfusion, usually associated with hypotension.
- Common classification: cardiogenic, hypovolemic, and septic.
- Shock is characterized by hypotension, tachycardia, tachypnea, altered mental status, decreased urine output, and lactic acidosis.

- Septic shock is often characterized by relatively warm extremities and normal or increased cardiac output.

To achieve a common terminology, the concept of systemic inflammatory response syndrome (SIRS) was introduced for findings of fever or hypothermia, tachycardia, hyperventilation, and leukocytosis or leukopenia regardless of cause. "Sepsis" is defined as SIRS in the setting of a known or presumed source of infection, and "severe sepsis" is defined as sepsis associated with organ system dysfunction and systemic effects, including hypotension, decreased urine output, or metabolic acidosis. "Septic shock" refers to persistent signs of organ hypoperfusion despite adequate fluid resuscitation.

After a rapid initial assessment, treatment of shock is directed at the presumed source, for example, volume (blood loss, hypovolemia), vasodilator or inotropic therapy (cardiogenic), or fluids, antibiotics, and drainage of any infected space (sepsis). If the response to the initial therapy is inadequate, and especially if intravascular volume status is uncertain clinically, pulmonary artery catheterization may be useful. For example, if the wedge pressure remains less than 12 to 15 mm Hg, additional volume should be administered. A recent prospective trial of "early goal-directed therapy" stressing volume resuscitation beginning in the emergency department showed improved hospital survival compared with standard therapy. If the wedge pressure is greater than 18 to 20 mm Hg and there is evidence of cardiac dysfunction, a vasodilator (nitroprusside) and diuretic therapy may be considered. If "hyperdynamic" indices are observed, that is, increased cardiac output and low peripheral resistance, fluids should first be given to achieve a high-normal wedge pressure. Low doses of dopamine, 2 to 5 µg/kg per minute, may improve renal perfusion. *After* volume support has been given and if tissue perfusion remains inadequate, careful administration of vasoconstrictors (e.g., norepinephrine) may improve organ perfusion. Recently, low-dose vasopressin has been reported to be beneficial in the hemodynamic support of patients with septic shock.

Multisystem organ failure, or multiple organ dysfunction syndrome (MODS), is usually defined as acute dysfunction of two or more organ systems lasting more than 2 days. Sepsis is the most common cause. The pathogenesis is attributed to the hemodynamic and immunologic effects of endotoxin, cytokines (tumor necrosis factor [TNF-α]), interleukins (IL-1, IL-2, IL-6, IL-8), platelet-activating factor, arachidonic acid metabolites, polymorphonuclear leukocyte-derived toxic products, and myocardial depressant factors. Corticosteroids have no known benefit and potential adverse effects in patients with sepsis syndrome, with or without ARDS. An exception is the use of relatively low doses of hydrocortisone or methylprednisolone in patients with documented adrenal insufficiency in the setting of severe sepsis, for which benefit has been reported.

Recently, a controlled, prospective trial of recombinant human activated protein C (drotrecogin alfa), administered intravenously over 96 hours, reported a 19% relative reduction (6% absolute decrease) in mortality among patients with severe sepsis. Activated protein C has anti-inflammatory and profibrinolytic properties that may contribute to this benefit. The main adverse effect of recombinant human activated protein C is bleeding.

- Sepsis syndrome typically is defined by a known or presumed source of infection associated with fever (or hypothermia) and leukocytosis (or leukopenia) and evidence of systemic effects (hypotension, decreased urine output, metabolic acidosis).
- Treatment is directed at the presumed source.
- Septic shock commonly is associated with multiorgan injury.
- Multisystem organ failure: acute dysfunction of two or more organ systems lasting >2 days.
- High-dose corticosteroid treatment is of no known benefit.
- Replacement therapy may be of benefit for patients with adrenal insufficiency.
- Recombinant human activated protein C is the first specific therapy to decrease mortality from severe sepsis.

Mortality of patients with sepsis and multiorgan failure may be greater than 70% to 90%. Adverse risk factors include age older than 65 years, continued systemic signs of sepsis, persistent deficit in oxygen delivery, and preexisting renal or liver failure. Physiologic scoring systems (e.g., APACHE) may predict outcome more accurately for subgroups of patients.

- Mortality of patients with sepsis and multiorgan failure may be >70% to 90%.

DISEASE SEVERITY SCORING SYSTEMS

The use of a severity-of-illness scoring system is increasingly prevalent in the ICU. These systems may define quantitative overall risks for *populations* of patients. An accurate quantifiable description of the pretreatment status of critically ill patients can allow improved precision in the evaluation and implementation of new therapies (i.e., clinical research). Furthermore, these systems can be of great use in quality improvement efforts. In most systems, however, the role in individual case management is unclear. The types of clinical scoring systems have ranged from simple counts of failing organs to highly sophisticated methods that incorporate (acute and chronic) clinical and physiologic parameters into proprietary logistic regression prediction equations derived from large databases.

The Glasgow Coma Scale (GCS) was developed in the early 1970s as a triage tool for patients with head injury. This scoring system assigns a weighted point score for three behavioral responses: eye opening (1 to 4 points), best verbal response (1 to 5 points), and best motor response (1 to 6 points). Thus, GCS scores range from 3 to 15 points: severe dysfunction = 3 to 8 points, moderate dysfunction = 9 to 12 points, and mild dysfunction = 13 to 14 points. The GCS system has been shown to correlate with mortality and the level of ultimate brain function in patients with traumatic brain injury. Because of its efficacy and simplicity, the GCS has been used within other scoring systems.

Several multisystem scoring systems have been developed for use in critically ill patients. Although a detailed review of these systems is beyond the scope of this text, they include the Acute Physiology and Chronic Health Evaluation (APACHE) system, Simplified Acute Physiology Score (SAPS), the Mortality Probability Model (MPM), Project IMPACT, and the Therapeutic Intervention Scoring System (TISS).

- Severity scoring systems attempt to quantify overall risk for *populations* of patients.
- Severity scoring systems can be of great use in clinical research and quality assurance functions.
- The best role for most scoring systems in the care of *individual* patients is undefined.

ETHICS IN THE ICU

The principles listed in Table 4-7 provide a framework for assessing ethical issues in the ICU. However, the potential for conflict frequently arises because patients often are unable to participate in their own care, many family members may be involved, and the medical staff may disagree about the prognosis and proposed interventions.

Recent legal opinions have supported the concept that a competent person may refuse life-sustaining therapy. Decision making for incompetent patients is more controversial, and living-will legislation has been designed partly to address such conflicts.

- A competent person may refuse life-sustaining therapy.
- Decision making for incompetent patients is more controversial; living-will legislation has been designed partly to address such conflicts.

"Do Not Resuscitate" orders have become increasingly common and important in recent years. The guidelines of the American Medical Association include

1. Consent to cardiopulmonary resuscitation is presumed unless the patient (or patient's surrogate) has expressed in advance the wish not to be resuscitated or if, in the judgment of the treating physician, an attempt to resuscitate the patient would be futile. Resuscitation efforts

Table 4-7 Principles for Assessing Ethical Issues in Intensive Care Units

Beneficence—acting in the patient's benefit by sustaining life, treating illness, and relieving pain

Nonmaleficence—do no harm

Autonomy—fundamental right to self-determination

Informed consent—providing factual and adequate information for competent patients to make decisions about their care

Substituted judgment—ability of a family member, guardian, or other surrogate to make decisions on behalf of the patient on the basis of what he or she believes the patient would have chosen if competent

Social justice—allocation of medical resources according to need (note that this concept implies overt health care rationing and may conflict with perceived individual rights)

Advance directives—living will: designed for persons to express their wishes regarding life-sustaining treatment at such time when they are deemed terminally ill and no longer able to participate in such decisions; typically there is provision or request for denial of specific life-support measures and designation of a surrogate decision maker

should be considered futile if they cannot be expected either to restore cardiac or respiratory function or to achieve the expressed goals of the patient.

2. The appropriateness of cardiopulmonary resuscitation should be discussed with patients at risk for cardiopulmonary arrest, preferably in the outpatient setting or early during hospitalization, and the resuscitation status should be reassessed periodically.

3. The physician is ethically obligated to honor the resuscitation preferences of the patient or surrogate except when this would mandate use of futile therapeutic efforts (potential conflicts may arise in the application of this principle).

4. "Do Not Resuscitate" orders should be entered in the medical record.

5. "Do Not Resuscitate" orders affect the administration of cardiopulmonary resuscitation only; other therapeutic interventions should not be influenced by the order.

Withholding Life Support Versus Withdrawal of Existing Support

Recent deliberations and court rulings have supported the concept that withholding and withdrawing of life support are essentially equivalent. In general, an irreversible or terminal illness is considered a prerequisite for withdrawal of support, but the interpretation may vary widely.

Critical Care Medicine Pharmacy Review
Philip J. Kuper, PharmD, Lance J. Oyen, PharmD

Review of Drugs Commonly Used in the ICU That Potentially Can Cause Delirium

Analgesics
  Opiates
  NSAIDs

Anesthetics & sedatives
  Benzodiazepines
  Bupivacaine
  Ketamine
  Lidocaine
  Propofol

Anticonvulsants
  Barbiturates
  Carbamazepine
  Phenytoin

Antifungals & antivirals
  Acyclovir
  Amphotericin
  Ketoconazole

Antihypertensives
  Captopril
  Clonidine
  Diltiazem
  Enalapril
  Hydralazine
  Methyldopa
  Nifedipine
  Nitroprusside
  Verapamil

Antimicrobials
  Aminoglycosides
  Cephalosporins
  Carbapenems
  Macrolides
  Metronidazole
  Monobactams
  Penicillins
  Quinolones
  Tetracyclines
  Trimethoprim-sulfamethoxazole
    (Cotrimoxazole)

Miscellaneous cardiac drugs
  Antiarrhythmics
  Atropine
  β-Blockers
  Digoxin

Miscellaneous
  Antihistamines
  Corticosteroids
  Theophylline
  Tricyclic antidepressants
  H_2 blockers

ICU, intensive care unit; NSAIDs, nonsteroidal anti-inflammatory drugs.
Data from McGuire BE, Basten CJ, Ryan CJ, et al: Intensive care unit syndrome: a dangerous misnomer. Arch Intern Med 2000;160:906-909, and Fish DN: Treatment of delirium in the critically ill patient. Clin Pharm 1991;10:456-466.

Critical Care Medicine Pharmacy Review (continued)

Review of Drugs Commonly Used in the ICU for Agitation With Ventilation

Drug	Comments	
	Pros	Cons
Benzodiazepines Midazolam Lorazepam Diazepam	Useful for anxiety-related agitation, inexpensive, minimal hemodynamic effects	Risk of oversedation and accumulation, especially prolonged use; depress respiratory drive; potential withdrawal with long-term use
Anesthetic Propofol	Predictable, short-term sedative/ hypnotic effects, no accumulation	Hypotension risk, depresses respiratory drive, high expense, deaths associated with acidosis
Neuroleptic Haloperidol	Specific for delirium, no effect on respiratory drive	Cardiac toxicity and hypotension risks, lowers seizure threshold
Sedative Dexmedetomidine	Pain and anxiolytic properties, does not depress ventilation	Short-term use only (until further research completed), potential withdrawal reaction
Opiates/analgesics Fentanyl Hydromorphone Methadone Morphine	Useful for pain-induced agitation (accurate history for pain important)	May contribute to delirium and confusion, may contribute to hypotension due to histamine release

ICU, intensive care unit.

Critical Care Medicine Pharmacy Review (continued)

Clinically Important Toxic Overdoses and Management

Drug overdose	Clinical syndrome	Basic treatment
Acetaminophen (paracetamol)	0.5-24 h: Nausea, vomiting 24-72 h: Nausea, vomiting, RUQ pain, increased LFTs and PT 72-96 h: Liver necrosis, coagulation defects, jaundice, renal failure, hepatic encephalopathy 4 d-2 wk: Resolution of liver dysfunction	Elimination: Gastric lavage (if <1 h after ingestion), activated charcoal (if <4 h after ingestion) (both longer if sustained-release product) Treatment: *N*-acetylcysteine for toxic ingestion based on Rumack-Matthew nomogram
Amphetamines	Hypertension, tachycardia, arrhythmias, myocardial infarction, vasospasm, seizures, paranoid psychosis, diaphoresis, tachypnea	Elimination: Activated charcoal for oral ingestion Agitation/seizures: Benzodiazepines Hypertension: Control agitation, α-antagonists (phentolamine), vasodilators (nitroglycerin, nitroprusside, nifedipine) Hyperthermia: Control agitation, external cooling
Iron	0.5-6 h: Nausea, vomiting, GI discomfort, GI bleed, drowsiness, hypoglycemia, & hypotension 6-24 h: Latency/quiescence (may not occur in severe ingestions) 6-48 h: Shock, coma, seizures, coagulopathy, acidosis, cardiac failure 2-7 d: Hepatoxicity & coagulopathy, metabolic acidosis, renal insufficiency 1-8 wk: GI disorders, achlorhydria	Elimination: Gastric lavage and/or whole bowel irrigation with polyethylene glycol electrolyte solution, especially with tablets (radiopaque) present on KUB Shock: IV fluids and blood (if hemorrhage present); vasopressors if needed Antidote: Deferoxamine to chelate iron, when iron levels >500 µg/dL or severe ingestion suspected (will change urine to "vin rosé" color)
Salicylate	Respiratory alkalosis (initially), metabolic acidosis (after substantial absorption), pulmonary edema, platelet dysfunction, nausea, vomiting, hearing loss, agitation, delirium	Elimination: Activated charcoal, hemo-dialysis (for severe poisoning), alkalinization of urine Agitation/delirium: Alkalize blood (acidemia enhances transfer into tissue, especially brain) with IV bicarbonate
Tricyclic antidepressants	Wide-complex tachyarrhythmias, hypotension, seizures	Tachyarrhythmias: Alkalizing blood (pH 7.5-7.55) with IV bicarbonate reduces binding to sodium channel Seizures: Benzodiazepines Hypotension: Fluid resuscitation, vasopressors

GI, gastrointestinal; IV, intravenous; KUB, radiograph of kidneys, ureters, bladder; LFT, liver function test; PT, prothrombin time; RUQ, right upper quadrant.

QUESTIONS

Multiple Choice (choose the one best answer)

1. A 65-year-old man, weighing 85 kg, is intubated for respiratory failure following a flulike illness and pneumonia. A chest film shows diffuse bilateral pulmonary infiltrates. Mechanical ventilation is initiated with assist/control mode, tidal volume 800 mL, rate 15/min, FIO_2 0.5, PEEP 5 cm. Arterial blood gases show PaO_2 55 mm Hg, $PaCO_2$ 48 mm Hg, and pH 7.35. Which one of the following is the best ventilator setting change?
   a. Increase respiratory rate to 20/min, FIO_2 to 0.8
   b. Decrease tidal volume to 500 mL, increase PEEP to 12 cm
   c. Change to pressure control ventilation set at 35 cm above PEEP of 15 cm
   d. Increase FIO_2 to 1.0, increase tidal volume to 900 mL
   e. Change to pressure control ventilation 10 cm and increase PEEP to 10 cm

2. A 55-year-old woman has been in the intensive care unit (ICU) for 3 weeks after surgery for bowel perforation, complicated by sepsis and acute lung injury. Vital signs are satisfactory, and an echocardiogram is normal. Mechanical ventilation has been discontinued, and she is able to walk with assistance, although she is short of breath with exertion. Laboratory studies show a hemoglobin concentration of 7.9 g/dL. Which one of the following is true in this setting?
   a. Erythropoietin therapy is associated with shortened ICU stay
   b. Red blood cell transfusion will improve hospital survival in sepsis
   c. Hemoglobin concentration should be maintained above 9 g/dL
   d. Red blood cell transfusion at this level of hemoglobin is not associated with improved hospital survival
   e. Red blood cells that have been stored for 30 days will still provide normal oxygen delivery

3. A 25-year-old man is admitted to the ICU after evaluation in the emergency department for dyspnea and confusion. He has a history of depression and illegal drug use. On examination, he is obtunded and responds minimally to painful stimuli. Arterial blood gases with the patient breathing room air show the following: PaO_2 80 mm Hg, $PaCO_2$ 50 mm Hg, pH 7.20, and bicarbonate 19 mEq/L. The serum level of sodium is 140 mEq/L, potassium 3.8 mEq/L, and chloride 89 mEq/L. Which of the following combined drug ingestions would best account for these findings?
   a. Sertraline plus codeine

   b. Acetaminophen plus methanol
   c. Aspirin plus oxycodone
   d. Diphenhydramine plus ethanol
   e. Cocaine plus methamphetamine

4. A 70-year-old man is transferred to the ICU for exacerbation of severe chronic obstructive pulmonary disease (COPD). He was admitted to the hospital 1 day earlier for increased cough, dyspnea, and production of discolored sputum. A chest film showed hyperinflation, but the lung fields were otherwise clear. He has been treated with intravenous antibiotics and methylprednisolone and inhaled bronchodilators. Arterial blood gases on 28% closed face mask oxygen showed the following: PaO_2 80 mm Hg, $PaCO_2$ 80 mm Hg, and pH 7.29. Which one of the following is true regarding this patient?

   a. Predicted 1-year mortality would be less than 25%
   b. Noninvasive positive pressure ventilation may avoid the need for intubation
   c. Inhaled corticosteroids will shorten hospital length of stay
   d. Antibiotics should be continued for 2 weeks
   e. Outcome is improved if corticosteroid taper is carried out over 4 weeks

5. A 21-year-old woman is intubated for severe respiratory distress due to asthma. She is sedated, and the mechanical ventilator is set assist/control mode, rate 20/min, tidal volume 700 mL, PEEP 5 cm, and FIO_2 0.4. The inspiratory-to-expiratory (I:E) ratio is 1:2. Over the course of 30 minutes, progressive tachycardia and hypotension develop. A chest film shows hyperinflation with clear lung fields and no pneumothorax. Arterial blood gas values are PaO_2 120 mm Hg, $PaCO_2$ 50 mm Hg, and pH 7.32. Which of the following is the most appropriate intervention?

   a. Decrease the respiratory rate
   b. Begin dopamine
   c. Increase tidal volume
   d. Decrease PEEP
   e. Decrease sedation

6. A 46-year-old woman is admitted for abdominal pain, nausea, and vomiting. At surgery, a ruptured gallbladder is removed. That evening, fever, hypotension, tachycardia, and oliguria develop. The hemoglobin concentration is 11 g/dL, leukocyte count 7×10^9/L, and platelet count 226×10^9/L. Coagulation studies are within normal limits. She is intubated and receiving fluids, antibiotics, and vasopressors intravenously. Which one of the following

is true about the use of recombinant human activated protein C in this setting?

a. Contraindicated if there is evidence of disseminated intravascular coagulation and a platelet count of 70 $\times 10^9$/L
b. Shown to decrease the frequency of acute respiratory distress syndrome
c. Shown to decrease the likelihood of acute renal failure
d. Associated with approximately a 20% relative improvement in hospital survival
e. Associated with decreased likelihood of coagulopathy and bleeding complications

7. A 75-year-old man with a 30 pack-year smoking history is admitted for pneumonia and respiratory failure. He is intubated and receiving full support by mechanical ventilation as well as intravenous antibiotics and nebulized bronchodilators. After 5 days, he is sedated but responding to stimuli. A chest film shows improvement in lower lobe infiltrates. Which of the following is the best method for assessing readiness for discontinuation of mechanical ventilation?

a. Switch to low intermittent mandatory ventilation rate with pressure support
b. Immediate 2-hour T-piece trial
c. Two-hour periods of spontaneous breathing with 5-cm pressure support, followed by "rest periods" of full ventilator support
d. Immediate extubation and use of noninvasive positive pressure ventilation
e. Decrease sedation and assess spontaneous tidal volume and respiratory rate

ANSWERS

1. Answer b.

The findings of diffuse pulmonary infiltrates and hypoxemia in the setting of pneumonia satisfy diagnostic criteria for acute respiratory distress syndrome. A recent multicenter, randomized trial showed that a tidal volume of 6 mL/kg ideal body weight and maintenance of plateau pressure below 30 cm H_2O were associated with decreased mortality compared with a tidal volume of approximately 12 mL/kg (31% vs. 39.8% mortality). This strategy is favored even if alveolar ventilation decreases, so-called permissive hypercapnia.

2. Answer d.

Prospective, controlled trials have indicated that a transfusion threshold of approximately 7.0 g/dL in anemic ICU patients is as safe as a threshold of 10 g/dL and may be associated with fewer adverse effects. Exceptions include active bleeding and unstable cardiovascular disease. Erythropoietin may decrease the transfusion requirement in chronically anemic patients, but the effect on ICU outcomes is unknown.

3. Answer c.

The blood gas values show the combination of respiratory acidosis and metabolic acidosis. Salicylate overdose in an adult typically is associated with a metabolic acidosis plus respiratory alkalosis, beyond that expected in compensation for the metabolic effect. For a combined overdose of aspirin and narcotic, hyperventilation is blunted, resulting in the combined acidosis. The other agents listed might be expected to result in hypoventilation or metabolic acidosis, but none of the other drugs would account for this combined acidosis.

4. Answer b.

ICU admission for COPD exacerbation is a marker of severe disease for which outcome studies have found hospital mortality approximately 25% and 1-year mortality approximately 50%. Treatments that have shown benefit in clinical trials include oxygen, bronchodilators, antibiotics, and systemic corticosteroids. The ideal duration of antibiotic treatment is unknown, but 3 to 5 days appears to be adequate in the absence of a clear diagnosis of bronchitis or pneumonia. A tapering course of corticosteroids over 8 weeks has shown no benefit over a 2-week schedule. Inhaled corticosteroids may reduce the frequency of outpatient treatment failure but do not affect hospital outcome. Noninvasive positive pressure ventilation in the setting of acute respiratory failure may decrease the work of breathing, improve alveolar ventilation, and provide support adequate to avoid the need for intubation in some patients.

5. Answer a.

The patient shows signs of severe asthma with air trapping and hyperinflation. At a respiratory rate of 20 breaths/min, each cycle is 3 seconds, and the I:E ratio indicates that the tidal volume is delivered in 1 second, allowing 2 seconds for expiration. Because her passive expiratory time is likely much longer than this, there is worsening hyperinflation or "breath-stacking." Options for ventilator management include lengthening expiratory time or decreasing overall respiratory rate. This probably would require increased sedation and possibly the use of muscle relaxants. The mild increase in Pco_2 should not be of immediate concern.

6. Answer d.

After early and appropriate antibiotic treatment, recombinant human activated protein C represents the first specific treatment shown to improve survival of patients with severe sepsis. A large scale, multicenter trial found an absolute decrease of 6% (25% vs. 31%) and relative decrease of 19% in mortality for patients receiving recombinant human activated protein C compared with controls. The major adverse effect is the risk of bleeding. Evidence of intravascular coagulation alone is not a contraindication, but the agent is not recommended if there is active bleeding or the platelet count is less than 30×10^9/L. Data are not yet available for the use of recombinant human activated protein C and the relative risk of other organ failures, including acute respiratory and renal failure.

7. Answer e.

In this case scenario, the patient's condition may be improving, but he continues to receive full ventilator support. The most sensitive and specific indicators of the readiness for extubation are the respiratory rate and tidal volume during spontaneous breathing. The rapid shallow breathing index (RSBI), measured as the respiratory rate divided by the tidal volume in liters, has become a common bedside assessment. An RSBI <80-100 is a favorable marker of readiness for extubation. Sedation should be decreased or discontinued before ventilator support is removed.

CHAPTER 5
DERMATOLOGY

Marian T. McEvoy, M.D.

GENERAL DERMATOLOGY

Skin Cancer

Nonmelanoma skin cancers (basal cell, squamous cell) are the most common malignancies in the United States. There are about 1,000,000 cases annually, and the cure rate is 90% with early detection and treatment. The incidence of nonmelanoma skin cancer is increasing because of a combination of increased exposure to ultraviolet light, changes in clothing style, increased longevity, and atmospheric ozone depletion.

Both basal cell and squamous cell carcinomas occur on sun-exposed skin areas. Basal cell carcinomas are usually slow growing and locally invasive. They may invade vital structures and can cause considerable disfigurement. Basal cell carcinomas rarely metastasize to regional lymph nodes. In contrast, squamous cell carcinomas can metastasize to regional lymph nodes, and approximately 2% of all squamous cell carcinomas lead to death.

- Basal cell carcinoma and squamous cell carcinoma occur on sun-exposed skin.
- Cure rate is 90% with early detection and treatment.

Malignant Melanoma

It is estimated that in 2003 there were 55,000 newly diagnosed *invasive* melanomas and 7,500 deaths from melanoma. The incidence of malignant melanoma is increasing in the United States. The estimated lifetime risk of invasive melanoma is about 1% for Americans born in the 1990s.

Risk factors for the development of malignant melanoma include fair skin, blond hair, freckling, intermittent sunlight exposure with blistering sunburns during childhood or adolescence, and genetic predisposition. The "familial atypical mole-melanoma syndrome" is transmitted by an autosomal dominant gene. Patients with either familial or nonfamilial dysplastic nevi have an increased risk for development of malignant melanoma. Other risk factors that have been identified include a personal or family history of melanoma or nonmelanoma skin cancer, a large number of benign pigmented nevi, giant pigmented congenital nevus, immunosuppression, human immunodeficiency virus (HIV) positivity, and the use of tanning beds. Many primary melanomas occur on non–sun-exposed sites such as the back, scalp, and subungual skin.

The key to improved survival with malignant melanoma is early diagnosis. The most important prognostic feature of malignant melanoma is tumor thickness (Table 5-1). The 5-year survival rate is approximately 36% in patients with lymph node metastasis and 5% in patients with extranodal metastasis. Other factors such as sex and anatomical site have sometimes been cited as criteria of independent prognostic importance.

- The key to improved survival with malignant melanoma is early diagnosis.
- Most important prognostic feature is tumor thickness.

Stage I malignant melanoma consists of the cutaneous lesion without lymph node involvement, stage II consists of the primary skin lesion plus lymph node involvement, and stage III represents distant metastasis. Surgical management is recommended to treat stage I malignant melanoma and consists of excision with tumor-free margins of 1 to 3 cm. Elective lymph node dissection does not improve outcome in patients with stage I disease. For stage II disease, excision of the primary skin lesion and regional lymph node

Table 5-1 Survival in Malignant Melanoma, by Tumor Thickness

Tumor, mm	5-y survival, %
≤0.75	100
0.76-1.50	94
1.51-2.25	84
2.26-3.00	77
>3.00	46

dissection are usually recommended. No form of adjuvant therapy has been shown to improve survival in patients with advanced disease.

- Surgical management of stage I malignant melanoma consists of excision with tumor-free margins of 1-3 cm.

Sentinel node biopsy, whereby the draining lymph node is identified (by dye injection) and sampled, improves the prognostic accuracy for intermediate and thick melanomas on the limbs. With melanomas on the head and neck and trunk, sampling of the sentinel node is complex and needs to be individualized on the basis of melanoma thickness and other prognostic factors.

Prevention of Melanoma and Nonmelanoma Skin Cancer

Dermatologists encourage regular use of sunscreens with a sun protection factor (SPF) of at least 15. Sunlight exposure during the first 18 years of life accounts for up to 80% of cumulative lifetime sun exposure. Persons with light skin types and outdoor workers need to be particularly vigilant with sun protection.

Cutaneous T-Cell Lymphoma

Cutaneous T-cell lymphoma occurs as mycosis fungoides and Sézary syndrome. Mycosis fungoides generally presents with discrete or coalescing patches, plaques, or nodules on the skin. Mycosis fungoides may progress to involve lymph nodes and viscera. Once extracutaneous involvement is recognized, the median duration of survival has been estimated at 2.5 years. The course of patients with patch- or plaque-stage cutaneous lesions, without extracutaneous disease, is less predictable, but the median duration of survival is approximately 12 years. Sézary syndrome is characterized by generalized erythroderma, keratoderma of the palms and soles, and a Sézary cell count of more than 1,000/mm^3 in the peripheral blood. Most patients have severe pruritus.

- Mycosis fungoides and Sézary syndrome are forms of cutaneous T-cell lymphoma.
- Mycosis fungoides may progress to involve lymph nodes and viscera.
- The median survival for patients with mycosis fungoides is 12 years, but it decreases to 2.5 years with extracutaneous involvement.

Both mycosis fungoides and Sézary syndrome are characterized by the presence of Sézary cells (lymphocytes with hyperchromatic and convoluted nuclei) involving the epidermis (epidermotrophism) and dermis. Immunohistochemical stains of cutaneous lesions demonstrate that these neoplastic T cells usually express CD3 and CD4 antigens, and molecular genetic studies reveal clonal rearrangement of the T-cell receptor gene in lymphocyte populations from skin biopsy, lymph node, and peripheral blood specimens of patients with cutaneous T-cell lymphoma.

- Mycosis fungoides and Sézary syndrome are T-cell lymphomas characterized by the presence of Sézary cells in skin and peripheral blood.

Treatment of cutaneous T-cell lymphoma includes topical nitrogen mustard, psoralen with ultraviolet-A light (PUVA), radiotherapy (electron beam, orthovoltage), and systemic chemotherapy. Interferon, retinoids, and other agents also have been used. Most recently, extracorporeal photopheresis (ingestion of 8-methoxypsoralen, after which the patient's leukocytes are exposed to ultraviolet light A and then reinfused) has been used in the treatment of cutaneous T-cell lymphoma.

Psoriasis

Psoriasis occurs in approximately 1% to 2% of the U.S population. Onset of lesions is most common in the third decade of life, and about a third of patients have a family history of psoriasis. The psoriasis most commonly presents with papules and plaques covered with a silvery scale. Patterns of psoriasis include psoriasis vulgaris that presents with large plaque-like lesions on the trunk and limbs and classic psoriasis involving the elbows and knees. Guttate psoriasis is an acute form of psoriasis which often follows streptococcal throat infection and presents with small lesions (5-10 mm in diameter) of psoriasis on the trunk and limbs. Other, less common forms of psoriasis include pustular psoriasis, which may be localized to the hands and feet or may be generalized. Approximately 50% of patients with psoriasis have nail abnormalities, most commonly onycholysis, pitting, and oil spots. Lesions of psoriasis may occur at previous sites of trauma.

- The onset of psoriasis most often occurs in the third decade of life.
- One-third of patients have a family history of psoriasis.
- About 50% of patients have nail abnormalities.

The treatment of psoriasis includes topical corticosteroids, topical tar preparations, and phototherapy. Newer forms of treatment of localized psoriasis include a topical synthetic vitamin D analogue, calcipotriene, and a topical retinoid, tazarotene.

Systemic agents used in the treatment of resistant psoriasis include methotrexate, acitretin, and cyclosporine.

Targeted Therapy in Psoriasis

Research into the pathogenesis of psoriasis has shown that the disease is T-cell–mediated. This has led to the development of several targeted therapies. Alefacept (LFA3TIP) was approved recently by the Food and Drug Asministration for the treatment of psoriasis. Infliximab and etanercept, currently approved for the treatment of rheumatoid arthritis, have been reported to be effective in the treatment of psoriasis.

Ultraviolet Light

Natural sunlight contains ultraviolet-B (UVB, 280-320 nm), ultraviolet-A (320-400 nm), and visible light. UVB radiation causes sunburn reaction. UVB has been used most commonly in combination with tar for treating inflammatory dermatoses, as in the Goeckerman therapy of psoriasis. UVB also may benefit atopic dermatitis, lichen planus, and certain other inflammatory dermatoses.

Narrow-Band UVB

The wavelength of UVB with therapeutic effect for treating psoriasis has been identified in the 311-nm range. Light units producing this wavelength have been developed (narrow-band UVB) and have been shown to be more effective than traditional UVB for the treatment of psoriasis.

PUVA

PUVA consists of ingestion of psoralen followed by exposure of the skin to ultraviolet-A light. PUVA has been used most commonly for therapy of generalized psoriasis, but it is also effective in the treatment of lichen planus, mycosis fungoides, urticaria pigmentosa, and vitiligo. PUVA therapy is associated with minimal systemic side effects but is associated with an increased risk (>12 times) of cutaneous squamous cell carcinoma in patients who have received long-term therapy.

- PUVA is commonly used for therapy of generalized psoriasis.
- PUVA is associated with minimal systemic side effects.
- The main side effect with PUVA is an increased risk of cutaneous squamous cell carcinoma.

Atopic Dermatitis

Atopy is manifested by the following: atopic dermatitis, asthma, and allergic rhinitis or conjunctivitis. Atopic dermatitis often presents in the neonatal period with scaling and erythema of the scalp and face, later spreading to the trunk. The distribution is often extensor in the older infant, and by the age of approximately 3 years the more classic flexural distribution is observed. In adolescence, facial involvement (perioral, eyelid, and forehead) is common. Generalized flares of eczema can occur at any age.

Disturbances in cell-mediated immunity lead to an increased incidence of bacterial and viral infections. Secondary infection with *Staphylococcus aureus* presents as a weeping, crusting dermatitis (impetiginization). Eczema herpeticum is the term used to describe a secondary infection with the herpes simplex virus, which may be generalized. Infections with the human papillomavirus and molluscum contagiosum are also more common and the lesions are more numerous in patients with atopic dermatitis.

- Eczema herpeticum, a generalized herpes simplex virus infection, may occur in patients with atopic dermatitis.

For many years, emollients and topical corticosteroids have been the mainstay of treatment in atopic dermatitis. Topical calcineurin inhibitors (tacrolimus, pimecrolimus) have been approved for the treatment of atopic dermatitis. These medications have the advantage that they do not induct atrophy or striae, have no systemic side effects, and are not associated with tachyphylaxis.

Allergic Contact Dermatitis

Allergic contact dermatitis is a form of localized or generalized dermatitis that results from exposure to an antigen. This is a type 4 hypersensitivity reaction (delayed, cell-mediated). Recognition of antigens by T lymphocytes requires participation of Langerhans cells, which are the "antigen-presenting" cells of the epidermis. One must consider the anatomical location of the cutaneous lesions and environmental exposure to allergens, including occupational, household, and recreational contactants.

- Allergic contact dermatitis is a type 4 hypersensitivity reaction (delayed, cell-mediated).
- Langerhans cells are the "antigen-presenting" cells of the epidermis.

Patch testing is performed by applying substances to the patient's back; each substance is placed under a small aluminum disk covered with adhesive tape. These are left on the patient's back for 48 hours, and the results are interpreted at 48 and 96 hours. Positive reactions occur most often to the following antigens: nickel sulfate, potassium dichromate, thimerosal, paraphenylenediamine, ethylenediamine, neomycin sulfate, benzocaine, thiuram, and formaldehyde.

Nickel sulfate allergies are mainly associated with jewelry. Paraphenylenediamine is present in hair dyes and other cosmetics; *para*-aminobenzoic acid (PABA) in sunscreens is immunologically related to paraphenylenediamine. Potassium dichromate sensitivity is one of the most common types of occupational allergic contact dermatitis and occurs in construction workers exposed to cement, leathers, and certain paints. Formaldehyde is a common preservative in cosmetics and shampoos. Neomycin sulfate and benzocaine are components of many topical antimicrobial and analgesic preparations. Thimerosal is a commonly used preservative in contact lens solutions and in some intramuscular injections. Thiuram is a rubber accelerator and fungicide and therefore may correlate with occupational dermatitis or dermatitis related to wearing shoes containing rubber.

- Nickel sulfate allergies are associated with jewelry.
- Potassium dichromate sensitivity occurs in construction workers exposed to cement, leathers, and certain paints.
- Formaldehyde is a common preservative in cosmetics and shampoos.

Acne Vulgaris

Acne vulgaris is one of the most common problems seen in clinical dermatology. Acne occurs physiologically at puberty with varying degrees of severity but may persist into the second and third decades of life. The pathogenesis of acne is multifactorial; inheritance, increase in sebaceous gland activity, hormonal influences, disturbances of keratinization, and bacterial infection have all been implicated. The primary lesions of acne are noninflammatory and include microcomedones, closed comedones (whiteheads), and open comedones (blackheads). The secondary or inflammatory lesions include papules and pustules, nodules, and cysts. Treatment options for acne are given in Table 5-2.

Systemic Retinoids

Isotretinoin (13-*cis*-retinoic acid) is a synthetic vitamin A derivative used primarily for the treatment of severe nodulocystic acne vulgaris. The mechanism of action of 13-*cis*-retinoic acid in acne is probably multifactorial, including improvement in keratinization, decrease in sebum production, and decrease in inflammation. A 20-week course at a

Table 5-2 Treatment of Acne Vulgaris

Type of acne	Treatment
Comedonal	Topical tretinoin (Retin A), benzoyl peroxide
Papular or pustular	Same as above, plus topical or systemic antibiotics
Cystic	Systemic antibiotics; if severe, isotretinoin (Accutane)

dosage of approximately 1 mg/kg per day is the standard regimen.

- Isotretinoin is used for the treatment of severe acne vulgaris.

The greatest risk associated with use of systemic retinoids is teratogenicity. Before isotretinoin is prescribed, female patients must be counseled on this side effect and use reliable contraception during therapy and for at least 1 month after use of the drug is discontinued.

- The greatest risk with the use of systemic retinoids is teratogenicity.

The systemic retinoids are associated with various side effects, including xerosis (dry skin), dermatitis, cheilitis, sticky skin, peeling skin, epistaxis, conjunctivitis, hair loss, and nail dystrophy. Symptoms of arthralgias and myalgias also may occur. Hyperlipidemia, including both hypertriglyceridemia and hypercholesterolemia, develops in most patients. Other *potential* laboratory abnormalities include increased liver enzyme values and leukopenia. Skeletal hyperostosis may occur, particularly in association with long-term use.

- Side effects of systemic retinoids include xerosis, dermatitis, cheilitis, sticky skin, peeling skin, epistaxis, conjunctivitis, hair loss, and nail dystrophy.

Acitretin is effective for the treatment of pustular psoriasis, erythrodermic psoriasis, and generalized chronic plaque-type psoriasis. It has been used successfully as a single agent and in combination with PUVA therapy. Because of the risk of teratogenicity, conception is not recommended for at least 3 years after acitretin therapy.

Autoimmune Bullous Diseases

Bullous pemphigoid is the most common autoimmune bullous disease. The disease predominantly occurs in elderly patients and usually presents with large, tense bullae on erythematous bases with a predilection for flexural areas (Plate 5-1). Lesions are often generalized but may be localized.

- Bullous pemphigoid is the most common autoimmune bullous disease.
- It occurs predominantly in elderly patients.
- It presents as large, tense bullae with a predilection for flexural areas.

Immunofluorescence testing is important for the diagnosis of bullous pemphigoid. Direct immunofluorescence testing of perilesional skin shows deposition of C3 in a linear pattern at the basement membrane zone in almost all cases and of IgG in more than 90%. Indirect immunofluorescence testing of serum demonstrates IgG anti–basement-membrane zone antibodies in approximately 70% of cases.

- Immunofluorescence testing is important for the diagnosis of bullous pemphigoid.
- Almost all cases have deposition of C3 and IgG in a linear pattern at the basement membrane zone.

Treatment of bullous pemphigoid includes systemic corticosteroids, dapsone, azathioprine, and cyclophosphamide. In general, bullous pemphigoid requires less immunosuppressive therapy than does pemphigus and, in contrast to pemphigus, the titer of circulating antibodies does not correlate with disease activity.

Epidermolysis bullosa acquisita is another subepidermal bullous disease. It is characterized clinically by blisters or erosions induced by trauma, which predominantly occur on distal locations. A small subset of patients have generalized lesions, which clinically may be difficult to distinguish from bullous pemphigoid.

- Epidermolysis bullosa acquisita is characterized by blisters or erosions induced by trauma.
- It occurs predominantly on distal sites.

Direct immunofluorescence testing in epidermolysis bullosa acquisita reveals a pattern similar to that in bullous pemphigoid, namely, deposition of IgG and C3 in a linear pattern at the basement membrane zone. In contrast to bullous pemphigoid, C3 may be absent or IgG may be the dominant immunoreactant. Indirect immunofluorescence testing of serum demonstrates IgG anti–basement-membrane zone antibodies in 25% to 50% of patients. Epidermolysis bullosa acquisita tends to be resistant to immunosuppressive therapy.

- On direct immunofluorescence, epidermolysis bullosa acquisita shows deposition of IgG and C3 in a linear pattern at the basement membrane zone.
- Epidermolysis bullosa acquisita tends to be resistant to immunosuppressive therapy.

Cicatricial pemphigoid is characterized by mucosal lesions, with limited or no cutaneous lesions. The disease predominantly affects oral and ocular mucous membranes, and less frequently the genital, pharyngeal, or upper respiratory mucosa. This disease is also known as benign mucous membrane pemphigoid, which is often a misnomer because untreated ocular involvement may lead to blindness. Patients may present with oral erosions or diffuse gingivitis.

- Cicatricial pemphigoid affects oral and ocular mucous membranes, and less frequently genital, pharyngeal, or upper respiratory mucosa.

Treatment of cicatricial pemphigoid is similar to that of bullous pemphigoid, with systemic corticosteroids, dapsone, azathioprine, or cyclophosphamide. Cyclophosphamide has been used particularly in patients with ocular involvement.

Herpes gestationis, also referred to as pemphigoid gestationis, consists of intensely pruritic urticarial papules, plaques, or blisters usually occurring in the latter half of pregnancy. The lesions are histologically characterized by a subepidermal bulla with eosinophils.

- Herpes gestationis consists of intensely pruritic urticarial papules, plaques, or blisters.

Direct immunofluorescence testing is particularly useful because the other dermatoses of pregnancy (such as pruritic urticarial papules and plaques of pregnancy, PUPP) are negative by immunofluorescence testing. The serum from approximately half of patients with herpes gestationis contains the "HG factor," which is a complement-fixing IgG anti–basement-membrane zone antibody. The circulating antibody crosses the placenta, and the baby born to a mother with herpes gestationis may have a transient blistering eruption develop during the neonatal period.

- In herpes gestationis, direct immunofluorescence is useful because the other dermatoses of pregnancy are negative with such testing.

Linear IgA bullous dermatosis is characterized by vesicles or blisters on erythematous bases in a generalized distribution with a high rate of mucosal involvement. There is no association with gluten-sensitive enteropathy. This disease is characterized by the direct immunofluorescence finding of IgA deposition in a linear pattern at the basement membrane zone, with or without C3 or IgG deposition.

- In linear IgA bullous dermatosis, direct immunofluorescence shows IgA deposition in a linear pattern at the basement membrane zone.

Dermatitis herpetiformis (Plate 5-2) is characterized by extremely pruritic, grouped vesicles occurring predominantly over the elbows, knees, buttocks, back of the neck and scalp, and low back, usually beginning in the third or fourth decade of life. Virtually all patients have some degree of gluten-sensitive enteropathy, although it is usually low-grade and subclinical. This association is important in terms of management of dermatitis herpetiformis. Dermatitis herpetiformis is also associated with thyroid disease.

- In dermatitis herpetiformis, virtually all patients have some degree of gluten-sensitive enteropathy.

The hallmark of the diagnosis of dermatitis herpetiformis is the direct immunofluorescence finding of IgA deposits in a stippled, granular, or clumped pattern along the basement membrane zone. It is recommended that skin biopsy specimens be obtained from an area 0.5 to 1 cm from an active lesion. IgA deposits tend to persist in the skin over time. A small percentage of patients who strictly adhere to a gluten-free diet may show diminution in IgA deposits after many years, but IgA deposits in the skin are unaffected by pharmacologic therapy. The serum of patients with dermatitis herpetiformis may contain IgA anti-reticulin and IgA anti-endomysial antibodies. IgA anti-endomysial antibodies and IgA anti-reticulin antibodies are found in approximately 70% of patients with dermatitis herpetiformis or celiac disease and in close to 100% of such patients who have grade 3 or 4 gluten-sensitive enteropathy. Testing for IgA anti-endomysial antibodies is useful for both diagnosis and management of dermatitis herpetiformis, although these antibodies correlate with the degree of gluten-sensitive enteropathy rather than the skin lesion per se.

- In dermatitis herpetiformis, direct immunofluorescence shows IgA deposits in a stippled, granular, or clumped pattern.
- Testing for IgA anti-endomysial antibodies is useful for diagnosis and management.

The mainstay of treatment of dermatitis herpetiformis consists of dapsone and a gluten-free diet. Patients who strictly adhere to a gluten-free diet may have a decreased need for dapsone. Patients must adhere to the diet for at least 8 months before its effect is seen. The titer of IgA anti-endomysial antibodies decreases during strict adherence to a gluten-free diet. Systemic corticosteroids are not helpful for the treatment of dermatitis herpetiformis.

- Treatment of dermatitis herpetiformis: dapsone and a gluten-free diet.

Bullous eruption of systemic lupus erythematosus shares clinical and histologic features with dermatitis herpetiformis. The blisters were therefore originally thought to represent the coexistence of dermatitis herpetiformis and lupus erythematosus, but they are now established as a distinct subset of lupus.

Direct immunofluorescence testing demonstrates deposition of IgG, IgM, IgA, or C3 in a linear or granular pattern at the basement membrane zone, similar to the classic "lupus band."

- In bullous eruption of systemic lupus erythematosus, direct immunofluorescence shows deposition of IgG, IgM, IgA, or C3 in a linear or granular pattern at the basement membrane zone.

The clinical variants of *pemphigus* include pemphigus vulgaris and pemphigus foliaceus (with subsets pemphigus erythematosus and fogo selvagem, the latter being an endemic form of pemphigus that occurs in South America). There is also a drug-induced variant of pemphigus, particularly associated with D-penicillamine, captopril, or other thiol-containing medications.

More than 50% of patients with pemphigus vulgaris present with oral lesions, and more than 90% have oral mucosal involvement at some point in the course of the disease. Pemphigus vulgaris is characterized by coalescing blisters and erosions, often with generalized involvement. In contrast, pemphigus foliaceus, considered to represent the "superficial" variant of pemphigus, may present with superficial scaling-crusting lesions of the head and neck area (in a seborrheic dermatitis-like pattern) or generalized distribution (Plate 5-3).

- Pemphigus vulgaris: coalescing blisters and erosions.
- Pemphigus foliaceus: superficial scaling-crusting lesions of the head and neck.

All types of pemphigus are characterized by the deposition of IgG and C3 at the intercellular space (epidermal cell surface) on direct immunofluorescence testing (intercellular substance [ICS] antibody). Indirect immunofluorescence testing demonstrates IgG anti-ICS antibodies in approximately 90% of cases. The titer of IgG anti-ICS antibodies is useful in both diagnosis and management of pemphigus. IgG in pemphigus is predominantly IgG4.

- All types of pemphigus are characterized by the direct immunofluorescence finding of IgG and C3 deposition at the epidermal cell surface.
- The titer of IgG anti-ICS antibodies is useful in diagnosis and management.

Pemphigus antibodies are pathogenic in that they have been demonstrated to induce acantholysis in vitro and in animal models.

- Pemphigus antibodies induce acantholysis.

High-dose corticosteroids generally are required to control pemphigus. Various "steroid-sparing" immunosuppressive agents have been used, including azathioprine, cyclophosphamide, gold, and dapsone.

- High-dose corticosteroids generally are required to control pemphigus.

Erythema Multiforme

This is an acute, usually self-limited eruption of maculopapular, urticarial, occasionally bullous lesions characterized by "iris" or "target" morphology (Plate 5-4). A subset of patients with erythema multiforme may have recurrent lesions. When erythema multiforme presents with extensive cutaneous and mucosal lesions, it is referred to as Stevens-Johnson syndrome. Various etiologic factors have been implicated in erythema multiforme. The most commonly cited precipitating factor is viral infection, particularly herpes simplex virus. This is responsible for a considerable percentage of recurrent erythema multiforme. Other infectious agents that have been noted to cause erythema multiforme include *Mycoplasma pneumoniae* and *Yersinia enterocolitica*. Drugs have been reported to induce erythema multiforme, particularly sulfonamides, barbiturates, and anticonvulsants. Erythema multiforme also may be associated with underlying connective tissue disease or malignancy. A small subset of patients with erythema multiforme have disease limited to the oral mucosa. Erythema multiforme tends to involve the lips, buccal mucosa, and tongue, in contrast to pemphigus vulgaris, which typically involves the pharynx, buccal mucosa, and tongue, and pemphigoid, which most often involves gingivae. Neither pemphigus nor pemphigoid involves the lips.

- The most commonly cited precipitating factor for erythema multiforme is viral infection, particularly herpes simplex.
- Other infectious agents: *Mycoplasma pneumoniae* and *Yersinia enterocolitica*.
- Drugs also induce erythema multiforme: sulfonamides, barbiturates, anticonvulsants.

Erythema Nodosum

Erythema nodosum typically presents as tender, erythematous, subcutaneous nodules localized to the pretibial areas. The lesions may be acute and self-limited or chronic, lasting for months up to years. The most common cause is streptococcal pharyngitis. Other infectious agents that have been implicated in the development of erythema multiforme include *Yersinia enterocolitica*, *Coccidioides*, and *Histoplasmosis*. Drug-induced erythema nodosum is most often associated with oral contraceptives and sulfonamides. Other associations with erythema nodosum include sarcoidosis, inflammatory bowel disease, and Behçet syndrome.

- The most common cause of erythema nodosum is streptococcal pharyngitis.
- Drug-induced erythema nodosum is most often associated with oral contraceptives and sulfonamides.
- Other associations: sarcoidosis, inflammatory bowel disease, Behçet syndrome.

Drug Reactions

The morphologic spectrum of reactions that may be induced by medications is broad, and hundreds of drugs may produce a given cutaneous reaction. Types of cutaneous lesions induced by drugs include maculopapular eruptions, acne-folliculitis, necrotizing vasculitis, vesiculobullous lesions, erythema multiforme, erythema nodosum, fixed drug eruptions, lichenoid reactions, photosensitivity reactions, pigmentary changes, and hair loss.

Approximately 2% of hospitalized patients have cutaneous drug reactions, and penicillin, sulfonamides, and blood products are responsible for approximately two-thirds of such reactions. The most common types of clinical presentations (in descending order of frequency) are exanthematous or morbilliform eruptions, urticaria or angioedema, fixed drug eruptions, and erythema multiforme. Stevens-Johnson syndrome, exfoliative erythroderma, and photosensitive eruptions are less common. Table 5-3 outlines the types of cutaneous reactions to drugs.

- About 2% of hospitalized patients have cutaneous drug reactions.
- Penicillin, sulfonamides, and blood products are responsible for about two-thirds of drug reactions.

Table 5-3 Cutaneous Reactions to Drugs

Type of skin reaction	Cause
Urticarial	Aspirin, penicillin, blood products
Photoallergic	Sulfonamides, thiazides, griseofulvin, phenothiazines
Phototoxic	Tetracyclines
Slate-gray discoloration	Chlorpromazine
Slate-blue discoloration	Amiodarone
Yellow or blue-gray pigmentation	Antimalarials

- Urticarial drug reactions are most often related to aspirin, penicillin, and blood products.
- Photoallergic reactions are most often associated with sulfonamides, thiazides, or phenothiazines.
- Phototoxic reactions may be induced by tetracyclines.

Exanthematous or morbilliform eruptions are the most common type of cutaneous drug reaction. This type of eruption usually begins within a week of onset of therapy, but it may occur more than 2 weeks after initiation of the therapy or up to 2 weeks after use of the drug has been discontinued. Ampicillin, penicillin, and cephalosporins are commonly associated with morbilliform eruptions. A fixed drug eruption is one or several lesions that recur at the same anatomical location on rechallenge with the medication. The genital and facial areas are common sites of involvement. Phenolphthalein, barbiturates, salicylates, and oral contraceptives have been implicated in the cause of fixed drug eruptions.

- Exanthematous or morbilliform eruptions are the most common cutaneous drug reaction.
- A fixed drug eruption is one or several lesions that recur at the same location on rechallenge.
- Phenolphthalein, barbiturates, salicylates, and oral contraceptives are implicated in fixed drug eruptions.

Lichenoid drug eruptions are morphologically similar to lichen planus (with violaceous papules of the skin) and most often have been associated with gold and antimalarial drugs, although various medications may induce this type of reaction.

CUTANEOUS SIGNS OF UNDERLYING MALIGNANCY

Cutaneous metastasis occurs in 1% to 5% of patients with metastatic neoplasms. The types of malignancy metastatic to the skin are lung, breast, kidney, gastrointestinal, melanoma, and ovary. Lesions usually present on the scalp, face, or trunk.

- Cutaneous metastasis occurs in 1%-5% of patients with metastatic neoplasms.
- Lesions usually present on the scalp, face, or trunk.

Paget disease of the nipple is an erythematous, scaly, or weeping eczematous eruption of the areola. Virtually all patients with Paget disease have an underlying ductal carcinoma of the breast. In contrast, *extramammary Paget disease*, a morphologically similar eruption that usually occurs in the anogenital region, is associated with underlying carcinoma in only about 50% of cases. Extramammary Paget disease may be associated with underlying cutaneous adnexal carcinoma or with underlying visceral carcinoma (particularly of the genitourinary or distal gastrointestinal tracts).

- Patients with Paget disease have underlying ductal carcinoma of the breast.
- Extramammary Paget disease may be associated with underlying carcinoma in only 50% of cases.

Acanthosis nigricans (Plate 5-5) consists of velvety hyperpigmentation of the intertriginous regions, particularly the axillae and groin. It has been associated with adenocarcinoma of the gastrointestinal tract, particularly the stomach. It also occurs with insulin-resistant diabetes. Acanthosis nigricans also may be associated with obesity or certain medications (such as prednisone and nicotinic acid). There is an autosomal-dominant variant of acanthosis nigricans.

- Acanthosis nigricans is associated with adenocarcinoma of the gastrointestinal tract, particularly the stomach.
- It also may be associated with obesity, certain medications, and insulin-resistant diabetes.

Pyoderma gangrenosum (Plate 5-6) consists of ulcers with irregular, undermined, inflammatory, violaceous borders that heal with cribriform scarring. The lesions are most commonly associated with inflammatory bowel disease or rheumatoid arthritis. The bullous form of pyoderma gangrenosum is associated with malignancy of the hematopoietic system, particularly leukemia.

- Pyoderma gangrenosum is most commonly associated with inflammatory bowel disease or rheumatoid arthritis.
- The bullous form is associated with leukemia.

The skin lesions of *glucagonoma syndrome (necrolytic migratory erythema)* (Plate 5-7) consist of erosions, crusting, and peeling involving the perineum and perioral areas, but may be generalized. The syndrome also includes stomatitis, glossitis (beefy tongue), anemia, diarrhea, and weight loss. It is associated with an islet cell (α) tumor of the pancreas.

- Glucagonoma syndrome consists of erosions, crusting, and peeling involving the perineum and perioral areas.
- It is associated with an islet cell tumor of the pancreas.

Gardner syndrome is a hereditary (autosomal dominant) form of colonic polyposis. Clinical features include adenomatous polyps of the colon, osteomas of the skull and face, scoliosis, soft tissue tumors (including dermoids, lipomas, and fibromas), and sebaceous (epidermal inclusion) cysts of the face and scalp. There is a high incidence of colonic carcinoma.

In approximately 60% of patients, adenocarcinoma of the colon develops by age 40 years, and malignancies of other sites have been associated with this syndrome, including adrenal, ovarian, and thyroid.

- Gardner syndrome is a hereditary (autosomal dominant) form of colonic polyposis.
- Clinical features: soft tissue tumors, sebaceous cysts of the face.
- There is a high incidence of colonic carcinoma.

Acquired ichthyosis most often has been associated with Hodgkin disease, but it has been reported with other types of lymphoma, multiple myeloma, and various carcinomas.

- Acquired ichthyosis is associated with Hodgkin disease.

Hirsutism may reflect androgen excess due to an adrenal or ovarian tumor.

Hypertrichosis is an increase in hair unrelated to androgen excess, such as hypertrichosis lanuginosa acquisita (growth of soft downy hair). It has been associated with carcinoid tumor, adenocarcinoma of the breast, lymphoma, gastrointestinal malignancy, and other types of neoplasms.

Sweet syndrome (acute febrile neutrophilic dermatosis) has skin lesions that consist of erythematous plaques and nodules, most commonly located on the extremities and face. The association is with leukemia, particularly acute myelocytic or acute myelomonocytic leukemia, although many other diseases also have been associated.

- Sweet syndrome is associated with leukemia.

Generalized pruritus is the presentation for many cutaneous and systemic disorders. Pruritus may be the presenting symptom in lymphoma.

- Pruritus may be the presenting symptom in lymphoma.

In *dermatomyositis*, the pathognomonic skin lesions are Gottron papules (Plate 5-8) involving the skin over the joints of the fingers, elbows, and knees. Poikilodermatous lesions or erythematous maculopapular eruptions may diffusely involve the face, particularly the periorbital area ("heliotrope rash" [Plate 5-9]), and the trunk and extremities. The cutaneous lesions are photosensitive. The disease is characterized by proximal myositis. Although creatine kinase and aldolase levels usually are increased in patients with myositis, it is important to verify the diagnosis by obtaining an electromyogram and a muscle biopsy specimen. Dermatomyositis is associated with an increased incidence of underlying malignancy.

- Dermatomyositis may involve the periorbital area ("heliotrope rash") or the dorsal aspect of the hands (Gottron papules).
- The lesions are photosensitive.
- Dermatomyositis is characterized by proximal myositis.

Cutaneous amyloidosis may present clinically as macroglossia (Plate 5-10), waxy papules on the eyelids or nasolabial folds, pinch purpura, and postproctoscopic purpura (Plate 5-11). Multiple myeloma may be associated with amyloid.

- Amyloidosis may be associated with multiple myeloma.

Tylosis is a rare disorder characterized by palmar-plantar keratoderma associated with esophageal carcinoma. It has autosomal dominant inheritance.

- Tylosis is associated with esophageal carcinoma.

The *autoimmune bullous diseases* are a heterogeneous group of disorders characterized by antibody deposition at the basement membrane zone or epidermis. An association with malignancy has been found in several of these disorders.

- Pemphigus is associated with thymoma with or without myasthenia gravis.
- Paraneoplastic pemphigus presents with clinical and histologic features of pemphigus and erythema multiforme and is associated with lymphoma and leukemia.
- Intestinal lymphoma rarely develops in patients with dermatitis herpetiformis.
- Epidermolysis bullosa acquisita is associated with amyloidosis and multiple myeloma.
- Bullous pemphigoid has not been associated with an increased risk of underlying malignancy.

DERMATOLOGY: AN INTERNIST'S PERSPECTIVE

Respiratory

The skin is involved in 15% to 35% of patients with *sarcoidosis*. Lesions may present as 1) lupus pernio (erythematous swelling of the nose), 2) translucent papules around the eyes and nasolabial folds, 3) annular lesions with central atrophy, 4) nodules on the trunk and extremities, and 5) scar sarcoid. Acute sarcoidosis may present with a combination of erythema nodosum, bilateral hilar lymphadenopathy, fever, and arthralgias (Löfgren syndrome).

- The skin is involved in 15%-35% of patients with sarcoidosis.

- Lesions may present as lupus pernio (erythematous swelling of the nose).

Erythema nodosum (Plate 5-12) is a reactive condition that may be associated with acute sarcoidosis. Erythema nodosum typically presents as tender, erythematous, subcutaneous nodules localized to pretibial areas. The lesions may be acute and self-limited or chronic, lasting for months up to years.

- Erythema nodosum may be associated with acute sarcoidosis.

In *Wegener granulomatosis*, cutaneous involvement occurs in more than 50% of patients and is manifested by cutaneous infarction, ulceration, hemorrhagic bullae, purpuric papules, or urticaria. A skin biopsy may show hypersensitivity vasculitis or granulomatous vasculitis.

- In Wegener granulomatosis, cutaneous involvement occurs in >50% of patients.
- Manifestations: ulceration, hemorrhagic bullae, purpuric papules, urticaria.

Churg-Strauss granulomatosis (allergic granulomatosis) is characterized by a combination of adult-onset asthma, peripheral eosinophilia, and pulmonary involvement with recurrent pneumonia or transient infiltrates. Skin lesions have been reported in up to 60% of patients and consist of palpable purpura, cutaneous infarcts, and subcutaneous nodules.

- Skin lesions of Churg-Strauss granulomatosis occur in up to 60% of patients.
- Skin lesions include palpable purpura, cutaneous infarct, and subcutaneous nodules.

In *relapsing polychondritis*, there is episodic destructive inflammation of cartilage of the ears, nose, and upper airways. There may be associated arthritis and ocular involvement. In the acute stage, the ears may be red, swollen, and tender. Later, they become soft and flabby. Nasal chondritis may lead to saddle-nose deformities. Relapsing polychondritis is mediated by antibodies to type II collagen.

- Relapsing polychondritis: episodic destructive inflammation of cartilage of ears, nose, upper airways.
- Nasal chondritis may lead to saddle-nose deformities.

Cardiovascular

Pseudoxanthoma elasticum may be transmitted by autosomal dominant or autosomal recessive inheritance. Yellow xanthoma-like papules are seen on the neck (plucked-chicken skin),

axillae, groin, and abdomen. Angioid streaks may be seen in the fundus. Skin biopsy shows degeneration of elastic fibers. Systemic associations include stroke, myocardial infarction, peripheral vascular disease, and gastrointestinal hemorrhage.

- Pseudoxanthoma elasticum is associated with stroke, myocardial infarction, peripheral vascular disease, and gastrointestinal hemorrhage.

Ehlers-Danlos syndrome includes 10 subgroups that vary in severity and systemic associations. Cutaneous findings are skin hyperextensibility with hypermobile joints and fish-mouth scars. Angina, peripheral vascular disease, and gastrointestinal bleeding may be associated.

- Ehlers-Danlos syndrome is associated with angina, peripheral vascular disease, and gastrointestinal bleeding.

Erythema marginatum is one of the diagnostic criteria for acute rheumatic fever. This uncommon eruption occurs on the trunk and is characterized by erythematous plaques with rapidly mobile serpiginous borders.

- Erythema marginatum is one of the diagnostic criteria for acute rheumatic fever.

Gastrointestinal

Osler-Weber-Rendu syndrome (hereditary hemorrhagic telangiectasia), with autosomal dominant inheritance, is manifested by cutaneous and mucosal telangiectasias. Frequent nosebleeds and gastrointestinal bleeds may be a presenting feature. Pulmonary arteriovenous malformations and central nervous system angiomas are also features of this syndrome.

- Osler-Weber-Rendu syndrome has autosomal dominant inheritance.
- Features: nosebleeds, gastrointestinal bleeds, pulmonary arteriovenous malformations, central nervous system angiomas.

Acrodermatitis enteropathica is an inherited (autosomal recessive) or acquired disease characterized by zinc deficiency (failure of absorption or failure to supplement). The clinical features include angular cheilitis, a seborrheic dermatitis-like eruption, erosions, blisters, and pustules, with skin lesions particularly involving the face, hands, feet, and perineum. Alopecia and diarrhea are other features of this syndrome.

- Acrodermatitis enteropathica: inherited (autosomal recessive) or acquired disease.

● Characterized by zinc deficiency (failure of absorption or failure to supplement).

Peutz-Jeghers syndrome is an inherited (autosomal dominant) syndrome of intestinal polyposis. Patients have hamartomas, mostly involving the small bowel, and a slightly increased risk for carcinoma. Cutaneous lesions include macular pigmentation (freckles) of the lips, periungual skin, fingers, and toes and pigmentation of the oral mucosa.

● Peutz-Jeghers syndrome is an inherited (autosomal dominant) syndrome of intestinal polyposis.
● An increased risk for carcinoma was recognized recently.

Dermatitis herpetiformis (Plate 5-2) is an immune-mediated bullous disease that presents with intensely itchy vesicles on extensor surfaces (elbows, knees, buttocks, scapulae). Gluten-sensitive enteropathy occurs in up to 70% of patients.

● Dermatitis herpetiformis is an immune-mediated bullous disease.
● Gluten-sensitive enteropathy occurs in up to 70% of patients.

Extensive *aphthous ulceration* may be associated with Crohn disease or gluten-sensitive enteropathy.

● Aphthous ulceration may be associated with Crohn disease or gluten-sensitive enteropathy.

Pyoderma gangrenosum (Plate 5-6) presents with ulceration, predominantly on the lower extremities, with inflammatory undermined borders. The lesions heal with cribriform scarring. The phenomenon whereby lesions occur at sites of trauma is known as pathergy—the occurrence of the disease at sites of trauma is classic. Systemic disease associations include inflammatory bowel disease (ulcerative colitis more commonly than Crohn disease), rheumatoid arthritis, and paraproteinemia.

● Pyoderma gangrenosum occurs at sites of trauma.
● Associated diseases are inflammatory bowel disease (ulcerative colitis more than Crohn disease), rheumatoid arthritis, and paraproteinemia.

Cutaneous Crohn disease may present as skin nodules with granulomatous histology. Other manifestations include pyostomatitis vegetans (granulomatous inflammation of the gingivae), granulomatous cheilitis, oral aphthous ulceration, perianal skin tags, and perianal fistulae.

● Manifestation of Crohn disease: pyostomatitis vegetans (granulomatous inflammation of gingivae).

Bowel bypass syndrome presents with a flu-like illness with fever, malaise, arthralgias, myalgias, and inflammatory papules and pustules on the extremities and upper trunk. The disease is recurrent and episodic and occurs in up to 20% of patients after jejunoileal bypass. The condition responds to antibiotics or to reversal of the bypass procedure.

● Bowel bypass syndrome: flu-like illness, inflammatory papules and pustules.
● Occurs in up to 20% of patients after jejunoileal bypass.

Gardner syndrome and *glucagonoma syndrome* are described earlier in this chapter.

Nephrology
Partial lipodystrophy is associated with C3 deficiency and the nephrotic syndrome.
Uremic pruritus is associated with end-stage renal disease and responds to ultraviolet B therapy.

Neurocutaneous
Fabry disease is an X-linked recessive disorder due to deficiency of the enzyme α-galactosidase A. The skin changes consist of numerous vascular tumors (angiokeratomas) that develop during childhood and adolescence. Corneal opacities are present in 90% of patients. Systemic manifestations include paresthesias and pain due to involved peripheral nerves, renal insufficiency, and vascular insufficiency of the coronary and central nervous system.

● Fabry disease is a recessive disorder due to deficiency of α-galactosidase A.
● Systemic manifestations: paresthesias, renal insufficiency, vascular insufficiency.

The clinical features of *ataxia-telangiectasia* include cutaneous and ocular telangiectasia, cerebellar ataxia, choreoathetosis, IgA deficiency, and recurrent pulmonary infections.

Tuberous sclerosis may be inherited in an autosomal dominant pattern (25%) or may occur sporadically (new mutation). Predominant cutaneous lesions include hypopigmented macules, adenoma sebaceum, subungual or periungual fibromas, and shagreen patch (connective tissue nevus) (Plate 5-13). This syndrome is associated with epilepsy (80%) and mental retardation (60%). Rhabdomyomas may occur in the heart in childhood. Angiomyolipomas occur in the kidneys in up to 80% of adults with this syndrome.

● Tuberous sclerosis may be inherited in an autosomal dominant pattern or be sporadic.

- It is associated with epilepsy (80%) and mental retardation (60%).
- Angiomyolipomas occur in kidneys in up to 80% of affected adults.

Neurofibromatosis (von Recklinghausen disease) (Plate 5-14) occurs in 1 in 3,000 births. Inheritance is autosomal dominant, and approximately 50% of cases are new mutations. The major signs of the disease are café au lait spots, axillary freckling (Crowe sign), neurofibromas, and Lisch nodules of the iris.

- Neurofibromatosis is autosomal dominant.
- Major signs: café au lait spots, axillary freckling, neurofibromas.

The associated central nervous system tumors include acoustic neuromas, optic gliomas, and meningiomas. Other associated tumors include pheochromocytoma, neuroblastoma, and Wilms tumor. Café au lait spots and neurofibromas frequently occur in the absence of neurofibromatosis. The diagnostic criteria for neurofibromatosis include two or more of the following:

1. Six or more café au lait macules more than 0.5 cm in greatest diameter in prepubertal patients, or more than 1.5 cm in diameter in adults.
2. Two or more neurofibromas of any type, or one plexiform neurofibroma.
3. Freckling of skin in axillary or inguinal regions.
4. Optic gliomas.
5. Lisch nodules.
6. An osseous lesion such as sphenoid dysplasia or thinning of long bone cortex with or without pseudarthrosis.
7. A first-degree relative with neurofibromatosis that meets the above diagnostic criteria.

Sturge-Weber-Dimitri syndrome is characterized by capillary angioma (port-wine stain) in the distribution of the upper or middle branch of the trigeminal nerve. There may be associated meningeal angioma in the same distribution. Intracranial tramline calcification, mental retardation, epilepsy, contralateral hemiparesis, and visual impairment may be associated.

- Sturge-Weber-Dimitri syndrome is characterized by capillary angioma in the distribution of the upper or middle branch of the trigeminal nerve.
- Associated features: intracranial calcification, mental retardation, epilepsy, contralateral hemiparesis, visual impairment.

Rheumatology: Cutaneous Associations of Arthritis

Psoriatic arthritis occurs in 4% to 5% of patients with psoriasis. Several different patterns of arthritis are seen and are well summarized in the Moll and Wright classification. An asymmetric oligoarthritis occurs in 70% of patients. This group includes patients with "sausage digits" and monoarthritis. The second most common presentation is a symmetric arthritis clinically similar to rheumatoid arthritis, which occurs in 15% of patients with psoriatic arthritis. Distal interphalangeal involvement, arthritis mutilans, and a spinal form of arthritis similar to ankylosing spondylitis each occurs in 5% of patients with psoriatic arthritis.

- Psoriatic arthritis occurs in 4%-5% of patients with psoriasis.
- Asymmetric oligoarthritis is most common.
- 5% of patients have ankylosing spondylitis.

Reiter syndrome consists of the triad of urethritis, conjunctivitis, and arthritis. The disease usually affects young men. Two-thirds of patients have skin lesions, namely, circinate balinitis, consisting of erythematous plaques of the penis, and keratoderma blennorrhagicum, a pustular psoriasiform eruption of the palms and soles. Most patients are HLA-B27 positive.

- Reiter syndrome triad: urethritis, conjunctivitis, arthritis.
- Most patients are HLA-B27 positive.

Erythema chronicum migrans is an annular, sometimes urticarial, erythematous lesion presenting as a manifestation of Lyme disease. The lesion develops subsequent to and surrounding the site of a tick bite. Lesions are single in 75% of patients and multiple in 25%. Other acute features of Lyme disease include fever, headaches, myalgias, arthralgias, and lymphadenopathy. The tick *Ixodes dammini* contains a spirochete, *Borrelia burgdorferi*, that is responsible for the syndrome. Arthritis is a late complication of Lyme disease. Weeks or months after the initial illness, meningoencephalitis, peripheral neuropathy, myocarditis, atrioventricular node block, or destructive erosive arthritis may develop.

- Erythema chronicum migrans presents as a manifestation of Lyme disease.
- The lesion develops subsequent to and surrounding the site of a tick bite.
- Lesions are single in 75% of patients and multiple in 25%.

In *rheumatoid arthritis*, nodules may occur over the extensor surfaces of joints, most commonly on the dorsal aspects of the hands and elbows. Rheumatoid vasculitis with ulceration may occur in the setting of rheumatoid arthritis with a high circulating rheumatoid factor.

During the late stages of *gout*, tophi (urate deposits with surrounding inflammation) occur in the subcutaneous tissues.

Improved methods of treatment account for the decrease in the incidence of tophaceous gout in recent years.

- Gouty tophi may occur in subcutaneous tissues.

In *lupus erythematosus* (LE), cutaneous abnormalities occur in approximately 80% of patients. LE can be classified into acute cutaneous LE (malar rash, generalized maculopapular eruption, or bullous LE), subacute cutaneous LE, and chronic cutaneous LE (localized discoid LE, generalized discoid LE, and lupus panniculitis).

- In LE, cutaneous abnormalities occur in 80% of patients.

Skin lesions are present in up to 85% of patients with acute systemic LE. A butterfly rash with erythema involving the nose and cheeks is characteristic. Erythematous papules and plaques also may occur on the dorsal aspect of the hands, and the skin overlying the interphalangeal and metacarpal phalangeal joints is spared. Maculopapular erythema also may occur on sun-exposed areas.

Subacute cutaneous LE (Plate 5-15) usually presents with generalized annular or polycyclic plaques. The lesions may appear papulosquamous or vesiculobullous. Subacute cutaneous LE is characterized by the presence of anti-Ro (anti-SSA) antibodies in serum and photosensitivity. These antibodies cross the placenta, and children born to mothers with subacute cutaneous LE may develop congenital heart block or a transient photodistributed skin eruption during the neonatal period.

- Subacute cutaneous LE presents with annular or polycyclic plaques.
- Subacute cutaneous LE is characterized by the presence of anti-Ro (anti-SSA) antibodies and photosensitivity.

Discoid LE (Plate 5-16) is characterized by erythematous papules and plaques with follicular hyperkeratosis and scaling. Localized discoid LE is usually not associated with systemic LE. Generalized discoid LE or disseminated discoid LE refers to lesions involving the head and neck area or the trunk and extremities. Discoid LE most commonly affects the face, scalp, and ears. Although most patients with discoid LE lack manifestations of systemic LE, approximately 25% of patients with systemic LE have had cutaneous lesions of discoid LE at some point during the course of their illness.

- Discoid LE is characterized by erythematous papules and plaques with follicular hyperkeratosis and scaling.
- Discoid LE most commonly affects the face, scalp, and ears.

- 25% of patients with systemic LE have had cutaneous manifestations of discoid LE.

Circulating antinuclear antibodies are demonstrable in most patients with systemic LE and subacute cutaneous LE, but they are present in only a small percentage of patients with discoid LE. A homogeneous antinuclear antibody pattern tends to correlate with the diagnosis of systemic LE, peripheral (rim) pattern correlates with lupus nephritis, speckled anticentromere pattern is associated with the CREST variant of scleroderma (CREST: calcinosis cutis, Raynaud phenomenon, esophageal dysmotility, sclerodactyly, and telangiectasia), nucleolar pattern usually correlates with the diagnosis of scleroderma and uncommonly with lupus, and the particulate pattern is associated with various connective tissue diseases, including LE. In addition to association with subacute cutaneous LE, anti-Ro (anti-SSA) antibodies are associated with Sjögren syndrome, LE with C2 deficiency, and neonatal LE.

The term "scleroderma" encompasses a spectrum of diseases ranging from generalized multisystem disease to localized cutaneous disease. The systemic end of the spectrum is represented by progressive systemic sclerosis and the CREST syndrome. The middle area of the spectrum is represented by eosinophilic fasciitis and linear scleroderma, which may have systemic involvement. Localized scleroderma (also known as morphea) may be a single plaque or may be multiple plaques in a generalized distribution.

Systemic scleroderma consists of diffuse sclerosis associated with smoothness and hardening of the skin, with masklike face and microstomia. Sclerodactyly, periungual telangiectasia, hyperpigmentation, and cutaneous calcification may be observed. Esophageal, pulmonary, renal, and cardiac involvement may be associated with systemic scleroderma. The CREST syndrome (Plate 5-17) is associated with circulating anticentromere antibodies.

- Systemic scleroderma may include sclerodactyly, periungual telangiectasia, hyperpigmentation, and cutaneous calcification.

Eosinophilic fasciitis manifests as tightly bound thickening of the skin and underlying soft tissues of the extremities. Other features include arthralgias, hypergammaglobulinemia, and peripheral blood eosinophilia.

- Eosinophilic fasciitis manifests as tightly bound thickening of the skin and underlying soft tissue of the extremities.

Morphea manifests as discrete sclerotic plaques with a white, shiny center and erythematous or violaceous periphery. Localized or linear scleroderma may have various presentations depending on extent, location, and depth of sclerosis. Most lesions are characterized by sclerosis and atrophy associated with depression or "delling" of the soft tissue; underlying bone may be affected in linear scleroderma.

- Morphea manifests as discrete sclerotic plaques with a white, shiny center.
- Underlying bone may be affected in linear scleroderma.

Hematologic

Graft-versus-host disease (GVHD) most commonly occurs after bone marrow transplantation and represents the constellation of skin lesions, diarrhea, and liver enzyme abnormalities. GVHD occurs in 60% to 80% of patients who undergo allogeneic bone marrow transplantation.

- GVHD commonly occurs after bone marrow transplantation.
- GVHD includes skin lesions, diarrhea, liver enzyme abnormalities.

GVHD generally occurs in two phases. Acute GVHD begins 7 to 21 days after transplantation, and chronic GVHD begins within months to 1 year after transplantation. One or both phases may occur in the same patient. Acute GVHD results from attack of donor immunocompetent T lymphocytes and null lymphocytes against host histocompatibility antigens. Chronic GVHD results from immunocompetent lymphocytes that develop in the recipient.

The cutaneous abnormalities of acute GVHD include pruritus, numbness or pain of the palms and soles, an erythematous maculopapular eruption of the trunk, palms, and soles, and blisters that, when extensive, resemble toxic epidermal necrolysis. Acute GVHD also includes intestinal abnormalities resulting in diarrhea and liver function changes.

- Cutaneous abnormalities of GVHD: pruritus, numbness or pain of palms and soles, erythematous maculopapular eruption of trunk, palms, and soles.

Chronic GVHD mainly affects skin and liver. Early chronic GVHD is characterized by a lichenoid reaction consisting of cutaneous and oral lesions that resemble lichen planus, with coalescing violaceous papules on the skin and white reticulated patches on the buccal mucosa. Late chronic GVHD is characterized by cutaneous sclerosis, poikilodermatous-reticulated lesions, and scarring alopecia. The cutaneous infiltrate is composed predominantly of suppressor/cytotoxic T cells.

- Chronic GVHD: lichenoid reaction consisting of cutaneous and oral lesions.

Mastocytosis (mast cell disease) can be divided into four groups, depending on the age at onset and the presence or absence of systemic involvement: 1) urticaria pigmentosa arising in infancy or adolescence without substantial systemic involvement, 2) urticaria pigmentosa in adults without substantial systemic involvement, 3) systemic mast cell disease, and 4) mast cell leukemia.

The cutaneous lesions may be brown to red macules, papules, nodules, or plaques that urticate on stroking. Less commonly, the lesions may be bullous, erythrodermic, or telangiectatic. The systemic manifestations are due to histamine release and consist of flushing, tachycardia, and diarrhea.

- Cutaneous lesions of mastocytosis: brown to red macules, papules, nodules, or plaques that urticate on stroking.
- Systemic manifestations are due to histamine release.

Necrobiotic xanthogranuloma—indurated plaques with associated atrophy and telangiectasia with or without ulceration—may occur on the trunk or periorbital areas. Serum electrophoresis shows an IgG κ paraproteinemia or multiple myeloma.

Endocrine

Diabetes Mellitus

Several dermatologic disorders have been described in diabetes.

Necrobiosis lipoidica diabeticorum (Plate 5-18) classically occurs on the shins and presents as yellow-brown atrophic telangiectatic plaques that occasionally ulcerate. Two-thirds of patients with this skin disorder have diabetes.

- Necrobiosis lipoidica diabeticorum occurs on the shins.
- Two-thirds of patients have diabetes.

Granuloma annulare is an asymptomatic eruption consisting of small, firm, flesh-colored or red papules in an annular configuration (Plate 5-19) (less commonly nodular or generalized). The association with diabetes is disputed.

- Granuloma annulare consists of small, firm, flesh-colored or red papules in an annular configuration.

Rarely, patients with poorly controlled diabetes present with spontaneously occurring *subepidermal blisters* (bullosa diabeticorum) on the dorsal aspects of the hands and feet.

The *stiff hand syndrome* has been reported in juvenile-onset insulin-dependent diabetes. Patients have limited joint mobility and tight waxy skin on the hands. There is an increased risk of subsequent renal and retinal microvascular disease.

- Stiff hand syndrome: increased risk of subsequent renal and retinal microvascular disease.

In *scleredema*, there is an insidious onset of thickening and stiffness of the skin on the upper back and posterior neck. The condition is more common in middle-aged men with diabetes. The diabetes is often long-standing and poorly controlled.

- Scleredema is more common in middle-aged men with diabetes.
- Diabetes is often long-standing and poorly controlled.

Thyroid

Pretibial myxedema and thyroid acropachy are cutaneous associations of Graves disease.

Metabolic

The *porphyrias* are a group of inherited or acquired abnormalities of heme synthesis. Each type is associated with deficient activity of a particular enzyme. The porphyrias are usually divided into three types: erythropoietic, hepatic, and mixed.

Erythropoietic porphyria is a hereditary form (autosomal recessive) characterized by marked photosensitivity, blisters, scarring alopecia, hirsutism, red-stained teeth, hemolytic anemia, and splenomegaly. The skin lesions are severely mutilating. Onset is in infancy or early childhood.

- Erythropoietic porphyria is autosomal recessive.
- Skin lesions are severely mutilating.

Erythropoietic protoporphyria is an autosomal dominant syndrome that usually begins during childhood. It is characterized by variable degrees of photosensitivity and a marked itching, burning, or stinging sensation that occurs within minutes after sun exposure. It is associated with deficiency of ferrochelatase.

- Erythropoietic protoporphyria is autosomal dominant.
- It is associated with deficiency of ferrochelatase.

Porphyria cutanea tarda, one of the hepatic porphyrias, is an acquired or hereditary (autosomal dominant) disease associated with a defect in uroporphyrinogen decarboxylase. The disease may be precipitated by exposure to toxins (such as chlorinated phenols or hexachlorobenzene), alcohol, estrogens, iron overload, hemochromatosis, and infection with hepatitis C. Porphyria cutanea tarda usually presents in the third or fourth decade of life. Clinical manifestations include photosensitivity, skin fragility, erosions and blisters (particularly on dorsal surfaces of the hands) (Plate 5-20), hyperpigmentation, milia, hypertrichosis, and facial suffusion.

Sclerodermoid skin changes develop in some patients. The diagnosis is confirmed by the finding of elevated porphyrin levels in the urine. Treatment includes phlebotomy and low-dose chloroquine.

- Porphyria cutanea tarda is acquired or inherited (autosomal dominant).
- It is associated with a defect in uroporphyrinogen decarboxylase.
- It may be precipitated by exposure to toxins or infection with hepatitis C.

Acute intermittent porphyria lacks skin lesions and is characterized by acute attacks of abdominal pain or neurologic symptoms.

- Acute intermittent porphyria lacks skin lesions.
- It involves acute attacks of abdominal pain or neurologic symptoms.

Variegate porphyria (mixed porphyria) also follows autosomal dominant inheritance. Variegate porphyria is characterized by cutaneous abnormalities that are similar to those of porphyria cutanea tarda and by acute abdominal episodes, as in acute intermittent porphyria. Variegate porphyria tends to be precipitated by drugs such as barbiturates and sulfonamides.

- Variegate porphyria is autosomal dominant.
- It tends to be precipitated by drugs such as barbiturates and sulfonamides.

NAIL CLUES TO SYSTEMIC DISEASE

Onycholysis consists of distal and lateral separation of the nail plate from the nail bed. Onycholysis may be due to psoriasis, infection (such as *Candida* or *Pseudomonas*), a reaction to nail cosmetics, or a drug reaction. Drugs that have been noted to induce onycholysis include tetracycline and chlorpromazine. Association with thyroid disease (hyperthyroidism more than hypothyroidism) has also been observed.

- Onycholysis may be due to psoriasis, infection (*Candida* or *Pseudomonas*), nail cosmetics, or a drug reaction.

Pitting is a common feature of psoriatic nails. Pits have also been associated with alopecia areata.

Terry nails consist of whitening of the proximal or entire nail as a result of changes in the nail bed. This abnormality is associated with cirrhosis.

- Terry nails are associated with cirrhosis.

Muehrcke lines consist of white parallel bands associated with hypoalbuminemia.

● Muehrcke lines are associated with hypoalbuminemia.

"Half-and-half" nails (*Lindsay nails*) are nails in which the proximal half is white and the distal half is red. This abnormality may be associated with renal failure.

● "Half-and-half" nails may be associated with renal failure.

Yellow nails are associated with chronic edema, pulmonary disease, pleural effusion, chronic bronchitis, bronchiectasis, and lung carcinoma.

Beau lines are transverse grooves in the nail associated with high fever, systemic disease, and drugs.

Koilonychia (spoon nails) is associated with iron deficiency anemia, but it may also be idiopathic, familial, or related to trauma.

● Koilonychia is associated with iron deficiency anemia.

Blue-colored lunula is associated with hepatolenticular degeneration (Wilson disease) and argyria.

Mees lines are white bands associated with arsenic.

● Mees lines are associated with arsenic.

CUTANEOUS MANIFESTATIONS OF HIV INFECTION

Primary infection with human immunodeficiency virus (HIV) results in a flu-like illness and an exanthem in 30% to 60% of patients. The exanthem may be morbilliform or pityriasis rosea-like. Oral ulceration and erosions and erosive esophagitis also may occur at this stage. The acute exanthem and enanthem are self-limited and often go undiagnosed.

In the early stage of the disease, cutaneous manifestations include genital warts, genital herpes, psoriasis, and mild seborrheic dermatitis. With symptomatic HIV infection (CD4 count of 200-400/mm^3), both infections and inflammatory dermatoses occur more frequently. These include psoriasis, oral hairy leukoplakia, candidiasis, herpes zoster, herpes simplex, tinea pedis, and onychomycosis. In patients with a family history of atopy, atopic dermatitis may be a manifestation at this stage.

As the CD4 count decreases to less than 200/mm^3, patients present with a disseminated fungal infection, herpes zoster, persistent herpes simplex, bacillary angiomatosis, and molluscum contagiosum. *Bacillary angiomatosis* consists of one or more vascular papules or nodules caused by a *Rickettsia*-like organism related to *Rochalimaea quintana*. Eosinophilic folliculitis, a pruritic eruption primarily involving the head, neck, trunk, and proximal extremities, is characteristic of symptomatic HIV infection.

With advanced HIV infection (CD4 counts of <50/mm^3), overwhelming infection is characteristic. Infectious agents include cytomegalovirus, *Cryptococcus*, *Acanthamoeba*, and extensive molluscum contagiosum.

Oral hairy leukoplakia is caused by Epstein-Barr virus infection of the oral mucosa and usually occurs in patients with advanced HIV infection.

Molluscum contagiosum, a common viral infection of otherwise healthy children, has been observed in 10% to 20% of patients with HIV infection.

● Molluscum contagiosum is observed in 10%-20% of patients with HIV infection.

Epidemic Kaposi sarcoma usually presents as oval papules or plaques oriented along skin lines of the trunk, extremities, face, and mucosa. This presentation is in contrast to that of classic Kaposi sarcoma in elderly patients, which occurs predominantly on the distal lower extremities. Kaposi sarcoma–herpes simplex virus (human herpesvirus 9) has been identified in tissue from patients with both epidemic and classic Kaposi sarcoma.

● Epidemic Kaposi sarcoma: oval papules or plaques along skin lines of the trunk, extremities, face, mucosa.

● It is most commonly associated with HIV infection.

Dermatology Pharmacy Review
Susan V. McCluskey, RPh

Drug	Toxic/adverse effects[*]	Drug interactions[†]
Systemic antibacterials		
Cephalosporins	Nausea, vomiting, diarrhea Anaphylaxis Hemolytic anemia Nephrotoxicity Neutropenia, thrombocytopenia Pseudomembranous colitis Rash, erythema multiforme	
Clindamycin	Nausea, vomiting, diarrhea, abdominal pain Granulocytopenia, neutropenia Hypotension Pseudomembranous colitis Rash, Stevens-Johnson syndrome	
Fluoroquinolones (ciprofloxacin, gatifloxacin, levofloxacin, lomefloxacin, moxifloxacin, norfloxacin, ofloxacin, sparfloxacin, trovafloxacin)	Nausea, vomiting, diarrhea, abdominal pain Increased liver enzymes Increased serum creatinine Nephrotoxicity Phototoxicity Pseudomembranous colitis Rash, erythema multiforme, toxic epidermal necrolysis	Cardiac arrythmias: amiodarone, bepridil, bretylium, disopyramide, erythromycin, phenothiazine, procainamide, quinidine, sotalol, tricyclic antidepressants Increased cardiovascular side effects: cisapride Increased levels or effects: astemizole, terfenadine Increased toxicity: cyclosporine
Macrolides (azithromycin, clarithromycin, dirithromycin, erythromycin)	Abdominal pain, nausea, diarrhea Oral candidiasis Increased liver enzymes Pseudomembranous colitis Anaphylaxis	Cardiotoxicity: astemizole, terfenadine, cisapride, pimozide, quinolones (gatifloxacin, sparfloxacin, moxifloxacin) Increased levels or effects: warfarin, carbamazepine, digoxin, ergot alkaloids, vinblastine, cyclosporine, tacrolimus, methylprednisolone Severe myopathy, rhabdomyolysis: HMG-CoA reductase inhibitors (atorvastatin, lovastatin, simvastatin, cerivastatin)
Penicillins	Nausea, vomiting, mild diarrhea Anaphylaxis Acute interstitital nephritis Hemolytic anemia Pseudomembranous colitis	Decreased penicillin effects: tetracyclines (demeclocycline, doxycycline, minocycline, oxytetracycline, tetracycline)
Sulfonamides	Nausea, vomiting, diarrhea Hematologic reactions Hepatitis Nephrotoxicity Rash, photosensitivity, Stevens-Johnson syndrome	Increased effect: warfarin Increased nephrotoxicity and decreased effect: cyclosporine Bone marrow suppression: methotrexate

Dermatology Pharmacy Review (continued)

Drug	Toxic/adverse effects[*]	Drug interactions[†]
Systemic antibacterials (continued)		
Tetracyclines (doxycycline, minocycline, tetracycline)	Photosensitivity Nausea, diarrhea Acute renal failure Exfoliative dermatitis Discoloration of teeth (young children)	Decreased effects: penicillin Increased levels: digoxin Risk of pseudotumor cerebri: isotretinoin Renal toxicity: methoxyflurane
Systemic immunomodulators and antiproliferatives		
Azathioprine	Nausea, vomiting, diarrhea Malignancies Rash Thrombocytopenia, leukopenia, anemia Veno-occlusive disease	Increased effects: allopurinol
Corticosteroids	Increased appetite, fluid retention Insomnia Hirsutism, hyperpigmentation Glucose intolerance Cataracts Osteoporosis	Antagonized effects: neostigmine, pyridostigmine Decreased steroid effects: rifampin, phenytoin Increased steroid effects: macrolides
Cyclophosphamide	Alopecia Sterility Nausea, vomiting, stomatitis Hemorrhagic cystitis Malignancies Thrombocytopenia, anemia, leukopenia Stevens-Johnson syndrome, toxic epidermal necrolysis	Cardiac toxicity potentiated: anthracyclines
Cyclosporine	Nausea, diarrhea, gum hyperplasia Hypertension Psoriasis Hirsutism, hypertrichosis Increased triglycerides Nephropathy Headache Tremor	Increased risk of rhabdomyolysis: atorvastatin, cerivastatin, lovastatin, pravastatin, simvastatin Increased toxicity: digoxin Decreased cyclosporine concentrations: phenytoin, orlistat, rifampin, sulfonamides Increased renal failure: foscarnet Increased nephrotoxicity: sulfonamides
Dapsone	Hemolytic anemia, methemo-globinemia, leukopenia, agranulocytosis Skin rash, exfoliative dermatitis Hepatitis Peripheral neuropathy Psychosis	Increased levels of both drugs: trimethoprim Increased hematologic reactions: pyrimethamine Decreased dapsone effects: rifampin

Dermatology Pharmacy Review (continued)

Drug	Toxic/adverse effects[*]	Drug interactions[†]
Systemic immunomodulators and antiproliferatives (continued)		
Gold compounds (auranofin, aurothioglucose, gold sodium thiomalate)	Rash Stomatitis Conjunctivitis Proteinuria Alopecia Hematuria Eosinophilia, leukopenia, thrombocytopenia Hepatotoxicity	Increased levels: phenytoin
Interferons	Flu-like symptoms Hypertension Psychiatric disturbances Rash Hypocalcemia, hyperglycemia Aplastic anemia Acute renal failure	
Methotrexate	Nausea, vomiting Vasculitis Stomatitis Leukopenia, thrombocytopenia Renal failure Rash, photosensitivity Hepatotoxicity	Increased methotrexate toxicity: penicillins, salicylates, nonsteroidal anti-inflammatory drugs, probenecid Increased bone marrow suppression: sulfonamides, trimethoprim Decreased levels: phenytoin
Psoralen (methoxsalen, trioxsalen)	Nausea Pruritus, erythema Painful blistering Depression	Other photosensitizing agents
Retinoids (isotretinoin, acitretin)	Teratogenicity Hirsutism, alopecia Photoallergic reactions Rash, vasculitis Lipid abnormalities Visual disturbances Psychiatric disorders Osteoporosis Hepatotoxicity Hearing impairment	Increased risk of pseudotumor cerebri: tetracyclines Hepatotoxicity: methotrexate Additive toxic effects: vitamin A
Thalidomide	Teratogenicity Stevens-Johnson syndrome Somnolence, headache Permanent nerve damage Acute renal failure Leukopenia	Increased sedation: barbiturates, chlorpromazine, reserpine

Dermatology Pharmacy Review (continued)

Drug	Toxic/adverse effects[*]	Drug interactions[†]
Topical antibacterials		
Azelaic acid	Pruritus, burning, peeling	
	Depigmentation	
Bacitracin	Allergic dermatitis	
Benzoyl peroxide	Excessive drying	Skin irritation: tretinoin
	Dermatitis	
Clindamycin	Dryness, peeling of skin	Antagonism: erythromycin
Erythromycin	Skin irritation	Antagonism: clindamycin
		Cumulative irritant effect with topical acne therapies
Metronidazole	Skin irritation	
Mupirocin	Skin irritation	
	Contact dermatitis	
	Headache	
Neomycin	Contact dermatitis (>10% of users)	
Sodium sulfacetamide	Skin irritation	
	Stevens-Johnson syndrome, toxic epidermal necrolysis	
Tetracycline	Skin irritation	
	Temporary follicular staining	
Topical immunomodulators and antiproliferatives		
Anthralin	Skin irritation	Before use, allow 1 week after use of topical steroids, due to rebound phenomenon of psoriasis
	Contact allergic reactions	
	Stains skin, hair	
	Should not be applied to eyes, mucous membranes, or intertriginous skin areas	
Calcipotriene	Skin irritation	
	Hypercalcemia	
	Worsening of psoriasis	
	Skin atrophy, hyperpigmentation	
Coal tar	Skin irritation	
	Contact dermatitis	
	Folliculitis	
	Phototoxicity	
	Psoriasis	
	Staining of skin	
Corticosteroids	Systemic absorption	
	Local irritation	
	Skin atrophy	
	Skin infection	
Mechlorethamine	Contact sensitivity	
	Hyperpigmentation	
	Irritant dermatitis	
	Telangiectases	

Dermatology Pharmacy Review (continued)

Drug	Toxic/adverse effects[*]	Drug interactions[†]
Topical immunomodulators and antiproliferatives (continued)		
Retinoids (adapalene, tretinoin, alitretinoin, tazarotene, bexarotene)	Skin irritation Photosensitivity	Considerable skin irritation: topical sulfur, resorcinol, benzoyl peroxide, salicylic acid Increased phototoxicity: thiazides, tetracyclines, fluoroquinolones, phenothiazides, sulfonamides
Tacrolimus, pimecrolimus	Carcinogenesis Increased risk of viral infections Phototoxicity Skin burning, pruritus	
Topical keratolytics		
Masoprocol	Local irritation Allergic contact dermatitis	Do not use with other skin care products or makeup
Resorcinol	Mild irritant Hyperpigmentation Methemoglobinemia Green discoloration of urine	Considerable skin irritation: retinoids
Salicylic acid	Local irritation	Increased irritation of skin: other medications
Sulfur	Skin irritation	Increased irritation of skin: other topical medications

HMG-CoA, 3-hydroxy-3-methylglutaryl coenzyme A.

[*]Toxic/adverse effects: focus is on dermatologic, very common, or life-threatening effects.

[†]Drug interactions: focus is on other dermatology drugs, very common, or life-threatening interactions.

QUESTIONS

Multiple Choice (choose the one best answer)

1. A 34-year-old man who is positive for human immunodeficiency virus presents for evaluation of pigmented lesions (Figure). He has been noncompliant with antiretroviral therapy. His CD4 count is 124 cells/mm^3. His viral load is more than 20,000. He has generalized lymphadenopathy (Figure). This lesion would be expected to respond to which one of the following?
   a. Reinstitution of antiretroviral therapy
   b. Oral doxycycline
   c. Wide local excision
   d. Interferon alfa
   e. Orthovoltage x-ray therapy

2. A 44-year-old woman is admitted to the coronary care unit with recent onset of chest pain and dyspnea at rest. On examination, her blood pressure is 80/45 mm Hg, her pulse is 128 beats per minute at low volume, her jugular venous pressure is increased at 14 cm, her apex beat is not palpable, and her heart sounds are distant. No added sounds are heard by the examining resident. On inspection, she has a rash involving her face and hands (Figure). Which one of the following is the most likely diagnosis?
   a. Scleroderma
   b. Sarcoidosis
   c. Dermatomyositis
   d. Systemic lupus erythematosus
   e. Behçet syndrome

3. A 60-year-old woman presents for evaluation of recent onset of weakness. She has difficulty climbing stairs and getting out of the bathtub. On examination, she had mottled erythema on the chest, arms, and upper part of the back and facial swelling (Figure). Which tumor is most likely associated with this scenario?
   a. Ovarian carcinoma
   b. Meningioma
   c. Rhabdomyosarcoma
   d. Hypernephroma
   e. Malignant melanoma

4. A 50-year-old alcoholic woman passed out in a park on a summer's day. When brought to the emergency department, she had a blood alcohol content of 0.2 mg/dL, aspartate aminotransferase value of 90 U/L, alanine aminotransferase of 105 U/L, and γ-glutamyltransferase of 300 U/L. Chest radiography revealed aspiration pneumonia. As you start intravenous therapy, you notice blisters and crusted lesions on her hands (Figure). What additional diagnostic test do you order?
   a. IgA endomysial antibody test
   b. Serum indirect immunofluorescence
   c. Serum niacin determination
   d. 24-Hour urine porphyrin studies
   e. α_1-Antitrypsin determination

5. An 18-year-old college student presents with weight loss and malaise. She has frequent bowel movements with pale-colored stools. On examination, she is pale and thin with lanugo hair on the upper part of the back. She has excoriations on the buttocks and elbows (Figure). What is the most likely diagnosis?
   a. Laxative abuse
   b. Anorexia nervosa
   c. Crohn disease
   d. Gluten-sensitive enteropathy with dermatitis herpetiformis
   e. Ulcerative colitis

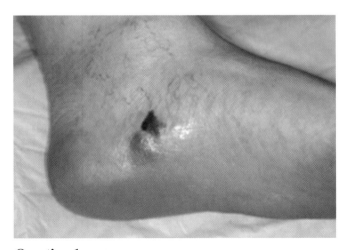

Question 1

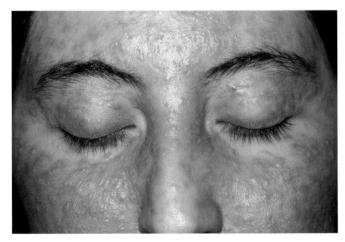

Question 2

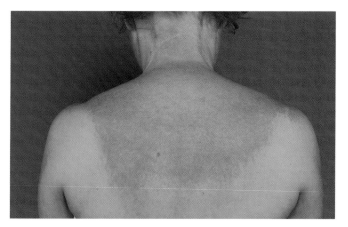

Question 3

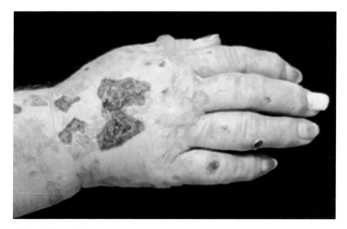

Question 4

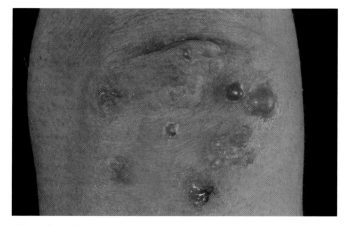

Question 5

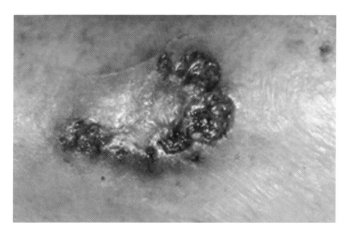

Question 6

6. A 36-year-old female flight attendant presents for evaluation of a leg ulcer. She is married and has no children. Her past history is significant for one previous deep venous thrombus and Crohn disease, which is currently inactive. The ulcer on the anterior shin started after trauma (Figure). On the basis of your clinical examination, which one of the following is the most likely diagnosis?
   a. Pyoderma gangrenosum
   b. Lupus anticoagulant syndrome
   c. Cryoglobulinemia
   d. Recluse spider bite
   e. Necrobiosis lipoidica diabeticorum

7. A 74-year-old white man undergoes resection of an abdominal aortic aneurysm. He has a complicated postoperative course and is transferred to the intensive care unit for treatment of adult respiratory distress syndrome. He requires ventilation over an extended period. After 2 weeks, parenteral nutrition is started. After 4 weeks in the intensive care unit, you notice a rash in the perianal area. He also has some scaly patches on the face, hands,

and legs (Figure). On the basis of your clinical examination, what additional test would you order?
   a. Potassium hydroxide examination
   b. Scabies preparation
   c. Serum magnesium determination
   d. Skin biopsy
   e. Serum zinc determination

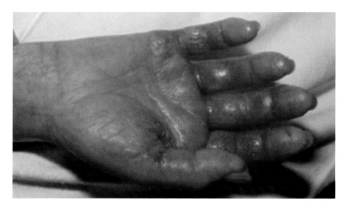

Question 7

ANSWERS

1. Answer c.

The lesion is a malignant melanoma. Wide local excision is the treatment of choice. At this site, sentinel node biopsy also is recommended for lesions more than 1 mm in thickness. The incidence of melanoma is increased in persons with acquired immunodeficiency syndrome. The other therapies listed are expected to be beneficial in Kaposi sarcoma (answers a, d, e) and bacillary angiomatosis (answer b).

2. Answer d.

The patient has a characteristic malar rash of systemic lupus erythematosus. The clinical scenario is one of pericarditis with pericardial effusion. The dermatologic finding in scleroderma is acrosclerosis. The cardiac findings consist of heart failure due to pulmonary or systemic hypertension. The cutaneous findings of sarcoidosis are granulomatous inflammation with possible associated cardiomyopathy. Cardiac disease is rare in dermatomyositis and Behçet disease.

3. Answer a.

Dermatomyositis is associated with an increased incidence of underlying malignancy. Of the tumors listed, ovarian carcinoma is the most common in a female patient.

4. Answer d.

This patient has porphyria cutanea tarda in addition to the acute medical problems. Known precipitants include alcohol excess, hepatitis C, estrogen therapy, and hemochromatosis.

5. Answer d.

A young patient with malnutrition, pruritus, and this clinical picture has gluten-sensitive enteropathy until proved otherwise. The other conditions listed might give rise to the malnutrition but not to the skin findings.

6. Answer a.

The clinical picture of an ulcer on the shin with cribriform scarring and undermined borders is consistent with a diagnosis of pyoderma gangrenosum. Affected patients have pathergy with ulceration developing at sites of trauma. Patients with lupus anticoagulant as a basis for ulceration present with stasis-type ulceration. Ulceration with cryoglobulinemia would be more distal and have an infarctive appearance. In ulcerative necrobiosis lipoidica diabeticorum (NLD), the ulcer is surrounded by skin with changes of NLD.

7. Answer e.

Zinc deficiency may occur in the setting of parenteral nutrition with inadequate or no zinc supplementation. The cutaneous findings are of periorificial dermatitis with acral involvement. The skin findings resolve with zinc replacement.

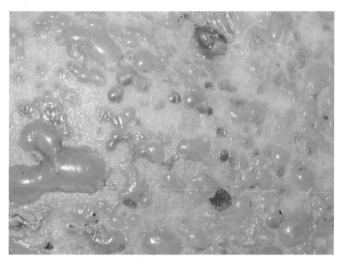

Plate 5-1. Bullous pemphigoid.

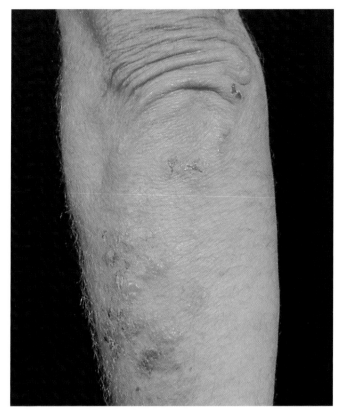

Plate 5-2. Dermatitis herpetiformis.

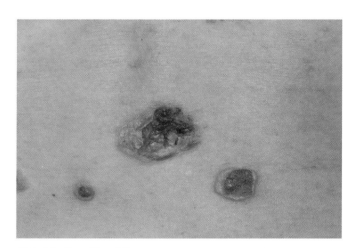

Plate 5-3. Pemphigus foliaceus.

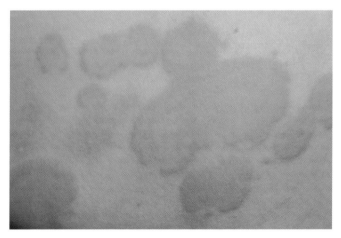

Plate 5-4. Erythema multiforme.

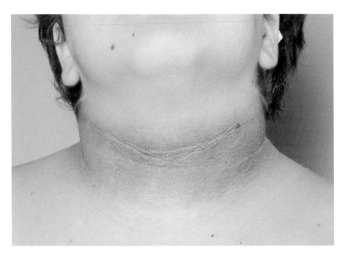

Plate 5-5. Acanthosis nigricans.

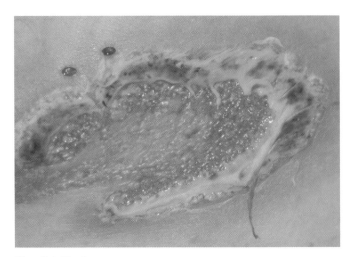

Plate 5-6. Pyoderma gangrenosum.

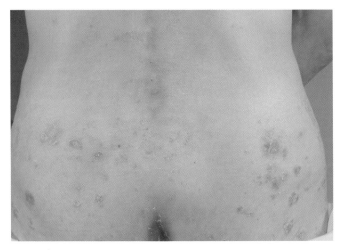

Plate 5-7. Glucagonoma syndrome (necrolytic migratory erythema).

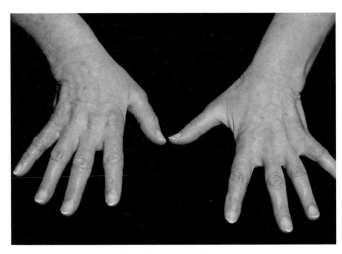

Plate 5-8. Dermatomyositis: Gottron papules.

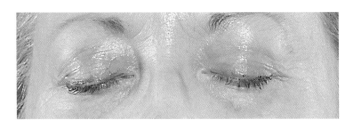

Plate 5-9. Dermatomyositis: heliotrope discoloration.

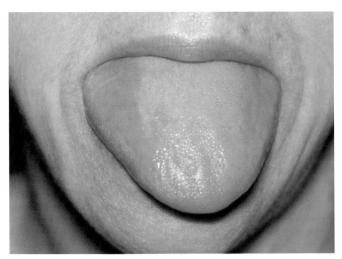

Plate 5-10. Amyloidosis: macroglossia.

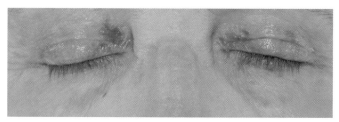

Plate 5-11. Amyloidosis: postproctoscopic purpura.

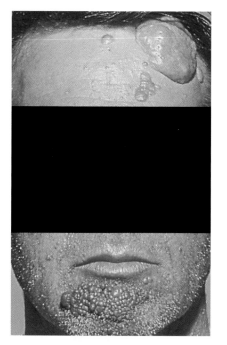

Plate 5-13. Tuberous sclerosis: adenoma sebaceum and forehead plaque.

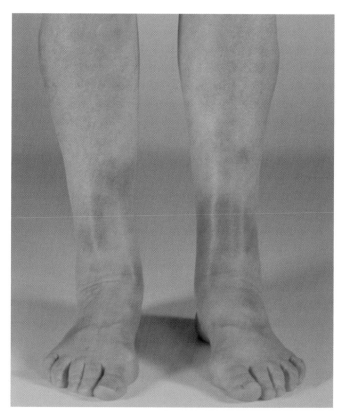

Plate 5-12. Erythema nodosum.

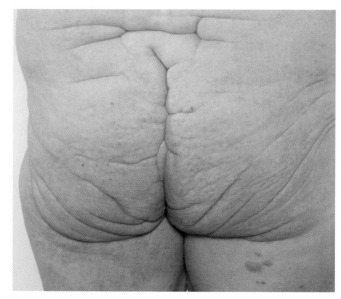

Plate 5-14. Neurofibromatosis: plexiform neurofibroma.

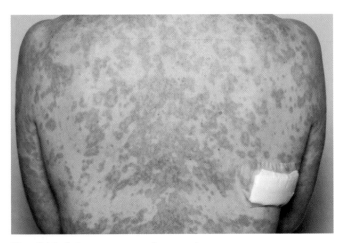

Plate 5-15. Subacute cutaneous lupus erythematosus.

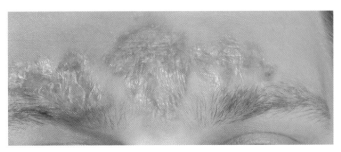

Plate 5-16. Discoid lupus erythematosus.

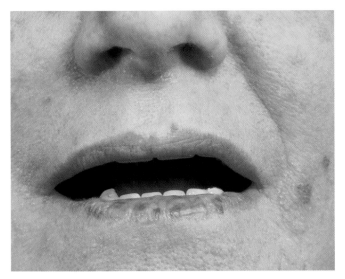

Plate 5-17. Scleroderma: CREST syndrome.

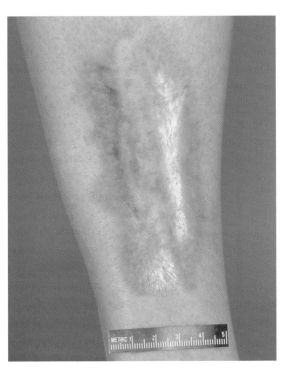

Plate 5-18. Necrobiosis lipoidica diabeticorum.

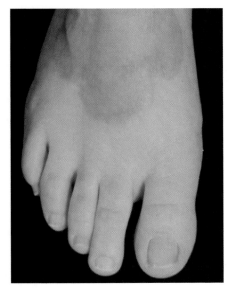

Plate 5-19. Granuloma annulare.

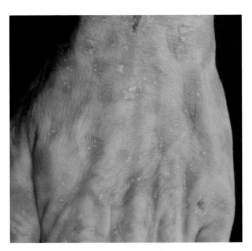

Plate 5-20. Porphyria cutanea tarda.

CHAPTER 6
ENDOCRINOLOGY

Adrian Vella, M.D.
Neena Natt, M.D.

BASIC PRINCIPLES OF ENDOCRINOLOGY

Myriad chemical messages control various functions at the level of cells, organs, and organ systems. Such messages may be autocrine (the chemical message directly affects the cell producing it), paracrine (the message has local effects), or endocrine (the message has distant sites of action). Typically, endocrine effects are caused by hormones that are produced by special organs.

Hormones may act at the cell surface or within the cell, or in both places. For example, steroid hormones exert effects on most cells in the body by acting through nuclear hormone receptors and regulate gene transcription and protein synthesis. In contrast, hormones such as adrenocorticotropic hormone (ACTH) act through specific cell surface receptors that in turn produce rapid effects through second messenger systems. Typically, hormones in the latter group exert their effects rapidly, whereas hormones that act through nuclear hormone receptors produce slower responses. Because of this lag in response, the serum concentrations of these hormones measured at any given time may not truly reflect the amount of "signal" that nuclear receptors have been exposed to over the preceding hours.

Most hormone systems require the interaction of multiple hormones secreted by different tissues. For example, the thyroid gland produces thyroxine (T_4), which in effect is the system's active or "end hormone" that exerts the physiologic effects. However, the secretion of T_4 is stimulated by a hormone, thyroid-stimulating hormone (TSH), produced by the pituitary gland. TSH, an example of a "trophic hormone," is secreted in response to decreasing levels of T_4, and its secretion is suppressed by increasing levels of T_4. This is an example of negative-feedback control, which in this case serves to maintain a constant concentration of T_4.

It is important to recognize that in certain situations endocrine dysfunction may be a manifestation rather than a cause of severe systemic illness. For example, with extreme weight loss, such as anorexia nervosa, secretion of the trophic hormones that regulate gonadal function is decreased or absent. This is not a result of primary endocrine disease but is a physiologic response to the depletion of the body's energy reserves (fat) necessary for successful reproduction. Treatment is directed at the underlying cause.

An important principle to remember in the evaluation of patients with suspected endocrine disease is to properly document endocrine dysfunction before proceeding with imaging studies. Imaging studies performed in isolation may be misleading because of the propensity of modern, detailed imaging studies to detect incidental abnormalities of endocrine glands that have no functional significance and often reflect normal variation or aging.

- Hormones typically act through membrane-bound receptors or nuclear receptors.
- Hormone systems are finely regulated by the interaction between trophic hormones and end hormones.
- Endocrine dysfunction may be a manifestation of systemic disease.

HYPOTHALAMIC-PITUITARY DISORDERS

The pituitary and hypothalamus control various peripheral hormone systems. The hypothalamus contains various centers vital to the regulation of sleep/wake cycles, appetite, and thirst. It is an integrator for many neural and endocrine inputs and, through a portal system running down the pituitary stalk, directly controls pituitary function. The pituitary can be divided anatomically and physiologically into the "anterior pituitary" and the "posterior pituitary."

The anterior pituitary secretes various trophic hormones. Disease of this region may result in syndromes of hormone excess or deficiency. The posterior pituitary is not a gland but the terminus of axons of neurons in the supraoptic and paraventricular nuclei of the hypothalamus. It is a storehouse or the site of release for the hormones vasopressin and oxytocin. The main consequence of posterior pituitary disease is disordered water homeostasis.

Pituitary or hypothalamic lesions may cause symptoms from local effects on the visual pathway or the cavernous sinus (with lesions of cranial nerves III, IV, and VI) as well as from effects on hypothalamic centers, leading to disordered appetite and sleep/wake cycles.

Hypopituitarism

Etiology

Anterior pituitary diseases can result in hypopituitarism, with deficiency of one or more or all the anterior pituitary hormones. Causes of hypopituitarism include primary pituitary disease, hypothalamic disease, interruption of the pituitary stalk, and extrasellar disorders. Hypopituitarism can be functional and result from suppression of hypothalamic regulation of the anterior pituitary gland. Common causes include suppression of the hypothalamic-pituitary-adrenal axis following the use of exogenous corticosteroids or suppression of gonadotropin-releasing hormone (GnRH) related to extreme weight loss, exercise, or systemic illness.

An extrasellar lesion such as craniopharyngioma or Rathke cleft cyst may impinge on and impair the function of the hypothalamic-pituitary unit.

- Hypopituitarism may be functional. Treatment is aimed at the underlying cause.
- Anterior pituitary hormone deficiency can be total, multiple, or selective.
- The most common causes of hypopituitarism are pituitary tumors, pituitary operations, and radiotherapy.
- Exogenous corticosteroid use or extreme weight loss can lead to functional suppression of hypothalamic regulation of the anterior pituitary gland.
- The commonest extrasellar cause of hypopituitarism is craniopharyngioma.

Clinical Presentation in Adults

Hypopituitarism can present with the features of deficiency of one or more anterior pituitary hormones. The clinical presentation depends on the age at onset, the hormone(s) affected, and the extent, speed of onset, and duration of the deficiency (Table 6-1). Hypopituitarism commonly presents as a chronic process of insidious onset. The manifestations are not related directly to anterior pituitary hormone deficiency (with the exception of prolactin) but to secondary deficiency of end hormones.

Gonadotropin Deficiency

In women, this leads to oligomenorrhea or amenorrhea, loss of libido, vaginal dryness and dyspareunia, and loss of secondary sex characteristics (estrogen deficiency). In men, gonadotropin deficiency leads to loss of libido, erectile dysfunction, infertility, loss of secondary sex characteristics, atrophy of the testes, and, occasionally, gynecomastia (testosterone deficiency).

ACTH Deficiency

The resultant hypocortisolism leads to malaise, anorexia, weight loss, gastrointestinal disturbances, and hyponatremia. Because ACTH helps maintain skin pigmentation, patients often have a pale complexion and are unable to tan or maintain a tan. Patients do not have features of mineralocorticoid deficiency because aldosterone secretion is unaffected.

TSH Deficiency

This leads to secondary hypothyroidism and an atrophic thyroid gland.

Prolactin Deficiency

The only clinical consequence of prolactin deficiency is the inability to lactate postpartum, which often is the first manifestation of Sheehan syndrome.

Growth Hormone Deficiency

In adults, growth hormone (GH) deficiency is often asymptomatic. However, some patients may complain of fatigue, decreased exercise tolerance, abdominal obesity, and loss of muscle mass.

- Gonadotropin deficiency manifests as hypogonadism and infertility.
- ACTH deficiency results in glucocorticoid deficiency without mineralocorticoid deficiency.
- TSH deficiency leads to secondary hypothyroidism.
- Prolactin deficiency manifests as a failure of lactation in the postpartum period.
- In adults, GH deficiency leads to an ill-defined syndrome of asthenia, weakness, and malaise.
- Typical clinical scenario for hypopituitarism: A patient has an insidious onset of signs and symptoms due to the particular end-hormone deficiency.

Hypopituitarism may present acutely with cortisol deficiency. This can occur after withdrawal of prolonged glucocorticoid therapy that has caused suppression of the hypothalamic-pituitary-adrenal axis. Acute destruction of the pituitary by trauma, surgical procedure, or hemorrhage may also present in this fashion. Medical or surgical illness or thyroid hormone replacement therapy in a patient with unrecognized ACTH deficiency also exacerbates cortisol deficiency.

Diagnosis

It is essential to document the degree of endocrine dysfunction and to determine the cause of hypopituitarism.

Table 6-1 Hypothalamic-Pituitary Hormones: Functions and Clinical Syndromes

Hormone	GH	PRL	LH/FSH	ACTH/LPH/END	TSH	ADH
Anterior pituitary cell type	Somatotroph	Lactotroph	Gonadotroph	Corticotroph	Thyrotroph	Supraoptic and para-ventricular nuclei
Regulation (*the dominant regulators are italicized*)	*GHRH (+)* GHRIH (−)	*DA (−)* TRH, VIP (+)	*GnRH (+)* DA, opioids (−)	*CRH (+)* AVP (+)	*TRH (+)* GHRIH, DA (−)	Plasma osmolality (osmo-receptors) and blood volume (volume & baro-receptors)
Secretion	Episodic Sleep-related surge	Episodic Sleep-related surge	Phasic in life Episodic Cyclic in women of reproductive age	Episodic Diurnal Stress-responsive	Episodic Minimal diurnal change	Exquisitely sensitive to changes in plasma osmolality
Physiologic functions	IGF-I–mediated growth Intermediary metabolism	Lactogenesis Others (?)	Initiation & maintenance of sexual/ reproductive functions	ACTH: Initiation & maintenance of cortisol production by adrenal cortex Pigmentary effects LPH/END	Initiation & main-tenance of T_4/T_3 secretion by thyroid	Maintenance of plasma osmolality Maintenance of blood volume & pressure
Deficiency in adult	Syndrome of GH deficiency?	Loss of postpartum lactation	Hypogonado-tropism	Secondary cortisol deficiency	Secondary hypo-thyroidism	Central diabetes insipidus
Deficiency in child	Shortness of stature Hypoglycemia	Not recognized	Hypogonado-tropism in adolescent	Secondary cortisol deficiency	Secondary hypo-thyroidism	Central diabetes insipidus
Hypersecretion in adult	Acromegaly	Hyperpro-lactinemic syndrome	No distinct syndrome	Cushing disease	TSH-induced hyper-thyroidism	SIADH
Hypersecretion in child	Gigantism	Hyperpro-lactinemic syndrome in adolescent	Precocious puberty	Cushing disease	TSH-induced hyper-thyroidism	SIADH

ACTH, corticotropin; ADH, antidiuretic hormone; CRH, corticotropin-releasing hormone; DA, dopamine; END, β-endorphin; FSH, follicle-stimulating hormone; GH, growth hormone; GHRH, GH-releasing hormone; GHRIH, GH-releasing inhibiting hormone or somatostatin; GnRH, gonadotropin-releasing hormone; LH, luteinizing hormone; LPH, β-lipotropin; PRL, prolactin; SIADH, syndrome of inappropriate ADH secretion; TRH, thyrotropin-releasing hormone; TSH, thyrotropin; VIP, vasoactive intestinal polypeptide.

Functional causes of hypopituitarism must be excluded before searching for an organic cause.

Endocrine Evaluation

Gonadotropin Axis—Deficiencies in this axis are manifested as a low serum concentration of testosterone or estradiol, with low or inappropriately normal levels of luteinizing hormone (LH) and follicle-stimulating hormone (FSH). The menstrual cycle is a sensitive indicator of hypothalamic-pituitary-gonadal function. Thus, a woman with a normal menstrual cycle can be assumed to have normal gonadotropin secretion.

ACTH-Adrenocortical Axis—A normal plasma level of cortisol does not confirm that the pituitary can secrete sufficient ACTH during conditions of stress. An ACTH stimulation test (cosyntropin test) may provide additional information. With chronic ACTH deficiency, the adrenal cortices are atrophic and typically do not show a cortisol secretory response to exogenous ACTH. A response may be seen if ACTH deficiency is partial or of recent onset. The cosyntropin test cannot distinguish between ACTH deficiency and primary adrenal insufficiency. Therefore, it is important to measure ACTH levels: a low or inappropriately normal ACTH level is consistent with pituitary dysfunction, whereas an increased ACTH level is consistent with primary adrenal disease. Other provocative tests include the use of insulin-induced hypoglycemia or metyrapone to stimulate ACTH secretion.

TSH-Thyroid Axis—Low serum levels of free thyroxine (FT_4) and an inappropriately normal or low serum level of TSH support the diagnosis of central hypothyroidism.

GH—Random determinations of GH concentrations are not useful in the evaluation of GH deficiency. Low serum concentrations of insulin-like growth factor (IGF)-I suggest the diagnosis. Provocative testing with insulin-induced hypoglycemia is the standard way to stimulate GH secretion. However, this is contraindicated for the elderly and for patients with ischemic heart disease. The combined arginine plus growth hormone-releasing hormone (GHRH) stimulation test has a diagnostic accuracy similar to that of insulin-induced hypoglycemia and, in the near future, will likely become the test of choice for diagnosing GH deficiency in adults.

Prolactin—Deficiency is suggested by low serum concentrations. Note that interruption of the pituitary stalk often increases prolactin concentrations through the release of lactotrophs from tonic inhibition by dopamine.

Structural Evaluation

This requires imaging of the hypothalamic-pituitary region, preferably with magnetic resonance imaging (MRI). If a space-occupying lesion in the region of the sella is detected, the visual fields need to be assessed.

Therapy in Adults

Therapy includes correction, if possible, of the cause (functional or structural) and administration of the deficient hormone(s) of the target gland(s) or, in selected cases, pituitary hormones.

ACTH Deficiency—Glucocorticoid replacement is essential. Hydrocortisone should be given twice daily. An average daily dose is 10 to 20 mg in the early morning and 5 to 10 mg in the early afternoon. Alternatively, a longer acting corticosteroid such as prednisone 5 mg once daily is sufficient. Patients must be instructed to double or triple the steroid dose during times of acute illness. For patients with combined deficiency of ACTH and TSH, glucocorticoid replacement should be initiated before thyroid hormone replacement therapy to avoid precipitation of an acute adrenocortical crisis.

TSH Deficiency—The drug of choice is L-thyroxine (T_4). Serum FT_4 must be monitored to ensure the adequacy of replacement therapy in these patients.

Gonadotropin Deficiency—If fertility is not desired, conjugated estrogens in combination with progesterone (on a cyclical or continuous basis) are prescribed for women with an intact uterus. In males, testosterone can be delivered intramuscularly or with transdermal patches or applied topically. For the restoration of fertility, gonadotropin therapy is indicated.

GH Deficiency—GH therapy may be considered for symptomatic patients with documented hypothalamic-pituitary disease and evidence of a suboptimal response to provocative testing. The goal of therapy is to restore serum IGF-I to normal levels and to avoid side effects. In the short term, GH therapy may enhance the sense of well-being and increase muscle strength, exercise tolerance, and bone mineral density. Currently, the long-term effects of this therapy are not known.

- Instruct patients about glucocorticoid dose modification during acute illness.
- For the combined deficiency of ACTH and TSH, initiate glucocorticoid therapy before thyroid hormone replacement therapy.
- Use FT_4 to monitor the adequacy of therapy in secondary hypothyroidism.

Pituitary Tumors

Pituitary tumors can be sporadic or part of multiple endocrine neoplasia type I (MEN I). They may present with the clinical features of a mass effect or endocrine dysfunction or they may be discovered incidentally when the head is imaged for other reasons. Tumors smaller than 1 cm are termed "microadenomas" and those 1 cm or larger are "macroadenomas." Evaluation of a pituitary tumor should address three questions:

Is the Tumor Causing a Local Mass Effect?

Superior extension of the tumor may compromise the optic pathways, leading to impaired visual acuity and visual field defects. Less frequently, it may produce a hypothalamic syndrome, with disturbed thirst, satiety, sleep, and temperature regulation. Lateral extension of the tumor may compress cranial nerves III, IV, V, and VI, leading to diplopia. Extension of the tumor inferiorly may lead to cerebrospinal fluid (CSF) rhinorrhea. Ophthalmologic evaluation, including assessment of visual acuity, visual fields, and optic disks, is important, particularly if there is suprasellar extension of the tumor.

Is Hypopituitarism Present?

Hypopituitarism may be caused by destruction of the pituitary gland or interruption of the pituitary stalk by tumor growth. Rarely, pituitary tumors can present acutely with pituitary apoplexy, which may be the first clinical expression of the underlying tumor. Endocrine evaluation is essential (see below, *Hypopituitarism*).

Is There Evidence of Hormone Excess?

From 30% to 40% of pituitary tumors are nonfunctioning. The rest are hyperfunctioning: prolactinomas (40%-50%), GH tumors resulting in acromegaly (10%-15%), ACTH tumors resulting in Cushing disease (10%-15%), and TSH tumors resulting in hyperthyroidism (<5%). An increase in FT_4 and an increased or inappropriately normal TSH may indicate a TSH-secreting pituitary adenoma. IGF-I levels and 24-hour urine free cortisol should be measured if indicated by the clinical history and examination findings.

A nonfunctioning tumor in the sella may not necessarily represent a pituitary tumor; for example, it could be metastatic disease.

- Ophthalmologic evaluation is important, particularly with suprasellar extension of a tumor.
- Endocrine evaluation should determine hormonal excess or deficiency.

Treatment

Generally, the first-line treatment for pituitary tumors (except prolactinomas) is surgical excision. Drug therapy is available for some functional tumors (see below). Simple observation is an option if the tumor is small, does not have a local mass effect, and is nonfunctional.

- Treatment includes surgical excision, irradiation, or medical therapy.
- Observation: This is an option when the tumor is small and nonfunctioning or, in the case of a microprolactinoma, when it is not associated with clinical features that affect quality of life.

Surgery

Transsphenoidal surgery is the operation of choice for most pituitary tumors (except prolactinoma). Rarely, craniotomy is performed on tumors with marked suprasellar extension. Both operations require considerable neurosurgical expertise. The morbidity (bleeding, infection, transient diabetes insipidus, CSF rhinorrhea, and anterior pituitary dysfunction) associated with transsphenoidal surgery is less than 1% for microadenomas and less than 4% for macroadenomas, and mortality is less than 1%. Persistence or recurrence rate of the tumor is less than 20% to 30% for microadenomas but is 50% to 70% for macroadenomas.

Radiotherapy

Radiotherapy is reserved for pituitary macroadenomas after surgical or medical therapy fails or as primary therapy for patients who are poor surgical candidates or who refuse operation. Radiotherapy may be delivered by conventional external beam radiation or stereotactic gamma knife radiosurgery. The latter delivers a single highly focused beam of radiation and is reserved for the treatment of small-volume pituitary adenomas or smaller macroadenomas that may involve the cavernous sinus. Both forms of radiotherapy have a long latent period (from a few months to years) before the onset of action, and postradiation hypopituitarism may occur (30%-40% of patients receiving conventional therapy).

Drug Therapy

Dopamine agonists (bromocriptine or cabergoline) are used for the management of prolactinomas. The somatostatin analogue octreotide may be used for the management of GH- or TSH-producing tumors.

Follow-Up

Follow-up to monitor tumor size and function is essential in managing pituitary tumors and determining the development of hypopituitarism, especially in patients who had surgical treatment or radiotherapy.

Prolactinoma

Pituitary tumors associated with hyperprolactinemia may be prolactinomas or nonfunctioning tumors with a suprasellar extension that produces a "stalk effect." In the latter situation, the impingement of the tumor on the pituitary stalk interferes with the tonic inhibition of lactotrophs by dopamine (secreted by the hypothalamus), leading to excess secretion of prolactin by normal lactotrophs.

- Pituitary tumors associated with hyperprolactinemia are prolactinomas or any tumor or mass lesion with a suprasellar extension and stalk effect.

Clinical Features

Women typically present with galactorrhea and oligomenorrhea or amenorrhea. In men, the recognition of hyperprolactinemia is often delayed because symptoms of hypogonadism, including decreased libido, may be attributed to other factors. For this reason, men are more likely to present with a macroprolactinoma. Galactorrhea is unusual in men because of the absence of estrogen priming of the breast.

Clinical features of prolactinoma:
- In women, ovulatory/menstrual dysfunction and galactorrhea.
- In men, decreased libido and impotence. Galactorrhea is rare.

Diagnosis

Differential Diagnosis

Pituitary tumors are not the only cause of hyperprolactinemia. Physiologic causes of hyperprolactinemia include pregnancy, the postpartum state, and stressful conditions such as surgery or seizure. Stalk disruption may occur with infiltrative disorders, including lymphoma and hypophysitis, which lead to disinhibition of prolactin secretion by normal lactotrophs.

Medications are a common cause of hyperprolactinemia. Neuroleptic agents, antidepressants, cimetidine, and verapamil are all associated with hyperprolactinemia. The mechanism of action is interference with the synthesis, secretion, or action of dopamine. In primary hypothyroidism, hyperprolactinemia is often encountered because of the stimulatory effect of thyrotropin-releasing hormone (TRH) on the synthesis and secretion of prolactin. Chest wall lesions such as herpes zoster, thoracotomy, or trauma increase prolactin concentrations possibly through stimulation of thoracic nerve terminals that eventually signal the hypothalamus. Hyperprolactinemia occurs in renal failure and cirrhosis because of delayed metabolism of the hormone. Organic hypothalamic disorders that produce hyperprolactinemia include surgery or irradiation, sarcoidosis or histiocytosis X, or neoplastic disorders such as craniopharyngioma or metastatic disease.

- Physiologic hyperprolactinemia occurs in pregnancy and in the postpartum period.
- Pathologic hyperprolactinemia occurs with prolactinomas or conditions that interrupt the pituitary stalk.
- Functional disorders leading to hyperprolactinemia include neuroleptics, primary hypothyroidism, chest wall lesions, and chronic renal or liver failure.

A Diagnostic Approach to Hyperprolactinemia:

- Rule out pregnancy. This is the commonest cause of amenorrhea and galactorrhea in females of reproductive age.
- Measure TSH to rule out primary hypothyroidism.
- Review medications.
- Image the hypothalamus and pituitary with computed tomography (CT) or MRI if other causes of hyperprolactinemia have been ruled out.
- If a tumor is present, evaluate other pituitary functions and visual fields if necessary.

The major diagnostic dilemma is to differentiate a macroprolactinoma from a nonfunctioning tumor that causes a stalk effect. This has therapeutic implications because medical therapy is the first-line treatment for a prolactinoma, whereas nonfunctioning tumors with suprasellar extension are resected surgically. A serum level of prolactin greater than 200 ng/mL supports the diagnosis of prolactinoma, and a level less than 75 ng/mL is more consistent with a stalk effect, particularly in macroadenomas. If the value is between 75 and 200 ng/mL, a trial of dopamine agonist therapy is reasonable. Regression of the tumor mass and a decrease in prolactin concentrations with this therapy support the diagnosis of prolactinoma.

If, after a thorough evaluation, a discernible cause of hyperprolactinemia is not found, follow-up is necessary because some patients may harbor a microadenoma or other hypothalamic-pituitary space-occupying lesion that is below the limit of radiographic detection, and follow-up examinations may show evidence of a mass. The serum level of prolactin should be checked every 6 to 12 months, and CT or MRI should be repeated in 1 or 2 years or earlier if deemed necessary by the development of new symptoms.

Therapy

Treatment is indicated for the management of infertility, hypogonadism, or galactorrhea. Medical treatment with a dopamine agonist is usually the first choice. Transsphenoidal surgery is usually reserved for patients who are intolerant or resistant to dopamine agonist therapy or who require urgent decompression of the sella turcica for visual field defects that have not responded to a trial of dopamine agonist.

Dopamine Agonists

Dopamine agonists (bromocriptine or cabergoline) are very effective in the treatment of hyperprolactinemia caused by prolactinoma. In most cases, these agents lead to rapid shrinkage of the tumor and a decrease in prolactin levels. Thus, these medications are indicated as first-line therapy even for large prolactinomas that cause a visual field defect. Frequent assessment of the visual fields and tumor size is indicated in such cases. Tumor size or the degree of increase in prolactin does not predict tumor response. Side effects are usually minor and include nausea, fatigue, nasal stuffiness, and postural hypotension. Long-term therapy with a dopamine agonist may lead to tumor fibrosis and shrinkage. Withdrawal of dopamine agonist therapy and remeasurement of prolactin levels should be considered in patients with prolactinomas (particularly microadenomas) because the disorder may resolve spontaneously.

Restoration of gonadal function and fertility is a major goal of drug therapy. In pregnancy, the risk of growth for microprolactinomas is less than 5% and for macroprolactinomas, 20% to 40%. Patients should be observed closely with clinical and visual field evaluations, especially if they have a macroprolactinoma. If tumor growth is suspected, the head should be examined with MRI. Although treatment with dopamine agonists usually is discontinued during pregnancy, it is reasonable to continue maintenance therapy if the patient has a macroprolactinoma. An increase in tumor size may be an indication for surgical excision.

- The treatment of choice for prolactinomas is medical therapy with a dopamine agonist.
- During pregnancy, the risk of growth for microprolactinomas is <5% and for macroprolactinomas, 20%-40%.
- If marked tumor growth complicates pregnancy, consider surgical excision.

Surgical Treatment for Prolactinomas

The surgical cure rates for microadenomas and macroadenomas are 60% to 80% and 0% to 30%, respectively.

GH Tumors: Acromegaly

GH-producing pituitary tumors account for more than 99% of cases of acromegaly. Rarely, acromegaly may be caused by ectopic GH-producing tumors or hypothalamic or extrahypothalamic GHRH-producing tumors. It is essential to diagnose acromegaly early because the disease is associated with considerable morbidity and premature mortality.

Clinical Features

The clinical features of acromegaly are due to excess IGF-I and the mass effects of the pituitary tumor. In adults, characteristic features are prominent supraorbital ridges, macroglossia, prognathism, and increase in hand and foot size. Patients may complain of excessive sweating, increased skin oiliness, headache, and symptoms of carpal tunnel syndrome. The prevalence of colon polyps is increased threefold among patients with acromegaly, who also are at increased risk for the development of colon cancer. Currently, it seems prudent to perform colonoscopy on all patients when acromegaly is diagnosed. Cardiovascular disease is the most common cause of premature death. Many patients have hypertension and glucose intolerance. Sleep apnea is a common feature that may resolve or improve with successful treatment of acromegaly.

- Acromegaly is associated with an increased risk of premalignant colon polyps and colon cancer.
- Other common features include hypertension, glucose intolerance, and sleep apnea.

Diagnosis

Biochemical Diagnosis

IGF-I is the best screening test for acromegaly (physiologic increases can occur in pregnancy and adolescence and with sleep apnea). If the IGF-I serum level is mildly to moderately increased, it is best to proceed with an oral glucose tolerance test to document nonsuppressible GH secretion. GH levels do not suppress to less than 1 ng/mL in active acromegaly. A random serum level of GH is not helpful because of the pulsatile secretion of GH.

Radiologic Diagnosis

After the diagnosis has been confirmed biochemically, the sella should be examined with MRI. If a pituitary tumor is not delineated (a rare event) or diffuse pituitary hypertrophy is noted, measure the serum level of GHRH to exclude a GHRH-producing tumor and search for evidence of an ectopic GH-producing tumor.

- Serum IGF-I is increased in all patients with active acromegaly.
- Failure of GH to suppress to <1 ng/mL with an oral glucose tolerance test is diagnostic of acromegaly.
- A random GH level is not helpful.

Therapy

Surgical excision of the GH-secreting tumor is the usual first treatment of choice. Excision may be curative (40%-80% of cases depending on the size of the tumor and the degree of lateral extension) and facilitates adjunctive therapy. For persistent disease, treatment with octreotide or gamma knife radiosurgery (plus interim octreotide) is used to control GH secretion.

Radiotherapy has a cure rate of 70% after 10 years; hypopituitarism can occur in up to 50% of patients at 10 years, but other morbidity is rare. The major disadvantage of radiotherapy is the long latent period (months to years) before disease activity is controlled. While awaiting the full effects of radiotherapy, pharmacologic therapy is needed.

Octreotide is an effective therapeutic option. Treatment should be initiated with short-acting octreotide administered subcutaneously three times daily to assess tolerance. This can be switched quickly to the long-acting depot form of octreotide administered monthly. Octreotide can normalize GH/IGF-I in 80% of patients and produce shrinkage of the tumor in 30% to 50%. Side effects include nausea, flatulence, orthostatism, headache, cholelithiasis (10% of patients), and impairment of glucose tolerance. Pegvisomant (GH-receptor antagonist) has recently become available and is indicated for patients who do not have a response to or cannot tolerate octreotide therapy.

- Surgical excision is the treatment of choice.
- For persistent disease after excision, pharmacologic therapy or radiotherapy should be considered.
- Pharmacologic therapy is required while awaiting the full effects of adjunctive radiotherapy.

ACTH-Producing Tumors

These are discussed below in the section on Cushing syndrome.

Gonadotropin-Producing Tumors

These tumors constitute the largest fraction of nonfunctioning pituitary tumors. Although more than 80% of such tumors are able to synthesize gonadotropins or their subunits (or both), increased serum levels of FSH, LH, or their subunits are found in less than 35% of patients. Clinically, the tumors are macroadenomas at presentation. They may occur at any age but usually present in middle-aged or elderly persons and predominantly in males. Mass effects dominate the clinical features, and some degree of hypopituitarism is usually present together with hyperprolactinemia caused by a stalk effect. Currently, no effective medical therapy is available. Surgical excision is required.

TSH-Producing Tumors

Primary TSH tumors may present with diffuse goiter and mild hyperthyroidism. Laboratory evaluation demonstrates an increased or inappropriately normal TSH level with an increased concentration of FT_4. The α-glycoprotein subunit levels are high, and there is no TSH response to stimulation with TRH. Often such tumors cosecrete growth hormone. Treatment options include excision, pharmacologic therapy with octreotide, and ancillary measures for the management of thyrotoxicosis.

Pituitary Incidentaloma

With advances in the resolution of imaging modalities, pituitary incidentaloma is increasingly recognized. Autopsy studies suggest that approximately 10% of persons harbor small pituitary tumors. Evaluation should determine whether the tumor affects pituitary endocrine function (hypopituitarism and hyperfunction) or causes a mass effect (or both). Screening tests should include the measurement of prolactin, FT_4, testosterone (in men), and cortisol. The finding of a functioning pituitary tumor that can cause morbidity or mortality or an incidentaloma larger than 1 cm in diameter dictates active

intervention. Otherwise, observe and repeat the imaging study in 6 to 12 months and at less frequent intervals thereafter.

Miscellaneous Pituitary Disorders

Craniopharyngioma

Craniopharyngioma is a slow-growing encapsulated squamous cell tumor that originates from remnants of Rathke pouch. It is the most common tumor in the pituitary region in childhood but can present at any age. Two-thirds of the tumors are suprasellar, and one-third originate in or extend into the sella. Most are cystic, and some have solid and cystic areas. Calcification is often present within the tumor. Mass effects and the consequences of hypopituitarism dominate the clinical presentation.

Surgical excision is possible for only small craniopharyngiomas. Treatment is often complicated by panhypopituitarism and diabetes insipidus. Larger craniopharyngiomas are decompressed. Radiotherapy should be considered for persistent or recurrent disease.

Pituitary Apoplexy

Pituitary apoplexy is a clinical syndrome produced by sudden hemorrhage or infarction of the pituitary gland. Apoplexy usually occurs in a gland with a preexisting cyst or adenoma, but it has been described in normal pituitary glands. The onset of symptoms may be acute or subacute. The majority of patients present with headache, visual field defects, ophthalmoplegia, and, often, altered mental status. The immediate threat to the patient's life is from cortisol deficiency. Therapy includes neurosurgical decompression and hormonal support.

Lymphocytic Hypophysitis

This is presumed to be autoimmune in origin. Classically, it occurs in women during the postpartum period. The clinical presentation may be due to a mass effect (a sellar mass) but more commonly to deficiency of one or more anterior pituitary hormones (ACTH deficiency is the commonest). Corticosteroid therapy is often used in an attempt to shrink the sellar mass, but its effects are often disappointing. In many cases, the diagnosis is made only postoperatively because the process may be radiologically indistinguishable from a pituitary adenoma. Hormonal replacement therapy is given as needed.

Diabetes Insipidus

Etiology

Central diabetes insipidus may result from granulomatous infiltration of the posterior pituitary and the pituitary stalk (sarcoidosis, tuberculosis, or histiocytosis X), closed head trauma or neurosurgery, or primary neoplasms such as craniopharyngioma or metastatic neoplasms primarily from the breast or lung. Idiopathic hypothalamic diabetes insipidus is probably the commonest cause of the syndrome and may be an autoimmune disorder. Nephrogenic diabetes insipidus may be caused by chronic renal disease, electrolyte abnormalities (hypercalcemia or hypokalemia), and drugs such as lithium and demeclocycline, which antagonize the effects of antidiuretic hormone (ADH) on the renal tubules.

- Diabetes insipidus may result from decreased production of ADH or lack of renal responsiveness to the hormone.

Clinical Features

Patients typically present with polyuria and polydipsia, often with a preference for ice-cold water. Nocturia is usually present, and enuresis may be the presenting complaint of children. The absence of nocturia, intermittent symptoms, and a 24-hour urine output greater than 18 L suggest psychogenic polydipsia. It is important to remember that because patients with diabetes insipidus rely solely on their thirst mechanism to regulate water balance, lack of access to water or loss of the sensation of thirst will lead to extreme hyperosmolar dehydration.

Cortisol and, to a lesser extent, thyroid hormones are necessary for the excretion of a water load. In patients with central diabetes insipidus, the development of hypopituitarism may mask the symptoms of diabetes insipidus, which become apparent only after adequate cortisol replacement therapy.

- Diabetes insipidus is characterized by polyuria and polydipsia.
- The absence of nocturia suggests psychogenic polydipsia.
- When thirst sensation is impaired or access to water is restricted, hyperosmolar dehydration may ensue.
- Cortisol is necessary for the kidney's ability to excrete a water load.

Diagnosis

Endocrine Diagnosis

The diagnosis of diabetes insipidus is often complicated by the disorder being partial and also because prolonged periods of polyuria, regardless of the primary cause, may decrease the maximal urine-concentrating ability of the kidney.

In a patient with polyuria and dilute urine, a random plasma osmolality greater than 295 mOsm/kg suggests the diagnosis of diabetes insipidus. Plasma osmolality less than 280 mOsm/kg implies psychogenic polydipsia. If plasma osmolality is between 280 and 295 mOsm/kg, a water deprivation test is indicated. A random plasma osmolality greater than 295 mOsm/kg (or at the end of a water dehydration test) and urine osmolality less than 300 mOsm/kg exclude primary polydipsia and confirm diabetes insipidus. To differentiate between central and nephrogenic diabetes insipidus, 1 μg desmopressin (DDAVP) is injected subcutaneously and urine osmolality is measured at 30, 60, and 120 minutes. A postinjection urine osmolality more than 150% the preinjection osmolality is consistent with central diabetes insipidus.

A partial response to water deprivation, with urine osmolality greater than 300 mOsm/kg, can occur in partial central or nephrogenic diabetes insipidus as well as in primary polydipsia. In these circumstances, it is also necessary to collect plasma for ADH levels at the end of the water deprivation test.

- A random plasma osmolality >295 mOsm/kg suggests diabetes insipidus.
- A random plasma osmolality <280 mOsm/kg, in an untreated patient, suggests psychogenic polydipsia.
- Central diabetes insipidus can be distinguished from nephrogenic diabetes insipidus by the response to exogenous desmopressin.
- The absence of response to water deprivation (urine osmolality <300 mOsm/kg) is diagnostic of diabetes insipidus.

Etiologic Diagnosis

Imaging of the hypothalamus and neurohypophysis as well as the sella is essential. Systemic diseases involving the hypothalamus or pituitary stalk must be considered.

Therapy

The underlying cause should be treated. However, in central diabetes insipidus, treatment seldom restores ADH secretion. There is no need for intervention in patients with mild diabetes insipidus (urine output, 2-5 L daily) who have free access to water. For greater degrees of central diabetes insipidus, which interfere with the patient's sleep, desmopressin is the drug of choice. It is administered by nasal spray (5-10 μg once or twice daily) or orally (0.1-0.8 mg daily in divided doses). For patients who are unconscious or allergic to nasal desmopressin, the drug can be given parenterally (1-2 μg subcutaneously or intravenously 1 or 2 times daily). Thiazides may be useful in treating nephrogenic diabetes insipidus. Psychiatric assessment is needed for patients with psychogenic polydipsia.

The Syndrome of Inappropriate ADH Secretion

Etiology

The syndrome of inappropriate ADH secretion (SIADH) occurs when ADH is secreted in the absence of a hyperosmolar or a hypovolemic or hypotensive (or both) stimulus. SIADH may be a consequence of 1) central nervous system or hypothalamic disorders (including trauma) or inflammatory, degenerative, vascular, or neoplastic disorders, 2) the use of drugs that enhance ADH secretion or action (chlorpropamide, carbamazepine, vincristine, vinblastine, cyclophosphamide, phenothiazines, monoamine oxidase inhibitors, and tricyclic antidepressants), 3) neurogenic influences such as pain or nausea, and 4) benign pulmonary disorders (pneumonia, lung abscess, empyema) as well as malignancies such as mesothelioma and small cell lung carcinoma.

Pathophysiology

SIADH leads to hyponatremia, with low serum osmolality and inappropriately concentrated urine. The expansion of the extracellular fluid volume leads to natriuresis (from an increase in glomerular filtration rate, atrial natriuretic hormones, and suppression of the renin-angiotensin-aldosterone axis). Natriuresis exacerbates plasma hypo-osmolality, thus explaining the absence of edema despite an expanded extracellular fluid volume.

- Physiologic or appropriate ADH hypersecretion occurs in response to plasma hyperosmolality or hypovolemia or hypotension.
- SIADH is characterized by hypervolemia, hyponatremia, and hypo-osmolality of body fluids and inappropriately concentrated urine. No edema is present.

Clinical Features

The clinical features depend on the degree and rapidity of the development of hyponatremia. Patients with SIADH may be asymptomatic if the hyponatremia develops gradually over weeks and months. Symptoms include lethargy, malaise, nausea and vomiting, and confusion. Severe or rapidly developing hyponatremia can lead to alterations in mental status or seizures.

- Clinical features depend on the degree and rapidity of the development of hyponatremia.

Diagnosis

The diagnosis of SIADH is one of exclusion. Pseudohyponatremia due to hyperlipidemia (normal plasma osmolality) and hyperosmolar states due to water loss, as in hyperglycemia (increased plasma osmolality), must be excluded. Exclude diseases in which excess ADH is appropriate (congestive heart failure, ascites, nephrosis, hypovolemia, hypothyroidism, and hypocortisolism).

The major diagnostic challenge is to differentiate SIADH from subclinical hypovolemia. In subclinical hypovolemia, the urine concentration of sodium is less than 20 mEq/L (in the absence of diuretic use) and the serum levels of creatinine and uric acid are increased, as are plasma renin activity and plasma aldosterone.

- The major diagnostic challenge is to differentiate SIADH from subclinical hypovolemia. Determination of urinary sodium and serum creatinine, uric acid, plasma renin activity, and aldosterone may be useful.

Therapy

Therapy for SIADH includes treating the underlying disorder. Water intake is restricted to 800 to 1,000 mL daily. If necessary, an ADH antagonist (demeclocycline, 900-1,200 mg daily) can be given. If acute neurologic sequelae are present, hypertonic saline is administered intravenously, 200 to 300 mL of 5% NaCl over 3 to 4 hours, to achieve a gradual increase in serum sodium (do not exceed 0.5 mEq/h or 12 mEq/24 h). Rapid correction of hyponatremia can lead to central pontine myelinolysis.

- Identify and treat the underlying disorder.
- Therapy for hyponatremia consists of water restriction and, if needed, demeclocycline.
- In the presence of acute neurologic sequelae, administer hypertonic saline to increase serum sodium by 0.5 mEq/ h.
- Rapid correction of hyponatremia can lead to potentially fatal central pontine myelinolysis.

DISORDERS OF THE THYROID GLAND

Laboratory Assessment of Thyroid Function

Several thyroid tests are available to determine thyroid function and structure. Abnormal test results can be obtained in euthyroid patients with nonthyroidal illness. Thus, the history and physical examination are as important as laboratory investigation in the evaluation of thyroid disease. The interpretation of thyroid function tests is as follows:

- Total T_4. Serum total T_4 concentration is a measurement of T_4 bound to thyroid hormone–binding proteins such as thyroxine-binding globulin (TBG). Therefore, conditions that affect TBG concentration affect total T_4 measurements. Androgens, anabolic steroids, glucocorticoids, chronic liver disease, niacin, or familial TBG deficiency decreases total TBG. Estrogens, pregnancy, acute hepatitis, and familial TBG excess increase TBG and, thus, total T_4 concentrations.
- Total triiodothyronine (T_3). Serum total T_3 concentration is decreased in hypothyroidism, nonthyroidal illness, and caloric deprivation and by drugs such as propranolol, amiodarone, and glucocorticoids. Serum T_3 levels are increased in thyrotoxicosis and peripheral hormone resistance. Serum T_3 concentrations should be measured to establish or exclude the diagnosis of T_3 thyrotoxicosis in a patient

with a suppressed TSH level and a normal serum concentration of FT_4.

- FT_4. FT_4 is decreased in hypothyroidism and nonthyroidal illness and increased in hyperthyroidism, nonthyroidal illness, and peripheral hormone resistance.
- Thyroid hormone-binding proteins. These can be measured directly by radioimmunoassay or, more commonly, with the T_3 resin uptake test, which provides an indirect measurement of unoccupied T_4 binding sites on binding proteins. The normal range is 30%-40%. A decrease in T_4 binding sites, and thus an increase in T_3 resin uptake, is seen in hyperthyroidism, in low TBG states, and in the presence of binding inhibitors, as in nonthyroidal illness or with the use of certain drugs (see above). An increase in T_4 binding sites, and thus a decrease in T_3 resin uptake, is seen in hypothyroidism and high TBG states.
- Free thyroxine index (FTI). FTI represents the product of serum T_4 and T_3 resin uptake. It is an indirect measurement of FT_4 and correlates well with FT_4 concentrations.
- Serum TSH. Current third-generation TSH assays can measure TSH concentrations as low as 0.05 mU/L, allowing clinicians to differentiate low-normal values from suppressed values. TSH is increased in primary hypothyroidism, during recovery from nonthyroidal illness, and with peripheral resistance to thyroid hormones. TSH is suppressed in hyperthyroidism of any cause (except that due to TSH-producing tumors), in nonthyroidal illness, and by drugs such as somatostatin, dopamine, and glucocorticoids. TSH is the best test of thyroid function. However, TSH is unreliable in cases of pituitary disease because values can be "inappropriately" normal relative to thyroid hormone concentrations. Thus, TSH levels may be normal or increased with TSH-producing tumors and normal or decreased in central hypothyroidism.
- Thyroid scanning. This may be performed with pertechnetate or radioactive iodine. Thyroid scanning is reserved for the documentation of toxic thyroid nodules, ectopic thyroid tissue in struma ovarii, and metastatic disease in the postoperative evaluation and follow-up of patients with differentiated thyroid cancer.
- Radioactive iodine (I 131) uptake (RAIU). The normal range for 24-hour uptake depends on the dietary iodine intake in a given population. In the U.S. population, the normal range is 10%-25%. A 24-hour RAIU study is indicated during the evaluation of hyperthyroidism to distinguish low-uptake states from high-uptake states and to aid in dose calculations when radioactive iodine is used to treat Graves disease.
- Serum thyroglobulin. Thyroglobulin is used mainly as a tumor marker in follow-up evaluations of patients with differentiated thyroid carcinoma. It also may be useful in the differential diagnosis of suppressed TSH with low radioactive iodine uptake (lymphocytic thyroiditis or exogenous hyperthyroidism). Serum thyroglobulin levels are usually elevated in lymphocytic thyroiditis and low in exogenous hyperthyroidism.
- TSH receptor–stimulating immunoglobulins (TSI). Measurement of these immune markers of Graves disease is important in the differential diagnosis of hyperthyroidism in pregnant women who cannot undergo RAIU. TSI levels may help to predict the possible occurrence of neonatal thyrotoxicosis in infants born to women with a history of or with active Graves disease. TSI measurement is also helpful in the diagnosis of euthyroid Graves ophthalmopathy.
- Antithyroglobulin and antimicrosomal (antiperoxidase) antibodies. These are used as markers of autoimmune thyroid disease. The absence of these antibodies does not exclude the presence of autoimmune thyroid disease. Conversely, the presence of these antibodies is not diagnostic of autoimmune thyroid disease; they can be found in otherwise healthy persons. High titers occur in more than 90% of patients with Hashimoto thyroiditis, and modestly increased titers are found in primary atrophic hypothyroidism and Graves disease. Antithyroglobulin antibodies, when present, make measurement of thyroglobulin unreliable for follow-up of thyroid malignancies.
- Thyroid ultrasonography. This is best reserved for the follow-up of patients with thyroid cancer and to assess local recurrence or cervical lymph node metastatic disease.

Hyperthyroidism

Etiology

Primary thyroid disorders that cause hyperthyroidism can be divided into those characterized by increased production and release of T_4 (high RAIU) and those characterized by unregulated release of T_4 due to gland destruction (suppressed RAIU) (Table 6-2).

The commonest cause of hyperthyroidism in iodine-sufficient areas is Graves disease. Other frequent causes include toxic nodular goiter, lymphocytic and subacute thyroiditis, and exogenous hyperthyroidism.

Clinical Features

Typical symptoms include heat intolerance, palpitations, increased sweating, diarrhea, weight loss, menstrual irregularities, insomnia, nervousness, irritability, and emotional lability. In severe, prolonged hyperthyroidism, proximal muscle weakness may be present. Ocular manifestations include findings due to sympathetic overactivity from hyperthyroidism of any cause (retraction of the upper lid, stare, and lid lag) or findings unique to Graves disease (puffiness of the lids, conjunctival

Table 6-2 Causes of Increased and Suppressed 24-Hour Radioactive Iodine Uptake (RAIU)

High RAIU	Low RAIU
Graves disease	Lymphocytic thyroiditis (postpartum thyroiditis)
Autonomous nodular goiter	Subacute thyroiditis
HCG-dependent hyperthyroidism of trophoblastic disease	Exogenous hyperthyroidism
TSH-secreting pituitary adenoma	Recent iodine load (e.g., contrast dye)
Metastatic follicular thyroid carcinoma	Struma ovarii (if RAIU measured over thyroid only)
Selective pituitary resistance to thyroid hormones	

HCG, human chorionic gonadotropin; TSH, thyroid-stimulating hormone.

injection and chemosis, proptosis, and extraocular muscle weakness). Patients with Graves ophthalmopathy may complain of a gritty sensation in the eyes, excessive lacrimation, photophobia, and diplopia. Most patients with hyperthyroidism have a small, firm goiter.

Atypical presentations of hyperthyroidism, particularly in the elderly, include apathy, weight loss, supraventricular tachycardia, atrial fibrillation, and congestive heart failure. Young adult males may develop gynecomastia.

- The clinical features of hyperthyroidism reflect the effects of excess thyroid hormone. However, some features, such as Graves ophthalmopathy, may be specific to the underlying cause.
- The presence of goiter and its characteristics vary according to the cause.
- Atypical presentations of hyperthyroidism in the elderly include weight loss, apathy, atrial fibrillation, and congestive heart failure.

Diagnosis of Hyperthyroidism

The biochemical diagnosis of hyperthyroidism rests on the demonstration of a suppressed TSH and increased serum level of FT_4. Normal FT_4 values should prompt the measurement of serum T_3 concentrations to determine the presence of T_3 toxicosis. Increased or inappropriately normal TSH in the presence of increased FT_4 indicates hyperthyroidism due to pituitary TSH-secreting tumors or selective pituitary resistance to thyroid hormones. A low level of serum TSH by itself is not diagnostic of hyperthyroidism and can be encountered in nonthyroidal illness, glucocorticoid therapy, dopamine therapy, and secondary hypothyroidism.

Etiology

Graves Disease

Graves disease is characterized by the triad of hyperthyroidism, ophthalmopathy, and dermopathy, which may occur singly or in combination. Management of hyperthyroidism does not influence the clinical course of eye or skin manifestations. The hyperthyroidism is caused by autoantibodies with TSH-like activity (TSI). Although Graves disease occurs most often in young females, it can occur at any age and in either sex. The disease exhibits a tendency to relapse and remit spontaneously. Usually, the thyroid is diffusely enlarged and smooth, with a firm consistency.

- Hyperthyroidism, ophthalmopathy, and dermopathy characterize Graves disease.
- Hyperthyroidism is caused by the production of TSI.

Painless Lymphocytic Thyroiditis (Postpartum Thyroiditis)

Painless lymphocytic thyroiditis is usually a self-limiting disease that occurs most commonly in the postpartum period and tends to recur with subsequent pregnancies. Patients with a history of lymphocytic thyroiditis also have an increased incidence of chronic autoimmune thyroiditis. It classically presents with a triphasic pattern of thyroid function: an initial hyperthyroid phase (suppressed TSH, low RAIU, increased FT_4) is followed by a hypothyroid phase and subsequent recovery of normal thyroid function. However, patients may present at any stage of the disorder or may have thyroid recovery without having a hypothyroid phase.

β-Blockers may be prescribed in the hyperthyroid phase for symptomatic tachycardia or tremor. There is no indication for antithyroid medications or radioactive iodine therapy because the hyperthyroidism is due to the release of preformed thyroid hormone into the circulation and not to increased production of thyroid hormone. Temporary thyroid hormone replacement therapy may be necessary for symptomatic patients during the hypothyroid phase. In some cases, the hypothyroidism may be permanent.

- Painless lymphocytic thyroiditis may occur in both sexes, but it is more common in the postpartum period.

- Patients typically present with transient hyperthyroidism, followed by transient hypothyroidism before thyroid recovery.
- Treatment is symptomatic: β-blockers for hyperthyroid symptoms and temporary thyroid hormone replacement therapy for hypothyroidism.
- Two-thirds of women with postpartum thyroiditis have recurrence of disease with subsequent pregnancies.

Subacute Painful Thyroiditis (de Quervain Thyroiditis)

Subacute painful thyroiditis is characterized by a painful, tender goiter. Patients often complain of fever, malaise, myalgia, and a history of upper respiratory tract infection. Odynophagia may be a prominent symptom. Transient hyperthyroidism (low RAIU) is often present at diagnosis and may be followed by transient hypothyroidism. The erythrocyte sedimentation rate is invariably increased.

The differential diagnosis includes hemorrhage into a thyroid nodule. In the latter, the onset of pain is similarly abrupt, but the features of a systemic illness are absent and a tender nodule can often be palpated. Thyroid function usually is unaffected, and the erythrocyte sedimentation rate is normal. Treatment options include nonsteroidal anti-inflammatory drugs (NSAIDs) for mild to moderate disease and corticosteroid therapy for severe disease. The response to corticosteroid therapy is dramatic, and patients typically experience relief of symptoms within 24 hours.

- Subacute thyroiditis is characterized by a tender thyroid gland.
- The erythrocyte sedimentation rate is markedly increased.
- Symptomatic therapy includes NSAIDs or corticosteroid therapy.

Multinodular Goiter

Toxic multinodular goiter occurs in patients with a longstanding nodular goiter in which autonomous nodules develop. The hyperthyroidism is usually mild, and cardiovascular manifestations may dominate the clinical features. The goiter is large, nodular, and asymmetrical. The thyroid may be difficult to palpate in some patients because of substernal extension or a short neck.

- Toxic multinodular goiter occurs in patients with nodular goiter.
- Hyperthyroidism may be characterized by organ-specific manifestations, particularly cardiovascular ones.
- A goiter may be difficult to palpate because of a short neck or substernal extension.

Toxic Adenoma

A hyperfunctioning autonomous follicular adenoma ("toxic adenoma"), found most often in middle-aged women, may lead to hyperthyroidism. The solitary nodule is usually larger than 3 cm, is easy to palpate, and has a firm consistency. A radioisotope scan demonstrates intense uptake in the nodule, with suppressed uptake in the rest of the gland.

- A radioisotope scan demonstrates intense uptake in the nodule, with suppressed uptake in the rest of the gland.
- Most solitary hyperfunctioning nodules are >3 cm.

Exogenous Hyperthyroidism

Exogenous hyperthyroidism can result from the use of T_4 or T_3 (or both). Factitial thyrotoxicosis should be suspected in thyrotoxic patients who do not have a palpable goiter and do not have suppressed RAIU. Low serum levels of thyroglobulin help to differentiate this disorder from painless lymphocytic thyroiditis.

- The absence of goiter and absence of suppressed RAIU in a thyrotoxic patient should prompt consideration of factitial thyrotoxicosis.

Therapy

Thionamides

Methimazole and propylthiouracil are used to treat the hyperthyroidism of Graves disease. They act by blocking thyroid hormone synthesis and may have immunomodulating properties that decrease the production of TSI. At very high doses, propylthiouracil decreases the peripheral conversion of T_4 to T_3. The effect of thionamides is temporary, and hyperthyroidism often recurs after discontinuation of treatment. Therefore, these drugs are used in Graves disease to control hyperthyroidism with the hope of spontaneous remission of the disease during therapy. Treatment is given for 12 to 18 months and then discontinued. More than 50% of patients experience disease relapse within the first 3 to 6 months. Adverse effects are uncommon (<5%) but potentially serious and include agranulocytosis and hepatitis. Agranulocytosis can develop abruptly within a few hours; commonly, it initially manifests with an extreme sore throat. Thionamides can cross the placenta and, in high doses, can block thyroid hormone synthesis in the fetal thyroid. For pregnant women, the lowest dose that controls symptoms is used.

- Thionamides block thyroid hormone synthesis and may decrease production of TSI.
- Agranulocytosis can develop abruptly within a few hours.
- Thionamides can cross the placenta and affect the fetal thyroid.

Radioactive Iodine

Radioactive iodine therapy is effective in ablating the thyroid gland and is commonly used to treat the hyperthyroidism of Graves disease or toxic multinodular goiter. This therapy has not been associated with long-term risks, but pregnancy and breast-feeding are contraindications. Most physicians avoid administering radioactive iodine to very young patients. The goal of therapy is to render the patient hypothyroid. The maximal effect from radioactive iodine is apparent within 2 to 3 months. Treatment of toxic multinodular goiter requires higher doses of radioactive iodine and often more than one course of treatment. Painful thyroiditis may develop within a week after treatment, as can transient worsening of hyperthyroidism. Currently, it is debated whether radioactive iodine therapy may worsen Graves ophthalmopathy. It has been suggested that this risk is decreased if corticosteroid treatment is given before radioactive iodine therapy to patients with symptomatic ophthalmopathy.

- Pregnancy and breast-feeding are contraindications to treatment with radioactive iodine.
- Radioactive iodine therapy may be given in Graves disease or toxic multinodular goiter.
- The dose of radioactive iodine is intended to make the patient hypothyroid.
- Radiation-induced enlargement of the gland may worsen obstructive symptoms, particularly in patients with a substernal goiter.

Surgery

Subtotal thyroidectomy is rarely performed to treat Graves disease but is indicated in certain situations, including a large obstructive gland and pregnancy. Thyrotoxic patients with thyroid nodules that look suspicious on fine-needle aspiration should be referred for surgery. To prevent a thyroid storm as well as excessive bleeding from the overactive friable gland, it is customary to render the patient euthyroid with antithyroid drug therapy and then to give iodide for 7 to 10 days preoperatively. Damage to the recurrent laryngeal nerves or parathyroid glands is not common (<1% to 2%) with experienced surgeons.

- Subtotal thyroidectomy is indicated for thyrotoxic patients with large goiters or suspicious-looking nodules and for patients with Graves disease who are young or pregnant.

Supportive Therapy

β-Blockers are used to control the adrenergic manifestations of hyperthyroidism. Propranolol (a nonselective β-blocker) is prescribed most commonly. These drugs are administered to patients with severe symptomatic hyperthyroidism while awaiting the effects of more definitive therapy. β-Blockers should not be given alone in the preoperative preparation of thyrotoxic patients because they do not prevent thyrotoxic crisis.

Thyroid Storm

This is a state of severe hyperthyroidism seen in untreated or inadequately treated hyperthyroid patients undergoing surgical treatment or who have acute intercurrent illness. It is characterized by delirium, fever, tachycardia, hypotension, vomiting, diarrhea, and, eventually, coma. Treatment should be initiated immediately. Together with other supportive therapy, propylthiouracil is given to block thyroid hormone synthesis, sodium iodide is given to inhibit the release of thyroid hormones, and propranolol is given to control the adrenergic manifestations.

Thyrotoxicosis in Pregnancy

Antithyroid drug therapy is the first-line treatment for thyrotoxicosis during pregnancy. Surgical excision may be an option after the first trimester. Radioactive iodine is contraindicated because of its ablative effects on the fetal thyroid. Because antithyroid drugs cross the placenta, the lowest dose necessary to control the disease should be given.

Hypothyroidism

Hypothyroidism can be primary (intrinsic thyroid disease) or secondary (hypothalamic-pituitary disease). Primary hypothyroidism accounts for more than 90% of all cases. The commonest cause of primary hypothyroidism in iodine-replete areas of the world is Hashimoto thyroiditis. Other common causes include hypothyroidism that follows radioactive iodine treatment of hyperthyroidism, surgical thyroidectomy, and radiotherapy for neck malignancies. Hypothyroidism may be transient during the course of subacute or painless thyroiditis.

- The commonest cause of hypothyroidism is Hashimoto thyroiditis.

Hashimoto Thyroiditis

Hashimoto thyroiditis is an autoimmune disorder that tends to cluster in families. It is a common disease, particularly in middle-aged and elderly women.

Clinical Features

The clinical presentation of hypothyroidism depends on the degree and duration of the deficiency. Most patients are asymptomatic at diagnosis. Early symptoms include leg cramps, ankle swelling, dry skin, and dry hair. Patients often complain of fatigue, achiness, and mental slowing. Cold intolerance and a mild degree of weight gain are frequently present. The thyroid gland is typically rubbery, with a bosselated texture.

Uncommon manifestations include psychosis, deafness, and cerebellar ataxia. Some patients experience central hypoventilation and apnea because of respiratory depression. Macrocytic anemia, pernicious anemia (associated autoimmune disease), or microcytic anemia (iron deficiency due to menorrhagia) may be present. Patients with extreme increases in TSH may experience galactorrhea (TRH stimulates prolactin secretion). Hyponatremia due to SIADH may be present. Associated laboratory findings include hyperlipidemia and increased aspartate aminotransferase, lactate dehydrogenase, or creatine kinase.

Autoimmune thyroiditis may be a manifestation of polyglandular autoimmunity (Addison disease, type 1 diabetes mellitus, hypoparathyroidism, pernicious anemia). It also is associated with vitiligo.

Diagnosis

The TSH concentration is increased in primary hypothyroidism and low or inappropriately normal in secondary hypothyroidism. A low FT_4 or FTI confirms the diagnosis of hypothyroidism, provided nonthyroidal illness has been excluded. Serum measurements of T_3 are not helpful in the diagnosis and may be normal in hypothyroid patients.

Hashimoto thyroiditis is usually associated with a bosselated, firm goiter and a high titer of antimicrosomal antibodies. Hypothyroidism occurring after radioactive iodine therapy, thyroid surgery, or radiotherapy to the neck or occurring transiently during the course of subacute or silent thyroiditis is usually evident from a careful clinical evaluation. The diagnosis of central hypothyroidism should prompt imaging of the head and testing of pituitary function.

- Low FT_4 or FTI and increased TSH levels are diagnostic of primary hypothyroidism if nonthyroidal illness has been excluded.
- Low FT_4 or FTI and inappropriately normal or low TSH levels indicate central hypothyroidism. MRI of the head and pituitary function tests should be performed.
- Typical clinical scenario for Hashimoto thyroiditis: A 60-year-old woman complains of fatigue, achiness, dry skin, cold intolerance, and weight gain.

Therapy

Thyroid hormone replacement therapy is initiated with synthetic T_4. The usual daily replacement dose is 1.6 µg T_4/kg body weight. In patients with ischemic heart disease, treatment usually is initiated at a lower dose (e.g., 25 µg), with dosage increments every few weeks. The goals of therapy are to normalize TSH in primary hypothyroidism and to normalize FT_4 in central hypothyroidism.

Failure to normalize TSH concentrations may be indicative of poor compliance, malabsorption due to concomitant use of medications (cholestyramine, sucralfate, or ferrous sulfate), or gastrointestinal disease. Other reasons include progressive thyroid disease, pregnancy, or increased hormone clearance (phenytoin, rifampin). A suppressed TSH level in a patient treated for primary hypothyroidism may indicate

reduced T_4 requirements of aging or decreased clearance. It is important to assess TSH annually or as indicated by the patient's symptoms to ensure compliance and to determine whether dose adjustment is needed.

- Monitor TSH in primary hypothyroidism.
- Monitor FT_4 in central hypothyroidism.
- Avoid medications that may interfere with intestinal absorption for at least 4 hours after ingestion.

Miscellaneous Circumstances

Thyroxine Replacement Therapy in Pregnancy

Females who are receiving T_4 replacement therapy should be counseled about the importance of ensuring adequate replacement before conception. Most patients with primary hypothyroidism who are receiving an adequate dosage before pregnancy require an increased dose as the pregnancy progresses. TSH levels should be assessed periodically during pregnancy, and the T_4 dose should be adjusted as necessary to maintain a normal TSH.

Thyroxine Replacement Therapy in Patients With Angina

Hypothyroid patients with progressive, symptomatic ischemic heart disease should be evaluated by a cardiologist. Hypothyroidism does not contraindicate intervention (there is increased risk of hyponatremia). Replacement therapy typically is initiated with 25 µg daily, and the dose is increased gradually to the replacement dosage.

Subclinical Hypothyroidism

This is a condition in which serum TSH levels are increased in clinically euthyroid patients with normal FT_4 concentrations. It is a relatively common disorder and affects 5% to 15% of elderly persons. Patients are usually asymptomatic or have minimal nonspecific symptoms that are likely unrelated to hypothyroidism. A trial of replacement therapy is indicated for symptomatic patients and those at risk for progressive disease. The risk of progression to overt hypothyroidism increases with age, the presence of thyroid antibodies, and TSH levels greater than 10 IU/mL.

Myxedema Coma

This occurs in patients who have severe, untreated hypothyroidism, and although it may be spontaneous, it usually is precipitated by acute illness (e.g., infection, surgery, myocardial infarction), exposure to cold, or the use of sedatives or opiates. The mortality rate (20%-50%) is high. The onset is insidious, with progressive stupor culminating in coma. Seizures, hypothermia, hypotension, hypoventilation, hyponatremia, and hypoglycemia may be present.

Treatment should be initiated promptly with intravenous T_4. This is usually given as a single daily dose (50-100 μg). Aggressive treatment of associated conditions such as hypothermia should be initiated. The use of glucocorticoids in all cases of myxedema coma is controversial. The optimal approach is to administer corticosteroids if there is clinical and laboratory evidence of hypocortisolism. An effort should be made to conserve body heat; external warming is likely to cause cutaneous vasodilatation, with increased hypotension. Often, the prognosis is determined by the coexisting conditions.

Thyroid Nodules

Thyroid nodules are extremely common and increase with age. Nodules may be detected during a routine medical examination, noticed by the patient, or detected during neck ultrasonography performed for other reasons. With the discovery of a nodule, the primary concern is whether the underlying process is benign or malignant. In addition to considering primary thyroid malignancies, it is important to consider metastatic disease (renal cell carcinoma is the commonest malignancy metastatic to the thyroid). Benign adenomas and cysts may present as thyroid nodules, as may a multinodular goiter with a dominant nodule. Occasionally, Hashimoto thyroiditis may simulate a solitary thyroid nodule.

The likelihood of malignancy increases with the presentation of a nodular process at a young age and in patients with a history of irradiation to the head and neck (especially during childhood). The initial step in the evaluation of a thyroid nodule is measurement of TSH to determine whether autonomy is present. Thyroid malignancy is considered less likely if the TSH level is abnormal. If the TSH level is suppressed, a thyroid scan should be performed.

Following TSH measurement, fine-needle aspiration should be performed in a palpable nodule. To be truly useful, this procedure should be performed by an experienced physician and the slides read by an experienced cytopathologist. If the aspirate has benign characteristics, annual follow-up with palpation and measurement of TSH is adequate, provided no change is noted by the patient or physician in the size and characteristics of the nodule. A nondiagnostic aspirate requires repetition (under ultrasonographic guidance if needed). If the aspirate is interpreted as suspicious or compatible with malignancy, surgical intervention is required.

- Of palpable thyroid nodules, 95% are benign.
- TSH measurement is the first test in the evaluation of thyroid nodules.
- Fine-needle aspiration has high sensitivity and specificity for excluding malignancy if performed and interpreted by experienced personnel.

- A thyroid scan is not helpful in the evaluation of a thyroid nodule unless the TSH is suppressed and a hyperfunctioning nodule is suspected.

Thyroid Cancer

Differentiated Thyroid Cancer

Papillary thyroid carcinoma is the commonest type of thyroid cancer (50%-60% of cases). Its incidence peaks in early adulthood and again in late adulthood. Dissemination is generally via the lymphatics to lymph nodes; other sites of metastases include the lungs and bone. Typically, it presents as a thyroid nodule, as cervical lymphadenopathy, or as an incidental finding in an excised gland.

Follicular carcinoma (20% of cases) spreads preferentially by the hematogenous route. The usual presentation is as a thyroid mass or metastatic deposits to the lungs, bones, or brain. Rarely, especially if the tumor burden is large, follicular carcinoma can cause thyrotoxicosis.

Undifferentiated *anaplastic carcinoma* usually presents as a rapidly progressive thyroid mass with compressive local neck symptoms. It has an extremely poor prognosis, with a median survival of less than 6 months after diagnosis.

Conversely, among patients with differentiated cancer, the 20-year cause-specific mortality rate varies between less than 5% and 15%, with papillary cancer having the best prognosis. Factors associated with a poorer prognosis include age older than 55 at diagnosis, completeness of resection, degree of local invasiveness, large size of primary tumor, and the presence of distant metastases (metastases to the cervical lymph nodes do not affect prognosis).

Surgical excision is the therapy of choice for differentiated thyroid cancer. For anaplastic cancer, excision is sometimes undertaken to palliate extrinsic compression of the trachea and to prevent or delay asphyxiation. The extent of surgical excision in differentiated thyroid cancer is a subject of debate, but near total thyroidectomy is usually performed. The affected lymph nodes are selectively excised.

Patients at low risk for recurrent disease are treated with a dose of T_4 to maintain TSH between 0.1 and 0.4 mIU/L. Those at higher risk undergo radioactive iodine imaging at 4 to 6 weeks postoperatively. If necessary, a sufficient dose of radioactive iodine is administered to ablate the thyroid remnant. Suppressive therapy is initiated with the goal TSH being less than 0.1 mIU/L.

Reevaluation in 3 to 6 months and annually thereafter is required. Chest radiography, serum TSH and thyroglobulin, and neck ultrasonography are performed at each visit. Most differentiated thyroid malignancies synthesize and secrete thyroglobulin, which can be used as a marker of recurrent or persistent disease. If a patient has little or no thyroid tissue and is receiving suppressive T_4 therapy, the serum thyroglobulin level should be less than 5 to 10 ng/mL; a higher level implies persistent or recurrent disease. Radioactive iodine imaging is indicated for patients with evidence of recurrent or metastatic disease.

- Papillary cancer spreads via the lymphatics to the lymph nodes and has the best prognosis. It presents as a thyroid mass or cervical lymphadenopathy or is an incidental finding.
- Follicular carcinoma spreads preferentially by the hematogenous route. It presents as a thyroid mass or distant metastatic deposits.
- Anaplastic carcinoma presents with rapidly progressive local symptoms.
- Surgical excision is the definitive therapy for differentiated thyroid cancer.
- Follow-up evaluation requires TSH, thyroglobulin, neck ultrasonography, and chest radiography. Radioactive iodine imaging is performed if there is evidence of recurrent or persistent disease.
- Recurrences are treated, depending on location, with excision or radioactive iodine.

Miscellaneous Thyroid Disorders

Sick Euthyroid Syndrome

Patients who require hospitalization for a systemic illness, psychiatric disorder, or trauma frequently have thyroid function test abnormalities in the absence of identifiable intrinsic thyroid disease. The abnormalities resolve with recovery from the associated illness. Specific therapy is not required. During the acute illness, the TSH level may be normal or low (~ 0.01 µU/mL) because of the central effects of the illness. TSH levels may be increased during recovery.

The major challenge in sick hospitalized patients is to distinguish between nonthyroidal illness and intrinsic thyroid or pituitary disease. Helpful features in the differential diagnosis include the presence of goiter, extrathyroidal manifestations of Graves disease, hypothalamic-pituitary mass effects, or hypopituitarism. A high serum level of T_3 suggests hyperthyroidism, whereas a TSH level greater than 20 µU/mL supports the diagnosis of primary hypothyroidism.

Amiodarone and the Thyroid

Amiodarone is a class III antiarrhythmic agent. Iodine comprises 40% of the drug by weight. This drug can affect thyroid function in several ways, including causing a drug-induced thyroiditis. In persons with impaired thyroid autoregulation (underlying autoimmune thyroid disease or nodular goiter), iodide excess can lead to hyperthyroidism or hypothyroidism. When using amiodarone, it is important to monitor thyroid function, particularly in the elderly (consider the high prevalence of Hashimoto thyroiditis and nodular goiter and the difficulty with detecting thyroid dysfunction in this age group).

Lithium and the Thyroid

Lithium decreases the synthesis and secretion of thyroid hormones. Its use has been associated with the development of goiter and hypothyroidism, especially in patients who have underlying autoimmune thyroid disease.

DISORDERS OF CALCIUM AND BONE METABOLISM

Hypercalcemia

Clinically, the causes of hypercalcemia are best categorized as either parathyroid-dependent or parathyroid-independent.

Parathyroid-dependent Hypercalcemia

Primary Hyperparathyroidism

Etiology—Primary hyperparathyroidism is the commonest cause of hypercalcemia in ambulatory patients. It is more common in females. A single parathyroid adenoma is the cause in 80% of patients; multiple adenomas are present in 5% of patients and hyperplasia of all four glands in 15%. Rarely, parathyroid carcinoma presents as a neck mass, with hypercalcemia. In 6% to 10% of patients with hyperparathyroidism, the adenoma may be found in the thyroid, thymus, or mediastinum. The disease may be sporadic or familial. Familial hyperparathyroidism may be a manifestation of MEN I or MEN IIA. Parathyroid hyperplasia is usually present in familial hyperparathyroidism.

- Primary hyperparathyroidism is a common disorder that may be sporadic or familial.
- Parathyroid adenoma is the usual cause.
- Hyperplasia is common in the familial forms of hyperparathyroidism. It may be an isolated feature or occur in association with MEN I or MEN IIA.

Clinical Features—Most patients with primary hyperparathyroidism are asymptomatic, and the hyperparathyroidism is identified by routine laboratory testing. Symptomatic hypercalcemia may be manifested as polyuria and polydipsia. Hypercalciuria can cause nephrolithiasis. Nephrocalcinosis and band keratopathy may occur in severe disease. Nonspecific symptoms of fatigue, weakness, myopathy, and depression may be present. Skeletal manifestations include osteopenia or osteoporosis and, in severe disease, bone pain and pathologic fractures.

- Primary hyperparathyroidism is commonly asymptomatic.
- When the disease is symptomatic, symptoms may involve several organ systems, including the kidneys, skeleton, and nervous and cardiovascular systems.

Laboratory Features—Hypercalcemia is usually mild and often has existed for several years before diagnosis. In most cases, serum phosphate concentrations are normal, but with prolonged hyperparathyroidism, they may be low. The serum level of parathyroid hormone (PTH) is usually increased or it may be inappropriately normal for the degree of hypercalcemia. Urine calcium excretion is often increased or at the upper limits of normal. Its measurement is important not only to assess the risk of nephrolithiasis but also to exclude disorders characterized by low rates of calcium excretion (familial hypocalciuric hypercalcemia and thiazide use).

Radiographic Features—Primary hyperparathyroidism is associated with loss of cortical bone. Characteristic radiographic skeletal changes include subperiosteal bone resorption (visible on the radial borders of the phalanges), a "salt and pepper" appearance of the skull, and osteitis fibrosa cystica (fibrous replacement of the resorbed bone, which may present with bone pain, tenderness, deformity, or fracture). Brown tumors are collections of osteoclasts intermixed with poorly mineralized woven bone. Renal stones or nephrocalcinosis may be visible on abdominal radiographs.

- The principal laboratory findings are hypercalcemia and increased PTH or inappropriately normal PTH for the degree of hypercalcemia.
- Urine calcium measurement is important in the differential diagnosis and helps guide management.
- Characteristic skeletal findings in severe disease are subperiosteal bone resorption and cortical bone loss. A "salt and pepper" skull and osteitis fibrosa cystica may be present.

Therapy—Parathyroidectomy is the treatment of choice for primary hyperparathyroidism. All parathyroids should be inspected at the time of the operation. An isolated parathyroid adenoma requires resection. In patients with parathyroid hyperplasia, subtotal parathyroidectomy is performed, leaving about 50 mg of parathyroid tissue intact. Later, it may be necessary to remove this tissue if hypercalcemia persists or recurs. Reversible mild asymptomatic hypocalcemia is common in the early postoperative period. However, in patients with severe preexisting parathyroid-induced bone disease, correction of hyperparathyroidism may lead to marked and prolonged hypocalcemia.

Conservative therapy may be indicated for mild uncomplicated disease, especially in the elderly. Indications for excision include serum calcium level greater than 1 unit above the upper limit of normal, nephrolithiasis or pronounced hypercalciuria, osteopenia or osteoporosis, and symptomatic hypercalcemia. Imaging studies to localize the parathyroid neoplasm usually are reserved for patients with persistent or recurrent hyperparathyroidism. However, with the advent of minimally invasive parathyroid surgery, preoperative localization with sestamibi scanning is increasingly being used.

- Parathyroidectomy is the treatment of choice.
- Indications for parathyroidectomy are serum calcium greater than 1 unit above the upper limit of normal, nephrolithiasis, marked hypercalciuria, osteopenia, osteoporosis, and symptomatic hypercalcemia.

Familial Hypocalciuric Hypercalcemia

This autosomal dominant disorder results from an altered setpoint of the calcium-sensing receptor in the parathyroid glands and renal tubules. Characteristically, it presents as uncomplicated asymptomatic mild hypercalcemia in a patient with a normal or slightly increased level of PTH, low urinary calcium, and a positive family history. The diagnosis is strongly supported by a calcium-to-creatinine clearance ratio less than 0.01. Parathyroid surgery is not indicated because the complications of hyperparathyroidism do not develop.

- Familial hypocalciuric hypercalcemia is not associated with symptoms and does not require treatment.

Thiazide-induced Hypercalcemia

Mild hypercalcemia may occur in patients taking thiazide diuretics. The hypercalcemia is multifactorial (dehydration, decreased renal calcium clearance, and possibly increased PTH secretion). PTH levels are inappropriately normal or mildly increased. The hypercalcemia usually resolves within a few weeks after the discontinuation of drug therapy. Thiazide-induced hypercalcemia is more likely to occur in patients with underlying mild primary hyperparathyroidism.

Lithium

Lithium raises the threshold of inhibition of PTH secretion by serum calcium. PTH levels are inappropriately normal or mildly increased. The hypercalcemia resolves after discontinuation of lithium.

Parathyroid-independent Hypercalcemia

Hypercalcemia of Malignancy

Hypercalcemia of malignancy often develops acutely and may be severe and life-threatening. It is the commonest cause of hypercalcemia in hospitalized patients and may be due to the destructive effects of skeletal metastases or the paraneoplastic effect of a discrete neoplasm. Patients in the latter group have few or no skeletal metastases, and the hypercalcemia resolves after treatment of the malignancy. Most of these tumors secrete parathyroid hormone–related peptide (PTHrp), which mediates this humoral hypercalcemia of malignancy. Serum PTH is suppressed in all cases of hypercalcemia due to malignancy.

Vitamin D Intoxication

Hypercalcemia, hypercalciuria, renal insufficiency, and soft tissue calcification follow prolonged ingestion of toxic doses of vitamin D or its metabolites. Because vitamin D is stored in fat, the condition may persist for months after treatment has been discontinued. Hypercalcemia is also seen in vitamin A intoxication.

Sarcoidosis, Other Granulomatous Disorders, and Some Lymphomas

The hypercalcemia and hypercalciuria in these disorders are due to the presence of vitamin D–dependent granulomas and some lymphomas that express high concentrations of the 1α-hydroxylase enzyme and thus can autonomously generate 1,25-dihydroxyvitamin D from circulating 25-hydroxyvitamin D. The serum levels of 25-hydroxyvitamin D are normal, and those of 1,25-dihydroxyvitamin D are increased. The hypercalcemia is responsive to glucocorticoid therapy.

Miscellaneous Causes

Hyperthyroidism enhances bone turnover and may lead to net bone loss. Hypercalcemia and, more frequently, hypercalciuria may be present. The hypercalcemia resolves with the treatment of thyrotoxicosis. In an addisonian crisis, hypercalcemia is often present and may be symptomatic. It is related to dehydration and increased albumin concentration and is reversible with glucocorticoid therapy. Immobilization may result in hypercalcemia in patients with rapid bone turnover, as in Paget disease of bone.

- Hypercalcemia of malignancy may be due to skeletal metastases, the secretion of a humoral factor such as PTHrp, or to the production of 1,25-dihydroxyvitamin D (typically by lymphomas).

Management of Hypercalcemia

When feasible, treatment of the primary cause may be the most important intervention. Glucocorticoids are the drugs of choice for the hypercalcemia of granulomatous disorders. Humoral hypercalcemia of malignancy may be treated by complete resection of the tumor.

In severe hypercalcemia or hypercalcemia in which the primary cause is not immediately treatable, calcium concentrations should be decreased. Aggressive rehydration with volume expansion promotes calciuresis and has a transient hypocalcemic effect. Loop (but not thiazide) diuretics help promote renal calcium excretion but should only be given after volume expansion. Pamidronate (a bisphosphonate) given as a single intravenous dose of 30 to 90 mg inhibits bone resorption and mobilization of calcium from bone and has a marked and prolonged effect on calcium concentrations. Calcitonin is used rarely because of its modest effects and the rapid onset of tachyphylaxis.

- Volume expansion and calciuresis (saline diuresis) form the cornerstone of therapy. Loop diuretics are useful adjuncts after rehydration.
- Pamidronate decreases calcium concentrations by inhibiting bone resorption and has a marked and prolonged effect on calcium concentrations.
- Dialysis is reserved for patients with renal failure.

Hypoparathyroidism

Etiology

Hypoparathyroidism may be due to decreased PTH production by the parathyroid glands or to resistance of the target tissue to the actions of PTH. The parathyroid glands may be damaged during thyroidectomy or radical neck dissection or they may be excised completely for the treatment of primary hyperparathyroidism due to parathyroid hyperplasia. Hypoparathyroidism may be transient or permanent, and it may appear within hours after the operation. Hypocalcemia after neck surgery often is manifested by symptoms of neuromuscular excitability, for example, Chvostek and Tinel signs.

Hypoparathyroidism also may result from an autoimmune or infiltrative process (hemochromatosis or Wilson disease) or from defective formation of the branchial arches associated with thymic aplasia (DiGeorge syndrome). Hypomagnesemia (use of diuretics, malabsorption, and malnutrition) impairs the secretion and action of PTH.

Pseudohypoparathyroidism is characterized by end-organ resistance to the actions of PTH because of a receptor or postreceptor defect. Patients often have a characteristic appearance: short stature, round face, short metacarpals and metatarsals, calcification of the basal ganglia, and mild mental retardation. A defect in the G_s subunit of the receptor is commonly identified. Pseudopseudohypoparathyroidism is a variant of the disorder, and the patients have the same characteristic physical features but not the biochemical abnormalities.

- Hypoparathyroidism may result from surgical damage to the parathyroids or from an autoimmune, infiltrative, or congenital process.
- Hypomagnesemia is a cause of functional hypoparathyroidism.

Clinical Features

Hypoparathyroidism leads to decreased mobilization of calcium from bone, decreased renal distal tubular calcium reabsorption, decreased proximal renal tubular phosphate excretion, and decreased renal production of 1,25-dihydroxyvitamin D. This leads to hypocalcemia and hyperphosphatemia. In hypoparathyroidism, PTH is low or inappropriately normal in the presence of hypocalcemia. In contrast, PTH is increased in pseudohypoparathyroidism.

Symptoms reflect the degree as well as the rate of development of hypocalcemia and include paresthesias, carpopedal spasm, laryngeal stridor, and convulsions. Apathy and depression may occur. Calcification of the basal ganglia and benign intracranial hypertension also occur. Gastrointestinal manifestations include abdominal pain, nausea, vomiting, and malabsorption. A prolonged QT interval may be present. Hypoparathyroidism is also associated with the development of cataracts and alopecia. Mucocutaneous candidiasis may be a manifestation of DiGeorge syndrome.

- Symptoms of hypocalcemia reflect its degree and the rate of its development.
- Hypoparathyroidism is characterized by hypocalcemia and hyperphosphatemia in the presence of normal renal function.
- PTH is low in hypoparathyroidism and increased in pseudo-hypoparathyroidism.

Diagnosis

Differential Diagnosis

Hypoparathyroidism with resultant hypocalcemia must be differentiated from other causes of hypocalcemia. Hypocalcemia may result from decreased secretion of PTH, PTH resistance, decreased production of vitamin D, vitamin D resistance, and from disorders associated with decreased mobilization of calcium from bone or increased calcium deposition in tissues. Vitamin D deficiency may be caused by malnutrition, malabsorption, or liver or kidney disease. In vitamin D deficiency, hypocalcemia triggers secondary hyperparathyroidism with renal phosphate wasting. In acute or chronic renal failure, the pathogenesis of hypocalcemia is multifactorial, resulting from hyperphosphatemia and decreased production of 1,25-dihydroxyvitamin D.

Hypocalcemia may occur in osteoblastic metastases (e.g., prostate cancer) and in the hungry bone syndrome seen after parathyroidectomy for hyperparathyroidism with severe bone disease. Hypocalcemia and soft tissue calcification may occur in acute pancreatitis. Hypocalcemia is also associated with the use of loop diuretics.

Diagnostic Approach

When evaluating hypocalcemia, it is important to correct the total calcium for the prevailing albumin levels or to determine the level of ionized calcium. The next step is to measure the serum level of PTH. In a hypocalcemic patient, a low serum level of PTH is diagnostic of hypoparathyroidism. A high serum level of PTH suggests vitamin D deficiency or pseudohypoparathyroidism. Low plasma levels of 25-hydroxyvitamin D occur from poor nutrition, malabsorption, or liver disease. Low plasma levels of 1,25-dihydroxyvitamin D occur in renal failure. The measurement of serum concentrations of creatinine and magnesium will identify renal failure and magnesium deficiency states.

Therapy

For acute, severe hypocalcemia, urgent treatment with intravenous calcium is indicated to prevent tetany, laryngeal stridor, or convulsions. Calcium gluconate, 10 to 20 mL of a 10% solution (90 mg elemental calcium per 10 mL) is infused over 5 to 10 minutes. The serum calcium level is maintained between 7.0 and 8.5 mg/dL by a subsequent infusion of calcium (10-15 mg/kg infused over 4-6 hours). Continuous electrocardiographic monitoring is essential.

For chronic hypocalcemia, treatment is oral calcium supplements (2.0-3.0 g daily). Ergocalciferol is given as 50,000 to 100,000 IU daily. It has a slow onset and offset of action. An alternative is calcitriol (1,25-dihydroxyvitamin D). Thiazide diuretics may be given to decrease the risk of marked hypercalciuria, and oral phosphate binders may be given to control hyperphosphatemia.

It is critical to monitor therapy closely because patients are at risk for hypercalciuria, nephrolithiasis, and nephrocalcinosis. Therapeutic doses are adjusted to keep the serum level of calcium just below the lower limits of normal, around 8.5 mg/dL, and urine calcium less than 300 mg/24 hours.

- Severe, acute hypocalcemia requires treatment with intravenous calcium.
- Chronic hypocalcemia requires treatment with oral calcium and vitamin D.

Osteoporosis

Osteoporosis is the commonest skeletal disorder encountered in clinical practice. It is characterized by decreased bone mass, with thinning of the cortices and loss of trabeculae leading to increased bone fragility and risk of fracture. Bone density (and bone loss) can be quantified with dual energy X-ray absorptiometry. Osteopenia is defined as a bone mass 1.0 to 2.5 standard deviations below the mean peak bone mass of a sex- and height-matched control population. Osteoporosis is defined as a bone mass value more than 2.5 standard deviations below the peak bone mass of a sex- and height-matched control population.

Etiology

The commonest types of osteoporosis are postmenopausal osteoporosis, characterized by high turnover of bone, and senile osteoporosis, which occurs in older men and women. Osteoporosis may be secondary to hypogonadism, hyperparathyroidism, hyperthyroidism, or hypercortisolism. It is associated with malnutrition (calcium deficiency, protein malnutrition, vitamin C deficiency, and alcoholism), malabsorption, neoplastic disorders (multiple myeloma, leukemia, lymphoma, and systemic mastocytosis), and abnormalities of bone collagen (osteogenesis imperfecta). Drugs such as corticosteroids, heparin, methotrexate, and GnRH analogues all increase bone loss. Immobilization also promotes bone loss.

- Osteoporosis may be primary or secondary.
- Osteoporosis may be secondary to endocrine, nutritional, intestinal, neoplastic, or genetic disorders. It also may be induced by drugs or immobilization.

Clinical Features

Fractures can occur with minor trauma and be axial or appendicular. Osteoporotic fractures heal normally. Vertebral fractures lead to loss of height and spinal deformity (kyphoscoliosis and dowager's hump). Other osteoporotic fractures include those of the hip and distal radius (Colles fracture).

The serum levels of calcium, phosphate, and alkaline phosphatase are normal in osteoporosis. The serum level of alkaline phosphatase may be increased slightly during fracture healing.

Lateral spine radiographs show a loss of horizontal trabeculae and an apparent prominence of the vertical trabeculae, biconcave vertebrae, and a decrease in vertebral height. Bone mineral density can be assessed by dual energy x-ray absorptiometry of the lumbar vertebrae (although vessel wall calcification and vertebral deformity with advancing age can make this measurement unreliable) or the hip. A decrease of 1 standard deviation from peak bone density of a control population leads to a doubling of the fracture risk.

- Osteoporosis is characterized by the occurrence of fracture with minimal trauma and normal serum levels of calcium, phosphate, and alkaline phosphatase.

Diagnosis

The diagnosis of osteoporosis is based on the finding of low bone mass with or without fractures and the exclusion of other causes of osteopenia, such as osteomalacia, multiple myeloma, and metastatic disease. Bone densitometry should be used as a screening study for patients at risk for osteoporosis (e.g.,

postmenopausal women not taking preventive measures). Whether routine screening for baseline values should be performed for asymptomatic postmenopausal women who receive estrogen replacement therapy is debated. Bone densitometry is indicated for patients who have radiologic evidence of previous vertebral fracture. It also is helpful in determining the need for surgery in hyperparathyroidism.

During the evaluation of a patient who has a fracture, it is important to remember that osteomalacia may coexist with osteoporosis. Myeloma or metastatic disease should be excluded as a cause of pathologic fracture. Secondary causes of osteoporosis should be actively excluded during history taking and the physical examination as well as by appropriate laboratory and radiographic investigations. The evaluation should include serum levels of calcium (and, if necessary, PTH), 25-hydroxyvitamin D, and TSH. If indicated, the patient should undergo screening for Cushing syndrome with a 1-mg overnight dexamethasone suppression test or 24-hour urine free cortisol measurement. Measurement of testosterone is indicated for males.

- The diagnosis of osteoporosis requires the exclusion of other causes of low bone mineral density. Osteomalacia, malignancy, and other secondary causes of osteoporosis should be actively excluded by the judicious use of history taking, physical examination, and laboratory evaluation.

Prevention and Treatment of Osteoporosis

To a certain extent, bone loss can be prevented by timely estrogen replacement in women at and beyond menopause and by the provision of adequate calcium and vitamin D intake in all adults (in premenopausal women and men younger than 65, 1,000 mg daily of elemental calcium; in postmenopausal women and men older than 65, 1,500 mg daily). Other measures to ensure attainment (and maintenance) of adequate bone mass include regular weight-bearing exercise and avoidance of alcohol and tobacco abuse.

Estrogen replacement is considered the therapy of choice for the prevention and treatment of osteoporosis in women who do not have contraindications to it. It decreases bone resorption and has been shown in epidemiologic and retrospective studies to decrease the incidence of osteoporotic fractures. Estrogen can be given orally or transdermally. To decrease the risk of endometrial hyperplasia, progesterone is also administered in a cyclical or continuous fashion if the patient has an intact uterus.

Alendronate and risedronate are oral bisphosphonates that have potent antiresorptive effects; they prevent bone loss and increase bone density. They have been shown to reduce fracture risk and to be effective in preventing steroid-induced bone loss. Bisphosphonates should be prescribed for patients who cannot or do not wish to take estrogen. Side effects include dyspeptic symptoms and esophagitis, particularly if the medication is taken incorrectly. Oral bisphosphonates should be taken in the morning with a glassful of water and on an empty stomach (any food or other drink may interfere with intestinal absorption), and the patient should not lie down for 30 to 60 minutes after the dose. These medications are available as a once-weekly dose, which increases tolerability and compliance. Preliminary studies have shown that combination therapy with estrogen and alendronate may increase bone density more effectively than single-agent therapy. No decrease in fracture risk has been demonstrated.

Calcitonin is a weak antiresorptive agent and is administered by nasal spray. The advent of alternative medications with greater efficacy means that calcitonin is rarely indicated. The exception is for the management of painful vertebral fractures.

- Estrogen replacement is the therapy of choice for the prevention and treatment of osteoporosis in women who do not have a contraindication to it.
- Women receiving estrogen replacement therapy require a breast examination and mammography annually.
- Nasal calcitonin is a weak antiresorptive agent.
- Bisphosphonates are potent antiresorptive agents that decrease the incidence of fractures. Severe esophagitis is a potential side effect.

Recombinant PTH has recently become available as treatment for osteoporosis after clinical trials demonstrated the ability of this agent to increase bone formation and bone mass when given by daily subcutaneous injection. There is little experience with recombinant PTH outside clinical trials, and whether it is best given in conjuction with a bisphosphonate is not clear. Similarly, the optimal schedule and duration of treatment is not known.

Osteomalacia

In adults, osteomalacia is characterized by defective mineralization of newly formed bone matrix, with the accumulation of unmineralized osteoid. Normal mineralization of bone requires adequate calcium and phosphate concentrations in the extracellular fluid, functional osteoblasts, and optimal conditions for the mineralization of mature osteoid. Osteomalacia results when any or a combination of these prerequisites is not met.

Vitamin D deficiency is the commonest cause of osteomalacia and results from poor intake (chronic alcoholism and institutionalized patients), malabsorption (celiac disease), and decreased exposure to the sun. Other causes include decreased liver production of 25-hydroxyvitamin D due to liver disease or increased metabolism to inactive compounds (phenytoin or rifampin). Renal disease and vitamin D–dependent rickets type I lead to decreased production of 1,25-dihydroxyvitamin D.

Phosphate deficiency may result from malnutrition or increased renal losses. This is seen in hereditary X-linked hypophosphatemia, acquired tubular phosphate leak due to production of a phosphaturic substance from an occult mesenchymal tumor (oncogenic osteomalacia), and a generalized tubular defect (Fanconi syndrome) that may be hereditary or acquired.

- Osteomalacia is characterized by defective mineralization and accumulation of unmineralized osteoid.
- In the U.S., the common causes of vitamin D deficiency are malnutrition, malabsorption, and liver disease.

Clinical Features

In addition to fractures or pseudofractures, typical symptoms due to osteomalacia include diffuse bone pain and tenderness, muscle weakness, and a waddling gait. The serum level of alkaline phosphatase is usually increased in all cases of osteomalacia except for cases due to hypophosphatasia. In vitamin D deficiency, secondary hyperparathyroidism is usually present and 25-hydroxyvitamin D is decreased.

Radiography may not be helpful, although radiographic features of secondary hyperparathyroidism may be apparent. In later stages, there may be radiographic evidence of pseudofractures (Looser zones). These are narrow lines of radiolucency that are perpendicular to the cortical bone surface and are typically bilateral and symmetric. They are found most commonly in the pubic rami, the medial aspect of the femur near the femoral head, the scapulae, and the metatarsals.

Therapy

Effective therapy is based on identifying and treating the underlying disorder as well as providing adequate calcium and phosphate at the areas of mineralization. This usually is achieved with calcium, vitamin D, and, when indicated, phosphate supplementation. Calcium supplementation should provide 1,000 to 2,000 mg of elemental calcium daily, whereas the degree of vitamin D supplementation varies according to the underlying diagnosis. In nutritional deficiency, 2,000 to 4,000 IU daily of vitamin D_2 is given until healing occurs, and then 400 IU daily is given for maintenance. Higher doses (25,000-50,000 IU daily) are used to treat vitamin D deficiency caused by malabsorption.

The goals of therapy are to achieve bone healing and to normalize the serum concentrations of calcium, phosphate, and alkaline phosphatase. Complications of treatment include hypercalciuria, hypercalcemia, and renal impairment. Hypercalciuria is the first sign of overdosage.

- Diffuse bone pain, tenderness, and muscle weakness are typical symptoms of osteomalacia.

- Serum alkaline phosphatase is increased in all cases of osteomalacia except for cases due to hypophosphatasia.
- Vitamin D deficiency is characterized by a low or normal serum level of calcium and secondary hyperparathyroidism.
- Treatment is directed at the underlying cause and at providing adequate mineral and vitamin D supplementation.
- Complications of treatment include hypercalciuria, hypercalcemia, and renal impairment.

Paget Disease

Paget disease affects 3% of the population older than 45 years. It is a monostotic or polyostotic bone disorder characterized by the presence of abnormal osteoclasts, which lead to an increased rate of bone resorption and, subsequently, disorganized bone remodeling. This results in decreased tensile strength, skeletal pain, and bone deformities. Commonly affected sites include the sacrum, spine, femur, tibia, skull, and pelvis. Its pathogenesis is not fully understood.

Clinical Features

Most patients present with increased serum levels of alkaline phosphatase or a radiographic abnormality. The two main clinical features are pain and deformity. The pain may be related to pagetoid involvement, fracture, degenerative changes in adjoining joints, or, rarely, the development of osteosarcoma. Deformity may affect the long bones, skull, or spine. The serum level of alkaline phosphatase is the most useful marker of disease activity and its response to therapy.

Neurologic complications are caused by nerve entrapment or hydrocephalus due to the development of platybasia. High-output cardiac failure is rare but can occur when more than 20% of the skeleton is affected, because of the increased vascularity of affected bone. Hypercalciuria and hypercalcemia can occur in an immobilized patient.

Diagnosis

Paget disease should be suspected if serum alkaline phosphatase concentrations are increased and plasma calcium levels are normal. A bone scan is the most sensitive test for identifying pagetic bone lesions. Typical radiographic findings demonstrate the characteristic bone expansion, deformity, trabecular expansion, and sclerosis.

Therapy

Many patients require only monitoring of alkaline phosphatase levels. Indications for active therapy include the presence of pain, disease involving weight-bearing bones, disease in proximity to joints, neurologic complications, or marked increase in alkaline phosphatase level (>1,000 U/L). Medical therapy consists of bisphosphonates administered intravenously or orally. Alkaline phosphatase levels are used to monitor therapy. Orthopedic surgery may be needed to treat deformity, fracture, or degenerative joint disease. Pretreatment with an antiresorptive agent reduces bleeding and postoperative hypercalcemia. Neurosurgical intervention may be required for nerve entrapment syndromes.

- Typical findings include normal serum levels of calcium, phosphate, and 25-hydroxyvitamin D and increased serum levels of alkaline phosphatase.
- Pseudofractures are characteristic radiographic findings.
- Indications for active therapy include the presence of pain, disease involving weight-bearing bones, disease in proximity to joints, neurologic complications, or a marked increase in the alkaline phosphatase level (>1,000 U/L).

DISORDERS OF THE ADRENAL GLANDS

Adrenal Failure

Etiology

Primary Adrenal Failure

Primary adrenal failure is manifested clinically by glucocorticoid and mineralocorticoid deficiency. It may result from autoimmune adrenalitis (Addison disease); destruction of the adrenals by a granulomatous process such as tuberculosis; bilateral adrenal hemorrhage related to sepsis, anticoagulation therapy or a lupus anticoagulant; congenital adrenal enzyme deficiency; or the use of drugs such as aminoglutethimide or ketoconazole that inhibit steroidogenesis. Adrenal metastases are common in metastatic malignancies such as lung cancer. However, clinically pronounced adrenocortical failure is uncommon in this setting.

Secondary Adrenal Failure

Secondary adrenal failure is due to ACTH deficiency. Mineralocorticoid deficiency is not present. ACTH deficiency may occur alone (exogenous steroid use or lymphocytic hypophysitis) or, more often, in association with other features of hypopituitarism. Functional ACTH deficiency is the most common cause of secondary adrenal failure and is a consequence of the suppression of the hypothalamic-pituitary-adrenal axis by the prolonged use of pharmacologic doses of glucocorticoids.

- In the United States, the commonest cause of primary adrenocortical failure is autoimmune adrenalitis.
- Primary adrenal failure: deficiencies of cortisol, aldosterone, and adrenal sex steroids.
- Secondary adrenal failure: deficiencies of cortisol and adrenal sex steroids. Aldosterone secretion is intact.

Clinical Features

Adrenal failure usually has an insidious presentation, with fatigue, muscle weakness, anorexia, weight loss, nausea, vomiting, and diarrhea. Hyponatremia, lymphocytosis, and eosinophilia may be present. Aldosterone deficiency leads to hypovolemia, orthostatism, hyperkalemia, and a hyperchloremic acidosis. In females, the loss of adrenal androgens leads to decreased pubic hair. Because ACTH levels are increased (lack of negative feedback by cortisol), patients with primary adrenal failure become hyperpigmented, particularly on the elbows, knees, and buccal mucosa and on surgical scars. In contrast, patients with secondary adrenal failure are pale (low ACTH levels). Because aldosterone secretion is unaffected, hyperkalemia does not occur.

Acute Adrenocortical Failure or Adrenal Crisis

Adrenal crisis usually occurs in patients with unrecognized adrenal failure who develop an intercurrent illness such as pneumonia. They experience dehydration and hypotension out of proportion to the severity of the current illness. Abdominal pain in combination with nausea and vomiting may mimic an acute abdomen. Unexplained fever, hyponatremia, hyperkalemia, azotemia, hypercalcemia, and eosinophilia may all be present. Adrenal crisis may be the first manifestation of bilateral adrenal hemorrhage.

- Addison disease presents insidiously with both glucocorticoid and mineralocorticoid deficiency.
- Adrenal crisis may develop during intercurrent illness in a patient with unrecognized adrenal failure, with inadequate cortisol replacement, or after bilateral adrenal hemorrhage.

Diagnosis

Endocrine Diagnosis

The diagnosis of adrenal failure can be confirmed by the cosyntropin test, which assesses the cortisol response to synthetic ACTH (1 μg or 250 μg). An appropriate response to cosyntropin is an increase in plasma cortisol by more than 7 μg/dL from the baseline value (this may not be achieved in normal patients with a high basal level of cortisol) or to an absolute value greater than 18 μg/dL.

A high ACTH level suggests primary adrenal insufficiency, whereas a low or "inappropriately normal" level indicates secondary failure. A normal response to cosyntropin rules out Addison disease but does not completely exclude ACTH deficiency (although the 1-μg test is more sensitive in this regard) that is partial or of recent onset. If the diagnosis is still suspected, an insulin-hypoglycemia or metyrapone test may be performed; these test the ACTH response to hypoglycemia (insulin) or to inhibition of adrenal steroidogenesis (metyrapone).

- An abnormal cosyntropin test establishes the diagnosis of adrenal failure but cannot differentiate primary from secondary adrenal failure.
- A normal cortisol response excludes primary adrenal failure but does not completely exclude secondary adrenal failure that is partial or of recent onset.

Therapy

Primary adrenal failure requires glucocorticoid and mineralocorticoid replacement, whereas secondary adrenal failure requires only glucocorticoid replacement. Patients should be educated about the need to increase steroid dosage during acute illness and the use of injectable glucocorticoid when oral replacement therapy is not possible. Patients should always wear a medic-alert bracelet or necklace. Usually, glucocorticoid replacement is with hydrocortisone or prednisone. The adequacy of therapy can be assessed only by the patient's sense of well-being and the absence of manifestations of glucocorticoid excess. Mineralocorticoid replacement is provided by fludrocortisone. Dose adjustment is guided by the presence of orthostatism, edema, hyperkalemia or hypokalemia, and, if needed, plasma renin activity.

In mild-to-moderate acute illness, the glucocorticoid dosage is doubled or tripled for the duration of the illness. Dexamethasone (4 mg intramuscularly) is given when the patient cannot take oral medications (nausea or vomiting). Intravenous hydrocortisone is given in stress doses before and during recovery from surgery. The management of an adrenal crisis requires intravenous rehydration, electrolyte replacement, and hydrocortisone (usually 100 mg every 6 hours). The cortisol and serum ACTH levels should be checked, but management should not be delayed while awaiting results. A search should be undertaken for a precipitating illness.

- Primary adrenal failure requires both glucocorticoid and mineralocorticoid replacement, whereas secondary failure requires only glucocorticoid replacement.
- Patient education is a critical component of effective management.
- Glucocorticoid replacement needs to be modified in acute illness.

Cushing Syndrome

Etiology

The commonest cause of Cushing syndrome is the prolonged use of supraphysiologic doses of glucocorticoids. Endogenous Cushing syndrome is caused by overproduction of cortisol by the adrenal cortex. This may be the result of adrenal autonomy (ACTH-independent) or unregulated, excessive secretion of ACTH (ACTH-dependent). ACTH-independent disorders include autonomous adrenal adenomas, adrenal carcinoma (which also usually produces adrenal androgens), or, rarely, macronodular or micronodular adrenal hyperplasia. ACTH-dependent Cushing syndrome may be caused by a small pituitary corticotroph adenoma (Cushing disease) or ectopic secretion of ACTH. Ectopic ACTH-secreting tumors can be aggressive and malignant (e.g., squamous cell carcinoma of the lung) or indolent (e.g., pheochromocytoma, medullary carcinoma of the thyroid, or bronchial carcinoid). Very rarely, corticotropin-releasing hormone (CRH)-producing tumors such as a bronchial carcinoid cause pituitary hyperplasia and excess ACTH secretion.

- Exogenous glucocorticoid therapy is the most common cause of Cushing syndrome.
- Endogenous Cushing syndrome comprises ACTH-independent and ACTH-dependent disorders.
- The most common causes of endogenous Cushing syndrome are Cushing disease (60% of cases), adrenal tumors (25%), and ectopic ACTH-producing tumors (15%).

Clinical Features

Many of the clinical features of Cushing syndrome are nonspecific and include weight gain, diabetes mellitus, hypertension, and mood affect. Symptoms and signs that appear to be more specific for the disorder include central obesity, supraclavicular fat pads, thin skin, easy bruising, wide (>1 cm) purple striae, and proximal muscle weakness. In severe and rapidly progressive disease (usually ectopic ACTH production by a malignant tumor), the presentation is dominated by weight loss, weakness, secondary diabetes, and mineralocorticoid excess (hypertension, edema, and hypokalemia). Often, there is not sufficient time for the development of the classic features of cortisol excess.

Adrenal androgen excess may produce acne, hirsutism, and menstrual irregularities. However, in adrenal carcinoma, the overproduction of androgens may be more extreme and lead to virilization. When ACTH is produced in marked quantities, as in the syndrome of ectopic ACTH, hyperpigmentation may occur.

- The clinical picture of cortisol excess varies according to the rapidity of onset and the underlying disorder.
- Central obesity, supraclavicular fat pads, thin skin, easy bruising, wide purple striae, and proximal muscle weakness are the more specific features of the disease.

Diagnosis

Confirmation of Cushing Syndrome

The diagnosis of Cushing syndrome involves a two-step approach: biochemical confirmation of the disorder and determination of the underlying cause. The best screening test for Cushing syndrome is measurement of 24-hour urine free cortisol excretion. An increase in urine free cortisol suggests but does not confirm the diagnosis of Cushing syndrome (levels increased more than threefold the upper limit of normal in a 24-hour collection are considered diagnostic if the clinical suspicion for the disorder is high). The differential diagnosis includes pseudo-Cushing states (depression, alcohol use, and acute illness). If the clinical suspicion of Cushing syndrome is high, a normal urine free cortisol excretion does not rule out the disorder (of the 24-hour urine cortisol collections from 10% of patients with established Cushing syndrome, 1 in 4 are normal). In this situation, it is best to repeat the test in 1 month. The 1-mg dexamethasone suppression test is best reserved for screening for subclinical Cushing syndrome in a patient with an adrenal incidentaloma (see below). The 2-day low-dose dexamethasone suppression test (0.5 mg every 6 hours for 2 days) has limited usefulness in the diagnosis of Cushing syndrome (except for cases in which the clinical suspicion for the disorder is low). False-positive results may be obtained in patients with pseudo-Cushing states or those taking estrogen-containing medications that increase cortisol-binding globulin. False-negative results may also occur, particularly in the case of ACTH-producing pituitary adenomas, some of which show unusual suppressibility to dexamethasone. Therefore, the 2-day low-dose dexamethasone suppression test has been replaced by the dexamethasone-CRH test.

- The best screening test for Cushing syndrome is a 24-hour urine free cortisol level. A level increased more than threefold in 24 hours is considered diagnostic, particularly if the clinical features of the disorder are prominent.
- The 24-hour urine free cortisol level may be intermittently normal in some patients with Cushing syndrome. If clinical suspicion is high but the 24-hour urine free cortisol level is normal, the test should be repeated.
- The 24-hour urine free cortisol level may be increased in pseudo-Cushing states, including psychiatric disorders and acute illness. In these conditions, false-positive results may be obtained on a low-dose dexamethasone suppression test.
- The 2-day low-dose dexamethasone suppression test has limited usefulness in the diagnosis of Cushing syndrome and has been largely replaced by the dexamethasone-CRH test.

Cause of Cushing Syndrome

After the diagnosis of Cushing syndrome has been confirmed biochemically, the next step is to determine whether the disease is ACTH-dependent or ACTH-independent. A suppressed ACTH (<5 pg/mL) implies adrenal autonomy, and CT of the abdomen should be performed. A normal (10-80 pg/mL) or modestly increased (<200 pg/mL) concentration is observed in an ACTH-dependent process. Extreme increases in ACTH (>200 pg/mL) suggest—but do not confirm—ectopic ACTH secretion.

The differentiation of pituitary-dependent disease from ectopic ACTH production can be one of the most difficult evaluations in endocrinology. Most causes of ACTH-dependent disease are due to pituitary disease; thus, if the clinical features are consistent with pituitary disease (middle-aged woman, slow onset, progression of disease), MRI of the pituitary gland should be considered. A pituitary lesion larger than 4 mm is suggestive of an ACTH-producing pituitary tumor, and the patient may proceed directly to transsphenoidal exploration. The absence of a pituitary lesion on MRI does not rule out Cushing disease because 50% of the tumors are not visible on MRI. If no abnormality is found on imaging of the sella, sampling of the inferior petrosal sinuses (together with CRH provocative testing) should be performed. Documentation of a central-to-peripheral ACTH concentration gradient confirms that the source of excess ACTH is from a pituitary tumor. The 2-day high-dose dexamethasone suppression test was used to distinguish between pituitary-dependent disease and ectopic ACTH secretion. However, this test is considered obsolete when traditional criteria are used for interpretation because one-third of bronchial carcinoid tumors respond like pituitary adenomas. Also, the clinical presentation of bronchial carcinoids may be indistinguishable from that of pituitary-dependent disease.

- After biochemical confirmation of Cushing syndrome, the next step is to measure ACTH levels.
- If the ACTH level is <5 pg/mL, proceed to CT of the adrenal glands.
- If the ACTH level is >10 pg/mL, distinguish between a pituitary-dependent tumor and ectopic ACTH production.
- Clinically, bronchial carcinoid tumors may be indistinguishable from pituitary disease.
- Inferior petrosal sinus sampling is the "gold standard" test for distinguishing between pituitary disease and ectopic disease.
- The 2-day high-dose dexamethasone suppression test is considered obsolete in the differential diagnosis of ACTH-dependent Cushing syndrome.

Therapy

Removal of the source of ACTH secretion is the treatment of choice in ACTH-dependent Cushing syndrome. However, this is not always possible; transsphenoidal surgery has about a 30% failure rate, and an ectopic source of ACTH may not be resectable or detectable. In these cases, bilateral adrenalectomy is the treatment of choice.

In ACTH-independent Cushing syndrome, resection of the adrenal adenoma or carcinoma is indicated. In adrenal carcinoma, complete resection may not be possible and adjuvant treatment with inhibitors of steroidogenesis such as ketoconazole may be indicated.

In all cases, surgical excision of the causative tumor is followed by a period of cortisol deficiency because of suppression of the hypothalamic-pituitary-adrenal axis. This may take 1 year to recover, and glucocorticoid replacement is required during this time. Life-long replacement of glucocorticoid and mineralocorticoid is necessary after bilateral adrenalectomy.

- A period of suppression of the normal axis occurs after removal of the causative tumor and may last up to 1 year.

Primary Aldosteronism

Etiology

Primary aldosteronism results from autonomous (renin-independent) aldosterone production by the zona glomerulosa. It may be due to an aldosteronoma, idiopathic bilateral hyperplasia, adrenocortical carcinoma, or, rarely, familial glucocorticoid-remediable aldosteronism.

Clinical Features

Most patients present with hypertension and hypokalemia. The hypertension can be of variable severity. The hypokalemia is often mild and may be absent. However, it may be exacerbated by diuretic therapy. Most patients are asymptomatic, but a few experience myopathic symptoms and paresthesias due to hypokalemia and alkalosis. Edema is usually absent.

Diagnosis

The diagnosis of primary aldosteronism requires documentation of autonomous aldosterone secretion and, subsequently, definition of the underlying cause. Although hypokalemia is often present in primary aldosteronism, it is a nonspecific finding and may not occur in patients treated with angiotensin-converting enzyme inhibitors or potassium-sparing diuretics such as spironolactone. A urine potassium concentration greater than 30 mEq/L in a patient with hypokalemia suggests renal wasting of potassium and is suspicious for mineralocorticoid excess.

The measurement of the ratio of plasma aldosterone (PA in ng/dL) to plasma renin activity (PRA in ng/mL per hour) is used to screen for primary aldosteronism. It is important to measure plasma aldosterone after correction of hypokalemia because the latter decreases aldosterone secretion. Increased plasma aldosterone and suppressed plasma renin activity with a PA/PRA greater than 20 is suggestive of primary aldosteronism. The diagnosis is confirmed by the demonstration of a nonsuppressed 24-hour urine aldosterone in the salt-replete state (instruct patients to add salt to their food during the collection).

Hypertension caused by excess of a mineralocorticoid other than aldosterone is seen in deoxycorticosterone-producing tumors, congenital adrenal hyperplasia due to 11- or 17-hydroxylase deficiency, Cushing syndrome, and genetic or acquired (use of licorice or chewing tobacco) deficiency of 11β-hydroxysteroid dehydrogenase. This enzyme is present in the distal renal tubule and catalyzes the inactivation of cortisol. Inactivation of this enzyme potentiates the mineralocorticoid effect of cortisol.

- It is estimated that 30% of patients with primary hyperaldosteronism have normokalemia.
- If hypokalemia occurs with the use of diuretics, suspect primary hyperaldosteronism.
- Urine potassium concentration >30 mEq/L in a patient with hypokalemia suggests renal wasting of potassium and increases the suspicion for primary aldosteronism.
- A PA/PRA ratio >20 suggests primary aldosteronism.

The major challenge is to distinguish between an aldosterone-producing adenoma and bilateral adrenal hyperplasia. This is important because an aldosterone-secreting adenoma can be treated surgically. However, bilateral hyperplasia can be treated only medically. CT of the adrenals may be misleading because the functional tumor is small and may not be visualized. Furthermore, a visible adrenal mass may be an incidental finding or the mass may be a hyperplastic nodule superimposed on a background of bilateral adrenal hyperplasia. Selective adrenal venous sampling is the most useful localizing procedure; a unilateral aldosterone gradient helps direct surgical excision.

- An adrenal mass seen on CT may not represent an aldosteronoma.
- The most reliable localizing test is selective adrenal venous sampling.

Therapy

Unilateral adrenalectomy is indicated for aldosteronoma unless the patient is a poor surgical risk. Surgical resection corrects the hypokalemia (100%) and normalizes or markedly improves the hypertension in about 70% of patients. Persistent postoperative hypertension should be treated with standard antihypertensive therapy.

Medical treatment is indicated for the management of bilateral adrenal hyperplasia and for patients with aldosteronoma who are not candidates for surgery. Spironolactone, an aldosterone antagonist, restores potassium concentrations and normalizes blood pressure in most patients. Adverse effects include gastrointestinal upset, menstrual irregularity, and, in men, gynecomastia, decreased libido, and impotence. Women of childbearing age who take spironolactone should use effective contraception because the drug may cause feminization of the male fetus through its androgen-blocking effects. Alternative treatment includes amiloride or triamterene.

Pheochromocytoma

Etiology

Pheochromocytomas arise in chromaffin cells of neural crest origin in the adrenal medulla or, less frequently, along the sympathetic chain and rarely in sympathetic tissue in the walls of the urinary bladder. Of these tumors, 10% are malignant and 10% are familial. Familial pheochromocytomas are more likely to be intra-adrenal, bilateral, and malignant. Pheochromocytomas can secrete catecholamines continuously or episodically.

Clinical Features

Pheochromocytomas may present as an incidental finding on abdominal imaging performed for other reasons. More commonly, they are suspected because of the presence of hypertension that is paroxysmal, refractory to treatment, or associated with paroxysmal symptoms of palpitations, sweating, anxiety, and pallor. Some patients present with hypermetabolism that is manifested as heat intolerance, sweating, and weight loss. The tumor may be part of MEN IIA or IIB, von Hippel-Lindau disease, or neurofibromatosis. In most patients, the paroxysmal symptoms are stereotyped and vary only in severity or frequency.

- Pheochromocytomas can be asymptomatic and discovered incidentally.
- Common symptoms include headache, palpitations, and sweating. The symptoms may be paroxysmal.
- Some patients may have a family history of pheochromocytoma. The tumor may be a manifestation of MEN IIA or IIB.

Diagnosis

The diagnosis of pheochromocytoma requires documentation of increased urinary excretion of free catecholamines and metanephrines. Catecholamine-containing drugs, alpha-methyldopa, labetalol, and monoamine oxidase inhibitors cause falsely elevated concentrations. Severe stress, intercurrent illness, drug and food interaction with monoamine oxidase inhibitors, or excessive use of sympathomimetic amines also causes increased excretion of urinary catecholamines. Normal values in a hypertensive or otherwise symptomatic patient are sufficient to exclude the diagnosis. In patients with paroxysmal symptoms, the diagnostic yield is increased by collecting urine during or shortly after a paroxysm.

For screening purposes, 24-hour urine metanephrines are preferred over plasma metanephrine levels because the latter is a less specific test. Plasma catecholamines have limited usefulness in the diagnosis of pheochromocytoma.

- Normal urinary catecholamine values in a hypertensive patient exclude the diagnosis. In patients with paroxysmal symptoms, the diagnostic yield is increased substantially by initiating collection during or shortly after a paroxysm.
- Increased values in hypertensive patients establish the diagnosis only if other disorders associated with hypertension and catecholamine excess are excluded (severe stress, intercurrent illness, acute myocardial ischemia, certain medications, or abrupt withdrawal of clonidine).

CT or MRI of the abdomen (and, if indicated, the pelvis, thorax, and neck) is used to localize a pheochromocytoma. On MRI, pheochromocytomas have a high-intensity signal on T_2-weighted images. ^{123}I-metaiodobenzylguanidine (^{123}I-MIBG) is taken up by pheochromocytomas and is used as an adjunct to CT or MRI if metastatic disease is suspected.

- Radiographic localization of the pheochromocytoma is attempted only if the biochemical diagnosis is firm.
- Pheochromocytomas appear as a high-intensity signal on T_2-weighted MRI.
- ^{123}I-MIBG is used as an adjunct to CT or MRI if metastatic disease is suspected.

Therapy

Complete excision of a pheochromocytoma is curative. Medical treatment is used preoperatively to diminish perioperative morbidity and mortality. Ongoing treatment is required if resection is incomplete and if recurrent or metastatic disease is present. α-Adrenergic blockade should be instituted with phenoxybenzamine, starting with 10 mg twice daily. α-Adrenergic blockers may be necessary to control reflex tachycardia after maximal α-blockade has been achieved. If cure is achieved, urinary catecholamine concentrations return to normal within 2 weeks. Long-term follow-up is important to assess for persistent or recurrent disease.

- Surgical excision of the tumor is curative.
- α-Adrenergic blockade should be initiated when the diagnosis is made.
- β-Blockade may be necessary to control reflex tachycardia after effective α-blockade.

Adrenal Incidentaloma

Etiology

Small (1-6 cm) adrenal masses are found in about 10% of autopsies and increasingly are being detected on abdominal

CT performed for other reasons. Although most of them are nonfunctioning adenomas, a few are functioning adenomas or carcinomas of the adrenal gland. Also, metastatic disease to the adrenals may present in this way.

Evaluation

Evaluation should address the following two questions:
- Is the lesion benign or malignant?
- Is the lesion hyperfunctioning?

The size of the adrenal mass can help to distinguish between a benign and a malignant tumor. Most adenomas are smaller than 4 cm in diameter. The incidence of carcinoma exceeds 35% in masses larger than 6 cm. Needle biopsy cannot distinguish between a benign and a malignant adrenal neoplasm and should not be attempted if pheochromocytoma is suspected. Needle biopsy is useful to confirm a suspicion of disease metastatic to the adrenals.

For all patients, screen for pheochromocytoma (24-hour urine metanephrines) and subclinical Cushing syndrome (1-mg overnight dexamethasone suppression test). It is important to ascertain the functional status of the adrenal mass before surgical management. An unsuspected pheochromocytoma may provoke a hypertensive crisis. Similarly, removal of the cortisol-producing tumor may be followed by an adrenal crisis. Such patients need perioperative and postoperative cortisol replacement until the ACTH-adrenal axis recovers, and this may take up to 1 year. Also, screen for primary aldosteronism if the patient has hypertension. An androgen-producing or a feminizing adrenal tumor needs to be considered only when clinical findings suggest overproduction of sex steroids.

Therapy

A functioning tumor should be excised. Patients with nonfunctioning tumors smaller than 4 cm should have CT repeated in 3 months to assess for growth. If the size is stable after 3 months, additional scans are performed 1 year after the diagnosis. An adrenal mass larger than 4 cm in diameter or a mass that is increasing in size on serial observation should be excised.

- Laboratory investigation of an adrenal incidentaloma should include 24-hour urinary catecholamines, a 1-mg overnight dexamethasone suppression test, and, if the patient is hypertensive, determination of the aldosterone/renin ratio.
- Pheochromocytoma or subclinical cortisol production should be excluded before surgical excision.
- Needle biopsy of an adrenal incidentaloma is not indicated unless metastatic disease is suspected (first, rule out pheochromocytoma).

- Excision is indicated for a functioning tumor, a mass >4 cm, and a mass that is increasing in size on serial observation.

THE TESTIS

Male Hypogonadism

Etiology

Decreased testosterone production may be a result of testicular failure (hypergonadotropic hypogonadism or primary hypogonadism) or LH deficiency due to a hypothalamic or pituitary disorder (hypogonadotropic hypogonadism or secondary hypogonadism). Hypergonadotropic hypogonadism may result from Klinefelter syndrome, testicular trauma, radiotherapy or chemotherapy, autoimmune or infectious (mumps) disorders, or orchitis and degenerative disorders such as dystrophia myotonica. Hypogonadotropic hypogonadism may be due to a functional hypothalamic disorder, for example, constitutional delay in puberty, use of neuroleptic drugs, nutritional disorders, severe systemic illness, hyperprolactinemia, or thyroid or adrenal disorders. Organic disorders of the hypothalamus and pituitary can also lead to hypogonadism (e.g., a pituitary tumor).

Androgen resistance may be genetic or acquired. Genetic androgen resistance includes testicular feminization and 5α-reductase deficiency. Acquired androgen resistance may occur with the use of the androgen receptor blockers spironolactone or flutamide.

- Decreased testosterone production may result from primary testicular failure or a central hypothalamic or pituitary disorder.
- Central hypogonadotropism may result from functional or organic hypothalamic disorders or from organic diseases of the anterior pituitary gland.

Clinical Features

In adult males, hypogonadism presents as decreased libido and potency, decreased ejaculate volume, infertility, decreased stamina, decreased sexual hair growth, and gynecomastia. Hot flashes may occur if testosterone deficiency is rapid in onset. In men with chronic and severe testosterone deficiency, physical findings may include pallor, female pattern of fat distribution, testicular atrophy, and gynecomastia.

Hypogonadism in adolescents presents as delayed puberty and growth. Sexual infantilism is associated with the absence of a pubertal growth spurt, eunuchoid habitus (ratio of arm span to height is >1), high-pitched voice, poor muscle development, and a female pattern of fat distribution. The testes usually are small and soft. Small, firm testes in a hypogonadal male suggest Klinefelter syndrome, and the presence of anosmia in an adolescent with sexual infantilism suggests Kallmann syndrome.

Diagnosis

The diagnosis is confirmed by documenting low serum levels of testosterone. Measurement of LH and FSH helps to differentiate primary from secondary hypogonadism. Gonadotropin concentrations are increased in primary testicular failure, but they are decreased or inappropriately normal in secondary hypogonadism. Additional tests that may be indicated include karyotyping to confirm Klinefelter syndrome. Secondary hypogonadism requires exclusion of Kallmann syndrome, measurement of the serum concentration of prolactin, pituitary function testing, and MRI of the head to exclude organic hypothalamic-pituitary disease.

- Serum levels of LH and FSH help to differentiate primary from secondary hypogonadism.
- Hypogonadotropic hypogonadism mandates assessment of pituitary function and MRI of the head. Evaluate for the presence of midline defects or anosmia in adults (Kallmann syndrome).

Therapy

Androgen Therapy

In adults, androgen therapy is aimed at the restoration and maintenance of secondary sex characteristics. Testosterone replacement cannot stimulate spermatogenesis. In secondary hypogonadism, gonadotropins can be used to induce spermatogenesis and to restore fertility.

Androgens can be replaced by 17-hydroxyl esters of testosterone (e.g., testosterone enanthate) administered intramuscularly every 2 weeks. However, this mode of delivery produces a supraphysiologic level of testosterone shortly after the injection, but the level gradually decreases to a low level before the next injection. A more favorable mode of delivery is transdermal testosterone by means of a patch or gel applied to the skin. Also, 17α-alkylated derivatives of testosterone can be administered orally; however, they are associated with substantial hepatotoxicity and should not be used.

Testosterone replacement therapy is contraindicated in the presence of prostate cancer (the prostate-specific antigen [PSA] level should be checked before treatment is initiated) or psychosis, and it may worsen the symptoms of prostatism. Side effects include acne, edema, erythrocytosis, and exacerbation of obstructive sleep apnea.

- In adults, androgen therapy restores and maintains secondary sex characteristics.
- An annual prostate examination and serum PSA level are recommended for patients receiving testosterone replacement therapy.

Selected Disorders of Male Hypogonadism

Klinefelter Syndrome

Klinefelter syndrome is common (1:400-500) and arises because of the presence of one or more extra X chromosomes. The classic karyotype is 47,XXY. The disorder is characterized by hyalinization of the seminiferous tubules and dysfunction of the Leydig cells, which is manifested at puberty. The testes are small and firm, and gynecomastia is present. If more than one X chromosome is present, the incidence of mental retardation and somatic abnormalities is increased. In mosaicism, the clinical manifestations are less severe and if an XY line is present, fertility may be possible.

Patients with Klinefelter syndrome have a slightly increased incidence of diabetes mellitus, chronic obstructive pulmonary disease, autoimmune disorders, varicose veins, malignancy of the breast, lymphoma, and germ cell neoplasm. Therapy includes testosterone replacement. Breast reduction surgery is indicated if the patient's gynecomastia is a source of emotional distress.

- Klinefelter syndrome is due to one or more extra X chromosomes; the classic karyotype is 47,XXY.
- Characteristic findings include small, firm testes, gynecomastia, increased FSH levels, and various degrees of testosterone deficiency.

Kallmann Syndrome

This syndrome is characterized by secondary hypogonadism and anosmia. It is a congenital disorder, often familial, that is due to defective migration of GnRH-producing neurons during embryogenesis. Patients present with delayed puberty. Anosmia is present in 80% of patients. Other midline defects such as a cleft lip or palate, color blindness, cryptorchidism, and skeletal abnormalities may occur. Laboratory evaluation shows isolated hypogonadotropic hypogonadism. On MRI, the olfactory bulbs may be abnormal or absent, but the hypothalamic-pituitary region is normal. Therapy for Kallmann syndrome consists of testosterone replacement to allow for the development of secondary sex characteristics. The administration of gonadotropin is required for fertility.

- Kallmann syndrome is characterized by hypogonadotropic hypogonadism and anosmia.

Gynecomastia

Etiology

Gynecomastia, the most common disorder of the male breast, is caused by some degree of estradiol excess that can be 1) a relative estrogen excess due to decreased testosterone production or the use of an androgen receptor blocker (spironolactone, cimetidine, or flutamide) or 2) an absolute increase in estradiol production because of adrenal cancer, a Leydig cell tumor, or a human chorionic gonadotropin (HCG)–producing tumor. Androgen-secreting tumors or exogenous androgen use can produce gynecomastia through the peripheral conversion of testosterone to estrogen.

In young healthy pubertal males, gynecomastia is physiologic and tends to be transient. The use of anabolic steroids or Klinefelter syndrome may account for a small number of cases. All other causes are rare in this age group. In adults, the two common causes are drugs and alcohol-related liver disease. Ectopic HCG-producing tumors, feminizing adrenal and testicular tumors, and pituitary tumors are rare causes of gynecomastia. In about 10% of cases, the cause of gynecomastia is indeterminate.

- The basic mechanism underlying the development of gynecomastia is an increase in the estrogen/androgen ratio.
- In adults, the two most common causes of gynecomastia are drugs and alcoholic liver disease.
- In about 10% of cases, the cause of gynecomastia is indeterminate.

Clinical Features

Patients usually present with breast enlargement or tenderness (or both) that may be unilateral or bilateral. Rarely, a patient may complain of galactorrhea. Gynecomastia is firm, with a fine nodularity, and spreads radially with a well-defined outer border.

Diagnosis

The differential diagnosis includes pseudogynecomastia (bilateral fatty enlargement) and malignancy. A history of alcohol consumption and medications should be part of the initial evaluation. Endocrine tests should include measurement of testosterone, estradiol, LH and FSH, β-HCG, TSH, and prolactin levels. If indicated, karyotyping should be performed.

An increase in β-HCG implies the presence of an HCG-secreting tumor. A high level of estradiol should prompt evaluation for feminizing adrenal or testicular tumors. If LH, FSH, and sex steroid concentrations are normal, an underlying endocrine disorder is unlikely.

- If the gynecomastia is bilateral, consider pseudogynecomastia. If unilateral, exclude malignancy.
- Evaluation includes measurement of testosterone, LH, FSH, β-HCG, TSH, estradiol, and prolactin levels.

THE OVARY

Amenorrhea

Primary amenorrhea is present when menarche has not occurred by age 16 years in a young female who has normal secondary sex characteristics or by age 14 in the absence of secondary sex characteristics. Secondary amenorrhea is present when a woman with previously established menstrual function does not menstruate for a period longer than three of her previous cycle intervals or for 6 months.

Etiology

Amenorrhea may be physiologic, as in pregnancy or after menopause. Pathologic amenorrhea may result from a hypothalamic disorder that leads to the loss of cyclical GnRH production, a pituitary disorder resulting in hypogonadotropic hypogonadism, an ovarian disorder, or a uterine disorder or genital tract disorder that prevents the egress of shed endometrium. The common causes of primary amenorrhea are gonadal dysgenesis (45% of cases), constitutional delay of puberty (20%), and müllerian agenesis (15%). The common causes of secondary amenorrhea are hypothalamic dysfunction (40% of cases), polycystic ovarian syndrome (30%), pituitary disease (20%), and ovarian failure (10%).

- Amenorrhea can result from impaired function of any component of the hypothalamic-pituitary-gonadal axis or from an anatomical abnormality of the genital tract.
- The common causes of amenorrhea are physiologic, for example, pregnancy.

Primary Amenorrhea

Developmental anomalies that present as primary amenorrhea include imperforate hymen, isolated absence of the uterus, and vaginal atresia. Ovarian disorders account for most of the causes of primary amenorrhea. Functional suppression of the hypothalamic GnRH cell population by a nutritional or psychiatric disorder, prolonged heavy exercise, systemic illness, hyperprolactinemia, or thyroid or adrenal disorders also cause amenorrhea. Organic hypothalamic-pituitary disease is an uncommon cause of primary amenorrhea; in young adults, craniopharyngioma is more common than prolactinoma.

- Outflow tract disorders are uncommon causes of primary amenorrhea.
- Ovarian disorders are the most common cause of primary amenorrhea.
- Hypothalamic-pituitary disease may be functional or organic.

Secondary Amenorrhea

Polycystic ovary syndrome, autoimmune oophoritis, abdominal irradiation, chemotherapy with cyclophosphamide or vincristine, and ovarian tumors that secrete excessive androgen can all present as secondary amenorrhea.

Functional hypogonadotropism may be triggered by situational stress, weight loss, or systemic illness (e.g, hyperthyroidism). In organic hypothalamic-pituitary disorders, secondary hypogonadism occurs alone or in association with other pituitary function abnormalities. The incidence of postpartum pituitary necrosis (Sheehan syndrome), previously a common cause, has decreased with improved obstetric care.

Acquired outflow tract abnormalities are rare causes of secondary amenorrhea. Such disorders may be the result of postpartum endometritis or destruction of the basal layer of the endometrium by overzealous dilatation and curettage, with subsequent obliteration of the endometrial cavity (Asherman syndrome).

- Functional or organic hypothalamic-pituitary disorders are the common cause of secondary amenorrhea.
- Ovarian causes of secondary amenorrhea include polycystic ovary syndrome and autoimmune oophoritis.
- Acquired outflow tract abnormalities are uncommon causes of secondary amenorrhea.
- Hyperthyroidism may present as amenorrhea.

Clinical Features

In addition to amenorrhea, patients may experience symptoms of estrogen deficiency. These include vaginal dryness, hot flashes, and loss of secondary sex characteristics. Other findings are those related to the etiologic disorder, such as galactorrhea, hirsutism, shortness of stature, or features of Turner syndrome.

Diagnosis

Secondary Amenorrhea

The first step in the work-up of amenorrhea is to exclude pregnancy regardless of the patient's history of sexual activity or contraceptive use. The serum levels of prolactin and TSH should be measured to exclude hyperprolactinemia and thyroid dysfunction, respectively. Serum levels of estradiol, LH, and particularly FSH help to differentiate ovarian from hypothalamic-pituitary disorders. An increase in FSH in a patient with low estradiol levels confirms primary ovarian failure. If ovarian failure (chemotherapy or radiotherapy) has no readily apparent cause, autoimmune oophoritis is likely, and appropriate tests to exclude other autoimmune endocrine disorders are indicated. Inappropriately low levels of FSH and LH indicate a hypothalamic-pituitary disorder, and pituitary function testing and appropriate imaging should be performed. Hirsutism and acne suggest hyperandrogenism and should be investigated by measuring the serum concentration of testosterone and dehydroepiandrosterone sulfate (DHEAS).

- The evaluation of secondary amenorrhea should include measurement of HCG, prolactin, TSH, estradiol, FSH, LH, and, if indicated, testosterone and DHEAS.
- Low estradiol and increased FSH levels indicate primary ovarian failure.
- Low estradiol and inappropriately low FSH and LH levels indicate a hypothalamic-pituitary disorder: rule out functional and organic disease.

Primary Amenorrhea

If the appearance is that of an adult female and there is no evidence of pregnancy, consider outflow tract obstruction or androgen insensitivity (e.g., testicular feminization). A pelvic examination is an important part of the evaluation. Normal findings on pelvic examination should prompt an evaluation similar to that for secondary amenorrhea. The absence of a uterus should prompt measurement of testosterone; a normal female testosterone concentration supports the diagnosis of müllerian agenesis, whereas a high serum level of testosterone suggests androgen insensitivity.

If sexual infantilism is present, gonadotropins should be measured. An increase in FSH suggests primary gonadal failure and dictates karyotyping. Normal or low FSH levels suggest hypogonadotropic hypogonadism or delayed puberty.

- Adult female sex characteristics and a negative pregnancy test should lead to a consideration of genital tract anomalies or androgen insensitivity.
- The presence of sexual infantilism suggests a disorder of the hypothalamic-pituitary-gonadal axis or delayed puberty.

Therapy

Management is directed at the underlying disorder and restoration of normal gonadal function. However, if successful treatment of the underlying disorder is not possible, estrogen replacement therapy and, when feasible, restoration of fertility are indicated.

Estrogen Replacement Therapy

Estrogen replacement therapy is undertaken to help control hot flashes, prevent atrophic vaginitis, preserve secondary sex characteristics, and prevent osteoporosis. Estrogen therapy is contraindicated if the patient has an estrogen-dependent neoplasm, cholestatic liver disease, or a history of venous thrombosis. Progesterone replacement therapy is indicated only for women with an intact uterus. Estrogen and progesterone replacement therapy can be administered sequentially or in combination. Sequential therapy usually results in predictable cyclic withdrawal bleeding. The goal of combination therapy is to induce endometrial atrophy and amenorrhea and is preferred by patients who find cyclical withdrawal bleeding inconvenient.

Estrogen replacement therapy increases the risk of endometrial cancer (but this is prevented by progesterone), and it is associated with a slight increase in the risk of breast cancer.

Ovulation Induction

Hypogonadal women who desire fertility can be given clomiphene citrate, exogenous gonadotropin, or GnRH therapy. The treatment of choice for hyperprolactinemia is bromocriptine or cabergoline.

Selected Disorders Associated With Amenorrhea

Turner 45/XO Gonadal Dysgenesis

Turner syndrome is the most common cause of primary amenorrhea and affects 1 in 3,000 newborn females. It is characterized by a missing X chromosome, which leads to the development of streak gonads, primary ovarian failure, and sexual infantilism. Physical abnormalities associated with Turner syndrome include a webbed neck, low-set ears, micrognathia, a shield-like chest, short metacarpals and metatarsals, an increased carrying angle at the elbows, renal developmental abnormalities, and cardiovascular anomalies (including coarctation and aortic stenosis). Mosaics tend to have less severe manifestations of the syndrome, and the degree of ovarian dysgenesis varies depending on the ratio of XO to XX germ cells.

Anorexia Nervosa

This syndrome occurs almost exclusively in females younger than 25 years. It is characterized by a distorted perception of weight and body image that leads to poor nutrition. Patients deny the nature of the problem. Amenorrhea occurs in most females with anorexia nervosa and often precedes the weight loss. Other features of the disorder include bradycardia, hypotension, constipation, growth of lanugo hair, and, in severe cases, dependent edema. Endocrine findings include secondary hypogonadism, low IGF-I, increased reverse T_3, and increased serum cortisol concentrations that are suppressed in response to exogenous dexamethasone.

Androgens in Normal Females

Circulating androgens in adult females originate from the ovaries and adrenal cortex. Testosterone is synthesized by the ovaries and adrenals and from conversion of androstenedione in the peripheral tissues. Dehydroepiandrosterone (DHEA) is produced mainly by the adrenals and, to a lesser extent, the ovaries. DHEAS is derived almost exclusively from the adrenal cortex. Ovarian androgens are synthesized by thecal cells in an LH-dependent fashion. Adrenal androgens are synthesized in the zona fasciculata and zona reticularis in an ACTH-dependent manner. These androgens are metabolized to testosterone or dihydrotestosterone at their target tissues. In females, androgens mediate the growth of sex hair and maintain libido and muscle mass.

- Testosterone originates from the ovaries and adrenals, but DHEAS is produced almost exclusively by the adrenal cortex.
- Ovarian androgen production is LH-dependent. Adrenal androgen production is ACTH-dependent.

Hirsutism and Virilization

"Hirsutism" refers to excessive androgen-induced hair growth in the androgen-sensitive areas of the female body. "Virilization" refers to the masculinization of secondary sex characteristics and the sex organs and is the result of pronounced androgen stimulation. Although virilization always is associated with hirsutism, hirsutism frequently occurs without virilization.

Etiology

Androgen excess may result from increased production of androgens by the ovaries or adrenal cortex (or both). Ovarian (LH-dependent) disorders include polycystic ovarian syndrome. Adrenocortical (ACTH-dependent) disorders include congenital adrenal hyperplasia and ACTH-dependent Cushing disease. Hirsutism also can occur because of increased sensitivity of the hair follicles to androgen. Hirsutism and virilization may be the consequence of exposure to exogenous androgens, anabolic steroids, or to some progestational agents derived from testosterone.

Clinical Features

The clinical features depend on the severity of the hyperandrogenism. Manifestations include acne, hirsutism of androgen-sensitive areas (including the upper lip, chin, chest, and lower abdomen), menstrual abnormalities, and masculinization (temporal hair recession, deepening voice, increased muscle mass, and clitorimegaly).

Diagnosis

A benign cause is suggested by onset at puberty with an indolent, slowly progressive course. In contrast, rapid onset with a severe, progressive course suggests a malignant disorder.

A positive family history is often elicited in racial hirsutism, polycystic ovarian syndrome, and late-onset congenital adrenal hyperplasia. Generally, a young woman who has mild hirsutism of pubertal onset and normal menstrual function and who is without any major disorder does not need to undergo detailed endocrine testing. Hirsutism of pubertal onset associated with menstrual irregularity but no virilization may be due to polycystic ovaries or late-onset congenital adrenal hyperplasia.

Diagnostic testing should include testosterone, DHEAS, and the serum level of prolactin as well as screening for Cushing syndrome (overnight 1-mg dexamethasone suppression test or 24-hour urine free cortisol). If a neoplastic disorder is suspected (serum testosterone >200 ng/dL or plasma DHEAS >7 ng/dL), pelvic ultrasonography and abdominal CT are indicated. In selected patients, determination of the serum level of 17-hydroxyprogesterone, with or without ACTH stimulation, to confirm congenital adrenal hyperplasia may be necessary.

- The most important diagnostic clues are the time of onset, tempo of progression, and severity of hyperandrogenic state.
- DHEAS >7 ng/dL suggests an adrenal tumor.
- Serum testosterone >200 ng/dL suggests an ovarian neoplasm. Serum testosterone <200 ng/dL suggests polycystic ovarian syndrome.

Selected Hyperandrogenic States

Idiopathic Hirsutism

This is usually due to a modest increase in ovarian androgen production, with increased peripheral androgen production and increased sensitivity of hair follicles to androgens. The hyperandrogenicity is usually mild and LH-dependent. Onset occurs at puberty and progresses slowly. Menstrual cycles are regular and findings on pelvic examination are unremarkable. The serum levels of testosterone and DHEAS are normal.

Polycystic Ovarian Syndrome

This is the commonest cause of hyperandrogenism. The diagnosis is made when the following criteria are present: 1) oligomenorrhea or amenorrhea, 2) clinical or biochemical hyperandrogenism, and 3) exclusion of other causes of hyperandrogenism (e.g., Cushing syndrome or congenital adrenal hyperplasia). The onset of the disorder is at puberty, and progression is slow. Most patients experience some degree of infertility. The serum levels of testosterone are usually at the upper limits of normal or modestly increased (usually <200 ng/mL). DHEAS levels are normal or mildly increased in 25% of patients. Serum levels of estradiol are normal. Gonadotropin secretion is abnormal, and approximately 60% of patients have an increased LH/FSH ratio. In most patients, the ovaries have a characteristic appearance on ultrasonography, with multiple peripherally located cysts. This radiographic finding, however, is not specific for polycystic ovarian syndrome; it is seen also in women with other causes of hyperandrogenism and in nonhirsute women with normal menses.

Polycystic ovarian syndrome is also considered a metabolic disorder: most patients are obese and have insulin resistance. Patients are at increased risk for the development of glucose intolerance or type 2 diabetes mellitus. Treatment with metformin may be considered for patients with established glucose intolerance. Currently, the use of this agent or insulin-sensitizing agents to treat hirsutism in women with polycystic ovarian syndrome who have normal glucose levels is not routinely recommended. Studies have shown that these agents may result in resumption of ovulation; thus, the patient should be counseled about contraception.

- Hirsutism, menstrual abnormality, infertility, and anovulation characterize polycystic ovarian syndrome.
- Serum concentrations of testosterone are normal or modestly increased but usually <200 ng/mL.
- Ultrasonographic findings of polycystic-appearing ovaries are not sufficient to make the diagnosis.
- Patients are usually obese, have insulin resistance, and are at increased risk for glucose intolerance or type 2 diabetes mellitus.

Late-onset Congenital Adrenal Hyperplasia

Congenital adrenal hyperplasia (CAH) is due to an inherited (autosomal recessive) deficiency of one of the steroidogenic enzymes necessary for the synthesis of corticosteroid hormones by the adrenal gland. The disorder may present in a "classic" fashion in the neonatal or postnatal period. This usually occurs with severe enzyme deficiency. However, cases of mild enzyme deficiency can present after puberty. The commonest cause is 21-hydroxylase deficiency (90%), but deficiency of 11β-hydroxylase or 3β-hydroxysteroid dehydrogenase also leads to CAH. Such blocks in the steroidogenic pathway result in the accumulation of precursor molecules proximal to the site of block. These precursors are shunted into pathways that lead to the synthesis of androgens. The process is ACTH-dependent and, thus, can be suppressed by dexamethasone. In 21-hydroxylase deficiency, the concentration of 17-hydroxyprogesterone is usually increased (>300 ng/dL), and if it is normal, an ACTH stimulation test is indicated. A concentration of 17-hydroxyprogesterone greater than 1,200 ng/dL 30 minutes after stimulation is diagnostic.

Virilizing Tumors of the Ovary and Adrenal Gland

These tumors can occur at any age; they produce severe hyperandrogenism, with a rapid onset and progression. Adrenal tumors characteristically are associated with high levels of DHEAS, whereas ovarian tumors produce high levels of testosterone. Diagnosis requires appropriate imaging. Rarely, selective venous sampling is required to localize the source of androgen excess.

Therapy of Hirsutism

Oral contraceptives are used in the management of idiopathic hirsutism and polycystic ovarian syndrome. They act by suppressing LH production, which in turn decreases ovarian testosterone production. It is important to avoid agents with androgenic progestins. Spironolactone is an androgen receptor blocker. Because it causes menstrual dysfunction, it often is combined with an oral contraceptive agent (some form of contraception is required because spironolactone may cause abnormal development of genitalia in a male fetus). A patient who receives medical therapy should be counseled that an effect may not be seen for 6 months. Also, because treatment is not effective against established hair, some form of mechanical hair removal is desirable early during therapy.

- In hirsutism, medical therapy is used to decrease androgen production or to inhibit the effect of androgens on hair follicles.

HYPERLIPIDEMIAS

Disorders of lipoprotein metabolism predispose to premature ischemic heart disease and vascular disease. In some patients, an extreme increase in triglyceride concentrations can lead to acute pancreatitis.

Etiology

Increases in total cholesterol and triglyceride concentrations may be caused by a coexisting disorder (e.g., poorly controlled diabetes mellitus) or the use of drugs (e.g., corticosteroids). In the absence of precipitating factors, an increase in lipoprotein concentration is termed "primary hyperlipidemia." It is the result of genetic (e.g., absence of the low-density lipoprotein [LDL] receptor) or acquired defects (due to an interaction of aging, weight gain, poor diet, sedentary lifestyle, and genetic predisposition).

- Hyperlipidemias: genetic or acquired disorders that can result from increased production or reduced clearance (or both).

Some of the primary hyperlipidemias are outlined in Table 6-3, and the causes of secondary hyperlipidemia are outlined in Table 6-4.

Clinical Features

Most patients with hyperlipidemia have no physical findings attributable directly to increased concentrations of lipoprotein. Some patients have a corneal arcus (arcus senilis), but the significance of this finding decreases with increasing age. Patients with an extreme increase in LDL may exhibit tendon xanthomas or thickening of the Achilles tendon. Other patients

Table 6-3 Features of Primary Hyperlipidemias

Feature	Familial hypercholesterolemia	Familial combined hyperlipidemia	Familial dysbetalipoproteinemia	Familial hypertriglyceridemia	Severe hypertriglyceridemia	
					Early onset	Adult onset
Pathophysiology	Defective LDL receptor or defective apo B-100; impaired catabolism of LDL	Overproduction of hepatic VLDL-apo B-100 but not of VLDL-Tg	Defective or absent apo E; excess of CM-remnants and VLDL in fasting state	Overproduction of hepatic VLDL-Tg but not of apo B-100	Lipoprotein lipase deficiency Apo C-II deficiency; defect in CM & VLDL catabolism	Overproduction of VLDL triglyceride Delayed catabolism of chylomicrons and VLDL
Mode of inheritance	Autosomal codominant	Autosomal dominant	Autosomal recessive	Autosomal dominant	Autosomal recessive	Autosomal recessive
Estimated population frequency	1:500	1:50	1:5,000	1:50	<1:10,000	Rare
Risk of CAD	+++	++	+	+ in families in which HDL-C is deficient	−	+
Physical findings	Arcus senilis Tendinous xanthomas	Arcus senilis	Arcus senilis Tuboeruptive & palmar xanthomas	None	Lipemia retinalis Eruptive xanthomas	Milky plasma Lipemia retinalis Eruptive xanthomas Pancreatitis
Associated findings		Obesity Glucose intolerance Hyperuricemia HDL deficiency	Obesity Glucose intolerance Hyperuricemia	Obesity Glucose intolerance Hyperuricemia HDL deficiency	HDL deficiency Recurrent abdominal pain Pancreatitis Hepatosplenomegaly	Obesity Glucose intolerance Hyperuricemia HDL deficiency Pancreatitis
Treatment	Diet Niacin & resin Statin & resin Probucol & resin	Diet Drugs singly or in combination with niacin, statin, gemfibrozil, resin	Diet Niacin Gemfibrozil Statin	Diet Niacin Gemfibrozil Abstain from alcohol, estrogen	Diet Fish oil	Diet Control diabetes when present Avoid alcohol, estrogen Gemfibrozil Fish oil

C, cholesterol; CAD, coronary artery disease; CM, chylomicrons; HDL, high-density lipoprotein; LDL, low-density lipoprotein; Tg, triglyceride; VLDL, very-low-density lipoprotein; +++, very high; ++, high; +, moderate; −, no increased risk.

with an increase in intermediate-density lipoprotein (IDL) may have palmar tuboeruptive xanthomas. In hyperchylomicronemia, eruptive xanthomas may develop on the buttocks.

Increased LDL, increased IDL, increased Lp(a) lipoprotein, and decreased high-density lipoprotein (HDL) all confer an increased risk of atherosclerotic vascular disease. Increased HDL is associated with decreased atherogenic risk.

Hypertriglyceridemia may be atherogenic by inducing alterations in other lipoproteins (e.g., it may decrease HDL and increase small-density LDL, very-low-density lipoprotein [VLDL] remnants, and IDL) and, in addition, may have an unidentified direct atherogenic action. Pancreatitis may develop with increases in triglyceride-rich lipoproteins (>1,000 mg/dL).

Table 6-4   Causes of Secondary Hyperlipidemias

Increased LDL cholesterol	Increased triglycerides	Decreased HDL
Hypothyroidism	Obesity	Hypertriglyceridemia
Dysglobulinemia	Diabetes mellitus	Obesity
Nephrotic syndrome	Hypothyroidism	Diabetes mellitus
Obstructive liver disease	Sedentary life	Cigarette smoking
Progestins	Alcohol	Sedentary life
Anabolic steroids, glucocorticoid therapy	Renal insufficiency	β-Blockers
Anorexia nervosa	Estrogens	Progestins
Acute intermittent porphyria	β-Blockers	Anabolic steroids
	Thiazides, steroids	
	Dysglobulinemias	
	Systemic lupus erythematosus	

HDL, high-density lipoprotein; LDL, low-density lipoprotein.

- Clinical presentations: ischemic vascular disease, pancreatitis, or xanthomas.

Diagnosis

The Adult Treatment Panel of the National Cholesterol Education Program has recommended that all adults older than 20 be evaluated for hypercholesterolemia to identify those at risk for coronary artery disease. Lipid screening tests should not be performed during an acute illness or hospitalization. Plasma triglyceride concentrations vary considerably after meals and must be measured in the fasting state. Provided plasma triglyceride concentrations are less than 400 mg/dL, LDL can be reliably estimated by use of the Friedwald equation [LDL = total cholesterol − (HDL + 5 × triglycerides)].

Lp(a) lipoprotein is believed to be an independent risk factor for vascular disease. It should be measured only in patients with a strong family history of premature ischemic heart disease who do not have conventional risk factors or in patients with established coronary artery disease who have progressive disease despite control of conventional risk factors.

- Lipid screening tests should not be conducted during an acute illness or hospitalization.

Nonmodifiable risk factors for cardiovascular disease include age older than 45 for men and 55 for women. Note that a woman with premature menopause who is not receiving estrogen replacement therapy is at increased risk for premature cardiovascular disease. A family history of premature coronary artery disease (myocardial infarction or sudden death before age 55 of a parent or sibling) confers increased risk. Modifiable risk factors include smoking, hypertension, diabetes mellitus, and an HDL less than 35 mg/dL. An HDL greater than 60 mg/dL confers protection against cardiovascular disease.

- Assessment of other coronary risk factors is important for evaluating the overall atherogenic risk and planning effective management.

Therapy

The National Cholesterol Education Program Guidelines are used to guide therapy (Table 6-5). The target LDL level depends on the presence of ischemic heart disease (secondary prevention) or risk factors for ischemic heart disease (primary prevention). High-risk patients have two or more risk factors.

Treatment requires dietary and lifestyle modification and correction of secondary causes when feasible (e.g., treatment of hypothyroidism or diabetes mellitus) in conjunction with the appropriate use of lipid-lowering agents.

Diet Therapy

Dietary therapy is used to achieve and maintain a normal body weight. A typical healthy diet can be provided by following the American Heart Association step I diet, which provides for 30% or fewer calories from fat and 10% or fewer calories from saturated fat. Alcohol restriction often decreases triglyceride concentrations.

Behavior Modification

Weight reduction enhances the cholesterol-lowering effect of an appropriate diet, decreases triglycerides, increases HDL, decreases blood pressure, and improves glucose tolerance. Smoking cessation and regular exercise also increase HDL.

Drug Therapy

After drug therapy for hyperlipidemia has been instituted, it is likely to be lifelong. Therefore, drug therapy should be embarked upon only after vigorous efforts at dietary and lifestyle modification. Both the physician and the patient should be

Table 6-5 Overview of Therapy for Hyperlipidemias

Clinical risk assessment	Initiate diet	Initiate drug therapy	Goal of therapy
No CAD; less than two risk factors	>160 mg/dL	>190 mg/dL	<160 mg/dL
No CAD; two or more risk factors	>130 mg/dL	>160 mg/dL	<130 mg/dL
CAD step II AHA diet	>100 mg/dL	>130 mg/dL	<100 mg/dL

AHA, American Heart Association; CAD, coronary artery disease.

made aware of the potential risks associated with lipid-lowering agents. The teratogenic potential of most of these drugs should also be borne in mind when prescribing them for females of childbearing age. Patients should be monitored for potential side effects as well as for the efficacy of the medication in reaching the predetermined goals. Lipid concentrations should be checked approximately 3 months after therapy has been instituted. If the lipid goals are not achieved, the dose may need to be increased. However, combination therapy may need to be considered for some patients. Because of the increased risk of myositis or hepatitis (or both), combination therapy should be reserved for secondary prevention in established cardiovascular disease.

Treatment of Increased LDL

In most instances, a statin is the drug of choice for the treatment of increased concentration of LDL. In estrogen-deficient women, estrogen replacement therapy is effective in decreasing LDL and increasing HDL. However, oral estrogens should not be given to patients with hypertriglyceridemia; for these patients, a transdermal estrogen patch may be considered. It must be noted that recent studies of long-term estrogen use do not provide evidence of dramatic benefit in cardiovascular outcomes. Patients who do not reach their therapeutic goals will benefit from the addition of a resin (colesevelam or cholestyramine) to the statin. Niacin can also be used for the treatment of increased LDL. However, few patients are able to tolerate this medication long-term because of its side effects, most notably facial flushing and worsening of glucose tolerance.

Treatment of Hypertriglyceridemia

Extreme hypertriglyceridemia (>1,000 mg/dL) requires timely treatment to reduce the risk of pancreatitis. This includes cessation of oral estrogen or alcohol use, better control of diabetes, and restriction of caloric intake. Fibrates such as gemfibrozil or fenofibrate are the drugs of choice. Most patients with hypertriglyceridemia have glucose intolerance or diabetes. These disorders are a relative contraindication to niacin, which increases insulin resistance and may worsen glycemic control. Fish oil capsules (1 g) at a dose of 8 to 10 capsules daily may also be effective.

Treatment of Low HDL

In the absence of heart disease, lifestyle modification is the intervention of choice in conjunction with an attempt to discontinue drugs that can lower HDL (e.g., androgens). In the presence of ischemic heart disease, lowering LDL to less than 100 mg/dL is indicated. Drugs that can increase HDL include niacin, statins, and, to a lesser extent, fibrates. In postmenopausal women, estrogen replacement therapy can increase HDL concentrations.

Treatment of Increased Lp(a) Lipoprotein

There is no effective treatment for increased concentrations of Lp(a) lipoprotein. Niacin may produce some modest decrease. Some authorities advocate intervention to lower LDL to less than 100 mg/dL in patients with increased Lp(a) lipoprotein. Estrogen replacement therapy may be effective in postmenopausal women.

DIABETES MELLITUS

Etiology and Classification

Diabetes mellitus is a metabolic disorder characterized by increased fasting and postprandial concentrations of glucose. It is the commonest metabolic disorder and affects about 10% of the U.S. population. The classification of this disorder into two broad categories is somewhat artificial and the reader should recognize that a degree of overlap exists. Type 1 diabetes mellitus (T1D) is characterized by immune destruction of the insulin-producing beta cells in the islets of Langerhans. It affects 10% to 20% of the diabetic population and usually appears at a younger age. Most patients eventually lose all endogenous insulin secretion and are prone to the development of ketoacidosis.

A complex interaction between genes and the environment leads to the development of T1D. This is illustrated by the 50% concordance for the disease seen in monozygotic twins when one of the twin pair has T1D. This disease is associated frequently with certain histocompatibility antigen (HLA) types, with polymorphisms of the insulin gene and other variants in immune response genes with weak contributions to the pathogenesis of this disorder. Antibodies to islets or some constituent of the islets are frequently present, at least in the early stages of the disease (islet-cell antibodies and glutamic acid decarboxylase [GAD] antibodies) and help to differentiate T1D from type 2 diabetes mellitus (T2D). Often, a "honeymoon" period is observed, during which insulin requirements decrease dramatically after restoration of euglycemia. The duration of this phase is highly variable.

- T1D is characterized by immune destruction of the islets, which leads to insulin deficiency.
- Concordance is seen in 50% of monozygotic twins.

The pathogenesis of T2D is more complex. It is characterized by abnormalities of insulin secretion and insulin action in target tissues such as the liver, muscle, and adipose tissue. The ability of glucose to stimulate its own uptake and to suppress its own release is also defective. Impaired suppression of glucagon secretion after the ingestion of a meal also contributes to postprandial hyperglycemia in these patients. Although T2D usually appears in older, obese patients, it increasingly has been described in obese, sedentary children and adolescents. T2D is more common among certain ethnic groups. Monozygotic twins exhibit almost 100% concordance if one of the twins is affected. The overall genetic contribution to the pathogenesis of T2D is greater than in T1D. However, individual genes have a weaker contribution than in T1D, for example, HLA polymorphisms in T1D. Environmental factors such as obesity also have a definite role in the development of the disease.

- T2D is characterized by defective insulin secretion and action.
- Environmental factors such as obesity have an important role in the development of T2D.
- T2D can occur at any age.

Maturity-onset diabetes of the young (MODY) describes a group of single-gene disorders that present as diabetes at a young age. MODY is usually inherited as an autosomal dominant trait. Various mutations are responsible for this disorder, and the clinical expression is variable.

Clinical Features

The onset of T1D is usually quite dramatic, with weight loss, polyuria, and polydipsia. Often, it is precipitated by an infection or other severe physical stress because patients lack the reserve of endogenous insulin secretion to overcome the effects of counter-regulatory hormones (glucagon, cortisol, growth hormone, and epinephrine) on glucose

metabolism. Severe dehydration and ketoacidosis may be present. In very young children, nocturnal enuresis may signal the onset of disease.

T2D usually has an insidious onset. Often, the disease is diagnosed during routine laboratory testing by the presence of glycosuria or fasting hyperglycemia. Patients may complain of blurring of vision, myopia, episodes of recurrent skin infections, monilial vaginitis (females), and balanitis (males). Occasionally, patients may present with evidence of chronic diabetic complications (neuropathy, nephropathy, or retinopathy) but without symptoms related to glucose intolerance. Symptoms such as polyuria, polydipsia, and polyphagia may only develop in situations of increased insulin resistance such as pregnancy, infection, or steroid use. Also, patients occasionally present with hyperosmolar nonketotic coma.

- T1D has a dramatic onset related to abrupt severe insulin deficiency, with polyuria, polydipsia, weight loss despite polyphagia, severe dehydration, and ketoacidosis.
- T2D has an insidious onset and may present with complications. Under certain conditions, polyuria, polydipsia, and polyphagia may develop.

Diagnosis

The normal fasting plasma glucose concentration is less than 105 mg/dL. In adults (but not pregnant women), fasting values of 126 mg/dL or greater on two or more occasions confirm the diagnosis of diabetes mellitus. Fasting values between 110 mg/dL and 125 mg/dL encompass the class of impaired fasting glucose. In July 1997, the American Diabetes Association recommended lowering the level for diagnosis from 140 mg/dL to 126 mg/dL because epidemiologic data demonstrated a progressive increase in microvascular complications with progressive impairment in fasting glucose concentrations greater than 105 mg/dL.

- In adults (not pregnant women), fasting plasma glucose values >126 mg/dL on two or more occasions confirm the diagnosis of diabetes mellitus.

Oral Glucose Tolerance Test

Currently, the main utility of glucose tolerance testing is during pregnancy, when it is used to screen for gestational diabetes mellitus. Epidemiologic data have demonstrated that impaired glucose tolerance is a marker for increased cardiovascular morbidity (in some cohorts) and mortality. However, the clinical application of glucose tolerance testing in this situation is unknown. Current therapy does not adequately treat postprandial hyperglycemia without causing fasting hypoglycemia.

Therapy for T1D

Insulin replacement is the cornerstone of therapy for T1D. The optimal regimen allows the patient to maintain a healthy, active lifestyle, with optimal glycemic control and minimal hypoglycemia. This can be achieved with intensive insulin therapy, but it requires considerable commitment from the patient to self-monitor plasma glucose concentrations and to adjust insulin dosage accordingly. The Diabetes Control and Complications Trial has demonstrated conclusively that intensive therapy with tight glycemic control prevents or markedly decreases the risks of chronic microvascular complications of diabetes.

Nutrition

Intake should allow for maintenance of a reasonable weight and for growth in children and adolescents. Protein should comprise 10% to 20% of total calories, total fat should account for less than 30% of calories (saturated fat, for less than 10%), and complex carbohydrates should comprise the rest.

Exercise

The glycemic response to exercise varies depending on the duration and type of exercise, the fitness of the person, and the relationship of exercise to meals and insulin injections. Blood glucose levels should be monitored before and after exercise to determine the response to exercise and to prevent hypoglycemia. Patients should always carry appropriate identification and have access to glucose or glucagon (or both).

Insulin Therapy

Intensive insulin therapy allows the use of insulin in a fashion that mimics insulin secretion by the healthy pancreas. Short-acting insulin (regular or lispro) is injected at mealtimes to facilitate disposal of the meal, and a once-daily long-acting insulin (ultralente or glargine insulin) is taken to replace basal insulin secretion.

An insulin pump provides a continuous subcutaneous infusion of insulin in a programmed fashion. It also is used to provide meal-stimulated insulin secretion, and it allows the patient to change the infusion rate of "basal" insulin (during exercise or at night).

The insulin dosage required for a typical patient with T1D who is within 20% of ideal body weight and does not have intercurrent illness approximates 0.5 to 1.0 U/kg daily. The insulin requirements may increase markedly during intercurrent illness.

The glycemic goals are individualized according to the presence of intercurrent disease (ischemic heart disease or cerebrovascular disease), diabetic complications, and the ability to perceive hypoglycemia. If a female who has T1D is considering pregnancy or is pregnant, tighter control is important to decrease the risk of birth defects or macrosomia.

- Intensive insulin therapy attempts to simulate normal insulin secretion, with a combination of short-acting and long-acting insulin.
- An insulin pump allows the patient to adjust basal insulin levels as needed.

Glycemic Goals of Optimal Therapy

Blood glucose targets are as follows: fasting, 70 to 130 mg/dL, and bedtime, 100 to 140 mg/dL. Hemoglobin A_{1C} should be less than 7%. Higher target levels are required for patients at risk for hypoglycemia because of their inability to recognize hypoglycemic symptoms.

Monitoring

On most days, the blood glucose concentration should be self-monitored 4 times daily—before meals and at bedtime. If the patient has unexplained morning hypoglycemia or hyperglycemia, blood glucose should be measured at 2 AM to 4 AM. Hemoglobin A_{1C} should be measured every 2 to 3 months.

- Hemoglobin A_{1C} should be monitored every 2 to 3 months; the goal is <7%.
- The patient should self-monitor blood glucose at least 4 times daily. The goal is 70-130 mg/dL fasting and 100-140 mg/dL at bedtime.

Therapy for T2D

Most patients with T2D are obese and lead sedentary lifestyles. Often, they have multiple cardiovascular risk factors such as hypertension and dyslipidemia. Therapy should include appropriate modification of these risk factors, appropriate exercise and nutrition, and achievement of appropriate glycemic control with a near-normal hemoglobin A_{1C}.

Calorie restriction while consuming a healthy, balanced diet is appropriate to promote weight reduction. Exercise improves insulin action, facilitates weight loss, reduces cardiovascular risks (increases HDL, decreases VLDL-triglycerides), and increases a patient's sense of well-being. If the patient has preexisting coronary or peripheral vascular disease, exercise recommendations should be modified appropriately.

- The treatment goals for T2D include appropriate lifestyle modification, modification of cardiovascular risk factors, and optimal glycemic control.
- Calorie restriction is appropriate to promote weight reduction.
- A prudent exercise program facilitates weight reduction and improves insulin action, cardiovascular fitness, and the sense of well-being.

Drug Therapy for T2D

Sulfonylureas are insulin secretagogues. These agents bind to the sulfonylurea receptor on beta cells, causing closure of potassium channels, with the subsequent influx of calcium and exocytosis of insulin. The efficacy of these medications depends on the presence of endogenous insulin secretion. Primary failure occurs in the absence of endogenous insulin secretion. Secondary failure occurs with progression of disease, when sulfonylureas are no longer effective in achieving glycemic control.

Repaglinide and *nateglinide* belong to a new class of oral hypoglycemic agents that have an extremely short half-life and act in a fashion similar to sulfonylureas. These agents are taken before each meal (the dose is skipped if the meal is missed).

Metformin is a biguanide, a class of drugs that improves the liver action of insulin. Lactic acidosis is extremely rare if the specific exclusion criteria for the use of metformin are followed: 1) renal impairment—plasma creatinine value of 1.5 or greater for men and 1.4 for women, 2) cardiac or respiratory insufficiency that is likely to cause central hypoxia or reduced peripheral perfusion, 3) history of lactic acidosis, 4) severe infection that could lead to reduced tissue perfusion, 5) liver disease, 6) alcohol abuse with binge drinking, and 7) use of intravenous radiographic contrast agents. For hospitalized patients, it is prudent to withhold metformin therapy.

Thiazolidenediones chiefly improve peripheral insulin action. Troglitazone, the first member of the class to be used clinically, has been discontinued because of its association with severe hepatotoxicity. The newer members of the group, rosiglitazone and pioglitazone, do not contain a vitamin E moiety, which is thought to account for the hepatotoxicity associated with troglitazone. Nevertheless, it is recommended that liver function be monitored closely during treatment with these drugs. Thiazolidenediones can cause marked fluid retention and should not be prescribed if the patient has congestive heart failure.

- Sulfonylureas are insulin secretagogues. Their efficacy depends on the presence of some degree of endogenous insulin secretion.
- Metformin improves the action of insulin in the liver. Its use should be avoided in certain circumstances because of the risk of lactic acidosis.
- Thiazolidenediones improve peripheral insulin action but are associated with fluid retention.
- Repaglinide and nateglinide are short-acting agents that increase insulin secretion; they are taken before meals.

Insulin is reserved for patients with T2D in whom diet and oral agents (monotherapy and combination therapy) have failed to achieve adequate glycemic control. It is the preferred therapy during pregnancy and when patients are undergoing surgical treatment or are severely ill. Patients with T2D often have some degree of meal-stimulated endogenous insulin secretion, which allows treatment with simpler insulin regimens than for T1D. Once-daily injections of intermediate-acting insulin in combination with an oral agent or twice-daily injections of intermediate-acting insulin are commonly used to manage T2D. Insulin therapy is associated with some degree of weight gain in most patients. For this reason, insulin sometimes is given in combination with metformin to help limit weight gain. In patients who have a more severe insulin deficiency, an intensive insulin program or a split mix program may be used (e.g., NR-0-NR-0).

- Simple insulin regimens are useful for patients with T2D who have experienced secondary failure (e.g., intermediate insulin once or twice daily; supplement once daily dosing with an oral agent if necessary).
- Prescribe an intensive insulin program or split mix program (e.g., NR-0-NR-0) for patients with severe insulin deficiency.

Combination Therapy

Combination therapy is frequently prescribed for T2D if maximal therapy with a single agent fails to achieve adequate glycemic control. This takes advantage of the different mechanisms of action of oral agents. A commonly used regimen is the combination of a sulfonylurea with metformin.

- Combination therapy with metformin and a sulfonylurea significantly improves control when therapy with one agent fails.

Hypoglycemia in Diabetes

Hypoglycemia occurs when there is a mismatch between glucose availability and glucose requirements. This may be due to unplanned exercise, inappropriate dosing of insulin, or inadequate caloric intake. Patients with T1D are prone to the development of hypoglycemia unawareness, which develops after repeated neuroglycopenia. This may require appropriate adjustment of glycemic goals because the prevention of hypoglycemia has been shown to reverse or ameliorate hypoglycemia unawareness. Many episodes of severe hypoglycemia occur at night and may not be apparent if glucose is checked at bedtime and at breakfast. Occasionally, patients report symptoms such as nightmares, morning headache, or night sweats. It is important to emphasize the need for periodic self-monitoring of blood glucose between 1:00 AM and 3:00 AM. Preventive strategies for nocturnal hypoglycemia include increasing the bedtime snack or modifying the insulin regimen.

Patients with long-standing T1D also have defective counterregulation because they are unable to secrete glucagon and become dependent on the autonomic nervous system to respond to hypoglycemia. The use of β-blockers in these situations can abolish all acute responses to hypoglycemia.

Insulin clearance is delayed by renal impairment and by circulating insulin antibodies. Alcohol may interfere with gluconeogenesis as well as the perception of hypoglycemic symptoms. Hypoglycemia may be a manifestation of cortisol deficiency (patients with T1D are at increased risk for other autoimmune endocrinopathies).

- Patients with T1D are especially prone to hypoglycemia.
- Episodes of severe hypoglycemia may occur during the night—check the blood glucose level between 1:00 AM and 3:00 AM.
- Hypoglycemia may be precipitated by exercise, decreased caloric intake, renal insufficiency, and cortisol deficiency.

Acute Complications of Diabetes Mellitus

Diabetic Ketoacidosis

Diabetic ketoacidosis occurs in patients with T1D and may be the initial presentation of diabetes. It is characterized by polyuria, polydipsia, dehydration, anorexia, nausea and vomiting, abdominal pain, tachypnea, obtundation, and coma. The physical findings include clinical evidence of dehydration, decreased mentation, deep and rapid Kussmaul respiration, and a characteristic breath odor (acetone). Often, diabetic ketoacidosis is precipitated by a failure to take insulin or to increase insulin and consume extra fluids during acute illness, infection, or other intercurrent illness such as myocardial infarction, pancreatitis, stroke, or trauma.

The diagnosis is based on the demonstration of moderate to severe hyperglycemia, ketonemia, and metabolic acidosis. Associated biochemical abnormalities include hyponatremia, azotemia, and hyperamylasemia. Serum levels of potassium, phosphate, and magnesium (despite large body losses) may be normal. However, concentrations of these ions often decrease precipitously after the acidosis has been corrected.

- Diabetic ketoacidosis occurs in the presence of severe insulin deficiency and is often precipitated by intercurrent illness.
- It may be the initial manifestation of T1D.
- Diagnosis requires the presence of pronounced hyperglycemia, ketonemia, and metabolic acidosis.
- Serum levels of potassium may be normal despite large body losses.
- A thorough search for precipitating factors should be undertaken in all cases.

Treatment

Treatment of diabetic ketoacidosis requires correction of the metabolic state and electrolyte depletion. These goals are achieved by the administration of insulin, the replacement of fluid and electrolytes, and treatment of precipitating factors.

Insulin therapy—Insulin infusion is preferred over subcutaneous or intramuscular injection. A priming dose of 10 to 20 units intravenously is followed by insulin infusion (5-10 U/h). This allows suppression of lipolysis and ketogenesis and stimulates glucose uptake.

Fluids—Fluids are given intravenously to restore volume and to correct electrolyte and fluid losses. The average fluid deficit in adults is 5 to 8 L. Approximately 4 L should be replaced in the first few hours. As plasma glucose values approach 250 mg/dL, change to 0.45% saline in 5% dextrose in water. This allows maintenance of intravenous insulin while keeping the plasma glucose about 200 mg/dL during the first 12 hours, permitting correction of ketosis and avoiding a rapid decrease in osmolarity with its risk of cerebral edema.

Electrolytes—The potassium deficit is about 300 to 500 mEq. Regardless of the initial serum level of potassium, the total body stores of potassium are low. With correction of the acidosis, the serum level of potassium decreases. Potassium should be added to the intravenous fluids as soon as renal perfusion and urine flow are assured. Add 40 mEq of potassium, as potassium chloride, to each liter of intravenous fluid. Phosphate repletion is indicated by phosphate levels less than 1 mg/dL. Give phosphate in a dose of 0.08 mM/kg intravenously over 6 hours. (Neutral potassium phosphate: 1 ampule contains 3 mM phosphate and 15 mEq of potassium.) Monitor the serum level of phosphate carefully because of the risk of hypocalcemia, seizures, and death.

Prognosis

The mortality rate of diabetic ketoacidosis is 5% to 15% and, in most patients, is due to an associated precipitating illness such as myocardial infarction, stroke, or sepsis. After successful therapy, the goal is to avoid recurrence by educating the patient.

- Prognosis: 5%-15% mortality, usually from associated illness.
- After successful therapy, the goal is to avoid recurrence.

Hyperglycemic Hyperosmolar Nonketotic Coma

Hyperglycemic hyperosmolar nonketotic coma is characterized by hyperglycemia, hyperosmolar dehydration, and the absence of ketoacidosis. It usually occurs in poorly treated T2D when there is sufficient insulin to inhibit excess lipolysis and ketogenesis but not enough to suppress hepatic glucose production or to stimulate peripheral glucose uptake. High concentrations of urine glucose provoke an osmotic diuresis, with marked dehydration and subsequently decreased renal function. It often is precipitated by acute illness such as myocardial infarction, pancreatitis, pneumonia, or surgery.

Diagnosis

Hyperglycemic hyperosmolar nonketotic coma should be suspected in any patient with diabetes who presents with an altered level of consciousness and severe dehydration. Laboratory abnormalities include marked hyperglycemia (often >600 mg/dL), absence of ketones, and increased plasma osmolarity (>320 mOsm/L). A search for an underlying disorder is an integral part of the evaluation.

- Hyperglycemic hyperosmolar nonketotic coma is characterized by hyperglycemia and dehydration without ketoacidosis.
- The disorder should be suspected in any patient with diabetes who has altered sensorium and severe dehydration.
- Laboratory evaluation demonstrates marked hyperglycemia (>600 mg/dL), no significant ketosis, and plasma hyperosmolarity (>320 mOsm/L).
- Always search for a precipitating disorder.

Therapy

The objectives of treatment are to restore volume and osmolarity and to control the hyperglycemia. Fluid resuscitation with normal saline should be followed by 0.45% saline to correct the hyperosmolarity. Insulin is administered intravenously, but it is important to decrease the plasma glucose level gradually to a level between 200 and 300 mg/dL to avoid cerebral edema. At this stage, the infusion of insulin should be discontinued, and it should be given subcutaneously. Electrolyte replacement as outlined above for diabetic ketoacidosis is also important. Repeated neurologic evaluation is essential because focal deficits or seizures may become apparent during therapy. Complications include vascular events such as myocardial infarction or stroke, cerebral edema, and hypokalemia. The mortality rate is 50%.

- Treatment: fluid and electrolyte replacement and management of hyperglycemia.
- Hyperglycemic hyperosmolar nonketotic coma has a mortality rate of 50%.

Chronic Complications of Diabetes Mellitus

Microvascular Disease in Diabetes

Chronic hyperglycemia and other metabolic abnormalities associated with diabetes lead to damage of the microcirculation. This is manifested clinically as diabetic retinopathy,

nephropathy, and neuropathy. Some degree of diabetic retinopathy occurs in 50% to 70% of patients with T1D within 10 years after diagnosis and reaches a prevalence of 95% by 15 to 20 years; it is rare in those who have had T1D for less than 5 years. Diabetic retinopathy is present in 15% to 20% of patients at the time of diagnosis of T2D and reaches 50% by 15 years. Background diabetic retinopathy is characterized by microaneurysms, hard exudates, hemorrhages, and macular edema. Proliferative retinopathy occurs when areas of the retina are ischemic; this provides a stimulus to the growth of new vessels. These vessels are fragile and prone to hemorrhage, which can lead to loss of vision. Panretinal photocoagulation is used to treat proliferative retinopathy. The destruction of ischemic areas of the retina decreases the stimulus for neovascularization and progression of proliferative retinopathy. The treatment of hypertension, hyperglycemia, glaucoma, and dyslipidemia is also important in these circumstances. Patients should have an annual dilated ophthalmic examination by an experienced ophthalmologist to identify those at risk.

Infections and Diabetes

Cutaneous skin infections are often a presenting feature of poorly controlled T2D. Typical infections include candidiasis as well as furuncles and carbuncles (caused by *Staphylococcus aureus* infection). Malignant external otitis due to infection with *Pseudomonas* is peculiar to diabetes and is life-threatening.

Ischemic Heart Disease in Diabetes

Ischemic cardiovascular disease appears earlier and is more extensive in persons with diabetes than in the general population. Coronary artery disease accounts for about 70% of deaths among those with diabetes and may present as sudden cardiac death. Epidemiologic studies have shown that persons with T2D have the same risk of myocardial infarction as patients who have already had a myocardial infarction. For this reason, treatment of dyslipidemia is considered to be secondary prevention in diabetes. Ischemic heart disease may present in an atypical manner; angina may present with epigastric distress, heartburn, and neck or jaw pain; myocardial infarction may be silent (in 15% of patients) and may present with sudden onset of left ventricular failure.

Hyperlipidemia in Diabetes

In poorly controlled T2D, the concentrations of triglyceride-rich lipoproteins are increased because of an overproduction of VLDL together with decreased lipoprotein lipase activity. HDL levels are low, and levels do improve but usually do not normalize with control of glucose and triglyceride levels. Compositional changes in LDL (small, dense LDL) that increase the atherogenicity of these particles are more likely to occur in patients with T2D.

Diabetes and Pregnancy

Both fasting and postprandial glucose concentrations decrease in normal pregnancy. Because of an increase in the concentration of circulating hormones such as human placental lactogen, estrogen, progesterone, and cortisol (which increase insulin resistance), insulin secretion also increases. Glucose is a major metabolic substrate for the fetus and traverses the placenta by facilitated diffusion.

Pregnancy is a diabetogenic state and may worsen glucose control in women with established diabetes. Inadequate glycemic control early in pregnancy increases the risk of congenital malformations, whereas poor control in late pregnancy increases the risk of macrosomia, neonatal hypoglycemia, hypocalcemia, polycythemia, hyperbilirubinemia, and respiratory distress. Pregnancy may exacerbate diabetic retinopathy, and nephropathy may lead to pregnancy-induced hypertension and toxemia.

Gestational diabetes complicates 2% to 3% of all pregnancies. All pregnant women older than 25 years should be evaluated at 24 to 28 weeks with a 50-g oral glucose tolerance test. Plasma glucose levels higher than 140 mg/dL 1 hour after ingestion of the glucose drink require formal testing with a 100-g glucose drink. Gestational diabetes is diagnosed if glucose values exceed 105 mg/dL (fasting), 190 mg/dL (1 hour), 165 mg/dL (2 hours), and 145 mg/dL (3 hours).

- Early detection and optimal management of diabetes during pregnancy can prevent congenital malformations and decrease neonatal morbidity and mortality.
- Gestational diabetes complicates 2%-3% of all pregnancies.
- Screen all pregnant women older than 25 years at 24-28 weeks.

Treatment

Tight glycemic control is essential in pregnancy and before conception to decrease the risk of fetal malformations. The goals of therapy are to ensure tight control of diabetes (while avoiding hypoglycemia and fasting ketonemia) and adequate nutrition and optimal weight gain. Home monitoring for blood glucose and urine ketones is important. Because postprandial glucose concentrations are closely associated with malformations and macrosomia, they are often used to guide therapy. The blood glucose concentration should be between 60 and 90 mg/dL while fasting and 70 to 140 mg/dL 1 hour after a meal.

Women with gestational diabetes who become euglycemic in the postpartum state should be followed up periodically. They are at high risk for the development of T2D (60% develop the disease within 15 years after the diagnosis of gestational diabetes) and should be encouraged to exercise, consume an appropriate diet, and make an effort to lose weight.

- Periodic follow-up of patients with gestational diabetes is necessary because 60% develop T2D within 15 years.

HYPOGLYCEMIA IN NONDIABETIC PATIENTS

Etiology

Hypoglycemic disorders may be classified into "insulin-mediated" (insulin levels not appropriately suppressed) and "noninsulin-mediated" (insulin levels suppressed). Causes of insulin-mediated hypoglycemia include insulinoma, use of sulfonylurea or exogenous insulin, and autoimmune hypoglycemia mediated by insulin antibodies that bind insulin and prevent its degradation. Noninsulin-mediated hypoglycemia may be related to alcohol use, cortisol insufficiency, or GH deficiency in children. Renal failure, liver failure, and sepsis are the common causes of noninsulin-mediated hypoglycemia in hospitalized patients. Mesenchymal or epithelial tumors may cause hypoglycemia through production of an insulin-like growth factor such as IGF-II.

- Insulin-mediated causes of hypoglycemia include insulinoma, exogenous insulin use, sulfonylurea use, and autoimmune hypoglycemia.
- Noninsulin-mediated causes of hypoglycemia include alcohol use, cortisol deficiency, childhood GH deficiency, renal failure, liver failure, sepsis, and tumors secreting IGF-II.

Clinical Features

Hypoglycemia may result in hyperadrenergic and neuroglycopenic symptoms. Hyperadrenergic symptoms include palpitations, sweating, tremor, and nervousness. Neuroglycopenic symptoms include confusion, inappropriate affect, blurred vision, diplopia, seizures, and loss of consciousness. Often, confusion or inappropriate affect are recognized by the patient's family or work colleagues. Symptoms are relieved promptly after oral nutrient intake. Patients with fasting hypoglycemia often learn to reduce symptoms by increasing the frequency of their meals; they may gain weight.

- Hypoglycemia may cause symptoms related to activation of the sympathoadrenal system and neuroglycopenia.

Diagnosis

The first essential step in the evaluation of a patient with a history suggestive of hypoglycemia is to document a low level of plasma glucose (<50 mg/dL) in the presence of symptoms and the prompt resolution of symptoms when the plasma glucose level is increased to the normal range (the Whipple triad). This can be achieved during a spontaneous episode or after provocation of symptoms by fasting. Blood glucose monitoring devices are inaccurate and unreliable when used to record low blood glucose levels and should not be used to confirm hypoglycemia or the Whipple triad.

After hypoglycemia has been confirmed, the next step is to establish its mechanism (insulin-mediated vs. noninsulin-mediated). This is achieved by simultaneously measuring the beta-cell polypeptides, insulin, and C peptide during a hypoglycemic episode (spontaneous or provoked). In insulin-mediated hypoglycemia, insulin levels do not suppress appropriately (insulin = 6 mU/mL). In patients with hyperinsulinemia, C peptide is measured to determine whether the source of insulin is endogenous or exogenous. Endogenous insulin is secreted from the pancreas with equimolar concentrations of C peptide, whereas exogenous insulin does not contain C peptide. Thus, C peptide is not suppressed (C peptide = 200 pmol/L) in endogenous hyperinsulinemia and is undetectable in exogenous hyperinsulinemia. It is essential to measure plasma sulfonylurea levels when the person is hypoglycemic because beta-cell polypeptide levels in a patient taking sulfonylureas are indistinguishable from those associated with insulinoma. The use of sulfonylureas is not always surreptitious: it may also be the result of pharmacy error or the patient mixing up his or her medications with those belonging to a family member.

- It is essential to document the Whipple triad in all patients with suspected hypoglycemic disorder: low plasma glucose at the time of symptoms and prompt resolution of symptoms following normalization of plasma glucose level.
- Blood glucose monitors should not be used to confirm hypoglycemia or the Whipple triad.
- Plasma insulin levels should be measured to determine the mechanism of hypoglycemia: insulin is not appropriately suppressed in insulin-mediated causes of hypoglycemia.
- C-peptide levels distinguish between exogenous and endogenous insulinoma: if the patient is injecting insulin, C-peptide levels are undetectable.
- Endogenous hyperinsulinemic hypoglycemia caused by insulinoma is indistinguishable from sulfonylurea use: plasma sulfonylurea should be measured in all cases of insulin-mediated hypoglycemia (while the patient is hypoglycemic).

Insulinoma

The diagnosis of insulinoma is confirmed with the demonstration of endogenous hyperinsulinemic hypoglycemia in the absence of detectable sulfonylurea in the blood. Diagnostic criteria for insulinoma include plasma concentration of insulin 6 mU/mL or greater (radioimmunoassay) and C peptide of 200 pmol/L or greater when the plasma glucose level is less than 50 mg/dL. The next step in the evaluation is an attempt at preoperative localization of the insulinoma

with ultrasonography and spiral CT of the pancreas. This is not always successful because ultrasonography and CT have a detection rate for insulinoma of only 60%. The key to successful removal of an insulinoma in patients with both positive and negative preoperative localization studies is surgical exploration of the pancreas by an experienced surgeon in combination with intraoperative ultrasonography. Almost all insulinomas can be identified and excised in this manner. Patients with insulinoma who refuse surgical excision or have persistent or recurrent malignant insulinoma may be treated with diazoxide, which inhibits insulin secretion.

- Diagnostic criteria for insulinoma are plasma insulin = 6 mU/mL and C peptide = 200 pmol/L when plasma glucose is >50 mg/dL and plasma sulfonylurea is undetectable.
- Preoperative abdominal ultrasonography and spiral CT of the pancreas localize approximately 60% of insulinomas.
- Intraoperative ultrasonography of the pancreas is a useful localization tool.

Postprandial Hypoglycemia

This is defined as symptomatic hypoglycemia occurring 1 to 5 hours after a meal. It can occur in patients who have had gastrectomy or who have rapid gastric emptying of unknown cause. The mechanism is believed to be due to the rapid entry of glucose into the small bowel, causing a rapid increase in the plasma level of glucose and dramatic secretion of insulin. So-called reactive hypoglycemia is likely not a true clinical entity. This disorder has been diagnosed in many patients on the basis of the results of an oral glucose tolerance test. However, this test is not reliable: normal subjects may demonstrate low plasma levels of glucose after an oral glucose load and remain asymptomatic, symptomatic patients often do not have associated low plasma levels of glucose, and patients who have "hypoglycemia" after oral glucose frequently have normal glucose levels following a mixed meal test.

- The oral glucose tolerance test is not useful in the evaluation and diagnosis of postprandial hypoglycemia.

Therapy

Treatment is directed at the hypoglycemia and underlying cause. For patients unable to eat or drink, 50 mL of 50% dextrose should be given intravenously and repeated in 15 minutes if necessary. If this is not available, 1 mg of glucagon can be administered subcutaneously or intramuscularly to stimulate endogenous insulin production.

- Glucagon injected subcutaneously or intramuscularly may be used to treat hypoglycemia if the oral or intravenous routes are not available.

MULTIPLE ENDOCRINE NEOPLASIA

MEN I

MEN I is a syndrome characterized by neoplasms of the parathyroid, endocrine pancreas, and anterior pituitary. It is familial and inherited as an autosomal dominant trait with high penetrance. The gene for MEN I belongs to the family of tumor suppressor genes and is located on chromosome 11.

Primary Hyperparathyroidism

This is the most common manifestation of MEN I, and it exhibits almost 100% penetrance by middle age. Parathyroid hyperplasia is usually the underlying cause. The differential diagnosis includes familial hyperparathyroidism (positive family history with no other features of MEN I) and familial hypocalciuric hypercalcemia. Treatment requires removal of most parathyroid tissue. Half of one gland may be left in situ or transplanted to the forearm to facilitate reexploration if hypercalcemia recurs.

Islet Cell Neoplasia

This is the second most common neoplasm in MEN I. Tumors may secrete pancreatic polypeptide (75%-85% of tumors), gastrin (60%), insulin (25%-35%), vasoactive intestinal peptide (VIP) (3%-5%), glucagon (5%-10%), and somatostatin (1%-5%). Islet cell tumors may also secrete other peptide hormones, including ACTH, CRH, and GHRH. One-third of these tumors are malignant. Diagnosis depends on the clinical recognition and appropriate investigation of the characteristic syndromes.

Pituitary Tumors

More than 15% of patients with MEN I have pituitary tumors. The most common tumor is a prolactinoma. Acromegaly in MEN I may be due to a pituitary tumor that secretes GH or to ectopic secretion of GHRH. Similarly, Cushing syndrome in MEN I may be caused by an ACTH-secreting pituitary tumor or ectopic secretion of ACTH or CRH.

Other Manifestations of MEN I

These include carcinoid tumors (secretion of serotonin, calcitonin, or CRH), thyroid or adrenal adenomas, and subcutaneous or visceral lipomas.

Screening for MEN I

Family screening is best done by measuring the serum levels of calcium and PTH. Laboratory evaluation or imaging studies (or both) for pancreatic or pituitary tumors are not indicated in the absence of relevant symptoms. Currently, there is no evidence that aggressive screening decreases the morbidity and mortality of MEN I.

MEN II

MEN II is subdivided into MEN IIA (medullary carcinoma of the thyroid [MTC], pheochromocytoma, and primary hyperparathyroidism) and MEN IIB (MTC, pheochromocytoma, mucosal neuromas, and marfanoid habitus). These two familial syndromes are inherited in an autosomal dominant pattern with a high degree of penetrance.

MEN IIA

MTC is the most common manifestation (>90% of cases) and is preceded by C-cell hyperplasia. Pheochromocytomas occur in about 50% of patients, and one-half are bilateral. These tumors have an increased incidence of malignancy (20%-40%). Hyperparathyroidism develops in 15% to 20% of patients.

MEN IIB

This differs from MEN IIA because of the absence of hyperparathyroidism. Also, MTC develops earlier in life and appears to be more aggressive. Hypercalcemia may be indicative of bone metastases. Mucosal neuromas are the most distinctive feature of MEN IIB and may occur on the tongue, eyelids, or lips and along the gastrointestinal tract. Intestinal neuromas may cause intermittent obstruction or diarrhea.

Genetics of MEN II

MEN II is caused by mutations in the *RET* proto-oncogene, which is present in 95% to 98% of affected persons. Screening for *RET* mutations allows early identification of patients at risk for MTC. This should be undertaken as early as possible in childhood. The presence of an *RET* mutation in a family member of a proband with MEN II is an indication for thyroidectomy.

Endocrinology Pharmacy Review
Lisa K. Buss, PharmD

Drug	Toxic/adverse effects	Drug interactions
Oral hypoglycemic agents		
Insulin	Hypoglycemia, localized reaction at injection site	See following Table
Sulfonylureas Glipizide Glyburide Glimepiride	Hypoglycemia, GI effects (nausea, diarrhea), dermatologic effects (pruritus, erythema, urticaria, photosensitivity)	See following Table
Biguanides Metformin	GI effects (diarrhea, nausea, vomiting, abdominal cramping, flatulence), metallic/abnormal taste, lactic acidosis, decreased vitamin B_{12} levels	Cimetidine, ethanol, iodinated contrast media, cationic drugs (amiloride, digoxin, morphine, procainamide, quinine, quinidine, ranitidine, trimethoprim, vancomycin)
α-Glucosidase inhibitors Acarbose Miglitol	Flatulence, abdominal bloating & pain, diarrhea	Digoxin, digestive enzymes, intestinal absorbents, sulfonylureas
Thiazolidenediones Pioglitazone Rosiglitazone	Myalgias, respiratory effects (URI, pharyngitis, sinusitis), headache, edema	Oral contraceptives
Repaglinide	Hypoglycemia, GI effects (nausea, diarrhea), musculoskeletal effects (arthralgia, back pain), respiratory effects (URI, sinusitis), headache	See following Table
Nateglinide	Respiratory effects (URI, flu-like symptoms), back pain, dizziness	None reported
Osteoporosis*		
Calcium	Constipation	Decreased calcium absorption with fiber laxatives, fluoride, iron, phenytoin, quinolones, tetracyclines
Vitamin D	None unless dose exceeds physiologic requirements	Decreased vitamin D absorption with cholestyramine & mineral oil Decreased vitamin D concentration with phenytoin & barbiturates
Calcitonin—salmon	Nasal symptoms (irritation, redness, sores), taste disorders, rhinitis	
Bisphosphonates Alendronate Risedronate	Nausea, diarrhea, abdominal pain, esophagitis, constipation	Antacids, calcium, salicylates (increased risk of GI effects)
Raloxifene	Hot flashes, GI effects (nausea, dyspepsia), respiratory effects (sinusitis, pharyngitis, flu-like symptoms), musculoskeletal effects (arthralgia, myalgia), weight gain, depression, insomnia	Cholestyramine, warfarin, estrogen
Teriparatide	Arthralgia, asthenia, leg cramps, constipation, diarrhea, dizziness, syncope, increased cough, rhinitis, nausea, hyperuricemia, hypercalcemia	None identified

Endocrinology Pharmacy Review (continued)

Drug	Toxic/adverse effects	Drug interactions
Thyroid agents		
Thyroid replacement	Unusual if dose is appropriate	Antacids, antidiabetic agents, cholestyramine,
Levothyroxine	If overdosed: weight loss, increased	colestipol, iron, oral anticoagulants
Liothyronine	appetite, palpitations, tachycardia,	
Liotrix	increased pulse rate & blood pressure	
Thyroid, dessicated	may occur	
Antithyroid agents	Dermatologic effects (pruritus, rash,	Warfarin
Methimazole	arthralgia), GI effects (nausea,	
Propylthiouracil	vomiting), loss of taste, headache	
Male reproductive drugs		
Androgenic agents	Females: amenorrhea or oligo-	Anticoagulants
Danazole	menorrhea, virilism	Tricyclic antidepressants
Fluoxymesterone	Males: gynecomastia, changes in libido,	
Methyltestosterone	headache, depression, sleep apnea,	
Testosterone	acne, hirsutism, male pattern	
	baldness	
Erectile dysfunction agents		
Sildenafil	Headache, flushing, dyspepsia, priapism	Nitrates, cimetidine, erythromycin,
		antifungals, protease inhibitors
Alprostadil	Penile pain, penile fibrosis, priaprism,	None identified
	warmth/burning in urethra	
Papaverine	Priapism, penile fibrosis, pain at	
	injection site	
Phentolamine		
Contraception	Thrombosis, hypertension, increased risk	Antibiotics, anticoagulants, anticonvulsants,
Estrogens	of cervical cancer	antifungals, corticosteroids, tricyclic
Ethinyl estradiol	Estrogen-related: nausea, bloating,	antidepressants
Mestranol	migraine headache, breast tenderness,	
Progestins	edema, cervical discharge, melasma	
Ethynodiol diacetate	Progestin-related: increased appetite,	
Desogestrel	weight gain, fatigue, acne, hair loss,	
Drospirenone	hirsutism, depression, breast regression,	
Etonogestrel	hypomenorrhea	
Gestodene		
Levonorgestrel		
Norelgestromin		
Norethindrone		
Norethindrone acetate		
Norgestimate		
Norgestrel		

Endocrinology Pharmacy Review (continued)

Drug	Toxic/adverse effects	Drug interactions
Hormone replacement therapy	Breast tenderness, breast enlargement, increased risk of ovarian cancer, possible increased risk of breast cancer	No important interactions have been reported
Estrogens		
Conjugated estrogens		
Esterified estrogens	Estrogen-related: breakthrough bleeding, spotting, thromboembolism, increased risk of endometrial cancer if estrogen therapy is unopposed, increased risk of gallbladder disease	
Estradiol		
Estropipate		
Progestins		
Medroxyprogesterone	Progestin-related: menstrual periods may resume, breast tumors, abdominal cramping	
Micronized progesterone		
Antihyperlipidemic agents		
Bile acid sequestrants		
Cholestyramine	GI effects (bloating, constipation, flatulence)	Administer at least 4 h before or 2 h after other drugs
Colestipol	Same as cholestyramine	Same as cholestyramine
Colesevelam	Dyspepsia, constipation	Same as cholestyramine
HMG-CoA reductase inhibitors ("statins")		
Lovastatin	Headache, myalgia, increased liver enzymes, diarrhea, rhabdomyolysis	CYP3A4 inhibitors,[†] fibrates
Pravastatin	Same as lovastatin	Cholestyramine, colestipol, cyclosporine, fibrates
Simvastatin	Same as lovastatin	Same as lovastatin
Atorvastatin	Same as lovastatin	Same as lovastatin
Fluvastatin	Same as lovastatin	Potent inhibitor of CYP2C9, warfarin
Fibric acid derivatives		
Gemfibrozil	Dyspepsia, diarrhea, myopathy, hepatotoxicity, cholelithiasis	Warfarin, statins, sulfonylureas
Fenofibrate	Same as gemfibrozil	Same as gemfibrozil
		Cholestyramine and colestipol (decreased fenofibrate absorption)
Nicotinic acid (niacin)		
Immediate-release	GI distress, skin flushing, tingling & warmth, headache, hypotension, hyperglycemia, hyperuricemia	Statins, cholestyramine, colestipol
Extended-release	Hepatotoxicity (>2 g daily, increased risk with sustained-release form)	
Selective cholesterol absorption inhibitor		
Ezetimibe	Diarrhea, arthralgia, adominal pain, headache, fatigue	Cyclosporine, fibric acid derivatives

GI, gastrointestinal; URI, upper respiratory tract infection.

*Patients should be instructed to take medicine with a full glass of water on arising in the morning. They should not lie down, eat, drink, or take other medications for at least a half hour after taking the medicine.

†CYP3A4 inhibitors include azole antifungals, macrolide antibiotics, diltiazem, verapamil, cyclosporine, nefazodone, fluvoxamine, ritonavir, nelfinavir, indinavir, and grapefruit juice.

Endocrinology Pharmacy Review (continued)

Drugs That Affect Hypoglycemic Effect of Insulin

Decrease effect	Increase effect
Acetazolamide	ACE inhibitors
AIDS antivirals	Alcohol
Albuterol	Anabolic steroids
Asparaginase	Antidiabetic agents
Calcitonin	β-Blockers
Contraceptives, oral	Calcium
Corticosteroids	Chloroquine
Cyclophosphamide	Clonidine
Danazol	Disopyramide
Diazoxide	Fluoxetine
Diltiazem	Guanethidine
Diuretics	Lithium carbonate
Dobutamine	MAO inhibitors
Epinephrine	Mebendazole
Estrogens	Pentamidine
Isoniazid	Propoxyphene
Lithium	Pyridoxine
Morphine	Salicylates
Niacin	Sulfonamides
Nicotine	Tetracycline
Phenothiazine	
Phenytoin	
Terbutaline	
Thiazide diuretics	
Thyroid hormones	

ACE, angiotensin-converting enzyme; AIDS, acquired immunodeficiency
   syndrome; MAO, monoamine oxidase.

Drugs That Affect Hypoglycemic Effect of Oral Hypoglycemic Agents

Decrease effect	Increase effect
β-Blockers	Androgens
Calcium channel blockers	Anticoagulants
Cholestyramine	Azole antifungals
Contraceptives, oral	Gemfibrozil
Corticosteroids	H_2 antagonists
Diazoxide estrogens	Magnesium salts
Hydantoins	MAO inhibitors
Isoniazid	Methyldopa
Niacin	Probenecid
Phenothiazine	Salicylates
Rifampin	Sulfonamides
Sympathomimetics	Tricyclic antidepressants
Thiazide diuretics	Urinary acidifiers
Thyroid agents	

MAO, monoamine oxidase.

QUESTIONS

DIABETES/LIPIDS/HYPOGLYCEMIA

Multiple Choice (choose the one best answer)

1. A 35-year-old man is referred for evaluation of his lipid status 3 months after a myocardial infarction. His family history is remarkable for a sibling who died suddenly at age 28. Physical examination reveals arcus senilis and bilateral thickening of the Achilles tendons. Since his myocardial infarction, he has been taking 80 mg of simvastatin daily (he is also taking aspirin). Currently, the lipid profile is as follows: total cholesterol 290 mg/dL, triglycerides 88 mg/dL, high-density lipoprotein (HDL) 45 mg/dL, and calculated low-density lipoprotein (LDL) of 227 mg/dL. He is asymptomatic. Further management would include all the following *except*:
   a. Family screening and counseling
   b. Addition of colesevelam or cholestyramine to the treatment regimen
   c. Electron beam CT for coronary calcification
   d. Consideration for lipoprotein apheresis
   e. Meeting with a dietitian to institute a step II diet

2. Diabetes mellitus was diagnosed in a 72-year-old man 5 months earlier when, during the course of a routine medical examination, his fasting glucose was found to be 140 mg/dL; HbA$_{1C}$ was 6.2% (normal, 4.0%-6.3%). Dietary therapy and lifestyle modification were instituted. At follow-up, the fasting glucose is 175 mg/dL and HbA$_{1C}$ is 7.5%. He has lost weight (20 lb) but complains of weakness and malaise. He has no appetite. The next step in management should be:
   a. Referral to a dietitian to advise about caloric intake
   b. CT of the abdomen
   c. Commence treatment with glipizide
   d. Commence treatment with metformin
   e. Urge the patient to cut back on physical activity

3. Diabetes mellitus was diagnosed in a 72-year-old man 18 months earlier when, during the course of a routine medical examination, fasting glucose was found to be 140 mg/dL; HbA$_{1C}$ was 6.2% (normal, 4.0%-6.3%). Dietary therapy and lifestyle modification were instituted. He returns seeking advice for weakness and malaise that have developed insidiously over the past 3 months. He has no appetite and has lost 20 lb. Over the past month, he has required assistance with stairs and getting out of bed. Leg discomfort keeps him awake at night. Currently, his fasting glucose is 75 mg/dL and HbA$_{1C}$ is 5.8%. On further testing, what is the most likely finding?

   a. Absence of femoral pulses
   b. Atrophy of the quadriceps
   c. Anesthesia to light touch and pinprick below the knee
   d. Absence of joint position and vibration sense
   e. Cutaneous changes compatible with cholesterol embolization to the feet

4. You are asked to evaluate a 50-year-old woman who has newly diagnosed diabetes mellitus. She presented with polyuria and polydipsia. Her fasting glucose was 340 mg/dL, and HbA$_{1C}$ was 8.2% (normal, 4.0%-6.3%). Body mass index was 28.5 kg/m^2. Blood pressure was normal. The examination findings were otherwise unremarkable. Other laboratory investigations were remarkable for the presence of microalbuminuria (100 mg/24 h; normal, <30 mg/24 h) and creatinine of 1.4 mg/dL (normal, 0.7-1.2 mg/dL). The next step in management should be:
   a. Measurement of glutamic acid decarboxylase (GAD) and C peptide
   b. Perform a glucagon stimulation test
   c. Dilated pupil ophthalmic examination
   d. Commence treatment with metformin
   e. Commence treatment with insulin

5. A 32-year-old woman has a 1-year history of frequent episodes of light-headedness, sweating, tremor, and blurred vision. These symptoms tend to occur when she awakens in the morning and are relieved within 10 minutes after she drinks orange juice. Her husband states that she also has had episodes of inappropriate behavior in the morning. Before this, she had been well. She takes no medications. She has a family history of type 2 diabetes mellitus (her mother takes insulin). Investigations during a spell showed the following: plasma glucose 40 mg/dL, insulin 10 mIU/L, and C peptide 250 pmol/L. Following the ingestion of orange juice, plasma glucose was 82 mg/dL. CT of the abdomen was performed before referral and documented a 1.2-cm cystic lesion in the tail of the pancreas. Which of the following statements is correct?
   a. Laboratory findings are diagnostic of insulinoma, refer for surgery
   b. Further localization studies are needed to help direct the nature of surgical intervention for excision of the insulinoma
   c. Endoscopic ultrasonography is indicated because the patient may have multiple pancreatic tumors
   d. The presence of an insulinoma has not been proven conclusively
   e. All family members should have screening tests for multiple endocrine neoplasia (MEN)

6. A 40-year-old woman has a 3-month history of frequent episodes of light-headedness, sweating, tremor, and blurred vision. She has been treated for hypertension for 6 months. One afternoon, she had an episode of confusion at work, followed by loss of consciousness accompanied by twitching movements. She was taken to the emergency department. Capillary blood glucose was 60 mg/dL (plasma glucose available later was 40 mg/dL). She regained normal consciousness after being given an injection of 50 mL 10% dextrose (repeat plasma glucose was 95 mg/dL). Investigations obtained at the time of the first measurement of plasma glucose showed the following: insulin 10 mIU/L and C peptide 250 pmol/L. Which of the following is *not* a diagnostic possibility?
   a. Surreptitious sulfonylurea use
   b. Surreptitious insulin use
   c. Insulinoma
   d. Dispensing error
   e. Noninsulinoma pancreatogenous hypersecretion syndrome (NIPHS)

7. A 52-year-old man has had diabetes for 10 years. He has no known complications and has been treated with glyburide and metformin. At his annual physical examination, the following laboratory results were obtained: fasting glucose 340 mg/dL, HbA$_{1C}$ 9.5% (normal, 4.0%-6.3%), thyroid-stimulating hormone (TSH) 5.5, creatinine 1.3 mg/dL, cholesterol 260 mg/dL, triglycerides 725 mg/dL, and HDL 25 mg/dL. Treatment priorities are:
   a. Correction of persistent hyperglycemia
   b. Thyroid hormone replacement
   c. Therapy with gemfibrozil
   d. Therapy with an angiotensin-converting enzyme (ACE) inhibitor
   e. Therapy with niacin

THYROID & BONE

8. A 58-year-old man seeks medical attention because of a 6-month history of fatigue, palpitations, and shakiness. He states that he has no other symptoms except some daytime hypersomnolence. Physical examination demonstrates increased sweating, a fine tremor of outstretched hands, and a small nontender goiter. Laboratory investigations show the following: TSH 1.2 mIU/L and free thyroxine 2.1 ng/dL. Which of the following investigations is indicated?
   a. Thyroid autoantibodies
   b. Radioactive iodine uptake
   c. Urine for amiodarone metabolites
   d. Insulin-like growth factor (IGF)-1
   e. Urine iodine excretion

9. A 48-year-old woman undergoes a carotid Doppler study for a carotid bruit detected on physical examination. The study shows a 0.8-cm nodule in the right lobe of the thyroid gland. She is otherwise asymptomatic and says she does not have dysphagia or dyspnea. She has no history of thyroid disease and no history of external radiation treatment to the head or neck as a child. There is no family history of thyroid disease. Examination findings are unremarkable. No thyroid nodule is palpable. TSH is 1.2 mIU/L. What is the next step in the management of this patient?
   a. Perform a thyroid scan
   b. Perform a fine-needle aspiration (FNA) of the thyroid nodule under ultrasonographic guidance
   c. Begin levothyroxine therapy at a dose that suppresses TSH, and repeat the neck examination in 6 months
   d. Advise surgical removal of the nodule
   e. Arrange for a follow-up visit in 6 months to 1 year

10. A 54-year-old woman is referred to you because of concern about her strength and well-being. Over the past year, she has had increasing difficulty with climbing stairs and rising from a sitting position and has complained of generalized achiness. She is not taking any medication. Physical examination shows proximal muscle weakness and ankle edema. Relevant laboratory findings include hemoglobin 9 g/dL (normochromic, normocytic), aspartate aminotransferase 60 U/L, alanine aminotransferase 75 U/L, and creatine kinase 900 U/L. What is the next step in the management of this patient?
    a. TSH
    b. Electromyography
    c. Muscle biopsy
    d. MRI of the cervical spine
    e. Serum calcium level

11. A 45-year-old woman requests consultation because she is concerned about the sudden appearance of a neck mass. It developed over the course of 2 weeks and is associated with mild discomfort that is worse at night. There is no history of previous neck irradiation. Physical examination shows a firm, indurated 3-cm nodule in the right thyroid lobe. There is no lymphadenopathy or tracheal deviation. The patient states she does not have dysphagia or breathing difficulty. Which of the following is *not* in the differential diagnosis?
    a. Anaplastic thyroid carcinoma
    b. Hemorrhage into a thyroid cyst
    c. Thyroglossal duct cyst
    d. Papillary carcinoma of the thyroid
    e. Lymphoma

12. A 44-year-old man is referred for evaluation after a wrist fracture. Subsequent bone mineral density reveals a T score of −2.8 in the lumbar spine and −2.6 in the femoral neck. He had previously been healthy and is not taking any medications. His skin, body habitus, and muscle strength are normal. Physical examination reveals a tall man with bilateral atrophic testes. What is the next step in management?
    a. Serum testosterone level
    b. Serum follicle-stimulating hormone (FSH) level
    c. Karyotype
    d. Testicular biopsy
    e. MRI of the sella turcica

13. You are asked to evaluate a 64-year-old woman admitted with acute confusion. The serum level of calcium is elevated at 13.4 mg/dL. Confusion reportedly developed over the preceding 24 hours. Which test supports the diagnosis of hypercalcemia of malignancy?
    a. Serum level of calcium >12 mg/dL
    b. Parathyroid hormone (PTH) level <1 pmol/L
    c. Undetectable PTH-related peptide (PTHrp)
    d. 25-Hydroxyvitamin D >40 ng/mL
    e. 1,25-Dihydroxyvitamin D >70 pg/mL

14. You are asked to comment on the following laboratory results: PTH 35 pmol/L, ionized calcium 4.5 mg/dL (normal, 4.65-5.3), and alkaline phosphatase 650 U/L. The patient is a 38-year-old woman who complains of aches and frequent muscle cramps. She has complained of fatigue and heavy menses for several years and is taking iron supplements. However, her hemoglobin value has remained at about 9 g/dL. Physical examination shows proximal muscle weakness and a waddling gait. Which of the following is not indicated?
    a. Measurment of 25-hydroxyvitamin D
    b. Measurement of antigliadin and antiendomysial antibodies
    c. Parathyroid imaging
    d. Screen for other vitamin deficiency
    e. Jejunal biopsy

PITUITARY

15. A 55-year-old businessman requests evaluation for fatigue, which has been present for more than 6 months. His sleep has been poor, as has his appetite. There has not been a notable change in weight. He has increasingly complained of mild, tension-type headaches. On physical examination, he has a striking facial expression, a visible goiter, and increased diaphoresis. There is no tremor, and the heart rate is 65 beats/min. The patient is not taking any medication. The next step would be to:
    a. Refer the patient to specialist care for depression
    b. Measure TSH
    c. Measure IGF-1
    d. Measure urine iodine excretion
    e. Obtain overnight oximetry

16. A 30-year-old man with a previous history of migraine is awoken by a sudden, severe headache accompanied by mild photophobia. Because of the unusual severity of the headache, he goes to the local emergency department, where he complains of a "black spot" in his right eye. The patient is noted to be confused and disoriented. Further management would include all the following *except*:
    a. MRI of the head
    b. Neurosurgical consultation
    c. Intravenous administration of corticosteroids
    d. Bromocriptine
    e. Frequent monitoring of the level of consciousness

17. During evaluation for osteopenia associated with amenorrhea, a 45-year-old woman is found to have undetectable FSH and luteinizing hormone (LH). Further testing demonstrates the following: prolactin level increased at 90 mg/dL (normal, 4-30), IGF-1 normal at 145 ng/mL, and free thyroxine 1.2 ng/dL. MRI reveals a 3-cm pituitary tumor that elevates the optic chiasm but does not compress it. The next step would be:
    a. Treatment with a dopamine agonist
    b. Gonadotropin replacement therapy
    c. High-dose corticosteroid therapy
    d. Visual field assessment and neurosurgical consultation
    e. Estrogen replacement therapy

18. A 55-year-old housewife underwent MRI after experiencing symptoms of worsening headache. She has a history of obesity and type 2 diabetes. The family history is unremarkable. The MRI findings are unremarkable except for the presence of a 0.7-cm hypodense pituitary tumor. She is referred for an endocrine evaluation. The examination findings are unremarkable. Further management would include all the following *except*:
    a. 24-Hour urine cortisol
    b. Serum prolactin
    c. IGF-1
    d. Free thyroxine
    e. Neurosurgical consultation

19. A 24-year-old woman complains of fatigue and malaise. She gave birth to a healthy infant 4 months before

presentation. She did not breastfeed. Menses have subsequently been irregular and infrequent, representing a change from before pregnancy. The family history is notable for a sister who has Hashimoto thyroiditis. The pregnancy test is negative, and the serum level of prolactin is normal. Of interest, TSH is 0.9 mIU/L (normal, 0.3-5.0) and free thyroxine is 0.8 ng/dL (normal, 0.8-1.4). The results of MRI of the pituitary are reported as normal. The next step would be to:

a. Start thyroxine replacement therapy
b. Request a neurosurgeon to perform a biopsy of the pituitary
c. Perform a water deprivation test
d. Perform a 1-μg corticotropin (ACTH) stimulation test
e. Measure IGF-1

20. A 24-year-old woman complains of fatigue and malaise. She gave birth to a healthy infant 6 months before presentation. She did not breastfeed. Menses have subsequently been irregular and infrequent, representing a change from before pregnancy. Her family physician is concerned about an increased serum level of prolactin, 190 mg/dL (normal, 4-30). MRI of the pituitary is reported to show marked enlargment of the contents of the sella turcica but no discrete tumor or impingement on the chiasm is found. The next step would be to:

a. Start bromocriptine
b. Request neurosurgical consultation
c. Start an oral contraceptive to regularize menses
d. Pregnancy test
e. Request formal visual perimetry

21. During evaluation for erectile dysfunction in association with hypogonadism, a 45-year-old man is found to have undetectable FSH and LH. Further testing documents the following: elevated level of prolactin at 2,290 mg/dL (normal, 4-30), IGF-1 is normal at 145 ng/mL, and free thyroxine is 1.2 ng/dL. MRI shows a 3.5-cm pituitary tumor that elevates the optic chiasm but does not compress it. After neurosurgical consultation, medical therapy with a dopamine antagonist is initiated. Which of the following would *not* require surgical intervention?

a. Persistent nasal drip
b. Development of a visual scotoma
c. Prolactin level of 1,500 mg/dL after 3 months of therapy; evidence of hemorrhage in the tumor on routine follow-up MRI
d. Severe, sudden headache with evidence of hemorrhage in the tumor seen on MRI
e. Severe nausea and hypotension every time the patient takes a dopamine antagonist

ANSWERS

1. Answer c.

Considering the age of the patient and his personal and family history, it is likely he is a familial hypercholesterolemia heterozygote. Aggressive lipid-lowering therapy often requires a combination of high-dose statins, a cholesterol-binding resin, and, if tolerated, the addition of nicotinic acid or a fibrate. Because of the high incidence of adverse events and patient intolerance, lipoprotein apheresis may be necessary. Drug treatment will not be successful without appropriate dietary intervention. Electron beam CT is not indicated because the patient is known to have ischemic heart disease and is expected to have high coronary calcification scores.

2. Answer b.

Mild degrees of weight loss early in the course of diabetes can have remarkable effects on glycemic control. However, this does not seem to be the case in this patient; furthermore, the accompanying malaise and fatigue are worrisome. Pancreatic carcinoma often has this presentation and must be excluded before any other recommendation is made about treatment. It must be remembered that some patients practice extreme caloric restriction in a bid to avoid the need for additional treatment and this should be considered after pancreatic carcinoma has been excluded.

3. Answer b.

The presence of painful proximal muscle weakness with marked systemic symptoms in the presence of early onset, relatively well-controlled diabetes strongly suggests diabetic amyotrophy. This is an inflammatory condition seen most commonly in diabetics (and unrelated to glycemic control). Predominantly, motor fibers are involved. Usually, the knee jerk reflex is absent and the quadriceps muscles are atrophied.

4. Answer c.

The presence of microalbuminuria in a newly diagnosed normotensive diabetic with markedly elevated HbA_{1C} suggests that hyperglycemia has been present for some time and makes type 1 diabetes unlikely. However, the most pressing concern is whether the patient has diabetic retinopathy requiring immediate treatment. A glucagon stimulation test will not be helpful in deciding whether to use insulin or an oral agent (metformin would be a worrisome choice because of the creatinine level).

5. Answer d.

This patient is likely to have an insulinoma. However, the laboratory results obtained during hypoglycemia do not exclude the surreptitious use of sulfonylureas. Hypoglycemia with endogenous hyperinsulinemia and the absence of sulfonylureas will have to be documented before surgical referral. Because of the negative family history, MEN is unlikely and preoperative localization would be optional in this setting. The cystic lesion seen in the pancreas may be an incidental lesion.

6. Answer b.

This patient has endogenous, inappropriate hyperinsulinemia as evidenced by the elevated C peptide level at the time of hypoglycemia. The patient had been given a sulfonylurea instead of her antihypertensive medication when she recently had a prescription filled. Although exogenous insulin will produce hypoglycemia, C peptide will be suppressed in this situation.

7. Answer a.

Hypertriglyceridemia is often a manifestation of poor diet, alcohol abuse, or uncontrolled diabetes. The latter is the likely cause in this patient who will benefit from tighter glycemic control. Niacin is likely to worsen glycemic control in this patient, and although gemfibrozil and an ACE inhibitor are reasonable interventions, neither will improve glycemic control and the ACE inhibitor will not improve the lipid profile. Thyroid hormone therapy is not indicated on the basis of the laboratory results provided.

8. Answer d.

This patient has central hyperthyroidism given the presence of elevated free thyroxine and a nonsuppressed TSH. Increased iodine intake (as in amiodarone use) or autoimmune thyroiditis would not explain these findings, which likely are due to a pituitary tumor. Often, TSH-producing tumors cosecrete growth hormone, and this possibility must be excluded before embarking on treatment. Radioactive iodine uptake will be increased because of the action of TSH on the thyroid.

9. Answer e.

This is a thyroid incidentaloma that because of its size (<1.0 cm) and absence of radiation to the head and neck can be safely observed. Ultrasonographically guided FNA is indicated if there is any change in size or the incidentaloma is larger than 1 cm. Levothyroxine suppression therapy is controversial and, because of the risks of prolonged thyroid-stimulating hormone suppression, is not indicated.

10. Answer a.

This patient's limb weakness, increased creatine kinase level, anemia, and altered liver function are all manifestations of hypothyroidism (TSH was 94 U/L). Hypercalcemia of malignancy may produce similar symptoms, but the time course is much more rapid.

11. Answer d.

The likeliest diagnosis in this setting is hemorrhage into a thyroid cyst. Sometimes, fluid can rapidly accumulate in a thyroglossal duct. This can be identified by its central location and its upward movement when the tongue is protruded. Anaplastic thyroid carcinoma can also present as a neck swelling of recent onset. Lymphomas rarely present over a 2-week period, but such presentations have been described. Papillary thyroid cancers do not grow rapidly.

12. Answer c.

This patient had a gynecoid body habitus with an arm span longer than his height. Karyotype was consistent with Klinefelter syndrome. Testicular biopsy findings are characteristic but not necessarily pathognomonic, and it is easier to obtain a karyotype. Determining the FSH and testosterone levels and performing pituitary imaging will not be necessary if the karyotype is diagnostic (as in this case). Klinefelter syndrome can present late in life.

13. Answer b.

In an elderly patient admitted with symptomatic hypercalcemia, malignancy is the most likely cause and is rarely caused by an occult neoplasm. Hypercalcemia is usually caused by multiple skeletal lesions or the secretion of PTHrp. In such settings, PTH is suppressed in response to the increased serum level of calcium. Some lymphomas express 1α-hydroxylase and produce excess 1,25-dihydroxyvitamin D. However, hypercalcemia is usually mild and of gradual onset (asymptomatic). PTH is suppressed in such situations.

14. Answer c.

This patient has secondary hyperparathyroidism, which is an appropriate response to the prevailing hypocalcemia. Why is she hypocalcemic? In view of her age, iron deficiency, and symptoms and signs of osteomalacia, it is likely that she has malabsorption (although poor nutritional intake from an eating disorder is a possibility). Other than parathyroid imaging, all the tests that are suggested are reasonable choices.

15. Answer c.

Acromegaly presents in many ways. Typically, early symptoms include depression and fatigue caused by disordered sleep. The effects of increased levels of IGF-1 on the thyroid often result in a goiter, which together with the sweaty, doughy palms that are often present can lead to the mistaken diagnosis of thyroid disease (especially if TSH secretion is altered by the pituitary tumor). The suspicion of acromegaly in this case was confirmed by the presence of the increased level of IGF-1.

16. Answer d.

Because of his previous history, it may be tempting to attribute the patient's symptoms to migraine. However, this episode of headache seems to be different and is accompanied by an altered level of consciousness. Pituitary apoplexy often presents in this fashion, especially in a previously undiagnosed pituitary tumor. Intravenous corticosteroids may decrease any swelling around the chiasm but are necessary because most of these patients are hypocortisolemic. Neurosurgical intervention is necessary if the level of consciousness worsens or the visual pathway is compromised. Bromocriptine or other dopamine agonists are unlikely to be useful in this acute setting.

17. Answer d.

An increased level of prolactin in association with a pituitary tumor does not automatically make the diagnosis of prolactinoma. With the presence of a large tumor, the modest increase in prolactin level is likely to be the result of stalk compromise by a large nonfunctioning pituitary tumor. Because of the poor response of these tumors to dopamine agonists or to high-dose corticosteroid therapy, definitive treatment would require excision. The timing of excision would depend on whether or not the visual fields are compromised.

18. Answer e.

Headache is a common symptom, and often during an evaluation of patients such as this one, a pituitary tumor is discovered incidentally. Subsequent investigation of an incidentaloma should focus on the presence of hormonal excess or deficiency and impingement of the tumor on other structures. A 24-hour urine cortisol level is especially important in this setting because of the history of obesity and type 2 diabetes. The serum levels of prolactin, IGF-1, and free thyroxine should always be measured in such circumstances.

19. Answer d.

This is a typical presentation of lymphocytic hypophysitis. Patients are usually female and present during or after pregnancy. They often have a family history of autoimmune disease. Subtle changes in the pattern of enhancement on MRI may be present, but with an otherwise normal pituitary no biopsy is indicated. Gonadotrophs and corticotrophs are almost always involved, often to the exclusion of other cell types, hence, the need for a 1-μg ACTH stimulation test before further management.

20. Answer d.

This is an unusual way to diagnose pregnancy! The question is included here to remind readers that pituitary "enlargement" is often physiologic in young females, especially during pregnancy (recall the pathophysiology of Sheehan syndrome). Regardless of the duration of amenorrhea, an increased level of prolactin in a (potentially fertile) female should require a pregnancy test.

21. Answer c.

The presence of a persistent nasal drip in this setting is worrisome for the development of cerebrospinal fluid rhinorrhea, which results from sudden shrinkage of the tumor in response to medical therapy. The presence of glucose in the fluid would confirm the diagnosis. Inability to tolerate medical therapy, visual pathway involvement, or development of pituitary apoplexy are all indications for intervention. However, the presence of asymptomatic hemorrhage does not mandate intervention. It is often a consequence of tumor shrinkage in response to treatment with a dopamine antagonist. The decrease in the prolactin level over 3 months suggests a good response to medical therapy.

CHAPTER 7

GASTROENTEROLOGY AND HEPATOLOGY

Thomas R. Viggiano, M.D.
Robert E. Sedlack, M.D.
John J. Poterucha, M.D.

PART I

Thomas R. Viggiano, M.D.
Robert E. Sedlack, M.D.

ESOPHAGUS

Esophageal Function

The upper esophageal sphincter (or cricopharyngeus muscle) and the muscle of the proximal one-third of the esophagus are striated muscle under voluntary control. A transition from skeletal to smooth muscle occurs in the midesophagus. In the distal one-third of the esophagus, the muscle is smooth muscle that is under involuntary control. The lower esophageal sphincter is a zone of circular muscle located in the distal 2 to 3 cm of the esophagus. To transport food from the mouth through the negative pressure of the chest into the positive pressure of the abdomen, the esophagus must transport food against a pressure gradient. To prevent reflux of gastric contents, the lower esophagus has a sphincter for unidirectional flow. Normal esophageal motility accomplishes both transport of food and prevention of reflux.

- The esophagus must transport food against a pressure gradient and prevent reflux of gastric contents.

Normal Motility

After a person swallows, the upper esophageal sphincter relaxes within 0.5 second. A primary peristaltic wave then passes through the body of the esophagus at a rate of 1 to 5 cm/s, generating an intraluminal pressure of 40 to 100 mm Hg. Within 2 seconds after the swallow, the lower esophageal sphincter relaxes and stays relaxed until the wave of peristalsis passes through it. Next, the lower esophageal sphincter contracts again to maintain its resting tone. Two major symptom complexes result if the esophagus is unable to perform its

two major functions: dysphagia (transport dysfunction) and reflux (lower esophageal sphincter dysfunction).

- Dysphagia: transport dysfunction.
- Reflux: lower esophageal sphincter dysfunction.

Dysphagia

Dysphagia is the defective transport of food and is usually described as "sticking." Odynophagia is pain on swallowing. The three causes of dysphagia must be distinguished: mechanical (obstructed lumen), functional (motility disorder), and oropharyngeal (faulty transfer of a food bolus to the esophagus). Answers to three questions frequently suggest the diagnosis: 1) what type of food produces the dysphagia, 2) what is the course of the dysphagia, and 3) is there heartburn (Fig. 7-1)? Dysphagia with an intermittent course is caused by a ring, a web, or a motility disorder.

- Be able to distinguish mechanical dysphagia from functional dysphagia.
- Intermittent dysphagia is caused by a ring, a web, or a motility disorder.

Mechanical Cause

Mechanical obstruction occurs if the lumen diameter is less than 12 mm. With mechanical obstruction, the course is progressive; dysphagia for solids is greater than for liquids, and there is associated weight loss.

- Mechanical obstruction: progressive course, weight loss, dysphagia for solids is greater than for liquids.

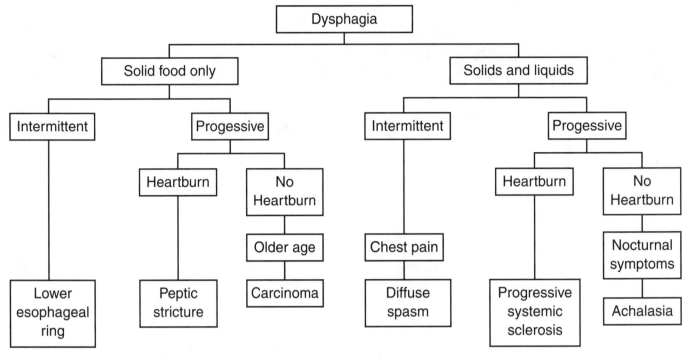

Fig. 7-1. Diagnostic scheme for dysphagia. Obtaining answers to three questions (see text) often yields the most likely diagnosis. (From MKSAP VI: part 1:44, 1982. American College of Physicians. By permission.)

Peptic stricture—This results from prolonged reflux and is usually a short (<2 to 3 cm long) narrowing in the distal esophagus.

- Peptic stricture results from prolonged reflux, usually in the distal esophagus.

Barrett esophagus—This is characterized by abnormal columnar epithelium that replaces the normal squamous mucosa in the distal esophagus. It can present as a stricture in the midesophagus that may occur with an ulcer; it increases the risk of the development of adenocarcinoma. Barrett esophagus is a complication of reflux and, thus, is acquired and not congenital.

- Barrett esophagus: abnormal columnar epithelium in the distal esophagus that is a complication of chronic reflux and predisposed to the development of adenocarcinoma.

Lye stricture—Alkali is more injurious to the esophagus than acid (in postgastrectomy patients, alkaline reflux can produce severe esophagitis). Do not induce vomiting after the ingestion of lye. Stricture tends to occur at the three physiologic narrowings where the initial passage of the corrosive may have been delayed. Bougienage after 3 or 4 weeks may prevent occurrence of stricture. There is increased incidence of squamous cell cancer.

- Postgastrectomy alkaline reflux can produce severe esophagitis.
- Do not induce vomiting after the ingestion of lye.
- Lye stricture is associated with an increased incidence of squamous cell cancer.

Benign tumor—Leiomyoma is the most common benign tumor. It is usually asymptomatic. Be able to recognize the appearance of this tumor on barium swallow fluoroscopy. Radiographically, a leiomyoma appears as a smooth filling defect with normal mucosa. It arises from the esophagus at a 90° angle, and its border is distinct from the esophageal wall. Perform endoscopy even if classic changes are seen on barium swallow.

Malignant tumor—Recognize the appearance of malignant tumors on barium swallow fluoroscopy. Also, know the conditions that predispose to esophageal squamous cell carcinoma: achalasia, lye stricture, Plummer-Vinson syndrome, human papillomavirus, tylosis, smoking, and alcohol. In the United States, 20% of malignant tumors are squamous and 80% are adenocarcinoma. Progressive dysphagia with weight loss is typical. The diagnosis is established by endoscopy with biopsy and cytology. *Prognosis*: the 5-year survival rate is only 7% to 15%; 28% of patients have lung metastases, and 25% have liver metastases. The prognosis is poor in the United States because of late detection of the tumor, but in China, the prognosis is excellent because of screening programs and early detection. *Treatment*: squamous cell carcinoma is more radiosensitive than adenocarcinoma. Surgery is difficult for proximal lesions. Surgery and preoperative irradiation are used for distal one-third lesions. *Palliation*: laser endoscopy, bougienage, and stent placement. *Chemotherapy*: no agents are known to be beneficial. Squamous cell carcinoma can produce ectopic parathyroid hormone; thus, hypercalcemia does not mean the tumor is unresectable.

- Know the radiographic appearance of leiomyoma and esophageal cancer.
- Conditions that predispose to esophageal squamous cell cancer: achalasia, lye stricture, Plummer-Vinson syndrome, human papillomavirus, tylosis, smoking, and alcohol. Barrett esophagus predisposes to adenocarcinoma.
- Esophageal malignancies are usually unresectable; palliative treatment.
- 5-Year survival is only 7%-15% in the U.S.

Ring—A lower esophageal ring (Schatzki ring) is a mucosal membrane that marks the junction of the esophageal and gastric mucosa. Muscular rings are rare. It presents as intermittent dysphagia for solids or as a sudden obstruction from a food bolus ("steak house syndrome"). Know the radiographic appearance. On radiographs, a lower esophageal ring is a thin annulus at the junction of the esophagogastric mucosa. Treatment is dilatation.

- Ring: presents as intermittent dysphagia and food bolus impaction.
- Know its radiographic appearance.
- Treatment is dilatation.

Web—A web is a membrane of squamous mucosa that occurs anywhere in the esophagus. It presents as intermittent dysphagia. Plummer-Vinson syndrome is a cervical esophageal web and iron deficiency anemia; it is associated with a 15% chance of oropharyngeal or esophageal squamous cell cancer.

- A web presents as intermittent dysphagia.
- Plummer-Vinson syndrome: cervical esophageal web, iron deficiency anemia, and a 15% chance of oropharyngeal or esophageal squamous cell cancer.
- Intermittent dysphagia is caused by rings, webs, or motility disorders.

Functional Cause

With functional obstruction (motility disorders), there is dysphagia for solids and liquids and an intermittent course; weight loss may or may not occur. The three important motor abnormalities of the esophagus are achalasia, diffuse esophageal spasm, and scleroderma.

- Functional obstruction: dysphagia for solids and liquids, intermittent course, with or without weight loss.

Achalasia—Achalasia results from esophageal denervation, specifically the degeneration of Auerbach ganglion cells. Chest radiography shows an air-fluid level. Barium swallow fluoroscopy shows a dilated esophagus with a beak-like tapering. *Motility pattern*: incomplete relaxation of the lower esophageal sphincter, hypertensive lower esophageal sphincter (usually does not have reflux), and aperistalsis in the body (most important). Always endoscopically examine patients who have achalasia because cancer of the esophagogastric junction may present with the radiographic appearance and motility pattern of achalasia (pseudoachalasia). A clue would be an older patient with dysphagia and heartburn. Treatment is pneumatic dilatation and not bougienage. Pneumatic dilatation is as effective as Heller myotomy. Botulinum toxin blocks the release of acetylcholine from presynaptic cholinergic neurons and decreases lower esophageal pressure for 3 to 12 months. Botulinum toxin provides short-term relief of symptoms and is safe and has few side effects. Currently, it is given to patients who are a high surgical risk and to the elderly.

In Brazil, the parasite *Trypanosoma cruzi* (Chagas disease) produces a neurotoxin that destroys the myenteric plexus. Esophageal dilatation identical to that of achalasia, megacolon, and megaloureter occurs in Chagas disease.

- Achalasia: a chest radiograph shows air-fluid level.
- Dilated esophagus with beak-like tapering on barium swallow fluoroscopy.
- Most important motility pattern in achalasia: aperistalsis.
- Always endoscopically examine patients who have achalasia.
- Treat achalasia with pneumatic dilatation and not with bougienage.
- Chagas disease has esophageal dysfunction identical to that of achalasia.

Diffuse esophageal spasm—Diffuse esophageal spasm usually presents as chest pain but may cause intermittent dysphagia, which is aggravated by stress and hot or cold liquids. Barium swallow fluoroscopy shows a corkscrew esophagus. *Motility*: simultaneous contractions of high amplitude in the body of the esophagus. If the patient is asymptomatic during the test, motility may be normal. The lower esophageal sphincter is hypertensive or has defective relaxation in one-third of patients. Medical treatment (nitrates, anticholinergic agents, nifedipine) has unpredictable results. Surgical treatment is long myotomy.

- Diffuse esophageal spasm usually presents as chest pain.
- It is aggravated by stress and hot or cold liquids.
- Barium swallow fluoroscopy shows a corkscrew esophagus.
- Medical treatment has unpredictable results.

Scleroderma—Esophageal involvement with scleroderma is associated with Raynaud phenomenon. Barium swallow fluoroscopy shows a common esophagogastric tube. *Motility*: aperistalsis in the body of the esophagus and incompetence of the lower esophageal sphincter, which causes severe reflux.

- Scleroderma: Raynaud phenomenon, aperistalsis, reflux.

Oropharyngeal Dysphagia

Oropharyngeal dysphagia is the result of faulty transfer of a food bolus from the oropharynx to the esophagus caused by structural abnormalities or disorders of either neural regulation or skeletal muscle (Table 7-1). Oropharyngeal dysphagia presents as high esophageal dysphagia associated with coughing, choking, or nasal regurgitation. After recognizing that oropharyngeal dysphagia is present, other associated symptoms may lead to the diagnosis of the underlying illness (e.g., a young person with oropharyngeal dysphagia, central scotoma, and neurologic symptoms has multiple sclerosis).

- Oropharyngeal dysphagia is the result of faulty transfer of a food bolus from the oropharynx to the esophagus caused by structural or neuromuscular disorders.
- It presents as cervical esophageal dysphagia associated with coughing, choking, or nasal regurgitation.

Gastroesophageal Reflux Disease

Reflux

The lower esophageal sphincter is the major barrier to reflux. This sphincter is a 2- to 4-cm–long specialized segment of circular smooth muscle in the terminal esophagus. The pressure of this sphincter varies markedly during the day, but the normal resting pressure is 15 to 30 mm Hg. Swallowing causes the pressure to decrease promptly (within 1 or 2 seconds after the onset of swallowing) and for the sphincter to remain relaxed until the peristaltic wave passes over it. The sphincter then contracts to maintain the increased resting pressure that prevents reflux. Pressure of the lower esophageal sphincter decreases markedly for 2 hours after a meal. Transient relaxations of the lower esophageal sphincter cause some gastroesophageal reflux to occur in everyone during the day but do not cause symptoms or esophagitis. Patients with clinically symptomatic reflux or inflammation show more frequent transient lower esophageal sphincter relaxations of unknown cause and have more frequent and longer lasting episodes of reflux.

- Lower esophageal sphincter pressure decreases for 2 hours after a meal.
- Patients with clinically symptomatic reflux show transient lower esophageal sphincter relaxations.

The degree of tissue damage is the real concern in gastroesophageal reflux disease (GERD). Several factors that determine whether reflux esophagitis occurs include the frequency of transient relaxations of the lower esophageal sphincter, the volume of gastric contents, the rate of gastric emptying (if delayed, reflux may develop), the potency of the refluxate (acid, pepsin, bile), the efficiency of esophageal clearance (motility, salivary bicarbonate), and the resistance of esophageal tissue to injury and ability to repair.

The evaluation of esophagitis is designed to answer four important questions (Table 7-2): Does the patient have reflux and, if so, how severe? Does the patient have esophagitis and, if so, to what extent? Are the patient's symptoms due to reflux? What is the mechanism of reflux?

Table 7-1 Causes of Oropharyngeal Dysphagia

Muscular disorders	Neurologic disorders	Structural causes
Amyloidosis	Amyotrophic lateral sclerosis[*]	Cervical osteophytes
Dermatomyositis[*]	Cerebrovascular accident	Cricopharyngeal dysfunction
Hyperthyroidism	Diphtheria	Goiter
Hypothyroidism	Huntington disease[*]	Lymphadenopathy
Myasthenia gravis[*]	Multiple sclerosis[*]	Zenker diverticulum
Myotonia dystrophica[*]	Parkinson disease	
Oculopharyngeal myopathy	Polio	
Stiff-man syndrome	Tabes dorsalis	
	Tetanus	

*Know the symptoms of these illnesses.

Table 7-2 Evaluation of Esophagitis

Question	Tests for reflux (the more sensitive one is listed first)
Is reflux present?	pH probe, isotope scan
Is esophagitis present?	Biopsy, endoscopy
Are symptoms due to reflux?	Acid perfusion (Bernstein test)
Mechanism of reflux?	Motility

Internists should know how to use tests that evaluate reflux in a cost-effective way. For most patients, the medical history is sufficiently typical to warrant a trial of therapy without expensive tests being conducted. Testing should be performed in patients who have an atypical medical history, refractory symptoms, long-standing reflux, dysphagia, weight loss, or possible complications of esophagitis.

Atypical symptoms of GERD include noncardiac chest pain, asthma, chronic cough, and hoarseness. Reflux is the most common cause of noncardiac chest pain. Asthmatic patients with coexisting reflux should receive treatment for reflux because it may improve control of respiratory symptoms. Reflux should be considered in asthmatic patients who have postprandial or nocturnal wheezing. Complications of reflux include ulceration, bleeding, stricture, aspiration, Barrett esophagus, and adenocarcinoma of the esophagus.

Barrett esophagus refers to a complication of chronic gastroesophageal reflux in which the normal esophageal squamous mucosa is replaced by columnar epithelium. Patients with Barrett esophagus are at increased risk for the development of carcinoma in the columnar epithelium. Although the matter is controversial, many experts recommend screening endoscopy with biopsy to look for dysplasia. There is no consensus on surveillance. Patients with Barrett esophagus should have aggressive antireflux treatment. If dysplasia is present, surgery should be considered. Photodynamic therapy could also be considered for patients who are not surgical candidates.

- For most patients, the medical history is sufficiently typical to warrant a trial of therapy without tests.
- Testing should be performed in patients who have an atypical medical history, refractory symptoms, long-standing reflux, dysphagia, iron deficiency anemia, weight loss, or possible complications of esophagitis. Test elderly patients who have onset of reflux.
- Atypical symptoms of gastroesophageal reflux: noncardiac chest pain, asthma, chronic cough, and hoarseness.
- Complications of gastroesophageal reflux: ulceration,

bleeding, stricture, aspiration, Barrett esophagus, and adenocarcinoma of the esophagus.

Tests for Reflux

Barium swallow fluoroscopy—Reflux is found in 60% of patients with esophagitis but also in 25% of control subjects. It is a qualitative test and does not distinguish between "normal" and abnormal reflux. Upper gastrointestinal radiography is used primarily as a screening test to exclude other diagnoses (e.g., ulcer) and to identify complications of reflux (e.g., strictures, ulcers, cancer or mass). Radiography may not detect Barrett esophagus.

- Reflux is found in 60% of patients with esophagitis but also in 25% of control subjects.

Esophagoscopy—This is the most definitive test if gross inflammation is present. However, 40% of patients may have symptomatic reflux with no gross inflammation. This is the preferred first test for long-standing cases of reflux to rule out Barrett esophagus. It is also the first test for patients with reflux without dysphagia.

- Esophagoscopy is the test preferred first for long-standing cases of reflux to rule out Barrett esophagus.
- It is the first test for patients with reflux without dysphagia.

Esophageal biopsy—In patients with reflux but without gross esophagitis, the basal cell layer and papillae are elongated. Esophagoscopy and biopsy are about 60% sensitive for detecting reflux. Eosinophilia in the biopsy specimen is 100% sensitive for the diagnosis of esophagitis. If Barrett esophagus is found, biopsy specimens should be obtained from along the length of Barrett epithelium as surveillance for dysplasia (premalignant changes) or malignancy.

- Biopsy may detect esophagitis when gross inflammation is not present.
- With Barrett esophagus, it is important to obtain biopsy specimens from along the length of the mucosa as surveillance for dysplasia (premalignant changes) or malignancy.

Twenty-four–hour pH monitoring—Monitoring the pH in the distal esophagus of patients during a 24-hour period of normal routine allows a more physiologic evaluation of reflux during daily activities. This test is valuable for patients with atypical symptoms, reflux symptoms refractory to therapy, a nondiagnostic evaluation, or pulmonary symptoms.

- 24-Hour pH monitoring allows a more physiologic evaluation of reflux during daily activities.

● This test is valuable for patients with atypical symptoms.

Acid perfusion (Bernstein test)—Saline perfusion for 10 minutes should not cause symptoms; next, switch to 0.1N HCl to determine whether the pain is reproduced. If heartburn and chest pain occur after acid instillation, treat for reflux.

● If heartburn and chest pain occur after acid instillation, treat for reflux.

Esophageal manometry—Manometry is reserved for patients with suspected esophageal motility disorders or for preoperative evaluation of surgical candidates.

● Esophageal manometry is reserved for suspected esophageal motility disorders.

Treatment of Reflux

Treatment of GERD is divided into three phases:

Phase 1 therapy—Lifestyle modifications: elevate the head of the bed 6 inches, modify the diet so it contains less fat and more protein, three meals a day, no eating for 3 hours before reclining, weight loss if overweight, and avoidance of specific foods (fatty foods, chocolate, alcohol, citrus juices, tomato products, coffee, carminatives). The patient should stop smoking and avoid alcohol. Avoid drugs that decrease lower esophageal sphincter pressure: anticholinergic agents, sedatives, tranquilizers, theophylline, progesterone or progesterone-containing birth control pills, nitrates, β-adrenergic agonists, and calcium channel blockers. Therapy is with antacids or alginic acid 30 minutes after meals and at bedtime.

Phase 2 therapy—Therapy includes drugs that decrease gastric acid output. All histamine (H_2) receptor antagonists are equally effective, and a twice daily dose is preferable for treating gastroesophageal reflux. Proton pump inhibitors are the most effective agents to relieve symptoms and to promote mucosal healing. It is best to treat gross esophagitis for 6 weeks. Long-term use of these agents is safe. Drugs that increase lower esophageal sphincter pressure and esophageal clearance—metoclopramide and bethanechol—have a limited role in treating reflux and often cause side effects.

Phase 3 therapy—This therapy includes antireflux surgery, which is reserved for patients who have reflux that is refractory to medical therapy or who develop complications. Nissen fundoplication is the preferred operation; fundoplication increases lower esophageal sphincter pressure. Although a new endoscopic suturing procedure has been developed, its long-term results are not available.

● Phase 1 therapy: modify lifestyle, avoid drugs that decrease lower esophageal sphincter pressure, and use antacids as

the first line of treatment.
● Phase 2 therapy: H_2-blockers or omeprazole.
● Phase 3 therapy: antireflux surgery is reserved for younger patients who want to avoid lifelong medical treatment and for patients who have reflux that is refractory to medical therapy or who develop complications.

Noncardiac Chest Pain

Chest pain is a frightening symptom, and patients are often referred to internists and gastroenterologists when the findings of a cardiac evaluation are not positive. Internists must understand the limitations of the diagnostic studies used to evaluate noncardiac chest pain. First, important cardiac disease must be ruled out. GERD is the most common cause of noncardiac chest pain, but esophageal pain may be due to a motor disorder (e.g., spasm) or esophageal inflammation (e.g., infection or injury). Esophageal spasm can closely mimic angina. Esophagogastroduodenoscopy rules out mucosal disease, that is, inflammation, neoplasms, and chemical injury. An esophageal motility study is performed to look for motor disorders (e.g., esophageal spasm and "nutcracker esophagus"), and 24-hour pH monitoring can be used to document the presence of reflux and its correlation with episodes of chest pain. Therapy for noncardiac chest pain includes avoidance of precipitants. Antacids, H_2 receptor antagonists, and proton pump inhibitors may be beneficial for patients with reflux. Sublingual nitroglycerin or calcium channel blockers are sometimes helpful in motor disorders, but their efficacy is unproven. If appropriate, reassure the patient that cardiac disease is not present.

● For noncardiac chest pain, rule out important cardiac disease.
● GERD is the commonest cause of noncardiac chest pain.
● Esophageal spasm can closely mimic angina.
● Esophagogastroduodenoscopy detects mucosal disease.
● Motility studies detect motility disorders.
● 24-Hour pH monitoring documents episodic reflux and correlation with symptoms.
● Sublingual nitroglycerin or calcium channel blockers are sometimes helpful.

Infections of the Esophagus

Patients with immunodeficiency disorders (acquired immunodeficiency syndrome [AIDS]), diabetes mellitus, malignancies (especially lymphoma and leukemia), or esophageal motility disorders are susceptible to opportunistic infections of the esophagus. These infections present as odynophagia. The most important infections to recognize are *Candida*, herpes, and cytomegalovirus. *Candida* infection: barium radiography shows small nodules in the upper one-third of the esophagus, and endoscopy shows cottage cheese–like plaques.

Diagnosis is made by seeing pseudohyphae on potassium hydroxide preparations. Treatment is with nystatin or clotrimazole for colonization and ketoconazole or fluconazole for esophagitis. Rarely, amphotericin B is used. Herpes infection: barium radiography and endoscopy show small discrete ulcers without plaques. Diagnosis is based on finding intranuclear inclusions (Cowdry type A bodies). Treatment is with acyclovir. Cytomegalovirus infection: radiography and endoscopy show severe inflammation with large ulcers. Intranuclear inclusions may be seen, but viral cultures are unreliable. Treatment is with ganciclovir or foscarnet (if ganciclovir-resistant).

- Opportunistic infections present as odynophagia in immunosuppressed patients.

Other Esophageal Problems

Medication-Induced Esophagitis

Medication-induced esophagitis presents as odynophagia or dysphagia and is more likely to occur if there is abnormal motility, stricture, or compression (left atrial enlargement). It is more common in the elderly and is recognized as inflammation in the midesophagus, with sparing of the distal esophagus. Medications commonly associated with esophagitis include tetracycline, doxycycline, quinidine, potassium supplements, bisphosphonates (alendronate, risedronate), ferrous sulfate, and ascorbic acid.

- Midesophageal inflammation is associated with abnormal motility, stricture, or compression and is more common in the elderly.
- Medicines responsible for esophagitis: tetracycline, doxycycline, quinidine, potassium supplements, bisphosphonates (alendronate, risedronate), ferrous sulfate, and ascorbic acid.

Mallory-Weiss Syndrome

Mallory-Weiss syndrome is mucosal laceration at the esophagogastric junction. It accounts for about 10% of cases of upper gastrointestinal tract bleeding: 75% of patients have a history of retching or vomiting before bleeding and 72% have diaphragmatic hernias. In 90% of patients, the bleeding stops spontaneously. Vasopressin, endoscopic injection, or electrocautery may control bleeding. Surgical treatment for persistent bleeding is rarely necessary. Angiography with intra-arterial infusion of vasopressin is successful in 70% of patients with continued bleeding.

- Mallory-Weiss syndrome: mucosal laceration at the esophagogastric junction.
- Accounts for about 10% of cases of upper gastrointestinal tract bleeding. Bleeding stops spontaneously in 90%.

- 75% of patients have a history of retching and vomiting before bleeding.

Esophageal Perforation

Esophageal perforation commonly occurs after dilatation in an area of stricture. Spontaneous perforation of the esophagus (Boerhaave syndrome) follows violent retching, often after an alcoholic binge. It also occurs after heavy lifting, defecation, seizures, and forceful labor (childbirth). The most common site of perforation is the left posterior part of the distal esophagus. If pleural fluid is present, it may have an increased concentration of amylase. Zenker diverticulum, cervical osteophytes (difficult intubations), and endoscopy (intubation) are causes of perforation of the cervical esophagus.

- Esophageal perforation commonly occurs after dilatation.
- Boerhaave syndrome follows violent retching, often after an alcoholic binge.

STOMACH AND DUODENUM

Peptic ulcers are defects in the gastric or duodenal mucosa that result from an imbalance between the digestive activity of acid and pepsin in the gastric juice and the host's protective mechanisms to resist mucosal digestion. Recent advances in our understanding of the pathogenesis of peptic ulcer have caused us to modify our presumption that idiopathic acid hypersecretion is a major etiologic factor. Newer classifications of peptic ulcers categorize ulcers as being associated with three possible etiologic factors: 1) *Helicobacter pylori*; 2) nonsteroidal anti-inflammatory drugs (NSAIDs), including aspirin; or 3) miscellaneous causes. Miscellaneous causes include ulcers due to hypersecretion from gastrinomas (Zollinger-Ellison syndrome), idiopathic hypersecretion, and duodenogastric reflux of gastric mucosal barrier–breaking agents such as bile salts or lysolecithin. Recent reports estimate that fewer than 5% of ulcers have a miscellaneous cause. Thus, at least 95% of peptic ulcers are due to either *Helicobacter pylori* or NSAIDs.

Helicobacter pylori

The Organism

H. pylori is a gram-negative, spiral-shaped microaerophilic bacillus that contains four to six unipolar, sheathed flagella. This fastidious organism resides beneath and within the mucus layer of the gastric mucosa and produces several enzymes such as urease and mucolytic proteases that are important for its survival and pathogenic effect. After it has been ingested, the organism moves into and through the mucus layer of the stomach. It has been postulated that several virulent factors are needed for successful colonization of the gastric mucosa, including the organism's motility, adhesins, proteases, phospholipases, cytokines, cytotoxins, and urease. Urease is thought to protect the organism from the acid environment. After colonization, the organism multiplies in the gastric mucus layer. Defense mechanisms may help control the infection, but unless treated, the organism remains in the gastric mucus layer for life.

H. pylori is a "slow" bacterium that causes persistent gastric infection and chronic inflammation. Ingestion of *H. pylori* can cause acute symptoms. Within weeks to months after infection, a chronic superficial gastritis develops, and after years to decades, chronic atrophic gastritis or gastric malignancy may develop.

Epidemiology

In the United States, *H. pylori* has an age-related prevalence, occurring in 10% of the general population younger than 30 and in 60% of those older than 60. *H. pylori* is present in 40% to 50% of the general population overall; it is more prevalent among blacks and Hispanics, poorer socioeconomic groups, and institutionalized persons. In developing countries such as India and Saudi Arabia, 50% of the population is infected by age 10 and 70% by age 20, and 85% to 95% of the population overall is infected. Evidence of person-to-person transmission includes clustering within families, higher than expected prevalence among institutionalized persons, transmission by endoscopy and biopsy, and a higher prevalence of infection among gastroenterologists. The fecal-oral route of transmission has been postulated, and indeed, *H. pylori* has been isolated from human feces.

Associated Diseases

Active Chronic Gastritis

H. pylori infection (type B gastritis) is found universally in patients with active chronic gastritis that is not associated with immunologic mechanisms (type A gastritis—pernicious anemia) or chemical injury (type C gastritis—alcohol, NSAIDs, aspirin, bile salts). *H. pylori*-induced active chronic gastritis is the most common type of chronic gastritis, and in some patients, it may progress to chronic atrophic gastritis. An important concept is that *H. pylori*-induced gastritis is the basic disease, and the development of duodenal or gastric ulcers or malignancy is a complication of the gastritis.

Duodenal Ulcer

H. pylori is found in 60% to 95% of patients with duodenal ulcers. The most important link between *H. pylori*-induced gastritis and the development of duodenal ulcers is the presence of gastric metaplasia in the duodenal bulb. Some data suggest that the metaplastic cells must be infected by *H. pylori*

to permit the development of duodenitis or duodenal ulcer. If *H. pylori*-positive patients with duodenal ulcer do not receive treatment, most have disease relapse within 1 year. However, if the infection is eradicated, the rate of relapse approaches zero. *H. pylori* infection causes an increase in basal and meal-stimulated gastrin release. Asymptomatic carriers of the bacillus may have a protective mechanism that prevents the hypersecretion of gastric acid. Enhanced gastric acid secretion occurs only in ulcer patients.

Gastric Ulcer

H. pylori is found in about 80% of patients with gastric ulcer. Eradication of the bacteria decreases the relapse rate of gastric ulcers.

Gastric Tumors

Adenocarcinoma—Studies from the United States and Great Britain have established a strong association between *H. pylori* infection (serum samples) and the emergence of noncardiac gastric adenocarcinoma. It has been postulated that *H. pylori* gastritis progresses to atrophic gastritis, and, in the presence of other risk factors, gastric adenocarcinoma eventually develops. This appears to be a rare occurrence. A cause-and-effect relationship remains to be established, and further studies are needed to determine the exact role of *H. pylori* in the development of gastric adenocarcinoma.

Mucosa-associated lymphoid tissue (MALT) lymphoma—*H. pylori* has also been associated with MALT lymphoma of the stomach. Of 450 patients with *H. pylori*-positive gastritis, 125 (28%) had mucosal lymphoid follicles and 8 (1.8%) had B lymphocytes infiltrating the epithelium, consistent with the development of early lymphoma.

Nonulcer Dyspepsia

Nonulcer dyspepsia is common, affecting about 20% of the U.S. population. Of those with functional dyspepsia, approximately 50% are infected with *H. pylori*, similar to the prevalence of *H. pylori* in asymptomatic persons. There is no convincing evidence that treatment of *H. pylori*-positive patients with nonulcer dyspepsia results in marked clinical improvement.

Diagnostic Tests for **H. pylori** Infection

Various diagnostic tests are available for determining whether *H. pylori* infection is present. The choice of which test to use is determined by the clinical setting and the cost.

Serology

H. pylori produces not only a local immune response but also a systemic immune response. Current detection methods exist for antibodies of the IgG, IgA, and IgM classes. Serologic testing is the most cost-effective, noninvasive way to diagnose primary *H. pylori* infection, but serologic results remain positive over time, which limits the usefulness of this test in follow-up evaluation. The sensitivity is 95%, the specificity is 90% to 95%, and the cost is $40 to $100.

Breath Test

A radiolabeled dose of urea is given orally to the patient. If *H. pylori* is present, the urease splits the urea and radiolabeled carbon dioxide is exhaled. The advantage of this test is that it is quick, easy to perform, and does not require endoscopy. As the breath test becomes more widely available, it will be the test of choice for follow-up evaluation. The sensitivity is 95% to 98%, the specificity is 95% to 98%, and the cost is $100 to $200.

Biopsy Urease Tests

A biopsy specimen is impregnated into agar that contains urea and a pH indicator. As the urea is split by *H. pylori*-produced urease, the pH of the medium changes the color of the agar from yellow to red. This test depends on bacterial urease, and the greater the number of organisms, the more rapidly the test becomes positive. The sensitivity is 95%, the specificity is 98%, and the cost is $20 (plus the cost of endoscopy to obtain tissue).

Stool Antigen Test

The *H. pylori* stool antigen test is simple and noninvasive and can be used to assess the success of eradication efforts. The sensitivity is 94%, and specificity is 92%.

Histology

An advantage of histology is being able to examine the underlying inflammatory reaction. *H. pylori* can be demonstrated with the Gram stain, hematoxylin and eosin stain, Giemsa stain, and Warthin-Starry (silver) stain. The sensitivity is 98%, the specificity is 98%, and the cost is $250.

Culture

Culturing *H. pylori* is tedious and expensive and should be reserved for special circumstances, for example, if an antibiotic-resistant organism is suspected or if virulence testing is being done. The sensitivity is 90% to 95%, the specificity is 100%, and the cost is $150.

Currently, because many symptomatic patients undergo endoscopy, histologic examination and biopsy urease tests are used most commonly in the initial evaluation. Newer, inexpensive serologic tests that can be performed in minutes are being investigated.

Treatment

The goal of treatment of an *H. pylori*-positive duodenal or gastric ulcer is to heal the ulcer and to eradicate (not suppress) the bacteria. Combination therapy with antisecretory agents and antimicrobial therapy for *H. pylori* is most effective. There is extensive research to determine the simplest and most efficacious agents for combination therapy, and specific recommendations for treatment regimens are constantly changing. The following general principles should guide treatment:

1. All patients with gastric or duodenal ulcer who are infected with *H. pylori* should receive combination therapy.
2. Patients with a well-documented ulcer who are infected with *H. pylori* but who are in remission with maintenance antisecretory therapy should receive combination therapy, then maintenance antisecretory therapy will not be necessary.
3. Maintenance antisecretory therapy is unnecessary except for patients with recurrent *H. pylori*-negative ulcers and for some patients with a previous history of bleeding from an ulcer.
4. Currently, treatment is not recommended for nonulcer dyspepsia and asymptomatic *H. pylori*-infected patients.

NSAID-Induced Ulcers

NSAIDs inhibit gastroduodenal prostaglandin synthesis, which results in decreased secretion of mucus and bicarbonate and reduced mucosal blood flow. NSAID-induced ulcers occur more commonly in the stomach than in the duodenum. They are located typically in the prepyloric area or antrum of the stomach.

The risk of peptic ulcer disease with NSAIDs is dose-dependent. It is important for physicians to understand that the anti-inflammatory properties of NSAIDs predispose to ulceration (prostaglandin inhibition) and there are different dose-response relationships for analgesia and anti-inflammatory properties of NSAIDs. The maximal analgesic effect plateaus well below the effective anti-inflammatory dose. Low doses of aspirin or NSAIDs give pain relief but have little anti-inflammatory activity. The newer NSAIDs have been marketed with more convenient (less frequent) dosing intervals and in dosages that have marked anti-inflammatory activity. Thus, the use of newer NSAIDs may subject the patient to an increased risk for ulcer without providing increased analgesia. Selective cyclooxygenase (COX)-2 inhibitors have been shown to decrease the rate of ulcer formation as well as ulcer complications such as bleeding, perforation, and pain. However, limited data suggest that even low-dose aspirin may reduce or eliminate any protective benefit of COX-2 drugs. In many instances, the use of NSAIDs can be discontinued and simple analgesic therapy with acetaminophen substituted. For patients who require NSAIDs, an attempt should be made to use the lowest possible dose. It also is important for physicians to know that the risk of peptic ulcer disease with NSAID use is maximal in the first month of treatment (ulcers may occur shortly after treatment is begun), and elderly patients and patients with a previous history of peptic ulcer disease are at highest risk.

The first step in the treatment of an NSAID-induced ulcer is to discontinue use of the drug. H_2-receptor antagonists and sucralfate are ineffective in preventing gastric ulcers and in decreasing the frequency of NSAID-induced mucosal erosions. Prostaglandin replacement with the synthetic prostaglandin misoprostol decreases the incidence of NSAID-induced gastric ulcers. However, diarrhea develops in many patients, thus limiting the usefulness of misoprostol. Proton pump inhibitors are effective in healing and preventing ulcers and have few side effects.

Duodenal Ulcer

H. pylori infection and associated antral gastritis occur in approximately 95% of patients with duodenal ulcer. However, only 10% to 20% of all patients who are infected with *H. pylori* ever develop an ulcer; therefore, other risk factors must be involved. Other risk factors that contribute to duodenal ulceration include NSAIDs, acid hypersecretion, cigarette smoking, cirrhosis, chronic pulmonary disease, and chronic renal disease. The use of NSAIDs is the second most common cause of duodenal ulcer. There is no evidence that diet, alcohol, corticosteroids, caffeine, or stress increases the risk of duodenal ulceration.

Gastric Ulcer

H. pylori infection and associated antral gastritis are present in 80% of patients with gastric ulcer. Most gastric ulcers occur in areas of gastritis on the lesser curvature of the stomach near the junction of the body and antrum. Because acid secretion is normal or low in patients with gastric ulcer, gastric ulceration is believed to occur when the gastric mucosal barrier of mucus and bicarbonate is damaged. The risk factors other than *H. pylori* that contribute to gastric ulceration include NSAIDs, bile reflux, and cigarette smoking. Bile reflux may occur from previous gastroduodenal surgery or from abnormal antral motility or pyloric sphincter function. Alcohol can cause gastritis, but there is no evidence that alcohol predisposes to gastric ulceration.

- 95% of duodenal ulcers are caused by *H. pylori* or NSAIDs, including aspirin.
- Risk factors for duodenal ulcers: *H. pylori*, NSAIDs, acid hypersecretion, cigarette smoking, cirrhosis, chronic pulmonary disease, and chronic renal disease.
- Risk factors for gastric ulcers are *H. pylori*, NSAIDs, bile reflux, and cigarette smoking.

Zollinger-Ellison Syndrome

Zollinger-Ellison syndrome is characterized by the triad of peptic ulceration, acid hypersecretion, and diarrhea caused by a gastrin-producing tumor. The tumor usually is located in the pancreas, but it can occur in the wall of the duodenum. Two-thirds of gastrinomas are malignant and can metastasize to regional lymph nodes and the liver. One-fourth of gastrinomas are related to a multiple endocrine neoplasia (MEN-I) syndrome and are associated with pituitary adenoma and hyperparathyroidism.

The most common clinical presentation is duodenal bulb ulceration, although multiple ulcers and postbulbar ulcers occur. The coexistence of a duodenal ulcer with diarrhea or a duodenal ulcer with hypercalcemia should raise the suspicion of Zollinger-Ellison syndrome. A duodenal ulcer that is not related to *H. pylori* infection or to NSAID use should also raise suspicion of Zollinger-Ellison syndrome. Gastrinoma also should be considered in patients with recurrent ulcers, intractable ulcers, a family history of ulcer disease or MEN-I syndrome, or evidence of gastric acid hypersecretion (enlarged rugal folds, dilated duodenum, increased acid output).

The serum level of gastrin should be determined if Zollinger-Ellison syndrome is suspected. Serum levels of gastrin greater than 1,000 pg/mL in patients who produce gastric acid are essentially diagnostic of gastrinoma. Increased serum levels of gastrin may also be seen in atrophic gastritis, pernicious anemia, postvagotomy states, proton pump inhibitor therapy, and renal failure because gastric acid output is low in these conditions. Basal and stimulated gastric acid secretory studies should be performed in all patients who have increased levels of gastrin. The basal acid output is more than 10 mEq per hour. When the laboratory results are equivocal, a secretin test should be performed. An intravenous bolus of secretin produces a paradoxical increase in the serum level of gastrin in patients with gastrinoma.

The test of choice to localize a gastrinoma is an octreotide scan. Almost all gastrinomas have somatostatin receptors, and radiolabeled octreotide, a somatostatin analogue, produces a positive scan in approximately 80% of cases. Endoscopic ultrasonography has been reported to localize approximately 70% of gastrinomas. Computed tomography (CT) of the abdomen localizes 50% of gastrinomas, and selective arteriography localizes 33%. In combination, these studies localize 80% to 85% of gastrinomas. If a tumor cannot be localized, surgical exploration is indicated in patients who do not have evidence of metastases or MEN-I.

Approximately 20% to 25% of gastrinomas can be completely removed surgically. If the tumor cannot be removed, some advocate a parietal cell vagotomy, which helps control acid secretion. Patients who are not candidates for surgery or who have an unresectable tumor can be managed medically with acid suppression and chemotherapy. High-dose, long-term treatment with proton pump inhibitors is safe and effective. Chemotherapy with streptozocin and 5-fluorouracil is effective in 50% of patients with metastatic disease.

- Zollinger-Ellison syndrome: peptic ulceration, acid hypersecretion, and diarrhea caused by a gastrin-secreting tumor.
- Rule out Zollinger-Ellison syndrome in patients with *H. pylori* and NSAID-negative duodenal ulcers, duodenal ulcers with diarrhea, or duodenal ulcers with hypercalcemia.
- Do not explore surgically if metastatic disease or MEN-I is present.

Stress Ulcers

Stress ulceration is caused by gastric mucosal ischemia due to an underlying illness. *H. pylori* is not an important pathogenic factor. The underlying conditions for stress ulcers are trauma, sepsis, and serious illness. Most of the hemorrhages occur 3 to 7 days after the traumatic event. Burns, especially those involving more than 35% of the body, may cause ulcers. Central nervous system trauma produces Cushing ulcer, which occurs in 50% to 75% of patients with head injury. This ulcer tends to be deep and perforate more often than other ulcers.

- Underlying conditions for stress ulcers: trauma, sepsis, serious illness.
- Hemorrhaging occurs 3-7 days after the traumatic event.
- Burns involving >35% of the body may produce ulcers.
- Stress ulcers occur in 50%-75% of patients with head injury (Cushing ulcers).

Prophylaxis against bleeding is to maintain intragastric pH greater than 4.0. Antacids clearly decrease the incidence of bleeding compared with placebo. H_2 receptor antagonists are as effective as antacids and sometimes easier to use. Sucralfate is as effective as antacids and H_2- blockers, according to some studies. Also, sucralfate may decrease nosocomial pneumonia in ventilator-dependent patients because gastric pH is not decreased (decreased bacterial overgrowth). Prostaglandins may have a role in prophylaxis. Enteral feedings can maintain intragastric pH greater than 3.5. If antacids cannot be used, give H_2-blockers or sucralfate; combination treatment may be helpful.

- Prophylaxis: maintain intragastric pH >4.0.
- Antacids, H_2 receptor antagonists, and sucralfate decrease the incidence of bleeding.
- Sucralfate may decrease nosocomial pneumonia in ventilator-dependent patients.

Medical therapy for bleeding, acute gastric mucosal ulcers: correct the underlying predisposing condition. Generally, upper gastrointestinal tract bleeding stops spontaneously about 85% of the time. Angiographic therapeutic techniques include intra-arterial vasopressin and transcatheter embolization.

Endoscopic techniques include epinephrine injection and electrocautery (bicap heater probe) or laser photocoagulation. Surgical therapy for bleeding, acute gastric mucosal ulcers must be considered when the blood requirement is more than 4 to 6 units per 24 to 48 hours. The mortality rate for all forms of surgical therapy is 30% to 40%.

Nonerosive Nonspecific Chronic Gastritis

Chronic gastritis is divided into type A and type B. Type A, or autoimmune, gastritis involves the body and fundus of the stomach. A subset of patients develops atrophic gastritis (inflammation of the gland zone with variable gland loss). Pernicious anemia with hypochlorhydria or achlorhydria and megaloblastic anemia may result. Antiparietal cell antibodies are found in 90% of patients. Intrinsic factor antibodies are detected less commonly. Other autoimmune diseases such as Addison disease and Hashimoto thyroiditis are often present. The serum levels of gastrin are increased. Gastric carcinoid tumors rarely develop. Gastric polyps occur, and intestinal metaplasia may be a precursor to gastric adenocarcinoma.

- Type A gastritis is associated with pernicious anemia and other autoimmune disorders.
- The serum levels of gastrin are increased.
- Type A gastritis is associated with gastric carcinoids, polyps, and adenocarcinoma.

Type B gastritis involves the antrum and is associated with *H. pylori* infection. Serum levels of gastrin are normal or increased. Gastric ulcers and duodenal ulcers occur commonly, and the incidence of gastric adenocarcinoma is increased.

- Type B gastritis is associated with *H. pylori* infection.
- The serum levels of gastrin are normal or increased.
- Type B gastritis is associated with gastric and duodenal ulcers and adenocarcinoma.

Gastric Cancer

In the 1940s, gastric cancer was the most common malignant disease in the United States. Since then, the decrease in incidence has been dramatic. Japan has the highest mortality rate from gastric cancer. Migration studies show a decrease in incidence among migrants from high-risk to low-risk areas and a suggestion of increased risk among persons moving from low-risk to high-risk areas. Environmental factors include diet—increased association with starch, pickled vegetables, salted fish and meat, smoked foods, and nitrate and nitrite consumption and increased salt consumption. The population at risk is persons older than 50. The male-to-female ratio is as high as 2:1. Also, gastric cancer is more common in lower socioeconomic groups.

- The incidence of gastric cancer has decreased dramatically in the United States since the 1940s.
- The incidence decreases among migrants from high-risk areas.
- Increased association with consumption of starch, pickled vegetables, salted fish and meat, smoked foods, and nitrate and nitrite and increased consumption of salt.
- A two- to threefold greater incidence among relatives.

Possible Precancerous Lesions or Situations

1) *H. pylori* infection, chronic atrophic gastritis, and intestinal metaplasia are frequently found in patients with gastric cancer; however, all three conditions are found frequently in older persons without gastric carcinoma. 2) Chronic benign gastric ulcer rarely progresses to cancer. 3) Pernicious anemia—previous autopsy studies showed a prevalence of 10%. An endoscopic screening study of 123 patients with pernicious anemia showed a prevalence of gastric neoplastic lesions of 8.1%. 4) The risk is minimally increased after gastrectomy, but surveillance endoscopy is not necessary.

- *H. pylori*-positive chronic atrophic gastritis is found frequently in patients with gastric cancer.
- Chronic benign gastric ulcer rarely progresses to cancer.
- Pernicious anemia: prevalence of 10%.
- Postgastrectomy: minimal increased risk, but endoscopy screening is not necessary.

Clinical Aspects

Gastric cancer is often asymptomatic, but abdominal discomfort and weight loss are the common presenting complaints. Physical examination is often unrevealing, but up to 30% of patients have an epigastric mass. Perform endoscopy, with multiple (seven or eight) biopsies and CT of the abdomen (to identify extragastric extension).

- Abdominal discomfort and weight loss are common presenting complaints.
- Up to 30% of patients have an epigastric mass.
- Perform endoscopy, with multiple (seven to eight) biopsies.

Treatment and Prognosis

For local disease—Resection often requires total gastrectomy for tumor-free margins. The omentum and spleen (splenic hilar nodes) are often removed in curative resection.

For disseminated disease—Surgical treatment is necessary only for palliation. Response to chemotherapy is generally poor. The only consistent factor is extent of disease. Five-year survival is 90% if the tumor is confined to the mucosa and submucosa, 50% if the tumor is through the serosa, and 10% if the tumor involves lymph nodes.

Gastric Polyps

Gastric polyps are rare; a 0.5% prevalence has been reported in an autopsy series. The two types of polyps are hyperplastic and adenomatous. Hyperplastic polyps are more common and not premalignant. No therapy is needed. Adenomatous polyps are premalignant, especially if larger than 2 cm. They occur most often in achlorhydric stomachs, that is, pernicious anemia, and are usually localized to the antrum. If pedunculated, the polyp can be removed endoscopically.

- Hyperplastic polyps are more common and not premalignant.
- Adenomatous polyps are premalignant, especially if larger than 2 cm.

Gastroduodenal Dysmotility Syndromes

Symptoms of abnormal gastric motility may include nausea, vomiting, bloating, early satiety, dyspepsia, heartburn, anorexia, weight loss, and food avoidance. The specific cause of abnormal gastric motor function is unknown but is believed to be related to autonomic neuropathy. Diabetes mellitus is probably the most common medical cause of symptomatic gastric motor dysfunction. Conditions causing gastroparesis are listed in Table 7-3.

- Nausea, vomiting, bloating, early satiety, dyspepsia, heartburn, anorexia, weight loss, and food avoidance may suggest abnormal gastric motility.
- It is believed to be related to autonomic neuropathy.
- Diabetes mellitus: the most common medical cause of symptomatic gastric motor dysfunction.

Treatment

Currently, several prokinetic drugs are available in the United States. These drugs augment motility, thus enhancing the movement of luminal contents. Metoclopramide is a dopamine antagonist and a cholinergic agonist that increases the rate and amplitude of antral contractions. It crosses the blood-brain barrier and frequently causes such side effects as drowsiness,

Table 7-3 Conditions Causing Gastroparesis

Acute conditions	Chronic conditions
Anticholinergic drugs	Amyloidosis
Hyperglycemia	Diabetes mellitus
Hypokalemia	Gastric dysrhythmias
Morphine	Pseudo-obstruction
Pancreatitis	Scleroderma
Surgery	Vagotomy
Trauma	

athetosis, and the release of prolactin. Domperidone is a selective dopamine antagonist that works only on peripheral receptors in the gut. It has no cholinergic effects and fewer side effects than metoclopramide. Bethanechol is a systemic cholinergic agonist with side effects. It may be useful in low dosage in combination with other agents. Erythromycin stimulates both cholinergic and motilin receptors.

- Metoclopramide is a dopamine antagonist and cholinergic agonist.
- Domperidone is a selective dopamine antagonist.
- Erythromycin stimulates both cholinergic and motilin receptors.

SMALL INTESTINE

Diarrhea

Patients use the term "diarrhea" to refer to any increase in the frequency, fluidity, or volume of the stool or any change in its consistency. Normally, stools are generally solid and brown, but these features may vary with diet. The frequency of stools varies among persons, from one to three daily to two or three stools weekly. Blood, pus (leukocytes), and oil are not present in normal stools (Table 7-4).

Diarrhea is defined as an increase in stool weight or volume. Because a stool is 65% to 80% water, stool weight is proportional to stool water. Because dietary fiber content influences the water content of the stool, stool weight can vary according to the diet of a culture. In the United States, normal daily stool weight is less than 200 g per day and normal stool volume is less than 200 mL per day (compared with <400 g/d and 400 mL/d in rural Africa).

It is important to understand normal daily intestinal fluid balance. Each day, 9 or 10 L of isotonic fluid is presented to the proximal small intestine (2 L, diet; 8 L, endogenous secretions). The small bowel absorbs most of the fluid (7-9 L), and the colon absorbs all the 1 or 2 L presented to it each day except for less than 200 mL and forms a soft, solid stool. There is considerable reserve, because the maximal absorptive capacity is 12 L per day for the small bowel and 4 to 6 L per day for the colon.

Table 7-4 Normal Stool Composition

Feature		Electrolytes, mEq/L	
Weight	<200 g	Na^+	40
Percent water	65-80	K^+	90
Fat	<7 g	Cl^-	15
Nitrogen	<2.5 g	HCO_3^-	30

Mechanisms of Diarrhea

Osmotic diarrhea occurs when water-soluble molecules are poorly absorbed, remain in the intestinal lumen, and retain water in the intestine. Osmotic diarrhea follows ingestion of an osmotically active substance and stops with fasting. Stool volume is less than 1 L per day, and the stool has an osmolar gap—stool osmolality is greater than the sum of electrolyte concentrations. Stool osmolar gap = 290 – 2 (stool Na + K). A normal stool osmotic gap is less than 50. Often, stool pH is less than 7.0. Clinical causes of osmotic diarrhea that produce an osmolar gap greater than 50 include lactase deficiency, sorbitol foods, saline cathartics, and antacids.

- In osmotic diarrhea, stool volume is <1 L/d.
- Diarrhea stops with fasting.
- Stool has an osmolar gap.
- Causes of osmotic diarrhea: lactase deficiency, sorbitol foods, and antacids.

In secretory diarrhea, fluid and electrolyte transport is abnormal, that is, the intestine secretes rather than absorbs fluid. Stool volume is greater than 1 L per day, and its composition is similar to that of extracellular fluid, so there is no osmolar gap. The diarrhea persists despite fasting and often presents with hypokalemia. Causes of secretory diarrhea include bacterial toxins, hormone-secreting tumors, surreptitious ingestion of laxative, bile acid diarrhea, and fatty acid diarrhea.

- In secretory diarrhea, stool volume is >1 L/d.
- There is no osmolar gap.
- Diarrhea persists despite fasting.
- Causes of secretory diarrhea: bacterial toxins, hormone-secreting tumors, surreptitious ingestion of laxative, bile acid diarrhea, and fatty acid diarrhea.

In exudative diarrhea, membrane permeability is abnormal and serum proteins, blood, or mucus is exuded into the bowel from sites of inflammation, ulceration, or infiltration. The diarrhea is small in volume and may be associated with bloody stools. Examples include invasive bacterial pathogens (e.g., *Shigella* and *Salmonella*) and inflammatory bowel disease.

- Exudative diarrhea: abnormal membrane permeability.
- Diarrhea is small in volume.
- Causes: invasive bacterial pathogens (*Shigella*, *Salmonella*) and inflammatory bowel disease.

Motility disorders—Both rapid transit (inadequate time for chyme to contact the absorbing surface) and delayed transit (bacterial overgrowth) can cause diarrhea. Rapid transit occurs after gastrectomy and intestinal resection and in hyperthyroidism and carcinoid syndrome. Delayed transit occurs with structural defects (strictures, blind loops, small-bowel diverticula) or underlying illnesses that cause visceral neuropathy (diabetes) or myopathy (scleroderma), that is, pseudo-obstruction.

- Rapid transit: diarrhea results from malabsorption.
- Delayed transit: diarrhea results from bacterial overgrowth.

Mixed mechanisms—Many disease processes may have more than one mechanism for causing diarrhea; for example, generalized malabsorption has osmotic and secretory components (fatty acids cause secretion in the colon).

Clinical Approach

It is useful to differentiate small-bowel ("right-sided") diarrhea from colonic ("left-sided") diarrhea (Table 7-5). Right-sided diarrhea is large in volume, with a modest increase in the number of stools. Symptoms attributed to inflammation of the rectosigmoid are absent, and proctoscopic examination findings are normal. Left-sided diarrhea presents as frequent small-volume stools with obvious evidence of inflammation, and proctosigmoidoscopic examination usually confirms inflammation. Left-sided diarrhea usually suggests an exudative mechanism, whereas the mechanism for right-sided diarrhea is nonspecific.

Acute Diarrhea

Acute diarrhea is abrupt in onset and usually resolves in several days (3-10 days). It is self-limited, and the cause (viral?) usually is not found. No evaluation is necessary unless the stools are bloody and fever or infection is suspected (e.g., travel history or common source outbreak). If these conditions exist, do not treat with antimotility agents. Begin the work-up with stool studies for bacterial pathogens, ova, and parasites and

Table 7-5 Right-Sided and Left-Sided Diarrhea: Contrasts in Clinical Presentation

Right-sided, or small-bowel, diarrhea	Left-sided, or colonic, diarrhea
Reservoir capacity intact	Reservoir capacity decreased
Large stool volume	Small amounts of stool
Modest increase in number of stools	Large increase in number of stools
No urgency	Urgency
No tenesmus	Tenesmus
No mucus	Mucus
No blood	Blood

proctosigmoidoscopy. Recognize the common situations that predispose to specific infections (see below, Infectious Diarrheas).

- For acute diarrhea, no evaluation is necessary unless the stools are bloody and fever or infection is suspected.
- Do not administer antimotility agents if the stools are bloody and fever or infection is suspected.

Chronic Diarrhea

Chronic diarrhea is an initial episode lasting longer than 4 weeks or diarrhea that recurs after the initial episode. The most common cause of chronic diarrhea is irritable bowel syndrome, but always rule out lactase deficiency. Be able to differentiate organic diarrhea from functional diarrhea (Table 7-6).

- The most common cause of chronic diarrhea is irritable bowel syndrome.
- Always rule out lactase deficiency in suspected irritable bowel syndrome.
- Differentiate organic diarrhea from functional diarrhea.

Chronic Watery Diarrhea

The evaluation of chronic watery diarrhea usually requires distinguishing between secretory diarrhea and osmotic diarrhea (Table 7-7). This can be done by collecting stools and measuring volume, osmolality, and electrolyte content and observing the patient's response to fasting.

- Evaluation of chronic watery diarrhea requires distinguishing between secretory diarrhea and osmotic diarrhea.

Anatomy of Nutrient Absorption

The sites of nutrient, vitamin, and mineral absorption are the following: 1) the duodenum absorbs iron, calcium, magnesium, folate, water-soluble vitamins, and monosaccharides; 2) the jejunum absorbs fatty acids, amino acids, monosaccharides, and water-soluble vitamins; and 3) the ileum absorbs monosaccharides, fatty acids, amino acids, fat-soluble vitamins (A, D, E, K), vitamin B_{12}, and conjugated bile salts.

The distal small bowel can adapt to absorb nutrients. The proximal small bowel cannot adapt to absorb vitamin B_{12} or bile salts. Fat absorption is the most complex process. Dietary fat consists mostly of triglycerides that must be digested by pancreatic lipase to fatty acids and glycerol, which are solubilized by micelles for absorption. The fatty acids and monoglycerides are reesterified by intestinal epithelial cells into chylomicrons that are absorbed into the circulation by lymphatic vessels (Table 7-8). Medium-chain triglycerides are absorbed directly into the portal vein and do not require micellar solubilization.

Table 7-6 Features Differentiating Organic Diarrhea From Functional Diarrhea

Feature	Organic diarrhea	Functional diarrhea
Weight loss	Often present	Not present
Duration of illness	Variable (weeks to years)	Usually long (>6 mo)
Quantity of stool	Variable but usually large (>200 g/24 h)	Usually small (<200 g/24 h)
Presence of blood in stool	May be present	Never present (unless from hemorrhoids)
Timing when diarrhea occurs	No special pattern	Usually in the morning but rarely wakes patient
Fever, arthritis, skin lesions	May be present	Not present
Emotional stress	No relation to symptoms	Usually precedes or coincides with symptoms
Cramping abdominal pain	Often	May be present

From Matseshe JW, Phillips SF: Chronic diarrhea: a practical approach. Med Clin North Am Jan 1978;62:141-154. By permission of WB Saunders Company.

Table 7-7 Features Differentiating Osmotic Diarrhea From Secretory Diarrhea

Feature	Osmotic diarrhea	Secretory diarrhea
Daily stool volume, L	<1	>1
Effect of 48-hour fasting	Diarrhea stops	Diarrhea continues
Fecal fluid analysis		
Osmolality, mOsm	400	290
Na + K × 2,[*] mEq/L	120	280
Solute gap[†]	>100	<50

[*]Multiplied by 2 to account for anions.

[†]Calculated by subtracting ([Na] + [K]) × 2 from osmolality.

From Krejs GJ, Hendler RS, Fordtran JS: Diagnostic and pathophysiologic studies in patients with chronic diarrhea. *In* Secretory Diarrhea. Edited by M Field, JS Fordtran, SG Schultz. Bethesda, MD, American Physiological Society, 1980, pp 141-151. By permission of publisher.

- The distal small bowel can adapt to absorb nutrients.
- The proximal small bowel cannot adapt to absorb vitamin B_{12} or bile salts.

Suspect malabsorption if the medical history suggests steatorrhea or if there is diarrhea with weight loss (especially if intake is adequate), chronic diarrhea of indeterminate nature, or nutritional deficiency (know the signs and symptoms of malabsorption) (Table 7-9).

- Diarrhea with iron deficiency anemia (evaluation for blood loss is negative) = proximal small bowel, e.g., sprue.
- Diarrhea with metabolic bone disease = decreased calcium and protein, thus, proximal small bowel.
- Hypoproteinemia with normal fat absorption suggests protein-losing enteropathy. If eosinophilia is present, eosinophilic gastroenteritis; if lymphopenia is present, intestinal lymphangiectasia.

- Oil droplets (neutral fat) or muscle fibers (undigested protein) present in stool = pancreatic insufficiency (maldigestion).
- Serum levels of calcium, magnesium, and iron are usually normal in pancreatic insufficiency. Serum levels of albumin may also be normal.
- Howell-Jolly bodies (if there is no history of splenectomy) or dermatitis herpetiformis suggests celiac sprue (small-bowel biopsy is not diagnostic for sprue, but the response to a gluten-free diet is).
- Fever, arthralgias, neurologic symptoms = Whipple disease.

Helpful hints in the medical history, physical examination, or laboratory results may suggest the possibility of diarrhea or malabsorption (Table 7-10). Other hints in the history might include 1) age—youth suggests lactase deficiency, inflammatory bowel disease, or sprue; 2) travel—parasites, toxigenic agents (exposure to contaminated food or water); 3) drugs—laxatives, antacids, antibiotics, colchicine, lactulose; and 4)

Table 7-8   Mechanisms of Fat Malabsorption

Alteration	Mechanism	Disease state
Defective digestion	Inadequate lipase	Pancreatic insufficiency
Impaired micelle formation	Duodenal bile salt concentration	Common duct obstruction or cholestasis
Impaired absorption	Small-bowel disease	Sprue and Whipple disease
Impaired chylomicron formation	Impaired β-globulin synthesis	Abetalipoproteinemia
Impaired lymphatic circulation	Lymphatic obstruction	Intestinal lymphangiectasia and lymphoma

Table 7-9   Causes of Symptoms in Malabsorption

Extragastrointestinal symptom	Result of
Muscle wasting, edema	Decreased protein absorption
Paresthesias, tetany	Decreased vitamin D and calcium absorption
Bone pain	Decreased calcium absorption
Muscle cramps	Weakness, excess potassium loss
Easy bruisability, petechiae	Decreased vitamin K absorption
Hyperkeratosis, night blindness	Decreased vitamin A absorption
Pallor	Decreased vitamin B_{12}, folate, or iron absorption
Glossitis, stomatitis, cheilosis	Decreased vitamin B_{12} or iron absorption
Acrodermatitis	Zinc deficiency

family history—celiac sprue, inflammatory bowel disease, polyposis coli, lactase deficiency.

- Medical history: previous surgery (short-bowel syndrome, dumping syndrome, blind loop syndrome, postvagotomy diarrhea, and ileal resection), irradiation, systemic disease.

Diseases Causing Diarrhea

Osmotic Diarrhea

Lactase deficiency—Lactose is normally split by lactase into glucose and galactose, which are absorbed in the small bowel. In lactase deficiency, lactose is not absorbed in the small intestine but enters the colon, where it is fermented in the lumen by bacteria to lactic acid and hydrogen is liberated. The result is diarrhea of low pH and increased intestinal motility. The most common disaccharidase deficiency is lactase deficiency. "Acquired" lactase deficiency (genetic?) is common in Orientals, blacks, Eskimos, and people from the Middle East. Diarrhea, abdominal cramps, and flatulence occur after ingestion of dairy products. There is improvement with diet. The pH of the stool is less than 6.0. Lactose tolerance test—

Blood sugar increases less than 20 mg/100 mL after ingestion of lactose. The hydrogen breath test may be abnormal. Jejunal biopsy results are normal (disaccharidase levels are decreased). Lactose intolerance can occur in any clinical setting in which the intestinal mucosa is damaged.

- Lactase deficiency: lactose is not absorbed in the small intestine.
- Diarrhea of low pH and increased intestinal motility.
- The most common disaccharidase deficiency is lactase deficiency.
- Diarrhea, abdominal cramps, and flatulence occur after ingestion of dairy products.
- The hydrogen breath test may be abnormal.
- Patients on a weight reduction diet who drink diet soda or chew sugarless gum may develop osmotic diarrhea from sorbitol.

Secretory Diarrhea

Watery diarrhea, hypokalemia, achlorhydria (WDHA) syndrome, or Verner-Morrison syndrome (also called "pancreatic cholera"), is a massive diarrhea (5 L daily) with dehydration and hypokalemia. (The patient may have numerous other

Table 7-10   Associated Symptoms of Systemic Illnesses Causing Diarrhea

Sign or symptom	Diagnosis to be considered
Arthritis	Ulcerative colitis, Crohn disease, Whipple disease, *Yersinia* infection
Marked weight loss	Malabsorption, inflammatory bowel disease, cancer, thyrotoxicosis
Eosinophilia	Eosinophilic gastroenteritis, parasitic disease
Lymphadenopathy	Lymphoma, Whipple disease
Neuropathy	Diabetic diarrhea, amyloidosis
Postural hypotension	Diabetic diarrhea, Addison disease, idiopathic orthostatic hypotension
Flushing	Malignant carcinoid syndrome
Proteinuria	Amyloidosis
Peptic ulcers	Zollinger-Ellison syndrome
Hyperpigmentation	Whipple disease, celiac disease, Addison disease, pancreatic cholera, eosinophilic gastroenteritis

From Fine KD, Krejs GJ, Fordtran JS: Diarrhea. *In* Gastrointestinal Disease: Pathophysiology, Diagnosis, Management. Fourth edition. Edited by MH Sleisenger, JS Fordtran. Philadelphia, WB Saunders Company, 1989, pp 290-316. By permission of publisher.

endocrine tumors [hypercalcemia or hyperglycemia].) This diarrhea is associated with a non–beta islet cell tumor of the pancreas. Vasoactive intestinal peptide is the most common mediator, followed by prostaglandin, secretin, and calcitonin. It is diagnosed with pancreatic scan or angiography and measurement of hormone levels. Treatment is with somatostatin or surgery.

- Pancreatic cholera: massive diarrhea, dehydration, and hypokalemia.
- Patients may have other multiple endocrine tumors.
- It is associated with a non–beta islet cell tumor of the pancreas.

Carcinoid Syndrome

Carcinoid tumors arise from enterochromaffin cells of neural crest origin. About 90% of the tumors are in the terminal ileum. There is episodic facial flushing (lasting up to 10 minutes), watery diarrhea, wheezing, right-sided valvular disease (endocardial fibrosis), and hepatomegaly. If the gut is normal, look for bronchial tumors or gonadal tumors. Dietary tryptophan is converted into serotonin (causes diarrhea, abdominal cramps [intestinal hypermotility], nausea, and vomiting), histamine (responsible for the flushing), and other chemicals (bradykinin, corticotropin). Intestinal tumors are usually asymptomatic because of the high hepatic first-pass clearance of these mediators. Carcinoid syndrome arises when these mediators are released into the systemic bloodstream; this suggests that liver metastases or bronchial tumors are present. The diagnosis of carcinoid syndrome is made by finding increased urinary levels of 5-hydroxyindoleacetic acid (5-HIAA) and by liver biopsy. This syndrome is not associated with hypertension, as in pheochromocytoma. Treatment is with octreotide.

Laxative Abuse

Of the population older than 60 years, 15% to 30% take laxatives regularly. This is laxative abuse. With the surreptitious ingestion of laxatives, patients complain of diarrhea but do not admit taking laxatives. In referral centers, this is the commonest cause of watery diarrhea. Proctoscopy shows melanosis coli. Barium enema demonstrates "cathartic colon," that is, dilated, hypomotile, and lacking haustra. Laxatives that cause melanosis coli include anthracene derivatives (senna, cascara, aloe). Diagnosis: stool phenolphthalein. Address the underlying emotional problems.

- Proctoscopy shows melanosis coli.
- Barium enema shows "cathartic colon," i.e., dilated, hypomotile, and lacking haustra.
- Address underlying emotional problems.

Bile Acid Malabsorption

Bile acid malabsorption is caused by ileal resection or disease. The diarrhea due to bile acid malabsorption may produce two different clinical syndromes, each requiring a different treatment. 1) Limited resection (<100 cm)—Malabsorbed bile acids enter the colon and stimulate secretion. Liver synthesis can compensate, so bile acid concentration in the upper small bowel is sufficient to achieve the critical micelle concentration and allow for normal fat absorption. There is no steatorrhea. Fecal fat is less than 20 g/24 hours. Treat with cholestyramine, which binds excess bile acids. 2) Extensive resection (>100 cm)—Bile acids are severely malabsorbed, and enterohepatic circulation is interrupted. This limits synthesis, and the liver cannot compensate. Bile acid concentration is decreased in the upper small bowel, micelles cannot be formed, and fat malabsorption results. The malabsorbed fatty acids themselves stimulate secretion in the colon. Fat-soluble vitamins (A, D, E, and K) may be malabsorbed. Additionally, excess fatty acids bind intestinal calcium; this allows an increase in oxylate absorption, which increases the risk of oxylate renal stones. Treat bile acid malabsorption with a low fat diet (<50 g daily) rich in medium-chain triglycerides. Cholestyramine would further decrease bile acid concentration and increase steatorrhea.

- Limited resection: treat with cholestyramine.
- Extensive resection: treat with a low fat diet rich in medium-chain triglycerides.

Bacterial Overgrowth

The proximal small intestine is usually sterile, and its major defense mechanisms are gastric acid, normal peristalsis (the most important defense), and intestinal IgA. When defenses are altered, bacterial overgrowth results. The mechanism of steatorrhea is deconjugation of bile acids by bacteria that normally do not occur in the proximal intestine. Deconjugation of the bile acids changes the ionization coefficient, and the deconjugated bile acids can be passively absorbed in the proximal small bowel. Normally, conjugated bile acids are actively absorbed distally in the ileum. As a result, the critical micellar concentration is not reached, and mild steatorrhea results from the intraluminal deficiency of bile acids.

- Normal peristalsis is the most important defense in the proximal small bowel.
- Deconjugated bile salts can be absorbed passively.
- Mild steatorrhea results from the intraluminal deficiency of bile acids.

Clinical features of bacterial overgrowth are steatorrhea (10-20 g daily), vitamin B_{12} malabsorption (macrocytic anemia),

positive jejunal cultures (>10^5 organisms), increased folate levels from bacterial production, and abnormal bile acid breath test. Breath test—bile acid breath test—^{14}C-labeled bile acids release $^{14}CO_2$ when deconjugated by bacteria in the gut. This test has low sensitivity (a 20%-30% false-negative rate).

Associated conditions—Postoperative (blind loops, enteroenterostomy, gastrojejunocolic fistula), structural (diverticula, strictures, fistulas), motility disorders (scleroderma, pseudo-obstruction), achlorhydria (atrophic gastritis, gastric resections; achlorhydria corrects with antibiotics), and impaired immunity. Two types of the latter are hypogammaglobulinemic sprue (no plasma cells in the lamina propria and flat villi seen in small-bowel biopsy specimens) and nodular lymphoid hyperplasia associated with IgA deficiency (know the radiographic appearance), which predisposes to *Giardia lamblia* infection.

- Diarrhea, vitamin B_{12} deficiency, and the above conditions suggest bacterial overgrowth.

Infectious Diarrheas

The toxigenic and invasive causes of bacterial diarrhea and the associated features are outlined in Tables 7-11 and 7-12.

Noninvasive Bacterial Diarrhea (Toxicogenic)

Staphylococcus aureus—The diarrhea is of rapid onset and lasts for 24 hours. There is no fever, vomiting, or cramps. The toxin is ingested in egg products, cream, and mayonnaise. Treatment is supportive.

Clostridium perfringens ("church picnic diarrhea")—The toxin is ingested in precooked foods, usually beef and turkey. Heat-stable spores produce toxins. Although the bacteria are killed and the toxin is destroyed, the spores survive. When food is rewarmed, the spores germinate, producing toxin. The diarrhea is worse than the vomiting and is later in onset. It lasts 24 hours. Treatment is supportive.

Escherichia coli ("traveler's diarrhea")—The toxin is ingested in water and salads. It is a plasmid-mediated enterotoxin.

Table 7-11   Causes of Bacterial Diarrhea: Toxigenic

Organism	Onset, h	Mediated by cyclic AMP	Fever	Intestinal secretion
Staphylococcus aureus	1-6	+	-	+
Clostridium perfringens	8-12	-	±	+
Escherichia coli	12	+	+	+
Vibrio cholerae	12	+	Due to dehydration	++++
Bacillus cereus	1-6	+	-	+

AMP, adenosine monophosphate.

Table 7-12   Causes of Bacterial Diarrhea: Invasive

Organism	Fever	Bloody diarrhea	Bacteremia	Antibiotic effective
Shigella	+	+	+	+
Salmonella	+	-	-	-
Vibrio parahaemolyticus	+	+	-	+(?)
Escherichia coli	+	-	-	-
Staphylococcus aureus (enterocolitis)	+	+	±	+
Yersinia enterocolitica	+	+	+	?
Campylobacter	+	+	±	+
Vibrio vulnificus	+	+	+	+

Treatment is rehydration with correction of electrolytes and ciprofloxacin, norfloxacin, or trimethoprim-sulfamethoxazole. *E. coli* may be important in nursery epidemic diarrhea.

Vibrio cholerae—The toxin is ingested in water. It is the only toxigenic bacterial diarrhea in which antibiotics clearly shorten the duration of the disease. Treatment is with tetracycline.

Bacillus cereus—The source of the toxin is fried rice in Oriental restaurants. One type has rapid onset and resembles *S. aureus* infection; the other type has a slower onset and resembles *C. perfringens* infection. The diagnosis is made by isolating the organism from contaminated food and by the medical history. Treatment is supportive.

Other toxigenic bacteria—*C. botulinum* produces a neurotoxin that is ingested in improperly home-processed vegetables, fruits, and meats. It interferes with the release of acetylcholine from peripheral nerve endings. *C. difficile*—See below, Antibiotic Colitis.

- Toxigenic bacterial diarrhea: watery, no fecal leukocytes.
- *S. aureus*: rapid onset.
- *C. perfringens*: "church picnic diarrhea," precooked foods, later in onset.
- *E. coli*: "traveler's diarrhea."
- *B. cereus*: fried rice in Oriental restaurants.

Invasive Bacterial Diarrhea

Shigella—It is often acquired outside the United States. Bloody diarrhea is characteristic, and fever and bacteremia occur. Diagnosis is based on positive stool and blood cultures. Treatment is with ampicillin. Resistant strains are emerging for which chloramphenicol is an alternative. (Plasmids are responsible for antibiotic deactivation resistance.)

Salmonella (non-*typhi*)—In the United States, *Salmonella typhimurium* is the most common agent. The toxin is ingested with poultry. Fever is present. The absence of bloody diarrhea is the main characteristic that distinguishes it from *Shigella* infection. Diagnosis is based on positive stool culture. Treatment is supportive. Treat only severe symptoms with ciprofloxacin. Treating mild symptoms with other antibiotics may result in a prolonged carrier state.

V. parahaemolyticus—The toxin is ingested with undercooked shellfish. This infection is increasing in frequency in the United States (it is common in Japan). Fever and bloody diarrhea are the chief characteristics. Diagnosis is based on positive stool culture. Antibiotics are of questionable value in treating this infection, but erythromycin may be most effective.

E. coli—In the United States, enteroinvasive *E. coli* is a rare cause of diarrhea. Enteroinvasive *E. coli* involves the colon and presents with fever, bloody diarrhea, and profound toxicity (similar to *Shigella* infection). Enterohemorrhagic *E. coli* (serotype O157:H7) produces a cytotoxin that damages vascular endothelial cells. *E. coli* O157:H7 can cause sporadic or epidemic illness from contaminated meat and raw milk. Enterohemorrhagic *E. coli* infection should be suspected when bloody diarrhea occurs after eating hamburger and when bloody diarrhea is complicated by hemolytic uremic syndrome or thrombotic thrombocytopenic purpura. Antibiotic treatment has not been effective and is not recommended because it may increase the risk for the development of hemolytic uremic syndrome or thrombotic thrombocytopenic purpura from the rapid release of toxin during bacterial death.

S. aureus (enterocolitis)—Diagnosis is based on positive stool culture or Gram stain, which shows a predominance of gram-positive cocci and a paucity of other organisms.

- Invasive bacterial diarrhea: fever, bloody stools, and fecal leukocytes.
- *Shigella*: bloody diarrhea.
- *Salmonella typhimurium*: no bloody diarrhea, treat with antibiotics only if blood cultures are positive.

- *V. parahaemolyticus*: undercooked shellfish, bloody diarrhea.
- *E. coli*: bloody stools, abdominal pain but no fever. Follows from eating hamburgers; may cause hemolytic uremic syndrome and thrombotic thrombocytopenic purpura.

"Newer" Enteric Bacterial Pathogens

Yersinia enterocolitica—The spectrum of disease includes acute enteritis and chronic enteritis. Acute enteritis is similar to shigellosis and usually lasts 1 to 3 weeks. It is characterized by fever, diarrhea, leukocytosis, and fecal leukocytes. Chronic enteritis is found especially in children. There is diarrhea, failure to thrive, hypoalbuminemia, and hypokalemia. Other features are acute abdominal pain (mesenteric adenitis), right lower quadrant pain, tenderness, nausea, and vomiting. It mimics appendicitis or Crohn disease. This gram-negative rod is hardy and can survive in cold temperatures. It grows on special medium (cold enriched). It is an invasive pathogen, with fecal-oral transmission in water and milk.

Extraintestinal manifestations are nonsuppurative arthritis and ankylosing spondylitis (in HLA-B27). Skin manifestations are erythema nodosum and erythema multiforme. Thyroid manifestations are Graves disease and Hashimoto disease. Multiple liver abscesses and granulomata are present.

Treatment is with aminoglycosides or trimethoprim-sulfamethoxazole (Bactrim). The bacteria are variably sensitive to tetracycline and chloramphenicol. β-Lactamases are frequently produced, making penicillin resistance common.

- *Y. enterocolitica* infection: acute abdominal pain (differential diagnosis includes appendicitis and Crohn disease).
- Fecal-oral transmission in water and milk.
- Manifestations include nonsuppurative arthritis and ankylosing spondylitis (in HLA-B27).

Campylobacter jejuni—These are comma-shaped, motile, microaerophilic gram-negative bacilli. Transmission is linked to infected water, unpasteurized milk, poultry, sick dogs, and infected children. The incubation period is 2 to 4 days before invasion of the small bowel. Infection results in the presence of blood and leukocytes in the stool. It may mimic granulomatous or idiopathic ulcerative colitis. It also may mimic small-bowel secretory diarrhea, with explosive, frequent watery diarrhea due to many species that produce a cholera-type toxin. The diarrhea usually lasts 3 to 5 days but may recur. Antibiotic treatment is with erythromycin when severe, but treatment often is not needed. Postdiarrheal illnesses are hemolytic uremic syndrome and postinfectious arthritis.

- *Campylobacter jejuni*: transmission is linked to infected water, unpasteurized milk, poultry, sick dogs, and infected children.

- It may mimic granulomatous or idiopathic ulcerative colitis.
- Diarrhea: usually lasts 3-5 days but may recur.

V. vulnificus (noncholera)—The organisms are extremely invasive and produce necrotizing vasculitis, gangrene, and shock. They are routinely isolated from seawater, zooplankton, and shellfish along the Gulf of Mexico and both coasts of the United States, especially in the summer. Two clinical syndromes are 1) wound infection, cellulitis, fasciitis, or myositis after exposure to seawater or cleaning shellfish and 2) septicemia after the ingestion of raw shellfish (oysters). Patients at high risk for septicemia include those with liver disease, congestive heart failure, diabetes mellitus, renal failure, an immunosuppressive state, or hemochromatosis. Treatment is with tetracycline.

- *V. vulnificus* is extremely invasive, producing necrotizing vasculitis, gangrene, and shock.
- Wound infection, cellulitis, fasciitis, or myositis occurs after exposure to seawater or cleaning shellfish.
- Septicemia occurs after the ingestion of raw shellfish (oysters).

Aeromonas hydrophila—Previously, the pathogenicity of the bacteria was questioned. Although the infection is often mistaken for that of *E. coli*, *A. hydrophila* is now recognized as an increasingly frequent cause of diarrhea after a person has been swimming in fresh or salt water. The organism produces several toxins. Treatment is with trimethoprim-sulfamethoxazole and tetracycline.

Malabsorption Due to Diseases of the Small Intestine

Celiac Sprue

Celiac sprue is a gluten-sensitive enteropathy. It presents in children as growth retardation and in adults as an iron deficiency that is unresponsive to iron taken orally. Osteomalacia can be present without steatorrhea if the proximal small bowel is involved. Splenic atrophy and abnormal blood smear with Howell-Jolly bodies may be clues to the diagnosis in 10% to 15% of patients. The skin manifestation is dermatitis herpetiformis. The measurement of circulating antigliadin and endomysial and tissue transglutaminase antibodies is useful for noninvasive screening. If the results are positive, a small-bowel biopsy should be performed. If the result of the endomysial antibody test is negative, another diagnosis should be considered. Small-bowel biopsy findings are not diagnostic, but response to a gluten-free diet is diagnostic. If the patient is unresponsive to the diet, review the diet for inadvertent gluten ingestion. If symptoms recur after 10 to 15 years of successful dietary management, rule out small-bowel lymphoma (especially if there is also abdominal pain).

- Celiac sprue: iron deficiency that is unresponsive to iron taken orally; osteomalacia with or without steatorrhea.
- Splenic atrophy and abnormal blood smear with Howell-Jolly bodies may be clues to the diagnosis in 10%-15% of patients.
- Lymphoma is a late complication.

Tropical Sprue

In tropical sprue, diarrhea occurs 2 to 3 months after travel to the tropics. After 6 months, megaloblastic anemia develops because of folate deficiency and possible coexisting vitamin B_{12} deficiency. Although somewhat controversial, the infectious agents are likely *Klebsiella* and *E. coli*. Small-bowel biopsy specimens show blunted villi similar to those in celiac sprue. Treatment is with tetracycline (250 mg four times daily) and folate with or without vitamin B_{12}.

- Tropical sprue: diarrhea and megaloblastic anemia after travel to the tropics.
- Cause: controversial; coliform bacteria (*Klebsiella* more than *E. coli*).
- Treatment: tetracycline (250 mg four times daily) and folate with or without vitamin B_{12}.

Whipple Disease

Whipple disease is a systemic infectious disease involving the central nervous system (CNS), heart, kidneys, and small bowel. It is caused by gram-positive bacilli. Small-bowel biopsy specimens show periodic acid-Schiff (PAS)–positive granules in the macrophages. Suspect Whipple disease in patients who have recurrent arthritis, pigmentation, adenopathy, or CNS symptoms (dementia, myoclonus, ophthalmoplegia, visual disturbances, coma, seizures). Treatment is with trimethoprim-sulfamethoxazole or tetracycline for 1 year.

- Suspect Whipple disease in patients who have recurrent arthritis, pigmentation, adenopathy, or CNS symptoms.
- Small-bowel biopsy specimens show PAS-positive granules in the macrophages.
- Treatment: trimethoprim-sulfamethoxazole or tetracycline for 1 year.

Eosinophilic Gastroenteritis

Patients with eosinophilic gastroenteritis have a history of allergies (e.g., asthma) and food intolerances and episodic symptoms of nausea, vomiting, abdominal pain, and diarrhea. Laboratory findings include eosinophilia, iron deficiency anemia, and steatorrhea or protein-losing enteropathy. Small-bowel radiographs show coarse folds and filling defects, and biopsy specimens show infiltration of the mucosa by eosinophils and, occasionally, absence of villi. Rule out parasitic infection. Treatment with corticosteroids produces a rapid response.

- Mucosal eosinophilic gastroenteritis: allergies, food intolerances, eosinophilia, and episodic intestinal symptoms.
- Rule out parasitic infection.
- Corticosteroids produce a rapid response.

Systemic Mastocytosis

Systemic mastocytosis is a proliferation of mast cells in the skin (urticaria pigmentosa), bones, lymph nodes, and parenchymal organs. Histamine is released, and 50% of patients have gastrointestinal symptoms, that is, diarrhea and peptic ulcer. "Bath pruritus" (itching after a hot bath) is a clue to the diagnosis.

- Systemic mastocytosis causes urticaria pigmentosa.
- 50% of patients have gastrointestinal symptoms.
- "Bath pruritus" is a clue to the diagnosis.

Intestinal Lymphangiectasia

Intestinal lymphangiectasia is a disorder caused by lymphatic obstruction. Hypoplastic lymphatics cause lymph to leak into the intestine. The clinical features are edema (often unilateral leg edema), chylous peritoneal or pleural effusions, and steatorrhea or protein-losing enteropathy. Laboratory findings include lymphocytopenia (average, 0.6×10^9/L) due to enteric loss. All serum proteins are decreased, including immunoglobulins. Small-bowel radiographs show edematous folds, and small-bowel biopsy specimens show dilated lacteals and lymphatics in the lamina propria that may contain lipid-laden macrophages. The same biopsy findings are seen in obstruction of mesenteric nodes (lymphoma, Whipple disease, Crohn disease) and obstruction of venous inflow to the heart (constrictive pericarditis, severe right heart failure). Diagnosis is based on abnormal small-bowel biopsy findings and documented enteric protein loss by increased $alpha_1$-antitrypsin levels in the stool. Treatment is with a low fat diet and medium-chain triglycerides (they enter the portal blood rather than the lymphatics). Occasionally, surgical excision of the involved segment is useful if the lesion is localized.

- Intestinal lymphangiectasia: unilateral lymphedema of the leg and chylous peritoneal or pleural effusions.
- Lymphocytopenia is universal.
- Decreased serum proteins.
- Small-bowel biopsy specimens show dilated lacteals and lymphatics.
- Treatment: low fat diet and medium-chain triglycerides.

Amyloidosis

Systemic amyloidosis is characterized by a diffuse deposition of an amorphous eosinophilic extracellular protein polysaccharide complex in the tissue. The major sites of amyloid deposition are the walls of blood vessels and the mucous membranes and muscle layers of the intestine. Any portion of the gut can be involved. Amyloid damages tissues by infiltration (muscle and nerve infiltration causes motility disorders and malabsorption) and ischemia (obliteration of vessels causes ulceration and bleeding). Intestinal dysmotility can produce diarrhea, constipation, pseudo-obstruction, megacolon, and fecal incontinence. Clinical findings in amyloidosis include macroglossia, hepatomegaly, cardiomegaly, proteinuria, and peripheral neuropathy. Pinch (post-traumatic) purpura or periorbital purpura after proctoscopic examination may occur. *Diagnosis*—Small-bowel radiography shows symmetrical, sharply demarcated thickening of the valvulae conniventes. Fat aspirate confirms the diagnosis in 80% of patients and rectal biopsy stained with Congo red in 70%.

Miscellaneous Small-Bowel Disorders

Meckel Diverticulum

Meckel diverticulum, the persistence of the vitelline duct, is the most frequent developmental abnormality of the gut. It usually occurs within 100 cm from the ileocecal valve on the antimesenteric border of the ileum. It contains all layers of the intestinal wall and so is a true diverticulum. The mucosa is usually ileal but may be gastric (pancreatic or intestinal). Complications include obstruction due to intussusception and volvulus around the band that fixes the diverticulum to the bowel wall. Benign (leiomyomas) and malignant (carcinoids or leiomyosarcoma) tumors have been found in diverticula. Diverticulitis is uncommon. Incarceration in an indirect inguinal hernia (Littre hernia) and perforation that causes peritonitis may occur. Hemorrhage is the common complication and results from ulceration of the ileal mucosa adjacent to the gastric mucosa. This accounts for 50% of the cases of lower gastrointestinal tract bleeding in children and young adults. Radiography usually is not helpful in making the diagnosis. A nuclear scan (parietal cells concentrate technetium) may show the diverticulum, but false-positive and false-negative results can occur.

- Meckel diverticulum is the most frequent developmental abnormality of the gut.
- It accounts for 50% of the cases of lower gastrointestinal tract bleeding in children and young adults.

Aortoenteric Fistula

A history of gastrointestinal tract bleeding in a patient who has had a previous aortic graft demands immediate evaluation to rule out an aortoenteric fistula. If the patient presents with massive bleeding, do not attempt endoscopy or arteriography. Emergency surgery is indicated.

- If a patient presents with massive bleeding, do not attempt endoscopy or arteriography. Emergency surgery is indicated.

Chronic Intestinal Pseudo-Obstruction

Pseudo-obstruction is a syndrome characterized by the clinical findings of mechanical bowel obstruction but without occlusion of the lumen. The two types are primary and secondary. The primary type, also called "idiopathic pseudo-obstruction," is a visceral myopathy or neuropathy. The secondary type is due to an underlying systemic disease or precipitating causes.

Idiopathic (primary) pseudo-obstruction is associated with recurrent attacks of nausea, vomiting, cramping abdominal pain, distention, and constipation, which are of variable intensity and duration. If it is a familial cause, the patient will have a positive family history and the condition will be present at a young age. Esophageal motility is abnormal (achalasia) in most patients. Occasionally, urinary tract motility is abnormal, and diarrhea or steatorrhea results from bacterial overgrowth. Upper gastrointestinal tract and small-bowel radiographs show dilatation of the bowel and slow transit (not mechanical obstruction).

- Idiopathic pseudo-obstruction is due to a familial cause or to a sporadic visceral myopathy or neuropathy.
- Recurrent attacks have variable frequency and duration.
- Abnormal esophageal motility occurs in most patients.
- Steatorrhea is caused by bacterial overgrowth.

Secondary pseudo-obstruction is due to underlying systemic disease or precipitating causes. These causes include the following (important causes to remember are in italics):

1. Diseases involving the intestinal smooth muscle: *amyloidosis*, scleroderma, systemic lupus erythematosus, myotonic dystrophy, and muscular dystrophy.
2. Neurologic diseases: *Parkinson disease*, Hirschsprung disease, Chagas disease, and familial autonomic dysfunction.
3. Endocrine disorders: *myxedema* and hypoparathyroidism.
4. Drugs: *antiparkinsonian medications (L-dopa)*, phenothiazines, tricyclic antidepressants, ganglionic blockers, clonidine, and narcotics.

Approach to the Patient With Chronic Intestinal Pseudo-Obstruction

First, rule out a mechanical cause for the obstruction. Second, look for an underlying precipitating cause such as metabolic abnormalities, medications, or an underlying associated disease. If a familial idiopathic cause is suspected, assess esophageal motility. Suspect scleroderma if intestinal radiography shows large-mouth diverticula of the small intestine.

Suspect amyloidosis if the skin shows palpable purpura and if proteinuria and neuropathy are present.

- Secondary pseudo-obstruction is due to an underlying systemic disease or precipitating cause.
- Scleroderma presents as large-mouth diverticula of the intestine.
- Amyloidosis presents with palpable purpura, proteinuria, and neuropathy.

Inflammatory Bowel Disease

"Idiopathic inflammatory bowel disease" refers to two disorders of unknown cause: chronic ulcerative colitis and Crohn disease. Other possible causes of inflammation, especially infection, should be excluded before making the diagnosis of idiopathic inflammatory bowel disease.

Ulcerative colitis is a mucosal inflammation involving only the colon. Crohn disease is a transmural inflammation that can involve the gastrointestinal tract anywhere from the esophagus through the anus. The rectum is involved in about 95% of patients with ulcerative colitis and in only 50% of those with Crohn disease. Ulcerative colitis is a continuous inflammatory process that extends from the anal verge to more proximal colon (depending on the extent of the inflammation). Crohn disease is a segmental inflammation in which inflamed areas alternate with virtually normal areas. Ulcerative colitis usually presents as frequent bloody bowel movements with minimal abdominal pain, whereas Crohn disease presents with fewer bowel movements, less bleeding, and, more commonly, abdominal pain. Crohn disease is associated with intestinal fistula, fistula from the intestine to other organs, and perianal disease. Ulcerative colitis does not form fistulas and perianal disease is uncommon. Strictures of the intestine are common with Crohn disease but rare in ulcerative colitis (when they are present, they suggest cancer).

- Ulcerative colitis involves only the colon.
- Crohn disease can involve the gastrointestinal tract anywhere from the esophagus through the anus.
- Ulcerative colitis is a continuous process.
- Crohn disease is a segmental inflammation.
- Ulcerative colitis has frequent bloody bowel movements.
- Crohn disease has fewer bowel movements, less bleeding, and more abdominal pain.
- Crohn disease is associated with intestinal fistula, strictures, and perianal disease.

Extraintestinal Manifestations of Inflammatory Bowel Disease

Arthritis occurs in 10% to 20% of patients, usually monarticular or pauciarticular involvement of large joints. Peripheral joint symptoms mirror bowel activity: joint symptoms flare when colitis flares and joint symptoms improve as colitis improves. Also, axial joint symptoms such as ankylosing spondylitis (relationship with HLA-B27) and sacroiliitis—which are usually progressive and do not improve when colitis improves—can develop.

- The peripheral joint symptoms mirror bowel activity.
- Axial joint symptoms such as ankylosing spondylitis and sacroiliitis can develop and have a progressive course independent of bowel activity.

Skin lesions occur in 10% of patients. The three types of lesions are erythema nodosum, pyoderma gangrenosum, and aphthous ulcers of the mouth. Erythema nodosum and aphthous ulcers usually improve with treatment of colitis, whereas pyoderma gangrenosum has an independent course. Severe, refractory skin disease is an indication for surgical treatment.

- The skin lesions are erythema nodosum, pyoderma gangrenosum, and aphthous ulcers of the mouth.

Eye lesions occur in 5% of patients. The lesion is usually episcleritis or uveitis (or both). Episcleritis usually mirrors inflammatory bowel disease activity, but uveitis does not.

Liver disease also occurs in 5% of patients. Primary sclerosing cholangitis is more common in chronic ulcerative colitis than in Crohn disease. If the alkaline phosphatase level is increased in a patient with inflammatory bowel disease, the work-up for primary sclerosing cholangitis includes ultrasonography, endoscopic retrograde cholangiopancreatography, and liver biopsy.

- If increased alkaline phosphatase occurs with inflammatory bowel disease, rule out primary sclerosing cholangitis.
- Central (axial) arthritis, pyoderma gangrenosum, primary sclerosing cholangitis, and uveitis usually follow a course independent of bowel disease activity.

Renal stones occur in 5% to 15% of patients. In Crohn disease with malabsorption, calcium oxalate stones occur. In chronic ulcerative colitis, uric acid stones are due to dehydration and loss of bicarbonate in the stool, leading to acidic urine.

Indications for Colonoscopy

Colonoscopy is indicated for evaluating the extent of the disease and for stricture (biopsy) and filling defect (biopsy). It is also indicated for differentiating Crohn disease from ulcerative colitis when the two are otherwise indistinguishable. Another indication is for monitoring by random mucosal biopsy the development of dysplasia or cancer in patients who have had ulcerative colitis or Crohn disease for more than 8 years.

● Know the indications for colonoscopy in inflammatory bowel disease.

Toxic Megacolon

In patients with active inflammation, avoid the causes of toxic megacolon, including aerophagia, opiates, anticholinergic agents, hypokalemia, and barium enema.

● In patients with active inflammation, avoid the causes of toxic megacolon.

Treatment of Ulcerative Colitis

Sulfasalazine—5-Aminosalicylic acid (ASA) (the active agent) is bound to sulfapyridine (vehicle). Colonic bacteria break the bond and release 5-ASA, which is not absorbed but stays in contact with the mucosa and exerts its anti-inflammatory action. The efficacy of 5-ASA may be related to its ability to inhibit the lipoxygenase pathway of arachidonic acid metabolism or to function as an oxygen free radical scavenger (further studies are needed). It is effective in acute disease and in maintaining remission. The side effects (male infertility, malaise, nausea, pancreatitis, rashes, headaches, hemolysis, impaired folate absorption, hepatitis, aplastic anemia, and exacerbation of colitis) are related to the sulfapyridine moiety and occur in 30% of patients who take sulfasalazine.

Other aminosalicylates—The 5-ASAs are a group of new drugs that deliver 5-ASA to the intestine in various ways. They eliminate sulfa toxicity but are more expensive than sulfasalazine. Two of these drugs are mesalamine and olsalazine. Mesalamine can be given topically (Rowasa suppositories, Rowasa enema) or orally (Asacol, 5-ASA coated with acrylic polymer that releases 5-ASA in the terminal ileum, and Pentasa, ethyl cellulose coating releases 50% of the 5-ASA in the small bowel). Olsalazine consists of two 5-ASA molecules conjugated with each other. Bacteria break the bond, releasing 5-ASA into the colon.

Aminosalicylates are used for mild to moderately active ulcerative colitis and for Crohn disease. Topical forms are useful for proctitis or left-sided colitis; systemic forms are used for pancolitis. Of the patients who do not tolerate sulfasalazine, 80% to 90% tolerate oral 5-ASA preparations. Side effects include hair loss, pancreatitis (often in patients who developed pancreatitis while taking sulfasalazine), reversible worsening of underlying renal disease, and exacerbation of colitis.

● Sulfasalazine and other aminosalicylates can induce remission in 80% of patients with mild-moderate ulcerative colitis and are effective maintenance therapy for 50%-75% of patients with ulcerative colitis.
● Sulfasalazine: side effects occur in 30% of patients.

● Other aminosalicylates are equally effective but more expensive; they are useful in 80%-90% of patients intolerant of sulfasalazine.

Corticosteroids—Topical preparations should be used twice daily by patients with active mild-to-moderate disease that is limited to the distal colon. Corticosteroids should be added to the regimen of patients with more proximal disease if sulfasalazine does not control the attacks. Up to 50% of the dose can be absorbed (depending on the preparation used and its vehicle). Oral preparations are indicated in active pancolonic disease of moderate severity in doses of 40 to 60 mg once daily or 20 to 40 mg daily in cases of mild disease that are unresponsive to topical corticosteroids and sulfasalazine. Prednisolone, the active metabolite, is the preferred form of drug for patients with cirrhosis (these patients may not be able to convert inactive prednisone to prednisolone). For patients who have a prompt response to oral corticosteroids, the dose may be tapered gradually at a rate not to exceed a 5-mg decrease in the total dose every 3 to 7 days. Intravenous preparations should be given in large doses (prednisolone, 100 mg in divided doses) for up to 10 to 14 days to severely ill patients. If at that time improvement occurs, it should be possible to convert the medication to oral corticosteroids (60-100 mg daily). If there is no improvement, surgical intervention (colectomy) is required. Because corticosteroids are not believed to prevent relapse, they should not be prescribed after the patient has complete remission and is symptom-free.

● Prescribe topical preparations twice daily for patients with active mild-moderate disease that is limited to the distal colon.
● Corticosteroids should be added to the regimen of patients with more proximal disease if systemic steroids and sulfasalazine have not controlled the attacks.
● Oral preparations are useful in active pancolonic disease of moderate severity.
● Intravenous preparations are given to severely ill patients.
● Corticosteroids are useful in remission induction for ulcerative colitis but are not effective in maintenance of remission.

Total parenteral nutrition does not alter the clinical course of an ongoing attack. Indications for its use include severe dehydration and cachexia with marked fluid and nutrient deficits, excessive diarrhea that has failed to respond to standard therapy for chronic ulcerative colitis, and debilitated patients undergoing colectomy. Opiates (or their synthetic derivatives) and anticholinergic agents are contraindicated in chronic ulcerative colitis because they are ineffective and can contribute to the development of toxic megacolon.

● Total parenteral nutrition does not alter the clinical course of the ongoing attack.

- Use of opiates and anticholinergic agents is contraindicated in chronic ulcerative colitis.

Surgical—Surgical treatment is curative in chronic ulcerative colitis. Indications for colectomy include severe intractable disease, acute life-threatening complications (perforation, hemorrhage, or toxic megacolon unresponsive to treatment), symptomatic colonic stricture, and suspected or documented colon cancer. Other indications are intractable moderate-to-severe colitis, refractory uveitis or pyoderma gangrenosum, growth retardation in pediatric patients, cancer prophylaxis, or inability to taper a regimen to low doses of corticosteroid (i.e., <15 mg daily) over a period of 2 to 3 months. Procedures include proctocolectomy with ileoanal anastomosis, Koch pouch, and conventional Brooke ileostomy.

- Surgical treatment is curative in chronic ulcerative colitis.

Treatment of Crohn Disease

Medical—For sulfasalazine, see above, Treatment of Ulcerative Colitis. This drug is more effective for colonic disease than for small-bowel disease, although 5-ASA products designed to be released and activated in the small bowel may prove to be effective in the colon. Sulfasalazine does not have an additive effect or a steroid-sparing effect when given with corticosteroids, nor does it maintain remission in Crohn disease as it does in ulcerative colitis. None of the aminosalicylates are effective for the prophylaxis of Crohn disease.

- Sulfasalazine is more effective for colonic disease than for small-bowel disease.
- It does not have an additive effect or sparing effect when given with corticosteroids.
- It does not maintain remission in Crohn disease.

Corticosteroids—See above, Treatment of Ulcerative Colitis. The agents that most quickly control an acute exacerbation of Crohn disease are corticosteroids. They are the most useful drugs for treating acute small-bowel Crohn disease and for achieving rapid remission.

Azathioprine and 6-mercaptopurine (the active metabolite of azathioprine) have steroid-sparing effects. Their use should be reserved for patients with active disease who are taking steroids and whose corticosteroid dose needs to be reduced (or a given dose needs to be maintained in the face of worsening disease activity).

- 6-Mercaptopurine is the active metabolite of azathioprine.
- Azathioprine and 6-mercaptopurine are effective as maintenance therapy for Crohn disease.
- Both agents have a steroid-sparing effect.

Metronidazole (at a dose of 20 mg/kg) is effective for treating perianal disease. Six weeks may be needed for the therapeutic effect to become manifest. Recurrences are frequent when the drug dose is tapered or discontinued, leading to chronic therapy. It is as effective as sulfasalazine for disease of the colon. If the disease is unresponsive to sulfasalazine, it is worthwhile switching to metronidazole, but not vice versa. It is less effective for small-bowel disease. Side effects include glossitis, metallic taste, vaginal and urethral burning sensation, neutropenia, dark urine, urticaria, disulfiram (Antabuse) effect, and paresthesias.

- Metronidazole is effective for treating perianal disease.
- Recurrences are frequent when the drug dose is tapered or discontinued.
- It is as effective as sulfasalazine for disease of the colon.

Infliximab (Remicade) is a chimeric monoclonal antibody directed against tumor necrosis factor-alpha. This intravenously administered anti-inflammatory agent is effective in treating moderately to severely active Crohn disease refractory to conventional therapy and in treating fistulizing Crohn disease. Infliximab is a steroid-sparing agent that is effective in maintaining remission of Crohn disease. Infusion reactions consisting of pruritus, dyspnea, or chest pain may occur. The drug is associated with an increased risk of infection, including perianal abscesses and respiratory infections. Rarely, subsequent infusions of infliximab may be associated with delayed hypersensitivity reactions.

- Infliximab is effective in treating moderately to severely active Crohn disease refractory to conventional therapy and in treating fistulizing Crohn disease.
- Infliximab is associated with acute infusion reactions, delayed hypersensitivity reactions, and an increased risk of infections.

Nutrition—Bowel rest per se does not have any role in achieving remission in Crohn disease. However, providing adequate nutritional support does help facilitate remission; any form of nutritional support is acceptable as long as the amount is adequate. Adequate nutrition can be essential in maintaining growth in children who have severe Crohn disease.

Surgical—If Crohn disease is present during exploration for presumed appendicitis, the acute ileitis should be left alone (many of these patients do not develop chronic Crohn disease). Appendectomy can be performed if the cecum and appendix are free of disease. Of the patients with Crohn disease who have surgical treatment, 70% to 90% require reoperation within 15 years (many within the first 5 years after the initial operation). The anastomotic site is the most likely site for recurrence of disease. Indications for surgical treatment include intractable symptoms, acute life-threatening complications, obstruction, unhealed fistulas that cause complications, abscess formation, and malignancy.

- 70%-90% of patients with Crohn disease operated on require reoperation within 15 years.
- The anastomotic site is the most likely site for disease recurrence.

GASTROINTESTINAL MANIFESTATIONS OF AIDS

Gastrointestinal tract symptoms occur in 30% to 50% of North American and European patients with AIDS and in nearly 90% of patients in developing countries. The most frequent gastrointestinal tract symptom is diarrhea, which is often chronic and associated with weight loss. Dysphagia, odynophagia, abdominal pain, and jaundice are less frequent. Gastrointestinal tract bleeding is rare. The goal of evaluation is to identify treatable causes of infection or symptoms.

- The majority of AIDS patients with diarrhea have one or more identifiable pathogens.
- Some have no identifiable cause despite extensive evaluation. This may represent idiopathic AIDS enteropathy or as yet unidentified pathogens.

The gastrointestinal tract in AIDS is predisposed to a spectrum of viral, bacterial, fungal, and protozoan pathogens.

Viral

Cytomegalovirus

Cytomegalovirus is one of the most common and potentially serious opportunistic pathogens. It most commonly affects the colon and esophagus, although the entire gut, liver, biliary tract, and pancreas are susceptible. There is a patchy or diffuse colitis that may progress to ischemic necrosis and perforation. *Symptoms*: watery diarrhea and fever; less commonly, hematochezia and abdominal pain. Odynophagia may be present if the esophagus is involved. *Diagnosis*: biopsy specimens show cytomegalic inclusion cells with surrounding inflammation (owl's eye). *Treatment*: ganciclovir, 5 mg/kg twice daily for 14 to 21 days. If resistant, use foscarnet.

Herpes Simplex Virus

The three gastrointestinal tract manifestations of herpes simplex virus infection in patients with AIDS are perianal lesions (chronic cutaneous ulcers), proctitis, and esophagitis. The organs affected are the colon and esophagus.

Symptoms: perianal lesions are painful; proctitis causes tenesmus, constipation, and inguinal lymphadenopathy; and esophagitis causes odynophagia, with or without dysphagia. *Diagnosis*: cytologic identification of intranuclear (Cowdry type A) inclusions in multinucleated cells. The diagnosis is confirmed with viral cultures. *Treatment*: acyclovir given orally or intravenously.

Adenovirus

Adenovirus reportedly causes diarrhea. The organ affected is the colon. *Symptoms*: watery, nonbloody diarrhea. *Diagnosis*: culture and biopsy. *Treatment*: none.

Bacteria

Mycobacterium avium-intracellulare

Infection of the gut occurs in patients with disseminated disease. The small intestine is affected more commonly than the colon. *Symptoms*: fever, weight loss, diarrhea, abdominal pain, and malabsorption. *Diagnosis*: acid-fast organisms in the stool and tissue confirmed by culture from stool and biopsy specimens. *Treatment*: multiple drug therapy with ethambutol, rifampin, ciprofloxacin, and clarithromycin.

Other Bacteria

Salmonella (*typhimurium* and *enteritidis*)—Treatment is with amoxicillin, trimethoprim-sulfamethoxazole, or ciprofloxacin.

Shigella flexneri—Treatment is with trimethoprim-sulfamethoxazole, ampicillin, or ciprofloxacin.

Campylobacter jejuni—Treatment is with erythromycin or ciprofloxacin.

In patients with AIDS, *Salmonella*, *Shigella flexneri*, and *Campylobacter jejuni* have a substantially higher incidence of intestinal infection, bacteremia, and prolonged or recurrent infections because of antibiotic resistance or compromised immune function or both.

Fungi

Candida albicans

In patients with AIDS, *Candida* causes locally invasive mucosal disease in the mouth and esophagus. Disseminated candidiasis is rare because neutrophil function remains relatively intact. The presence of oral candidiasis in persons at risk for AIDS should alert the physician to possible human immunodeficiency virus (HIV) infection. If oral candidiasis is present, endoscopy is required to confirm esophageal involvement. *Symptoms*: odynophagia suggests esophageal involvement. *Diagnosis*: histologic examination shows hyphae, pseudohyphae, or yeast forms. *Treatment*: nystatin, ketoconazole, fluconazole, or amphotericin.

Histoplasma capsulatum

Histoplasma capsulatum is an important opportunistic infection in AIDS patients who reside in endemic areas. Colonic involvement is more common than small-bowel involvement. *Symptoms*: diarrhea, weight loss, fever, and abdominal pain. *Diagnosis*: established by culture. Colonoscopy may show inflammation and ulcerations, and histologic examination with Giemsa staining shows intracellular yeast-like *Histoplasma capsulatum* within lamina propria macrophages. *Treatment*: amphotericin or itraconazole.

Protozoa

Cryptosporidium

Cryptosporidium is among the commonest enteric pathogens, occurring in 10% to 20% of patients with AIDS and diarrhea in the United States and in 50% of those in developing countries. The organs affected are the small and large intestine and the biliary tree. *Symptoms*: voluminous watery diarrhea, severe abdominal cramps, weight loss, anorexia, malaise, and low-grade fever. Biliary tract obstruction has been reported. *Diagnosis*: microscopic identification of organisms in stool specimens with modified acid-fast staining or stains specific for *Cryptosporidium*. Organisms may also be identified in biopsy specimens or in duodenal fluid aspirates. *Treatment*: paromomycin reduces the diarrhea.

Isospora belli

Isospora belli is the more common cause of diarrhea in developing countries. It resembles *Cryptosporidium* oocysts. The small intestine is primarily affected, but the organisms can be identified throughout the gut and in other organs. *Symptoms*: watery diarrhea, cramping abdominal pain, weight loss, anorexia, malaise, and fever. *Diagnosis*: oval oocysts in stool seen with a modified Kinyoun carbolfuchsin stain. Biopsy specimens from the small intestine may show organisms in the lumen or within cytoplasmic vacuoles in enterocytes. *Isospora belli* oocysts contain two sporoblasts and differ from *Cryptosporidium* oocysts, which are small, round, and contain four sporozoites. *Treatment*: trimethoprim-sulfamethoxazole.

Microsporida (Enterocytozoon bieneusi)

These organisms are emerging as an important pathogen; they have been identified in up to 33% of AIDS patients who have diarrhea. The organ affected is the small intestine. *Symptoms*: watery diarrhea with gradual weight loss but no fever or anorexia. *Diagnosis*: based on electron microscopic identification of round-to-oval meront (proliferative) and sporont (spore-forming) stages of Microsporida in the villous but not crypt epithelial cells of the duodenum and jejunum. There are reports of positive stool specimens with Giemsa staining. *Treatment*: none known.

Other Protozoa

Entamoeba histolytica—Treatment is with metronidazole.
Giardia lamblia—Treatment is with metronidazole.
Blastocystis hominis—Because there is no evidence that *Blastocystis hominis* is pathogenic, it does not need to be treated.

The rates of symptomatic infection with *Entamoeba histolytica*, *Giardia lamblia*, and *Blastocystis hominis* are not markedly higher than in patients who do not have AIDS. *Entamoeba histolytica* is a nonpathogenic commensal in most patients with AIDS. Giardiasis may require prolonged treatment, as in other immunocompetent persons.

DIAGNOSTIC EVALUATION OF PATIENTS WITH AIDS WHO HAVE DIARRHEA

Initial studies include examination for stool leukocytes; stool cultures for *Salmonella* species, *Shigella flexneri*, and *Campylobacter jejuni* (at least three specimens); stool examination for ova and parasites (using saline, iodine, trichrome, and acid-fast preparations); and stool assay for *Clostridium difficile* toxin. Additional studies include 1) gastroscopy to inspect tissue, to aspirate luminal material, and to obtain biopsy specimens; 2) examination of duodenal aspirate for parasites and culture; 3) culture of duodenal biopsy specimens for cytomegalovirus and mycobacteria; 4) colonoscopy to inspect tissue and to obtain biopsy specimens; 5) culture of biopsy specimens for cytomegalovirus, adenovirus, mycobacteria, and herpes simplex virus; and 6) staining biopsy specimens with hematoxylin-eosin for protozoa and viral inclusion cells, with methenamine silver or Giemsa stain for fungi, and with Fite method for mycobacteria.

Whether further evaluation is needed if the studies listed above do not yield a diagnosis is a matter of controversy. Most experts advocate empiric treatment with loperamide (Imodium). Others recommend that biopsy specimens from the duodenum be examined with electron microscopy for Microsporida or from the colon for adenovirus. We favor empiric treatment with loperamide because there is no treatment for either Microsporida or adenovirus.

COLON

Pseudomembranous Enterocolitis

This is a necrotizing inflammatory disease of the intestines characterized by the formation of a membrane-like collection of exudate overlying a degenerating mucosa. Precipitating factors include colon obstruction, uremia, ischemia, intestinal surgery, and all antibiotics (except vancomycin).

Antibiotic Colitis

The symptoms of antibiotic colitis are fever, abdominal pain, and diarrhea (mucus and blood), which usually occur 1 to 6 weeks after antibiotic therapy. Sigmoidoscopy shows pseudomembranes and friability. Biopsy specimens show inflammation and microulceration with exudation. The condition usually remits, but it recurs in 15% of patients. Complications include perforation and megacolon. *Pathogenesis*: the antibiotic alters colonic flora so there is overgrowth of *Clostridium difficile*. The toxin produced by *C. difficile* is cytotoxic, causing necrosis of the epithelium and exudation (pseudomembranes). *Diagnosis*: a toxin assay is positive in 98% of patients, and cultures are positive in about 75%. Radiography shows pseudomembranes. Proctoscopic findings may be normal or show classic pseudomembranes. *Treatment*: discontinue use of antibiotics and provide general supportive care (e.g., fluids). Avoid use of antimotility agents. If no response, metronidazole (250 mg three times daily) is 80% effective and inexpensive. Vancomycin (125 mg four times daily) is also 80% effective but expensive. If the patient is very ill, cholestyramine binds toxin. For a first recurrence, the same antibiotic can be used or the drug can be switched. For multiple recurrences, add cholestyramine and prolong the course of treatment with antibiotics.

- Antibiotic colitis: symptoms include fever, abdominal pain, diarrhea 1-6 weeks after antibiotic therapy.
- A toxin assay is positive in 98% of patients.
- Culture is positive in 75%.
- Metronidazole is the initial treatment.
- 15% of patients have recurrence.

Radiation Colitis

Irradiation injury usually affects both the colon and the small bowel. Endothelial cells of small submucosal arterioles are very radiosensitive and respond to large doses of irradiation by swelling, proliferating, and undergoing fibrinoid degeneration. The result is an obliterative endarteritis. Disease spectrum— *Acute disease* occurs during or immediately after irradiation; the mucosa fails to regenerate, and there is friability, hyperemia, and edema. *Subacute disease* occurs 2 to 12 months after irradiation. Obliterative endarteritis produces progressive inflammation and ulceration. *Chronic disease* consists of fistulas, abscesses, strictures, and bleeding from intestinal mucosal vessels. Predisposing factors include other diseases that produce microvascular insufficiency (e.g., hypertension, diabetes mellitus, atherosclerosis, and heart failure) because they accelerate the development of vascular occlusion, total irradiation dose of 40 to 50 Gy, previous chemotherapy, adhesions, previous surgery and pelvic inflammatory disease, and age (the elderly are more susceptible). Radiography of acute disease shows fine serrations of the bowel, and radiography of chronic dis-

ease shows stricture of the rectum. Endoscopy shows atrophic mucosa with telangiectatic vessels. *Treatment*: endoscopic coagulation is effective for bleeding. Surgery may be required for fistulas, strictures, or abscesses.

- Radiation colitis involves both the colon and small bowel.
- The endothelial cells of the small submucosal arterioles are very radiosensitive.
- The result is obliterative endarteritis.
- Predisposing factors: hypertension, diabetes mellitus, atherosclerosis, chemotherapy, and >40 Gy of irradiation.
- The rectum is involved most commonly.

Ischemia

Review of Vascular Anatomy

The celiac trunk supplies the stomach and duodenum. The superior mesenteric artery supplies the jejunum, ileum, and right colon. The inferior mesenteric artery supplies the left colon and rectum.

Acute Ischemia

The symptoms of acute ischemia are sudden severe abdominal pain, vomiting, and diarrhea (with or without blood). Early in the course of ischemia, physical examination findings are normal despite complaints of severe abdominal pain, but later findings indicate peritonitis. Risk factors include severe atherosclerosis, congestive heart failure, atrial fibrillation (source of emboli), hypotension, and oral contraceptives.

There are several syndromes.

1. Acute mesenteric ischemia is due to embolic obstruction of the superior mesenteric artery in 80% of patients. Most (95%) emboli lodge in this artery because of laminar flow, vessel caliber, and the angle it takes off from the aorta. The clue to search for emboli is atrial fibrillation. This syndrome results in a loss of small bowel and produces short-bowel syndrome. Radiography shows ileus, small-bowel obstruction, and, later, gas in the portal vein. The treatment is embolectomy.

2. Ischemic colitis is due to a transient decrease in perfusion pressure in a setting of chronic, diffuse mesenteric vascular disease. This decrease occurs in severe dehydration or shock and results in ischemia of the gastrointestinal tract. It commonly involves areas of the colon between adjacent arteries, that is, "watershed areas," such as the splenic flexure and rectosigmoid. This syndrome presents with abdominal pain and rectal bleeding. The characteristic radiographic feature is thumbprinting of watershed areas. The treatment is supportive and, if the condition deteriorates, surgical resection.

3. Nonocclusive ischemia is due to poor tissue perfusion caused by inadequate cardiac output. It can involve both the small and large bowel. Its distribution does not conform to an area

supplied by a major vessel. It occurs in patients with cardiac failure or anoxia or in patients who are in shock. It is questioned whether digitalis causes mesenteric vasoconstriction.

- Acute superior mesenteric artery syndrome is usually due to emboli.
- Ischemic colitis: diagnosis is based on the radiographic finding of thumbprinting of watershed areas.

Chronic Ischemic Colitis (Intestinal Angina)

Chronic ischemic colitis is uncommon. Symptoms include postprandial pain and fear of eating (weight loss). At least two of three major splanchnic vessels must be occluded. It is associated with hypertension, diabetes mellitus, and atherosclerosis. Abdominal bruit is a clue to the diagnosis. Angiography is diagnostic in about 50% of cases and shows a stenotic area in two of three major vessels. The treatment is surgical revascularization.

Occlusion of the superior mesenteric vein accounts for approximately 10% of cases of bowel ischemia. Risk factors include hypercoagulable states such as polycythemia vera, liver disease, pancreatic cancer, intra-abdominal abscess, and portal hypertension. It presents as abdominal pain that gradually becomes severe. Diagnosis is based on angiographic findings. The treatment is surgical.

- Chronic ischemic colitis is associated with hypertension, diabetes mellitus, and atherosclerosis.
- Mesenteric venous thrombosis occurs with hypercoagulable states.

Amebic Colitis

The colon is the usual site of the disease initially. Symptoms vary from none to explosive bloody diarrhea with fever, tenesmus, and abdominal cramps. Proctoscopy shows discrete ulcers with undermined edges and normal adjacent mucosa. If an exudate is present, swab and make wet mount preparations for trophozoites. Indirect hemagglutination is useful for invasive disease. Radiography shows concentric narrowing of the cecum in 90% of cases. Treat with metronidazole. *Entamoeba histolytica* is the only pathogenic ameba in humans.

- The colon is the initial site of disease.
- Proctoscopy shows discrete ulcers with undermined edges.
- Radiography shows concentric narrowing of the cecum in 90% of cases.
- *Entamoeba histolytica* is the only pathogenic ameba in humans.

Tuberculosis

Tuberculosis presents as diarrhea, a change in bowel habits, and rectal bleeding. The ileocecal area is the most commonly involved site. Radiography shows a contracted cecum and ascending colon and ulceration. Proctoscopy demonstrates deep and superficial ulcers. The rectum may be spared. A hypertrophic ulcerating mass may be seen. Biopsy samples stained with Ziehl-Neelsen stain are positive for acid-fast bacilli. All cases are associated with pulmonary or miliary tuberculosis.

- Tuberculosis is associated with diarrhea, change in bowel habits, and rectal bleeding.
- The ileocecal area is commonly involved.
- Deep and superficial ulcers are characteristic findings.
- All cases are associated with pulmonary or miliary tuberculosis.

Streptococcus bovis Endocarditis

This is associated with colon disease (diverticulosis or cancer). The colon should be evaluated.

Irritable Bowel Syndrome

The term "irritable bowel syndrome" is used for symptoms that are presumed to arise from the small and large intestines. It refers to a well-recognized complex of symptoms arising from interactions of the intestine, the psyche, and, possibly, luminal factors. Most patients have abdominal pain that is relieved with defecation or associated with a change in the frequency or consistency of the stool. Other associated symptoms include abdominal bloating and passage of excessive mucus with the stool.

Patients with irritable bowel syndrome usually have a long duration of symptoms, symptoms associated with situations of stress, and no weight loss, no intestinal bleeding, and no associated organic symptoms (e.g., arthritis or fever). Irritable bowel syndrome is a diagnosis of exclusion: the diagnosis is confirmed by an appropriate medical evaluation that does not reveal any organic illness. Always ask if the patient's symptoms are related to ingestion of dairy foods because lactase deficiency must be ruled out. Patients who have upper abdominal discomfort and bloating may require an ultrasonographic examination of the abdomen and esophagogastroduodenoscopy. Patients with lower abdominal discomfort or with a change in bowel habits may require stool studies, proctoscopic examination, and colon radiography or colonoscopy.

The treatment of irritable bowel syndrome is reassurance, stress reduction, high fiber diet, or the use of fiber supplements. The use of antispasmodics to control abdominal pain or antimotility agents to control diarrhea should be reserved for patients who do not have a response to a high fiber diet.

Nontoxic Megacolon (Pseudo-Obstruction)

Acute pseudo-obstruction of the colon occurs postoperatively (nonabdominal operations) and with spinal cord injury, sepsis, uremia, electrolyte imbalance, and drugs (narcotics, anticholinergics, and psychotropic agents). When the cecum is more than 13 or 14 cm in diameter, the risk of perforation increases. Obstruction should be ruled out with Hypaque enema. Treatment includes placement of a nasogastric tube, discontinuation of drug therapy, correction of metabolic abnormalities, and, if needed, colonoscopic decompression or cecostomy.

Chronic pseudo-obstruction of the colon is seen in disorders that cause generalized intestinal pseudo-obstruction.

Congenital Megacolon

Congenital megacolon (Hirschsprung disease) occurs in 1 in 5,000 births. There is increased incidence with Down syndrome. Congenital megacolon usually becomes manifest in infancy; however, it can present in adulthood. There is a variable length of aganglionic segment from the rectum to the proximal colon (usually confined to the rectum or rectosigmoid). The diagnosis is usually made at birth because of meconium ileus or obstipation. If the diagnosis is made in an adult, the patient has a history of chronic constipation. Colon radiography shows a characteristically narrowed distal segment and a dilated proximal colon. Rectal biopsy shows aganglionosis. Anorectal manometry shows loss of the anorectal inhibitory reflex. Treatment is with sphincter-saving operations.

- Congenital megacolon: increased incidence with Down syndrome.
- In adults, chronic constipation.
- Colon radiography shows a characteristically narrowed distal segment and dilated proximal colon.
- Rectal biopsy shows aganglionosis.
- Motility: absence of anorectal inhibitory reflex.

Lower Gastrointestinal Tract Bleeding

The evaluation of rectal bleeding should begin with a digital examination, anoscopy, and proctosigmoidoscopy. If a definitive diagnosis cannot be made, perform a barium enema or arteriography, depending on the nature of the bleeding. The inability to cleanse the colon appropriately during active bleeding makes the barium enema difficult to perform and interpret. Some advocate the use of nuclear scanning if the activity of the bleeding is uncertain. With active bleeding, angiography is the diagnostic procedure of choice. It is also indicated for patients with recurrent episodes of rectal bleeding who have had normal results on previous standard tests, that is, barium enema or colonoscopy. Colonoscopy is not useful if bleeding in the lower gastrointestinal tract is torrential, but it may be of some benefit if there is a slower rate of bleeding. Colonoscopy is valuable for evaluating patients who have unexplained rectal bleeding and persistently positive findings on tests for occult blood in the stool.

- Initial evaluation of rectal bleeding: digital examination, anoscopy, and proctosigmoidoscopy.
- If activity of bleeding is uncertain, try a nuclear scan.
- Colonoscopy is not useful if there is torrential bleeding in the lower gastrointestinal tract.
- Angiography is the procedure of choice for active bleeding.

The important causes of lower gastrointestinal tract bleeding are the following:

- Angiodysplasia: it usually involves the right colon and small bowel and may respond to endoscopic treatment.
- Diverticular disease: usually bleeding without other symptoms.
- Inflammatory bowel disease (colitis): 5% of patients present with this.
- Ischemic colitis: painful and bloody diarrhea.
- Cancer: rarely causes marked bleeding.
- Meckel diverticulum: the commonest cause of lower gastrointestinal tract bleeding in young patients. It is usually painless.
- Hemorrhoids: are usually present as rectal outlet bleeding.

Evaluation of lower gastrointestinal tract bleeding—Stabilize the patient, perform proctoscopy to rule out rectal outlet bleeding, and obtain a nasogastric tube aspirate or use esophagogastroduodenoscopy to rule out upper gastrointestinal tract bleeding. A radionuclide-tagged red blood cell scan may help determine whether bleeding is occurring, but it may not localize precisely the bleeding site. If there is active bleeding, perform angiography. If bleeding stops or occurs at a slow rate, perform colonoscopy. If the patient is young, perform a Meckel scan.

Treatment—If angiography localizes the bleeding site, infusion of vasopressin or embolization may be useful. If colonoscopy demonstrates bleeding, injection of epinephrine, electrocoagulation, or laser coagulation may be useful. If bleeding is massive or if marked bleeding continues, surgical management is needed.

Diverticular Disease of the Colon

Definitions

"Diverticula" are acquired herniations of the mucosa and submucosa through the muscular layers of the colonic wall. "Diverticulosis" is the mere presence of uninflamed diverticula of the colon. "Diverticulitis" is the inflammation of one or more diverticula. The diagnosis and management of the complications of diverticular disease are outlined in Table 7-13.

Diverticulitis

Microperforation or macroperforation of the diverticulum with subsequent peridiverticular inflammation is necessary to

Table 7-13 Diagnosis and Management of Complications of Diverticular Disease

Complication	Signs and symptoms	Findings	Treatment
Diverticulitis	Pain, fever, and constipation or diarrhea (or both)	Palpable tender colon, leukocytosis	Liquid diet, with or without antibiotics, or elective surgery
Pericolic abscess	Pain, fever (with or without tenderness), or pus in stools	Tender mass, guarding leukocytosis, soft tissue mass on abdominal films or ultrasonograms	Nothing by mouth, intravenous fluids, antibiotics, early surgical treatment with colostomy
Fistula	Depends on site: dysuria, pneumaturia, fecal discharge on skin or vagina	Depends on site: fistulogram, methylene blue	Antibiotics, clear liquids, colostomy, and, later, resection
Perforation	Sudden severe pain, fever	Sepsis, leukocytosis, free air	Antibiotics, nothing by mouth, intravenous fluids, immediate surgical treatment
Liver abscess	Right upper quadrant pain, fever, weight loss	Tender liver, tender bowel or mass, leukocytosis, alkaline phosphatase, lumbosacral scan (filling defect)	Antibiotics, surgical drainage, operation for bowel disease
Bleeding	Bright red or maroon blood or clots	Blood on rectal exam, sigmoidoscopy, colonoscopy, angiography	Conservative: blood transfusion if needed, with or without operation

produce diverticulitis. The severity of the clinical symptoms depends on the extent of the inflammation. Free perforation is infrequent (diverticula are invested by longitudinal muscle and mesentery). Local perforations may dissect along the colon wall and form intramural fistulas. The clinical presentation is left lower quadrant pain, fever, abdominal distention, constipation, and, occasionally, a palpable tender mass. Treatment includes resting the bowel or using a low fiber diet and antibiotics and obtaining an early surgical consultation. Indications for surgical treatment during the acute phase include the development of generalized peritonitis, an enlarging inflammatory mass, fistula formation, colonic obstruction, inability to rule out carcinoma in an area of stricture, or recurrent episodes of diverticulitis.

- Diverticulitis: the clinical symptoms depend on the extent of inflammation.
- Free perforation is infrequent.
- Clinical presentation: left lower quadrant pain, fever, abdominal distention, constipation, and, occasionally, a palpable tender mass.
- Treatment: bowel rest and antibiotics; obtain a surgical consultation.

Angiodysplasia

Angiodysplasia is a common and increasingly recognized cause of lower gastrointestinal tract bleeding in elderly patients. Acquired vascular ectasias are believed to be associated with aging. Angiodysplasia is associated with cardiac disease, especially aortic stenosis. It usually involves the cecum and ascending colon. There are no associated skin or visceral lesions. The ectasias appear to be due to the chronic, partial, intermittent, and low-grade obstruction of submucosal veins where they penetrate the colon. Obstruction is from muscle contraction and distention of the cecum. Colon radiography is of no diagnostic value. Angiography localizes the extent of involvement. Colonoscopy may show lesions. Apply cautery.

- Acquired vascular ectasias are associated with aging.
- Angiodysplasia is associated with cardiac disease, especially aortic stenosis.
- It usually involves the cecum and ascending colon.
- Colonoscopy may show lesions. Apply cautery.

Colon Polyps

Types of epithelial polyps include hyperplastic, hamartomatous, inflammatory, and adenomatous polyps. Hyperplastic polyps are metaplastic, completely differentiated glandular elements; they are benign. Hamartomatous polyps are a mixture of normal tissues; they are benign. Inflammatory polyps are an epithelial inflammatory reaction; they are benign. Adenomatous polyps represent a failure of differentiation of glandular elements. They are the only neoplastic (premalignant) polyp. The three types of adenomatous polyps are tubular adenoma, mixed (tubulovillous) adenoma, and villous adenoma (syndrome of hypokalemia, profuse mucus). The risk of cancer in any adenomatous polyp depends on two features: size larger than 1 cm and the presence of villous elements. If a polyp is found on flexible sigmoidoscopy and biopsy shows a hyperplastic polyp, no further work-up is needed. If biopsy shows an adenomatous polyp, perform colonoscopy to look for additional polyps and to perform polypectomy.

- Adenomatous polyps are the only neoplastic (premalignant) polyp; there are three types.
- The risk of cancer in any adenomatous polyp depends on size >1 cm and the presence of villous elements.
- If biopsy shows an adenomatous polyp, perform colonoscopy.

Hereditary Polyposis Syndromes

Only those polyposis syndromes associated with adenomatous polyps have a risk of cancer.

Familial Polyposis

This is adenomatous polyps of the colon. More than 95% of the patients develop colorectal carcinoma. There are no extra-abdominal manifestations except for bilateral congenital hypertrophy of the retinal pigment epithelium. Diagnosis is based on family history and documentation of adenomatous polyps. Screening is indicated for all family members, and colectomy is indicated before malignancy develops.

- More than 95% of patients with familial polyposis develop colorectal carcinoma.
- There are no extra-abdominal manifestations except for bilateral congenital hypertrophy of the retinal pigment epithelium.
- Colectomy is indicated before malignancy develops.

Gardner Syndrome

This is adenomatous polyps involving the colon, although rarely the terminal ileum and proximal small bowel are involved. More than 95% of patients develop colorectal cancer. Extraintestinal manifestations include congenital hypertrophy of the retinal pigment epithelium; osteomas of the mandible, skull, and long bones; supernumerary teeth; soft tissue tumors; thyroid and adrenal tumors; and epidermoid

and sebaceous cysts. Screening is indicated for family members, and colectomy should be performed before malignancy develops.

- More than 95% of patients with Gardner syndrome develop colorectal cancer.
- There are extraintestinal manifestations.
- Screening is indicated for family members.

Turcot-Despres Syndrome

This is adenomatous polyps of the colon associated with malignant gliomas and other brain tumors. The inheritance is autosomal recessive.

Polyposis Syndromes Not Associated With Risk of Cancer

Peutz-Jeghers Syndrome

This is hamartomas of the small intestine and, less commonly, of the stomach and colon. Pigmented lesions of the mouth, hands, and feet are associated with ovarian sex cord tumors and tumors of the proximal small bowel.

- Peutz-Jeghers syndrome: hamartomas of the small intestine.
- Pigmented lesions of the mouth, hands, and feet are associated with ovarian sex cord and proximal small bowel tumors.

Juvenile Polyposis

This is hyperplastic polyps involving the colon and, less commonly, the small intestine and stomach. It presents as gastrointestinal tract bleeding or intussusception with obstruction.

- Only adenomatous polyps are premalignant.
- Perform colectomy for diffuse polyposis only if the polyps are adenomatous.
- Screening is indicated for patients with heritable polyposis syndromes only if the polyps are adenomatous.
- All the above syndromes are autosomal dominant except Turcot-Despres syndrome.

Colorectal Cancer

Epidemiology

Epidemiology is important in etiologic theories. Colorectal carcinoma is the second most common cancer in the United States, with 100,000 new cases and 60,000 deaths annually. Colon cancer eventually develops in 6% of Americans. The mortality rate has not decreased since the 1930s. The incidence varies widely among different populations; it is highest in "westernized" countries. Compared with past rates, rates for cancer of the right colon and sigmoid colon have increased but have decreased for the rectum: cecum/ascending colon, 25%; sigmoid, 25%; rectum, 20%; transverse colon, 12%; rectosigmoid, 10%; and descending colon, 6%.

- Colorectal cancer is the second most common cancer in the United States.
- Rates for cancer of the right colon and sigmoid colon have increased.

Etiology

The role of the environment as a cause of colorectal cancer is supported by regional differences and migrant studies of incidence. A high fat diet increases the risk and may enhance the cholesterol/bile acid content of bile, which is converted by colonic bacteria to compounds that may promote tumors. A high fiber diet is protective. Increased stool bulk may dilute carcinogens/promoters and decrease exposure by decreasing transit time. Fiber components may bind carcinogens or decrease bacterial enzymes that form toxic compounds. Charbroiled meat or fish and fried foods contain possible mutagens. Antioxidants (vitamins A and C), selenium, vitamin E, yellow-green vegetables, and calcium may protect against cancer.

- A high fat diet increases the risk of colorectal cancer.
- A high fiber diet has a protective effect.
- Charbroiled meat or fish and fried foods contain possible mutagens.

Genetic Factors

Certain oncogenes amplify or alter gene products in colon cancer cells. Aneuploidy is characteristic of more aggressive tumors. The carbohydrate structure of colonic mucus is altered in colon cancer. Cell-cell interaction possibly has a role in cancer development. Also, genetic predisposition has a role in many patients with colon cancer. Familial adenomatous polyposis syndromes are autosomal dominant. Most colon cancer arises in adenomatous polyps. Hereditary nonpolyposis colon cancer (Lynch syndrome) is an autosomal dominant disease that may account for up to 5% of cases of colon cancer. Genetic susceptibility in the general population also has a role, for example, a threefold increased risk of colorectal cancer in first-degree relatives of patients with sporadic colorectal cancer.

- Aneuploidy is characteristic of more aggressive tumors.
- Genetic predisposition to cancer exists in many patients with colon cancer.
- Familial adenomatous polyposis is autosomal dominant.
- There is a threefold increased risk of colorectal cancer in first-degree relatives of patients with sporadic colorectal cancer.

Risk Factors for Colorectal Cancer

The risk factors for colorectal cancer include the following: Age older than 40—the risk increases sharply at age 40, doubles each decade until age 60, and peaks at age 80. Personal history of adenoma or colon cancer—the risk increases with the number of adenomas; from 2% to 6% of patients with colon cancer have synchronous colon cancer and 1.1% to 4.7% have metachronous colon cancer. Inflammatory bowel disease—dysplasia precedes cancer. The cancer rate begins to increase after 7 years of chronic ulcerative colitis and increases 10% per decade of disease. After 25 years, the risk is 30%. The risk is greatest for universal colitis. The risk is delayed a decade in left-sided colitis and is negligible in ulcerative proctitis. Cancer risk is not related to the severity of the first attack, disease activity, or age at onset. The rate of colon cancer is also increased 4 to 20 times in Crohn disease or ileocolitis. A family history of colon cancer is a risk factor, and a personal history of female genital or breast cancer carries a twofold increased risk of colon cancer.

- Colorectal cancer risk factor: age older than 40.
- Risk increases with the number of adenomas.
- From 2%-6% of patients with colon cancer have synchronous colon cancer and 1.1%-4.7% have metachronous colon cancer.
- Cancer rate begins to increase after 7 years of chronic ulcerative colitis.
- After 25 years, the risk is 30%.
- The risk is greatest for universal colitis.
- Crohn disease: the rate of colon cancer is increased 4-20 times.

Pathology and Prognostic Indicators

Cancer arises in the epithelium and invades transmurally to penetrate the bowel wall; it then enters the regional lymphatics to reach distant nodes. Hematogenous spread is through the portal vein to the liver.

Surgical-pathologic stage of primary tumor—The depth of invasion and the extent of regional lymph node involvement are important in determining prognosis.

Modified Dukes classification demonstrates that survival is determined by the extent of the invasion—A, mucosa, submucosa (95% 5-year survival); B1, into, not through, the muscularis propria without nodal involvement (85%); B2, through the bowel wall without regional nodal involvement (70%-85%); C1, with regional nodes involved (45%-55%); C2, with regional nodes involved (20%-30%); and D, distant metastases (<1%).

The extent of regional node involvement and prognosis: 1 to 4 nodes, 35% recur; more than 4 nodes, 61% recur.

Other pathologic features and prognosis include 1) an ulcerating/infiltrating tumor is worse than an exophytic/polypoid tumor; 2) poorly differentiated histologic features are worse than highly differentiated ones; 3) venous/lymphatic invasion has a poor prognosis, as does aneuploidy.

Clinical features and prognosis—A high preoperative level of carcinoembryonic antigen is associated with a high recurrence rate and a shorter time before recurrence develops. The prognosis is poor if obstruction or perforation is present. The prognosis is worse for younger than for older patients.

- The depth of invasion and the extent of regional lymph node involvement are important in determining prognosis.
- A high preoperative level of carcinoembryonic antigen is associated with high recurrence and a shorter time before recurrence.
- The prognosis is poor if obstruction or perforation is present.
- The prognosis is worse for younger than for older patients.

Diagnosis

The clinical presentation is that of a slow growth pattern. Disease may be present for 5 years before symptoms appear. The symptoms depend on the location of the disease. A tumor in the proximal colon may present with symptoms of anemia, abdominal discomfort, or a mass. The left colon is narrower, and patients may present with obstructive symptoms, change in bowel habits, and rectal bleeding.

If cancer is suspected, perform an air-contrast barium enema and flexible sigmoidoscopy or colonoscopy. If cancer is detected with an air-contrast barium enema or flexible sigmoidoscopy, colonoscopy is needed to rule out synchronous lesions.

A metastatic survey includes physical examination, evaluation of liver-associated enzymes, and chest radiography. Image the liver if the levels of liver-associated enzymes are abnormal. The preoperative level of carcinoembryonic antigen is helpful for assessing prognosis and for follow-up.

- Proximal colon disease: presenting symptoms may be anemia, abdominal discomfort, or mass.
- Left colon disease: obstructive symptoms, change in bowel habits, and rectal bleeding.
- Preoperative level of carcinoembryonic antigen is helpful for assessing prognosis and for follow-up.

Treatment

For most cases, surgical resection is the treatment of choice. This includes wide resection of the involved segment (5-cm margins), with removal of lymphatic drainage. In rectal carcinoma, a low anterior resection is performed if an adequate distal margin of at least 2 cm can be achieved; this rectal sphincter-saving operation does not make the prognosis worse in comparison with abdominal perineal resection. The tumor may require resection to prevent obstruction or bleeding even if distant metastases are present.

- For most cases, surgical resection is the treatment of choice.

Postoperative Management—No Apparent Metastases

A single colonoscopy either preoperatively or within 6 to 12 months postoperatively is needed to exclude synchronous lesions. If the findings are negative, colonoscopy is repeated every 3 years.

Adjuvant chemotherapy—5-Fluorouracil and levamisole decrease recurrence by 41% and mortality by 33% in colonic stage C; they may be beneficial for stage B2. Radiotherapy plus 5-fluorouracil decreases the recurrence rate in rectal cancer stages B2 and C, but it is not clear if there is any survival advantage.

- A single colonoscopy to exclude synchronous lesions and then colonoscopy every 3 years if the findings are negative.
- Annually test for occult blood in the stool.
- 5-Fluorouracil and levamisole decrease recurrence by 41% and mortality by 33% in colonic stage C.

Prevention of Colorectal Carcinoma

Primary prevention—The steps to be taken in primary prevention are not known, although epidemiologic data indicate that a high fiber, low fat diet is reasonable. Secondary prevention—Identify and eradicate premalignant lesions and detect cancer while it is still curable. Screening includes occult blood screening and sigmoidoscopy. With occult blood screening, earlier stage lesions are detected, but this has not decreased mortality. The Hemoccult test has a 20% to 30% positive predictive value for adenomas and 5% to 10% for carcinomas. With sigmoidoscopy, earlier stage lesions are detected, and the removal of adenomas results in a lower than expected incidence of rectosigmoid cancer, but none show decreased mortality. Flexible sigmoidoscopy detects 2 to 3 times more neoplasms than rigid proctoscopy.

Recommendations for screening—1) For average risk (i.e., anyone not in the high-risk group): annual rectal examination after age 40; annual occult blood test plus sigmoidoscopy every 3 to 5 years after age 50. Alternatively, colonoscopy every 10 years after age 50 can replace sigmoidoscopy and occult blood testing. 2) For previous adenoma or carcinoma: annual occult blood testing; colonoscopy every year until normal for 2 years, then every 3 years. 3) For familial adenomatous polyposis: annual sigmoidoscopy beginning at puberty until polyposis is diagnosed, then colectomy. 4) For hereditary nonpolyposis cancer syndromes: colonoscopy at age 20, then annual occult blood testing and colonoscopy every 3 years. 5) For first-degree relative with colorectal cancer: annual occult blood testing and periodic sigmoidoscopy beginning at age 40. 6) For a woman with breast or genital cancer: annual occult blood testing and periodic sigmoidoscopy. 7) For ulcerative colitis: annual colonoscopy and multiple biopsies starting after 7 years of universal chronic ulcerative colitis or after 15 years of left-sided chronic ulcerative colitis; dysplasia indicates the need for more frequent endoscopic follow-up and may lead to colectomy.

- Earlier stage lesions can be detected, but early detection has not been shown to decrease mortality.
- Flexible sigmoidoscopy detects 2-3 times more neoplasms than rigid proctoscopy.

PANCREAS

Embryology

The pancreas develops in week 4 of gestation as a ventral and dorsal outpouching or bud from the duodenum. Each bud has its own duct. As the duodenum rotates, the buds appose and join, and the ducts anastomose. "Pancreas divisum" results from the failure of the ducts of the dorsal and ventral pancreas to fuse. It is debated whether this may predispose to acute or recurrent pancreatitis. In "annular pancreas," part of the ventral pancreas encircles the duodenum (usually the second part, proximal to the ampulla) and causes obstruction.

- Pancreas divisum: failure of the dorsal and ventral pancreas to fuse. Might predispose to acute pancreatitis. Be able to recognize this condition on radiographs.
- Annular pancreas: part of the ventral pancreas encircles the duodenum (usually the second part, proximal to the ampulla) and causes obstruction. Be able to recognize this on radiographs.

Classification of Pancreatitis

Acute pancreatitis is a reversible inflammation. The two varieties are interstitial and necrotizing pancreatitis. Interstitial pancreatitis accounts for 80% of cases. Perfusion of the pancreas is intact. It is less severe than necrotizing pancreatitis, with less than 1% mortality. Necrotizing pancreatitis accounts for 20% of cases. It is more severe, with 10% mortality if sterile and 30% if infected.

Chronic pancreatitis is irreversible (i.e., structural disease, with endocrine or exocrine insufficiency). It is documented by pancreatic calcifications on abdominal radiography, parenchymal and ductal abnormalities on endoscopic ultrasonography (EUS), or by ductal abnormalities on endoscopic retrograde cholangiopancreatography (ERCP), by scarring on pancreatic biopsy, or by endocrine insufficiency (diabetes mellitus) or exocrine insufficiency (malabsorption).

- Acute interstitial pancreatitis: perfusion is intact, mortality is <1%.
- Acute necrotizing pancreatitis: perfusion is compromised, mortality is 10% if sterile and 30% if infected.

- Chronic pancreatitis is documented by pancreatic calcifications, ductal abnormalities, endocrine insufficiency (diabetes), and exocrine insufficiency (malabsorption).

Acute Pancreatitis

In acute pancreatitis, activation of pancreatic enzymes causes autodigestion of the gland. The clinical features are abdominal pain, nausea and vomiting ("too sick to eat"), ileus, peritoneal signs, hypotension, and abdominal mass.

Etiologic Factors

Alcohol is the most common cause and gallstones the second most common cause. The third most common cause is idiopathic (approximately 10% of cases). The following drugs cause pancreatitis: azathioprine, 6-mercaptopurine, L-asparaginase, hydrochlorothiazide diuretics, sulfonamides, sulfasalazine, tetracycline, furosemide, estrogens, valproic acid, pentamidine (both parenteral and aerosolized), and the antiretroviral drug didanosine (ddI). Know these drugs.

The evidence that the following drugs may also cause pancreatitis is less convincing and not definite: corticosteroids, NSAIDs, methyldopa, procainamide, chlorthalidone, ethacrynic acid, phenformin, nitrofurantoin, enalapril, erythromycin, metronidazole, and nonsulfa-linked aminosalicylate derivates (such as 5-aminosalicylic acid and interleukin-2).

Other causes—Hypertriglyceridemia may cause pancreatitis if the triglyceride level is usually greater than 1,000. Look for types I, IV, and V hyperlipoproteinemia and for associated oral contraceptive use. Hypertriglyceridemia may mask hyperamylasemia. Hypercalcemia may also cause pancreatitis; look for underlying multiple myeloma, hyperparathyroidism, or metastatic carcinoma. In immunocompetent patients, mumps and coxsackievirus cause acute pancreatitis. In AIDS patients, acute pancreatitis has been reported with cytomegalovirus infection. Ductus divisum, or incomplete fusion of the dorsal and ventral pancreatic ducts, may predispose to acute pancreatitis in some people, although this is a controversial matter.

- In nonalcoholic patients with acute pancreatitis, review all medications, check lipid and calcium levels, and rule out gallstones.
- Know which medications definitely cause acute pancreatitis.

Clinical Presentation

Pain—It may be mild to severe; it is usually sudden in onset and persistent. The pain is located typically in the upper abdomen and radiates to the back. Relief may be obtained by bending forward or sitting up. The ingestion of food or alcohol commonly exacerbates the pain. The absence of pain is a poor prognostic feature because these patients usually present with shock.

Fever—If present, it is low grade, rarely exceeding 101°F in the absence of complications.

Volume depletion—Most patients are hypovolemic because fluid accumulates in the abdomen.

Jaundice—Patients with pancreatitis may have a mild increase in total bilirubin, but they usually are not clinically jaundiced. When jaundice is present, it generally represents obstruction of the common bile duct by stones, compression by pseudocyst, or inflamed pancreatic tissue.

Dyspnea—A wide range of pulmonary manifestations may be seen. In more than half of all cases of acute pancreatitis, some degree of hypoxemia is present. This is usually from pulmonary shunting. Patients often have atelectasis and may develop pleural effusions.

- Fever >101°F suggests infection.

Diagnosis of Acute Pancreatitis

Serum amylase—Determining the serum level of amylase is the most useful test for acute pancreatitis. The level of amylase increases 2 or 3 hours after an attack and remains increased for 3 or 4 days. The magnitude of the increase does not correlate with the clinical severity of the attack. Serum amylase levels may be normal in some (<10%) patients because of alcohol or hypertriglyceridemia. A persistent increase suggests a complication, for example, pseudocyst, abscess, or ascites. Serum amylase is cleared by the kidney. The urine amylase level remains elevated after the serum amylase level returns to normal. Isoenzyme identification may aid in distinguishing between salivary (nonpancreatic) and pancreatic sources. Serum lipase may help distinguish between pancreatic hyperamylasemia and an ectopic source (lung, ovarian, or esophageal carcinoma). Lipase levels are also increased for a longer time than amylase levels after acute pancreatitis.

Nonpancreatic hyperamylasemia—Parotitis; renal failure; macroamylasemia; intestinal obstruction, infarction, perforation; ruptured ectopic pregnancy; diabetic ketoacidosis; drugs (such as morphine); burns; pregnancy; and neoplasms (lung, ovary, esophagus).

- If the presentation for pancreatitis is classic but the amylase value is normal, repeat the amylase test, check urine amylase and serum lipase levels, and scan the abdomen.
- Persistent hyperamylasemia suggests a complication.
- If the amylase level is mildly elevated and there is a history of vomiting but no signs of obstruction, perform esophagogastroduodenoscopy to rule out a penetrating ulcer.

Physical findings include the following: 1) Vital signs—tachycardia and orthostasis. 2) Skin—fat necrosis and xanthelasmas. The Grey Turner sign (flank discoloration) and Cullen sign (periumbilical discoloration) suggest retroperitoneal hemorrhage. 3) Abdomen—the findings often are less impressive than the amount of pain the patient is experiencing.

- Be able to recognize metastatic fat necrosis.
- The Grey Turner sign and Cullen sign suggest retroperitoneal hemorrhage.

Laboratory findings—1) Chest radiography: an isolated left pleural effusion strongly suggests pancreatitis. Infiltrates may represent aspiration pneumonia or adult respiratory distress syndrome. 2) Abdominal flat plate: look for the sentinel loop (a dilated loop of bowel over the pancreatic area) and colon cutoff sign (abrupt cutoff of gas in the transverse colon). Pancreatic calcifications indicate chronic pancreatitis. 3) Ultrasonography: the procedure of choice for acute pancreatitis, although in the presence of ileus, air in the bowel may obscure visualization of the pancreas. Ultrasonographic examination gives information about the pancreas and is the best method for delineating stones. However, it is not a good method to use if the patient is obese. 4) CT: if visualization of the pancreas is poor with ultrasonography, CT is the next step. It gives the same information as ultrasonography, is slightly less sensitive in detecting stones and texture abnormalities, involves irradiation, and is more expensive. CT is indicated for critically ill patients to rule out necrotizing pancreatitis and is the better imaging choice for obese patients. 5) ERCP: it has no role in the diagnosis of acute pancreatitis and should be avoided because it may cause infection. When acute pancreatitis is associated with jaundice and cholangitis, endoscopic papillotomy is indicated.

- An isolated left pleural effusion on chest radiography is strongly suggestive of acute pancreatitis.
- On an abdominal flat plate, be able to recognize the sentinel loop sign, colon cutoff sign, and pancreatic calcifications.
- Ultrasonography is the procedure of choice for patients with mild acute pancreatitis and for thin patients and to rule out gallstones.
- CT is indicated for obese patients and seriously ill patients to rule out necrotizing pancreatitis.
- ERCP has no role in the diagnosis of acute pancreatitis.

Treatment

Supportive care is the backbone of treatment, with monitoring for and treatment of complications when they occur.

Fluids—Restore and maintain intravascular volume; this usually can be accomplished with crystalloids and peripheral intravenous catheters. Monitor blood pressure, pulse, urine output, daily intake and output, and weight. Eliminate medications that may cause pancreatitis. The use of a nasogastric tube does not shorten the course or severity of pancreatitis, but it should be used in case of ileus or severe nausea and vomiting.

Analgesics—Meperidine (Demerol), 75 to 125 mg given intramuscularly every 3 or 4 hours, is preferred, especially over morphine, because it causes less spasm of the sphincter of Oddi. The efficacy of antisecretory drugs such as H_2-blockers, anticholinergic agents, somatostatin, or glucagon has not been documented. Total parenteral nutrition is unnecessary in most cases of pancreatitis. Peritoneal dialysis does not change the overall mortality, although it may decrease early mortality in severe pancreatitis.

- Supportive care is the backbone of treatment.
- Eliminate medications that may cause pancreatitis.
- The use of a nasogastric tube does not shorten the course or severity of pancreatitis.
- Meperidine (Demerol) is preferred because it causes less spasm of the sphincter of Oddi.

Complications

A local complication is phlegmon, a mass of inflamed pancreatic tissue. It may resolve. Pseudocysts, a fluid collection within a nonepithelial-lined cavity, should be expected if there is persistent pain and persistent hyperamylasemia. In 50% to 80% of patients, this resolves within 6 weeks without intervention. A pancreatic abscess usually develops 2 to 4 weeks after the acute episode and presents as fever (>101°F), persistent abdominal pain, and persistent hyperamylasemia. If a pancreatic abscess is not drained surgically, the mortality rate is virtually 100%. Give antibiotics that are effective for gram-negative and anaerobic organisms. Jaundice is due to obstruction of the common bile duct. Pancreatic ascites results from disruption of the pancreatic duct or a leaking pseudocyst.

- A local complication of pancreatitis should be suspected if fever, persistent pain, or persistent hyperamylasemia occurs.

A systemic complication is respiratory distress syndrome, a well-recognized complication of acute pancreatitis. Circulating lecithinase probably splits fatty acids off lecithin, producing a faulty surfactant. Pleural effusions occur in approximately 20% of patients with acute pancreatitis. If aspirated, a high amylase content is found. Fat necrosis may be due to increased levels of serum lipase.

- Adult respiratory distress syndrome is a complication of acute pancreatitis.
- Pleural effusions occur in approximately 20% of patients with acute pancreatitis and have a high amylase content.

Assessment of Severity

Most patients with acute pancreatitis recover without any sequelae. The overall mortality rate of acute pancreatitis is 5% to 10%, and death is due most often to hypovolemia and shock, respiratory failure, pancreatic abscess, or systemic sepsis. The Ranson criteria are reliable for predicting mortality in acute pancreatitis (Table 7-14). Mortality is as follows: fewer than three signs, 1%; three or four signs, 15%; five or six signs, 40%; and seven or more signs, 100%.

- Most patients with acute pancreatitis recover without any sequelae.

Chronic Pancreatitis

Chronic use of alcohol (at least 10 years of heavy consumption) is the most common cause of chronic pancreatitis. Gallstones and hyperlipidemia usually do not cause chronic pancreatitis.

Hereditary pancreatitis is caused by a mutation in the cationic trypsinogen gene, which is inherited as an autosomal dominant trait with variable penetrance. Onset is before age 20, although 20% of patients may present later than this. It is marked by recurring abdominal pain, positive family history, and pancreatic calcifications. It may increase the risk of pancreatic cancer.

Trauma with pancreatic ductal disruption causes chronic pancreatitis. Protein calorie malnutrition is the commonest cause of chronic pancreatitis in Third World countries.

- Chronic pancreatitis is commonly caused by alcohol but seldom by gallstones or hyperlipidemia.
- Hereditary pancreatitis is seen in young people with a positive family history and pancreatic calcifications.

Table 7-14 Ranson Criteria

Admission	48 Hours
Age >55 y	pO_2 <60 mm Hg
Leukocyte count >15 × 10^9/L	Hematocrit decrease >10%
Glucose >200 mg/dL	Albumin <3.2 g/dL
Aspartate aminotransferase >250 U/L	Blood urea nitrogen increase >5 mg/dL
Lactate dehydrogenase >350 U/L	Calcium <8 mg/dL
	Estimated fluid sequestration >4 L

Modified from Ranson JHC: Acute pancreatitis: surgical management. *In* The Exocrine Pancreas: Biology, Pathobiology, and Diseases. Edited by VLW Go, JD Gardner, FP Brooks, et al. New York, Raven Press, 1986, pp 503-511. By permission of publisher.

- Protein calorie malnutrition is the commonest cause of chronic pancreatitis in Third World countries.

Triad of Chronic Pancreatitis

The triad consists of pancreatic calcifications, steatorrhea, and diabetes mellitus. Pancreatic calcifications—Diffuse calcification is due to heredity, alcohol, or malnutrition. Local calcification is due to trauma, islet cell tumor, or hypercalcemia. By the time steatorrhea occurs, 90% of the gland has been destroyed and lipase output has decreased by 90%.

- Chronic pancreatitis presents as abdominal pain, pancreatic calcification, steatorrhea, and diabetes mellitus.

Laboratory Diagnosis

Amylase and lipase levels may be normal. Stool fat may be normal. If malabsorption is present, then stool fat is more than 10 g per 24 hours on a 48- to 72-hour stool collection while the patient is on a 100-g fat diet.

For the cholecystokinin (CCK)/secretin stimulation test of pancreatic function, secretin and CCK are injected intravenously and then the contents of the small bowel are aspirated and the concentration of pancreatic enzymes determined.

In the bentiromide test, para-aminobenzoic acid (PABA) conjugated with *N*-benzoyl tyrosine (bentiromide) is given orally. If chymotrypsin activity is adequate, the molecule is cleaved and PABA is absorbed and excreted in the urine. This test requires a normal small intestine (normal D-xylose test) and is useful only in severe steatorrhea.

CT shows calcifications, irregular pancreatic contour, dilated duct system, or pseudocysts.

ERCP shows protein plugs, segmental duct dilatation, and alternating stenosis and dilatation, with obliteration of branches of the main duct.

- Amylase and lipase levels may be normal, but evidence for structural disease or endocrine or exocrine insufficiency is present.
- For steatorrhea to occur, 90% of the gland must be damaged.

Pain

The mechanism of the pain is not clearly defined; it may be due to ductular obstruction. One-third to one-half of patients have a decrease in pain after 5 years. The possibility of coexistent disease such as peptic ulcer should be considered. Abstinence from alcohol may relieve the pain. Analgesics, aspirin, or acetaminophen is used occasionally with the addition of codeine (narcotic addiction is a frequent complicating factor). Celiac plexus blocks relieve pain for 3 to 6 months, but long-term efficacy is disappointing. A trial of pancreatic enzyme replacement for 1 or 2 months

should be tried. Women with idiopathic chronic pancreatitis are most likely to have a response. Surgical treatment should be considered only after conservative measures have failed. Patients with a dilated pancreatic duct may have a favorable response to a longitudinal pancreatojejunostomy (Puestow procedure).

- Abstinence from alcohol may relieve pain.
- Narcotic addiction is a frequent complicating factor.
- A 1- or 2-month trial of pancreatic enzyme replacement is worthwhile. Women are more likely to have a response.
- Surgical treatment: only after conservative measures have failed.

Malabsorption

Patients have malabsorption not only of fat but also of essential fatty acids and fat-soluble vitamins. The goal of enzyme replacement is to maintain body weight. Diarrhea will not resolve. Enteric-coated or microsphere enzymes are designed to be released at an alkaline pH, thus avoiding degradation by stomach acid. The advantage is that they contain larger amounts of lipase. The disadvantages are that they are expensive and bioavailability is not always predictable.

Pancreatic Carcinoma

Pancreatic carcinoma is more common in men than in women. It usually presents between the ages of 60 and 80 years. The 5-year survival rate is less than 2%. Risk factors include diabetes mellitus, chronic pancreatitis, hereditary pancreatitis, carcinogens, benzidine, cigarette smoking, and high fat diet. Pancreatic carcinoma usually presents late in the course of the disease. Patients may have a vague prodrome of malaise, anorexia, and weight loss. Symptoms may be overlooked until the development of pain or jaundice.

- Courvoisier sign: painless jaundice with a palpable gallbladder suggests pancreatic cancer.
- Trousseau sign: recurrent migratory thrombophlebitis is associated with pancreatic cancer.
- Recent-onset diabetes and nonbacterial (thrombotic) "marantic" endocarditis.

Routine laboratory blood analysis has limited usefulness. Patients may have increased levels of liver enzymes, amylase, and lipase or anemia, although this is variable. Tumor markers are also nonspecific. Abdominal ultrasonography and CT are both approximately 80% sensitive in localizing pancreatic masses. Either imaging method may be used in conjunction with fine-needle aspiration or biopsy to make a tissue diagnosis. ERCP and EUS are used if the abdominal ultrasonographic or CT results are inconclusive. Both

ERCP and EUS have a sensitivity greater than 90%. ERCP also allows aspiration of pancreatic secretions for cytologic analysis. The "double duct" sign is a classic presentation, with obstruction of both the pancreatic and the bile ducts. Biopsy specimens from suspect lymph nodes may be taken at EUS.

- Abdominal ultrasonography and CT are 80% sensitive in localizing pancreatic masses.
- ERCP and EUS have a sensitivity >90%.

Surgical treatment is the only hope for cure; however, most lesions are nonresectable. The criteria for resectability are a tumor smaller than 2 cm, absence of lymph node invasion, and absence of metastasis. Survival is the same for total pancreatectomy and the Whipple procedure: 3-year survival, 33%; 5-year survival, 1%; and operative mortality, 5%.

Radiotherapy may have a role as a radiosensitizer in unresectable cancer. However, survival is unchanged. The results of chemotherapy have been disappointing, and studies have not consistently shown improved survival.

Cystic Fibrosis

Because patients with cystic fibrosis are living longer, internists should know the common intestinal complications of this disease. Exocrine pancreatic insufficiency (malabsorption) is the common (85%-90% of patients) and most important complication. Endocrine pancreatic insufficiency (diabetes) occurs in 20% to 30% of patients. Rectal prolapse occurs in 20% of patients, and a distal small-bowel obstruction from thick secretions occurs in 15% to 20%. Focal biliary cirrhosis develops in 20% of patients.

- Pancreatic insufficiency occurs in 85%-90% of patients.

Pancreatic Endocrine Tumors

Zollinger-Ellison syndrome is a non–beta cell islet tumor of the pancreas that produces gastrin and causes gastric acid hypersecretion. This results in peptic ulcer disease (see above, Stomach and Duodenum).

Insulinoma is the most common islet cell tumor—a beta cell islet tumor that produces insulin, which causes hypoglycemia. The diagnosis is based on finding increased fasting plasma levels of insulin and hypoglycemia. CT, EUS, or arteriography may be useful in localizing the tumor.

Glucagonoma is an alpha cell islet tumor that produces glucagon. It presents with diabetes, weight loss, and a classic skin rash (migratory necrolytic erythema). The diagnosis is based on finding increased glucagon levels and failure of blood glucose to increase after the injection of glucagon.

Pancreatic cholera is a pancreatic tumor that produces vasoactive intestinal polypeptide (VIP), which causes watery diarrhea (see above, Secretory Diarrhea).

Somatostatinoma is a delta cell islet tumor that produces somatostatin, which inhibits insulin, gastrin, and pancreatic enzyme secretion. The result is diabetes mellitus and diarrhea. The diagnosis is based on finding increased plasma levels of somatostatin.

Octreotide is useful in treating pancreatic endocrine tumors except for somatostatinomas. Octreotide prevents the release of hormone and antagonizes target organ effects.

- Zollinger-Ellison syndrome: non–beta cell islet tumor of the pancreas.
- Insulinoma: commonest islet cell tumor.
- Pancreatic cholera: pancreatic tumor that produces VIP, which causes secretory diarrhea.
- Octreotide prevents hormone release and antagonizes hormone effects.

PART II

John J. Poterucha, M.D.

INTERPRETATION OF ABNORMAL LIVER TESTS

The evaluation of patients who have abnormal liver tests includes many clinical factors: the chief complaints of the patient, patient age, risk factors for liver disease, personal or family history of liver disease, medications, and physical examination findings. Because of these many factors, designing a standard algorithm for the evaluation of liver test abnormalities is difficult and often inefficient. Nevertheless, with basic information, liver test abnormalities can be evaluated in an efficient, cost-effective manner.

COMMONLY USED LIVER TESTS

Aminotransferases

Aminotransferases are found in hepatocytes and are markers of liver cell injury or hepatocellular disease. Hepatocellular injury causes these enzymes to "leak" out of the liver cells, and increased levels of these enzymes are detected in the serum within a few hours after liver injury. The aminotransferases consist of alanine aminotransferase (ALT), also known as serum glutamate pyruvate transaminase (SGPT), and aspartate aminotransferase (AST), also known as serum glutamic-oxaloacetic transaminase (SGOT). ALT is relatively specific for liver injury, whereas AST is found not only in hepatocytes but also in skeletal and cardiac muscle and other organs. Because some automated blood tests assay only for AST, it is useful to determine the serum level of ALT before embarking on an evaluation for liver disease.

Alkaline Phosphatase

Alkaline phosphatase is found on the hepatocyte membrane that borders the bile canaliculi (the smallest branches of the bile ducts). Because alkaline phosphatase is also found in bone and placenta, an isolated increase in the level of this enzyme should prompt further testing to determine whether the increase is from the liver or other tissues. Determination of alkaline phosphatase isoenzymes is one method of doing this. Another is the determination of γ-glutamyl transpeptidase (GGT), an enzyme of intrahepatic biliary canaliculi that is more sensitive than alkaline phosphatase. Other than to confirm the hepatic origin of an increased level of alkaline phosphatase, GGT has little role in the diagnosis of diseases of the liver because its

synthesis can be induced by many medications, thus reducing its specificity for *clinically important* liver disease.

Bilirubin

Bilirubin is the water-insoluble product of heme metabolism that is taken up by the hepatocyte and conjugated with glucuronic acid to form monoglucuronides and diglucuronides. Conjugation makes bilirubin water soluble, allowing it to be excreted in the bile. When bilirubin is measured in the serum, there are direct (conjugated) and indirect (unconjugated) fractions. Diseases characterized by overproduction of bilirubin, such as hemolysis or resorption of a hematoma, are characterized by hyperbilirubinemia that is less than 20% conjugated. Hepatocyte dysfunction or impaired bile flow produces hyperbilirubinemia that is usually more than 50% conjugated. Because conjugated bilirubin is water soluble and may be excreted in the urine, patients with liver disease and hyperbilirubinemia have dark urine. In these patients, the stools have a lighter color because of the absence of bilirubin pigments.

Prothrombin Time and Albumin

Prothrombin time (PT) and serum level of albumin are true markers of liver synthetic function. Abnormalities of PT and albumin imply severe liver disease and should prompt an immediate evaluation. PT is a measure of the activity of factors II, V, VII, and X, all of which are synthesized in the liver. Because these factors are also dependent on vitamin K for synthesis, deficiencies of vitamin K also produce abnormalities of PT. Vitamin K deficiency can result from the use of antibiotics during a period of prolonged fasting, small-bowel mucosal disorders such as celiac disease, and severe cholestasis, with an inability to absorb fat-soluble vitamins. True hepatocellular dysfunction is characterized by an inability to synthesize clotting factors even when stores of vitamin K are adequate. A simple way to distinguish between vitamin K deficiency and liver dysfunction in a patient with a prolonged PT is to administer vitamin K. A 10-mg dose of oral vitamin K for 3 days or 10 mg of subcutaneous vitamin K normalizes the PT within 48 hours in a vitamin K-deficient patient but has no effect on the PT in a patient with decreased liver synthetic function.

Because albumin has a half-life of 21 days, decreased serum levels due to liver dysfunction do not occur acutely. However, the serum level of albumin can decrease relatively quickly in a severe systemic illness such as bacteremia. This rapid decrease likely results from the release of cytokines and the accelerated metabolism of albumin. A chronic decrease of albumin in a patient without overt liver disease should prompt a search for albumin in the urine.

HEPATOCELLULAR DISORDERS

Diseases that primarily affect hepatocytes are termed "hepatocellular disorders" and are characterized predominantly by increases in aminotransferases. The disorders are best considered as "acute" (generally <3 months) or "chronic." Acute hepatitis may be accompanied by malaise, anorexia, abdominal pain, and jaundice. Common causes of acute hepatitis are listed in Table 7-15.

Diseases that produce a sustained (>3 months) increase in aminotransferase levels are in the category of chronic hepatitis. The increase (usually two- to fivefold) in aminotransferases is more modest than in acute hepatitis. Patients are usually asymptomatic but occasionally complain of fatigue and right upper quadrant pain. The differential diagnosis of chronic hepatitis is relatively lengthy; the more important and common disorders are listed in Table 7-16.

CHOLESTATIC DISORDERS

Diseases that predominantly affect the biliary system are called "cholestatic diseases." They can affect the microscopic ducts (e.g., primary biliary cirrhosis), large bile ducts (e.g., pancreatic cancer causing obstruction of the common bile duct), or both (e.g., primary sclerosing cholangitis). Generally, the predominant abnormality in these disorders involves alkaline phosphatase. Although diseases that cause an increase in bilirubin are often referred to as "cholestatic," it is important to remember that severe hepatocellular injury, as in acute hepatitis, also produces hyperbilirubinemia because of hepatocellular dysfunction. The common causes of cholestasis are listed in Table 7-17.

JAUNDICE

Evaluation of a patient with jaundice is an important diagnostic skill (Fig. 7-2). Jaundice is visibly evident hyperbilirubinemia and occurs when the bilirubin concentration is greater than 2.5 mg/dL. It is important to differentiate conjugated from unconjugated hyperbilirubinemia. A common disorder that produces unconjugated hyperbilirubinemia is Gilbert syndrome. Total bilirubin is generally less than 3.0 mg/dL and

Table 7-15 Common Causes of Acute Hepatitis

Disease	Clinical clue	Diagnostic test
Hepatitis A	Exposure history	IgM anti-HAV
Hepatitis B	Risk factors	HBsAg, IgM anti-HBc
Drug-induced hepatitis	Compatible medication/timing	Improvement after withdrawal of the agent
Alcoholic hepatitis	History of alcohol excess, AST:ALT >2, AST <400	Liver biopsy, improvement with abstinence
Ischemic hepatitis	History of severe hypotension	Rapid improvement of aminotransferase levels
Acute duct obstruction	Abdominal pain, fever	Cholangiography

ALT, alanine aminotransferase; AST, aspartate aminotransferase; HAV, hepatitis A virus; HBc, hepatitis B core; HBsAg, hepatitis B surface antigen.

Table 7-16 Common Causes of Chronic Hepatitis

Disease	Clinical clue	Diagnostic test
Hepatitis C	Risk factors	Anti-HCV, HCV RNA
Hepatitis B	Risk factors	HBsAg
Nonalcoholic steato-hepatitis	Obesity, diabetes mellitus, hyperlipidemia	Ultrasonography, liver biopsy
Hemochromatosis	Arthritis, diabetes mellitus, family history	Iron studies, gene test, liver biopsy
Alcoholic liver disease	History, AST:ALT >2	Liver biopsy
Autoimmune hepatitis	ALT 200-1,500, usually female, other autoimmune disease	Antinuclear or anti-smooth muscle antibody, liver biopsy

ALT, alanine aminotransferase; AST, aspartate aminotransferase; HBsAg, hepatitis B surface antigen; HCV, hepatitis C virus.

Table 7-17   Common Causes of Cholestasis

Disease	Clinical clue	Diagnostic test
Primary biliary cirrhosis	Middle-aged woman	Antimitochondrial antibody
Primary sclerosing cholangitis	Association with ulcerative colitis	Cholangiography (ERCP)
Large bile duct obstruction	Jaundice and pain are common	Ultrasonography, ERCP
Drug-induced	Compatible medication/timing	Improvement after withdrawal of the agent
Infiltrative disorder or malignancy	History of malignancy, sarcoidosis, amyloidosis	Ultrasonography, computed tomography
Inflammation-associated cholestasis	Symptoms of underlying inflammatory state	Blood cultures, appropriate antibody tests

ERCP, endoscopic retrograde cholangiopancreatography.

direct bilirubin 0.3 mg/dL or less. The concentration of bilirubin is generally higher in the fasting state or when the patient is ill. A presumptive diagnosis of Gilbert syndrome can be made in an otherwise well person with unconjugated hyperbilirubinemia and normal levels of hemoglobin (to exclude hemolysis) and normal liver enzymes (to exclude liver disease).

Direct hyperbilirubinemia is a more common cause of jaundice than indirect hyperbilirubinemia. Patients with direct hyperbilirubinemia can be categorized as those with nonobstructive conditions and those with obstruction. Abdominal pain, fever, or a palpable gallbladder (or a combination of these) suggests obstruction. Risk factors for viral hepatitis, a bilirubin concentration greater than 15 mg/dL, and persistently high aminotransferase levels suggest that the jaundice is due to hepatocellular dysfunction. A sensitive, specific, and noninvasive test to exclude obstructive causes of cholestasis is hepatic

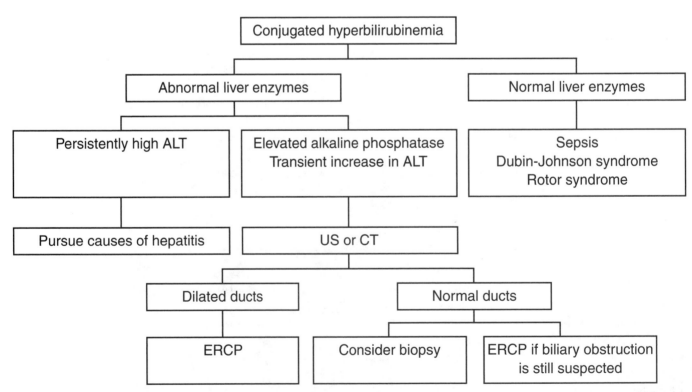

Fig. 7-2. Evaluation of conjugated hyperbilirubinemia. ALT, alanine aminotransferase; CT, computed tomography; ERCP, endoscopic retrograde cholangiopancreatography; US, ultrasonography. (From Poterucha JJ: Evaluation of the patient with abnormal liver tests. *In* Mayo Clinic Gastroenterology and Hepatology Board Review. Edited by SC Hauser. Mayo Clinic Scientific Press, Rochester, Minnesota, and CRC Press, Boca Raton, Florida, 2004, pp 303-308. By permission of Mayo Foundation for Medical Education and Research.)

ultrasonography. Diseases characterized by obstruction of a large bile duct generally demonstrate intrahepatic bile duct dilatation, especially if the bilirubin concentration is greater than 10 mg/dL and the patient has had jaundice for more than 2 weeks. Acute large bile duct obstruction, usually from a stone, may not allow time for the bile ducts to dilate. An important clue to the presence of an acute large duct obstruction is a marked but very transient increase in the levels of aminotransferases. If the clinical suspicion for obstruction of the bile duct is still strong despite negative ultrasonographic results, endoscopic retrograde cholangiography should be considered. Uncomplicated gallbladder disease, such as cholelithiasis with or without cholecystitis, does not cause jaundice or abnormal liver tests unless a common bile duct stone or sepsis is present.

ALGORITHMS FOR PATIENTS WITH ABNORMAL LIVER TESTS

Algorithms for the management of patients with abnormal liver tests are at best guidelines and at worst misleading. The patient's clinical presentation should be considered in interpreting abnormal liver tests. In general, patients with abnormal liver tests that are less than twice the normal value can be followed unless the patient is symptomatic or the albumin level, PT, or bilirubin concentration is abnormal. Persistent

abnormalities should be evaluated. Algorithms for the management of patients with increased levels of ALT or alkaline phosphatase are shown in Figures 7-3 and 7-4, respectively.

SPECIFIC LIVER DISEASES

Viral Hepatitis

Hepatitis A

Hepatitis A virus (HAV) accounts for 20% to 25% of cases of acute hepatitis in developed countries. The disease generally is transmitted by the fecal-oral route and has an incubation period of 15 to 50 days. Spread is more common in overcrowded areas with poor hygiene and poor sanitation. Hepatitis caused by HAV is generally mild in children, who often have a subclinical or nonicteric illness. Infected adults are more ill and usually develop jaundice. The prognosis is excellent, although HAV can rarely cause fulminant hepatitis. Chronic liver disease does not develop from HAV. Serum IgM anti-HAV is present during an acute illness and generally persists for 2 to 6 months. IgG anti-HAV appears slightly later, persists for life, and offers immunity from further infection. Immune serum globulin should be given for household contacts of infected patients. When a common source of food-borne infection is identified, immune serum globulin should be given

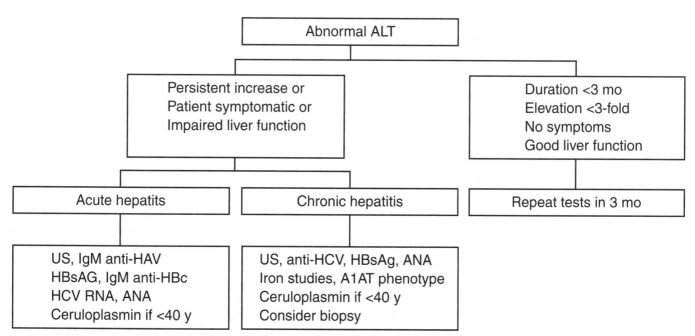

Fig. 7-3. Evaluation of abnormal alanine aminotransferase (ALT) levels. A1AT, a1-antitrypsin; ANA, antinuclear antibody; anti-HAV, hepatitis A virus antibody; anti-HBc, hepatitis B core antibody; anti-HCV, hepatitis C virus antibody; HBsAg, hepatitis B surface antigen; HCV, hepatitis C virus; US, ultrasonography. (From Poterucha JJ: Evaluation of the patient with abnormal liver tests. In Mayo Clinic Gastroenterology and Hepatology Board Review. Edited by SC Hauser. Mayo Clinic Scientific Press, Rochester, Minnesota, and CRC Press, Boca Raton, Florida, 2004, pp 303-308. By permission of Mayo Foundation for Medical Education and Research.)

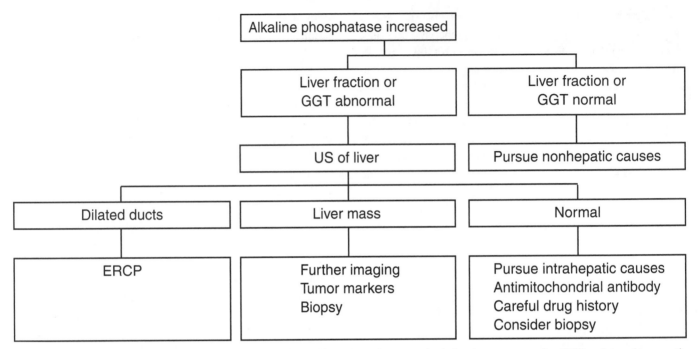

Fig. 7-4. Evaluation of increased levels of alkaline phosphatase. ERCP, endoscopic retrograde cholangiopancreatography; GGT, γ-glutamyl transpeptidase; US, ultrasonography. (From Poterucha JJ: Evaluation of the patient with abnormal liver tests. *In* Mayo Clinic Gastroenterology and Hepatology
Board Review. Edited by SC Hauser. Mayo Clinic Scientific Press, Rochester, Minnesota, and CRC Press, Boca Raton, Florida, 2004, pp 303-308. By permission of Mayo Foundation for Medical Education and Research.)

to those exposed. Hepatitis A vaccine is recommended for
U.S. citizens traveling to highly endemic areas, homosexual
men, intravenous drug users, recipients of clotting factor concentrates, and patients with chronic liver disease. In addition,
hepatitis A vaccine should be administered to those who are
given immune globulin as prophylaxis against hepatitis A.

- HAV is transmitted by the fecal-oral route.
- The incubation period is 15-50 days.
- The prognosis is excellent.
- Chronic liver disease does not develop.
- IgM anti-HAV is present during the acute illness.
- Give immune serum globulin for household contacts.
- Hepatitis A vaccine should be given to persons at high risk
  for infection and to patients with chronic liver disease.

Hepatitis B

Hepatitis B virus (HBV) is a DNA virus that is transmitted
parenterally or by sexual contact. In high-prevalence areas,
for example, certain areas of Asia and Africa, infants may
acquire infection from the mother during childbirth. High-
risk groups in the United States include injection drug users,
persons with multiple sexual contacts, and health care workers. The clinical course of HBV infection varies. Many infections in adults are subclinical, and even when symptomatic, the
disease resolves within 6 months. During acute hepatitis,

symptoms (when present) are generally more severe than those
of HAV infection. Jaundice rarely lasts longer than 4 weeks.
Some patients may have preicteric symptoms of "serum sickness," including arthralgias and urticaria. These symptoms
may be related to immune complexes, which can also cause
polyarteritis and glomerulonephritis.

- HBV is transmitted parenterally or by sexual contact.
- Infants may acquire infection from the mother.
- High-risk groups: injection drug users, persons with mul-
  tiple sexual contacts, and health care workers.
- Most infections in adults are subclinical.
- Jaundice rarely lasts >4 weeks.

A brief guide to the interpretation of serologic markers of
hepatitis B is found in Table 7-18. Viral markers in the blood
during a self-limited infection with HBV are shown in Figure
7-5. Note that IgM hepatitis B core antibody (anti-HBc) is
nearly always present during acute hepatitis B. Some patients
with acute hepatitis B, particularly those with fulminant hepatitis B, may lack hepatitis B surface antigen (HBsAg). Hepatitis
B e antigen (HBeAg) and HBV DNA levels greater than 10^5
copies/mL correlate with ongoing viral replication and indicate high infectivity. Spontaneous conversion from an HBeAg-
positive state to HBeAg-negativity with the appearance of
hepatitis B e antibody (anti-HBe) may be accompanied by an

Table 7-18   Hepatitis B Serologic Markers

Test	Interpretation
Hepatitis B surface antigen (HBsAg)	Current infection
Antibody to hepatitis B surface (anti-HBs)	Immunity (immunization or resolved infection)
IgM antibody to hepatitis B core (IgM anti-HBc)	Usually recent infection, occasionally "reactivation" of chronic infection
IgG antibody to hepatitis B core (IgG anti-HBc)	Remote infection
Hepatitis B e antigen (HBeAg) and/or HBV DNA >10^5 viral copies/mL	Active viral replication (high infectivity)
Antibody to hepatitis B e (anti-HBe)	Remote infection

Modified from Poterucha JJ: Chronic viral hepatitis. *In* Mayo Clinic Gastroenterology and Hepatology Board Review. Edited by SC Hauser. Mayo Clinic Scientific Press, Rochester, Minnesota, and CRC Press, Boca Raton, Florida, 2004, pp 317-325. By permission of Mayo Foundation for Medical Education and Research.

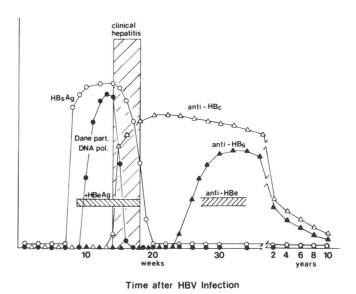

Time after HBV Infection

Fig. 7-5. Viral markers in blood during self-limited hepatitis B virus infection. Anti-HBc, hepatitis B core antibody; anti-HBe, hepatitis B e antibody; anti-HBs, hepatitis B surface antibody; HBeAg, hepatitis B e antigen; HBsAg, hepatitis B surface antigen. (From Robinson WS: Biology of human hepatitis viruses. *In* Hepatology: A Textbook of Liver Disease. Vol 2. Second edition. Edited by D Zakim, TD Boyer. Philadelphia, WB Saunders Company, 1990, pp 890-945. By permission of publisher.)

increase in the level of aminotransferases. Patients with hepatitis B mutants may have high HBV DNA levels but lack HBeAg. Commonly encountered serologic patterns of HBV are shown in Table 7-19.

Ten percent of patients who acquire HBV as adults and 90% of those infected as neonates do not clear HBsAg from the serum within 6 months and, thus, become chronically infected. Chronicity occurs more commonly in patients with a defect of the immune system. Patients with chronic hepatitis B but normal findings on liver tests and liver biopsy have inactive chronic hepatitis B and are sometimes called "healthy carriers." They have a good prognosis. Patients with active chronic hepatitis B have increased levels of ALT, the presence of HBeAg or HBV DNA levels greater than 10^5 copies/mL, and histologic inflammation. These patients are at higher risk for cirrhosis, liver failure, and hepatocellular carcinoma than patients with HBV infection who lack these features. Patients with chronic hepatitis B and cirrhosis are at high risk for the development of hepatocellular carcinoma and, every 6 to 12 months, liver ultrasonography should be performed and the alpha-fetoprotein level determined. Patients with neonatal acquisition of hepatitis B may develop hepatocellular carcinoma even in the absence of cirrhosis.

- IgM anti-HBc is nearly always present during acute hepatitis B.

- HBV DNA level >10^5 copies/mL and HBeAg correlate with ongoing viral replication and indicate high infectivity.
- 10% of patients acquiring HBV as adults and 90% of those infected as neonates do not clear HBsAg.
- Healthy carriers of HBsAg have essentially a normal liver histologically and a good prognosis.
- Chronic hepatitis due to HBV may lead to cirrhosis.
- Patients with HBV-induced cirrhosis are at high risk for the development of hepatocellular carcinoma.

Patients with chronic hepatitis B, an abnormal ALT level, and active viral replication (HBeAg or HBV DNA level >10^5 copies/mL) are potential candidates for therapy. Treatment with interferon alfa results in a 30% to 40% response rate as measured by loss of HBeAg and HBV DNA and the appearance of anti-HBe. A few patients also clear HBsAg. Patients more likely to respond to interferon therapy include those with a relatively recent diagnosis of chronic hepatitis B, high serum levels of aminotransferases, active hepatitis without evidence of cirrhosis on biopsy, and low serum levels of HBV DNA. Patients with HBV infection who have a response to interferon therapy may have a transient increase in aminotransferase levels after about 8 weeks of treatment. An acute hepatitis syndrome may be precipitated and interferon should be given with caution, if at all, to patients with cirrhosis. Lamivudine and adefovir are oral agents that decrease HBV DNA levels and

Table 7-19   Interpretation of Hepatitis B Serologic Patterns

HBsAg	Anti-HBs	IgM anti-HBc	IgG anti-HBc	HBeAg	Anti-HBe	HBV DNA, viral copies/mL	Interpretation
+	-	+	-	+	-	+	Acute infection
-	+	-	+	-	-/+	-	Prior infection with immunity
-	+	-	-	-	-	-	Vaccination with immunity
+	-	-	+	-	+	$<10^5$	Chronic hepatitis B without replication
+	-	-	+	+	-	$>10^5$	Chronic hepatitis B with replication
+	-	-	+	-	+	$>10^5$	Chronic hepatitis B with precore mutant

Anti-HBc, hepatitis B core antibody; anti-HB e, hepatitis B e antibody; anti-HBs, hepatitis B surface antibody; HBeAg, hepatitis B e antigen; HBsAg, hepatitis B surface antigen; HBV, hepatitis B virus.

Modified from Poterucha JJ: Chronic viral hepatitis. In Mayo Clinic Gastroenterology and Hepatology Board Review. Edited by SC Hauser. Mayo Clinic Scientific Press, Rochester, Minnesota, and CRC Press, Boca Raton, Florida, 2004, pp 317-325. By permission of Mayo Foundation for Medical Education and Research.

may result in clinical improvement. About 20% to 30% of patients who take lamivudine or adefovir have seroconversion to antibodies to hepatitis B e (anti-HBe). Lamivudine-resistant mutations occur in 30% of patients who have received treatment for 1 year, but the mutations are less virulent than the wild-type strain. Adefovir resistance is less common than lamivudine resistance, and both drugs are safer than interferon for patients with cirrhosis because flares of hepatitis and infectious complications are uncommon.

Hepatitis D

Hepatitis D virus (HDV), or delta agent, is a small RNA particle that requires the presence of HBsAg to cause infection. HDV infection can occur simultaneously with acute HBV infection (coinfection) or HDV may infect a chronic HBsAg carrier (superinfection). HDV is strongly associated with injection drug abuse in the United States. Infection with HDV should be considered only in patients with HBsAg; it is diagnosed by anti-HDV seroconversion.

- HDV requires the presence of HBsAg to cause infection.
- HDV is strongly associated with injection drug abuse.
- HDV infection is diagnosed by anti-HDV seroconversion.

Hepatitis C

Hepatitis C virus (HCV), an RNA virus, is the most common chronic blood-borne infection in the United States. Although the number of new cases of hepatitis C infection is decreasing, the propensity of the virus to cause chronic infection continues to result in an increasing number of deaths. HCV has a role in 40% of all cases of chronic liver disease and is the number one indication for liver transplantation. HCV is a parenterally transmitted virus. The most common risk factor is illicit drug use. Persons with a history of transfusion of blood products before 1990 (when routine testing of blood products for HCV was introduced) are also at considerable risk for infection with HCV. Sexual transmission of HCV occurs but seems to be inefficient, and only about 2% of long-term spouses of patients with chronic hepatitis C have serologic evidence of HCV infection. The risk of transmission of HCV to health care workers by percutaneous (needlestick) exposure is also low, approximately 2%. For a health care worker who has a needlestick exposure from a patient with hepatitis C, baseline testing for anti-HCV and ALT is recommended. Follow-up testing can be with HCV RNA at 4 to 6 weeks or anti-HCV and ALT at 4 to 6 months (or both). Prophylactic treatment with immune globulin or anti-hepatitis C therapy is not recommended.

Antibodies to HCV (anti-HCV) indicate exposure to the virus and are not protective. The presence of anti-HCV can indicate either current infection or a previous infection with subsequent clearance. The presence of anti-HCV in a patient with an abnormal ALT level and risk factors for hepatitis C acquisition is strongly suggestive of current HCV infection. The initial test used for anti-HCV determination is enzyme-linked immunoassay (EIA). Although this test is very sensitive (few false-negative results), its specificity is variable. If the anti-HCV by EIA is negative, the patient is unlikely to have

Table 7-20 Interpretation of Anti-HCV Results

Anti-HCV by EIA	Anti-HCV by RIBA	Interpretation
Positive	Negative	False-positive EIA, patient does not have true antibody
Positive	Positive	Patient has antibody*
Positive	Indeterminate	Uncertain antibody status

EIA, enzyme-linked immunoassay; HCV, hepatitis C virus; RIBA, recombinant immunoblot assay.
*Remember that anti-HCV does not necessarily indicate current hepatitis C infection (see text).

hepatitis C. The specificity of EIA is improved with the addition of the recombinant immunoblot assay (RIBA) for anti-HCV. A guide to interpretation of anti-HCV tests is given in Table 7-20.

The reference standard for the diagnosis of HCV infection is the presence of HCV RNA, as determined with the polymerase chain reaction (PCR). Quantitative HCV RNA tests measure the *amount* of HCV RNA present but are not as sensitive as HCV RNA determination with PCR. HCV levels do not correlate with disease severity, and the major use of quantitative assays is to stratify the response to therapy.

- HCV is a parenterally transmitted virus and a common cause of chronic hepatitis.
- Common modes of transmission are illicit drug use and transfusion of blood products before 1990.
- HCV RNA by PCR is the reference standard for diagnosis.

Infection with HCV rarely presents as acute hepatitis. The natural history of hepatitis C is summarized in Figure 7-6. About 60% to 85% of persons acquiring hepatitis C develop a chronic infection, and subsequent spontaneous loss of the virus is rare.

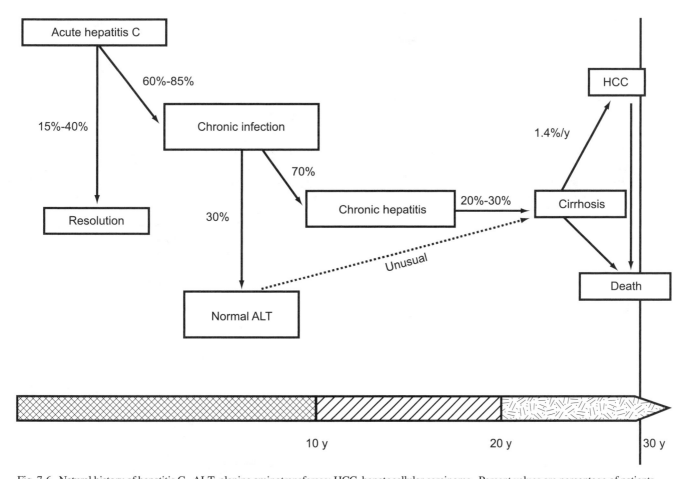

Fig. 7-6. Natural history of hepatitis C. ALT, alanine aminotransferase; HCC, hepatocellular carcinoma. Percent values are percentage of patients.

Consequently, most patients with hepatitis C present with chronic hepatitis with mild to moderate increases in ALT levels. Some patients have fatigue or vague right upper quadrant pain. Patients may also come to medical attention because of complications of end-stage liver disease or, rarely, extrahepatic complications such as cryoglobulinemia or porphyria cutanea tarda. Up to 30% of patients chronically infected with HCV have a persistently normal ALT level. Because the majority of patients with hepatitis C are asymptomatic, treatment is generally aimed at preventing future complications of the disease. About 20% to 30% of patients with chronic hepatitis C develop cirrhosis over a 10- to 20-year period. Patients with cirrhosis due to HCV generally have had disease for more than 20 years.

Pegylated interferon alfa in combination with ribavirin is the current standard of care for patients with hepatitis C who are deemed candidates for treatment. This combination, given for 6 to 12 months, results in sustained clearance of HCV RNA from the serum in 60% of patients. Patients with genotype 2 or 3 and without clinical or biochemical evidence of advanced liver disease have an 80% to 90% chance of a sustained response to therapy and, thus, may be treated without liver biopsy. Patients with genotype 1 or 4 usually will have a liver biopsy to aid in the decision about treatment because response rates are less than 50% and the potential risks of therapy may outweigh benefits. On the basis of the natural history of hepatitis C and the response to therapy, an algorithm for patients without any contraindication to treatment can be proposed, although deviations are common because of patient preference or transmission issues (Fig. 7-7). These guidelines apply generally to the large percentage of patients with hepatitis C who are asymptomatic or have nonspecific symptoms such as fatigue. Therapy should be recommended to patients with extrahepatic manifestations of hepatitis C, such as vasculitis related to cryoglobulinemia.

Patients who are not candidates for treatment should be evaluated annually with routine liver tests. Patients with cirrhosis are at increased risk for hepatocellular carcinoma, particularly if there is a history of alcohol excess. The risk of hepatocellular carcinoma complicating hepatitis C with cirrhosis is 1% to 4% per year. Screening with alpha fetoprotein and liver ultrasonography every 6 to 12 months is advised for patients who are potential candidates for treatment with modalities such as liver transplantation or percutaneous ablation.

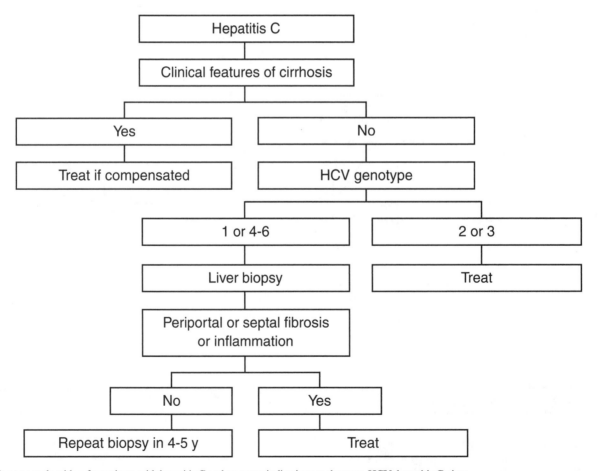

Fig. 7-7. Treatment algorithm for patients with hepatitis C and no contraindications to therapy. HCV, hepatitis C virus.

Patients with HCV infection and decompensated cirrhosis should be considered for liver transplantation.

- Symptomatic, clinically recognized acute hepatitis C is unusual.
- 60%-85% of patients who acquire HCV remain chronically infected.
- 20%-30% of patients develop cirrhosis over 20 years.
- The combination of pegylated interferon alfa and ribavirin results in sustained clearance of HCV RNA in approximately 60% of patients.
- Patients with cirrhosis due to hepatitis C are at increased risk for hepatocellular carcinoma, particularly if there is also a history of alcohol excess.

Hepatitis E

Hepatitis E virus (HEV) is an enterically transmitted RNA virus that causes acute hepatitis in patients from endemic areas (India, Pakistan, Mexico, and Southeast Asia) and in travelers returning from these regions. Clinically, hepatitis E resembles hepatitis A. There is a high risk of fulminant hepatitis E in women who acquire the infection during pregnancy. Chronic hepatitis E does not occur.

- HEV is an enterically transmitted RNA virus that clinically resembles hepatitis A.
- There is a high risk of fulminant hepatitis E in women who acquire the infection during pregnancy.

Miscellaneous

Epstein-Barr virus, cytomegalovirus, and herpes viruses have been implicated as causes of acute viral hepatitis, which may be most serious in immunocompromised patients. Patients with infectious mononucleosis syndromes commonly have abnormal liver tests and mild increases in bilirubin levels, although clinically recognized jaundice is unusual.

Autoimmune Hepatitis

"Autoimmune hepatitis" was previously called "autoimmune *chronic* active hepatitis" because the diagnosis required 3 to 6 months of abnormal liver enzyme tests. However, 40% of cases of autoimmune hepatitis present as an acute hepatitis. Autoimmune hepatitis can affect patients of any age, predominantly females. The onset is usually insidious, and an initial liver biopsy specimen may show cirrhosis.

By definition, patients with autoimmune hepatitis should not have a history of drug-related hepatitis, HBV, HCV, or Wilson disease. Immunoserologic markers, including antinuclear antibody (ANA), smooth muscle antibody, soluble liver antigen antibodies, or antibodies to liver/kidney microsomal (LKM) antigens, are usually detected. Patients with autoimmune hepatitis may have other autoimmune diseases, including Hashimoto thyroiditis. Marked increases in serum levels of gamma globulin are common, and aminotransferase levels are generally 4 to 20 times normal. Corticosteroids (30-60 mg daily) produce improvement in the majority of patients, and the improvement in liver tests and gamma globulin is often dramatic. Azathioprine may be added to allow the use of lower doses of prednisone. Immunosuppressive doses should be decreased to control symptoms and to maintain the serum level of aminotransferases below five times normal. Even after an excellent response to corticosteroids, relapse often occurs and the control of autoimmune hepatitis usually requires maintenance therapy.

- Autoimmune hepatitis is a chronic condition but may present as an acute hepatitis.
- There should not be a history of drug-related hepatitis, HBV, HCV, or Wilson disease.
- Immunoserologic markers are often detected.
- Marked increases in serum levels of gamma globulin are common.
- Most patients have improvement with corticosteroid therapy, and the improvement in liver tests and gamma globulin is often dramatic.
- The control of autoimmune hepatitis usually requires maintenance therapy.

Alcoholic Liver Disease

Alcoholic Hepatitis

Alcoholic hepatitis is characterized histologically by fatty change, degeneration and necrosis of hepatocytes (with or without Mallory bodies), and an inflammatory infiltrate of neutrophils. Almost all patients have fibrosis, and they may have cirrhosis. Clinically, patients may be asymptomatic or icteric and critically ill. Common symptoms include anorexia, nausea, vomiting, abdominal pain, and weight loss. The most common sign is hepatomegaly, which may be accompanied by ascites, jaundice, fever, splenomegaly, and encephalopathy. The level of AST is increased in 80% to 90% of patients, but it is almost always less than 400 U/L. Aminotransferase levels greater than 400 U/L are not a feature of alcoholic liver disease, and a search for other causes (e.g., ingestion of acetaminophen) should be pursued. The AST:ALT ratio is frequently greater than 2. Leukocytosis is commonly present, particularly in severely ill patients. Although the constellation of symptoms may mimic biliary disease, the clinical features are characteristic in an alcoholic patient. Because cholecystectomy carries a high morbidity in patients with alcoholic hepatitis, the clinical distinction is important and empiric cholecystectomy is contraindicated.

- Alcoholic hepatitis is characterized by fatty change, degeneration and necrosis of hepatocytes (with or without Mallory bodies), and an inflammatory infiltrate of neutrophils.
- Common symptoms include anorexia, nausea, vomiting, abdominal pain, and weight loss.
- Common signs are hepatomegaly, ascites, jaundice, fever, splenomegaly, and encephalopathy.
- The level of AST is increased (almost always <400 U/L) in 80%-90% of patients.
- The AST:ALT ratio is frequently >2.
- Leukocytosis occurs in severely ill patients.

Poor prognostic markers of alcoholic hepatitis include encephalopathy, spider angiomata, ascites, renal failure, prolonged PT, and a bilirubin concentration greater than 20 mg/dL. Many patients have progression to cirrhosis, particularly if alcohol intake is not curtailed. Corticosteroid therapy may be beneficial as an acute treatment of alcoholic hepatitis in patients with severe disease characterized by encephalopathy and a markedly prolonged PT. A discriminant function greater than 32 helps to identify patients with a poor prognosis.

Discriminant function = 4.6 ($PT_{patient} - PT_{control}$) + bilirubin (mg/dL)

- Poor prognostic markers: encephalopathy, ascites, renal failure, prolonged PT, and bilirubin >20 mg/dL.
- Corticosteroid therapy may be beneficial in severe disease.

Alcoholic Cirrhosis

Cirrhosis is defined histologically by septal fibrosis with nodular parenchymal regeneration. Only 60% of patients with alcoholic cirrhosis have signs or symptoms of liver disease, and most patients with cirrhosis have no history of alcoholic hepatitis. Liver enzymes may be relatively normal in cirrhosis without alcoholic hepatitis. Concomitant HCV infection is common in patients with alcoholic liver disease. The prognosis of alcoholic cirrhosis depends on whether patients continue to consume alcohol and whether there are signs (jaundice, ascites, gastrointestinal bleeding) of chronic liver disease. The 5-year survival rate for patients without ascites, jaundice, or hematemesis and who abstain from alcohol is 89% and for those with signs and who continue to consume alcohol, 34%. Liver transplantation is an option for patients with end-stage alcoholic liver disease if they maintain abstinence from alcohol.

- Only 60% of patients with alcoholic cirrhosis have signs or symptoms of liver disease.
- Liver enzymes may be relatively normal.

- The 5-year survival for patients without ascites, jaundice, or hematemesis and who abstain from alcohol is 89%.
- The 5-year survival for those with symptoms and who continue to consume alcohol is 34%.
- Liver transplantation is an option for patients who can demonstrate a pattern of abstinence from alcohol.

Nonalcoholic Fatty Liver Disease

Nonalcoholic fatty liver disease is a common cause of abnormal liver function tests. A subset of nonalcoholic fatty liver disease is nonalcoholic steatohepatitis (NASH), which is characterized histologically by fatty change and inflammation. Characteristically, patients with nonalcoholic fatty liver disease are obese or have hyperlipidemia or diabetes mellitus. The aminotransferase levels are mildly abnormal, and the alkaline phosphatase level is increased in about one-third of patients. NASH accounts for some cases of "cryptogenic" cirrhosis. The pathogenesis of NASH is unknown, and the effect of weight loss and control of hyperlipidemia and hyperglycemia is variable. In 20% to 30% of patients, NASH progresses to cirrhosis, and the risk factors for more advanced disease are advanced age, marked obesity, and diabetes. Other than to control risk factors, there is no effective therapy for NASH. In patients with fat in the liver, it is important to rule out other diseases that result in steatosis, including hepatitis C, celiac disease, Wilson disease, alcoholic liver disease, and rapid weight loss.

Chronic Cholestatic Liver Diseases

Primary Biliary Cirrhosis

Primary biliary cirrhosis is a chronic, progressive, cholestatic liver disease that primarily affects middle-aged women. Its cause is unknown but appears to involve an immunologic disturbance resulting in small bile duct destruction. In many patients, the disease is identified by an asymptomatic increase in alkaline phosphatase. Common early symptoms are pruritus and fatigue. Patients may have Hashimoto thyroiditis or sicca complex. Biochemical features include increased levels of alkaline phosphatase and IgM. Later, the concentration of bilirubin increases, the serum level of albumin decreases, and PT is prolonged. Steatorrhea may occur because of progressive cholestasis. Fat-soluble vitamin deficiencies and metabolic bone disease are common.

Antimitochondrial antibodies are present in 90% to 95% of patients with primary biliary cirrhosis. The classic histologic lesion is granulomatous infiltration of septal bile ducts. Ursodiol treatment benefits patients who have this disease by improving survival and delaying the need for liver transplantation. Cholestyramine and rifampin may be beneficial in the management of pruritus.

- Primary biliary cirrhosis primarily affects middle-aged women.
- Common early symptoms: pruritus and fatigue.
- Alkaline phosphatase and IgM levels increase.
- Fat-soluble vitamin deficiencies and metabolic bone disease are common.
- Antimitochrondrial antibodies are present in 90% to 95% of patients.
- Classic histologic lesion: granulomatous infiltration of septal bile ducts.
- Treatment: ursodiol.

Primary Sclerosing Cholangitis

Primary sclerosing cholangitis (PSC) is a chronic cholestatic liver disease characterized by obliterative inflammatory fibrosis of extrahepatic and intrahepatic bile ducts. An immune mechanism has been implicated. Patients may have an asymptomatic increase in alkaline phosphatase or progressive fatigue, pruritus, and jaundice. Bacterial cholangitis may occur in patients with dominant strictures or in whom instrumentation has been performed. Cholangiography establishes the diagnosis of PSC, showing short strictures of bile ducts with intervening segments of normal or slightly dilated ducts, producing a beaded appearance. This cholangiographic appearance may be mimicked by acquired immunodeficiency syndrome (AIDS) cholangiopathy (due to cytomegalovirus or cryptosporidium) and ischemic cholangiopathy after intra-arterial infusion of fluorodeoxyuridine.

- PSC: obliterative inflammatory fibrosis of extrahepatic and intrahepatic bile ducts.
- Asymptomatic increase in alkaline phosphatase.
- Cholangiography establishes the diagnosis.
- AIDS cholangiopathy mimics the cholangiographic appearance of PSC.

Seventy percent of patients with PSC have ulcerative colitis, which may antedate, accompany, or even follow the diagnosis of PSC. Proctocolectomy performed for ulcerative colitis has no effect on the development or clinical course of PSC. Patients with PSC are at higher risk for cholangiocarcinoma; its development may be manifested by rapid clinical deterioration, jaundice, weight loss, and abdominal pain. There is no effective medical therapy for PSC, and many patients have progressive liver disease and require liver transplantation. Percutaneous or endoscopic balloon dilatation of bile duct strictures may offer palliation, especially in patients with recurrent cholangitis.

- 70% of patients with PSC have ulcerative colitis.
- Proctocolectomy has no effect on the development of PSC.

- PSC patients are at higher risk for cholangiocarcinoma.
- Treatment for PSC is generally supportive.
- Many patients require liver transplantation.

Hereditary Liver Diseases

Genetic Hemochromatosis

Genetic hemochromatosis is an autosomal recessively transmitted disorder characterized by iron overload. The physiologic defect appears to be an inappropriately high absorption of iron from the gastrointestinal tract. The gene for genetic hemochromatosis has been identified and termed "*HFE*." In the general population, the heterozygote frequency is 10%. Only homozygotes manifest progressive iron accumulation.

- Genetic hemochromatosis is a disorder of iron metabolism.
- Characteristic: high absorption of iron from the gastrointestinal tract.
- Autosomal recessive transmission.
- Only homozygotes have progressive iron accumulation.

Patients often present with end-stage disease, although an increased sensitivity to screening is aiding in earlier diagnosis. The peak incidence of clinical presentation is between the ages of 40 and 60 years. Iron overload is manifested more often and earlier in men than in women because women are protected by the iron losses of menstruation and pregnancy. Clinical features include arthropathy, hepatomegaly, skin pigmentation, diabetes mellitus, cardiac dysfunction, and hypogonadism. Hemochromatosis should be considered in patients presenting with symptoms or diseases such as arthritis, diabetes, cardiac arrhythmias, or sexual dysfunction. Routine liver biochemistry studies generally show little disturbance. The serum level of iron is increased, the transferrin saturation is greater than 50%, and the serum levels of ferritin are high. Increased levels of iron and ferritin occur in other liver diseases, particularly advanced cirrhosis. Testing for mutations in the *HFE* gene and liver biopsy with quantification of hepatic iron concentration are standard methods for diagnosing hemochromatosis. Of patients with hemochromatosis, 80% to 90% are homozygous for the C282Y mutation that is the basis for genetic testing. Generally, hepatic iron levels in hemochromatosis are greater than 10,000 µg/g dry weight. A diagnostic algorithm is shown in Figure 7-8.

- Iron overload is more common in men.
- Clinical features: arthropathy, hepatomegaly, skin pigmentation, diabetes mellitus, cardiac dysfunction, and hypogonadism.
- Iron saturation and serum levels of ferritin are high.

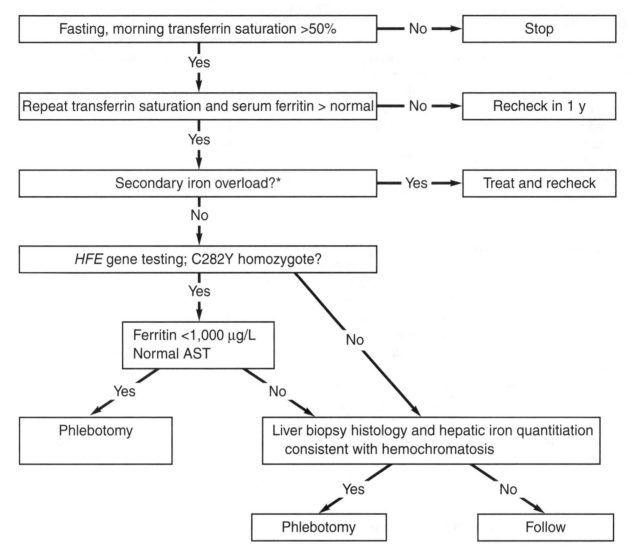

Fig. 7-8. Diagnostic algorithm for hereditary hemochromatosis. AST, aspartate aminotransferase. *Anemias with ineffective erythropoiesis, multiple blood transfusions, oral/parenteral iron supplement. (From Brandhagen DJ, Gross JB Jr: Metabolic liver disease. *In* Mayo Clinic Gastroenterology and Hepatology Board Review. Edited by SC Hauser. Mayo Clinic Scientific Press, Rochester, Minnesota, and CRC Press, Boca Raton, Florida, 2004, pp 381-392. By permission of Mayo Foundation for Medical Education and Research.)

● Standard tests for making the diagnosis: genetic testing and liver biopsy with hepatic iron concentration.

Hemochromatosis is treated with removal of iron by repeated phlebotomies. The standard recommendation is to remove 500 mL weekly to the point of mild anemia. A maintenance program of four to eight phlebotomies annually is then required. When initiated in the precirrhotic stage, removal of iron can render the liver normal and may improve cardiac function and diabetes mellitus. Treatment does not reverse arthropathy or hypogonadism, nor does it eliminate the increased risk (30%) of hepatocellular carcinoma if cirrhosis has already developed. All first-degree relatives of patients should be evaluated for hemochromatosis.

● Hemochromatosis is treated with repeated phlebotomies.
● Treatment does not reverse arthropathy or hypogonadism or eliminate the increased risk of hepatocellular carcinoma.
● First-degree relatives should be tested for hemochromatosis.

Wilson Disease

Wilson disease is an autosomal recessive disorder characterized by increased amounts of copper in tissues. The basic defect involves an inability of the liver to prepare copper for biliary excretion. The liver is chiefly involved in children, whereas neuropsychiatric manifestations are more prominent in older patients. The Kayser-Fleischer ring is a brownish pigmented ring at the periphery of the cornea. It is not invariably present and is more frequent in patients with neurologic manifestations.

Hepatic forms of Wilson disease include fulminant hepatitis (often accompanied by hemolysis and renal failure), chronic hepatitis, and insidiously developing cirrhosis. The development of hepatocellular carcinoma is rare. Neurologic signs include tremor, rigidity, altered speech, and changes in personality. Fanconi syndrome and premature arthritis may occur.

- Wilson disease: an autosomal recessive disorder characterized by increased copper in tissues.
- Basic defect: inability of the liver to prepare copper for biliary excretion.
- Kayser-Fleischer ring: brownish pigmented ring at the periphery of the cornea.
- Hepatocellular carcinoma is rare.
- Neurologic signs: tremor, rigidity, altered speech, and changes in personality.

Evidence of hemolysis (total bilirubin increased out of proportion to direct bilirubin), a low or normal level of alkaline phosphatase, and a low serum level of uric acid (due to Fanconi syndrome) suggest Wilson disease. The diagnosis is established on the basis of a low level of ceruloplasmin and an increased urinary concentration of copper. Ceruloplasmin levels may be misleading—they may be increased by estrogen or biliary obstruction and decreased by liver failure of any cause. High concentrations of copper in the liver are found in Wilson disease, although similarly high values can also occur in cholestatic syndromes. The treatment of choice is penicillamine, which chelates and increases the urinary excretion of copper. Trientine is an alternative to penicillamine. Zinc inhibits absorption of copper by the gastrointestinal tract and can be used as adjunctive therapy. All siblings of patients should be evaluated for Wilson disease. Liver transplantation corrects the metabolic defect of the disease.

- Diagnosis: low ceruloplasmin and increased urinary concentration of copper.
- Treatment: penicillamine or trientine; zinc.
- Liver transplantation corrects the metabolic defect.

Alpha₁-Antitrypsin Deficiency

Alpha₁-Antitrypsin Deficiency

Alpha₁-antitrypsin is synthesized in the liver. The gene is on chromosome 14. M is the common normal allele, and Z and S are abnormal alleles. Intrahepatic accumulation of alpha₁-antitrypsin in the ZZ phenotype causes liver disease; however, disease occurs in only 10% to 20% of patients with the ZZ phenotype. During the first 6 months of life, patients often have a history of cholestatic jaundice that resolves. In later childhood or adulthood, cirrhosis may develop. Patients with alpha₁-antitrypsin–induced liver disease often have no clinically important lung disease. The prevalence of cirrhosis in patients with the MZ

phenotype is likely increased, but the risk is small. Hepatocellular carcinoma may complicate alpha₁-antitrypsin deficiency, especially in males. The diagnosis of alpha₁-antitrypsin deficiency is made by determining the alpha₁-antitrypsin phenotype. The serum levels of alpha₁-antitrypsin may vary and be unreliable. Liver transplantation corrects the metabolic defect and changes the recipient's phenotype to that of the donor.

- Intrahepatic accumulation of alpha₁-antitrypsin causes liver disease.
- The diagnosis is made by determining the alpha₁-antitrypsin phenotype.
- Hepatocellular carcinoma can complicate alpha₁-antitrypsin deficiency, especially in males.
- Liver transplantation corrects the metabolic defect.

Fulminant Hepatic Failure

Fulminant hepatic failure is defined as hepatic failure with encephalopathy developing less than 8 weeks after the onset of jaundice in patients with no history of liver disease. The common causes are listed in Table 7-21. Poor prognostic markers include a drug-induced (other than acetaminophen) cause, older age, grade 3 or 4 encephalopathy, acidosis, and PT greater than 3.5 international normalized ratio (INR). Treatment is supportive, and patients should be transferred to a medical center where liver transplantation is available.

- Fulminant hepatic failure: hepatic failure with encephalopathy developing <8 weeks after the onset of jaundice and in patients with no history of liver disease.

Table 7-21   Common Causes of Fulminant Hepatic Failure

Infective
    Hepatitis virus A, B, C(?), D, E
    Herpesvirus
Drug reactions and toxins
    Acetaminophen
    Antituberculous agents
    Mushroom poisoning
Vascular
    Ischemic hepatitis ("shock" liver)
    Acute Budd-Chiari syndrome
Metabolic
    Wilson disease
    Fatty liver of pregnancy
Miscellaneous (rare)
    Massive malignant infiltration
    Autoimmune hepatitis

- Poor prognostic markers: drug-induced (not acetaminophen), older age, grade 3 or 4 encephalopathy, PT >3.5 INR.

Drug-Induced Liver Disease

Drugs cause toxic effects in the liver in different ways, often mimicking naturally occurring liver disease. Most drug-induced liver disorders are idiosyncratic and not dose-related; 2% of the cases of jaundice in hospitalized patients and 25% of the cases of fulminant hepatitis are drug-induced. Consequently, all drugs that have been used by a patient with liver disease must be identified.

Acetaminophen toxicity may occur at relatively low doses in alcoholics because alcohol induces hepatic microsomal P450 enzymes, which metabolize acetaminophen to its toxic metabolite. Disulfiram also can cause fulminant hepatitis. Amoxicillin/clavulanate causes severe cholestatic hepatitis, and valproic acid, tetracycline, and zidovudine may cause severe microvesicular steatosis associated with encephalopathy. Hepatotoxicity due to amiodarone may have histologic features that mimic those of alcoholic hepatitis. Methotrexate in a total dose of more than 2 g may cause hepatic fibrosis; some physicians advocate periodic liver biopsy in patients receiving long-term methotrexate treatment for psoriasis or rheumatoid arthritis. Intravenous cocaine may cause massive necrosis and death, probably because of ischemia. Antituberculous agents, including isoniazid, rifampin, and ethambutol, may cause acute hepatitis.

- Most drug-induced liver disorders are idiosyncratic, not dose-related.
- 2% of cases of jaundice (hospitalized patients) and 25% of cases of fulminant hepatitis are drug-induced.
- Identify all drugs that have been used by a patient with liver disease.
- In alcoholics, acetaminophen toxicity may occur at relatively low doses.
- Amoxicillin/clavulanate causes severe cholestatic hepatitis.
- Amiodarone may cause hepatotoxicity that histologically mimics alcoholic or nonalcoholic steatohepatitis.
- A total dose of methotrexate >2 g may cause hepatic fibrosis.
- Intravenous cocaine can cause massive necrosis.

Liver Tumors

Hepatocellular Carcinoma

The risk of hepatocellular carcinoma is increased in cirrhosis of nearly any cause but particularly if due to HBV, HCV, hemochromatosis, or alcohol. Alpha fetoprotein is increased in only 50% of patients with hepatocellular carcinoma; however, a level of alpha fetoprotein greater than 400 ng/mL in a cirrhotic patient with a liver mass is diagnostic of hepatocellular carcinoma. Common metastatic sites are lymph nodes, lung, bone, and brain. Paraneoplastic syndromes include anemia, fever, hypercalcemia, hypoglycemia, and clubbing. Liver transplantation is an option for patients with three or fewer lesions (largest <3 cm) or a single lesion smaller than 5 cm. Transplantation is advised particularly for patients with cirrhosis who may not tolerate resection because of poor liver reserve. Percutaneous alcohol ablative techniques such as alcohol injection or radiofrequency ablation may be useful for small tumors.

- The risk of hepatocellular carcinoma is increased in cirrhosis of nearly any cause.
- Alpha fetoprotein is increased in 50% of patients with hepatocellular carcinoma.
- Common metastatic sites: lymph nodes, lung, bone, and brain.
- Paraneoplastic syndromes: anemia, fever, hypercalcemia, hypoglycemia, and clubbing.
- Liver transplantation: an option for selected patients.

Cholangiocarcinoma

The incidence of cholangiocarcinoma is increased in patients with PSC, *Opisthorchis* infection, and a history of choledochal cysts. Cholangiocarcinoma may be difficult to diagnose, especially in patients with PSC. For most patients, surgical resection is the treatment of choice, although resection is not possible in many patients.

Adenoma

Adenomas are associated with the use of oral contraceptives or estrogen. Patients can present with acute right upper quadrant pain and hemodynamic compromise because of bleeding.

Cavernous Hemangioma

Cavernous hemangioma is the most common benign tumor of the liver. Computed tomography (CT) with contrast agent is often diagnostic, demonstrating peripheral enhancement of the lesion.

Metastases

Metastases are more common than primary tumors of the liver. Frequent primary sites are the colon, stomach, breast, lung, and pancreas. Surgical resection of isolated colon cancer metastases has a limited effect on long-term survival.

Complications of End-Stage Liver Disease

Ascites

The pathogenesis of ascites is disputed but probably involves a combination of decreased effective circulatory blood volume and inappropriate renal sodium retention with expansion of plasma volume. The initial event may be vasodilatation. Patients with ascites generally have a low urinary concentration of sodium. The treatment of ascites involves sodium restriction, diuretics, and (occasionally) fluid restriction. Generally, spironolactone (100-200 mg daily) is given initially, although a low dose of furosemide (20-40 mg) is often added. The goal is to increase urinary sodium and to allow the loss of 1 L of ascitic fluid (1 kg weight) per day. Paracentesis is indicated for diagnostic purposes and should be performed therapeutically in patients with tense ascites or with respiratory compromise from abdominal distention. Large-volume or even total paracentesis in combination with 6 g of albumin per liter of ascitic fluid removed is safe and well tolerated.

- The pathogenesis of ascites probably involves a combination of decreased effective circulatory blood volume and inappropriate renal sodium retention with expansion of plasma volume.
- Patients generally have a low urinary concentration of sodium.
- Treatment: sodium restriction, diuretics.
- Large-volume paracentesis is safe and well tolerated.

Pleural effusion (hepatic hydrothorax) occurs in 6% of patients with cirrhosis and is right-sided in 67%. Edema usually follows ascites and is related to hypoalbuminemia and possibly increased pressure on the inferior vena cava by the intra-abdominal fluid. The sudden onset of ascites should raise the possibility of hepatic venous outflow obstruction (Budd-Chiari syndrome). Tests most useful for determining the cause of ascites are measurements of total protein and the serum–ascitic fluid albumin gradient (SAAG), which is calculated by [albumin (serum) – albumin (ascites)]. SAAG greater than 1.1 g/dL indicates portal hypertension. Ascites due to portal hypertension induced by congestive heart failure can be distinguished from cirrhotic ascites because congestive heart failure usually has an ascitic fluid protein greater than 2.5. Ascites from cancer or tuberculosis generally has an ascitic fluid protein greater than 2.5 and an albumin gradient less than 1.1 (Table 7-22).

Refractory ascites is uncommon. Most physicians advocate therapeutic paracentesis as needed. Transjugular intrahepatic portosystemic shunt (TIPS) is effective in some patients with refractory ascites and is particularly useful for cirrhotic patients with pleural effusion as the major manifestation of fluid retention. Peritoneovenous shunts are complicated by disseminated intravascular coagulation and shunt malfunction and are rarely performed.

- Pleural effusion occurs in 6% of patients with cirrhosis and is right-sided in 67%.

Table 7-22 Use of Serum–Ascites Albumin Gradient (SAAG) and Ascites Protein to Determine the Cause of Ascites

SAAG	Ascites protein <2.5 mg/dL	Ascites protein ≥2.5 mg/dL
≥1.1	Portal hypertension due to cirrhosis	Portal hypertension due to hepatic venous outflow obstruction (including right heart failure)
<1.1	Nephrotic syndrome	Malignancy, tuberculosis

- The sudden onset of ascites raises the possibility of hepatic venous outflow obstruction (Budd-Chiari syndrome).
- An albumin gradient >1.1 g/dL almost always indicates portal hypertension.

Spontaneous Bacterial Peritonitis

Spontaneous bacterial peritonitis (SBP) occurs in 10% to 20% of patients with cirrhosis who have ascites. It is defined as a bacterial infection of ascitic fluid without any intra-abdominal source of infection. Fever, abdominal pain, and abdominal tenderness are classic symptoms; however, many patients have few or no symptoms. SBP should be suspected in any patient with cirrhotic ascites. For all patients, diagnostic paracentesis is advisable as an initial step. Coagulopathy and thrombocytopenia are not contraindications for diagnostic paracentesis. A cell count and culture of ascitic fluid should be performed for all patients. Bedside inoculation of blood culture bottles with ascitic fluid increases the diagnostic yield. SBP is more common in patients with large-volume ascites and those with a low ascitic fluid protein (<1.5 g/dL). Also, blood from all patients with SBP should be cultured because almost 50% of these cultures will be positive. Variants of SBP are listed in Table 7-23.

SBP and culture-negative neutrocytic ascites should be treated, usually with a third-generation cephalosporin. The response to antibiotics should be assessed by repeat paracentesis 48 hours after the initiation of therapy. The polymorphonuclear count should decrease by 50%, and cultures should be sterile. The hospital mortality rate for SBP is 50% to 70%. If a patient survives hospitalization, the 1-year mortality rate is 60% to 80%. A polymicrobial infection of ascitic fluid should prompt a search for an intra-abdominal focus of infection; SBP nearly always involves a single organism. The presence of bacterascites is thought to be due to contamination, and repeat paracentesis is advised.

Table 7-23   Variants of Spontaneous Bacterial Peritonitis

| Condition | Ascitic fluid | | |
	Polymorpho-nuclear cells/mL	Cultures	Management
Spontaneous bacterial peritonitis	>250	Positive	Antibiotics
Culture-negative neutrocytic ascites	>250	Negative	Antibiotics
Bacterascites	<250	Positive	Repeat paracentesis for cell count and cultures

Patients with an episode of SBP are at high risk for recurrence, and prophylactic therapy with norfloxacin is recommended. Prophylactic therapy for 7 days is also advised for any patient with cirrhosis who is hospitalized for gastrointestinal tract bleeding regardless of whether ascites or SBP is present.

- SBP occurs in 10%-20% of patients with cirrhosis who have ascites.
- Classic symptoms: fever, abdominal pain, and abdominal tenderness.
- Many patients have few or no symptoms.
- Bedside inoculation of blood culture bottles with ascitic fluid increases the diagnostic yield.
- SBP is more common in cases of large-volume ascites and in patients with low ascitic fluid protein (<1.5 g/dL).
- Spontaneous bacterial peritonitis nearly always involves only one organism.

- Prophylactic therapy is advised for patients with a previous episode of SBP.

Hepatorenal Syndrome

Hepatorenal syndrome, or functional renal failure, consists of renal failure with normal tubular function in patients with portal hypertension. The differential diagnosis is given in Table 7-24. Hepatorenal syndrome is difficult to differentiate from prerenal azotemia; thus, a brief trial of colloid expansion may be indicated. Hepatorenal syndrome is often precipitated by vigorous diuretic therapy. Treatment is supportive, although vasoconstrictors, octreotide with albumin infusion, and TIPS may be useful. After liver transplantation is performed, renal function returns to normal.

- Hepatorenal syndrome: renal failure with normal tubular function in a patient with portal hypertension.
- It is difficult to differentiate from prerenal azotemia.
- It is often precipitated by vigorous diuretic therapy.
- After liver transplantation, renal function returns to normal.

Portal Systemic Encephalopathy

Portal systemic encephalopathy is a reversible decrease in the level of consciousness of patients with severe liver disease. Disturbed consciousness, personality change, intellectual deterioration, and slowed speech are common manifestations. The electroencephalogram is frequently abnormal, and patients often demonstrate asterixis (flapping tremor). The grading system commonly used for this condition is given in Table 7-25.

The sudden development of portal systemic encephalopathy in patients with stable cirrhosis should prompt a search for bleeding, infection (especially SBP), or electrolyte disturbances; however, simple precipitating events may include increased dietary protein, constipation, or sedatives. Serum and arterial levels of ammonia are usually increased. Lactulose

Table 7-24   Differential Diagnosis for Hepatorenal Syndrome

Variable	Prerenal azotemia	Hepatorenal syndrome	Acute renal failure
Urinary sodium concentration, mEq/L	<10	<10	>30
Urine-to-plasma creatinine ratio	>30:1	>30:1	<20:1
Urinary osmolality	At least 100 mOsm > plasma osmolality	At least 100 mOsm > plasma osmolality	Equal to plasma osmolality
Urinary sediment	Normal	Unremarkable	Casts, debris

From Epstein M: Functional renal abnormalities in cirrhosis: pathophysiology and management. *In* Hepatology: A Textbook of Liver Disease. Vol 2. Second edition. Edited by D Zakim, TD Boyer. Philadelphia, WB Saunders Company, 1990, pp 493-512. By permission of publisher.

Table 7-25 Grading System for Portal Systemic Encephalopathy

Grade of encephalopathy	Level of consciousnesss
0	Normal
1	Trivial lack of awareness
	Personality change
	Day-night reversal
2	Lethargic
	Inappropriate behavior
3	Asleep but arousable
	Confused when awake
4	Unarousable

Modified from Schafer DF, Jones EA: Hepatic encephalopathy. *In* Hepatology: A Textbook of Liver Disease. Vol 1. Second edition. Edited by D Zakim, TD Boyer. Philadelphia, WB Saunders Company, 1990, pp 447-460. By permission of publisher.

has a laxative effect that decreases the nitrogenous compounds presented to the liver and is the first-line treatment for hepatic encephalopathy. Oral neomycin or protein restriction (or both) is considered for patients refractory to lactulose.

- Portal systemic encephalopathy: reversible decrease of the level of consciousness in patients with severe liver disease.
- Patients often have asterixis or flapping tremor.
- Sudden development of portal systemic encephalopathy: look for bleeding, infection, or electrolyte disturbances.
- Treatment: lactulose.

Variceal Hemorrhage

Esophageal varices are collateral vessels that develop because of portal hypertension. Varices also can occur in other parts of the gut. Isolated gastric varices without esophageal varices can occur with sinistral (left-sided) portal hypertension due to splenic vein thrombosis. Most patients with cirrhosis who have varices do not hemorrhage, but a first hemorrhage has a 10% to 30% mortality. For patients who have cirrhosis but have not had bleeding, endoscopy to assess for the presence of varices is advised. Patients with moderate or large-sized varices, especially if there are red marks on the varices, should be treated with nadolol or propranolol to prevent bleeding.

Bleeding from esophageal varices is generally massive. For patients with acute bleeding, early endoscopy is indicated for diagnosis and treatment. Endoscopic therapy consists of band ligation or, less commonly, sclerotherapy. Octreotide decreases portal venous pressure and should also be given for acute variceal bleeding.

- Esophageal varices are collateral vessels that result from portal hypertension.
- Most patients with cirrhosis who have varices do not hemorrhage.
- First hemorrhage: 10%-30% mortality.
- Bleeding is generally massive.
- Early endoscopy is indicated for diagnosis and treatment.

Of patients with esophageal varices, 80% to 100% have recurrent bleeding within 2 years after the first episode. Oral propranolol or nadolol may prevent rebleeding, although most physicians advocate endoscopic variceal ligation until the varices have been obliterated. Patients with refractory bleeding are candidates for shunting procedures. Surgical shunts have a high rate of mortality and morbidity and are complicated by portal systemic encephalopathy. TIPS is effective in controlling bleeding and has the advantage of avoiding an operation. The incidence of portal systemic encephalopathy after TIPS is 10% to 40%, but this complication usually can be controlled with medical therapy.

- Rebleeding occurs in 80%-100% of patients.
- Patients with refractory bleeding are candidates for shunting.
- The incidence of portal systemic encephalopathy after transjugular intrahepatic portal systemic shunting is 10%-40%.

Biliary Tract Disease

Gallstones and Cholecystitis

The two types of gallstones are cholesterol and pigment. Cholesterol gallstones occur when bile is supersaturated with cholesterol relative to bile salts. Excessive cholesterol secretion (females, obesity, exogenous estrogens) or deficient bile acid secretion (bile acid sequestrant therapy) may lead to cholesterol gallstones. Pigment stones are a manifestation of hemolysis or cirrhosis, although there usually is no identifying cause. Ultrasonography is 90% to 97% sensitive for detecting gallstones. Cholecystitis may be suggested by gallbladder contraction, marked distention, surrounding fluid, or wall thickening. Ultrasonography also offers the opportunity to detect dilated bile ducts. If performed during an episode of pain, radionuclide biliary scanning is helpful in diagnosing cystic duct obstruction with cholecystitis. Positive test results are marked by nonvisualization of the gallbladder despite biliary excretion of radioisotope.

Asymptomatic gallstones require no therapy, even in high-risk patients. Patients with episodes of biliary colic or acute cholecystitis should have cholecystectomy. High surgical risk patients may undergo percutaneous cholecystostomy. Stone dissolution with ursodiol should be used for only small

CT-radiolucent cholesterol stones, but this requires 6 to 24 months of treatment and is seldom used.

- Cholesterol gallstones occur when bile is supersaturated with cholesterol.
- Pigment stones can occur with hemolysis or cirrhosis.
- Ultrasonography is 90%-97% sensitive for detecting gallstones.
- Radionuclide biliary scanning helps diagnose cystic duct obstruction with cholecystitis.
- Asymptomatic gallstones require no therapy.

Bile Duct Stones

Most bile duct stones originate in the gallbladder, although a few patients have primary duct stones. CT and ultrasonography are relatively insensitive for common bile duct stones, and diagnosis generally requires cholangiography, usually accomplished via endoscopic retrograde cholangiopancreatography (ERCP). Magnetic resonance cholangiopancreatography or endoscopic ultrasonography may also be useful to diagnose common bile duct stones, although neither one, unlike ERCP, offers therapeutic potential.

Patients with bile duct stones can have minimal or no symptoms or they can have life-threatening cholangitis with abdominal pain, fever, and jaundice. Common bile duct stones should be removed. In 90% of patients, this can be performed with ERCP. The urgency of the procedure depends on the clinical presentation. Patients with minimal symptoms can have elective ERCP, but those with cholangitis and fever unresponsive to antibiotics should have urgent endoscopic treatment. Patients with gallbladder stones who have a sphincterotomy and clearance of their duct stones have only a 10% chance of having additional problems with their gallbladder stones; thus, cholecystectomy can be avoided in patients who are at high risk for complications with surgery.

- Most bile duct stones originate in the gallbladder.
- Diagnosis of common bile duct stones usually requires cholangiography.
- Common bile duct stones should be removed.
- Urgent endoscopic treatment is needed if cholangitis and fever are unresponsive to antibiotics.

Malignant Biliary Obstruction

Malignant biliary obstruction is usually the result of carcinoma of the head of the pancreas, bile duct cancer, or metastatic malignancy to hilar nodes. If the disease is unresectable, palliative endoscopic or percutaneous stenting is as effective as surgical bypass. One exception is impending duodenal obstruction, at which time operation offers the opportunity for bypass of both biliary and duodenal obstruction.

Gallbladder Carcinoma

Gallbladder carcinoma has a strong association with calcified (porcelain) gallbladder. For this reason, cholecystectomy is advised for patients with porcelain gallbladder.

Sphincter of Oddi Dysfunction

Sphincter of Oddi dysfunction is a poorly defined entity characterized by right upper quadrant pain without any structural cause. Patients with typical biliary-type pain, increased values on liver tests during the pain, a dilated common bile duct, and delayed drainage of contrast after cholangiography often have improvement after sphincterotomy. Patients without each of these criteria generally have a poor response to sphincterotomy.

Gastroenterology Pharmacy Review

Virginia H. Thompson, RPh, Alma N. Adrover, RPh, MS

Review of H$_2$ Receptor Antagonists, Proton Pump Inhibitors, and Antacids

Drug	Indication	Dosage	Toxic/adverse effects	Comments
H$_2$ receptor antagonists[*]				
Cimetidine	Duodenal ulcer, active phase	800 mg po qhs[†] × 4-6 wk	Adjust dose in severe liver and renal disease	Absorption may be affected by antacids (avoid simultaneous administration)
	Duodenal ulcer, maintenance	400 mg po qhs[†]	Reduces liver metabolism of drugs metabolized via cytochrome P450 pathway. Multiple drug interactions. May cause CNS side effects	
	Gastric ulcer, active phase	800 mg po qhs[†] × 6 wk, or 300 mg po qid × 6 wk		Injectable form available
	Gastric ulcer, maintenance	400 mg po qhs[†]		
	GERD	800 mg po bid × 12 wk		
	Heartburn (OTC)	100 mg po prn, max 400 mg/d		
Famotidine	Duodenal ulcer, active phase	40 mg po qhs[†] × 4-6 wk or 20 mg po bid × 4-6 wk	Adjust dose in renal insufficiency (CrCl <50 mL/min)	Absorption may be affected by antacids (avoid simultaneous administration) Does not inhibit cytochrome P450 pathway Injectable form available
	Duodenal ulcer, maintenance	20 mg po qhs[†]		
	Gastric ulcer, active phase	40 mg po qhs[†] × 8 wk		
	Gastric ulcer, maintenance	20 mg po qhs[†]		
	GERD	20 mg po bid × 6 wk		
	Heartburn (OTC)	10 mg po prn, max 20 mg/d		For heartburn, take 1 h before eating or drinking anything suspected of causing GI distress
Nizatidine	Duodenal ulcer, active phase	300 mg po qhs[†] or 150 mg po bid	Adjust dose in moderate-to-severe renal disease May cause CNS side effects	Absorption may be affected by antacids (avoid simultaneous administration)
	Duodenal ulcer, maintenance	150 mg po qhs[†]		Does not inhibit cytochrome P450 pathway
	Benign gastric ulcer	300 mg po qhs[†] or 150 mg po bid		For heartburn take 1 h before eating or drinking anything suspected of causing GI distress
	GERD	150 mg po bid × 6 wk		
	Heartburn (OTC)	75 mg po prn, max 150 mg/d		

Gastroenterology Pharmacy Review (continued)

Review of H$_2$ Receptor Antagonists, Proton Pump Inhibitors, and Antacids (continued)

Drug	Indication	Dosage	Toxic/adverse effects	Comments
H$_2$ receptor antagonists[*] (continued)				
Ranitidine	Duodenal ulcer, active phase	150 mg po bid or 300 mg po qhs[†]	Adjust dose in renal insufficiency (CrCl <50 mL/min)	"Efferdose" available: dissolve in 6-8 oz water before drinking
	Duodenal ulcer, maintenance	150 mg po qhs[†]	May cause CNS side effects	Binds only weakly to cytochrome P450
	Gastric ulcer, active	150 mg po bid		Injectable form available
	Gastric ulcer, maintenance	150 mg po qhs[†]		
	GERD	150 mg po bid × 6 wk		
	Heartburn (OTC)	75 mg po prn, max 100 mg/d		
Proton pump inhibitors[‡]				
Omeprazole	Duodenal ulcer	20 mg po qd × 4-8 wk	No dose adjustment needed in severe renal disease	Take 1 h before meals
	H. pylori	20 mg po qd[§]		Swallow whole; do not chew, crush, or split capsule
	Gastric ulcer	40 mg po qd × 4-8 wk	Dose adjustment suggested in severe liver disease	
	GERD	20 mg po qd × 4-8 wk		Available in generic version
Esomeprazole	H. pylori	40 mg po qd[§]		Isomer of omeprazole
	GERD	20 mg po qd × 4-8 wk		Take 1 h before meals
				Swallow whole; do not chew or crush capsule (may open capsule & mix with applesauce)
Lansoprazole	Duodenal ulcer	15 mg po qd × 4 wk	Consider dose reduction in severe liver disease	Take 1 h before meals
	H. pylori	30 mg po qd[§]		Swallow whole; do not chew or crush capsule
	Gastric ulcer	30 mg po qd for up to 8 wk		(may open capsule & mix with applesauce)
	GERD	15 mg po qd × 8-16 wk		Oral suspension packets available
Rabeprazole	Duodenal ulcer	20 mg po qd after morning meal for up to 4 wk	Does not appear to interact with hepatic cytochrome P450	Swallow whole; do not chew, crush, or split tablet
	Gastric ulcer	20 mg po qd × 6 wk		
	H. pylori	20 mg po bid × 7 d[§]		
	GERD	20 mg po qd × 4-8 wk		

Gastroenterology Pharmacy Review (continued)

Review of H$_2$ Receptor Antagonists, Proton Pump Inhibitors, and Antacids (continued)

Drug	Indication	Dosage	Toxic/adverse effects	Comments
Proton pump inhibitors[‡] (continued)				
Pantoprazole	Duodenal ulcer	40 mg po qd × 8 wk	Does not appear to interact with hepatic cytochrome P450	May be taken with/without food
	Gastric ulcer	40 mg po qd × 8 wk		Not affected by concomitant administration of antacids
	GERD	40 mg po qd for up to 8 wk		Swallow whole; do not chew, crush, or split tablet
				Injectable form available
Antacids[//]				
Aluminum hydroxide	500-1,500 mg po 3-6 × qd	Binds with phosphate ions May cause constipation Use with caution in Alzheimer disease Careful with accumulation in renal disease		May have cytoprotective effect Useful in biliary reflux
Calcium carbonate	500-1,500 mg po prn	Milk-alkali syndrome		40% elemental calcium
Magaldrate	30 mL po prn			Chemical entity of aluminum & magnesium hydroxide
Magnesium hydroxide	30 mL po prn	Cathartic effect at higher doses Careful with accumulation in renal disease		May have cytoprotective effect
Sodium bicarbonate	300-2,000 mg po 1-4 × qd	Avoid sodium overload Milk-alkali syndrome		Most rapidly acting antacid
Sodium citrate	30 mL po qd	Increases absorption of aluminum from aluminum-containing antacids, potentiating aluminum toxicity in renal disease Conversion to bicarbonate may be impaired in liver disease		May chill & dilute with water before using

bid, twice daily; CNS, central nervous system; CrCl, creatinine clearance; GERD, gastroesophageal reflux disease; GI, gastrointestinal; NSAID, nonsteroidal anti-inflammatory drug; OTC, over-the-counter (nonprescription); po, orally; prn, as needed; qd, daily; qhs, at bedtime.

*Indicated for phase 2 therapy in the treatment of reflux disease and for the prevention of bleeding associated with stress ulcers. Ineffective in preventing gastric ulcers and in decreasing the frequency of NSAID-induced mucosal erosions.

[†]Nocturnal acid secretion may be better controlled with 6 p.m. administration instead of 10 p.m. because highest acid production starts at 7 p.m.

[‡]Indicated for healing and prevention of NSAID-induced gastric ulcers. Class of drugs that provides the most complete control of acid production and better overall symptom control and mucosal healing. Most effective in treatment of GERD. Proton pump inhibitors may interact with drugs for which gastric pH is important determinant of bioavailability, ie, ketoconazole, ampicillin, iron, digoxin, cyanocobalamin.

[§]Used in combination as described in section on *Helicobacter pylori* treatment.

[//]All antacids should be administered 30 minutes after meals and at bedtime. Coadministration of antacids with fluoroquinolones may result in crystalluria and nephrotoxicity. Give 2 hours before or 8 hours after antacid. Antacids reduce absorption of ketoconazole and tetracyclines. Do not give antacids within 3 hours of these drugs. Coadministration of enteric-coated drugs (such as bisacodyl) and antacids may cause coating to dissolve too rapidly, resulting in gastric or duodenal irritation.

Gastroenterology Pharmacy Review (continued)

Review of Adjuvants for Treating Gastrointestinal Disorders

Drug name	Dosage	Toxic/adverse effects	Comments
Anticholinergics			
Atropine	0.4-0.6 mg po	Drowsiness, dizziness, dry mouth, blurred vision, urinary retention	Take 30-60 min before meals
L-Hyoscyamine	0.125-0.25 mg po tid-qid	Susceptibility to heat stroke	
Belladonna alkaloids	0.18-0.3 mg po tid-qid		Need to increase dental hygiene because of decreased salivary secretion
Scopolamine	0.4-0.8 mg po qd Patch, 1.5 mg for 3 d	Vision changes, drowsiness	Inhibits excessive motility of GI tract Used for motion sickness
Glycopyrrolate	1-2 mg po bid-tid		
Antispasmodics			
Dicyclomine	20-40 mg po qid	Drowsiness, dizziness, dry mouth	
Antiflatulents			
Simethicone	40-120 mg po prn		Take after meals & before bedtime Defoaming action—chew tablets completely
Charcoal	520 mg after meals po prn	Can adsorb other drugs from GI tract	Limit use to no more than 2 d
Prokinetic			
Metoclopramide	10 mg po up to qid	Extrapyramidal symptoms may occur Dizziness, drowsiness, crosses BBB Avoid in depressed or epileptic patients	Take before meals & before bedtime Effective in decreasing symptoms but not in healing Injectable form available
Bethanechol	25 mg po qid after meals		Useful in combination with other agents Increases lower esophageal sphincter tone Increases esophageal clearance Injectable form available
Cytoprotective agents			
Misoprostol	200 µg po qid with food	Diarrhea, cramping Do not use in pregnant women or women of child-bearing age without prior pregnancy test	Abortifacient properties Used to prevent NSAID-induced gastric ulcers & to treat duodenal ulcers

Gastroenterology Pharmacy Review (continued)

Review of Adjuvants for Treating Gastrointestinal Disorders (continued)

Drug name	Dosage	Toxic/adverse effects	Comments
Cytoprotective agents (continued)			
Sucralfate	Active duodenal ulcer—1 g po qid × 4-8 wk	Use with caution in renal failure— possible aluminum accumulation Do not give antacids within 30 min of administration	Local action, not absorbed systemically Adheres to damaged mucosa and protects it against acid, pepsin, and bile salts Give 1 h before meals & before bedtime May decrease nosocomial pneumonia in ventilator-dependent patients

BBB, blood-brain barrier; bid, twice daily; GI, gastrointestinal; NSAID, nonsteroidal anti-inflammatory drug; po, orally; prn, as needed; qd, daily; qid, 4 times daily; tid, 3 times daily.

Gastroenterology Pharmacy Review (continued)

Review of Drugs for Treating Diarrhea, Constipation, and Ulcerative Colitis, Crohn Disease, and Irritable Bowel Syndrome (IBS)

Drug name	Dosage	Toxic/adverse effects	Comments
Diarrhea			
Bismuth subsalicylate	2 tab or 30 mL po prn up to 8 doses/24 h	Salicylate toxicity Decreases bioavailability of tetracycline Discoloration of tongue/stools Avoid in renal failure	Antacid & adsorbent properties Used to prevent traveler's diarrhea Do not use in patients with influenza or chicken pox because of risk of Reye syndrome
Diphenoxylate with atropine	5 mg po qid, max 20 mg/d	Dizziness, drowsiness, dry mouth, miosis	Diphenoxylate = meperidine congener without analgesic properties
Loperamide	4 mg po × 1, then 2 mg po prn; max 16 mg/d	Drowsiness	Slows intestinal motility Effective for traveler's diarrhea
Cholestyramine	4 g po qd-tid	Steatorrhea Long-term use may decrease absorption of iron, calcium, folic acid	Binds bile acids Mix powder with fluids Administer other medicines 1-2 h before or 6 h after
Octreotide	50-250 µg sq tid	Flushing, bradycardia, dizziness	Somatostatin analogue Useful for secretory diarrhea
Constipation			

Fiber (bulk producing)
  Methylcellulose
  Polycarbophil
  Psyllium
	
	5 mL po up to tid
	2-4 tab po qd
	5 mL po up to tid
		Bloating, flatulence, iron and calcium malabsorption
		Decreases effects of digoxin, coumadin, salicylates, tetracyclines, nitrofurantoin
		Watch for esophageal obstruction in elderly patients
		Contraindicated in patients with intestinal ulceration & stenosis
			Recommended initial treatment for most forms of constipation
			Increases stool bulk
			Decreases transit time
			Drink a full glass of liquid with each dose

Stool softeners Docusate (sodium, calcium, potassium)	 100 mg po bid	Avoid taking with mineral oil	Best agent for constipation prevention Surfactant
Hyperosmolar agents Glycerin	 1 suppository per rectum prn	Local irritation if used rectally	
Lactulose* Sorbitol	30 mL po qd 15-30 mL po qd	} Abdominal cramps Use with caution in diabetic patients & in renal impairment }	Sweet taste

Gastroenterology Pharmacy Review (continued)

Review of Drugs for Treating Diarrhea, Constipation, and Ulcerative Colitis, Crohn Disease, and Irritable Bowel Syndrome (IBS) (continued)

Drug name	Dosage	Toxic/adverse effects	Comments
Constipation (continued)			
Stimulants		Rectal irritation (rectal bisacodyl)	Limit use to not more than a
Bisacodyl	10 mg po or per rectum qd	Urine discoloration (senna)	week
Senna	2 tab po qd		Avoid coadministration with antacids, H$_2$ receptor antagonists & milk products (oral bisacodyl)
Cascara	5 mL po qd		
Castor oil	30 mL po qd		
Saline			
Milk of magnesia	} 30 mL po qd	Contraindicated in renal disease and CHF	Limit use to not more than a week
Magnesium citrate		Watch for symptoms of magnesium toxicity	
		May alter fluid and electrolyte balance	
Polyethylene glycol (PEG) saline lavage	17 g po qd	Do not use in patients with suspected GI obstruction or perforation	For occasional use only Dissolve in 8 oz of liquid before taking
Emollient/Lubricant			
Mineral oil	15-45 mL po qd	Lipid pneumonia Malabsorption of lipid-soluble vitamins Reduces absorption of anticoagulants, oral contraceptives, and digoxin	Not for routine use
Ulcerative Colitis, Crohn Disease, and IBS			
Mesalamine (5-ASA)	2.4-4 g po qd 1 g qd per rectum (suppository or retention enema)	Overdose: symptoms of salicylate toxicity; if patient develops chest pain, consider pericarditis	Effective in treatment of mild to moderate active phases Swallow tablets whole May give oral & rectal therapy concurrently Available as Asacol and Pentasa that release 5-ASA in the terminal ileum and small bowel, respectively
Olsalazine	1 g po qd in divided doses	Monitor for renal abnormalities Causes diarrhea	Take with food Biconverted to 5-ASA in colon Effective in treatment of mild to moderate active phases

Gastroenterology Pharmacy Review (continued)

Review of Drugs for Treating Diarrhea, Constipation, and Ulcerative Colitis, Crohn Disease, and Irritable Bowel Syndrome (IBS) (continued)

Drug name	Dosage	Toxic/adverse effects	Comments
Ulcerative Colitis, Crohn Disease, and IBS (continued)			
Sulfasalazine	3-4 g po qd	Use with caution in asthmatic patients & patients with glucose-6-phosphate dehydrogenase deficiency Cross-sensitivity with sulfonamides May impair folic acid absorption Orange-yellow discoloration of the urine, skin, & soft contact lenses	Effective in treating acute disease & maintenance of remission of ulcerative colitis Does not maintain remission in Crohn disease Swallow whole Metabolized to sulfapyridine and 5-ASA by intestinal bacteria Slow/fast acetylators exhibit differences in metabolism Maintain adequate fluid intake
Balsalazide	675 g po qd in divided doses	Monitor for renal abnormalities	Bioconverted to 5-ASA in colon
Prednisone	40-60 mg po qd Use topically on mild to moderate active disease of distal colon	Osteoporosis Cushingoid appearance Muscle weakness Adrenal suppression	Most effective in maintenance of remission of ulcerative colitis Most effective in acute exacerbation of Crohn disease Use prednisolone in patients with cirrhosis
Azathioprine	2-5 mg/kg po qd	Immunosuppression	Metabolized to 6-mercaptopurine Drug interaction with allopurinol Injectable form available
6-Mercaptopurine	2.5-5 mg/kg po qd		Steroid-sparing effect
Metronidazole (perianal disease)	20 mg/kg po qd	Metallic taste, dark urine	Recurrence with discontinuation
Infliximab (Crohn disease)	5 mg/kg IV infusion over 2 h	Associated with severe acute infusion reaction, delayed hypersensitivity, & increased risk of infection	For moderate to severe active Crohn disease refractory to conventional therapy & in fistulizing Crohn disease
Tegaseroid (IBS)	6 mg po bid before meals for 4-6 wk	Not recommended in severe hepatic or renal impairment or symptomatic gallbladder disease	For treatment of women with IBS, constipation predominant

bid, twice daily; CHF, congestive heart failure; GI, gastrointestinal; IBS, irritable bowel syndrome; IV, intravenously; NSAID, nonsteroidal anti-inflammatory drug; po, orally; prn, as needed; qd, daily; qhs, at bedtime; qid, 4 times daily; sq, subcutaneously; tab, tablets; tid, 3 times daily.

*Also indicated in treatment of portal systemic encephalopathy.

Gastroenterology Pharmacy Review (continued)

Review of *Helicobacter pylori* Treatment Regimens

Regimen	Drug combinations	Dosage, mg orally	Duration, d
A	Amoxicillin[*]	1,000 bid	10-14
	Clarithromycin[†]	500 bid	
	Lansoprazole[‡]	30 bid	
B	Amoxicillin[*]	1,000 bid	10-14
	Clarithromycin[†]	500 bid	
	Omeprazole[‡]	20 bid	
C	Clarithromycin[†]	500 bid	14
	Metronidazole[§]	500 bid	
	Omeprazole[‡]	20 bid	
D	Clarithromycin[†]	500 bid	14
	Metronidazole[§]	500 bid	
	Lansoprazole[‡]	30 bid	
E	Tetracycline[//]	500 qid	14
	Metronidazole[§]	250 qid	
	Bismuth subsalicylate[¶]	525 qid	
	H_2-receptor antagonist in ulcer treatment doses for 28 days		

bid, twice daily; qid, 4 times daily.

[*]Be aware of penicillin allergy; may cause nausea and diarrhea.

[†]Metallic taste; drug interaction with terfenadine, astemizole, cisapride.

[‡]Do not crush or alter capsules.

[§]Avoid alcohol use; may cause nausea and diarrhea.

[//]Reduces effectiveness of oral contraceptives. Absorption reduced in presence of divalent and trivalent cations (Ca, Mg, Fe, Al).

Photosensitivity (avoid exposure to sunlight).

[¶]Darkening of tongue and stools.

Data from ASHP therapeutic position statement on the identification and treatment of *Helicobacter pylori*-associated peptic ulcer disease in adults. Am J Health Syst Pharm 2001;58:331-337.

QUESTIONS

Multiple Choice (choose the one best answer)

1. You are asked to see a 54-year-old man in consultation because he is having difficulty swallowing. For 6 months, he has had increasing difficulty swallowing solids, especially meats, and he has lost 10 lb. Otherwise, he has been in excellent health and has no other complaints. He has smoked 1 pack of cigarettes daily for 30 years and has taken medications for chronic heartburn for 20 years. An upper gastrointestinal radiograph shows a narrowing of the esophageal lumen in the mid esophagus, with a small ulcer present. Which of the following is the most likely explanation of these findings?
   a. Achalasia
   b. Diffuse esophageal spasm
   c. Esophageal ring
   d. Barrett esophagus
   e. Nonspecific esophageal motility disorder

2. You are called to the emergency department to evaluate a 27-year-old woman. Four hours ago, while eating turkey, she felt something "stick" in the lower part of her chest. She has been unable to vomit and has attempted to swallow water but has not been able to swallow anything. During the past 2 years, she has had multiple episodes of solid food sticking in the lower part of her chest but has been able to "throw up," and the episodes resolved. She states that she does not have heartburn or weight loss and is otherwise healthy. The physical examination results are normal. Which of the following is the most likely explanation of her findings?
   a. Achalasia
   b. Diffuse esophageal spasm
   c. Lower esophageal ring
   d. Peptic stricture
   e. Nonspecific esophageal motility disorder

3. A 37-year-old woman has difficulty swallowing. During the past 4 years, she has had several episodes of food sticking in the lower esophagus which were relieved by drinking water. For the past 6 months, she has had difficulty swallowing both solids and liquids and has lost 10 lb. An upper gastrointestinal radiograph shows smooth, beaklike tapering of the distal esophagus and dilatation of the proximal esophagus. The results of esophagogastroduodenoscopy are normal. Which of the following is the most likely explanation of her symptoms?
   a. Peptic stricture
   b. Lower esophageal ring
   c. Achalasia

   d. Diffuse esophageal spasm
   e. Nonspecific motility disorder

4. A 49-year-old executive is referred to you for evaluation of chest pain that has been present for 4 months. He describes several episodes of a deep substernal chest pain lasting 30 to 60 minutes that resolves spontaneously. He exercises regularly and says he has no exertional chest pain. The results of a cardiology evaluation, including resting and exercise electrocardiography and coronary angiography, are normal, as is esophagogastroduodenoscopy with biopsy of the lower esophagus. The patient's father died of cardiac disease, and he is very worried about this pain. Which of the following is the next best step in the evaluation of this patient?
   a. Upper gastrointestinal radiography
   b. Computed tomography of the chest
   c. Magnetic resonance imaging of the chest
   d. Bernstein test (acid perfusion test)
   e. Esophageal motility study

5. A 39-year-old woman complains of coughing and choking with swallowing and food sticking in the neck. Occasionally, she has had regurgitation of swallowed liquids into her nose. All the following conditions could explain her symptoms *except*:
   a. Achalasia
   b. Zenker diverticulum
   c. Myasthenia gravis
   d. Multiple sclerosis
   e. Amyotrophic lateral sclerosis

6. A 27-year-old man with acquired immunodeficiency syndrome (AIDS) has had painful swallowing for 1 week. He states that he does not have heartburn or sticking of food when swallowing. He is taking zidovudine (AZT), indinavir, and lamivudine. Upper gastrointestinal endoscopy shows diffuse ulceration of the esophagus, and biopsy specimens of the esophageal mucosa show intranuclear inclusions in endothelial cells and fibroblasts. Which of the following is the most likely explanation for these findings?
   a. Autoimmune aphthous ulcers
   b. Medication esophagitis
   c. Infection with cytomegalovirus
   d. Infection with *Candida albicans*
   e. Bullous pemphigoid

7. Odynophagia developed 3 days previously in a 77-year-old woman who is taking multiple medications. She states that she does not have heartburn but has noticed some dysphagia with solids, which is relieved by drinking liquids. Upper gastrointestinal radiography shows inflammation in the mid

esophagus, with sparing of the distal esophagus. All the following medications may explain these findings *except*:
a. Potassium supplements
b. Tetracycline
c. Nonsteroidal anti-inflammatory drugs (NSAIDs)
d. Calcium channel blockers
e. Ascorbic acid

8. A 39-year-old man comes to the free clinic with abdominal discomfort and frequent indigestion. He is a migrant worker, and his eating habits are irregular. Two previous upper gastrointestinal radiographic studies showed duodenal ulcers. He states that he does not take NSAIDs or aspirin and does not drink alcohol. A rapid serologic test is positive for *Helicobacter pylori*. Which of the following is the most appropriate next step in his management?
a. Refer for esophagogastroduodenoscopy
b. Perform esophagogastroduodenoscopy and biopsy for *H. pylori*
c. Determine serum level of gastrin
d. Treat with antisecretory agents
e. Treat with antibiotics and antisecretory agents

9. A 44-year-old woman has chronic indigestion. Several years ago duodenal ulcer was documented with endoscopy. She has continued to have dyspepsia, and diarrhea recently developed. She states that she does not take NSAIDs, aspirin, or alcohol. Her father and brother have had operations for ulcers. The results of physical examination are normal. Laboratory test results, including a complete blood count and chemistry profiles, are normal, except for a calcium value of 10.8 mg/dL. A rapid serologic test is negative for *H. pylori*. Which of the following is the most likely explanation for her symptoms?
a. Nonulcer dyspepsia
b. Gastroesophageal reflux
c. Peptic ulcer disease due to alcohol
d. Peptic ulcer disease due to *H. pylori* infection
e. Zollinger-Ellison syndrome

10. A 70-year-old man comes to your office with progressive dysphagia with solids and a 20-lb weight loss over 2 months. He has no previous history of heartburn. Esophagogastroduodenoscopy shows an ulcerated narrowing in the mid esophagus, and biopsy findings are consistent with squamous cell carcinoma. All the following clinical conditions could predispose to esophageal squamous cell carcinoma *except*:
a. Alcohol ingestion
b. Smoking
c. Gastroesophageal reflux disease

d. Achalasia
e. Human papillomavirus

11. A 43-year-old business executive comes to the outpatient clinic with diarrhea that has been present for 3 days. She has just returned from a business trip to Mexico, and she noticed her first loose stool on the flight home. She has been having 6 to 7 loose, watery stools daily with no blood. She says she does not have a fever but has lost 2 lb. She is in excellent health otherwise and takes no medication. The physical examination results are normal. Which of the following is the most appropriate course of action at this time?
a. Metronidazole, 250 mg three times daily
b. Amoxicillin, 250 mg four times daily
c. Ciprofloxacin, 500 mg twice daily
d. Obtain stool for culture and sensitivity, ova, parasites, and *Clostridium difficile* toxin assay
e. Check stool osmolality

12. A 26-year-old woman is evaluated for diarrhea that has been present for 1 month. She has had three or four loose, watery, nonbloody stools daily for 1 month. She says she does not have a fever and has not been traveling or camping. She has lost 8 lb intentionally by strictly adhering to a diet during the past month. She has been drinking a lot of diet soda and chewing sugarless gum. The physical examination results are normal. The patient appears well hydrated and has no orthostatic blood pressure or pulse changes. Her stools are loose and brown. No fecal leukocytes are present. Which of the following is the most likely explanation of her symptoms?
a. Secretory diarrhea from a toxigenic bacterium
b. Secretory diarrhea from a hormone-producing tumor
c. Osmotic diarrhea from lactase deficiency
d. Osmotic diarrhea from sorbitol ingestion
e. Diarrhea from a bacterial pathogen

13. A 54-year-old executive complains of diarrhea that has been present for 3 months. He has been having two or three loose brown stools daily for 3 months. He states that he does not have a fever and has not lost weight, and he has never observed blood in his stools. He says he has not traveled other than a fishing trip to remote areas of Canada. He is otherwise in excellent health, and the results of physical examination are normal. Which of the following is the most appropriate course of action?
a. Advise him to drink fluids, and offer an antimotility agent
b. Obtain stool for culture and sensitivity, ova, and parasites
c. Amoxicillin, 250 mg four times daily

d. Ciprofloxacin, 500 mg three times daily
e. Metronidazole, 250 mg three times daily

14. A 22-year-old medical student comes to the emergency department passing bright red blood from the rectum. He is in excellent health; however, he has had two similar episodes previously, at ages 16 and 19 years. Previous evaluations, including stool studies and colonoscopy, have not disclosed a bleeding source. He has been told he has hemorrhoidal bleeding. The physical examination findings are normal. Rectal examination shows bloody red, liquid stools. No hemorrhoids are found. Which of the following is the most likely explanation for his symptoms?
a. Crohn disease involving the terminal ileum
b. Juvenile polyps
c. Meckel diverticulum
d. Ulcerative colitis
e. Aortoenteric fistula

15. A 34-year-old schoolteacher is referred to you because of edema that has been present for 2 years. He first noticed swelling of his left leg, but for the past 3 months both legs have "become swollen" and the edema has increased. He also has noticed dyspnea on exertion for 1 month. Physical examination demonstrates 4+ pitting edema of both legs. Examination of the chest reveals dullness and decreased breath sounds at both bases. Laboratory evaluation includes a complete blood count, which shows 4×10^9/L leukocytes, with 65% segmented neutrophils, 3% eosinophils, 3% band forms, 1% basophils, 5% lymphocytes, and 7% monocytes. Total protein value is 4.0 g/dL, and albumin is 2.5 g/dL. Urinalysis results are normal, and no urine protein is present. Which of the following is the most likely explanation of these findings?
a. Bacterial overgrowth of small intestine
b. Crohn disease
c. Abetalipoproteinemia
d. Idiopathic cyclic edema
e. Intestinal lymphangiectasia

16. An 18-year-old college freshman comes to the outpatient clinic with nausea, abdominal pain, and diarrhea that have been present for 3 to 4 weeks. Her symptoms follow meals; however, she has not been able to identify specific foods that cause worse symptoms. She says she does not have a fever and has not been traveling or camping. She is allergic to pollens, dusts, and mold but has had no recent symptoms of allergic rhinitis, and she is not taking any medications. She acknowledges that the demands of school and playing on the basketball team have been stressful. Results of physical examination are normal.

Laboratory evaluation includes a normal complete blood count. The leukocyte count is 9.6×10^9/L, with 60% segmented neutrophils, 4% band forms, 15% eosinophils, and 24% lymphocytes. Stool studies for ova and parasites and culture and sensitivity are negative. Which of the following is the most likely explanation for her symptoms?
a. Irritable bowel syndrome
b. Infection with *Giardia lamblia*
c. Infection with *Entamoeba histolytica*
d. Eosinophilic gastroenteritis
e. Chronic pancreatitis

17. A 40-year-old woman presents with osteomalacia and iron deficiency anemia. Stool studies are negative for occult blood and show a stool fat value of 20 g/24 hours. She has had no previous operation. In addition to hypochromic microcytic red blood cells, the peripheral blood smear shows Howell-Jolly bodies. Which of the following is the most likely explanation for this woman's condition?
a. Whipple disease
b. Intestinal lymphangiectasia
c. Tropical sprue
d. Celiac sprue
e. Bacterial overgrowth

18. A 70-year-old man complains of diarrhea and four episodes of arthritis during the past 3 months. His family thinks he is becoming more forgetful. On examination, he appears hyperpigmented and has generalized lymphadenopathy. Stool fat value is 20 g/24 hours. Small-bowel biopsy shows PAS-positive granules in macrophages in the lamina propria of the small intestine. What is the most likely cause of this patient's condition?
a. Tropical sprue
b. Intestinal lymphangiectasia
c. Abetalipoproteinemia
d. Whipple disease
e. *Vibrio vulnificus* infection

19. A 50-year-old man has a 3-month history of diarrhea and a 10-lb weight loss. He has not traveled. Physical examination shows a large tongue with furrowed edges, a systolic murmur along the left sternal border that increases with inspiration, hepatomegaly, and diminished vibratory sensation in both feet. A complete blood count and chemistry screening profile are normal, and urinalysis shows 4+ proteinuria. Which of the following is the most likely explanation for these findings?
a. Celiac sprue
b. Whipple disease
c. Progressive systemic sclerosis

d. Amyloidosis

e. Intestinal lymphangiectasia

20. A 64-year-old woman presents with pain in the left lower quadrant of the abdomen and constipation. On physical examination, her temperature is 38.3°C (101°F), and a tender mass is palpable in the left lower quadrant of the abdomen. Laboratory studies include a normal abdominal radiograph and a complete blood count showing 15×10^9/L leukocytes with a left shift. What is the most appropriate management?

a. Obtain stool and blood for cultures and perform flexible sigmoidoscopy

b. Obtain stool for culture and schedule a return visit in 2 days for review of the culture report

c. Obtain stool for culture, begin therapy with oral antibiotics, and instruct the patient to schedule a return appointment if her symptoms do not improve

d. Admit the patient to the hospital, do not allow her to have oral intake, begin treatment with intravenous fluids and antibiotics, and obtain a surgical consultation

e. Emergency operation

21. A 65-year-old woman presents with recurrent red rectal bleeding. Results of physical examination are normal except for aortic stenosis. Flexible sigmoidoscopy to 30 cm, colon radiography, and upper gastrointestinal endoscopy results are also normal. What is the most appropriate next step in her diagnostic evaluation?

a. Radionuclide bleeding scan

b. Angiography

c. Colonoscopy

d. Small-bowel radiography

e. Small-bowel endoscopy

22. A 75-year-old woman presents with lower abdominal pain and bloody diarrhea. Results of proctoscopic examination to 30 cm are normal, and colon radiography shows "thumbprinting" of the splenic flexure. Risk factors for the development of her condition include all the following *except*:

a. Hypertension

b. Diabetes mellitus

c. Diverticulosis

d. Atherosclerosis

23. A 64-year-old man comes to the outpatient clinic with fever, abdominal pain, and diarrhea that have been present for 2 days. He was dismissed from the hospital 3 weeks ago after a 4-day admission for treatment of pyelonephritis. Two days ago, he started to have 3 or 4 loose, watery brown stools with a small amount of blood and mucus.

He then noticed a mild cramping in the left lower quadrant and had a temperature of 99.6°F. There is mild tenderness over the left lower quadrant. Laboratory examination includes normal results of urinalysis, complete blood count, and abdominal radiography. Sigmoidoscopy shows discrete areas of well-demarcated white exudate-like material. Which of the following is the best next step in this patient's management?

a. Obtain stool for ova and parasites

b. Obtain stool for culture and sensitivity

c. Obtain stool for *Clostridium difficile* toxin assay

d. Colonoscopy with biopsy

e. Colon radiography

24. A 62-year-old man comes to the emergency department with abdominal pain, vomiting, and diarrhea that have been present for 12 hours. He describes the sudden onset 12 hours ago of a mid-abdominal pain that has increased in severity. He passed three stools; the last stool, passed 1 hour ago, was bloody. He vomited shortly after arrival in the emergency department. He has a past medical history of stable class II angina and nephrolithiasis, but he is otherwise healthy. On physical examination, the man is in obvious distress because of abdominal pain. His vital signs are normal except for an irregular pulse at a rate of 126 beats/min. A complete blood count, urinalysis results, and electrolyte and creatinine values are normal, as is chest radiography. Electrocardiography shows atrial fibrillation, with no evidence for acute ischemia. Abdominal radiography shows a small distended loop of small intestine in the mid abdomen. The serum amylase value is 196 U/L. Which of the following is the most likely explanation of these findings?

a. Acute pancreatitis

b. Acute cholecystitis

c. Acute ileus

d. Acute mesenteric ischemia

e. Nephrolithiasis

25. A 55-year-old man is evaluated for a 4-month history of diarrhea and weight loss. He describes his stool as pale and light-colored, with oil droplets present. He has lost 26 lb. His appetite has been good. He denies recent abdominal pain. He takes no medication, does not smoke, and drinks alcohol "socially." The physical examination results are normal. Laboratory evaluation includes normal electrolyte and creatinine values, and blood glucose is 150 mg/dL, albumin 2.8 g/dL, and serum amylase 114 U/L. Which of the following is the most likely explanation for these findings?

a. Pancreatic ductal adenocarcinoma

b. Acute pancreatitis due to alcohol

c. Acute pancreatitis due to gallstones

d. Chronic pancreatitis due to alcohol

e. Chronic pancreatitis due to gallstones

26. A 52-year-old man comes to your office because his family has thought he looked "yellow" for several weeks. He says he has no abdominal pain, has no previous history of liver disease, and is not taking any medication. Physical examination shows scleral icterus and jaundice. An abdominal examination reveals a nontender palpable gallbladder. The results of laboratory evaluation are a total bilirubin value of 7 mg/dL, direct bilirubin 4 mg/dL, and amylase 115 U/L. A complete blood count and electrolyte and creatinine values are normal. Ultrasonography of the abdomen shows dilated intrahepatic ducts and an enlarged gallbladder. Which of the following is the most likely explanation for these findings?

a. Acute cholecystitis

b. Choledocholithiasis (common duct stone)

c. Acute pancreatitis

d. Chronic pancreatitis

e. Pancreatic cancer

27. A 49-year-old pharmacist comes to your office because of chronic diarrhea. For 10 years, he has had episodes of loose stool. He states that he has not lost weight and has not had any intestinal bleeding, and he has had some normal bowel movements and episodic constipation. He has not traveled and has no specific food intolerances. He was evaluated in the past and was given no explanation for his problem. The most likely explanation of these findings is:

a. Diverticulosis of the colon

b. Ulcerative colitis

c. Hirschsprung disease

d. Granulomatous colitis

e. Irritable bowel syndrome

28. A 23-year-old medical student is asymptomatic but comes to your office because of a family history of colon cancer. His father died of colon cancer at age 46 years. He is the oldest of five children. Colonoscopic examination demonstrates several hundred small polyps distributed throughout the colon, and biopsy shows benign tubular adenomas with moderate dysplasia. All the following are indicated in this patient's management *except*:

a. Screening upper gastrointestinal endoscopy

b. Screening of siblings

c. Genetic counseling

d. Treatment with sulindac and follow-up colonoscopy annually

e. Surgical consultation for proctocolectomy

29. A 50-year-old woman is undergoing a comprehensive health evaluation and she is interested in whether she needs colon cancer screening. For assessment of the patient's risk of colon cancer, it is appropriate to ask her about all the following *except*:

a. Family history of colon cancer

b. History of colon polyps

c. History of *H. pylori* infection

d. History of breast cancer

e. History of female genital cancer

30. A 46-year-old man presents with a 25-lb weight loss despite an excellent appetite. He also has noticed an increased number of greasy, foul-smelling bowel movements. Physical examination shows mild muscle wasting. Laboratory evaluation is notable for microcytic anemia, low ferritin value, twofold increase in the alkaline phosphatase value, and normal values for bilirubin, aspartate aminotransferase (AST), and alanine aminotransferase (ALT). Liver ultrasonography, colonoscopy, and three stools to test for occult blood have normal results. Which of the following would be the most appropriate next test?

a. Abdominal computed tomography

b. Repeat colonoscopy

c. Endoscopic retrograde cholangiopancreatography

d. Small-bowel biopsy

e. Liver biopsy

31. A 40-year-old man comes for evaluation of fatigue that has been present for 6 months. The past medical history is notable only for an episode of gonococcal urethritis 10 years previously. The results of physical examination are unremarkable. Laboratory findings are notable for a twofold increase in ALT. Serologic test results are positive for hepatitis B surface antigen (HBsAg), IgG antibody to hepatitis B core antigen, hepatitis B e antigen (HBeAg), and hepatitis B virus DNA (HBV DNA) and negative for IgM antibody to hepatitis B core antigen (IgM anti-HBc), antibody to hepatitis D virus, and antibody to hepatitis C virus (anti-HCV). Which one of the following is the most likely diagnosis?

a. Chronic hepatitis B

b. Acute nonfulminant hepatitis B

c. Acute fulminant hepatitis B

d. Chronic hepatitis C

e. Autoimmune hepatitis

32. A 23-year-old woman is brought by her boyfriend for evaluation because she has had jaundice for 2 weeks and somnolence for 24 hours. The boyfriend is known to be positive for HBsAg and HBeAg, and the couple became sexually

active 8 weeks previously. On examination, the woman is jaundiced and disoriented and has asterixis. Laboratory findings are notable for an ALT of 2,431 U/L, total bilirubin 12.5 mg/dL, conjugated bilirubin 7.4 mg/dL, and prothrombin time 2.4 international normalized ratio. Laboratory tests for which one of the following would confirm your diagnosis?

a. Anti-HBs
b. Anti-HCV
c. IgM anti-HBc
d. Anti-HBe
e. Antinuclear antibody

33. A 44-year-old man has had an abnormal level of ALT for 6 months. He used intravenous drugs 30 years ago. Examination is notable for splenomegaly and spider angiomata. Laboratory tests are notable for an ALT of 83 U/L, AST 62 U/L, platelets 66×10^9/L, albumin 3.2 g/dL, and prothrombin time 1.4 international normalized ratio. Anti-HCV is positive. Which one of the following statements is most correct?

a. A bone marrow biopsy should be performed because of the thrombocytopenia
b. The patient is at considerable risk for hepatocellular carcinoma, and screening is advised
c. Splenectomy should be performed to treat thrombocytopenia
d. Most patients infected with hepatitis C virus ultimately have clearing of the virus
e. The anti-HCV result is likely false-positive

34. A 76-year-old man has chronic hepatitis C. During the past 3 months he has noted progressive abdominal distention and peripheral edema. The examination is notable for spider angiomata, abdominal distention consistent with ascites, and peripheral edema. Paracentesis shows an ascitic fluid protein value of 0.9 g/dL and albumin 0.4 g/dL. The serum albumin value is 2.9 g/dL. Which one of the following would be the best next step?

a. Treatment with sodium restriction and diuretics
b. Transjugular intrahepatic portosystemic shunt
c. Peritoneovenous shunt
d. Echocardiography
e. Laparoscopy to exclude peritoneal carcinomatosis

35. A 43-year-old asymptomatic man has chronic hepatitis C. Combination therapy for 12 months with interferon and ribavirin failed to clear the virus. Laboratory results are notable for an ALT of 65 U/L and normal values for bilirubin, albumin, and prothrombin time. A liver biopsy specimen shows a mild lymphocytic portal infiltrate but no

fibrosis. Which of the following statements about this patient is true?

a. He should be given lamivudine
b. He should have screening for hepatocellular carcinoma with both ultrasonography and determination of alpha fetoprotein every 6 months
c. He should have endoscopy to determine whether esophageal varices are present
d. He should be referred for liver transplantation
e. He should receive the hepatitis A and B vaccines if he is not already immune

36. A 43-year-old woman complains of fatigue. Her past medical history is notable for hypothyroidism, and her only medication is thyroid hormone replacement. The physical examination results are unremarkable. Laboratory results are notable for an ALT of 423 U/L, AST 284 U/L, and gamma globulin 4.5 g/dL. Alkaline phosphatase and thyroid-stimulating hormone values are normal. At followup 3 months later, her symptoms and test results are unchanged. The test with the highest yield to determine the cause of the patient's abnormal liver enzyme values is which one of the following?

a. Urine screen for alcohol
b. Antimitochondrial antibody
c. Endoscopic retrograde cholangiography
d. Antinuclear antibody
e. IgM anti-hepatitis A virus

37. A 60-year-old woman with long-standing diabetes presents with an asymptomatic twofold increase in AST and ALT. Results of other liver tests are normal. The patient's only medications are insulin and transdermal estrogen. She denies alcohol intake or a family history of liver disease. Physical examination findings are notable for mild obesity and hepatomegaly. Ultrasonography shows gallstones and changes consistent with fatty infiltration of the liver. Which one of the following is true about the most likely cause of the increased liver test values?

a. Associated with hyperlipidemia
b. Liver biopsy will always exclude alcoholic liver disease
c. The condition progresses to cirrhosis in less than 1% of patients
d. Liver enzyme values will improve after cholecystectomy
e. The increases should resolve with discontinuation of transdermal estrogen

38. A 53-year-old man has cirrhosis due to alpha$_1$-antitrypsin deficiency. He is being managed with diuretics for ascites

but has had increasing abdominal distention. His wife now brings him for evaluation because of confusion and low-grade fever. On examination, he has a temperature of 38.7°C and is confused, although he is able to complain of mild abdominal pain. Laboratory results are notable for a platelet count of 46×10^9/L, leukocyte count of 14×10^9/L, hemoglobin 13.4 g/dL, and prothrombin time 1.6 international normalized ratio. Which one of the following would be the best next step?

a. Fresh frozen plasma, then paracentesis
b. Platelet transfusion, then paracentesis
c. Paracentesis
d. Esophagogastroduodenoscopy
e. Abdominal computed tomography

39. A patient comes to you because a friend told her she should have cholecystectomy. She is 44 years old and in good general health. For the past 7 months she has had epigastric burning that occurs nearly daily, particularly if she leans forward or lies down after a large meal. The symptoms improve with antacids. A flat plate obtained to follow kidney stones demonstrated gallbladder stones. Which one of the following statements is true?

a. Cholecystectomy is advised
b. Ursodiol will likely dissolve the stones
c. Abdominal computed tomography is advised
d. A trial of acid suppression is warranted
e. Endoscopic retrograde cholangiography should be performed

ANSWERS

1. Answer d.

This patient has progressive dysphagia with solids and chronic heartburn. The history suggests a mechanical narrowing or stricture that is most likely due to gastroesophageal reflux. The chronicity of symptoms suggests that Barrett esophagus may be a complication, and the presence of a stricture and an ulcer in the mid esophagus strongly suggests that Barrett esophagus is present. Esophageal rings occur in the distal esophagus and usually cause intermittent dysphagia or food bolus impaction. Motility disorders such as achalasia and diffuse esophageal spasm or nonspecific motility disorders usually present as intermittent dysphagia with solids and liquids, and upper gastrointestinal radiography does not show a stricture.

2. Answer c.

The history of intermittent dysphagia and a sudden food bolus impaction strongly suggest a lower esophageal ring. Intermittent dysphagia also may be caused by an esophageal web or a motility disorder. However, food bolus impactions that do not pass after drinking liquids are unusual in these conditions.

3. Answer c.

Intermittent dysphagia with solids which has progressed to dysphagia with both solids and liquids suggests a chronic motility disorder. The smooth, beaklike tapering on upper gastrointestinal radiography is classic for achalasia. Sometimes achalasia may not be appreciated on an endoscopic examination. A motility study would confirm the diagnosis.

4. Answer e.

This man presents with noncardiac chest pain. The most common cause of noncardiac chest pain is esophageal reflux; however, reflux has been ruled out by the normal results on endoscopy and biopsy of the lower esophagus. The second most likely cause of noncardiac chest pain is diffuse esophageal spasm, and that is the most likely diagnosis in this case. An esophageal motility study is indicated.

5. Answer a.

Cervical esophageal dysphagia associated with coughing, choking, or nasal regurgitation that occurs with the act of swallowing suggests oropharyngeal dysphagia. Oropharyngeal dysphagia may be caused by neurologic, muscular, or structural disorders of the swallowing mechanism. Myasthenia gravis, multiple sclerosis, and amyotrophic lateral sclerosis can cause oropharyngeal dysphagia. Structural causes include Zenker diverticulum, cervical lymphadenopathy, goiter, cricopharyngeal dysfunction, and cervical osteophytes. Achalasia is denervation of the lower esophageal sphincter, and this can cause dysphagia that is localized to the mid or lower part of the chest and is not associated with coughing, choking, or nasal regurgitation. Achalasia also does not cause cervical dysphagia or dysphagia related to the act of swallowing.

6. Answer c.

Odynophagia (pain on swallowing) is caused by inflammation, spasm, or distention of the esophagus. In an immunocompromised patient, odynophagia suggests the presence of infection with an opportunistic agent. *Candida*, herpes, and cytomegalovirus are common causes of odynophagia in immunodeficient patients. Bullous pemphigoid can cause odynophagia but does not occur in immunodeficient patients. Medication esophagitis is usually present in the elderly or in patients with esophageal motility disorders. The upper gastrointestinal endoscopy and biopsy findings are consistent with a viral infection. Thus, cytomegalovirus infection is the correct answer.

7. Answer d.

This patient presents with medication-induced esophagitis. Medications commonly associated with esophagitis include tetracycline, doxycycline, NSAIDs, quinidine, potassium supplements, ferrous sulfate, and ascorbic acid.

8. Answer e.

This man has two previously documented duodenal ulcers, is infected with *H. pylori*, and has never been treated with antibiotics and antisecretory agents. No further evaluation for *H. pylori* or active ulcer disease is necessary. This patient should be treated and followed to determine whether symptoms have resolved. A serum gastrin study should be done when hypersecretion is suspected, when peptic ulcer disease is not associated with *H. pylori* infection, or when NSAIDs, aspirin, or alcohol has been ingested. Treatment with antisecretory agents will relieve symptoms but will not prevent recurrence.

9. Answer e.

The history of a previously documented ulcer in a person who is not infected with *H. pylori* and not taking aspirin, alcohol, or NSAIDs should increase suspicion for a possible hypersecretory syndrome. The family history and increased serum calcium value also suggest hypersecretory syndrome due to multiple endocrine neoplasia. Given this unusual clinical scenario, Zollinger-Ellison syndrome is the most likely diagnosis.

10. Answer c.

The clinical conditions that predispose to squamous cell carcinoma of the esophagus include achalasia, lye stricture, Plummer-Vinson syndrome, human papillomavirus, smoking, alcohol ingestion, and a rare genetic condition called tylosis. Gastroesophageal reflux disease predisposes to Barrett esophagus and the development of adenocarcinoma of the esophagus.

11. Answer c.

This woman presents with acute diarrhea related to traveling to Mexico. The most likely cause of her diarrhea is infection with a toxigenic *Escherichia coli*. Fluoroquinolone antibiotics, with or without an antimotility agent, shorten the course of traveler's diarrhea due to toxigenic *E. coli*. Laboratory studies are not cost-effective unless the diarrhea is prolonged or associated with fever.

12. Answer d.

This woman's diarrhea stopped with fasting, suggesting that an osmotic mechanism caused her diarrhea. She has been dieting and ingesting both diet soft drinks and chewing gum that contain sorbitol. The most likely explanation for her symptoms is osmotic diarrhea related to sorbitol ingestion.

13. Answer b.

Chronic diarrhea is diarrhea that lasts longer than 1 month or diarrhea that recurs. Stool studies are the first step in the evaluation of chronic diarrhea. The history of traveling suggests the possibility of an infectious diarrhea. These symptoms would not be uncommon for giardiasis. It is appropriate to obtain a stool for culture and parasite study.

14. Answer c.

Meckel diverticulum is the most common cause of lower gastrointestinal tract bleeding in young adults. This is the third episode of bleeding for this young person, who has had negative results on intestinal evaluation previously. However, the studies that were performed would not find a Meckel diverticulum. A nuclear scan is indicated to rule out this diagnosis.

15. Answer e.

This man presents with edema, exertional dyspnea, and clinical evidence for bilateral pleural effusions. All the serum protein values are low, but there is no loss of protein into urine. These findings are consistent with a protein-losing enteropathy. A protein-losing enteropathy with lymphocytopenia strongly suggests the presence of intestinal lymphangiectasia.

16. Answer d.

This young woman has nausea, abdominal pain, and diarrhea that follow the ingestion of food. The history of previous allergies and the presence of eosinophilia suggest the possibility of eosinophilic gastroenteritis. Protozoa, such as *Entamoeba histolytica*, do not cause eosinophilia, and the results of stool cultures and parasite study are normal.

17. Answer d.

This young woman presents with malabsorption, iron deficiency anemia, and metabolic bowel disease. Malabsorption is usually due to a small intestinal or pancreatic cause. Iron and calcium are absorbed in the proximal small intestine, and this history suggests a disorder that occurs in the proximal small intestine (which is supplied by the celiac artery). These findings in combination with the presence of Howell-Jolly bodies in a patient who has not had a previous splenectomy strongly suggest celiac sprue as the cause of malabsorption.

18. Answer d.

The presence of malabsorption, central nervous system symptoms, arthritis, hyperpigmentation, and lymphadenopathy strongly suggests Whipple disease. The small-bowel biopsy findings confirm this diagnosis.

19. Answer d.

Systemic amyloidosis can involve any portion of the intestine. Amyloid is deposited in the blood vessels and mucous membranes of the intestine and can cause malabsorption, motility disorders, or ischemia with intestinal ulceration and bleeding. Clinical findings include macroglossia, hepatomegaly, cardiomegaly, peripheral neuropathy, and proteinuria. The diagnosis can be confirmed by fat aspirate study.

20. Answer d.

Acute diverticulitis is a clinical diagnosis that can be made in elderly patients who present with fever and pain and tenderness in the left lower quadrant of the abdomen with or without a palpable mass. This patient has marked fever and leukocytosis. The most appropriate course of action would be to rest the intestine and begin therapy with intravenous fluids and antibiotics. A surgical consultation should be obtained to help with the management of her illness and because she most likely will have recurrent diverticulitis and ultimately require surgical management.

21. Answer c.

The most likely explanation for recurrent red rectal bleeding in an older person who does not have diverticulitis is angiodysplasia of the colon. The best test to detect angiodysplasia is colonoscopy. Colonoscopy also offers therapeutic potential if the vascular malformations are localized and amenable to endoscopic coagulation.

22. Answer c.

This elderly woman with lower abdominal pain, bloody diarrhea, and "thumbprinting" of the colon at the splenic flexure has ischemic colitis. Chronic intestinal ischemia usually occurs in patients with pronounced arteriosclerotic vascular disease. Risk factors for the development of atherosclerosis are hypertension and diabetes mellitus. Diverticulosis occurs in elderly patients but does not increase the risk for ischemic colitis.

23. Answer c.

This patient presents with diarrhea, mild abdominal pain, and fever. After an illness that required antibiotics for management, there is no evidence of recurrent urinary tract infection, and proctoscopic examination is strongly suggestive of pseudomembranous colitis. Antibiotic-related pseudomembranous colitis is most often caused by *Clostridium difficile*, and the most sensitive test to document antibiotic-related pseudomembranous colitis is toxin assay of the stool.

24. Answer d.

Ischemia should be considered as a cause of abdominal pain when the pain begins suddenly and is followed by other symptoms of gastrointestinal dysfunction. Ischemia also should be considered in patients with underlying arteriosclerotic vascular disease. The sudden onset of abdominal pain in a patient who is in atrial fibrillation should raise the suspicion for an embolic event. The mild ileus and low increase in serum amylase concentration are not consistent with acute pancreatitis, acute hepatobiliary disease, or ileus. The most likely explanation for this patient's findings is acute mesenteric ischemia from an embolic event.

25. Answer d.

This patient presents with evidence for malabsorption, in that he has diarrhea with pale stools and weight loss. The presence of oil droplets implies that ingested fat in the form of triglycerides has not been broken down by pancreatic lipase and is strongly suggestive for pancreatic insufficiency caused by chronic pancreatitis. Gallstones rarely or never cause chronic pancreatitis but are a common cause of acute pancreatitis. This man, who admits drinking "socially," most likely has chronic pancreatitis, with pancreatic insufficiency caused by alcohol ingestion.

26. Answer e.

Painless jaundice with a palpable nontender gallbladder is the Courvoisier sign and strongly suggests the presence of pancreatic cancer. Acute cholecystitis, choledocholithiasis, and acute pancreatitis usually present with abdominal pain. It is unusual for chronic pancreatitis to present without abdominal pain, and it is also unusual for chronic pancreatitis to present with jaundice. Although chronic pancreatitis could explain these findings, pancreatic cancer more commonly presents with them.

27. Answer e.

The history of long-standing alternating diarrhea, constipation, and normal bowel movements suggests irritable bowel syndrome. In irritable bowel syndrome, there is usually no weight loss, no intestinal bleeding, and no symptoms to suggest other systemic disease. Always rule out lactase deficiency, and remember that irritable bowel syndrome is a diagnosis of exclusion, that is, the diagnosis is confirmed by an appropriate medical evaluation with negative results.

28. Answer d.

This patient has familial adenomatous polyposis, which is associated with a virtually 100% risk for colon cancer. The presence of dysplasia suggests that this patient is at high risk for malignancy. Total proctocolectomy should be performed. Familial adenomatous polyposis is an autosomal dominant condition, and thus siblings should be screened and the family should have genetic counseling. Because there is a small risk of coexistent polyps in the duodenum, upper gastrointestinal endoscopy should be performed. Although there are reports of sulindac retarding the growth of polyps, it would be inappropriate to use sulindac in this high-risk situation.

29. Answer c.

The high-risk conditions for colorectal cancer include a previous history of adenomas or carcinoma, familial adenomatous polyposis, history of colon cancer in a first-degree relative, women with breast or genital cancer, patients with ulcerative colitis for more than 7 years, and families with hereditary nonpolyposis cancer syndrome. Patients with all these high-risk conditions should have aggressive screening for colorectal cancer. *H. pylori* infection is not associated with a higher risk of colon cancer.

30. Answer d.

This man presents with weight loss, stool changes that suggest steatorrhea, iron deficiency without evidence of gastrointestinal blood loss, increase of the alkaline phosphatase value, and normal values for other liver enzymes. When evaluating "liver" enzyme increases, remember to first document that the enzyme increase is from the liver. In a patient with an abnormal alkaline phosphatase value and normal values for other liver enzymes, determination of alkaline phosphatase isoenzymes or γ-glutamyltransferase is advised. The clinical features of this patient suggest malabsorption due to small-bowel disease, and celiac sprue should be considered. A small-bowel biopsy should be performed, perhaps in conjunction with testing serum for antiendomysial or antigliadin antibodies. In this patient, sprue is associated with an increased value for bone alkaline phosphatase (due to osteomalacia associated with malabsorption), although occasionally sprue also can be associated with nonspecific liver enzyme abnormalities that improve with a gluten-free diet.

31. Answer a.

The chronic symptoms and mild nature of the increase in the ALT are consistent with chronic hepatitis. Common causes of chronic hepatitis are hepatitis B, hepatitis C, autoimmune hepatitis, nonalcoholic steatohepatitis, and alcoholic liver disease. The history of sexually transmitted disease puts the patient at risk for other sexually transmitted diseases, including hepatitis B, a diagnosis that is confirmed by the positive result for HBsAg. This patient also has markers of active viral replication (HBeAg and HBV DNA) and, thus, would be a possible treatment candidate. IgM anti-HBc would more likely be positive in *acute* hepatitis B. Patients with chronic hepatitis C nearly always are positive for anti-HCV, and autoimmune hepatitis typically presents with more prominent aminotransferase increases.

32. Answer c.

This patient presents with fulminant hepatic failure, defined as liver failure with encephalopathy developing less than 8 weeks after the onset of jaundice in a patient with no history of liver disease. Common causes are hepatitis A and B, drugs, Wilson disease, or toxins. Her boyfriend has hepatitis B and is highly infectious because of the presence of HBeAg. Patients with fulminant hepatitis B may present in the "window" period, after HBsAg has been cleared and before anti-HBs appears. Such patients will be positive for IgM anti-HBc. Anti-HBe becomes positive several months after the initial infection. Hepatitis C and autoimmune hepatitis are unusual causes of fulminant hepatic failure and would be unlikely in this patient.

33. Answer b.

This patient presents with a hepatitis C antibody and clinical findings of chronic liver disease with portal hypertension (spider angiomata and splenomegaly). He has a risk factor for hepatitis C. Therefore, it is extremely unlikely that the anti-HCV result is false-positive. Patients with hepatitis C and cirrhosis are at considerable risk for hepatocellular carcinoma, and screening is advised for patients who are candidates for treatment such as liver transplantation. Once a patient becomes chronically infected with hepatitis C virus, spontaneous clearance is rare. Splenomegaly with mild pancytopenia is common in patients with portal hypertension, and a bone marrow biopsy is not necessary. Splenectomy should be avoided in patients with cirrhosis and portal hypertension.

34. Answer a.

Ascites due to portal hypertension is characterized by a fluid protein value less than 2.5 g/dL and a serum ascites albumin gradient (calculated by subtracting the ascitic fluid albumin value from the serum albumin value) more than 1.1. Therefore, one can be confident that the ascites in this patient is due to portal hypertension, and treatment with sodium restriction and diuretics is advised. Only if this fails would a transjugular portosystemic shunt be considered. Peritoneovenous shunts are complicated by shunt dysfunction and disseminated intravascular coagulation and are used only as a last resort. Ascites due to heart failure and peritoneal carcinomatosis is characterized by a fluid protein value more than 2.5 g/dL.

35. Answer e.

In patients with chronic liver disease, severe liver failure may develop if they contract an acute viral hepatitis; therefore, they should be vaccinated against hepatitis A and B if they are not already immune. Patients with hepatitis C and cirrhosis are at considerable risk for hepatocellular carcinoma, and screening is advised. Endoscopy to search for varices (so that primary prophylaxis with β-adrenergic blockers can be considered) and early referral for liver transplantation would also be considered for patients with cirrhosis. The patient described in the question does not have cirrhosis, so none of these steps are indicated. Lamivudine is effective against hepatitis B but not against hepatitis C.

36. Answer d.

This patient presents with fatigue, chronic hepatitis with a 10-fold increase in ALT, and hypergammaglobulinemia. These findings are suggestive of autoimmune hepatitis, and most patients will be positive for antinuclear antibody. Many patients with autoimmune hepatitis will also have a history of other autoimmune disorders such as hypothyroidism. Alcoholic liver disease may present with chronic hepatitis, but the AST value is usually more than the ALT value and the enzyme levels are generally lower than those found in this patient. Antimitochondrial antibody testing would be useful to diagnose primary biliary cirrhosis, which would typically present with a cholestatic enzyme profile (i.e., increased alkaline phosphatase). Hepatitis A does not result in chronic liver disease. There is no indication for endoscopic retrograde cholangiography.

37. Answer a.

This patient likely has nonalcoholic steatohepatitis. Affected patients are characterized by increased values on liver tests (usually aminotransferases) and often have a predisposing factor such as obesity, diabetes, or hyperlipidemia. Mild hepatomegaly is also common. Liver biopsy demonstrates features of fatty infiltration with hepatocyte necrosis, which can mimic alcoholic steatohepatitis. About 10% to 20% of patients with nonalcoholic steatohepatitis have progression to cirrhosis. Cholecystectomy is advised only for symptomatic patients with gallstones. Estrogen replacement is rarely associated with cholestatic liver enzyme increases.

38. Answer c.

New-onset encephalopathy in a patient with cirrhosis should prompt a search for bleeding, infection, or electrolyte disturbances. Patients with ascites should undergo paracentesis to exclude spontaneous bacterial peritonitis. Diagnostic paracentesis is a safe procedure that can be performed even in a patient with coagulopathy and thrombocytopenia. Fluid should be sent for a cell count and differential, and blood culture bottles should be inoculated with fluid at the bedside. Spontaneous bacterial peritonitis is usually monomicrobial, although about 20% of cultures are negative because of a low inoculum of bacteria in the peritoneal fluid. The cell count will reveal an ascitic fluid polymorphonuclear leukocyte count of more than 250 cells/mL. Abdominal computed tomography would be necessary only if a secondary cause for peritonitis is being considered (such as a patient with polymicrobial peritonitis).

39. Answer d.

The patient described has the typical pain of gastroesophageal reflux and should respond to acid suppression. Gallstones cause disease by producing biliary pain, acute cholecystitis, or choledocholithiasis with cholangitis or pancreatitis. Biliary pain is hard, steady epigastric or right upper quadrant pain that usually lasts hours, often awakens the patient from sleep, and is associated with nausea. The pain may radiate into the right scapular area. Cholecystitis is accompanied by inflammation, abdominal tenderness, fever, and an increased leukocyte count in the blood. Most patients with gallbladder disease have gallstones demonstrated on ultrasonography, although "sludge" occasionally may cause disease and be evident only by microscopically examining a bile specimen obtained at the time of endoscopy. Acalculous cholecystitis usually occurs in sick patients hospitalized for other reasons. Asymptomatic gallstones should not be treated. Operation is the mainstay of treatment for gallstones, although small, *uncalcified* stones can be dissolved with 6 to 12 months of treatment with ursodeoxycholic acid (ursodiol).

CHAPTER 8

GENERAL INTERNAL MEDICINE

Scott C. Litin, MD

The goal of this chapter is to discuss important topics that have not been covered thoroughly in other chapters. The interpretation of diagnostic tests and results of therapy must be well understood by internists because these skills are used every day in practice. Frequently, internists are asked to make a preoperative risk assessment of a medical patient about to have a noncardiac operation. Managing patients who are receiving anticoagulants, assessing risk and treating patients who have hyperlipidemia, and managing other disorders frequently encountered in the office are also important. This chapter discusses these topics.

INTERPRETATION OF DIAGNOSTIC TESTS

Diagnostic tests are tools that either increase or decrease the likelihood of disease. When a diagnostic test is applied to a population at risk for a particular disease, patients in the studied population can be assigned to one of four groups on the basis of disease status and the test result. A table can be designed illustrating the concept (Table 8-1):

True-positive (TP) = disease present, abnormal test result
False-positive (FP) = disease absent, abnormal test result
False-negative (FN) = disease present, normal test result
True-negative (TN) = disease absent, normal test result

By convention, the four possible groups are assigned the shorthand letters "a," "b," "c," and "d" (Table 8-2). On the basis of this table (called a "2 × 2 table"), the following test

Table 8-1   2 × 2 Table

		Disease	
		Present	Absent
Test	Positive	True-positive (TP)	False-positive (FP)
	Negative	False-negative (FN)	True-negative (TN)

characteristics can be defined:

1. Sensitivity

    Positive (test) in disease (PID)

    True positivity rate—proportion of patients with the disease who have a positive test result

    $$\text{Sensitivity: } \frac{TP}{TP + FN}$$

    The 2 × 2 table definition: a/(a + c)

    Rules to remember:

    "SN out"—if a test has 100% sensitivity, a negative test rules **out** the disorder

    Screening tests attempt to maximize sensitivity to avoid missing a person who has the disease

    Characteristic of test—not affected by the prevalence of disease in the population

2. Specificity

    Negative (test) in health (NIH)

    True negativity rate—proportion of patients without the disease who have a negative test result

    $$\text{Specificity: } \frac{TN}{TN + FP}$$

    The 2 × 2 table definition: d/(b + d)

    Rules to remember:

    "SP in"—if a test has 100% specificity, a positive test rules **in** the disorder

    Confirmatory tests used in follow-up of screening try to maximize specificity to avoid incorrectly labeling a healthy person as having disease

    Characteristic of test—not affected by the prevalence of disease in the population

3. Positive predictive value

    When a patient's illness is evaluated by interpreting a diagnostic test, the 2 × 2 table is read horizontally, not vertically. Thus, in judging the value of a diagnostic test, it is not essential to know its sensitivity and specificity. One really wants to

Table 8-2 2×2 Table

		Target disorder		
		Present	Absent	
Diagnostic test result	Positive	TP a	FP b	a+b
	Negative	c FN	d TN	c+d
		a+c	b+d	a+b+c+d

Prevalence = (a+c)/(a+b+c+d)

Test characteristics

    Sensitivity = a/(a+c)

    Specificity = d/(b+d)

Frequency-dependent properties

    PPV = a/(a+b)

    NPV = d/(c+d)

know whether a patient with positive test results actually has the disease, that is, how well the test results predict a disease compared with the reference standard for that disease. Thus, the horizontal properties of the diagnostic test are of primary interest. Among all patients with a positive diagnostic test result (TP + FP), in what proportion, $\frac{TP}{TP+FP}$, has the diagnosis been predicted correctly or ruled in? This proportion is the positive predictive value (PPV).

- PPV is the proportion of patients who have the disease among all the patients who test positive for the disease.
- This provides information most useful in clinical practice.
- PPV is affected by the prevalence of the disease in the population.
- The 2×2 table definition: PPV $= \frac{TP}{TP+FP} = a/(a + b)$.

4. Negative predictive value

It is also important to know the percentage of patients with a negative test result (FN + TN) who actually do not have the disease. This proportion, $\frac{TN}{FN+TN}$, is the negative predictive value (NPV).

- NPV is the proportion of patients who do not have the disease of interest among all the patients who test negative for the disease.
- NPV is affected by the prevalence of disease in the population.
- The 2×2 table definition, NPV $= \frac{TN}{FN+TN} = d/(c + d)$.

5. Prevalence

Prevalence is defined as the proportion of persons with the disease in the population to whom the test has been applied. In the 2×2 table, prevalence is written

$$\frac{TP + FN}{TP + FP + FN + TN} = \frac{a + c}{a + b + c + d}$$

How to Construct a 2×2 Table

The sensitivity, specificity, and predictive values of normal and abnormal test results can be calculated with even a limited amount of information. For example, assume that a new diagnostic test is positive in 90% of patients who have the disease and is negative in 95% of patients who are disease-free. The prevalence of the disease in the population to which the test is applied is 10%. This provides the following information:

    Sensitivity = 90%

    Specificity = 95%

    Prevalence = 10%

This test is now ready to be applied to a group of patients by filling in a 2×2 table (Table 8-3). The calculation is often made easier if the test is applied to a large number of patients, for example, 1,000, so a + b + c + d = 1,000.

Because the prevalence of the disease is 10%, 100 patients have the disease ($0.1 \times 1,000 = 100$, or a + c = 100). Of the patients, 90%, or 900, are disease-free ($0.9 \times 1,000 = 900$, or b + d = 900).

Because the sensitivity of the test is 90%, 90% of the 100 patients with disease have a positive test result ($a = 0.9 \times 100 = 90$) and 10% have a negative result ($c = 0.1 \times 100 = 10$).

Specificity of 95% means that 95% of the 900 patients who are disease-free have a negative test result ($d = 0.95 \times 900 = 855$) and 5% have a positive test result ($b = 0.05 \times 900 = 45$).

The 2×2 table (Table 8-3) shows that 135 patients (a + b) have a positive test result; however, only 90 of these 135 patients actually have the disease. Therefore, the PPV of a positive test is $\frac{a}{a+b} = \frac{90}{135} = 66.7\%$, that is, only two-thirds of all patients with a positive test result will actually have the disease. Similarly, one can determine that 865 patients (c + d) have a negative test result: 855 of these 865 patients are disease-free. Therefore, the NPV of the test is $\frac{d}{c+d} = \frac{855}{865} = 98.8\%$.

Clinicians should be able to perform these simple calculations. Clinical decision making by internists is more likely to depend on the PPV and NPV of test results for a given population than on the sensitivity or specificity of the test.

For example, if the prevalence of the disease in the clinician's population is 2% instead of 10%, the PPV and NPV can be recalculated. The PPV of abnormal test results falls to 26.9%, quite different from the 66.7% above, although the sensitivity and specificity of the test (90% and 95%, respectively) have not changed (Table 8-4).

- An important factor in interpreting a patient's test result is knowledge of the prevalence of the disease in the population being tested.

Table 8-3 2 × 2 Table for Test With 90% Sensitivity, 95% Specificity, and 10% Prevalence

		Disease present	Disease absent	
Diagnostic test result	Positive	90 \ a	45 \ b	135 \ a+b
	Negative	c	d	c+d
		10	855	865
		a+c	b+d	a+b+c+d
Total		100	900	1,000

Prevalence = (a+c)/(a+b+c+d) = 100/1,000 = 10%
Test characteristics
  Sensitivity = a/(a+c) = 90/100 = 90%
  Specificity = d/(b+d) = 855/900 = 95%
Frequency-dependent properties
  PPV = a/(a+b) = 90/135 = 66.7%
  NPV = d/(c+d) = 855/865 = 98.8%
Likelihood ratio (LR) for a positive test result:
  LR+ = Sensitivity/(1 − Specificity) = 90%/5% = 18
Likelihood ratio for a negative test result:
  LR− = (1 − Sensitivity)/Specificity = 10%/95% = 0.11
Pretest Odds = Prevalence/(1 − Prevalence) = 10%/90% = 0.11
Posttest Odds = Pretest Odds × Likelihood Ratio
Posttest Probability = Posttest Odds/(Posttest Odds + 1)

Table 8-4 2 × 2 Table for Test With 90% Sensitivity, 95% Specificity, and 2% Prevalence

		Disease present	Disease absent	
Test result	Positive	18 \ a	49 \ b	67 \ a+b
	Negative	c	d	c+d
		2	931	933
		a+c	b+d	a+b+c+d
Total		20	980	1,000

Prevalence = (a+c)/(a+b+c+d) = 20/1,000 = 2%
Test characteristics
  Sensitivity = a/(a+c) = 18/20 = 90%
  Specificity = d/(b+d) = 931/980 = 95%
Frequency-dependent properties
  PPV = a/(a+b) = 18/67 = 26.9%
  NPV = d/(c+d) = 931/933 = 99.8%

- High-risk populations (high prevalence of disease) tend to improve the PPV of an abnormal test result.
- Low-risk populations (screening tests) make the NPV of a normal test result look impressive.

Use of Odds and Likelihood Ratios

Some physicians prefer interpreting diagnostic test results by using the likelihood ratio. This ratio takes properties of a diagnostic test (sensitivity and specificity) and makes them more helpful in clinical decision making. It helps the clinician determine the probability of disease in a specific patient after a diagnostic test has been performed.

The formula for a likelihood ratio for a positive test result (LR+) is

- $LR+ = \dfrac{+\text{Test in Disease}}{+\text{Test in No Disease}} = \dfrac{\text{Sensitivity}}{1 - \text{Specificity}}$

The formula for a likelihood ratio for a negative test result (LR−) is

- $LR- = \dfrac{-\text{Test in Disease}}{-\text{Test in No Disease}} = \dfrac{1 - \text{Sensitivity}}{\text{Specificity}}$

For example, if test A has a sensitivity of 95% and a specificity of 90%

$$LR+ = \frac{\text{Sensitivity}}{1 - \text{Specificity}} = 95/10 = 9.5$$

$$LR- = \frac{1 - \text{Sensitivity}}{\text{Specificity}} = \frac{5}{90} = 0.06$$

However, if test B has a sensitivity of 20% and a specificity of 80%, then

$$LR+ = \frac{\text{Sensitivity}}{1 - \text{Specificity}} = \frac{20}{20} = 1$$

$$LR- = \frac{-\text{Sensitivity}}{\text{Specificity}} = \frac{80}{80} = 1$$

As a general rule, diagnostic tests with an LR+ greater than 10 or an LR− less than 0.1 have a greater influence on the posttest probability of disease (i.e., are better tests) than diagnostic tests with likelihood ratios between 10 and 0.1. In the two examples above, test A is more likely to rule in or rule out disease than test B.

Sample likelihood ratios are provided in the example below and in Table 8-5.

Example

A 40-year-old white man is admitted to the hospital for pneumonia. He admits to consuming 2 six-packs of beer each week. On the basis of this history and your clinical judgment, you assume that he has a pretest probability of 20% for a diagnosis of alcoholism. You perform the CAGE questionnaire and his responses are positive for all four questions. You notice that the LR+ for three or more CAGE questions is 250.

Table 8-5 Examples of Symptoms, Signs, and Tests and the Likelihood Ratio (LR)

Target disorder	Symptom, sign, test		Patient population	Health care setting	LR
Alcohol abuse or dependency	Yes to ≥3 questions on CAGE		Patients admitted to orthopedic or medical services over a 6-month period	Teaching hospital in U.S.	250
Sinusitis (by further investigation)	Maxillary toothache or purulent nasal secretion or poor response to nasal decongestants or abnormal trans-illumination or history of colored nasal discharge	4+ signs or symptoms	Patients with nasal complaints	Teaching hospital in U.S.	6.4
		3 signs or symptoms			2.6
		2 signs or symptoms			1.1
		1 sign or symptom			0.5
		None			0.1
Ascites	Presence of fluid wave (done by internal medicine residents)		Male veteran patients	Veterans' hospital in U.S.	9.6

Data from Bush B, Shaw S, Cleary P, et al: Screening for alcohol abuse using the CAGE questionnaire. Am J Med 1987;82:231-235; Williams JW Jr, Simel DL: Does this patient have sinusitis? Diagnosing acute sinusitis by history and physical examination. JAMA 1993;270:1242-1246; Williams JW Jr, Simel DL, Roberts L, et al: Clinical evaluation for sinusitis. Making the diagnosis by history and physical examination. Ann Intern Med 1992;117:705-710; Williams JW Jr, Simel DL: Does this patient have ascites? How to divine fluid in the abdomen. JAMA 1992;267:2645-2648; Simel DL, Halvorsen RA Jr, Feussner JR: Quantitating bedside diagnosis: clinical evaluation of ascites. J Gen Intern Med 1988;3:423-428.

At this point, you have two choices. The first is to use a nomogram (Fig. 8-1) and take a straightedge and connect the pretest probability of 20% and the LR+ of 250 to the posttest probability. This shows that the posttest probability for a diagnosis of alcoholism is 99%.

The second option should be used when there is no nomogram for performing this simple calculation. Without a nomogram, the following must be done: 1) convert the pretest probability to pretest odds, 2) multiply the pretest odds by the likelihood ratio to obtain the posttest odds, and 3) convert the posttest odds to posttest probability.

Probability and odds can be converted somewhat interchangeably with the following formulas:

$$\text{Odds} = \frac{\text{Probability}}{1 - \text{Probability}}$$

$$\text{Probability} = \frac{\text{Odds}}{1 + \text{Odds}}$$

In the example, step 1 involves converting pretest probability to pretest odds. In this case, you estimated that the pretest probability of alcoholism is 20%. With the formulas above, pretest odds $= \frac{0.20}{1 - 0.20} = 0.25$. Therefore, the pretest odds of having the condition are 0.25. Step 2 involves determining the posttest odds for a positive test. This can be determined by multiplying the pretest odds (0.25) by the LR+ for 3 or more positive questions on the CAGE questionnaire (250): $0.25 \times 250 = 62.5$. Step 3 allows conversion of posttest odds to posttest probability by placing the numbers in the formula:

$$\text{Probability} = \frac{\text{Odds}}{1 + \text{Odds}}$$

$$\text{Posttest Probability} = \frac{62.5}{63.5} = 98.4\%$$

In conclusion, the posttest probability for the diagnosis of alcoholism for this patient is 98.4%, which is close to the value obtained from the nomogram.

Interpretation of Therapeutic Results

Physicians often make treatment decisions on the basis of the results of randomized controlled trials (RCTs). To understand if the results of such trials are impressive, the physician is required to translate these results into language understandable to both physicians and patients. This terminology can also be used to compare various therapies for the disease of

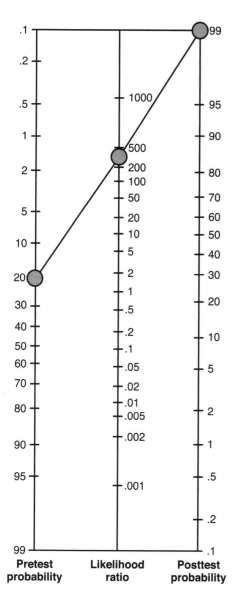

Fig. 8-1. Nomogram.

referred to as the "experimental event rate" (EER), because they received a particular therapy.

The traditional measure often used to report the difference between the treated and untreated groups is the "relative risk reduction" (RRR), which is calculated as $\frac{CER - EER}{CER}$. This measure relates the reduction in risk for the outcome event with the intervention compared with the baseline risk rate (CER). In this example, the RRR is $\frac{5\% - 2\%}{5\%} = 60\%$. Therefore, anticoagulant therapy reduced the yearly risk of developing stroke in patients with atrial fibrillation by 60% compared with the baseline risk of developing a stroke with no therapy. However, the RRR often is not clinically helpful because the number itself does not provide information about the baseline risk rate (i.e., CER). For example, even if only a very small number of control patients (0.005%) and patients receiving anticoagulation (0.002%) experience stroke, the RRR is unchanged, $\frac{0.005\% - 0.002\%}{0.005\%} = 60\%$. Therefore, the RRR often is not useful to the clinician or patient, although a large RRR can be used to make a dramatic endorsement for therapy by proponents of that therapy.

- RRR = $\frac{CER - EER}{CER}$
- Often RRR is not clinically useful because it does not provide information about the baseline risk rate.

Absolute Risk Reduction

In the example above, it would be very useful for the physician and patient to know the absolute difference in rates of stroke between the control group and the atrial fibrillation group given anticoagulants (CER – EER). This measure is called the "absolute risk reduction" (ARR). In the combined Stroke Prevention in Atrial Fibrillation (SPAF) trials, the ARR or (CER – EER) = (5% – 2%) = 3% per year.

- ARR = (CER – EER)
- ARR is clinically more useful to interpret therapeutic results.

Number Needed to Treat

The physician and patient often want to know the number of patients needed to be treated (NNT) with a therapy to prevent one additional bad outcome. That number can be calculated with $\frac{1}{ARR}$. Therefore, the NNT to prevent one stroke by using the adjusted dose of warfarin in patients with atrial fibrillation would be $\frac{1}{3\%} = \frac{1}{0.03} = 33$. Therefore, the NNT would be 33 patients; that is, 33 patients would need to be treated with warfarin (INR 2.0-3.0) for 1 year to prevent one additional stroke.

- NNT identifies the number of patients who need to be treated with a therapy to prevent one additional bad outcome.
- NNT = $\frac{1}{ARR}$

interest. Sackett and others have coined terms and derived useful equations to help physicians make sense of RCTs concerned with therapy.

Relative Risk Reduction

The results of RCTs of anticoagulant therapy to prevent stroke in patients with atrial fibrillation have been published and summarized. In primary prevention studies, the average 1-year risk for stroke in the placebo group was 5% per year. Because no therapy was administered to that group, this can be called the "control event rate" (CER). In these studies of patients with atrial fibrillation treated with adjusted-dose warfarin (international normalized ratio [INR] 2.0-3.0), the approximate stroke risk was reduced to 2% per year. This can be

Number Needed to Harm

Conversely, if the rate of adverse events caused by the experimental therapy is known and compared with the rate of adverse events in the placebo group, the number needed to harm (NNH) can be calculated. This useful number tells the physician how many treated patients it takes to produce one additional harmful event. In the studies dealing with stroke prevention in atrial fibrillation, the average risk of intracranial hemorrhage for the group given warfarin was 0.3% per year, compared with 0.1% per year for the placebo group. Therefore, the NNH can be calculated by taking the reciprocal of the absolute risk increase (ARI). The ARI can be calculated by subtracting the harm CER from the harm EER or, in this case, $0.3\% - 0.1\% = 0.2\%$. In this example, the NNH is $\frac{1}{0.2\%} = \frac{1}{0.002} = 500$. Therefore, 500 patients would need to be treated with anticoagulant for 1 year to cause one additional intracranial hemorrhage, compared with the control group.

- NNH identifies how many treated patients are needed to produce one additional harmful event.
- $NNH = \frac{1}{\text{Harm EER} - \text{Harm CER}}$

PREOPERATIVE MEDICAL EVALUATION

The Art of Medical Consultation

Recommendations have been made to guide internists in advising surgeons on assessing preoperative risk and managing perioperative problems (J Gen Intern Med 2:257-269, 1987). The following guidelines will help internists to optimize compliance with the advice they give:

1. Limit the number of recommendations to five or fewer.
2. Focus on crucial recommendations and avoid diluting the management plan with trivial suggestions.
3. Be specific, especially about drug dosages. Recommend not only which drug to use but also specify the dose and frequency of administration.
4. Advice about therapy (i.e., initiating or discontinuing drug therapy) is heeded more often than diagnostic suggestions (i.e., ordering tests).
5. Labor-intensive advice that requires the surgeon to do something (look at a blood smear, perform a procedure) is poorly heeded. If such tasks must be performed, the medical consultant should do them personally.
6. Oral communication with a surgeon usually enhances compliance.
7. Follow-up visits and notes further improve compliance.

Successfully communicating one's assessment and plan is an art. A three-step approach of "diagnosis–treatment–prognosis" is often helpful.

1. Diagnosis—the internist creates a problem list that is a table of contents for anyone involved in the care of the patient. It is particularly useful to anesthesiologists and surgeons.
2. Treatment—the internist offers recommendations that will diminish the surgical risks associated with the patient's problem. The emphasis is on therapeutics aimed only at diminishing surgical risk.
3. Prognosis—the internist states the surgical and anesthetic risk for each problem (often available in published literature). When this information is lacking, the internist has to substitute personal judgment.
4. The internist should comment on the cumulative risk for a patient with multiple medical problems, such as cardiac, pulmonary, and liver disease. The risk in such patients may become prohibitive.

- Diagnosis—a problem list.
- Treatment—recommendations only for decreasing surgical risk.
- Prognosis—surgical and anesthetic risk for each problem.
- The internist should comment on the cumulative risk for a patient with multiple medical problems.

Risks of Anesthesia and the Operation

Operative deaths are uncommon because of the many technical advances that have been made in surgery and anesthesia and the assessment of the risk. The risk of dying during the perioperative period (i.e., intraoperatively or within 48 hours postoperatively) is about 0.3% when all operations are considered. For major surgical procedures, the mortality risk is less than 1% for patients younger than 65 years but increases to about 5% for those between 65 and 80 years. Deaths occur during three time periods: anesthetic induction (10%), intraoperatively (35%), and during the first 48 hours postoperatively (55%). Postoperative mortality between 48 hours and 6 weeks is usually due to pneumonia, sepsis, cardiac arrest, pulmonary embolus, or renal failure. The American Society of Anesthesiologists (ASA) has published a classification scheme to aid clinicians (Table 8-6). This classification is subjective, and many physicians favor a systematic assessment instead of a global impression. However, ASA class IV and V patients have roughly 100 times the mortality of class I patients for a surgical procedure. In addition, an emergency procedure almost doubles the risk in any ASA classification of patients.

- The risk of dying during the perioperative period is 0.3% for all operations.
- Three periods during which deaths occur: anesthetic induction (10%), intraoperatively (35%), and within 48 hours postoperatively (55%).

Table 8-6 American Society of Anesthesiologists Classification of Anesthetic Mortality Within 48 Hours Postoperatively

Class	Physical status	48-Hour mortality
I	Normal healthy person <80 years old	0.07%
II	Mild systemic disease	0.24%
III	Severe but not incapacitating systemic disease	1.4%
IV	Incapacitating systemic disease that is a constant threat to life	7.5%
V	Moribund patient not expected to survive 24 hours, regardless of surgery	8.1%
E	Suffix added to any class indicating emergency procedure, e.g., IE, IIE, IIIE	Doubles risk

From MKSAP IX: Part C, Book 4, 1991. American College of Physicians. By permission.

Many physicians have mistakenly assumed that spinal anesthesia is safer than general anesthesia for high-risk patients. From a cardiopulmonary standpoint, this is not the case. Spinal anesthesia may be associated with wide fluctuations in blood pressure, anxiety, and less control of the airway and ventilation. Thus, it is inappropriate for the internist to write, "Patient too ill for general anesthesia; okay if done under spinal." The final decision about the type of anesthesia is ultimately the responsibility of the anesthesiologist.

- From a cardiopulmonary point of view, spinal anesthesia is not safer than general anesthesia.
- Spinal anesthesia may be associated with wide fluctuations in blood pressure.
- The final decision about the type of anesthesia is the responsibility of the anesthesiologist.

The type of operation performed is an important determinant of cardiovascular morbidity and mortality (Table 8-7).

However, the importance of associated disease in determining surgical risk may outweigh the nature of the procedure or the type of anesthesia used in predicting outcome. The following sections discuss risk assessment and management strategies grouped by organ system.

Pulmonary Risks and Management

Pulmonary complications (hypoventilation, atelectasis, and pneumonia) develop in about one-third of patients postoperatively and account for 50% of overall perioperative mortality. Patients with probable increased risk include those older than 70 whose duration of anesthesia is longer than 2 hours or who currently have a respiratory infection.

- Pulmonary complications account for 50% of overall perioperative mortality.

- Patients at definite risk for pulmonary complications include smokers and those who have chronic obstructive pulmonary disease, obesity, thoracic surgery, or upper abdominal surgery.
- Age older than 70 and anesthesia lasting longer than 2 hours are risk factors.

Preoperative pulmonary function testing should be part of the evaluation of high-risk patients. The interpretation of these tests regarding risk assessment is controversial. However, most authors agree that the simple spirometric measurement of forced expiratory volume in 1 second (FEV_1) is probably as good a predictor as any of surgical risk.

- FEV_1 is a good predictor of surgical risk.
- FEV_1 >2 L, patient can safely undergo procedure.
- FEV_1 <1 L, high risk of postoperative pulmonary complication.

Several measures have been advocated for decreasing pulmonary risks.

- Preoperative measures include instruction in respiratory maneuvers, cessation of smoking, use of bronchodilators, antibiotic treatment of chronic bronchitis, and chest physiotherapy.
- Postoperative measures include chest physiotherapy and inspiratory maneuvers, minimization of postoperative narcotic analgesia, and early mobilization of elderly patients.

Cardiac Risks and Management

Annually, of every 10 U.S. citizens, about 1 undergoes a noncardiac operation. Because of the increasing prevalence of surgical procedures in the elderly, about one-third of all noncardiac surgical patients are at risk for cardiac morbidity or mortality after taking into account the prevalence of coronary

Table 8-7 Cardiac Risk* Stratification for Noncardiac Surgical Procedures

Risk	Procedure
High	
Reported cardiac risk often >5%	Emergent major operations, particularly in the elderly
	Aortic and other major vascular procedures
	Peripheral vascular procedures
	Anticipated prolonged surgical procedures associated with large fluid shifts and/or blood loss
Intermediate	
Reported cardiac risk generally <5%	Carotid endarterectomy
	Head and neck operations
	Intraperitoneal and intrathoracic procedures
	Orthopedic procedures
	Prostate operations
Low†	
Reported cardiac risk generally <1%	Endoscopic procedures
	Superficial procedure
	Cataract extraction
	Breast operation

*Combined incidence of cardiac death and nonfatal myocardial infarction.

†Do not generally require further preoperative cardiac testing.

From Report of the American College of Cardiology/American Heart Association Task Force on Practice Guidelines (Committee to Update the 1996 Guidelines on Perioperative Cardiovascular Evaluation for Noncardiac Surgery): Guidelines on perioperative cardiovascular evaluation for noncardiac surgery. Circulation 2002;105:1257-1267. By permission of American College of Cardiology.

artery disease or the high-risk status in this population. Patients with known or suspected cardiac disease commonly are referred for assessment before a noncardiac procedure is performed. Important questions are posed during these consultations:

1. How can a high-risk patient be identified?
2. What selective testing needs to be performed (if any) to further define risk?
3. What intervention or perioperative management is appropriate to decrease cardiac-related morbidity and mortality during noncardiac surgical procedures?

In an attempt to allow clinicians to estimate cardiac risk after clinical assessment, a risk factor index, the Goldman index, was devised through a prospective analysis of patients older than 40 who were undergoing noncardiac general surgery (N Engl J Med 297:845-850, 1977). This scale has been validated prospectively and has formed the framework of preoperative cardiac evaluation (Tables 8-8 and 8-9).

In addition, the American College of Cardiology/American Heart Association (ACC/AHA) Task Force has published updated guidelines to instruct physicians in the perioperative cardiovascular evaluation of patients for noncardiac surgical procedures (Circulation 105:1257-1267, 2002). These guidelines go beyond the Goldman index in presenting the framework for determining which patients are candidates for cardiac testing. The physician must consider several interacting variables and assess appropriate weight. Because no adequately controlled or randomized clinical trials have defined this process, a collection of outcome data and expert opinion is the basis of the algorithmic approach shown in Figure 8-2.

● Information needed to determine appropriate preoperative cardiac assessment: the risk of the surgical procedure, clinical predictors, and functional status of the patient.

Myocardial infarction (MI) is the most feared perioperative complication. Of perioperative MIs, 50% are fatal and 60% are not accompanied by anginal pain. The risk of perioperative MI peaks 24 to 48 hours postoperatively. Patients who have had an MI recently are at greatest risk for perioperative MIs. The risk of perioperative MI without cardiac disease is 0.2%. In retrospective studies, the risk of perioperative MI in patients with a recent MI (<3 months) is 27%; if the MI occurred 3 to 6 months earlier, 11%; and if the MI was more than 6 months earlier, 5%. With hemodynamic catheters and

Table 8-8 The Goldman Cardiac Risk Index for Noncardiac Surgery

Clinical variable	Point assessment
History	
Age >70 y	5
Recent myocardial infarction (≤6 mo)	10
Physical examination	
Ventricular gallop or jugular venous pressure ≥12 cm H_2O	11
Important valvular aortic stenosis	3
Electrocardiogram	
Rhythm other than sinus or atrial ectopy on preoperative tracing	7
More than 5/min ectopic ventricular beats on any tracing preoperatively	7
Poor general medical condition (any of the following)	
Po_2 <60 mm Hg or Pco_2 >50 mm Hg	
Serum potassium <3.0 mEq/L or bicarbonate <20 mEq/L	
Blood urea nitrogen >50 mg/dL or creatinine >3.0 mg/dL	3
Chronic liver disease	
Noncardiac debilitation	
Surgical procedure	
Intraperitoneal, intrathoracic, aortic	3
Emergency	4
Maximum score	53

Modified from Goldman L, Caldera DL, Nussman SR, et al: Multifactorial index of cardiac risk in noncardiac surgical procedures. N Engl J Med 1977;297:845-850. By permission of the Massachusetts Medical Society.

Table 8-9 Cardiac Complications Stratified by the Goldman Risk Index

Risk index class	Point score	No or minimal complications, %	Severe complications, %	Cardiac death, %
I	0-5	99	0.6	0.2
II	6-12	96	3	1
III	13-25	86	11	3
IV	≥26	49	12	39

Modified from Goldman L, Caldera DL, Nussman SR, et al: Multifactorial index of cardiac risk in noncardiac surgical procedures. N Engl J Med 1977;297:845-850. By permission of the Massachusetts Medical Society.

aggressive intensive care management, the perioperative MI rate for patients with a recent MI can be markedly decreased (MI <3 months = 5.7%; MI 4-6 months = 2.3%). Traditional teaching has recommended that nonemergent surgery be delayed for at least 6 months after an MI. However, it has become possible to risk-stratify MI patients during convalescence (Fig. 8-2). If a recent stress test has shown no residual myocardium at risk, the likelihood of reinfarction after noncardiac surgery would be low. Thus, it may be possible to perform surgery in selected MI patients 4 to 6 weeks after the infarction.

- Of perioperative MIs, 50% are fatal and 60% are silent.
- The risk of perioperative MI peaks 24-48 hours postoperatively.
- Patients with a recent MI are at greatest risk for perioperative MI.
- Standard recommendation—delay nonemergent surgery for at least 6 months after MI.
- If a stress test has shown no residual myocardium at risk, the likelihood of reinfarction is low and the patient could be considered for elective surgery 4-6 weeks after the infarction.

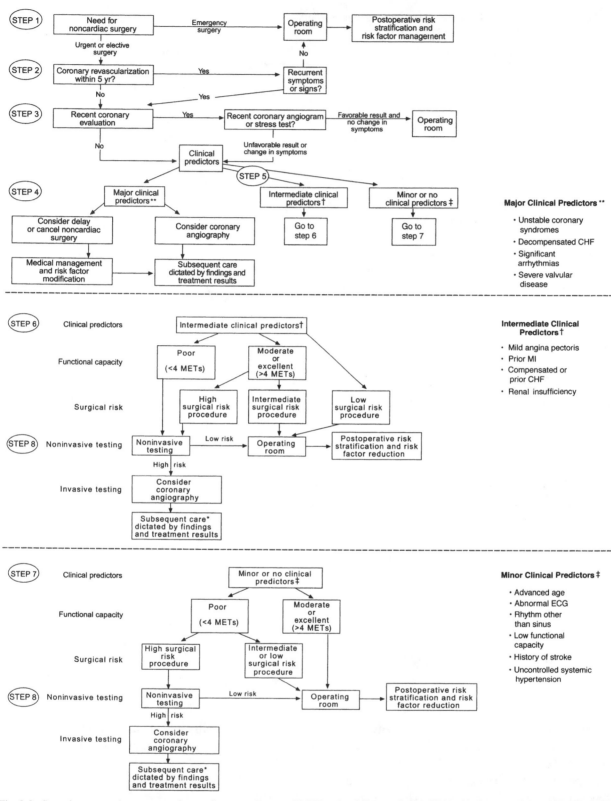

Fig. 8-2. Stepwise approach to preoperative cardiac assessment. >4 METs: the ability to climb a flight of stairs or walk up a hill. The ability to walk on level ground at 4 miles/h or run a short distance. The ability to do heavy housework, e.g., scrubbing floors or lifting or moving heavy furniture. High-, intermediate-, and low-risk surgical procedures are defined in Table 8-7. *Subsequent care may include cancellation or delay of surgery, coronary revascularization followed by noncardiac surgery, or intensified care. CHF, congestive heart failure; ECG, electrocardiogram; METs, metabolic equivalents; MI, myocardial infarction. (From Report of the American College of Cardiology/American Heart Association Task Force on Practice Guidelines [Committee on Perioperative Cardiovascular Evaluation for Noncardiac Surgery]: Guidelines for perioperative cardiovascular evaluation for noncardiac surgery. J Am Coll Cardiol 1996;27:910-948. By permission of American College of Cardiology.)

Perioperative Medical Therapy

Studies suggest that appropriately administered β-blockers reduce perioperative ischemia and may reduce cardiac events in high-risk patients. Ideally, treatment with β-blockers should be started a few days before elective surgery, with the dose titrated to achieve a resting heart rate between 50 and 60 beats/minute. β-Blocker therapy required in the recent past to control symptoms of angina, symptomatic arrhythmias, or hypertension should be restarted or continued. Treatment with β-blockers should be instituted preoperatively in appropriate candidates with untreated hypertension or known coronary artery disease (CAD) or those at major risk for CAD.

- β-Blocker therapy required in the recent past to control symptoms of angina, symptomatic arrhythmias, or hypertension should be restarted or continued.
- β-Blockers should be started preoperatively in appropriate candidates with untreated hypertension or known CAD or those at major risk for CAD.

Monitoring for Perioperative Myocardial Ischemia

In high-risk patients undergoing noncardiac operations, early postoperative myocardial ischemia is an important correlate of adverse cardiac outcomes. Subgroups of patients who are at high risk for postoperative ischemia and who might benefit most from intensive Holter monitoring in the postoperative period can be identified preoperatively: left ventricular hypertrophy, CAD, diabetes mellitus, hypertension, and digoxin therapy. By identifying high-risk patients and monitoring them postoperatively with real-time monitors with alarms triggered by ST-segment depression, ischemia theoretically could be identified instantaneously so that rapid intervention could potentially prevent clinical ischemia. However, this hypothesis has not been studied and has not been proved. These interventions, if performed in all at-risk patients, would drive up costs tremendously. For patients at increased risk for perioperative myocardial ischemia, the ACC/AHA guidelines recommend electrocardiography (ECG) preoperatively, immediately postoperatively, and daily for the first 2 days after the operation.

- Early postoperative myocardial ischemia is an important correlate of adverse cardiac outcome in high-risk noncardiac surgical patients.

Valvular Heart Disease

Patients with valvular heart disease present specific risks in noncardiac surgery. Marked aortic stenosis is associated with a "fixed" cardiac output that cannot increase in response to surgical stress. Although these patients have minimal risk with local anesthesia, spinal anesthesia increases the risk because of the frequent induction of vasodilatation, which can cause cardiovascular collapse. General anesthesia can be performed with acceptable risks in selected hemodynamically monitored patients with severe aortic stenosis, but conventional wisdom is to repair the valve preoperatively (when possible) in patients with critical aortic stenosis.

- Marked aortic stenosis is associated with a "fixed" cardiac output that cannot increase with surgical stress.
- Although selected patients with severe aortic stenosis can tolerate general anesthesia, the valve should be repaired preoperatively when possible in those with critical aortic stenosis.

When mitral or aortic valve regurgitation is present, the status of left ventricular function is of primary importance. Patients with regurgitant valvular disease and preserved left ventricular function tolerate vasodilatation.

- Patients with valvular regurgitation and preserved left ventricular function tolerate vasodilatation.
- Patients with valvular heart disease should receive prophylactic treatment for endocarditis in accordance with the standard recommendations of the AHA.

Anticoagulation Issues in Patients With Mechanical Prosthetic Heart Valves Undergoing Noncardiac Operations

No randomized controlled trials have been conducted on anticoagulation in noncardiac surgical patients who have mechanical heart valves. However, the following suggestions are offered.

1. Consult with the surgeon to determine whether the intensity of anticoagulation needs to be altered. Procedures such as dental extractions, cataract removal, and other minor operations may often be performed safely with minimal or no decrease in the intensity of anticoagulation.
2. Many factors must be considered when determining a risk-to-benefit assessment of continuous anticoagulation in patients with mechanical prosthetic cardiac valves. Mitral prosthetic valves are more thrombogenic than aortic prostheses, regardless of the type of valve that has been used. Generally, the older caged-ball valves (Starr-Edwards) are more thrombogenic than bileaflet valves (St. Jude Medical). Bioprosthetic valves are the least thrombogenic. Associated factors such as atrial fibrillation, severely impaired left ventricular function, or a history of previous thromboembolism also increase the risk of thromboembolism.
3. After a risk-to-benefit assessment has been completed, one of the following strategies can be chosen: a) discontinue

warfarin therapy for several days before the procedure to allow the INR to decrease to less than 1.5 (a level at which it is considered safe to perform surgery) in an outpatient setting; b) decrease the dose of warfarin (outpatient setting) to maintain the intensity of anticoagulation in a lower or subtherapeutic range during the procedure (discuss this with the surgeon); c) discontinue warfarin therapy and institute unfractionated heparin therapy coverage (inpatient setting)—administration of heparin can be discontinued 4 hours before the operation and reinstituted, in conjunction with oral anticoagulant therapy, postoperatively, when it is considered safe; or d) discontinue warfarin therapy and institute coverage with low-molecular-weight heparin (LMWH) (outpatient setting)—discontinuing the LMWH 12 to 24 hours before the operation and then postoperatively reinstituting it in conjunction with oral anticoagulant therapy when it is considered safe.

In many situations, strategy a or b may be undertaken safely at considerable cost advantage (because of the need for fewer hospitalization days or heparin-related costs) without an appreciable increase in risk to the patient. Preoperative heparin therapy during warfarin withdrawal is recommended for those situations in which the risk of operative bleeding with anticoagulant therapy and the risk of thromboembolism without anticoagulant therapy are high (e.g., major surgical procedure in a patient with mitral valve prosthesis, cardiomyopathy, and previous thromboembolism). Reinstitution of anticoagulant therapy as early as safely possible is appropriate for all the strategies mentioned above.

- Usually, tooth extractions, cataract operations, and other minor procedures may be performed safely with therapeutic levels of anticoagulation.
- Prosthetic valves in the mitral position are more thrombogenic than aortic prostheses.
- Older caged-ball valves are more thrombogenic than bileaflet valves.
- Bioprosthetic valves are least thrombogenic.
- Anticoagulation in patients with mechanical prosthetic cardiac valves substantially decreases the incidence of thromboemboli but never eliminates it entirely.

Congestive Heart Failure

Patients with congestive heart failure (CHF) have an incidence of perioperative pulmonary edema ranging from 3% (New York Heart Association class I) to 25% (class IV). Patients with a history of CHF but no preoperative evidence of this disorder have a 6% incidence of perioperative pulmonary edema. Preoperative CHF is the greatest risk factor for the development of pulmonary edema; however, 50% of those who develop this complication have no history of CHF. In

most patients in whom CHF develops perioperatively, it does so in the first hour after the termination of anesthesia. CHF should be treated aggressively preoperatively, and therapy for chronic compensated CHF should be maintained during the perioperative period.

- The incidence of perioperative pulmonary edema among patients with CHF is from 3% to 25%.
- The greatest preoperative risk for developing pulmonary edema is CHF.
- If CHF develops perioperatively, it usually does so in the first hour after anesthesia is terminated.
- Treat CHF aggressively preoperatively, and in the perioperative period, maintain therapy for chronic compensated CHF.

Hypertension

Ideally, patients should have well-controlled hypertension (i.e., ≤140/90 mm Hg) for several months preoperatively to minimize lability of intraoperative blood pressure as well as postoperative and neurologic complications. However, studies have shown that when hypertension is stable and diastolic blood pressure is 110 mm Hg or less, no benefit is derived from postponing elective procedures to achieve better control. If the diastolic blood pressure is greater than 110 mm Hg, it should be stabilized preoperatively to diminish risk. Although the systolic blood pressure is less well studied, most medical consultants suggest that systolic blood pressure be controlled to less than 180 mm Hg before the induction of anesthesia for elective procedures. β-Blockers are particularly effective agents to use. In the perioperative period, antihypertensive agents should be continued. Parenteral agents should be substituted for oral medications in patients who are unable to take pills by mouth or nasogastric tube.

- If diastolic blood pressure is >110 mm Hg, blood pressure should be stabilized preoperatively.

Hematologic Risks and Management

Patients with poorly controlled polycythemia vera have a high rate of surgical morbidity and mortality because of an excess of thromboembolic events and decrease in oxygen transport from high blood viscosity. In polycythemia vera, phlebotomy should be performed to decrease the hematocrit to less than 47% before elective operations. Platelet counts less than 50×10^9/L (50,000/mm^3) or greater than $1,000 \times 10^9$/L (1,000,000/mm^3) should be evaluated preoperatively. A platelet count of 50×10^9/L (50,000/mm^3) usually provides adequate hemostasis for most surgical procedures. If the count is less than 20×10^9/L (20,000/mm^3), spontaneous bleeding is a common complication. Bleeding time, activated partial thromboplastin time (APTT), prothrombin time (PT), and fibrinogen level should be determined preoperatively only if the medical history and physical examination results indicate increased bleeding risk, such as previous bleeding with a major or minor surgical procedure, easy bruisability, or a family history of bleeding disorder.

- Patients with poorly controlled polycythemia vera have a high rate of surgical morbidity and mortality due to thromboembolic events and high blood viscosity.
- In polycythemia vera, perform phlebotomy to decrease hematocrit to <47% before an elective operation.
- A platelet count of 50×10^9/L (50,000/mm^3) usually provides adequate hemostasis for most operations.
- Preoperatively, determine the bleeding time, APTT, fibrinogen level, and PT only if the medical history and physical examination findings indicate increased bleeding risk.

Liver Risks and Management

Patients with chronic liver disease, particularly those with progressive hepatic failure, have a considerable operative risk. Preoperatively, one should concentrate on correcting electrolyte abnormalities and abnormal clotting variables, reducing ascites, treating encephalopathy, and improving the patient's nutritional status.

Endocrinologic Risks and Management

Patients who are thyrotoxic are at high risk for surgical complications, such as arrhythmias, high output CHF, and death. Thyroid storm occurs in 20% to 30% of these patients. Thus, elective surgery should be postponed and treatment (antithyroid drugs or radioiodine) should be given for at least 3 months until the patient is euthyroid. If an operation is emergent, a patient who is thyrotoxic should be pretreated with propranolol and propylthiouracil. A patient who is hypothyroid may undergo a surgical procedure at very low risk. Patients with severe myxedema should be given thyroxine replacement therapy and receive careful monitoring and supportive therapy, including free water restriction and diuretics.

- Patients who are thyrotoxic are at high risk for surgical complications.
- This condition should be treated for 3 months or until the patient is euthyroid before any elective operation is performed.
- In the case of an emergency operation, pretreatment with propranolol and propylthiouracil.

Patients with diabetes mellitus have a greater risk of surgical complications due to underlying cardiovascular and cerebrovascular disease. It is preferable to have the patient in moderate diabetic control preoperatively to diminish the risk of infection. During the perioperative period, the patient may not be able to recognize the signs and symptoms of hypoglycemia. Therefore, oral hypoglycemic agents are withheld and the insulin dose is cut in half on the day of the operation. Metformin, a nonsulfonylurea oral hypoglycemic agent, is discontinued before the operation to avoid possibly inducing lactic acidosis in situations in which renal function may fluctuate unpredictably. The serum glucose level should be maintained in the 150 to 250 mg/dL range during the perioperative period.

- In cases of diabetes mellitus, there is greater risk of surgical complications because of underlying cardiovascular and cerebrovascular disease.
- Withhold oral hypoglycemic agents, cut insulin dose in half on the day of the operation, and maintain the serum glucose level at 150 to 250 mg/dL during the perioperative period.

Adequate preoperative and perioperative corticosteroid replacement preparation should be given to any patient who has received suppressive doses of corticosteroids for 2 weeks or longer during the past year.

Nutrition

Perioperatively, malnourished patients have increased complications related to wound infection, pneumonia, respiratory insufficiency, and adversely affected cellular and humoral immune function. In a nutritional assessment, clinical judgment of malnutrition is as accurate as objective measurements. Thus, detailed laboratory measurements of albumin and other substances are not usually required. There is some rationale for giving preoperative nutritional supplementation to malnourished patients and continuing support through the perioperative period.

Thromboembolism Prophylaxis

Although all surgical patients are at some risk for venous thromboembolic disease, certain patients form a high-risk subset, including those who are elderly, have prolonged anesthesia or a prolonged operation, previous venous thromboembolic disease, hereditary disorders of thrombosis, or prolonged immobilization or paralysis, malignancy, obesity, varicosities, or estrogen use. Reasonable guidelines for thromboembolism prophylaxis in surgical patients to decrease the overall risk of deep venous thrombosis or pulmonary embolism are given in Table 8-10.

Perioperative Antibiotic Prophylaxis

Antibiotics are given perioperatively to prevent infection of normal sterile tissues by direct contamination during the surgical procedure. The risk of wound infection depends

Table 8-10 Prevention of Venous Thromboembolism

Patient characteristics	Recommended therapy
Low-risk general surgery patients	Early ambulation
Moderate-risk general surgery patients	LDUH, LMWH, IPC, or ES
Higher risk general surgery patients	LDUH or higher dosage LMWH
Higher risk general surgery patients prone to wound complications, e.g., hematomas and infection	IPC is an alternative
Very high-risk general surgery patients with multiple risk factors	LDUH or LMWH, combined with IPC
Selected very high-risk general surgery patients	Perioperative warfarin (goal INR 2.5; range, 2.0-3.0)
Patients undergoing total hip replacement surgery[*]	LMWH, started 12 to 24 h after surgery; or warfarin, started before or immediately after surgery (goal INR 2.5; range, 2.0-3.0); or adjusted-dose heparin, started preoperatively; possible adjuvant use of ES or IPC[†]
Patients undergoing total knee replacement surgery[*]	LMWH, warfarin, or IPC
Patients undergoing hip fracture surgery	LMWH or warfarin (goal INR 2.5; range, 2.0-3.0) started preoperatively or immediately after surgery
High-risk patients undergoing orthopedic surgery	IVC filter placement, only if other forms of anticoagulant-based prophylaxis are not feasible because of active bleeding; this should rarely be necessary
Patients undergoing intracranial neurosurgery	IPC with or without ES: LMWH and LDUH may be acceptable alternatives; consider IPC or ES, with LMWH or LDUH, for high-risk patients
Patients with acute spinal cord injury	LMWH; although ES and IPC appear ineffective when used alone, ES and IPC may have benefit when used with LMWH, or if anticoagulants are contraindicated; during rehabilitation, consider continuation of LMWH or conversion to full-dose oral anticoagulation
Trauma patients with an identifiable risk factor for thromboembolism	LMWH, as soon as considered safe; consider initial prophylaxis with IPC if administration of LMWH will be delayed or is contraindicated; in high-risk patients with suboptimal prophylaxis, consider screening with duplex ultrasonography, or filter placement in the IVC
Patients with MI	LDUH or full-dose anticoagulation; IPC and possibly ES may be useful when heparin is contraindicated
Patients with ischemic stroke and lower-extremity paralysis	LDUH or LMWH; IPC with ES also is probably effective
General medical patients with clinical risk factors for venous thromboembolism, particularly those with CHF or chest infections	LDUH or LMWH
Patients with long-term indwelling central vein catheters	Warfarin (1 mg daily) or LMWH daily to prevent axillary-subclavian venous thrombosis
Patients having spinal puncture or epidural catheters placed for regional anesthesia or analgesia	LMWH should be used with caution and guidelines followed

CHF, congestive heart failure; ES, elastic stockings; INR, international normalized ratio; IPC, intermittent pneumatic compression; IVC, inferior vena cava; LDUH, low-dose unfractionated heparin; LMWH, low-molecular-weight heparin; MI, myocardial infarction.

[*]Optimal duration of prophylaxis is uncertain; 7 to 10 days are recommended with LMWH or warfarin; 29 to 35 days with LMWH may offer additional protection.

[†]LDUH, aspirin, dextran, and IPC reduce the overall incidence of venous thromboembolism but are less effective.

Data from Geerts WH, Heit JA, Clagett GP, et al: Prevention of venous thromboembolism. Chest 2001;119 (suppl):132S-175S.

mainly on the type of operation. "Clean" operations are ones in which the gastrointestinal, genitourinary, and respiratory tracts are not entered and there is no surrounding inflammation. Previously, antibiotic prophylaxis was not required for this type of procedure because the risk of infection was only about 5%, as compared with a much higher risk for other procedures that required prophylactic treatment with antibiotics to prevent wound infection (clean-contaminated, contaminated, and dirty operations). However, antibiotic prophylaxis, cefazolin 1 g intravenously, is now recommended for simple clean procedures such as inguinal hernia repair and breast surgery. A short course of prophylactic therapy (one dose of antibiotic 1 to 2 hours preoperatively and no more than one dose postoperatively) is as effective as longer regimens and is less likely to be associated with toxicity or development of resistant organisms in clean or clean-contaminated operations. Technically, the antibiotics used in dirty or contaminated procedures are for treatment of established infection rather than for prophylaxis and are often continued for 5 to 10 days postoperatively.

Preoperative Laboratory Tests

Few laboratory tests should be ordered solely because an operation is planned. In the absence of symptoms, signs, or risk factors for a disease, results of routinely ordered tests are usually normal, and when abnormal, they are often ignored. Authors who have evaluated specific preoperative tests have suggested that chest radiography, ECG, PT, APTT, and bleeding time are not justified as "routine" preoperative tests for young healthy persons. Tests should be performed for specific clinical indications and not because a patient is being evaluated in the outpatient clinic, hospital, or operating room (Table 8-11).

Because ECG abnormalities increase with age and certain abnormalities are related to major perioperative morbidity, most physicians suggest that a routine ECG be performed before an elective operation in all patients older than 50 years. Although the relationship between chest radiographic findings and perioperative morbidity is not well defined, postoperative chest radiography is frequently needed for elderly patients because of pulmonary complications, and a baseline preoperative radiograph is helpful if the patient is older than 60.

- Chest radiography, ECG, PT, APTT, and bleeding time are not "routine" preoperative tests for young healthy persons.
- Tests should be performed for specific clinical indications.

Geriatric Surgical Patients

The number of surgical procedures performed on elderly patients has steadily increased. Elderly patients comprise 15% of the population but account for one-third of all surgical procedures, one-half of all emergency surgical procedures, and three-fourths of overall surgical mortality. Age is an independent risk factor for perioperative cardiovascular morbidity. Most elderly patients have at least one associated chronic medical illness. This and the pathophysiologic effects of aging on the cardiovascular and pulmonary systems probably explain why geriatric patients have a higher perioperative mortality rate than younger patients. Intervention aimed at meticulously looking for and treating perioperative complications (anemia, infection, pneumonia) leads to improved outcomes (less postoperative delirium, fewer hospital days) in geriatric patients.

- Elderly patients account for one-third of all surgical procedures.
- Age is an independent risk factor for perioperative cardiovascular morbidity.
- Geriatric patients have a much higher prevalence of CAD.
- Geriatric patients have a higher perioperative mortality rate.

Table 8-11   Indications for Standard Preoperative Tests in Nonemergency Situations

Test	Indications
Hematocrit	All women; men >60 years; anticipated blood loss
Electrolytes	Patients >60 years or with renal disease or diabetes, or who take diuretics, steroids, bowel preparations
Prothrombin and partial thromboplastin times, platelet count	Patients with liver disease, bleeding, or malignancy, or who take anticoagulants
Electrocardiography	Patients >50 years or with cardiovascular disease, lung disease, peripheral vascular disease, or diabetes
Chest radiography	Patients >60 years or with pulmonary or cardiovascular disease or acute pulmonary symptoms

Modified from MKSAP X: Part A, Book 3, 1994. American College of Physicians. By permission.

Perioperative Medication Management

The internist tailors perioperative drug therapy to individual circumstances, with particular attention to three factors:

1. Have the indications and doses for the specific drug been clearly defined?
2. What are the likely anesthetic and surgical interactions and complications?
3. Is a clinically important withdrawal syndrome likely, and how can it be managed safely?

Most drugs used to manage chronic medical conditions can and should be continued through the perioperative period. Often, patients can receive medications with sips of water on the morning of the operation and resume oral medications or parenteral substitution later in the day. Should particular questions occur about the continuation of a specific drug, communication with an anesthesiologist is important.

● Most drugs for chronic medical conditions should continue to be taken through the perioperative period.

CURRENT CONCEPTS IN ANTICOAGULANT THERAPY

INR

What Are Recommended INR Therapeutic Ranges for Oral Anticoagulant Therapy?

The recommended INR therapeutic ranges are summarized in Table 8-12. In short, an INR of 2.0 to 3.0 is used for most indications except for the few high-risk conditions (e.g., mechanical prosthetic heart valves) in which a slightly higher INR is suggested.

Antithrombotic Therapy for Venous Thromboembolic Disease

Guidelines for anticoagulation in patients with venous thromboembolic disease are summarized in Table 8-13.

Anticoagulation in Prosthetic Heart Valves

What Are the Recommendations for Anticoagulation in Patients With Mechanical Prosthetic Heart Valves?

It is strongly recommended that all patients with mechanical prosthetic heart valves receive warfarin. Levels of warfarin that prolong the INR to 2.5 to 3.5 are recommended in most situations. Patients with bileaflet valves in the aortic position and no other risk factors may have an INR of 2.0 to 3.0. Levels of warfarin producing an INR less than 1.8 have a high risk of thromboembolic events, and levels that increase the INR to more than 4.5 have a high risk of excessive bleeding.

Table 8-12 Recommended Therapeutic Range for Oral Anticoagulant Therapy

Indication	INR
Prophylaxis for venous thrombosis (high-risk surgery)	2.0-3.0
Treatment of venous thrombosis	2.0-3.0
Treatment of pulmonary embolism	2.0-3.0
Prevention of systemic embolism	
Tissue heart valves*	2.0-3.0
Acute myocardial infarction (to prevent systemic embolism)†	2.0-3.0
Valvular heart disease	2.0-3.0
Atrial fibrillation	2.0-3.0
Antiphospholipid-antibody syndrome (secondary prevention)	2.5-3.5
Mechanical prosthetic heart valves	
AVR and no risk factors‡	
Bileaflet valve	2.0-3.0
Other disk valve or Starr-Edwards	2.5-3.5
AVR and risk factor§	2.5-3.5
MVR§	2.5-3.5

AVR, aortic valve replacement; INR, international normalized ratio; MVR, mitral valve replacement.

*Treatment usually for 3 months unless other risk factors continue.

†If oral anticoagulant therapy is elected to prevent recurrent myocardial infarction, an INR of 2.5 to 3.5 is recommended, consistent with Food and Drug Administration recommendations.

‡Risk factors: atrial fibrillation, left ventricular dysfunction, previous thromboembolism, hypercoagulable state.

§Consider addition of ASA 80 to 100 mg once daily to decrease embolic risk.

Modified from Litin SC, Gastineau DA: Current concepts in anticoagulant therapy. Mayo Clin Proc 1995;70:266-272, and data from Bonow RO, Carabello B, de Leon AC Jr, et al: ACC/AHA guidelines for the management of patients with valvular heart disease: executive summary. A report of the American College of Cardiology/American Heart Association Task Force on Practice Guidelines (Committee on Management of Patients With Valvular Heart Disease). Circulation 1998;98:1949-1984.

For high-risk patients, aspirin (80-100 mg daily) in addition to warfarin further decreases the risk of thromboembolism without increasing the risk of major bleeding, although minor bleeding is increased.

● All patients with mechanical prosthetic heart valves should receive warfarin.
● In most cases, use warfarin levels that prolong the INR to 2.5-3.5.
● Warfarin levels that 1) decrease the INR <1.8 have a high risk of thromboembolic events or 2) increase the INR >4.5 have a high risk of excessive bleeding.

Table 8-13 Guidelines for Anticoagulation in Adults With Venous Thromboembolic Disease

Deep venous thrombosis or pulmonary embolus	Guidelines for anticoagulation
Suspected	Obtain baseline APTT, PT, CBC Check for contraindication to heparin therapy Give unfractionated heparin, 5,000 U IV, and order imaging study
Confirmed	Rebolus with heparin, 80 U/kg IV, and start maintenance infusion at 18 U/kg per hour* or use appropriate regimen of subcutaneous fixed-dose LMWH Start warfarin therapy on first day at 5 mg and then administer warfarin daily at estimated maintenance dose Discontinue LMWH or unfractionated heparin when it has been administered jointly with warfarin for at least 4 or 5 days and the INR ≥2.0 for 2 consecutive days Anticoagulate with warfarin for at least 3 months at an INR of 2.0 to 3.0 (longer treatment should be given to patients with ongoing risk factors or recurrent thrombosis)

APTT, activated partial thromboplastin time; CBC, complete blood count; INR, international normalized ratio; IV, intravenous; LMWH, low-molecular-weight heparin; PT, prothrombin time.

*If unfractionated heparin is used, check APTT at 6 hours to keep APTT between 1.5 and 2.5 times control (anti-Xa heparin level of 0.3-0.7 IU/mL) and check platelet count daily.

● In patients with prosthetic heart valves, a low dose of aspirin plus warfarin may have an additive benefit without causing major bleeding (increases minor bleeding).

What Is Recommended if a Patient With a Prosthetic Heart Valve Has a Systemic Embolism Despite Adequate Therapy With Warfarin (INR 2.5-3.5)?

These patients may respond to a slight increase in the warfarin dose, thus increasing the INR to 3.5 to 4.5. Also, aspirin (80-100 mg daily) could be added to the regimen.

● No regimen ever totally eliminates the risk of systemic embolization or the risk of bleeding.

What Are the Recommendations for Anticoagulation in Patients With Bioprosthetic Heart Valves?

It is recommended that all patients with bioprosthetic valves in the mitral position receive warfarin therapy (INR, 2.0-3.0) for the first 3 months. Anticoagulant therapy is also reasonable during the first 3 months for patients with bioprosthetic valves in the aortic position who are in sinus rhythm. Certain patients with bioprosthetic valves have underlying conditions (i.e., atrial fibrillation, left atrial thrombosis) that require long-term warfarin therapy to prevent systemic emboli. For patients with bioprosthetic heart valves who are in sinus rhythm, long-term therapy with aspirin (325 mg daily) may offer protection against thromboembolism and appears reasonable for those without contraindication.

● Patients with bioprosthetic valves receive warfarin therapy (INR, 2.0-3.0) for 3 months.
● Patients with bioprosthetic valves who have atrial fibrillation or left atrial thrombus require long-term warfarin therapy to prevent systemic emboli.
● Long-term therapy with aspirin may protect patients with bioprosthetic heart valves who are in sinus rhythm against thromboembolism.

Hemorrhagic Complications of Anticoagulation

When the Anticoagulant Effect of Warfarin Needs to Be Reversed, What Is the Best Way to Do This?

The anticoagulant effect of warfarin can be reversed by stopping treatment, administering vitamin K, or, in urgent situations with pronounced bleeding, replacing vitamin K-dependent coagulation factors with fresh frozen plasma. When warfarin therapy is discontinued, no marked effect is seen on the INR for 2 days or more because of the half-life of warfarin (36-42 hours) and the delay before newly synthesized functional coagulation factors replace dysfunctional coagulation factors.

Administering vitamin K rapidly lowers the INR, depending on the dosage of vitamin K and the severity of the anticoagulant effect. When high doses of vitamin K are administered, reversal occurs in about 6 hours. The disadvantage is that patients often remain resistant to warfarin for up to a week, making continued warfarin treatment difficult. This problem can be overcome by giving much lower dosages of vitamin K orally, subcutaneously, or by slow intravenous infusion.

- The anticoagulant effect of warfarin can be reversed by stopping treatment, giving vitamin K, or replacing vitamin K-dependent coagulation factors with fresh frozen plasma.
- In cases of life-threatening bleeding or serious warfarin overdosages, replacement of vitamin K-dependent coagulation factors with fresh frozen plasma produces an immediate effect and is the treatment of choice.
- In nonurgent situations, a low dose of vitamin K (1-2.5 mg) may be given orally to decrease the INR and avoid warfarin resistance.

Are There Certain Patient Characteristics That Increase the Risk of Hemorrhagic Complications of Anticoagulant Treatment?

A strong relationship between the intensity of anticoagulant therapy and the risk of bleeding has been reported in patients receiving treatment for deep venous thrombosis and prosthetic heart valves. The concurrent use of drugs that interfere with hemostasis and produce gastric erosions (aspirin, nonsteroidal anti-inflammatory drugs) increases the risk of serious upper gastrointestinal tract bleeding. Other drugs such as trimethoprim-sulfamethoxazole inhibit the clearance of warfarin, thus potentiating its effect. Physicians should consider any medication a potential source of interaction until proven otherwise. Several existing disease states associated with increased bleeding during warfarin therapy include treated hypertension, renal insufficiency, hepatic insufficiency, and cerebrovascular disease.

- The relationship between the intensity of anticoagulant therapy and the risk of bleeding is strong.
- The concurrent use of drugs that interfere with hemostasis and produce gastric erosions increases the risk of serious upper gastrointestinal tract bleeding.
- Trimethoprim-sulfamethoxazole, amiodarone, and omeprazole potentiate the effect of warfarin and increase bleeding risk.

COMMON CLINICAL PROBLEMS IN GENERAL INTERNAL MEDICINE

Treatment of Hyperlipidemia

Case

A 55-year-old man with stable class II angina is referred for consideration of drug treatment for hyperlipidemia. He is otherwise healthy. He quit smoking cigarettes 2 years previously and has no other known risk factors for CAD. He has closely followed the advice of a dietitian for the past 6 months, but his cholesterol levels have shown no marked decrease. His most recent values are total cholesterol, 240 mg/dL; high-density lipoprotein cholesterol (HDL-C), 35 mg/dL; and triglycerides, 75 mg/dL.

Discussion

Evidence has shown that lowering increased low-density lipoprotein cholesterol (LDL-C) levels is associated with both primary and secondary prevention of coronary events. Moreover, several angiographic trials have shown consistent decreases in progression and increases in regression of atherosclerotic plaques that have been followed up for several years.

The third report of the National Cholesterol Education Program's Adult Treatment Panel (ATP III) identified patients with definite CAD or CAD risk equivalents (clinical atherosclerotic disease, diabetes mellitus) to be at very high risk (>20% events per 10 years) and suggested aggressive treatment.

In ATP II, the risk level was assigned by counting risk factors to identify the patient with multiple (2+) risk factors. The risk factors employed were those that are used to modify LDL-cholesterol goals. In ATP III, the risk level is assigned by a combination of risk factor counting, followed by a 10-year risk assessment (Framingham risk scoring) in the multiple-risk-factor patient. The risk factors used for modifying LDL-C goals include:

- Cigarette smoking.
- Hypertension (blood pressure ≥140/90 mm Hg or taking antihypertensive medication).
- Low HDL-C (<40 mg/dL).
- Family history of premature CAD (CAD in male first-degree relative ≤55 years old; CAD in a female first-degree relative ≤65 years old).
- Age (men ≥45 years old; women ≥55 years old).
- If a patient has a high HDL-C (≥60 mg/dL), one risk factor is subtracted from the count.

LDL-C is used to monitor patients with hypercholesterolemia and is calculated from the following formula:

$$LDL\text{-}C = (\text{Total Cholesterol}) - (\text{HDL-C}) - \frac{\text{Triglycerides}}{5}$$

In this patient, LDL-C = (240) − (35) − (75/5) = 190 mg/dL.

Secondary causes of hyperlipidemia should be ruled out in all patients. Secondary causes of hyperlipidemia may be due to diseases (hypothyroidism, diabetes, nephrotic syndrome, renal failure, obstructive liver disease), drugs (corticosteroids, progestins, thiazides, β-blockers), or diet (alcohol abuse, increased saturated fats).

● Rule out secondary causes for hyperlipidemia in all patients: diseases, drugs, and diet.

After secondary causes have been ruled out, the next line of treatment involves weight reduction for overweight patients, increased physical activity, and dietary therapy. Both weight reduction and exercise not only promote lowering of cholesterol levels but have other benefits, such as decreasing triglycerides, increasing HDL-C, decreasing blood pressure, and decreasing the risk of diabetes mellitus.

Therapeutic lifestyle changes (weight reduction, physical activity, intensive diet therapy) are initiated for patients without CAD or risk equivalents if LDL-C is 160 mg/dL or greater, for patients without CAD but who have at least two risk factors if LDL-C is 130 mg/dL or greater, and for patients with CAD or CAD risk equivalents if LDL-C is greater than 100 mg/dL. Strategies for LDL-C management by CAD risk are summarized in Table 8-14.

If hypolipidemic drugs are prescribed, the choice of drug depends on the mechanism of action, side-effect profile, efficacy, and cost. The following discussion considers the most common classes of drugs used in the treatment of hyperlipidemia.

Bile acid sequestrants (e.g., cholestyramine, colestipol, and colesevelam)—Clinical trials have documented their benefit and safety. Their mechanism of action involves removing plasma LDL by depleting the bile acid pool, which causes an increase in liver LDL receptors. These drugs are often given alone (to patients with mild increases in LDL-C levels) or in combination with other drugs (to patients with greater increases in LDL-C levels). Side effects include gastrointestinal symptoms, binding of other concurrently administered drugs, constipation, and increased triglyceride levels, especially in patients who begin with increased levels.

Nicotinic acid (niacin)—This agent is effective in decreasing total cholesterol and triglyceride levels as well as increasing HDL-C levels. Side effects are common and limit the use of this drug in many patients. Side effects can include flushing, nausea, abdominal discomfort, and skin itching. Also, the levels of plasma glucose, uric acid, and liver enzymes may increase. Slow-release preparations reduce the side effect of flushing, but the incidence of liver dysfunction increases markedly, especially with higher doses. Small doses of aspirin taken before niacin may block flushing.

HMG-CoA reductase inhibitors, or statins (e.g., lovastatin, pravastatin, simvastatin, and atorvastatin)—These drugs are highly effective in decreasing LDL-C by blocking liver cholesterol synthesis, which causes an increase in LDL liver receptors. They have few side effects, although myalgias, myopathy, and an increase in liver enzymes may occur. Myopathy can increase with concurrent use of cyclosporine, niacin, erythromycin, and fibrates (fibric acid derivatives). Primary prevention studies have shown decreased mortality risks with the use of statins. In large secondary prevention trials, statin drugs have been shown to reduce total mortality, cardiac mortality, and the incidence of stroke. They are effective in treating severe forms of hypercholesterolemia.

Table 8-14 LDL Cholesterol Goals and Cutpoints for Therapeutic Lifestyle Changes and Drug Therapy in Different Risk Categories

Risk category	LDL goal, mg/dL	LDL level at which to initiate therapeutic lifestyle changes, mg/dL	LDL level at which to consider drug therapy, mg/dL
CAD or CAD risk equivalents (10-year risk >20%)	<100	≥100	≥130 (100-129: drug optional)*
2+ Risk factors (10-year risk ≤20%)	<130	≥130	10-year risk 10%-20%: ≥130 10-year risk <10%: ≥160
0-1 Risk factor†	<160	≥160	≥190 (160-189: LDL-lowering drug optional)

CAD, coronary artery disease; LDL, low-density lipoprotein.

*Some authorities recommend use of LDL-lowering drugs in this category if an LDL cholesterol level of <100 mg/dL cannot be achieved by therapeutic lifestyle changes. Others prefer use of drugs that primarily modify triglycerides and HDL, e.g., nicotinic acid or fibrate. Clinical judgment also may call for deferring drug therapy in this subcategory.

†Almost all people with 0-1 risk factor have a 10-year risk <10%; thus, 10-year risk assessment in people with 0-1 risk factor is not necessary.

From Expert Panel on Detection, Evaluation, and Treatment of High Blood Cholesterol in Adults: Executive Summary of the Third Report of the National Cholesterol Education Program (NCEP) Expert Panel on Detection, Evaluation, and Treatment of High Blood Cholesterol in Adults (Adult Treatment Panel III). JAMA 2001;285:2486-2497.

Fibrates (e.g., gemfibrozil and fenofibrate)—These are the drugs of choice for decreasing isolated increased levels of triglycerides. In some patients, these drugs slightly lower LDL-C and raise HDL-C levels. Fenofibrate is more effective than gemfibrozil in lowering LDL-C. Side effects are rare and related mostly to the gastrointestinal tract. These drugs also may increase the risk of gallstones. Therapeutically, they are most useful for disorders of hypertriglyceridemia, especially in patients with diabetes mellitus.

All the above-mentioned drugs have the potential to interact with warfarin (bile acid sequestrants can bind the drug, thus decreasing the INR, and the other hypolipidemic drugs may potentiate warfarin, thus increasing the INR). Therefore, when they are prescribed for patients taking anticoagulants, close monitoring is indicated.

Generally, the following drugs alone or sometimes in combination are recommended:

1. For patients with increased levels of LDL-C: bile acid sequestrants, HMG-CoA reductase inhibitors, and nicotinic acid.
2. For patients with increased levels of LDL-C and triglycerides: nicotinic acid, fibrates, and HMG-CoA reductase inhibitors.
3. For patients with isolated hypertriglyceridemia if treatment is indicated: fibrates and nicotinic acid.

Drug therapy for hyperlipidemia must be individualized. In general, a positive effect is obtained and fewer side effects are experienced by starting therapy with low doses of medication and increasing the dose slowly, if necessary.

Tobacco Abuse

Case

A 60-year-old woman comes to your office for her annual mammogram, breast examination, and pelvic examination. You note from the preexamination questionnaire that she is a current smoker and has smoked one pack per day for 30 years. Examination of the lungs shows scattered rhonchi and wheezes with a prolonged expiratory phase. You broach the subject of smoking cessation with the patient, but the patient quickly and defensively counters with a number of statements, including "after 30 years of smoking, the damage is done" and "there's no sense quitting." The patient also fears gaining weight after quitting and says that when she did try to quit several years ago, she quickly became so nervous and edgy that she could not sleep and was unpleasant to be around. How might you devise a plan to deal effectively with this patient's tobacco abuse problem?

Discussion

Tobacco use is the leading cause of preventable premature death in the United States. It accounts for about 20% of all-cause mortality in the United States annually. In addition to being the causative factor for nearly 90% of all cases of lung cancer, smoking is associated with cancer of the oral cavity, larynx, esophagus, stomach, pancreas, uterine cervix, and genitourinary tract. However, among ex-smokers abstinent for 15 years or longer, the increase in lung cancer mortality is decreased to rates nearly those of nonsmokers.

Smokers are two to six times as likely to have an MI as nonsmokers, and 20% of all deaths due to cardiovascular disease are attributable to smoking. After several years of abstinence, the cardiovascular risk of ex-smokers is not significantly different from that of those who have never smoked.

Compared with smokers, ex-smokers have less phlegm production and wheezing, greater FEV_1 and vital capacity, better immune function, and lower mortality rates from pulmonary infections, bronchitis, and emphysema. Although some lung damage is irreversible, ex-smokers have marked improvement in their pulmonary function during the first year of cessation. After that, the decline in lung function stabilizes at a nonsmoker's rate. Smokers continue to show a decline in lung function at many times the rate of ex-smokers.

Often, one of the most compelling arguments for a patient to stop smoking is that it harms others. It is estimated that in the United States more than 50,000 people die annually of medical complications of passive smoking. Most of these deaths are from accelerated heart disease, although the number of lung cancer deaths is also substantial. Studies have estimated that nonsmoking spouses of smokers have an all-cancer risk about 1.5 times that of nonsmoking spouses of nonsmokers.

The Public Health Service Clinical Practice Guideline advises physicians to use an easy-to-remember five-step approach in counseling their patients in smoking cessation.

1. **Ask**—Systematically identify all tobacco-users at every visit. The physician should question patients about smoking at any new encounter, inquiring not only if they smoke but how much they smoke. It is also helpful to ask whether they have ever tried to stop smoking, and if so, what happened.
2. **Advise** all smokers to quit. Make this a strong and personalized message. Fewer than two-thirds of physicians report advising their patients to stop smoking, and only two-thirds of patients report receiving smoking cessation advice from their physician. This counsel can often be an influential message to patients. The physician should state the advice clearly; for example, "As your physician, I must advise you to stop smoking now." It helps to personalize the "quit smoking" message by referring to other illnesses the patient has, family history, passive smoking issues, and so forth.
3. **Assess** each person's willingness to make a quit attempt. If a person is willing to make a quit attempt, move on to

step 4 (assist). If the patient desires intensive treatment, provide a referral. Some patients are unwilling to make a quit attempt. For them, provide a motivational intervention.

4. **Assist** the patient in stopping to smoke. Set a quit date with the patient. Try to do it within 4 weeks, acknowledging with the patient that the time never is ideal. Provide self-help materials. Recommend or prescribe nicotine gum, nicotine patches, intranasal nicotine spray, nicotine inhaler, or bupropion, especially for any patient who smokes more than 10 cigarettes daily and is motivated to attempt smoking cessation. Consider signing a stop-smoking contract with the patient.

5. **Arrange** follow-up visits. Set up a follow-up visit within 1 or 2 weeks after the quit date. Counseling programs and behavioral therapy programs can be effective in smoking cessation. A transdermal nicotine patch together with behavioral therapy results in significantly higher cessation rates than transdermal nicotine alone. If during follow-up visits you discover the patient has relapsed, advise him or her that this is not uncommon. Encourage the patient to try again immediately.

Pharmacologic therapy to aid in smoking cessation should be recommended to most patients. In clinical trials, smoking cessation rates at 6 to 12 months are more than doubled among those using active therapy, as compared with placebo treatment. Two categories of pharmacologic smoking cessation treatment are available: nicotine replacement therapy and non-nicotine therapy. Nicotine replacement therapy is available in several forms. A transdermal nicotine patch releases nicotine at a steady rate for 16 to 24 hours and is associated with higher patient compliance because of its once-a-day dosing schedule. Nicotine gum, nicotine nasal spray, and nicotine inhaler are immediate-release forms of nicotine replacement and are effective in smoking cessation treatment but must be used several times each day. They have the advantage of allowing patients to use them in response to smoking urges. Currently, bupropion is the only non-nicotine therapy available that has proven efficacy for smoking cessation. It should not be used if the patient has seizure risk; otherwise, it is appropriate for any smoker who is motivated to stop smoking. Bupropion may have the added advantage of attenuating postcessation weight gain.

Several other important concerns that patients have can be addressed and answered. For those who worry about weight gain with smoking cessation, it is useful to let them know that although the majority of patients do gain weight, the average is about 3 kg, and this can be anticipated and dealt with effectively. For patients who have noted difficulties with nervousness and poor sleep after smoking cessation, advise them that these symptoms are related to nicotine withdrawal and usually resolve after 2 or 3 weeks. Nicotine replacement therapies can often help control these symptoms. Some patients notice an increase in coughing after they stop smoking. This can be explained as a temporary response caused by an increase in the lung's ability to remove phlegm and, thus, represents recovery of the lung's own defense mechanisms. After cessation has been achieved, the patient should be advised to refrain from having even an occasional cigarette, because nicotine addiction seems to be triggered quickly in most ex-smokers.

Acute Low Back Pain

Case

A 55-year-old man comes to your office with a 3-day history of severe low back pain in the lumbosacral area. The patient does not recall any specific trauma, and the review of systems is negative for fever, weight loss, or other constitutional symptoms. The patient does not complain of numbness, tingling, or weakness in his legs, and he has no bladder or bowel symptoms. The patient works in a factory, and his job requires some minor lifting and bending. Make a diagnostic assessment, therapeutic plan, and suggestions about levels of activity.

Discussion

The Agency for Health Care Policy and Research published clinical practice guidelines relating to adult patients with acute low back problems. The following discussion focuses on suggestions from these guidelines.

Acute low back problems are one of the most common reasons for patients to visit a physician's office. Acute low back problems are defined as "activity intolerance due to lower back or back-related leg symptoms of less than 3 months' duration." It is important to know that 90% of patients with acute low back problems have a spontaneous recovery and return to previous levels of activity within 1 month. On the initial assessment of such a patient, a focused medical history and physical examination should be performed so that a potentially dangerous underlying condition is not overlooked. On the basis of this evaluation, low back symptoms can be classified into one of three working categories:

1. *Potentially serious spinal conditions*—This category includes tumor, infection, fracture, or major neurologic disorder. One should look for "red flags" in the history or examination that would point to these conditions, that is, a history of trauma (fracture) or cancer (spinal epidural metastases), risk factors for spinal infection or fever/chills (infection), and saddle anesthesia or bladder and bowel dysfunction (cauda equina syndrome).

2. *Sciatica*—This category includes back-related lower limb symptoms suggestive of lumbosacral nerve root compromise. Sciatica would be further suggested by a positive straight leg raise, as defined by pain below the knee at less than 70° of leg elevation, aggravated

by dorsiflexion of the ankle. Crossover pain (i.e., eliciting pain in the leg with sciatica by straight raising of the unaffected leg) is an even stronger indication of nerve root compression. Correlative findings on sensory examination, specific muscle strength loss, and reflex changes can be used to further diagnose sciatica and to localize the nerve root suspected to be involved.

3. *Nonspecific back symptoms*—This category includes low back pain without signs or symptoms of a serious underlying condition or nerve root compression.

The patient in the case example appears to have nonspecific back discomfort. After this diagnosis is made, the physician could educate the patient about this problem, reassuring him that the evaluation results do not suggest a dangerous problem and that rapid recovery can be expected. Should the patient not recover within a month, a more extensive evaluation may be needed, including radiography and special studies.

In the interim, the physician must address the need for symptom control measures. This can include oral medications. The safest effective medication for acute low back problems appears to be acetaminophen, which has a low side-effect profile. Nonsteroidal anti-inflammatory drugs can also be prescribed, but the disadvantages are cost and side-effect profile (gastrointestinal tract irritation and ulceration). Muscle relaxants are reported to be no more effective than nonsteroidal anti-inflammatory drugs in treating low back symptoms, and they can produce marked drowsiness. A combination of relaxants and nonsteroidal anti-inflammatory drugs has not demonstrated an increased benefit. Muscle relaxants may produce marked drowsiness. Opioids appear no more effective than safer analgesics and should be avoided if possible. If opioids are chosen, they should be prescribed for only short periods and the patient must be warned of the potential side effects of drowsiness, cloudy mentation, and constipation and the potential for dependency.

Physical methods are often used in the treatment of acute back problems; however, most of these methods, including traction, massage, ultrasound, and trigger point injections, have not been proven to be effective in studies of patients with symptoms. Spinal manipulation is safe and might be effective for appropriate patients who have acute low back symptoms in the absence of a radiculopathy.

Activity alteration is a balance between avoiding undue back irritation and preventing debility due to inactivity. Most patients do not require bed rest. In fact, it has been shown that patients with acute low back pain who continue ordinary activities within the limits permitted by the pain recover more rapidly than those treated with bed rest or back-mobilizing exercises. If bed rest is used, it should be used for only 2 or 3 days, because prolonged bed rest has a potential debilitating effect and its efficacy in treatment is unproven. Generally, bed rest is reserved for patients with severe limitations caused by sciatica. Certain postures and activities can increase stress on the back and aggravate the symptoms. Patients must be taught to minimize the stress of lifting by keeping the object being lifted close to the body at the level of the navel. Lifting with the legs as opposed to the back must be emphasized. Prolonged sitting may sometimes aggravate problems, and patients should be encouraged to change their position frequently. Until the patient returns to normal activity, aerobic conditioning may be recommended to help avoid debilitation from inactivity. When requested, it may be appropriate for the physician to offer specific instructions about activity at work for patients with acute limitations due to low back symptoms. The physician should make it clear to both the patient and the employer that even moderately heavy unassisted lifting may aggravate back symptoms and that any restrictions are intended to allow for spontaneous recovery or for time to build activity tolerance through exercise.

General Internal Medicine Pharmacy Review
John G. O'Meara, PharmD

Antihyperlipidemic Agents

Drug (trade name)	Dose	Side effects	Drug interactions	Comments
Bile acid sequestrants				No systemic absorption, may be given to pregnant women; decrease LDL, modestly increase HDL & triglycerides
Cholestyramine (Questran, Prevalite, Locholest)	4-16 g/d in 2 or more divided doses	Bloating, constipation, flatulence	Take at least 4 h before or 2 h after other drugs	
Colestipol (Colestid)	2-16 g/d (tablet) or 5-30 g/d (powder) as single dose or divided twice daily	Same as cholestyramine	Same as cholestyramine	
Colesevelam (Welchol)	3.8 g/d as single dose or divided twice daily	Dyspepsia, constipation	Fewer drug interactions than with cholestyramine & colestipol	Least GI side effects in this class; take with a meal
HMG-CoA reductase inhibitors ("statins")				Most effective agents in lowering LDL All statins: Pregnancy category X
Lovastatin (Mevacor)	20-80 mg once daily with evening meal or divided twice daily	Headache, myalgia, increased liver enzymes, diarrhea, rhabdomyolysis (rare)	CYP3A4 inhibitors—azole antifungals (itraconazole, fluconazole, ketoconazole), macrolide antibiotics (erythromycin, clarithromycin), diltiazem, verapamil, cyclosporine, nefazodone, fluvoxamine, grapefruit juice, ritonavir, nelfinavir, indinavir—increase serum levels of lovastatin, simvastatin, and, to lesser extent, atorvastatin Fibrates (increased risk of myopathy)	Generic formulations of lovastatin are available

General Internal Medicine Pharmacy Review (continued)

Antihyperlipidemic Agents (continued)

Drug (trade name)	Dose	Side effects	Drug interactions	Comments
HMG-CoA reductase inhibitors ("statins") (continued)				
Pravastatin (Pravachol)	10-40 mg once daily at bedtime	Same as lovastatin	Cholestyramine, colestipol (decreased pravastatin absorption), amprenavir & cyclosporine (increased pravastatin serum levels), fibrates (increased risk of myopathy)	Not metabolized extensively by cytochrome system (thus, reduced potential for drug interactions)
Simvastatin (Zocor)	10-80 mg once daily at bedtime	Same as lovastatin	Same as lovastatin	
Atorvastatin (Lipitor)	10-80 mg once daily (anytime during day, $t_{1/2} \sim 14$ h)	Same as lovastatin	Same as lovastatin	Most potent statin
Fluvastatin (Lescol, Lescol XL)	20-80 mg once daily at bedtime	Same as lovastatin	Potent CYP2C9 inhibitor, warfarin (increased hypoprothrombinemic effect via inhibition of warfarin metabolism)	Least potent statin
Fibric acid derivatives				Primary effects: decrease triglycerides, increase HDL
Gemfibrozil (Lopid)	1,200 mg/d in 2 doses 30 min before morning & evening meal	Dyspepsia, diarrhea, myopathy, hepatotoxicity, cholelithiasis	Warfarin (increased risk of bleeding), statins (increased risk of myopathy), sulfonylureas (increased risk of hypoglycemia)	
Fenofibrate (Tricor)	67-201 mg once daily with a meal	Same as gemfibrozil	Same as gemfibrozil, cholestyramine & colestipol (decreased fenofibrate absorption)	
Clofibrate (Atromid-S)	1-2 g/d in 2-4 divided doses	Same as gemfibrozil	Same as gemfibrozil	"Black box warning"— liver tumorigenicity in rodents, possible increased risk of malignancy and cholelithiasis in humans, no evidence for beneficial effect on cardiovascular mortality

General Internal Medicine Pharmacy Review (continued)

Antihyperlipidemic Agents (continued)

Drug (trade name)	Dose	Side effects	Drug interactions	Comments
Nicotinic acid (niacin)				Most effective agent in increasing HDL
Immediate-release (Niacor)	2-6 g/d in 2 or more divided doses	GI distress, skin flushing, tingling & warmth, headache, hypotension, hepato-toxicity (>2 g/d, increased risk with extended-release formulation), hyperglycemia, hyperuricemia	Statins (increased risk of myopathy), chole-styramine & colestipol (decreased niacin absorption)	Aspirin 325 mg 30 min before niacin may decrease flushing reaction (prostaglandin-mediated)
Extended-release (Niaspan)	1-2 g once daily at bedtime			Immediate-release niacin: start low & titrate dose upward slowly to minimize side effects
Cholesterol absorption inhibitor				
Ezetimibe (Zetia)	10 mg once daily; take at least 2 h before or 4 h after a bile acid sequestrant	Similar to placebo in clinical trials	Cholestyramine (decreased absorption of ezetimibe), cyclosporine (increased ezetimibe levels)	Not recommended for patients with moderate or severe hepatic insufficiency No increase in myopathy or rhabdomyolysis when taken with statins
Combination agent				
Extended-release niacin/lovastatin (Advicor)	Starting dose 500/20 mg once daily at bedtime, titrate every 4 wk by 500 mg (nicotinic acid component), maximum daily dose 2,000/40 mg	See nicotinic acid and lovastatin	See nicotinic acid and lovastatin	See nicotinic acid and lovastatin

GI, gastrointestinal; HDL, high-density lipoprotein; LDL, low-density lipoprotein.

General Internal Medicine Pharmacy Review (continued)
Kari L. Beierman, PharmD

Summary of Drugs for Smoking Cessation

Drug	Toxic/adverse effects	Drug interactions	Comments
Nicotine replacement		Drug metabolism may be altered by use/nonuse of nicotine Monitor clinical outcomes	Do not smoke while taking nicotine replacement
Nicotine gum	Taste alteration, mouth/throat irritation, headache		2-mg dose (NTE 30 pieces/d) 4-mg dose (NTE 20 pieces/d)
Nicotine inhaler	Taste alteration, mouth/throat irritation, cough, headache		Usual dose is 6-16 cartridges/d; do not use >6 mo
Nicotine lozenge	Taste alteration, nausea, heartburn, hiccups, cough, headache		2- & 4-mg lozenges, start with 2 mg if first cigarette is >30 minutes after waking up and with 4 mg if first cigarette is within 30 minutes after waking up, not to exceed 20 lozenges daily of either strength
Nicotine nasal spray	Nasal/throat irritation, runny nose, watery eyes, sneezing, congestion, taste alteration, headache	Nasal vasoconstrictors	Dose is 1 mg (2 sprays, 1/nostril) to a maximum 40 mg (80 sprays daily) Irritation decreases with use
Nicotine patch	Redness, itching, & burning at application site; nervousness, headache		Apply to clean, healthy, non-hairy skin, rotate sites of application every 24 h
Nonnicotine replacement Bupropion (Zyban)	Dry mouth, insomnia, headache, nausea	MAOIs, TCAs, SSRIs, levodopa	Contraindicated for patients with previous seizure history; may be taken with/without nicotine replacement

MAOI, monoamine oxidase inhibitor; NTE, not to exceed; SSRI, selective serotonin reuptake inhibitor; TCA, tricyclic antidepressant.

General Internal Medicine Pharmacy Review (continued)

Summary of Anticoagulants

Drug	Toxic/adverse effects	Drug interactions	Comments
Warfarin (Coumadin) PO	Hemorrhage, bruising, skin lesions/necrosis	Many interactions (cytochrome P-450 enzymes), more frequent monitoring advised when new medications started/stopped	Dose based on INR Pregnancy category X
Heparin IV, SQ	Hemorrhage, hypersensitivity, thrombocytopenia	Many interactions, monitor patients closely, especially when receiving other anticoagulants	Monitor APTT, platelet counts, dose usually based on weight
Low-molecular-weight heparin, SQ 　　Dalteparin (Fragmin) 　　Enoxaparin (Lovenox) 　　Tinzaparin (Innohep)	Hemorrhage, pain/bruising at injection site	Increased bleeding risk when given with oral anticoagulants, platelet inhibitors, & thrombolytic agents	Use with caution in patient with history of heparin-induced thrombocytopenia, dosed per treatment guidelines

APTT, activated partial thromboplastin time; INR, international normalized ratio; IV, intravenous; PO, orally; SQ, subcutaneous.

Lipid-Lowering Drugs

Drug	General side effects	Hypersensitivity	Pregnancy
Colesevelam	Constipation, dyspepsia, myalgia		Effect on absorption of vitamins has not been studied
Ezetimibe (Zetia)	Diarrhea, taste disturbances, tongue paresthesias	Angioedema, rash	Safety is unknown (C)

QUESTIONS

Multiple Choice (choose the one best answer)

1. You work in an urgent care facility and know from previous data analysis that the prevalence of deep vein thrombosis among patients coming to your facility complaining of unilateral leg swelling is 20%. You also know that a quantitative latex D-dimer assay can help identify patients with blood clots, with a quoted sensitivity of 95% and a specificity of 50%. If you used this latex D-dimer assay to screen for deep vein thrombosis in everyone who presents to your facility with unilateral leg swelling, what percentage of those who test positive will actually have deep vein thrombosis?
   a. 98%
   b. 95%
   c. 50%
   d. 32%
   e. 5%

2. In question 1, what percentage of patients with a *negative* latex D-dimer assay will *not* have deep vein thrombosis?
   a. 98%
   b. 95%
   c. 50%
   d. 32%
   e. 5%

3. A well-done randomized, blinded, placebo-controlled trial evaluated the efficacy of once-daily subcutaneously injected parathyroid hormone (PTH) versus placebo in preventing vertebral fractures in osteoporotic postmenopausal women. The study duration was 20 months. During that time, 15% of the women in the placebo group had new vertebral fractures compared with 5% of those in the injected PTH group. On the basis of this information, what is the number of patients who need to be treated for 20 months with subcutaneously injected PTH to prevent one additional vertebral fracture?
   a. 3
   b. 5
   c. 10
   d. 15
   e. 33

4. A 67-year-old man is referred for perioperative cardiac risk assessment. He is scheduled to have aortobifemoral vascular bypass grafting to correct symptoms of lower extremity claudication that occur after he walks half a block. He quit smoking 8 months ago. He has no history of angina, myocardial infarction, diabetes mellitus, or congestive heart failure. He leads a fairly sedentary lifestyle. What should be the next step in perioperative evaluation and management of this patient?
   a. Treadmill exercise test
   b. Dipyridamole thallium study
   c. Computed tomography of the chest to assess for coronary calcification
   d. Coronary angiography
   e. No further testing is needed, so the patient may proceed directly to the operating room for vascular surgery

5. A 76-year-old woman is referred for a preoperative cardiac evaluation before anticipated breast biopsy of a suspicious area of calcification identified on a screening mammogram. She has a rather complex medical history that includes insulin-dependent diabetes mellitus, asthma (controlled with inhaler therapy and occasional short courses of prednisone), and an episode compatible with heart failure 2 years ago. At that time, echocardiography demonstrated a left ventricular ejection fraction of 45%. Currently, she states that she has no symptoms of angina or congestive heart failure. Current medications include inhalers, furosemide 40 mg daily, and lisinopril 10 mg daily. She does very little exertional activity. Chest radiography shows mild cardiomegaly, and no acute changes are noted on electrocardiography. What is the most appropriate next step in the perioperative evaluation and management of this patient?
   a. Treadmill exercise test
   b. Dipyridamole thallium study
   c. Exercise echocardiography
   d. Coronary angiography before the planned procedure
   e. No further testing is needed, so the patient may proceed directly to the operating room for breast biopsy

6. Ultrasonography has confirmed a new thrombus in the superficial femoral vein of a 60-year-old woman. She is otherwise healthy and states that she has not had recent trauma to the leg or serious medical illness. Her only medication is Premarin, 0.625 mg daily, for a history of hot flashes. She previously had a total abdominal hysterectomy. She states that she does not have a personal or family history of venous thromboembolism, and she does not have bleeding risks. She weighs 80 kg. What is the most appropriate next step in the management of this patient?
   a. Leg elevation and anti-inflammatory drugs until she has recovered
   b. Outpatient enoxaparin 80 mg subcutaneously every 12 hours
   c. Hospitalization and treatment with unfractionated heparin

d. Her use of oral estrogen therapy should not have increased the risk of deep vein thrombosis, and it should be continued

e. Request computed tomography of the chest and abdomen to look for occult carcinoma

7. A 54-year-old woman with diabetes mellitus who is receiving sulfonylurea therapy is referred for management of hyperlipidemia. Her past medical history includes vaginal hysterectomy. Her total cholesterol is 240 mg/dL. High-density lipoprotein (HDL) cholesterol is 40 mg/dL and the triglyceride level is 250 mg/dL. Similar values were noted 6 months ago when she met with a dietitian. The patient states that she has been compliant with diet therapy. The hemoglobin A_{1C} level is at the upper limit of normal. Which one of the following is the most appropriate next step in the management of this patient's hyperlipidemia?

a. Continue diet and exercise

b. Ask the dietitian to reinstruct this patient, and ask the patient to return in 6 months so the lipid values can be determined again

c. Begin treatment with an HMG-CoA reductase inhibitor

d. Begin treatment with gemfibrozil because she has diabetes and an increased level of low-density lipoprotein (LDL) cholesterol

e. Initiate estrogen therapy

ANSWERS

1. Answer d.

A 2×2 table must be constructed to determine the positive predictive value for the D-dimer test among patients being evaluated for deep vein thrombosis. The correct answer is $\frac{a}{a+b}$, or $\frac{190}{590} = 32\%$.

Diagnostic test result		Disease present	Disease absent	
	Positive	190 a	400 b	590 a+b
	Negative	c 10	d 400	c+d 410
		a+c 200	b+d 800	a+b+c+d 1,000

2. Answer a.

The negative predictive value of the D-dimer test is $\frac{d}{c+d}$ or $\frac{400}{410} = 98\%$.

3. Answer c.

You are asked to determine the number needed to treat (NNT) in a randomized controlled trial showing that the PTH-treated group had an event rate of 5%, or EER = 5%. The placebo group had an event rate of 15%, or CER = 15%. The formula for NNT $= \frac{1}{ARR}$. ARR = (CER − EER) or, in this case, 15% − 5% = 10%. Therefore, NNT $= \frac{1}{0.25} = 10$.

4. Answer b.

Although this patient has no history concerning clinical predictors, he has poor functional status (<4 METs). Therefore, according to the American College of Cardiology/American Heart Association Stepwise Approach, he should have noninvasive testing before proceeding with a high-risk surgical procedure such as major vascular surgery. On the basis of the results of treatment, he could either go to the operating room or undergo further invasive testing.

5. Answer e.

The patient has intermediate clinical predictors (diabetes mellitus and compensated congestive heart failure). She also has poor or indeterminate exercise tolerance. However, the intended procedure has a low surgical risk, and according to the American College of Cardiology/American Heart Association Stepwise Approach, she can proceed directly to the operating room without further testing.

6. Answer b.

The superficial femoral vein is in the deep venous system; therefore, conservative treatment is not appropriate. Outpatient low-molecular-weight heparin has been approved by the U.S. Food and Drug Administration for the treatment of deep venous thrombosis. Enoxaparin (one of the approved low-molecular-weight heparin agents) is dosed at 1 mg/kg subcutaneously every 12 hours for treatment of deep venous thrombosis. Therefore, the correct dose of enoxaparin for this patient would be 80 mg subcutaneously every 12 hours. There appears to be no indication for hospitalization in this case. Oral estrogen therapy is associated with an increased risk of deep venous thrombosis. One might consider discontinuing treatment with this drug or replacing it with transdermal estrogen, which may have less of a procoagulant effect. It is not recommended to go on a "witch-hunt" and look for occult malignancy in patients who present with idiopathic venous thrombosis. Routine age-appropriate cancer screening is recommended, but this would not include computed tomography of the chest and abdomen.

7. Answer c.

The patient has a coronary artery disease risk equivalent, that is, diabetes mellitus. In this circumstance, the LDL level at which to consider drug therapy is ≥130 mg/dL. Because of this, her failure on diet and a calculated LDL cholesterol of 150 mg/dL, it is appropriate to initiate lipid-lowering drug therapy. An HMG-CoA reductase inhibitor is the drug of choice for patients with diabetes. Gemfibrozil is a consideration, but because of the potential drug interaction with sulfonylureas, it would not be a good choice. Oral estrogen could increase triglyceride values (not lower them) and has not been proven to decrease the risk of coronary artery disease.

CHAPTER 9

GENETICS

Virginia V. Michels, M.D.

Genetic factors play a role in the development of many types of human disease. Genetic determinants may be chromosome abnormalities, single gene defects, mitochondrial mutations, or epigenetic or multifactorial factors.

CHROMOSOME ABNORMALITIES

Approximately a sixth of all birth defects and cases of congenitally determined mental retardation are due to chromosome abnormalities. Chromosome abnormalities occur in about 1 in 180 live births. One-third of these abnormalities involve an abnormal number (aneuploidy) of non-sex chromosomes (autosomes). Factors known to result in a higher-than-average risk for having a child with autosomal aneuploidy are maternal age 35 years or older and having previously had an affected child. Prenatal diagnosis by karyotyping of fetal cells obtained by amniocentesis or chorionic villus sampling can be offered to pregnant women who are at increased risk.

- Chromosome abnormalities occur in 1 in 180 live births.
- Risk factors for autosomal aneuploidy: maternal age ≥35 years and having had an affected child.

Down Syndrome

The most common autosomal aneuploidy syndrome in term infants is Down syndrome (incidence, 1 in 880). The most serious consequence of Down syndrome is mild-to-moderate mental retardation (average IQ, about 50). Forty percent of patients with Down syndrome have a congenital heart defect, most frequently ventricular septal defect or atrioventricular canal defect, although other congenital heart defects may occur. Thyroid disease is frequent, and Alzheimer disease develops at a relatively early age in many. A few patients have hypoplasia of the odontoid process, which is important to diagnose before participation in certain sports. Males with Down syndrome are usually sterile, but affected females are fertile and have a very high risk of having an affected child. Most persons with Down syndrome have trisomy 21 as a result

of a new mutation nondisjunctional event; in these cases, the risk to the parents of having another affected child is 1% to 2% or higher, depending on maternal age. In 3% of persons with Down syndrome, a translocation chromosome abnormality is present, in which the extra chromosome 21 is attached to another chromosome, most commonly 14 (Fig. 9-1). These translocation chromosomes may be inherited in an *unbalanced* form from a parent carrying a *balanced* form of the translocation; these parents have a 5% to 15% risk of having another affected child. Even if the parents have completed their childbearing, the karyotype of the affected individual should be determined so that other relatives (e.g., adult siblings) can be counseled. The same principles are presumed to be true for other autosomal aneuploidy syndromes.

- The most serious consequence of Down syndrome is mild-to-moderate mental retardation.
- The most frequent heart defect in Down syndrome is ventricular septal defect or atrioventricular canal defect.
- Males with Down syndrome are usually sterile, but females are fertile.
- Most persons with Down syndrome have trisomy 21.
- Early-onset Alzheimer disease is common in adults with Down syndrome.

Sex Chromosome Aneuploidy Syndromes

Approximately 35% of chromosome abnormalities in live-born infants involve sex chromosome aneuploidy. These infants may have an additional X or Y chromosome or be lacking one. Patients with 47,XXX or 47,XYY karyotypes usually have no major birth defects or mental retardation, although the mean IQ may be 90 rather than 100. Patients with a 47,XXY karyotype (Klinefelter syndrome) have small testes, infertility, and a tall eunuchoid body habitus. They are at increased risk for breast cancer and leg ulcers. Patients with a 45,X karyotype (Turner syndrome) or its variants—one structurally abnormal X, such as 46,X,i(X)q (Fig. 9-2)—or mosaicism for an X or Y chromosome—such as 45,X/46,XX—usually are mentally normal.

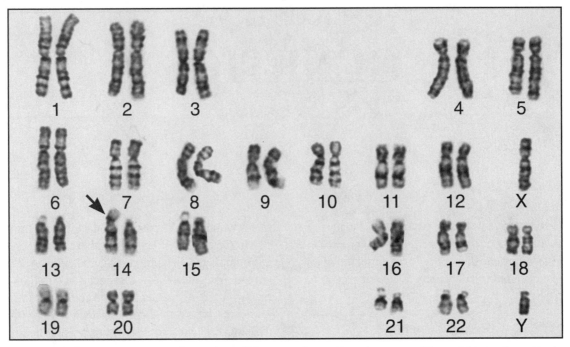

Fig. 9-1. Karyotype 46,XY,−14,+t(14;21)(p11;q11) from patient with Down syndrome. Extra chromosome 21 material is translocated to chromosome 14 (*arrow*). Result is robertsonian translocation. (Karyotype courtesy of G. Dewald, Ph.D.)

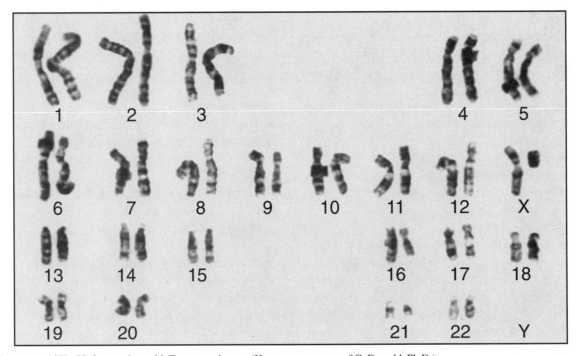

Fig. 9-2. Karyotype 46,X,r(X) from patient with Turner syndrome. (Karyotype courtesy of G. Dewald, Ph.D.)

Fluorescent in situ hybridization probes can be used to distinguish a marker X versus Y, a distinction that is important for determining risk of gonadal malignancy (increased with Y chromosome material). Streak gonads are usually present. Patients have a risk of approximately 30% for a bicuspid aortic valve with or without coarctation of the aorta. Women with Turner syndrome are at increased risk for ascending aortic aneurysm formation, and thus periodic echocardiographic monitoring is recommended. Short stature, webbed neck, increased number of pigmented nevi, failure to develop secondary sexual characteristics, short 4th or 5th metacarpals or metatarsals, renal malformations, and increased risk for thyroid disease are also variably present.

- Typical case of 47,XXY karyotype (Klinefelter syndrome): small testes, infertility, tall eunuchoid body habitus.
- Typical case of 45,X karyotype (Turner syndrome): short stature, lack of secondary sex characteristics, usually mentally normal, 30% risk of bicuspid aortic valve or aortic coarctation.
- Risk for ascending aortic aneurysm is increased in Turner syndrome.

Other Chromosome Abnormalities

Thirty-four percent of chromosome abnormalities involve structural changes such as deletions, duplications, inversions, or translocations. They may be detected by peripheral blood karyotype or, for more subtle alterations, by subtelomeric fluorescent in situ hybridization probes (Fig. 9-3). The translocations may be balanced (no net loss or gain of genetic material) or unbalanced. People with balanced translocations are usually phenotypically normal and healthy but may be at increased risk for miscarriages or their children may have birth defects. Patients with net loss or gain of genetic material by any of the mechanisms listed above have phenotypic abnormalities that usually include mental subnormality and frequently other major or minor birth defects. Parents of all patients with a structural chromosome abnormality should have chromosome analyses to determine whether they are carriers of a balanced translocation.

- Parents of all patients with a structural chromosome abnormality should have chromosome analyses.

Fragile X-Linked Mental Retardation

The fragile X-linked mental retardation syndrome occurs in about 1 in 1,000 males. It is characterized by a visible fragile site on the long arm of an X chromosome at band q27 when the lymphocytes are cultured in media deficient in folic acid (Fig. 9-4). The fragile site is never observed in all cells, and the frequency may be as low as 4%. Some carrier females do not express the fragile site cytogenetically. Affected males may be physically normal or have a long, thin face with prominent jaw, large simplified ears, and enlarged testes. Carrier females are phenotypically normal or mildly retarded and dysmorphic. The degree of mental retardation ranges from mild to profound.

- Males with fragile X: may be physically normal or have a long, thin face, prominent jaw, large ears, enlarged testes, mild to profound mental retardation.

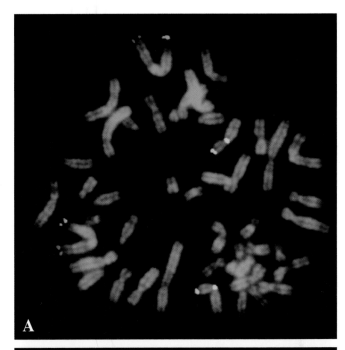

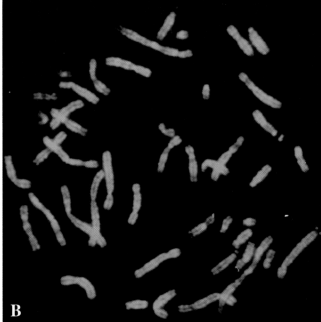

Fig. 9-3. Fluorescent DNA probes for subtelomeres of each p and q arm of all chromosomes, except acrocentric p arms, are used to analyze a complete set of subtelomere regions. *A*, A normal pattern of 1 p in green, 1 q in orange, and Xp in yellow (fusion of green and orange) and X centromere in aqua (used as control). *B*, Chromosomes 16p in green and 16q in orange have a normal pattern but, in addition, 16q probe is present on 4q. Thus, this chromosome 4 is derivative so that 4p probe is deleted (not shown) and 16q subtelomere region is duplicated. (Photograph courtesy of S. Jalal, Ph.D.)

- Carrier females: phenotypically normal or mildly retarded and dysmorphic.

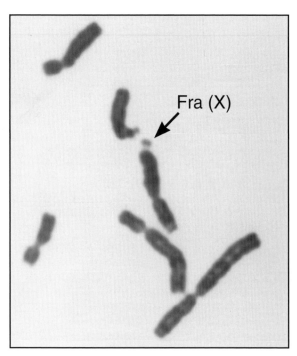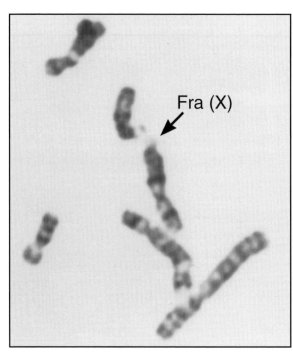

Fig. 9-4. Chromosome analysis from patient with fragile X syndrome. Fragile site is visible on long arm of X chromosome at band q27 when lymphocytes are cultured in media deficient in folic acid. (Photograph courtesy of G. Dewald, Ph.D.)

PATTERNS OF INHERITANCE

Autosomal Dominant

In autosomal dominant inheritance, the responsible gene is located on one of the autosomes and one copy of the gene is sufficient for the trait to be expressed or for the disease to be present (i.e., heterozygotes have the disease). There is a 50% chance that any child born to an affected person will inherit the abnormal gene.

● Autosomal dominant inheritance: responsible gene is located on autosome.
● There is a 50% chance that a child of an affected person will inherit the abnormal gene.

The severity of the disease caused by the abnormal gene may be uniform for some conditions, such as achondroplasia, but the severity may be variable for other conditions, such as neurofibromatosis and Marfan syndrome. This difference of severity is referred to as "variable expression." In contrast, "incomplete penetrance" means that some persons who have inherited the gene show no signs of it. Obviously, the clinical decision regarding whether a person has signs of the gene defect depends on the thoroughness of the examination and on the sensitivity of the investigative techniques. For example, many families with hypertrophic cardiomyopathy were thought to include members with incomplete penetrance until asymptomatic relatives were examined with echocardiography.

Although transmission of a disease through members of either sex through multiple generations of a family strongly suggests autosomal dominant inheritance, it is important to remember that autosomal dominant diseases can occur without a positive family history. This can occur because of incomplete penetrance, new mutation, somatic mosaicism, or incorrect assignment of paternity. New mutation events represent changes in the genetic material of the individual egg or sperm that give rise to the fetus. Although the risk for siblings of a person whose disease arose by new mutation is not increased over that of the general population, the risk for offspring still is 50%. Somatic mosaicism refers to the possibility that one of the parents has the gene defect in only some cells, including the reproductive cells (germinal mosaicism), such that the person has no or few signs of the disease but potentially can transmit the disease to one or more children.

● In autosomal dominant inheritance, disease severity may be uniform or variable.
● Incomplete penetrance: no signs of abnormal gene in a person who has inherited it.
● Somatic mosaicism: person has gene defect in only some cells.

Some of the diseases with autosomal dominant inheritance are listed in Table 9-1 and summarized on the following pages.

Imprinting is an epigenetic phenomenon that can influence the observed pattern of disease occurrence within families with single gene defects. For imprinted genes, the gene's activity (i.e., expression) in an individual differs depending on the parent (mother or father) from whom the gene was inherited. At the molecular level, these differences may result from methylation status and possibly other factors. An example of imprinting occurs in autosomal dominant familial paragangliomas due to *SDHD* gene mutations. Paragangliomas can develop in a person who inherits the defective gene from his or her father, but they do not develop in a person who inherits the defective gene from his or her mother. Regardless of whether or not a paraganglioma develops, the defective gene can be transmitted to the next generation.

Ehlers-Danlos Syndromes

There are at least seven forms of Ehlers-Danlos syndrome. Type I, or gravis type, serves as a prototype for discussion of

Table 9-1 Diseases With Autosomal Dominant Inheritance

Achondroplasia
Amyloidosis (many types)
Ehlers-Danlos syndrome, types I, II, III, VIII, some type IV, VI, and VII
Hereditary spherocytosis
Huntington disease
Hypertrophic cardiomyopathy
LEOPARD* syndrome
Low-density lipoprotein (LDL) receptor deficiency (hypercholesterolemia)
Marfan syndrome
Multiple endocrine neoplasia, types I, IIa, and IIb
Myotonic dystrophy
Neurofibromatosis, types 1 and 2
Noonan syndrome†
Osler-Weber-Rendu disease (hereditary hemorrhagic telangiectasia)
Osteogenesis imperfecta, types I and IV, most type II
Polycystic kidney disease (some forms are autosomal recessive)
Porphyria (several types)
Pseudoxanthoma elasticum (some forms are autosomal recessive)
Tuberous sclerosis
Von Hippel-Lindau disease
Von Willebrand disease

---

*Lentigenes (multiple), electrocardiographic conduction abnormalities, ocular hypertelorism, pulmonary stenosis, abnormalities of genitalia, retardation of growth, deafness.
†Most cases are sporadic, but there is good evidence that they have new mutation autosomal dominant disease.

this group of genetically heterogeneous disorders. The syndrome is inherited as an autosomal dominant condition. The basic defect in type I disease has been defined for some cases as a defect in the α-1 or α-2 chain of type V collagen. The disorder is characterized by velvety textured, hyperextensible, fragile skin that bruises and splits easily and heals poorly, resulting in wide, thin scars. Many tissues are friable, which is an important consideration when surgical procedures are needed. Even fetal membranes are affected and frequently rupture before term, resulting in premature birth. Wrinkled, redundant skin may develop over the knee and elbow joints. Small fat- or mucin-containing spherules may be present in the subcutaneous tissue and may be calcified. The joints are hyperextensible and prone to dislocations. Pes planus, scoliosis, degenerative arthritis, visceral diverticulosis, and spontaneous pneumothorax may occur. Mitral valve prolapse may occur in 50% of patients. Dilatation of the aortic root or pulmonary artery and prolapse of the tricuspid valve may occur. Vascular rupture is relatively rare.

- Ehlers-Danlos type I is an autosomal dominant condition.
- Features: velvety textured, hyperextensible, fragile skin.
- Joints are hyperextensible and prone to dislocation.
- Associated conditions: pes planus, scoliosis, degenerative arthritis, visceral diverticulosis, spontaneous pneumothorax.
- Mitral valve prolapse occurs in 50% of patients.
- Vascular rupture is relatively rare in types I and II.

Hypertrophic Cardiomyopathy

Hypertrophic cardiomyopathy frequently is inherited as an autosomal dominant disorder. Penetrance ranges from more than 60% to 100% in different families when relatives are studied with electrocardiography and echocardiography. Investigation of first-degree relatives is necessary. Even if parents are normal by echocardiography, the possibility of new mutation cannot be excluded, and children born to an affected parent must be considered at risk and should be evaluated.

- Hypertrophic cardiomyopathy is autosomal dominant.
- Investigation of first-degree relatives is necessary.
- Children of affected parents are at risk.

The course of the disease may be variable, even within a family; therefore, the age at onset cannot be predicted precisely.

- The course of the disease is variable.
- The age at onset cannot be predicted.

Molecular defects that can cause hypertrophic cardiomyopathy include the β cardiac myosin heavy-chain gene, cardiac troponin T, troponin I, α-tropomyosin, myosin-binding protein

C, ventricular myosin essential light chain, ventricular myosin-regulating light chain, cardiac actin, γ2 regulatory subunit of adenosine monophosphate-activated kinase, and possibly others that remain unidentified.

Marfan Syndrome

The Marfan syndrome has an incidence of 1 in 10,000. It is an autosomal dominant disorder with variable expression, and approximately 20% of cases arise by new mutation. There are no well-documented instances of nonpenetrance.

- Marfan syndrome is relatively common—1 in 10,000.
- It is an autosomal dominant disorder.
- About 20% of cases arise by new mutation.

Marfan syndrome involves the musculoskeletal, ocular, and cardiovascular systems. Skeletal abnormalities include tall stature, a low upper:lower segment ratio (limbs are relatively long compared with the trunk), scoliosis or kyphosis, and pectus deformities. Increased joint laxity and hyperextensibility are common, but occasionally patients have limited extension of fingers and elbows. The face may be long and the palate highly arched. This "marfanoid habitus" may be present in patients with other disorders such as other connective tissue dysplasias, multiple endocrine neoplasia type IIb, Stickler syndrome, and homocystinuria. The characteristic body habitus is never sufficient evidence for making the diagnosis of Marfan syndrome in the absence of other criteria.

- Marfan syndrome involves the musculoskeletal, ocular, and cardiovascular systems.
- Typical case: tall stature, low upper:lower segment ratio, scoliosis or kyphosis, pectus deformities, lens subluxation, aortic regurgitation due to aortic root dissection.
- Increased joint laxity and hyperextensibility are common.

The ocular abnormalities associated with Marfan syndrome may include subluxation of the lenses, myopia, and retinal detachment. Dislocation of the lenses occurs in 50% to 80% of patients; the lens frequently is displaced upward. Gross dislocations may be evident without the aid of special equipment, but lesser degrees of dislocation may be evident only by slit-lamp examination. Therefore, all patients suspected of having Marfan syndrome must have a complete ophthalmologic evaluation. Patients with Marfan syndrome should have frequent ophthalmologic examinations to permit early detection of complications such as retinal detachment or glaucoma.

- Ocular abnormalities of Marfan syndrome: subluxation of lenses, myopia, retinal detachment.
- Dislocations occur in 50%-80% of cases.

- All patients must have ophthalmologic evaluation.

The life expectancy of patients with Marfan syndrome is shortened because of cardiovascular disease. The most common manifestation is mitral valve prolapse with or without mitral regurgitation. Prophylactic antibiotic therapy for bacterial endocarditis is warranted. Acute onset of severe mitral regurgitation due to rupture of chordae tendineae may occur even in childhood. Mitral valve prolapse in a patient with a "marfanoid" body habitus is not a sufficient basis for the diagnosis of Marfan syndrome in the absence of a positive family history of Marfan syndrome or other characteristic findings. Patients with some forms of Ehlers-Danlos syndrome and nonspecific connective tissue dysplasias can have a similar body habitus, joint laxity, and mitral valve prolapse.

- Life expectancy in Marfan syndrome is shortened by cardiovascular disease.
- Mitral valve prolapse in Marfan syndrome is progressive.
- Prophylactic antibiotic for bacterial endocarditis is warranted.

Dilatation of the ascending aorta is the next most common cardiovascular disorder; it may lead to aortic regurgitation, aortic rupture, or dissecting aneurysm. Although less than 70% of patients have evidence of cardiovascular disease on physical examination, more than 80% have abnormalities detected by echocardiography.

- Most common cardiovascular manifestations are mitral valve prolapse and dilatation of ascending aorta.
- More than 80% of patients have abnormalities found on echocardiography.

Although surgical risks are increased in patients with Marfan syndrome because of tissue friability, surgical treatment frequently is successful for mitral and aortic regurgitation and for aortic dissection.

- Surgical risks are increased in Marfan syndrome.
- Surgical treatment is often successful for mitral and aortic regurgitation and aortic dissection.

Additional features sometimes associated with Marfan syndrome include decreased amounts of subcutaneous tissue, skin striae, inguinal hernias, pneumothorax, and degenerative joint disease.

The basic cause of Marfan syndrome is a defect in fibrillin; the gene encoding fibrillin is on chromosome 15q15-21. Presymptomatic and prenatal diagnosis is possible in some families. However, because of limitations in molecular genetic testing, clinical criteria remain the appropriate basis for diagnosis.

- The cause of Marfan syndrome is a defect in fibrillin.

Myotonic Dystrophy

Myotonic dystrophy, the most common form of muscular dystrophy in adults, has an incidence of approximately 1 per 8,000 to 20,000. The inheritance pattern is autosomal dominant with extremely variable expression. Although the average age at onset is in the second to third decade of life, the disease may be evident at birth or may first be noticed in the seventh decade. The disease is characterized by myotonia, muscle atrophy and weakness, ptosis of the eyelids, and expressionless facies resulting from particularly severe involvement of facial and temporal muscles. The rate of progression of the disease is variable, but disability is usually severe within 15 to 20 years after onset. Associated abnormalities may include premature frontal baldness, testicular atrophy or menstrual irregularities, gastrointestinal symptoms related to smooth muscle involvement, and cardiac disease. Distinctive refractile posterior subcapsular cataracts often are evident by slit-lamp examination. Although glucose intolerance is common, overt diabetes mellitus occurs in only about 6% of patients.

- Myotonic dystrophy is the most common form of muscular dystrophy in adults.
- The incidence is 1 in 8,000-20,000.
- The inheritance pattern is autosomal dominant with extremely variable expression.
- The age at onset is usually the second to third decade of life.
- Typical case of myotonic dystrophy: myotonia, muscle atrophy and weakness, ptosis of eyelids, expressionless facies, and premature frontal baldness.
- Disability is severe within 15-20 years after onset.
- Associated abnormalities: testicular atrophy or menstrual irregularities, gastrointestinal symptoms.
- Diabetes mellitus occurs in 6% of patients.

The diagnosis is based on clinical findings and a typical electromyographic pattern characterized by prolonged rhythmic discharges. The gene for myotonic dystrophy is located on chromosome 19q13, and genetic counseling is warranted for the patient and family. First-degree relatives should be investigated. The risk for children born to an affected parent is 50%. The molecular basis of most cases of myotonic dystrophy is expansion of a CTG trinucleotide repeat sequence affecting a gene encoding a protein kinase. Thus, direct DNA-based diagnosis of the disease is possible in most cases.

- The diagnosis of myotonic dystrophy is based on clinical and electromyographic findings or DNA analysis.
- Genetic counseling is warranted for patients and family members with myotonic dystrophy.

- First-degree relatives should be investigated.

Cardiac disease is present in approximately two-thirds of patients with myotonic dystrophy, and sudden death may occur.

- Cardiac disease occurs in two-thirds of patients with myotonic dystrophy, and sudden death may occur.

Neurofibromatosis

Type 1

Neurofibromatosis 1 is an autosomal dominant disorder with an incidence of approximately 1 in 3,500. Approximately 50% of patients have the disease because of a new mutation. The disorder has markedly variable expression but very high penetrance. The diagnosis is based on two or more of the following clinical criteria: six or more café-au-lait macules of 1.5 cm or more in diameter (in a child, five or more that are 0.5 cm), axillary or inguinal freckling, two or more Lisch nodules of the iris, two or more neurofibromas or one plexiform neurofibroma, a definitely positive family history, or one of these and one of the uncommon characteristic manifestations such as orbital or sphenoid wing dysplasia, optic or other central nervous system glioma, renal artery dysplasia with or without abdominal aortic coarctation, or tibial pseudofracture. Additional, less specific signs of the disease may include pheochromocytoma and scoliosis. Malignancy, often neurofibrosarcoma, develops in fewer than 10% of patients. Patients should have, at minimum, an annual physical examination, including blood pressure check and thorough neurologic assessment. The gene has been identified and is a GTPase-activating protein involved in the ras signaling process. The gene is very large, and multiple different mutations have been identified. Therefore, DNA-based testing for direct diagnosis is difficult. Linkage analysis can be used for presymptomatic or prenatal diagnosis in informed families (see below, *Linkage Analysis*).

- Neurofibromatosis 1 is autosomal dominant.
- The incidence is 1 in 3,500.
- The disorder has markedly variable expression but very high penetrance.
- Malignancy (often neurofibrosarcoma) develops in fewer than 10% of patients.
- Multiple different mutations have been identified.

Type 2

Neurofibromatosis 2 is an autosomal dominant disorder that is genetically distinct from neurofibromatosis 1. It is characterized by bilateral vestibular schwannomas (commonly referred to as "acoustic neuroma" in the past) or a family history of neurofibromatosis 2 with a unilateral vestibular schwannoma, or two of the following: meningioma, glioma, neurofibroma, schwannoma, or posterior subcapsular lenticular opacities. Café-au-lait macules may or may not be present. The gene has been identified and is localized to the long arm of chromosome 22. It has been referred to as either "merlin" or "schwannomin." In addition to occurring in the germline of patients with neurofibromatosis 2, acquired mutations in this gene occur in some sporadic meningiomas and schwannomas. DNA-based diagnosis is available by linkage analysis in some familial cases or, preferably, by direct mutation analysis in many patients. Patients should have an annual physical examination with thorough neurologic assessment, monitoring of hearing, and magnetic resonance imaging of the head with gadolinium. Magnetic resonance imaging of the spine should be done in patients with newly diagnosed disease or patients with symptoms referable to the spinal cord.

- Neurofibromatosis 2 is autosomal dominant.
- Characteristics: vestibular schwannomas, sometimes nervous system gliomas, subcapsular cataracts, café-au-lait macules.

Osteogenesis Imperfecta

Osteogenesis imperfecta is characterized by multiple bone fractures, and some patients have opalescent teeth, blue sclerae, and hearing loss. Some patients have increased bruisability.

Tuberous Sclerosis

Tuberous sclerosis is an autosomal dominant disorder with variable expression and high penetrance. Approximately 50% of cases arise by new mutation. Tuberous sclerosis is characterized by cortical or retinal tubers, seizures, mental retardation in less than 50%, depigmented "ash leaf" macules, facial angiofibromas, dental pits, subungual or periungual fibromas, shagreen patches, and renal cysts or angiomyolipomas. Cardiac rhabdomyomas are more frequent in the fetus and infant and often resolve with age. Pulmonary fibrosis resulting in a "honeycomb" appearance on radiography or computed tomography is more frequent in young women and tends to progress rapidly. Central nervous system astrocytomas may occur. There is non-allelic heterogeneity, with one gene defect that causes tuberous sclerosis on chromosome 9 and another on chromosome 16. The gene on chromosome 9 is referred to as hamartin; that on chromosome 16 is called tuberin. Both act as tumor suppressor genes.

- Tuberous sclerosis is autosomal dominant and has high penetrance.
- About 50% of cases arise by new mutation.
- Typical case: cortical or retinal tubers, seizures, mental retardation in <50%, "ash leaf" macules, angiofibromas,

subungual or periungual fibromas, shagreen patches, and renal cysts or angiomyolipomas.

Von Hippel-Lindau Disease

Von Hippel-Lindau disease is characterized by retinal, spinal cord, and cerebellar hemangioblastomas; cysts of the kidneys, pancreas, and epididymis; and renal cancers. Other manifestations include hemangioblastomas of the medulla oblongata, cysts and hemangiomas of other visceral organs, pancreatic cancer, and pheochromocytomas. Retinal hemangioblastomas may be the earliest manifestation.

- Typical case: retinal, spinal cord, and cerebellar hemangioblastomas; cysts of kidneys, pancreas, and epididymis.
- Retinal hemangioblastomas may be the earliest manifestation of von Hippel-Lindau disease.

Hemangioblastomas of the central nervous system in von Hippel-Lindau disease are benign, and associated morbidity is due to space-occupying effects. They occur most frequently in the cerebellum and spinal cord but also can be in the medulla oblongata and rarely in the cerebrum.

Renal cysts, hemangiomas, and benign adenomas are usually asymptomatic. Renal clear cell cancers are bilateral or multiple in 40% to 87% of cases. They are the leading cause of death, which occurs at a mean age of 44 years.

- Renal cysts, hemangiomas, and benign adenomas are usually asymptomatic in von Hippel-Lindau disease.
- Renal cancer is a major cause of death.

Inheritance is autosomal dominant, and the risk for any child born to an affected person is 50%. Expression is variable, and penetrance is high in thoroughly evaluated families. Males and females are affected equally.

- Von Hippel-Lindau disease is autosomal dominant.

The gene that causes von Hippel-Lindau disease is localized to chromosome 3p25-26. The normal gene has a key role in cellular response to hypoxia and acts as a tumor suppressor. Presymptomatic and prenatal diagnosis by direct mutation analysis is possible for most patients.

Autosomal Recessive

Autosomal recessive disease occurs because of abnormal genes that are located on the autosomes. However, one copy of the abnormal gene is not sufficient to cause disease, and heterozygotes (carriers) are not clinically different from the general population. When two persons who are heterozygotes for a given gene defect mate, the children are at 25% risk of inheriting the abnormal gene from both parents and, thus, of having the disease.

- Autosomal recessive inheritance: abnormal genes are located on autosomes, but one copy of the abnormal gene is not sufficient to cause disease.
- Heterozygotes (carriers) are not clinically different from the general population.

Because the heterozygous state may be transmitted silently through many generations before the chance mating of two heterozygotes occurs, it is not surprising that there rarely is a family history of the disease in previous generations. The occurrence of multiple affected siblings within a family suggests autosomal recessive inheritance; however, because of the small average family size in this country, many autosomal recessive diseases seem to occur as isolated cases.

The risk for the children of a person who has an autosomal recessive disease depends on the frequency of the abnormal gene in the population. Except for common diseases such as cystic fibrosis or sickle cell anemia, the risk is usually small, provided that this person does not marry a relative or a person who has a family history of the same disease.

Many diseases that are caused by an identified metabolic defect, such as homocystinuria, are autosomal recessive diseases due to an enzyme deficiency. When the enzymatic defect is established, carrier testing and prenatal diagnosis sometimes are possible.

Some of the diseases with autosomal recessive inheritance are listed in Table 9-2 and summarized on the following pages.

Friedreich Ataxia

This is an autosomal recessive disorder. The first sign of the disease is ataxic gait. The mean age at onset is approximately 12 years. Dysarthria, hypotonic muscle weakness, loss of vibration and position senses, and loss of deep tendon reflexes develop subsequently. In some patients, diabetes mellitus, nystagmus, optic atrophy, dementia, respiratory dysfunction due to kyphoscoliosis, and decreased sensory nerve conduction velocities also develop. The major cause of death is cardiomyopathy. Since detection of the gene defect, many atypical cases have been recognized, such as with preservation of deep tendon reflexes.

- Friedreich ataxia is autosomal recessive.
- Typical clinical scenario: A 12-year-old child presents with an ataxic gait, dysarthria, hypotonic muscle weakness, loss of vibration and position senses, and loss of deep tendon reflexes develop subsequently.
- The major cause of death is cardiomyopathy.

Table 9-2 Diseases With Autosomal Recessive Inheritance

Alkaptonuria
α_1-Antitrypsin deficiency
Cystic fibrosis
Familial Mediterranean fever
Friedreich ataxia
Gaucher disease
Glycogen storage disease, types I, II, III, IV, V, VII
Hemochromatosis
Homocystinuria
Oculocutaneous albinism
Phenylketonuria
Pseudoxanthoma elasticum (some forms are autosomal
   dominant)
Refsum disease
Sickle-cell disease
Tay-Sachs disease
α- and β-Thalassemia
Wilson disease

In one series, 60 of 82 patients with Friedreich ataxia had clinical evidence of cardiac dysfunction 4 months to 4 years before death, and 56% died of heart failure. The mean age at death was 36.6 years. Cardiac arrhythmias, particularly atrial fibrillation, were common and occurred in 50% of fatal cases.

- Cardiac arrhythmias occur in 50% of fatal cases of Friedreich ataxia.

The risk for a sibling being affected is 25%. The gene involved, localized to chromosome 9q12-21.1, has been named frataxin, and the mechanism of mutation is most frequently expansion of GAA trinucleotide repeat.

- The risk of Friedreich ataxia in a sibling of an affected person is 25%.

Gaucher Disease

Gaucher disease is an autosomal recessive disorder due to deficiency of the enzyme glucocerebrosidase, which results in lipid storage in the spleen, liver, bone marrow, and other organs. Type 1 (nonneuronopathic) disease is most frequent in Ashkenazi Jews (carrier frequency, 1 in 10). The disease may be asymptomatic at any age or present in childhood or adulthood with splenomegaly, hepatosplenomegaly, thrombocytopenia, anemia, degenerative bone disease, osteoporosis, or pulmonary disease. Type 2 (infantile, neuronopathic) has no ethnic predisposition, and type 3 (juvenile form) has intermediate clinical signs. The first sign of neurologic involvement in types 2 and 3 is supranuclear ophthalmoplegia. Enzyme replacement therapy is effective for nonneuronopathic Gaucher disease.

- Gaucher disease is autosomal recessive.
- The disease is due to deficiency of the enzyme glucocerebrosidase.
- Type 1 is most frequent in Ashkenazi Jews.
- Type 2 has no ethnic predisposition.
- The first sign of neurologic involvement in types 2 and 3 is supranuclear ophthalmoplegia.
- Enzyme replacement therapy is effective for nonneuronopathic Gaucher disease.

Glycogen Storage Diseases

Glycogen storage disease type I is due to deficiency of the enzyme glucose-6-phosphatase. It is characterized by hypoglycemia, hypercholesterolemia, hyperuricemia, lactic acidosis, short stature, hepatomegaly, and delayed onset of puberty. In adults with this disease, malignant hepatomas, premature coronary disease, pancreatitis, gout, and renal disease may develop.

- Glycogen storage disease type I is due to deficiency of the enzyme glucose-6-phosphatase.
- Characteristics: hypoglycemia, hypercholesterolemia, hyperuricemia, lactic acidosis, short stature, hepatomegaly, delayed puberty.

Glycogen storage disease type II (Pompe disease) is an autosomal recessive disorder due to deficiency of the lysosomal enzyme α-1,4-glucosidase (acid maltase). The infantile form is characterized by hypotonia, macroglossia, and progressive cardiomyopathy resulting in death within the first year of life.

- Glycogen storage disease type II is autosomal recessive.
- The disease is due to deficiency of the enzyme α-1,4-glucosidase.
- Characteristics of infantile form: hypotonia, macroglossia, progressive cardiomyopathy.

Juvenile and adult forms of glycogen storage disease type II also exist. The presenting characteristic is skeletal muscle weakness, and cardiac involvement usually is absent or minimal.

- Characteristics of juvenile and adult forms of glycogen storage disease: skeletal muscle weakness, minimal or absent cardiac involvement.

Glycogen storage disease type III is due to an autosomal recessively inherited deficiency of amylo-1,6-glucosidase (debrancher) activity. The enzyme is deficient in the liver, and in some patients also in skeletal muscle, cultured skin fibroblasts, and leukocytes. Clinically, the disorder is characterized by hepatomegaly and growth retardation that resolves at puberty. There may be hypoglycemia and hyperlipidemia. Skeletal muscle weakness may develop in adult life. Cardiomyopathy, when present, may be life-threatening and mimic hypertrophic cardiomyopathy. Histologic evaluation of cardiac tissue reveals increased intracellular glycogen with no disarray of myofibers or myofibrils. Deficiency of the enzyme has been documented in cardiac muscle.

- Glycogen storage disease type III is autosomal recessive.
- The disease is due to deficiency of amylo-1,6-glucosidase activity.
- Characteristics: hepatomegaly and growth retardation that resolves at puberty.

Homocystinuria

The classic form of homocystinuria is due to an autosomal recessively inherited deficiency of cystathionine β-synthase. The incidence of the disease is approximately 1 per 200,000. Clinically, it is characterized by tall stature with a low upper segment:lower segment ratio, pectus deformities, scoliosis, genu valgum, pes planus, and a highly arched palate. Lens dislocation is progressive, and the direction of displacement is usually, but not always, downward. Myopia, retinal detachment, secondary glaucoma, fair hair and skin, cutaneous flushing, and hernias may be present.

- The incidence of homocystinuria is about 1 per 200,000.
- Typical case: tall stature, pectus deformities, scoliosis, genu valgum, pes planus, highly arched palate, lens dislocation.
- Lens dislocation is progressive.

Cardiovascular abnormalities include arterial or venous thrombosis, angina pectoris, coronary occlusions at a young age, renal artery narrowing resulting in hypertension and renal atrophy, cerebrovascular accidents, thrombophlebitis, and pulmonary emboli. Dilatation of the pulmonary artery and left atrial endocardial fibroelastosis have been reported. Thrombi are particularly likely to occur after operation, venipuncture, or catheterization.

- Cardiovascular abnormalities of homocystinuria: arterial or venous thrombosis, angina pectoris, and coronary occlusions at a young age.
- Thrombi are likely after operation, venipuncture, or catheterization.

Histologic examination of the arteries reveals marked fibrous thickening of the intima. Aortic intimal fibrosis may be severe enough to mimic coarctation. Medial changes consist of thrombosis and dilatation with widely spaced, frayed muscle fibers. The elastic fibers of the large arteries may be fragmented, and dilatation of the ascending aorta has been observed. No consistent platelet defect has been noted.

The disease sometimes may be diagnosed from positive results of urinary nitroprusside test and confirmed by quantitative urinary homocysteine determination. Levels of plasma homocysteine and its precursor, methionine, are increased. Testing of the plasma homocysteine level is the most sensitive, with levels of 50 to 200 μmol/L. This should not be confused with the lesser increases that occur in hyperhomocysteinemia. The goal of treatment is to lower the plasma homocysteine level, which seems to result in slower progression and fewer symptoms of the disease; 50% of patients respond to pyridoxine therapy (25-1,000 mg/day). Supplemental folate also should be given because patients who are potentially capable of responding to pyridoxine may not do so in the presence of folate deficiency. A low-protein, low-methionine diet can be useful, but adults find it difficult to comply with this. For infants, a low-methionine formula is available. Betaine also has been reported to be of benefit in decreasing plasma homocysteine levels.

- In homocystinuria, levels of plasma homocysteine and its precursor, methionine, are increased.
- The goal of treatment is to lower the plasma homocysteine level.

Mild hyperhomocystinemia, sometimes associated with polymorphisms in methylenetetrahydrofolate reductase, is believed to be a risk factor for atherosclerosis but is a different condition.

Pseudoxanthoma Elasticum

There are two hereditary forms of pseudoxanthoma elasticum: autosomal dominant and autosomal recessive. Both forms are characterized by yellowish skin papules, especially on the neck and flexural areas, angioid streaks and choroiditis of the retina, and vascular complications, including angina pectoris, claudication, calcification of peripheral arteries, and renal vascular hypertension. The defective gene is *ABCC6* located on chromosome 16p13.1.

- Two hereditary forms of pseudoxanthoma elasticum: autosomal dominant and autosomal recessive.
- Characteristics: yellowish skin papules, angioid streaks and choroiditis of retina, and vascular complications.

Refsum Disease

Refsum disease is an autosomal recessive neurodegenerative disease characterized by cerebellar ataxia, hypertrophic

polyneuropathy, and retinitis pigmentosa. Deafness, ichthyosis, and cardiac conduction defects are frequently present.

- Refsum disease is autosomal recessive.
- Typical case: cerebellar ataxia, hypertrophic polyneuropathy, retinitis pigmentosa.
- Frequently present: deafness, ichthyosis, cardiac conduction defects.

Phytanic acid is a fatty acid present in dairy products and fat from grazing animals. Patients with Refsum disease are deficient in the catabolic enzyme phytanic acid α-hydroxylase, which results in accumulation of ingested phytanic acid in fatty deposits in the involved organ systems.

- Patients with Refsum disease are deficient in phytanic acid α-hydroxylase.

Dietary restriction of phytanic acid results in clinical improvement and stabilization of the disease. Electrocardiographic changes sometimes resolve after treatment. Plasmapheresis removes phytanic acid from the body and may allow liberalization of the diet; it can be extremely valuable in the management of acutely ill patients.

Tay-Sachs Disease

Tay-Sachs disease is an autosomal recessive disease due to deficiency of hexosaminidase A. The classic infantile form of the disease is rapidly fatal and is due to storage of ganglioside GM$_2$ in neural tissue. It is particularly common in people of Ashkenazi Jewish ancestry; the carrier frequency is 1 in 30. Therefore, screening for carriers by determination of enzyme activity in serum (or leukocytes, particularly in pregnant women, in whom the serum level is unreliable) is recommended in this population. Prenatal diagnosis is available when both the mother and the father are carriers.

- Tay-Sachs disease is autosomal recessive.
- The disease is due to deficiency of hexosaminidase A.

X-Linked Recessive

X-linked recessive diseases are caused by abnormal genes located on the X chromosome. Female heterozygotes who have one abnormal gene on one X chromosome and one normal gene on the other X chromosome usually are clinically normal. Exceptions may occur because of the phenomenon of lyonization, in which one X chromosome is inactivated at random early in fetal life; if the normal gene is inactivated in a critical number of cells, the woman may have symptoms or clinical signs of the disease. However, the disease usually is less severe than in males. The likelihood of clinical signs of the disease developing in a female varies by disease. For example, it is rare for female carriers of hemophilia A (factor VIII deficiency) to have severe bleeding problems, but it is relatively common for carriers of ornithine carbamoyltransferase (ornithine transcarbamoylase) deficiency to have intermittent symptoms.

- X-linked recessive diseases are caused by abnormal genes on the X chromosome.
- The development of clinical signs of the disease in a female varies by disease.

Males who inherit the abnormal gene have no corresponding genetic loci on the Y chromosome and therefore are referred to as "hemizygotes." Any male child born to a heterozygous female is at 50% risk for having the disease; female children are at 50% risk for inheriting the gene and being carriers. All the daughters of affected males are carriers, and all the sons are unaffected (i.e., male-to-male transmission cannot occur).

- Males with the abnormal gene are called "hemizygotes."
- A male child of a heterozygous female has a 50% risk of having the disease.
- A female child is at 50% risk of inheriting the gene.

X-linked recessive diseases also may arise by new mutation affecting either the mother or the afflicted son. Genetic counseling is difficult in these situations because if the mother represents the new mutation the risk for her future male children is 50%. However, if the child represents the new mutation, there is no significant risk for siblings of that child. New advances in DNA-based diagnosis have resulted in opportunities for carrier detection for some diseases, which circumvent problems created by lyonization.

Some of the conditions with X-linked recessive inheritance are listed in Table 9-3 and summarized on the following pages.

Duchenne and Becker Muscular Dystrophies

Duchenne muscular dystrophy is one of the most common types of muscular dystrophy; its incidence is approximately 1 in 3,500 newborn males. Approximately a third of the cases arise by new mutation. Progressive skeletal weakness beginning at 2 to 5 years of age, with death in the late teens or 20s, is characteristic. The diagnosis is made on the basis of clinical findings and a markedly increased creatine kinase level. The muscle biopsy findings are relatively nonspecific. Becker muscular dystrophy has later onset.

- The incidence of Duchenne muscular dystrophy is 1 in 3,500 newborn males.
- Duchenne muscular dystrophy is X-linked recessive.
- Skeletal weakness at 2-5 years of age is characteristic.

Table 9-3 X-Linked Recessive Conditions

Adrenoleukodystrophy ("X-linked" form)
Chronic granulomatous disease (many cases; autosomal recessive forms are less common)
Color blindness
Duchenne and Becker muscular dystrophies
Fabry disease
Glucose-6-phosphate dehydrogenase deficiency
Hemophilia A and B
Ocular albinism
Rickets, hypophosphatemic
Testicular feminization

The genetic defect that results in both Duchenne and Becker muscular dystrophies involves the dystrophin gene located on chromosome X at band p2l. Approximately two-thirds of patients have a submicroscopic partial gene deletion, and the rest have undetected deletions, duplications, or other abnormalities. The dystrophin gene is very large, consisting of at least 60 exons and 1,800 kilobases. The protein product of this gene, dystrophin, is a rod-shaped cytoskeletal protein that is predominantly localized to the surface membrane of striated muscle cells. Identification of the molecular defect has resulted in improved ability to determine carrier status in female relatives by DNA analysis. This is a considerable improvement over carrier testing by measurement of creatine kinase levels, because levels are increased in only 70% of obligate carriers. DNA analysis also can be used for prenatal diagnosis. All mothers, sisters, and children of patients with Duchenne or Becker muscular dystrophy should have genetic counseling.

- Mothers, sisters, and children of patients with Duchenne or Becker muscular dystrophy need genetic counseling.

The heart disease in patients with Duchenne muscular dystrophy is characterized by extensive changes in systolic time intervals, suggestive of compromised left ventricular function. There are histologic changes characterized by multifocal dystrophic areas with fibrosis and loss of myofilaments. These changes are most marked in the posterobasal segment and contiguous lateral and inferior walls of the left ventricle. Some families with dystrophin defects have dilated cardiomyopathy without serious skeletal muscle weakness.

- The heart disease in Duchenne muscular dystrophy involves changes in systolic time intervals.

Fabry Disease

Fabry disease is a lysosomal storage disease due to deficiency of α-galactosidase A. Females may have less severe signs of the disease than males. Glycosphingolipids accumulate in the endothelium, perithelium, and smooth muscle of blood vessels. There is also accumulation in ganglion cells, myocardial cells, reticuloendothelial cells, and connective tissue cells.

- Fabry disease is due to deficiency of α-galactosidase A.
- The disease is X-linked recessive.
- Females may have less severe signs of the disease than males.

The first signs of the disease may be telangiectatic angiokeratomas of the skin and mucous membranes. Acroparesthesias and episodes of severe burning pain in the palms and soles with proximal radiation also may occur in childhood and adolescence. Sweating is impaired and patients may have recurrent abdominal pain with fevers. Whorl-shaped corneal opacities and cataracts develop. In adulthood, cardiovascular and renal diseases are the major causes of morbidity and mortality.

- The first signs of Fabry disease may be telangiectatic angiokeratomas of skin and mucous membranes.
- Acroparesthesias may occur in childhood and adolescence.
- Whorl-shaped corneal opacities and cataracts develop.
- In adults, cardiovascular and renal diseases develop.

MITOCHONDRIAL MUTATIONS

Mitochondria each contain several circular copies of their own genetic material, mitochondrial DNA. This mitochondrial DNA is approximately 16,000 base pairs in length and encodes for transfer RNAs and several proteins involved in the mitochondrial respiratory chain. Many mitochondrial enzymes, including some others of the respiratory chain complex, are encoded by nuclear DNA and transported into the mitochondria. Mitochondrial DNA mutations cause Leber optic atrophy and the multisystem syndromes of mitochondrial myopathy, encephalopathy, episodes of lactic acidosis, and stroke (MELAS), myoclonic epilepsy with ragged red fibers (MERRF), and neuropathy, ataxia, and retinitis pigmentosa (NARP). Many cases of Kearns-Sayre syndrome (cardiomyopathy and ophthalmoplegia) are due to mitochondrial mutations. Mitochondrial disorders can arise as new mutations or be maternally inherited; in most cases, only the egg contributes mitochondria that persist in the zygote, and the sperm usually does not. Mitochondrial mutations may be homoplasmic (present in all mitochondrial DNA) or heteroplasmic (present in only some of the mitochondrial DNA).

- Mitochondrial DNA mutations cause Leber optic atrophy and multisystem syndromes.
- Many cases of Kearns-Sayre syndrome are due to mitochondrial mutations.
- Usually, only the egg contributes mitochondria that persist in the next generation.

MULTIFACTORIAL CAUSATION

Multifactorial means that the disease or trait is determined by the interaction of environmental influences and a polygenic (many gene) predisposition. Human conditions that may have multifactorial causation include many common birth defects—such as congenital heart defects, cleft lip and palate, and neural tube defects—and many common diseases—such as diabetes mellitus, asthma, hypertension, and coronary artery atherosclerosis.

- Multifactorial causation: disease or trait is due to environmental influences and a polygenic predisposition.
- Birth defects that may have multifactorial causation: congenital heart defects, cleft lip and palate, neural tube defects.
- Diseases that may have multifactorial causation: diabetes mellitus, asthma, hypertension, coronary artery atherosclerosis.

The multifactorial model predicts that there will be a tendency for familial aggregation of the condition but without a strict mendelian pattern of inheritance. Familial aggregation also can be due to common environmental factors, so familial aggregation by itself is not sufficient to prove multifactorial causation.

Because familial aggregation exists for multifactorial disorders, it is implicit that the occurrence risk will be increased for members of an affected family over that of the general population. As expected, the risk is highest for first-degree relatives (parents, siblings, children), who have half of their genes in common. The risk is less for second-degree relatives (grandparents, aunts, uncles, grandchildren, nephews, nieces), who share one-quarter of their genes. The risk decreases exponentially thereafter; third-degree relatives (great-grandparents, cousins, great-grandchildren) share only one-eighth of their genes. Empiric (observed) risk figures for some well-studied multifactorial disorders fit well with the predicted risks.

The genetic liability in multifactorial causation is due to the cumulative effect of many genes, each having a small effect, rather than to the effect of one major gene. These genes create a liability that presumably is continuously distributed within the population. If the genetic liability is strong enough, under an unfortunate set of environmental circumstances the disorder will occur.

- Genetic liability in multifactorial causation is due to cumulative effect of many genes.

For many multifactorial conditions, there is a difference in predilection between males and females which could result directly from genetic differences or from different internal (e.g., hormonal) or external environmental factors. Furthermore, if a member of the less commonly affected sex has the condition, his or her genetic liability was probably greater and therefore the risk for his or her relatives is greater. Similarly, if a person has a more severe form of the disease, the risk for relatives is higher. For disorders in which disease frequency increases with age, earlier onset sometimes implies a greater risk for relatives. Finally, the greater the number of affected individuals within the family, the higher the risk for other relatives. There also are racial differences in the frequency of many disorders of multifactorial causation.

When the inheritance pattern of any disease is being determined, the possibility of genetic heterogeneity always must be considered. For example, there are both autosomal dominant and multifactorial causes of atrial septal defect which may be indistinguishable clinically. Failure to recognize that different genetic diseases can cause the same or similar clinical entities can result in confusion when determining risks.

Table 9-4 lists some conditions of multifactorial causation.

DIAGNOSIS OF GENETIC DISEASE BY DNA ANALYSIS

Diagnosis of genetic diseases with peripheral blood specimens or specimens obtained by amniocentesis or chorionic villus sampling has become a routine part of clinical practice because of the identification of the basic genetic defect underlying numerous mendelian conditions and the capability for direct DNA diagnosis. In addition, even when the causative genetic defect has not yet been identified, knowledge of the involved gene may allow for diagnosis by linkage analysis. Because individual

Table 9-4 Conditions of Multifactorial Causation

Atherosclerosis
Atopic disease or allergy
Cancer
Cardiac defects (congenital)
Cleft lip or palate
Diabetes mellitus
Hypertension
Neural tube defects
Schizophrenia

---

genes are too small to be seen microscopically, standard chromosome analysis generally is not helpful even when the gene has been localized to a specific chromosome region.

The DNA-based laboratory procedures used for diagnosis, the limitations of the tests, and the importance of an accurate clinical diagnosis and family history are described below. A discussion of the prenatal diagnosis of Duchenne muscular dystrophy (DMD) provides an excellent example of these issues. Although the following examples describe prenatal diagnosis, the same principles apply to diagnosis of an affected or presymptomatic individual.

Importance of an Accurate Clinical Diagnosis and Family History

The importance of a correct diagnosis in the index patient when diagnosis by DNA analysis is being contemplated cannot be overemphasized. This criterion is in contrast to many instances of genetic diagnosis by chromosome analysis in which the cytogeneticist usually can be relied on to note most abnormalities (fragile X and subtle deletions are examples of exceptions) regardless of the exact indication for the study. This approach is possible because the procedure of chromosome analysis involves examination of all 46 chromosomes in a given cell to look for gross structural changes. In contrast, it is impossible to systematically examine each of a person's 30,000 or more genes to detect all abnormalities.

- It is impossible to systematically examine each of a person's 30,000 genes.

The laboratory's process of detection of even one abnormal gene must be directed by the precise clinical diagnosis. The DNA-based assays are specific for the disease being studied, and abnormalities elsewhere in the genome will not be detected. Thus, if the incorrect assay is chosen because of an incorrect clinical diagnosis, the disease-causing mutation will not be detected. For example, if a pregnant woman's brother and uncle are believed to have DMD but the correct diagnosis is X-linked Emery-Dreifuss muscular dystrophy, the wrong DNA analysis will be performed and may result in an erroneous prediction as to whether the fetus is affected. It is the responsibility of the physician to obtain medical records or to arrange for one of the affected relatives to be examined to confirm the reported diagnosis, and the physician may want the assistance of a medical geneticist or other specialist in this process.

In addition to confirmation of the diagnosis, an accurate family pedigree is necessary. It is important to know whether the index patient represents a sporadic case or whether other family members also are affected. This information must be considered in determination of whether DNA diagnosis is possible and in interpretation of the results of DNA analysis.

● An accurate family pedigree is necessary for diagnosis.

In sporadic cases, the diagnosis often can be established only for diseases for which direct DNA diagnosis is possible. In contrast, in families with multiple affected members, direct DNA diagnosis is the first choice when possible, followed by linkage analysis if the mutation cannot be directly identified. For example, in DMD, approximately 60% of patients have a deletion identifiable by techniques in routine use for clinical testing. If a deletion is detected in a sporadic patient with DMD, it usually is possible to determine whether the mother is a carrier, and, if so, direct DNA diagnosis can be applied for her male fetuses. If a deletion cannot be detected in a sporadic patient with DMD, then specific prenatal diagnosis is not possible for the mother's future children, although exclusion of a disease may still be possible by use of linked markers. The mother of a sporadic patient with DMD has a prior risk for being a carrier of approximately 2 in 3, and the options include fetal sex determination followed by termination of all male fetuses, although at least 2 of 3 would be expected to be unaffected, or termination of fetuses that inherited the same markers as the index patient, in which at least 1 of 3 would be unaffected.

● In families with multiple affected members, direct DNA diagnosis is the first diagnostic choice.

Alternatively, if multiple family members are affected with DMD, the issue of new mutation is not a concern. If a deletion is detected in these multiplex families, this is the simplest approach for testing male fetuses of female carriers within the family. However, if a deletion is not detected, then blood specimens can be collected from multiple family members for linkage analysis (Fig. 9-5).

Linkage Analysis

Linkage analysis is based on the biologic fact that individual units of genetic material (genes) are situated in linear order on one of the 24 types of chromosomes (22 autosomes plus the X and Y chromosomes). The word "alleles" refers to the different forms of genetic material at the same gene locus, for example, the A and B alleles at the ABO blood group locus. Genes located on different chromosomes segregate independently, so there is a 50% chance that an individual egg or sperm will contain the same or different alleles encoded within these two chromosomal loci (Fig. 9-6).

● "Alleles" are different forms of genetic material at the same gene locus.

Genes located on the same chromosome are syntenic. During the pairing of homologous chromosomes during

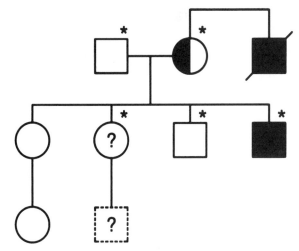

Fig. 9-5. Sample pedigree of family with males with Duchenne muscular dystrophy (shaded symbols). Carrier females are shown with half-shaded symbols. Members for whom blood was requested for DNA linkage analysis are marked with an asterisk. Squares, males; circles, females; line through square indicates that person is deceased; dashed-line square indicates male fetus. Note that blood for DNA from pregnant woman's father and unaffected brother is helpful for DNA linkage studies. Most laboratories offering these tests assist the referring physician in determining which family members need testing.

meiosis, crossovers can occur between genes even if they are located on the same chromosome. The average number of crossovers per chromosome per meiosis is two. Genes located far apart on the same chromosome are more likely to be separated by crossovers than are genes located close together. If the genes are so far apart that they are separated by crossovers at least 50% of the time, then these genes are not linked even though they are syntenic, and they exhibit random segregation (Fig. 9-7).

● Genes located on the same chromosome are syntenic.

Of course, linkage is not an all-or-none phenomenon. There is the potential for crossover to occur between any two gene loci, and this could happen in 20% of meioses, 2% of meioses, or 0.2% of meioses, for example, depending on the "distance" between them. Although physical distance is correlated with the likelihood of crossover, other factors such as location of the genes adjacent to the chromosome centromere and sex of the individual also influence the likelihood of crossover. Therefore, a measure of the functional likelihood of crossover, a centimorgan (cM), is used to describe the observed recombination rate. Thus, if crossovers occur in 10% of meioses, the loci are said to be 10 cM apart. On average, 1 cM corresponds to approximately 1,000 kilobases of DNA. The degree of linkage of specific genes must be generated from clinical observations in numerous families.

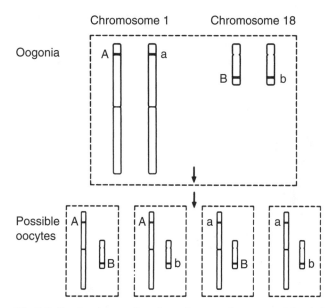

Fig. 9-6. Random segregation of gene locus on chromosome 1 in relation to gene locus on chromosome 18. There is a 50% chance that allele A will segregate with allele B or allele b. These loci are not syntenic and do not demonstrate linkage.

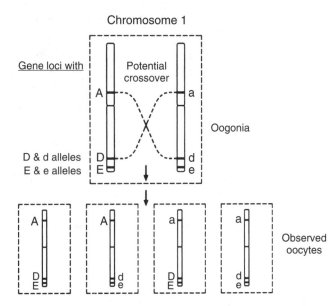

Fig. 9-7. Three gene loci on chromosome 1. Locus with allele A and allele a is located at sufficient distance from loci with alleles D/d and E/e that random segregation occurs. However, loci with alleles D/d and E/e always show D and E together or d and e together (not drawn to scale). Loci for D/d and E/e do not show random segregation and thus are linked.

For tests used in clinical practice, it is important to know the frequency of crossovers occurring between the disease gene and the marker gene, because this is one factor that limits the accuracy of the test. If the disease gene and the marker gene are 2 cM apart, it is important for the patient to know that the accuracy will be less than 98%. The use of flanking markers, that is, markers on both sides of the gene, if available, can help circumvent the problem of undetected crossovers. Although known genes sometimes are used for markers, more commonly DNA segments of unknown function are used for markers. These "anonymous" DNA segments, like genes themselves, can be highly variable in their nucleotide sequence. These normal variations are located extensively throughout the genome and can be recognized by one of many different kinds of bacterial enzymes that cut DNA at specified sites or by polymerase chain reaction. DNA polymorphisms located within the gene of interest are less likely to show recombination with the mutation site than those located adjacent to the gene (Fig. 9-8).

- The accuracy of linkage-based diagnosis is variable from one disease to another, depending on how tightly the disease gene and marker DNA are linked.

The size of the DNA fragments generated by these cutting enzymes varies among individuals because of normal variations in our DNA sequences. These different-sized fragments are referred to as restriction fragment length polymorphisms. These can be separated by size by electrophoresis on a gel.

Once separated by size, the DNA fragments can be transferred to a nylon membrane as part of the procedure known as Southern blot analysis.

Southern Blot Procedure

After a patient's DNA has been extracted from peripheral blood lymphocytes, subjected to enzyme cutting, and electrophoresed to separate different sizes of DNA fragments, a radioactive probe for the disease gene or for the marker DNA segments is applied and hybridizes to the complementary DNA sequences of interest. The fragments then can be visualized on x-ray film. An example of linkage analysis by Southern blotting in a family with DMD is shown in Figure 9-9.

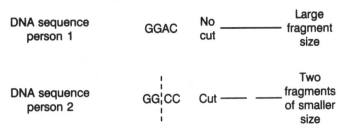

Fig. 9-8. Bacterial restriction enzyme *Hae* III. There are hundreds of types of bacterial enzymes that recognize and cleave specific DNA sequences. An appropriate enzyme that provides the most information for DNA markers near the disease gene of interest will be selected by the laboratory performing the test. Resulting fragments of differing sizes in different persons are restriction fragment length polymorphisms.

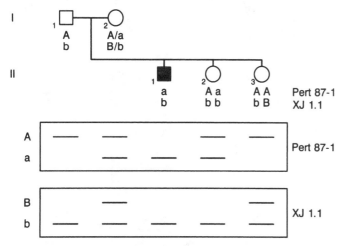

Fig. 9-9. Representation of a family segregating for Duchenne muscular dystrophy and data for two probes that detect restriction fragment length polymorphism, Pert 87-1 and XJ 1.1. Bottom half of figure represents Southern blot analysis of these two probes with arbitrary designation of alleles A/a for Pert 87-1 and B/b for XJ 1.1. Square, normal male; circle, female; shaded symbol, affected individual. Sister II.3 of affected male II.1 inherited Ab haplotype from her father and AB haplotype from her mother. Because her brother has ab haplotype, it can be predicted that she is not a carrier and her fetus is not at increased risk. Although sister II.2 did inherit the ab haplotype, it cannot be determined with certainty that she is a carrier because it is not known whether the mutation arose in the brother or whether the mother is a carrier. Sister II.2 could elect prenatal diagnosis, with the realization that males who inherit the ab haplotype might be affected or unaffected, whereas those who inherit the Ab haplotype would most likely be unaffected.

In addition to linkage analysis, Southern blotting can be used in some cases for direct detection of deletion or duplication types of mutations, or for single-base mutations if the enzyme restriction site is directly altered by the mutation. An example of direct detection of a deletion in a patient with DMD is shown in Figure 9-10.

Polymerase Chain Reaction

Another method of DNA diagnosis that has had great impact on clinical practice is polymerase chain reaction (PCR). PCR involves replication of a specific, relatively small segment of DNA in an exponential fashion, so that up to a billion copies are produced. One uses known DNA sequences from within the area of interest, and these known DNA sequences allow creation of synthetic oligonucleotides that serve as primers to hybridize with the patient's DNA sequence to initiate the amplification process (Fig. 9-11).

The multiple copies of the DNA segment that are produced by PCR then can be identified by various techniques, including direct visualization after gel electrophoresis. This allows detection of mutations in the patient's DNA. For example, PCR can be used for detection of mutations in specific regions of the dystrophin gene for the diagnosis of DMD and other diseases.

Diseases Amenable to DNA Diagnosis

The number of diseases that can be diagnosed with DNA analysis is increasing as additional disease genes are localized or identified and cloned. The physician who encounters a clinical situation for the first time which may be amenable to DNA-based diagnosis should discuss the testing procedure and its limitations with the laboratory personnel or a geneticist familiar with the details of the specific disease testing before a detailed discussion of the presymptomatic or prenatal diagnosis with the patient. Ideally, these discussions should take place before a woman becomes pregnant. For example, if a woman provides a family history of a brother with DMD and she is deciding whether to have a child, it would be prudent to confirm the diagnosis and get a detailed family history to determine whether prenatal diagnosis seems feasible rather than simply stating that prenatal diagnosis is possible. This woman would be in a difficult situation if she became pregnant while assuming that prenatal diagnosis was possible, only to find out later that prenatal diagnosis was not possible because her brother was a sporadic case or is deceased and she has no detectable deletion. Parenthetically, deletions can be much more difficult to detect in a woman heterozygous for an X-linked disease than in a hemizygous affected male. Another potential pitfall in presymptomatic prenatal diagnosis by DNA analysis is genetic heterogeneity. For example, most patients with autosomal dominant polycystic kidney disease have a gene defect in *PKD1* on chromosome 16. However, up to 10% of families have a phenotypically similar disease due to a different, nonallelic genetic mutation. Thus, if a person who has a parent with polycystic kidney disease wants to know if he or she has inherited the gene defect, it should first be established whether the exact mutation can be found in the affected parent. There are numerous other examples of this type of genetic heterogeneity, including retinitis pigmentosa, spinocerebellar ataxias, and Charcot-Marie-Tooth disease.

It is anticipated that the rapid advances made in molecular genetics in the past several years will accelerate as the genetic bases of additional diseases are identified and newer techniques for molecular diagnosis become available.

- Genetic heterogeneity can confound DNA studies.
- DNA-based diagnoses cannot be used for all families, even when DNA tests for a specific disease are available.

An example of an X-linked disease has been used throughout this discussion, but the same general principles apply to autosomal dominant and recessive diseases.

Diagnosis by Fluorescent In Situ Hybridization

Fluorescent in situ hybridization (FISH) is a cytogenetic technique that is being used with increasing frequency for

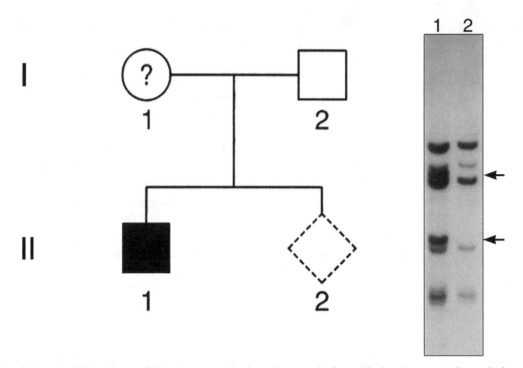

Fig. 9-10. Mother (I.1) of this patient (II.1) with sporadic Duchenne muscular dystrophy wanted to know whether she was a carrier or whether a new mutation had occurred in her son because of her concern for the risk for future children. Southern blot analysis detected a deletion in her son (II.1) (lane 2 as compared with control in lane 1). By densitometry, the mother seemed to have less than the expected amount of DNA (not shown) corresponding to her son's deletion. Thus, she was determined to be a carrier for the dystrophy and can be offered specific prenatal diagnosis. If no deletion had been detectable (by various methods), then her carrier status could not have been determined.

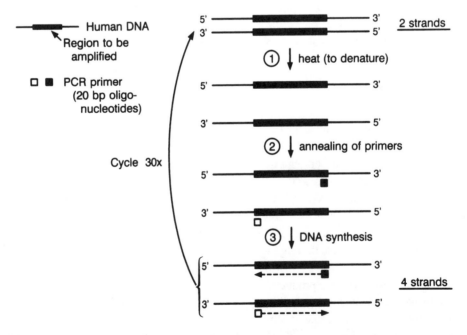

Fig. 9-11. Polymerase chain reaction (PCR) is used to make multiple copies of a short segment of the DNA of interest. DNA from the patient is denatured to single-stranded DNA in the presence of oligonucleotide primers. DNA sequences of these primers are made to specification to anneal with DNA sequences on both sides of the DNA segment of interest. DNA between these primers is then synthesized, and the entire process can be repeated automatically.

diagnosis of certain congenital and malignant disorders. The technique uses DNA probes homologous to the DNA area of interest within the chromosome so the probe binds the DNA segment of interest. The DNA probe is labeled with a fluorophore so it can be visualized under the microscope. The probe can be designed to bind to a discrete region of a chromosome, as in the case of Sphrintzen velocardiofacial syndrome. This syndrome is caused by a microdeletion (i.e., a deletion otherwise too small to be seen under the microscope) (see Fig. 9-3). It is relatively common with an estimated frequency of approximately 1 in 4,000. This syndrome is characterized by a variable combination of subaverage intellect, a characteristic facial appearance, velopharyngeal incompetence resulting in nasal speech, cleft palate, mild-to-moderate hearing loss, predisposition to dental caries, congenital heart defect (especially tetralogy of Fallot), and increased risk for hypocalcemia. Many patients are so mildly affected that the syndrome is not diagnosed until they have a more severely affected child.

DNA probes also can be designed to "paint" an entire chromosome (whole chromosome paints) and are helpful for defining complex chromosome rearrangements, as can occur in some malignancies. Less commonly, DNA FISH probes can be used to identify single gene defects such as hereditary neuropathy with liability to pressure palsies due to deletion of peripheral myelin protein 22 on chromosome 17p11.2, or Charcot-Marie-Tooth disease type I due to a duplication of this gene.

GLOSSARY

Autosome: A chromosome other than a sex chromosome.

Chromosome: Long strands of double-stranded DNA that encode genes and that are associated with a protein framework. A normal human has 46 chromosomes per cell.

Deletion: Structural abnormality in which part of a chromosome is missing.

Duplication: Structural abnormality in which an extra copy of part of a chromosome is present.

Epigenetic: Effect on the phenotype or gene expression that does not involve the DNA sequence.

Gene: A portion of DNA molecule that codes for a specific RNA or protein product.

Hemizygote: A person who has a gene form on one chromosome but no homologous chromosome with a corresponding gene site. The term usually refers to males because they have only one X chromosome.

Heterozygote: A person who has different gene forms at a given site on two homologous chromosomes.

Homozygote: A person who has the same gene forms at a given site on two homologous chromosomes.

Inversion: Structural abnormality characterized by reversal of a segment within the chromosome.

Karyotype: The chromosome complement of an individual person.

Linkage (genetic linkage): Physical proximity of two gene loci on the same chromosome such that segregation is nonrandom.

Phenotype: The observable biochemical or physical characteristics of an individual as determined by genetic material and environment.

Proband: The index patient.

Recurrence: Occurrence of another case of a specific condition in the same family.

Translocation: Structural abnormality characterized by transfer of a piece of one chromosome to another chromosome.

QUESTIONS

Multiple Choice (choose the one best answer)

1. A 60-year-old man with recent onset of loss of balance and tremor notices that these conditions have worsened during the past year. He had worked as an engineer, but then memory problems developed. He had been healthy and athletic, and his review of systems is unremarkable. He is married and has two healthy daughters. One of his grandsons has mental subnormality. The family history is negative for any other neurologic problems. On physical examination, a widely based gait, intention tremor, and mild dysarthria are noted. A paraneoplastic antibody panel is normal. MRI of the head shows increased T2 signal intensity in the middle cerebellar peduncles, with no evidence of infarct. Is this history consistent with a genetic defect, and what is the next best test?
   a. The family history is negative for ataxia so a genetic defect is an unlikely cause
   b. The late age at onset makes a genetic defect unlikely
   c. You consider a genetic cause and order a chromosome analysis
   d. You consider a genetic cause and order a molecular DNA diagnostic panel for the spinocerebellar ataxia and for fragile X
   e. You consider a genetic cause and order a molecular DNA diagnostic panel only for the spinocerebellar ataxia but not for fragile X because the patient had been intellectually normal

2. A 45-year-old woman with Down syndrome is brought for a routine medical evaluation by a caretaker of the group home where the patient lives. Records reveal a 47,XX,+21 karyotype from 1984. The patient has lived in the home for 5 years and seemed to have adjusted well. The patient works as a housekeeper in a supervised setting through a local agency that employs persons with handicaps. The caretaker wonders whether the patient is sick because lately she has seemed less verbal and unable or unwilling to perform her job. The present illness and review of systems is negative for weight loss or gain, hair loss, or change in bowel pattern. Her appetite is good, and she is sleeping well. The physical examination is normal except for the external stigmata of Down syndrome and the mental subnormality. The patient is able to speak but responds only to "yes" or "no" questions. You order basic laboratory tests, including blood count, electrolyte test, liver and thyroid function tests, creatinine and glucose tests, urinalysis, chest radiography, and stool test for hemoglobin, all of which have normal results. What is the next step in the evaluation and management?

   a. You reassure the caretaker that the patient is healthy and probably is just being difficult
   b. You diagnose depression and prescribe an antidepressant
   c. You consider a diagnosis of Alzheimer disease and prescribe a trial of donepezil hydrochloride
   d. You repeat the chromosome analysis before doing anything further because of the advances in genetic diagnostic techniques
   e. You perform molecular DNA diagnostic testing before doing anything further to confirm the diagnosis of Down syndrome

3. A 27-year-old woman with Turner syndrome presents for a preemployment physical examination. She is a teacher who provides an accurate history of her medical care. She reports that her karyotype is 45,X and that she has been on hormone replacement therapy since preadolescence. She states that she had echocardiography, performed when she was a child, that did not show coarctation of the aorta. She has no history of urinary tract infections. On physical examination, she is normotensive and of short stature. The remainder of her examination is unremarkable. Which special test, if any, is reasonable to perform?
   a. Echocardiography to look for bicuspid aortic valve or aortic dilatation
   b. Mammography to begin surveillance for breast cancer
   c. Ultrasonography of the renal arteries to look for stenosis
   d. Ultrasonography of the thyroid to look for nodules
   e. No special tests are needed

4. A 28-year-old man with normal intellect presents with a deep vein thrombosis. There was no history of preceding trauma or immobilization. He is 6 feet 1 inch tall and has mild pectus carinatum. Except for a few skin striae over the back and the acute changes in his leg compatible with thrombosis, his physical examination is normal. He has normal vision without the need for corrective lenses. He has no anemia or red blood cell macrocytosis. A coagulation profile is essentially normal except for a plasma homocysteine level of 80 μmol/L (normal, <13). What is the appropriate clinical diagnosis?
   a. Single gene disorder, Marfan syndrome
   b. Chromosome anomaly, Klinefelter syndrome
   c. Single gene disorder, Ehlers-Danlos syndrome
   d. Multifactorial, hyperhomocysteinemia
   e. Single gene disorder, homocysteinemia

5. A 58-year-old woman is asymptomatic but reports that her brother has Gaucher disease. The brother had marked thrombocytopenia and had his spleen removed at age 20

years "because it was enlarged." Your patient has minimal enlargement of the spleen but reports that she had "the flu" last week. She has a slightly low hemoglobin value of 11 g/dL with normal indices, and her platelet count is 110,000×10⁹/L (normal, 150-450). What is the next course of action?

a. On the basis of her brother's severe course, she does not need to be tested for Gaucher disease despite a genetic risk

b. She should be tested for Gaucher disease on the basis of her evaluation and 50% risk

c. She should be tested for Gaucher disease on the basis of her evaluation and 25% risk

d. Only males are affected by Gaucher disease, so she cannot be affected

e. She does not need to be tested despite her genetic risk because she is asymptomatic

6. A 30-year-old man presents with a long-standing rash on his buttocks and genitalia which is increasing in severity. He also reports feeling "run down." On physical examination, his blood pressure is 145/95 mm Hg. His rash is characterized by reddish-purplish, 1- to 3-mm papules that do not blanch. His creatinine value is 1.4 mg/dL. You initiate further evaluation and include which of the following diagnostic tests?

a. Mitochondrial DNA analysis

b. DNA-based linkage analysis

c. Chromosome analysis with fluorescent in situ hybridization probes

d. Serum iron, total iron-binding capacity, and percent saturation test

e. α-Galactosidase A test

7. A 24-year-old woman presents because of headaches. Her father has von Hippel-Lindau disease. She is aware of but is not interested in gene testing at this time. Her physical examination, including blood pressure, is completely normal. Her ophthalmologic examination and MRI of the head with gadolinium are normal. You can inform the patient that:

a. Her normal evaluation indicates she has not inherited the abnormal *VHL* gene

b. Her headaches are not related to von Hippel-Lindau disease but she still should have imaging of her kidneys

c. Her headaches are not related to von Hippel-Lindau disease and she does not need other tests at this time

d. The only way to find the cause of her headaches is to have the gene test for von Hippel-Lindau disease

e. Her headaches are not related to von Hippel-Lindau disease but it is imperative for her to have the gene test for the disease

ANSWERS

1. Answer d.

A negative family history and later age at onset never exclude diagnosis of a genetic disorder. These are only two of many factors to consider. It is unlikely that a man who had been healthy and of normal intelligence until older age would have a chromosome abnormality visible under the microscope to explain the disorder. Genetic disorders that one could consider and easily test for include a DNA panel for spinocerebellar ataxias and for fragile X. The patient's MRI findings are believed to be relatively specific for the fragile X premutation tremor ataxia syndrome. Males with this premutation are not mentally retarded and the frequency of premutation carrier males in the general population is estimated at 1 in 813. The proportion of affected males who will go on to have this neurologic syndrome is unknown.

2. Answer c.

Patients with Down syndrome are predisposed to early-onset Alzheimer disease. Although a diagnosis of depression also could be considered in this case, the fact that the patient has a good appetite and is sleeping well is somewhat against this, and there is no increased frequency of depression as far as is known in patients with Down syndrome. A chromosome analysis would not yield any further information. Although techniques have improved since 1984, an extra chromosome would have been clearly visible and identifiable and there would be no increased information from this or from any DNA diagnostic testing.

3. Answer a.

Patients with Turner syndrome are at increased risk for renal malformations, but in a person of this age with no history of urinary tract infection or hypertension, serious renal malformation would not be anticipated. Although the patient is at increased risk for thyroid disease, your physical examination does not suggest anything to cause consideration of thyroid ultrasonography. However, patients with Turner syndrome can have bicuspid aortic valve, which in previous years and even now is sometimes difficult to determine except by very careful echocardiography. Furthermore, regardless of bicuspid or tricuspid valve, patients with Turner syndrome are at increased risk for aortic dilatation and thus echocardiography is currently recommended every 5 years.

4. Answer e.

The patient has a considerably increased homocysteine level and has some features on physical examination suggestive of a diagnosis of autosomal recessive homocystinuria (homocysteinemia), such as the pectus deformity and striae. Such patients are predisposed to phlebitis, and not all patients have dislocated lenses or mental subnormality. The patient does not have a simple multifactorial predisposition to hyperhomocysteinemia, in which levels are usually, at most, increased twofold more than the normal range. Rather, it is most likely that the patient has a single gene disorder due to a cystathionine β-synthase deficiency, the most common of the causes of homocystinuria. The treatment is different, so the distinction is important. Not only do they benefit from vitamin B_{12} and folate treatment but also, most importantly, some of these patients are B_6-responsive because B_6 is a specific cofactor for this enzyme. Furthermore, some patients are not vitamin-responsive and will benefit from treatment with betaine.

5. Answer c.

Gaucher disease is an autosomal recessive disorder, and it is extremely variable even within the same family. Thus, the fact that this patient has minimal findings compared with her severely affected brother does not exclude the diagnosis. The chance that she inherited the genetic defect is 25%, although her slightly enlarged spleen and decreased platelet count make this diagnosis even more likely. Thus, enzyme testing is recommended for cerebroside β-galactosidase.

6. Answer e.

The patient's cutaneous findings and an increased creatinine value are almost pathognomonic for Fabry disease. The most direct way to make this diagnosis in a male is with the serum or leukocyte α-galactosidase A value. This is an important diagnosis to make because therapeutic enzyme replacement is likely to be available soon on a clinical basis. Furthermore, all daughters of an affected male will be carriers.

7. Answer b.

Von Hippel-Lindau disease has variable manifestations at various ages. Normal examination at age 24 years does not exclude the diagnosis. In some patients, signs or symptoms do not develop until as late as 60 years. However, patients with von Hippel-Lindau disease are predisposed to renal cysts and malignancies, and these may occur as early as young adulthood. Therefore, all patients at risk should have, at a minimum, careful ultrasonography of the kidney. CT and MRI are more sensitive. However, because the scans have to be repeated annually, one would want to avoid CT in a 24-year-old woman because of the amount of radiation that would be incurred over the years. Although the patient may want to consider gene testing further, this should be her own decision based on any concerns she may have for psychosocial and insurance issues, for example.

CHAPTER 10
GERIATRICS

Darryl S. Chutka, M.D.

GERIATRIC ASSESSMENT

The assessment of elderly patients should be different from that of the general examination of younger adults. The overall function of elderly patients depends on factors other than their medical problems. In addition to the medical problems of elderly patients, it is important to assess their functional status, cognitive capacity, and economic situation and whether their environment is safe and appropriate for their needs. It also is wise to address advance directives with all geriatric patients. Appropriate preventive screening should be a part of the assessment of the elderly who are in good health.

In addition to evaluating for conditions common to the geriatric population, such as heart disease, hypertension, diabetes mellitus, arthritis, and renal insufficiency, it is important to assess for conditions that can have a negative effect on function, such as impairment of vision or hearing (or both), mobility status, urinary incontinence, risk of falling, nutrition, and cognitive status. A thorough review of medications taken (prescription, herbal, and over-the-counter) is important.

- The overall function of elderly patients depends on factors other than medical problems.
- It is important to assess functional status, cognitive capacity, and economic situation and whether the environment is safe and appropriate for their needs.

Because the assessment of geriatric patients includes additional spheres of evaluation, the physician needs to become more efficient in the evaluation process. Previous medical records, paraprofessional interviews, screening tests, and patient questionnaires become valuable tools necessary to improve the efficiency of geriatric assessment. These tools can decrease substantially the time required by the physician to obtain a thorough history, thus allowing the physician to concentrate on the physical examination and patient education about maintaining and improving function. A thorough geriatric assessment should include the following:

Vision—Essentially all elderly patients have presbyopia, and the physician should determine whether the patient has access to proper assistive devices (reading glasses, magnifiers, and adequate light) to read. Assessment for other major eye diseases should be performed, including glaucoma, macular degeneration, and cataracts, because all these conditions increase in frequency with age and can markedly impair functional status.

Hearing—Impaired hearing is common among the elderly. There is considerable potential for improving hearing. In addition to periodic audiometric testing, it is important to ask the spouse or other family members if they are aware of the patient having any marked hearing loss. Patients often deny or minimize the symptoms of hearing impairment. Hearing impairment in the elderly is associated with decreased physical, social, and cognitive function. Improved hearing through the use of amplification devices improves the functional status of elderly persons.

Nutrition—Both undernutrition and overnutrition (obesity) are common nutritional problems among the elderly and have considerable potential for increased risks of morbidity, mortality, and reduced functional status. Elderly patients should be asked about any weight changes over the past 3 months, and they should be weighed at every physician visit. Height should be checked annually. This will allow the physician to calculate the body mass index (weight in kilograms/height in meters squared). Laboratory markers that reflect undernutrition and have been correlated with increased mortality among the elderly include hypoalbuminemia and low serum levels of cholesterol.

Urinary incontinence—Urinary incontinence is common among the elderly, especially older women. Incontinence has been shown to importantly impair social function and is a common reason for nursing home placement. Most elderly will not bring up the issue of urinary incontinence with their physician and assume that it is an expected result of aging. Therefore, it is important for physicians to ask patients about urinary incontinence.

Mobility and balance—Impaired balance and mobility can reduce functional independence and are major risks for falls. Falls may also signify cardiac or neurologic dysfunction and may have serious sequelae. The patient should be asked about any recent falls and the circumstances surrounding them. The physician can perform simple tests of balance and gait. Lower extremity range of motion and strength should be assessed.

Medications—Polypharmacy is common among the elderly and can lead to serious drug-drug interactions and complications from adverse drug reactions. Patients should be asked about the medications they take, including prescription and nonprescription drugs and herbal products. Patients should be instructed to bring with them to the office all the medications they currently are taking or have taken recently so the physician can review them. The need for the medication, its dosage frequency, and potential to cause harm or to interact with other medications should be assessed. Also, consider whether one medication may be substituted for two or more drugs.

Cognitive status—Although cognitive impairment is obvious in some elderly, it may be difficult to diagnose in others, especially when mild. Cognitive impairment is more common with advancing age, and the screening yield is highest among those older than 85 years, among whom the prevalence of Alzheimer disease can exceed 40%. Several screening tests are available. Most commonly used is the Mini-Mental State Examination (MMSE), a 30-point assessment of several components of cognitive function. Other screening tests include clock drawing and making change. Because these are screening tests, a normal result does not definitively rule out the possibility of dementia (but makes it less likely that the patient has marked cognitive impairment). If cognitive impairment is suspected but the results of mental status testing are normal, the patient should have formal psychometric cognitive testing, which is more sensitive.

Affect assessment—Depression is common among the elderly and potentially can reduce functional status. It also may result in considerable morbidity and mortality. Several effective screening tests, such as the Geriatric Depression Scale, are available. Unexplained weight loss may be a clue to depression.

Functional assessment—How an elderly person functions in the environment is an important component of the assessment. Functional status represents a combination of the person's medical condition and his or her interactions with the social environment. It is important to remember that an elderly person's functional state may change quickly, and various illnesses or prolonged hospitalization may cause a dramatic decline in functional status. The functional state is evaluated in three tiers: The basic activities of daily living (BADL) are the most simple activities required to remain independent, such as eating, bathing, dressing, transferring, and toileting. The instrumental activities of daily living (IADL) are the more complex activities required to maintain a household, such as shopping, driving, managing finances, and performing routine household chores. The advanced activities of daily living (AADL) are the ability to function in the community and include the ability to hold a job or to participate in recreational activities. The environment of the patient should be assessed to determine if the patient's functional state allows him or her to live safely in that environment.

Support assessment—If an elderly patient has a compromised functional state, the degree of social support available for him or her should be determined. The physician needs to ascertain who is available to help with various tasks to keep the individual safe in an independent environment. This usually includes family (most often an adult daughter), friends, and community services. A financial assessment should be made to determine whether the patient can afford treatments recommended by the physician or whether he or she qualifies for financial assistance from the government. A referral to social services may be needed to determine whether the patient meets the criteria for the benefits or services available.

Advance directives—Advance directives should be discussed early with each elderly patient. It is important for the caregiver to know the patient's preferences should the patient become unable to make independent decisions because of an incapacitating illness. Living wills and a durable power of attorney for health care should be discussed and the directives reviewed periodically to determine if the patient thinks they continue to reflect his or her wishes. These directives also should be reviewed any time a major change occurs in the medical or functional status of the patient.

- A thorough geriatric assessment should include an assessment of vision, hearing, nutrition, continence, mobility and balance, medications, cognitive status, affect, functional state, available support, and advance directives.

FALLS

Falls are a common cause of morbidity and an important contribution to mortality among the elderly. Because falls increase in frequency with advancing age, the likelihood of injury from falls also increases. It is estimated that three-fourths of all deaths related to falls occur in persons older than 65 years. The increased frequency of falls among the elderly reflects multiple age-related changes, including decreased strength from loss of muscle mass, decreased visual and hearing acuity, decreased proprioception, and slowed reaction time. These changes can produce an alteration of gait and decreased balance in an elderly person.

Most falls (70%) occur in the person's home. An accident, usually related to hazards in the environment (throw rugs, slippery floors, lack of grab bars in bathtubs, and inadequate lighting), is the most common cause of falls among the elderly who live independently. Most accidental falls occur while the person is performing typical daily activities such as walking or changing position (e.g., sitting to standing). An important percentage (10%) occur on stairs, more commonly while the person is descending the stairs. Falls that occur in nursing homes are more likely related to medical problems such as gait abnormalities, impaired balance, weakness, and confusion and are less likely to be caused by an environmental hazard. The common risk factors for falls include weakness of the legs (stroke or neuropathy), gait instability (Parkinson disease), balance disorder (vertigo or orthostatism), cognitive impairment (dementia), and the use of multiple medications. Medications that may contribute to falls include antihypertensive agents, diuretics, tricyclic antidepressants (which may produce orthostatic hypotension), sedative-hypnotics, ethanol, and neuroleptics (which may impair balance).

- Falls among the elderly usually reflect decreased strength from loss of muscle mass, decreased visual and hearing acuity, decreased proprioception, and slowed reaction time.
- Most falls (70%) occur in the person's home.
- Falls that occur in nursing homes are more likely related to medical problems.

Evaluation of Falls

A thorough medical history is the most important component of the assessment of a fall. If the reason for the fall is not known after the patient's history has been taken, it is unlikely that the cause will be found on physical examination or laboratory testing. The history should include the patient's perception of the cause of the fall, any warning symptoms the patient experienced before the fall, and any associated symptoms that occurred with the fall. The patient also should be questioned about how he or she felt immediately after the fall. Loss of consciousness may suggest a cardiac or neurologic event (arrhythmia, seizure, or cerebrovascular event).

The physical examination should include a neurologic examination that tests gait, balance, reflexes, sensory impairment, and extremity strength. Any sensory impairment should be noted. Because falls may be associated with acute illnesses, patients should be assessed for infections, myocardial infarction, and gastrointestinal tract hemorrhage. Orthostatic hypotension, although common among the elderly, may also indicate a medication effect or hypovolemia from hemorrhage or dehydration.

- A thorough medical history is the most important component of the assessment.

- The physical examination should include a neurologic examination that tests gait, balance, sensory impairment, and extremity strength.

Prevention and Treatment of Falls

The goal of the assessment of a fall is to decrease the likelihood of subsequent falls. The treatment plan is based on the findings of the assessment. However, more than one factor is often identified as contributing to falls. Potential interventions for the prevention of falls may include the following:

- Reduction in environmental hazards—provide adequate lighting, remove obstacles from floors, eliminate slippery floors, use appropriate footwear, eliminate bed side rails.
- Physical therapy—improve gait, balance, and strength, especially in the lower extremities.
- Assistive devices—improve gait and balance.
- Review of the medication program—avoid drug-drug interactions and eliminate potentially offending drugs.
- Treat medical problems that may contribute to falls (cataracts, postural hypotension, postprandial hypotension, Parkinson disease).

SYNCOPE

"Syncope" is defined as a transient loss of consciousness with loss of postural tone. It becomes more common with advancing age and has many causes. Although the cause of the syncopal spell itself is usually benign, several serious consequences can result from the fall, including bone fracture and subdural hematoma. Regardless of the cause of syncope, the underlying mechanism is inadequate cerebral blood perfusion. It has been estimated that as many as one-third of the cases of syncope have a cardiac cause. These include valvular heart disease (aortic stenosis, mitral regurgitation, and mitral stenosis), hypertrophic cardiomyopathy, myocardial infarction, or cardiac arrhythmias (tachyarrhythmias or bradyarrhythmias). An orthostatic decrease in blood pressure is also common in the elderly because of changes in baroreceptor function. In addition, several disease states can be associated with orthostatic hypotension, including peripheral neuropathy, Parkinson disease, and Shy-Drager syndrome. Also, various medications can produce hypotension, including antihypertensive agents, tricyclic antidepressants, neuroleptics, and diuretics. Although vasovagal syncope is more common in younger persons, it can occur in the elderly. Carotid sinus hypersensitivity, an exaggerated hypotensive reflex that occurs in response to carotid sinus massage, also can cause syncope. Other exaggerated cardiovascular reflexes that can result in syncope include micturition, defecation, and coughing. Seizures, hypoxemia (pulmonary embolism or respiratory failure), severe hypoglycemia, and anemia can also produce syncope.

The medical history is the most important part of the evaluation of syncope; the physical examination should focus on the signs related to cardiovascular or neurologic disease. Orthostatic blood pressure should be measured. Findings from the history and physical examination should guide the selection of tests to be performed. Tests that may be of value are electrocardiography (ECG) and, occasionally, ambulatory cardiac monitoring when a cardiac arrhythmia is suspected. Rarely, electrophysiologic studies should be considered. When neurologic abnormalities are found on examination, an imaging study (computed tomography [CT] or magnetic resonance imaging [MRI]) of the head may yield important information. Electroencephalography (EEG) is useful when a seizure disorder is thought to cause syncope. Laboratory blood tests do not commonly give the diagnosis for syncope; however, several of these tests may be helpful in certain circumstances. Blood count and electrolyte and creatinine determinations can give information about volume status. Measurement of cardiac enzymes may be useful if a recent myocardial infarction is suspected. Echocardiography should be performed if there is evidence of structural cardiac disease.

- It has been estimated that as many as one-third of the cases of syncope have a cardiac cause.
- Changes in baroreceptor function can result in an orthostatic decrease in blood pressure.
- The medical history is the most important part of the evaluation of syncope.

VISION CHANGES

A combination of anatomical and physiologic changes related to aging and various disease states common in the elderly frequently cause decreased vision. Vision loss increases with advancing age, and more than one-quarter of those older than 85 years report marked visual impairment. More than 90% of the elderly wear eyeglasses. It has been estimated that at least 25% of nursing home residents are legally blind. The most common eye problem in the elderly is presbyopia, difficulty with close focus. Presbyopia is the result of decreased lens flexibility, which occurs with aging. Cataracts are also more common with advancing age; they begin forming early in life, but the progression varies from person to person. The prevalence of cataracts is approximately 50% in those between 65 and 74 years old and up to 70% in those older than 75. Typically, cataracts produce a gradual reduction in visual acuity and represent opacities of the crystalline lens. In those with early cataracts, near vision may actually improve; however distant vision becomes blurred. This occurs because of an increase in the convexity of the lens. Although cataracts are usually bilateral, one eye may be affected more than the other. Cataract surgery with intraocular lens

implantation is effective in restoring visual acuity. The decision about the surgical treatment of cataracts should be individualized and based on the patient's disability.

Glaucoma is the most common cause of blindness worldwide and is characterized by increased intraocular pressure and associated optic nerve damage, manifested by cupping of the optic disk, atrophy of the optic nerve, and an associated reduction in the visual field. The two major types of glaucoma are chronic open-angle and angle-closure. Open-angle glaucoma is more common and occurs in up to 70% of adults with glaucoma. Chronic open-angle glaucoma produces a slow, progressive loss of peripheral vision that often is not appreciated by the patient until a considerable amount of vision is lost. Glaucoma is more common among African Americans than whites and is the most common cause of blindness in African Americans. In those with the disease, a positive family history of glaucoma is very common. Open-angle glaucoma is associated with partial obstruction of aqueous humor flow through the trabecular meshwork. Funduscopic examination shows atrophy and cupping of the optic disk. Visual field testing documents typical peripheral field defects. A small number of patients with funduscopic or visual field changes of glaucoma have normal intraocular tension. If the physician routinely checks for glaucoma, it can be diagnosed and treated effectively before pronounced loss of vision occurs. The decision to treat glaucoma is not based only on the degree of increased ocular tension. Treatment is started when there is evidence of loss of vision or physical evidence of ocular damage.

Several options are available for the treatment of glaucoma, including surgery and medication. Medications are effective in decreasing the production of aqueous humor or in increasing its outflow. Pilocarpine causes pupillary constriction and opens the trabecular meshwork, resulting in increased flow of aqueous humor. β-Blockers such as timolol decrease the production of aqueous humor, as do carbonic anhydrase inhibitors. Epinephrine decreases the production of aqueous humor and increases its flow. The goal of surgical treatment is to increase the flow of aqueous humor. Laser trabeculectomy is performed occasionally for open-angle glaucoma and usually is successful in increasing the outflow of aqueous humor.

Acute angle-closure glaucoma is much less common than chronic open-angle glaucoma and represents about 5% of glaucoma cases. It often presents after pupillary dilation. It results from the obstruction of aqueous humor as it flows from the anterior chamber of the eye through the canal of Schlemm. This obstruction abruptly increases intraocular pressure. Patients with acute angle-closure glaucoma present with symptoms of intense eye pain, blurred vision with halos around lights, headache, and nausea. Physical examination reveals a slightly dilated pupil unresponsive to light. Urgent treatment is necessary to prevent permanent loss of vision.

Macular degeneration is the most important disease of the retina in the elderly. It is the leading cause of blindness in those older than 50. Macular degeneration is associated with the gradual and progressive loss of central vision, with sparing of peripheral vision. In addition to advanced age, macular degeneration has several risk factors, including a family history of macular degeneration, hyperopia, a light color of the iris, and chronic tobacco use. Although it initially tends to develop in one eye, it eventually becomes bilateral in many patients. It results in atrophy of the pigmented retinal epithelium. Impaired function of the photoreceptors eventually occurs, resulting in the characteristic loss of central vision and sparing of peripheral vision. The breakdown of the epithelium causes the deposition of drusen. The pathologic changes of macular degeneration generally can be seen on funduscopic examination. Laser treatment can be beneficial in some types of macular degeneration; however, the management of most patients with macular degeneration consists of devices used to assist vision, such as increased lighting and magnifying lenses.

- The most common eye problem in the elderly is presbyopia.
- Glaucoma is the most common cause of blindness worldwide. It is characterized by increased intraocular pressure and associated optic nerve damage.
- Chronic open-angle glaucoma is the most common form of glaucoma and produces a slow, progressive loss of peripheral vision.
- Macular degeneration is associated with the gradual and progressive loss of central vision and the sparing of peripheral vision.

HEARING CHANGES

Notable hearing loss in the elderly is common and usually due to a central auditory processing disorder, which causes difficulty with speech perception. The ability to discriminate speech is worse than predicted for the amount of pure tone lost. The prevalence of hearing loss, especially of high frequencies (presbycusis), increases markedly among persons older than 65 years and approaches 50% in those older than 80. Presbycusis is typically bilateral and associated with a high-frequency hearing loss. The cause is not known. Noise-induced hearing loss produces a similar high-frequency hearing loss. Elderly patients with a high-frequency hearing loss usually have the most difficulty with appreciating consonant sounds. A pronounced hearing impairment is thought to be present when there is a loss of 25 decibels or more at 500, 1,000, or 2,000 Hz. Speech typically occurs between 1,000 and 3,000 Hz.

Causes of conductive hearing loss include cerumen impaction, perforation of the tympanic membrane, cholesteatoma, Paget disease, and otosclerosis. Hearing aids may be beneficial, and many improvements have been made in these devices. Some models of hearing aids are able to select the optimal frequency amplification for the specific environment, and others can be programmed to amplify the specific frequencies that the patient has lost. A less complex version amplifies the higher frequencies, the frequencies most commonly lost with aging. Hearing aids are most beneficial when used in an environment with minimal background noise, for example, a one-on-one conversation in a quiet room. They are least helpful when used in crowds with extensive background noise.

- The prevalence of hearing loss, especially of high frequencies (presbycusis), increases markedly in the elderly.
- Causes of conductive hearing loss include cerumen impaction, perforation of the tympanic membrane, cholesteatoma, Paget disease, and otosclerosis.

RHEUMATOLOGIC PROBLEMS

Rheumatologic problems are among the commonest complaints of the elderly. These diseases tend to be chronic and often accumulate with time. Although most of these diseases are not life-threatening, they commonly cause an alteration in lifestyle and lead to substantial disability. Osteoarthritis is extremely common among the elderly and is present to some degree in more than 80%. It produces joint symptoms that vary with time and degree of activity. Osteoarthritis usually can be differentiated from rheumatoid arthritis by the medical history and physical examination findings. Osteoarthritis tends not to produce systemic symptoms, which are common in rheumatoid arthritis. Joint inflammation can occur in osteoarthritis, but it is more pronounced in rheumatoid arthritis. Although disease activity varies, acute worsening of a specific joint should make one suspicious of a superimposed crystalline arthritis (gout or pseudogout) or septic arthritis, which occasionally is found in patients with underlying chronic joint disease.

Osteoarthritis

Osteoarthritis has a predilection for the hands (distal and proximal interphalangeal joints and first carpometacarpal joint of the thumb), knees, hips, and feet (first tarsometatarsal joint), with relative sparing of the elbow, wrist, metacarpophalangeal joints, and ankle. It has a typical radiographic appearance that includes asymmetrical narrowing of the joint space, presence of osteophytes, subchondral sclerosis, and cystic changes in the bone. Systemic symptoms do not occur. Joint pain is common with joint use and weight-bearing activity. Rest usually provides relief from the pain. The treatment of osteoarthritis includes adequate rest, local heat, and exercise to strengthen periarticular muscles, occasionally the injection of corticosteroids into the joint space when inflammation is present, and analgesics. Because only joint inflammation is rarely marked in osteoarthritis, an analgesic such as acetaminophen should be tried initially for pain relief. Once this has been tried and thought to be ineffective in managing the pain, more aggressive treatment should be used. Nonsteroidal anti-inflammatory drugs (NSAIDs) can be quite effective; however, they carry a risk of important adverse effects, especially when taken chronically. If NSAIDs are not tolerated or are ineffective, alternative treatment may include tramadol or codeine. Combinations of these drugs with low doses of acetaminophen may be helpful. Occasionally, corticosteroid may be injected into individual joints for temporary relief of pain. Some patients with knee osteoarthritis receive relief with injections of hyaluronic acid.

- Osteoarthritis usually can be differentiated from rheumatoid arthritis by the medical history and physical examination findings.
- Marked joint inflammation in osteoarthritis is uncommon.
- Radiographic findings in osteoarthritis include asymmetrical narrowing of the joint space, osteophytes, subchondral sclerosis, and cystic bone changes.

Rheumatoid Arthritis

Rheumatoid arthritis is often found in elderly patients, most commonly as a chronic disease that was acquired earlier in life. It also can develop later in life and has two presentations. As in younger persons, it may present with symmetrical distal joint inflammation, positive rheumatoid factor, and a tendency to progress with time. The second presentation is common in the elderly and consists of the acute onset of proximal joint pain and stiffness, which can be very similar to polymyalgia rheumatica. Testing for rheumatoid factor often gives negative results, and rheumatoid nodules are often absent. In contrast to osteoarthritis, patients with rheumatoid arthritis have systemic symptoms. Extra-articular manifestations are occasionally present with rheumatoid arthritis and include potential involvement of the skin (rheumatoid nodules), lung (fibrosis, rheumatoid nodules, and pleural effusions), blood vessels (vasculitis), nervous system (mononeuritis multiplex), and hematologic system (Felty syndrome). Sjögren syndrome (splenomegaly and leukopenia) also occasionally accompanies rheumatoid arthritis. Radiographs of joints involved by rheumatoid arthritis characteristically show symmetrical narrowing of the joint space. Demonstrating inflammatory, symmetrical arthritis on physical examination usually makes the diagnosis. Laboratory tests can often be misleading in the elderly. Testing for rheumatoid factor is often negative in many elderly patients with rheumatoid arthritis. The test result can be false-positive in many elderly patients who do not have the disease, although the rheumatoid factor usually is of low titer.

Elderly patients with rheumatoid arthritis receive the same therapeutic agents as younger patients: NSAIDs, chloroquine, methotrexate, gold, and low doses (5-7.5 mg daily) of corticosteroids.

- Patients with rheumatoid arthritis often have systemic symptoms.
- Extra-articular manifestations are occasionally present.
- Radiographically, rheumatoid arthritis characteristically shows symmetrical narrowing of the joint space.
- The elderly with rheumatoid arthritis receive the same therapeutic agents as younger patients.

Crystalline Arthropathy

Crystalline arthropathy is common among the elderly. Whereas gout tends to be more common in men and to involve more distal joints (especially the great toe), pseudogout is more common in women and tends to involve more proximal joints (especially the knee and wrist).

Gout is usually a monoarticular arthritis, although uncommonly presents as a polyarticular disease. It is caused by intra-articular deposition of uric acid crystals. It is associated with hyperuricemia, which may be produced by thiazide diuretics. Gouty attacks may be precipitated by stressful events such as surgery, severe illnesses, or trauma. Although gout usually is diagnosed on the basis of the medical history and physical examination, the diagnosis is confirmed by microscopic evaluation of the synovial fluid from an affected joint. Urate crystals are long and needle-shaped and negatively birefringent with polarizing microscopy. Treatment for an acute attack of gout includes NSAIDs. Colchicine, orally or intravenously, may be given to patients who should not receive NSAIDs. In some circumstances, intra-articular or systemic corticosteroids may be necessary. This may be preferred for some elderly patients because of the high incidence of gastrointestinal or renal adverse effects. Long-term suppressive therapy usually is not initiated until several acute episodes of gout have occurred. Suppressive therapy may include allopurinol or probenecid daily or low doses of oral colchicine. Treatment of asymptomatic hyperuricemia is rarely necessary, although it is initiated in patients with uric acid renal stones or, occasionally, when starting chemotherapy for various hematologic malignancies.

- Gout tends to be more common in men and to involve more distal joints.
- Urate crystals are needle-shaped and negatively birefringent with polarizing microscopy.
- Treatment for an acute attack of gout includes NSAIDs, colchicine, or, in some cases, intra-articular or systemic corticosteroids.

Pseudogout (calcium pyrophosphate deposition disease) is usually a monoarticular arthritis that most frequently involves the knee or wrist. As with gout, an acute attack can occur with a stressful event such as surgery, trauma, or illness. Radiographs of joints with pseudogout often show linear articular calcification, although approximately 25% of the elderly have articular calcification with no clinical evidence of the disease. Calcium pyrophosphate crystals are rectangular and exhibit positive birefringence with polarizing microscopy. An acute attack is treated with NSAIDs or corticosteroids injected into the affected joints. Daily therapy with a low dose of colchicine may decrease the frequency of acute attacks.

- Pseudogout is usually a monoarticular arthritis, most commonly involving the knee or wrist.
- Calcium pyrophosphate crystals are rectangular and exhibit positive birefringence with polarizing microscopy.
- An acute attack is treated with NSAIDs or corticosteroids injected into the affected joints.

Polymyalgia Rheumatica and Temporal Arteritis

Polymyalgia rheumatica and temporal arteritis occur more commonly in women than in men and in persons older than 50 years. Patients with polymyalgia rheumatica describe stiffness, aching, and weakness of proximal muscles (shoulders and hips), especially in the morning. This is thought to be due to synovitis of the shoulder or hip joint (or both). The clinical presentation of polymyalgia rheumatica may be very similar to that of rheumatoid arthritis in the elderly. Patients also may complain of nonspecific malaise, fatigue, low-grade fever, and anorexia with weight loss. Although patients commonly describe weakness, muscle strength is normal when tested. The diagnosis usually is suspected from the classic history obtained from the patient; no specific laboratory test is diagnostic for the disease. Patients usually have an increased erythrocyte sedimentation rate and, occasionally, mild anemia. The levels of muscle enzymes (creatine kinase and aspartate aminotransferase) are not increased. The response to treatment is very characteristic and often can be used to support the diagnosis. Treatment with low doses of oral corticosteroids (prednisone, 15-20 mg daily) produces dramatic improvement in symptoms, often within 24 hours. After treatment has been initiated, the corticosteroid dose can be tapered gradually, using the patient's clinical response and erythrocyte sedimentation rate as indicators of disease activity.

- Patients with polymyalgia rheumatica describe stiffness, aching, and weakness of proximal muscles.
- Patients usually have an increased erythrocyte sedimentation rate and, occasionally, mild anemia.
- Treatment with low doses of oral corticosteroids produces dramatic improvement in symptoms.

Temporal arteritis develops in about 15% of patients with polymyalgia rheumatica. Pathologically, there is inflammation of medium-sized arteries, which arise from the aortic arch. Systemic symptoms include low-grade fever and fatigue; anorexia with weight loss is also common. A majority of patients have a unilateral or bilateral headache, usually in the temporal area. Many also have scalp tenderness and jaw claudication due to facial artery involvement with disease. Loss of vision, including unilateral or bilateral visual blurring, visual field loss, diplopia, or blindness caused by ischemic optic neuritis, may occur and is the most worrisome symptom. As with polymyalgia rheumatica, temporal arteritis usually is suspected on the basis of the patient's description of the symptoms. Few findings are documented on physical examination. Some patients have tender, swollen, or pulseless temporal arteries. Rarely, bruits may be heard over medium-sized arteries involved by the disease. Although no diagnostic laboratory test is specific for temporal arteritis, almost all patients have a markedly increased erythrocyte sedimentation rate, often greater than 100 mm/h. Mild anemia may also be present. After temporal arteritis is suspected, the diagnosis should be confirmed with temporal artery biopsy. A 4- to 5-cm piece of temporal artery should be obtained, initially on the side of the patient's symptoms. If the pathologic findings are negative, a similar biopsy should be performed on the opposite side. The inflammatory changes in the artery may be spotty or confined to a small portion of the artery, occasionally causing difficulty in confirming the diagnosis pathologically. Temporal artery biopsy should not be performed routinely in those with polymyalgia rheumatica without symptoms of temporal arteritis. Treatment consists of prednisone, 60 mg daily, and may be started before the biopsy sample is obtained, assuming the biopsy is to be performed within 48 hours. The prednisone dose should be tapered on the basis of an assessment of the patient's clinical response to treatment as well as the response of the erythrocyte sedimentation rate.

- Temporal arteritis develops in about 15% of patients with polymyalgia rheumatica.
- Symptoms include low-grade fever, fatigue, anorexia with weight loss, unilateral or bilateral headache, scalp tenderness, and jaw claudication.
- The diagnosis should be confirmed with temporal artery biopsy.
- Treatment consists of high doses of corticosteroids.

THYROID DISEASE

Thyroid disease becomes more common with advancing age. Most elderly patients with hyperthyroidism present with typical findings. A small but important percentage have atypical symptoms. Some elderly persons develop anorexia with weight loss, altered stool frequency (either diarrhea or constipation), or cardiovascular abnormalities, including hypertension, increased angina, myocardial ischemia, congestive heart failure, and atrial fibrillation. Other symptoms that may develop include apathy, depression, tremor, and myopathy. Decrease in bone density is accelerated with hyperthyroidism. Ophthalmopathy, lid lag, tachycardia, and increased perspiration are relatively more uncommon in the elderly than in younger patients. The development of a goiter with hyperthyroidism is noted in about 60% of the elderly. The commonest cause of hyperthyroidism in the elderly is Graves disease. Radioiodine therapy is the treatment of choice for hyperthyroidism in elderly patients.

- Most elderly patients with hyperthyroidism present with the typical findings, although they may develop apathy, depression, tremor, and myopathy.
- The commonest cause of hyperthyroidism in the elderly is Graves disease.
- Radioiodine therapy is the treatment of choice for hyperthyroidism.

The diagnosis of hypothyroidism in elderly patients is usually made by finding an increased sensitive thyroid-stimulating hormone (sTSH) on laboratory testing of asymptomatic patients. The common symptoms of hypothyroidism are vague (constipation, cold intolerance, and dry skin) and often attributed to the many "symptoms of aging." Almost all these cases of hypothyroidism are due to primary thyroid failure rather than to pituitary or hypothalamic insufficiency. The commonest cause of hypothyroidism in the elderly is Hashimoto thyroiditis. Treatment should begin with a low dose of thyroid supplement (25-50 µg daily) that is increased by 25 µg every 3 to 4 weeks. Patients with coronary artery disease should receive an even lower starting dose and more gradual dose increments because if thyroid replacement is too rapid, it can precipitate cardiac ischemia. It takes approximately 6 to 8 weeks for a given dose of thyroid supplement to equilibrate; therefore, the sTSH should not be checked before this time to assess whether the dose of thyroid supplement is correct. Thyroid hormone requirements decrease with advancing age, and most elderly require 75 to 100 µg daily; however, some require as little as 50 µg daily. Subclinical hypothyroidism can be found in approximately 15% of the elderly. These patients are clinically euthyroid and have a low-normal total (serum) thyroxine (T_4) level and a slightly increased sTSH level. Whether to treat these patients is a matter of controversy. Patients with an sTSH less than 6 mU/L and negative microsomal antibodies rarely have progression to clinical hypothyroidism. Most physicians choose to observe patients who have modest increases in sTSH (<10 mU/L) unless symptoms of hypothyroidism develop or the sTSH level continues to increase.

- The common symptoms of hypothyroidism are vague and often attributed to symptoms of aging.
- The commonest cause of hypothyroidism in the elderly is Hashimoto thyroiditis.
- Treatment of hypothyroidism should begin with a low dose of thyroid supplement (25-50 µg daily) that is increased by 25 µg every 3 to 4 weeks.

Euthyroid sick syndrome is common in elderly hospitalized patients. Patients are clinically euthyroid but have low serum levels of triiodothyronine (T_3) and T_4 and a low-normal level of sTSH. Laboratory values tend to return to normal after the patient has recovered from the illness. The syndrome may be caused by a decreased amount of thyroid-binding protein and a substance that inhibits T_4 binding.

- Patients with euthyroid sick syndrome are clinically euthyroid but have low serum levels of T_3 and T_4 and a low-normal level of sTSH.

SEXUAL FUNCTION AND SEXUALITY

Multiple physical and social changes occur with aging that can result in changes in the desire and capacity of an older person for sexual activity. Although there is evidence that interest in sexuality is retained well into older age, for several reasons the frequency of sexual activity tends to be reduced with aging. Whereas this is true for the elderly population in general, there is great variability in sexual interest and activity from one elderly person to another. One of the most important factors that may determine whether a person is sexually active is the availability of a partner who is capable of sexual activity. The setting in which the elderly live may also have a role in whether a person is sexually active. Many elderly live in an environment in which sexual activity is difficult or not condoned, for example, in a nursing home or in the home of their children. Because privacy may not be possible in these settings, intimacy is unlikely to occur.

Little is known about the influence of sex hormones on libido for either the male or female. Although it is not thought that estrogen or progestin has a role in sexual desire in females, evidence suggests that androgens increase sexual interest. Lack of estrogen can produce reduced vaginal lubrication and mucosal atrophy, which can cause dyspareunia. Painful conditions such as osteoarthritis also may contribute to diminishing desire for sexual activity. Erectile dysfunction increases in frequency with advancing age and is the most common reason for a man to reduce his degree of sexual activity. It may be related to psychosocial as well as to physical factors. An erection is the result of a combination of neurologic and vascular activity, which may be impaired with aging.

With age, testosterone levels tend to decrease in males. This age-related change does not appear to be related to erectile dysfunction; however, it may decrease interest in sexual activity. Many cases of erectile dysfunction are associated with complications of atherosclerotic disease such as coronary artery disease, peripheral arterial disease, and stroke. Hypertension and antihypertensive medications also have been associated with erectile dysfunction. Diabetes mellitus is associated with a high incidence of erectile dysfunction, which may be secondary to the vascular or neurologic complications (or both) of diabetes.

The evaluation of a patient with erectile dysfunction begins with a medical history. The patient's libido should be determined, as should the frequency and quality of erections. Hypogonadism should be suspected when a marked reduction in libido has occurred. This may also be caused by depression. The medications that are taken and the amount of alcohol use also need to be reviewed carefully. Medications that have been associated with erectile dysfunction include antihypertensive agents, phenothiazines, antidepressants, H_2-receptor antagonists, digoxin, and clofibrate. Symptoms of medical problems such as diabetes mellitus, peripheral neuropathy, peripheral arterial disease, hypertension, thyroid disease (both hypothyroidism and hyperthyroidism), and uremia should be sought. The physical examination should concentrate on findings that would suggest the presence of hypogonadism, peripheral arterial disease, or peripheral neuropathy. Appropriate laboratory tests should include sTSH, fasting blood glucose, and total and bioavailable testosterone. When hypogonadism is suspected, luteinizing hormone (LH) and prolactin levels should be determined. Nocturnal penile tumescence testing is considered unreliable and does not reliably distinguish between psychogenic and organic causes. A duplex scan of the penile arteries can be useful to assess blood flow to the penis. This test can be performed before and after vasodilator therapy and can predict the response to this therapy.

Treatment for erectile dysfunction includes both mechanical and pharmacologic therapies. Appropriate treatment for specific medical disorders that can be associated with erectile dysfunction should be started. Patients with hypogonadism should be given androgens. Androgens alone should not be expected to reverse erectile dysfunction. Vacuum devices are safe and relatively effective for any cause of erectile dysfunction. Intracorporeal injection of prostaglandin E_1 is also effective in producing a sustained erection. Patients tend to lose their enthusiasm for injections with time, probably because of the relatively invasive nature of the treatment. Sildenafil was the first oral medication approved for the treatment of erectile dysfunction. It is effective in up to 70% of patients regardless of the underlying cause. It inhibits the breakdown of cyclic guanosine monophosphate and improves blood flow to the penis. Because of the potential for hypotension, it is contraindicated for persons receiving nitrate therapy. Also, there may be increased risk of adverse effects in those with coronary artery disease.

- One of the most important factors that may determine whether a person is sexually active is the availability of a partner.
- With age, testosterone levels tend to decrease in males and do not appear to be related to erectile dysfunction.
- Treatment for erectile dysfunction includes both mechanical and pharmacologic therapies.

DEMENTIA

Dementia is an acquired cognitive impairment that affects all spheres of the intellect. It is a gradually progressive disorder and becomes more common with increasing age. Approximately 10% of the population older than 65 years have some degree of dementia. The number increases with age and has been reported to be as high as 50% among those older than 90 years. Dementia involves considerably more than the loss of memory. Other cognitive functions that are affected include judgment, abstract thinking, attention, ability to learn new material, and, eventually, the recognition and production of speech. Personality changes frequently accompany dementia. The commonest form of irreversible dementia is Alzheimer disease (50%-70% of cases), followed by vascular dementia (15%-25%). In the recent past, the prevalence of reversible dementias was thought to be as high as 30%. Currently, it is believed that in most patients with some reversibility in cognitive impairment, the improvement is only transient and most of the patients eventually develop irreversible dementia. The prevalence of truly reversible dementia is quite low, from 1% to 2%. The most common causes of potentially reversible dementia include the following: depression, selected drugs, metabolic disorders (hypothyroidism, hyperthyroidism, hyperparathyroidism), toxic agents (heavy metals, pesticides, alcohol, various organic solvents), nutritional deficiencies (vitamin B_{12}, niacin, thiamine), normal-pressure hydrocephalus, subdural hematoma, central nervous system (CNS) tumors, and CNS infections (neurosyphilis, chronic fungal or bacterial meningitis, and human immunodeficiency virus [HIV] infection).

Alzheimer Disease

The diagnosis of Alzheimer disease cannot be confirmed until postmortem examination: no laboratory test or radiologic evaluation, including CT or MRI of the head, is specific for diagnosis of the disease. The diagnosis is made primarily on the basis of the history, usually from family members, and a determination of the cognitive status of the patient. The accuracy of clinicians in diagnosing Alzheimer disease is as high as 95%. The disease is a gradually progressive impairment of cognition. It is characterized by gradually progressive difficulty learning new tasks and information. Loss of memory begins with recent events and eventually includes memory of distant events. Both receptive and expressive language difficulty develop in which the patient has difficulty naming familiar objects and understanding language. Patients may easily become lost, even in familiar surroundings. Calculation skills decline, and patients may no longer be capable of such tasks as balancing a checkbook. Eventually behavioral problems develop in many patients, including the tendency to wander and to develop paranoia, agitation, delusions, or hallucinations (or a combination of these). Typically, patients with Alzheimer disease have little insight into the disease process and are often brought to the physician by a family member. Pathologically, the CNS findings include neuronal plaques, which represent extracellular deposits of protein containing amyloid, and neurofibrillary tangles, which are intracellular protein bound to microtubules. Neuronal plaques and neurofibrillary tangles are also found in non-demented persons but in much smaller amounts. Alzheimer disease is associated with a decreased amount of CNS neurotransmitters such as acetylcholine, norepinephrine, and serotonin. Acetylcholine deficiency is especially prominent, as is a decrease in choline acetyltransferase activity.

The evaluation of a demented patient establishes the existence and degree of cognitive impairment, ruling out reversible dementias. Screening mental status examinations (such as the MMSE) often identify those who may not have obvious cognitive impairment. If cognitive impairment is suspected but the mental status examination findings are normal, formal psychometric studies should be conducted. Normal findings on mental status examinations do not rule out dementia. The MMSE is also used to follow future deterioration. The medical evaluation consists of a medical history and physical examination (including neurologic examination) and general laboratory tests. Accepted laboratory tests include a complete blood count; electrolyte panel; liver function tests; blood urea nitrogen; serum levels of creatinine, calcium, glucose, and vitamin B_{12}; thyroid function; syphilis serology; chest radiography; and ECG. Although some form of brain imaging study (CT or MRI) is usually performed, there are arguments for and against this practice. An imaging study is performed to rule out various types of potentially reversible CNS lesions such as mass lesions, normal-pressure hydrocephalus, or previous strokes and not to examine for cerebral atrophy. If the patient has had dementia for an extended period, has no focal findings on neurologic examination, has

no history of head trauma, and has no headache, an imaging study may not be cost-effective. EEG, HIV testing, and lumbar puncture are performed only in unusual circumstances and are rarely necessary.

Until recently, the treatment of Alzheimer disease has been limited to controlling abnormal behavior (agitation, delusions, hallucinations, and paranoia) with various neuroleptic drugs (sedative-hypnotics and major tranquilizers). None of the neuroleptic medications commonly used improve cognitive function, and very often, they worsen memory and orientation. Major tranquilizers may also cause movement disorders (tardive dyskinesia) and can contribute to falls. The recent availability of tacrine, donepezil, rivastigmine, and galantamine acetylcholinesterase inhibitors has given clinicians the first real options for treating Alzheimer disease. Although acetylcholinesterase inhibitors are not considered disease-modifying drugs, they may transiently delay cognitive decline and should be considered for patients who have mild to moderate dementia. The major benefit of these drugs is their potential to delay institutionalization, although there have been reports of improvement in abnormal behaviors associated with dementia with the use of these drugs. The high prevalence of liver toxicity associated with tacrine has not been found with the other acetylcholinesterase inhibitors. Evidence suggests that vitamin E and selegiline may slow the progression of Alzheimer disease through their antioxidant activity. NSAIDs may protect against the development of Alzheimer disease by suppressing the inflammation and immune response present in the brains of patients with Alzheimer disease. These agents are not given routinely for prevention because of the risk of adverse effects. Estrogen therapy has not been consistently shown to be of benefit in the prevention or treatment of Alzheimer disease.

- The diagnosis of Alzheimer disease is established on the basis of the history, usually from family members, and a determination of the cognitive status of the patient.
- Screening mental status examinations often identify patients who may not have obvious cognitive impairment.
- Accepted laboratory tests include a complete blood count; electrolyte panel; liver function tests; blood urea nitrogen; serum levels of creatinine, calcium, glucose, and vitamin B_{12}; thyroid function; syphilis serology; chest radiography; and ECG. A brain imaging study (CT or MRI) is usually performed.
- Acetylcholinesterase inhibitors may transiently delay cognitive decline.

Diseases other than Alzheimer disease may cause dementia. At times, it may be difficult to differentiate one from the other, although subtle differences often are present clinically.

Vascular Dementia

Vascular dementia tends to affect older persons and is due to repeated cerebral infarcts. It is the second most common cause of dementia and can be difficult to differentiate from Alzheimer disease. The patient usually demonstrates a stepwise progression of cognitive impairment consistent with the multiple ischemic infarcts, often with focal neurologic deficits also produced by the ischemic CNS events. Several types of vascular dementias are possible, including cortical multi-infarcts, subcortical multi-infarcts due to small-vessel thrombosis (lacunar strokes), and deep white matter small-vessel ischemia with demyelination (Binswanger disease). Amyloid angiopathy may cause cognitive impairment and is associated with cerebral hemorrhages. The presentation depends on which portion of the brain is affected by the ischemic insults. CNS imaging usually shows evidence of multiple strokes or white matter ischemia. Treatment consists of management of risk factors for cerebrovascular disease such as hypertension, diabetes mellitus, and hyperlipidemia. Also, antiplatelet therapy is usually given.

- Patients with vascular dementia usually demonstrate a stepwise progression of cognitive impairment.

Dementia With Lewy Bodies

Patients with this cortical dementia have cognitive impairments similar to those of Alzheimer disease. Pathologically, Lewy bodies are cytoplasmic inclusion bodies, and they can be found in subcortical brain tissue. Patients have findings of parkinsonism with bradykinesia, extremity rigidity, and postural instability. Absence of a resting tremor is common (unlike Parkinson disease). The ability of patients to maintain attention is poor. Also, they show marked day-to-day changes in cognitive status and may develop hallucinations (visual and auditory). Patients are very sensitive to the effects of antipsychotic medications and frequently have adverse extrapyramidal reactions, which may be life-threatening.

- Dementia with Lewy bodies is associated with cognitive impairment and findings of parkinsonism.
- Patients typically show marked day-to-day changes.

Dementia With Parkinson Disease

Up to 40% of patients with Parkinson disease develop dementia, and many are indistinguishable from those with Alzheimer disease. These patients have the features typical of Parkinson disease, including resting tremor, rigidity, and bradykinesia, in addition to the intellectual impairments of dementia, which tend to be very slowly progressive. For some patients, effective treatment of Parkinson disease with dopamine improves cognitive status, but not for those with more severe dementia.

- Up to 40% of patients with Parkinson disease develop dementia.

Frontotemporal Dementia

Frontotemporal dementia is characterized by changes in personality and behavior due to prominent frontal lobe involvement. It has less effect on cognitive status and memory impairment. Onset of the disease tends to be somewhat earlier than for Alzheimer disease, often in the 50s and 60s. Patients frequently have poor personal hygiene and disinhibition and may demonstrate hypersexual behavior. Urinary incontinence is also common. Physical examination usually shows prominent frontal reflexes. CNS imaging demonstrates the typical frontal and temporal lobe involvement. One variety of frontotemporal dementia is Pick disease, characterized pathologically by intraneuronal inclusion bodies known as "Pick bodies." Management of the behavioral disturbance is the most challenging aspect of the treatment of this condition.

- Pick disease is characterized by prominent changes in personality and behavior.

Creutzfeldt-Jakob Disease

Creutzfeldt-Jakob disease is an uncommon cause of dementia. It has an earlier onset than Alzheimer disease, usually in the sixth decade. The progression of the disease is rapid, eventually producing a vegetative state and the development of myoclonic jerks and seizures. Most patients die within 1 year after disease onset. The cause is thought to be infectious and due to prions.

- Creutzfeldt-Jakob disease is a rapidly progressive dementia associated with myoclonic jerks and seizures.

Other Dementias

Huntington disease is an autosomal dominant disorder with early onset of symptoms (usually in the fourth or fifth decade). Eventually, choreiform movements develop. Cognitive impairment is severe and progressive. Acquired immunodeficiency syndrome (AIDS) dementia affects up to 50% of persons with AIDS. It can produce a subcortical dementia, and it is gradually progressive. Currently, AIDS dementia is uncommon among the elderly. Also, dementia can occur as a chronic complication of Lyme disease years after onset of the infection.

Delirium

Delirium is an acute confusional disorder frequently mistaken for dementia. It is associated with a decreased level of consciousness, hallucinations, and delusions. Its several causes are listed in Table 10-1. It is important to differentiate delirium from dementia because of the potential for reversibility of cognitive

Table 10-1   Causes of Delirium

Drugs
    Sedative-hypnotics
    Anticholinergic agents
    NSAIDs
    β-Blockers
    Antipsychotic agents
Metabolic disturbances
    Hyperglycemia
    Hypoglycemia
    Hypercalcemia
Hypoxia
Hypotension
Common medical illnesses in patients with limited organ
  reserve function or organ failure
    Urinary tract infection
    Sepsis
    Pneumonia

NSAID, nonsteroidal anti-inflammatory drug.

impairment associated with delirium. Patients with delirium frequently have a preexisting mild (often unrecognized) dementia.

- Delirium is a reversible cause of cognitive impairment and may be related to medications or acute medical conditions.

PREOPERATIVE ASSESSMENT OF THE ELDERLY

Elderly patients commonly undergo anesthesia and surgery, and age alone should not be a contraindication for a surgical procedure. Most elderly persons have some increased risk of perioperative complications because of a combination of normal physiologic changes of aging and, more importantly, various disease states. Most perioperative deaths result from cardiac or respiratory complications. It can be difficult to determine preoperatively if an elderly patient has marked cardiac or respiratory disease. The high prevalence of inactivity among the elderly commonly masks the presence of coronary or pulmonary disease because symptoms may be present only with exercise. Usually, an older patient who is active, without symptoms, at low risk for cardiorespiratory disease, and scheduled for a nonvascular operation does not require further testing. However, asymptomatic patients who are inactive and have several risk factors for cardiorespiratory disease may benefit from noninvasive cardiac or pulmonary testing (or both).

The patient's medications should be reviewed preoperatively. Because of the increased risk of postoperative bleeding, aspirin should be discontinued at least 1 week before the operation. NSAIDs also can increase the risk of bleeding and should be discontinued preoperatively. Because of a shorter antiplatelet effect, NSAIDs may be taken up to 48 hours before the operation. Oral hypoglycemic medications should not be given the morning of the operation because of the risk of hypoglycemia. The blood glucose level can be managed by the administration of regular insulin if needed. Other medications that the patient takes daily should be given the morning of the operation. Cardiovascular medications, especially β-blockers and clonidine, should not be discontinued abruptly. If corticosteroids have been taken recently in doses capable of suppressing adrenal function, they should be given preoperatively.

In addition to the questions typically asked of younger patients during a preoperative assessment, functional ability and cognitive status should be assessed in the elderly. The MMSE is an adequate screening test for cognitive impairment. Patients with cognitive impairment preoperatively are at increased risk for postoperative delirium. They also may have difficulty completing a physical therapy program. It is not unusual for the functional status of an elderly person to deteriorate markedly after an operation, especially with a prolonged hospital stay. It is wise to prepare for assistance in the home or to consider temporary nursing home placement for possible strength rehabilitation to prevent even longer hospitalization.

- Most elderly persons have some increased risk of perioperative complications because of both normal physiologic changes of aging and various disease states.
- Most perioperative deaths result from cardiac or respiratory complications.

PREVENTIVE GERIATRICS

For many disease states, there is evidence to recommend continuing screening tests with advancing age. In other areas, data are not sufficient about whether screening is beneficial for the elderly. In these situations, clinical judgment (taking into account the patient's functional status and estimated life expectancy) is important in deciding whether certain screening tests should be performed. Before a screening test is indicated, several basic principles must be considered, including the following: The incidence of the disease is high enough to warrant performing screening tests. There must be a period during which the disease is present but the patient is asymptomatic and the disease can be diagnosed with a screening test. Effective treatment is available for the disease. Early treatment of the disease has a better outcome than it would if the diagnosis is made after symptoms develop. The screening test has a reasonable sensitivity and specificity and is relatively inexpensive and safe.

Cardiovascular Disease

- High low-density lipoprotein (LDL) cholesterol and low high-density lipoprotein (HDL) cholesterol carry predictive value in the elderly for coronary artery disease. Many organizations now recommend checking for hyperlipidemia in persons older than 65 years, especially those who have an established diagnosis of coronary artery disease or multiple risk factors.
- The risks of hypertension as well as the benefits of treatment extend to the elderly, and it is recommended that screening for hypertension be performed in the elderly.
- Routine screening for carotid artery disease in the elderly is not recommended.
- Routine screening with a resting or exercise ECG is not recommended for the elderly.

Malignancy

- Because breast cancer continues to increase in incidence with age, continued annual screening with mammography is recommended. For patients older than 75 years, clinical judgment should be used. If appropriate, it is reasonable to continue mammography as long as the patient's life expectancy exceeds 5 years.
- Although colon cancer is common among the elderly, screening recommendations require clinical judgment. Tests with an acceptable sensitivity and specificity (e.g., colonoscopy) are difficult for many elderly and have some associated risks. Simple tests such as digital rectal examination or fecal occult blood tests have a low sensitivity and specificity. The American Cancer Society recommends several options for colon cancer screening. According to these recommendations, annual fecal occult blood testing, with flexible sigmoidoscopy every 5 years, is preferable. Colonoscopy should be performed if the results of either test are abnormal. For those at increased risk for colorectal cancer, such as a history of colorectal adenomatous polyps, screening with colonoscopy should be performed. The Preventive Health Services Task Force recommends screening with fecal occult blood testing or sigmoidoscopy or both.
- If cervical Papanicolau smears have been performed appropriately at younger ages and the results have been negative, performing the smears may be discontinued at age 65. For the elderly who did not have regular screening with cervical Papanicolau smears, the incidence of cervical cancer is notable. Screening is recommended for older women who have not previously had a screening test or if information about previous screening is unavailable or if screening is unlikely to have occurred in the past.
- Although prostate cancer is common in males, screening tests are controversial. The U.S. Preventive Task Force considers the evidence inadequate to recommend for or against screening for prostate cancer with the prostate-specific antigen test or digital rectal examination. The American Cancer Society recommends that a digital rectal examination and prostate-specific antigen test be offered annually to men older than 50 if they have a life expectancy of at least 10 years.
- Screening tests for lung cancer, including chest radiography, chest CT, or sputum cytology, are not recommended for either smokers or nonsmokers.
- No test has been recommended for the early detection of ovarian cancer.

PULMONARY CHANGES

Pulmonary function decreases with advancing age, likely because of a combination of normal anatomical and physiologic changes, injury from exposure to various environmental toxins (tobacco and air pollution), and disease states that affect the lung. Changes in the shape of the thorax also contribute to changes in pulmonary physiology. The apical-to-base length of the lungs decreases as the anterior-to-posterior length increases with age. The bronchioles and alveolar ducts increase in diameter, decreasing alveolar surface area. The aging lungs also have reduced compliance because of decreased lung elasticity. These anatomical and physiologic changes result in reduced airflow rates, decreased efficiency of air exchange, and alterations in lung volumes. Changes that occur with aging in pulmonary physiology include a decrease in mucociliary clearance, vital capacity, 1-second forced expiratory volume (FEV_1), maximal breathing capacity, and diffusing capacity (DLCO). The lung residual volume and alveolar-arterial oxygen gradient (AaO_2) increase with age. Aging has no effect on total lung capacity.

- Pulmonary function decreases with advancing age because of a combination of anatomical and physiologic changes, exposure to environmental toxins, and disease states that affect the lung.

RESPIRATORY DISEASE

Pneumonia is one of the top 10 causes of death among the elderly and is the cause of death of 15% of nursing home residents. The bacterial organisms that cause pneumonia change with advancing age. The elderly have an increased number of gram-negative bacteria as part of their normal oral flora. They also have an increased likelihood of aspirating oral secretions, which contributes to the increased incidence of pneumonia caused by gram-negative and anaerobic bacteria. The likely cause of pneumonia depends on the setting in which the elderly patient acquired the infection. Overall, *Streptococcus pneumoniae* is the commonest etiologic organism. *Haemophilus influenzae*, other gram-negative bacteria, and anaerobes are common among the elderly in nursing homes and hospitals. Organisms such as *Legionella, Chlamydia,* and *Moraxella catarrhalis* are also found occasionally in the elderly. Treatment for pneumonia should reflect the most likely etiologic agent. Recently, a large percentage of *S. pneumoniae* organisms have become penicillin-resistant. Appropriate empirical treatment of pneumonia acquired by an elderly patient in an outpatient setting is a second-generation cephalosporin. An extended-spectrum macrolide (clarithromycin or azithromycin) would also be acceptable. For hospital-acquired pneumonia, additional coverage is needed for gram-negative and atypical bacteria. Acceptable treatment includes a third-generation cephalosporin, with erythromycin given intravenously. An extended-spectrum quinolone could also be given. Nursing home-acquired pneumonia can be quite serious; however, if the patient's condition is not toxic and appears stable and the patient is able to take adequate oral fluids, the pneumonia can be treated in the nursing home if the patient is observed closely. Generally, a third-generation cephalosporin given intramuscularly or an extended-spectrum quinolone is the treatment of choice for these patients.

- The elderly have an increased number of gram-negative bacteria as part of their normal oral flora and an increased likelihood of aspirating oral secretions.
- *Streptococcus pneumoniae* is the commonest etiologic organism of pneumonia.
- Pneumonia due to *Haemophilus influenzae*, other gram-negative bacteria, or anaerobes is common in nursing homes and hospitals.

Tuberculosis, after decreasing in frequency for many years, is increasing in frequency. The number of reported cases has increased 20% over the past 10 years. Tuberculosis is more common with advancing age, with the elderly having two to four times the case rate of those younger than 65 years. Persons residing in nursing homes have from two to six times the case rate of the general population. Most cases of tuberculosis in the elderly are due to reactivation of a previous infection rather than being newly acquired disease. It is thought that about 10% of patients with a positive tuberculin skin test (PPD) eventually develop active tuberculosis (4% in the first 2 years). Tuberculosis is suspected on the basis of clinical findings, which can be subtle and include fatigue, anorexia with weight loss, and cough. Chest radiographic findings may be helpful in assessing whether disease is present. Confirmation of the disease requires evaluation of sputum and gastric washings for the presence of the acid-fast organisms. Although culture results usually are available within 2 weeks, cultures may take up to 8 weeks to become positive. An increasing number of multidrug-resistant *Mycobacterium tuberculosis* organisms are being detected; however, these organisms are not commonly seen in the elderly because most cases are due to reactivation of the disease acquired many years ago when there were fewer drug-resistant organisms.

Without symptoms, the PPD is the best test available to determine the possibility of tuberculosis. Intermediate-strength tuberculin (5 TU) is administered intradermally, and the degree of induration (not erythema) is determined.

On admission to a nursing home, the patient should have a two-stage PPD. The second test is administered on the seventh day if the patient has less than 10 mm of induration. The second test is interpreted 2 days after it is applied. Up to 15% of additional patients with a positive reaction are identified with this method. If the PPD is positive, chest radiography should be performed. If the findings are negative and the patient is asymptomatic, no treatment should be initiated unless it can be shown that the patient has had conversion to a positive PPD within the last 2 years. If the chest radiographic findings are abnormal, sputum and gastric washings should be obtained and cultured.

Up to one-third of all new patients admitted to a nursing home may have a positive PPD. Chemoprophylaxis is not recommended for all elderly with a positive PPD. Toxicity from isoniazid (INH), especially hepatotoxicity, is very common in the elderly. Evidence of active tuberculosis should be excluded before chemoprophylaxis is given. Elderly patients receiving isoniazid treatment should have close follow-up for symptoms of hepatotoxicity. Isoniazid-induced hepatotoxicity is common with advancing age and develops in up to 5% of those older than 65 years. The baseline level of aspartate aminotransferase should be determined and checked periodically in elderly patients taking isoniazid. These patients also should receive vitamin B_6 (pyridoxine) supplements (10-25 mg daily) to prevent peripheral neuropathy.

IMMUNIZATIONS

Pneumococcal pneumonia vaccine is effective against 23 strains of *S. pneumoniae*, which accounts for 80% of the strains that commonly cause pneumonia. Because of decreasing effectiveness, revaccination should be considered after 6 years for those who received their initial vaccination before age 65. The influenza vaccine is changed on a yearly basis, depending on the prevalent strain. It should be given in late autumn, and it should be given annually to high-risk persons, persons older than 65, and those in frequent close contact with the elderly. After the vaccine has been injected, it takes about 2 to 3 weeks before immunity to influenza develops. Any of the elderly who are unvaccinated during an influenza epidemic should be given amantadine or rimantadine.

- Pneumococcal pneumonia vaccine is effective against 80% of the bacterial strains that commonly cause pneumonia.
- Influenza vaccine should be given annually to high-risk persons, persons older than 65, and those in frequent close contact with the elderly.

OSTEOPOROSIS

Osteoporosis and its complications are extremely common among the elderly. Osteoporosis results in a loss of bone density, with a normal bone-to-mineral ratio. Hip, wrist, and vertebral compression fractures are common causes of morbidity and mortality. Peak bone density is achieved at about age 30, with men having a greater bone density than women at all ages. After age 30, bone density gradually decreases. In women, loss of estrogen, either because of surgery (bilateral oophorectomy) or menopause, causes a more rapid decrease in bone density.

- Hip, wrist, and vertebral compression fractures are common causes of morbidity and mortality from osteoporosis.
- No simple laboratory tests are available that can confirm the diagnosis of osteoporosis. The diagnosis is usually made clinically. The following help in establishing the diagnosis:
  1. The presence of multiple risk factors, including advanced age, female sex, white, low calcium intake through much of one's lifetime, thin build, a history of corticosteroid or tobacco use, history of previous fracture (especially vertebral), northern European ancestry, prolonged inactivity, and family history positive for osteoporosis
  2. Ruling out secondary causes (glucocorticoid excess, hypogonadism, hyperthyroidism, hyperparathyroidism, osteomalacia, myeloma)
  3. Physical examination findings (loss of height, increased thoracic kyphosis)
  4. Radiographic findings of osteopenia or vertebral compression fractures

- The diagnosis of osteoporosis is usually made clinically.

Bone density can be measured with several techniques, the most common of which is dual X-ray absorptiometry. Bone density is determined to assess the risk of fracture, to follow the progression of disease, or to evaluate the response to treatment.

- Bone density is determined to assess the risk of fracture, to follow the progression of disease, or to evaluate the response to treatment.

Previously, the treatment of osteoporosis was disappointing and was aimed at prevention. Currently, several therapeutic options are available that can provide effective treatment for established osteoporosis. The initial treatment for osteoporosis in postmenopausal women should be adequate calcium intake, weight-bearing exercise, and adequate vitamin D (600-800 IU daily). Premenopausal women require 1,000 mg daily of elemental calcium, and postmenopausal women require 1,500 mg daily. Calcium carbonate is adequate for most, and it is the least expensive form of calcium supplementation. Calcium citrate should be used if the patient has a lack of gastric acid. Pharmacologic therapy is effective in increasing bone density as well as decreasing the risk of bone fractures. Although hormonal therapy has been shown to stabilize the decrease in bone density and, in some cases, to increase bone density slightly, alternative pharmacologic treatment is more effective and has fewer adverse effects. The bisphosphonates alendronate and risedronate increase bone density and decrease the risk of hip and vertebral fractures. Compliance with these medications can be a problem, although both are now available in once-weekly dosing. They are poorly absorbed and bind to food and calcium and, thus, must be taken with tap water before food is ingested. Also, they have been associated with esophagitis. To minimize this, the patient must remain upright for at least 30 minutes after taking the medication.

Calcitonin increases vertebral bone density, but more data are needed to know whether it decreases the risk of hip fracture. Calcitonin appears to have an analgesic effect and may be helpful in patients with painful osteoporotic vertebral compression fractures. Raloxifene is a selective estrogen receptor modulator that reduces bone resorption. Although it has estrogen-like effects on bone, it acts as an estrogen antagonist in the breast and uterus. It can cause a modest increase in bone mineral density in the hip and spine. Teriparatide is a synthetic polypeptide consisting of the biologically active *N*-terminal portion of human parathyroid hormone. It has recently been released and approved for the treatment of osteoporosis. Unlike all other treatment options for osteoporosis, parathyroid hormone increases bone formation rather than decreasing bone resorption. It appears to produce a greater increase in bone density than other pharmacologic treatments for osteoporosis; however, its high cost may be prohibitive for many patients. Also, it must be administered daily by subcutaneous injection.

- Initial treatment of osteoporosis in postmenopausal women should be adequate calcium intake, weight-bearing exercise, adequate vitamin D (600-800 IU/d), and hormonal replacement therapy.
- Bisphosphonates increase bone density and decrease the rate of hip and vertebral fractures.

- Calcitonin appears to have an analgesic effect and may be helpful in patients with painful osteoporotic vertebral compression fractures.
- Raloxifene is a selective estrogen receptor modulator that reduces bone resorption and produces a modest increase in bone mineral density in the hip and spine.
- Teriparatide may be an option for a select group of patients with osteoporosis.

OSTEOMALACIA

Osteomalacia is the result of defective bone mineralization and is caused most commonly by a deficiency of vitamin D. It may be due to inadequate intake of vitamin D, lack of exposure to the sun, malabsorption, chronic liver disease, or chronic renal disease. Radiographically, the bone appears osteopenic and can resemble osteoporosis. Unlike osteoporosis, several abnormal laboratory findings are associated with osteomalacia, including decreased levels of calcium, phosphorus, and 1,25-dihydroxyvitamin D and increased levels of alkaline phosphatase. Defective bone mineralization may also be caused by very low levels of phosphate. This can be due to excessive use of aluminum-containing antacids, tumor effect, or renal tubule disorders.

- Osteomalacia is the result of defective bone mineralization and is most commonly caused by a deficiency of vitamin D.
- Osteomalacia is associated with decreased levels of calcium, phosphorus, and 1,25-dihydroxyvitamin D and increased levels of alkaline phosphatase.

PRESSURE ULCERS

Seventy percent of pressure ulcers occur in persons older than 70 years. Approximately 60% of pressure ulcers develop during hospitalization, 18% in nursing homes, and the rest at home. They are especially common among the elderly in intensive care units. The most important risk factor for the development of a pressure ulcer is immobility. Nutritional deficiencies, age-related changes in the skin, and urinary incontinence are also contributing risk factors. Most pressure ulcers occur below the waist. The common sites include the sacrum, greater trochanter, ischial tuberosity, calcaneus, and lateral malleolus of the ankle. Four factors are thought to be important in the development of pressure ulcers: pressure, shearing force, friction, and moisture. When the persistent pressure of skin overlying a bony prominence exceeds the capillary pressure, the blood supply to the tissues is impaired. After approximately 2 hours, tissue ischemia can occur and result in skin ulceration. This is the basis for rotating patients at least every 2 hours when they are incapable of turning themselves. Friction

and shearing forces are contributing factors when the patient is dragged across a bed or chair. This has the effect of causing angulation and occlusion of subcutaneous blood vessels and producing ischemia of the underlying tissue. Chronic skin moisture produces tissue maceration and promotes skin breakdown. This tends to magnify skin damage.

- Risk factors for the development of pressure ulcers are immobility, nutritional deficiencies, age-related changes in the skin, and urinary incontinence.

Pressure ulcers can be classified into one of four stages (I-IV). They tend to be understaged because often the underlying tissue damage is not immediately apparent.

Stage I: Nonblanchable erythema of intact skin. There may be associated edema.

Stage II: Partial-thickness skin loss involving the epidermis or dermis or both. The ulcer is superficial and may present as an abrasion, a blister, or a shallow crater.

Stage III: Full-thickness skin loss with damage or necrosis of subcutaneous tissue. The damage may extend to the fascia. The ulcer is a deep crater.

Stage IV: Full-thickness skin loss with extensive destruction, tissue necrosis, or involvement of muscle, bone, or tendons. Sinus tracts may be present.

The most important component of the treatment of pressure ulcers is prevention. Preventive strategies include repositioning patients at least every 2 hours to minimize tissue ischemia over sites at risk. Several commercial devices are available to help reduce contact pressure. The use of pressure-reducing mattresses can decrease the pressure over a given area of tissue. Minimizing head elevation and lifting the patient instead of dragging will prevent friction and shearing force. Keeping the patient as dry as possible when incontinent and keeping the skin moisturized help maintain skin integrity.

After a pressure ulcer has developed, the basic strategy for its treatment includes the following:

- Relieving pressure over the ulcer.
- Debridement of nonviable tissue.
- Optimizing the wound environment (preventing wound maceration and avoiding friction and shearing forces) to promote the formation of granulation tissue.
- Management of other conditions (malnutrition or infection when present) that may delay wound healing.

Stages II, III, and IV pressure ulcers should be debrided of necrotic tissue when present. Stage II ulcers can be debrided mechanically with wet-to-wet (saline) gauze dressings changed every 6 hours. Also, several enzymatic debriding agents are available and effective. Surgical debridement may be useful, especially for deeper ulcers (stages III and IV). This should be done with caution in patients with lower extremity ulcers and arterial disease. Water debridement (whirlpool) is useful for larger ulcers. A moist wound environment is optimal for wound healing. Heat lamps dry the ulcer and should not be used. Several products are available to help maintain a moist wound environment, including semipermeable polyurethane films and foams, hydrocolloid dressings, and hydrophilic polymer gels. Topical iodine-povidone, hydrogen peroxide, and acetic acid compounds can impair wound healing and should not be used on pressure ulcers. Infection commonly complicates the healing of pressure ulcers. Infected ulcers require treatment with systemic antibiotics. Topical antibiotics have little penetration into deeper tissue and can promote the development of resistant bacteria. Culturing the surface of an ulcer does not represent accurately the bacteria involved in an infected ulcer; all skin ulcers develop surface bacterial colonization. An accurate determination of the bacteria involved requires deep tissue cultures.

An ulcer that does not heal should alert the physician to the presence of osteomyelitis. Bone radiographs and bone scans are often performed in patients with suspected osteomyelitis, but they have a rather high incidence of false-negative and false-positive results. MRI is an effective diagnostic test when osteomyelitis is suspected; however, bone biopsy with culture is the best confirmatory test.

Platelet-derived growth factor is occasionally useful in stimulating the healing of pressure ulcers. For large or very deep ulcers, surgical treatment may be necessary. The use of skin grafts or rotation flaps using neighboring subcutaneous tissue and muscle may be the best option for these patients.

- Stages II, III, and IV pressure ulcers should be debrided of necrotic tissue.
- A moist wound environment is optimal for wound healing.
- Infected ulcers require treatment with systemic antibiotics.
- Bone biopsy with culture is the best confirmatory test for osteomyelitis.

URINARY INCONTINENCE

Urinary incontinence is common among the elderly, affecting at least 15% of those living independently and about 50% of those in institutions. It is much more common in females than in males. It causes numerous medical, social, and economic complications and is a common reason for nursing home placement. These complications include urinary tract infection, skin breakdown, social isolation, and depression. Understanding urinary incontinence requires knowledge of the anatomy of the urinary tract and the physiology of normal micturition. Failure to appreciate this information can result in inaccurate diagnosis and ineffective treatment.

Anatomy

The detrusor muscle consists of three muscular layers. Its functions include urine storage (relaxed detrusor) and urine emptying (detrusor contraction). Both sympathetic and parasympathetic nerves innervate the detrusor muscle. Stimulation of the sympathetic nerves results in relaxation of the detrusor muscle, and stimulation of the parasympathetic nerves produces contraction of the detrusor muscle. The internal sphincter is a smooth muscle under involuntary (sympathetic innervation) control. Sympathetic stimulation produces increased internal sphincter tone. The external sphincter is striated muscle and under voluntary (pudendal innervation) control. It contracts in response to transient increases in intra-abdominal pressure (e.g., cough or sneeze) but fatigues rapidly.

Stretch receptors in the wall of the detrusor muscle send information to the CNS. The spinal cord transmits sensory signals to the brain and motor signals to the bladder. The brain causes stimulation of the sympathetic nerves and inhibition of the parasympathetic nerves when urine storage is desired (relaxation of the detrusor muscle and contraction of the internal sphincter) and stimulation of the parasympathetic nerves and inhibition of the sympathetic nerves when bladder emptying is desired (contraction of the detrusor muscle and relaxation of the internal sphincter).

- Both sympathetic and parasympathetic nerves innervate the detrusor muscle.
- Stimulation of the sympathetic nerves results in relaxation of the detrusor muscle, and stimulation of the parasympathetic nerves produces contraction of the detrusor muscle.

Effects of Age

Changes in the urinary system that occur with age do not cause urinary incontinence: incontinence is not a normal result of aging. However, the changes that occur can contribute to the problem of incontinence. These changes include smaller bladder capacity, early contractions of the detrusor muscle, decreased ability to suppress contractions of the detrusor muscle and to postpone urination, and increased nocturnal production of urine.

Medications Affecting Urination and Continence

Many medications can have an effect on urinary continence. They may alter the ability of the brain to appreciate bladder fullness or the ability of the internal sphincter to contract and relax, or they may interfere with the function of the bladder. These medications include potent diuretics that cause brisk filling of the bladder, anticholinergic agents that can impair contraction of the detrusor muscle, sedative-hypnotics that may cause confusion, narcotics that impair contraction of the detrusor muscle, α-adrenergic agonists that increase internal sphincter tone, α-adrenergic antagonists that decrease internal sphincter tone, and calcium channel blockers that decrease detrusor muscle tone.

Established Incontinence

Patients are more likely to have reversible incontinence if the incontinence is of recent onset. Although established incontinence is more difficult to treat, it can be managed with substantial benefit to the patient. The four types of established incontinence are overactive bladder (urge incontinence), outlet incompetence (stress incontinence), overflow incontinence, and functional or iatrogenic incontinence.

Overactivity of the detrusor muscle (urge incontinence, overactive bladder) is a common cause of established incontinence, accounting for 40% to 70% of cases. It tends to be most common in middle-aged and older women and men. It causes early detrusor contractions at low bladder volumes. Symptoms include urinary frequency and urgency, with losses of small-to-moderate urine volumes. Nocturia often occurs. At times, detrusor overactivity is seen with CNS disease (mass lesions, Parkinson disease, stroke) or bladder irritation (urinary tract infection, benign prostatic hyperplasia, fecal impaction, atrophic urethritis). There is no association between chronic asymptomatic bacteriuria and urinary incontinence.

- Overactivity of the detrusor muscle is a common cause of established incontinence.
- Symptoms include urinary frequency and urgency, with losses of small-to-moderate urine volumes and nocturia.

Outlet incompetence (stress incontinence) is common in middle-aged women and rare in men (unless internal sphincter damage has occurred). It is caused by inadequate resistance of urinary outflow and worsened by laxity of pelvic floor musculature and lack of bladder support. This may be caused by hypermobility of the urethra or intrinsic urinary sphincter insufficiency. The symptoms include losses of small amounts of urine with transient increases in intra-abdominal pressure (e.g., cough, sneeze, laugh, or change in position). Some patients describe a combination of urgency incontinence and stress incontinence. This is known as "mixed urinary incontinence." In these patients, the history can be confusing.

- Outlet incompetence (stress incontinence) is common in women.
- Symptoms include losses of small amounts of urine with transient increases in intra-abdominal pressure.

Overflow incontinence is uncommon. It is seen with urinary outflow obstruction (benign prostatic hyperplasia, prostate cancer, or pelvic tumor) or detrusor underactivity-hypotonic bladder (autonomic neuropathy). This often occurs transiently postoperatively in the elderly. Symptoms are difficulty emptying the bladder, with low urine flow, and frequent urinary dribbling. Patients give a history of difficulty starting urination and a weak urinary stream, with stream hesitancy.

Functional incontinence is the inability of normally continent patients to reach toilet facilities in time. Often, it is due to various medications (e.g., potent diuretics and α-adrenergic antagonists) and some limitation of mobility (restraint use, arthritis, or hemiparesis).

- Overflow incontinence is uncommon and due to urinary outflow obstruction or detrusor underactivity-hypotonic bladder.
- An atonic or hypotonic bladder often occurs transiently postoperatively.

Evaluation of Incontinence

The evaluation of urinary incontinence includes a thorough medical history, physical examination, and several simple selected laboratory tests. The history is most important and should include the amount of urine lost, duration of symptoms, precipitating factors, whether symptoms of obstruction exist, and the patient's functional status. Also, symptoms of neurologic disease, associated disease states, menstrual status and parity, and medications taken should be documented.

Physical examination of the abdomen should evaluate bladder distention and possible abdominal masses. In examining the pelvis, assess for uterine, bladder, or rectal prolapse; atrophic vaginitis; and pelvic masses. The rectal examination should document any masses, fecal impaction, sphincter tone, and prostate enlargement or nodules. A neurologic examination should be performed to search for disease of the brain or spinal cord, autonomic nerves, or peripheral nerves.

Laboratory tests commonly ordered in the investigation of urinary incontinence include urinalysis and urine culture to check for infection, pyuria, and hematuria; blood urea nitrogen and creatinine determination to assess renal function; calcium and glucose measurements to assess polyuric states; occasionally, intravenous pyelography or renal ultrasonography (or both) to check for hydronephrosis, which may occur with chronic bladder outlet obstruction; and postvoid residual bladder volume to estimate the degree of bladder emptying.

Urodynamic studies are occasionally necessary to establish the diagnosis of incontinence, but the results are not always consistent with the clinical picture and, thus, can be misleading. Urodynamic studies are indicated when patients have medically confusing histories or more than one type of urinary incontinence (mixed incontinence). Cystometry measures bladder volume and pressure and can be used to detect uninhibited detrusor muscle contractions, lack of bladder contractions, and bladder sensation. Voiding cystourethrography measures the urethrovesical angle and residual urine volume. Uroflow measures urinary flow rate, and electromyography evaluates the external sphincter and detects detrusor-sphincter dyssynergia.

- The medical history is the most important part of the incontinence evaluation.
- Urodynamic studies are occasionally necessary to establish the diagnosis of incontinence, but the results can be misleading in some patients.

Treatment of Incontinence

The treatment of urinary incontinence is usually successful to some degree. All patients should be encouraged to drink an adequate volume of fluid, 40 to 60 oz daily. Patients should complete a voiding diary that records fluid intake, types of fluids ingested, and voidings (both continent and incontinent). The treatment of detrusor overactivity is aimed at suppressing the early contractions of the detrusor muscle. Behavioral training should be the initial treatment attempted. Often, it is successful in decreasing incontinent episodes. It includes eliminating bladder irritants (especially caffeine), urge suppression techniques, scheduled toileting, and prompted voiding. When behavioral training is ineffective, pharmacologic therapy may be added. Medications that inhibit parasympathetic stimulation of the bladder muscle (anticholinergics) are often effective. Drugs with anticholinergic activity that are most commonly used include oxybutynin and tolterodine. Tricyclic antidepressants have also been used, but they have a higher risk of anticholinergic adverse effects (dry mouth, constipation, blurred vision). Topical estrogen therapy may also be effective in some women when atrophic urethritis is the cause of early contractions of the detrusor muscle.

- The treatment of detrusor overactivity is aimed at suppressing early detrusor contractions.
- Nonpharmacologic therapy should be attempted initially.
- Medications that inhibit parasympathetic stimulation of the bladder muscle (anticholinergics) are often effective.
- Topical estrogen therapy may also be effective.

The treatment of outlet incompetence should also begin with behavioral therapy. Patients should be instructed in pelvic floor exercises (Kegel exercises). This often is more effective with the assistance of biofeedback. Although pelvic floor exercises are useful, they must be performed for several months before any benefit is recognized. Increasing the tone of the internal sphincter with α-adrenergic agonists (pseudoephedrine or imipramine) may be of limited short-term benefit. Tolerance to these medications develops quickly, and the beneficial effect disappears. Hormonal therapy (topical estrogen) has been used for outlet incompetence in an attempt to restore the mucosa of the urethra, increasing its resistance, but the results have been disappointing. Pessaries are occasionally used for outlet incompetence, but chronic use is difficult because of potential vaginal irritation. Urethral plugs are available and can provide temporary relief of symptoms. However, they potentially can produce urethral irritation.

For selected patients, surgical therapy may be effective. Internal sphincter bulking agents such as collagen may provide substantial benefit for up to 2 years. Occasionally a surgical procedure to provide an artificial urinary sphincter may be considered. For patients who have more severe symptoms of outlet incompetence, surgical suspension of the bladder and bladder neck sling therapy can restore continence.

- Patients with outlet incompetence should be instructed in pelvic floor exercises.
- Pharmacologic treatment has limited short-term benefit.
- For selected patients, surgical therapy may be effective.

The treatment of overflow incontinence is aimed at providing complete drainage from a bladder that either is not contracting adequately or has marked outflow obstruction. For a hypotonic bladder, treatment can be tried with medications that increase the tone of the detrusor muscle, including the cholinergic agonist bethanechol. This may be effective for short-term use, for example, for a transient hypotonic bladder postoperatively; however, adverse effects are common in the elderly and limit its long-term use. Treatment of obstruction includes operation (transurethral resection of the prostate) and use of α-adrenergic antagonists (terazosin, doxazosin, or tamsulosin), which decrease the tone of the internal sphincter. An external (condom) urinary catheter is of little benefit because it does not provide adequate drainage of the bladder. Occasionally, an indwelling catheter or intermittent catheterization is necessary. When a patient is expected to regain contractile function of the bladder, intermittent catheterization is performed at a frequency determined by the residual urine volume. If outflow obstruction is a chronic condition and not expected to improve, indefinite self-catheterization or an indwelling catheter may become necessary.

- Medications that increase the tone of the detrusor muscle can be tried for transient hypotonic bladder.
- Surgery is often necessary to relieve bladder outlet obstruction from benign prostatic hypertrophy.
- An indwelling catheter or indefinite catheterization is occasionally necessary.

Urologic Consultation

In most elderly patients, the diagnosis of urinary incontinence can be established without the need for evaluation by a urologist. The following conditions indicate the need for urologic evaluation: high postvoid residual urine volume, symptoms of urinary outflow obstruction, marked uterine or bladder prolapse, abnormal findings on prostate examination, recurrent urinary tract infection, hematuria, unknown diagnosis, or failure to improve with treatment.

Use of Urinary Catheters

External (condom) catheters have a slight risk of infection, and problems with penile skin breakdown limit long-term use. They also have minimal benefit in overflow incontinence. Intermittent catheterization has a small risk of infection with each catheter insertion (from 1% in those who are ambulatory and otherwise healthy to 20% in those who are frail and have multiple chronic illnesses). It is useful for temporary incontinence, as in postoperative transient hypotonic bladder. Postvoid residual volumes should be used as a guide in determining the frequency of catheterization. Intermittent catheterization is of limited use in the management of chronic incontinence in nursing home patients because of catheter expense and in those living independently if they have limited manual dexterity or poor vision.

Essentially all patients with indwelling catheters eventually develop marked bacteriuria. Other than maintaining a closed urinary collection system, nothing has been found to prevent or even substantially delay the onset of bacteriuria. Neither urethral cleansing nor bladder irrigation has been shown to be effective. The chronic use of suppressive antibiotics is not recommended because it does not prevent long-term suppression of bacteriuria and eventually results in infections caused by resistant organisms. Antibiotic treatment should be reserved for symptomatic infections only, although it may be difficult to determine when a symptomatic urinary tract infection is present in a catheterized elderly patient.

- Essentially all patients with indwelling catheters eventually develop marked bacteriuria.
- Chronic use of suppressive antibiotics is not recommended.

URINARY TRACT INFECTION

Urinary tract infection becomes more common with advancing age and causes a wide spectrum of disease. It is the most common infection in nursing home residents and the most common cause of sepsis in the elderly. It also may produce the syndrome of asymptomatic bacteriuria. Incomplete emptying of the bladder, which is common in the elderly (cystocele, benign prostatic hyperplasia, or hypotonic bladder), urinary

instrumentation, and chronic catheterization all predispose the elderly to urinary tract infection. The elderly have various bacterial organisms that typically produce urinary tract infections. *Escherichia coli*, the most common organism to cause urinary tract infections in the younger population, causes about half of these infections in the elderly. Other gram-negative organisms such as *Enterococcus* sp, *Proteus* sp, *Klebsiella* sp, and *Pseudomonas* sp are common in the elderly. Because of the variety of organisms, the urine usually should be cultured when evaluating an elderly patient who has a urinary tract infection. Treatment may be started with typical antibiotics (e.g., trimethoprim/sulfamethoxazole, amoxicillin, or cephalosporins), pending the results of urine culture. Those who have potential for resistant organisms (recent antibiotic use, hospitalization, or indwelling urinary catheter) should receive an antibiotic with a wider spectrum of coverage, such as a quinolone, pending the results of the culture.

Asymptomatic bacteriuria becomes more common with age and has been associated with increased mortality; however, the mortality appears to be unrelated to the bacteriuria and is likely a marker for increased severity of illness, frailty, and debility. Asymptomatic bacteriuria should not be treated unless there is a history of chronic urinary obstruction. Asymptomatic bacteriuria is common in patients with indwelling urinary catheters. Most of these patients eventually develop bacteriuria, and the bacterial organisms change with time. Routine surveillance cultures should not be performed, and the bacteriuria should not be treated unless the patient is symptomatic. In patients who have had urinary catheters removed, bacteriuria should be treated if the urine remains bacteriuric for more than 48 hours. In many cases, the bacteriuria will resolve with removal of the urinary catheter alone.

- Urinary tract infection is the most common infection in nursing home residents and the most common cause of sepsis in the elderly.
- Because of the variety of organisms, the urine should be cultured when evaluating an elderly patient who has a urinary tract infection.
- Asymptomatic bacteriuria should not be treated unless there is a history of chronic urinary obstruction.

USE OF MEDICATIONS IN THE ELDERLY

More than 30% of all prescriptions are written for persons older than 65 years. Medications are a common cause of iatrogenic disease in the elderly and are handled differently in the elderly because of various changes in pharmacokinetics and pharmacodynamics. Overall, the activity of many drugs has a longer duration, lower doses often achieve desired therapeutic effects, adverse drug effects are more frequent, drug-drug interactions are more frequent, and the likelihood of drug toxicity is greater in the elderly.

Pharmacokinetics includes drug absorption, distribution, metabolism, and elimination. Age-related changes have an effect on each of these variables, affecting some more than others. Age-related changes that have an effect on drug absorption include decreased blood supply to the small bowel (the site of most drug absorption), villous atrophy resulting in decreased surface area for the absorption of drugs, and decreased gastric acidity. Little evidence supports any marked reduction in drug absorption with increasing age. Drug absorption is the least important of the pharmacokinetic changes associated with aging. Drug distribution has a major role in altered pharmacokinetics and changes significantly with age. This is due to age-related alterations in the various volumes of distribution in the elderly. These changes include an increase in adipose tissue, a decrease in total body water and lean body mass, and, for many, a change in levels of plasma protein. The result of increased adipose tissue is an increase in the volume of distribution for lipid-soluble drugs, which can result in an increase in drug half-life (e.g., highly lipid-soluble benzodiazepines). The decrease in body water creates a smaller volume of distribution for water-soluble drugs, potentially leading to a higher than expected drug concentration (e.g., ethanol). A decrease in plasma protein (e.g., albumin) results in less protein-bound (inactive) acidic drugs and a greater amount of free (active) drug. This can produce a greater than anticipated drug effect. α_1-Acid glycoproteins are acute phase reactants and increase in patients with inflammatory conditions. This can cause an increase in basic drug (lidocaine, propranolol) protein binding and less free drug and may result in a less than anticipated drug effect.

Drug metabolism occurs primarily in the liver. With advanced age, the ability of the liver to metabolize drugs decreases because of various factors, including a decrease in the number of functioning hepatocytes, reduced hepatic blood flow, and reduced hepatic enzymatic activity. Phase I metabolism involves the oxidation or reduction of a drug by the cytochrome P450 system. This type of metabolism produces active metabolites and slows with age. Phase II metabolism involves acetylation and produces inactive metabolites. It shows no changes with advancing age. A patient's ability to metabolize a specific drug is extremely difficult to predict because no simple test is available that provides this information.

Drug elimination refers primarily to the ability of the renal system to excrete drugs from the circulation. Generally, renal function decreases with age, with both decreased renal plasma flow and glomerular filtration rate (up to 30%), although the variability among elderly persons is great. The serum level of creatinine is not a good measure of renal function in the elderly and tends to underestimate the degree of renal insufficiency.

Creatinine is a product of muscle breakdown. Because lean body mass decreases with advancing age, less creatinine is produced. Thus, an elderly patient who has as much as a 30% reduction in renal function may have a normal serum level of creatinine. A more accurate estimate of renal function is the following:

$$\text{Creatinine clearance} = \frac{(140 - \text{Age}) \times \text{Weight (kg)}}{72 \times \text{Creatinine}} \; (\times 0.85 \text{ for Women})$$

- Age-related changes occur in pharmacokinetics involving drug absorption, distribution, metabolism, and elimination.
- Drug distribution has a major role in altered pharmacokinetics.
- The ability of the liver to metabolize drugs decreases in most elderly patients.
- Because of decreased renal function with age, elimination of many drugs is delayed in the elderly.

Pharmacodynamic changes also occur with aging and have an effect on the action of medications. The term "pharmacodynamics" refers to drug sensitivity, which can change with age. These changes may reflect an alteration of receptor number or receptor sensitivity to drug or an altered receptor response to a drug. Less is known about age-related altered pharmacodynamics than about pharmacokinetics; however, the pharmacodynamic changes for several drugs have been identified. There is a reduced responsiveness of β-adrenergic drugs (e.g., less tachycardia with isoproterenol, less bradycardia with β-blockers), increased sedation with benzodiazepines, greater analgesia with opiates, and greater anticoagulant activity with warfarin.

Adverse drug effects are common in the elderly and frequently cause serious complications. Elderly patients often have limited organ reserve function and are unable to respond as younger persons can to an adverse effect. Drug-drug effects tend to occur more commonly in the elderly and tend to be more serious. The likelihood of a drug-drug effect is related to the number of medications taken.

- Pharmacodynamic changes result in an alteration in a given drug effect with age.
- Adverse drug effects tend to occur more often and are often more severe in the elderly, primarily because of reduced organ reserve capacity with age.

As a result of altered pharmacokinetics and pharmacodynamics with aging, medications need to be prescribed carefully for the elderly, avoiding polypharmacy whenever possible and watching for evidence of adverse drug effects and drug-drug interactions, both of which increase in frequency with age. Medications have been identified that have potentially greater risks in the elderly. These drugs should be prescribed with great caution for older patients. Some of these medications are discussed in the following paragraphs.

Long-acting benzodiazepines (diazepam, chlordiazepoxide, and flurazepam) are highly lipid-soluble and, thus, have a very long half-life in elderly patients. They also have active metabolites. These drugs can easily accumulate in the elderly and possibly produce drug toxicity. Barbiturates also are highly lipid-soluble and have very long half-lives in the elderly. Drug accumulation may occur; also, tolerance develops quickly to their sedating activity. Diphenhydramine is available over-the-counter and is often used to induce sleep. It potentially can cause cognitive impairment in the elderly. Propoxyphene is a weak analgesic with little therapeutic advantage over acetaminophen; yet, it has all the risks and adverse effects of narcotics. Pentazocine is a mixed agonist and antagonist oral narcotic that has significant potential for adverse effects on the CNS, including confusion and hallucinations.

Meperidine is a weak analgesic with an unpredictable rate of oral absorption. Its metabolites can accumulate in patients with renal insufficiency; seizures or respiratory depression may manifest toxicity. Tricyclic antidepressants have the potential for various adverse effects because of their nonselective neurochemical blockade. α-Adrenergic antagonist activity can produce orthostatic hypotension, antihistamine activity can lead to sedation, and anticholinergic effects can cause urinary obstruction in men and delirium, constipation, and blurred vision. Monoamine oxidase inhibitors and antidepressants have marked potential for serious adverse effects, such as hypertension, when they interact with tyramine-containing products. Chlorpropamide, an oral hypoglycemic agent, is a first-generation sulfonylurea and has an extremely long half-life; thus, it has a substantial risk of causing prolonged hypoglycemia.

Geriatrics Pharmacy Review
Robert W. Hoel, RPh, PharmD, Jamie M. Gardner, PharmD

Drug	Toxic/adverse effects	Considerations in the elderly
Glaucoma agents	Burning, itching eyes	Many nonprescription ophthalmics exacerbate narrow-angle glaucoma (decongestants, antihistamines)
Endocrine agents		
Insulin, oral hypoglycemic agents	Monitor for excess hypoglycemia	Administer judiciously if patient exhibits anorexia, avoid first-generation sulfonylureas (chlorpropamide)
Thyroid agents Levothyroxine (Levothroid, Synthroid)	Symptoms of hyperthyroidism (tachycardia, palpitations, weight loss, insomnia, sweating), excess worsens CHF	Bioequivalence possible problem if switching between different products; stay with same brand
Psychotropic agents*		
Antipsychotic agents	Generally do not improve dementia, but modify behavioral responses	In elderly, start with dose 1/4-1/3 of standard dosages. Use in dementia is unlabeled.
Haloperidol	Tardive dyskinesia, extrapyramidal or parkinsonian-like symptoms, sedation	Less orthostasis, cardiovascular, and anti-cholinergic effects than with phenothiazines
Phenothiazines (chlorpromazine, thioridazine, etc.)	Sedation, orthostatic hypotension, dizziness, increased falls, anticholinergic & extrapyramidal effects	Consider using newer agent (risperidone, olanzapine) with fewer of nearly all side effects (less hypotension, less anticholinergic & extrapyramidal effects)
Risperidone, olanzapine, quetiapine	Less sedation, orthostasis, extra-pyramidal effects than others	
Antidepressants		
Tricyclic agents (imipramine, amitriptyline)	Anticholinergic, dysrhythmias, drowsiness	Avoid except nortriptyline or desipramine, which has favorable side effect profile
SSRIs	Overall, less severe side effects, but no more effective than tricyclics	
Paroxetine, sertraline	Nausea, weight loss, mental status changes (especially sedation), sexual dysfunction	
Fluoxetine	In addition to the above, hallucinations, anxiety, anorexia	Often worsens anxious behavior
Nefazodone, trazodone	Sedation, anticholinergic, orthostasis, less sexual dysfunction, agitation, or weight change	Trazodone—sedation (with low dose), weak antidepressant effect
Mirtazapine	Sedation, weight gain	
Sedative-hypnotics		
Benzodiazepines	Sedation, confusion	Use short half-life agents. Lorazepam, oxazepam, & temazepam are preferred because no phase I metabolism
Zolpidem	Sedation	Indicated only for short-term (7 days) treat-ment of insomnia
Diphenhydramine	Sedation, anticholinergic effects, urinary retention	Worsens narrow-angle glaucoma, very susceptible to sedation, anticholinergic effects, & confusion; avoid

Geriatrics Pharmacy Review (continued)

Drug	Toxic/adverse effects	Considerations in the elderly
Cognitive agents	Nausea, insomnia, fatigue	Dose adjustments may be indicated and as tolerated
Tacrine, donepezil	Donepezil is better tolerated	Cholinergic effects (incontinence, diaphoresis)
Cardiovascular agents		
Digoxin	Dysrhythmias, confusion, visual disturbances, anorexia, nausea, vomiting, diarrhea at toxic levels	Many drugs decrease clearance (NSAIDs, etc), monitor K^+ and toxicity, which is frequent
Nitrates	Hypotension & orthostasis, dizziness, syncope, headache	Tolerance to beneficial effects may be alleviated with 8-12 h nitrate-free interval
ACE inhibitors (or ARB)	Can worsen renal function, especially in renal artery stenosis	Proven long-term benefits in CHF, may protect against renal effects of diabetes, substitute ARB if ACE inhibitor not tolerated
Calcium channel blockers	(See Cardiovascular chapter)	
Verapamil	Constipation, negative inotropic effects, atrioventricular node blocking effect	
Dihydropyridines	Peripheral edema	
β-Blockers	Bronchoconstriction with agents having β_2 effect or high doses of all agents, depression, orthostasis, glucose intolerance, block warning signs of hypoglycemia	Proven long-term benefits in CHF, MI, but increase dose gradually
Diuretics (see Cardiovascular agents)	Electrolyte imbalances, dehydration, orthostasis	Elderly especially prone to orthostatic problems, but low-dose thiazide is still first-line therapy
Antihypertensive agents (see Cardiovascular agents)	Additive orthostatic hypotension occurs with many common drugs	Orthostasis increases likelihood of falls
Anticoagulants		
Warfarin	Monitor INR (PT) and bleeding	Review changes in entire drug regimen for interactions; elderly who are prone to falls may have risk of bleeding but show greatest therapeutic benefit
Gastrointestinal (GI) drugs		
H_2 antagonists	Confusion occasionally	Do not necessarily prevent NSAID-induced GI ulcers
Proton pump inhibitors	No more side effects than in younger adults	Do not necessarily prevent NSAID-induced GI ulcers
Respiratory agents		
Theophylline	Tachycardia, insomnia, anxiety; narrow therapeutic index necessitates monitoring drug levels	Overall, side effects not tolerated well; disease usually can be controlled with other agents (i.e., inhaler therapy)

Geriatrics Pharmacy Review (continued)

Drug	Toxic/adverse effects	Considerations in the elderly
Osteoporosis agents		
Calcium (Ca) salts	Constipation; H_2 antagonists & proton pump inhibitors inhibit absorption of Ca salts except Ca citrate	Elderly & postmenopausal women need 1,500 mg elemental Ca daily, smoking cessation, HRT, weight-bearing exercise
Vitamin D		400-800 IU vitamin D daily with Ca
Alendronate, risedronate	Erosive esophagitis	Must take before meals and other medicine with full glass of water & remain upright for 30 min
Calcitonin, salmon (200 units nasal spray)		Efficacy data are weaker than for bisphosphonates or HRT
HRT	Abnormal vaginal bleeding, thromboembolism, DVT	Estrogen with progestin to prevent endometrial cancer
Raloxifene	Thromboembolism, DVT, hot flashes	Effective osteoporosis prevention, but not menopausal symptoms
Incontinence agents		
Oxybutynin, flavoxate, imipramine, tolterodine	Drowsiness, confusion, anticholinergic effects inhibit early detrusor contractions, hesitancy	Additive effects lead to confusion, falls, retention
Rheumatologic agents		
NSAIDs	Nausea, ulcer, fluid retention, nephrotoxicity if renal disease present	Use lowest dose possible to reduce side effects after a trial of scheduled acetaminophen
COX-2 inhibitors	Nephrotoxicity similar to NSAIDs	Good alternative, but potential for side effects, possibly less potential for GI bleeding
Hydroxychloroquine	Muscle weakness, retinal damage, visual disturbances, nausea	Long time to benefit; stop if no benefit in 6 mo; need eye exam twice yearly
Methotrexate	Myelosuppression, nausea, hypotension	Start with lowest dose, increase as tolerated
Corticosteroids	Nausea, ulcers, weight gain, blood glucose fluctuations, osteoporosis; taper to avoid adrenal suppression	Taper to lowest effective dose that decreases symptoms; consider osteoporosis therapy
Colchicine	Nausea, myelosuppression	Toxicity with accumulation as renal clearance decreases
Impotence agents		
Sildenafil	Headache, flushing, dyspepsia, hypotension	Not for those receiving nitrate therapy
Prostaglandin E_1	Penile pain, urethral burning	Available in suppository or injection

ACE, angiotensin-converting enzyme; ARB, angiotensin receptor blocker; CHF, congestive heart failure; DVT, deep venous thrombosis; HRT, hormone replacement therapy; INR, international normalized ratio; MI, myocardial infarction; NSAID, nonsteroidal anti-inflammatory drug; PT, prothombin time; SSRI, selective serotonin reuptake inhibitor.

*Use of antipsychotics, sedative-hypnotics, and anxiolytics in a nursing facility in treating behaviors associated with dementia is regulated, surveyed, and requires specific supporting documentation in the patient's chart.

QUESTIONS

Multiple Choice (choose the one best answer)

1. A 72-year-old woman who has lived alone since the death of her husband 1 year ago complains of difficulty with her memory. She frequently forgets appointments, shopping items, and the names of people she has recently met. She also frequently misplaces objects and is unable to recall where they are. The patient describes some loss of appetite, with a 20-lb weight loss over the past 3 months. On physical examination, the heart rate is 84 beats/min and blood pressure is 148/86 mm Hg. No focal abnormalities are found on neurologic examination. Deep tendon reflexes are equal and symmetric. Balance is slightly decreased. The patient scores 20/30 on the Mini-Mental State Examination. The next step in the evaluation and management of this patient's cognitive complaints should be:
   a. CT or MRI of the head to confirm the diagnosis of Alzheimer disease
   b. A 3-month trial of donepezil
   c. Further studies to evaluate depression
   d. Further studies to evaluate for occult malignancy
   e. A 3-month trial of a tricyclic antidepressant

2. An 85-year-old obese man who is a nursing home resident is evaluated for urinary incontinence. He has advanced dementia and is unable to give a history. The nursing home staff indicate he is incontinent throughout the day and night and is constantly found wet. His medical record indicates that he has hypertension, benign prostatic hyperplasia, and diabetes mellitus. Currently, he is taking diltiazem, furosemide, and glipizide. What is the next step in evaluating and managing this patient's incontinence?
   a. Initiate scheduled toileting
   b. Perform urodynamic studies
   c. Use an external (condom) catheter
   d. Use an indwelling catheter
   e. Measure the postvoid residual urine volume

3. A 65-year-old woman complains of urinary incontinence. She indicates that she loses urine when she coughs or walks down a flight of stairs and occasionally when she arises from a sitting position. These symptoms have become gradually worse over the past several years. The patient has had four vaginal deliveries. Which of the following would be of *least benefit* for this patient's symptoms of incontinence?
   a. Pelvic floor exercises
   b. Oxybutynin
   c. Topical estrogen
   d. Pseudoephedrine
   e. Vaginal pessary

4. A 68-year-old man is brought to the clinic by his daughter. The family is concerned about the behavior of their father, who lives alone. He has been increasingly forgetful and has frequently misplaced various objects around the house and has lost several social security checks. The other day he left the water running in the bathtub, flooding the bathroom and causing considerable damage. The patient denies any problem and feels that his family is "fussing" too much. The patient has a history of coronary artery disease, diabetes mellitus, and mild-to-moderate renal insufficiency. He is taking metoprolol, glipizide, and captopril. On physical examination, it is noted that the patient has lost approximately 15 lb since last year. The patient scores 29/30 on a Mini-Mental State Examination (MMSE). No important abnormalities are noted on examination. What is the next best course of action to take with this patient?
   a. Start donepezil for Alzheimer disease
   b. Start sertraline for depression
   c. Reassure the family that at this time their father is fine
   d. Perform formal psychometric testing
   e. Discontinue metoprolol therapy

5. An 84-year-old woman who is a nursing home resident with a history of renal insufficiency, congestive heart failure, and chronic atrial fibrillation is noted to be more lethargic, confused, and less communicative than previously. She responds slowly to commands. She is taking multiple medications, including atenolol, furosemide, diltiazem, lisinopril, and digoxin for her medical problems. On physical examination, her heart rate is 45 beats/min with a regular rhythm and blood pressure is 84/50 mm Hg. Which of the following medications is most likely to account for the patient's condition?
   a. Atenolol
   b. Furosemide
   c. Diltiazem
   d. Lisinopril
   e. Digoxin

6. A 65-year-old man is brought to the outpatient clinic by his son. The patient has lived with his son and daughter-in-law since his wife died 3 years ago. The son states that his father has developed some confusion and has been having occasional hallucinations. He will describe seeing other people in his room. On some days, he is minimally symptomatic. Physical examination reveals notable rigidity of the upper extremities, bradykinesia, and difficulty maintaining attention. This patient is most likely demonstrating which disease process?
   a. Alzheimer disease

b. Parkinson disease
c. Dementia with Lewy bodies
d. Frontotemporal dementia
e. Multistroke dementia

7. Two days after a 68-year-old man had elective total hip arthroplasty, a fever of 38.6°C and right knee pain developed. Physical examination findings include degenerative arthritis of the distal interphalangeal joints of both hands and degenerative changes in both knees. There is increased warmth of the knee and a moderate knee effusion. Pertinent laboratory findings include a leukocyte count of 11×10^9/L (11,000/mm^3). Radiography of the knee shows linear calcification and a knee effusion. Which of the following is the *most correct* statement about this patient?
   a. Treatment should be started with an antibiotic given intravenously for a septic joint
   b. Arthrocentesis should be performed
   c. Allopurinol should be started to prevent future episodes
   d. Examination of the synovial fluid with polarizing microscopy is likely to show negatively birefringent crystals
   e. Treatment should be started with indomethacin

ANSWERS

1. Answer c.

This patient describes symptoms of cognitive impairment. She also has considerable insight into her memory problem and has had a marked weight loss. The recent death of her husband should raise the suspicion of depression. Of the options listed, further evaluation for depression is most appropriate. Neither CT nor MRI of the head is used to prove Alzheimer disease; the finding of cerebral atrophy is not specific for this disease. Imaging studies of the head are performed to rule out reversible causes of cognitive impairment such as a subdural hematoma, central nervous system tumor, or normal-pressure hydrocephalus. A 3-month trial of donepezil therapy would not be expected to be of much benefit for this patient. If the patient has Alzheimer disease and the medication is effective, she would be expected to show stability in her cognitive decline. A 3-month trial is too short to assess the effectiveness of this medication. Without specific symptoms, an evaluation for malignancy is unlikely to help with diagnosis. If depression is diagnosed, a trial of an antidepressant is reasonable. In the elderly, tricyclic antidepressants have considerably more risk for adverse effects than a selective serotinin reuptake inhibitor, which would be the class of antidepressants preferred to treat the elderly population.

2. Answer e.

It is difficult to determine what type of urinary incontinence this patient has because the patient is unable to furnish a reliable history. Because the patient is known to be wet throughout the day and night, the possibility of overflow incontinence must be considered. Occasionally, a palpable distended bladder can be found on physical examination, but this may be difficult to detect in an obese patient. The initial evaluation for this patient should include measurement of the postvoid residual urine volume and determination of the completeness of bladder emptying. This may be done by in-and-out bladder catheterization or by bladder ultrasonography. A markedly increased residual urine volume would strongly suggest overflow incontinence. This may be secondary to either bladder outlet obstruction or inadequate bladder contractions (hypotonic bladder). Although scheduled toileting may be useful for many patients with urinary incontinence, it would not be effective for those with overflow incontinence. Tolterodine is an anticholinergic medication and can inhibit early detrusor contractions. This may be helpful for overactive bladder, but it can worsen overflow incontinence. Although urodynamic studies would certainly reveal the diagnosis for this patient, the test requires a cooperative patient. An external catheter would not be expected to be of benefit in this patient. Because the problem with overflow incontinence is inadequate bladder drainage, the catheter would not provide this. Also, long-term use of an external catheter tends to cause skin irritation.

3. Answer b.

This patient has stress urinary incontinence. Effective treatment for this condition can include pelvic floor exercises, which if performed correctly can be very effective. Pharmacologic therapy can be used, but the results are usually disappointing. Imipramine and pseudoephedrine are occasionally helpful because of their α-adrenergic agonist activity, increasing the tone of the internal sphincter; however, tolerance usually develops quickly to these medications. The mechanism of action for topical estrogen is a direct effect on the urethral mucosa. This can improve atrophic urethritis and can occasionally be effective in urinary stress incontinence. Again, results are often disappointing. A vaginal pessary can be effective by increasing the resistance at the bladder outlet, but many patients find them difficult to insert or uncomfortable to wear long-term. Oxybutynin would not be effective in treating urinary stress incontinence because its main effect is on the detrusor. It is useful in suppressing early bladder contractions in persons with an overactive bladder.

4. Answer d.

This patient very likely has early dementia. His cognitive change has been noticed by members of his family. It is not unusual for patients with dementia to deny they have any cognitive problems. Although the patient scored in the normal range on the MMSE, this is not a definitive test. The MMSE is a screening test that may not detect early cognitive impairment, especially in those with advanced education. Formal psychometric testing should be performed to give a more accurate evaluation of the patient's cognitive status. Starting treatment with donepezil is reasonable for a patient with early Alzheimer disease, but first the diagnosis needs to be established. Depression could cause the patient's symptoms, but the diagnosis has not been established. It is not appropriate to reassure the family that their father is fine at this point, because a negative MMSE does not rule out dementia. Although β-blockers can have adverse effects on the central nervous system in the elderly, it is not wise to discontinue this medication for this patient because he has known coronary artery disease. Stopping this treatment could precipitate a worsening of cardiac symptoms.

5. Answer e.

This patient has a history of chronic atrial fibrillation; however, on examination, the cardiac rhythm is regular. This may indicate that the patient has converted to sinus rhythm; however, digitalis toxicity must also be considered. Her regular rhythm and bradycardia suggest a junctional rhythm, which can be seen in digitalis toxicity. A heart rate of 45 beats/min is slower than would be caused by a β-blocker. Of the medications listed, diltiazem has been associated with digitalis toxicity. Calcium channel antagonists can impair the renal elimination of digitalis. Her history of renal insufficiency increases her risk for digitalis toxicity due to further impairment of digitalis elimination.

6. Answer c.

This patient has dementia with Lewy bodies. Patients with this condition typically develop dementia with parkinsonian features, including bradykinesia, rigidity, and gait instability. Unlike patients with Parkinson disease, those with Lewy body dementia do not typically develop a resting tremor. Both auditory and visual hallucinations are common. The patients also commonly have difficulty maintaining concentration and show marked day-to-day variation in the severity of their symptoms. Patients with Lewy body dementia often show a marked increased sensitivity to the extrapyramidal effects of neuroleptic drugs such as haloperidol.

7. Answer b.

This patient has an acute monoarticular arthritis likely due to either crystalline or septic arthritis. Both may produce the clinical syndrome described. The knee is a common location for calcium pyrophosphate deposition disease (CPDD), or pseudogout, although gout may present in the knee. Allopurinol can prevent recurrent attacks of gout. Linear articular cartilage calcification is seen with CPDD but can also be seen in radiographs of the knee of many normal, asymptomatic persons. Arthrocentesis should be performed in this patient to analyze the synovial fluid to determine the cause of the arthritis. Finding negatively birefringent, needle-like crystals in the synovial fluid is consistent with gout, whereas positively birefringent, rectangular crystals are found in CPDD. Starting treatment with indomethacin could be effective for either gout or CPDD, although occasionally indomethacin is not well tolerated by elderly patients.

CHAPTER 11
HEMATOLOGY

Thomas M. Habermann, M.D.

ANEMIAS

Evaluation of Anemias

The causes of anemia are complex. The World Health Organization (WHO) defined the lower limit of normal for venous hemoglobin concentration in males older than 14 years living at sea level as 13 g/dL and in nonpregnant females, 12 g/dL. However, accurate interpretation requires the use of an appropriate age-, sex-, and race-adjusted reference range. An organized approach to the anemias is essential. Because the initial evaluation of anemia after the history and physical examination begins with a complete blood count (CBC), anemias can be classified on the basis of mean corpuscular volume (MCV): microcytic, macrocytic, and normocytic anemia.

The CBC is the most commonly ordered blood test. The measured values of the CBC include the total counts for red blood cells (RBCs), platelets, and white blood cells (WBCs) and the volumes of RBCs, platelets, WBCs, and hemoglobin. The calculated values include the hematocrit, MCV, mean corpuscular hemoglobin, mean corpuscular hemoglobin concentration, and red cell distribution width.

The most common anemias are microcytic anemias (Tables 11-1 and 11-2). The differential diagnosis of hypochromic microcytic anemias includes iron deficiency, thalassemic syndromes, anemia of chronic disease, sideroblastic anemias, hemoglobin E, unstable hemoglobins, and lead poisoning. Vitamin B_6 deficiency may cause a microcytic anemia. The causes of iron deficiency include blood loss, increased requirements (as in pregnancy), and decreased absorption (partial gastrectomy and malabsorption syndromes). The following are associated with blood loss: gastrointestinal disorders (ulcers, malignancy, telangiectasia, arteriovenous malformations, hiatal hernia, and long-distance runner's anemia), respiratory disorders (malignancy, pulmonary hemosiderosis), menstruation, phlebotomy (blood donor, diagnostic phlebotomy, polycythemia rubra vera, and self-inflicted), trauma, and surgery.

Iron deficiency is the most common cause of anemia in the world. In the United States, iron deficiency occurs in 11% of adolescent females and women of childbearing age and iron deficiency anemia in 3% to 5%. In a nonreferral practice, iron deficiency may be the cause of up to 90% of all hypochromic microcytic anemias (Plate 11-1). Of the remaining 10%, thalassemic syndromes are more common than the other rare forms of hypochromic microcytic anemias. However, the incidence and prevalence of anemia of chronic disease vary, depending on whether the setting is inpatient or outpatient and whether a community-based or a referral center. The CBC and other laboratory values provide additional information for differentiating these entities (Table 11-2). These laboratory studies often provide the major clues to the type of anemia. Blood loss should be considered in the differential diagnosis of any patient with anemia. The evaluation of stool for blood loss is essential in the initial work-up and may also provide clues to a combined anemia. A laboratory approach to microcytic anemias is outlined in Figures 11-1 and 11-2. The serum ferritin test is the most useful initial test for documenting iron deficiency, but the values obtained may be increased in the presence of iron deficiency and coexistent inflammatory states (rheumatoid arthritis), liver disease, hepatocellular carcinoma, and malignancy.

Confusing problems in iron deficiency include patient compliance with iron treatment, incorrect dosage schedules, treatment with enteric-coated iron preparations, diminished

Table 11-1 Differentiation of Microcytic Anemias on the Basis of Blood Values

Variable	Type of anemia	
	Thalassemia	Iron deficiency
RBC count	$>5.0\times10^{12}/L$	$<5.0\times10^{12}/L$
Red cell distribution width	<16	>16
MCV-RBC $(5 \times Hb) - 3.4$	Negative	Positive

Hb, hemoglobin; MCV, mean corpuscular volume; RBC, red blood cell.

Table 11-2 Comparison of Hypochromic Microcytic Anemias

Disease state	MCV	Red blood cells	TIBC, µg/dL	% transferrin saturation	Ferritin, µg/L	Marrow iron
Iron deficiency anemia	Decreased	Decreased	>300	<9	Low	Absent
Anemia of chronic disease	Normal or decreased	Decreased	<300	>15 or normal	Normal or increased	Normal or increased
Thalassemia minor	Decreased	Usually increased	<300	Normal	Normal or increased	Normal

MCV, mean corpuscular volume; TIBC, total iron-binding capacity.
Modified from Savage RA: Cost-effective laboratory diagnosis of microcytic anemias of complex origin. ASCP check sample H84-10(H-153). By permission of American Society of Clinical Pathologists.

absorption (previous operation or mucosal disease of the small bowel), competitive interference with antacids, blood loss in excess of treatment, other causes of anemia, and physician impatience with response. Oral replacement therapy is the treatment of choice for iron deficiency. Ferrous sulfate three times daily at a dose of 325 mg orally 1 hour before or 2 hours after meals is the initial treatment. A CBC should be performed again 4 weeks after the initiation of iron therapy.

Correction of the anemia would be anticipated in 6 weeks. Treatment for another 6 months is necessary to replenish bone marrow reserves. Indications for intravenous iron therapy include patients on renal dialysis, bloodless medical treatment, and bloodless surgery for patients who decline blood transfusions because of religious beliefs. Treatment is with iron dextran (InFeD), with the risk of anaphylactoid reactions, or ferric gluconate for renal dialysis patients.

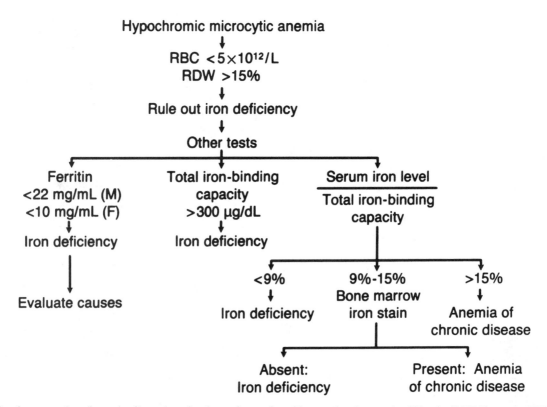

Fig. 11-1. Algorithm for approach to diagnosis of hypochromic microcytic anemias with normal or decreased red blood cell (RBC) counts. RDW, red cell distribution width. (Modified from Savage RA: Cost-effective laboratory diagnosis of microcytic anemias of complex origin. ASCP check sample H84-10[H-153]. By permission of American Society of Clinical Pathologists.)

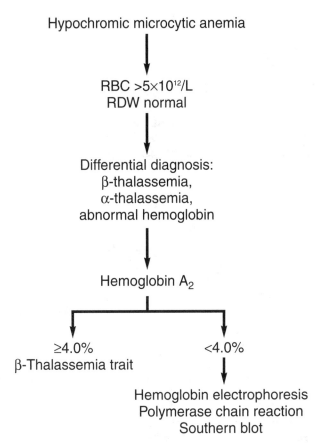

Fig. 11-2. Algorithm for approach to diagnosis of hypochromic microcytic anemias with an increased total red blood cell (RBC) count. RDW, red cell distribution width. (Modified from Savage RA: Cost-effective laboratory diagnosis of microcytic anemias of complex origin. ASCP check sample H84-10[H-153]. By permission of American Society of Clinical Pathologists.)

● Typical clinical scenario: An elderly patient with a history of abdominal pain and weakness presents with microcytic hypochromic anemia. The serum level of ferritin is low. The RBC count is low. The RBC distribution width index is increased. The diagnosis is iron deficiency anemia. A likely cause is colon cancer producing chronic blood loss. Upper and lower gastrointestinal endoscopy is indicated.

Thalassemia is the most common single gene disorder in the world. β-Thalassemia results when β-globulin chains are decreased (heterozygous) or absent (homozygous), resulting in an excess of α-globulin chains in the RBCs. Patients with the β-thalassemia trait have a mild anemia and marked microcytosis. β-Thalassemia can be identified with simple screening methods (Tables 11-1 and 11-2 and Fig. 11-2). However, if iron deficiency coexists, the hemoglobin A_2 level may be normal. The risks of β-thalassemia include having offspring with thalassemia major or heterozygous hemoglobinopathies and iatrogenic iron overload when the disorder is misdiagnosed as iron deficiency.

The normal population has two α-chain loci but only one β-chain locus per haploid genome. Thus, the absence of one or two of four α-globin genes does not cause symptomatic abnormality (α-thalassemia silent carrier, α-thal minor). Patients with α-thalassemia minor characteristically have a low-normal MCV, with a normal concentration of hemoglobin. The α-thalassemia trait may be confirmed with a polymerase chain reaction-based assay. However, most cases may be managed without laboratory confirmation. Genetic counseling is indicated after the diagnosis of α- or β-thalassemia has been established.

● Typical clinical scenario: An African American person (or person of Mediterranean or Southeast Asian ancestry) has mild anemia and is asymptomatic. The RBC count is disproportionately normal or increased compared with the hemoglobin level. The RBC distribution width index is normal. The concentration of hemoglobin A_2 is increased (β-thalassemia) or normal (α-thalassemia).

The differential diagnosis of macrocytic anemias includes vitamin B_{12} deficiency, folate deficiency, drugs, myelodysplasia, liver disease, alcohol abuse, hypothyroidism, cold agglutinin disease, tobacco, and hemolysis. A laboratory approach to macrocytic anemias is outlined in Figure 11-3. The pathophysiology of drug-induced macrocytosis includes marrow toxicity from interference with folate metabolism (alcohol) and from other drugs (zidovudine) and altered folate metabolism from anticonvulsants (phenytoin, primidone, and phenobarbital) and other drugs (oral contraceptives, triamterene, sulfasalazine, and sulfamethoxazole). Common causes of macrocytosis are chemotherapy drugs that inhibit purine or pyrimidine synthesis (azathioprine and 5-fluorouracil), deoxyribonucleotide synthesis (hydroxyurea and cytarabine [cytosine arabinoside]), and dihydrofolate reductase (methotrexate).

Patients with achlorhydria of any cause do not absorb vitamin B_{12} because hydrochloric acid is required to free vitamin B_{12} from food. A normally functioning pancreas is required. The many causes of vitamin B_{12} deficiency include pernicious anemia, total or partial gastrectomy, ileal resection, bacterial overgrowth syndromes, achlorhydria, and chronic pancreatitis.

The symptoms and signs of vitamin B_{12} deficiency include a beefy and atrophic tongue, diarrhea, and neurologic signs (paresthesias, gait disturbance, mental status changes ["B_{12} madness"], vibratory/position sense impairment [dorsal column "dropout"], and the absence of ankle reflexes and extensor plantar responses). The MCV is increased, and Howell-Jolly bodies are typically present, as are hypersegmented neutrophils. A serum level of vitamin B_{12} less than 200 pg/mL is suggestive of the diagnosis of vitamin B_{12} deficiency. Vitamin B_{12} levels of 100 to 200 pg/mL are not diagnostic of a deficiency state.

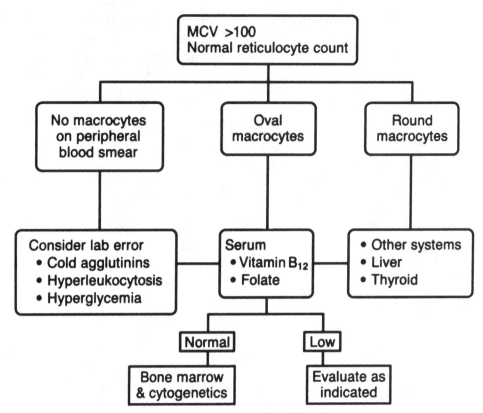

Fig. 11-3. Laboratory approach to macrocytic anemias. MCV, mean corpuscular volume. (Modified from Colon-Otero G, Menke D, Hook CC: A practical approach to the differential diagnosis and evaluation of the adult patient with macrocytic anemia. Med Clin North Am May 1992;76:581-597. By permission of WB Saunders Company.)

Urinary methylmalonic acid is increased in vitamin B_{12} deficiency. An abnormal intrinsic factor antibody confirms the diagnosis of pernicious anemia. Of patients with pernicious anemia, 60% have a positive blocking antibody test. The serum level of vitamin B_{12} may rarely be normal in pernicious anemia. Serum gastrin levels are high in pernicious anemia.

The Schilling test may be required after testing for intrinsic factor blocking antibody. The Schilling test confirms a defect in intestinal absorption (sprue, inflammatory bowel disease). In part I of the test, radiolabeled vitamin B_{12} is administered orally, nonradioactive vitamin B_{12} is administered intramuscularly within 1 to 2 hours, and the urine and serum levels are measured. Normal urinary excretion rates after a flushing dose of nonradioactive vitamin B_{12} in the first 24 to 72 hours are greater than 7%. Low urine radioactivity with normal renal function means decreased absorption. The differential diagnosis of an abnormal finding in part I includes pernicious anemia, small-bowel disease interfering with absorption, and bacterial competition for vitamin B_{12}. True-negative results in part I of the Schilling test include dietary deficiency and cobalamin-binding protein abnormalities. False-negative results occur in food-bound malabsorption due to achlorhydria. In part II of the test, intrinsic factor is added.

Patients with pernicious anemia have normal results. False-positive results occur in cases attributable to mucosal megaloblastosis. Antibiotics are given in part III of the Schilling test, and the differential diagnosis of a positive result includes ileal malabsorption and defective intrinsic factor in the test. A negative test result occurs in the blind loop syndrome secondary to bacterial competition for vitamin B_{12}.

The treatment of pernicious anemia is vitamin B_{12}, 1,000 µg intramuscularly for 5 days, followed by 500 to 1,000 µg intramuscularly every month. Alternatively, vitamin B_{12} may be given orally at a dose of 500 to 1,000 µg daily. Lifelong treatment is required. Vitamin B_{12} levels are spuriously low in pregnancy and in persons receiving oral contraceptive treatment. In the elderly and patients with low WBC counts, the serum levels of methylmelonic acid are increased in vitamin B_{12} deficiency but are normal during pregnancy and when taking oral contraceptives.

- Typical clinical scenario: An elderly diabetic patient has weakness and fatigue, and laboratory evaluation suggests macrocytic anemia. The vitamin B_{12} level is low. The serum level of methylmalonic acid is increased. Anti-intrinsic factor and anti-parietal cell antibody tests are positive.

Megaloblastic anemia caused by folate deficiency develops in 1 to 3 years, in contrast to 3 years for vitamin B_{12} deficiency, because of the low storage levels of folic acid in tissues and the relatively high dietary requirement. Morphologically, this anemia is indistinguishable from vitamin B_{12} deficiency. Folate is absorbed in the proximal small bowel. Deficiency states are associated with increased requirements (pregnancy and hemolytic anemia), poor intake (alcoholics), diseases of the small intestine (sprue), and interference with the recycling of folate from liver stores to tissue (alcohol). The possibility of concomitant vitamin B_{12} and iron deficiency (sprue) should be considered if the response to replacement therapy is not optimal. The serum homocysteine level is increased in folate deficiency because of impaired folate-dependent conversion of homocysteine to methionine.

- Typical clinical scenario: Macrocytic anemia is diagnosed in a person who is alcoholic.

The normochromic normocytic group of disorders present the greatest challenge in differential diagnosis. Both iron and vitamin B_{12} deficiencies are possible causes and should be excluded. The differential diagnosis includes stem cell dysfunction (aplastic anemia and red cell aplasia), marrow replacement (malignancy and fibrosis), kidney disease, hemolysis, acute hemorrhage, mixed nutritional deficiency, myelodysplastic syndromes, chemotherapy, anemia of acute disease, anemia of chronic disease characterized by a low total iron-binding capacity (acute infections, chronic infections, neoplasia, rheumatoid arthritis, polymyalgia rheumatica), and erythropoietin deficiency. The anemia of renal failure and liver disease is important in this differential diagnosis. The anemia of kidney disease may be related to decreased erythropoietin level or shortened RBC survival. It is important to obtain a reticulocyte count to exclude hemolysis early in the evaluation of patients with normochromic normocytic anemia. It is essential to exclude blood loss from the gastrointestinal tract that may be acute and not manifested by features of microcytic blood. No blood test confirms anemia of chronic disease or of acute disease. The soluble transferrin receptor differentiates iron deficiency anemia (the receptor is usually increased in iron deficiency) from the anemia of chronic disease (the receptor is usually normal).

- Typical clinical scenario for anemia of chronic disease: The patient has renal insufficiency (or human immunodeficiency virus [HIV] infection or other serious medical problem) and microcytic hypochromic anemia. The ferritin level is normal or high. The RBC count is low, and there is no evidence of hemolysis. The erythopoietin level is inappropriately low, given the presence of anemia.

Erythropoietin

Erythropoietin is a glycoprotein that acts through specific receptors on RBC precursors; 90% is produced in the kidneys and a small amount in the liver. There are no preformed stores. Erythropoietin production increases with hypoxia. Hypoxic signals include anemia, hypoxemia, decreased oxygen release (high oxygen-affinity hemoglobinopathies), and decreased renal blood flow (renal artery stenosis). Regulation is linked to an oxygen sensor, not to peripheral catabolism. The serum levels of erythropoietin are not influenced by age or sex. The higher hemoglobin value in men appears to be due to androgenic steroids. The toxicity profile is low. Recombinant human erythropoietin is identical to native erythropoietin. Hypertension may develop or progress in patients receiving renal dialysis.

The serum levels of erythropoietin are low, never absent, in chronic renal failure, polycythemia rubra vera, rheumatoid arthritis, and HIV infection. Zidovudine can increase the serum levels. High erythropoietin levels are present in marrow hypofunction (pure red cell aplasia), deficiency states (iron deficiency), tumor, autonomous production (hepatocellular carcinoma), and high altitude.

Approved indications for erythropoietin therapy include anemia of malignancy, anemia caused by neoplastic agents, anemia caused by renal insufficiency, and anemia due to HIV infection in patients who are taking zidovudine. For patients undergoing an operation and donating autologous blood, erythropoietin may increase the amount of blood donated by about 40%. The ferritin concentration should be greater than 100 µg/L or the transferrin saturation greater than 20%. The erythropoietin level should be less than 500 U/L. Recombinant erythropoietin is recommended for chemotherapy patients when the hemoglobin level is less than 10 g/dL. Two preparations are available: epoetin alfa (150 U/kg three times a week or 40,000 U a week) and darbepoetin alfa (2.25 µg/kg a week).

- Erythropoietin: a glycoprotein produced in the kidney; production increases with hypoxia.
- The erythropoietin level is low in renal failure, polycythemia rubra vera, rheumatoid arthritis, and HIV infection.
- Its level is high in pure red cell aplasia, iron deficiency, tumors, and at high altitude.
- Indications for erythropoietin therapy include end-stage renal disease, anemia of HIV infection, anemias of malignancy and neoplastic agents, after bone marrow transplantation, and for patients undergoing an operation donating autologous blood.

Patients must have adequate iron stores to respond to erythropoietin. If erythropoietin is given to a healthy person, the hematocrit can increase dramatically. As the hematocrit increases above 60%, the viscosity of the blood rapidly increases. Thus, hypertension, myocardial infarction, or stroke may occur with the misuse of erythropoietin. Doping with erythropoietin for sporting events has been associated with cerebrovascular events due to marked increases in the hematocrit. Patients who have iron deficiency, vitamin B_{12} and folate deficiency, hyperparathyroidism, or aluminum toxicity will not have a response to erythropoietin.

- Typical clinical scenario: A patient receiving chemotherapy presents to a primary care physician with fatigue and a hemoglobin concentration of 8.5 g/dL. Treatment with recombinant erythropoietin is indicated.

Hemolytic Anemia

In the initial evaluation of suspected hemolysis, it is essential to determine the presence of hemolytic anemia as manifested by laboratory evidence of an increased rate of erythropoiesis and increased RBC destruction. Evidence of increased erythropoiesis includes an increased reticulocyte count, and evidence of increased catabolism and destruction includes an increase in indirect bilirubin and lactate dehydrogenase (LDH) in the initial screening tests. Avoiding this step results in the ordering of unnecessary laboratory tests. If these tests suggest hemolytic anemia, specific causes should be sought. Hemolytic anemias may be Coombs-negative or Coombs-positive.

The initial evaluation includes a history and physical examination, CBC, morphology, and reticulocyte count. Conditions found during the work-up that can be mistaken for hemolysis include hemorrhage, recovery from deficiency states, metastatic carcinoma, and myoglobinuria. Studies of a family's hematologic history are important. The differential diagnosis of hemolytic anemia is outlined in Figure 11-4.

Inheritance Patterns

Membrane defects and unstable hemoglobin diseases are autosomal dominant. Most enzymopathies are autosomal recessive. However, the most common enzymopathy, glucose-6-phosphate dehydrogenase deficiency, is sex-linked, as is phosphoglycerate kinase deficiency.

- Membrane defects and unstable hemoglobin diseases are autosomal dominant.
- Most enzymopathies are autosomal recessive.
- Glucose-6-phosphate dehydrogenase deficiency is sex-linked.

Laboratory Findings

The bilirubin value is usually 1 to 5 mg/dL and almost exclusively unconjugated or indirect. Direct bilirubin should be less than 15% of the total if the bilirubin value is greater than 4 mg/dL. The haptoglobin concentration is usually low, with no compensatory increased rate of synthesis, and the LDH level is increased. CBC abnormalities in autoimmune hemolytic anemia include anemia, thrombocytosis, or thrombocytopenia. The presence of autoimmune hemolytic anemia and autoimmune thrombocytopenia is called "Evans syndrome." The reticulocyte value usually is persistently increased, reflecting an enhanced bone marrow response.

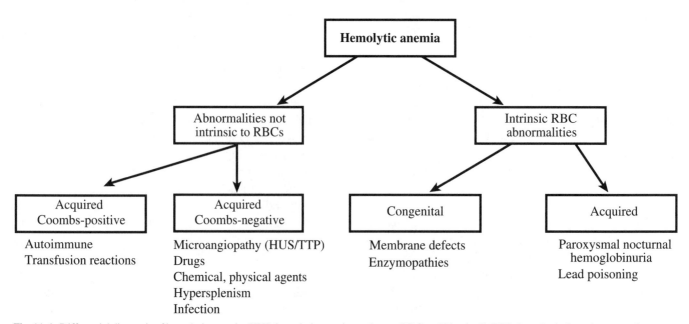

Fig. 11-4. Differential diagnosis of hemolytic anemia. HUS, hemolytic uremic syndrome; RBC, red blood cell; TTP, thrombotic thrombocytopenic purpura.

Peripheral Smear (Differential Diagnosis)

Spherocytes (Plate 11-2) are associated with hereditary spherocytosis, alcohol burns, *Clostridium* infections, autoimmune hemolytic anemia, and hypophosphatemia. Basophilic stippling occurs in lead poisoning, β-thalassemia, and arsenic poisoning. Hypochromia occurs in thalassemia and lead poisoning. Target cells are present in thalassemia, hemoglobin C and E, obstructive jaundice, hepatitis, lecithin–cholesterol-acyltransferase deficiency, and the splenectomy state (Plate 11-3). Agglutination is present in cold agglutinin disease (Plate 11-4). Stomatocytes are associated with acute alcoholism and also occur as an artifact. Spur cells (acanthocytes) (Plate 11-5) are present in chronic liver disease, abetalipoproteinemia, malabsorption, and anorexia nervosa. Burr cells (echinocytes) occur in uremia. Heinz bodies are present in glucose-6-phosphate dehydrogenase deficiency. Howell-Jolly bodies (the result of fragmentation of the nucleus) indicate hyposplenism and megaloblastic anemia.

Differential Diagnosis of Intravascular Hemolysis

The differential diagnosis includes transfusion reactions from ABO antibodies, microangiopathic hemolytic anemia, paroxysmal nocturnal hemoglobinuria, paroxysmal cold hemoglobinuria, autoimmune hemolytic anemia (uncommon), cold agglutinin syndrome, immune-complex drug-induced hemolytic anemia, infections (including falciparum malaria and clostridial sepsis), and glucose-6-phosphate dehydrogenase deficiency.

- Most hemolysis is extravascular.

In intravascular hemolysis, hemoglobin is released into the plasma, where it combines rapidly with haptoglobin, which transports it to the liver. When haptoglobin is depleted, hemoglobinemia results and the plasma turns pink-red at concentrations of 50 to 100 mg/dL.

Hemoglobinuria occurs when the plasma hemoglobin is less than 25 mg/100 mL. The urine may become pink, red, brown, or black. Other causes of red urine include beets, phenazopyridine (Pyridium), porphyrinuria, and myoglobinuria. Hemosiderin is an insoluble form of iron consisting of breakdown products of ferritin. Hemosiderinuria is the result of desquamation of renal tubular cells.

Coombs-Positive Hemolytic Anemia

Positive results with a direct Coombs test indicate the presence of C3 or IgG (or both) on the surface of RBCs. The three most common causes of Coombs-positive hemolytic anemias are idiopathic, drugs, and malignancy, including chronic lymphocytic leukemia, non-Hodgkin lymphoma, and ovarian carcinoma. The Coombs test gives positive results in 8% to 15% of all hospitalized patients, and studies have not demonstrated

the cause in 95% of these patients. Hemolytic transfusion and drug-related reactions are important causes of a positive Coombs test.

- Coombs test: detects the presence of C3 or IgG (or both) on RBCs.
- The cause of positive findings on the Coombs test is unknown for 95% of hospitalized patients.
- Transfusion-related and drug-related reactions are important causes of a positive Coombs test.

Drug-Induced Hemolytic Anemia (Mechanisms)

Autoantibody Mechanism

The autoantibody mechanism associated with methyldopa is dose-related, and hemolysis develops in about 0.3% to 0.8% of patients. Hemolysis occurs 18 weeks to 4 years after ingestion of the drug. The direct Coombs test becomes positive in 3 to 6 months and is IgG in high titer. There is no anamnestic response to rechallenge. Discontinuation of use of the drug usually leads to a rapid reversal in hemolysis. The mechanism of action is related to an altered cellular immune system, with a block in the activation of suppressor T cells. Methyldopa induces the formation of anti-Rh antibodies. Other drugs with a similar mechanism known to cause autoimmune hemolytic anemia include procainamide, ibuprofen, and cimetidine.

Drug Adsorption Mechanism

In drug adsorption (hapten) immunohemolytic anemia (penicillin, cephalosporin), the drug binds to the RBC membrane and antibody forms against the drug membrane–antigen complex. This complication requires high doses of drug for more than 7 days. The onset is subacute at 7 to 10 days. A high titer of penicillin antibody is always present in the serum. A positive Coombs test develops in 3% of patients and is dose-related in that 30% of patients are positive at 2 million U/day and 100% at 10 million U/day. Penicillin allergy is not necessarily present. Drug-adsorption immunohemolytic anemia may be fatal if not detected early. Other drugs, including cephalosporins, tetracycline, quinidine, tolmetin, and cisplatin, may cause autoimmune hemolytic anemia through the same mechanism.

Immune-Complex Mechanism

In the immune-complex, "innocent bystander," mechanism (quinine, rifampin, and stibophen), the antidrug antibody forms first and reacts with the drug to form an immune complex. The antidrug–antibody complex is then absorbed on the RBCs. The cell-bound complex may activate complement, causing intravascular hemolysis. The Coombs test is positive because of the complement on the RBC surface. Clinically, a small quantity of drug is sufficient to cause autoimmune hemolytic anemia if there was previous exposure. Acute intravascular hemolysis with hemoglobinemia and hemoglobinuria is the usual clinical course. Drugs implicated in this type of autoimmune hemolytic anemia include quinidine, quinine, phenacetin, acetaminophen, para-aminosalicylate (PAS), isoniazid (INH), streptomycin, rifampin, methadone, probenecid, insulin, sulfonylureas, hydralazine, hydrochlorothiazide, sulfa drugs, triamterene, and melphalan. Immune hemolytic anemia and renal failure are found in patients taking captopril, hydrochlorothiazide, rifampin, dipyrone, and mitomycin C.

- Autoantibody mechanism: methyldopa.
- Drug adsorption mechanism: penicillin.
- Immune-complex mechanism: stibophen, quinine, and quinidine.
- Some drugs produce autoimmune hemolytic anemia by more than one mechanism.
- Typical clinical scenario: A patient has evidence of hemolysis (increased reticulocyte count, LDH, and indirect bilirubin), positive Coombs test with or without splenomegaly, and jaundice, with a positive drug history.

The first general principle in the treatment of warm autoimmune hemolytic anemia is to treat the underlying disease and to discontinue the use of drugs that have been implicated in hemolysis. If the patient's condition is stable clinically, do not transfuse blood. Avoid transfusion for patients with autoimmune hemolytic anemia. If the patient is symptomatic and studies show improvement in symptoms if the hemoglobin concentration is greater than 8 g/dL, transfuse packed RBCs only if angina, cardiac decompensation, or neurologic symptoms (e.g., lethargy, weakness, confusion, or obtundation) are present. If transfusion is required, transfuse the most compatible RBCs by crossmatch with type-specific ABO and Rh blood. The major risk of transfusion is the formation of autoantibodies to foreign RBC antigens.

Corticosteroids are indicated for the treatment of idiopathic autoimmune hemolytic anemia and are considered in the treatment of disease-associated autoimmune hemolytic anemia. In drug-related warm autoimmune hemolytic anemia, treatment usually is limited to discontinuing the implicated drug. The dose of prednisone should be 1 mg/kg daily. Most patients have a response in 7 days. Patients should have supplementation with oral folate (1 mg daily). If the patient has a relapse during tapering of the drug, return to the previous dose. Splenectomy is required for about 60% of patients with idiopathic autoimmune hemolytic anemia. Immunosuppressive drugs such as cyclophosphamide, danazol (400-800 mg daily), and high-dose intravenous gamma globulin are the next lines of therapy.

Cold Agglutinin Syndrome (Primary Cold Agglutinin Disease)

Cold agglutinin syndrome is characterized by agglutination, hemolytic anemia, a positive Coombs test, chronic anemia, and a "monotonous" prognosis. Autoantibodies are maximally reactive at low temperatures. The degree of hemolysis depends on the thermal amplitude: the higher the titer, the more likely to bind complement. The clinical signs and symptoms are related to small-vessel occlusion and include acrocyanosis of the ears, tip of the nose, toes, and fingers. Hepatosplenomegaly is uncommon. The skin is dusky blue and then turns normal or blanches. All digits may be affected equally. This should be differentiated from Raynaud phenomenon, in which the skin of one or two fingers turns white to blue to red.

The peripheral blood smear shows agglutination of RBCs that disappears if prepared at 37°C (Plate 11-4). Agglutinated RBCs clump together. In rouleaux, the cells stack up on one another (Plate 11-6). The anemia is mild to moderate, and the Coombs test is positive. The cold agglutinin titer is greater than 1:1,000. Therapy includes avoidance of the cold. Oral danazol (200 mg twice daily) or subcutaneous interferon alfa may be given as initial therapy. Some patients may respond to immunosuppressive drugs such as cyclophosphamide or chlorambucil. Plasma exchange is not very effective but should be considered if the patient is acutely ill, because IgM is intravascular.

- Cold agglutinin syndrome: agglutination and hemolytic anemia.
- Positive Coombs test response and cold agglutinin titer >1:1,000.
- Typical clinical scenario: The patient has acrocyanosis of the ears, tip of the nose, toes, and fingers. The diagnosis of cold agglutinin syndrome is made by finding, on a peripheral blood smear, agglutinated RBCs that disappear if the smear is prepared at 37°C. Differentiate from Raynaud phenomenon with Coombs-positive hemolytic anemia.

Immunology of Cold Agglutinins

An IgM antibody exhibits a reversible thermal-dependent equilibrium reaction with the I or i antigen, which is related to the ABO on RBCs and is favored at lower temperatures. A monoclonal κ protein is found in cold agglutinin syndrome, chronic lymphocytic leukemia, multiple myeloma, lymphoma, and Waldenström macroglobulinemia. In secondary diseases, there is a polyclonal light chain reaction with a high thermal cold agglutinin of anti-I specificity (*Mycoplasma pneumoniae*) or anti-i specificity (infectious mononucleosis, cytomegalovirus, and lymphoma).

Mycoplasma pneumoniae (anti-I)

Of the patients with *Mycoplasma pneumoniae*, 50% have cold agglutinins greater than 1:64, most have splenomegaly, and acrocyanosis is unusual. The course of this complication generally resolves in 2 or 3 weeks, but fatalities have been reported. Treatment includes keeping the patient warm and treating the infection with tetracycline or erythromycin.

Infectious Mononucleosis (anti-i)

Of patients with infectious mononucleosis, 40% to 50% have cold agglutinins and 3% have autoimmune hemolytic anemia. The onset occurs by 13 days in 67% of patients. The duration of hemolysis is less than 1 month in 75% of patients and 1 to 2 months in 25%. Hepatosplenomegaly is present in 71% of patients. Corticosteroids are of distinct value in treating this disorder, as may be splenectomy.

Paroxysmal Cold Hemoglobinuria (Complement-Mediated Lysis)

Paroxysmal cold hemoglobinuria is the least common cause of autoimmune hemolytic anemia. Results of the Donath-Landsteiner test are positive. This condition can be idiopathic or secondary. The secondary causes include syphilis (congenital and late), mononucleosis, mycoplasma, chickenpox, mumps, and measles. Measles is the most common secondary cause. Clinical manifestations include shaking chills, fever, malaise, abdominal pain, back pain, and leg pain. There is rapid and severe anemia. The prognosis is good. This condition resolves after the infection clears. Treatment includes protection from the cold, treatment of the underlying disease, and possibly a short course of corticosteroids.

Coombs-Negative Hemolytic Anemias

The differential diagnosis includes the enzymopathies (glucose-6-phosphate dehydrogenase deficiency and pyruvate kinase deficiency), paroxysmal nocturnal hemoglobinuria, hereditary spherocytosis, Wilson disease, and thrombotic thrombocytopenic purpura.

Glucose-6-Phosphate Dehydrogenase Deficiency

This is the most common RBC enzyme deficiency. It causes decreased glutathione, which is an antioxidant. It is inherited on the X chromosome and is sex-linked. All enzymopathies are autosomal recessive except glucose-6-phosphate dehydrogenase and phosphoglycerate kinase deficiencies, which are sex-linked. It is present in 12% of African Americans (70% G6PD B+, the wild type), and 20% of African American females carry the G6PD A− variant. The variant in people of Mediterranean origin is G6PD B− and is associated with the ingestion of uncooked fava beans and may cause hemolysis. In females, one X chromosome is inactivated, and the gene is present on both, so the activity ranges from 0% to 100%, with a mosaic population. Glucose-6-phosphate dehydrogenase deficiency confers some protection against falciparum malaria.

Protection extends to both males and heterozygous females. This selective advantage has been attributed to the inhibition of parasite growth and replication through the mechanism of increased oxidant stress.

The oxidation of hemoglobin leads to the formation of methemoglobin, and sulfhemoglobin may be a product, with precipitation, condensation, and attachment of the denatured portion to the inside of the membrane-forming Heinz bodies. The normal enzyme has a half-life of 62 days, but reticulocytes have a half-life of 124 days and aged cells have a half-life of 31 days. Therefore, in an acute hemolytic state, the glucose-6-phosphate level may be within normal limits because sensitive old RBCs are destroyed and younger RBCs with higher enzyme activity are resistant. Therefore, in the African American variant, the hemolysis is self-limited. There is individual variability to oxidant stress. It is not possible to stimulate the enzyme with methylene blue or ascorbic acid to counteract the formation of methemoglobin; these drugs may actually exacerbate the anemia.

In the steady state, there is no anemia or RBC defect. There is an increased risk of hemolysis in patients with concurrent kidney or liver disease, viral or bacterial infection, diabetic acidosis, viral hepatitis, and low levels of blood glucose. Even a mild infection can produce hemolytic anemia; this is more common than drug provocation. The organisms commonly associated with this complication are *Salmonella*, *E. coli*, pneumococcus, and *Rickettsia*. Favism is found only in whites, not in blacks.

Drugs that commonly cause hemolytic anemia in glucose-6-phosphate dehydrogenase deficiency include antimalarial agents (primaquine and chloroquine), dapsone, sulfonamides (sulfanilamide, sulfamethoxazole, sulfapyridine, and sulfasalazine), nitrofurantoin, diazoxide, high-dose aspirin, probenecid, and nitrites (which are derived from nitrates from nitroglycerin, fertilizer-contaminated home wells, and amyl nitrite).

Abnormal laboratory findings include intravascular hemolysis, methemoglobinemia, and methemalbuminemia (highly specific for intravascular hemolysis). Supravital staining for Heinz bodies is a good screening test, but the absence of these bodies does not rule out the diagnosis. Reticulocytosis rarely masks the deficiency in whites, but it may in blacks and heterozygous females. The glucose-6-phosphate dehydrogenase assay is the definitive test. Therapy includes treating the underlying infection and withdrawing use of the offending drug.

- Glucose-6-phosphate dehydrogenase deficiency: the most common RBC enzyme deficiency; it is inherited on the X chromosome.
- Falciparum malaria provides some protection.

- Half-life: normal enzyme, 62 days; reticulocytes, 124 days; and aged cells, 31 days.
- No anemia or RBC defect occurs in the steady state.
- Important to look for cause, particularly drugs.
- Infection is more common than drug provocation.
- A good screening test: Heinz bodies seen on supravital staining of the peripheral blood.
- Treat underlying infections and withdraw the use of offending drugs.
- Typical clinical scenario: Acute symptomatic anemia in an African American following infection or drug ingestion. There is evidence of intravascular hemolysis (including an increase in the LDH level), urinary hemoglobinuria, and hemosiderinuria and a decrease in haptoglobin levels. The Heinz body test is positive. The Coombs test is negative.

Other Enzymopathies

The most common deficiency states are glucose-6-phosphate dehydrogenase and pyruvate kinase. In a referral population, only 35% of patients who were referred for an enzyme deficiency work-up had an identifiable enzyme deficiency.

Paroxysmal Nocturnal Hemoglobinuria

Paroxysmal nocturnal hemoglobinuria is an acquired clonal chronic hematologic stem cell disorder. Patients with this condition have a median survival of 10 years. It is a clonal disorder in which blood cells are unusually sensitive to activated complement and are lysed. Hemolysis occurs at night because this is when plasma becomes more acidotic. The disorder is characterized by abnormal pluripotent stem cells, reticulocytopenia, leukopenia, or thrombocytopenia due to lysis by complement. Normal and abnormal cells occur simultaneously in most patients.

A distinct class of membrane proteins is selectively deleted from the plasma membranes of maturing cells. The abnormal cells in paroxysmal nocturnal hemoglobinuria have decreased glycosylphosphatidylinositol (GPI)-linked proteins in erythroid, granulocytic, megakaryocytic, and, in some cases, lymphoid cells, the result of a somatic mutation in the *PIG-A* gene. Flow cytometric studies can detect the presence or absence of these GPI-linked proteins, which include CD14, CD16, CD24, CD55, and CD59. This disease involves deficiencies in the surface molecules that normally regulate activation of C3B and C5 to C9 in the complement cascade. There is a decrease in a membrane protein (decay-accelerating factor [CD55]) and homologous restriction factor that regulates the alternate complement pathway on normal blood cells. Also, the activity of RBC acetylcholinesterase is decreased.

Clinically, paroxysmal nocturnal hemoglobinuria is characterized by a chronic hemolytic anemia with hemoglobinuria and hemoglobinemia (intravascular hemolysis). Venous thrombosis of the portal system, brain, and extremities is associated with 50% of the deaths in paroxysmal nocturnal hemoglobinuria. Episodes of severe pain may occur in the abdomen and back in conjunction with painful or difficult swallowing.

Complications include acute nonlymphocytic leukemia in 5% to 10% of patients (paroxysmal nocturnal hemoglobinuria clone disappears), aplastic anemia (the association of aplastic anemia, splenomegaly, and relative reticulocytosis suggests the diagnosis), and venous thrombosis (Budd-Chiari syndrome is the major cause of death). Budd-Chiari syndrome is manifested by abdominal pain, tender hepatomegaly, nausea, vomiting, fever, and increased levels of LDH, serum glutamic-oxalacetic transaminase, γ-glutamyltransferase, and conjugated bilirubin. Liver ultrasonography and venography are important in making the diagnosis. Treatment includes emergent heparinization, a long-term course of anticoagulation, and fibrinolytic therapy.

The most useful assay is flow cytometry to establish the absence of the GPI-linked antigens (this has replaced the sucrose hemolysis test and the Ham test [acid hemolysis test]).

Up to 60% of patients benefit from prednisone treatment. Prednisone (alternate-day therapy, 20-40 mg every other day) may inhibit activation of complement by the alternate pathway. Prednisone is of no benefit if the bone marrow is hypoplastic or there is mild hemolysis. Corticosteroid treatment should be discontinued if no effect occurs in 6 weeks. Danazol may be effective. Transfuse packed RBCs. If complicated by hemolysis, washed or frozen RBCs should be given. A hemolytic crisis may be initiated by infections. Treatment may include corticosteroids, transfusion, and hydration to prevent renal failure. For venous thrombosis, the treatment of choice is heparin, which may activate the alternate pathway of complement. Painful episodes are managed with narcotics and rehydration. Bone marrow transplantation is indicated for severe aplastic anemia. Antithymocyte globulin is effective in the management of paroxysmal nocturnal hemoglobinuria with aplastic anemia.

- Paroxysmal nocturnal hemoglobinuria: a chronic disease caused by an unidentifiable RBC defect.
- Venous thrombosis is associated with 50% of deaths.
- Intravascular hemolysis with hemoglobinuria and hemoglobinemia.
- Leukemia occurs in 5%-10%; aplastic anemia.
- Diagnosis: Ham test, sucrose hemolysis test, and flow cytometry studies.
- Typical clinical scenario: A patient has pancytopenia, Coombs-negative anemia, dark urine, abdominal pain, absence of stainable iron in the marrow, and unusual venous thrombosis.

Hereditary Spherocytosis

Hereditary spherocytosis most commonly is an autosomal dominant disorder in which splenomegaly is invariably present. It is caused by an underlying defect in the RBC membrane cytoskeleton due to a partial deficiency in one or more of the components ankyrin, spectrin and ankyrin, band 3, and protein 4.2. Osmotic fragility of RBCs is increased. The results of the incubated osmotic fragility test—the most reliable diagnostic test—are almost always abnormal. The clinical features include jaundice, splenomegaly, negative results on the Coombs test, spherocytes, and increased osmotic fragility. Gallstones are present in 43% to 85% of patients. Treatment is splenectomy, which invariably causes a reduction in hemolysis. It should be performed after the first decade of life.

- Hereditary spherocytosis: autosomal dominant (75%) as well as autosomal recessive or sporadic.
- Splenomegaly is invariably present; cholelithiasis occurs in 55%-75% after the 5th decade.
- Other features: negative results on the Coombs test and increased osmotic fragility.
- Treatment: splenectomy after the first decade of life for patients with moderate or severe hemolysis. Asymptomatic adults with a hemoglobin concentration >11 g/dL and reticulocyte count <6% may be observed.
- Typical clinical scenario: A patient presents with extravascular hemolysis, spherocytosis, splenomegaly, and premature gallstones.

THROMBOTIC MICROANGIOPATHIES: DIFFERENTIAL DIAGNOSIS

In microangiopathic hemolytic anemia, the RBCs are fragmented and deformed in the peripheral blood (Plate 11-7). The fragmentation is caused by fibrin deposits in small blood vessels that lead to mechanical hemolysis. The results of the Coombs test are negative. Patients with microangiopathic hemolytic anemia are often thrombocytopenic. The associated disorders are characterized by widespread microvascular thrombosis leading to end-organ injury.

Microangiopathic hemolytic anemia is associated with thrombotic thrombocytopenic purpura, hemolytic uremic syndrome, malignant hypertension, pulmonary hypertension, acute glomerulonephritis, acute renal failure, renal allograft rejection, HELLP syndrome (hemolysis, elevated liver function tests, and low platelet count), pregnancy (last trimester), postpartum, disseminated intravascular coagulopathy, collagen vascular diseases (scleroderma, systemic lupus erythematosus, Wegener syndrome, periarteritis nodosa), cardiac valve hemolysis, carcinomatosis, small gastric carcinomas, hemangiomas, Kasabach-Merritt syndrome, viral infections (HIV), bacterial infections (*E. coli* O157:H7), drugs (mitomycin C, quinine, ticlopidine, tacrolimus, cisplatin, and cyclosporine), acute radiation nephropathy, post-bone marrow transplantation (total body irradiation and allogeneic bone marrow transplantation more than autologous marrow transplantation), and post solid-organ transplantation.

Thrombotic Thrombocytopenic Purpura

Idiopathic thrombotic thrombocytopenic purpura is a syndrome rather than a disease. Classically, it is characterized by the pentad of anemia, thrombocytopenia, neurologic signs, fever, and kidney abnormalities. The primary criteria are thrombocytopenia and microangiopathy, and these are sufficient to establish the diagnosis. The anemia is normochromic normocytic, with microangiopathic hemolytic features (Plate 11-7). The serum LDH levels are increased and often high. The Coombs test gives negative results. The results of coagulation studies are normal or only mildly abnormal, in contrast to disseminated intravascular coagulopathy. The cause of this syndrome is unknown in more than 90% of patients. It is related to pregnancy and the use of oral contraceptives.

Clinically, thrombocytopenia is associated with bleeding in 96% of patients and includes petechiae, purpura, retinal bleeding, hematuria, gingival bleeding, melena, menorrhagia, hematemesis, and hemoptysis. Neurologic signs consist of remittent and frequent changes, including headache, coma, mental changes, paresis, seizure/coma, aphasia, syncope, visual symptoms, dysarthria, vertigo, agitation, confusion, and delirium. Kidney abnormalities include a creatinine level greater than 1.5 mg/dL (in less than 20% of patients). Azotemia is an unfavorable prognostic sign. An abnormal urinary sediment with proteinuria, hematuria, pyuria, or casts was present in 82% of patients in one series. Coagulation studies, including activated partial thromboplastin time (APTT), prothrombin time (PT), and fibrinogen, are characteristically normal.

The pathologic findings are characterized by widespread intraluminal hyaline vascular occlusions with platelet aggregates and fibrin, with no inflammatory changes in the microvasculature (terminal arterioles or capillaries) in virtually any organ. The preferred biopsy site is the bone marrow. Other sites to consider for biopsy are the gingiva, skin, petechial spot, muscle, and lymph nodes. Systemic endothelial damage is the result of apoptosis in the microvasculature. This causes the release of von Willebrand factor (vWF), which is believed to participate in platelet agglutination and thrombus formation. Patients with thrombotic thrombocytopenic purpura are deficient in the vWF-cleaving protease ADAMTS13 that reduces the size of the large vWF multimers. A severe deficiency of ADAMTS13 is detected in patients with acquired or congenital thrombotic thrombocytopenic purpura. Large multimers of vWF appear to be the aggregating agents of thrombotic thrombocytopenic purpura. Patients who have had a single acute episode of thrombotic thrombocytopenic purpura have little if any plasma vWF-cleaving protease activity, and an IgG antibody accounts for the lack of protease activity in the sporadic form.

Without treatment, more than 90% of patients die of multiorgan failure, but with treatment, 70% to 80% survive the disease and have few or no sequelae. The treatment of choice is plasma exchange (plasmapheresis with infusion of fresh frozen plasma or the supernatant fraction from cryoprecipitate preparations [cryosupernatant]). The deficiency of ADAMTS13 as the cause of thrombotic thrombocytopenic purpura explains why plasma infusion or exchange is effective. This is the only treatment at many centers. Other ancillary treatments with unknown value include dipyridamole (400-600 mg daily), aspirin (from 300 mg twice weekly to 600-1,200 mg daily), and prednisone (60 mg/kg daily). The overall response rate to therapy is 80% to 90%. The projected 10-year risk of relapse in the Canadian Apheresis Group Trial is 36%. The management of refractory disease includes intravenous vincristine, splenectomy, and intravenous high-dose gamma globulin. Platelet transfusions should be used only when required for an invasive procedure.

- Thrombotic thrombocytopenic purpura: the pentad of anemia, fever, thrombocytopenia, neurologic signs, and renal abnormalities.
- Its cause is unknown; exclude oral contraceptives and pregnancy as etiologic factors.
- Features: Coombs test gives negative results, microangiopathy, normal PT, normal APTT, and normal fibrinogen.
- The treatment of choice is plasmapheresis, with the replacement of fresh frozen plasma.
- Typical clinical scenario: A patient has anemia, thrombocytopenia, neurologic signs or symptoms, renal abnormalities, and fever. Peripheral blood smear shows schistocytes. Clotting times (PT and APTT) are normal.

Hemolytic Uremic Syndrome

Hemolytic uremic syndrome is characterized by microangiopathic hemolytic anemia (anemia and thrombocytopenia) and renal microangiopathy, with a creatinine level greater than 3 mg/dL. Fever and neurologic signs are not part of this syndrome. The pathologic findings are similar to those in thrombotic thrombocytopenic purpura but are limited to the kidneys. It is often preceded by an acute infectious process. The morbidity and mortality rates are much higher for adults than for children. A recurrent illness may be caused by defective production of the complement control protein factor H. Adult hemolytic uremic syndrome is best managed with plasma

exchange. The syndrome may be associated with *E. coli* O157:H7 diarrhea, as is the classic association in children. Other associations include various *E. coli* serotypes and *Shigella dysenteriae*. Hemolytic uremic syndrome is usually not associated with a decrease in ADAMTS13 activity. The management of the hemolytic-uremic syndrome with this complication is supportive. Dialysis may be necessary. Corticosteroids may be incorporated in the management.

SICKLE CELL DISORDERS

The sickle cell disorders include sickle cell anemia (homozygous sickle gene), sickle cell trait (heterozygous), and other forms of sickle cell disease (sickle cell–hemoglobin C disease, sickle cell thalassemia).

Sickle cell anemia is the most common heritable hematologic disease affecting humans. The gene for the β chain must be inherited from both parents. It occurs in black Africans and rarely in whites. About 8% of African Americans carry the sickle cell gene, with disease occurring in 1/625 individuals. The sickle cell trait offers a selective advantage because, in *Plasmodium falciparum* malaria, the parasitized cells preferentially sickle. Sickle cell anemia is an example of a balanced polymorphism (a common mutation) that provides a selective advantage but also has the potential to produce a disease state. In the heterozygous state, there is protection against malaria. In the homozygous state, sickle cell anemia is a serious, life-shortening disease. Hemoglobin S is different from hemoglobin A in the substitution of valine for glutamic acid at the sixth position of the β chain. Deoxygenated hemoglobin S aggregates into rigid polymers that essentially fill the cell and distort it into a sickle shape. The end result of the polymerization is a permanently altered membrane protein. Vaso-occlusion is a function of decreased erythrocyte deformability, increased viscosity, and increased RBC adherence to the endothelium at the capillary level. Two-thirds of the RBCs are removed by extravascular mechanisms.

Vaso-occlusion occurs in arterioles and larger arteries, not capillaries. Polymorphonuclear leukocytes release activators.

Sickling is inhibited by hemoglobin F, which is a potent inhibitor of polymerization. Polymerization leads to sickling. Sickling is promoted by low oxygen tension, low pH, high cellular concentration of hemoglobins, loss of cell water, hemoglobin D, and hemoglobinopathy.

Symptoms are not present until the patient is older than 6 months. Vaso-occlusive disease develops between the ages of 12 months and 6 years. Acute crises are due to recurrent obstruction of the microcirculation by intravascular sickling. Laboratory testing is not helpful. Atypical symptoms should suggest pneumonia, pulmonary infarct, acute pyelonephritis, or cholecystitis.

Bone and joint pain crises are characterized by gnawing pain and swelling of the elbows and knees. Pain prevalence is highest between ages 19 and 39 years. The average duration is 10 days. Radiographs may show bone infarcts and periostitis, but these do not appear until symptoms subside. Infarcts and periostitis may be documented with bone scans. Abdominal crises are due to small infarcts of the mesentery and abdominal viscera, with symptoms lasting for 4 or 5 days. This is a nonsurgical problem if bowel sounds are present. Associated signs and symptoms include fever, tenderness, hypertension, tachycardia, tachypnea, nausea, and vomiting. Treatment includes bed rest, folate supplementation, heating pads, tub baths, analgesics, intravenous narcotics, antihistamines, aggressive intravenous hydration, and correction of hypoxia and acidosis.

The Cooperative Study of Sickle Cell Disease reported that the incidence of hemorrhagic stroke was highest among patients 20 to 29 years old, with a mortality rate of 26% in the first 2 weeks and no deaths after infarctive strokes. The frequency of stroke is 10% to 15% among children and young adults. Transient ischemic attack is a strong risk factor for infarctive stroke. Angiographic procedures should not be performed unless the patient has been prepared with RBCs. The management for these crises is immediate exchange transfusion to decrease hemoglobin S levels to less than 30% and maintain the hematocrit at less than 33% to 35%. In a randomized study of chronic transfusion, therapy decreased the risk of recurrence of a cerebrovascular event. Chronic transfusion therapy is indicated for this complication to maintain hemoglobin S higher than 30%, because the risk of recurrent episodes is more than 46% to 90%. Multivariate analysis found that low steady-state hemoglobin concentration and high leukocyte concentration were not factors for hemorrhagic stroke. This complication clusters in families and is associated with a risk of recurrence of up to 90%.

In pulmonary crises, acute chest syndrome accounts for up to 25% of deaths in sickle cell disease and the risk is 25%. Clinical aspects include fever, chest pain, tachypnea, increased WBC count, and pulmonary infiltrates. Age is a factor in cause. In children, infected segments enhance local sickling, so sickling is a secondary phenomenon. The causative organisms include pneumococcus, *Mycoplasma*, *Haemophilus*, *Salmonella*, and *E. coli*. In adults, sickling tends to be a primary event, with no sign of infection. In a cooperative study, 13% of patients required ventilator support, 11% had neurologic events, and the mortality rate was 9%. With multifactorial causes (thromboembolism and fat embolism), chronic lung disease is a long-term complication. Acute management includes supportive measures, which include decreasing the level of hemoglobin S to 20% to 30%.

Aplastic crises usually follow a febrile illness, with the disappearance of reticulocytes and normoblasts. B19 parvovirus infections are more common in adults than in children. Other organisms include *Salmonella*, *Streptococcus pneumoniae*, and Epstein-Barr virus. The aplastic crisis lasts 5 to 10 days. Hemolytic crises may occur in patients with concomitant glucose-6-phosphate dehydrogenase deficiency, hereditary spherocytosis, and mycoplasmic pneumonia.

Infectious crises are the most frequent cause of death of patients younger than 5 years. The organisms include *Streptococcus pneumoniae* of the blood and cerebrospinal fluid (70% of patients). Normally, 80% of the cases of meningitis in this age group are caused by *Haemophilus influenzae*. At ages older than 5 years, gram-negative bacteria predominate, with osteomyelitis caused by *Salmonella*, *Staphylococcus*, and pneumococcus. Bone infarction is more common than osteomyelitis. In contrast to bone infarction, osteomyelitis presents with high fever, a left shift with an increased leukocyte count, an increased erythrocyte sedimentation rate, and positive blood cultures. The causes of infections/infectious crises include decreased IgM, defective alternate pathway, deficiency phagocytosis-promoting peptide tuftsin, and impaired splenic function. The challenge with *Streptococcus pneumoniae* is not followed by appropriate opsonin production. Supportive care measures include prophylactic penicillin therapy and immunization. High-risk patients should be hospitalized (fever $\geq 40°C$, WBC $<6\times10^9/L$ or $>30\times10^9/L$, or pulmonary infiltrates).

The chronic manifestations of sickle cell anemia are multiple. Anemia is the most common manifestation. There is a progressive lag in growth and development after the first decade of life and a chronic destruction of bone and joints, with ischemia and infarction of the spongiosa. The vertebrae become fish-mouthed. Avascular necrosis is common in multiple joints, and the incidence of femoral and humeral necrosis increases with advanced age. Ocular manifestations include retinopathy with stasis and occlusion of small vessels that is nonproliferative or proliferative. The small vessels may require laser photocoagulation.

Cardiovascular manifestations include cardiomegaly, flow murmurs, and a pansystolic murmur with a click that mimics mitral regurgitation. Restrictive lung disease may develop. Hepatobiliary manifestations include hepatomegaly (present clinically in 40%-80% of patients; in autopsy series, 80%-100%) with the pathologic features of distended sinusoids, periportal fibrosis, and hemosiderin pigment. Marked hyperbilirubinemia may be due to hepatitis, intrahepatic sickling, choledocholithiasis, or coexistent glucose-6-phosphate dehydrogenase deficiency. Hemochromatosis is a complication. There is an increased incidence of pigmented gallstones in 30% to 60% of adults, with symptoms in 10% to 15%. Elective laparoscopy is recommended. Hepatic crises occur and resolve in 1 to 3 weeks. Renal manifestations include papillary necrosis, hyposthenuria by age 6 to 12 months (disruption of the countercurrent multiplier system, nocturia, enuresis), hematuria (ulcer in renal pelvis, urate stones), nephrotic syndrome caused by focal segmental glomerulo-nephropathy, tubular damage from small infarcts, and priapism. Chronic renal insufficiency is common (25%-75% of patients). Leg ulcers are painful and may be complicated by infection.

Although disease manifestations do not increase during pregnancy, maternal mortality increases 5% to 8% and fetal mortality, 20%. Early complications of pregnancy include thrombophlebitis, pyelonephritis, and hematuria. Late complications include preeclampsia, toxemia, congestive heart failure, postpartum endometritis, and major infarcts of the lung, kidney, and brain. Prophylactic exchange transfusions are not recommended.

Laboratory findings include anemia (range, 5.5-9.5 g/dL), sickled cells, cigar cells, ovalocytes, target cells, basophilic stippling, polychromatophilia, reticulocytosis (3%-12%), and hyposplenia with Howell-Jolly bodies. A persistent increase in the WBC count of 12 to 15×10^9/L is characteristic. Evidence of chronic hemolysis may be present. Values on liver function tests are often increased. On hemoglobin electrophoresis, hemoglobin S moves more slowly than hemoglobin A. Routine diagnostic tests include the sickle solubility test and cellulose acetate gel electrophoresis.

The primary treatment is prevention. Infection, fever, dehydration, acidosis, hypoxemia, cold, and high altitude should be avoided. Immunizations, penicillin prophylaxis, and education are essential. Acetaminophen is indicated for fever because aspirin contributes to an acid load. A temperature higher than 105°F (40.6°C) means infection (infection is uncommon if the temperature is lower than 102°F [38.9°C]). Prophylactic use of penicillin is beneficial. Vaccines, including pneumococcal, influenza A, and *Haemophilus*, are indicated, as is folate supplementation, especially during pregnancy. Iron chelation is recommended if the transfusion requirement is high. Splenectomy is recommended for children who survive the initial splenic sequestration crisis. This is the only indication for splenectomy.

Blood transfusion and exchange transfusions are the most effective means of treatment available. Hemoglobin S fractions of less than 30% have been recommended for life-threatening complications. Post-transfusion increases in hemoglobin of more than 10 g/dL should be avoided. These modalities are indicated especially for the following: history of cerebrovascular accidents, recurrent acute chest syndrome, progressive retinopathy, renal or cardiac decompensation preoperatively, and pregnancy (multiple gestations, history of fetal loss, and severe disease). At 30 to 34 weeks, maintain the hemoglobin concentration above 10 g/dL. Short-term transfusion therapy is indicated in acute chest syndrome. Other indications for transfusion are priapism, protracted hematuria, and chronic skin ulcers. High-risk patients should be given transfusion to achieve a hemoglobin concentration greater than 10 g/dL for laparotomy or thoracotomy. In vaso-occlusive crises, the cornerstone of treatment includes fluids and correction of urinary sodium losses.

Other important considerations are treatment of infections: penicillin for children and coverage for *Staphylococcus* in adults. Analgesics are essential. Blood transfusions do not modify the course. Prenatal diagnosis may be made by analysis of amniotic fluid or chorionic villi biopsy, which is preferred to fetal blood sampling. New approaches that inhibit potassium and water loss from sickle cell RBCs include low-dose clotrimazole and magnesium. In the Multicenter Study of Hydroxyurea in Sickle Cell Anemia, which was a double-blind, placebo-controlled trial, hydroxyurea decreased the frequency of painful vaso-occlusive crises by about 50%. In patients with severe recurrent episodes, the frequency of the acute chest syndrome was decreased and patients required fewer transfusions. Hydroxyurea increases fetal hemoglobin. Side effects include readily reversible myelosuppression. In addition, hydroxyurea causes slight neutropenia and decreases the reticulocyte count, which may contribute to the efficacy of the drug.

Hematopoietic stem cell transplantation with marrow or umbilical cord blood from HLA-identical siblings has demonstrated that sickle cell disease can be cured. The present indications are stroke and recurrent chest syndrome. Gene therapy studies are beginning. Related cord blood transplantation offers a good probability of success and has a low risk of graft-versus-host disease.

The Cooperative Study of Sickle Cell Disease reported in a prospective analysis that 50% of patients with sickle cell anemia survive beyond the fifth decade. Few patients survive into their 60s. Symptomatic patients had the highest early mortality. A high level of fetal hemoglobin predicted improved survival of young patients. Acute chest syndrome, renal failure, seizures, a baseline WBC count greater than 15×10^9/L, and a low level of fetal hemoglobin were associated with the risk of early death in patients 20 years or older. Of adult patients, 78% died during an acute sickle cell crisis. Acute pain and chest syndrome were the most common causes of death, and stroke was the next most common cause. This was followed by infection (*E. coli*, *Staphylococcus aureus*, HIV, tuberculosis, malaria, pneumococcus, and hepatitis). In children younger than 5 years, the cause of infection nearly always is pneumococcal sepsis.

Sickle cell trait occurs in 8% of African Americans. There is no anemia, RBC abnormalities, increased risk of infections, or increased mortality; 35% to 45% of hemoglobin is hemoglobin S. Associations with sickle cell trait include hematuria, splenic infarction at high altitude (higher than 10,000 feet), hyposthenuria, bacteriuria, pyelonephritis in pregnancy, pulmonary embolism, glaucoma, and decreased mortality from *P. falciparum* infection.

In sickle cell–hemoglobin C disease, patients have hemoglobin S and C, with an absence of hemoglobin A and normal or increased levels of hemoglobin F. Patients with sickle cell–hemoglobin C survive longer than those with sickle cell anemia. Sickle cell–hemoglobin C disorder is less severe than sickle cell disease, with four exceptions: proliferative retinopathy, retinal detachment, aseptic necrosis of the head of the femur, and acute chest syndrome due to fat emboli in the final months of pregnancy. There is mild anemia; in 10% of patients, the hemoglobin concentration is less than 10 g/dL. Sickle cells are rare on the peripheral blood smear, and 50% of the cells in the peripheral blood are target cells. Splenic hypofunction occurs at an older age.

Hemoglobin S/β-thalassemia is less severe than sickle cell disease. Both affect the β chain. The spleen remains functional, but retinopathy is more common. The protective effect of α-thalassemia is due largely to improvement in hemoglobin concentration.

- Hydroxyurea decreases the frequency of painful vaso-occlusive crises by 50%.
- Acute chest syndrome, renal failure, seizures, a baseline WBC count >15×10⁹/L, and a low level of fetal hemoglobin are associated with the risk of early death in adults.
- Death is associated with acute pain and chest syndrome, stroke, and infection.
- Patients with sickle cell–hemoglobin C survive longer than those with sickle cell anemia.
- High WBC counts are a risk factor for severe pain, acute chest syndrome, and mortality from a hemorrhagic cerebrovascular event.
- The best method of prenatal diagnosis is to sample either from the amniotic sac or chorionic villi and to test for an abnormal endonuclease cleavage pattern.
- Hemoglobin S levels of less than 30% are recommended for life-threatening complications.
- A post-transfusion increase in hemoglobin of more than 10 g/dL should be avoided.
- Typical clinical scenario: An African American patient has pain, fevers, stroke, or infection and evidence of Coombs-negative hemolytic anemia with Howell-Jolly bodies on a peripheral blood smear. The diagnosis is made with hemoglobin electrophoresis.

MALIGNANCIES

Chronic Lymphocytic Leukemia

Chronic lymphocytic leukemia is a lymphoproliferative disorder of mature lymphocytes (Plate 11-8). The clinical diagnosis requires an absolute lymphocytosis greater than 5,000 mature-appearing lymphocytes per microliter and more than 30% lymphocytes in the bone marrow. It is the commonest

form of leukemia in patients 60 years and older in the Western world (90% of patients are older than 50), and it accounts for 30% of all leukemias at any one time. It is more common in men and is rare in Asia.

Chronic lymphocytic leukemia is more of an accumulative than a proliferative disorder of long-lived immunologically incompetent cells. B-cell chronic lymphocytic leukemia is the only major adult leukemia not associated with exposure to ionizing radiation, drugs, or chemicals. The two staging classifications are outlined in Tables 11-3 and 11-4.

Low-risk patients have a normal hemoglobin, low lymphocyte count, nondiffuse bone marrow infiltration pattern, and a lymphocyte doubling time of more than 1 year, which identify patients with Rai stage 0 or 1 or Binet stage I disease. New prognostic factors for a better prognosis which determine a risk-adapted approach include a normal karyotype, deletion 13q, hypermutated *IGVH* gene, nonexpression of CD38, and expression of ZAP-70.

Poor risk factors include advanced stage, unmutated *IGVH* genes, expression of CD38, atypical lymphocyte morphology, trisomy 12, deletion of q23, deletion of 17p or 11q, and loss or mutation of the *p53* gene.

The clinical course is chronic in 60% of patients. Complications include recurrent infection; 50% of patients have hypogammaglobulinemia. Fever is due to infection and not to chronic lymphocytic leukemia, except in Richter syndrome. Autoimmune and immunodeficiency complications include autoimmune hemolytic anemia (in 10% of patients), monoclonal gammopathy (in 5%), immune-mediated thrombocytopenia (occurs in 2% and is IgG-mediated and treated with corticosteroids), pure RBC aplasia, hypogammaglobulinemia, impaired delayed-type hypersensitivity, increased susceptibility to microorganisms, and second malignancies.

- In chronic lymphocytic leukemia, fever is not related to the disease but to infection, except in Richter syndrome.
- Hypogammaglobulinemia occurs in 50% of patients with recurrent infection.
- Autoimmune hemolytic anemia occurs in 10%.
- Thrombocytopenia occurs in <5%.
- Prophylactic intravenous gamma globulin is indicated for gamma globulin levels <0.3 g/dL with or without previous infection.
- Typical clinical scenario: A middle-aged or older patient has an increased WBC count, lymphocytosis, and lymphadenopathy. Peripheral blood lymphocyte flow cytometry shows the presence of mature CD23+ B lymphocytes that aberrantly express the T-cell marker CD5. The cells are also "dimly" positive for surface immunoglobulin that is "light chain restricted" (i.e., almost all the cells express one type of light chain, κ or λ).

Table 11-3 Staging: Rai Classification

Stage	Characteristics	No. of patients	Median survival time, mo	No. of patients[*]	Median survival time, mo
0	Peripheral lymphocytosis ($>15\times10^9$/L), bone marrow lymphocytosis (>40%)	22	>150	79	129
I	Lymphocytosis, lymphadenopathy	29	101	154	74.4
II	Lymphocytosis, splenomegaly	39	71	203	58.2
III	Lymphocytosis, anemia with hemoglobin <11 g/dL excluding AIHA	21	19	127	28.1
IV	Lymphocytosis, thrombocytopenia	14	19	105	19.3

AIHA, autoimmune hemolytic anemia.

[*]Six combined series.

Data from Rai KR, Sawitsky A, Cronkite EP, et al: Clinical staging of chronic lymphocytic leukemia. Blood 1975;46:219-234.

Table 11-4 Classification of International Workshop on Chronic Lymphocytic Leukemia

Clinical stage	Features
A	No anemia or thrombocytopenia and fewer than three areas of lymphoid enlargement. (Spleen, liver, and lymph nodes in cervical, axillary, and inguinal regions.) A(0), A(I), or A(II).
B	No anemia or thrombocytopenia with three or more involved areas. B(I) or B(II).
C	Anemia (<10 g/dL) and/or thrombocytopenia regardless of the number of areas of lymphoid enlargement. C(III) or C(IV).

From International Workshop on CLL: Chronic lymphocytic leukaemia: proposals for a revised prognostic staging system. Br J Haematol 1981;48:365-367. By permission of Blackwell Scientific Publications.

The major hematologic malignancies associated with chronic lymphocytic leukemia include Richter syndrome, which is chronic lymphocytic leukemia that has transformed into diffuse large cell lymphoma and is characterized by fevers, massive asymmetrical adenopathy, splenomegaly, and a poor outcome. Chronic lymphocytic leukemia is associated with an increased incidence of solid tumors of the lung and skin (basal cell, squamous cell). Patients may develop secondary drug-induced acute nonlymphocytic leukemia. Infectious complications include *Staphylococcus aureus*, pneumococci, *Pseudomonas*, *Klebsiella*, *Pneumocystis*, cytomegalovirus, *Candida*, herpes simplex, and herpes zoster.

Findings that establish the diagnosis include blood lymphocytosis greater than 5,000 mature-appearing lymphocytes (<55% prolymphocytes) per microliter, "smudged" cells on the peripheral blood smear, and a characteristic phenotype (CD19+, CD20+, CD23+, coexpression of the T-cell marker CD5+, and faint monoclonal light chain restriction). The neoplastic cells usually express high levels of bcl-2 protein, rendering them resistant to programmed cell death (apoptosis). Chromosomal abnormalities are found in more than 50% of patients.

For chronic lymphocytic leukemia, the standard practice is to withhold treatment until the disease is active or progressive.

A French study compared treatment with no treatment in early-stage disease and found no difference in survival. In contrast, survival of patients with advanced-stage disease is better if the disease responds to treatment, with a median response duration of 4 years, compared with 1 year if no response. Chlorambucil with or without prednisone versus fludarabine is the initial treatment of choice. The complete remission rate and median duration of remission are higher with fludarabine. The risk of life-threatening infections is higher with fludarabine. In three different trials, no survival advantage has been shown for patients treated with fludarabine. Fludarabine may be the initial choice for patients who clinically need a rapid and sustained remission. Most patients have disease relapse within 3 years. Bone marrow transplantation is being evaluated in chronic lymphocytic leukemia. Prednisone alone may be indicated for isolated immune-related anemia and thrombocytopenia. Fludarabine is the treatment of choice for patients who have disease relapse after treatment with chlorambucil.

Fludarabine induces an overall response rate of 32% to 60% in previously treated patients and approximately 80% in previously untreated patients, with a median response duration of 33 months. The major toxic effects of fludarabine are myelosuppression and immunosuppression, which predispose to opportunistic infections due to a quantitative suppression in T-helper (CD4) lymphocytes.

A large randomized trial has demonstrated the usefulness of recombinant erythropoietin in increasing hemoglobin levels in patients with chronic lymphocytic leukemia who have anemia. Splenectomy may be indicated for patients with refractory immune anemia and thrombocytopenia, massive splenomegaly, and hypersplenism. An alternative is to include systemic chemotherapy with CAP (cyclophosphamide, doxorubicin [Adriamycin], and prednisone). With each relapse, the disease becomes more resistant to treatment.

Chemoimmunotherapy regimens are being evaluated, for example, FCR (fludarabine, cyclophosphamide, and rituximab), and show promise.

Treatment guidelines—Rai classification:

Stage 0—No treatment.

Stage I and stage II—The NCI-Working Group recommended treatment if active disease was present and included the presence of disease-related symptoms (weight loss ≥10% in 6 months, fatigue, performance score of 2 or more, fevers without overt infection, or night sweats), massively enlarged nodes or spleen, progressive or rapid rate of increase (<12 months) in the peripheral blood lymphocyte count, autoimmune anemia or thrombocytopenia and repeated infections with or without hypogammaglobulinemia.

Stage III and stage IV—Short median life expectancy, invariably symptomatic. Treat all patients to alleviate symptoms and to improve life expectancy.

Treatment guidelines—International Workshop classification:

Stage A—Observe.

Stage B—Some patients will need treatment, as outlined in stages I and II indications above.

Stage C—Treat all patients.

- Observe patients with stage 0 or stage A disease.
- Treat all patients with Rai stages III and IV disease and International Workshop stage C.
- The optimal treatment of choice is chlorambucil with or without prednisone or fludarabine.
- Fludarabine is the treatment of choice for patients who have disease relapse after treatment with chlorambucil or prednisone (or both).
- Typical clinical scenario: A 60-year-old patient has lymphocytosis and lymphadenopathy. Peripheral blood lymphocyte flow cytometry shows mature CD23+ B lymphocytes that aberrantly express the T-cell marker CD5. The cells are also "dimly" positive for surface immunoglobulin that is "light-chain restricted" (i.e., almost all the cells express one type of light chain, κ or λ).

Patients who have disease relapse may be followed without therapy until they experience disease-related symptoms or progressive disease, with deterioration of blood cell counts, discomfort from lymphadenopathy or hepatosplenomegaly, recurrent infections, or associated autoimmune disorders.

Hairy Cell Leukemia

Hairy cell leukemia is characterized by an insidious onset of cytopenias without constitutional symptoms. At some time during the course of the disease, 90% of patients have splenomegaly. The hairy cell cytoplasmic projections are "hairy," with multiple thin or blunt projections (Plate 11-9). The cells contain tartrate-resistant acid phosphatase (positive tartrate-resistant acid phosphatase [TRAP] stain). Most are B cells in nature and clonal, as demonstrated by light- and heavy-chain immunoglobulin gene rearrangements. Hairy cell leukemia accounts for less than 2% of all cases of leukemia. The male-to-female ratio is 4:1. The cause is not known.

- Hairy cell leukemia: cytopenias.
- Splenomegaly is common.
- Hairy cells have cytoplasmic projections.
- B-cell in nature and clonal.
- Constitutes <2% of all cases of leukemia.

The symptoms are related to cytopenias, infections, and splenomegaly. Laboratory findings demonstrate anemia, thrombocytopenia, neutropenia, and pancytopenia. More than 75% of patients have anemia, thrombocytopenia, and neutropenia. The bone marrow yields a dry tap on bone marrow aspiration; biopsy specimens are hypercellular with diffuse infiltration. Hairy cells may or may not be seen in the peripheral blood.

- Cytopenias in >75% of patients with hairy cell leukemia.
- Bone marrow: dry tap.
- Hairy cells may not be seen in a peripheral blood smear.
- Infection is related to granulocytopenia and impaired cell-mediated immunity.
- Typical clinical scenario: A patient has cytopenias and splenomegaly. Malignant cells in bone marrow biopsy specimens contain TRAP.

Infection is the major cause of death. Infection should be considered when a patient who previously had a stable condition develops new symptoms. Fever is not a manifestation of the disease but indicates an underlying infection. Localized pyogenic infections are more common, for example, bacterial pneumonia, urinary tract infections, and infections of the skin. Impaired cell-mediated immunity predisposes patients to other infections. The incidence of atypical mycobacterial infections is increased. There is a higher incidence of viral infections, fungal infections, parasitic diseases, toxoplasmosis, histoplasmosis, and coccidiosis. Bleeding and vasculitis (skin, joint, erythema nodosum) are other complications.

- Hairy cell leukemia: infection is the major cause of death.
- Fever denotes infection.
- Atypical mycobacterial infections.

Observation may be indicated only for patients who are asymptomatic with a normal CBC or very mild cytopenias. Indications for intervention include masked cytopenia, serious or recurrent infections associated with neutropenia, bleeding due to thrombocytopenia, splenic infarction, vasculitis, and an increasing number of hairy cells. Treatment with 2-chlorodeoxyadenosine produces durable complete remission rates in 85% to 88% of patients after a single 7-day continuous, intravenous infusion. Other treatments include interferon alfa-2a or 2b recombinant, which produces a 13% complete remission rate after 18 months of subcutaneous treatments and a partial remission rate of 66%. Pentostatin produces complete remission rate in 75% of patients. Patients now have a survival rate similar to that of the normal population. Splenectomy only improves peripheral blood cell counts and has no effect on the bone marrow. The only indications for splenectomy are a very large spleen and patchy bone marrow involvement in a young patient, splenic infarct, and profound life-threatening bleeding due to thrombocytopenia.

- 2-Chlorodeoxyadenosine is the treatment of choice for hairy cell leukemia.
- Other treatments include pentostatin, interferon alfa-2a or 2b recombinant, and splenectomy.
- Typical clinical scenario: A 50-year-old man presents with pancytopenia and cells in the peripheral blood that have projections.

Infectious Mononucleosis

The outcomes of infectious mononucleosis include acute infectious mononucleosis, asymptomatic primary infection, symptomatic chronic infection, chronic infectious mononucleosis syndrome, malignant lymphoproliferative disorders, hypogammaglobulinemia, and death (200 deaths/10 years). Ninety percent of patients have fever of 38°C to 39°C for 10 to 14 days and 70% to 90% develop a sore throat, with an exudative tonsillitis in 30% to 50%. Lymphadenopathy occurs in 80% to 90% of patients, splenomegaly in 50% to 60%, hepatomegaly in 10% to 15%, and rash in 5% to 15%. From 50% to 90% of patients are asymptomatic carriers. Laboratory abnormalities include leukocytosis in 70% of patients, lymphocytosis in 50% (variant lymphocytosis and transient increase in suppressor T cells) (Plate 11-10), mild thrombocytopenia in 50%, and increased values on liver function tests in 80% to 90%. Complications of infectious mononucleosis include fulminant infections in immunodeficient hosts, severe tonsillar hypertrophy, splenic rupture, upper airway obstruction, neurologic syndromes (Guillain-Barré syndrome), myocarditis, and bleeding due to thrombocytopenia. Malignant diseases associated with Epstein-Barr viral infections include Burkitt lymphoma, nasopharyngeal carcinoma, post-transplantation lymphoproliferative disorders, HIV-related non-Hodgkin lymphoma, and Hodgkin disease. Hematologic complications include autoimmune hemolytic anemia and autoimmune thrombocytopenic purpura.

Hodgkin Lymphoma

With therapy, 75% of patients with Hodgkin lymphoma are cured. Untreated, the 5-year survival rate is less than 5%. Since 1973, Hodgkin lymphoma has ranked second in decreased survival rates among cancer patients in the United States. The age at presentation has a bimodal distribution, with the first peak at a median age of about 25 years. Hodgkin lymphoma usually presents as a locally limited disease that progresses in an orderly manner. The typical finding at presentation is lymph node enlargement, but virtually any organ or tissue may be involved (lung, bone marrow, liver, and bone). Less common presentations include pruritus, cytopenias, abnormal findings on liver function tests, and jaundice (extrahepatic biliary obstruction, autoimmune hemolytic anemia, or, rarely, intrahepatic cholestasis). Patients with Hodgkin lymphoma have impaired cell-mediated immunity and are predisposed to herpes zoster and cytomegalovirus infections. A low hemoglobin concentration and a low serum level of albumin are the two most important prognostic factors.

The diagnosis of Hodgkin lymphoma is based on the presence of Reed-Sternberg cells, which typically have two or more nuclei with prominent nucleoli that give the cells the appearance of owl's eyes (Plate 11-11).

Disease stage is the principal factor in selecting treatment (Tables 11-5 and 11-6). In the United States, up to 50% of patients have mediastinal disease on computed tomography (CT) of the chest that may not be detectable on a standing posterior-anterior chest radiograph. Lymphangiography complements CT and is used infrequently. Special nonroutine procedures include formal staging laparotomy, magnetic resonance imaging (MRI), gallium scan, bone scan, and liver/spleen scan.

Before treatment is started, male patients should be advised to store sperm if they intend to have children and female patients are advised not to become pregnant for 2 years after therapy because 75% of relapses occur during this period.

Radiotherapy is a consideration in the management of Hodgkin disease emergencies, including acute superior vena cava syndrome, airway obstruction, pericardial tamponade, and epidural spinal cord compression.

The preferred treatment for pathologic stage I or IIA Hodgkin disease had been radiotherapy, at a dose of 35 to 44 Gy, to a mantle (fields extending to include all nodes above the diaphragm)

and upper abdominal field. The corresponding rates of freedom from progression and survival at 14 years are 93% and 83%. Currently, the treatment of choice is a short course of chemotherapy with ABVD (doxorubicin [Adriamycin], bleomycin, vinblastine, and dacarbazine [DTIC]) and lower doses of radiotherapy. The treatment of choice for stages IIIA, IIIB, IVA, and IVB is combination chemotherapy (Table 11-7). Although somewhat controversial, stages IB and IIB are also treated with combination chemotherapy. Chemotherapy is given if the disease is only infradiaphragmatic. The cure rates are up to 65% for patients with advanced disease. There is less sterility and secondary leukemia than with MOPP (mechlorethamine, vincristine [Oncovin], procarbazine, and prednisone) chemotherapy. Stanford V, a 12-week dose-intensive chemotherapy with 36 Gy radiotherapy, is currently being evaluated. Increased-dose BEACOPP (bleomycin, etoposide, doxorubicin [Adriamycin], cyclophosphamide, vincristine [Oncovin], procarbazine, and prednisone) resulted in improved disease-resurvival and overall survival.

Relapse patterns are relatively predictable in Hodgkin disease. After irradiation, relapse occurs in the first 2 years and usually involves nonirradiated sites adjacent to the treated fields. Relapse after chemotherapy occurs at sites of bulky disease. Patients who have relapse after radiotherapy have about a 66% chance of cure with salvage chemotherapy. Those who have relapse after chemotherapy currently are offered

Table 11-5   The Cotswolds Staging Classification of Hodgkin Disease

Classification	Description
Stage I	Involvement of a single lymph node region or lymphoid structure
Stage II	Involvement of two or more lymph node regions on the same side of the diaphragm (the mediastinum is considered a single site, whereas hilar lymph nodes are considered bilaterally)
Stage III	Involvement of lymph node regions or structures on both sides of the diaphragm
Stage III-1	With or without involvement of splenic, hilar, celiac, or portal nodes
Stage III-2	With involvement of para-aortic, iliac, and mesenteric nodes
Stage IV	Involvement of one or more extranodal sites in addition to a site for which the designation "E" has been used
	Designations applicable to any disease stage
A	No symptoms
B	Fever (temperature >38°C), drenching night sweats, unexplained loss of >10% of body weight within the preceding 6 months
X	Bulky disease (a widening of the mediastinum by more than 1/3 or the presence of a nodal mass with a maximal dimension >10 cm)
E	Involvement of a single extranodal site that is contiguous or proximal to the known nodal site
CS	Clinical stage
PS	Pathologic stage (as determined by laparotomy)

From Lister TA, Crowther D: Staging for Hodgkin's disease. Semin Oncol 1990;17:696-703. By permission of WB Saunders Company.

Table 11-6 Staging Procedures for Hodgkin Disease

History and examination: identification of B symptoms

Imaging procedures: plain chest radiography; computed tomography of thorax, abdomen, and pelvis; bipedal lymphangiography

Hematologic procedures: full blood cell count with differential, determination of erythrocyte sedimentation rate, and bilateral bone marrow aspiration and biopsy

Biochemical procedures: tests of liver function and measurement of serum albumin, lactate dehydrogenase, and calcium

Special procedures: laparotomy, ultrasonographic scanning, magnetic resonance imaging, gallium scanning, technetium bone scanning, and liver-spleen scanning

Staging laparotomies: are not performed

Modified from Lister TA, Crowther D: Staging for Hodgkin's disease. Semin Oncol 1990;17:696-703. By permission of WB Saunders Company.

autologous stem cell or bone marrow transplantation. In a study that compared autologous bone marrow transplantation with conventional chemotherapy for recurrent or refractory disease, the 3-year event-free survival was 53% for the transplantation group and 10% for the chemotherapy group.

Late complications of Hodgkin disease are substantial. The risks include infertility, amenorrhea, pneumococcal sepsis in 7% of patients following splenectomy, hypothyroidism, thyroid carcinoma, avascular necrosis, cardiomyopathy due to doxorubicin or radiotherapy, radiation pneumonitis, radiation-induced constrictive pericarditis, pulmonary fibrosis, and secondary malignancies. The secondary malignancies include acute non-lymphocytic leukemia, myelodysplastic syndromes, non-Hodgkin lymphoma, and solid tumors. ABVD is less leukemogenic than MOPP. Patients at highest risk are those who have received multiple courses of chemotherapy. The risk of non-Hodgkin lymphoma is 4% at 10 years. Radiotherapy increases the risk of solid tumors. After 15 years, the risk of secondary solid tumors is 13%; these tumors include malignancies of the stomach, breast, lung, thyroid, skin, and head and neck.

- Polymerase chain reaction detects Epstein-Barr virus in 60%-80% of cases of Hodgkin disease.
- Disease stage is the principal factor in selecting treatment for Hodgkin disease.
- Of patients who have relapse after radiotherapy, 66% are in long-term remission after chemotherapy.
- The treatment of choice for patients with pathologic stage IIB, IIIA2, IIIB, or IV disease: ABVD or Stanford V chemotherapy is administered two cycles beyond a complete remission.

- Autologous bone marrow or peripheral blood stem-cell transplantation is indicated after a first relapse from any front-line chemotherapy for Hodgkin disease.
- Complications of survival include acute nonlymphocytic leukemia, solid tumors, and cardiomyopathy.
- Typical clinical scenario: A patient has asymptomatic lymphadenopathy or mediastinal mass. Lymph node biopsy shows the presence of large binucleated or multinucleated cells with prominent nucleoli (Reed-Sternberg cells).

Non-Hodgkin Lymphoma

Non-Hodgkin lymphomas are clinically, pathologically, cytogenetically, and immunologically a diverse group of lymphoproliferative disorders. The prognosis depends on the histologic subtype, stage, and other clinical and laboratory features. The Working Formulation for Clinical Usage, which groups non-Hodgkin lymphomas by natural history and response to therapy, had been the most widely used scheme in the United States. This scheme was based on morphologic patterns only. These morphologic patterns have characteristically associated cytogenetic abnormalities and oncogene associations. The most recent classification is the WHO Classification of Neoplastic Diseases of the Hematopoietic and Lymphoid Tissues. This classification is an adaptation of the Revised European-American Lymphoma (REAL) classification; it subtracted some entities (follicular subsets and large-cell subsets), added some new entities (mantle cell, mucosa-associated lymphoid tissue [MALT], monocytoid B cell, and anaplastic large cell), and recognized peripheral T-cell non-Hodgkin lymphomas and new subsets (intestinal T cell) (Table 11-8).

The low-grade non-Hodgkin lymphomas, which include follicular histologic features, are a group of lymphoproliferative disorders that are not curable (unless pathologic stage I disease), are most commonly present with advanced stage III and IV disease, are very treatable with simple programs, occur in older patients, and have long survival (median, 8 years). The paradox of non-Hodgkin lymphomas is that low-grade non-Hodgkin lymphomas are not curable, but patients live for a long time even after disease relapse. In contrast, the intermediate and high-grade lymphomas are potentially curable, but the length of survival is short if the patient does not have remission. The disease may progress to a more aggressive lymphoma, with a risk that ranges from 10% to 70% in reported series, depending on the frequency of new biopsies at the time of progression, follow-up duration, and postmortem data.

Because low-grade non-Hodgkin lymphomas are not curable, the most reliable end points are progression-free survival and overall survival. Achievement of complete remission is not a viable end point in low-grade lymphomas. In patients who have been deemed to be in remission, immunoglobulin κ/λ light-chain restriction studies of peripheral blood and bone

Table 11-7 Suggested Initial Therapy of Hodgkin Disease Based on Clinical Stage of Disease

Stage	Treatment—no. of monthly cycles of chemotherapy and dose of radiotherapy (RT)
IA	
Limited high neck (0, 1 risk factor*)	Involved or extended field RT 20-24 Gy
Nonbulky	ABVD × 3 + involved field RT 20-24 Gy
Bulky mediastinal or >2 risk factors*	ABVD × 6-8 + involved field RT 24-30 Gy
IB	
Nonbulky and ≤2 risk factors*	ABVD × 6-8
Bulky mediastinal disease or >2 risk factors*	ABVD × 6-8 + involved field RT 24-30 Gy
IIA	
Nonbulky and ≤2 risk factors*	ABVD × 4-6: +/− involved field RT 20-24 Gy
Bulky mediastinal disease or >2 risk factors*	ABVD × 6-8 + involved field RT 24-30 Gy
IIB	
Nonbulky	ABVD × 6-8
Bulky mediastinal or other bulky disease plus extranodal disease or >2 risk factors*	ABVD × 6-8 + involved field RT 24-30 Gy
IIIA	ABVD × 6-8
IIIB	ABVD × 6-8
IVA	ABVD × 6-8
IVB	ABVD × 6-8

ABVD, doxorubin (Adriamycin), bleomycin, vinblastine, and DTIC.

*Risk factors: serum albumin <4 g/dL, hemoglobin <10.5 g/dL, male sex, age ≥45 years, stage IV, leukocyte count ≥15,000/μL, and lymphocytes <8% of total leukocyte count and/or <600 /μL (<0.6×10^9/L). (Hasenclever D, Diehl V for the International Prognostic Factors Project on Advanced Hodgkin's Disease. N Engl J Med 1998;339:1506-1514.)

From Habermann TM, Colgan JP: Hodgkin's disease. *In* Clinical Hematology and Oncology: Presentation, Diagnosis, and Treatment. Edited by Furie B, Cassileth PA, Atkins MB, et al. Philadelphia, Churchill Livingstone, 2003, pp 615-635. By permission of Elsevier.

marrow with flow cytometry demonstrate malignant cells in the peripheral blood after treatment, and polymerase chain reaction studies have demonstrated persistent abnormal cell populations in patients believed to be in complete remission.

Most patients with low-grade non-Hodgkin lymphoma have stage III or IV disease, which is not curable with standard treatment regimens. Observation is the initial treatment of choice for asymptomatic patients. The Stanford group reported on 83 patients with advanced disease who were not treated initially and had an actuarially predicted survival of 82% at 5 years and 73% at 10 years. At median follow-up of 50 months, 51 of the 83 patients (61%) required therapy at a median interval of 3 years from the time of diagnosis. Spontaneous regression was observed in 19 patients, partial remission in 13, and complete remission in 6. Treatment with more aggressive regimens has not improved survival.

For patients with symptoms, bulky disease, or progressive disease, options with the goal of achieving complete remission include oral chlorambucil taken daily, intravenous CVP (cyclophosphamide, vincristine, and prednisone), CVP with total lymphoid irradiation, or CHOP (cyclophosphamide, doxorubicin [hydroxydaunomycin], vincristine [Oncovin], and prednisone). CVP or chlorambucil is considered the standard treatment of choice. New treatments include fludarabine and the incorporation of interferon.

Anti-B-cell antibody therapies have been developed. Anti-CD20 antibody therapy, rituximab, has been approved for patients who have had relapse and is being evaluated as an initial treatment regimen. Anti-CD20 conjugated to yttrium 90 (Zevalin) and anti-CD22 conjugated to iodine-131 tositumomab produce high remission rates in patients with advanced follicular lymphoma who have had multiple relapses and are refractory to chemotherapy (Table 11-9).

Gastric MALT lymphomas have clonal gene rearrangements and are associated with *Helicobacter pylori* infections. This is the first malignant lymphoproliferative disorder to respond to an antimicrobial approach. Up to 70% of patients have a response to a regimen such as amoxicillin, metronidazole, and omeprazole. Subsequent treatment approaches include radiotherapy or oral chlorambucil.

Table 11-8 Classification of Tumors of Hematopoietic and Lymphoid Tissues

B-cell neoplasms	**T-cell and natural killer (NK)-cell neoplasms**
Precursor B-cell neoplasm	Precursor T-cell neoplasms
Precursor B lymphoblastic leukemia/lymphoma	Precursor T lymphoblastic leukemia/lymphoma
Mature B-cell neoplasms	Blastic NK-cell lymphoma
Chronic lymphocytic leukemia/small cell lymphocytic lymphoma	Mature T-cell and NK-cell neoplasms
B-cell prolymphocytic leukemia	T-cell prolymphocytic leukemia
Lymphoplasmacytic lymphoma	T-cell large granular lymphocytic leukemia
Splenic marginal zone lymphoma	Aggressive NK-cell leukemia
Hairy cell leukemia	Adult T-cell leukemia/lymphoma
Plasma cell myeloma	Extranodal NK/T-cell lymphoma, nasal type
Solitary plasmacytoma of bone	Enteropathy-type T-cell lymphoma
Extraosseous plasmacytoma	Hepatosplenic T-cell lymphoma
Extranodal marginal zone B-cell lymphoma of mucosa-associated lymphoid tissue (MALT-lymphoma)	Subcutaneous panniculitis-like T-cell lymphoma
	Mycosis fungoides
Nodal marginal zone B-cell lymphoma	Sézary syndrome
Follicular lymphoma	Primary cutaneous anaplastic large cell lymphoma
Mantle cell lymphoma	Peripheral T-cell lymphoma, unspecified
Diffuse large B-cell lymphoma	Angioimmunoblastic T-cell lymphoma
Mediastinal (thymic) large B-cell lymphoma	Anaplastic large cell lymphoma
Intravascular large B-cell lymphoma	T-cell proliferation of uncertain malignant potential
Primary effusion lymphoma	Lymphomatoid papulosis
Burkitt lymphoma/leukemia	**Hodgkin lymphoma**
B-cell proliferations of uncertain malignant potential	Nodular lymphocyte predominant Hodgkin lymphoma
Lymphomatoid granulomatosis	Classic Hodgkin lymphoma
Post-transplant lymphoproliferative disorder, polymorphic	Nodular sclerosis classic Hodgkin lymphoma
	Lymphocyte-rich classic Hodgkin lymphoma
	Mixed cellularity classic Hodgkin lymphoma
	Lymphocyte-depleted classic Hodgkin lymphoma

Modified from Jaffe ES, Harris NL, Stein H, et al (Eds): World Health Organization Classification of Tumours. Pathology and Genetics of Tumours of Haematopoietic and Lymphoid Tissues. Lyon, IARC Press, 2001, pp 120, 190, 238. By permission of the International Agency for Research on Cancer.

In patients with the histologic features of intermediate-grade non-Hodgkin lymphoma or diffuse large cell lymphoma, anthracycline chemotherapy (CHOP) regimens are the hallmark of therapy, with complete remission rates of 60% to 80% for stage II to IV disease and long-term disease-free survival as predicted by the International Prognostic Factor Index. Currently, trials are comparing standard treatment with the incorporation of autologous bone marrow transplantation as primary treatment. CHOP is the current reference standard of treatment for intermediate-grade non-Hodgkin lymphoma. In one study, CHOP with anti-CD20 was superior to CHOP alone. The long-term complete remission rates are 30% to 86%.

In nonrandomized studies of patients with relapsed disease who received high doses of chemotherapy with or without radiotherapy and autologous bone marrow transplantation, the overall cure rates have been reported to be 20%. For patients who had disease relapse after complete remission and who are sensitive to retreatment with standard chemotherapy regimens, the reported cure rates are 35% to 40%. An international study, the PARMA study, randomly assigned patients who were initially in complete remission but subsequently in first or second relapse to DHAP (cisplatin, cytosine arabinoside, and dexamethasone) chemotherapy or high-dose therapy, followed by autologous bone marrow transplantation. Autologous bone marrow transplantation increased the event-free and overall survival. Autologous bone marrow transplantation is considered the standard treatment for intermediate-grade and high-grade non-Hodgkin lymphoma in sensitive relapse. Currently, the role of autologous bone

Table 11-9 Treatment Strategies for Non-Hodgkin Lymphomas (NHL)

	Follicular NHL	Diffuse large B-cell NHL	Gastric MALToma *H. pylori*-positive
Initial treatment	Observation CVP	Rituxan/CHOP	Antibiotic therapy (triple therapy)
Treatment for first relapse	Anti-CD20 monoclonal antibody	Peripheral blood stem cell transplantation	Radiotherapy Oral chlorambucil

CHOP, cyclophosphamide, doxorubicin (hydroxydaunomycin), vincristine (Oncovin), prednisone; CVP, cyclophosphamide, vincristine, prednisone; MALT, mucosa-associated lymphoid tissue.

marrow transplantation as part of the initial management of non-Hodgkin lymphomas is being evaluated in randomized studies.

Prognostic factors are important in lymphoma. The International Prognostic Factor Index is based on clinical pretreatment characteristics and the relative risk of death. Clinical features that were associated with survival included age (≤60 vs. >60 years), LDH (normal or greater), performance status (0, 1 vs. 2-4), stage (I/II vs. III/IV), and extranodal involvement (≤1 site vs. >1 site). Patients were divided into different risk groups based on the number of risk factors, with predicted 5-year survivals in the low-risk group (with zero or one factor) of 73%; in the low-intermediate group (with two factors), 51%; in the high-intermediate group (with three factors), 43%; and in the high group (with four or five factors), 26%.

- Non-Hodgkin lymphomas are diverse.
- The WHO classification is now the most commonly used classification scheme.
- The Ann Arbor Staging System has traditionally been used for lymphoma.
- Currently, the most predictive pretreatment characteristics for the risk of death are age, LDH, performance status, stage, and extranodal involvement (the International Prognostic Factor Index).
- Exceptions to the standard management programs in non-Hodgkin lymphoma include MALT, primary bone, isolated gastric, central nervous system, testicular, bowel, orbital, pulmonary, and cutaneous T- and B-cell lymphomas.
- In most patients, low-grade lymphoma is not curable but survival time is long.
- Of patients with the histologic features of diffuse large cell advanced intermediate-grade non-Hodgkin lymphoma, 30%-40% are cured of disease with anthracycline regimens. CHOP chemotherapy had been the standard treatment of choice. However, CHOP plus anti-CD20 is superior to CHOP.

- Patients with HIV-related lymphoproliferative disorders with a CD4 count <200/mL have a poor response to standard treatment.
- Low-grade lymphomas may transform into intermediate-grade and high-grade lymphomas.
- Lymphoblastic lymphoma and Burkitt lymphoma have a higher risk of central nervous system involvement and tumor lysis syndrome.
- Death rates in non-Hodgkin lymphoma have increased since 1973.
- Typical clinical scenario for follicular lymphomas: a 65-year-old patient has asymptomatic cervical and axillary lymphadenopathy. Lymph node biopsy shows involvement with lymphoma, predominantly small cell, with relative preservation of follicular architecture. Bone marrow biopsy findings are also positive. In the absence of symptoms, observation is reasonable.
- Lymphomas are managed with different treatments (Table 11-9).
- Typical clinical scenario for diffuse large B-cell lymphoma: A patient with abdominal pain, fever, and weight loss is found to have bulky retroperitoneal adenopathy. A biopsy specimen demonstrates diffuse replacement of the lymph node with large lymphoma cells. The usual treatment is staging evaluation, followed by chemotherapy such as CHOP.

Monoclonal Gammopathies

The differential diagnosis of monoclonal gammopathies includes monoclonal gammopathies of undetermined significance (MGUS) and malignant monoclonal gammopathies. The malignant gammopathies include multiple myeloma (IgG, IgA, IgD, IgE, and free light chains), overt multiple myeloma, smoldering multiple myeloma, plasma cell leukemia, nonsecretory myeloma, osteosclerotic myeloma, plasmacytoma (solitary plasmacytoma of bone, extramedullary plasmacytoma), malignant lymphoproliferative diseases (Waldenström [primary] macroglobulinemia, malignant lymphoma), heavy chain diseases, and amyloidosis (primary, with myeloma).

Monoclonal Gammopathies of Undetermined Significance

In MGUS, the monoclonal (M)-protein level is less than 3 g/dL in the serum and there are fewer than 10% plasma cells in the bone marrow. The serum level of creatinine is normal, and the urine has either a small amount of or no M protein. The serum level of calcium is normal. No anemia and no osteolytic bone lesions are present. MGUS may be a precursor to multiple myeloma. Twenty-three percent of patients may have progression to a malignant monoclonal gammopathy. Population-based studies have demonstrated that 1% of adults older than 50 years and 3% of those older than 70 have an M protein in the serum. Of monoclonal gammopathies, 60% are IgG, 20% are IgM, 10% are IgA, and 7% are free light chains. In most patients, serum protein electrophoresis should be repeated initially at 6 months and then at 12-month intervals indefinitely if there is no progression or symptoms. Patients with MGUS should be observed. Unnecessary treatment can lead to development of a myelodysplastic syndrome or acute leukemia. Annually, approximately 1% of cases of MGUS progress to multiple myeloma or a related lymphoproliferative disorder.

- MGUS is the most common dysproteinemia.
- M protein is ≤3 g/dL; <10% plasma cells in the bone marrow; normal concentrations of hemoglobin, creatinine, and calcium.
- Asymptomatic.
- Stable M-protein measurements.
- Patients are safely observed, with no chemotherapy.
- Typical clinical scenario: A patient without symptoms has a serum M spike <3 g/dL and bone marrow plasma cells <10%. The CBC, serum creatinine level, and bone radiographs are normal. Observe, with no therapy.

Multiple Myeloma

Multiple myeloma is a result of the insidious accumulation in the marrow of neoplastic plasma cells that produce homogeneous immunoglobulin in the serum (85%) or in the urine (or in both); it accounts for 1% of all malignancies. Osteoclast-activating activity due to exaggerated expression of specific cytokine results in osteolytic bone lesions. Interleukin-6 may be involved in the pathogenesis of myeloma. The median age at onset of multiple myeloma is 65 years. It is more common in males and African Americans. Ten percent or more plasma cells are found in the bone marrow (Plate 11-12). At least one of the following must be present: M protein in the serum greater than 3 g/dL (in 80% of patients), M protein in the urine (light chain only in 20%), anemia, hypercalcemia, renal failure, or osteolytic bone lesions. M protein is detected in the serum or urine of 98% of patients.

Clinical features include weakness, fatigue, bone pain (66% of patients), anemia (initially about 66%, eventually all), renal insufficiency (50%), hypercalcemia (20%), and spinal cord compression (5%). Back and chest pain is characteristically exacerbated by movement. Patients are at higher risk for infections with encapsulated gram-positive organisms such as *Streptococcus pneumoniae*. The incidence of gram-negative infections and herpes zoster is also increased. The CBC findings are similar to those of normochromic normocytic anemia. Radiographs show punched-out lytic lesions, osteoporosis, and fractures in 75% of patients at diagnosis. Bone scans are rarely helpful. MRI may be helpful if plain radiographs do not show abnormality, especially spine lesions.

The median survival has been about 3 years. This may be improving with peripheral blood stem cell transplantation and newer treatment regimens. A beta$_2$-microglobulin level greater than 2.7 mg/mL and a bone marrow plasma cell labeling index of 0.8% or greater are adverse prognostic factors. If these values are low, the median survival is 6 years. Patients with smoldering myeloma (M protein >3 g/dL, more than 10% plasma cells in the bone marrow, no lytic bone lesions, and no other manifestations of myeloma) should be observed.

Because multiple myeloma is not curable, treatment may be delayed until evidence of disease progression develops, the patient becomes symptomatic, or treatment is necessary to prevent imminent complications. Two randomized trials have demonstrated that patients with anemia or small osteolytic lesions may be observed. The median overall survival for patients with multiple myeloma is about 36 months. The standard treatment for patients older than 70 years, poor performance status, pronounced renal failure, or other comorbid conditions is melphalan and prednisone given for 7 days every 6 weeks; the objective response rate is 50% to 60%; the median survival is 3 years. Palliative radiotherapy at a dose of 20 to 30 Gy is effective in the management of disabling focal pain unresponsive to analgesic therapy.

Autologous peripheral stem cell transplantation is the initial treatment of choice. Before an autologous peripheral stem cell harvest, treatment with high-dose dexamethasone alone or in combination with thalidomide is effective in the management of patients younger than 70 years; it does not have the toxic effects that melphalan has on stem cells. VAD (vincristine, doxorubicin [Adriamycin], and dexamethasone) is an alternative to melphalan and prednisone. The overall response rate to thalidomide is about 32%. Side effects include sedation, fatigue, constipation, and peripheral neuropathy. High-dose dexamethasone produces a response rate of 45% and does not cause stem cell damage. High-dose therapy followed by an autologous stem cell transplantation improves the response rate and survival in patients with multiple myeloma, but it is not curable. The overall response rates are 75% to 90%, and the complete response rate is 20% to 40%. Most patients have disease relapse. Oral thalidomide is effective in treating a relapse of multiple myeloma. Studies have demonstrated that interferon alfa-2a or 2b recombinant is capable of prolonging the duration of remission, in comparison with no maintenance therapy, but overall survival differences have not been demonstrated. Anemia responds to erythropoietin in 50% of patients. Bisphosphonate therapy, such as pamidronate and zoledronic acid, delays the onset of skeletal-related events, reduces bone pain, and modestly extends survival. The proteozome inhibitor bortezomib (PS-341) is effective in pretreated patients with relapsed disease or refractory multiple myeloma patients.

Renal failure may be caused by hypercalcemia, dehydration, and light chain nephropathy (myeloma kidney). Cast nephropathy may respond to plasmapheresis.

- Plasma cells: <10% in MGUS and >10% in myeloma.
- Serum M protein: <3 g/dL in MGUS and usually >3 g/dL in myeloma.
- Multiple myeloma: usually has a urine M protein.
- Myeloma: bone pain (66% of patients), renal dysfunction (50%), hypercalcemia (30%), spinal cord compression (5%).
- Myeloma: punched-out lytic bone lesions, pneumococcal infection.
- Multiple myeloma patients are at increased risk for infections due to encapsulated organisms, including *Streptococcus pneumoniae*.
- Patients with low-risk disease, including a plasma cell labelling index of ≤0.8% or beta₂-microglobulin of ≤2.7 mg/mL, have longer overall survival.
- The principal organisms causing infection are *Streptococcus pneumoniae* and *Haemophilus influenzae*. Vaccination is recommended.
- Typical case scenario: A patient presents with back and bone pain that is exacerbated by movement. The patient is discovered to have anemia with or without renal insufficiency and hypercalcemia. A bone survey shows lytic bone lesions, and serum and urine protein electrophoresis demonstrate M protein. Bone marrow biopsy specimens contain >10% plasma cells. Recombinant erythropoietin may improve the anemia.

Solitary Plasmacytomas

Solitary plasmacytomas may occur without other evidence of multiple myeloma. These extramedullary lesions are potentially curable with irradiation.

- Severe back pain may be a manifestation of spinal cord compression, requiring immediate MRI or CT, dexamethasone treatment, irradiation, and possible surgical decompression.

Waldenström Macroglobulinemia

Waldenström macroglobulinemia is characterized by an increase in the IgM paraprotein usually greater than 3.0 g/dL, lymphadenopathy, anemia, or hepatosplenomegaly. Retinal "sausage" formation may be present. The bone marrow is populated with well-differentiated plasmacytoid lymphocytes. Bence Jones proteinuria may be present in 80% of patients, and hyperviscosity syndrome occurs in 15%. Other features include cryoglobulinemia, sensorimotor peripheral neuropathy, cold agglutinin hemolytic anemia, and renal disease (nephrotic syndrome).

Many patients have only an IgM MGUS, with no signs or symptoms, and should be observed without initial treatment.

Hyperviscosity syndrome is characterized by fatigue, dizziness, blurred vision, bleeding from mucous membranes, sausage-shaped retinal veins, and papilledema. The plasma volume is expanded, with an increase in serum viscosity. Because 80% of IgM is intravascular, the initial treatment of choice is plasmapheresis with albumin and saline replacement, followed by chemotherapy. This disorder has been treated most commonly with chlorambucil (6-8 mg daily) and prednisone (40 mg/m² for 10 days at 6-week intervals); 60% of patients have a response, with a median survival of 5 years. The treatment of choice is 2-chlorodeoxyadenosine. For patients who have not had a response to this agent, an alternative treatment is chlorambucil and prednisone. Fludarabine is also being evaluated for newly diagnosed disease. Anti-CD20 monoclonal antibody therapy is effective for relapsed disease. Transfusion with packed RBCs should not be given solely on the basis of the hemoglobin concentration, because the increased plasma volume produces spuriously low values.

- IgM paraprotein >3.0 g/dL.
- Hyperviscosity syndrome.
- Treatment of choice is chlorambucil, 2-chlorodeoxyadenosine, or fludarabine.
- Typical clinical scenario: A 65-year-old patient has fatigue, bleeding from oral and nasal areas, and visual and neurologic symptoms. Serum protein electrophoresis demonstrates an IgM M protein, and bone biopsy shows a lymphoplasmacytic infiltration.

Amyloidosis

Amyloidosis is a group of diseases with extracellular deposition of pathologic insoluble fibrillar proteins, which stain with Congo red, in organs and tissues. The amyloid fibrils in primary amyloidosis are fragments of the variable portions of the immunoglobulin light chains. Patients with amyloidosis present with fatigue, weight loss, hepatomegaly, macroglossia, renal insufficiency, proteinuria, nephrotic syndrome, congestive heart failure, orthostatic hypotension, carpal tunnel syndrome, and peripheral neuropathy. Amyloidosis is classified as primary (light-chain related; 90% of patients in the United States), secondary (chronic infections, autoimmune disease), familial (associated with positive transthyretin) (prealbumin stain), associated with aging (senile), localized (skin, bladder, other organs), and dialysis (associated with beta$_2$-microglobulin). Most commonly, patients with primary amyloidosis have kidney involvement, followed by congestive heart failure due to an infiltrative cardiomyopathy (25% of patients), carpal tunnel syndrome (20% of patients), peripheral neuropathy, and orthostatic hypotension.

Generally, the diagnosis of primary amyloidosis is first established by finding M protein in the serum or urine. The bone marrow usually has less than 20% plasma cells, and there are no lytic bone lesions. Initial biopsies should include fat aspiration of the abdominal wall (80% positive), rectum (75%), or bone marrow (56%). Nearly 90% of patients with primary systemic amyloidosis have a detectable M protein in the serum or urine, which is lambda in two-thirds of patients. This is the most important screening test when the diagnosis is expected. The bone marrow usually has plasma cells that have a clonal predominance of a light chain isotype. Four of 10 patients present with nephrotic syndrome, 1 in 6 with right-sided congestive heart failure that worsens with calcium channel blockers, and about 1 in 7 with a sensorimotor peripheral neuropathy. Unexplained hypercholesterolemia may be a manifestation of the nephrotic syndrome. The electrocardiogram may show low voltage or a pattern consistent with myocardial infarction. The echocardiogram is abnormal in 60% of patients with concentrically thickened ventricles. The neuropathy is progressive, painful, symmetrical, and demyelinating. Peripheral neuropathy is often associated with autonomic failure, as manifested by diarrhea, pseudo-obstruction, or orthostatic syncope. About 50% of patients with amyloid neuropathy have carpal tunnel syndrome. Other symptoms and signs include fatigue, weight loss, change in voice, macroglossia, submandibular swelling, and post-proctoscopic purpura. Acquired inhibitors for thrombin and factor X deficiency may occur.

The median survival for all patients with primary amyloidosis is 13 months; for those with overt congestive heart failure, less than 6 months; with nephrotic syndrome, 27 months; and with peripheral neuropathy, 42 months.

Oral chemotherapy produces superior results compared with colchicine. Treatment with melphalan and prednisone is effective. Treatment with 4′-iodo-4′-deoxyrubicin (IDOX), which binds to amyloid fibrils, is being studied. Treatment with high-dose intravenous melphalan with autologous blood stem cell support results in remission of both the plasma cell dyscrasia and clinical signs and symptoms in 50% to 65% of patients treated; this treatment is being studied.

Patients with amyloidosis are unusually sensitive to digitalis. In congestive heart failure, salt restriction and diuretics are the mainstay of treatment.

The pathologic characteristics are as follows: primary amyloidosis consists of the variable region of immunoglobulin light chains; secondary amyloidosis consists of protein A.

- Typical clinical scenario: A 64-year-old man with weakness, weight loss, congestive heart failure, carpal tunnel syndrome, peripheral neuropathy, and orthostatic hypotension has a λ light chain M spike detected on serum electrophoresis.

Acute Leukemias

The cause of acute leukemia is unknown in most cases, but there are many associations: idiopathic aplastic anemia, paroxysmal nocturnal hemoglobinuria, myeloproliferative disorders, myelodysplastic syndromes, radiation, benzene, chemotherapy (alkylating agents, topoisomerase II inhibitors [etoposide]), Down syndrome, Fanconi syndrome, and ataxia-telangiectasia. The classic syndrome of patients who have been exposed to alkylating agents (melphalan, cyclophosphamide, chlorambucil) is pancytopenia in 10 to 36 months, with the chromosome abnormalities of monosomy 5 and 7. This condition is refractory to standard treatment regimens.

- Alkylating agents should be prescribed only for benign diseases, with consideration of the risk of development of acute myelogenous leukemia, non-Hodgkin lymphoma, bladder cancer, and other solid tumors.
- Recently described secondary leukemias are related to topoisomerase II inhibitor agents (etoposide).

Acute Nonlymphocytic Leukemia (Acute Myelogenous Leukemia)

The median age of patients with acute nonlymphocytic leukemia (Plate 11-13) is 65 years. Fifty percent of patients have symptoms for more than 3 months. Good prognostic signs include age younger than 40 years; chromosome abnormalities of t(8;21), t(15;17), inversion 16, or normal chromosomes; and achieving complete remission with one cycle of induction chemotherapy. Poor prognostic signs include age older than 40 years; preleukemic phase; chromosome abnormalities of monosomy 5, monosomy 7, trisomy 8, 11q−, and complex cytogenetic patterns; and poor general physical condition or underlying health problems.

For patients who present with extreme leukocytosis (WBC >100×10^9/L) with acute leukemia, the initial complication of most concern is cerebral hemorrhage. Emergency treatment includes hydration, alkalinization of urine, allopurinol (600 mg), hydroxyurea (6-8 g orally), cranial irradiation (4-6 Gy), and leukapheresis, followed by the treatment of the specific type of leukemia.

- Acute nonlymphocytic leukemia: median age of patients is 65 years; 50% have symptoms >3 months.
- Good prognosis: patients <40 years old; chromosomal abnormalities t(8;21), t(15;17), inv 16, or normal chromosomes; and achieving complete remission with one cycle of induction chemotherapy.
- Typical clinical scenario for acute leukemia: A 40-year-old patient has fever, sore throat, bleeding gums (thrombocytopenia), and anemia. The WBC count is 50×10^9/L. A peripheral blood smear shows numerous immature WBC precursors ("blasts"). Differentiation between acute myelogenous and acute lymphoblastic leukemia requires evaluation of bone marrow biopsy specimens with special stains and immunophenotyping.
- Typical clinical scenario for acute promyelocytic leukemia (M3): A patient who has acute leukemia presents with disseminated intravascular coagulation. Cytogenetics show t(15;17) translocation.
- Typical clinical scenario for secondary acute myelogenous leukemia: Cytopenias are demonstrated in a patient who has received chemotherapeutic agents for a previous malignancy. Cytogenetic studies show monosomy 5 or 7.

Therapeutic interventions include the following: platelet and RBC transfusions are required throughout the course of treatment. Early empiric broad-spectrum antibiotic coverage for fever is essential.

Induction chemotherapy includes cytarabine (cytosine arabinoside) and an anthracycline agent (daunorubicin or idarubicin). The complete remission rate is about 65% for patients 60 years or younger and 35% to 50% for those older than 60 years, with the potential for cure in 20% of patients. Despite substantial recent advances, most patients with acute myelogenous leukemia eventually have relapse, and most have it within 1 year. Of patients who have relapse after induction and consolidation therapy, 30% to 50% achieve a second remission. Remission rates have been reported to be higher with idarubicin.

All-*trans*-retinoic acid (ATRA) is the treatment of choice in M3 acute promyelocytic leukemia (promyelocytic acute nonlymphocytic leukemia) (Plate 11-14) with a t(5;17) translocation. These patients then need to be treated with cytarabine or a daunorubicin-type program. This is the first malignancy in which a chromosomal alteration has served as the target for induction chemotherapy. ATRA improves the overall survival and treatment at induction, and maintenance therapy may be superior. Arsenic trioxide (Trisenox) has now been approved by the U.S. Food and Drug Administration as second-line

treatment for acute promyelocytic leukemia. Gemtuzumab (Mylotarg), an anti-CD33 antibody, was approved recently for the treatment of CD33+ acute nonlymphocytic leukemia in patients older than 60 years experiencing a first relapse.

The three types of postremission therapy are maintenance, consolidation, and intensification. Maintenance therapy uses low doses of chemotherapy, which avoids severe bone marrow suppression. Consolidation therapy uses regimens similar to those used for induction therapy. Intensification therapy uses more intensive therapy than that used during remission induction. Postremission therapy includes chemotherapy and autologous or allogeneic transplantation. Low-dose combination cytarabine and 6-thioguanine are superior to no additional treatment in prolonging disease-free survival after complete remission has been achieved. High-dose cytarabine improves the duration of remission in patients younger than 60 years, as compared with conventional-dose cytarabine with or without 6-thioguanine.

The following generalizations may be made about allogeneic bone marrow transplantation in acute nonlymphocytic leukemia. Generally, after 2 years of complete remission, the risk of relapse is lower. Transplantation in cases of relapse is age-dependent: patients younger than 30 years have a better prognosis than those 30 or older. Allogeneic bone marrow transplantation in early relapse or in second remission is almost as efficacious as transplantation during the first complete remission. If the patient is younger than 55 years, bone marrow transplantation should be considered for those in first remission if they have an HLA match and poor prognostic factors, which include poor-risk cytogenetic features and antecedent hematologic disease. For patients without poor risk factors and not part of a formal study, transplantation should be considered in early relapse or second remission. Currently, the disease-free survival at 5 years for patients having allogeneic transplantation during the first remission is 50%; during the first relapse, 30%; and during the second remission, 28%. Early results of autologous transplantation are encouraging. Chemotherapy treatment and autologous transplantation are equivalent.

Acute Lymphoblastic Leukemia

Acute lymphoblastic leukemia (Plate 11-15) is most common in children; complete remission rates are greater than 90%, and 60% to 70% of patients have long-term disease-free survival. In adults, this leukemia is less common, with remission rates of up to 75%; however, most patients have disease relapse. Of adult acute lymphocytic leukemia, 80% of cases are B cell in origin, 20% have T-cell markers, and 1% or 2% express surface immunoglobulin. Most B-cell leukemias express CD10, the common ALL antigen (cALLa). Patients with early pre-B-acute lymphocytic leukemia, also called "null acute lymphocytic leukemia," are cALLa negative.

One-third of patients present with bleeding, and 25% have symptoms for more than 3 months. Bone pain, lymphadenopathy, splenomegaly, and hepatomegaly are more common in acute lymphoblastic leukemia than in acute non-lymphocytic leukemia. Splenomegaly, lymphadenopathy, and hepatomegaly occur in three-fourths of the patients (compared with one-half of those with acute myelogenous leukemia).

The best prognosis is for children 3 to 10 years old. After the age of 20, survival time continues to decrease with increasing age and the duration of complete remissions is shorter. Poor prognostic factors include age, WBC count greater than 30×10^9/L, null cell phenotype, specific chromosome abnormalities, and achievement of remission after more than 4 weeks of intensive chemotherapy.

From 80% to 90% of adults have chromosome abnormalities. Those with normal chromosomes have the best prognosis. The poorest prognosis is associated with t(9;22); t(4;11); t(8;14); and t(1;19). These patients have lower complete remission rates, shorter duration of remission, and very poor survival. Also, t(9;22) has less than 15% survival at 5 years and is present in 25% of adults but in only 2% to 3% of children. Chromosome abnormalities are independent of age, WBC count, and immunophenotype.

The three agents commonly used in induction therapy include vincristine, prednisone, and anthracyclines in combination with one or more of the following: L-asparaginase, cytarabine, methotrexate, or cyclophosphamide. The complete remission rate is 70% to 90%. The addition of L-asparaginase, cytarabine, or cyclophosphamide may improve the duration of remission.

Intensification/postinduction therapy is commonly used. The long-term relapse-free survival in adults is 10% to 42%. The use of allogeneic bone marrow transplantation in the first complete remission results in a 21% to 71% disease-free survival at 2 to 10 years, with relapse rates of 10% to 40%. Allogeneic transplantation is recommended for patients with t(9;22) and t(4;11). Trials are under way for evaluating autologous bone marrow transplants and matched unrelated transplants.

In relapse, allogeneic or autologous bone marrow transplants are of benefit in patients who achieve a second complete remission. After a second complete remission and then an allogeneic transplant, the disease-free survival ranges from 26% to 54% at various times. At second complete remission and then autologous transplant, the disease-free survival ranges from 23% to 31% for various times.

Recent results of unrelated allogeneic donor transplants have shown a 45% leukemia-free survival for patients in the first remission, but there are significant logistical and age restrictions. Trials are under way to evaluate autologous transplantation. Indications for bone marrow transplantation include high-risk cytogenetic abnormalities in the first remission and patients in a second or subsequent remission.

In a study that compared bone marrow and peripheral blood allogeneic transplantation in acute leukemia, myelodysplasia, and chronic myeloid leukemia, the use of peripheral blood led to faster hematologic recovery and improved survival.

Chronic Myeloid Disorders
Myelodysplastic Syndromes

Chronic myeloid disorders include myelodysplastic syndromes, chronic myeloid leukemia, chronic myeloproliferative disease, and atypical myeloproliferative disorders.

Myelodysplastic disorders are characterized by dysplastic bone marrow hyperplasia associated with various degrees of peripheral blood cytopenias with or without chromosome changes. They are typically heterogeneous and biologically diverse. Myelodysplastic syndromes, as classified by the French-American-British Group (with median survival time), are refractory anemia (26 months), refractory anemia with ringed sideroblasts (34 months), refractory anemia with excess blasts (9 months), refractory anemia with excess blasts in transformation (5 months), and chronic myelomonocytic leukemia (12 months). These disorders present with anemia and other cytopenias. The course of the disease is complicated by hemorrhage in 20% of patients and infection in 40%. Clonal karyotypic abnormalities have been reported in 30% to 70% of patients, predominantly deletions, as compared with acute myelogenous leukemia, which has balanced translocations. Del(5q), del(20q), and −y are the only abnormalities that confer a favorable prognosis, and these patients frequently present with anemia that requires transfusions. The most life-threatening complication is transformation to acute leukemia. This occurs in 12% of patients with refractory anemia, in 8% with refractory anemia with ringed sideroblasts, in 44% with refractory anemia with excess blasts, in 14% with chronic myelomonocytic leukemia, and in 60% with refractory anemia with excess blasts in transition. A large proportion of patients die of cytopenic complications, most commonly leukopenia.

The standard of care for most patients is supportive, with RBC transfusions, erythropoietin, and antibiotics for infection. Patients younger than 55 years should be considered for allogeneic bone marrow transplantation if the patient has an HLA match. Antileukemic chemotherapy regimens have a complete remission rate of 47% to 66%, with disease-free survival of 30% to 45%. New treatment approaches include 5-azacytidine, antithymocyte globulin, and amifostine. Granulocyte-colony stimulating factor (G-CSF) increases the absolute neutrophil count in 90% of patients.

Chronic Myelogenous Leukemia (Chronic Granulocytic Leukemia)

Chronic myelogenous leukemia constitutes 20% of all leukemias and is characterized by an acquired defect of clonal origin at the pluripotential cell level. There is a pool of granulocyte precursors with the capacity for normal maturation (Plate 11-16). The Philadelphia chromosome, t(9;22), is the hallmark of this disease in 95% of patients and is identified with karyotypic or fluorescent in situ hybridization or polymerase chain reaction of peripheral blood or bone marrow specimens. The translocation results in the fused *bcr-abl* oncogene. The hyperproliferation of the *bcr-abl* clone results in production of an upregulated tyrosine kinase enzyme. The myeloid compartment is expanded and normal hematopoiesis is suppressed. New chromosomal abnormalities appear and reappear. The diseases are preleukemic and terminate in a maturation block or blast crisis. Different cell types can be seen, including myeloblasts (50%-60% of patients), megakaryoblasts (15%), B lymphoblasts, erythroblasts (10%), monoblasts, myelomonocytic blasts, and basophilic blasts.

Before the advent of allogeneic bone marrow transplantation and interferon alfa-2a or 2b recombinant, the median survival was 3.5 years after diagnosis. Prognostic factors are different in multiple series. In one study, a good prognosis (61-month median survival vs. 34 months) was associated with a spleen size of 0 to 6 cm and 0% to 10% circulating blasts. A poor prognosis was associated with an age older than 45 years and a platelet count greater than 700×10^9/L. The presence of chromosome abnormalities other than t(9;22) is an adverse prognostic factor. The chronic phase is characterized by fewer than 10% blasts in blood and bone marrow and typically has a median duration of 4 years.

Symptoms include malaise, dyspnea, anorexia, fever, night sweats, weight loss, abdominal fullness, easy bruising, bleeding, gout, priapism, and hypermetabolism. Splenomegaly is present in 85% of patients.

Characteristic laboratory findings include leukocytosis, with fewer than 10% blasts in the chronic phase of the disease, and WBC counts of 100×10^9/L are common. Granulocytes in all stages of maturation are present on peripheral blood smear, with basophilia and eosinophilia and a characteristic myelocyte bulge. The number of platelets is increased, with large bizarre forms found in peripheral blood smears. The hemoglobin concentration ranges from 9 to 12 g/dL. The leukocyte alkaline phosphatase score is low or zero. The differential diagnosis of a low or zero leukocyte alkaline phosphatase score also includes paroxysmal nocturnal hemoglobinuria, infectious mononucleosis, and aplastic anemia. The vitamin B_{12} level is increased because of increased transcobalamin I. Other findings include pseudohyperkalemia, pseudohypoglycemia, and false-positive increase in acid phosphatase in the serum. The bone marrow is hyperplastic, with myelofibrosis in 10% to 40% of patients.

- Chronic myelogenous leukemia: acquired defect of clonal origin.

- Philadelphia chromosome, t(9;22), is the hallmark of the disease.
- Increased WBC count; granulocytes in all stages of maturation.
- Bone marrow shows hyperplasia; myelofibrosis in 10%-40% of patients.
- The leukocyte alkaline phosphatase score is low or zero in chronic myelogenous leukemia, paroxysmal nocturnal hemoglobinuria, infectious mononucleosis, and aplastic anemia.
- Increased vitamin B_{12}; increased acid phosphatase.
- Typical clinical scenario: A patient without symptoms presents with a high WBC count, myeloid bulge, basophilia, and splenomegaly. Cytogenetic studies show a t(9;22) translocation.

There is little evidence that any patient has been cured with conventional therapy. The initial treatment of chronic myelogenous leukemia includes hydroxyurea, interferon alfa, allogeneic bone marrow transplantation, autologous bone marrow transplantation, and imatinib mesylate (STI-571 [Gleevec]).

Hydroxyurea has been used more commonly, with response rates of 85% to 90%. One study demonstrated that both overall and post-transplant survival are inferior for patients treated with busulfan compared with those given hydroxyurea. Hydroxyurea is the treatment of choice for high blast counts and leukostasis lesions, and it is safe in thrombocytopenia. Continued maintenance therapy is necessary. Megaloblastic RBCs appear in the peripheral blood. Hydroxyurea should be considered for patients who are candidates for bone marrow transplantation.

Recombinant interferon alfa-2a or 2b suppresses the Philadelphia chromosome. Hematologic responses are 40% to 80%, with cytogenetic remissions in the range of 10% to 40%. Prospective randomized trials have demonstrated an improvement in survival and duration of remission in patients treated with interferon alfa-2a or 2b recombinant, in comparison with hydroxyurea. The addition of cytarabine to interferon reportedly improves survival and cytogenetic responses.

Imatinib is an oral agent that inhibits the *bcr-abl* protein product. Preliminary studies demonstrated high remission rates for those who have had disease relapse after treatment with oral interferon, for accelerated phase disease, and in untreated patients. This is the standard first-line therapy for chronic myelogenous leukemia. In a randomized trial that compared interferon and cytarabine versus imatinib (STI-571), there were higher hematologic response rates for imatinib. In addition, the cytogenetic response rates were superior (76% vs. 12%).

The treatment of "blast crisis" includes allopurinol, fluids, hydroxyurea, cranial irradiation, and leukocyte apheresis.

- Accelerated phase at 30-36 months; the chronic phase converts to an accelerated or blast phase (75% of patients), which is characterized by blast counts >20%; increase in anemia, thrombocytopenia, basophilia, and leukocyte alkaline phosphatase score; splenomegaly; lymphadenopathy; bone pain; cerebral hemorrhage; fever; headache; and myelofibrosis. Cytogenetic abnormalities precede the condition by 6 months.
- Blast transformation occurs in 13% of patients in the first 2 years, and the annual risk is then 25%.
- Imatinib (STI-571) is the treatment of choice.

Currently, the only curative regimen is high-dose chemotherapy with total body irradiation, followed by transplantation of allogeneic bone marrow from HLA-compatible siblings. Allogeneic bone marrow transplantation should be performed in the chronic phase, preferably within the first 12 months in young patients who have an HLA-identical match or an identical twin. Hematologic relapse occurs in 10% to 20% of patients receiving a transplant in the chronic phase. The long-term disease-free survival rates approach 80% if the patient has favorable factors (age <30 years, related donor, HLA-identical match) and transplant occurs less than 1 year after diagnosis. Otherwise, long-term survival may be less than 30%.

- Currently, the only curative regimen is HLA-compatible allogeneic bone marrow transplantation.

Because only 15% of all new cases of chronic myelogenous leukemia have an HLA sibling donor, studies are evaluating HLA-matched unrelated volunteer donor bone marrow transplantation protocols and autologous bone marrow transplantation. Autologous bone marrow transplantation can improve survival, but there is no evidence of cure.

- Typical clinical scenario: A 45-year-old woman presents with anemia and leukocytosis. The spleen is palpable 3 cm below the costal margin. The leukocyte differential count demonstrates basophilia, myelocytes, and metamyelocytes. The blast count is not increased. The treatment of choice is imatinib.

Myeloproliferative Disorders

Myeloproliferative disorders include polycythemia rubra vera, agnogenic myeloid metaplasia, essential thrombocythemia, and chronic granulocytic leukemia. These are clonal processes with a multipotent stem cell origin that are characterized clinically by peripheral blood and bone marrow proliferation. Their characteristic features are listed in Table 11-10. These disorders are interrelated: polycythemia rubra vera converts to agnogenic myeloid metaplasia in 10% of patients, and essential thrombocythemia converts to agnogenic myeloid metaplasia in 5%. Acute myelogenous leukemia is a complication of polycythemia rubra vera (10% of patients), essential thrombocythemia (<5%), agnogenic myeloid metaplasia (10%-20%), and chronic myelogenous leukemia (70%-90%). In each of these disorders, overall survival is less than that of age-matched controls. There is also a risk of thrombosis and hemorrhagic complications, especially in polycythemia rubra vera and essential thrombocythemia.

- Myeloproliferative disorders include polycythemia rubra vera, agnogenic myeloid metaplasia, essential thrombocythemia, and chronic granulocytic leukemia.
- Myeloproliferative disorders are interrelated.

Myelofibrosis With Myeloid Metaplasia, Agnogenic Myeloid Metaplasia, Post-Polycythemic and Post-Thrombocytic Myeloid Metaplasia

Splenomegaly occurs in 100% of the patients and is the hallmark of agnogenic myeloid metaplasia. Other features are a leukoerythroblastic peripheral blood smear (96% of patients), dacrocytes (teardrop cells), and hypocellular marrow (85% of patients) (Plate 11-17). The basic event is the fibroblastic proliferation in bone marrow. Anemia may be caused by expanded plasma volume, ineffective erythropoiesis, blood loss, or hemolysis.

The bone marrow shows panhyperplasia with modest fibrosis to osteosclerosis. The spleen is characterized by extramedullary hematopoiesis in the sinusoids of red pulp. Hepatomegaly may occur in 70% of patients because of engorgement by blood, extramedullary hematopoiesis, or hemosiderosis.

- The median survival approaches 5 years.
- Agnogenic myeloid metaplasia: its hallmark is splenomegaly.
- Leukoerythroblastic peripheral blood smear in 96% of patients.
- Teardrop cells.
- Basic event: fibroblastic proliferation of bone marrow.

Twenty percent of patients are asymptomatic and should be observed; 80% are still asymptomatic at 5 years. Medical therapy for anemia with symptoms includes transfusion with packed RBCs if the RBC mass is low. Androgens (fluoxymesterone, 50 mg twice daily, or danazol) and prednisone 30 mg daily improve anemia in one-third to one-half of patients. Corticosteroids may be of benefit in one-third of patients with hemolysis or thrombocytopenia. In the evaluation of anemia, check stool for occult blood loss from esophageal varices and microinfarcts of the gut and treat vitamin B_{12} and folate deficiency if indicated.

Table 11-10 Characteristic Features of Chronic Myeloproliferative Disorders

Characteristic	Polycythemia rubra vera	Agnogenic myeloid metaplasia	Primary thrombocythemia	Chronic granulocytic leukemia
Increased red cell mass	Yes	No	No	No
Myelofibrosis	Later	Yes	Rare	Later
Thrombocytosis	Variable	Variable	Yes	Variable
bcr-abl Oncogene	No	No	No	Yes

From Petitt RM, Silverstein MN: Current clinical management of primary thrombocythemia. Contemp Intern Med Jan 1991, pp 46-52. By permission of Aegean Communications.

Pressure symptoms occur in 23% of patients and may be managed with hydroxyurea or splenic irradiation. Hydroxyurea is indicated for symptomatic hepatosplenomegaly, leukocytosis, and thrombocytosis.

Bleeding with or without thrombocytopenia is managed with platelet transfusions.

Treat disseminated intravascular coagulopathy appropriately if present (may be present in up to 40% of patients).

Splenectomy may be of benefit in major hemolysis, pressure symptoms, life-threatening thrombocytopenia, portal hypertension, and refractory thrombocytopenia. Splenectomy is contraindicated in disseminated intravascular coagulopathy.

Bone marrow transplantation may be helpful in some young patients. The prognosis is good if the patient is asymptomatic, the hemoglobin concentration is more than 10 g/dL, the platelet count is greater than 100×10^9/L, and the liver is less than 5 cm below the costal margin.

- Typical clinical scenario: A 58-year-old woman presents with fatigue and anemia. The differential blood cell count included two nucleated RBCs, 4 myelocytes, and 2 metamyelocytes. RBC morphology demonstrates dacrocytes. The bone marrow is fibrotic.

Essential Thrombocythemia (Primary Thrombocythemia)

Essential thrombocythemia is a clonal hematologic disorder in which patients present with asymptomatic thrombocytosis, thrombotic disorders, or hemorrhage. Patients have a near-normal life expectancy. The overall risk of bleeding is 3% and of thrombosis, 20%. The risk factors for these include age older than 60, previous thrombosis, and short remission. Young females have a higher risk of miscarriage. The risk of acute leukemic transformation is less than 2%.

The diagnosis of essential thrombocythemia includes a platelet count greater than 600×10^9/L, megakaryocytic hyperplasia and stainable iron in the bone marrow, splenomegaly, absence of the Philadelphia chromosome or M*bcr* rearrangement (100% of patients), normal RBC mass (100%), and no collagen fibrosis. Also, there is no reactive thrombocytosis. Clinical findings that suggest reactive thrombocytosis include a recent normal manual platelet count, a clinical condition associated with reactive thrombocytosis, and no clinical features of a myeloproliferative disorder. The secondary causes include acute or chronic inflammatory disease, acute or chronic bleeding, iron deficiency, chronic bone marrow stimulation (e.g., hemolysis), rebound after thrombocytopenia, disseminated malignancy, splenectomy or congenital asplenia or functional hyposplenism, postoperative state, intense exercise, parturition, trauma, and epinephrine. An increased C-reactive protein level in patients with thrombocytosis suggests a reactive process.

Treatment depends on the clinical situation. Platelet apheresis should be used for emergent management of acute bleeding or thrombosis. Treatment of patients younger than 30 years is controversial. They may be observed if there are no hemorrhagic or thrombotic problems, no important trauma, and no emergency or elective surgery. Platelet apheresis is indicated in cases of elective surgery for patients of any age and in pregnant women during the course of delivery. Treatment is recommended for patients with thrombotic symptoms, a previous history of thrombotic events, and cardiovascular risk factors and for those older than 60 years who have a platelet count higher than 600×10^9/L. Currently, hydroxyurea is the treatment of choice for most patients. Anagrelide is a therapeutic alternative for patients who cannot tolerate hydroxyurea or who are younger than 65. Patients who are asymptomatic and have a platelet count less than 600×10^9/L and patients who are asymptomatic and of childbearing age may be observed. Chronic treatments available for the management of essential thrombocythemia include hydroxyurea, anagrelide, antiaggregating agents for mild thrombotic symptoms (including aspirin and dipyridamole), radioactive phosphorus at a dose of 2.7 mCi/m^2, and interferon alfa-2a or 2b recombinant.

Erythrocytosis

An increased hematocrit due to a decreased plasma cell volume and normal RBC mass is "relative polycythemia." Absolute erythrocytosis is almost always present with a hemoglobin concentration in males of 18 g/dL and in females, 16.5 g/dL. The history, physical examination, CBC, arterial blood gases, leukocyte alkaline phosphatase score, and bone marrow examination can indicate the diagnosis of polycythemia in a high percentage of patients (Table 11-11).

The differential diagnosis of erythrocytosis with a normal oxygen saturation value and normal leukocyte alkaline phosphatase score includes the following: hypernephroma, renal adenoma, hydronephrosis, renal cyst, transplantation, Bartter syndrome, cerebellar hemangioblastoma, adrenal cortical adenoma or hyperplasia, ovarian carcinoma, hepatoma, pheochromocytoma, uterine fibroids, and hemoglobinopathies. The administration of erythropoietin or androgens to healthy persons may cause erythrocytosis. Other causes include exogenous administration of erythropoietic drugs, post-renal transplant erythropoiesis, and congenital polycythemia. Patients with unexplained erythrocytosis should have intravenous pyelography or CT of the abdomen to exclude hypernephroma.

- Polycythemia rubra vera: very low erythropoietin.
- Cerebral blood flow decreases at a hematocrit >46%.
- Smoking 1.5 packs of cigarettes a day can increase the hematocrit to 60% (check carboxyhemoglobin).
- RBC mass returns to normal when the person stops smoking.

Polycythemia Rubra Vera

Polycythemia rubra vera is a myeloproliferative disorder of undetermined cause. Its clinical features include postbathing pruritus, weakness, erythromelalgia (acral dysesthesias, erythema), headache, dizziness, weight loss, joint symptoms, dyspnea, and epigastric distress. More than 50% of patients have leukocytosis and thrombocytosis. Thrombosis is a presenting feature in 12% to 49% of patients and occurs in more than 40% during the course of the disease. The classification according to the Polycythemia Vera Study Group includes the following:

Category A—increased RBC mass, splenomegaly, normal arterial oxygen saturation.

Category B—platelet count greater than 400×10^9/L, WBC count greater than 12×10^9/L (no fever or infection), leukocyte alkaline phosphatase score higher than 100, serum level of vitamin B_{12} greater than 900 ng/L. The presence of all three criteria in category A establishes the diagnosis. If the patient has an increased RBC mass (category A) with either of the other two category A criteria, then two of the four category B criteria are necessary to establish the diagnosis. These are no longer considered prerequisites for the diagnosis of polycythemia rubra vera. Unfavorable prognostic signs are previous thrombotic disease, age older than 60 years, diabetes mellitus, vascular disease, and hypertension.

New approaches to diagnosis include only the use of the serum erythropoietin level and the bone marrow examination in the diagnostic algorithm rather than the diagnostic criteria after it has been established that the hemoglobin and hematocrit are higher than the 95th percentile and polycythemia vera-related features are present (thrombocytosis, leukocytosis, microcytosis, iron deficiency, splenomegaly, pruritus, erythromelalgia, and unusual thrombosis). The erythropoietin level, which is usually low in polycythemia rubra vera, may be normal, but the estimated specificity is greater than 90%.

Bone marrow findings typically demonstrate trilineage hyperplasia but are normal in up to 10% of patients. From 90% to 95% of bone marrow specimens have an absence of iron stores even if the patient is not phlebotomized. Cytogenetic abnormalities are present in 13% to 18% of patients. The bone marrow is negative for the Philadelphia chromosome. Morphologically, the bone marrow findings may resemble those of chronic myelogenous leukemia in 10% to 40% of patients. The leukocyte alkaline phosphatase score is increased. Other morphologic abnormalities are present.

- The leukocyte alkaline phosphatase score may be increased in polycythemia rubra vera, leukemoid reactions, agnogenic myeloid metaplasia, idiopathic thrombocytopenic purpura, pregnancy, pyogenic infections, and stress erythrocytosis.
- Laboratory evaluation for polycythemia rubra vera: previous results to document interval change, low or normal erythropoietin level, and bone marrow evaluation (hypercellularity, atypical megakaryocytic hyperplasia, decrease in iron stores, reduced expression of the thrombopoietin receptor [c-Mpl]).
- Erythropoietin is increased in secondary erythrocytosis.
- Typical clinical scenario for polycythemia rubra vera: A hemoglobin concentration >18 g/dL in a white male or >2 g/dL that is documented and persistent, microcytosis, absence of iron stores, and splenomegaly. Other features include postbathing pruritus, unusual thrombosis, and erythromelalgia. The erythropoietin level is low.

The mainstay of treatment for all patients with polycythemia rubra vera is phlebotomy. However, there is no consensus about the optimal therapy for this disorder. Phlebotomy improved median survival by more than 10 years by decreasing the risk of thrombosis. Treatment for patients who are asymptomatic is phlebotomy to maintain the hematocrit below 42% in women and 45% in men. Patients are phlebotomized long term every 2 to 4 months, because there is 250 mg of iron in 1 pint of blood. If the normal daily absorption is 4 mg, then phlebotomizing every 2 months will maintain the hematocrit in the appropriate

Table 11-11 Differential Diagnosis of Erythrocytosis

	Polycythemia rubra vera	Relative or stress polycythemia (Gaisböck syndrome)	Anoxic polycythemia	Tumor
History	Multiple symptoms	Nervousness Hypertension Obesity	High-altitude COPD Fibrosis Congenital heart disease Sleep apnea Hemoglobinopathy	Renal cancer Uterine leiomyoma Pheochromo- cytoma Meningioma
Gout	Occasionally	Occasionally		
Other history	Postbathing pruritus*			
Examination	Plethora skin, mucous membrane Distention of retinal vein Hepatomegaly (50%) Splenomegaly (75%)*	±Plethora	Cyanosis Clubbing*	No cyanosis, clubbing, or COPD Mass in left upper quadrant
Laboratory				
Oxygen saturation	Normal	Normal	<88% (±88%-92%)*	Normal
LAP score	+++ (almost invariably)*	Normal	Normal	Normal
Red blood cell mass	++	Normal	+ to ++	+ to ++
Plasma volume	Normal or slightly increased	Reduced	Normal	Normal
Excretory urogram	Normal	Normal	Normal	Tumor
Erythrocyte sedimentation rate	0-1*	Normal	Normal, low	
Bone marrow	Pancytosis	Erythrocytosis	Erythrocytosis	Erythrocytosis
Platelets	+ to ++ (50%)	Normal	Normal	±Normal

COPD, chronic obstructive pulmonary disease; LAP, leukocyte alkaline phosphatase.
*Most important differentiating factors.
Modified from Dameshek W: Comments on the diagnosis of polycythemia vera. Semin Hematol 1966;3:214-215. By permission of WB Saunders Company.

range. A phlebotomy program starts at 500 mL every day if the patient is symptomatic and, if asymptomatic and at low risk, 3 to 6 phlebotomies weekly. The goal is to maintain the hematocrit at 42% to 45%. In the elderly, start phlebotomies at 250 mL. The risk of arterial and venous thrombosis is 20%. In older patients who have vascular lesions, the risk of thrombosis is related to the rate and volume of phlebotomy. Also, there is a risk of recurrent thrombosis in patients with a history of thrombosis. Low-dose aspirin therapy is indicated for all patients who do not have a contraindication to this therapy.

For patients who are symptomatic or who are at risk for thrombosis, hydroxyurea, interferon alfa, anagrelide, and phosphorus 32 are the treatments. Hydroxyurea is the treatment of choice for older patients. Anagrelide and interferon alfa are alternative therapies and the treatment of choice for younger patients. Interferon alfa is the treatment of choice for younger patients and women of childbearing age. Erythromelalgia in polycythemia rubra vera is managed with aspirin and by normalizing the platelet count. Interferon alfa may reduce the pruritus in polycythemia rubra vera in up to 81% of patients. All patients 60 years and younger with cardiovascular risk factors or a previous history of thrombosis should be considered for treatment. With phosphorus 32, the number of platelets decreases in 2 weeks and the number of RBCs decreases in 1 month. This treatment is an alternative for patients older than 60. Treatment of younger patients with phosphorus 32 increases the risk of acute nonlymphocytic leukemia 2.3-fold. Chlorambucil is not indicated because of a 5.3-fold risk of the development of acute nonlymphocytic leukemia when compared with phlebotomy.

The management of thrombosis and bleeding includes heparin, warfarin, hydroxyurea, platelet apheresis if the platelet count is greater than 800×10^9/L, phlebotomy, and allopurinol.

- Sequence of ordering tests in erythrocytosis—if the hematocrit is >58% in males or >52% in females, proceed with an erythrocytosis evaluation. If the arterial oxygen saturation is >92%, check carboxyhemoglobin concentration (smoker's polycythemia). If the arterial blood gases are normal, measure the erythropoietin level.
- For polycythemia rubra vera, phlebotomy is the cornerstone of treatment.
- For patients older than 60 years with or without a history of thrombosis, add hydroxyurea or anagrelide.

Oncogenesis

The hallmark of neoplastic disease is clonal proliferation of cells. Balanced reciprocal translocations affect specific sites on the genome (Table 11-12).

- Viral associations with hematologic malignancies: HTLV-I in adult T-cell leukemia; Epstein-Barr virus in Burkitt lymphoma, Hodgkin disease, and post-transplantation lymphoproliferative disorders.

COAGULATION

Prolonged Bleeding Time

The coagulation mechanism does not participate in bleeding time. An abnormal bleeding time reflects vascular defects, quantitative disorders of platelets (including thrombocytopenia and thrombocytosis), functional disorders of platelets, or operator error. Qualitative platelet defects result in abnormal bleeding time but normal partial thromboplastin time (PTT), PT, thrombin time, and platelet count (except in von Willebrand disease and disseminated intravascular coagulopathy).

- For prolonged bleeding time, the differential diagnosis includes Glanzmann thrombasthenia, von Willebrand disease, Bernard-Soulier syndrome, disseminated intravascular coagulopathy, thrombocytopenia, storage pool disease, drugs (aspirin and others), and uremia.

von Willebrand Disease

von Willebrand disease is the most common inherited bleeding disorder. Different subtypes have been described. In most subtypes, the inheritance pattern is autosomal dominant with incomplete penetrance (parent of either sex). The bleeding usually is mucocutaneous. The most common bleeding symptoms are epistaxis, skin ecchymoses, cutaneous hematomas, prolonged bleeding from trivial wounds, oral cavity bleeding, bleeding from tooth extractions, and menorrhagia. Bleeding may be exacerbated by aspirin. Hemarthroses are rare.

To understand von Willebrand disease, it is helpful to review endothelial interactions. The steps are platelet adhesion and then platelet aggregation. Collagen and vWF antigen are involved in both steps. vWF is a multimeric protein that circulates in blood plasma and is stored in endothelial cells and platelets. It is found in plasma, platelets, and endothelial regions and is detected functionally by its ability to cause aggregation of washed platelets when ristocetin is administered. Aggregation requires adenosine diphosphate (ADP) and thromboxane A_2. The activation of the clotting mechanism and generation of thrombin seem to result from the activation of the platelet membrane during adhesion and aggregation. Platelets make available platelet factor III phospholipid and catalyze the activation of other coagulation factors. The vWF/factor VIII complex is composed of the following: 1) factor VIII:C, the coagulant activity that is missing in hemophiliac plasma; this is decreased in hemophilia and von Willebrand disease and circulates in the plasma with vWF. 2) Factor VIII vWF antigen (vWF:Ag); vWF is a carrier protein for factor VIII, protecting it from rapid proteolytic destruction, and is the mediator of the initial adhesion of platelets to the blood vessel wall. The adhesive function is contained mainly within large multimers. 3) vWF activity: ristocetin cofactor, the activity necessary for ristocetin-induced platelet aggregation that is not present in von Willebrand disease. The ristocetin cofactor is the closest measurement of vWF activity. This is decreased in von Willebrand disease and is normal in hemophilia. vWF has an essential role in the adhesion of platelets to the subendothelium. Factor VIII coagulant activity and vWF activity reside in two separate molecules that are noncovalently bound in the plasma. Therefore, von Willebrand disease represents a defect in hemostasis involving the interaction of the platelet membrane glycoprotein, subendothelial tissues, and vWF. There is decreased synthesis, decreased release, or abnormal production of vWF. Defects in vWF may cause bleeding because platelets cannot adhere to sites of vascular injury. vWF has three functions: platelet adhesion, platelet-to-platelet aggregation, and a carrier for factor VIII.

The many distinct variants of von Willebrand disease can be divided into three subtypes. This classification is intended to reflect differences in the pathophysiology of the von Willebrand disease phenotypes. Type 1 is characterized by a partial *quantitative* abnormality in vWF. It is the most common type (75% of patients) and is autosomal dominant. The total amount of circulating vWF multimers is 50% or less. The distribution and function of vWF are normal. The definitive diagnosis of type 1 von Willebrand disease requires documentation of bleeding, low levels of qualitatively normal vWF, and inheritance.

Table 11-12 Chromosome Rearrangement and Increase of Specific Oncogenes

Disease	Rearrangement	Oncogene	Gene product
Burkitt lymphoma	t(8,14)	c-*myc*	Cell cycle progression
	t(8,22)		Translocation into transcriptionally active immunoglobulin heavy or light chain loci
Chronic myelogenous leukemia	t(9,22)	c-*abl*	Tyrosine kinase
Follicular small cleaved cell lymphoma	t(14,18)	*bcl*-2	Anti-apoptosis
Diffuse large cell non-Hodgkin lymphoma	---	*bcl*-6	Transcriptional repression
Mantle cell lymphoma	t(11,14)	*bcl*-1	Overexpression of PRAD1 Increase in cyclin D1

Patients who do not meet all three criteria may have "possible" von Willebrand type 1 disease. The broad normal ranges for vWF levels and the variation in levels over time may complicate the diagnosis of vWF type 1. Type 2 disease (A, B, M, and N) is characterized by a *qualitative* dysfunctional abnormality in vWF. In type 3 von Willebrand disease, there is virtually no detectable von Willebrand protein. Heterozygous von Willebrand disease (1% of the population) is characterized clinically by mild to moderate bleeding. It is autosomal dominant in inheritance pattern. The laboratory diagnosis of von Willebrand disease includes abnormal APTT and PT; prolonged bleeding time; decrease in factor VIII, vWF antigen (vWF:Ag), and vWF activity (ristocetin cofactor activity); normal platelet aggregation except in the presence of ristocetin; and mildly prolonged PTT. A normal APTT does not exclude the diagnosis of von Willebrand disease.

- vWF has three functions in hemostasis: adhesion and aggregation of platelets and the transportation and stabilization of factor VIII in the plasma.
- The tests for the diagnosis and exclusion of von Willebrand disease are vWF antigen and ristocetin cofactor activity (vWF:Rco).
- Supplementary tests that may be needed for the type of von Willebrand disease include APTT, bleeding time, platelet count, vWF multimer analysis, and ristocetin-induced platelet aggregation response.
- Typical clinical scenario: A patient with recurrent mucosal bleeding has a prolonged APTT.

The goal of treatment is to correct the coagulant defect, the result of subnormal vWF levels. Restoration of vWF levels results in control of hemorrhage in the absence of a consistent correction of the bleeding time. Mild and moderate cases of

von Willebrand disease require treatment only at the time of an operation or bleeding. For menorrhagia, birth control pills are effective (estrogen use may increase vWF and mask mild von Willebrand disease). For dental extractions, local hemostasis and local fibrinolytic agents with or without desmopressin (DDAVP) are effective. In pregnancy, there is no need to transfuse in mild to moderate cases of the disease because the levels of vWF increase with the duration of pregnancy. The mainstays of treatment are desmopressin and factor VIII concentrates rich in vWF. Desmopressin causes the release of preformed vWF multimers from the subendothelium and is useful in type 1 von Willebrand disease. Side effects include facial flushing, headache, mild decrease in blood pressure, mild tachycardia, and hyponatremia. Repeated doses at intervals shorter than 24 hours may result in a decrease or loss of response (tachyphylaxis). Desmopressin may be delivered intranasally, subcutaneously, or intravenously. A trial should be conducted before it is used as primary therapy. The levels increase for 4 to 8 hours. This agent usually is effective only in type 1 von Willebrand disease. For patients with type 2B or 3 von Willebrand disease or for those with type 1 disease that has become transiently unresponsive to desmopressin, viral-inactivated factor VIII preparations rich in high-molecular-weight multimer vWF are recommended. Humate-P (antihemophilic factor [human], pasteurized) has been approved by the U.S. Food and Drug Administration. Cryoprecipitate from carefully selected and repeatedly tested donors is more desirable than cryoprecipitate from random donors, but the risk of transmission of viral diseases is higher.

- Desmopressin is the treatment of choice for mild disease.
- Preparations rich in high-molecular-weight multimer vWF are recommended for types 2B and 3 disease and for type 1 disease transiently unresponsive to desmopressin.

Glanzmann Thrombasthenia

Glanzmann thrombasthenia results from a defect in the first phase of platelet aggregation because of a marked decrease in or absence of platelet glycoproteins IIb/IIIa. It is autosomal recessive in inheritance pattern. Early hemorrhagic complications occur in the neonatal period, and epistaxis, purpura, petechiae, and ecchymoses persist throughout life. Laboratory findings include no clumping of platelets on the peripheral blood smear, normal platelet number and morphology, and no aggregation with ADP, epinephrine, thrombin, or collagen. Aggregation does occur with ristocetin. Treatment consists of nasal packing, local measures, and cryoprecipitate, with or without platelets, when local measures are not successful. Leukocyte-depleted, single-donor platelet concentrates are preferable to reduce the risk of alloimmunization.

Bernard-Soulier Syndrome

Bernard-Soulier syndrome is the result of the absence of glycoprotein Ib/IX complexes on the surface of human platelets that mediate ristocetin-induced vWF-dependent platelet aggregation. Glycoprotein Ib/IX is the platelet receptor for vWF. These platelets are unable to react with subendothelial vWF. It is more common in whites and blacks and is autosomal recessive in inheritance pattern. This disorder is characterized by moderate to severe bleeding with surgery and menstruation. Bleeding typically is from mucous membranes, the gums, and the gastrointestinal tract. Bleeding time is markedly prolonged. Characteristically, there is thrombocytopenia with giant platelets. The aggregation pattern is the opposite of that of Glanzmann thrombasthenia, with normal platelet aggregation with ADP, collagen, epinephrine, and thrombin but no aggregation with ristocetin. No specific treatment is available for Bernard-Soulier syndrome other than local measures and platelets.

Storage Pool Disease

Normally, adenosine triphosphate (ATP), ADP, serotonin, and calcium are stored by platelets and released from them. In storage pool disease, there is a marked decrease in platelet ADP and a lesser decrease in ATP. Because of the profound decrease in ADP, the amount released from the platelets is insufficient to bring uninvolved platelets into larger aggregates.

Disseminated Intravascular Coagulopathy

Disseminated intravascular coagulopathy is characterized by a dynamic process caused by many diseases with microvascular clotting due to thrombin deposition. The laboratory findings vary. No single laboratory test can confirm or exclude the diagnosis, which depends on the clinical setting and laboratory findings. The manifestations vary from patient to patient and from time to time in the same patient. These may be of little clinical significance or cause life-threatening bleeding or clotting.

The mortality rates of severe disseminated coagulopathy range from 50% to 85%.

The pathophysiologic mechanism of disseminated intravascular coagulopathy is complex. Thrombin is formed in the vascular system and alters platelets. The platelets aggregate, agglutinate, and secrete many products, resulting in thrombocytopenia and platelets that do not function well. As plasmin circulates, it systematically degrades fibrin and fibrinogen, creating the D-dimer and X, Y, D, and E fragments known as "D-fibrinogen degradation products." Thrombin cleaves fibrinopeptides A and B from fibrinogen to form fibrin monomers. The complex of fibrin degradation products and fibrin monomers is called "soluble fibrin monomer." Fibrin degradation products interfere with fibrin monomer polymerization. Fibrin degradation products and D-dimer induce interleukin-1 and interleukin-6. Thrombin induces the release of other factors, including proinflammatory cytokines. These monomers may complex with fibrinogen (polymerization) to form insoluble fibrin, which is deposited in capillaries and small blood vessels, resulting in microangiopathy. Activated factor XIII cross-links fibrin to make it more resistant to fibrinolysis. Thrombin increases the activity of factors V and VIII. Therefore, thrombin accounts for the decrease in fibrinogen, platelets, and factors II, V, VIII, and XIII. Secondary fibrinolysis may occur. Bleeding occurs because the coagulation factors are depleted or fibrinolysis with vessel damage results in a decrease in control proteins, such as antithrombin III and protein C. Activated factor XII leads to kallikrein production, resulting in the conversion of plasminogen to plasmin (the global proteolytic enzyme), which is capable of digesting fibrinogen, clotting factors, and complement. The clinical picture depends on a balance: if thrombin activity is greater than plasmin activity, thrombosis occurs; if plasmin activity is greater than thrombin activity, hemorrhage occurs.

The following occur in acute disseminated intravascular coagulopathy: bleeding from wounds and perivenipuncture sites, ecchymoses, petechiae, hematomas, hematuria, intracranial hemorrhage, intrapleural hemorrhage, intraperitoneal hemorrhage, hemoptysis, vaginal bleeding, melena, and hematemesis. Thromboembolic complications, as manifested by necrotic skin lesions, pulmonary emboli, acute arterial occlusions, ischemia, stroke, and myocardial infarction, may occur in 8% of patients. Thrombosis is more common than bleeding in chronic disseminated intravascular coagulopathy.

Disseminated intravascular coagulopathy has many causes. Malignancy is the most common cause: prostate, breast, lung, leukemia (acute progranulocytic [M3]), pancreas, or lymphoma. Infection is the second most common cause (gram-negative [30%-50% of patients] and gram-positive organisms, e.g., *Staphylococcus*, *Streptococcus*, pneumococcus, typhoid, *Rickettsia*, viral, fungal, histoplasmosis, *Aspergillus*), and surgery or trauma is the third. Other causes are liver disease, obstetrical (amniotic fluid, embolism, abruptio placenta), acute renal failure associated with cardiogenic shock, gunshot wounds, endothelial injury (giant hemangiomas [Kasabach-Merritt syndrome], aortic aneurysms, angiography), hemolytic transfusion reactions, burns, crush injuries, acidosis, alkalosis, reactions to toxins (snake venom), and transfusion reactions.

The optimal screening study results are thrombocytopenia in 90% of patients, increased PT in 50% to 75%, and hypofibrinogenemia in 70% of those with severe disease. The best available confirmatory test is the fibrin D-dimer assay, a test that is specific for fibrin degradation products and detects fibrinogen fragments formed by the lysis of cross-linked fibrin. More sensitive techniques include detection of products of fibrinolysis or fibrin degradation products (D-dimer products) and coagulation activation (soluble fibrin monomers). The values obtained with these two tests may be increased in the postoperative state and in patients with recent thrombi because of fibrinolysis that may not reflect a pathologic state.

- Screening tests for disseminated intravascular coagulopathy: thrombocytopenia (90% of patients), increased PT (50% to 75% of patients), and hypofibrinogenemia (70% of patients with severe disease).

The first goal is to treat the underlying disease. Next, the approach depends on the clinical situation. If the patient has a low level of fibrinogen, low platelet count, or low levels of clotting factor and is not bleeding or undergoing a surgical procedure, no treatment is necessary. If the patient is bleeding or undergoing a surgical procedure, treat with cryoprecipitate, fresh frozen plasma, and platelets. Monitoring the effect of replacement therapy with platelet and fibrinogen levels 30 minutes to 1 hour after transfusion and every 4 to 6 hours thereafter provides a guide to further replacement therapy. If the patient continues to bleed and the above measures do not cause an increase in coagulation factors, it may be necessary to continue factor and platelet replacement therapy and to start a continuous infusion of heparin. Heparin is contraindicated if there is a central nervous system lesion. If there is evidence of fibrin deposition or thrombosis (such as dermal necrosis in purpura fulminans, acral ischemia, livedo reticularis, or venous thromboembolism), heparin therapy is indicated. Full-dose therapy (a loading dose of 5,000 U, followed by 1,000 U/h), low-dose continuous infusion heparin (300 to 500 U/h), and subcutaneous heparin have been advocated. Monitoring is a problem. The initial approach is to monitor the PT, fibrinogen level, and platelet count. A heparin assay to achieve a level of 0.2 to 0.4 µ/mL is an alternative approach that is not advocated as routine practice. The thrombotic events of disseminated intravascular coagulopathy in solid tumor malignancy can be treated effectively with heparin, but warfarin anticoagulation may not be as effective. Other instances in which heparin is indicated are retained dead fetus with hypofibrinogenemia before induction of labor, excessive bleeding associated with giant hemangioma, promyelocytic leukemia, and mucinous adenocarcinoma. For more than 95% of patients, heparin is not indicated. Antithrombin III is a supportive therapeutic option in severe disseminated intravascular coagulopathy.

Chronic disseminated intravascular coagulopathy is common. Routine tests of hypercoagulability are abnormal in a substantial number of patients with cancer. Increased levels of fibrinogen are common. The syndrome of coexisting cancer and thrombotic disease is called "Trousseau syndrome," which is associated with mucin-producing neoplasms.

Coagulation and Liver Disease

The most important factor is the condition of the blood vessels. There is no tendency to bleed unless and until blood vessels are damaged, such as by a needle, a surgical procedure, or gastric acid. The three main coagulation patterns are 1) portal hypertension, which is characterized by thrombocytopenia and normal coagulation factor synthesis; 2) cholestasis, which results in impaired absorption of fat-soluble vitamins, with vitamin K deficiency and an increase in PT and APTT; and 3) acute and chronic hepatocellular disease, which is characterized by a normal fibrinogen level (until late in the course of the disease), thrombocytopenia, and an increase in PT and APTT because of multiple factor deficiencies. Liver disease is compared with disseminated intravascular coagulopathy and vitamin K deficiency in Table 11-13.

Factor-Deficiency States

The causes of an isolated elevated APTT include factor deficiencies (XII, XI, IX, and VIII) and antiphospholipid antibodies (lupus anticoagulant and anticardiolipin antibodies). Mixing studies result in correction in factor deficiencies and no correction on initial mixing at 2 hours in the case of antiphospholipid antibodies.

Factor XIII Deficiency

Factor XIII deficiency is characterized by normal blood tests but marked bleeding. There is a history of umbilical cord bleeding, ecchymoses, and prolonged hemorrhage from cuts. It is autosomal recessive in inheritance pattern. All routine clotting tests, including bleeding time, may give normal results. Treatment is with cryoprecipitate. The causes of an isolated elevated APTT include factor deficiencies (XII, XI, IX, and VIII) and antiphospholipid antibodies (lupus anticoagulant and anticardiolipin antibodies). Mixing studies result in correction of factor deficiencies and no correction on initial mixing at 2 hours in antiphospholipid antibody syndrome.

Table 11-13 Differences in Laboratory Findings in Liver Disease, Disseminated Intravascular Coagulopathy, and Vitamin K Deficiency

Tests	Liver disease	Disseminated intravascular coagulopathy	Vitamin K deficiency
Thrombocytopenia	Mild, decreased in 50% of patients, $<50\times10^9$/L platelets uncommon	90% of patients	No
Increased prothrombin time	Common	90% of patients	Common
Decreased fibrinogen	Late in disease	70% of patients	No
Factor V	Decreased	Regularly decreased	Normal
Factor VIII	Normal	Regularly decreased	Normal
Factors VII, X	Decreased	Normal	Decreased

Factor XII Deficiency

Factor XII deficiency is an autosomal recessive disorder in which thromboembolic complications occur. It is often associated with a very high APTT; PT is normal.

Factor XI Deficiency (Hemophilia C)

Factor XI deficiency is a rare autosomal recessive disorder that occurs predominantly in Ashkenazi Jews. This is a mild bleeding disorder that usually becomes manifest after surgery or trauma or with the initiation of treatment with antiplatelet agents or anticoagulants. The indications for replacement therapy depend on several variables. Treatment options include fresh frozen plasma and virally inactivated factor XI concentrate.

Factor IX Deficiency (Christmas Disease, Hemophilia B)

This X-linked disorder accounts for 15% of all cases of hemophilia. It is clinically indistinguishable from factor VIII deficiency. The laboratory abnormalities include an abnormal PTT. Patients who undergo a surgical procedure or who have major bleeding could receive purified factor IX concentrates. Recombinant factor IX products (nonacog alfa [BeneFix]) developed from a monoclonal antibody-purifying process are available. They are safe from contamination with the acquired immunodeficiency syndrome (AIDS) virus, and the risk of hepatitis is markedly decreased. Rare thrombotic episodes have been reported with recombinant factor IX.

Factor VIII Deficiency (Hemophilia A)

This disease results from a defect in factor VIII:C, is X-linked recessive in inheritance pattern, and accounts for 85% of cases of hemophilia. If a hemophiliac male has children from a normal female, all daughters are obligatory carriers and all sons are normal. If a normal male marries a carrier, each daughter has a 50% chance of being a carrier and each son has a 50% chance of having hemophilia. At birth, there are no bleeding manifestations; however, 50% of males bleed at the time of circumcision. Bleeding occurs in 75% of severely affected infants by age 18 months. The severity of hemophilia runs true in families. Persons with severe hemophilia have less than 1% factor VIII and clinically have hemarthroses, atrophied muscles, subcutaneous hematomas in the tongue and neck, and hematomas in the genitourinary and gastrointestinal tracts. Those with mild hemophilia have factor VIII levels of 5% to 25% and may bleed heavily, even fatally, postoperatively or after dental extractions unless the factor is adequately replaced.

Laboratory studies show an abnormal PTT, abnormal factor VIII, normal PT, normal bleeding time, and normal thrombin time.

Treatment options include desmopressin, plasma-derived clotting factor concentrates, and recombinant clotting factor concentrates. Desmopressin may establish adequate hemostatic levels in mild hemophilia.

Factor VIII concentrate has a half-life of 8 to 12 hours. Current factor VIII concentrates are regarded to be safe from HIV transmission. However, three highly purified products, all produced by monoclonal antibodies, are available and no cases of AIDS or hepatitis B or C have been reported with their use. No seroconversions to HIV have been reported with any of the products in the United States, including products that have been heated in aqueous solution, solvent-detergent treated, or immunoaffinity purified. Heat- and solvent-detergent–treated concentrates appear to be free from transmission of hepatitis B, hepatitis C, and HIV. Hepatitis A and parvovirus are not inactivated by these techniques. Recombinant factor VIII products (Recombinate, Kogenate, Helixate FS [albumin-free]) are available and appear to be free from human virus transmission and are the standard treatment of choice. A recombinant factor VIII manufactured without human or antiviral protein is now available (Refacto).

The management of patients with factor VIII inhibitors is complex. Porcine factor VIII should be considered in the initial management if the patient does not have an inhibitor to this factor. When porcine factor VIII cannot be used, prothrombin complex concentrates (I, VII, IX, and X) may be administered to bypass the need for factor VIII. These agents have a risk of thrombotic complications. Recently, recombinant factor VIIa has become available. Always check the Bethesda unit assay before any general surgical procedure is performed in a patient with hemophilia. From 5% to 20% of persons with hemophilia develop inhibitors (IgG antibodies) that inactivate factor VIII:C (Bethesda units). If the inhibitor is less than 3 Bethesda units/mL, treat with higher doses or replacement therapy. If the value is higher (>10 Bethesda units), one can attempt to use prothrombin complex concentrates (II, VII, IX, X) to "bypass." Hemophilia A is compared with von Willebrand disease in Table 11-14.

- Factor VIII and factor IX deficiencies are X-linked.
- Management of hemophilia A: a trial of desmopressin should be undertaken in cases of mild to moderate hemophilia A.
- For other patients, use factor VIII products that are heat-treated, solvent-detergent–treated, immunoaffinity purified, or produced by recombinant techniques.
- Recombinant techniques appear to be free from human virus transmission and are the treatment of choice.
- Typical clinical scenario: A male patient has bleeding into the joints and a prolonged APTT. PT and bleeding time are normal.

Acquired factor VIII deficiency states may occur and have the following causes: idiopathic, postpartum, collagen vascular diseases (rheumatoid arthritis, systemic lupus erythematosus, temporal arteritis), drug hypersensitivity (penicillin, sulfonamides), malignancies (lymphoproliferative, solid tumors), and

Table 11-14 Differences Between Hemophilia A and von Willebrand Disease

	Hemophilia A	von Willebrand disease
Inheritance	Sex-linked	Autosomal
Bleeding time	Normal	Prolonged
Factor VIII:C	Decreased	Decreased
vWF	Normal	Decreased
Ristocetin cofactor	Normal	Decreased

vWF, von Willebrand factor.

old age. Clinically, bleeding is intramuscular, retropharyngeal, retroperitoneal, and cerebral. Also, hematuria occurs. Treatment is difficult and requires the combination of corticosteroids, cyclophosphamide, plasmapheresis, prothrombin-complex concentrate, activated prothrombin-complex concentrate, and porcine factor VIII. The combination of cyclophosphamide and prednisone may be effective in an outpatient setting for patients with an acquired factor VIII inhibitor.

Factor VII Deficiency

Factor VII deficiency is characterized clinically by epistaxis, gingival bleeding, bleeding after trauma, menorrhagia, and hemarthroses. The APTT is normal, and PT is abnormal.

Factor X Deficiency

Factor X deficiency is characterized by bleeding that is the same as that in factor VII deficiency. An acquired factor X deficiency state may occur in amyloidosis. The APTT and PT are abnormal.

Factor V Deficiency

Factor V deficiency may be acquired in myeloproliferative disorders. Bruising occurs with severe bleeding postoperatively and at the onset of menstruation. Treatment consists of administering platelets and fresh frozen plasma.

Causes of an increased thrombin time include heparin, heparin-like anticoagulants, increase in fibrin degradation products, and decreased or defective fibrinogen.

The hemorrhagic disorders are summarized in Table 11-15.

Treatment of Factor-Deficiency States

Circulatory overload problems must be taken into consideration when patients receive transfusion with materials used to treat deficiency states. To control major bleeding or to prepare patients for a surgical procedure, it is advised that the plasma level of factor VIII be increased to 60% in patients with factor VIII deficiency. The number of factor VIII units is calculated by multiplying the patient's weight in pounds by 12 (e.g., 160 lb × 12 = 1,920 units of factor VIII).

Fresh frozen plasma is a good source of all factors. It has been used in treating congenital deficiencies in factors II, V, VII, IX, X, XI, and XIII and multiple coagulation deficiencies, including oral anticoagulant overdose, liver disease, massive transfusion, disseminated intravascular coagulopathy, plasmapheresis, and vitamin K deficiency. Multiple coagulation factor deficiencies should be suspected in patients with prolonged PT and partial thromboplastin times greater than 1.5 times normal if not due to known coagulation factor deficiency or circulating lupus-like anticoagulant. In dosing fresh frozen plasma, 1 or 2 units usually is not sufficient to replace coagulation factors, as in patients with liver disease, which

Table 11-15 Summary of Test Results in Hemorrhagic Disorders and Anticoagulant Therapy

	Prothrombin time	APTT	Thrombin time	Fibrinogen	Bleeding time
Classic hemophilia A	Normal	Abnormal	Normal	Normal	Normal
von Willebrand disease	Normal	Normal or abnormal	Normal	Normal	Abnormal
Afibrinogenemia	Abnormal	Abnormal	Abnormal	Absent	Normal
Hypofibrinogenemia	Normal	Normal	Normal	Low	Normal
Dysfibrinogenemia	Normal or abnormal	Normal or abnormal	Abnormal	Normal	Normal
Factor XIII deficiency	Normal	Normal	Normal	Normal	Normal
Heparin	Slightly abnormal	Abnormal	Abnormal	Normal	Normal or abnormal
Warfarin (Coumadin)	Abnormal	Normal or abnormal	Normal	Normal	Normal

APTT, activated partial thromboplastin time.

requires 3 to 9 units. The maximal effect declines 2 to 4 hours after transfusion. Purified antihemophilic concentrates are derived from fresh frozen plasma of paid donors and are lyophilized or freeze-dried in form. Complications include hepatitis and factor VIII inhibitors. Cryoprecipitate is a good source of factors V, VIII, and fibrinogen. The activity per gram of protein is 12 to 60 times that of fresh frozen plasma. One bag increases the factor VIII level 2.5% or one bag per 6 kg of body weight twice a day in factor VIII deficiency. Factor IX complex contains factors II, VII, IX, and X. Activated factor IX-complex products include Konyne and anti-inhibitor coagulant complex, heat treated (Autoplex T). This is indicated for severe factor IX deficiency and in the management of factor VIII inhibitors. Complications include hepatitis, disseminated intravascular coagulopathy, and thrombosis.

Thrombophilia: The Hypercoagulable States

Thrombophilia refers to the hereditary or acquired tendency to have recurrent venous or arterial thromboembolism. Clinical indications of hypercoagulable states include a family history of thrombosis, recurrent thrombosis without other precipitating risk factors, thrombosis at unusual sites, and postpartum thrombosis. The clinical features of familial thrombophilia include venous or arterial thrombosis at an early age, family history of venous thromboembolism, recurrent venous thromboembolism, unusual sites of thromboembolism (cerebral, mesenteric, and renal), thrombosis during pregnancy, and idiopathic venous or arterial thromboembolism. With the congenital states, the initial episode of venous thromboembolism is rare before the age of 18 years and uncommon after the age of 50 and occurs in high-risk situations.

Venous thromboembolism, deep venous thrombosis, and pulmonary embolism are major causes of morbidity, affecting more than 2 million patients annually in the United States. The annual mortality rate is 50,000, higher than that for breast cancer. Deep venous thrombosis and pulmonary embolism affect otherwise healthy patients as a major complication of surgery and hospitalization. Risk factors for thrombosis are noncongenital, congenital, and acquired. Noncongenital risk factors include age, trauma, obesity, immobilization, pregnancy, diabetes mellitus, and oral contraceptive pills. Mutations or polymorphisms in antithrombotic and prothrombotic factors, the thrombophilias, are the genetic factors. Congenital risk factors include the deficiency states of protein S, protein C, prothrombin 20210A gene abnormality (factor II G20210A), hyperhomocystinemia, plasminogen deficiency, antithrombin III deficiency, and congenital resistance to activated protein C (APC). Of all cases of APC resistance, 90% are caused by heterozygosity or homozygosity for a single point mutation in the factor V gene, factor V Leiden. Acquired conditions include lupus anticoagulant, disseminated intravascular coagulopathy, paroxysmal nocturnal hemoglobinuria, pregnancy, malignancy, inflammatory bowel disease, myeloproliferative disorders, cryoglobulinemia, and aberrant blood flow.

Resistance to APC is an autosomal dominant disorder resulting from a point mutation in the gene encoding coagulation factor V, commonly known as the factor V "Leiden" mutation. Normally, protein C inactivates factor Va. An alteration interferes and increases the risk of venous thrombosis. This mutation renders factor V resistant to proteolytic down-regulation by APC, and so the clotting mechanism continues to generate the clotting enzyme thrombin. The heterozygous mutation has a prevalence of 5% to 7% in the white population. There is approximately a tenfold increased prevalence (20%-50%) among persons with familial or recurrent venous thromboembolism and a 20% increased prevalence among those with deep venous thrombosis. Homozygotes have an 80-fold increased risk for venous thromboembolism. The risk of venous thromboembolism is increased 30-fold among heterozygotes receiving oral contraceptive therapy. The diagnosis is established by an APTT-based APC resistance ratio or DNA-based testing. DNA-based testing is recommended for patients with an abnormal APTT-based APC resistance ratio, for patients with an abnormally prolonged APTT (lupus-like anticoagulant), and for those taking anticoagulants. Of patients with hereditary APC resistance, 90% have a single nucleotide mutation of the coagulation factor V gene, the *R506Q* gene. Asymptomatic patients with APC resistance should have prophylactic intervention when clinical thrombosis risk factors are present. An initial deep venous thrombosis in an APC-resistant person is managed in a standard fashion. Those who are homozygotes or heterozygotes with additional thrombophilic predispositions should be considered for lifelong anticoagulation prophylaxis. These patients do not need a higher than required international normalized ratio (INR).

- Typical case scenario for protein S or C deficiency: A 40-year-old person has venous thrombosis.

Protein S deficiency is more common than protein C or antithrombin III deficiency. Routine coagulation assays fail to detect these patients. A 50% decrease in either protein S or C increases thrombotic tendencies. Family studies are required. Assays are available for all three deficiency states. Protein S is a vitamin K-dependent factor that is required for expression of APC anticoagulant activity. There is an increased incidence of thrombosis, with venous complications greater than arterial. APC destroys activated factors V and VIII and, thus, is a potent plasma anticoagulant. APC requires a second vitamin K-dependent factor, or cofactor, protein S. Antithrombin III deficiency is an uncommon cause of venous thromboembolism. The management of protein S deficiency, protein C deficiency, and antithrombin III deficiency requires heparin and oral anticoagulant agents. There is an increased incidence of warfarin necrosis that is a rare complication in nonhospitalized patients and occurs 2 to 10 days after treatment with warfarin is initiated. Other causes of protein S and protein C deficiency include liver disease, oral anticoagulation, and oral contraceptives.

The antiphospholipid antibodies, which are identified by immunoassays instead of functional testing, include anticardiolipin antibodies, lupus anticoagulants, protein-phospholipid reactivity, and anti-reagin antibodies. Antiphospholipid antibodies are immunoglobulins (IgG or IgM) that interfere with in vitro phospholipid steps of coagulation, causing a prolonged clotting time in the APTT, dilute Russell viper venom time, or plasma clot time. Antiphospholipid antibodies are heterogeneous. Some prolong phospholipid-dependent clotting reactions (lupus anticoagulant detected by increased APTT and prolonged dilute Russell viper venom time) and others bind to cardiolipin or β_2-glycoprotein 1 bound to phospholipids (anticardiolipin antibodies detected by IgG and IgM serum anticardiolipin antibodies).

Activation of protein C is phospholipid-dependent. Therefore, interference with this reaction may create a prothrombotic state. Patients with antiphospholipid antibodies are at higher risk for thrombosis. This is an interfering inhibitor of APTT that does not correct with equal volumes of normal plasma. The screening test is prolonged APTT. Clinically, venous thrombosis of the lower extremities is more common than arterial thrombosis. The clinical approach to lupus anticoagulant and antiphospholipid antibody syndrome is as follows. The APTT does not correct with a 1:1 mixture of normal plasma. The best confirmatory test is the dilute Russell viper venom time (addition of exogenous phospholipid) or the platelet neutralization procedure (addition of phospholipid to the APTT system in the form of platelets). The dilute Russell viper venom time is also abnormal in patients receiving heparin.

Other assays for antiphospholipid antibody include β_2-glycoprotein 1 antibodies and antithrombin antibodies. If there is no history of thrombotic disease, check the APC-resistant factor Va, antithrombin III, protein C, and protein S. If normal, observe. Prophylactic anticoagulant therapy is indicated for times of increased risk, such as postoperative state and long-bone fracture. Alternatives to oral contraceptives should be considered. If the patient develops thrombosis and is receiving heparin, follow heparin levels or the anti-Xa test. Alternatively, low-molecular-weight heparin obviates the need for monitoring. If the patient requires oral warfarin, regulate with an arbitrary INR of 2.5 to 3.5 or with the prothrombin-proconvertin test. After thrombotic events, long-term warfarin is indicated.

The clinical syndromes of the antiphospholipid antibody include major (venous and arterial thromboses, spontaneous abortions, and thrombocytopenia) and minor (livedo reticularis, multistroke dementia, and chorea) components. The thrombotic manifestations are venous (deep venous thrombosis, cutaneous thrombosis, renal vein thrombosis, and Budd-Chiari syndrome) or arterial (central nervous system, coronary thrombosis, and renal artery or vein thrombosis). Hematologic associations include thrombocytopenia, hemolysis, and hypocomplementemia. Obstetrical associations are maternal (deep venous thrombosis, chorea, eclampsia, and pulmonary embolus) and fetal (spontaneous abortion, fetal death, and second and third trimester premature birth).

There is no indication for the treatment of asymptomatic patients without a history of associated conditions. For thrombosis, initially treat with heparin, followed by anticoagulation with warfarin, with an INR greater than 3.0. Low doses of aspirin and heparin are recommended for the management of pregnant women. Pregnant women with a previous history of venous thromboembolism may be followed with active clinical surveillance or actively prophylaxed with heparin treatment.

Who should be tested? Patients who should be considered for further testing include persons younger than 40 years with thrombotic events and those with a strong family history of thrombosis, recurrent thromboses at different sites, skin necrosis, recurrent fetal loss, and thrombosis at unusual sites (sagittal sinus thrombosis, mesenteric thrombosis). Pregnancy increases the risk of venous thromboembolism about fivefold that of the general population and if a patient has had venous thromboembolism in the past, there is a transient, approximately threefold increase in the risk. Pulmonary embolism is the most common medical cause of maternal deaths associated with live births.

Asymptomatic carriers do not need treatment. Asymptomatic family members do not need treatment. Patients with their first venous thromboembolism who have persistent clinical risk factors and reduced coronary reserve and patients with recurrent venous thromboembolism who are homozygotes or compound/double heterozygotes are candidates for long-term anticoagulation.

- Typical clinical scenario for antiphospholipid antibody syndrome: A patient with recurrent events in the same vascular location has an abnormal APTT. Laboratory testing shows that the prolonged APTT is corrected by the addition of platelet-rich plasma.

Anticoagulants

There are different anticoagulation targets. Procoagulant proteins may be depleted (warfarin). Procoagulant proteins may be inhibited indirectly (unfractionated heparin and low-molecular-weight heparin [LMWH], e.g., fondaparinux, ardeparin, dalteparin, danaproid, enoxaparin, and tinzaparin). Procoagulant proteins may be inhibited directly (hirudin, lepirudin, bivalirudin, argatroban). The fibrinolytic system may be enhanced (thrombolytic therapy).

Warfarin

Warfarin is a vitamin K antagonist, which limits the gamma-carboxylation of the vitamin K-dependent coagulation proteins II, VII, IX, and X and anticoagulant proteins C and S, impairing their biologic function in blood coagulation. This drug is contraindicated in pregnancy. Warfarin derivatives,

direct thrombin inhibitors, and hirudin cross the placenta and are contraindicated. Unfractionated heparin, LMWH, and danaproid do not cross the placenta. Complications include embryopathy. Other relative contraindications for warfarin include a hemorrhagic tendency such as thrombocytopenia or coagulation factor abnormalities, diastolic blood pressure greater than 110 mm Hg, gastrointestinal tract lesions liable to bleed, severe liver disease, severe renal disease, malabsorption, subacute bacterial endocarditis, diverticulosis, or colitis. It is also contraindicated if a surgical procedure was performed recently on the central nervous system or eye.

In venous thromboembolism, warfarin treatment should be started within 24 hours after the initiation of heparin. The appropriate dose of warfarin for preventing systemic embolism and myocardial infarction, for prophylaxis for venous thrombosis, and for treating venous thrombosis and pulmonary embolism is that which maintains PT at an INR of 2 or 3, which corresponds to a PT ratio of 1.3 to 1.5. A loading dose of 5 mg avoids the development of a potential hypercoagulable state caused by a precipitous decrease in the levels of protein C. Patients should receive 3 months of warfarin treatment if at low risk. However, for patients with unproved venous thromboembolism and persistent risk factors, the duration of anticoagulation is debated. Patients with metastatic cancer who have venous thromboembolism are candidates for long-term therapy, as are those with recurrent thromboembolism. Warfarin has been demonstrated to be efficacious in atrial fibrillation. A target range for the INR of 2.5 to 3.5 is recommended for tilting disk valves, bileaflet aortic valves in the mitral position, bileaflet aortic valves, atrial fibrillation, caged ball valves, and disk valves.

Bleeding occurs in 2% to 4% of patients. In patients with a prolonged PT with or without bleeding, use of the drug should be stopped for 24 to 72 hours. Available information suggests that patients taking warfarin with an INR greater than 8 are at a substantially increased risk for bleeding. In patients who have taken a suicidal dose or have a suspected cerebral hemorrhage and who need no further anticoagulation, vitamin K given intravenously at a dose of 20 to 30 mg may be administered with fresh frozen plasma. Fresh frozen plasma alone may be administered to patients taking warfarin who require continued anticoagulation but who have life-threatening bleeding by the National Institutes of Health consensus. Drugs that potentiate warfarin include those that prolong PT, such as phenylbutazone, metronidazole, sulfinpyrazone, trimethoprim-sulfamethoxazole, and disulfiram. Gingko may increase the risk of hemorrhage of a person taking warfarin. Drugs that inhibit platelet function, such as aspirin, also may potentiate the toxic effects of warfarin. Some drugs antagonize warfarin; for example, cholestyramine decreases its absorption. Other drugs, such as barbiturates, carbamazepine, and rifampin, increase the clearance of warfarin. Acetaminophen may be a cause of overanticoagulation in the outpatient setting.

Unfractionated Heparin

Heparin inhibits thrombin by binding to antithrombin III and forming a heparin-antithrombin III complex, which interrupts the clotting cascade by deactivating thrombin (factor IIa) and factor Xa. The heparin is then reused. In the initial treatment of deep venous thrombosis or pulmonary embolism, the goal is to prolong APTT at a level of 1.5 to 2.5 times normal within the first 24 hours of treatment. A plasma level of heparin of 1.2 to 0.4 IU/mL is necessary. If this is not accomplished, the risk of recurrent thromboembolism is 15-fold, and the risk persists for weeks. Heparin and warfarin may be given simultaneously and be overlapped for 5 days, after which treatment should be warfarin alone. Heparin should be administered for a minimum of 4 days (range, 5-7 days) and not be discontinued until the INR has been in the therapeutic range for 2 consecutive days, because of the half-lives of the vitamin K-dependent factors. Warfarin treatment should be maintained for 3 months if there are no risk factors. Prolonged treatment may be indicated when risk factors such as prolonged immobilization, hypercoagulable state, and recurrent deep venous thrombosis exist.

Heparin is indicated for the treatment of venous thrombosis and pulmonary embolism. It also is given to *prevent* venous thrombosis and pulmonary embolism (prophylactic doses of 5,000 units subcutaneously every 8 to 12 hours in cases of abdominal surgery or for medical patients with a history of thrombosis, prolonged bed rest, congestive heart failure, or cancer). The common duration for the postoperative period is 7 days or with hospital dismissal. A dose of 12,000 units is administered subcutaneously twice daily for the prevention of mural thrombosis after myocardial infarction. Heparin is indicated for the prevention of coronary artery rethrombosis after thrombolysis, and it is the treatment of choice for venous thrombosis and pulmonary embolism in pregnancy (17,500 units subcutaneously twice daily). Impedance plethysmography, ultrasonography, or venography may document this complication of pregnancy. (Warfarin is contraindicated in pregnancy because of the risks of embryopathy, including nasal hypoplasia and central nervous system abnormalities.) Heparin is indicated after thrombolytic therapy. The normal dose is a 5,000-unit bolus (or loading dose of 80 U/kg), followed by 12,000 U per hour (18 U/kg per hour) by continuous infusion, with the goal of achieving a therapeutic APTT of 1.5 times control. Side effects include hemorrhage (which occurs in 6.8% of patients receiving continuous infusion), osteoporosis, and skin necrosis. A hypersensitivity reaction may convert antithrombin III from a slow inhibitor to a very rapid inhibitor.

Resistance to heparin is defined as the need for more than 40,000 U daily. The thrombotic process may be reactivated when heparin therapy is discontinued. Heparin resistance is due to increased plasma concentrations of factor VIII and heparin-binding proteins. Approaches include monitoring the plasma heparin concentration or LMWH.

Low-Molecular-Weight Heparin

LMWH has advantages over unfractionated heparin; its more predictable dose response allows fixed doses without laboratory monitoring. Also, the risk of heparin-induced thrombocytopenia is lower because nonspecific binding of heparin to other proteins and cells causes variability. Furthermore, about 50% of all patients with venous thrombosis can be treated with LMWH without hospitalization. LMWH does not cause a marked change in the measured APTT because of the propensity toward factor Xa inhibition over thrombin inhibition. In most circumstances, blood monitoring is not required. If monitoring is necessary, the heparin assay (anti-factor Xa) may be performed 4 hours after the dose. Levels should be measured. Indications for monitoring include prolonged use (pregnancy, extremes of body weight, i.e., <46 kg or >100 kg), and renal insufficiency. Generally, twice-daily dosage should give better coverage for prophylaxis and treatment, although single dosage for prophylaxis is adequate for dalteparin and enoxaparin. Subcutaneous dosages for prophylaxis for the available LMWHs include ardeparin, enoxaparin, dalteparin, tinzaparin, and danaparoid. LMWH can be used as an effective alternative to warfarin therapy. The dosage of LMWH may vary with the indication (prophylaxis vs. therapeutic) and the type of preparation. Certain situations present a high risk of bleeding (obesity, long duration of therapy, and renal insufficiency [creatinine >2.0 or creatinine clearance ≤30]). Protamine is partially effective in reversing LMWH. Contraindications for LMWH include a previous heparin-induced thrombocytopenia and severe renal dysfunction. Clinical trials have demonstrated that LMWH is at least as effective as unfractionated heparin for venous thromboembolism and recurrent venous thromboembolism and for the prevention of venous thromboembolism. LMWH is more effective than placebo, unfractionated heparin, warfarin, or aspirin for thromboprophylaxis for orthopedic surgery. LMWH is contraindicated in heparin-associated thrombocytopenia. LMWH therapy is safe during pregnancy because it does not cross the placenta.

Direct Thrombin Inhibitors

The direct thrombin inhibitors are hirudin, lepirudin, bivalirudin, and argatroban. Lepirudin is a recombinant form of hirudin. An APTT ratio of 1.5 to 2.5 has been associated with highest efficacy. The thrombin-specific inhibitors prolong the PT as well as APTT, with APTT as the recommended test.

However, at higher doses and concentrations, APTT is not reliable and is associated with an increased risk of bleeding. Currently, the main use of direct thrombin inhibitors is for type II heparin-induced thrombocytopenia.

Thrombolytic Therapy

The thrombolytic agents are streptokinase, urokinase, recombinant tissue plasminogen activator (t-PA), alteplase (Activase), and reteplase (Retevase), a small t-PA molecule. Fibrin is the major target of thrombolytic therapy. Anticoagulation does *not* dissolve or prevent the growth of thrombi (even at recommended doses), eliminate the source of subsequent emboli in the deep veins during an acute attack, alleviate hemodynamic problems, prevent valvular damage, prevent persistent venous hypertension, or prevent persistent pulmonary hypertension. The primary role of anticoagulation is prophylaxis against further propagation of the clot.

Thrombolytic therapy lyses thrombi and emboli and restores circulation to normal, normalizes hemodynamic disturbances, reduces morbidity, decreases systemic and mean pulmonary artery pressures at 72 hours, prevents venous vascular damage and subsequent venous hypertension in the lower extremities, and prevents permanent damage to the pulmonary vascular bed, decreasing the likelihood of persistent pulmonary hypertension. Residual emboli usually persist with heparin therapy alone. Although t-PA, tenecteplase, and reteplase have a relative fibrin specificity, considerable fibrinolysis and bleeding may occur. The initial fibrinolysis of the plug is followed by proteolysis of fibrinogen and factors V and VIII. Venous thrombi generally are rich in fibrin and are potentially more suitable than platelet thrombi for fibrinolytic therapy. The age of the thrombus is also important because it is essential to start treatment with these agents within 48 hours in cases of pulmonary emboli and in less than 7 days in cases of deep venous thrombosis. In cases of pulmonary emboli, thrombolytic therapy improves hemodynamics and pulmonary perfusion; it may be indicated with the involvement of more lobar pulmonary arteries or an equivalent amount of emboli in other vessels with or without shock or submassive emboli accompanied by shock, impending shock, or persistent hypotension. In deep venous thrombosis, these agents may minimize valvular dysfunction and decrease the risk of recurrent and postphlebitic syndrome. Currently, thrombolytic agents are not recommended for routine use in managing pulmonary emboli and deep venous thrombosis. Thrombolytic treatment should be restricted to and considered for patients with extensive iliofemoral venous thrombosis with a low risk of bleeding and patients with hemodynamic compromise due to pulmonary embolism.

If the timing is appropriate, thrombolytic agents may be administered in thrombosis of the hepatic, renal, mesenteric, cerebrovenous, sinus, and central retinal veins. Of arterial disorders, acute myocardial infarction has been studied most extensively. The SCAT 1 trial demonstrated that mortality was significantly lower among patients randomly assigned to heparin after thrombolytic therapy for acute myocardial infarction. The GUSTO-1 trial showed that rapid infusion of t-PA with intravenously given heparin was slightly more beneficial than streptokinase. The GUSTO-3 trial compared t-PA and reteplase, and there was no significant difference. Reteplase is easier to administer. In ongoing trials studying acute myocardial infarction, the thrombotic occlusion is a fibrin-based plug attached to a fissured atherosclerotic plaque. Other fibrin-specific agents under evaluation include tenecteplase and staphylokinase.

Thrombolytic therapy is monitored with fibrinogen levels. The absolute contraindications to this therapy include active internal bleeding and a cerebrovascular accident within the preceding 2 weeks and surgery within less than 1 month. Relatively major contraindications include the following if they have occurred within less than 10 days: major surgical procedure, obstetrical delivery, pregnancy, the first 10 days postpartum, organ biopsy, burns, skin grafts, previous puncture of noncompressible vessels, thoracentesis, paracentesis, gastrointestinal tract bleeding, ulcerative colitis, diverticulosis, serious trauma, systolic blood pressure greater than 180 mm Hg, diastolic pressure greater than 100 mm Hg, intracranial neoplasms, or thrombocytopenia. Relatively minor contraindications include a high likelihood of left-sided heart thrombus such as mitral stenosis with atrial fibrillation, subacute bacterial endocarditis, severe liver or kidney disease, age older than 75 years, diabetic hemorrhagic retinopathy, active and progressive cavitating lung lesions, ulcerative cutaneous and mucous membrane lesions, and a recent intra-arterial diagnostic procedure except measurement of arterial blood gases. Bleeding may be superficial or internal; it occurs because of the indiscriminate lysis of fibrin. Because thrombolytic agents are not substitutes for heparin and warfarin, the morbidity is additive. Approaches to hemorrhage control include volume replacement, manual techniques, and RBC transfusions. If bleeding is massive, replace with cryoprecipitate and fresh frozen plasma and discontinue treatment with heparin. With central nervous system bleeding, discontinue fibrinolytic therapy, administer cryoprecipitate and fresh frozen plasma, and avoid anticoagulants and antiplatelet agents.

Aplastic Anemia

Aplastic anemia is most often acquired and may develop as a consequence of a defect in the stem cell population, defective marrow microenvironment, or immunologic factors, including antibody-mediated bone marrow suppression, cellular cytolytic suppressive T-cell mechanisms, and bone marrow suppression by cytokines. This group of disorders of failure of hematopoiesis is characterized by peripheral pancytopenia, bone marrow hypocellularity, and the absence of malignant or myeloproliferative diseases at the time of diagnosis. The pathogenesis is heterogeneous and mostly undefined. The differential diagnosis of pancytopenia and hypercellular bone marrow includes aplastic anemia, myelodysplastic syndrome, T-cell clonal disorders, paroxysmal nocturnal hemoglobinuria, and Fanconi anemia. The criteria for the diagnosis of aplastic anemia include less than 25% marrow cellularity and two of the following: neutrophil count less than 0.5×10^9/L, platelet count less than 20×10^9/L, a corrected reticulocyte count less than 1%, and normal cytogenetic findings.

Before the use of allogeneic bone marrow transplantation and antithymocyte globulin, 80% of patients with severe aplastic anemia were not alive at 1 or 2 years and 20% had partial recovery. The only curative treatment available for aplastic anemia is allogeneic stem cell transplantation.

- Aplastic anemia: pancytopenia, hypocellular bone marrow, and absence of primary disease of hematopoietic tissue (myelodysplastic syndrome).
- Full recovery is uncommon without allogeneic bone marrow transplantation or antithymocyte globulin.

The clinical features of aplastic anemia include weakness, fatigue, easy bruising or bleeding, fever, and infections. Lymphadenopathy and splenomegaly are uncommon. In 40% to 70% of patients, the cause of aplastic anemia is idiopathic. An idiopathic cause is more frequent in adults. Drugs are the second most common cause of aplastic anemia. These include chloramphenicol, phenylbutazone, methylphenylethylhydantoin, trimethadione, sulfonamides, gold, and benzene. Paroxysmal nocturnal hemoglobinuria (positive CD59 and CD58 cell surface markers on flow cytometry studies of bone marrow) and infections are the third and fourth most common causes, respectively. Infectious hepatitis is the most common infection to cause aplastic anemia. Non-A, non-B, non-C hepatitis and hepatitis A are the most common types of hepatitis to cause aplastic anemia. Hepatitis B is the type of hepatitis that least often causes aplastic anemia. Other infectious agents that cause aplastic anemia include Epstein-Barr virus, influenza virus, HIV, parvovirus, and mycobacteria. Ionizing radiation may also be a cause.

Patients with aplastic anemia should undergo HLA typing. If transfusion is needed, select nonrelated donors and use cytomegalovirus-negative, leukocyte-poor RBC transfusions and single-donor platelet transfusions to maintain the platelet count greater than 10×10^9/L. Transfusions to maintain the hemoglobin concentration greater than 7 g/dL should be given with considerable care and concern. Family members should not be donors because they are more likely to sensitize the patient to minor histocompatibility antigens present in the donor but absent in the patient. Outcomes of patients undergoing allogeneic bone marrow transplantation for aplastic anemia are significantly adversely affected by previous transfusion. A search for unrelated HLA-matched donors should be considered for patients younger than 30 years without an HLA match.

Immunosuppression is the treatment of choice for patients older than 40 years and includes antithymocyte globulin and corticosteroids and cyclosporine. These agents are not curative. In a trial with patients who had moderate to severe aplastic anemia, 11 of the 21 treated with antithymocyte globulin alone had sustained improvement, compared with none of the 21 patients in the control group. For patients not eligible for bone marrow transplantation, treatment with antithymocyte globulin, methylprednisolone, and cyclosporine has been reported to result in 65% to 70% partial recovery of the peripheral blood counts, with overall long-term responses of 30% to 75%. Blood count recovery usually is not complete; however, transfusions are not required, and the absolute neutrophil count is at a level to protect against infectious complications. About 30% of patients have relapse, and clonal myeloid disorders develop in 25% of patients. Toxic effects of antithymocyte globulin include anaphylaxis, fever, urticaria, thrombocytopenia, and serum sickness. Side effects of long-term cyclosporine therapy include hypertension, renal insufficiency, seizures, and hypomagnesemia. In contrast to stem cell transplantation, patients are not cured.

The allogeneic HLA-matched bone marrow transplantation success rate is 40% to 90% for young patients. This is the therapy of choice for all patients with a homozygous twin and should be considered immediately for all patients younger than 20 years. It also should be considered for high-risk patients between the ages of 20 and 40 with an HLA match. A trial of immunosuppressive therapy is indicated for patients older than 40 years, including those with moderate disease. Graft failure rates are about 10%, and chronic graft-versus-host disease complicates 40% of cases.

Cyclosporine or corticosteroids, at a dose of 0.2 to 1.0 mg/kg daily, and androgens are other treatments. Androgens are not effective in severe aplastic anemia. The toxic effects include virilization and liver toxicity. The 17-alpha derivative is responsible for hepatic adenomas and hepatocellular carcinoma. Mismatched family and unrelated donors have survival rates ranging from 0% to 54%.

- With severe aplastic anemia, transfuse judiciously.
- If the patient is younger than 40 years and has an HLA-matched donor or identical twin, consider bone marrow transplantation with cyclophosphamide alone or cyclophosphamide plus irradiation as preconditioning for patients who previously had transfusion. If the patient is older and has no HLA match, treat with a combination of antithymocyte globulin and methylprednisolone with or without cyclosporine.

● Long-term survival of patients with severe disease has increased from <25% for those given androgens to 75% for those given intensive immunosuppressive therapy and to 66% for those who had bone marrow transplantation.

Neutropenia

The differential diagnosis of nonmalignant acute neutropenia includes decreased production, ineffective granulopoiesis (vitamin B_{12} deficiency, folate deficiency), drugs, infections (HIV, parvovirus, and hepatitis), hematologic disorders (cyclic neutropenia and aplastic anemia), increased destruction, autoimmune neutropenia (Felty syndrome, rheumatoid arthritis, systemic lupus erythematosus, and Sjögren syndrome), hypersplenism, ulcerative colitis, hemodilution, and hematologic disorders (cyclic neutropenia and aplastic anemia). Drug-induced neutropenia is associated with sulfonamides, semisynthetic penicillins (nafcillin, ampicillin), phenothiazines, nonsteroidal anti-inflammatory drugs (indomethacin, phenylbutazone), antithyroid medications (propylthiouracil, methimazole), allopurinol, anticonvulsants, and diuretics (chlorthiazide). Drug-induced neutropenia becomes manifest 1 to 2 weeks after initial drug exposure or sooner following a recent repeat exposure. The treatment of choice is to discontinue the drug. Corticosteroids characteristically are not efficacious.

The differential diagnosis of chronic neutropenia includes cyclic neutropenia and chronic idiopathic neutropenia. Cyclic neutropenia, characterized by oscillations in the neutrophil counts every 19 to 23 days, is a disorder of neutrophil production at a regulation phase. The typical clinical syndrome is manifested as furuncles, cellulitis, chronic gingivitis, and abscesses. Patients can predict the timing of successive episodes. Treatment involves timely antibiotics, avoidance of dental and surgical work at nadirs, oral hygiene, and dental care. G-CSF (filgrastim) may be effective in increasing the neutrophil count in cyclic neutropenia and chronic idiopathic neutropenia.

In the adult population, the recommended dose of G-CSF is 5 µg/kg daily subcutaneously.

The 1999 American Society of Clinical Oncology colony-stimulating factor guidelines emphasized the following: primary prophylaxis is recommended when the incidence of febrile neutropenia is greater than 40% of the control group. Therefore, in general, for previously untreated patients receiving most chemotherapy regimens, primary administration of colony-stimulating factors should not be used routinely. Special circumstances for patients who might benefit from these agents include preexisting neutropenia due to disease, extensive previous chemotherapy, previous irradiation to the pelvis, a history of recurrent febrile neutropenia while receiving earlier chemotherapy, and conditions that potentially enhance the risk of infection (poor performance status, decreased immune function, open wounds, or active tissue infections). There is evidence that colony-stimulating factors can decrease the probability of febrile neutropenia in subsequent cycles of chemotherapy after a documented occurrence in a previous cycle. These agents are effective adjuncts in progenitor-cell transplantation. The data are inadequate to support the routine use of these agents in afebrile patients or the routine use of them in dose-intensity programs. Colony-stimulating factors should be avoided with concomitant chemotherapy or radiotherapy. Granulocyte-macrophage colony-stimulating factor is another available growth factor, but the lack of randomized trials precludes definitive recommendations.

Neutropenia is common among blacks, and if patients are asymptomatic, this need not be evaluated further. Other causes of neutropenia include autoimmune neutropenia (which is due to an antibody), antigens, rheumatoid arthritis, and chronic active hepatitis.

Thrombocytopenia

The causes of isolated thrombocytopenia in adults are numerous and broadly include autoimmune idiopathic thrombocytopenic purpura, drug-induced thrombocytopenia, pseudothrombocytopenia, refractoriness to platelet transfusion therapy, post-transfusion purpura, and hereditary and secondary causes. Secondary causes include pregnancy, antiphospholipid antibodies syndrome, chemotherapy drugs, autoimmune systemic lupus erythematosus (in which 14%-26% of patients develop thrombocytopenia), infections (HIV, hepatitis C, rubella, infectious mononucleosis), chronic lymphocytic leukemia, non-Hodgkin lymphoma, sarcoidosis, ovarian carcinoma, acute alcohol toxicity, and purpura of septicemia. Thrombocytopenia occurs in microangiopathic hemolytic anemias and hypersplenism.

The diagnosis of pseudothrombocytopenia should be excluded with examination of a peripheral blood smear. Causes of pseudothrombocytopenia include EDTA-induced platelet clumping, platelet satellitosis, hereditary disorders (May-Hegglin anomaly, Bernard-Soulier syndrome, and Alport syndrome), and large platelets in myeloproliferative disorders.

A spuriously low platelet count may be reported in EDTA-induced platelet agglutination. This is an antibody-mediated phenomenon caused by antibodies that bind to the patient's platelets after withdrawal of calcium in the test tube. The platelet count is spuriously low with automated techniques only; on the peripheral blood smear, the number is normal because the platelets are clumped or rarely adhere to neutrophils.

Idiopathic thrombocytopenic purpura is an autoimmune disease characterized by thrombocytopenia with a normal WBC count and hemoglobin concentration (Table 11-16). The American Society of Hematology guidelines for this

Table 11-16 Idiopathic Thrombocytopenic Purpura

Characteristics	Acute	Chronic
Presentation	Abrupt onset of petechiae, purpura, mucosal bleeding	Insidious petechiae, menorrhagia
Usual age	Children (2-6 years old)	Adults (20-40 years old)
Sex	Male = female	Female:male = 3:1
Antecedent infection	Common 85%	Uncommon
	Typically an upper respiratory tract infection	
Platelet count, ×10^9/L	<20	30-80
Duration	2-6 weeks	Months to years
Spontaneous remission	80% within 6 months	Uncommon, fluctuates

From Lee GR, Bithell TC, Foerster J, et al: Wintrobe's Clinical Hematology. Vol 2. Ninth edition. Philadelphia, Lea & Febiger, 1993, p 1331. By permission of publisher.

disorder were published in 1996. This group defined idiopathic thrombocytopenic purpura as "isolated thrombocytopenia with no clinically apparent conditions." The diagnosis of idiopathic thrombocytopenic purpura is a diagnosis of exclusion. Patients with risk factors should be tested for HIV antibody. The clinical manifestations include purpura, mucous membrane hemorrhage, and cerebromeningeal bleeding. From 7% to 28% of children and up to 40% to 60% of adults have progression to a chronic state of idiopathic thrombocytopenic purpura. In most patients, the platelet count is less than 50×10^9/L and in 30%, less than 10×10^9/L. The mean platelet volume is increased. Only 10% of patients have splenomegaly. If it is present, one should think of other causes. Bone marrow examination shows a normal to increased number of megakaryocytes. Antibodies to specific platelet-membrane glycoproteins, usually the IIb/IIIa complex, and platelet IgG (erroneously called "antiplatelet-antibody tests") are detected in most patients but are not necessary for diagnosis or treatment. Up to 10% of patients with chronic idiopathic thrombocytopenic purpura may have accessory spleens. The absence of Howell-Jolly bodies on a peripheral blood smear of patients who have previously had splenectomy suggests the diagnosis, which is confirmed by radionuclide imaging or CT. Surgical removal may be beneficial. The measurement of bleeding time is not helpful because it is abnormal, with a platelet count less than 75×10^9/L.

The American Society of Hematology guidelines for treatment are as follows: patients with platelet counts of 50×10^9/L or higher do not routinely require treatment. Those with a platelet count less than 50×10^9/L but greater than 30×10^9/L should be treated if there is mucous membrane bleeding or risk factors for bleeding, including hypertension, peptic ulcer disease, and vigorous lifestyle. Patients with platelet counts less than 30×10^9/L should be treated. Prednisone is the mainstay of initial treatment; initially, 70% of patients have a response, with about a 40% chance of long-term remission at the initial dose of prednisone of 1 mg/kg daily for up to 1 month. Corticosteroids decrease antibody production in the reticuloendothelial system and decrease reticuloendothelial clearance. Patients with severe bleeding should be treated with intravenous immunoglobulin and platelets and transfusion alone or in combination with high-dose intravenous corticosteroids (methylprednisolone, 1 g daily for 2-3 consecutive days; the initial response rate is 80%).

The management of disease that does not respond completely to these measures is difficult and controversial. The American Society of Hematology had no formal recommendations. Splenectomy, the treatment of choice for steroid-refractory idiopathic thrombocytopenic purpura, removes the predominant site of antibody production and platelet destruction; the likelihood of long-term remission is 50% to 75%. Pneumococcal, meningococcal, and *Haemophilus influenzae* vaccines should be administered before splenectomy. Dexamethasone (40 mg daily for 4 sequential days every 28 days for 12 months) is an option for the treatment of resistant idiopathic thrombocytopenic purpura or disease relapse. Danazol decreases the number of phagocytic cell IgG Fc receptors. A slow infusion of vincristine or vinblastine may be given to patients who do not have a response to the above measures. Other agents used in refractory cases include azathioprine (Imuran), cyclophosphamide, colchicine, cyclosporine, and immunoadsorption apheresis on staphylococcal protein A columns.

- Spontaneous bleeding may occur with platelet counts less than 10×10^9/L.
- Idiopathic thrombocytopenic purpura is a diagnosis of exclusion.

- The diagnosis rests on the history, screen for drugs and alcohol, physical examination, and the CBC.
- Examine the peripheral blood smear (exclude microangiopathy).
- Consider discontinuing any drug that may cause the disease.
- A bone marrow examination is appropriate to establish the diagnosis of idiopathic thrombocytopenic purpura in patients older than 60 years and in patients considered candidates for splenectomy.
- In idiopathic thrombocytopenic purpura with severe bleeding, intravenous immunoglobulin is the treatment of choice, with platelet transfusions and high-dose corticosteroids.

In drug-induced thrombocytopenia, the pathophysiologic mechanism is related to haptens bound to a carrier protein. Clinically, there is acute bleeding, with a hemorrhage syndrome characterized by bleeding from mucous membranes, petechiae, and oozing after brushing the teeth. These problems subside after use of the drug is discontinued. Drug-induced thrombocytopenia subsides in 4 to 14 days except for gold, which may take much longer. In contrast, viral-induced thrombocytopenia resolves in 2 weeks to 3 months. The drugs most commonly implicated include heparin, quinidine, quinine, valproic acid, gold, trimethoprim-sulfamethoxazole, amphotericin B, carbamazepine, chlorthiazide, chlorpropamide, procainamide, rifampin, and vancomycin. Glycoprotein IIb/IIIa antagonists, drugs that inhibit the interaction with fibrinogen and platelet interaction, may cause thrombocytopenia (abciximab [ReoPro], eptifibatide [Integrilin], tirofiban [Aggrastat]) and may cause acute (within 24 hours) or delayed (up to 14 days after initiating chronic therapy) thrombocytopenia in 0.5% to 2.0% of patients secondary to antibodies.

Heparin-induced thrombocytopenia (HIT) is a clinicopathologic syndrome that has a variable incidence of 1% to 7.8% and is patient-population dependent. Type I HIT occurs early, is associated with intravenous heparin, and is a common transient nonimmunologic event of no clinical relevance due to direct heparin-induced platelet aggregation. Type II HIT is an immunologic reaction caused by IgG antibodies to an antigen (platelet factor 4 bound to heparin) that activates platelets through their Fc receptors. The platelet counts usually decrease 50% or more, and such a decrease should raise clinical suspicion, even if the count is greater than 150×10^9/L. The coagulation system may be activated, increasing the production of thrombin. Thrombosis occurs in 10% of patients. HIT may develop in patients who were exposed to heparin in the previous 120 days, with thrombocytopenia developing within hours after rechallenge. HIT thrombosis can occur 5 to 19 days after the cessation of heparin therapy. Venous thrombosis (deep venous thrombosis and pulmonary embolus) is more common than arterial thrombosis. Other clinical events include warfarin-induced venous limb damage, acute platelet activation syndromes (fevers, chills, or transient amnesia) 5 to 30 minutes after an intravenous bolus of heparin, or skin lesions at the site of injection of heparin (necrosis or erythematous plaques). The diagnosis may be confirmed by functional assays (serotonin release assay) or antigen assays (antibody against platelet factor 4).

The treatment of HIT is complex. Heparin should be discontinued. The subsequent risk of thrombosis with discontinuing heparin or substituting warfarin is as high as 50%. It is monitored by the APTT (1.5-3.0 times normal). Thromboembolectomy may be considered. LMWH cannot be used because of the high cross reactivity of the antibody with the LMWH/platelet factor IV complex. Alternatives to heparin include a low-molecular-weight heparinoid (danaparoid, 750 anti-Xa units twice daily) or a thrombin inhibitor (lepirudin) or argatroban. In the intensive care unit, infusion of factor VIIa at a dose of 90 mg/kg may be considered in the initial management because thrombin inhibitors do not immediately reverse anticoagulation. Argatroban is the treatment of choice for patients on dialysis because it is not excreted by the kidneys.

The risk varies with the dose of heparin, the type of heparin (unfractionated > LMWH > porcine > bovine) and clinical associations (higher risk for surgical than for medical patients). HIT is usually mild, and the patients are asymptomatic. It develops 3 to 15 days (median, 10 days) after therapy. It is not dose-related and can occur at very low doses. There are no reliable risk factors. Patients are at higher risk if there is a history of this problem. It is essential to pay attention to any substantial decrease in platelet number while patients are taking heparin.

- From 6% to 8% of pregnant women at term and 25% of women with preeclampsia have mild thrombocytopenia with platelets $>80\times10^9$/L.
- Drug-induced thrombocytopenia subsides in 4-14 days, except for gold.
- Viral-induced thrombocytopenia resolves in 2 weeks to 3 months.
- Heparin is the drug that most commonly causes thrombocytopenia.

The management of idiopathic thrombocytopenic purpura in pregnancy is complex. The American Society of Hematology consensus panel recommended intravenous immunoglobulin for pregnant women with severe and symptomatic thrombocytopenia. The recommendations for percutaneous umbilical sampling, fetal scalp vein monitoring at the time of delivery, and the route of delivery are controversial. Neonatal hemorrhagic complications are low. After delivery, infant platelet counts should be followed for 4 days. Intravenous immunoglobulin is recommended for platelet counts less than 20×10^9/L, and brain imaging of the infant is recommended for platelet counts less than 50×10^9/L.

For chemotherapy-associated thrombocytopenia, the threshold for platelet transfusion is 10,000 cells/μL. Interleukin-11 is the only pharmacologic agent that is approved in the United States. It is modestly effective and associated with cytokine toxicities.

Thrombocytopenia in Pregnancy

The most common cause of thrombocytopenia in pregnancy is incidental thrombocytopenia of pregnancy, which occurs in 5% of pregnancies and accounts for 75% of cases and is not associated with adverse maternal or fetal outcomes. The diagnosis is one of exclusion. No treatment is required.

Other common causes include preeclampsia, idiopathic autoimmune thrombocytopenia (idiopathic thrombocytopenic purpura), HIV infection, and thrombotic thrombocytopenic purpura. Of women with preeclampsia, 50% are thrombocytopenic. No specific therapy is required, and platelet recovery occurs 72 hours after delivery. Thrombocytopenia may occur in 3% of pregnant women with HIV infection. Intravenous immunoglobulin is effective therapy.

Other causes of thrombocytopenia in pregnancy include acute fatty liver of pregnancy, drugs (quinine/quinidine, cocaine, and heparin), folate deficiency, infections (cytomegalovirus), and antiphospholipid antibody-related thrombocytopenia. HELLP syndrome is a variant of preeclampsia. Disseminated intravascular coagulopathy develops in up to 38% of pregnant women. The primary treatment of HELLP syndrome is stabilization of the patient's condition and delivery of the fetus.

Post-Transfusion Purpura

In post-transfusion purpura, thrombocytopenia occurs 5 to 8 days after blood transfusion in patients alloimmunized against the platelet antigen HPA-1a. The treatment of choice is intravenous administration of immunoglobulin and corticosteroids.

Postsplenectomy State

Postsplenectomy complications include sepsis due to pneumococcus, meningococcus, *Haemophilus influenzae*, *E. coli*, and *Staphylococcus aureus*. Hematologic features include such RBC abnormalities as Howell-Jolly bodies present on the peripheral blood smear. The leukocyte count has a postsplenectomy surge and then returns to normal. Platelets also show a postsplenectomy surge; the value usually returns to normal in 1 month. If there is a history of splenectomy but no Howell-Jolly bodies on a peripheral blood smear, suspect an accessory spleen and confirm it with a liver-spleen scan.

Spontaneous Splenic Ruptures

Spontaneous splenic ruptures have been reported to occur in infectious mononucleosis, cytomegalovirus infections, acute and chronic myelogenous leukemia, acute and chronic lymphocytic leukemia, myeloproliferative diseases, and non-Hodgkin lymphoma.

Transfusion Reactions

The primary cause of transfusion-related deaths is medical error, which includes bypassed safeguards, similar patient names, and verbal or faxed communications. The major transfusion reactions include acute hemolytic transfusion reactions, transfusions associated with anti-IgA antibodies, transfusion-associated adult respiratory distress syndrome, delayed hemolytic transfusion reactions, febrile transfusion reactions, urticarial transfusion reactions, and circulatory overload (Table 11-17).

Acute hemolytic transfusion reactions are the most life-threatening. These occur within minutes to hours and are caused by preexisting RBC antibodies in the recipient. The most common cause is human error, especially when blood is released on an emergency basis, and these are due to ABO mismatches. Of fatal transfusion reactions, 85% involve ABO incompatibility. Other causes include antibodies not detected before transfusion, such as Kell, Duffy (Jk^a), and Kidd (Fy^a). ABO mismatches are less frequent than with Kell, Duffy, and

Table 11-17 Risks of Complications From Transfusions in the United States

Complication	Risk per unit
Minor allergic reaction	3/100
Circulatory overload	Unknown
Febrile, nonhemolytic	3/100
Delayed hemolytic transfusion reaction	1/4,000
Transfusion-related acute lung injury (TRALI)	1/10,000
Acute hemolytic transfusion reaction	1/250,000-1/1.0 million
HIV infection	1/1.4-1/2.0 million
Hepatitis B	1/60,000-1/200,000
Hepatitis C	1/800,000-1/2.0 million
HTLV I/II infection	1/200,000
Bacterial infections	1/2,000-1/500,000
IgA-related anaphylaxis	1/100,000
Graft-versus-host disease	Rare
Immunosuppression	Unknown
Post-transfusion purpura	Rare

HIV, human immunodeficiency virus; HTLV, human T-cell leukemia virus.

Kidd and have virtually disappeared from transfusion reaction complications, but clerical error may be a factor in the occurence of these reactions. Intravascular hemolysis is caused by problems related to ABO, Kell, Duffy, and Kidd. Females are at greater risk than males, because sensitization through pregnancy leads to a higher frequency of preformed antibodies. The recipient's preexisting antibodies, usually IgM, bind to the donor's RBCs and cause complement-mediated hemolysis. Obstetrical complications with massive bleeding also predispose females to acute hemolytic transfusion reactions. Age is a factor because older people receive more transfusions. Transfusion of large amounts of blood products given urgently also increases the risk. Clinically, there is pain at the intravenous site, apprehension, back pain, abdominal pain, fever, chills, chest pain, hypotension, nausea, flushing, and dyspnea. The Coombs test gives positive results in all but anti-A.

Complications include oliguria in 33.3% of patients, acute postischemic renal failure, and disseminated intravascular coagulopathy in 4%. The mortality rate is about 20%. Treatment includes immediate termination of the transfusion, intravenous access, vigorous administration of fluids, and furosemide to increase renal cortical blood flow. It is difficult to distinguish between an acute hemolytic transfusion reaction and a febrile nonhemolytic transfusion reaction at the time fever occurs. Therefore, fevers occurring during transfusion should be worked up for hemolysis.

Transfusion reactions associated with anti-IgA antibodies and anaphylactic reactions are due to IgA deficiency, the development of a class-specific anti-IgA antibody, normal IgA levels with anti-IgA antibodies acquired through pregnancy or previous transfusions, and ataxia-telangiectasia, in which 44% of patients have class-specific anti-IgA antibodies. The pathogenesis is due to anti-IgA antibodies of IgG type that are capable of binding complement. Clinically, patients develop apprehension, hives, hypotension, chest pain, abdominal pain, lumbar pain, flushing of the face and neck, dyspnea, and cyanosis. Wheezing, diarrhea, vomiting, unconsciousness, and chills may occur. Fevers are uncommon. Treatment includes stopping the transfusion and giving antihistamines and conventional anti-anaphylactic drugs. Transfusion policies for patients include an IgG anti-IgA antibody, washed RBCs, frozen RBCs, and IgA-deficient plasma.

Transfusion-associated adult respiratory distress syndrome or transfusion-related acute lung injury (TRALI) is a complication of transfusion that is often undiagnosed and ranks third among causes of transfusion-related deaths. It is characterized by respiratory distress in 1 to 6 hours after transfusion, hypotension, bilateral pulmonary infiltrates, normal or low pulmonary capillary wedge pressure, and fever. Recovery is rapid, occurring in 24 to 48 hours. Most blood donors implicated in this complication have had multiple pregnancies.

Possible mechanisms include leukoagglutinins in plasma or HLA-specific lymphocytotoxic antibodies passively transfused from the donor to the recipient, resulting in polymorphonuclear leukocyte-complement–triggered microvascular injury and pulmonary edema. The treatment is supportive. Essentially all patients require oxygen. Many patients require a ventilator with positive end-expiratory pressure and dopamine. This disorder may be misdiagnosed as circulatory overload. From 5% to 8% of patients die of complications of the pulmonary injury.

Delayed hemolytic transfusion reactions (1/4,000 transfusions) occur because of the inability to detect clinically significant recipient antibodies before transfusion. This transfusion reaction, which usually occurs 5 to 10 days after transfusion, is less dramatic and less dangerous than acute hemolytic reactions and is more common in females. The recipient's plasma already contains antibody before transfusion because of previous transfusion or previous pregnancy. It usually involves the Rh or Kidd system. The antibodies become undetectable because of low antibody titers and increase quickly in titer on rapid stimulation. Results of the Coombs test are positive. There is evidence of hemolysis. One-third of patients are asymptomatic, and the others present with anemia, chills, jaundice, and fever. Management consists of monitoring hemoglobin concentration and renal output.

Urticarial reactions are a complication in 3% of transfusions. Glottal edema and asthma are rarely associated with urticarial transfusion reactions. The cause is an antibody in the recipient against foreign-donor serum proteins. Treatment consists of stopping the transfusion, which is not absolutely necessary, and giving antihistamines (premedication with antihistamines if the patient had a previous reaction).

Febrile reactions are characterized by chills and fever an hour after the transfusion starts, with accompanying flushing, headache, tachycardia, and discomfort lasting 8 to 10 hours. This occurs in 1% of all transfusions. The causes include cytokines from WBCs and platelets against donor antigens and antiserum protein antibodies. Treatment consists of stopping the transfusion to evaluate the problem further; initially, a febrile reaction cannot be distinguished from a hemolytic transfusion reaction because both conditions may present with fever. Preventive methods include blood filters.

Circulatory overload may cause tightness in the chest, dry cough, and acute edema in patients with an already increased intravascular volume or decreased cardiac reserve. This is a frequently overlooked diagnosis. Symptoms generally develop within several hours after transfusion. Management includes slowing the transfusion to 100 mL an hour, placing the patient in the sitting position, and giving diuretics.

Post-transfusion purpura is a rare syndrome characterized by the abrupt onset of severe thrombocytopenia 5 to 10 days after blood transfusion; the estimated mortality is 10% to 15%. Most cases involve patients whose platelets lack the P1A1 antigen and who have developed an antibody from a previous pregnancy or transfusion. Therapy usually is successful. Intravenous immunoglobulin at a dose of 400 to 500 mg/kg is the treatment of choice. Plasma exchange and corticosteroids are alternative treatments.

Pathogen transmission may occur with transfusions. These risks are summarized in Table 11-17.

- The most common cause of acute hemolytic transfusion reaction is clerical error.
- The risk of HIV transmission via transfusion is <1/500,000-1/1.5 million.

Thrombopoietin

Thrombopoietin and interleukin-11 have been approved for secondary prophylaxis against chemotherapy-induced thrombocytopenia. In clinical practice, even severe treatment-related thrombocytopenia only rarely leads to death or life-threatening illness because transfusion of platelet concentrates ensures that very few patients with thrombocytopenia die of hemorrhage.

Gaucher Disease

Adults have type 1 Gaucher disease, with no neurologic symptoms, splenomegaly, and no symptoms; 50% have anemia or thrombocytopenia. Bone lesions are present in 75% of patients, with the femur most commonly having an Erlenmeyer flask deformity. Avascular necrosis and pathologic fractures may occur. The pathogenesis is related to an accumulation of glucosylceramide from deficient β-glucuronidase. The Gaucher cell is large and has an eccentric nucleus and fibrillar cytoplasm that is wrinkled like tissue paper (Plate 11-18). Treatment options include alglucerase (Ceredase) (an enzyme replacement therapy that is extraordinarily expensive), hemisplenectomy, and allogeneic bone marrow transplantation.

- The differential diagnosis of asymptomatic massive splenomegaly includes Gaucher disease, agnogenic myeloid metaplasia, chronic myelogenous leukemia, portal hypertension, splenic cyst, non-Hodgkin lymphoma, and hairy cell leukemia.

Porphyria

The porphyrias are enzyme disorders that are autosomal dominant with low disease penetrance, except for congenital erythropoietic porphyria, which is autosomal recessive, and porphyria cutanea tarda, which may be acquired. Most persons remain biochemically and clinically normal throughout life. Clinical expression is linked to environmental and acquired factors.

Disease manifestations depend on the type of excess porphyrin intermediate. When there is an excess of the earlier precursor molecules (δ-aminolevulinic acid and porphobilinogen), the clinical manifestations are neuropsychiatric. These symptoms include autonomic dysfunction (abdominal pain, vomiting, constipation, tachycardia, and hypertension), psychiatric symptoms, fever, leukocytosis, syndrome of inappropriate antidiuretic hormone, and neurologic symptoms (proximal paresis and paresthesias). If the excess is in the distal intermediates (uroporphyrins, coproporphyrins, and protoporphyrins), the manifestations are cutaneous (photosensitivity, blister formation, facial hypertrichosis, and hyperpigmentation). If the excess is early and late, there are neuropsychiatric and cutaneous manifestations. Porphobilinogen production and excretion are invariably increased during marked symptoms caused by the three neuropathic porphyrias, which include acute intermittent porphyria, hereditary coproporphyria, and porphyria variegata. In hereditary coproporphyria and porphyria variegata, there is an accumulation of coproporphyrinogen/coproporphyrin or protoporphyrinogen/protoporphyrin and a concomitant increase in δ-aminolevulinic acid and porphobilinogen. In the acute porphyrias, urinary porphobilinogen is increased during the attacks. Acute intermittent porphyria lacks skin lesions. It is important to check fecal porphyrins in protoporphyria, porphyria variegata, and coproporphyria. The porphyrias are compared in Table 11-18. Secondary coproporphyrinuria has many causes, including impaired hepatobiliary transport of coprophyrin (steroids) or increased liver or erythroid synthesis (alcohol, liver disease, or hemolytic anemia).

- Determine the 24-hour urinary porphobilinogen during the acute episode.

Cardiac Toxicity of Chemotherapeutic Agents

Doxorubicin has the greatest potential for cardiac toxicity. It is dose-limited at a dose of 450 mg/m^2 to 500 mg/m^2. The course is characterized by cardiomyopathy to congestive heart failure to death. The pathologic features are characterized by a diffuse patchy myocardial cell degeneration that antedates any alteration in left ventricular function. Risk factors include age older than 70 years, coronary artery disease, hypertension, combination chemotherapy and previous or concomitant mediastinal radiotherapy, and the use of other cardiotoxic agents. Weekly and prolonged continuous infusion schedules may decrease the risk of toxicity. Acutely, there may be transient and reversible nonspecific ST-segment changes, a decrease in ejection fraction, or arrhythmias. The dilated cardiomyopathy is dose-dependent: a 3.5% risk at a total dose of 400 mg/m^2, 7% at a dose of 500 to 550 mg/m^2, and 36% at a total dose of 600 mg/m^2 or greater. The clinical features of the cardiomyopathy vary widely. Follow-up examination requires evaluating left

Table 11-18   Comparison of Porphyrias

Porphyria cutanea tarda	Acute intermittent porphyria	Porphyria variegata
Features		
Most common Iron overload Skin lesions on light-exposed areas Hypertrichosis Increased uroporphyrins in urine No neuropathic features Most common of porphyrias	Increased urinary δ-aminolevulinic acid and porphobilinogen Triad: abdominal pain of 3-5 days' duration, neurologic problems of polyneuropathy & motor paresis, psychiatric problems with hallucinations, confusion, psychosis, seizures Decreased porphobilinogen deaminase Normal protoporphyrin & coproporphyrin in stool	Clinically: skin, sun-exposed, mechanical fragility; abdominal pain; neurologic problems (e.g., acute intermittent porphyria) Increased protoporphyrin & coproporphyrin in stool
Associations		
Alcoholic liver disease Estrogens: females, males treated for prostatic carcinoma Hexachlorobenzene	Drugs: sulfonamides, barbiturates, alcohol Menstrual cycle Infection Inadequate nutrition Stress: infections, surgery	Common in South Africa, Holland
Treatment		
Phlebotomy, to remove iron Chloroquine Low-dose antimalarials	Avoid prolonged fasting & crash diets Large amounts of carbohydrate (400 g daily) Intravenous hematin Luteinizing hormone-releasing hormone agonists	

ventricular ejection fraction by radionuclide ventriculography or echocardiography. The former is more sensitive.

- Doxorubicin has the greatest potential for cardiac toxicity.
- The incidence of cardiomyopathy is dose-dependent.
- Age >70 years, coronary artery disease, and previous irradiation may potentiate toxicity.

Superior Vena Cava Syndrome

Most cases (78%) of superior vena cava syndrome are caused by malignancy. Extrinsic compression of the thin superior vena cava, which has a low intravascular pressure, in a rigid compartment is the pathophysiologic basis of this syndrome. The causes include bronchogenic carcinoma (75% of cases, with small cell and squamous cell carcinoma most common), lymphoma (15%), testicular carcinoma (consider this if biopsy shows anaplastic or undifferentiated carcinoma; check the β-subunit of human chorionic gonadotropin and alpha fetoprotein), carcinoma, and adenocarcinoma of undetermined primary. The symptoms include suffusion of the face and conjunctiva, dyspnea, facial swelling, other swelling, cough, dysphagia, syncope, orthopnea, stridor, and lethargy. Physical examination demonstrates thoracic vein distention, neck vein distention, facial edema, cyanosis, edema of the upper extremities, paralyzed vocal cord, Horner syndrome, and heart murmurs. The diagnosis is established by the history and physical examination findings. Superior vena cava venography is not useful. A tissue diagnosis is essential to establish the diagnosis precisely. Mediastinotomy is the safest way to obtain a histologic diagnosis. If the syndrome is rapid in onset, treatment must be rapid. For patients with lymphoma, testicular carcinoma, or small cell carcinoma of the lung, treat the underlying disease initially with chemotherapy. If life-threatening problems are present, such as tracheal obstruction or increased intracranial pressure, emergency radiotherapy may be necessary in any disorder presenting with superior vena cava syndrome. Steroids may be helpful. Initial treatment with irradiation is indicated for solid tumors, with a total dose of 30 to 50 Gy or a single dose of 7 to 12 Gy. Anticoagulation is indicated only if a blood clot has been implicated in the pathophysiology. Diuretics and surgical decompression are not indicated.

- For superior vena cava syndrome, establish a tissue diagnosis.
- Features: edema of the face and neck and venous engorgement of the upper torso.
- It is a medical emergency in certain situations; immediate irradiation may be required.

Hypercalcemia

Virtually any malignancy may lead to hypercalcemia. Specific causes include carcinomas of the breast and lung (squamous and large cell carcinoma are common causes and adenocarcinoma and small cell carcinoma are uncommon causes), hypernephroma, other tumors (head and neck, cervix, prostate, neuroblastoma, hepatoma, and melanoma), lymphoma, Burkitt lymphoma, multiple myeloma, Hodgkin disease, chronic myelogenous leukemia, and Waldenström macroglobulinemia.

The signs and symptoms include lassitude, somnolence, weakness, anorexia, nausea, vomiting, constipation, abdominal pain, peptic ulcer, pancreatitis, polyuria, polydipsia, poor intake, renal failure, hyporeflexia, Babinski sign, myopathy, stupor, coma, occasional localizing signs, visual abnormalities, psychotic behavior, bradycardia, tachycardia, shortened QT interval, digitalis sensitivity, arrhythmias, hypertension, fractures, pain, skeletal deformities, loss of height, poor skin turgor, calcinosis, and band keratopathy. It is misdiagnosed as terminal disease, brain metastases, drug toxicity, renal failure, diabetes insipidus, acute abdomen, and intractable peptic ulcer disease. The diagnosis can be confirmed by measuring serum levels of parathyroid hormone (PTH). These levels are low in malignancy and increased in primary hyperparathyroidism.

- Misdiagnoses include terminal disease, brain metastases, drug toxicity, renal failure, diabetes insipidus, acute abdomen, and intractable peptic ulcer disease.

The mechanisms of action of hypercalcemia are multiple. Osteolytic metastases may produce accelerated skeletal resorption. Osteoclast activating factors are associated with multiple myeloma, lymphoma, and Burkitt non-Hodgkin lymphoma. Other factors include dehydration, mobilization, adrenal

insufficiency due to tumor metastases, estrogens, androgens, progestins, and tamoxifen.

Most hypercalcemia is related to increased bone resorption. Intestinal absorption is low or low-normal in most cases. There usually is no increase in renal tubular reabsorption, but the kidney may be involved in hyperparathyroidism, breast cancer, metabolic alkalosis, and salt depletion. The course is short and rapidly progressive. There may be moderate to severe weight loss and no renal calculi; pancreatitis is rare. The serum level of calcium is greater than 14 mg/dL in 75% of patients. The serum level of alkaline phosphatase may be increased, normal, or decreased. Anemia and metabolic alkalosis may be present. The alkaline phosphatase level is increased in 50% of patients but can be increased in primary hyperparathyroidism. Hypophosphatemia can occur whether or not there is a PTH-secreting tumor. Hypoalbuminemia must be considered, and for every gram of albumin below 4, add 1 g to the ionized calcium.

Treatment is multifaceted. The use of such precipitating factors as vitamins A and D, lithium, thiazides, absorbable antacids, and estrogens should be discontinued. The patient should be mobilized. Also, the patient should be hydrated with a minimum of 2.5 to 4 L of fluid in the first 24 hours. To each liter of normal saline, add 20 to 40 mEq of potassium chloride and 10 to 20 mEq of magnesium. Experimentally, if the sodium is increased from 25 mEq to 250 mEq, calcium excretion is increased threefold and is not related to the glomerulofiltration rate. Treat the underlying disease.

Glucocorticoids are efficacious in multiple myeloma and non-Hodgkin lymphomas. The typical dose is 80 mg of prednisone in divided doses daily. The mechanisms of action include antitumor effects, an antivitamin D effect, inhibition of prostaglandin synthesis or release, inhibition of osteoclast-activating factor production, anti-PTH activity, and an inhibitory effect on osteoprogenitor cells. Furosemide should be administered after 2 L of fluid. The dosages are variable, ranging from 20 to 40 mg up to every 4 hours. Furosemide blocks the tubular reabsorption of calcium, depletes sodium, depletes potassium, and depletes magnesium. The bisphosphonates have an inhibitory effect on osteoclast function and viability. Etidronate at a dose of 7.5 mg/kg over 4 hours is given intravenously up to 7 days. This decreases calcium within 2 days. Pamidronate is given by intravenous infusion at a dose of 15 to 45 mg daily for up to 6 days. Alternatively, 90 mg may be given over 24 hours or it may be administered orally at a dose of 1,200 mg for up to 5 days. In general, the bisphosphonates are more potent than calcitonin and less toxic than plicamycin. Plicamycin inhibits RNA synthesis in osteoclasts. There may be subjective improvement within 12 hours and improvement in the serum levels of calcium in 36 hours. The dose is 25 µg/kg over 4 hours and may be repeated once if necessary. Side effects include thrombocytopenia, hemorrhage, renal complications, increased liver enzymes, sudden arterial occlusion, and toxic epidermal necrolysis. Contraindications include thrombocytopenia and coagulopathy. The use of phosphate should be restricted to extreme life-threatening hypercalcemia. Calcium phosphate complexes are deposited in vessels, lungs, and kidneys.

HEMOCHROMATOSIS

Hemochromatosis is the end result of a pathologic process that evolves over years and is due to the excessive absorption of dietary iron. The causes of hemochromatosis include hereditary hemochromatosis (idiopathic), secondary anemia and ineffective erythropoiesis (thalassemia major, thalassemia minor), hereditary spherocytosis, idiopathic refractory sideroblastic anemia and myelodysplasia, oral intake of iron (medicinal), liver disease (alcoholic cirrhosis, portal caval anastomosis), drugs (isoniazid, chloramphenicol), and copper deficiency. Patients with end-stage disease present with endocrine complications and hepatic fibrosis.

Hereditary hemochromatosis is a potentially fatal disorder that is among the most common deleterious genes in whites of North America and Europe and is as prevalent as the sickle cell gene in African Americans. The prevalence is 1:300. The gene for hereditary hemochromatosis has been identified and designated the *HFE* gene. This is detectable with a polymerase chain reaction assay. The HLA-linked HFE protein is present within most cells of the body, where it interacts with the transferrin receptor. Mutations in the protein alter the regulatory functions, resulting in unimpeded iron uptake by duodenal mucosal cells. These homozygotes typically develop clinical evidence of hemochromatosis. Family studies are essential because a substantial number of homozygous relatives of patients with hemophilia have complications of hemochromatosis yet to be detected. It is inherited as an autosomal recessive trait. Males present with the disease in the fourth to fifth decade.

About half of the persons who are homozygous for *HFE* have no signs or symptoms. Nearly every organ system can be involved. Initial symptoms include fatigue, impotence (males), amenorrhea (females), abdominal pain, and atrial fibrillation. The transferrin saturation (serum iron/total iron-binding capacity) is greater than 50% even early in life and before tissue iron loading occurs. Screening appears to be effective and should be considered at about age 30 for men. For a young woman, it is necessary to ascertain whether or not she is taking oral contraceptives, which may increase the transferrin saturation. This should be repeated after iron therapy has been discontinued, when the patient is not taking oral contraceptive pills, and when the patient is fasting, and it should be repeated with a ferritin assay to evaluate the total iron-binding content.

The screening test advocated most for homozygotes is a transferrin saturation greater than 50%. Urine iron is increased in the range of 5 to 20 mg per 24 hours (normal, <2 mg per 24 hours). Liver biopsy defines the degree of iron overload and the status of the liver (fibrosis, cirrhosis, and hepatitis). The reference standard for diagnosis is liver biopsy, and hepatic iron by dry weight is markedly increased at 200 to 1,800 µg/100 ng dry weight (normal, 30 to 140). Supporting evidence is also provided by the amount of iron removed by venesection therapy (>5 g) and pedigree studies. Family members, including all first-degree relatives (parents, siblings, and children), should have screening tests. DNA analysis is recommended and may be a reasonable alternative to liver biopsy in asymptomatic patients.

The goal of treatment is to improve prognosis and the clinical course in patients with established liver damage. The mainstays of treatment are phlebotomy and chelation until the ferritin level is less than 20 µg/L; 200 to 250 mg of iron are removed per phlebotomy unit. Patients initially have venesection once to twice weekly until the ferritin concentration is less than 20 µg/L. Maintenance phlebotomies are required, typically every 3 months. Iron chelation therapy is not appropriate because of cost and inconvenience. Deferoxamine (10 mg daily by continuous infusion) is the chelation agent used most often.

Timely diagnosis and therapy can prevent irreversible organ failure. Features not altered by chelation include arthropathy, hormonal inefficiencies, liver cirrhosis, development of hepatocellular carcinoma, and diabetes mellitus. Adverse prognostic factors include cirrhosis and diabetes mellitus. Liver transplantation has a role in the management of these patients. Patients who begin treatment before end-organ damage have a normal life span. The risk to siblings is 25%; thus, all of them should have screening tests for iron or genetic testing.

- Endocrine dysfunction: 50% with diabetes mellitus at presentation and a minority have vascular sequelae; hypogonadism (decreased libido, impotence, and amenorrhea); hypopituitarism.
- Cardiac: congestive heart failure and arrhythmias.
- Skin: bronze, "slate gray."
- Arthropathy: chondrocalcinosis, bone cysts, and irregularity.
- Hepatomegaly, abdominal pain, cirrhosis, and hepatocellular carcinoma; 30% of patients with cirrhosis develop hepatocellular carcinoma.
- Transferrin saturation >50% on at least two occasions should raise clinical suspicion.
- After an index case is identified, first-degree relatives must have screening tests.
- The gene for hereditary hemochromatosis and two mutations, C282Y and H63D, have been defined: *HFE*.

- About 82% of patients with clinically severe hereditary hemochromatosis of European descent are homozygous for the hemoglobin HFE mutation.
- The molecular genetics of non-HLA-linked African hemochromatosis has not been elucidated.
- Treatment: phlebotomy.
- Typical clinical scenario: The patient is asymptomatic but has fatigue, impotence, amenorrhea, abdominal pain, and atrial fibrillation. The ferritin level and iron-binding capacity are increased.

HEMATOLOGY OF ACQUIRED IMMUNODEFICIENCY

In AIDS, lymphocytopenias are the hallmark of the disease. There is an absolute decrease of T4 lymphocytes, with a relative reduction of the T4:T8 ratio. Also, T4 lymphocytes are functionally impaired. Whereas T8 lymphocytes may increase early in the disease during infection, they decrease in number late in the disease. Neutropenia occurs in 50% of the patients. Natural killer cells are normal in number but altered in function. Neutropenia may be due to autoimmune destruction with antigranulocyte antibodies in two-thirds of patients, decreased production, zidovudine (AZT), ganciclovir, trimethoprim-sulfamethoxazole, pentamidine, coexisting infections, non-Hodgkin lymphoma, or antineoplastic chemotherapy. Neutrophil dysfunction is also manifested by decreased chemotaxis, granulation, and phagocytosis.

Anemia occurs in 70% of HIV-infected patients. Most commonly, the anemia is normochromic normocytic. The degree of anemia is a prognostic factor. Anemia occurs in 10% of asymptomatic HIV-positive patients, in 50% of patients with AIDS-related complex, and in more than 75% of patients with overt AIDS. HIV-associated RBC problems include decreased RBC production; 70% of AIDS patients have decreased erythropoietin levels. Approximately 25% of patients have positive results on the Coombs test, but marked hemolysis is not common. Of patients treated with zidovudine, 30% develop pronounced anemia, which is characteristically macrocytic. Decreased RBC production is a principal cause. Erythropoietin has been given successfully to those with an erythropoietin level less than 500 IU/mL. Clinical studies have demonstrated that transfusions may decrease survival and increase the risk of cytomegalovirus infection. Anemia is also associated with infections from *Mycobacterium avium* complex, parvovirus B19, *M. tuberculosis*, and *Histoplasma* species. Anemia may be malignancy-related. Decreased vitamin B_{12} levels are detected in 20% of HIV-infected patients and are due to altered serum transport of vitamin B_{12} and not to a deficiency in body stores unless there has been prolonged malabsorption. Microangiopathic hemolytic anemia is milder than with other causes of this disorder. Plasmapheresis with plasma exchange is the treatment of choice. Vincristine may be efficacious in refractory cases.

Thrombocytopenia occurs in 40% of HIV-infected patients and is often detected early in the disease. Platelet survival is decreased in HIV-infected patients. The serum and cell-bound antibodies are frequently positive. Circulating complexes are either the cause of or are associated with immune cytopenias. Idiopathic thrombocytopenic purpura is usually accompanied by platelet-associated antibodies and responds to zidovudine (80% of patients), prednisone (90%), danazol, dapsone (60%), immunoglobulin given intravenously, and splenectomy (80%). Other HIV associations include thrombotic thrombocytopenic purpura, decreased platelet production, and peripheral platelet sequestration. Other and non-HIV associations include therapy, infection, and malignancy. Coagulation disorders may complicate HIV disorders. The lupus-like anticoagulant is present in 20% of HIV patients, usually in association with opportunistic infections, and is rarely associated with thrombosis or bleeding. Vitamin K deficiencies due to nutritional abnormalities, drugs, or liver dysfunction may occur. Other problems include increased level of vWF:Ag (with a poor prognosis if >200%), increased level of t-PA (with a poor prognosis if >20 ng/mL), and increased level of fibrinogen.

Non-Hodgkin lymphoma is the second most common HIV-associated malignancy, occurring in 2.9% of patients. Extranodal disease occurs in 66% of patients. Up to one-third of patients with lymphoma may have bone involvement. There is also an increased risk of Hodgkin disease among HIV patients, but this is not one of the diagnostic criteria for AIDS.

Microangiopathic hemolytic anemia is milder than with other causes of this disorder. Plasmapheresis with plasma exchange is the treatment of choice. Vincristine may be efficacious in refractory cases.

PARVOVIRUS INFECTION

Parvovirus infection (B19), or fifth disease, is a highly contagious disease in children. Adults with this infection may develop a polyarthralgia syndrome or cytopenia. Abnormalities in the erythroid line include severe anemia, reticulocytopenia, and RBC hypoplasia in the bone marrow. Pancytopenia may occur. Immunoglobulin therapy administered intravenously is the treatment of choice.

Hematology Pharmacy Review
Robert C. Wolf, PharmD, Darryl C. Grendahl, RPh, Thomas M. Habermann, MD

Drug	Toxic/adverse effects	Comments
Alkylating agents		
Carmustine	Delayed marrow suppression, nausea, vomiting, pulmonary, hepatotoxicity, secondary leukemia	Cumulative marrow suppression, crosses blood-brain barrier
Busulfan	Pulmonary fibrosis, hepatic veno-occlusive disease, skin hyperpigmentation	Liver metabolism, renal excretion
Carboplatin	Marrow suppression, nausea & vomiting, less nephrotoxicity & neurotoxicity than cisplatin	Renal excretion
Chlorambucil	Pulmonary, secondary leukemia, myelosuppression	Hepatic metabolism
Cisplatin	Nephrotoxicity, peripheral neuropathy, ototoxicity, magnesium depletion	Renal excretion, Raynaud phenomenon
Cyclophosphamide	Acute nonlymphocytic leukemia & dysmyelopoietic syndromes (monosomy 5 and 7), bladder cancer, leukopenia, hemorrhagic cystitis, pulmonary fibrosis, SIADH, alopecia, nausea, vomiting	Liver metabolism to active compound, renal excretion, lower dose with renal failure, late transitional cell carcinoma of bladder
Dacarbazine	Marrow suppression, flu-like syndrome, severe nausea & vomiting, fever	
Melphalan	Marrow suppression, secondary leukemia, stomatitis (high dose)	Absence of renal clearance allows use of high-dose melphalan in patients with renal failure, erratic oral absorption
Nitrogen mustard	Marrow suppression, nausea & vomiting, sterility, secondary leukemia	
Streptozocin	Diabetes, marrow suppression, severe nausea & vomiting, renal	Leads to pancreatic & endocrine insufficiency
Procarbazine	Secondary leukemia, sterility	
Ifosfamide	Myelosuppression, CNS toxicity (lethargy, confusion), cystitis	Liver metabolism, renal elimination

Hematology Pharmacy Review (continued)

Drug	Toxic/adverse effects	Comments
Antibiotics		
Bleomycin	Pulmonary fibrosis (threshold 400 µg/lifetime) but may recur at lower doses, fever and chills, myalgias, skin pigmentation, alopecia, adult respiratory distress syndrome with oxygen	Lower dose with renal insufficiency
Dactinomycin	Marrow suppression, radiation recall, nausea and vomiting, mucositis, alopecia	
Daunorubicin	Marrow suppression, radiation recall, cardio-myopathy, mucositis, nausea & vomiting, alopecia, acute nonlymphocytic leukemia	Decrease dose by 50% if bilirubin >1.5 mg/dL or by 75% if bilirubin >3.0 mg/dL
Doxorubicin	Dose-related cardiomyopathy, marrow suppression, alopecia, nausea & vomiting, stomatitis, radiation recall, acute nonlymphocytic leukemia	Liver metabolism, biliary excretion, decrease dose by 50% if bilirubin >1.5 mg/dL or by 75% if bilirubin >3.0 mg/dL
Idarubicin	Myelosuppression, alopecia	
Mitomycin C	Delayed marrow suppression, nausea & vomiting, alopecia, hepatotoxicity, microangiopathic hemolytic anemia	Vesicant, alkylator, forms free radicals
Mitoxantrone	Marrow suppression, cardiac toxicity, nausea & vomiting, mucositis, alopecia, blue sclera & urine	
Hormones		
Corticosteroids	Diabetes, hepatotoxicity, aseptic necrosis, adrenal insufficiency, myopathy, infection, osteoporosis, peptic ulcer disease, hypokalemia, psychosis, cataract	
Plant Derivatives		
Etoposide (VP-16)	Acute nonlymphocytic leukemia, t(11q23), myelosuppression, hypotension, mucositis	
Vincristine	Neurotoxicity (peripheral, autonomic, cranial)	
Vinblastine	SIADH, myelosuppression	

Hematology Pharmacy Review (continued)

Drug	Toxic/adverse effects	Comments
Antimetabolites		
2'-Deoxycoformycin Fludarabine 2-Chlorodeoxyadenosine	Myelosuppression & immunosuppression Opportunistic infections	
Methotrexate	Myelosuppression, mucositis, hepatotoxicity	Drug interactions: NSAIDs, probenecid
Cytarabine	Myelosuppression, neurotoxicity (high dose), conjunctivitis (high dose)	
Other agents		
Alemtuzumab	Fever, chills/rigors, opportunistic infections	Monoclonal antibody to CD52
Bortezomib	Sensory peripheral neuropathy, orthostatic hypertension, fever, thrombocytopenia, neutropenia	Proteasome inhibitor
Asparaginase PEG-asparaginase	Hypersensitivity, hemorrhage/thrombosis, hyperglycemia, pancreatitis, increased LFT, somnolence/confusion	
Hydroxyurea	Myelosuppression (rapid), anorexia, hyperpigmentation	
Tretinoin	Retinoic acid syndrome; xerostomia, cheilitis; skin desquamation; dry, irritated eyes; myalgias; hyperleukocytosis; teratogenic; hypertriglyceridemia	Pulmonary infiltrates, fluid retention, hypotension (responsive/preventable with dexamethasone)
Thalidomide	Sedation, peripheral neuropathy, constipation, rash, teratogenic	
Arsenic trioxide	Acute promyelocytic leukemia differentiation syndrome, QT interval prolongation, myelosuppression, targeted therapy	Fever, dyspnea, weight gain, pleural or pericardial effusion ± leukocytosis
Targeted therapy		
Rituximab	Fever, chills/rigors, headache, hypotension, anaphylactoid symptoms	Monoclonal antibody to CD20
Imatinib (STI571)	Myelosuppression, fluid retention, nausea, muscle cramps, diarrhea, headache, myalgia, arthralgia	Tyrosine kinase inhibitor Multiple potential drug interactions via cytochrome P450-3A4 pathway
Immunotherapy		
Interferon alfa	Fatigue, flu-like symptoms, myelosuppression, increased LFTs	Cytochrome P-450 inhibitor (multiple potential drug interactions)
Filgrastim (G-CSF)	Bone pain, fever	
Sargramostim (GM-CSF)	Bone pain, fever	
Oprelvekin (interleukin 11)	Fluid retention, tachycardia, fatigue	
Gemtuzumab ozogamicin	Myelosuppression, fever, chills/rigors, hypotension, increased LFTs	Monoclonal antibody to CD33 conjugated to calicheamicin (antitumor antibiotic)

CNS, central nervous system; LFT, liver function tests; NSAID, nonsteroidal anti-inflammatory drug; SIADH, syndrome of inappropriate antidiuretic hormone.

Hematology Pharmacy Review (continued)

Hematologically Active Agents Used in Cardiology

Drug	Toxic/adverse effects	Hypersensitivity	Pregnancy
Argatroban	Hemorrhage, hypotension	Coughing, dyspnea, rash	B
Bivalirudin	Hemorrhage, GI symptoms	None	B
Lepirudin	Hemorrhage, heart failure	Anaphylactoid, angioedema (rare), cough, bronchial spasm, stridor, rash	B
Cilostazol	Headache, diarrhea, flushing, hypotension, tachycardia	Rash	C
Ximelagatran	Hemorrhage, elevated LFTs	Unknown	Unknown

GI, gastrointestinal; LFT, liver function test.

QUESTIONS

Multiple Choice (choose the one best answer)

1. A 55-year-old woman presented with a history of anemia since childhood. She required transfusions during pregnancy. Seven years ago, the folate level was 0.9 μg/L (normal, 2.0-14). A complete blood count showed the following: hemoglobin 10.2 g/dL, mean corpuscular volume 68 fL, and erythrocytes 3.59×10^{12}/L. The ferritin level was <1 μg/L (normal, 20-200). The folate level was 1.2 μg/L (normal, 2.0-14). Fecal hemoglobin levels were within normal limits. The most likely diagnosis is:
   a. Iron deficiency anemia
   b. Arteriovenous malformation of the small bowel
   c. Glucose-6-phosphate dehydrogenase deficiency
   d. Celiac sprue
   e. Pernicious anemia

2. A 60-year-old woman presented with a 4-month history of progressive dyspnea. Fourteen years ago, she had a diagnosis of diffuse large B-cell non-Hodgkin lymphoma. A complete blood count showed the following: hemoglobin 7.5 g/dL, mean corpuscular volume 68.6 fL, and erythrocytes 3.45×10^{12}/L. The ferritin level was 3 μg/L (normal, 20-300). The most likely diagnosis is:
   a. Iron deficiency anemia
   b. Arteriovenous malformation of the small bowel
   c. Glucose-6-phosphate dehydrogenase deficiency
   d. Celiac sprue
   e. Pernicious anemia

3. An 18-year-old woman presents with a 3-year history of anemia. On physical examination, she is icteric. The results of a complete blood count are as follows: hemoglobin 6.3 g/dL, mean corpuscular volume 97 fL, leukocytes 3.2×10^9/L, platelets, 97×10^9/L, and reticulocytes 27.7%. The peripheral blood smear shows regeneration with no spherocytes. Total bilirubin is 4.8 mg/dL, with a direct bilirubin of 0.3 mg/dL. Lactate dehydrogenase is 10 times the upper limit of normal. What would you do next?
   a. Upper gastrointestinal tract endoscopy to exclude peptic ulcer disease
   b. Extended upper gastrointestinal tract endoscopy to exclude arteriovenous malformation of the small bowel
   c. Flow cytometry for paroxysmal nocturnal hemoglobinuria
   d. Radiographic study of the small bowel to exclude celiac sprue
   e. Determine vitamin B_{12} level

4. A 63-year-old man with a history of type 2 diabetes mellitus presents with a 27-lb weight loss. On physical examination, he has a fissure of the tongue and decreased vibratory sensation distally in the extremities. Pertinent laboratory values include the following: hemoglobin 10.1 g/dL, erythrocytes 2.49×10^{12}/L, and mean corpuscular volume 124 fL. What would you do next?
   a. Consider a laboratory error and not pursue further evaluation
   b. Request a fasting blood glucose test
   c. Request a sensitive thyroid-stimulating hormone test
   d. Determine the vitamin B_{12} level
   e. Determine the serum folate level

5. A 28-year-old woman started having intermittent headaches 2 weeks ago. One week ago, she had petechiae, bruises, and low-grade fevers. One day ago, left-sided weakness, lethargy, and confusion developed. A complete blood count shows hemoglobin of 9.7 g/dL and a normal mean corpuscular volume. The reticulocyte count is 24%, and bilirubin is 3.6 mg/dL, all indirect. The peripheral blood smear shows schistocytes. The platelet count is 5.5×10^9/L. Urinalysis shows +2 protein. Serum creatinine is 1.8 mg/dL. What is the next best management step?
   a. Heparin
   b. Platelets, cryoprecipitate, and fresh frozen plasma
   c. Plasmapheresis
   d. Plasmapheresis with replacement with fresh frozen plasma
   e. Corticosteroids

6. A 30-year-old homeless man seropositive for human immunodeficiency virus (HIV) who takes multiple unknown medications is evaluated for fatigue, skin nodules, lymphadenopathy, and weight loss. No medical records are available for review. A complete blood count shows the following: hemoglobin 12.0 g/dL, mean corpuscular volume 106 fL, leukocytes 5,600/mm³ (5.6×10^9/L), and platelets, 200,000/mm³ (200×10^9/L). The most likely cause of the macrocytosis is:
   a. Vitamin B_{12} deficiency
   b. Zidovudine
   c. Folate deficiency
   d. Liver disease
   e. Myelodysplasia

7. A 50-year-old African American man had an L5 hemilaminectomy 5 days ago. He subsequently experienced right thigh pain, left shoulder pain, diffuse chest pain,

dyspnea, and diffuse abdominal pain. The peripheral blood smear shows sickle cells. The most common cause of death in this clinical situation is:

a. Acute pain and chest syndrome
b. Human immunodeficiency virus infection
c. Pulmonary embolus
d. Pneumococcal sepsis
e. Hemorrhagic stroke

8. A 69-year-old woman presents with asymptomatic bilateral cervical lymphadenopathy. The leukocyte count is 9.5×10^9/L, with an absolute lymphocyte count of 5,700/mm^3 (5.7×10^9/L). The platelet count is 190,000/mm^3 (190×10^9/L). Hemoglobin is 13.5 g/dL. The treatment of choice is:

a. Observation
b. Prednisone
c. Chlorambucil/prednisone or fludarabine
d. 2-Chlorodeoxyadenosine (2-CDA)
e. CHOP (cyclophosphamide, doxorubicin, vincristine [Oncovin], prednisone)

9. A 49-year-old man presents with a 5-day history of progressive costovertebral angle pain and thoracic back pain, with fevers to 103°F. The spleen is palpable 18 cm below the costal margin. The leukocyte count is 3.2×10^9/L, with an absolute neutrophil count of 800. The platelet count is 56×10^9/L. Hemoglobin concentration is 11.9 g/dL. On the peripheral blood smear, the lymphocytes have cytoplasmic "projections." The therapy of choice is:

a. Observation
b. Prednisone
c. Chlorambucil/prednisone or fludarabine
d. 2-CDA
e. CHOP

10. A 68-year-old woman presents with asymptomatic cervical lymphadenopathy. The complete blood count and lactate dehydrogenase values are normal. Computed tomography of the abdomen demonstrates mild lymphadenopathy. A lymph node biopsy demonstrates B-cell follicular (grade 1) small cleaved cell non-Hodgkin lymphoma. The therapy of choice is:

a. Observation
b. Oral chlorambucil
c. CVP (cyclophosphamide, vincristine, prednisone)
d. Anti-CD20 antibody therapy
e. CHOP

11. A 68-year-old man presented to the emergency department with abdominal pain. Computed tomography of the abdomen showed an abdominal mass that was 15 by 18 cm. The mass was resected. The biopsy specimen shows diffuse large B-cell non-Hodgkin lymphoma. The lactate dehydrogenase level and findings on bilateral bone marrow examination are normal. There is no remaining disease. The treatment of choice is:

a. Observation because there is no remaining disease
b. Oral chlorambucil
c. CVP
d. Anti-CD20 antibody therapy
e. CHOP with anti-CD20 therapy

12. A 27-year-old woman presents with a cough of 2 months' duration. Chest radiography shows a mediastinal mass that was 8 cm in maximal diameter with a maximal thoracic diameter of 32 cm. A biopsy specimen shows large abnormal cells with an "owl's eye" appearance. Computed tomography demonstrates axillary lymphadenopathy and celiac and inguinal adenopathy. Examination of the bone marrow does not show any abnormality. The treatment of choice is:

a. CHOP
b. MOPP (mechlorethamine, vincristine [Oncovin], procarbazine, prednisone)
c. ABVD (doxorubicin [Adriamycin], bleomycin, vinblastine, dacarbazine)
d. Autologous bone marrow transplant
e. Total nodal irradiation plus ABVD

13. A 64-year-old man presents with a 20-lb weight loss, fatigue, peripheral edema, and peripheral neuropathy. He had no lymphadenopathy or hepatosplenomegaly. The complete blood count was normal. Echocardiography shows a left ventricular ejection fraction of 19%. The results of serum protein electrophoresis are normal. The next best test is:

a. Bone marrow biopsy
b. Cardiac biopsy
c. Fat aspirate
d. Peripheral nerve biopsy
e. Small-bowel biopsy

14. A 42-year-old man has an IgG κ monoclonal protein of 1.5 g/dL in the gamma region. The complete blood count and serum levels of creatinine and calcium are normal. The initial treatment of choice is:

a. Observation
b. Melphalan/prednisone
c. Interferon alfa recombinant
d. Dexamethasone
e. Thalidomide and dexamethasone

15. A 49-year-old woman presents with menorrhagia of 5 months' duration. The spleen is not palpable. The leukocyte count is 26,000/mm^3 (26×10^9/L), with a differential of 72% neutrophils, 11% lymphocytes, 2% basophils, 3% monocytes, 8% metamyelocytes, and 12% myelocytes. The platelet count is 440,000/mm^3 (440×10^9/L). The next test in the evaluation of this patient is:
    a. Bone marrow biopsy with cytogenetic studies
    b. Peripheral blood cytogenetic studies
    c. Erythrocyte sedimentation rate
    d. Leukocyte alkaline phosphatase (LAP) score
    e. *Bcr-abl* molecular genetic studies

16. A 60-year-old man presents for an examination. The patient notes postbathing pruritus. He has splenomegaly. A complete blood count shows the following: hemoglobin 12.6 g/dL, hematocrit 38%, mean corpuscular volume 74 fL, total erythrocytes 5.40 million/mm^3 (5.4×10^{12}/L), platelets 550,000/mm^3 (550×10^9/L), and leukocytes 17,000/mm^3 (17×10^9/L). The differential count is within normal limits. The erythrocyte sedimentation rate is 0. What is the most likely diagnosis?
    a. Polycythemia rubra vera
    b. Stress erythrocytosis
    c. Anoxic polycythemia
    d. Hypernephroma
    e. Pheochromocytoma

17. A 68-year-old man presents with frequent episodes of epistaxis, petechiae, and rectal bleeding. He bled after a tonsillectomy at age 19, and dental surgery has been complicated by bleeding. He has no medical records with him. The prothrombin time is normal. The partial thromboplastin time is 80 seconds (normal, 45-60). There was correction with 1/10 volumes. The next best test is:
    a. Determine the bleeding time
    b. Determine factor VIII level and von Willebrand factor antigen and ristocetin cofactor activity
    c. Determine hemophilia B factor IX level
    d. Glanzmann thrombasthenia platelet function studies
    e. Disseminated intravascular coagulopathy D-dimer assay

18. A 58-year-old man had a radical retropubic prostatectomy. Postoperatively, the hemoglobin concentration decreased from 11 to 9.6 g/dL. He was treated with erythrocytes, fresh frozen plasma, and cryoprecipitate. The hemoglobin concentration decreased to 6.6 g/dL, with a prothrombin time (PT) of 15 seconds (normal, up to 12 seconds) and an international normalized ratio (INR) of 1.5. The fibrinogen level was 58 mg/dL, and the platelet count was 40×10^9/L. After vigorous transfusion support,

the hemoglobin concentration continued to decrease, the INR did not correct, and the fibrinogen was low. The treatment of choice is:
    a. Transfusion with erythrocytes, platelets, and fresh frozen plasma and cryoprecipitate
    b. Transfusion with erythrocytes and platelets
    c. Plasmapheresis with replacement with fresh frozen plasma
    d. Transfusion with erythrocytes and platelets and intravenous administration of heparin
    e. Intravenous administration of heparin

19. A 38-year-old woman presents with menorrhagia. The prothrombin time is normal. The activated partial thromboplastin time is 49 seconds (normal, 25-40). Factor VIII coagulant activity is 27%. Factor VIII antigen is decreased. What is the treatment of choice for the long-term management of this patient?
    a. Humate-P
    b. Recombinant factor VIII
    c. Heat-treated factor VIII concentrate
    d. Solvent-detergent–treated factor VIII
    e. Desmopressin (DDAVP) if an initial trial demonstrates a response

20. A 72-year-old man is evaluated in consultation for multiple medical problems. He has received heparin treatment for recent deep venous thrombosis. Which one of the following profiles would be most consistent with full-dose heparin therapy?
    a. Normal PT, activated partial thromboplastin time (APTT), thrombin time (TT), fibrinogen, and bleeding time
    b. Abnormal APTT only
    c. Abnormal PT, APTT, TT, and fibrinogen
    d. Slightly abnormal PT, abnormal APTT, abnormal TT, normal fibrinogen, and normal or abnormal bleeding time
    e. Abnormal APTT and thrombin time only in all cases

21. A 50-year-old woman has a history of progressive splenomegaly and cytopenias. She presents at this time with the sudden onset of pain in the left upper quadrant. The spleen is palpable 5 cm below the left costal margin. A complete blood count discloses the following: hemoglobin 8.6 g/dL, leukocytes 4.2×10^9/L, and platelets 1,670×10^9/L. A peripheral blood smear shows nucleated red cells, 4.5% myelocytes, 1% metamyelocytes, and 1% blasts. A red blood cell smear shows dacryocytes. The most likely diagnosis is:
    a. Chronic myelogenous leukemia

b. Hypernephroma

c. Agnogenic myeloid metaplasia

d. Acute nonlymphocytic leukemia

e. Polycythemia rubra vera

22. A 56-year-old man presents with a history of recurrent pulmonary emboli, recurrent deep venous thromboses, and thrombocytopenia. The antinuclear antibody (ANA) assay is positive. The next best test is:

a. Protein S assay

b. Antiphospholipid antibody assay

c. Antithrombin III assay

d. Protein C assay

e. Factor V Leiden assay

23. A 64-year-old man presents with acute onset of a left-sided headache and left footdrop. He fell 6 weeks ago while training a horse. On physical examination, a lump is noted on his right temple. He has had a 12-year history of thrombocytopenia. At this time, the platelet count is 16×10^9/L. Computed tomography of the head shows a subdural hematoma. The initial medical management of choice is:

a. Oral prednisone

b. Intravenous immunoglobulin, platelets, and intravenous methylprednisolone, 1 g daily for 3 days

c. Platelet transfusions alone from a single donor

d. Intravenous immunoglobulin

e. Intravenous high-dose corticosteroids

24. A 27-year-old gravida 2, para 1 woman is evaluated in the late second trimester. Her blood pressure is normal, and the platelet count is 105,000/mm^3 (105×10^9/L). The optimal management is:

a. Oral prednisone

b. Cesarean section after fetal maturation is documented

c. Observation

d. Bone marrow examination

e. Antiplatelet antibody tests

25. A 52-year-old man had a valvuloplasty at age 3 years. Four years ago, cardiac surgery was repeated, and 15 days ago, aortotomy was performed. During this procedure, 3 units of packed erythrocytes were transfused. During reexploration 14 days ago, 5 units of packed erythrocytes were transfused. The hemoglobin concentration decreased to 8.4 g/dL. The Coombs test was positive. The indirect bilirubin value was 1.8 mg/dL, and the reticulocyte count was 8.72% (normal, 0.6%-1.83%). The most likely diagnosis is:

a. Acute hemolytic transfusion reaction

b. Blood loss

c. Infection

d. Transfusion reaction associated with IgA antibodies

e. Delayed hemolytic transfusion reaction

26. A 50-year-old woman is admitted to the coronary care unit with congestive heart failure and cardiac arrhythmia. She has a long history of lethargy. The work-up documents cardiomyopathy, diabetes mellitus, and amenorrhea. Family members should have which one of the following screening tests?

a. Serum ferritin

b. Transferrin saturation

c. Molecular studies for hemoglobin H mutation

d. Complete blood count, glucose, and liver function tests

e. Liver biopsy

27. A 68-year-old man who has the diagnosis of diffuse large cell non-Hodgkin lymphoma received his first cycle of CHOP chemotherapy. On the seventh day of the second cycle of treatment, the leukocyte count was 0.5×10^9/L, and the absolute neutrophil count was 250×10^9/L. The patient has been checking his temperature, and he is afebrile. The management of this patient should be:

a. Observation

b. Oral ciprofloxacin

c. Trimethoprim-sulfamethoxazole

d. Granulocyte colony-stimulating factor (G-CSF)

e. No more chemotherapy

28. A 49-year-old man has been receiving chemotherapy for Hodgkin disease. After the fifth cycle, cough, dyspnea, and fevers developed. Chest radiography shows bilateral infiltrates. The leukocyte and absolute neutrophil counts are normal. A transbronchoscopic lung biopsy specimen does not show evidence of infection or active Hodgkin disease. What would you do next?

a. Discontinue nitrogen mustard

b. Discontinue doxorubicin (Adriamycin)

c. Discontinue prednisone

d. Discontinue bleomycin

e. Discontinue vincristine

ANSWERS

1. Answer d.

The low mean corpuscular volume and ferritin level are consistent with iron deficiency. This and the low folate concentration suggest small-bowel disease. Small-bowel radiographs and biopsy findings confirmed the diagnosis of celiac sprue.

2. Answer a.

The low mean corpuscular volume, decreased total red blood cell count, and decreased ferritin level are consistent with iron deficiency. The colonoscopic findings were negative. Upper gastrointestinal endoscopy demonstrated gastric antral erosions with Cameron ulcers. This resolved after the patient received iron replacement therapy.

3. Answer c.

The patient has normochromic normocytic anemia. The reticulocyte count is increased. Fecal hemoglobin is normal, indirect bilirubin is increased, and the Coombs test is negative. The patient has a Coombs-negative hemolytic anemia with pancytopenia. The most likely diagnosis is paroxysmal nocturnal hemoglobinuria. Flow cytometry is the next best test.

4. Answer d.

This is macrocytic anemia in a diabetic patient. Of the listed responses, vitamin B_{12} deficiency would be the most likely diagnosis. The vitamin B_{12} level was <50 ng/mL (normal, 200-1,000). The intrinsic factor blocking antibody was positive.

5. Answer d.

The patient has thrombotic thrombocytopenic purpura. The treatment of choice is plasmapheresis with replacement with fresh frozen plasma.

6. Answer b.

All the answers listed are causes of macrocytosis. This patient has acquired immunodeficiency syndrome with Kaposi sarcoma and is taking zidovudine (AZT). Zidovudine is the most likely cause in this clinical situation.

7. Answer a.

The clinical scenario is consistent with sickle cell anemia and acute chest syndrome with pulmonary crisis. The most common cause of death in sickle cell anemia is acute pain and chest syndrome.

8. Answer a.

The patient has Rai stage I or International Workshop on Chronic Lymphocytic Leukemia stage A disease. The treatment of choice is observation.

9. Answer d.

The patient has splenomegaly with pancytopenia, the most characteristic presentation of hairy cell leukemia. The treatment of choice is 2-CDA.

10. Answer a.

The patient has stage III low-grade non-Hodgkin lymphoma with no evidence of bulky disease or symptoms. The treatment of choice is observation. Early treatment has not been shown to be beneficial.

11. Answer e.

This patient has diffuse large cell non-Hodgkin lymphoma, which is potentially curable. Even though no disease is present, therapeutic intervention is indicated. CHOP with anti-CD20 is the treatment of choice.

12. Answer c.

The patient has stage IV Hodgkin disease. The treatment of choice is ABVD. Autologous bone marrow transplantation or peripheral stem cell transplantation is the treatment of choice for relapse of the disease.

13. Answer c.

The results of serum protein electrophoresis may be normal in up to 20% of patients with primary amyloidosis. A fat aspirate is the next best and least invasive test to diagnose primary amyloidosis.

14. Answer a.

The patient has monoclonal gammopathy of undetermined significance, as manifested by a monoclonal protein level <3 g/dL and normal calcium, hemoglobin, and creatinine values. Malignancy (multiple myeloma, amyloidosis, lymphoma) may develop in 23% of these patients. This patient should have observation with serum protein electrophoresis studies.

15. Answer d.

The differential diagnosis in this case is leukemoid reaction versus chronic myelogenous leukemia. The palpable spleen suggests the latter. The LAP score differentiates these two disorders. In this case, the score was 28 (normal, 40-100). The next best test after the LAP score is bone marrow biopsy with cytogenetic studies.

16. Answer a.

An erythrocyte sedimentation rate of 0 is consistent with polycythemia rubra vera. The decreased mean corpuscular volume is consistent with iron deficiency anemia associated with polycythemia rubra vera.

17. Answer b.

Prolonged APTT and normal PT with prolonged bleeding time are all compatible with von Willebrand disease. A workup showed that the von Willebrand factor antigen and ristocetin cofactor were both abnormal.

18. Answer e.

The patient has disseminated intravascular coagulopathy. Replacement of all the missing factors and products is the initial treatment of choice. If these measures fail, heparin therapy is indicated. Plasmapheresis with replacement with fresh frozen plasma is the treatment of choice for thrombotic thrombocytopenic purpura (TTP). This patient does not have TTP because prothrombin time and fibrinogen are very abnormal.

19. Answer e.

The findings, including the factor VIII level, are consistent with mild von Willebrand disease. Patients with mild-to-moderate von Willebrand disease should have a trial of desmopressin. If there is a response, desmopressin should be used in the long-term management of the disease.

20. Answer d.

Slightly abnormal PT, abnormal APTT, abnormal TT, normal fibrinogen, and normal or abnormal bleeding time are characteristic findings in patients receiving heparin intravenously.

21. Answer c.

This patient has the classic findings of agnogenic myeloid metaplasia—splenomegaly, leukoerythroblastic blood smear, and dacryocytes in the peripheral blood smear.

22. Answer b.

The most likely diagnosis for this patient with recurrent venous thrombi, thrombocytopenia, and a positive ANA is antiphospholipid antibody syndrome. In this patient, the antiphospholipid antibody was 2.2 (normal, <1.0).

23. Answer b.

The patient has life-threatening bleeding due to idiopathic thrombocytopenic purpura that should be treated with intravenous immunoglobulin and platelets in combination with high-dose methylprednisolone.

24. Answer c.

The patient most likely has incidental thrombocytopenia of pregnancy. Although she should be followed up, no further work-up or treatment is necessary at this time.

25. Answer e.

The patient has a positive Coombs test, indirect hyperbilirubinemia (1.8 mg/dL), and a reticulocyte count of 8.72% (normal, 0.6%-1.83%). An antibody to the Kidd system was detected. This antibody developed after the previous transfusion. Antibodies to the Rh or Kidd systems may become undetectable over time. The subsequent transfusion resulted in a rapid stimulation of the antibody.

26. Answer b.

The patient has hemochromatosis. The most accepted screening test is transferrin saturation.

27. Answer a.

The patient should be observed and not treated with G-CSF at this time. The patient has afebrile neutropenia. The current American Society of Clinical Oncology practice guidelines and randomized studies do not support the routine use of G-CSF in this situation. To date, randomized trials with oral antibiotics have not supported the use of G-CSF in this situation. Myelosuppression is an expected toxic effect of CHOP chemotherapy in potentially curable diffuse large cell non-Hodgkin lymphoma. CHOP is usually given for six to eight cycles. In this situation, treatment should be continued, with potential dose modifications, because the patient has a potentially curable disease.

28. Answer d.

ABVD is the chemotherapeutic treatment most commonly given for Hodgkin disease. Bleomycin is the drug that most commonly causes pulmonary toxic effects.

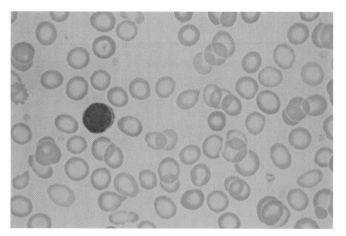

Plate 11-1. Hypochromic microcytic anemia. Small cells, <6 μm in diameter, with increased central pallor and assorted aberrations in size (anisocytosis) and shape (poikilocytosis). (Courtesy of Curtis A. Hanson, M.D., Mayo Clinic.)

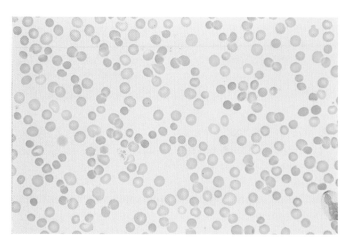

Plate 11-2. Spherocytes. Smooth, small, and spheroidal darkly stained cells with minimal or no central pallor. (Courtesy of Curtis A. Hanson, M.D., Mayo Clinic.)

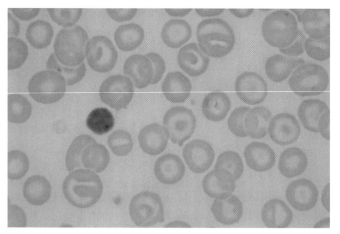

Plate 11-3. Target cells. Red blood cells with a broad diameter and dark center. (Courtesy of Curtis A. Hanson, M.D., Mayo Clinic.)

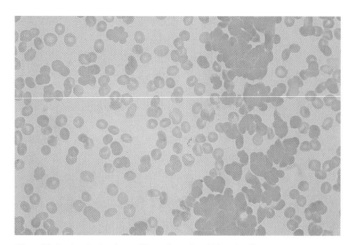

Plate 11-4. Agglutination. Clumping of red blood cells.

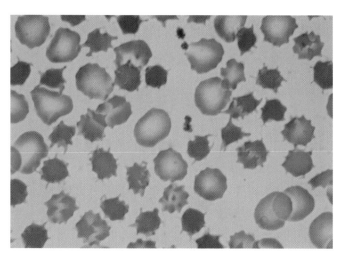

Plate 11-5. Spur cells (acanthocytes). Note the thin, thorny, or finger-like projections. (Courtesy of Curtis A. Hanson, M.D., Mayo Clinic.)

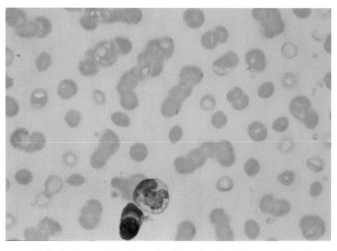

Plate 11-6. Rouleaux. Stacking of red blood cells. (Courtesy of Curtis A. Hanson, M.D., Mayo Clinic.)

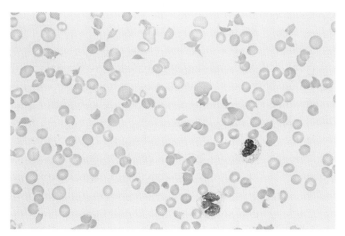

Plate 11-7. Schistocytes. Fragmented red blood cells shaped like helmets, triangles, or kites. (Courtesy of Curtis A. Hanson, M.D., Mayo Clinic.)

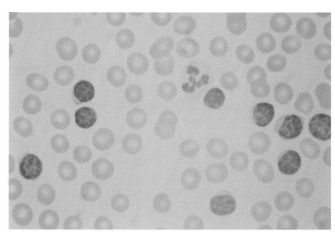

Plate 11-8. Chronic lymphocytic leukemia. Large number of small and agranular mature lymphocytes with nuclei approximately the same size as red blood cells.

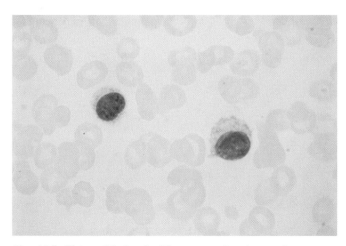

Plate 11-9. Hairy cell leukemia. These mature lymphocytes have eccentrically placed nuclei, pale cytoplasm, and characteristic projections.

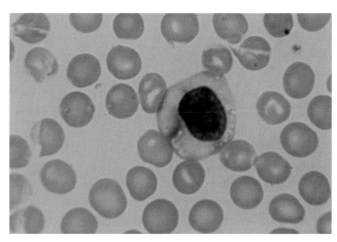

Plate 11-10. Infectious mononucleosis. Large atypical lymphocyte has a large oblong nucleus and a large amount of pale cytoplasm, which may be vacuolated.

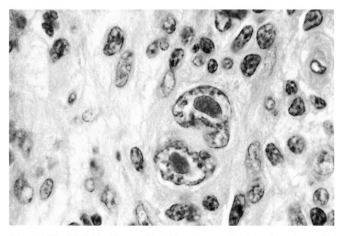

Plate 11-11. Hodgkin disease. Reed-Sternberg cell, a large binuclear cell. (Courtesy of Curtis A. Hanson, M.D., Mayo Clinic.)

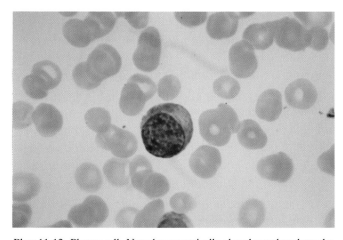

Plate 11-12. Plasma cell. Note the eccentrically placed round nucleus; the copious, dark blue cytoplasm has a characteristic pale-staining area adjacent to the nucleus.

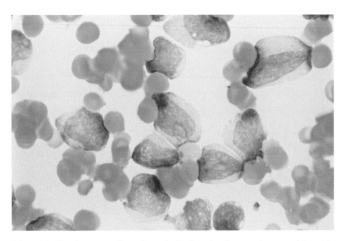

Plate 11-13. Acute nonlymphocytic leukemia. Large pleomorphic cells with large nuclei and a barely visible nuclear membrane.

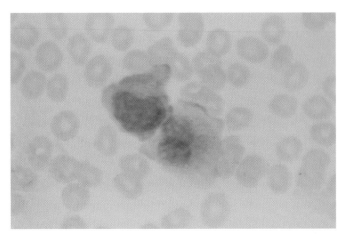

Plate 11-14. Acute promyelocytic leukemia. Note the large nuclei; more than half of the leukemic cells have large atypical granulations. (Courtesy of Curtis A. Hanson, M.D., Mayo Clinic.)

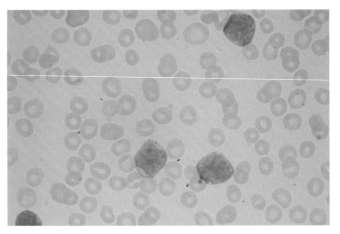

Plate 11-15. Acute lymphoblastic leukemia. Large, rounded, and indented nuclei with diverse shapes and scant, darker blue cytoplasm.

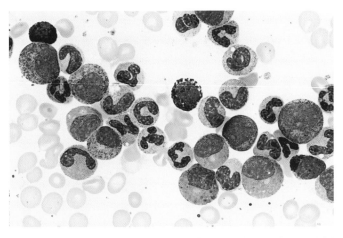

Plate 11-16. Chronic myelogenous leukemia. Normal-appearing myeloid cells representing all stages of maturation, with a decreased number of erythropoietic cells and one basophil precursor in the center. (Courtesy of Curtis A. Hanson, M.D., Mayo Clinic.)

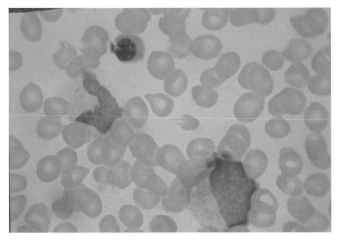

Plate 11-17. Agnogenic myeloid metaplasia. The peripheral blood smear is leukoerythroblastic with dacryocytes.

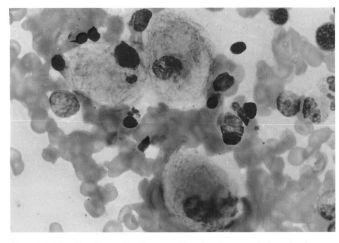

Plate 11-18. Gaucher cells. Large cells with characteristic pale, foamy, and fibrillar cytoplasm. (Courtesy of Curtis A. Hanson, M.D., Mayo Clinic.)

CHAPTER 12

HIV INFECTION

Zelalem Temesgen, M.D.

Human immunodeficiency virus (HIV) belongs to the family Retroviridae, subfamily Lentiviridae. Retroviridae organisms share a distinct biologic characteristic: an initial stage of primary infection followed by a relatively asymptomatic period of months to years and a final stage of overt disease.

There are two types of HIV: HIV-1 and HIV-2. Most reported cases of HIV disease around the world are caused by HIV-1. HIV-1 is further classified into subtypes M, N, and O, referred to as clades. Subtype M (main) is the collective name for a group of clades designated "A" to "K." For example, clade "B" is responsible for most HIV infections reported in the United States. HIV-2 is found predominantly in western Africa. Although HIV-1 and HIV-2 are clinically indistinguishable and have identical modes of transmission, HIV-2 appears to be less easily transmitted than HIV-1 and slower to progress to acquired immunodeficiency syndrome (AIDS).

- There are two types of HIV: HIV-1 and HIV-2.
- Most reported cases of HIV disease are caused by HIV-1.

EPIDEMIOLOGY

The AIDS epidemic is currently in its third decade and continues to affect a large number of people throughout the world. According to "The AIDS Epidemic Update: December 2003" released by the joint United Nations Program on HIV/AIDS (UNAIDS), the AIDS epidemic claimed more than 3 million lives in 2003, and an estimated 5 million people acquired HIV in 2003—bringing to 40 million the number of people globally living with HIV.

Sub-Saharan Africa continues to be the world's region most affected by the HIV/AIDS epidemic. In 2003, an estimated 26.6 million people in this region were living with HIV, including the 3.2 million who became infected during the past year. Approximately 2.3 million people died as a result of AIDS in 2003. Beyond sub-Saharan Africa, more recent epidemics continue to grow in China, Indonesia, Papua New Guinea, Viet Nam, several central Asian republics, the Baltic States, and North Africa.

The Centers for Disease Control and Prevention (CDC) estimates that 800,000 to 900,000 people are currently living with HIV in the United States and approximately 40,000 new HIV infections occur each year in the United States. Ethnic minorities are disproportionately affected by the HIV epidemic. Although African Americans make up only about 12% of the U.S. population, half of the new HIV infections overall and 43% of HIV cases reported among men in 2001 were in African Americans. Similarly, nearly 20% of the total number of new cases of AIDS in the United States occur in Hispanics, but they make up only 13% of the general U.S. population. The availability of potent antiretroviral drugs and their use in three or more combination regimens—highly active antiretroviral therapy—have led to a dramatic decline in the morbidity and mortality associated with HIV and AIDS in the United States. During 1998-2002, the estimated number of deaths among persons with AIDS declined 14%. This decline was noted in all racial and ethnic groups.

- Globally, 40 million people are living with HIV; in the United States, 900,000 have the disease.
- Ethnic minorities are disproportionately affected by the HIV epidemic.
- AIDS-related death declined 14% in the United States from 1998-2002.

TRANSMISSION

HIV is transmitted sexually, perinatally, by parenteral inoculation (intravenous drug injection, occupational exposure), through blood products, and, less commonly, through donated organs or semen. Sexual transmission is the most common means of infection. Some of the conditions that may increase the risk of sexually acquiring HIV infection are traumatic intercourse (such as receptive anal); ulcerative genital infections such as syphilis, herpes simplex, and chancroid; and lack of circumcision. The use of latex condoms, especially if used properly, reduces the risk of HIV transmission.

- HIV is transmitted sexually, perinatally, by parenteral inoculation, through blood products, and through donated organs or semen.

In the United States, all blood donations have been routinely tested for HIV-1 antibody since early 1985. Since June 1, 1992, all U.S. blood centers test for antibodies to both HIV-1 and HIV-2. The estimated risk of acquiring HIV through blood transfusion is 1 in 450,000 to 1 in 600,000.

- In the United States, all blood donations have been routinely tested for HIV-1 antibody since early 1985.

LABORATORY DIAGNOSIS

The enzyme-linked immunosorbent assays and enzyme immunoassays (ELISA, EIA) are the most common assays used as a screening test for HIV-1 infection. They detect specific HIV antibodies. They have high (>99%) sensitivity and specificity but low positive predictive values in low-prevalence populations. For this reason, positive results require verification with an additional test. False-positive results can occur for several reasons. These include the presence of cross-reacting antibodies in certain patients (such as multiparous women, patients with multiple transfusions) and participation in HIV vaccine studies. Causes of false-negative results include testing during the pre-seroconversion (window) period, use of replacement transfusions, bone marrow transplantation, agammaglobulinemia, seroreversion in late-stage disease, unusual HIV subtypes (HIV-2, clade O and N), and atypical immune response. Technical or laboratory error can be a cause of both false-positive and false-negative results.

Individuals with positive or indeterminate results of ELISA/EIA should have the test repeated. If results are repeatedly positive, the patient should undergo additional confirmatory testing, usually Western blot testing. The Western blot test detects specific viral proteins, such as *gag* (p18, p24, p55), *pol* (p31, p51, p66), and *env* (gp41, gp120/gp160) gene products. The CDC guidelines for interpretation of the Western blot are as follows. The presence of antibody against any two of the three major viral gene products (p24, gp41, or gp120/gp160) is classified as positive. A Western blot result is classified as negative if no bands are present. Results that cannot be classified as positive or negative on the basis of these criteria are categorized as indeterminate. If results are indeterminate, the clinician should assess the risk of HIV infection in the patient and retest in 3 to 6 months (Fig. 12-1). HIV-RNA assays may be of additional help in these cases. The risk of HIV infection is extremely low in patients with repeatedly indeterminate results of Western blot testing.

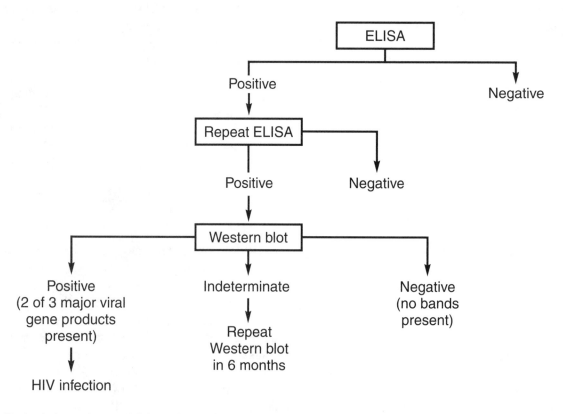

Fig. 12-1. Testing for human immunodeficiency virus (HIV). ELISA, enzyme-linked immunosorbent assay.

- ELISA/EIA should be repeated in persons with positive or indeterminate results.
- Western blot testing is used to confirm the results of ELISA/EIA.

PATHOGENESIS

Contrary to previously held beliefs, HIV is not dormant during the so-called clinical latency period. There is active virus application at all stages of disease. As many as 10 billion viral particles are produced and cleared daily in an HIV-infected person throughout all stages of disease. Concurrent with this rapid turnover of the HIV virus, more than 2 billion CD4 lymphocytes are produced every day.

- HIV is not dormant during the so-called clinical latency period.

Primary HIV Infection

Synonyms for this syndrome are acute HIV infection and acute retroviral syndrome. Within days to weeks after exposure to HIV, upwards of 40% of infected individuals present with a brief illness that may last for a few days to a few weeks. This period of illness is associated with a huge amount of circulating virus, a rapid decline in the CD4 cell count, and a vigorous immune response. Patients usually present with a mononucleosis-like illness, but the clinical manifestations may be protean (Table 12-1). An atypical lymphocytosis is present in approximately 50% of patients. Results of ELISA may be negative (window period), whereas p24 antigen, HIV culture, or polymerase chain reaction results may provide the diagnosis. The differential diagnosis includes infection due to Ebstein-Barr virus, cytomegalovirus, primary herpes simplex virus, toxoplasmosis, rubella, viral hepatitis, secondary syphilis, and drug reactions. Currently, treatment with the most potent antiretroviral combination regimen available is recommended with the hope of intervening before the HIV infection is fully established, when the viral population is relatively homogeneous and the host immune system is relatively intact.

- Acute HIV infection occurs within days to weeks after exposure to HIV.
- Patients usually present with a mononucleosis-type illness.
- Results of ELISA may be negative for HIV.
- HIV p24 antigen, HIV culture, and HIV polymerase chain reaction results may provide the diagnosis.
- Treatment is with the most potent antiretroviral combination regimen.

INFECTIONS ASSOCIATED WITH HIV INFECTION

Pneumocystis Pneumonia

Pneumocystis pneumonia is one of the most common opportunistic infections in patients with AIDS. The onset of illness is insidious, with several weeks of fever, weight loss, malaise, and night sweats. Chest radiography typically shows bilateral interstitial pulmonary infiltrates, but a lobar distribution and spontaneous pneumothoraces may occur. Arterial blood gas analysis usually shows hypoxia and respiratory alkalosis. A wide A-a gradient (>35 mm Hg) and low PO_2 (<70 mm Hg) are associated with increased mortality. Several methods are used for the diagnosis of *Pneumocystis* pneumonia. Staining for *Pneumocystis* pneumonia in hypertonic saline-induced expectorated sputum is 30% to 85% sensitive. The sensitivity improves with liquefaction and the use of monoclonal antibody staining, and it may decrease with the use of *Pneumocystis* pneumonia prophylaxis. Bronchoalveolar lavage is 85% to 90% sensitive. In rare circumstances, transbronchial lung biopsy may be needed to make the diagnosis. Open lung biopsy is even less commonly required.

Table 12-1   Clinical Manifestations of Primary Human Immunodeficiency Virus Infection

General	Neuropathic	Dermatologic	Gastrointestinal
Fever	Headache, retro-orbital pain	Maculopapular rash	Oral candidiasis
Pharyngitis	Meningoencephalitis	Roseola-like rash	Nausea, vomiting
Lymphadenopathy	Peripheral neuropathy	Diffuse urticaria	Diarrhea
Myalgia	Radiculopathy	Desquamation	
Lethargy	Guillain-Barré syndrome	Alopecia	
Anorexia, weight loss	Cognitive impairment	Mucocutaneous ulceration	

From Tindall B, Imrie A, Donovan B, Penny R, Cooper DA: Primary HIV infection. *In* The Medical Management of AIDS. Third edition. Edited by MA Sande, PA Volberding. Philadelphia, WB Saunders Company, 1992, pp 67-86. By permission of publisher.

- *Pneumocystis* pneumonia is one of the most common opportunistic infections in AIDS.
- Bronchoalveolar lavage is 85%-90% sensitive for the diagnosis of *Pneumocystis* pneumonia.

The treatment of choice for both severe and mild-to-moderate disease is trimethoprim-sulfamethoxazole, 15 mg/kg per day (trimethoprim component) in 3 or 4 equally divided doses for 21 days. If there is no improvement 5 to 7 days after treatment is begun, switching to or adding another drug should be considered. Alternative treatment options are listed in Table 12-2. Controlled studies have shown that adjunctive corticosteroid therapy increases survival in patients with moderate-to-severe disease. Benefit was shown when the PaO_2 in room air was less than 70 mm Hg or the alveolar-arterial PO_2 difference (A-a gradient) was more than 35 mm Hg. When indicated, adjunctive corticosteroid therapy should be started immediately; a delay may compromise its effectiveness.

- The treatment of choice for severe and mild-to-moderate disease is trimethoprim-sulfamethoxazole.
- Adjunctive corticosteroid therapy increases survival in patients with moderate-to-severe disease and is indicated for *Pneumocystis* pneumonia with hypoxia (PO_2 <70 mm Hg).

Primary prophylaxis of *Pneumocystis* pneumonia is indicated in all HIV-infected patients with a CD4 count less than 200 cells/mm^3 or a history of oropharyngeal candidiasis. Persons who have a history of an AIDS-defining illness but who would not otherwise qualify and those with CD4$^+$ T-lymphocyte percentage of less than 14% should be considered for prophylaxis.

Drugs used for prophylaxis are listed in Table 12-3. The agent of choice is trimethoprim-sulfamethoxazole, which has the additional benefit of potential protection against other infectious agents (*Nocardia, Toxoplasma gondii, Staphylococcus aureus, Streptococcus pneumoniae, Haemophilus influenzae, Listeria monocytogenes, Isospora belli*) and prevention of extrapulmonary pneumocystosis. Primary prophylaxis may be able to be discontinued if patients have a CD4$^+$ T-lymphocyte count of more than 200 cells/µL sustained for at least 3 to 6 months and, preferably, a sustained reduction in viral load also.

- Typical clinical scenario: A 50-year-old patient with known HIV presents with shortness of breath and a 2-week history of fever and night sweats. Chest radiography shows bilateral pulmonary infiltrates. Arterial blood gas study reveals a PO_2 of 60 mm Hg on room air. An increased A-a gradient is found.
- *Pneumocystis* pneumonia prophylaxis is indicated with a CD4 count <200 cells/mm^3 or a history of oropharyngeal candidiasis.

Tuberculosis

The resurgence of tuberculosis in the United States is not entirely explained by the HIV epidemic. Factors such as socioeconomic conditions, immigration, breakdown of the public health infrastructure, and lack of interest of the medical and scientific community in tuberculosis all play a role. In addition to the impact of HIV on the incidence of tuberculosis, there are other important interactions between HIV infection and *Mycobacterium tuberculosis*: tuberculosis may accelerate the course of HIV infection; unlike many of the opportunistic infections in patients with HIV infection, tuberculosis can be

Table 12-2 Drugs Used for the Treatment of *Pneumocystis* Pneumonia

Trimethoprim-sulfamethoxazole
Trimethoprim PO 15 mg/kg per day + dapsone PO 100 mg/day
Clindamycin IV 600 mg every 8 h (or PO 300-450 mg every 6 h) + primaquine PO 30 mg base/d
Pentamidine IV 4 mg/kg per day
Atovaquone suspension 750 mg twice daily
Trimetrexate IV 45 mg/m^2 per day + leucovorin (folinic acid) IV 20 mg/m^2 every 6 h
Prednisone* 40 mg PO twice daily for 5 days, followed by 40 mg PO daily for 5 days, then 20 mg PO daily until completion of therapy

IV, intravenously; PO, orally.
*If PaO_2 is less than 70 mm Hg or A-a gradient is more than 35 mm Hg.

Table 12-3 Drugs Used for Prophylaxis of *Pneumocystis* Pneumonia

Trimethoprim-sulfamethoxazole
1 Double-strength tablet each day
1 Double-strength tablet 3 times per week
1 Single-strength tablet daily
Dapsone 100 mg PO daily
Aerosolized pentamidine 300 mg inhaled monthly with Respirgard II nebulizer
Dapsone 50 mg PO daily + pyrimethamine* 50 mg orally 3 times a week
Dapsone 200 mg PO weekly + pyrimethamine* 75 mg orally weekly
Atovaquone 1,500 mg PO daily

PO, orally.
*Plus leucovorin (folinic acid) 25 mg orally weekly.

cured if diagnosed promptly and treated appropriately; and tuberculosis can be prevented. Tuberculosis may occur relatively early in HIV infection. When it occurs later, it tends to have atypical features, such as extrapulmonary disease, disseminated disease, and unusual chest radiographic appearance (lower lung zone lesions, intrathoracic adenopathy, diffuse infiltrations, and lower frequency of cavitation). Outbreaks of multiple drug-resistant tuberculosis have been reported. Patients may have a fulminant course with high mortality (>70%) and a rapid course to death in 2 to 3 months.

- Tuberculosis can occur early in HIV infection.
- Tuberculosis that occurs late in HIV infection tends to have atypical features.

The management of HIV-infected patients taking antiretroviral agents and undergoing treatment for active tuberculosis is complex. Protease inhibitors and nonnucleoside reverse transcriptase inhibitors (NNRTIs) have substantive interactions with the rifamycins (rifampin, rifabutin, and rifapentine) used to treat mycobacterial infections. Protease inhibitors and NNRTIs not only are substrates for but also may inhibit or induce the cytochrome P-450 system. Rifamycins, however, induce cytochrome P-450 and may substantially decrease blood levels of the antiretroviral drugs. Compared with rifampin, rifabutin has substantially less activity as an inducer of cytochrome P-450, and when used in appropriately modified doses it might not be associated with a clinically important reduction of protease inhibitors or NNRTIs. Thus, the substitution of rifabutin for rifampin in treatment regimens for tuberculosis has been proposed as a practical choice for patients who are also undergoing therapy with protease inhibitors or with the NNRTIs nevirapine or efavirenz. Rifampin may still be used when 1) the antiretroviral regimen includes the NNRTI efavirenz and two nucleoside analogue reverse transcriptase inhibitors (NRTIs), 2) the antiretroviral regimen includes the protease inhibitor ritonovir and one or more NRTIs, or 3) the antiretroviral regimen includes the combination of two protease inhibitors. A 6-month course may still be used for the treatment of tuberculosis that is susceptible to all first-line antituberculosis drugs. However, clinicians should consider the factors that increase a person's risk for a poor clinical outcome (e.g., lack of adherence to tuberculosis therapy, delayed conversion of *M. tuberculosis* sputum cultures from positive to negative, and delayed clinical response) when deciding the total duration of tuberculosis therapy. Directly observed therapy should be strongly considered.

- Antituberculosis drugs interact with anti-HIV drugs.
- A 6-month course of rifampin may be used for tuberculosis that is susceptible to all first-line antituberculosis drugs.

Optimal regimens for multiple drug-resistant tuberculosis are unknown. Recently, paradoxical reactions have been reported with the concurrent administration of antiretroviral and antituberculosis therapy. These reactions are attributed to recovery of the patient's delayed hypersensitivity response and include hectic fevers, lymphadenopathy, worsening of chest radiographic manifestations of tuberculosis (e.g., miliary infiltrates, pleural effusions), and worsening of original tuberculous lesions. Changes in antituberculosis or antiretroviral therapy are rarely needed. If the symptoms are severe, a short course of corticosteroids to suppress the enhanced immune response can be attempted while continuing with antituberculous and antiretroviral therapy. Prophylaxis is recommended for all patients who are HIV-positive and have skin reactions of more than 5 mm to 5 tuberculin units of purified protein derivative and who do not have active tuberculosis. Drug regimens recommended for the prophylaxis of tuberculosis are listed in Table 12-4.

- Optimal regimens for multiple drug-resistant tuberculosis are unknown.
- Prophylaxis for tuberculosis is recommended for all patients who are HIV-positive and have skin reactions of more than 5 mm to 5 tuberculin units of purified protein derivative and who do not have active tuberculosis.

Mycobacterium avium Complex

Mycobacterium avium complex causes infection when immunosuppression is severe (CD4 cell count <50/mm^3). Disseminated *M. avium* complex infection is the most common systemic bacterial infection in patients with HIV infection. Common presentations include low-grade fever, night sweats, weight loss, fatigue, abdominal pain, and diarrhea. Blood cultures are usually positive; however, organisms also can be isolated from stool, respiratory tract secretions, bone marrow, liver, and other biopsy specimens.

Table 12-4 Drugs Used for the Prophylaxis of Tuberculosis

Isoniazid 300 mg PO daily for 9 mo
Isoniazid 300 mg PO daily for 6 mo
Isoniazid 900 mg twice weekly for 9 mo
Isoniazid 900 mg twice weekly for 6 mo
Rifampin 600 mg PO + pyrazinamide 15-20 mg/kg PO daily for 2 mo
Rifampin 600 mg PO + pyrazinamide 50 mg/kg PO twice weekly for 2-3 mo
Rifampin 600 mg PO daily for 4 mo

PO, orally.

- *Mycobacterium avium* complex causes infection when immunosuppression is severe (CD4 cell count <50/mm^3).
- *M. avium* complex is the most common systemic bacterial infection in HIV-infected patients.

The organism is resistant to conventional antimycobacterial agents. Treatment involves multiple drugs with many side effects. Symptoms often can be ameliorated, and some studies have shown an increase in survival with treatment. The current recommended treatment regimen includes one of the newer macrolides (clarithromycin, azithromycin), ethambutol, and one or two additional drugs with activity against *M. avium* complex. These include rifabutin, ciprofloxacin, amikacin, rifampin, and clofazimine. Rifabutin is thought to be the best option for a third agent. Treatment with full therapeutic doses is continued for life.

- *M. avium* complex is resistant to conventional antimycobacterial drugs.
- Treatment of *M. avium* complex is for life, with full therapeutic doses of multiple agents.

For patients with AIDS whose CD4 cell count is less than 50 cells/mm^3, prophylaxis with clarithromycin 500 mg twice daily or azithromycin 1,200 mg weekly is recommended. Rifabutin 300 mg daily is an alternative if these are not tolerated. The detection of *M. avium* complex organisms in the respiratory or gastrointestinal tract when a blood culture is negative is not, in itself, an indication for prophylaxis. Primary prophylaxis may be discontinued in patients with CD4$^+$ T-lymphocyte counts of more than 100 cells/µL and a sustained suppression of HIV plasma RNA for more than 3 to 6 months. An immune reconstitution syndrome consisting of focal lymphadenitis and fever without bacteremia has been described in patients who have responded to antiretroviral therapy.

- Prophylaxis for *Mycobacterium avium* complex is indicated for patients with AIDS whose CD4 cell count is less than 50 cells/mm^3.

Cryptococcus neoformans

Cryptococcus neoformans is a round or oval yeast that is acquired from the environment. It is inhaled into the lungs, where it usually causes asymptomatic infection, but it has a strong propensity for dissemination to the central nervous system. Other sites for potential dissemination include skin, bone, and the genitourinary tract. The most common manifestation of *C. neoformans* disease is cryptococcal meningitis, which usually occurs when the CD4 count is less than 50 cells/mm^3. The onset is insidious, symptoms are nonspecific (fever, headache, malaise), and symptoms may have a waxing and waning course. Meningismus may not be present. Brain imaging studies are also nonspecific; cerebral atrophy and ventricular enlargement are the most common findings. Cerebrospinal fluid findings may be minimal or include an increased opening pressure, mild mononuclear pleocytosis, and increased protein value. The India ink preparation is positive in more than 70% of cases. The serum and cerebrospinal fluid cryptococcal antigen test has a sensitivity of 93% to 99%. Cultures of cerebrospinal fluid are usually positive. In up to 80% of patients, results of blood cultures are positive for *C. neoformans*. Adverse prognostic factors include altered mental status on presentation and high fungal burden (positive result of India ink test, high antigen titers, and extraneural disease).

- *Cryptococcus neoformans* has a strong propensity for dissemination to the central nervous system.
- The most common manifestation of *C. neoformans* disease is cryptococcal meningitis.
- The India ink preparation is positive in more than 70% of cases.

Initial therapy includes amphotericin B with or without flucytosine for at least 2 weeks, followed by fluconazole 400 mg daily for a total of 8 to 10 weeks. Fluconazole (200 mg daily) is more effective than amphotericin B (1 mg/kg weekly) and itraconazole for chronic suppression. Persistence of infection in the prostate may be a cause of relapse of infection. Although fluconazole and itraconazole can reduce the frequency of cryptococcal disease, routine primary prophylaxis is not recommended for several reasons. These include cost, the relative infrequency of cryptococcosis, the possibility of drug interactions, and the potential for development of drug resistance.

- Typical clinical scenario: A patient with known HIV and a CD4 count of 20 cells/mm^3 presents with fever and headache. Computed tomography of the head shows mild cerebral atrophy but no specific lesions. Cerebrospinal fluid examination shows increased cerebrospinal fluid pressure, mild lymphocytosis, and increased protein concentration.
- Initial therapy for *C. neoformans* infection in HIV includes amphotericin B with or without flucytosine followed by fluconazole.
- Routine primary prophylaxis for *C. neoformans* disease is not recommended.

Cytomegalovirus

Cytomegalovirus disease usually affects persons with advanced HIV disease (CD4 cell count <100/mm^3). Chorioretinitis is the most common clinical manifestation of cytomegalovirus disease. The usual symptoms are floaters, visual field deficits, and painless loss of vision. Funduscopic examination reveals yellowish white granules with perivascular exudates and hemorrhages. Cytomegalovirus gastrointestinal disease most commonly involves the esophagus and colon and manifests with abdominal pain, dysphagia, and bloody diarrhea. Cytomegalovirus also can cause hepatitis, pneumonitis, sclerosing cholangitis, encephalitis, adrenalitis, polyradiculopathy, and myelopathy. Agents used for the treatment of cytomegalovirus disease and their general characteristics are listed in Table 12-5. After an induction course of therapy for 2 to 3 weeks or until clinical stability, maintenance therapy is continued with a reduced dose to prevent relapse. For gastrointestinal disease, maintenance therapy can be deferred until relapse is actually shown. Relapses generally are treated with reinduction courses of the initial agent. If this fails or if the progression is rapid, treatment with an alternative agent or combination regimens (e.g., ganciclovir plus foscarnet) should be considered.

- Typical clinical scenario: A patient with known advanced HIV disease presents with painless loss of vision in both eyes. Fundal examination reveals yellowish white granules, exudates, and hemorrhages. Therapy with ganciclovir or other effective cytomegalovirus agents should be initiated promptly.
- Cytomegalovirus disease usually affects persons with advanced HIV disease.
- In HIV, cytomegalovirus can cause chorioretinitis, gastrointestinal disease, hepatitis, and other organ involvement.
- Maintenance therapy is indicated after treatment of initial cytomegalovirus infection.

Syphilis

Sexually transmitted diseases, including syphilis, that cause genital ulceration may be cofactors for acquiring HIV infection. There are reports of false-negative and false-positive serologic tests for syphilis in patients with HIV. Neurosyphilis has been reported to occur earlier and more frequently in patients with AIDS than in HIV-negative patients. Patients with AIDS also have been reported to have unusually severe manifestations of all stages of syphilis. Recent studies, however, suggest that these phenomena are rare. In general, serologic response to infection seems to be the same in HIV-positive and HIV-negative persons and there are no specific clinical manifestations of syphilis that are unique to HIV. Penicillin-based regimens, whenever possible, are recommended by the CDC for all stages of syphilis in HIV-infected persons.

- Neurosyphilis occurs earlier and more frequently in patients with AIDS than in HIV-negative patients.
- Patients with AIDS have unusually severe manifestations of all stages of syphilis.

Toxoplasmosis

Toxoplasma gondii, a protozoan, is the most common cause of focal central nervous system lesions in patients with AIDS. The most common symptoms of *Toxoplasma* encephalitis include headache and confusion; fever may be absent. Focal neurologic deficits occur in 69% of cases. The median CD4 cell count at diagnosis is 50/mm^3. Multiple ring-enhancing lesions usually are noted on brain imaging studies. Magnetic resonance imaging is more sensitive than computed tomography for identifying lesions.

Table 12-5   Induction Treatment of Cytomegalovirus Retinitis

Drug	Dose	Major adverse effect
Ganciclovir intraocular release device*	Every 6 mo	Retinal detachment
Ganciclovir IV	5 mg/kg twice daily	Bone marrow suppression
Foscarnet IV	60 mg/kg three times daily or 90 mg/kg twice daily	Renal toxicity
Cidofovir IV[†]	5 mg/kg weekly for 2 weeks, followed by 5 mg/kg every 2 weeks	Renal toxicity
Ganciclovir intravitreal injection*	2,000 µg in 0.05-0.1 mL	Bone marrow suppression
Foscarnet intravitreal injection*	1.2-2.4 mg in 0.1 mL	Renal toxicity

IV, intravenously.

*Local anti-cytomegalovirus therapy should be accompanied by systemic therapy, such as oral ganciclovir, to avoid the risk of involvement of the other eye and extraocular diseases.

[†]Vigorous hydration and coadministration of probenecid are required to limit renal toxicity.

- *Toxoplasma gondii* is the most common cause of focal central nervous system lesions in patients with AIDS.
- Multiple ring-enhancing lesions usually are noted on brain imaging studies.

Empiric antitoxoplasmosis therapy is indicated in patients with AIDS and positive *Toxoplasma* serologic testing who present with multiple intracranial lesions. Effective treatment should result not only in amelioration of symptoms but also in a reduction of the number, size, and contrast enhancement of the brain lesions. If the patient is seronegative for *Toxoplasma*, has a single mass lesion on both computed tomography and magnetic resonance imaging, or did not achieve the desired response after an empiric course of antitoxoplasmosis therapy for 10 to 14 days, the presumptive diagnosis of *Toxoplasma* encephalitis becomes doubtful and a diagnostic brain biopsy is indicated. Drugs used for the treatment of HIV-associated toxoplasmosis are listed in Table 12-6. Lifelong suppressive therapy (secondary prophylaxis), with the same agents used for primary therapy but at a reduced dose, is necessary to prevent relapse. All HIV-infected persons with a CD4+ lymphocyte count of less than $100/mm^3$ who are seropositive for *Toxoplasma* should receive primary prophylaxis against *Toxoplasma* encephalitis. The agent of choice for this is trimethoprim-sulfamethoxazole (1 double-strength tablet daily); dapsone plus pyrimethamine is an alternative regimen. Atovaquone with or without pyrimethamine also may be considered.

- Lifelong suppressive therapy is needed to prevent relapse of HIV-associated toxoplasmosis.
- The agent of choice for primary prophylaxis against *Toxoplasma* encephalitis is trimethoprim-sulfamethoxazole.

HIV-infected patients should be tested for IgG antibody to *Toxoplasma* as part of their initial work-up; if the result is negative, they should be counseled about the various potential sources of *Toxoplasma* infection, such as raw or undercooked meat and handling of cat litter.

The differential diagnosis of central nervous system mass lesions in patients with AIDS includes toxoplasmosis, lymphoma, and bacterial brain abscesses and infections caused by *C. neoformans*, *Coccidioides immitis*, *M. tuberculosis*, and *Nocardia asteroides*, among others.

- Typical clinical scenario: A patient with known HIV disease presents with headache and confusion. There is evidence of upper and lower extremity weakness. Computed tomography shows multiple ring-enhancing lesions on brain imaging studies.

Table 12-6 Drugs Used for the Treatment of HIV-Associated Toxoplasmosis

Preferred regimens

Pyrimethamine* 200 mg PO loading dose followed by 50-75 mg PO daily plus sulfadiazine 1 g PO every 6 h

Pyrimethamine* 200 mg PO loading dose followed by 50-75 mg PO daily plus clindamycin 600 mg IV or PO every 6 h

Alternative regimens

Trimethoprim-sulfamethoxazole IV or PO 5 mg/kg every 6 h

Pyrimethamine* 200 mg PO loading dose followed by 50-75 mg PO daily plus clarithromycin 1,000 mg PO every 12 h

Pyrimethamine* 200 mg PO loading dose followed by 50-75 mg PO daily plus azithromycin 600-1,800 mg PO daily

Pyrimethamine* 200 mg PO loading dose followed by 50-75 mg PO daily plus dapsone 100 mg PO daily

IV, intravenously; PO, oral, orally.
*With folinic acid 10-20 mg daily.

AIDS Dementia Complex

This consists of a triad of cognitive, motor, and behavioral dysfunction. In its mildest form, it may begin early in the course of HIV disease, but it is otherwise a late manifestation of HIV disease. It can progress from subtle cognitive impairment to severe dementia with marked motor dysfunction. Computed tomography and magnetic resonance imaging of the brain show diffuse atrophy. No specific therapy has proved to be effective. Its prevalence may have been reduced by antiretroviral therapy.

- AIDS dementia complex triad: cognitive, motor, and behavioral dysfunction.
- AIDS dementia complex is a late manifestation of HIV disease.
- Diffuse atrophy is shown on imaging studies.

Progressive Multifocal Leukoencephalopathy

This is a demyelinating disease caused by JC virus. Symptoms and signs are variable and consist of focal neurologic deficits without altered sensorium or a systemic toxic state. Fever is usually absent. Symptoms evolve over weeks to months. Diagnosis is based on clinical findings and magnetic resonance imaging, which shows characteristic white matter changes (bright areas on T2-weighted images) without contrast enhancement or mass effect. Routine cerebrospinal fluid studies are generally nondiagnostic, but identification of JC virus DNA in the cerebrospinal fluid by polymerase chain reaction may confirm the diagnosis. Prognosis is poor, and there is no proven effective treatment.

- Progressive multifocal leukoencephalopathy is caused by the JC virus.
- The diagnosis is based on clinical findings and on white matter changes on magnetic resonance imaging.
- There is no proven effective therapy.

Candida albicans

Mucocutaneous disease (such as oral thrush or recurrent vaginitis) is common. Esophagitis is also frequent and is a common cause of dysphagia. Systemic candidal infection, including candidemia, is rare unless additional risk factors for disseminated fungal infection such as severe neutropenia and indwelling catheters are involved. Candidal esophagitis is an AIDS-defining condition. For mucocutaneous disease, initial treatment with clotrimazole troches or nystatin may be adequate. Fluconazole or itraconazole is used for the treatment of candidal esophagitis and topical treatment failures. Amphotericin B can be used for azole failures.

- Mucocutaneous disease is common.
- Systemic candidal infection is rare.

Enteric Infections

Initial evaluation of patients with AIDS who have abdominal pain, large-volume diarrhea, and weight loss should include stool cultures for bacteria, three separate stool specimens for ova and parasites, and specific examination for cryptosporidiosis, isosporiasis, microsporidiosis, and *Cyclospora*, as indicated. *Cytomegalovirus* or *M. avium-intracellulare* should be considered in the differential diagnosis, particularly in patients with advanced HIV infection. If no diagnosis is made, upper and lower gastrointestinal endoscopy and biopsy may yield pathogens that are treatable.

Salmonella Infections

In contrast to immunocompetent persons, HIV-infected persons are more likely to have *Salmonella* infection that is severe, invasive, and widespread. Bacteremia is common and constitutes an AIDS-defining diagnosis. Salmonellosis presents with fever, severe diarrhea, abdominal pain, or typhoidal illness with little diarrhea or gastrointestinal symptoms. Ciprofloxacin is used for treatment for 10 to 14 days; however, recurrence is common and maintenance therapy may be needed.

- HIV-infected persons are more likely to have *Salmonella* infection that is severe, invasive, and widespread.
- Ciprofloxacin is used for treatment of *Salmonella* infection.

Cryptosporidiosis

Cryptosporidium parvum is a protozoal organism that causes massive, watery diarrhea, crampy abdominal pain, anorexia, flatulence, and malaise. Fever and bloody diarrhea are uncommon, but malabsorption and dehydration are common. Cryptosporidiosis is diagnosed by identification of *C. parvum* oocysts in fecal samples or biopsy specimens. The specimens are stained with either a modified acid-fast procedure or a fluorescent assay that uses monoclonal antibodies to *Cryptosporidium* antigens. Biliary tract involvement may occur with cryptosporidiosis. If the CD4 cell count is more than $180/mm^3$, cryptosporidium infection is usually self-limited (<4 weeks); if it is less than $140/mm^3$, persistent disease develops in 80% to 90%. In adults, there are no proven regimens for the treatment of cryptosporidiosis, but paromomycin, a nonabsorbable aminoglycoside used for the treatment of *Entamoeba histolytica*, has been effective in some patients. More recently, a new drug, nitazoxanide, was approved by the Food and Drug Administration for the treatment of diarrhea caused by *C. parvum* and *Giardia lamblia* in pediatric patients (1-11 years old).

- *Cryptosporidium parvum* causes massive, watery diarrhea, crampy abdominal pain, anorexia, flatulence, and malaise.
- Cryptosporidiosis is diagnosed by identification of *C. parvum* oocysts in fecal samples or biopsy specimens.
- Paromomycin has been effective in some patients.

Isosporiasis

Isospora belli causes illness similar to that caused by *C. parvum*: profuse diarrhea without blood or fever but accompanied by abdominal pain and malabsorption. Isosporiasis is endemic in developing countries. The organism is identified with a modified acid-fast stain on fecal or biopsy specimens. Trimethoprim-sulfamethoxazole DS (160 mg of trimethoprim and 800 mg of sulfamethoxazole) four times daily for 10 days is effective for the treatment of *I. belli* infections, but lifelong suppressive therapy may be required.

- Isosporiasis: profuse diarrhea without blood or fever but accompanied by abdominal pain and malabsorption.
- Trimethoprim-sulfamethoxazole DS is effective treatment for isosporiasis.

Microsporidiosis

Two species of Microsporida, *Enterocytozoon bieneusi* and *Encephalitozoon intestinalis*, cause enteric and biliary disease in patients with AIDS. Infection with these organisms resembles infection with *C. parvum*, with perhaps less voluminous diarrhea. Electron microscopy of biopsy specimens and special stains are required for diagnosis. Currently, there is no effective therapy for microsporidiosis, but albendazole has shown promise in some studies, especially in the treatment of disease caused by *E. intestinalis.*

- Microsporida species cause enteric and biliary disease in patients with AIDS.
- Electron microscopy of biopsy specimens and special stains are required for diagnosis.
- There is no effective therapy for microsporidiosis.

Cyclospora

Cyclospora cayetanensis organisms are protozoal and cause gastrointestinal disease similar to cryptosporidiosis. Symptoms include watery diarrhea, fatigue, anorexia, myalgia, abdominal cramps, flatus, and nausea. Dehydration and weight loss are common. Biliary tract involvement is possible. Standard ova and parasite testing cannot detect the organisms; special staining techniques or electron microscopy may be required for diagnosis. Trimethoprim-sulfamethoxazole is effective for the treatment of *Cyclospora.* Chronic prophylaxis may be necessary.

- Symptoms of *Cyclospora*: watery diarrhea, fatigue, anorexia, myalgia, abdominal cramps, flatus, nausea, dehydration, and weight loss.
- Special staining or electron microscopy may be required for diagnosis.
- Trimethoprim-sulfamethoxazole is effective treatment.

Bacillary Angiomatosis

Bacillary angiomatosis was first described in 1983, and the causative organisms, *Bartonella quintana* and *Bartonella henselae*, were isolated for the first time in 1992. Bacillary angiomatosis is characterized by vascular proliferative lesions that can involve any organ in the body. The most commonly involved site is the skin, where it may present as nodules or plaques that are sometimes difficult to differentiate from those of Kaposi sarcoma. Other sites include bone, lymph nodes, brain, respiratory tract, and gastrointestinal tract. Characteristic fluid-filled spaces occasionally are noted in the liver and spleen and are called peliosis hepatis or peliosis splenis. Diagnosis is established by biopsy, demonstration of the organism on Warthin-Starry stain, and cultivation of the causative organisms. Results of blood culture (lysis centrifugation technique) also may be positive if incubation is prolonged. Treatment is with erythromycin or doxycycline.

- Bacillary angiomatosis is characterized by vascular proliferative lesions in skin and other organs.
- Differential diagnosis: Kaposi sarcoma.
- The diagnosis is based on positive results of Warthin-Starry stain and cultivation of the causative organism.
- Treatment is with erythromycin or doxycycline.

AIDS-ASSOCIATED MALIGNANCIES

Kaposi Sarcoma

Kaposi sarcoma is a tumor of uncertain origin; vascular proliferation is its most prominent feature. It is the most common neoplasm affecting HIV-infected persons. It is most common in the homosexual and bisexual population with AIDS. Herpes-like DNA sequences have been identified in AIDS-associated Kaposi sarcoma. These are thought to represent a new human herpesvirus, now designated human herpesvirus 8 (HHV-8). Seroepidemiologic studies have made a strong association between HHV-8 and Kaposi sarcoma. In addition, HHV-8 was found to be associated with all forms of Kaposi sarcoma, and its seroconversion precedes the appearance of Kaposi sarcoma in HIV-infected persons. Clinical manifestations include nodules, plaques, lymph node enlargement, and signs and symptoms of visceral involvement. Skin, lung, and the gastrointestinal tract are the commonly affected organs. Lung involvement may mimic infection. Treatment options include local therapy (radiotherapy, intralesional chemotherapy, cryotherapy) and systemic therapy (chemotherapy, interferon-α). Liposome-encapsulated anthracycline chemotherapeutic agents recently have become available, potentially enabling delivery of higher doses of effective drug with fewer toxic side effects.

- Kaposi sarcoma is the most common neoplasm in HIV-infected persons.
- It is most common in the homosexual and bisexual population with AIDS.
- Kaposi sarcoma is possibly related to HHV-8 infection.
- Clinical manifestations include nodules, plaques, lymph node enlargement, and signs and symptoms of visceral involvement.

Non-Hodgkin Lymphoma

In contrast to most other HIV-associated opportunistic conditions and Kaposi sarcoma, highly active antiretroviral therapy has not been associated with a substantial decline in the incidence of HIV-related lymphoma. The vast majority of non-Hodgkin lymphomas in patients with HIV are of B-cell origin. Intermediate- or high-grade B-cell non-Hodgkin lymphoma is a CDC-defined AIDS diagnosis. As patients with AIDS live longer, this complication will become more frequent. It commonly presents with constitutional symptoms (fever, night sweats, weight loss), lymphadenopathy, and involvement of extranodal sites such as the central nervous system, bone marrow, gastrointestinal tract, and liver. Involvement of the brain can be as an isolated disease (primary central nervous system lymphoma) or as leptomeningeal involvement in the context of spread of lymphoma elsewhere.

The optimal treatment of HIV-associated non-Hodgkin lymphoma has not been well defined. It has become clear, however, that high-intensity chemotherapeutic regimens do not necessarily translate into better outcome when compared with lower-dose regimens, especially in patients with profound immunosuppression. Factors that have been associated with poor treatment outcome include a $CD4^+$ count less than 100 cells/mm^3, advanced HIV infection, a history of AIDS-defining conditions, older age (older than 35 years), injection drug use, and increased serum lactate dehydrogenase value.

- The vast majority of non-Hodgkin lymphomas in patients with HIV are of B-cell origin.
- Non-Hodgkin lymphoma in HIV commonly presents with constitutional symptoms (fever, night sweats, weight loss), lymphadenopathy, and involvement of extranodal sites.
- Non-Hodgkin lymphoma in HIV can present as isolated central nervous system lymphoma.
- High-intensity chemotherapy regimens may not produce better outcomes than low-dose regimens.

Primary Central Nervous System Lymphoma

This is associated with Epstein-Barr virus in almost 100% of cases, is a complication of advanced AIDS (CD4 count <50/mm^3), and occurs in 1% to 3% of all patients with AIDS. Clinical presentation includes headache, focal neurologic deficits, and seizure. Brain imaging studies show single or multiple contrast-enhancing lesions. Biopsy is required for diagnosis. Whole-brain radiation is the primary treatment of primary central nervous system lymphoma. Radiation therapy to the brain has been associated with some return in neurologic function, but the median survival time has not been substantially increased.

- Typical clinical scenario: A patient with known HIV disease and a CD4 count of 30 cells/mm^3 presents with headache and weakness of the right upper and lower extremities. Imaging shows two contrast-enhancing lesions in the left frontoparietal lobe.
- Primary central nervous system lymphoma is associated with Epstein-Barr virus.
- Clinical presentation includes headache, focal neurologic deficits, and seizure.
- Biopsy is required for diagnosis.

ANTIRETROVIRAL AGENTS

Before November 1995, the antiretroviral drugs available and approved for clinical use in the United States consisted of only four nucleoside analogue reverse transcriptase inhibitors: zidovudine (Retrovir, ZDV, AZT), zalcitabine (Hivid, ddC), didanosine (Videx, ddI), and stavudine (Zerit, d4T). Since then, three new classes of agents and 16 new agents have been approved.

The Replication Cycle of HIV

A working knowledge of the HIV replication cycle is essential for understanding the mechanism of action of antiretroviral agents (Plate 12-1). The human immunodeficiency virus is an enveloped virus that contains two copies of viral genomic RNA and associated transfer RNA molecules in its core. In addition to the copies of RNA, the viral core also contains various *gag* and *pol* protein products. The first step in the HIV replication cycle is the interaction between the envelope proteins of the virus and specific surface receptors (e.g., CD4 receptor) of the host cell, leading to the binding of the viral envelope and the host cytoplasmic membrane. Recently, additional cell surface proteins, so-called co-receptors, that are required for the virus entry into the host cell have been identified. After entry into the cell, the viral reverse transcriptase enzyme catalyzes the conversion of viral RNA into DNA. This viral DNA enters the nucleus and becomes inserted into the chromosomal DNA of the host cell (integration). This integrated DNA may remain in an unexpressed form (e.g., in resting lymphocytes) and persist in a latent state for a long period. In acutely infected cells, however, expression of the viral genes leads to production of viral proteins. The precursor *gag* and *gag-pol* proteins, as well as viral RNA, are assembled at the cell surface into new viral particles and leave the host cell by a process called budding. During the process of budding, they acquire the outer layer and envelope. At this stage, the protease enzyme cleaves the precursor *gag* and *gag-pol* proteins into their mature products. If this final phase of the replication cycle does not take place, the released viral particles are noninfectious and not competent to initiate the replication cycle in other susceptible cells. The various steps in the HIV replication cycle (e.g., viral entry, integration) are being investigated as potential sites of action for antiretroviral therapy.

At the time of this writing, four classes of antiretroviral drugs have received approval by the U.S. Food and Drug Administration: nucleoside/nucleotide analogue reverse transcriptase inhibitors, nonnucleoside analogue reverse transcriptase inhibitors, protease inhibitors, and fusion inhibitors.

Four classes of antiretroviral drugs are approved by the U.S. Food and Drug Administration: nucleoside/nucleotide analogue reverse transcriptase inhibitors, nonnucleoside analogue reverse transcriptase inhibitors, protease inhibitors, and fusion inhibitors.

Nucleoside/Nucleotide Analogue Reverse Transcriptase Inhibitors (NRTIs)

NRTIs were the first antiretroviral agents to be developed. These agents are structurally similar to the building blocks of nucleic acids (RNA, DNA) but differ from their natural analogues by the replacement of the hydroxy (-OH) group in the 3′ position by another group that is unable to form the 5′ to 3′ phosphodiester linkage essential for DNA elongation. NRTIs block reverse transcriptase activity by competing with the natural substrates and incorporating into viral DNA to act as chain terminators in the synthesis of proviral DNA. To exert their antiviral activity, NRTIs must first be intracellularly phosphorylated to their active 5′-triphosphate forms by cellular kinases.

- NRTIs are structurally similar to the building blocks of nucleic acids.
- NRTIs block reverse transcriptase activity.

Resistance to NRTIs is associated with mutations in the *pol* gene that codes for the enzyme reverse transcriptase. Specific mutations that confer resistance to individual agents have been identified. High-level zidovudine resistance has been associated with broad cross-resistance to other nucleoside analogues. Other mutations that confer cross-resistance to several agents also have been observed. The M184V mutation, associated with resistance to lamivudine, has a complex effect on other nucleoside analogues. This mutation may confer limited cross-resistance to didanosine and zalcitabine. It also may delay the development of zidovudine resistance and restore zidovudine activity once resistance emerges. This "ZDV resensitization" effect also has been noted with the L74V mutation, selected for by didanosine.

- Resistance to NRTIs is associated with mutations in the *pol* gene that codes for the enzyme reverse transcriptase.

There have been reports of a rare and potentially fatal syndrome consisting of severe hepatomegaly with steatosis and lactic acidosis in the absence of hypoxemia. This syndrome can occur with any of the NRTIs. When recognized, treatment with nucleoside analogues should be suspended.

- A rare and potentially fatal syndrome of severe hepatomegaly with steatosis and lactic acidosis in the absence of hypoxemia has been reported in association with NRTIs.

Hypersensitivity reactions have been reported in approximately 5% of patients receiving abacavir. Symptoms consist of rash accompanied by systemic signs and symptoms such as fever, fatigue, nausea, vomiting, diarrhea, or abdominal pain. These symptoms usually appear within the first 6 weeks of treatment. The rash is usually maculopapular but can be variable in appearance. Hypersensitivity reactions also may occur without a rash. Symptoms usually resolve rapidly when use of the drug is discontinued. Once use of abacavir has been discontinued, it should not be reintroduced. More severe symptoms, including death, have been reported when use of abacavir is reinstituted.

The general characteristics of the currently available NRTIs are listed in Table 12-7.

Nonnucleoside Reverse Transcriptase Inhibitors (NNRTIs)

NNRTIs bind directly and noncompetitively to the enzyme reverse transcriptase. Although the drugs differ chemically from each other, they all bind to the same site, a site distinct from the substrate (dNTP) binding site. They block DNA polymerase activity by causing conformational change and disrupting the catalytic site of the enzyme. Unlike nucleoside analogues, NNRTIs do not require phosphorylation to become active and are not incorporated into viral DNA. They also have no activity against HIV-2.

- NNRTIs bind directly and noncompetitively to the enzyme reverse transcriptase.
- NNRTIs block DNA polymerase activity.
- NNRTIs do not require phosphorylation.
- NNRTIs are not active against HIV-2.

When NNRTIs are administered as a single agent or as a part of an inadequately suppressive treatment regimen, resistance emerges rapidly. Mutations conferring resistance to one drug in this class generally confer cross-resistance to most other NNRTIs. Cross-resistance to nucleoside analogues or protease inhibitors has not been observed. However, the Y181C mutation, selected for by nevirapine, reverses zidovudine resistance when introduced into isolates that carry the major zidovudine resistance mutations. Nevirapine and efavirenz are inducers of the hepatic cytochrome P-450 system. Delavirdine, however, inhibits P-450. Through this interaction with the P-450 enzyme system, NNRTIs may change the metabolism of and thus lower (nevirapine, efavirenz) or increase (delavirdine) the plasma levels of coadministered drugs that are metabolized by the cytochrome P-450 system. Similarly, drugs that induce or inhibit cytochrome P-450 activity may have an effect on the plasma concentrations of NNRTIs. Malformations of the fetus have been noted in primates exposed to efavirenz. Therefore, efavirenz is contraindicated in pregnant women.

- Mutations conferring resistance to one drug in NNRTIs generally confer cross-resistance to most other NNRTIs.

The general characteristics of the three NNRTIs currently approved for clinical use are listed in Table 12-8.

Table 12-7 General Characteristics of Currently Available Nucleoside/Nucleotide Analogue Reverse Transcriptase Inhibitors

	Zidovudine	Didanosine EC	Zalcitabine	Stavudine	Lamivudine	Abacavir	Emtricitabine	Tenofovir
Dose	300 mg twice daily	400 mg daily	0.75 mg three times daily	40 mg twice daily	150 mg twice daily	300 mg twice daily	200 mg daily	300 mg daily
Bioavail-ability, %	64	42	80	86	82	83	50-95	25
CSF pene-tration, %	60	21	20	30-40	<10	30	4	NA
Serum half-life, h	1.1	1.6	1.2	1.0	3-6	1.5	2.5-7	17
Intracellu-lar half-life, h	3	25-40	3	3.5	12	>12	20	10-50
Protein binding, %	34-38	5	<4	0	<36	50	NA	0.7-7.2
Major toxicity	Bone marrow suppres-sion	Pancreatitis, peripheral neuropathy	Stomatitis, peripheral neuropathy	Peripheral neuropathy	Minimal	Hyper-sensitivity	Minimal	Minimal, emerging reports of renal toxicity
Food restriction	None	Empty stomach	None	None	None	None	None	With food

CSF, cerebrospinal fluid; NA, not available.

Protease Inhibitors

Protease inhibitors exert their antiviral effect by inhibiting HIV-1 protease. HIV-1 protease is a complex enzyme composed of two identical halves (i.e., a symmetrical dimer) with an active site located at the base of the cleft. It is responsible for the cleavage of the large viral *gag* and *gag-pol* polypeptide chains into smaller, functional proteins, thus allowing maturation of the HIV virion. This process takes place in the final stages of the HIV life cycle. Inhibition of the protease enzyme results in the release of structurally disorganized and noninfectious viral particles. Protease inhibitors have antiviral activity in both acutely and chronically infected cells. Protease inhibitors are metabolized by the cytochrome P-450 system and are themselves, to varying degrees, inhibitors of this system. This leads to a considerable number of interactions with drugs that are inducers, inhibitors, or substrates of this system. General characteristics of currently available protease inhibitors are listed in Table 12-9.

- Protease inhibitors exert their antiviral effect by inhibiting HIV-1 protease.
- Protease inhibitors have antiviral activity in both acutely and chronically infected cells.

- Protease inhibitors have considerable interactions with drugs that are metabolized through the P-450 system.

Protease inhibitors have had potent antiretroviral, immunologic, and clinical benefits in HIV-infected persons, but their long-term efficacy and safety have not been completely elucidated. In fact, new side effects have become manifest with the continued widespread use of these drugs. Metabolic complications of these drugs have included hyperglycemia, frank diabetes mellitus, and abnormalities of lipid metabolism and lipid deposition. These complications were noted even in patients who responded well virologically to treatment and were otherwise in improved health. The biochemical and physiologic basis of protease inhibitor-related metabolic complications has, as of yet, not been adequately investigated and remains obscure. Of note, similar metabolic abnormalities have been reported in patients taking antiretroviral regimens that do not contain protease inhibitors.

- The long-term efficacy and safety of protease inhibitors have not been completely elucidated.
- Metabolic complications of protease inhibitors have included hyperglycemia, frank diabetes mellitus, and abnormalities of lipid metabolism and lipid deposition.

Table 12-8 General Characteristics of Currently Available Nonnucleoside Reverse Transcriptase Inhibitors

	Nevirapine	Delavirdine	Efavirenz
Dose	200 mg twice daily	400 mg three times daily	600 mg daily
Bioavailability, %	90	>80	Unknown
Protein binding, %	60	98	99.5-99.75
CSF penetration, %[*]	45	<1	0.26-1.19
Major adverse effects	Rash	Rash	Rash, CNS symptoms, fetal malformations in primates
Food effects	No substantial effect[†]	No substantial effect[†]	Avoidance of high-fat meals
Effect on P-450	Induction	Inhibition	Induction and inhibition

CSF, cerebrospinal fluid; CNS, central nervous system.
[*]As percentage of concurrent serum levels.
[†]No substantial effect means drug can be taken without regard to food.
From Temesgen Z, Wright AJ: Antiretrovirals. Mayo Clin Proc 1999;74:1284-1301. By permission of Mayo Foundation for Medical Education and Research.

Table 12-9 General Characteristics of Currently Available Protease Inhibitors

	Saquinavir (Fortovase)	Ritonavir	Indinavir	Nelfinavir	Amprenavir	Lopinavir-ritonavir
Dose	1,200 mg three times daily	600 mg twice daily	800 mg every 8 h	750 mg three times daily	1,200 mg twice daily	400/100 mg twice daily
Bioavailability, %	12	75	60	20-80	60-80	80
Protein binding, %	98	98-99	?	>98	90	98-99
Adverse effects	Gastrointestinal	Gastrointestinal, paresthesia, taste perversion (liquid)	Gastrointestinal, nephrolithiasis, hyperbilirubinemia	Diarrhea	Gastrointestinal, rash, paresthesias	Gastrointestinal, diarrhea Hyperlipidemia
Food effects	With fatty snacks or full meal	With meals	On empty stomach or with light snack	With meals	With or without, but high-fat meals should be avoided	With food
P-450 inhibition	+	++++	++	++	++	++++

Spontaneous bleeding has been reported in patients with hemophilia A and B treated with protease inhibitors, but a causal relationship between these incidents and protease inhibitor therapy has not been established.

The issue of resistance among protease inhibitors is complex and incompletely understood. Mutations that confer drug resistance have been identified in protease genes. Several of these mutations have been found to be key for individual protease inhibitors. Nevertheless, accumulation of several mutations is necessary for high-level resistance to occur, and cross-resistance is common among the various protease inhibitors that are currently in use. There is no cross-resistance between protease inhibitors and reverse transcriptase inhibitors.

Dual Protease-Inhibitor Regimens

The inhibitory effect of protease inhibitors on each other's metabolism has led to the evaluation of specific combinations that may delay or prevent the onset of resistance and allow for dose reductions, more convenient dosing regimens, and less toxicity. Currently, the ritonavir-saquinavir combination is the one for which the most data are available and is the only one recommended by the U.S. Department of Health and Human Services guidelines. Other combinations, including ritonavir-indinavir, indinavir-nelfinavir, ritonavir-nelfinavir, nelfinavir-saquinavir, and amprenavir-based regimens, are currently being evaluated. The long-term safety and efficacy of these combinations are unknown. Recently, this pharmacokinetic property of protease inhibitors has been exploited to produce a combination drug known as Kaletra. Kaletra contains two protease inhibitors: lopinavir and ritonavir. Ritonavir is present at a low dose, sufficient to inhibit the cytochrome P-450 system. This results in a susbstantial increase in lopinavir concentrations that exceed the in vitro inhibitory concentrations (IC_{50} or IC_{95}) for wild-type or even drug-resistant strains of HIV.

Fusion Inhibitors

Enfuvirtide (T-20) is the only fusion inhibitor that is currently approved by the U.S. Food and Drug Administration. It binds a region of the HIV envelope glycoprotein gp41 and prevents viral fusion with the target cell membrane. Enfuvirtide is administered by subcutaneous injection. The standard dosage is 90 mg twice daily. Enfuvirtide is packaged in powder form in single-dose vials and must be reconstituted with sterile water. The current indication for enfuvirtide is for the treatment of patients who have experienced multiple regimen failures. There are three important toxic effects that have been found in clinical trials of enfuvirtide. Almost everyone experienced injection-site reactions, typically erythematous nodules, mild-to-moderate in severity, rarely causing discontinuation of use of the drug. Much less frequent were hypersensitivity reactions. Third, bacterial pneumonia occurred at a higher frequency in enfuvirtide-treated patients than in patients in the comparator arms. The explanation for the pneumonia and its clinical importance are unknown.

HIV can become resistant to enfuvirtide, but there is no cross-resistance to the other currently approved antiretroviral drugs. Although resistance mutations selected by enfuvirtide may confer resistance to other fusion inhibitors, HIV isolates with demonstrated resistance to enfuvirtide may retain susceptibility to T-1249, another fusion inhibitor that is now currently in development.

Guidelines for Use of Antiretroviral Therapy for HIV Infection

Advances in the management of HIV infection have made earlier state-of-the-art treatment guidelines and recommendations obsolete. In recent months, guidelines addressing the issue of antiretroviral therapy in different populations and situations have become available.

Guidelines for Use of Antiretroviral Agents in HIV-Infected Adults and Adolescents

A panel of leading AIDS specialists, convened by the U.S. Department of Health and Human Services in collaboration with the Henry J. Kaiser Family Foundation, developed recommendations for use of antiretroviral agents in HIV-infected adults and adolescents. There is general consensus for treating patients with the acute HIV syndrome, those within 6 months of seroconversion, and those with symptoms ascribed to HIV infection. However, the HIV RNA or the CD4 level that should trigger initiation of treatment in an asymptomatic HIV-infected person with a high CD4 cell count continues to be debated. In general, the decision to treat asymptomatic patients should be based on the willingness and readiness of an individual to begin therapy, the degree of existing immunodeficiency as determined by the $CD4^+$ T-cell count, the risk of disease progression as determined by the $CD4^+$ T-cell count and level of plasma HIV RNA, the potential benefits and risks of initiating therapy in asymptomatic individuals, and the likelihood, after counseling and education, of adherence to the prescribed treatment regimen. The panel recommends that treatment should be offered to HIV-infected persons with a CD4 count less than 350 $CD4^+$ T cells/mm^3 or plasma HIV RNA levels exceeding 55,000 copies/mL (by reverse transcriptase polymerase chain reaction or bDNA assay). Additionally, patients must actively participate in all therapeutic decisions, understand the benefits and risks of treatment, and make an informed commitment to complex long-term treatment. Treatment should be offered to all patients with symptoms ascribed to HIV infection.

- Recommendation for use of antiretroviral agents: treat patients with acute HIV syndrome, those within 6 months of seroconversion, those with symptoms ascribed to HIV infection.

The goal of treatment is maximal viral suppression for as long as possible. Response to treatment is evaluated with plasma HIV RNA (viral load) levels. HIV RNA testing should be performed at baseline and repeated every 3 to 4 months during therapy, or at more frequent intervals if the situation warrants. A minimal change in plasma viremia is considered to be a three-fold or 0.5-$\log_{10}$ increase or decrease. A substantial decrease in $CD4^+$ T-lymphocyte count is a decrease of more than 30% from baseline for absolute cell numbers and a decrease of more than 3% from baseline in percentages of cells. In general, successful regimens are expected to decrease the plasma HIV RNA level by at least 1 log (10-fold) at 2 to 8 weeks and to less than 50 copies/mL at 4 to 6 months. In cases of therapy failures, a new regimen consisting of at least two new agents, without cross-resistance to the drugs in the failed regimen, should be substituted. Resistance testing (genotyping or phenotyping) has been found useful for making the appropriate drug selection for incorporation into a salvage treatment regimen.

- The goal of treatment is maximal viral suppression for as long as possible.
- Successful treatment decreases the HIV RNA level 10-fold at 2-8 weeks and to <50 copies/mL at 4-6 months.

Antiretroviral Drug Resistance Testing

Many studies have shown a strong correlation between the presence of drug resistance and treatment failure. Genotyping assays detect drug resistance mutations that are present in the relevant viral genes (e.g., reverse transcriptase and protease genes). They can be performed fairly rapidly, and results are available within 1 to 2 weeks. Interpretation of test results requires knowledge of mutations that are selected for by various antiretroviral drugs and their effect on the susceptibility of the virus to those and related drugs. Phenotyping assays measure the ability of HIV to grow in various concentrations of antiretroviral drugs. Compared with genotypic assays, phenotyping assays are more costly and have a longer turnaround time (2-3 weeks). Results are reported as the "-fold" increase in the median inhibitory concentration (IC_{50}) (the concentrations of drugs that inhibit 50% of viral replication). One should be aware of the limitations of resistance testing. Current genotyping and phenotyping assays are insensitive for minor viral species (species that constitute less than 10%-20% of the circulating virus population). These viral populations will not be detectable by current assays. In addition, currently available assays lack uniform quality assurance.

- There is a strong correlation between the presence of drug resistance and treatment failure.

Recently, several trials have found that resistance testing, in the setting of virologic failure, may help to maximize the benefits of antiretroviral therapy. Current guidelines recommend the use of antiretroviral drug resistance testing in cases of virologic failure during highly active antiretroviral therapy and suboptimal suppression of viral load after initiation of antiretroviral therapy. One should also consider resistance testing in acute HIV infection, in which such testing may help determine whether drug-resistant virus was transmitted.

Recommendations for Use of Antiretroviral Drugs in Pregnant Women

In the past few years, perinatal transmission of HIV has dramatically decreased in the United States. This decrease is a result of recommendations from the U.S. Public Health Service for universal prenatal HIV counseling and testing with consent for all pregnant women and the use of zidovudine for reduction of perinatal HIV transmission. These recommendations were based on the results of Pediatric AIDS Clinical Trial Group Protocol 076. This trial showed that zidovudine, when administered to the mother during the antepartum and intrapartum periods and to the newborn for the first 6 weeks of life, reduces the perinatal transmission of HIV by two-thirds. The advances in understanding the pathogenesis of HIV and the changes in antiretroviral therapy and monitoring of disease have made the establishment of new guidelines necessary. Consequently, the U.S. Public Health Service has updated its recommendations for the use of antiretroviral drugs in pregnant women.

- Perinatal transmission of HIV has decreased dramatically in the United States.
- Zidovudine is used for reduction of perinatal HIV transmission.

The recommendations note that health care providers of pregnant HIV-infected women must address two separate but related issues: treatment of the mother's HIV infection and reduction of the risk for HIV transmission to the fetus. The benefits of therapy must therefore be weighed against the potential risk for adverse events to the fetus or newborn. Decisions regarding initiation or alterations in therapy should involve the same factors as those used for women who are not pregnant, with the additional consideration of the potential impact of such therapy on the fetus and infant. HIV-infected pregnant women should be provided with the most complete and current information regarding the use of antiretroviral therapy, mode of delivery, and other issues and should be allowed to make their own decisions. The woman's autonomy in decision making should be respected. In its guidelines, the U.S. Public Health Service presents various clinical scenarios and recommendations and discussions relevant to these scenarios.

Several studies have shown that cesarean delivery (elective or scheduled) performed before the onset of labor and rupture of membranes is associated with a 55% to 80% decrease in perinatal HIV-1 transmission compared with other types of delivery. Thus, in the updated guidelines, elective or scheduled cesarean section is an option, particularly for HIV-infected women presenting in late pregnancy (after about 36 weeks of gestation) but not receiving antiretroviral therapy, as well as for HIV-infected women receiving highly active combination antiretroviral therapy but with HIV RNA levels that remain substantially more than 1,000 copies/mL at 36 weeks of gestation. However, cesarean section, compared with vaginal delivery, does present an increased risk of complications, such as increased rates of postoperative infection and anesthesia risks, and these risks must be balanced against the uncertain benefit of cesarean section.

- Cesarean delivery (elective or scheduled) performed before the onset of labor and rupture of membranes is associated with a 55%-80% decrease in perinatal HIV-1 transmission.

Recommendations for Postexposure Prophylaxis

Numerous studies have estimated that the average risk for HIV transmission is approximately 0.3% after percutaneous exposure to HIV-infected blood and 0.09% after mucous membrane exposure. A retrospective case-control study of health care workers documented that the use of zidovudine was associated with a 79% decrease in the risk for HIV transmission. Results of that study, as well as results from studies in animals and data from the Pediatric AIDS Clinical Trial Group on the efficacy of zidovudine for preventing perinatal transmission of HIV, prompted the U.S. Public Health Service to issue recommendations for prophylaxis in health care workers after occupational exposure to HIV. With the availability of new drugs and the accumulation of more knowledge, these 1996 guidelines were recently updated.

- In health care workers, the use of zidovudine is associated with a 79% decrease in the risk for HIV transmission.

The risk of infection is a function of the type of exposure and the infectivity of the exposure source. The guidelines provide an algorithm to guide clinicians in assessing risk and deciding when to offer postexposure prophylaxis. Systems, including written protocols, should be in place to prompt reporting and facilitate management of exposed health care workers. For most HIV exposures, a 4-week regimen of two antiretroviral drugs (zidovudine and lamivudine) is recommended. The addition of a protease inhibitor (indinavir or nelfinavir) is recommended for exposures with an increased risk of transmission or when resistance to one of the recommended drugs is known or suspected. Individual clinicians may, of course, prefer other antiretroviral drugs or combinations because of local knowledge and experience.

These recommendations are based on information available at the time they were developed. A mechanism has been put in place, through the HIV/AIDS Treatment Information Service Web site (*http://www.aidsinfo.nih.gov*), to regularly refine and update the recommendations in tandem with the evolution of knowledge about HIV infection.

- The risk of infection is a function of the type of exposure and the infectivity of the exposing source.
- For most HIV exposures, a 4-week regimen of two antiretroviral drugs (zidovudine and lamivudine) is recommended.
- A protease inhibitor is added to the regimen for exposures with an increased risk of transmission or when resistance to a recommended drug is known or suspected.

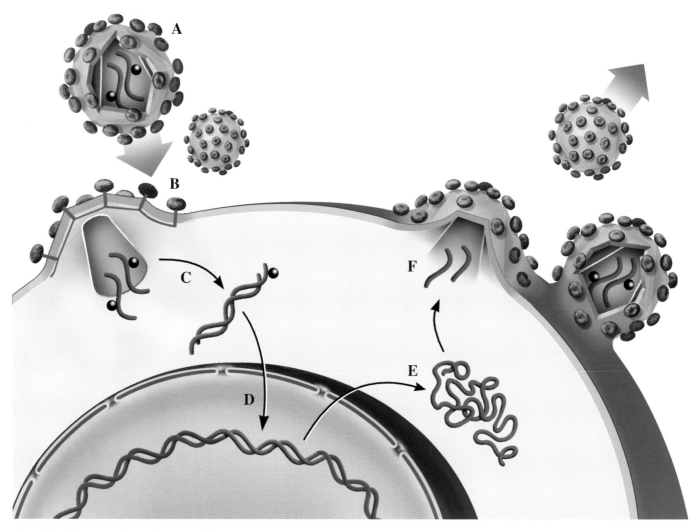

Plate 12-1. Life cycle of human immunodeficiency virus.

A, The virus is an enveloped virus that contains viral genomic RNA and various *gag* and *pol* protein products. *B*, The interaction between the envelope proteins of the virus and CD4 receptor and other receptors of the host cell leads to the binding of the viral envelope and the host cytoplasmic membrane. *C*, The viral reverse transcriptase enzyme catalyzes the conversion of viral RNA into DNA. *D*, The viral DNA enters the nucleus and becomes inserted into the chromosomal DNA of the host cell. *E*, Expression of the viral genes leads to production of viral RNA and proteins. *F*, These viral proteins, as well as viral RNA, are assembled at the cell surface into new viral particles and leave the host cell by a process called budding. During the process of budding, they acquire the outer layer and envelope. At this stage, the protease enzyme cleaves the precursor *gag* and *gag-pol* proteins into their mature products.

HIV Infection Pharmacy Review
Lynn L. Estes, PharmD

Drug (trade name)	Normal adult dosage*	Dosing instructions	Toxic/adverse effects	Drug interactions[†]
Nucleoside/nucleotide reverse transcriptase inhibitors (NRTIs)				
Abacavir (Ziagen)	300 mg twice daily	Take with or without food Alcohol increases abacavir levels	Hypersensitivity reaction usually occurs within days to 6 wk of initiation: fever, malaise, abdominal cramping, nausea, diarrhea, with or without rash, may be associated with increased values on LFTs and of creatine kinase. Hypersensitivity reactions also may present with respiratory symptoms such as cough, dyspnea, or pharyngitis. Rechallenge after a hypersensitivity reaction is *contraindicated* and can have severe or fatal consequences. Severe or fatal reactions also have been noted in patients who had a therapy interruption for reasons unrelated to hypersensitivity, followed by re-initiation of abacavir Other side effects include N/V/D, fever, malaise, headache, rare bone marrow suppression, increased values on LFTs NRTI class: fat redistribution, lactic acidosis, and hepatomegaly with steatosis have been reported with NRTIs	Potentially can inhibit or be affected by other drugs that inhibit alcohol dehydrogenase or UDP-glucuronyl transferase Alcohol increases abacavir levels
Abacavir, lamivudine, and zidovudine (Trizivir)	>40 kg: 1 tablet twice daily Not recommended in patients <40 kg or patients with creatinine clearance ≤50 mL/min	Take without regard to food	Abacavir: Hypersensitivity reaction usually occurs within days to 6 wk of initiation: fever, malaise, abdominal cramping, nausea, diarrhea, with or without rash, may be associated with increased values on LFTs and of creatine kinase. Hypersensitivity reactions also may present with respiratory symptoms such as cough, dyspnea, or pharyngitis. Rechallenge after a hypersensitivity reaction is contraindicated and can have severe or fatal consequences. Other side effects include N/V/D, fever, malaise, headache, rare bone marrow suppression	Abacavir Metabolized by cytosolic alcohol dehydrogenase or by UDP-glucuronosyltransferase Potentially can inhibit or be affected by other drugs that inhibit alcohol dehydrogenase or UDP-glucuronosyltransferase

HIV Infection Pharmacy Review (continued)

Drug (trade name)	Normal adult dosage*	Dosing instructions	Toxic/adverse effects	Drug interactions[†]
		Nucleoside/nucleotide reverse transcriptase inhibitors (NRTIs) (continued)		
			Lamivudine: Minor or infrequent: headache, nausea, diarrhea, abdominal pain, insomnia, pancreatitis in pediatric patients (rare in adults). Has activity against hepatitis B, and flares of hepatitis B may occur on discontinuation	
			Zidovudine: Major: 1) bone marrow suppression with anemia or neutropenia—frequency and severity related to dose, duration, and disease state; 2) malaise, GI intolerance, insomnia, or asthenia—dose-related and may resolve with continued therapy. Minor or infrequent: myopathy with increased CPK, hepatitis with increased transaminases (AST, ALT), hepatic failure, cardiomyopathy, fingernail discoloration, neurotoxicity	
			NRTI class: fat redistribution; lactic acidosis and hepatomegaly with steatosis have been reported with NRTIs	
Didanosine (ddI, Videx)	≥60 kg Tablets/EC capsules: 200 mg twice daily or 400 mg EC daily Powder: 250 mg twice daily <60 kg Tablets/EC capsules: 125 mg twice daily or 250 mg EC daily Powder: 167 mg twice daily	Take all formulations on empty stomach Buffered tablets and oral powder: Thoroughly chew, crush, or disperse in water or apple juice Do not mix with acidic juices Space apart 2 hours from drugs that may be chelated	Major: 1) peripheral neuropathy; 2) pancreatitis—increased risk with history of pancreatitis, advanced HIV, alcoholism, concurrent medications that cause pancreatitis (e.g., pentamidine), stavudine; 3) GI intolerance (nausea, diarrhea) Minor or infrequent: hyperuricemia, hepatitis, rash Fatal lactic acidosis has been reported in pregnant patients receiving a combination of stavudine and didanosine—avoid combination in pregnancy NRTI class: fat redistribution, lactic acidosis, and hepatomegaly	Space buffered tablets apart from drugs that are affected by increased gastric pH (e.g., itraconazole capsules) and drugs that may be chelated (e.g., quinolones, tetracyclines) Tenofovir can substantially increase didanosine concentrations—didanosine dose reduction recommended Ribavirin can increase didanosine exposure and risk of toxicity.

HIV Infection Pharmacy Review (continued)

Drug (trade name)	Normal adult dosage*	Dosing instructions	Toxic/adverse effects	Drug interactions[†]
Nucleoside/nucleotide reverse transcriptase inhibitors (NRTIs) (continued)				
		Pediatric formulation: Must mix with an antacid—see package insert	with steatosis have been reported with NRTIs	Use combination with caution Methadone can decrease didanosine levels—consider dose increase Hydroxyurea can increase potential for toxicity
Emtricitabine (Emtriva)	200 mg daily	Take without regard to food	Similar to lamivudine—generally well tolerated Most common: headache, diarrhea, nausea, and mild-to-moderate rash. Can cause skin discoloration (hyperpigmentation on palms or soles)—generally mild. Has activity against hepatitis B, and flares of hepatitis B may occur on discontinuation NRTI class: fat redistribution; lactic acidosis and hepatomegaly with steatosis have been reported with NRTIs	
Lamivudine (3TC, Epivir)	150 mg twice daily or 300 mg daily (<50 kg: 2 mg/kg twice daily)	Take without regard to food	Generally well tolerated Minor or infrequent: headache, nausea, diarrhea, abdominal pain, insomnia, pancreatitis in pediatric patients (rare in adults). Has activity against hepatitis B and flares of hepatitis B may occur on discontinuation NRTI class: fat redistribution; lactic acidosis and hepatomegaly with steatosis have been reported with NRTIs	
Lamivudine and zidovudine (Combivir)	1 tablet twice daily	Take without regard to food	Lamivudine: generally well tolerated Minor: headache, nausea, diarrhea, abdominal pain, insomnia; possible flares of hepatitis B on discontinuation Zidovudine Major: 1) bone marrow suppression with anemia or neutropenia—frequency and severity related to dose, duration, and disease state;	

HIV Infection Pharmacy Review (continued)

Drug (trade name)	Normal adult dosage*	Dosing instructions	Toxic/adverse effects	Drug interactions†
			Nucleoside/nucleotide reverse transcriptase inhibitors (NRTIs) (continued)	
			2) malaise, GI intolerance, insomnia, or asthenia—dose-related and may resolve with continued therapy Minor or infrequent: myopathy with increased CPK, hepatitis with increased transaminases (AST, ALT), hepatic failure, cardiomyopathy, fingernail discoloration, neurotoxicity Lamivudine has activity against hepatitis B and flares of hepatitis B may occur on discontinuation NRTI class: fat redistribution; lactic acidosis and hepatomegaly with steatosis have been reported with NRTIs	
Stavudine (d4t, Zerit)	≥60 kg: 40 mg twice daily <60 kg: 30 mg twice daily	Take without regard to food	Major: peripheral neuropathy Other: N/V/D, decreased appetite, headache, insomnia Rare: pancreatitis, anemia, hepatotoxicity, ascending neuromuscular weakness Fatal lactic acidosis has been reported in pregnant patients receiving a combination of stavudine and didanosine—avoid combination in pregnancy NRTI class: fat redistribution (may be more common with stavudine); lactic acidosis and hepatomegaly with steatosis have been reported with NRTIs	Possible increased pancreatitis, neuropathy, hepatotoxicity, lactic acidosis risk with didanosine or hydroxyurea
Tenofovir (Viread)	300 mg daily	Take without regard to food	Mild GI complaints, asthenia, headache, renal dysfunction (may be best to avoid in patients with renal dysfunction), osteomalacia Has activity against hepatitis B and flares of hepatitis B may occur on discontinuation NRTI class: fat redistribution; lactic acidosis and hepatomegaly with steatosis have been reported with NRTIs	Can substantially increase didanosine levels—didanosine dose reduction recommended Can decrease atazanavir levels—use of atazanavir plus ritonavir suggested Cidofovir, ganciclovir, and valganciclovir can compete for tubular secretion—monitor closely

HIV Infection Pharmacy Review (continued)

Drug (trade name)	Normal adult dosage*	Dosing instructions	Toxic/adverse effects	Drug interactions[†]
Nucleoside/nucleotide reverse transcriptase inhibitors (NRTIs) (continued)				
Zalcitabine (Hivid, ddC)	0.75 mg three times daily	Do not take with antacids	Major: peripheral neuropathy (15%-30%) Minor or infrequent: pancreatitis (about 1%), hepatotoxicity, arthralgia, oral & esophageal ulcers, myalgia, leukopenia, abdominal pain, N/V/D, headache, hypersensitivity NRTI class: fat redistribution; lactic acidosis and hepatomegaly with steatosis have been reported with NRTIs	
Zidovudine (AZT, ZDV, Retrovir)	200 mg three times daily or 300 mg twice daily	Take without regard to food	Major: 1) bone marrow suppression with anemia or neutropenia—frequency and severity related to dose, duration, and disease state; 2) malaise, GI intolerance, insomnia or asthenia—dose-related and may resolve with continued therapy Minor or infrequent: myopathy with increased CPK, hepatitis with increased transaminases (AST, ALT), hepatic failure, cardiomyopathy, fingernail discoloration, neurotoxicity NRTI class: fat redistribution; lactic acidosis and hepatomegaly with steatosis have been reported with NRTIs	Ribavirin can inhibit phosphorylation and activation of zidovudine—avoid if possible
Nonnucleoside reverse transcriptase inhibitors				
Delavirdine (Rescriptor)	400 mg three times daily	Take without regard to food	Rash is most common (can usually treat through this, but can be serious in some cases). Mild headache, fatigue, GI complaints, increased values on LFTs also may occur	Substrate for CYP 3A4[‡,§] (and 2D6) Can inhibit CYP 3A4,[//] 2D6, 2C9, and 2C19 Avoid histamine$_2$ blockers or proton pump inhibitors
Efavirenz (Sustiva)	600 mg daily (preferably at bedtime to start)	Take with or without food, except that a high-fat meal can increase bioavailability up to 50% and should be avoided	Major: rash (about 27%—can usually treat through this) and central nervous system symptoms, e.g., dizziness, light-headedness, nightmares, feeling of disengagement, impaired concentration—especially during first couple of weeks. Central nervous system symptoms can be minimized by	Substrate for CYP 3A4[‡,§] Can induce or inhibit CYP 3A4[//] (induction most common) In vitro also inhibits 2C9, 2C19 Can decrease methadone levels or effect—titrate dose

HIV Infection Pharmacy Review (continued)

Drug (trade name)	Normal adult dosage*	Dosing instructions	Toxic/adverse effects	Drug interactions[†]
		Nonnucleoside reverse transcriptase inhibitors (continued)		
			taking at bedtime, and they often subside after 2-4 wk	
			Can cause increased values on LFTs, especially in patients with hepatitis C. Teratogenic—avoid in pregnancy. Case reports of psychosis, delusional thoughts, suicidal ideation, and depression—more frequent in patients with history of mental illness. Modest increases of triglycerides and cholesterol possible. Can cause false-positive urine test for marijuana. Can increase cholesterol and triglyceride values by 10%-20% in some patients	
Nevirapine (Viramune)	200 mg daily ×14 d, then 200 mg twice daily	Start with 2-week lead-in of reduced dose to reduce incidence of rash Autoinduction occurs and stabilizes at 2-4 wk	Major: rash (29%), which often can be treated through if mild. Also, more rarely causes serious cutaneous reactions (Stevens-Johnson also reported). Rash occurs usually in first 28 days; decreased incidence with 14-day lower dose lead-in). Severe and fatal cases have been reported, particularly in first 12 weeks. Increased values on LFTs or history of hepatitis B or C may increase the risk of hepatotoxicity. If hepatitis occurs, therapy should be permanently discontinued. Other: nausea, headache, abdominal pain, diarrhea, mouth sores, somnolence During first 8 wk: patients should be intensively monitored for serious cutaneous reactions and signs of hepatotoxicity. Liver function should be monitored.	Substrate for CYP 3A4[‡,§] Induces CYP 3A4[//] Decreases methadone levels Decreases oral contraceptive levels—use alternative birth control

HIV Infection Pharmacy Review (continued)

Drug (trade name)	Normal adult dosage*	Dosing instructions	Toxic/adverse effects	Drug interactions[†]
		Protease inhibitors (PIs)		
Amprenavir (Argenerase)	>50 kg: 1,200 mg twice daily (total of 16 tablets a day); often combined with boosting doses of ritonavir and lower daily doses of amprenavir	Take with or without food but avoid a high-fat meal (can decrease absorption) 1,200 mg twice daily contains 1,744 IU of vitamin E; pediatric solution contains 46 IU/mL	Amprenavir is a sulfonamide and could have cross-allergenicity with other sulfonamides. Other adverse effects may include nausea, vomiting, headache, rash; question about long-term effects of large amounts of vitamin E (avoid extra vitamin E supplementation) Oral solution is contraindicated in infants and children <4 y, pregnant women, patients with liver or renal failure, and patients on disulfiram or metronidazole due to the high content of propylene glycol and potential accumulation PI class: diabetes or hyperglycemia, hemolytic anemia, and, in hemophiliacs, spontaneous bleeding or hematomas. Also can cause increased lipid values, and lipodystrophy (possibly somewhat less with amprenavir)	Substrate for CYP 3A4[‡,§] Can inhibit CYP 3A4[//] (potency similar to indinavir and nelfinavir) Decreases oral contraceptive levels—use alternative birth control Space from didanosine buffered tablets (not needed with EC formulation) Space apart from antacids
Atazanavir (Reyatez)	400 mg daily (can be combined with boosting doses of ritonavir in a dose of 300 mg atazanavir/100 mg ritonavir daily)	Take with food	Increased indirect bilirubin value, jaundice, GI effects, rash, prolonged PR interval or heart block in some patients PI class: diabetes or hyperglycemia (less likely with atazanavir), hemolytic anemia, and, in hemophiliacs, spontaneous bleeding or hematomas. Also can cause lipodystrophy. Atazanavir does not appear to increase lipid values, in contrast to other PIs	Substrate for CYP 3A4[‡,§] Can inhibit CYP 3A4[//], 1A2, 2C9 Tenofovir can decrease atazanavir levels—use of atazanavir plus ritonavir suggested Space from didanosine buffered tablets (not needed with EC formulation) Space apart from antacids, avoid use with histamine 2 and proton pump inhibitors if possible

HIV Infection Pharmacy Review (continued)

Drug (trade name)	Normal adult dosage*	Dosing instructions	Toxic/adverse effects	Drug interactions[†]
		Protease inhibitors (PIs) (continued)		
Indinavir (Crixivan)	800 mg every 8 h (often used in lower-dose twice-daily regimens in combination with ritonavir 100 or 200 mg)	Empty stomach preferred Alternatively, can take with liquids or a light meal Drink ≥48 oz water/d to decrease nephrolithiasis If given with ritonavir, can give without regard to food	Major: nephrolithiasis up to 4% (can decrease risk by drinking >48 ounces of liquids per day) ± hematuria. Asymptomatic increase in bilirubin without LFT elevations Infrequent: increased hepatic transaminase values, headache, N/V/D, metallic taste, fatigue, insomnia, blurred vision, dizziness, rash, thrombocytopenia, dry skin or lips, joint aches, ingrown toenails PI class: diabetes or hyperglycemia, hemolytic anemia, and, in hemophiliacs, spontaneous bleeding or hematomas. Also can cause lipodystrophy and increased lipid values	Substrate for CYP 3A[‡,§] Inhibits CYP 3A4[//] Space apart from didanosine buffered tablets Grapefruit juice substantially decreases indinavir levels, so should be avoided
Lopinivir and ritonavir (Kaletra)	>40 kg: 400/100 mg (3 capsules) twice daily; 4 capsules twice daily in combination with nevirapine and efavirenz	Take with food	Frequent: abnormal bowel movements, diarrhea, weakness or fatigue, headache, nausea, rash in children, higher incidence of increased triglyceride and cholesterol values than with other PIs Infrequent: worsening liver disease in patients with hepatitis B or C Oral solution contains alcohol— avoid with metronidazole or disulfiram PI class: diabetes or hyperglycemia, hemolytic anemia, and, in hemophiliacs, spontaneous bleeding or hematomas. Also can cause lipodystrophy and increased lipid values	Substrate for CYP 3A4[‡,§] Both are very potent inhibitors of CYP 3A4[//] Ritonavir inhibits CYP 2D6 Ritonavir inhibits or competes for CYP 2C9, 2C19 Ritonavir induces CYP 1A2 (decreases theophylline levels) Decreases methadone levels Decreases oral contraceptive levels—use alternative birth control Space apart from didanosine

HIV Infection Pharmacy Review (continued)

Drug (trade name)	Normal adult dosage*	Dosing instructions	Toxic/adverse effects	Drug interactions[†]
		Protease inhibitors (PIs) (continued)		
Nelfinavir (Viracept)	1,250 mg twice daily or 750 mg three times daily; can also be used with boosted regimens with low-dose ritonavir	Take with food	Frequent: mild diarrhea or soft stool Minor or infrequent: nausea, abdominal pain, flatulence, asthenia, rash Avoid powder formulation in patients with phenylketonuria PI class: diabetes or hyperglycemia, hemolytic anemia, and in hemophiliacs, spontaneous bleeding or hematomas. Also can cause lipodystrophy and increased lipid values	Substrate for CYP 3A4[‡,§] Inhibits CYP 3A4[//] (induces CYP 3A4 occasionally) Decreases oral contraceptive levels—use alternative birth control
Ritonavir (Norvir)	600 mg twice daily (taper up to this over 5-10 days); often used in combination with other PIs as a "boosting" agent at doses of 100-400 mg twice daily	Take with food May mix solution with chocolate milk or liquid nutritional supplement	Frequent: GI intolerance (dose-related, may resolve with continued therapy)—less common when used in low-dose boosting regimens Other: taste changes; dizziness, headache, somnolence, paresthesias (circumoral and extremities), hyperlipidemia, hypertriglyceridemia (increase >200%), increased CPK and uric acid, hepatotoxicity PI class: diabetes or hyperglycemia, hemolytic anemia, and, in hemophiliacs, spontaneous bleeding or hematomas. Also can cause lipodystrophy and increased lipid values; these may be more severe with ritonavir than with other PIs	Substrate for CYP 3A4[‡,§] Very potent inhibitor of CYP 3A4[//] Inhibits or competes for CYP 2C9, 2C19, 2D6 Induces CYP 1A2 (decreases theophylline levels) Can increase meperidine toxicity Decreases methadone levels Decreases oral contraceptive levels—use alternative birth control Space apart from didanosine
Saquinavir (Invirase, Fortovase)	1,200 mg Fortovase (Fortovase or Invirase often used at different doses in combination with ritonavir or nelfinavir)	Take with a full meal (or within 2 h afterward)	Frequent: dose-related GI intolerance (may subside with continued therapy), nausea, abdominal pain, diarrhea, headache, asthenia, mouth ulcers, paresthesias, rash, increased values on LFTs, increased lipid values PI class: diabetes or hyperglycemia, hemolytic anemia, and, in hemophiliacs, spontaneous bleeding or hematomas. Also can cause lipodystrophy and increased lipid values	Substrate for CYP 3A4[‡,§] Inhibits CYP 3A4[//] Dexamethasone decreases saquinavir levels Grapefruit juice increases saquinavir levels

HIV Infection Pharmacy Review (continued)

Drug (trade name)	Normal adult dosage*	Dosing instructions	Toxic/adverse effects	Drug interactions[†]
Fusion inhibitors				
Enfuvirtide (Fuzeon)	90 mg subcutaneously twice daily	Each 108-mg vial should be reconstituted 1:1 with sterile water for injection Reconstituted injection should be refrigerated and used within 24 h	Major: local injection site reactions Other: Possible increased rate of bacterial pneumonia, hypersensitivity reaction	

ALT, alanine aminotransferase; AST, aspartate aminotransferase; CNS, central nervous system; CPK, creatine phosphokinase; CYP, cytochrome P-450; GI, gastrointestinal; HIV, human immunodeficiency virus; LFTs, liver function tests; N/V/D, nausea, vomiting, diarrhea.

*Without substantial hepatic or renal dysfunction.

[†]Not all-inclusive and does not include drugs with overlapping toxic effects. See package insert and other resources for specific drug interactions.

[‡]Abbreviated list of CYP 3A4 inducers—can decrease levels or effect of substrates for CYP 3A4 (PIs, NNRTIs): rifampin (avoid with PIs except ritonavir), rifabutin, rifapentine, carbamazepine, phenobarbital, phenytoin, nevirapine, efavirenz, St. John's wort (avoid with PIs).

[§]Abbreviated list of CYP 3A4 inhibitors—can potentially increase levels or effect of substrates for CYP 3A4 (PIs, NNRTIs): PIs, erythromycin, azole antifungals, amiodarone, cimetidine.

[||]Abbreviated list of CYP 3A4 substrates—levels or effect can be increased by CYP 3A4 inhibitors such as PIs; levels potentially can be decreased by CYP 3A4 inducers such as nevirapine or efavirenz: benzodiazepines (avoid midazolam, triazolam; can use lorazepam with PIs), statins (avoid use of lovastatin, simvastatin with PIs; pravastatin does not interact and atorvastatin can be used with caution/monitoring), dihydropyridine calcium channel blockers, ergot alkaloids (avoid with PIs), sildenafil (dose reduction needed with PIs), some antidysrhythmics, warfarin may be inconsistently affected, cisapride (avoid with PIs), pimozide (avoid with PIs), rifabutin (may need dose alterations of one or both drugs), some antidepressants, anticonvulsants (carbamazepine, phenytoin, phenobarbital)—monitor levels, immunosuppressants (cyclosporine, tacrolimus, sirolimus), azole antifungals.

QUESTIONS

Multiple Choice (choose the one best answer)

1. A 28-year-old black man who is positive for human immunodeficiency virus (HIV) has had waxing and waning headache, irritability, and malaise during the past 6 weeks. He had been extensively treated with antiretrovirals in the past, but all regimens failed. He has a low-grade fever of 38.0°C and stable blood pressure and heart rate. He has no nuchal rigidity or neurologic deficits on examination. CT of the head shows no abnormalities except for mild cerebral atrophy. His CD4 cell count is 40/μL and HIV-1 RNA is 275,000 copies/mL. What is the next most appropriate diagnostic test?
   a. Stereotactic brain biopsy
   b. Positron emission tomography of the brain
   c. MRI of the brain
   d. Lumbar puncture and cerebrospinal fluid studies
   e. *Toxoplasma* serologic test

2. A 33-year-old white woman presents with complaints of fatigue, malaise, and sore throat of 2 weeks' duration. She is concerned about HIV infection because HIV infection was diagnosed in her husband 7 years ago. She was tested for HIV 6 months ago, and the result was negative. The couple is sexually active and uses condoms but not consistently. The husband is receiving antiretroviral therapy but there are problems with suppressing his HIV. On physical examination, the patient has a temperature of 38.1°C, blood pressure 140/75 mm Hg, heart rate 80 beats/min, and respiratory rate 20 breaths/min. She has a macular erythematous rash on her trunk and swollen cervical lymph nodes. Results of the rest of her examination, including lungs, heart, and abdomen, are unremarkable. Laboratory results are hemoglobin 13 g/dL, leukocyte count 9,600/μL, and platelet count 220,000/μL. Atypical lymphocytes are noted on peripheral smear. Serum creatinine value is normal (1.0 mg/dL). Liver function test values (aspartate aminotransferase, alanine aminotransferase, bilirubin, and alkaline phosphatase) were all within normal range. All of the following statements are true about her diagnosis *except*:
   a. Results of HIV antibody testing may be negative
   b. Antiretroviral therapy is indicated
   c. p24 antigen assay may help in making the diagnosis
   d. Polymerase chain reaction for HIV may help in making the diagnosis
   e. This presentation is rare

3. A 32-year-old black man who is HIV-positive presents to the emergency department with complaints of fever, shortness of breath, nonproductive cough, and night sweats. He is not receiving any antiretroviral treatment. He has a temperature of 38.7°C, and examination of the heart, lungs, and abdomen is normal. He has no skin lesions. Chest radiography shows bilateral interstitial infiltrates. On arterial blood gas analysis, the PO_2 is 60 mm Hg.

   Laboratory values are as follows:
   Hemoglobin 12 g/dL
   Leukocyte count 8,400/μL
   Platelet count 150,000/μL
   Serum creatinine 1.0 mg/dL
   CD4 cell count 105/μL

   What is the next most appropriate diagnostic test?
   a. Sputum test for bacteria and acid-fast bacilli
   b. Tuberculin skin test
   c. CT of the chest
   d. HIV-1 RNA assay
   e. Induced sputum with staining for *Pneumocystis carinii* pneumonia

4. A 28-year-old Hispanic man, known to be HIV-positive for the past 6 years, wants to discuss issues concerning antiretroviral therapy. He is not receiving this therapy currently. He has no complaints and his physical examination is unremarkable. His laboratory study results include hemoglobin 13.5 g/dL, leukocyte count 8,400/μL, and platelet count 200,000/μL. Serum creatinine value is 0.8 mg/dL. Liver function test values (aspartate aminotransferase, alanine aminotransferase, bilirubin, and alkaline phosphatase) are all within normal range. CD4 cell count is 490/μL, and HIV-1 RNA level is 20,000 copies/mL. What is the next appropriate step regarding antiretroviral therapy?
   a. No treatment is indicated at this time
   b. Two nucleoside analogue reverse transcriptase inhibitors (NRTIs) plus a protease inhibitor
   c. Two NRTIs plus a nonnucleoside analogue reverse transcriptase inhibitor (NNRTI)
   d. Three NRTIs
   e. Two NRTIs plus a boosted protease inhibitor

5. An HIV serodiscordant couple (HIV infection recently was diagnosed in the man, the woman is HIV-negative) want information about the risk of HIV transmission. They are also interested in having children. Each of the following statements regarding HIV transmission is correct *except*:
   a. The proper use of condoms greatly reduces the risk of HIV transmission

b. Traumatic intercourse increases the risk of HIV transmission
c. Ulcerative genital infections increase the risk of HIV transmission
d. The risk of HIV transmission from an HIV-infected mother to her infant (vertical transmission) is nearly 65%
e. Antiretroviral agents decrease the rate of vertical transmission

6. A 36-year-old white man with a known diagnosis of AIDS presents with right-sided weakness and gait difficulty, progressing during the past 6 weeks. His cognitive ability seems to be intact. On examination he is afebrile and no nuchal rigidity is noted, but he has considerable motor weakness on the right side with hyperactive reflexes. His CD4 cell count is 15/μL and HIV-1 RNA is 150,000 copies/mL. Testing for antitoxoplasma IgG antibody is negative, as is the serum crytococcal antigen test. CT of the brain shows hypodense white matter lesions without a mass effect on contrast enhancement. MRI of the brain shows multiple bright areas on T2-weighted images in the same locations. All the following statements can be made about this condition *except*:
   a. Antiretroviral treatment may help improve this condition
   b. There is no specific treatment
   c. It is caused by a human papovavirus

d. It also can occur in early HIV
e. Symptoms evolve over a protracted period—weeks to months

7. A 46-year-old black man with HIV infection presents with complaints of blurring and loss of vision. Examination reveals visual field deficits. Funduscopic examination shows retinal perivascular exudates and hemorrhages. The patient has been losing some weight, but otherwise his physical examination is unremarkable. He has never received antiretroviral therapy.

Laboratory values are as follows:
Hemoglobin 9.2 g/dL
Leukocyte count 3,500/μL
Platelet count 85,000/μL
Serum creatinine 0.6 mg/dL

All the following comments regarding his opportunistic infection are correct *except*:
   a. His CD4 count is likely less than 50 cells/μL
   b. His HIV RNA is likely high
   c. Intravenous ganciclovir is a preferred drug for treating this infection in this patient
   d. Intravenous foscarnet is a preferred drug for treating this infection in this paitent
   e. Antiretroviral therapy will help with the management of this infection

ANSWERS

1. Answer d.

The symptoms suggest a central nervous system process. In the absence of a focal mass on imaging studies, cryptococcal meningitis becomes prominent in the differential diagnosis and requires cerebrospinal fluid analysis for confirmation. Common findings include an increased opening pressure, mild mononuclear pleocytosis, and increased protein value. The India ink preparation is positive in more than 70% of cases. The serum and cerebrospinal fluid cryptococcal antigen test has a sensitivity of 93% to 99%. Cerebrospinal fluid cultures are the standard. Up to 80% of patients have blood culture results that are positive for *Cryptococcus neoformans*.

2. Answer e.

This is a case of primary HIV infection. It is a fairly common presentation of HIV in newly infected individuals. It is noted in upward of 40% of infected individuals who present with a brief illness that may last for a few days to a few weeks. This period of illness is associated with a huge amount of circulating virus, a rapid decline in the CD4 cell count, and a vigorous immune response. Patients usually present with a mononucleosis-like illness, but the clinical manifestations may be protean. An atypical lymphocytosis may be present in approximately 50% of patients. Results of enzyme-linked immunosorbent assay may be negative (window period), whereas p24 antigen, HIV culture, or polymerase chain reaction results may provide the diagnosis. Treatment with the most potent antiretroviral combination regimen available is recommended with the hope of intervening before the HIV infection is fully established, when the viral population is relatively homogeneous, and the host immune system is relatively intact.

3. Answer e.

This patient's presentation is most consistent with *Pneumocystis carinii* pneumonia. Staining for this in hypertonic saline-induced expectorated sputum is the initial diagnostic method of choice. If negative, staining of specimens obtained through bronchoalveolar lavage should be attempted. Open lung biopsy is rarely needed.

4. Answer a.

In general, patients with the acute HIV syndrome, those within 6 months of seroconversion, and those with symptoms ascribed to HIV infection should receive antiretroviral therapy. Treatment should be offered to asymptomatic HIV-infected individuals with a CD4 count less than 350 cells/mm^3 or plasma HIV RNA value more than 55,000 copies/mL. The regimen of choice for initiation of antiretroviral therapy is the combination of a protease inhibitor or efavirenz nonnucleoside analogue reverse transcriptase inhibitor in combination with two NRTIs. The combination of ritonavir plus saquinavir (boosted protease inhibitor) with one or two nucleoside analogue reverse transcriptase inhibitors is another option.

5. Answer d.

The risk of HIV transmission to infants born to HIV-infected mothers is 16% to 30%.

6. Answer d.

Symptoms of focal neurologic deficits without altered sensorium that evolve over weeks to months and show characteristic white matter changes on MRI strongly suggest progressive multifocal leukoencephalopathy. This is a demyelinating disease caused by JC virus, a human papovavirus, and occurs in patients with advanced acquired immunodeficiency syndrome. It has a very poor prognosis. There is no proven effective treatment.

7. Answer c.

The symptoms in this patient, the funduscopic findings, and the disease stage are consistent with a diagnosis of cytomegalovirus retinitis. Current agents available for the treatment of cytomegalovirus disease include intravenous ganciclovir, foscarnet, and cidofovir. However, in this patient, who has preexisting cytopenias, ganciclovir is not a preferred drug because of its well-known myelosuppressive adverse effects. As with most opportunistic infections and conditions, the treatment of HIV itself may ameliorate the condition.

CHAPTER 13

HYPERTENSION

Gary L. Schwartz, M.D.

HYPERTENSION

Definition

Because blood pressure is a continuously distributed trait in the population and the risk of cardiovascular disease associated with the level of blood pressure increases progressively as it exceeds 115 mm Hg systolic or 75 mm Hg diastolic, the definition of hypertension is somewhat arbitrary. Currently for adults, hypertension is defined as systolic blood pressure 140 mm Hg or higher or diastolic blood pressure 90 mm Hg or higher. Hypertension is further stratified into two stages on the basis of the highest level of either systolic or diastolic blood pressure (Table 13-1). Systolic blood pressure between 120 and 139 mm Hg or diastolic blood pressure between 80 and 89 mm Hg is in the prehypertensive range. Persons with blood pressure in this range are at increased risk for cardiovascular disease and progression to hypertension over time.

- Hypertension is defined as systolic blood pressure ≥140 mm Hg or diastolic blood pressure ≥90 mm Hg.

Table 13-1 Classification of Blood Pressure for Adults 18 Years and Older[*]

Category	Blood pressure level, mm Hg		
	Systolic		Diastolic
Normal	<120	and	<80
Prehypertension	120-139	or	80-89
Hypertension			
Stage 1	140-159	or	90-99
Stage 2	≥160	or	≥100

[*]Not taking antihypertensive drugs and not acutely ill. When systolic and diastolic blood pressures fall into different categories, the higher category should be selected to classify the person's blood pressure status.

Modified from The Seventh Report of the Joint National Committee on Prevention, Detection, Evaluation, and Treatment of High Blood Pressure: The JNC 7 report. JAMA 2003;289:2560-2571.

Isolated systolic hypertension, mainly a problem of people older than 55 years, is defined as systolic blood pressure 140 mm Hg or higher and diastolic blood pressure less than 90 mm Hg. Secondary causes of isolated systolic hypertension include disorders associated with either increased cardiac output (anemia, thyrotoxicosis, arteriovenous fistula, Paget disease of bone, and beriberi) or increased cardiac stroke volume (aortic insufficiency and complete heart block).

- Isolated systolic hypertension is defined as systolic blood pressure ≥160 mm Hg with diastolic pressure <90 mm Hg
- Isolated systolic hypertension mainly affects people older than 55 years.
- Secondary causes include increased cardiac output (anemia, thyrotoxicosis, arteriovenous fistula, Paget disease of bone, beriberi) and increased cardiac stroke volume (aortic insufficiency, complete heart block).

Epidemiology

Blood pressure increases with age. Systolic blood pressure increases through the seventh decade, but diastolic blood pressure plateaus in the fifth decade. Thus, both the incidence and prevalence of hypertension increase with age, and isolated systolic hypertension becomes the most common subtype in older persons. For a middle-aged person with normal blood pressure, the lifetime risk of developing hypertension is 90%.

In addition to age, other nonreversible factors associated with increased risk of developing hypertension include being African American or having a family history of hypertension. Reversible factors are having a blood pressure level in the prehypertensive range, being overweight, having a sedentary life style, ingesting a high sodium–low potassium diet, having excessive intake of alcohol, or having the metabolic syndrome. "Metabolic syndrome" is defined by the presence of three or more of the following conditions: abdominal obesity (waist circumference >40 inches in men or >35 inches in women), impaired fasting blood glucose (fasting glucose ≥110 mg/dL), blood pressure 130/85 mm Hg or higher, increased plasma level of triglycerides (≥150 mg/dL) or low high-density lipoprotein (HDL) cholesterol (<40 mg/dL in men or <35 mg/dL in women). Correcting reversible factors can lower blood pressure and prevent the development of hypertension.

In young adulthood and early middle age, hypertension is more common in men than in women. In people older than 60 years, the reverse is true. Hypertension is more common in African Americans than in whites at all ages, and in both races, it is more common in the economically disadvantaged.

Hypertension is a major risk factor for cardiovascular disease morbidity and mortality (myocardial infarction, congestive heart failure, stroke), progressive atherosclerosis, chronic kidney disease, and dementia. Although risk is continuous and proportionate over both systolic and diastolic blood pressure levels, diastolic blood pressure is the better predictor of risk in young people and systolic blood pressure is the dominant predictor of risk in people older than 50 years.

For any given level of blood pressure, the risk is greater in men than in women, in African Americans than in whites or other racial-ethnic groups, in older than in younger people, and in those with longer duration of hypertension, additional risk factors for cardiovascular disease, or target organ injury. It is estimated that 58 million Americans have hypertension or are taking medication to decrease blood pressure. In addition to definite hypertension, an additional 45 million Americans have prehypertension.

- Nonreversible risk factors for hypertension: older age, being African American, having a family history of hypertension.
- Reversible risk factors for hypertension: prehypertensive blood pressure level, overweight, sedentary lifestyle, high sodium–low potassium diet, excessive alcohol intake, and metabolic syndrome.
- Treatment of reversible risk factors can prevent the development of hypertension.
- Hypertension is a major risk factor for cardiovascular disease and dementia.
- Diastolic blood pressure is the best predictor of cardiovascular disease in young people.
- Systolic blood pressure is the dominant predictor of risk of cardiovascular disease in middle-aged and older people.
- Individual risk from hypertension is related to its level, duration, and the presence of other risk factors for cardiovascular disease or target organ injury.
- At any given level of blood pressure, African Americans and men are at the greatest risk.

For persons with hypertension, mortality is most often due to complications of coronary artery disease. Factors that add to this risk are tobacco use, hyperlipidemia, diabetes mellitus, obesity, sedentary lifestyle, sex (men and postmenopausal women), age older than 60 years, and a family history of premature cardiovascular disease (women <65 years, men <55 years). The presence of target organ damage (stroke, left ventricular hypertrophy, ischemic heart disease, congestive heart failure, renal disease, retinopathy, peripheral vascular disease, and dementia) increases the risk of cardiovascular disease events even if blood pressure is subsequently controlled. This fact argues for early identification and prompt treatment of hypertension to avoid the development of target organ injury.

- The most common cause of death of persons with hypertension is coronary artery disease.
- Other risk factors for coronary artery disease include tobacco use, hyperlipidemia, diabetes mellitus, obesity, sedentary lifestyle, male sex, postmenopausal state, older age, and family history of premature cardiovascular disease.
- Target organ damage increases the risk of cardiovascular disease events even if blood pressure is subsequently controlled.

Left ventricular hypertrophy is a strong predictor of sudden death and myocardial infarction in persons with hypertension. Other factors associated with increased left ventricular muscle mass include increasing age, obesity, and regular vigorous physical activity. Unlike increases in left ventricular mass associated with hypertension, obesity, and age, an increase due to vigorous physical activity is not associated with increased risk of cardiovascular disease (athletic heart). Echocardiography is more sensitive than electrocardiography in detecting left ventricular hypertrophy.

- Left ventricular hypertrophy is a strong predictor of sudden death and myocardial infarction in persons with hypertension.
- Echocardiography is more sensitive than electrocardiography in detecting left ventricular hypertrophy.

Diagnosis

The diagnosis of hypertension relies on several measures of blood pressure performed in a rigorous manner with a validated and well-maintained mercury or aneroid sphygmomanometer and with an appropriate-sized cuff (the bladder should encircle at least 80% of the arm). The person should be at rest in the seated position (back and feet supported) for at least 5 minutes before the measurement. Recent physical activity, use of tobacco or caffeine (within 30 minutes of the measurement), or a full urinary bladder can transiently increase blood pressure and should be avoided. The arm should be bare (no tight clothing constricting the upper arm) and positioned so the cuff is at the level of the heart. The diagnosis of hypertension in a person with an initially elevated blood pressure is confirmed by at least two office visits. At least two standardized measures of blood pressure should be made at each visit. For most persons, confirmation can occur over 1 to 2 months. If initial blood pressure is severely elevated or in the presence of additional risk factors for cardiovascular disease or clinical cardiovascular disease, confirmation should be made in a shorter time.

Some persons have elevated blood pressure when it is measured in the clinic environment but have normal blood pressure at all other times. This is called "office hypertension" or "white coat hypertension." Whether these persons develop the adverse consequences of sustained hypertension is uncertain; therefore, they usually require no treatment initially but need to be followed and periodically assessed for the development of hypertensive target organ damage. Self-measurement of blood pressure outside the office setting can identify white coat hypertension. However, the diagnosis is best confirmed with noninvasive ambulatory blood pressure monitoring. On average, self-recorded blood pressure at home or awake average blood pressure by ambulatory monitoring is lower than office measures and, therefore, values less than 135 mm Hg systolic and less than 85 mm Hg diastolic are considered elevated. Blood pressure devices for home use need to be validated at regular intervals (twice yearly) by the health care provider.

Older persons may have "pseudohypertension," a falsely increased systolic and diastolic blood pressure when measured by the cuff method; it is the result of a stiff vascular tree caused by atherosclerosis. Similar to persons with "white coat hypertension," persons with pseudohypertension may have marked elevations of blood pressure but lack expected target organ injury. They may also complain of symptoms that suggest low blood pressure with treatment. Pseudohypertension may exist if the radial artery remains palpable after the brachial artery is occluded by cuff inflation (Osler maneuver). However, the Osler maneuver is not a very sensitive screening method for pseudohypertension. Confirmation requires intra-arterial blood pressure measurement.

- The diagnosis of hypertension requires several blood pressure measurements made in a standardized fashion on different occasions.
- Recent physical exercise, use of tobacco or caffeine, or a full urinary bladder can transiently elevate blood pressure.
- Office (white coat) hypertension: elevated blood pressure only when measured in the clinic environment.
- Pseudohypertension: inaccurately high cuff blood pressure as a result of a stiff vascular tree in older persons.

Evaluation

After the diagnosis of hypertension has been established, 1) identify lifestyle factors that contribute to higher blood pressure, 2) identify other risk factors for cardiovascular disease,

3) assess for target organ damage, and 4) consider the possibility of secondary hypertension. Secondary hypertension accounts for approximately 5% to 10% of all cases of high blood pressure.

- Secondary hypertension accounts for 5%-10% of all cases of high blood pressure.

Clues to secondary hypertension are features that are inconsistent with essential hypertension. Classic features of essential hypertension are onset in the fourth or fifth decade of life, a positive family history for hypertension, initial blood pressure stage 1 elevated and easily controlled with one or two medications, no target organ damage, normal routine laboratory studies, and blood pressure that does not progress to higher levels over a short period of time. Factors inconsistent with essential hypertension are listed in Table 13-2.

- Consider secondary hypertension if the presenting features are inconsistent with those of essential hypertension.

Table 13-2   Factors Inconsistent With Essential Hypertension

General
  Age at onset—before 30 or after 50 years
  Blood pressure >180/110 mm Hg at diagnosis
  Significant target organ damage at diagnosis
    Hemorrhages and exudates on retinal examination
    Renal insufficiency
    Cardiomegaly
    Left ventricular hypertrophy
  Poor response to an appropriate three-drug program
Features suggesting specific secondary causes of hypertension
  Primary aldosteronism
    Unprovoked hypokalemia, Chvostek sign, Trousseau sign
  Pheochromocytoma
    Labile blood pressure with diaphoresis, tachycardia, headache, pallor, neurofibromas, orofacial neuromas (MEN II)
  Renovascular disease
    Abdominal bruit
  Cushing disease
    Truncal obesity, pigmented striae, impaired fasting glucose, hypokalemia
  Coarctation of the aorta
    Delayed or absent femoral pulses
  Polycystic kidney disease
    Abdominal or flank mass, family history of renal disease

MEN, multiple endocrine neoplasia.

Drugs

Certain drugs can cause or aggravate hypertension or interfere with the action of antihypertensive medications. These drugs and their mechanisms of action are listed in Table 13-3.

- Certain drugs can cause or aggravate hypertension or interfere with the action of antihypertensive medications.

- Oral contraceptives induce sodium retention, increase renin substrate, and facilitate the action of catecholamines.
- Nonsteroidal anti-inflammatory drugs induce sodium retention by blocking the formation of renal vasodilating natriuretic prostaglandins.
- Tricyclic antidepressants inhibit the action of centrally acting agents (methyldopa, clonidine).

Table 13-3   Drugs That Can Increase Blood Pressure or Interfere With Antihypertensive Therapy

Drug	Mechanism
Oral contraceptives (with high estrogenic activity)	Induce sodium retention Increase renin substrate Facilitate action of catecholamines
Alcohol (>1 oz daily)	Activation of sympathetic nervous system Increases cortisol secretion Increases intracellular calcium levels
Sympathomimetics and amphetamine-like substances (cold formulas, allergy medications, diet pills)	Increase peripheral vascular resistance Interfere with action of guanethidine and guanadrel
Nonsteroidal anti-inflammatory drugs	Induce sodium retention by blocking formation of renal vasodilating, natriuretic prostaglandins, thus interfering with action of diuretics, β-blockers, and angiotensin-converting enzyme inhibitors
Corticosteroids, ACTH	Iatrogenic Cushing disease
Tricyclic antidepressants	Block uptake of guanethidine Inhibit action of centrally acting drugs such as methyldopa and clonidine
Monoamine oxidase inhibitors (in combination with tyramine—found in aged cheeses and some red wines)	Prevent degradation and metabolism of norepinephrine released by tyramine-containing foods Increase blood pressure when combined with reserpine/guanethidine
Cocaine	Vasoconstriction Interferes with action of adrenergic inhibitors
Marijuana	Increases systolic blood pressure
Cyclosporine, tacrolimus	Renal and systemic vasoconstriction
Erythropoietin	Systemic vasoconstriction
Serotonin	Systemic vasoconstriction
Glycyrrhizinic acid (chewing tobacco, imported licorice, health food products)	Inhibitor of renal cortisol catabolism

ACTH, adrenocorticotropic hormone.

Laboratory Studies

Routine laboratory tests should include a complete blood count; measurements of sodium, potassium, glucose, creatinine or blood urea nitrogen, uric acid, calcium, cholesterol (total and HDL), and triglycerides; urinalysis, chest radiography, and electrocardiography. Additional studies should not be performed unless abnormalities are identified on initial screening tests or the history or examination suggests a secondary form of hypertension.

Treatment

The goal of therapy is to eliminate the morbidity and mortality of cardiovascular disease attributable to hypertension by decreasing blood pressure to less than 140/90 mm Hg. A lower goal of less than 130/80 mm Hg is appropriate for persons with diabetes mellitus or chronic kidney disease.

Lifestyle Modifications

Lifestyle modifications should be encouraged for all persons with prehypertension. They may be sufficient as initial therapy for some persons with stage 1 hypertension. They are adjunctive therapy for those with more severe hypertension.

Restriction of daily sodium intake to 100 mEq (2.4 g sodium, 6 g salt) decreases blood pressure in some but not all hypertensive persons. Although salt sensitivity is more common among persons who are African Americans, obese, or elderly or who have low renin hypertension, higher blood pressure levels, or renal failure, the antihypertensive effect of many medications is enhanced by sodium restriction. Also, sodium restriction minimizes diuretic-induced potassium losses.

The prevalence of hypertension is greater among those who are obese. An increase in blood pressure often parallels weight gain. Weight loss may decrease blood pressure. Weight reduction to within the normal range (bone mass index [BMI] 18.5-24.9) is the goal, although losses of as little as 10 lb may decrease blood pressure.

Restriction of daily alcohol intake to less than 1 oz (30 mL) of ethanol (<1/2 oz for women or lighter weight men) is often associated with a decrease in blood pressure. Alcohol is a source of calories, and its use is often associated with poor compliance with antihypertensive therapy. Excessive alcohol intake may cause labile hypertension that is difficult to control in association with other symptoms (flushing, tachycardia) that suggest pheochromocytoma.

Regular aerobic exercise may decrease blood pressure directly and indirectly by facilitating weight loss. At least 30 minutes of activity such as walking daily should be encouraged.

Consumption of a diet rich in fruits, vegetables, and low-fat dairy products with a reduced content of total and saturated fat (Dietary Approaches to Stop Hypertension [DASH] diet) is effective in lowering blood pressure in patients with prehypertension or stage 1 hypertension.

Because complications of coronary artery disease are the most common causes of mortality in hypertensive persons, all risks for cardiovascular disease must be addressed. The benefits of blood pressure reduction are diminished in smokers. Components of the metabolic syndrome coexist more often in hypertensive than in normotensive persons.

- Restrict daily sodium intake to 100 mEq.
- Reduce weight to within the normal range.
- Restrict alcohol intake to <1 oz daily.
- Exercise for at least 30 minutes daily.
- Follow the DASH diet.
- Address all risk factors for cardiovascular disease.

A diet deficient in potassium may increase blood pressure; therefore, an adequate intake of potassium should be encouraged. The DASH diet is a high potassium diet. There is little evidence to support a role for increased intake of calcium or magnesium. Studies do not support the use of biofeedback or relaxation therapies for blood pressure control.

A trial of lifestyle modifications alone for up to 12 months is appropriate for patients with stage 1 hypertension who do not have diabetes or other risk factors for cardiovascular disease, target organ involvement, or clinical cardiovascular disease. If lifestyle modifications fail to decrease blood pressure to less than 140/90 mm Hg, drug treatment should be initiated. For patients at increased risk because of additional risk factors for cardiovascular disease, drug treatment should be started if lifestyle modifications are ineffective after 3 to 6 months. Drug treatment should be considered initially in addition to lifestyle modifications for patients with stage 2 hypertension or for those with stage 1 hypertension who also have diabetes, target organ involvement, or clinical cardiovascular disease. Successful changes in lifestyle (weight loss, reductions in salt or alcohol intake, and exercise) may allow tapering of an established drug program.

- A trial of lifestyle modifications alone is appropriate initial therapy for stage 1 hypertension in the absence of diabetes, target organ involvement, or clinical cardiovascular disease.
- Stage 2 hypertension or stage 1 hypertension with concurrent diabetes, target organ damage, or clinical cardiovascular disease should be treated initially with both lifestyle modifications and drug therapy.

Pharmacologic Therapy

In more than 50% of persons with stage 1 hypertension, blood pressure can be controlled with single drug therapy. Important factors to consider when selecting a drug for initial therapy are its efficacy as monotherapy, side effects, and cost. Proper drug selection is important for maintaining long-term compliance.

Most patients with stage 2 hypertension, those with initial blood pressure more than 20/10 mm Hg above goal, or those targeted to lower blood pressure goals (chronic kidney disease or diabetes) will require more than one drug for blood pressure control. Consideration of initial therapy with a combination of two drugs (one of which is a diuretic appropriate for the level of renal function) should be considered.

Drugs appropriate for monotherapy are thiazide-type diuretics, β-blockers, calcium channel blockers (CCBs), angiotensin-converting enzyme inhibitors (ACEIs), and angiotensin II receptor blockers (ARBs). Low-dose combinations may also be used for initial therapy, as noted above. Thiazide diuretics should be considered as the initial therapy of choice for most patients with uncomplicated hypertension who lack clear indications for other choices. Other classes of drugs should be considered if diuretics are ineffective or contraindicated or in settings in which the efficacy of an alternative drug has been established (e.g., ACEIs in a hypertensive person with congestive heart failure [see indications for specific drugs below]). Centrally acting α-agonists (clonidine, methyldopa, guanabenz and guanfacine) and traditional vasodilators (hydralazine and minoxidil) may be associated with pseudotolerance. Pseudotolerance is reflex stimulation of the renin-angiotensin-aldosterone system or the sympathetic nervous system (or both systems) that results in fluid retention, an increase in vascular resistance, or an increase in cardiac output and loss of efficacy with prolonged use. Therefore, these drugs are not ordinarily used as monotherapy. Centrally acting α-agonists are appropriate when given in combination with diuretics, whereas traditional vasodilators are best as a third drug in combination with diuretics and adrenergic inhibitors. Additional important factors influencing drug selection include the recognition that certain drugs work better according to a person's age and race (diuretics and CCBs are more effective in African Americans and the elderly; β-blockers, ACEIs, and ARBs are more effective in whites and younger patients). If the first drug chosen fails to control blood pressure, increase the dose or discontinue it and substitute a drug from a different class or add a second drug. With combination therapy, make certain that the chosen drugs work in combination and that two drugs of the same class are not given simultaneously. Usually, one of the drugs in the combination should be a diuretic. Fatigue and impotence are potential side effects of all antihypertensive drugs.

- Drugs for monotherapy: diuretics, β-blockers, CCBs, ACEIs, and ARBs.
- Thiazide-type diuretics: the drug of choice for most patients with uncomplicated hypertension.

- Combination therapy with two drugs should be considered for stage 2 hypertension or if initial blood pressure is >20/10 mm Hg above the goal.
- Centrally acting α-agonists are not ordinarily used as monotherapy but are appropriate in combination with diuretics.
- Traditional vasodilators are best as a third drug in combination with diuretics and adrenergic inhibitors.

Thiazide Diuretics

Thiazide diuretics inhibit sodium reabsorption in the initial portion of the distal convoluted tubule of the nephron (where 5%-8% of filtered sodium is reabsorbed). Acute effects to lower blood pressure are due to volume contraction and decreased cardiac output, but chronically they cause a reduction in peripheral vascular resistance. In large group studies, diuretics are most effective in older persons and African Americans. They are recommended for the initial treatment of uncomplicated hypertension and isolated systolic hypertension in the elderly. Concomitant diseases for which these drugs should be considered are edema states and heart failure associated with congestion. Thiazides decrease the risk of osteoporotic fractures in postmenopausal women, lessen the risk of recurrent calcium nephrolithiasis, and are effective in lessening the risk for cardiovascular disease events in persons with diabetes or in those at high risk for coronary heart disease. They are effective in the secondary prevention of stroke. In addition to their role as initial therapy, thiazide diuretics potentiate the effect of most other antihypertensive drugs. Metabolic disturbances associated with their use include hypokalemia, hyperuricemia, hypercalcemia (thiazides decrease urinary calcium excretion), hypomagnesemia, hyponatremia, fasting hyperglycemia (insulin resistance), hypochloremic metabolic alkalosis, and increased levels of low-density lipoprotein (LDL) cholesterol and triglycerides. Long-term therapy increases the risk for diabetes. Because of these potential adverse effects, relative contraindications to the use of thiazide diuretics include diet-controlled type 2 diabetes, gout, hyperlipidemia, cardiac arrhythmias, and ischemic heart disease. The adverse metabolic effects of thiazide diuretics are dose-dependent and often of little consequence when low doses are used.

Drug interactions include potentiation of lithium toxicity (thiazides decrease the renal clearance of lithium), lessening of the anticoagulant effect of warfarin, and enhancement of digitalis toxicity, and the effects of skeletal muscle relaxants. Nonsteroidal anti-inflammatory drugs and high dietary sodium decrease the antihypertensive effect of thiazide diuretics. They are usually ineffective when the serum creatinine level is greater than 1.5 to 2.0 mg/dL (creatinine clearance, <30 mL/min). Under these circumstances, a more potent loop diuretic or metolazone is more effective. Volume expansion is often etiologically important in hypertension accompanying renal insufficiency. Thiazide diuretics have been associated with volume depletion, pancreatitis, vasculitis, mesenteric infarction, hepatitis, intrahepatic cholestasis, interstitial nephritis, and photosensitivity. Rarely, they cause blood dyscrasias.

- Important indications of thiazide diuretics: uncomplicated hypertension, heart failure with congestion, edema states, isolated systolic hypertension in the elderly, high risk for coronary artery disease, diabetes, or history of stroke.
- Thiazide diuretics increase the risk of diabetes but decrease the risk of osteoporosis-related fracture and recurrent calcium nephrolithiasis.
- Metabolic disturbances: hypokalemia, hyperuricemia, hypercalcemia, hypomagnesemia, hyponatremia, fasting hyperglycemia, hypochloremic metabolic alkalosis, and increased levels of LDL cholesterol and triglycerides.
- Adverse effects: pancreatitis, vasculitis, mesenteric infarction, hepatitis, and photosensitivity.
- Drug interactions: potentiation of lithium toxicity (increases lithium levels by enhancing proximal tubular reabsorption of the drug), lessening of anticoagulant effect of warfarin, and enhancement of digitalis toxicity and effects of skeletal muscle relaxants.

Loop Diuretics

Loop diuretics inhibit sodium reabsorption from the thick ascending portion of Henle's loop of the nephron (where 35%-45% of filtered sodium is reabsorbed).

1. Furosemide. The major indication for furosemide is hypertension associated with renal insufficiency. Because of its short duration of action, furosemide must be given twice daily to maintain a reduced body fluid volume essential for an antihypertensive effect. Similar to thiazide diuretics, furosemide can cause volume depletion, hypokalemia, hyperuricemia, fasting hyperglycemia, and hypochloremic alkalosis. Unlike thiazide diuretics, furosemide increases urinary calcium excretion. Potential adverse effects include reversible deafness, postural hypotension (especially in older persons), photosensitivity, pancreatitis, blood dyscrasias, nephrocalcinosis, and interstitial nephritis. Furosemide enhances salicylate clearance and the effects of skeletal muscle relaxants but is not associated with an increase in lithium level. It is synergistic when used with metolazone, and the combination is effective in states of resistant edema. Avoid administration with aminoglycosides or other ototoxic drugs. Nonsteroidal anti-inflammatory drugs and high dietary sodium reduce the antihypertensive effect of all diuretics.

- Important indication for furosemide: hypertension associated with renal insufficiency.

- Metabolic effects: hypokalemia, hyperuricemia, fasting hyperglycemia, hypochloremic alkalosis, and increased urinary calcium excretion.
- Adverse effects: reversible deafness and postural hypotension.

2. Bumetanide. The actions of bumetanide, including adverse effects, electrolyte alterations, and drug interactions, are identical to those of furosemide; however, bumetanide is a more potent diuretic on a milligram-per-milligram basis (1 mg is equivalent to 40 mg furosemide) and has twice the bioavailability of furosemide.

3. Ethacrynic acid. The actions of ethacrynic acid are similar to those of furosemide. Although permanent hearing loss is a risk, ethacrynic acid is an alternative diuretic for patients with sulfa sensitivity because it is not a sulfonamide derivative.

4. Torsemide. Torsemide is different from the other loop diuretics in that it is eliminated mainly by liver metabolism, which prolongs its duration of action as long as 12 hours. Otherwise, its actions are similar to those of other loop agents.

Potassium-Sparing Diuretics

1. Spironolactone. Spironolactone is an aldosterone antagonist given specifically to persons who have primary aldosteronism or severe secondary aldosteronism. Use of this drug in severe heart failure has been shown to decrease the risk of morbidity and death. Its diuretic effect is antagonized by the concomitant use of salicylates. Adverse effects include hyponatremia, hyperkalemia, hyperchloremic acidosis, gynecomastia (but not breast cancer), and skin rash. Spironolactone is often given in combination with thiazides to limit hypokalemia.

- Important indications for spironolactone: primary aldosteronism and states of secondary aldosteronism, especially severe heart failure.
- The diuretic effect is antagonized by the concomitant use of salicylates.
- Adverse effects: hyperkalemia, gynecomastia, and skin rash.

2. Eplerenone. Eplerenone is an aldosterone receptor antagonist similar to spironolactone, and its indications for use are the same as for spironolactone. This drug may lessen mortality in persons with heart failure following myocardial infarction. Eplerenone differs from spironolactone by having less affinity for progesterone and androgen receptors. Gynecomastia occurs less often; however, impotence and menstrual irregularities can occur. Hyperkalemia is the most common adverse effect. Inhibitors of the cytochrome P450 enzyme CYP3A4 may increase serum levels of eplerenone.

- Eplerenone may be better tolerated than spironolactone, primarily because of less risk for gynecomastia in men.

3. Triamterene. Triamterene inhibits renal potassium wasting independently of aldosterone. It is used most often in combination with thiazide diuretics to limit renal potassium wasting. Side effects include hyperkalemia and skin rash. Acute renal failure can occur if triamterene is used in combination with indomethacin. Triamterene can be excreted into the urine as crystals that can form stones, often containing calcium. The drug should not be used during pregnancy because it is a folic acid antagonist.

- Triamterene inhibits renal potassium wasting independently of aldosterone.
- Do not use in combination with indomethacin or during pregnancy.

4. Amiloride. Amiloride limits renal potassium wasting and is used most often in combination with thiazide diuretics. Its side effects are hyperkalemia, gastrointestinal distress, and skin rash.

Of the potassium-sparing diuretics, only spironolactone and eplerenone can cause gynecomastia. Except under special circumstances, potassium-sparing drugs should be avoided in cases of renal failure and when ACEIs or ARBs are used.

- In general, avoid potassium-sparing diuretics in renal failure and when ACEIs or ARBs are used.

Adrenergic Inhibitors

If a diuretic fails to control blood pressure, an adrenergic inhibitor can be added. Adrenergic inhibitors are divided into centrally acting and peripherally acting drugs.

1. Peripherally acting inhibitors.
   a. Reserpine. Reserpine blocks the transport of norepinephrine into storage granules in peripheral neurons, decreasing sympathetic nervous system tone. Side effects include depression, nasal congestion, and stimulation of gastric acid secretion; thus, contraindications for reserpine are a history of depression or peptic ulcer disease

- Major side effects of reserpine: depression, nasal congestion, and stimulation of gastric acid secretion.

   b. Guanethidine. Guanethidine is used only as part of a combination drug program to treat resistant hypertension. It decreases blood pressure by causing degranulation of catecholamine storage granules in nerve endings. It does not enter the central nervous system. It has a long half-life. The maximal hypotensive effect of a given dose may not be manifested

for 2 or 3 weeks. It should be given only once daily, and titration requires several weeks. Its major side effects are postural hypotension, fluid retention, diarrhea, and retrograde ejaculation. Tricyclic antidepressants, antihistamines, and ephedrine interfere with its action. Guanadrel sulfate, a short-acting form of guanethidine, is easier to titrate to an effective dose because it has a shorter half-life.

- An important indication for guanethidine is resistant hypertension.
- Major side effects: postural hypotension, fluid retention, diarrhea, and retrograde ejaculation.
- Tricyclic antidepressants, antihistamines, and ephedrine interfere with its action.

   c. α_1-Receptor blockers. These drugs block α_1-adrenergic receptors on vascular smooth muscle cells, impairing catecholamine-induced vasoconstriction. Because the initial dose can precipitate hypotension and syncope, it should be taken at bedtime. Longer acting peripheral α_1-receptor blockers (doxazosin, terazosin) allow single daily dosing. Prazosin, an older drug, must be taken at least twice daily. These drugs may lessen voiding symptoms associated with benign prostatic hypertrophy. In the elderly, the use of α_1-receptor blockers is frequently associated with orthostatic hypotension, but they do not have adverse metabolic side effects. Other side effects include gastrointestinal distress and, rarely, sedation, edema, and dry mouth. Because this class of drugs is less effective than diuretics in reducing the risk for congestive heart failure, it is no longer considered an option for the initial management of hypertension.

- α_1-Receptor blockers are no longer considered appropriate initial therapy for hypertension.
- Because the first dose can cause hypotension and syncope, it should be taken at bedtime.
- In the elderly, these drugs are often associated with orthostatic hypotension, but they have no adverse metabolic side effects and may lessen symptoms of prostatism.

   d. β-Blockers. Many β-blockers are available and differ in cardioselectivity (affinity for cardiac β_1 receptors is greater than for noncardiac β_2 receptors), lipid solubility, and whether they have partial intrinsic (agonist) sympathomimetic activity (ISA). Non-ISA β-blockers lower blood pressure by reducing cardiac output and inhibiting both renin release and central sympathetic outflow. β-Blockers with ISA activity do not reduce cardiac output but cause mild peripheral vasodilatation. As lipid solubility increases, the liver metabolizes more of the drug, more of it enters the brain, and its duration of action is shorter. As lipid solubility decreases, the drug is eliminated mainly by renal excretion, less of it enters the brain, and its duration of action is longer. Very lipid-soluble drugs are propranolol, penbutolol, and carvedilol. Intermediate lipid-soluble drugs are metoprolol, pindolol, and timolol. The least lipid-soluble drugs are atenolol, betaxolol, carteolol, celiprolol, esmolol, and nadolol.

- β-Blockers differ by lipid solubility.
- As lipid solubility increases, the liver metabolizes more of the drug, more of the drug enters the brain, and its duration of action is shorter.
- As lipid solubility decreases, the drug is eliminated mainly by renal excretion, less of the drug enters the brain, and its duration of action is longer.
- The most lipid-soluble drugs: propranolol, penbutolol, and carvedilol.
- The least lipid-soluble drugs: atenolol, betaxolol, carteolol, celiprolol, esmolol, and nadolol.

β_1-Cardioselective β-blockers are acebutolol, atenolol, betaxolol, bisoprolol, celiprolol, esmolol, metoprolol, and nebivolol. Cardioselectivity is relative; at high doses, all β-blockers are nonselective (i.e., they block both cardiac β_1 and noncardiac β_2 receptors). β-Blockers with ISA activity are pindolol, acebutolol, carteolol, celiprolol, and pentbutolol. Cardioselectivity is not associated with a difference in blood pressure–lowering effect. However, it may be associated with less adverse effects on lipids (β-blockers can increase triglycerides and lower HDL cholesterol) and may allow quicker recovery from hypoglycemia in diabetic patients. Paradoxical increases in blood pressure under stress are also less likely with cardioselective drugs.

β-Blockers are appropriate initial therapy for hypertension. In large group studies, they are most effective in younger persons and whites. Certain comorbid conditions suggest the use of these drugs. Three β-blockers—propranolol, timolol, and metoprolol—prevent sudden death and recurrent myocardial infarction after an initial event. Most persons with congestive heart failure should be receiving a β-blocker (metoprolol, bisoprolol, or carvedilol). Also, these drugs should be considered for patients with hypertension who have concomitant angina or hypertrophic cardiomyopathy. Other concomitant conditions that may benefit from the use of these drugs are supraventricular arrhythmias, glaucoma, migraine headache, and essential tremor. Noncardioselective drugs may be effective in preventing migraines and inhibiting essential tremor. Given preoperatively, β-blockers decrease the risk of postoperative myocardial infarction in persons at increased risk for coronary artery disease. Although severe or poorly controlled asthma is a contraindication for β-blockers, many persons with well-controlled or mild asthma or mild chronic obstructive pulmonary disease can tolerate low doses of cardioselective agents. Contraindications to β-blocker therapy are conduction system disease of the heart, angina due to coronary vasospasm, Raynaud phenomenon, severe (but not mild) occlusive peripheral vascular disease, pheochromocytoma (in absence of α-blockade), and depression. Because β-blockers may mask the symptoms of hypoglycemia and delay recovery from it, caution is required when these agents are given to patients with diabetes who are taking hypoglycemic drugs or insulin. Complete heart block can occur if a β-blocker is given in combination with verapamil. Side effects include cold extremities (non-ISA β-blockers), decreased exercise capacity, bronchospasm, dyslipidemia (elevated triglyceride level, lower HDL cholesterol [worse with lipid-soluble, non-ISA, noncardioselective drugs]), worsening of psoriasis, fatigue, insomnia, nasal congestion, and, possibly, depression.

- Cardioselectivity is relative; all β-blockers are nonselective at high doses.
- Propranolol, timolol, and metoprolol prevent sudden death and recurrent myocardial infarction in persons with an initial event.
- Most patients with congestive heart failure should be receiving a β-blocker.
- Contraindications: Severe reactive airway disease, conduction system disease of the heart, angina due to coronary vasospasm, Raynaud phenomenon, severe occlusive peripheral vascular disease, pheochromocytoma (before α-blockade), and depression.
- β-Blockers may mask hypoglycemia and delay recovery from it, so prescribe them carefully for diabetics who take insulin or oral hypoglycemic drugs.
- Side effects: cold extremities, fatigue, impaired exercise tolerance, bronchospasm, dyslipidemia, insomnia, nasal congestion, and, possibly, depression.

e. Labetalol. Labetalol is the combination of a non-selective β-blocker and a postsynaptic α_1-receptor blocker. The ratio of α- to β-blocking action is 1:4. The drug lowers blood pressure primarily by decreasing peripheral vascular resistance. Labetalol can be given intravenously to treat hypertensive crisis. All the precautions applying to β-blockers apply to this drug. Labetalol can cause liver dysfunction and an increase in antinuclear antibody and antimitochondrial antibody titers. Common side effects are orthostatic hypotension and scalp itching. Labetalol may interfere with metanephrine and catecholamine assays, resulting in a false-positive test for pheochromocytoma.

- Labetalol can be given intravenously for hypertensive crisis.
- All precautions applying to β-blockers apply to labetalol.
- Labetalol can cause an increase in liver function tests and in antinuclear and antimitochondrial antibody titers.
- Common side effects: orthostatic hypotension and scalp itching.
- Labetalol may result in a false-positive test for pheochromocytoma.

f. Carvedilol. Carvedilol is a weak β_1-selective blocker with α_1-blocking activity. This drug reduces the risk of death and hospitalization in persons with heart failure.

- Carvedilol is beneficial in heart failure.

2. Centrally acting α_{2a} agonists

These drugs stimulate central α-receptors that exert an inhibitory effect on sympathetic outflow. Blood pressure is reduced because of a decrease in cardiac output and peripheral vascular resistance. Norepinephrine and renin levels decrease. Fluid retention occurs; thus, these agents should be used in combination with diuretics. Side effects common to all these agents are orthostatic hypotension, sedation, and dry mouth. Sudden discontinuation of any of these agents can cause a sudden rebound rise in blood pressure.

a. Methyldopa. Doses should not exceed 3 g daily. Side effects include hepatitis, fever, positive Coombs test, hemolytic anemia, leukopenia, thrombocytopenia, and increased antinuclear antibody titers. Hemoglobin and liver enzymes should be checked periodically. Methyldopa potentiates lithium and haloperidol toxicity, increases prolactin levels with consequent breast stimulation, and interferes with

metanephrine assays. Because newer centrally acting agents are safer, this drug should not be used often. Currently, a major use for this drug is in the treatment of hypertension in pregnancy, for which its safety has been established.

- An important indication for methyldopa is hypertension in pregnancy.
- Methyldopa side effects: hepatitis, fever, positive Coombs test, hemolytic anemia, leukopenia, thrombocytopenia, and antinuclear antibody positivity.
- It potentiates lithium and haloperidol toxicity and increases prolactin levels.

b. Clonidine. In contrast to methyldopa, clonidine is not associated with liver toxicity or hematologic abnormalities. Because of the possibility of rebound hypertension with sudden discontinuation, as with all central agents, clonidine should be tapered and discontinued preoperatively if oral medications will not be allowed for several days postoperatively. An alternative with clonidine is conversion preoperatively to the transdermal form of the drug. Comorbid conditions that may benefit from clonidine include restless legs, menopausal hot flashes, and diabetic diarrhea.

- Clonidine is not associated with liver toxicity or hematologic abnormlities.
- An alternative to tapering the drug preoperatively is to switch to the transdermal form.
- Clonidine may help restless legs, menopausal hot flashes, and diabetic diarrhea.

c. Guanabenz. Guanabenz is similar in action to clonidine and methyldopa. It may also have weak peripheral neuronal blocking properties. Similar to clonidine and unlike methyldopa, it is not associated with liver toxicity or hematologic abnormalities. Also, unlike other central agents, guanabenz does not cause fluid retention.

- The side effects of guanabenz are similar to those of clonidine.
- It is the only central α-agonist that does not cause fluid retention.

d. Guanfacine. Guanfacine, a newer clonidine-like drug, can be given once daily and may have fewer central nervous system side effects. Similar to guanabenz and clonidine, it is not associated with liver toxicity or a positive Coombs test.

Traditional Vasodilators

The traditional vasodilators are usually given as a third agent in combination with a diuretic and an adrenergic inhibitor to persons with severe or resistant hypertension. They are used most properly only in combination with a diuretic and an adrenergic inhibitor because they cause stimulation of the sympathetic nervous system (increase in heart rate and cardiac output) and renin release (fluid retention).

1. Hydralazine. This drug decreases blood pressure by directly dilating arterioles. The daily dose should not exceed 200 mg. Its plasma half-life is prolonged in renal insufficiency. Side effects include headache, palpitations, tachycardia, fluid retention, lupus-like syndrome, and peripheral neuropathy. The liver enzyme *N*-acetyltransferase inactivates the drug. The level of this enzyme is genetically determined and persons are characterized as being "rapid acetylators" (high levels of the enzyme) or "slow acetylators" (low levels of the enzyme). Rapid acetylators require larger doses of the drug for an effect. Lupus-like syndrome is more common in slow acetylators. Hydralazine should not be used in the setting of recent cerebral hemorrhage, acute myocardial infarction, or a dissecting aortic aneurysm because of its tendency to increase cardiac output and cerebral blood flow.

● Hydralazine causes direct dilatation of arterioles.
● The daily dose should not exceed 200 mg.
● Side effects: headache, palpitations, tachycardia, fluid retention, lupus-like syndrome, and peripheral neuropathy.
● Do not use in the setting of recent cerebral hemorrhage, acute myocardial infarction, or dissecting aortic aneurysm.

2. Minoxidil. Minoxidil is a potent, direct vasodilator used to treat severe hypertension with or without renal insufficiency. Its side effects include substantial volume expansion with edema, hirsutism, and pericardial effusion. Often, high doses of both a loop diuretic and an adrenergic inhibitor are required to control reactive sympathetic stimulation and fluid retention.

● Minoxidil is a more potent vasodilator than hydralazine.
● Side effects: volume expansion with edema, hirsutism, and pericardial effusion.

Angiotensin-Converting Enzyme Inhibitors

ACEIs decrease blood pressure by inhibiting the enzyme that converts angiotensin I to angiotensin II, a potent vasoconstrictor. They also potentiate the activity of bradykinin, a vasodilator. Although they are vasodilators, ACEIs do not induce reactive fluid retention or sympathetic stimulation. They are appropriate initial therapy for hypertension and work well in combination with other antihypertensive agents, particularly diuretics. In large group studies, ACEIs have been most effective in younger persons and whites. ACEIs retard progression of nephropathy in type 1 diabetes mellitus and prevent the development of congestive heart failure and recurrent myocardial infarction in persons who have had an initial myocardial infarction complicated by reduced left ventricular function. ACEIs are an important treatment for established congestive heart failure and induce regression of left ventricular hypertrophy more effectively than other antihypertensive agents. ACEIs are antiproteinuric and slow the progression of nondiabetic proteinuric renal disease. Also, they decrease the risk of mortality, myocardial infarction, and stroke in high-risk persons (i.e., persons with known coronary artery disease, previous stroke, peripheral vascular disease, or diabetes with at least one additional risk factor).

The combination of an ACEI and a diuretic may prevent recurrent stroke. ACEIs increase insulin sensitivity and may lessen the risk of developing diabetes. Their use can be associated with hypoglycemia in diabetic patients. Captopril is the only sulfhydryl-containing ACEI. Unique side effects presumed to be due to the sulfhydryl group in captopril are skin rash, loss of taste, proteinuria with membranous glomerulonephropathy, and leukopenia. Leukopenia is more likely to occur in the presence of collagen vascular disease and renal insufficiency. Nonsulfhydryl-containing ACEIs are benazepril, enalapril, fosinopril, lisinopril, moexipril, perindopril, quinapril, ramipril, and trandolapril. The side effects shared by all ACEIs are orthostatic hypotension, hyperkalemia, cough, bronchospasm, angioedema, and loss of renal function. Anaphylactic reactions can occur in patients during dialysis or apheresis. In persons with bilateral renal artery stenosis, ACEIs can cause acute renal failure because of disruption of autoregulation of glomerular filtration in the presence of severe renal ischemia. The kidneys eliminate all ACEIs except fosinopril. Fosinopril has a balanced renal and hepatic elimination, with increased hepatic elimination in the setting of renal dysfunction. ACEIs are contraindicated in pregnancy because they can cause fetal toxicity.

● ACEIs inhibit the enzyme that converts angiotensin I to angiotensin II and is responsible for the metabolism of bradykinin.
● ACEIs are appropriate initial therapy for hypertension.
● ACEIs retard progression of nephropathy in patients with type 1 diabetes.
● ACEIs are anti-proteinuric and slow the progression of nondiabetic proteinuric renal disease.
● ACEIs are important in the treatment of congestive heart failure.
● ACEIs prevent recurrent myocardial infarction and the development of congestive heart failure in persons who have had a myocardial infarction complicated by reduced left ventricular function.

- ACEIs may lessen the risk of death, myocardial infarction, and stroke in persons who have known atherosclerotic vascular disease or diabetes plus one additional risk factor.
- The combination of an ACEI and a diuretic may prevent recurrent stroke.
- Except for fosinopril, dose reduction is necessary in renal insufficiency.
- Side effects of captopril: skin rash, loss of taste, proteinuria with membranous glomerulonephropathy, and leukopenia.
- Side effects of all ACEIs: orthostatic hypotension, hyperkalemia, cough, angioedema, and loss of renal function.
- ACEIs are contraindicated in pregnancy.

Calcium Channel Blockers

CCBs are direct vasodilators. They are divided into dihydropyridines (nifedipine, nicardipine, isradipine, felodipine, nisoldipine, and amlodipine) and nondihydropyridines (verapamil, diltiazem). Only long-acting forms are approved for use in hypertension. Verapamil (and, to a lesser extent, diltiazem) slows the heart rate, depresses cardiac contractility, and inhibits cardiac atrioventricular nodal conduction. The dihydropyridines have less effect on cardiac conduction and heart contractility. CCBs are appropriate for initial therapy of hypertension. In large group studies, CCBs have been most effective in older persons (especially with isolated septal hypertrophy) and African Americans. They should be considered for persons with concomitant ischemic heart disease and chronic, stable angina (amlodipine, nicardipine, nifedipine, diltiazem, and verapamil), variant angina due to coronary vasospasm (amlodipine, nifedipine, and diltiazem), supraventricular arrhythmias (verapamil and diltiazem), Raynaud phenomenon (nifedipine), and migraine headaches (verapamil). Verapamil decreases the risk of a subsequent myocardial infarction if the first one was not associated with pulmonary congestion. Diltiazem decreases the risk of a subsequent myocardial infarction after a non–Q-wave infarction. The long-term use of nifedipine delays the need for valve replacement in chronic aortic insufficiency and may lower pressure in primary pulmonary hypertension. Dihydropyridine CCBs lessen the risk of stroke in older persons with systolic hypertension.

Verapamil and diltiazem should be avoided in the presence of cardiac conduction system disease (sick sinus syndrome and second-degree or greater heart block) or when the left ventricular ejection fraction is less than 40%. All CCBs should be avoided in symptomatic heart failure, although dihydropyridine CCBs can be used safely in asymptomatic persons who require additional treatment to control blood pressure or angina. Verapamil in combination with β-blockers can lead to complete heart block and profound cardiodepression. Because it decreases the renal and nonrenal elimination of digoxin, verapamil increases the risk of digoxin toxicity. Quinidine and verapamil in combination can cause serious hypotension in persons with idiopathic hypertrophic subaortic stenosis.

- CCBs are direct vasodilators.
- Verapamil and diltiazem should not be used in sick sinus syndrome or heart block of second degree or greater.
- Avoid using verapamil in combination with β-blockers.
- Avoid verapamil if the left ventricular ejection fraction is <40%.
- Verapamil increases the risk of digoxin toxicity.
- All CCBs should be avoided in persons with symptomatic heart failure.

All CCBs can increase liver enzymes and cause hepatic necrosis. The most common side effect of verapamil is constipation, and the most serious side effect is heart block. Most of the side effects associated with dihydropyridine CCBs are related to peripheral vasodilation. These include headache, tachycardia, flushing, and dependent edema. The dependent edema associated with CCBs is not improved with diuretics but may be lessened by ACEIs. Gingival hyperplasia most commonly occurs with dihydropyridines. Rarely, serious cutaneous eruptions can occur with CCBs. Cimetidine and other drugs that decrease blood flow to the liver may increase the biologic effects of CCBs. CCBs increase cyclosporine blood levels. Unlike other antihypertensive agents, nonsteroidal anti-inflammatory drugs do not interfere with the blood pressure–lowering effect of CCBs and a high sodium diet may increase the blood pressure–lowering effect. The liver metabolizes all CCBs, and dose adjustments may be necessary if liver disease is present. CCBs can be used safely in renal insufficiency.

- The most common side effect of verapamil: constipation.
- The most serious side effect of verapamil: heart block.
- Common side effects: headache, tachycardia, flushing, and edema.
- CCBs can cause gingival hyperplasia.
- CCBs increase cyclosporine blood levels.
- CCBs can increase liver enzymes and cause hepatic necrosis.
- Nonsteroidal anti-inflammatory drugs and a high salt diet do not lessen the blood pressure–lowering effect of CCBs.
- All CCBs are metabolized in the liver, so dose adjustments are necessary if liver disease is present.

Angiotensin II Receptor Blockers

ARBs (losartan, valsartan, candesartan, irbesartan, eprosartan, telmisartan, and olmesartan) lower blood pressure by blocking the cell surface receptors (AT_1) that angiotensin II interacts with to produce all its known pressor effects. Similar to ACEIs, ARBs increase plasma renin activity (PRA), but unlike ACEIs, ARBs also increase (not decrease) angiotensin

II levels. However, unlike ACEIs, ARBs do not increase bradykinin levels. ARBs are appropriate initial therapy for hypertension, and in large group studies, they have been most effective in younger persons and whites. ARBs are generally effective in the same clinical settings as ACEI; thus, their major role is as an alternative to ACEIs when these agents are indicated but not tolerated. ARBs are antiproteinuric and have been shown to lessen the progression of nephropathy associated with type II diabetes (losartan and irbesartan). Unlike with ACEIs, special benefits of ARBs after myocardial infarction or in congestive heart failure have not been established. ARBs should not be given to persons with heart failure who are already taking β-blockers and ACEIs but should be considered for persons intolerant of ACEIs. Unlike ACEIs, ARBs do not cause cough (cough may be due to high levels of bradykinin).

The most common side effect of ARBs is dizziness. Diuretics or salt and volume depletion can potentiate their hypotensive effect. Similar to ACEIs, ARBs can cause fetal toxicity and should be avoided in pregnancy. They also can precipitate acute renal failure in persons with bilateral renal artery stenosis and can cause angioedema. In general, persons who experience angioedema with an ACEI should not be given an ARB. The risk of hyperkalemia may be less than with ACEIs. Losartan is the only ARB that is uricosuric. These drugs have no adverse effect on plasma lipids or glucose.

- ARBs inhibit the actions of angiotensin II by blocking its cell surface receptors.
- The major role for ARBs: a substitute for an ACEI when an ACEI is indicated but not tolerated.
- Side effects of ARBs: dizziness, hyperkalemia, acute renal failure, angioedema.
- ARBs do not cause cough.
- Avoid ARBs in pregnancy because of fetal toxicity.

CAUSES OF SECONDARY HYPERTENSION

Renovascular Hypertension

Renovascular hypertension is the most common form of potentially curable secondary hypertension. It occurs in 1% to 2% of the general hypertensive population, 10% of persons with resistant hypertension, and up to 30% of those with hypertensive crisis. Stenosis of a renal artery increases renin production from the ischemic kidney. Renin acts on circulating renin substrate to produce angiotensin I, which is converted to angiotensin II (a potent vasoconstrictor) by angiotensin-converting enzyme (ACE) in the lung and other tissues. In addition to vasoconstriction, angiotensin II stimulates aldosterone production, which causes renal sodium retention and volume expansion. Angiotensin II also stimulates the sympathetic nervous system and the release of vasopressin.

- Renovascular disease is the most common form of potentially curable secondary hypertension.
- Renal artery stenosis activates the renin-angiotensin system.
- Angiotensin II is a potent vasoconstrictor; it stimulates aldosterone production, sympathetic nervous system activity, and vasopressin release.
- Renovascular hypertension is due to extracellular volume expansion and increased peripheral vascular resistance.

Correcting renal ischemia eliminates the stimulus for excess renin release and often cures or lessens hypertension. In unilateral renal artery stenosis, prolonged hypertension eventually causes nephrosclerosis in the nonischemic kidney or ischemic injury to the involved kidney. If either occurs, relieving renal arterial stenosis may not cure hypertension. The longer the duration of hypertension before diagnosis, the greater the likelihood of these untoward renal events and the less the likelihood of cure of hypertension with intervention.

- Correcting renal ischemia eliminates excess renin release.
- The longer the duration of hypertension before diagnosis, the less likely correction of renal ischemia will be beneficial.

Fibromuscular disease is the most common cause of renovascular hypertension in younger persons, especially women between 15 and 50 years old. It accounts for 10% of renovascular hypertension in the population. Lesions usually affect the middle and distal portions of the main renal vessels, often extending into branches. Three subtypes have been defined on the basis of the portion of the arterial wall involved: 1) intimal fibroplasia (1%-2% of cases), 2) medial fibromuscular dysplasia (95% of cases), and 3) periadventitial fibrosis (1%-2% of cases). Medial fibromuscular dysplasia, the most common subtype in adults, has a classic string-of-beads appearance (representing aneurysmal dilatations) on angiography (Fig. 13-1) and progresses in 30% of cases. Medial fibromuscular dysplasia may also occur in other vessels branching off the aorta (e.g., the carotid and celiac arteries). The rare subtypes of intimal fibroplasia and periadventitial fibrosis can progress rapidly to severe stenoses. Dissection and thrombosis can occur and are seen more commonly with the rare subtypes. Occlusion of the renal artery is rare.

- Fibromuscular disease is the most common cause of renovascular hypertension in younger persons, especially women.
- Medial fibromuscular hyperplasia is the most common subtype.

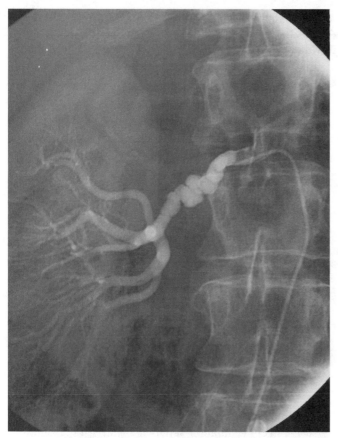

Fig. 13-1. Fibromuscular renal vascular disease (medial fibromuscular dysplasia).

Clues suggesting renovascular hyptertension include lack of a family history of hypertension, onset of hypertension before age 30 (consider fibromuscular dysplasia, especially in women), onset of hypertension after age 50 (consider atherosclerotic renovascular disease), presentation of accelerated or malignant hypertension, or sudden worsening of preexisting hypertension in a middle-aged or older person (renovascular hypertension superimposed on essential hypertension). The most important physical finding is an abdominal bruit, especially a high-pitched systolic-diastolic bruit in the upper abdomen or flank. However, 50% of persons with renovascular hypertension do not have this finding. Other physical clues are severe retinopathy of accelerated or malignant hypertension (hemorrhages, exudates, and papilledema) or evidence of atherosclerotic occlusive disease in other vascular beds. Laboratory abnormalities are hypokalemia (due to secondary aldosteronism), an increased serum level of creatinine, proteinuria (rarely in the nephrotic range), and a small kidney seen on an imaging study.

- For hypertension before age 30, especially in women, consider fibromuscular dysplasia.
- For hypertension after age 50, consider atherosclerotic renovascular disease.
- The most important physical finding is an abdominal bruit, present in only 50% of cases.

- Dissection or thrombosis of a renal artery: complications most commonly seen with rare subtypes.
- Renal artery occlusion is rare.

Atheromatous disease is the most common cause of renovascular hypertension in middle-aged and older persons. It accounts for 90% of renovascular hypertension in the population. The lesions usually are in the proximal third of the renal artery, often near the orifice (Fig. 13-2). Although atheromatous renal artery disease is common in older persons with hypertension (especially in diabetics or persons with evidence of atherosclerosis in other vascular beds), it causes or aggravates hypertension less often. The disease is bilateral in 30% of cases, and in 50% of cases, it progresses even if blood pressure is controlled. Atherosclerosis of the renal artery can progress to occlusion of the vessel. Progressive disease can cause end-stage renal disease.

- Atheromatous disease is the most common cause of renovascular hypertension in middle-aged or older persons.
- The disease is bilateral in 30% of cases and progressive in 50%.
- It can cause renal artery occlusion.

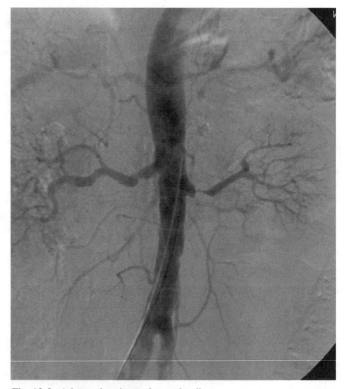

Fig. 13-2. Atherosclerotic renal vascular disease.

- Laboratory abnormalities: hypokalemia, increased serum level of creatinine, proteinuria, and a small kidney seen on an imaging study.

An acute decline in renal function either after the initiation of therapy with an ACEI or an ARB or with a drug-induced, sudden, severe decrease in blood pressure may indicate underlying bilateral renal artery stenosis. Other presentations of bilateral renal artery stenosis (i.e., ischemic nephropathy) include the sudden development of pulmonary edema accompanied by severe hypertension (flash pulmonary edema) or a subacute decline in renal function with or without worsening hypertension.

Atheroembolic renal disease may also present with a sudden onset or worsening of hypertension and a subacute decline in renal function. Historical clues (e.g., occurrence after angiography or aortic surgery), physical findings (distal livedo reticularis and peripheral emboli), and laboratory abnormalities (increased erythrocyte sedimentation rate, anemia, hematuria, eosinophilia, and eosinophiluria) help identify this disorder.

- A sudden decline in renal function with the use of an ACEI or ARB or an episode of pulmonary edema may indicate bilateral renal artery disease.
- The sudden onset or worsening of hypertension and subacute decline in renal function may also be due to atheroembolic renal disease.

In young persons who have hypertension (even if not severe) of short duration and suggestive clinical features, evaluation for renovascular disease is indicated. The identification and correction of renal artery stenosis in such persons can be performed with low risk of morbidity and mortality and is associated with a high probability of cure. Older persons should be evaluated for renovascular hypertension on a selective basis. Selection should be restricted to persons with suggestive clinical features in whom blood pressure cannot be controlled medically or who have an unexplained, observed decline in renal function and who are considered reasonable risks for (and are willing to undergo) interventional therapy.

- In young persons with hypertension of short duration, evaluate for renovascular disease.
- Older persons should be evaluated for renovascular hypertension on a selective basis.

Screening Tests

Intravenous Pyelography

Historically, intravenous pyelography (IVP) was the mainstay screening test for renovascular hypertension, but currently captopril radionuclide renal scan or duplex renal ultrasonography is the initial screening test of choice. Characteristic findings on IVP suggestive of renovascular disease are 1) unilateral decrease in renal size, with the pole-to-pole diameter of the smaller kidney decreased by 1.5 cm or more; 2) delayed appearance of contrast agent in the collecting system of the ischemic kidney; 3) hyperconcentration of contrast agent in the ischemic kidney on delayed films; 4) ureteral scalloping by collateral vessels; and 5) cortical thinning or irregularity. The sensitivity is 70% to 75%, and the specificity is 85%.

- Findings on IVP suggesting renovascular hypertension: unilateral reduction in renal size ($\geq$1.5-cm decrease in pole-to-pole diameter of the smaller kidney), delayed appearance of contrast in the collecting system of the ischemic kidney (hyperconcentration of contrast in the ischemic kidney), ureteral scalloping by collateral vessels, and cortical thinning or irregularity.

Captopril Radionuclide Renal Scan

Some consider captopril radionuclide renal scanning the screening test of choice. However, the sensitivity of captopril renography is only 75%, and the specificity is 85%. Pretest treatment of patients with captopril increases the sensitivity of the scan compared with that of standard renography. The rationale is that glomerular filtration in an ischemic kidney depends on the vasoconstricting effect of angiotensin II on the efferent arteriole of the nephron to maintain effective transglomerular filtration pressure. Treatment with an ACEI causes efferent arteriolar dilatation, with loss of filtration pressure in the nephron. This causes a decline of glomerular filtration in the ischemic kidney, with less of an effect on renal blood flow. These changes are identified with the scanning technique. The radionuclides used most commonly are iodine 131 orthoiodohippuric acid (OIH) and Tc-99m mercaptoacetyltriglycine (MAG3), which are markers for renal blood flow (they are excreted primarily by renal tubular secretion), and Tc-99m diethylenetriamine pentaacetic acid (DPTA), which is a marker for glomerular filtration rate (it is excreted primarily by glomerular filtration). Criteria for a positive test with DPTA are time to peak activity in the kidney of 11 minutes or more and a ratio of the glomerular filtration rate between the kidneys of 1.5 or more. The criterion for a positive test with OIH or MAG3 is residual cortical activity at 20 minutes of 30% or more of peak activity. The renal scan is safe for persons with a history of contrast allergy. The interpretive value is reduced by renal insufficiency (creatinine >2.0 mg/dL) or by bilateral or branch renal artery disease. Urinary outflow obstruction may mimic renal artery stenosis.

- Some consider the captopril radionuclide renal scan to be the screening test of choice.
- Sensitivity is 75%, and specificity is 85%.
- It is safe for persons with a history of contrast allergy.
- It is ineffective in renal insufficiency.
- Findings with unilateral urinary outflow obstruction are similar to those of renal artery stenosis.

Duplex Ultrasonography

Duplex ultrasonography is considered the screening test of choice by some, especially for persons with renal insufficiency. It is noninvasive and does not use contrast media. It should be considered in persons with renal insufficiency or a history of contrast allergy. This test identifies increases in blood flow velocity that occur with luminal narrowing of a renal artery. Criteria for a positive test are a ratio of peak flow velocity in the involved renal artery to peak flow velocity in the aorta greater than 3.5 and renal artery peak systolic flow of 180 cm/s or more. Calculation of the resistive index, a measure of small-vessel disease in the kidney, can identify persons more (low resistive index) or less (high resistive index) likely to benefit from interventional therapy. Overlying bowel gas or other technical problems limit complete study of both renal arteries in up to 50% of cases. Often, accessory or branch vessel disease is not identified. The sensitivity is 80% to 90%, and the specificity is 90%.

- Duplex ultrasonography is considered by many to be the screening test of choice.
- Consider it in persons with renal insufficiency or a history of contrast allergy.
- Sensitivity is 80%-90%, and specificity is 90%.
- Calculation of the resistive index can determine the likelihood of benefit from intervention.
- In up to 50% of persons, one or both renal arteries cannot be studied adequately.
- Accessory or branch vessel disease may not be identified.

Magnetic Resonance Angiography

This test visualizes the main renal arteries without use of a radiocontrast agent or exposure to radiation. It should be considered for persons with renal insufficiency or those with a history of radiocontrast allergy. Also, it is a good choice for persons who have severe, diffuse atherosclerosis and, thus, are at risk for atheroembolization with angiography. Field limitations may decrease the ability to see lesions in the distal main renal arteries or lesions in branch vessels (common sites of fibromuscular disease). Accessory renal arteries may not be identified. The degree of arterial stenosis may be overestimated by this method. Persons prone to claustrophobia may not tolerate being placed in the magnetic resonance

equipment. Renal stents cause imaging artifacts. This is an expensive screening test.

- Magnetic resonance angiography: visualizes the renal arteries without a radiocontrast agent or radiation exposure.
- Good choice for persons with renal insufficiency or radiocontrast allergy.
- Renal stents cause imaging artifacts.
- May cause claustrophobia.
- It is expensive.

Spiral Computed Tomographic Angiography

Spiral computed tomographic (CT) angiography offers excellent three-dimensional images but requires a considerable amount of radiocontrast agent and patient cooperation. This is an alternative for patients with normal renal function who do not have a contrast allergy. Renal stents do not cause imaging artifacts.

- Spiral CT requires considerable radiocontrast.
- Renal stents do not cause imaging artifacts.

Renal Arteriography

Renal arteriography is the standard method for identifying renal arterial lesions. Renal artery stenosis must be demonstrated in combination with clinical features. Because of shortcomings associated with screening tests, it is appropriate to proceed directly to arteriography in situations in which the clinical suspicion for renal vascular hypertension is high.

- Renal arteriography: the standard method for identifying renal arterial lesions.

Digital Venous Subtraction Angiography

Digital venous subtraction angiography uses contrast media, but access to the circulation is through a peripheral vein. With the advent of newer screening tests, it is used less often. This technique adequately visualizes the proximal main renal arteries (usual location of atherosclerotic disease) in 90% of persons but is less effective in visualizing distal portions of the main renal arteries or branches (the usual location of fibromuscular dysplasia). This technique is expensive, and in 20% to 30% of persons, neither renal artery is identified because of superimposition of abdominal vessels or patient motion. The sensitivity and specificity are both 85% to 90%.

- In current practice, digital venous subtraction angiography is used less often.
- Sensitivity and specificity are both 85%-90%.
- The proximal main renal arteries are visualized in 90% of persons.

- It is less effective for assessing distal main renal arteries or branches.
- It is expensive.
- At least one renal artery is not identified in 20%-30% of cases.

Captopril Test

Acute blockade of angiotensin II formation by ACEIs induces a reactive increase in PRA. The magnitude of this increase is usually greater in renovascular hypertension than in essential hypertension and is the basis for the captopril test. The use of antihypertensive drugs that influence the renin-angiotensin-aldosterone axis must be discontinued for several days before the test. PRA is measured at baseline and at 60 minutes after administering captopril orally. Criteria for a positive test are 1) post-captopril PRA more than 12 ng/mL per hour, 2) absolute increase in PRA over baseline of at least 10 ng/mL per hour, and 3) 150% or greater increase in PRA if the baseline PRA is more than 3 ng/mL per hour or 400% or greater if baseline PRA is less than 3 ng/mL per hour. The results are compromised if the person has renal insufficiency. The sensitivity is 39% to 100%, and the specificity is 72% to 100%. Because the results can be influenced by many factors that are difficult to identify and control, predictive accuracy is low.

- Captopril test: difficult to control all factors that influence test results.
- Sensitivity is 39%-100%, and specificity is 72%-100%.
- The test is unreliable in persons with renal insufficiency.

Renal Vein Renins

Lateralization of renal vein renins is a good predictor of a favorable outcome following intervention for unilateral renal artery stenosis; however, because many factors that influence renin secretion are difficult to identify and control (as noted for the captopril test), the predictive value of the test is low. It is invasive and expensive. Lateralization is present if the ratio of renin activity on the affected side compared with that on the normal side is 1.5:1.0 or greater. The sensitivity is 63% to 77%, and the specificity is 60% to 95%.

- Renal vein renins is an expensive and invasive test.
- Sensitivity is 63%-77%, and specificity is 60%-95%.
- Lateralization of renal vein renins is a good predictor of a favorable outcome following intervention for unilateral renal artery stenosis.

Therapy for Renovascular Hypertension

Options for the management of renovascular hypertension include medical and interventional therapies. Percutaneous balloon angioplasty, stent placement, and surgical procedures to relieve renal ischemia are the interventional treatments. Goals of interventional therapy are to cure or to improve hypertension and to preserve renal function. Medical therapy is reserved for patients not considered candidates for interventional therapy (because of the extent or location of the vascular lesions, high surgical risk, or uncertainty about the causative significance of the lesion).

Percutaneous transluminal angioplasty is the treatment of choice for amenable lesions caused by fibromuscular dysplasia and is an option with or without stent placement in some cases of atherosclerotic renovascular disease. Hypertension is cured in 60% of persons with fibromuscular dysplasia and in 30% of those with atherosclerosis. Complications of angioplasty include groin hematoma, dye-induced azotemia, dissection of the renal artery, renal infarction, and, rarely, rupture of the renal artery, with the potential for loss of the kidney and the need for immediate surgery. Cholesterol embolization is a risk in older persons with diffuse atherosclerosis.

- Angioplasty is the treatment of choice for amenable lesions caused by fibromuscular dysplasia and is an option for some lesions caused by atherosclerosis.
- Complications of angioplasty: groin hematoma, dye-induced azotemia, dissection of the renal artery, renal infarction, and, rarely, rupture of the renal artery.

Stent-supported angioplasty is an appropriate option for some patients with atherosclerotic renovascular disease. In the presence of aneurysmal or severe atherosclerotic disease of the aorta, surgical intervention is the treatment of choice. Kidneys 8 cm or less in pole-to-pole length should be removed—not revascularized—if intervention is indicated and removal will not jeopardize overall renal function.

- Stent-supported angioplasty is an option for some patients with atherosclerotic renovascular disease.
- Surgical treatment is best for cases of atheromatous renal artery disease associated with aneurysmal or severe atherosclerotic disease of the aorta.

The medical treatment of renovascular hypertension is not different from that of essential hypertension. Both volume retention (due to aldosterone) and vasoconstriction (due to activation of the sympathetic nervous system and angiotensin II) contribute to the elevation of blood pressure. ACEIs and ARBs can precipitate acute renal failure in the presence of bilateral renal artery stenosis. Medical treatment does not correct the underlying ischemia of the affected kidney, and decreases in systemic blood pressure may further aggravate loss of renal function. Progression of atherosclerotic renal artery disease can be slowed by control of all modifiable risk factors, including the use of statin drugs for aggressive cholesterol lowering.

- The medical treatment of renovascular hypertension is similar to that of essential hypertension.
- If there is bilateral renal artery stenosis, ACEIs and ARBs can precipitate acute renal failure.
- Medical treatment does not correct the underlying ischemia of the affected kidney.
- Management of all modifiable cardiovascular risk factors can lessen the risk of progression of atherosclerotic renovascular disease.
- Typical clinical scenario for renovascular hypertension due to fibromuscular dysplasia: A 30-year-old woman complains of new-onset headaches for the past 2 months. She has no past history of hypertension. On examination, blood pressure is 180/110 mm Hg. Retinal examination shows hemorrhages. On auscultation of the abdomen, a systolic-diastolic bruit is heard in the left upper quadrant.
- Typical clinical scenario for renovascular hypertension due to atherosclerosis: A 54-year-old man has a several-year history of mild hypertension that has been well controlled. He has a 30 pack-year history of cigarette smoking and hypercholesterolemia that is diet-controlled. He has a past history of coronary artery bypass graft surgery. Blood pressure suddenly worsens and is now 170/115 mm Hg. On auscultation of the abdomen, a systolic bruit is detected in the right upper quadrant. Bilateral femoral bruits are also noted.

Renal Parenchymal Disease

Renal parenchymal disease is the most common secondary cause of hypertension and is present in 3% to 5% of persons with elevated blood pressure. Also, hypertension is a common cause of chronic kidney disease and is the second most common cause of end-stage renal failure in the population. Persons with chronic kidney disease and hypertension are at high risk for the development of cardiovascular disease. Contributing to this increased risk is a loss of the normal nocturnal decline in blood pressure ("non-dipper") in persons with renal disease.

Regardless of the cause of chronic kidney disease, hypertension is associated with a more rapid loss of renal function. This may be due to transmission of higher pressures into the glomerulus as afferent renal artery resistance fails to limit transmission of higher systemic pressures into the nephron. Higher glomerular transcapillary pressures and flows injure glomerular cells by several mechanisms, ultimately leading to glomerulosclerosis. In addition, the degree of proteinuria is an independent predictor of progressive loss of renal function.

At least three major mechanisms are involved in the hypertension of renal disease: volume expansion from impaired renal elimination of salt and water, renin oversecretion, and decreased production of renal vasodilators (i.e., prostaglandins, kallikrein, or kinin). In addition, accumulation of mediators of oxidative stress, reducing the availability of the vasodilator nitric oxide, and increased levels of the vasoconstrictor endothelin may also contribute.

The goal blood pressure in chronic kidney disease is less than 130/80 mm Hg. Achieving goal blood pressure lessens the risk of progressive loss of renal function. Also, ACEIs may have additional benefits to slow progression of both diabetic and nondiabetic renal diseases. Treatment should begin with dietary sodium restriction. In addition, diuretic therapy is often necessary for blood pressure control. If serum creatinine is more than 2.0 mg/dL, the more potent loop agents or metolazone is necessary. In diuretic-resistant persons, the combination of a loop agent with a thiazide may be required. Oversecretion of renin occurs in only a small proportion of persons with chronic kidney disease. However, ACEIs reduce proteinuria and high glomerular transcapillary pressures by decreasing resistance in the efferent arteriole of the nephron. These actions retard further loss of renal function. ACEIs can cause hyperkalemia and an acute decline in renal function. Unless severe, modest acute declines in renal function should be tolerated because the acute decline is often followed by stabilization and preservation of renal function chronically. Acute, severe decline in renal function with ACEI therapy raises the possibility of bilateral renal artery stenosis. ARBs can be used if ACEIs are not tolerated and may be used instead of ACEIs in persons with type 2 diabetes and nephropathy. CCBs are effective blood pressure–lowering drugs in persons with chronic kidney disease. Non-dihydropyridine CCBs reduce proteinuria but dihydropyridine CCBs do not. In proteinuric renal disease not controlled with adequate doses of a diuretic and an ACEI, CCBs could be added as a third agent. β-Blockers should be considered if the person has angina or previously had a myocardial infarction. In advanced renal insufficiency, avoid the use of lipid-insoluble β-blockers, which rely on the kidney for excretion. Minoxidil should be considered for resistant hypertension.

- Renal parenchymal disease: the most common secondary cause of hypertension.
- Hypertension: the second most common cause of end-stage renal disease.
- Treatment of hypertension in renal disease should include sodium restriction, diuretics appropriate to level of renal function, and ACEIs.
- ACEIs slow the progression of proteinuric renal disease.
- In chronic kidney disease, ACEI therapy can cause hyperkalemia and acute declines in renal function.
- Minoxidil should be considered for resistant hypertension.

Primary Aldosteronism

Hypertension, hypokalemia (with renal wasting of potassium), suppressed plasma renin activity, and increased aldosterone levels characterize the syndrome of primary aldosteronism. Prevalence estimates range from 2% to 15% of the hypertensive population. Its main subtypes are unilateral aldosterone-producing adenoma (30%-40% of cases) and bilateral idiopathic zona granulosa adrenal hyperplasia (60%-70% of cases). Rarer subtypes are unilateral hyperplasia, glucocorticoid suppressible hyperplasia, and aldosterone-producing cortical carcinoma. Primary aldosteronism should be suspected in any hypertensive person who presents with spontaneous hypokalemia or marked hypokalemia precipitated by usual doses of diuretics (potassium <3.0 mEq/L). Other causes of hypokalemic hypertensive syndromes should be considered: diuretics, renovascular hypertension, exogenous steroids, Cushing disease, excess deoxycorticosterone, Liddle syndrome, 11β-hydroxylase deficiency, and ingestion of licorice containing glycyrrhizinic acid (renal cortisol catabolism inhibitor). Primary aldosteronism may be the cause of resistant hypertension even in the absence of hypokalemia because approximately 30% of cases are not associated with spontaneous hypokalemia. It also should be considered in persons who have hypertension and a known adrenal mass (in addition to Cushing disease and pheochromocytoma) or in persons who have hypokalemia despite taking ACEIs or ARBs for treatment of hypertension (in the presence or absence of concomitant diuretic use).

- Primary aldosteronism: hypertension, hypokalemia (with renal wasting of potassium), suppressed plasma renin, and increased aldosterone.
- Main subtypes: unilateral aldosterone-producing adenoma and bilateral adrenal hyperplasia.
- Suspect primary aldosteronism in persons with spontaneous hypokalemia, marked hypokalemia precipitated by usual doses of diuretics, resistant hypertension, hypertension and an adrenal mass, or hypokalemia despite use of ACEIs or ARBs.

Clinical Features

Clinical symptoms are uncommon. Most persons with primary aldosteronism cannot be differentiated from those with essential hypertension. Rarely, severe hypokalemia may cause muscle weakness, cramps, headache, palpitations, polydipsia, polyuria, or nocturia. Hypertension is usually moderate, but it may be severe and resistant to control. Retinal vascular changes of severe hypertension may be present. Rarely, the sign of Trousseau or Chvostek may be present if marked alkalosis is associated with the hypokalemia. Peripheral edema is rare.

- Clinical symptoms are uncommon.
- Severe hypokalemia may cause muscle weakness, cramps, headache, palpitations, polydipsia, polyuria, or nocturia.
- Peripheral edema is rare.

Laboratory Features

Characteristic laboratory abnormalities include hypokalemia, mild metabolic alkalosis (serum bicarbonate >31 mEq/L), and relative hypernatremia (serum sodium concentration >142 mEq/L). Relative hypernatremia is related to suppression of vasopressin as the result of volume expansion, resetting of the central osmostat for vasopressin release, altered thirst, and hypokalemia-induced suppression of vasopressin release or action. A mild increase in the fasting blood glucose level is detected in 25% of persons (hypokalemia suppresses insulin release). The electrocardiogram may show changes of hypokalemia (prolongation of the ST segment, U waves, and T-wave inversions) as well as left ventricular hypertrophy.

- Laboratory abnormalities in primary aldosteronism: hypokalemia, mild metabolic alkalosis, relative hypernatremia, and increased fasting glucose level.
- Electrocardiogram may show changes of hypokalemia (prolongation of the ST segment, U waves, T-wave inversions).

Diagnosis

The investigation for primary aldosteronism is divided into three phases: 1) screening, 2) confirmation of the diagnosis, and 3) determination of the subtype.

Screening studies should include measurement of serum sodium, potassium, and PRA. If the person is hypokalemic, a 24-hour urine collection for potassium should be obtained (>30 mEq of potassium in a person with hypokalemia defines renal wasting of potassium). A plasma aldosterone concentration (PAC) may be determined because some advocate calculating the ratio of PAC to PRA. A ratio greater than 20 (with PAC >15 ng/dL and PRA <2.0 ng/mL per hour) suggests the diagnosis of primary aldosteronism. Ideally, PRA and PAC should be measured in the morning after the discontinuation of drugs that could influence the measurements (diuretics, β-blockers, ACEIs, and ARBs).

In persons with positive screening test results, 24-hour urinary aldosterone excretion should be measured during the fourth day of a high salt diet. The diagnosis of primary aldosteronism rests on demonstrating renin suppression and inappropriately high aldosterone excretion in a sodium-replete state (24-hour sodium excretion >200 mEq) in hypertensive persons. Before a diagnostic evaluation is initiated, the use of potentially interfering drugs must be discontinued and plasma volume status assessed. Spironolactone influences the renin-angiotensin-aldosterone axis and must be discontinued for at least 6 weeks before investigation. Diuretics, ACEIs, and ARBs may increase and β-blockers may decrease PRA levels in persons with primary aldosteronism. If hypertension must be treated in the interim, guanadrel, α-blockers, or CCBs may be used. After a high salt diet for 3 days (and with concomitant vigorous potassium supplementation), persons should submit a 24-hour urine collection for measurement of sodium, potassium, creatinine, and aldosterone and the PRA should be measured. Creatinine can be used as an approximation of the adequacy of the collection. A 24-hour urine aldosterone greater than 12 to 14 μg (when urine sodium is >200 mEq) and a PRA less than 1.0 ng/mL per hour confirm the diagnosis of primary aldosteronism.

- In a hypokalemic, hypertensive person, a PAC:PRA ratio >20 suggests primary aldosteronism.
- Before diagnostic evaluation: discontinue drugs that could influence PRA or PAC levels and assess plasma volume status.
- After a 3-day high salt diet, measure the PRA and sodium, potassium, creatinine, and aldosterone in a 24-hour urine collection.
- 24-Hour urine aldosterone >12 to 14 μg (with concomitant urine sodium >200 mEq) and a PRA <1.0 ng/dL per hour confirm the diagnosis of primary aldosteronism.

The major subtypes to differentiate are unilateral aldosterone-producing adenoma and bilateral adrenal hyperplasia. Removing an aldosterone-producing adenoma normalizes blood pressure in approximately 30% of cases and relieves hypokalemia in 100%. Unilateral or bilateral adrenalectomy seldom corrects hypertension when bilateral adrenal hyperplasia is present. CT or magnetic resonance imaging (MRI) of the adrenal glands is the initial study for distinguishing between subtypes. CT is effective in localizing adenomas larger than 1 cm in diameter when the adrenal glands are imaged at 0.3-cm intervals. Generally, if a single adenoma larger than 1 cm in diameter is clearly identified, surgical treatment is the choice. If no mass is identified, assume the diagnosis of bilateral hyperplasia and prescribe spironolactone or other potassium-retaining diuretics. Often, additional medications are needed for blood pressure control.

- Removing an aldosterone-producing adenoma normalizes blood pressure in 30% of cases and hypokalemia in 100%.
- Unilateral or bilateral adrenalectomy seldom corrects hypertension in persons with bilateral adrenal hyperplasia.
- CT or MRI of the adrenal glands is the initial study for distinguishing between subtypes.
- If a single adenoma is >1 cm in diameter, the treatment is surgical.

- If no mass is seen, prescribe spironolactone, eplerenone, or other potassium-retaining diuretics and other medications as needed to control blood pressure.

If the results are equivocal or the gland opposite that containing the presumed adenoma is abnormal or if CT findings are normal in a person with severe hypertension, hypokalemia, and markedly elevated aldosterone (findings suggestive of an adenoma), sampling blood from the adrenal veins for aldosterone may distinguish between subtypes or identify an adrenal gland containing a small adenoma not visible on imaging. In these settings, subspecialty consultation should be sought.

- If the results are equivocal, sampling blood from the adrenal veins for aldosterone may distinguish between subtypes.
- Typical clinical scenario for primary aldosteronism: A 42-year-old man is evaluated for resistant hypertension. The physical examination findings are normal except for elevated blood pressure of 150/105 mm Hg despite treatment with an ACEI, β-blocker, and CCB. Initial laboratory values are sodium 144 mEq/L, potassium 2.9 mEq/L, glucose 110 mg/dL, and creatinine 1.0 mg/dL.

Pheochromocytoma

Pheochromocytomas are tumors of chromaffin cell origin that produce paroxysmal or sustained hypertension. The incidence in the general population is 2 to 8 cases per million persons per year. The prevalence is 0.5% for persons with hypertension and suggestive symptoms and 4% for hypertensive persons with an adrenal tumor. A "rule of 10" is often quoted for these tumors: 10% are extra-adrenal (90% are located in one or both adrenal glands); 10% occur in children (90% occur in adults between the third and fifth decades of life; equal occurrence in men and women); 10% are multiple or bilateral (familial tumors are more likely to be bilateral); 10% recur after the initial resection; 10% are malignant; and 10% are familial. Extra-adrenal pheochromocytomas may occur anywhere along the sympathetic chain and occasionally in aberrant sites (superior para-aortic region [46%], glomus jugulari, inferior para-aortic region [29%], bladder [10%], or thorax [10%]). Chromaffin cells synthesize catecholamines from tyrosine. Norepinephrine is the end product in all sites except the adrenal medulla, where 75% of norepinephrine is metabolized to epinephrine. Extra-adrenal tumors produce only norepinephrine, whereas adrenal tumors may produce an excess of one or both catecholamines. A person with a tumor that secretes predominantly epinephrine has mainly systolic hypertension, tachycardia, sweating, flushing, and tremulousness and may present with hypotension. A person with a tumor that secretes mainly norepinephrine has both diastolic and systolic hypertension, less tachycardia, and fewer paroxysms of anxiety and palpitations.

- Pheochromocytoma: remember the "rule of 10."
- Ninety percent are in one or both adrenal glands.
- It may occur anywhere along the sympathetic chain.
- It is malignant in up to 10% of cases.
- An extra-adrenal tumor produces only norepinephrine.
- An adrenal tumor can produce an excess of epinephrine or norepinephrine (or both).

Familial pheochromocytomas tend to be bilateral. Familial syndromes include the following:
1. A simple form inherited as an autosomal dominant trait unassociated with other glandular abnormalities
2. Multiple endocrine neoplasia type IIA (medullary carcinoma of the thyroid [increased plasma level of calcitonin], pheochromocytoma, hyperparathyroidism) and type IIB (pheochromocytoma, medullary carcinoma of the thyroid, mucosal neuromas, thickened corneal nerves, intestinal ganglioneuromatosis, marfanoid body habitus [Plates 13-1 and 13-2])
3. Neurofibromatosis (café au lait spots)
4. von Hippel-Lindau disease (pheochromocytoma, retinal hemangiomatosis, cerebellar hemangioblastomas, renal cell carcinoma)

- Familial pheochromocytomas tend to be bilateral.
- Pheochromocytoma is associated with neurofibromatosis, von Hippel-Lindau disease, and multiple endocrine neoplasia types IIA and IIB.

Symptoms

Symptomatic paroxysms of hypertension occur in fewer than 50% of persons; most have sustained hypertension. Paroxysms are characterized by headache, diaphoresis, palpitations, and pallor. A paroxysm is usually rapid in onset, rapid in offset, and may be triggered by exercise, bending, urination, defecation, induction of anesthesia, smoking, or infusion of intravenous contrast media. Some persons experience unintended weight loss and have signs and symptoms of hypermetabolism. Others have both hypertension and orthostatic hypotension or cardiomyopathy. Rarely, persons may present with catecholamine-induced cardiomyopathy, fever, or peripheral vasospasm. The hypertension can be severe, resistant to control, and associated with retinopathy of accelerated-malignant hypertension.

- Common symptoms of pheochromocytoma: headache, diaphoresis, palpitations, and pallor.

- Paroxysms can be induced by exercise, bending, urination, defecation, induction of anesthesia, smoking, or infusion of contrast media.
- Some persons experience unintended weight loss or peripheral vasospasm; others have both hypertension and orthostatic hypotension or cardiomyopathy.

Screening

Screening for pheochromocytoma should be selective. Candidates for screening are hypertensive persons with paroxysmal hypertension with or without suggestive symptoms, an adrenal mass, treatment-resistant hypertension, concomitant diabetes mellitus, unintended weight loss and other features of hypermetabolism, marked hypertension in response to anesthesia induction, neurocutaneous lesions, orthostatic hypotension, or a family history of pheochromocytoma, medullary carcinoma of the thyroid, or hyperparathyroidism.

Screening tests include measurement of catecholamines (epinephrine, norepinephrine, and dopamine) and their metabolites (metanephrine, normetanephrine, and vanillylmandelic acid) in the plasma and urine. Measurement of plasma free metanephrines is the most sensitive screening test. Measurement of the 24-hour urinary excretion of metanephrines is less sensitive but is associated with fewer false-positive results. Plasma free metanephrines is the screening test of choice if a familial syndrome is suspected, if the person has a previous history of pheochromocytoma, and if the clinical suspicion is high. A negative result for either plasma or urine metanephrines excludes the diagnosis in most cases.

Because of the low prevalence of pheochromocytoma, false-positive results outnumber true-positive results among persons screened for this disorder. Dietary factors, drugs, and physiologic stresses can interfere with screening test results. Some of these are listed in Table 13-4. In those with marginally positive results, the factors noted in Table 13-4, if present, should be eliminated and the screening test repeated.

- Screening for pheochromocytoma: history of paroxysmal hypertension with or without suggestive symptoms, hypertension and an adrenal mass, treatment-resistant hypertension, hypertension with diabetes mellitus, hypermetabolism and unintended weight loss, or marked hypertension in response to anesthesia induction.
- The most sensitive screening test is plasma free metanephrines.
- Dietary factors, drugs, and physiologic stresses can interfere with screening test results.

Diagnosis and Treatment

CT or MRI of the abdomen is the initial test used to locate a tumor (90% of all tumors are in one or both adrenal glands and 98% of all tumors are in the abdomen) and should only

Table 13-4   Drugs That Interfere With Measurement of
Catecholamines and Metabolites

Associated with increased values
   Amphetamines, buspirone, and most psychoactive agents
   Phenothiazines
   Cyclobenzaprine
   Labetalol
   Drugs containing catecholamines (e.g., decongestants)
   Levodopa
   Methyldopa
   Acetaminophen
   Coffee (including decaffeinated)
   Caffeine
   Withdrawal from clonidine or related drugs
   Benzodiazepines (and withdrawal)
   Ethanol (and withdrawal)
   Sotalol
   Tricyclic antidepressants
   Nicotine
   Dibenzyline
   Urapidil
Associated with decreased values
   Metyrosine
   Methylglucamine (iodinated contrast medium)

be performed after biochemical testing has confirmed the presence of the disorder. Specialized studies are occasionally necessary to identify extra-adrenal tumors not identified with CT or MRI (i.e., ^{131}I-MIBG scanning, positron emission tomography, or vena caval sampling for catecholamines). After the tumor has been identified, treatment is surgical. Preoperatively, administer α-blockers (phenoxybenzamine), followed by β-blockers if needed to control blood pressure and cardiac rhythm. Persons with hypertensive crisis can be given α-blockers or sodium nitroprusside intravenously. β-Blockers can be given if tachycardia is excessive. Because pheochromocytomas can recur in 10% of cases, long-term biochemical follow-up is required.

- Use CT or MRI of the abdomen to locate the tumor.
- The treatment is surgical.
- Preoperatively, administer α-blockers, followed by β-blockers.
- Typical clinical scenario for pheochromocytoma: A 25-year-old college student is evaluated for spells. These are sudden in onset and offset and last 25 to 35 minutes. Symptoms include frontal headache, diaphoresis, pounding pulse, and nausea. According to persons witnessing a

spell, the patient is pale. Since the onset of these spells, he has lost 20 lb. During a recent spell, his blood pressure was noted to be 220/160 mm Hg. He has no past history of hypertension. The examination findings are essentially normal except for evidence of weight loss, a resting pulse of 105 beats/min, and blood pressure of 160/110 mm Hg.

Coarctation of the Aorta

Coarctation of the aorta is a constriction of the vessel, commonly just beyond the takeoff of the left subclavian artery (see Chapter 3, Cardiology). It usually is detected in childhood, but occasionally the diagnosis is not made until adulthood. The classic feature is increased blood pressure in the upper extremities, with low or unobtainable blood pressure in the lower extremities. The mechanism of hypertension involves both volume expansion and inappropriate renin secretion. Symptoms of coarctation include headache, cold feet, and exercise-induced leg pain (claudication). Clinical signs include elevated blood pressure in the arms, murmurs in the front or back of the chest, visible pulsations in the neck or chest wall, and weak femoral pulses or delay when the radial and femoral pulses are palpated simultaneously. Chest radiography can be diagnostic. A characteristic "3 sign" due to dilatation above and below the constriction plus notching of the ribs (Fig. 13-3) by enlarged collateral vessels may be identified. The diagnosis is made with transesophageal echocardiography or MRI of the aorta.

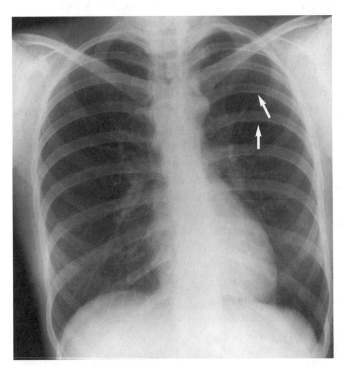

Fig. 13-3. Chest radiograph of a patient with coarctation of the aorta showing notching (*arrows*) of ribs from collateral vessels.

Traditionally, treatment has been surgical repair of the aorta. Balloon angioplasty with or without stenting is becoming the treatment of choice. After repair, hypertension is usually transient and may be associated with mesenteric vasculitis and bowel infarction. PRA levels are usually high. The recommended treatment for hypertension after repair is β-blockers or ACEIs.

- Coarctation of the aorta is usually just beyond the takeoff of the left subclavian artery.
- It usually is detected in childhood but may not be identified until adulthood.
- Classic feature: increased blood pressure in the upper extremities and low or unobtainable blood pressure in the lower extremities.
- Mechanism of hypertension: volume expansion and inappropriate renin secretion.
- Symptoms: headache, cold feet, and exercise-induced leg pain.
- Signs: Elevated blood pressure in the arms, murmurs in front or back of the chest, visible pulsations in the neck or chest wall, and weak femoral pulses.
- Transesophageal echocardiography or MRI makes the diagnosis.
- Treatment is with balloon angioplasty or surgery.

Other Causes of Hypertension

Cushing syndrome (see Chapter 6, Endocrinology) is often associated with hypertension and always should be considered in the hypertensive person who has impaired fasting glucose and unexplained hypokalemia. Hypothyroidism is associated with diastolic hypertension. It is a state of decreased cardiac output and contractility. Tissue perfusion is maintained by an increase in peripheral vascular resistance mediated by increased activity of the sympathetic nervous system. In contrast, hyperthyroidism is associated with systolic hypertension and a wide pulse pressure due to increased cardiac output and decreased peripheral vascular resistance.

Hyperparathyroidism may be associated with hypertension. Hypercalcemia may increase blood pressure directly by increasing peripheral vascular resistance and indirectly by increasing vascular sensitivity to catecholamines.

Approximately 35% of persons with acromegaly have hypertension, which is largely due to the sodium-retaining effects of growth hormone.

Obstructive sleep apnea is associated with hypertension that may be severe and resistant to control. Upper body obesity is a risk factor for obstructive sleep apnea and is common in hypertensive persons. Consider the diagnosis of obstructive sleep apnea in persons who are overweight, snore loudly, and complain of morning headaches and daytime sleepiness. Bed partners may observe breath-holding episodes at night. The mechanism of hypertension involves increased sympathetic nervous system activity. This condition can be associated with increased metanephrines.

Intracranial tumors, especially those occurring in the posterior fossa, may cause hypertension. Occasionally, hypertension is labile, with features suggesting pheochromocytoma.

Panic syndrome also may be associated with a labile increase in blood pressure and symptoms that suggest pheochromocytoma. Acute stress from various causes (emotional or physical) can increase blood pressure through intense stimulation of the sympathetic nervous system and the renin-angiotensin system (especially if volume contraction is present).

- Hypothyroidism can cause diastolic hypertension.
- Hyperthyroidism can cause systolic hypertension.
- Hyperparathyroidism and acromegaly may be associated with hypertension.
- Obstructive sleep apnea can cause hypertension and may increase metanephrines.
- Brain tumors in the posterior fossa and panic syndrome can cause labile hypertension, suggesting pheochromocytoma.
- Acute stress can increase blood pressure.

Hypertension in Pregnancy

Normally, blood pressure decreases early in pregnancy and then gradually increases to prepregnant levels toward term. During pregnancy, plasma angiotensinogen, renin activity, and aldosterone increase. Vessels are hyporesponsive to pressor agents, including norepinephrine and angiotensin II, perhaps because of prostaglandins produced by the uteroplacental unit. Although aldosterone levels increase, renal sodium retention is not marked, probably because progesterone and prostaglandins are natriuretic. Progesterone is also a vasodilator. Plasma volume and cardiac output increase 50% to 60% from baseline during normal pregnancy. Renal blood flow and glomerular filtration rate increase by 35%. Blood pressure decreases in normal pregnancy because of reduced peripheral vascular resistance. Systolic blood pressure is affected less than diastolic blood pressure because of increased cardiac output in response to vasodilatation. The usual nocturnal decrease in blood pressure is preserved during normal pregnancy. Other substances that increase during normal pregnancy are estrogen, deoxycorticosterone, and vasodilating prostaglandins produced by the uteroplacental unit.

- Blood pressure decreases early in pregnancy and gradually increases to prepregnant levels toward term.
- Angiotensinogen, renin activity, and aldosterone increase.
- During pregnancy, vessels are hyporesponsive to norepinephrine and angiotensin II.

- Renal sodium retention is not marked, probably because progesterone and prostaglandins are natriuretic.
- In normal pregnancy, blood pressure decreases because of reduced peripheral vascular resistance.

Definition

Hypertension during pregnancy is defined as systolic blood pressure 140 mm Hg or greater or diastolic blood pressure 90 mm Hg or greater. The diagnosis is confirmed by documentation of elevated blood pressure on two determinations made 6 hours apart.

Four major hypertensive syndromes in pregnancy are 1) chronic hypertension—hypertension known to be present before pregnancy or diagnosed before the 20th week of gestation, 2) preeclampsia-eclampsia (described below), 3) chronic hypertension with superimposed preeclampsia, and 4) gestational hypertension—hypertension that develops for the first time after 20 weeks' gestation without other findings of preeclampsia; it can evolve into preeclampsia. If gestational hypertension does not evolve into preeclampsia by delivery and blood pressure normalizes within 12 weeks post partum, it is called "transient hypertension of pregnancy." This is a predictor for the future development of essential hypertension. If blood pressure remains elevated, it is recognized retrospectively as "chronic hypertension" that was previously undiagnosed and masked by the decrease in blood pressure that occurs during early pregnancy.

- Hypertension during pregnancy: Blood pressure ≥140 mm Hg systolic or ≥90 mm Hg diastolic.
- Transient hypertension is a predictor of the future development of essential hypertension.

The pregnancy-specific syndrome of preeclampsia is characterized by hypertension (blood pressure ≥140/90 mm Hg) and proteinuria (24-hour urine protein excretion ≥0.3 g) that develops after the 20th week of gestation. Eclampsia is defined by seizures that occur in the presence of preeclampsia which cannot be attributed to other causes. Findings that increase the certainty of the diagnosis of preeclampsia (and increase the risk for eclampsia) and the need for close monitoring and consideration for delivery include headache, blurring of vision and other cerebral symptoms, epigastric pain, nephrotic range proteinuria (≥3.5 g/24 h), oliguria, systolic blood pressure 160 mm Hg or higher or diastolic blood pressure 110 mm Hg or higher, creatinine level greater than 1.2 mg/dL, platelet count less than 100×10^9/L, evidence of microangiopathic hemolytic anemia (abnormal blood smear or increased lactate dehydrogenase), elevated liver enzymes (aspartate and alanine aminotransferase [AST and ALT]), or pulmonary edema.

Preeclampsia occurs more commonly in African American women and women who are relatively young or old to be pregnant, who are having their first pregnancy or a twin pregnancy, who are obese, who have diabetes or insulin resistance, who have a family history of preeclampsia in their mother, who have had preeclampsia with a previous pregnancy, or who have renal disease, chronic hypertension, a collagen vascular disease, or a congenital thrombophilia disorder. Preeclampsia that develops before the 20th week of gestation suggests molar pregnancy, fetal hydrops, α-thalassemia, or renal disease.

- Preeclampsia: hypertension and proteinuria after the 20th week of gestation.
- Eclampsia: preeclampsia with seizures.
- Risk factors for preeclampsia: African American race, relatively young or old for pregnancy, first or twin pregnancy, obesity, diabetes mellitus or insulin resistance, family history of preeclampsia in the mother, preeclampsia with a previous pregnancy, renal disease, chronic hypertension, collagen vascular disease, or congenital thrombophilia disorder.

In preeclampsia, the endovascular trophoblastic cells of the placenta do not adequately invade the uterine spiral arteries. Consequently, the normally thick-walled muscular spiral arteries are not transformed into saclike flaccid vessels capable of accommodating the tenfold increase in uterine blood flow associated with normal pregnancy. This leads to underperfusion of the placenta. Circulating mediators produced by the hypoperfused placenta act on vascular endothelial cells, which then produce several factors (procoagulants, vasoconstrictors, and mitogens) that constrict and obstruct vascular beds, producing the characteristic pathologic changes (hemorrhage and necrosis) that may be seen in the brain, heart, and liver of women with preeclampsia. Preeclampsia is a disorder of systemic vasoconstriction.

Unlike normal pregnant women, those with preeclampsia are sensitive to the pressor effects of norepinephrine and angiotensin II. There is a marked increase in peripheral resistance. Renal blood flow and glomerular filtration rate are decreased (but may remain above nonpregnant levels). Vascular volume is decreased and is often associated with hemoconcentration. This may be due to extravasation of albumin into the interstitial space. Central venous pressure and pulmonary capillary wedge pressure are often low. Placental prostaglandin levels decrease. Renal fractional urate clearance decreases, and uric acid is most often increased. Hyperuricemia often distinguishes patients with preeclampsia from those with chronic hypertension in pregnancy. An increase in uric acid concentration and a decrease in the platelet count are the earliest laboratory findings associated with preeclampsia. The HELLP syndrome (**H**emolysis, **E**levated **L**iver enzymes, and **L**ow **P**latelet count) occurs when intravascular coagulation and liver ischemia develop in preeclampsia. The HELLP syndrome can rapidly develop into a life-threatening disorder of liver failure and worsening thrombocytopenia in the presence of only mild or moderate hypertension. The most serious complication of the HELLP syndrome is liver rupture (right upper quadrant abdominal pain), which is associated with high maternal and fetal mortality.

- Women with preeclampsia are sensitive to the pressor effects of norepinephrine and angiotensin II.
- With preeclampsia, peripheral vascular resistance markedly increases.
- Uric acid is most often increased; this distinguishes women with preeclampsia from those with chronic hypertension in pregnancy.
- An increase in uric acid and a decrease in the platelet count are the earliest laboratory abnormalities in preeclampsia.
- Laboratory evaluation for hypertension developing after 20 weeks' gestation: hemoglobin/hematocrit, platelet count, 24-hour urine protein, creatinine, uric acid level, AST/ALT, albumin, lactate dehydrogenase, blood smear, coagulation profile.

Treatment of Chronic Hypertension in Pregnancy

Most women with stage 1 or 2 hypertension and normal renal function will have good outcomes. As blood pressure decreases in early pregnancy, often control can be maintained with less or no medication. For previously untreated women or for those who have had their medications discontinued in early pregnancy, drug therapy should be considered if diastolic blood pressure is 100 mm Hg or higher or systolic blood pressure 150 mm Hg or higher in the second trimester or 160 mm Hg or higher in the third trimester or if target organ injury occurs (left ventricular hypertrophy, increased creatinine level). Methyldopa (most completely studied) is recommended as initial therapy. This is the only drug that has been shown to decrease perinatal mortality and for which long-term studies on the offspring are available.

If methyldopa is ineffective or not tolerated, other drugs can be considered. Except for ACEIs and ARBs, none of the currently available drugs are known to increase perinatal morbidity or mortality. ACEIs or ARBs are contraindicated because exposure to these agents in the second or third trimester of pregnancy can cause serious fetal abnormalities (limb defects, lung hypoplasia, craniofacial deformities, and renal dysplasia). There is evidence that α-β-blockers are safe and effective for treating chronic hypertension in pregnancy.

The use of β-blockers (atenolol) in the second trimester has been associated with intrauterine fetal growth retardation and low placental weight. Their use should be restricted to the third trimester. However, use in the third trimester can be associated with fetal bradycardia, impaired fetal compensatory response to hypoxia, and neonatal hypoglycemia.

Only limited data are available for CCBs. These drugs are potent tocolytics and can affect progression of labor. They can be associated with profound hypotension and circulatory collapse if magnesium sulfate is given concurrently for seizure prophylaxis in preeclampsia.

Because of theoretical concerns about diuretics decreasing vascular volume and placental blood flow, they are not considered first-line agents. However, if indicated (salt-sensitive hypertension or in the presence of renal or cardiac disease), they are considered safe, and they can potentiate the effects of other agents to lower blood pressure. They are contraindicated in preeclampsia and intrauterine growth retardation.

- Use drug therapy if diastolic blood pressure is ≥100 mm Hg or systolic blood pressure is ≥150 mm Hg in the second trimester or ≥160 mm Hg in the third trimester.
- Recommended initial therapy: methyldopa.
- ACEIs and ARBs are contraindicated during pregnancy.

Treatment of Preeclampsia-Eclampsia

Prevention strategies for preeclampsia have limited value. In recent studies, aspirin and calcium supplements have not been shown to lessen the risk for preeclampsia. It is important to identify the high-risk woman and to monitor her closely to identify preeclampsia early. Early recognition of preeclampsia is based primarily on diagnostic blood pressure increases in the late second or early third trimester. Proteinuria is an important sign of progression and usually warrants hospitalization. The woman should be kept at rest in bed. Monitor blood pressure, urine output, and fluid retention (weigh patient) daily. Periodically determine the platelet count, creatinine level, uric acid level, albumin level, and urine protein excretion. Evidence of central nervous system involvement (headache, disorientation, visual symptoms) or liver distention (abdominal pain, liver tenderness) are important findings that suggest progression of preeclampsia. Hepatic rupture is associated with 65% mortality and can be prevented only by delivery of the fetus. Evidence of progressive preeclampsia after the 30th week of gestation is an indication for delivery. When gestational age is critical (25-30 weeks), worsening maternal symptoms, laboratory evidence of end-organ dysfunction, or deterioration of the fetal condition indicates delivery. If a fetus is immature and preeclampsia is nonprogressive, a period of observation is warranted. Hypertension should be treated with drugs if diastolic blood pressure is 100 mm Hg or greater. The oral agent of choice is methyldopa. Reasonable alternatives are α-β-blockers, CCBs, or hydralazine. The intravenous agent of choice is hydralazine.

- Proteinuria is an important sign of progression and usually warrants hospitalization.
- Keep the woman at rest in bed.

- Central nervous system involvement or liver distention suggests progression of preeclampsia.
- Progressive preeclampsia after the 30th week of gestation is an indication for delivery.
- Worsening maternal symptoms, laboratory evidence of end-organ dysfunction, or deterioration of the fetal condition indicates delivery.
- If diastolic blood pressure is ≥100 mm Hg, treat with drugs.
- Oral agent of choice: methyldopa.
- Intravenous agent of choice: hydralazine.

Magnesium sulfate is the treatment of choice for impending eclampsia or for preventing recurrent seizures. It should be given as a continuous intravenous infusion during labor and delivery and for at least 24 hours post partum. Monitor the patient's patellar reflex, urine output, and respirations while giving magnesium. The usual loading dose can be given in the setting of marked renal dysfunction, but subsequent dosing must be guided by frequent monitoring of blood levels. Calcium gluconate is the treatment of choice for magnesium toxicity and should be kept at the bedside.

- Magnesium sulfate: treatment of choice for impending eclampsia or for preventing recurrent seizures.
- Calcium gluconate: treatment of choice for magnesium toxicity.

Treatment of Hypertensive Crisis

The drug of choice for the treatment of a hypertensive crisis during pregnancy is intravenous hydralazine. Treatment can be initiated with a 5- to 10-mg bolus, followed by 5 to 10 mg every 20 to 30 minutes until control is achieved and then repeated as needed (usually every 3 hours). Side effects include tachycardia and headache. For hypertension refractory to hydralazine, the α-β-blocker labetalol is recommended. Treatment can be initiated with a 20-mg intravenous bolus. If the response is inadequate, 40 mg can be given 10 minutes later and, if necessary, 80 mg can be given at 10-minute intervals for two additional doses. If blood pressure is not controlled, an alternative drug should be considered. Avoid giving hydralazine to women with congestive heart failure or asthma. Nifedipine can be used. The initial dose is 10 mg orally, and it is repeated in 30 minutes if necessary. It is important to note that the U.S. Food and Drug Administration has not approved rapidly acting nifedipine for the treatment of hypertension. Sudden and severe decreases in blood pressure can occur and be associated with untoward cardiovascular events. The concomitant use of magnesium sulfate may cause severe hypotension. Generally, sodium nitroprusside (cyanide poisoning in the fetus) should be avoided; rarely, however, it may be needed for hypertension

that does not respond to the drugs mentioned above. It also may be needed if hypertensive encephalopathy develops. An infusion can be started at a rate of 0.25 μg/kg per minute and increased as needed to a maximum rate of 5 μg/kg per minute. Risk of fetal toxicity increases with infusions that last longer than 4 hours.

- The drug of choice for treating hypertensive crisis: hydralazine administered intravenously.
- For hypertension refractory to hydralazine, give labetalol.
- Administer sodium nitroprusside only if blood pressure fails to respond to other drugs.

Hypertensive Emergencies and Urgencies

Acute, severe increases in blood pressure are a serious medical concern; prompt therapy may be lifesaving. Clinically, this situation can be classified as a hypertensive urgency or a hypertensive emergency (crisis).

Definitions

Hypertensive Emergency

The term "hypertensive emergency" is defined as severe hypertension with evidence of acute injury to target organs (brain, heart, kidney, vasculature, and retina). It implies the need for hospitalization to immediately lower blood pressure with parenteral therapy. Examples include malignant hypertension, hypertensive encephalopathy, aortic dissection, unstable angina, acute myocardial infarction, eclampsia, pulmonary edema, or acute renal failure. Malignant hypertension is a clinical syndrome associated with severe elevation of blood pressure that is frequently fatal if not treated promptly. It is characterized by a marked increase in peripheral vascular resistance due to systemic (angiotensin II) or locally generated (endothelin) vasoconstrictor substances. Any form of hypertension can progress to the malignant phase. Clinical features include severe hypertension (diastolic blood pressure >130 mm Hg), retinal hemorrhages and exudates, papilledema, oliguria, azotemia, nausea and vomiting, findings of heart failure, and encephalopathy. Encephalopathy is the result of cerebral edema due to breakthrough hyperperfusion of the brain caused by severely increased blood pressure. Manifestations include papilledema, headache, confusion, somnolence, stupor, gastrointestinal distress, visual loss, focal neurologic deficits, coma, and seizures.

Fibrinoid necrosis of arterioles is the characteristic vascular lesion of malignant hypertension. Arteriolar injury worsens ischemia and promotes further release of vasoactive substances, setting up a vicious cycle. Microangiopathic hemolysis with fragmentation of erythrocytes and intravascular coagulation may occur in the setting of fibrinoid necrosis.

- Hypertensive emergency: severely elevated blood pressure associated with acute injury to target organs.
- Hospitalization and parenteral therapy to decrease blood pressure immediately are required.
- Hypertensive encephalopathy: papilledema, headache, somnolence, confusion, stupor, gastrointestinal distress, visual loss, focal neurologic deficits, coma, and seizures.

Hypertensive Urgency

The term "hypertensive urgency" is defined as severe hypertension without evidence of acute target organ injury but occurring in a setting in which it is important to decrease blood pressure to safer levels over a 24- to 48-hour period. Oral therapy in the outpatient setting is often adequate. Examples include severe hypertension in a person with known coronary artery disease, an aneurysm of the aorta (or other site), or a history of congestive heart failure or severe hypertension immediately following major surgery. "Accelerated hypertension" is a subacute progressive increase in blood pressure associated with hemorrhages and exudates (but not papilledema) on retinal examination. If left untreated, it may progress to malignant hypertension.

- Hypertensive urgency: severe hypertension without acute target organ injury.
- Treatment is administered orally, and hospitalization usually is not required.
- Accelerated hypertension may progress to malignant hypertension if not treated.

Causes

The causes of hypertensive urgencies and emergencies include the development of accelerated-malignant hypertension on the background of neglected essential hypertension (approximately 7% of cases of untreated hypertension will progress to the malignant phase), sudden discontinuation of antihypertensive therapy (especially multidrug programs or programs containing clonidine and β-blockers), renovascular disease, collagen vascular diseases (especially scleroderma), eclampsia, acute glomerulonephritis, pheochromocytoma, monoamine oxidase inhibitors and tyramine-containing foods, intracerebral or subarachnoid hemorrhage, acute aortic dissection, acute head injury, and acute stroke. Approximately 50% of hypertensive crises occur in persons with preexisting hypertension.

- Common causes of hypertensive urgencies and emergencies: neglected essential hypertension, discontinuation of antihypertensive therapy, renovascular disease, scleroderma, pheochromocytoma, and stroke.
- Malignant hypertension: a rapidly progressive vasospastic disorder.

- Renin and angiotensin II levels are increased.
- If not reversed, blood vessel walls undergo necrosis.

Evaluation and Management

Persons with hypertensive emergencies should be hospitalized in an intensive care unit. An arterial catheter should be inserted to monitor blood pressure continuously. In addition to a focused history (compliance with previously prescribed medications, use of blood pressure–raising drugs), and examination (retinal examination is mandatory), initial laboratory studies should include chest radiography, electrocardiography, creatinine or blood urea nitrogen, urinalysis, glucose, sodium, potassium, hemoglobin, and blood smear (fragmented erythrocytes). Studies to determine the underlying cause should be deferred; however, a spot urine test for catecholamines is reasonable. The challenge of treating hypertensive emergencies is to lower blood pressure promptly without compromising the function of vital organs. Blood pressure should be lowered quickly to a diastolic level of approximately 110 mm Hg (decrease mean blood pressure by 20%), followed by careful monitoring for evidence of worsening cerebral, renal, or cardiac function. Blood pressure is then gradually decreased to a diastolic level of 90 to 100 mm Hg. Ischemic pancreatitis and intestinal infarction are potential serious complications.

Generally, sodium nitroprusside is the drug of choice. It must be given in an intensive care setting, with an arterial catheter in place. This balanced arterial and venous dilator decreases both preload and afterload. The dose is 0.25 to 10.0 μg/kg per minute by intravenous infusion. The infusion must be protected from light. Toxicity is related to the metabolism of nitroprusside to cyanide in erythrocytes (metabolic acidosis). Thus, thiocyanate levels should be monitored every 48 hours and therapy discontinued if the blood level is greater than 12 mg/dL. Sodium nitrite or hydroxocobalamin can be infused in case of toxicity. Side effects of sodium nitroprusside include nausea, vomiting, agitation, disorientation, psychosis, muscular twitching, coarse tremor, and flushing. Frequently, patients with malignant hypertension are volume-depleted because of pressure natriuresis. However, as blood pressure decreases, fluid retention occurs and the addition of a loop diuretic is often required.

- Sodium nitroprusside: the drug of choice for a hypertensive emergency.
- Toxicity is related to the metabolism of nitroprusside to cyanide in erythrocytes.
- Monitor thiocyanate levels every 48 hours.
- In case of toxicity, infuse sodium nitrite or hydroxocobalamin.
- Sodium nitroprusside side effects: nausea, vomiting, agitation, muscular twitching, coarse tremor, and flushing.

Several alternative parenteral agents are available for the management of hypertensive emergencies and urgencies.

Labetalol is a combination α-blocker and nonselective β-blocker with an onset of action of 5 to 10 minutes. It can be given in repetitive intravenous miniboluses of 20 to 80 mg or as a constant infusion at a dose of 0.5 to 2 mg/min. Its duration of action is 3 to 6 hours. It can be used in most situations except acute heart failure. It is especially useful for postoperative hypertension and in hypertensive crisis of pregnancy. The same cautions and contraindications apply to this drug as to other β-blockers. Adverse effects include scalp tingling, vomiting, heart block, and orthostatic hypotension.

Glyceryl trinitrate (nitroglycerin) is a direct arteriolar and venous vasodilator with an onset of action of 2 to 5 minutes and with a duration of action of 3 to 5 minutes. It is given as a constant infusion of 5 to 100 μg/min. This drug decreases myocardial oxygen demand by decreasing preload and afterload. It dilates epicardial coronary arteries and collaterals. Tolerance can develop with prolonged infusion. It is especially useful if acute coronary ischemia or acute congestive heart failure is present. Adverse effects include headache, flushing, nausea, and methemoglobinemia.

Hydralazine is a direct arteriolar vasodilator with an onset of action of 10 to 20 minutes if given intravenously and 20 to 30 minutes if given intramuscularly. The usual dose is 10 to 20 mg intravenously or 10 to 50 mg intramuscularly. Its duration of action is 3 to 8 hours. Hydralazine is used primarily to treat hypertensive crisis of pregnancy. Adverse effects include headache, flushing, nausea, vomiting, and myocardial ischemia. Hydrozones form when hydralazine is mixed with dextrose.

Esmolol is a cardioselective β-blocker with an onset of action of 1 to 2 minutes and a duration of action of 10 to 20 minutes. It is given as a constant intravenous infusion in a dose of 50 to 300 μg/kg per minute. Esmolol is useful in postoperative hypertension, aortic dissection, and ischemic heart disease. It is often used in combination with vasodilators for effective control of blood pressure. The cautions and contraindications that apply to β-blockers also apply to this drug. Adverse effects include nausea and bradycardia.

Enalaprilat is an ACEI with an onset of action of 15 minutes and a duration of action of 6 hours. It is given intravenously in doses of 1.25 to 5 mg every 6 hours, with a maximal dose of 20 mg in 24 hours and less if renal disease is present. It is useful in postoperative hypertension and in settings of acute heart failure. Adverse effects include ACEI side effects, a precipitous decrease in blood pressure in high renin states, and an acute decline in renal function if renal artery disease is present.

Nicardipine is a dihydropyridine CCB with an onset of action of 5 to 10 minutes and a duration of action of 1 to 4 hours. It is given as a constant intravenous infusion of 5 to 15 mg per hour. It is useful for postoperative hypertension. Nicardipine should not be given in the setting of acute heart failure. Adverse effects include headache, nausea, flushing, and phlebitis.

Phentolamine is an α-blocker that is administered intravenously in doses of 5 to 15 mg. It is most effective for states of catecholamine excess and is the drug of choice if pheochromocytoma is suspected. Adverse effects include tachycardia and flushing.

Fenoldopam is a dopamine receptor (D_1) agonist that is given by constant intravenous infusion of 0.1 to 1.6 μg/kg per minute. The onset of action is within 5 minutes and offset is over 30 to 60 minutes. This drug is useful in settings of impaired renal function because it increases renal blood flow and sodium excretion. Side effects are nausea, vomiting, headache, and flushing.

Diazoxide is considered obsolete with the availability of newer and safer drugs.

- Glyceryl trinitrate (nitroglycerin) is useful in acute congestive heart failure or coronary ischemia.
- Tolerance can develop to glyceryl trinitrate.
- Hydralazine is used for hypertensive crisis of pregnancy.
- Esmolol, enalaprilat, and nicardipine are useful for postoperative hypertension.
- Phentolamine is the drug of choice if pheochromocytoma is suspected.
- Fenoldopam increases renal blood flow and sodium excretion.

Conditions Requiring Avoidance of Specific Drugs

- Acute myocardial infarction or angina: hydralazine (increases cardiac work).
- Dissecting aortic aneurysm: hydralazine (increases cardiac output).

As soon as possible, initiate regular oral treatment and taper intravenous treatment. After blood pressure has been brought under control, a search should be conducted for secondary causes. This should include screening for renovascular disease, pheochromocytoma, and primary aldosteronism.

- Typical clinical scenario: A 54-year-old man has a 12-year history of hypertension. It was controlled with a combination of hydrochlorothiazide, clonidine, and amlodipine. Because of cost and side effects, the patient stopped all therapy abruptly 3 weeks ago. Over the past 2 days, he has developed a headache of increasing severity. His wife has noted that he is confused and his speech is slurred; this prompted his visit to the office. On examination, the patient is stuporous and confused. His speech is slurred. Blood pressure is 230/140 mm Hg and the pulse is 115 beats/min. Retinal hemorrhages and papilledema are noted. Rales are present in both lung bases. An S_3 gallop is noted on heart examination. A chest radiograph shows findings of pulmonary edema. The creatinine level is 2.4 mg/dL. Erythrocytes are noted on urinalysis.

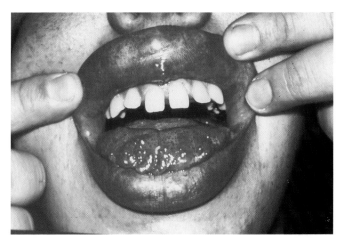

Plate 13-2. Oral neuromas associated with multiple endocrine neoplasia type IIB.

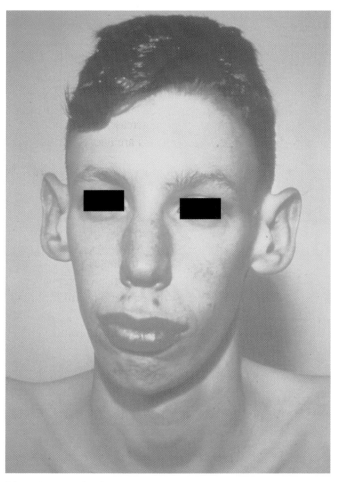

Plate 13-1. Marfanoid appearance of a patient with multiple endocrine neoplasia type IIB.

Hypertension Pharmacy Review

John G. O'Meara, PharmD, Jamie M. Gardner, PharmD, Todd M. Johnson, PharmD

Drug (brand name)	Daily dose, mg	Toxic/adverse effects	Drug interactions	Comments
Diuretics				
Thiazide-type (selected)		Glucose intolerance & insulin resistance, hyperlipidemia, hyperuricemia	Lithium (increased lithium levels), NSAIDs (decreased diuretic effectiveness), bile acid sequestrants (decreased thiazide absorption)	Preferred agents for isolated systolic hypertension
Hydrochlorothiazide (HydroDIURIL, Esidrix)	12.5-5 1-2/d			
Chlorthalidone (Hygroton)	12.5-5 1/d			Metolazone & indapamide may be effective in renally impaired patients
Indapamide (Lozol)	1.25-5 1/d			
Metolazone (Zaroxolyn, Diulo)	2.5-10 1/d			
Metolazone (MyKrox)	0.5-1 1/d			Lower doses avoid adverse metabolic effects
Loop		Similar to thiazide-type agents; hypocalcemia, dehydration, circulatory collapse	Similar to thiazides	Reserved for hypertensive patients with renal insufficiency
Bumetanide (Bumex)	0.5-4 2-3/d			
Ethacrynic acid (Edecrin)	25-100 2-3/d			
Furosemide (Lasix)	40-240 2-3/d			
Torsemide (Demadex)	5-100 1-2/d	Ototoxicity is potential adverse effect of all loop diuretics		
Potassium-sparing		Hyperkalemia	Potassium supplements, ACEIs, ARBs (all increase risk of hyperkalemia)	Weak diuretics alone, used in combination with other diuretics to avoid hypokalemia
Amiloride (Midamor)	5-10 1-2/d	Gynecomastia (spironolactone)		
Spironolactone (Aldactone)	25-100 1-2/d			
Triamterene (Dyrenium)	25-100 1-2/d			Avoid in renal impairment (serum creatinine >2.5 mg/dL)
Adrenergic inhibitors				
α_1-Blockers		Postural hypotension, tachycardia, dizziness, headache	Midodrine (decreased midodrine effectiveness)	Avoid "first-dose syncope" by starting with a low dose taken at bedtime
Doxazosin (Cardura)	1-16 1/d			
Prazosin (Minipress)	2-30 2-3/d			May have favorable effect on lipid profile, benign prostatic hypertrophy
Terazosin (Hytrin)	1-20 1/d			

Hypertension Pharmacy Review (continued)

Drug (brand name)	Daily dose, mg	Toxic/adverse effects	Drug interactions	Comments
Adrenergic inhibitors (continued)				
β-Blockers		Bronchospasm, brady-	Non-dihydropyridine	Acebutolol, carte-
Cardioselective		cardia, decreased	(non-DHP) calcium	olol, penbutolol,
Acebutolol (Sectral)	200-800 1-2/d	exercise tolerance,	channel blockers	pindolol possess
Atenolol (Tenormin)	25-100 1-2/d	may mask symptoms	(heart block),	ISA
Betaxolol (Kerlone)	5-20 1/d	of insulin-induced	sympathomimetics	Contraindications:
Bisoprolol (Zebeta)	2.5-10 1/d	hypoglycemia, im-	(unopposed	severe sinus
Metoprolol (Lopressor,	50-300 1-2/d	paired peripheral	α-adrenergic	bradycardia,
Toprol XL)		circulation, insomnia,	stimulation)	≥2nd-degree
Noncardioselective		fatigue, increased		heart block &
Carteolol (Cartrol)	2.5-10 1/d	triglycerides (except		cardiogenic
Nadolol (Corgard)	40-320 1/d	agents with ISA),		shock, asthma/
Penbutolol (Levatol)	10-20 1/d	decreased HDL		severe COPD
Pindolol (Visken)	10-60 2/d	cholesterol		
Propranolol (Inderal)	40-480 2/d			
Timolol (Blocadren)	20-60 2/d			
α-β-Blockers		Postural hypotension,	Rifampin (decreased	
Carvedilol (Coreg)	12.5-50 2/d	bronchospasm, hepato-	carvedilol plasma	
Labetalol (Normodyne,	200-1,200 2/d	toxicity (labetalol)	concentration)	
Trandate)				
Central α-agonists		Sedation, dry mouth,	β-Blockers, tricyclic	Avoid abrupt
Clonidine (Catapres)	0.2-1.2 2-3/d	withdrawal hyper-	antidepressants	withdrawal of
Clonidine (Catapres-TTS)	0.1-0.3 1/wk (patch)	tension (clonidine),	(decreased anti-	clonidine
Guanabenz (Wytensin)	8-32 2/d	depression	hypertensive	(rebound hyper-
Guanfacine (Tenex)	1-3 1/d	Hepatic & autoimmune	effectiveness)	tension)
Methyldopa (Aldomet)	500-3,000 2/d	disorders (methyldopa)		Methyldopa is
				preferred anti-
				hypertensive in
				pregnancy
Peripheral agents		Postural hypotension,	Tricyclic anti-	Reserpine contra-
Guanadrel (Hylorel)	10-75 2/d	diarrhea, depression,	depressants	indicated in
Guanethidine (Ismelin)	10-150 1/d	sedation, peptic ulcer	(decreased anti-	depression,
Reserpine (Serapsil)	0.05-0.25 1/d		hypertensive	active peptic
			effectiveness)	ulcer, ulcerative
				colitis
Calcium channel antagonists				
Dihydropyridines		Edema, headache,	CYP3A4 inhibitors	Immediate-release
Nisoldipine (Sular)	20-60 1/d	flushing, postural	(may increase CCB	nifedipine not
Nifedipine (Procardia XL,	30-120 1/d	dizziness, tachy-	serum concentrations)	recommended
Adalat CC)		cardia, gingival	Enzyme inducers (e.g.,	for severe
Nicardipine (Cardene)	60-120 2-3/d	hyperplasia	rifampin, carbamaze-	hypertension
Isradipine (DynaCirc)	5-20 2/d		pine, barbiturates)	Long-acting dihy-
Felodipine (Plendil)	2.5-10 1/d		may decrease effect-	dropyridines
Amlodipine (Norvasc)	2.5-10 1/d		iveness of CCBs	effective for
				isolated systolic
				hypertension

Hypertension Pharmacy Review (continued)

Drug (brand name)	Daily dose, mg	Toxic/adverse effects	Drug interactions	Comments
Calcium channel antagonists (continued)				
Nondihydropyridines		AV nodal block, brady-	Diltiazem & verapamil	Nondihydropyri-
Diltiazem (Cardizem,	120-540 1-2/d	cardia, worsening	(CYP3A4 inhibitors)	dines contraindi-
Tiamate, Tiazac,		systolic function;	increase serum concen-	cated in 2nd- or
Dilacor, Diltia)		constipation (verapa-	tration of benzodiaze-	3rd-degree AV
Verapamil (Calan, Isoptin,	120-480 1/d	mil), rash (diltiazem)	pines, carbamazepine,	block
Verelan, Covera HS)			tacrolimus, cyclosporine,	
			lovastatin, simvastatin,	
			pimozide, protease	
			inhibitors, rifabutin, &	
			ergoalkaloids	
Direct vasodilators				
Hydralazine (Apresoline)	40-200 2-4/d	Headache, palpitations,	Diuretics, hypotensive	Use both agents
		tachycardia, angina,	agents, MAO	with a β-blocker
		SLE	inhibitors	& diuretic to
Minoxidil (Loniten)	2.5-40 1-2/d	Hypertrichosis, sodium		minimize reflex
		& water retention,		tachycardia &
		tachycardia		fluid retention
ACEIs				
Benazepril (Lotensin)	10-40 1-2/d	Cough, dizziness, rash,	Potassium-sparing	Contraindicated in
Captopril (Capoten)	12.5-150 2-3/d	hyperkalemia, angio-	diuretics, potassium	pregnancy, renal
Enalapril (Vasotec)	2.5-40 1-2/d	edema (rare)	salts, lithium (in-	artery stenosis
Fosinopril (Monopril)	10-40 1-2/d		creased lithium	(bilateral or
Lisinopril (Zestril, Prinivil)	5-40 1/d		levels), NSAIDs	solitary kidney)
Moexipril (Univasc)	7.5-30 1-2/d			Start with lowest
Perindopril (Aceon)	4-8 1-2/d			dose available
Quinapril (Accupril)	5-80 1-2/d			for patients
Ramipril (Altace)	2.5-20 1-2/d			taking concurrent
Trandolapril (Mavik)	1-4 1/d			diuretic
				Preferred agents
				for hypertensive
				diabetics with
				proteinuria
Angiotensin II antagonists				
Losartan (Cozaar)	25-100 1-2/d	Similar to ACEIs, lower		Contraindicated in
Valsartan (Diovan)	80-320 1/d	incidence of cough		pregnancy, renal
Irbesartan (Avapro)	150-300 1/d			artery stenosis
Candesartan (Atacand)	2-32 1/d			(bilateral or
Telmisartan (Micardis)	40-80 1/d			solitary kidney),
Eprosartan (Teveten)	400-800 1-2/d			alternative for
Olmesartan (Benicar)	20-40 1/d			patients who
				have ACEI-
				induced cough

Hypertension Pharmacy Review (continued)

Drug (brand name)	Daily dose, mg	Toxic/adverse effects	Drug interactions	Comments
Aldosterone receptor antagonist				
Eplerenone (Inspra)	50-100 1-2/d	Hyperkalemia, hypertriglyceridemia	ACEIs, angiotensin II receptor antagonists, potassium supplements, potassium-sparing diuretics (increase risk of hyperkalemia), CYP3A4 inhibitors (increased levels of eplerenone)	Contraindications: serum potassium >5.5 mEq/L, type 2 diabetes with microalbuminuria, serum creatinine >2.0 mg/dL (males) or >1.8 mg/dL (females), creatine clearance <50 mL/min, concomitant use with potassium supplements/potassium-sparing diuretics, strong CYP3A4 inhibitors

ACEI, angiotensin-converting enzyme inhibitor; ARB, angiotensin receptor blocker; AV, atrioventricular; CCB, calcium channel blocker; COPD, chronic obstructive pulmonary disease; HDL, high-density lipoprotein; ISA, intrinsic sympathomimetic activity; MAO, monoamine oxidase; NSAID, nonsteroidal anti-inflammatory drug; SLE, systemic lupus erythematosus.

QUESTIONS

Multiple Choice (choose the one best answer)

1. A 44-year-old woman has a history of bipolar affective disorder effectively treated with lithium. At an office visit, her blood pressure is elevated. The diagnosis of hypertension is confirmed on follow-up visits over the next 2 months. A trial of lifestyle modifications does not lower her blood pressure, and you are considering initiation of drug therapy. She also complains of lower extremity edema and would like to start taking a diuretic. Renal function is normal. Which one of the following diuretics would be *most appropriate* for this patient?
   a. Hydrochlorothiazide
   b. Chlorthalidone
   c. Furosemide
   d. Spironolactone
   e. Metolazone

2. A 33-year-old woman has a history of hypertension controlled with lisinopril. She has recently married and informs you that she is now trying to get pregnant. Her blood pressure in the office is 132/84 mm Hg. What is the *most appropriate* recommendation for her antihypertensive drug therapy?
   a. Blood pressure is well controlled and no change is required
   b. Discontinue lisinopril and start hydrochlorothiazide
   c. Discontinue lisinopril and start atenolol
   d. Discontinue lisinopril and start methyldopa
   e. Discontinue lisinopril and start losartan

3. A 72-year-old woman is evaluated for worsening hypertension. She has a 40-year history of high blood pressure previously well controlled. About 4 weeks ago, she noted the sudden onset of severe dyspnea while doing routine housework. She was seen in the local emergency department. Blood pressure was markedly elevated at 220/120 mm Hg. Physical examination and chest radiographic findings were consistent with pulmonary edema. She was hospitalized. Myocardial infarction was excluded. A stress echocardiogram showed normal left ventricular function and was negative for ischemia. An adjustment in medications lowered the blood pressure and was associated with resolution of her symptoms. One week ago, she again became acutely short of breath. At the emergency department, blood pressure was elevated at 190/105 mm Hg, and she was noted to be in pulmonary edema. Myocardial infarction was excluded. She responded to further adjustment in medications. She has a past medical history of myocardial infarction, mild renal insufficiency, and hyperlipidemia

modified with a statin. Currently, blood pressure is 190/100 mm Hg. Examination findings are otherwise unremarkable. Urinalysis shows slight proteinuria. The serum creatinine level is 2.0 mg/dL (1.4 mg/dL 6 months ago). Current medications include furosemide 40 mg twice daily, metoprolol 50 mg twice daily, amlodipine 10 mg once daily, spironolactone 25 mg once daily, and isosorbide monohydrate 60 mg once daily. A recent trial of lisinopril was stopped because of a marked increase in serum creatinine level. What is the *most appropriate* next step in her evaluation?
   a. Increase amlodipine to 10 mg twice daily
   b. Start losartan 50 mg once daily
   c. Obtain a renal magnetic resonance angiogram (MRA)
   d. Obtain a captopril-mediated radionuclide renal scan
   e. Consider coronary angiography

4. A 70-year-old man has a long-standing history of poorly controlled hypertension. Currently, his blood pressure is 170/90 mm Hg. His current program consists of hydrochlorothiazide 25 mg once daily, atenolol 50 mg once daily, and hydralazine 25 mg twice daily. The serum creatinine level is 2.4 mg/dL. Urinalysis is negative except for proteinuria. A 24-hour urine protein is 1.5 g. What is the *most appropriate* approach for this patient?
   a. Set a goal blood pressure of <140/90 mm Hg; increase hydrochlorothiazide to 50 mg daily
   b. Set a goal blood pressure of <130/80 mm Hg; discontinue hydrochlorothiazide and substitute a loop diuretic; consider substituting an angiotensin-converting enzyme inhibitor (ACEI) for hydralazine and check creatinine and potassium
   c. Set a goal blood pressure of <140/90 mm Hg; substitute an ACEI for hydralazine and check creatinine and potassium
   d. Set a goal blood pressure of <130/80 mm Hg; discontinue atenolol and substitute an ACEI; discontinue hydralazine and substitute minoxidil
   e. Set a goal blood pressure of <140/90 mm Hg; increase hydralazine to 50 mg twice daily

5. A 36-year-old woman complains of spells consisting of frontal headache, diaphoresis, and nausea. The episodes are sudden in onset and offset and vary in duration from 15 to 25 minutes. A blood pressure of 210/160 mm Hg was measured during a recent spell. She has lost weight of approximately 7 kg over the last 6 months. Her family history is significant for pheochromocytoma in her mother. On examination, her blood pressure is 140/100 mm Hg and the pulse is 94 beats/min. Examination

findings are otherwise unremarkable. Currently, she is not taking any medications. Routine laboratory tests are also normal. What is the *most appropriate* next step in her evaluation?

a. Begin therapy with labetalol
b. Obtain a CT scan of the abdomen
c. Measure fractionated catecholamine levels in the urine
d. Measure plasma free metanephrines
e. Begin therapy with an ACEI and consider duplex ultrasonography of the renal arteries

6. A 53-year-old man is being evaluated for resistant hypertension. He has a 15-year history of high blood pressure. His current treatment program consists of hydrochlorothiazide/triamterene 25/50 mg once daily, atenolol 50 mg once daily, and lisinopril 20 mg once daily. He attempts a low salt diet. He is sedentary. He is taking no other medications and is a nondrinker. He does not smoke. There is no history of diabetes or dyslipidemia. He is uncertain of a family history of hypertension. Physical examination findings are normal except for a blood pressure of 160/105 mm Hg. Routine laboratory studies include the following: serum creatinine 1.1 mg/dL, sodium 144 mEq/L, potassium 3.0 mEq/L, and fasting glucose 94 mg/dL. Urinalysis shows trace protein and an electrocardiogram shows changes consistent with left ventricular hypertrophy. What is the *most appropriate* next step in evolution?

a. Discontinue hydrochlorothiazide/triamterene and substitute furosemide
b. Obtain plasma free metanephrines
c. Perform duplex ultrasonography of the renal arteries
d. Obtain plasma renin activity and plasma aldosterone concentration after drugs that can influence their values

have been discontinued and alternative drugs for blood pressure control have been started
e. Perform overnight oximetry to screen for sleep apnea

7. A 63-year-old woman comes to the emergency department complaining of headache, nausea, and blurred vision. Her husband says that she has been confused at times over the past 3 days. She has a history of hypertension but quit taking her medications 6 weeks ago when her prescriptions expired. She has been healthy otherwise except for a history of asthma, controlled with inhalers. On examination, blood pressure is 220/140 mm Hg. There are no focal neurologic findings. Retinal examination reveals hemorrhages and papilledema. Laboratory findings include the following: serum creatinine 2.0 mg/dL, sodium 135 mEq/L, and potassium 4.0 mEq/L. Chest radiography shows cardiomegaly. The electrocardiogram is normal. Urinalysis demonstrates red blood cells. What is the *most appropriate* next step in the evaluation or management of this patient?

a. Identify her previous antihypertensive therapy program and immediately restart the medications. If blood pressure and symptoms improve in the next hour, arrange close follow-up with her primary care physician
b. Give labetalol 20 mg intravenously over 5 minutes and observe the blood pressure response. If blood pressure and symptoms improve, dismiss her on oral labetalol and arrange close follow-up with her primary care physician
c. Admit the patient to the intensive care unit for parenteral antihypertensive therapy
d. Begin a 24-hour urine collection for metanephrines
e. Identify her previous antihypertensive therapy program and immediately restart the medications. Admit her to the medicine service for close observation.

ANSWERS

1. Answer c.

Thiazide diuretics (hydrochlorothiazide, chlorthalidone, and metolazone) impair the renal clearance of lithium and can precipitate lithium toxicity. Furosemide is not associated with increases in lithium levels and, thus, would be the preferred diuretic in this setting. Because of a short duration of action, furosemide must be given twice daily to lower blood pressure in persons with normal renal function. Spironolactone generally is not used as first-line therapy for essential hypertension.

2. Answer d.

ACEIs and angiotensin receptor blockers (ARBs) are the only two classes of antihypertensive drugs that are absolutely contraindicated in pregnancy. Because this patient is sexually active and is trying to get pregnant, it is probably best to discontinue lisinopril at this time, although the fetal abnormalities associated with ACEIs and ARBs occur during the second and third trimesters of pregnancy. Atenolol should not be used early in pregnancy because it can cause fetal growth retardation. Because hydrochlorothiazide can be associated with reduction in placental blood flow, theoretically increasing the risk for preeclampsia, it is not considered a first-line agent for the treatment of hypertension in pregnancy. Methyldopa is the first-line oral agent of choice for hypertension in pregnancy because it has been well studied and is not associated with fetal abnormalities.

3. Answer c.

This elderly woman with long-standing hypertension and hyperlipidemia has developed progressive hypertension and renal insufficiency with episodes of acute (flash) pulmonary edema. This presentation is highly suggestive of ischemic nephropathy due to bilateral atherosclerotic renal artery stenosis. The acute decline in renal function associated with exposure to the ACEI is consistent with this diagnosis. A renal MRA is an excellent study to assess the proximal renal arteries. It carries no risk of contrast nephropathy and would be the most appropriate study to identify ischemic nephropathy. Because bilateral renal artery disease is suspected, a renal scan that compares one side with the other would not be appropriate. In addition, the study is insensitive in the presence of renal insufficiency. Because the patient experienced an acute decline in renal function with an ACEI, she would likely experience the same complication with losartan. In the presence of marked bilateral renal artery stenosis, transcapillary pressure in the glomerulus is dependent on angiotensin II–induced constriction of the post-glomerular efferent arteriole. Use of an ACEI or an ARB interferes with this angiotensin II effect, leading to acute dilatation of the efferent arteriole with subsequent loss of transcapillary filtration pressure and reduction in the glomerular filtration rate. Amlodipine is being given at a maximum dose and further increases are unlikely to reduce blood pressure further. Coronary angiography could be a consideration if the renal MRA is normal. The negative stress echocardiogram decreases the likelihood that her episodes of pulmonary edema are due to critical coronary artery disease.

4. Answer b.

The goal blood pressure for persons with chronic kidney disease is <130/80 mm Hg, a more aggressive goal than for persons with uncomplicated hypertension. Inadequate control of extracellular volume is a common cause of lack of blood pressure control in persons with renal insufficiency. Moreover, hydrochlorothiazide is ineffective when the serum creatinine level is >2.0 mg/dL. Under these circumstances, a more potent loop diuretic or metolazone is more effective. ACEIs are effective in reducing proteinuria and preserving renal function in the setting of proteinuric renal disease and should be introduced as part of the treatment program. In the setting of renal insufficiency, creatinine and potassium need to be assessed after the introduction of ACEI therapy. Minoxidil is a potent vasodilator that is often effective in achieving blood pressure control in persons with resistant hypertension. Because minoxidil causes reflex stimulation of the sympathetic nervous system and extracellular fluid retention, it must be used in combination with an adrenergic inhibitor (usually a β-blocker) and a diuretic (usually a potent loop diuretic).

5. Answer d.

This presentation is highly suggestive of a familial pheochromocytoma. Plasma free metanephrines is the most sensitive screening test for this disorder and is the screening test of choice if a familial syndrome is suspected. Because 90% of pheochromocytomas are located in one or both adrenal glands and 98% are located in the abdomen, CT or MRI of the abdomen is the first test to identify a tumor. However, because incidental adrenal tumors are common, imaging should be performed only after biochemical confirmation. Once confirmed, initial antihypertensive therapy should be with an α-blocker. Because β-blocker therapy can cause a paradoxical rise in blood pressure, it should be used only to treat tachycardia that can develop with adequate α-blockade. Therefore, labetalol is not appropriate initial therapy for suspected pheochromocytoma. In addition, labetalol can interfere with screening test results.

6. Answer d.

This patient presents with hypertension and hypokalemia. The most common cause of hypokalemia in a hypertensive patient is diuretic treatment. Secondary causes of hypertension associated with hypokalemia are primary aldosteronism, renovascular disease, and Cushing syndrome. Primary aldosteronism should always be considered in a hypertensive patient who has hypokalemia while taking an ACEI with or without concomitant diuretic therapy. In the present case, the patient is hypokalemic despite receiving a potassium-sparing agent and an ACEI. If the plasma renin activity obtained to screen for primary aldosteronism is high, further evaluation for renovascular disease would be appropriate. If both the plasma renin activity and plasma aldosterone concentration are low, further evaluation for Cushing disease would be appropriate.

7. Answer c.

This patient presents with a hypertensive emergency that is defined as severely elevated blood pressure with evidence of acute target organ injury. She has findings of hypertensive encephalopathy and requires immediate hospitalization in an intensive care unit and blood pressure reduction with parenteral therapy. The most likely cause in this case is acute cessation of oral antihypertensive therapy. A work-up for secondary causes of hypertension is sometimes necessary if the cause of the hypertensive emergency is uncertain, but this evaluation should be deferred until blood pressure is controlled. Labetalol contains a non–cardioselective β-blocker and should be avoided in persons with asthma.

CHAPTER 14

INFECTIOUS DISEASES

William F. Marshall, M.D.
Abinash Virk, M.D.
Gregory D. Hart, M.D.
John W. Wilson, M.D.
Lynn L. Estes, Pharm.D.

PART I

William F. Marshall, M.D.
Abinash Virk, M.D.

This chapter approaches the field of infectious diseases from three perspectives. The first section reviews the characteristics of specific pathogenic organisms, the second covers clinical syndromes associated with various infections, and the third section reviews the antimicrobial drugs.

SPECIFIC MICROORGANISMS

GRAM-POSITIVE COCCI

Group A β-Hemolytic Streptococci: *Streptococcus pyogenes*

Infections

Group A streptococci are reemerging as an important cause of human disease. They are responsible for several different clinical syndromes. *S. pyogenes* is the most common cause of bacterial pharyngitis. Although the pharyngitis is usually self-limited, antibiotic therapy (penicillin) should be given to prevent acute rheumatic fever. Penicillin also will shorten the duration of symptoms if it is given within the first 24 hours of infection. Rapid diagnostic tests for streptococcal pharyngitis are easily administered and are specific but not as sensitive (50%-70%) as a throat culture for detecting *S. pyogenes*. Common complications of streptococcal pharyngitis include paratonsillar abscesses, otitis media, and sinusitis.

- Common complications of streptococcal pharyngitis include paratonsillar abscesses, otitis media, and sinusitis.

S. pyogenes is a virulent organism that is responsible for many skin and soft tissue infections. Several terms are used to differentiate these by the depth of infection and resulting clinical appearance.

Impetigo describes a superficial skin infection (Plate 14-1). Historically, *S. pyogenes* was the most common cause of impetigo. Since the 1980s, however, most cases of impetigo have been caused by *Staphylococcus aureus* or mixed infections with both *S. aureus* and β-hemolytic streptococci.

Erysipelas is an infection of the skin with involvement of cutaneous lymphatic vessels. It often occurs on the face and produces a raised, violaceous rash with a well-demarcated border. This infection is painful and most often occurs in the elderly. Recent reports have associated erysipelas with "toxic strep" syndrome.

In *cellulitis*, the infection involves the skin and subcutaneous tissue. Cellulitis is most common in tissue damaged by trauma and in extremities with impaired venous or lymphatic drainage (e.g., the arm after mastectomy or the leg after saphenous vein harvest for coronary artery bypass grafting). Minor inflammation or skin tears from tinea pedis may serve as a portal of entry for β-hemolytic streptococci.

Invasive Group A Streptococcal Infection

Since the mid 1980s, there have been increasing reports of severe group A streptococcal infection, including necrotizing fasciitis, myonecrosis, and a toxic shock–like syndrome. Suggested causes for the increase include the spread of virulent strains (especially M1 and M3), specific virulence factors (streptococcal pyogenic exotoxin and proteases), and a lack of immunity to these strains in the affected patients. In an outbreak of streptococcal necrotizing fasciitis in Minnesota, schoolchildren served as a reservoir for the responsible organism. Victims were mostly older and in poor health.

The overall mortality rate of streptococcal necrotizing fasciitis is 30%, even in previously healthy patients and with appropriate treatment. Many victims require amputation or extensive debridement of affected tissues. Effective treatment requires early recognition of the illness with prompt initiation of antibiotics, along with early and aggressive surgical debridement of devitalized tissue when indicated.

Unlike many other pathogens, group A streptococci remain exquisitely susceptible to the penicillins. The cephalosporins (first-generation) and vancomycin are effective alternative drugs. Erythromycin-resistant strains are reported but are so far uncommon in the United States. There is mounting evidence that clindamycin is the most effective antibiotic for treating streptococcal necrotizing fasciitis.

- Clindamycin is the most effective antibiotic for treating streptococcal necrotizing fasciitis.

Toxins

Group A streptococci produce many disease-causing exotoxins. Scarlet fever may develop in persons with no previous immunity to erythrogenic toxin. Production of hyaluronidase causes the rapidly advancing margins characteristic of cellulitis due to β-hemolytic streptococci. Streptococcal exotoxin A is similar to the toxin produced by *S. aureus* which causes toxic shock syndrome.

Nonsuppurative Complications

The nonsuppurative complications of group A streptococcal infection are *acute rheumatic fever* and *acute glomerulonephritis*. In the United States, there was a resurgence of acute rheumatic fever among children and military recruits during the 1980s. Rheumatic fever occurs only after streptococcal pharyngitis, never after skin infections. The diagnostic criteria for rheumatic fever are described in Table 14-1. Decreasing inflammation with aspirin (or corticosteroids) is the main therapy for acute rheumatic fever, although it will not prevent the development of chronic rheumatic heart disease.

- There was a resurgence of acute rheumatic fever among children and military recruits in the 1980s.

The risk for recurrent episodes of acute rheumatic fever with subsequent streptococcal infection is extremely high. Continuous antibiotic prophylaxis is effective for preventing these recurrences. Monthly injections of benzathine penicillin G and orally administered penicillin, sulfonamides, and erythromycin are effective for preventing recurrences of rheumatic

fever. If there was no carditis with the acute rheumatic fever episode and no attack within the previous 5 years, prophylaxis may be discontinued after the age of 25 years. For patients who had significant carditis with residual valvular disease, lifelong prophylaxis may be necessary. Endocarditis prophylaxis is a separate issue. Endocarditis prophylaxis is recommended for people with significant rheumatic valvular disease who undergo dental or medically invasive procedures.

Acute glomerulonephritis may occur after infection with nephritogenic strains of *S. pyogenes*. Both cutaneous infections and pharyngitis can result in acute glomerulonephritis.

- Continuous prophylactic antibiotics are used to prevent recurrent acute rheumatic fever.
- Acute glomerulonephritis may occur after either streptococcal skin infections or pharyngitis.
- Patients with significant rheumatic valvular disease require endocarditis prophylaxis for dental or medically invasive procedures.

Table 14-1   Jones Criteria for Diagnosis of Initial Attack of Rheumatic Fever[*] (1992 Update)

Major manifestations
    Carditis
    Polyarthritis
    Chorea
    Erythema marginatum
    Subcutaneous nodules
Minor manifestations
    Clinical findings
        Arthralgia
        Fever
    Laboratory findings
        Elevated acute-phase reactants (erythrocyte
            sedimentation rate, C-reactive protein)
        Prolonged PR interval
Supporting evidence of antecedent group A streptococcal
    infection
        Positive throat culture or rapid diagnostic test
        Elevated or rising streptococcal antibody titer

[*]If supported by evidence of recent *Streptococcus pyogenes* infection, then the presence of two major, or one major and two minor, criteria is enough for diagnosis. Exceptions in which the Jones criteria do not need to be fulfilled: 1) recurrent rheumatic fever (a single major or several minor criteria are sufficient if there is supporting evidence of a recent *S. pyogenes* infection), 2) isolated chorea, and 3) indolent carditis.

From Special Writing Group of the Committee on Rheumatic Fever, Endocarditis, and Kawasaki Disease of the Council on Cardiovascular Disease in the Young of the American Heart Association: Guidelines for the diagnosis of rheumatic fever: Jones Criteria, 1992 update. JAMA 268:2069-2073, 1992. By permission of American Medical Association.

Group B: *Streptococcus agalactiae*

This organism, part of the normal flora of the genital and gastrointestinal tracts, is an important cause of postpartum maternal and neonatal infections. The penicillins are the treatment of choice for infections caused by *S. agalactiae*. Meningitis, which most commonly occurs in neonates, is best treated with penicillin or ampicillin plus gentamicin. Prepartum vaginal culture for group B streptococcus may identify persons at highest risk for infection and allow eradication of the organism before delivery.

Group D Streptococci

Streptococcus bovis is the most clinically important of the group D streptococci. There is an association between *S. bovis* bacteremia and carcinoma of the colon or other colonic disease. *S. bovis* is clinically similar to the viridans group of streptococci and is generally susceptible to penicillin and the cephalosporins.

- Typical clinical scenario: A 59-year-old man with bacteremia and *S. bovis* endocarditis. Colonoscopy shows carcinoma of the colon. Penicillin (alone or with an aminoglycoside) is the treatment of choice for endocarditis caused by *S. bovis*.

Enterococci

The enterococci are an important cause of nosocomial infections. All enterococci are intrinsically resistant to many antimicrobial agents, including all of the cephalosporins. This resistance allows the organisms to proliferate and cause infections in the hospital setting. In fact, the enterococci are only inhibited, not killed, by the penicillins or vancomycin alone. Strains that are resistant to both the penicillins and vancomycin (vancomycin-resistant enterococci) are spreading worldwide. Linezolid and quinupristin/dalfopristin are two newer antibiotics that inhibit the growth of vancomycin-resistant enterococci. Neither agent is bactericidal against the enterococci. Quinupristin/dalfopristin is active against only *Enterococcus faecium*.

To achieve the bactericidal activity necessary to cure endocarditis due to enterococci, a combination of penicillin (or ampicillin) plus gentamicin or streptomycin is required. The choice of aminoglycoside depends on the results of susceptibility testing. The duration of therapy depends on how long the patient has been ill with endocarditis. Four weeks of therapy is adequate if the illness has been present for less than 3 months. When a patient is symptomatic for longer than 3 months, there is an unacceptable failure rate with the 4-week regimen. Therefore, 6 weeks of therapy is recommended. Vancomycin can be used in place of penicillin in the allergic patient, but it is considerably less effective. Optimal regimens for isolates resistant to both gentamicin and streptomycin are unknown. A valve replacement procedure may increase the chance for successfully treating subacute bacterial endocarditis due to drug-resistant enterococci.

- Enterococcal endocarditis is best treated with a combination of penicillin (or ampicillin) plus streptomycin or gentamicin.

Enterococcal urinary tract infections or simple bacteremia usually respond to treatment with either a penicillin or vancomycin alone, as long as the strains are susceptible in vitro. Alternatives for treatment of uncomplicated urinary tract infections in penicillin-allergic patients include the fluoroquinolones, nitrofurantoin, or vancomycin.

Streptococcus pneumoniae

S. pneumoniae (pneumococcus) is a leading cause of community-acquired infections such as pneumonia, meningitis, otitis media, and sinusitis. Like many organisms, it is becoming increasingly resistant to traditional antibiotics. Potential complications of pneumococcal pneumonia include empyema and pericarditis from direct extension of infection. Empyema should be suspected when fever persists despite appropriate antibiotic therapy of pneumococcal pneumonia.

S. pneumoniae is the most common cause of bacterial meningitis in adults (Plate 14-2), including those with recurrent meningitis due to cerebrospinal fluid leaks. Meningitis due to susceptible *S. pneumoniae* can still be treated successfully with high-dose penicillin G. However, given the spread of penicillin-resistant strains, meningitis should be treated with high-dose cefotaxime or ceftriaxone, possibly in combination with vancomycin while the results of susceptibility testing are awaited. Adjunctive treatment of meningitis with dexamethasone has been shown to be beneficial if started at the same time as the first dose of antibiotic.

- *S. pneumoniae* is the most common cause of bacterial meningitis in adults.
- Consider the possibility of a cerebrospinal fluid leak in patients with recurrent *S. pneumoniae* meningitis.

Asplenia predisposes individuals to severe infections with *S. pneumoniae* (and other encapsulated organisms). After splenectomy, fulminant, often fatal, pneumococcal bacteremia with disseminated intravascular coagulation is more common. Similarly, *S. pneumoniae* infections are more frequent and unusually severe in patients with sickle cell disease, multiple myeloma, alcoholism, or hypogammaglobulinemia.

S. pneumoniae is the leading cause of invasive bacterial respiratory disease in patients with human immunodeficiency virus (HIV) infection. Prophylaxis for *Pneumocystis carinii* pneumonia with trimethoprim-sulfamethoxazole may provide effective primary or secondary prophylaxis, but breakthrough infections with resistant organisms are not uncommon.

- Splenectomy predisposes to fulminant, often fatal, pneumococcal bacteremia with disseminated intravascular coagulation.
- *S. pneumoniae* infections are more frequent and unusually severe in patients with sickle cell disease, multiple myeloma, alcoholism, and hypogammaglobulinemia.
- *S. pneumoniae* is the leading cause of invasive bacterial respiratory disease in patients with HIV infection.

Infections due to *S. pneumoniae* have traditionally been treated with penicillin. However, the rate of penicillin resistance (minimal inhibitory concentration, >2 μg/mL) is increasing dramatically. As of 2002, 12% of pneumococcal isolates in Minnesota had high-level resistance to penicillin. Penicillin-resistant strains are often resistant to the effects of other antibiotics such as the cephalosporins. Penicillin resistance is conferred by an alteration of the penicillin-binding proteins which results in a decreased affinity of these cell wall components for the penicillins. Risk factors for development of infection due to penicillin-resistant pneumococci include previous use of β-lactam antibiotics, nosocomial acquisition, and multiple previous hospitalizations.

Penicillin-resistant strains of *S. pneumoniae* remain susceptible to vancomycin. High doses of cefotaxime, ceftriaxone, and imipenem also may be effective. Ciprofloxacin is usually not effective; however, the newer fluoroquinolones (levofloxacin, gatifloxacin, and moxifloxacin) are active against pneumococci. However, strains resistant to the quinolones already have been detected in Canada.

The pneumococcal vaccine is polyvalent, containing capsular polysaccharide from the 23 serotypes that most commonly cause pneumococcal infection. It is recommended for adults 65 years or older, those with chronic lung, kidney, or heart disease, and immunosuppressed and splenectomized persons. The vaccine can be given simultaneously with influenza virus vaccine. Pneumococcal vaccine booster is recommended 5 years after the initial dose in high-risk patients.

- Typical clinical scenario: Pneumococcal infection in a splenectomized patient presents with fulminant bacteremia with disseminated intravascular coagulation. The diagnosis is *S. pneumoniae* sepsis.

Viridans Streptococci

Several species of non-Lancefield typable streptococci are referred to as the "viridans group of streptococci." They are normal oral and enteric flora. This group of organisms is a common cause of subacute bacterial endocarditis, which should be suspected when viridans streptococci are found in blood cultures. Like the pneumococci, these organisms are increasingly likely to display resistance to penicillin. Viridans streptococcal bacteremia may be associated with shock and respiratory distress in neutropenic recipients of a bone marrow transplant.

One species of viridans streptococci, *Streptococcus milleri*, is more frequently associated with pyogenic abscesses. This is often a monomicrobial abscess and not necessarily associated with endocarditis.

- Typical clinical scenario: A 40-year-old man, 14 days after bone marrow transplantation, is neutropenic and has bacteremia with viridans streptococci, shock, and respiratory distress.

STAPHYLOCOCCI

Staphylococcus aureus (Coagulase-Positive *Staphylococcus*)

Toxins

Preformed enterotoxins produced by *S. aureus* are a common cause of food poisoning in the United States. The toxin is heat stable and, therefore, is not destroyed by cooking contaminated foods. Exfoliatins are exotoxins produced by *S. aureus* belonging to phage group II which cause "scalded skin syndrome," an erythematous rash that progresses to bullous lesions, most commonly in children. It can be differentiated from toxic epidermal necrolysis by skin biopsy. Toxic shock syndrome is due to an exotoxin (TSST-1) produced by *S. aureus* that may be causing an otherwise subclinical infection.

- Preformed enterotoxins produced by *S. aureus* are not destroyed by cooking food.
- Toxic shock syndrome is due to an exotoxin (TSST-1) produced by *S. aureus* that may be causing an otherwise subclinical infection.

Clinical Syndromes

S. aureus is the causative agent of several superficial infections, including folliculitis (infection of hair follicles without involvement of skin or subcutaneous tissues), furunculosis (a more extensive follicular infection often involving subcutaneous tissues), carbuncles (infection in thick inelastic tissues of the scalp or upper back), and impetigo (although this is most commonly caused by group A β-hemolytic streptococci). Surgical drainage of infected lesions occasionally is required.

S. aureus is the most common cause of osteomyelitis in adults. It is the second most common cause of prosthetic joint infection, the coagulase-negative staphylococci being the most common.

- *S. aureus* is a common cause of chronic osteomyelitis in adults.
- *S. aureus* is the second most common cause of prosthetic joint infection.

Most cases of community-acquired *S. aureus* bacteremia should be treated for 4 to 6 weeks with parenteral antibiotics because of the potential for metastatic abscesses and infective endocarditis. If nosocomial *S. aureus* bacteremia is caused by a removable focus of infection (such as an intravenous catheter), 10 to 14 days of therapy is usually sufficient. *S. aureus* infrequently causes community-acquired pneumonia, but it may develop as a complication of influenza. *S. aureus* is a common cause of nosocomial infection, including postoperative wound infections, line-associated bacteremias, and ventilator-associated pneumonia. Detection of *S. aureus* in the urine should raise concern for an underlying bacteremia with secondary seeding of the urinary tract.

- Cases of community-acquired *S. aureus* bacteremia should be treated for 4 to 6 weeks with parenteral antibiotics.
- *S. aureus* infrequently causes community-acquired pneumonia, but it may develop as a complication of influenza.

Mechanisms of Resistance

Most *S. aureus* strains produce β-lactamase and thus are resistant to penicillin G. The semisynthetic penicillins (nafcillin, oxacillin) and first-generation cephalosporins remain active against such strains. Since first encountered in the 1970s, strains of *S. aureus* with intrinsic resistance to the β-lactam antibiotics have spread worldwide. This resistance is caused by an alteration of the penicillin-binding proteins in the cell wall. These strains, referred to as MRSA ("methicillin-resistant *S. aureus*," or "multiple drug-resistant *S. aureus*"), are resistant to all β-lactam drugs and often to other classes of antibiotics.

Treatment

If *S. aureus* is penicillin-susceptible (approximately 5% of clinical isolates), penicillin G is the most active agent. For penicillin-allergic patients, effective alternatives include cefazolin and vancomycin. If the isolate is methicillin-susceptible, then nafcillin, oxacillin, cephalosporins (first-generation), vancomycin,

and imipenem are active. Vancomycin is the most reliably active drug for treating serious infections caused by MRSA. Linezolid and quinupristin/dalfopristin are newer drugs that are also active against MRSA. Occasional strains of MRSA may still be susceptible to trimethoprim-sulfamethoxazole, minocycline, or the macrolides. However, these antibiotics are mostly used for treatment of non–life-threatening infections.

S. aureus organisms commonly colonize the nares, which may predispose to invasive infections. Subclinical nasal colonization can result in nosocomial transmission of MRSA. Topical mupirocin ointment or other therapies (such as cotrimoxazole with or without rifampin) may temporarily eradicate the nasal colonization, but relapse is common.

- Vancomycin is the most reliably active drug for treating serious infections caused by MRSA.

Coagulase-Negative Staphylococci

Staphylococcus epidermidis is the most common of the coagulase-negative staphylococci, although many other staphylococcal species are included in this group. For clinical purposes, they are interchangeable. Coagulase-negative staphylococci are normal skin flora. They are opportunistic pathogens that commonly cause infections associated with medical devices. They rarely cause disease in otherwise healthy persons.

Clinical Syndromes

Coagulase-negative staphylococci are most commonly associated with intravascular device-related bacteremia, prosthetic valve endocarditis, osteomyelitis (usually after joint arthroplasty or other prosthetic implantations), and meningitis after neurosurgical procedures. Treatment usually requires removal of the foreign body and administration of appropriate antibiotics. Coagulase-negative staphylococci can cause peritonitis in patients undergoing chronic ambulatory peritoneal dialysis.

Staphylococcus saprophyticus is a unique species of coagulase-negative staphylococcus that is a common cause of urinary tract infections in young women.

Treatment

Coagulase-negative staphylococci are usually resistant to the β-lactam antibiotics. Unless in-vitro susceptibility testing shows other active agents, infections due to coagulase-negative staphylococci should be treated with vancomycin. The fluoroquinolones may be active against some strains, but resistance may emerge rapidly. *S. saprophyticus* is an exception because it is usually susceptible to the penicillins and many other antibiotics.

Determining the significance of blood cultures growing coagulase-negative staphylococci can be difficult. True infections generally result in multiple positive blood cultures, whereas single positive cultures usually are considered contaminants.

A regimen of vancomycin plus rifampin for 6 weeks, with gentamicin added for the first 2 weeks, is recommended for the treatment of prosthetic valve endocarditis caused by coagulase-negative staphylococci. Valve replacement may be necessary in recalcitrant cases.

- Unless in vitro susceptibility testing shows other active agents, infections due to coagulase-negative staphylococci should be treated with vancomycin.
- Typical clinical scenario: A 29-year-old woman with an indwelling intravascular catheter has fever of 102°F. The diagnosis was infection with coagulase-negative staphylococcus.

GRAM-NEGATIVE BACILLI

Escherichia coli Infections

E. coli organisms cause invasive disease as a result of ascending infection (such as in the urinary tract) or a break in a mucosal barrier (such as intra-abdominal infection). *E. coli* bacteremia is often related to focal infections such as intra-abdominal abscesses or pyelonephritis. *E. coli* is the most common cause of urinary tract infections and spontaneous bacterial peritonitis. Like most gram-negative bacilli, *E. coli* is variably susceptible to ampicillin, the cephalosporins (including first-generation agents), trimethoprim-sulfamethoxazole, aminoglycosides, and the fluoroquinolones.

E. coli O157:H7 produces a cytotoxic exotoxin that causes hemorrhagic colitis and may be complicated by hemolytic-uremic syndrome in approximately 10% of cases. This strain of *E. coli* is a normal part of bovine fecal flora that can contaminate undercooked hamburger, unpasteurized apple cider, and other food products. Treatment of *E. coli*-associated hemorrhagic colitis is supportive only. Antibiotics are actually contraindicated because their use will increase the risk for development of hemolytic-uremic syndrome.

- Antibiotics are contraindicated in the treatment of *E. coli* O157:H7-associated hemorrhagic colitis.

Klebsiella, Enterobacter, Serratia Infections

Klebsiella pneumoniae is an important cause of both community-acquired and nosocomial pneumonia and often is associated with alcoholism, diabetes mellitus, and chronic obstructive pulmonary disease. Red currant jelly-colored sputum is characteristic. Lung abscess and empyema are more frequent with *K. pneumoniae* than with other pneumonia-causing organisms. Cephalosporins are the drugs of choice for treating most types of *Klebsiella*. Strains of *Klebsiella* resistant to ceftazidime have emerged. This resistance is caused by a broad-spectrum β-lactamase. Susceptibility testing results for such strains may erroneously report that they are susceptible to cefotaxime. If resistant to ceftazidime, consider them resistant to all cephalosporins.

- Lung abscess and empyema are more frequent with *K. pneumoniae* than with other pneumonia-causing organisms.

Enterobacter and *Serratia* primarily are associated with nosocomial infections. *Enterobacter* species often are resistant to third-generation cephalosporins such as cefotaxime. Despite in vitro data suggesting susceptibility, β-lactamase production is induced when grown in the presence of cephalosporins. Carbapenems such as imipenem or meropenem, fluoroquinolones, cefepime, and trimethoprim-sulfamethoxazole are usually active against these strains.

- *Enterobacter* species often are resistant to third-generation cephalosporins such as cefotaxime, despite in vitro data suggesting susceptibility.

Pseudomonas aeruginosa

This organism predominantly causes nosocomial infection and is resistant to many common antibiotics. *P. aeruginosa*, together with *S. aureus*, is the most frequent cause of infections complicating severe burn injuries. Other infections caused by *P. aeruginosa* include folliculitis associated with hot tubs, osteomyelitis (particularly in injection drug users), malignant otitis externa in patients with diabetes mellitus, complicated urinary tract infections, ventilator-associated pneumonia, and pulmonary infections in patients with cystic fibrosis. Patients with neutropenia are also at particularly high risk for *Pseudomonas* infection, especially bacteremia. Hence, the febrile neutropenic patient should be treated empirically with antipseudomonal antibiotics while culture results are awaited. Ecthyma gangrenosum is a necrotizing skin lesion that may develop in neutropenic patients with bacteremia due to *P. aeruginosa*.

- *P. aeruginosa*, together with *S. aureus*, is the most frequent cause of infections complicating massive burns.
- Typical clinical scenarios: *P. aeruginosa* causes malignant otitis externa in patients with diabetes mellitus. Ecthyma gangrenosum is a necrotizing skin lesion that develops in neutropenic patients with bacteremia due to *P. aeruginosa*.

Agents active against most *P. aeruginosa* organisms include the extended-spectrum penicillins (piperacillin, ticarcillin), aminoglycosides, ceftazidime and cefepime (the only cephalosporins reliably active against this organism), aztreonam, imipenem, and ciprofloxacin. Administering two active drugs, usually a β-lactam and an aminoglycoside, is recommended when treating serious infections caused by *P. aeruginosa*. Antibiotic resistance frequently emerges during and after treatment.

Stenotrophomonas (Xanthomonas) maltophilia

This organism most commonly causes nosocomial infections. Its most notable trait is intrinsic resistance to imipenem and meropenem (as well as the aminoglycosides, quinolones, and most β-lactam drugs). *S. maltophilia* usually is susceptible to trimethoprim-sulfamethoxazole and ticarcillin-clavulanate.

- *S. maltophilia* is intrinsically resistant to imipenem and meropenem.

Salmonella

Salmonella infections are increasing in the United States. Well-identified outbreaks have been associated with food contamination. Undercooked chicken or eggs are often sources of infection. Gastroenteritis is the most common manifestation. However, more serious illnesses, including infections of atherosclerotic aortic aneurysms, may occur.

Salmonella typhi is rare in the United States. Patients with typhoid fever have relative bradycardia and rose spots (50%). The leukocyte count may be decreased. Blood cultures usually are positive within approximately 10 days of symptom onset, whereas stool cultures become positive later.

Salmonella choleraesuis causes chronic bacteremia and mycotic aneurysms. *Salmonella typhimurium* and *Salmonella enteritidis* produce gastroenteritis and occasionally bacteremia. Urinary tract infections caused by *Salmonella* occur in patients from the Middle East who are infected with *Schistosoma haematobium*.

- *Salmonella* causes infections of atherosclerotic aortic aneurysms.

As with many organisms, antimicrobial resistance is increasingly common with *Salmonella*. Most cases of *Salmonella* gastroenteritis resolve without therapy. In fact, treatment with antibiotics may actually prolong the duration of intestinal carriage and fecal shedding. Serious or invasive infections should be treated with a third-generation cephalosporin or fluoroquinolone while results of susceptibility testing are awaited.

- Most cases of *Salmonella* gastroenteritis should not be treated with antibiotics because treatment prolongs the carrier state.

Haemophilus influenzae

Widespread use of the vaccine against *H. influenzae* B has dramatically reduced the incidence of invasive disease in children. Non-typable strains of *H. influenzae* more commonly cause disease in adults (primarily respiratory infection). Infections caused by *H. influenzae* include pneumonia, meningitis, epiglottitis, and primary bacteremia. Chronic lung disease, pregnancy, HIV infection, splenectomy, and malignancy are risk factors for invasive disease.

- Chronic lung disease, pregnancy, HIV infection, splenectomy, and malignancy are risk factors for invasive disease due to *H. influenzae*.

Up to 40% of *H. influenzae* organisms recovered from adults with invasive disease are resistant to ampicillin by virtue of β-lactamase production. They can be treated with cotrimoxazole, third-generation cephalosporins, fluoroquinolones, or a β-lactam–β-lactamase inhibitor combination such as ampicillin-sulbactam.

- Approximately 40% of *H. influenzae* clinical isolates are resistant to ampicillin.

H. influenzae is an uncommon cause of meningitis in adults, although it can occur with hypogammaglobulinemia, asplenia, or cerebrospinal fluid leak. Third-generation cephalosporins (cefotaxime or ceftriaxone) are the drugs of choice for *H. influenzae* meningitis.

Other Haemophilus Species

Haemophilus parainfluenzae, *Haemophilus aphrophilus*, and *Haemophilus paraphrophilus* are normal oral flora. When these or other members of the HACEK (*Haemophilus aphrophilus*, *paraphrophilus*, and *parainfluenzae*; *Actinobacillus actinomycetemcomitans*; *Cardiobacterium hominis*; *Eikenella corrodens*; *Kingella* species) group of organisms are grown from blood cultures, their presence should always raise the suspicion for endocarditis. Large valvular vegetations with systemic emboli are common with HACEK endocarditis. Usual treatment is with ampicillin (if the organism is susceptible) or a third-generation cephalosporin for 3 weeks.

Bordetella pertussis

The incidence of whooping cough is increasing as immunization is neglected. Twelve percent of cases occur in persons more than 15 years of age. *B. pertussis* infection often results in persistent coughing in older children and adults. As many as 50 million adults are now susceptible to infection as a result of waning immunity. Whooping cough may cause severe lymphocytosis (>100 lymphocytes $\times 10^9$/L). Diagnosis of *B. pertussis* infection may be difficult. Culture or molecular testing of a nasopharyngeal aspirate is most sensitive. Early treatment of pertussis with a macrolide antibiotic is most effective. Aerosolized bronchodilators or corticosteroids may alleviate the persistent coughing.

- *B. pertussis* may cause severe lymphocytosis (>100 lymphocytes $\times 10^9$/L).
- *B. pertussis* can cause persistent coughing in older children and adults.

Brucella

Although rare in the United States, brucellosis may occur in meat handlers, persons exposed to livestock, or persons who drink unpasteurized milk. Most cases occur in four states (Texas, California, Virginia, and Florida). Brucellosis may cause a chronic granulomatous disease with caseating granulomas. Brucellosis (along with tuberculosis) is a cause of "sterile" pyuria. Chronic brucellosis is one of the infectious causes of fever of undetermined origin. Calcifications in the spleen may be an indication of the presence of infection (although histoplasmosis also causes splenic calcifications). Serologic testing, special blood cultures, and bone marrow cultures are helpful in making the diagnosis. Treatment is with doxycycline along with streptomycin or rifampin. Cotrimoxazole may be effective.

- Brucellosis may cause fever of unknown origin and is associated with animal exposures.

Legionella

Legionellae are fastidious gram-negative bacilli. *Legionella pneumophila* causes both community-acquired and nosocomial pneumonia, typically occurring in the summer months. Nosocomial legionellosis may be due to contaminated water supplies. Immunocompromised patients, especially those receiving chronic corticosteroid therapy, are especially susceptible to *Legionella* infections. Typical clinical features of legionellosis include weakness, malaise, fever, dry cough, diarrhea, pleuritic chest pain, relative bradycardia, diffuse rales bilaterally, and patchy bilateral pulmonary infiltrates.

Characteristic laboratory features of *Legionella* pneumonia include decreased sodium and phosphorus values, increased leukocyte level, and increased liver enzyme values. Legionellae organisms will not grow on standard media. Diagnosis depends on results of special culture, finding organisms by direct fluorescent antibody staining, or detecting an increase in anti-*Legionella* antibody titers. Urine antigen detection is a more sensitive (>80%) and simple diagnostic test for *L. pneumophila* infections.

Legionellae are intracellular parasites. As such, they are resistant to all β-lactam drugs and aminoglycosides in vivo.

Effective agents for treating *Legionella* include macrolides, fluoroquinolones, and, to a lesser extent, doxycycline. Some authorities recommend adding rifampin for severe infection.

- Immunocompromised patients, especially those receiving chronic corticosteroid therapy, are especially susceptible to *Legionella* infections.
- Laboratory features of legionellosis include decreased serum sodium and phosphorus values, increased leukocyte level, and increased liver enzyme values.
- Typical clinical scenario: A 63-year-old man who is receiving chronic corticosteroid therapy presents with fever, dry cough, diarrhea, and patchy bilateral infiltrates on chest radiography. Laboratory tests show hyponatremia and increased liver function values. Diagnosis is *Legionella* and can be established by special *Legionella* culture, serologic tests, and urinary antigen detection. Therapy is with macrolides or fluoroquinolones.

Tularemia

Francisella tularensis is spread by the bite of a tick or deer fly, by aerosol droplets, or by direct contact with tissues of infected animals (rabbits, muskrats, squirrels, beavers). Typically, infection causes an eschar at the site of inoculation, regional lymphadenopathy, and high fevers. Pneumonia also can occur. Streptomycin and gentamicin are the most effective therapies. Tetracycline is also active, but its use is associated with a 10% relapse rate. Tularemia has been identified as a potential bioterrorism agent.

- *F. tularensis* is spread by arthropod bite, aerosol droplets, or direct contact with tissues of infected animals.

Plague: *Yersinia pestis*

From 1950 to 1991, there were 336 cases in the United States, and more than 50% of these occurred after 1980. Plague is enzootic in the southwestern United States. New Mexico had 56% of cases, and 29% of cases are among American Indians. Rats and fleas are the vectors. Clinical presentations include 1) lymphadenopathy with septicemia—the most common form—and 2) the pneumonic form (high case-fatality rate). Treatment is with streptomycin or tetracycline. As with tularemia, there is concern that plague could be used for bioterrorism.

Pasteurella multocida

P. multocida is a common cause of cutaneous infection after a cat or dog bite. Onset of illness is typically within 24 hours of the bite. It causes local inflammation, a rapidly progressing cellulitis, and bacteremia. *P. multocida* is susceptible to penicillin, amoxicillin, amoxicillin-clavulanate, tetracyclines, and fluoroquinolones. First-generation cephalosporins (cephalexin) and the antistaphylococcal penicillins (such as nafcillin and oxacillin) are *not* active against *P. multocida* infections.

- Cephalexin and the antistaphylococcal penicillins should *not* be used to treat cat or dog bite wounds infected with *P. multocida*.
- Typical clinical scenario: A 35-year-old man presents with cutaneous infection after a dog or cat bite. It rapidly progresses to cellulitis and bacteremia.

Capnocytophaga (Formerly DF-2)

These gram-negative bacilli are difficult to grow on routine culture media. They are normal oral flora of domestic animals (especially dogs) and humans. *Capnocytophaga* causes bacteremia and fulminant sepsis, primarily in splenectomized persons. Dog and cat bites are associated with 50% of cases. Occasionally, bacteremia with human oral *Capnocytophaga* species occurs in neutropenic patients with mucositis. Treatment with a penicillin or a cephalosporin is most effective.

- *Capnocytophaga* causes bacteremia and fulminant sepsis, primarily in splenectomized persons.
- Dog and cat bites are associated with 50% of cases.

Cat-Scratch Disease

Bartonella henselae (formerly *Rochalimaea henselae*) is the primary causative agent of cat-scratch disease. The disease is characterized by a papule or pustule at the site of inoculation, followed by tender enlargement of the regional lymph nodes. Low-grade fever and malaise also may be present. Exposure to domestic cats (especially kittens) is the main risk factor. About 10% of patients may have extranodal manifestations. Disseminated infection can occur in patients with acquired immunodeficiency syndrome (AIDS).

Diagnosis of cat-scratch disease is based on the clinical picture and serologic evidence of antibodies to *B. henselae*. In biopsied tissue, the organisms can be seen with Warthin-Starry stain. Because the disease is usually self-limited, treatment is indicated only for patients with significant symptoms or bothersome adenopathy. Azithromycin appears to be the most effective antibiotic for treatment of cat-scratch disease.

Vibrio Species

In the United States, consumption of raw or undercooked shellfish such as oysters is the most common source of infection with pathogenic vibrios (e.g., *Vibrio parahaemolyticus*, *V. vulnificus*). Disease usually manifests as self-limited enteritis. Cholera, caused by *Vibrio cholerae*, continues to cause periodic pandemics, the most recent affecting South and Central America. Although indigenous cases are rare in the United States and Canada, cholera has developed in travelers returning from affected areas.

V. vulnificus is unique in that it causes a distinctive soft tissue infection in compromised hosts, especially those with underlying cirrhosis or hemochromatosis. Disease is usually acquired by the ingestion of raw oysters or via injury sustained in warm salt water. After the abrupt onset of fever and hypotension, multiple hemorrhagic bullae develop. Even with prompt therapy with ceftazidime or a tetracycline, mortality exceeds 30% for bacteremic *V. vulnificus* infection.

- Consumption of raw oysters is the most common source of vibrio infection in the United States.

GRAM-POSITIVE BACILLI

Listeria

Listeria monocytogenes is a small, motile, gram-positive, rod-shaped organism. Meningitis and bacteremia are the most common clinical manifestations of infection. *Listeria* may be difficult to visualize on Gram stain of spinal fluid. The elderly, neonates, pregnant women, and persons taking corticosteroids are at highest risk for disease due to *Listeria*. Epidemics have been associated with consumption of contaminated dairy products. Diarrhea may be a feature of epidemic listeriosis.

Penicillin and ampicillin are the most effective agents against *Listeria*. Combination with an aminoglycoside is often recommended for treatment of severe disease. *Listeria* is always resistant to the cephalosporins. Cotrimoxazole is an effective alternative for the penicillin-allergic patient. Treatment should be continued for 2 to 4 weeks to prevent relapse of disease.

- The elderly, neonates, pregnant women, and persons taking corticosteroids are at highest risk for disease due to *Listeria*.
- Epidemics mainly are associated with consumption of contaminated dairy products.
- Diarrhea may be a feature of epidemic listeriosis.

Corynebacterium diphtheriae

Diphtheria is a classic infectious disease that is easily prevented with vaccination. Epidemics of diphtheria recently occurred in states of the former Soviet Union. Diphtheria causes a focal infection of the respiratory tract (pharynx in 60%-70% of cases, larynx, nasal passages, or tracheobronchial tree). A tightly adherent, gray pseudomembrane is the hallmark of the disease, but disease can occur without pseudomembrane formation. Manifestations depend on the extent of involvement of the upper airway and the presence or absence of systemic complications due to toxin. Toxin-mediated complications include myocarditis (10%-25%), which causes congestive heart failure and arrhythmias, and polyneuritis (bulbar dysfunction followed by peripheral neuropathy). The respiratory muscles may be paralyzed.

- In diphtheria, toxin-mediated complications include myocarditis (10%-25%), which causes congestive heart failure and arrhythmias, and polyneuritis.
- Diphtheria may cause respiratory muscle paralysis.

The diagnosis of diphtheria is definitively established by culture with Löffler medium. Rapid diagnosis sometimes can be made with methylene blue stain or fluorescent antibody staining of pharyngeal swab specimens. Diphtheria is highly contagious. Equine antiserum is still the main therapy. Although there is no evidence that antimicrobial agents alter the course of disease, they may prevent transmission to susceptible hosts. Erythromycin and penicillin G are active against *C. diphtheriae*. Non-immune persons exposed to diphtheria should be evaluated and treated with erythromycin or penicillin G if culture results are positive. They should also be immunized with diphtheria-tetanus toxoid.

- Non-immune persons exposed to diphtheria should be evaluated and treated with erythromycin or penicillin G if culture results are positive.

Cutaneous infection with *C. diphtheriae* can occur in indigent persons and alcoholics. Preexisting dermatologic disease (most often in the lower extremities) is a risk factor. Lesions may appear "punched-out" and filled with a membrane, but they may be indistinguishable from other infected ulcers. Toxin-mediated complications (such as myocarditis and neuropathy) are uncommon. Diagnosis is established with methylene blue staining and culture of the lesion with Löffler medium.

- Cutaneous diphtheria is reported in indigent patients and alcoholics.

Bacillus Species

Bacillus species are increasingly recognized as causes of bacteremia in patients with indwelling catheters or prosthetic devices and in injection drug users. Other syndromes include ocular infections (posttraumatic endophthalmitis) and gastroenteritis. Anthrax (*Bacillus anthracis*) causes cutaneous disease in handlers of animal skins (also "wool-sorters' disease").

Although many strains of *Bacillus* are susceptible to penicillins and cephalosporins, infection should be treated with vancomycin or clindamycin while the results of susceptibility tests are awaited.

In 2001, several cases of inhalational and cutaneous anthrax followed the deliberate dissemination of *B. anthracis* spores through the mail. Inhalation anthrax is particularly deadly. It produces hemorrhagic mediastinitis, hemorrhagic meningitis, and bacteremia. Cutaneous anthrax usually manifests as a solitary papule that evolves into an eschar. The diagnosis of anthrax is confirmed by culture of blood, pleural fluid, cerebrospinal fluid, or a skin lesion. Sputum rarely reveals the organism. Nasal swab culture is useful for epidemiologic purposes but is not sufficiently sensitive to diagnose individual exposures.

B. anthracis is usually susceptible to penicillins, tetracyclines, clindamycin, vancomycin, rifampin, and the fluoroquinolones. Inhalational exposures should be treated for at least 60 days. Combination therapy with multiple active drugs is preferred for the treatment of inhalational anthrax.

GRAM-NEGATIVE COCCI

Moraxella

Moraxella catarrhalis (*Branhamella catarrhalis*) is a respiratory tract pathogen primarily causing bronchitis and pneumonia in persons with chronic obstructive pulmonary disease. It also may cause otitis media, sinusitis, meningitis, bacteremia, and endocarditis in immunosuppressed patients. Ampicillin resistance through β-lactamase production is common. Trimethoprim-sulfamethoxazole, the fluoroquinolones, and amoxicillin-clavulanate are effective for therapy.

Neisseria

Neisseria meningitidis and *N. gonorrheae* are discussed in the section Clinical Syndromes (Part II of this chapter).

ANAEROBIC BACTERIA

Bacteroides and *Provotella*

Bacteroides species are anaerobic gram-negative rods that are normal colonic flora (*Bacteroides fragilis* group). Related organisms also reside in the mouth (such as *Provotella melaninogenica*). Infections caused by these organisms are often polymicrobial and result from disruption or perforation of mucosal surfaces. These anaerobes often produce abscesses containing foul-smelling pus. *Bacteroides* species also are associated with pelvic infections, particularly in women (e.g., septic abortion, tubo-ovarian abscess, or endometritis). Anaerobic bacteremia usually is associated with focal infection elsewhere (such as intra-abdominal abscess). Osteomyelitis due to *Bacteroides* usually results from a contiguous source and is often polymicrobial (such as diabetic foot ulcer or osteomyelitis of the maxilla or mandible after dental infection). Pleuropulmonary infections include aspiration pneumonia and lung abscess, most commonly with *P. melaninogenica* and other oral anaerobes.

- *Bacteroides* species are associated with intra-abdominal and pelvic abscesses.
- Anaerobic bacteremia usually is associated with focal infection elsewhere (such as intra-abdominal abscess).
- Pleuropulmonary infections caused by *Bacteroides* and *Provotella* species include aspiration pneumonia and lung abscess.

Many strains of *Bacteroides* and *Provotella* produce penicillinase, making them resistant to penicillin. Metronidazole, ampicillin-sulbactam, and imipenem are active against most anaerobic gram-negative rods. Resistance to clindamycin is increasingly common. The third-generation cephalosporins and fluoroquinolones have little activity against the anaerobic gram-negative bacilli.

Peptococcus and *Peptostreptococcus*

These anaerobic streptococci often are involved in polymicrobial infection. Like *Bacteroides*, they are part of the normal flora of the mouth and colon and are associated with anaerobic pleuropulmonary infection and intra-abdominal abscess.

Both *Peptococcus* and *Peptostreptococcus* are exquisitely sensitive to the penicillins. For patients allergic to penicillin, the effective alternative therapies include clindamycin, vancomycin, and cephalosporins.

Clostridia

Clostridium tetani *and Tetanus*

C. tetani is a strictly anaerobic gram-positive rod that produces a neurotoxin (tetanospasmin). This neurotoxin, when produced by organisms in infected wounds, is responsible for the clinical manifestations of disease. Although rare in the United States, 200 to 300 cases still occur annually, mostly in elderly persons who have never been immunized.

The first muscles affected by tetanus are controlled by cranial nerves, resulting in trismus. Eye muscles (cranial nerves III, IV) rarely are involved. As the disease progresses, other muscles become involved (generalized rigidity, spasms, opisthotonos). Sympathetic overactivity is common (labile hypertension, hyperpyrexia, arrhythmias). The diagnosis of tetanus is based on clinical findings, although a characteristic electromyogram is suggestive.

- The diagnosis of tetanus is based primarily on clinical findings.

Treatment of tetanus includes supportive care, proper wound management, and administration of antiserum (human tetanus immune globulin). Penicillin G or metronidazole should be administered to eradicate vegetative organisms in the wound. Active tetanus does not induce protective immunity. Therefore, a primary tetanus immunization series should be given after an episode of tetanus.

- Active tetanus does not induce protective immunity to subsequent episodes of tetanus.

Botulism

Clostridium botulinum produces a heat-labile neurotoxin that inhibits acetylcholine release from cholinergic terminals at the motor end plate. Botulism usually is caused by the ingestion of contaminated food (home-canned products and improperly prepared or handled commercial foods). Wound botulism results from contaminated traumatic wounds. Neonatal botulism can result from consumption of contaminated honey.

- Neurotoxin of *C. botulinum* inhibits acetylcholine release from cholinergic terminals at the motor end plate.

The clinical symptoms of botulism include unexplained diplopia; fixed, dilated pupils; dry mouth; and descending flaccid paralysis with normal sensation. Patients are usually alert and oriented and have intact deep tendon reflexes. Fever is rare.

- Typical clinical scenario: In *C. botulinum* infection (botulism), a patient presents with unexplained diplopia; fixed, dilated pupils; dry mouth; and descending flaccid paralysis with normal sensation.

Treatment of botulism is primarily supportive although an equine antitoxin is available. In food-borne cases, purging the gut with cathartics, enemas, and emetics to remove unabsorbed toxin also may be of value. Antibiotic therapy does not affect the course of illness.

Other Clostridial Infections

Clostridium perfringens is one of the causes of food poisoning. Illness usually develops 7 to 15 hours after ingestion and manifests as diarrhea with abdominal cramps. *Clostridium difficile* is the primary cause of antibiotic-associated pseudomembranous colitis. Bacteremia or soft tissue infection with *Clostridium septicum* indicates a high probability of coincident occult colonic malignancy.

- *C. perfringens* may cause a food-associated illness.
- *C. difficile* causes antibiotic-associated diarrhea.
- In patients with *C. septicum* bacteremia, occult bowel carcinoma should be suspected.

ACTINOMYCOSIS

Actinomyces israelii, an anaerobic, gram-positive, branching, filamentous organism, is the most common cause of human actinomycosis. *A. israelii* is part of the normal flora of the mouth. Infections are associated with any condition that creates an anaerobic environment (such as trauma with tissue necrosis, pus). The pathologic characteristic is formation of "sulfur granules," which are clumps of filaments. Infection is not characterized by granuloma formation.

- The pathologic characteristic of actinomycosis is "sulfur granules" (clumps of filaments).

"Lumpy jaw" is caused by a paramandibular infection with *A. israelii*. It is characterized by a chronic draining sinus and may follow a dental extraction. Pulmonary actinomycosis develops when aspirated material reaches an area of lung with decreased oxygenation (such as in atelectasis). A chronic suppurative pneumonitis may develop and eventually result in a sinus tract draining through the chest wall. There may be subsequent perforation into the esophagus, pericardium, ribs, and vertebrae. Ileocecal perforation from focal actinomycosis has been reported. Appendicitis may be a predisposing factor.

- "Lumpy jaw" is caused by a paramandibular infection with *A. israelii*. It is characterized by a chronic draining sinus and may follow a dental extraction.

A. israelii also may be found in culture of tubo-ovarian abscesses and other pelvic infections. It is especially associated with pelvic inflammatory disease developing in a woman with an intrauterine device.

A prolonged course of therapy with penicillin is the preferred treatment for actinomycosis.

MYCOBACTERIAL DISEASES

Mycobacterium tuberculosis

Clinical Disease

Pulmonary tuberculosis can manifest as primary infection, reactivation of previously latent infection, or reinfection. Primary infection involves continuous uninterrupted mycobacterial proliferation without a period of involution or quiescence.

Primary disease commonly occurs in infants, children, and immunosuppressed adults. The radiographic findings of primary pulmonary disease include mid- or lower-zone parenchymal infiltrates with hilar adenopathy and pleural effusions. Reactivation-type pulmonary tuberculosis is the more common "classic" presentation in adults. Patients often present with symptoms such as prolonged cough (initially dry, later productive), fever, chills, night sweats, general fatigue, and weight loss. Hemoptysis and chest pain may occur. Chest radiographic abnormalities are variable but may include fibronodular infiltrates or cavitary disease, often found in the apical and posterior segments of the upper lobe or superior segments of the lower lobe. With cavitary disease, sputum samples are usually acid-fast bacillus smear-positive. Culture of respiratory specimens remains the standard for diagnosing tuberculosis and allows for drug susceptibility testing. However, in 10% to 15% of tuberculosis cases, the cultures will be negative and diagnosis is dependent on radiographic or clinical findings. Nucleic acid amplification through polymerase chain reaction offers a more rapid means for identification of *M. tuberculosis* than traditional culture. Tissue biopsy for histologic review often reveals classic caseating (necrotizing) granulomas with or without acid-fast organisms.

- In adults, reactivation-type pulmonary tuberculosis is the typical presentation.
- Symptoms of tuberculosis include prolonged cough, hemoptysis, fever, chills, night sweats, general fatigue, and weight loss
- Chest radiographs may show fibronodular or cavitary disease in the apical and posterior segments of the upper lobe or superior segments of the lower lobe.
- Culture is important for *M. tuberculosis* confirmation and susceptibility testing.

Treatment of Pulmonary Tuberculosis

Regimens for the treatment of pulmonary tuberculosis are outlined in Table 14-2. All 6-month regimens must contain isoniazid, rifampin, and an initial 2 months of therapy with pyrazinamide. All 9-month regimens must contain isoniazid and rifampin. Patient compliance is paramount to a successful treatment program, and directly observed therapy should be considered for most patients. Multidrug resistance is defined as resistance to both isoniazid and rifampin, although such strains are often also resistant to other drugs as well. Infections with multidrug-resistant tuberculosis are very difficult to treat and should be referred to an expert in tuberculosis management.

- Directly observed therapy is strongly recommended for most patients with tuberculosis.

Table 14-2 Treatment of Pulmonary Tuberculosis

Option 1
   Initiation: INH, RFP, PZA, EMB daily × 8 wk
   Continuation: INH, RFP daily or 2-3 times/wk DOT for
    16 wk
Option 2
   Initiation: INH, RFP, PZA, EMB daily × 2 wk, then INH,
    RFP, PZA, EMB 2 times/wk DOT × 6 wk
   Continuation: INH, RFP 2 times/wk DOT × 16 wk
Option 3
   INH, RFP, PZA, EMB 3 times/wk DOT × 6 mo
Special circumstances
   Intolerant to PZA: INH, RFP × 9 mo*
   Pregnancy†: INH, RFP, EMB × 9 mo

INH, isoniazid; RFP, rifampin; PZA, pyrazinamide; EMB, ethambutol; DOT, directly observed therapy. Ethambutol or streptomycin should be added to all regimens until susceptibility data are known or unless isoniazid resistance is less than 4% in that geographic area. Pyridoxine (vitamin B_6) should be given with all regimens containing isoniazid and during pregnancy.
*Twice/wk dosing can be given after 1 to 2 months if isolate is sensitive.
†Streptomycin and pyrazinamide are not recommended during pregnancy; streptomycin may be harmful to the fetus, and pyrazinamide has not been well studied during pregnancy.

Extrapulmonary Tuberculosis

Lymphatic tuberculosis (scrofula) is most commonly found in the head and neck region, including posterior cervical and supraclavicular chains. Although most cases of mycobacterial lymphadenitis in children are caused by *Mycobacterium avium* complex, more than 90% of cases in adults are from *M. tuberculosis* infection. Pleural tuberculosis commonly presents with a unilateral effusion. Pleural fluid analysis reveals a predominance of mononuclear cells and a low glucose level. Culture of the pleural fluid is usually negative, but pleural biopsy can increase the diagnostic yield to 90% to 95%. Genitourinary tuberculosis can involve the kidneys, ureters, bladder, and reproductive organs. Calcifications of renal parenchyma and ureteral strictures may be seen. Vertebral infection with tuberculosis (Pott disease) causes an anterior wedging and collapse of the vertebral body, producing a gibbus deformity. Tuberculous infection of the central nervous system manifests as a chronic meningitis with basilar arachnoiditis, cranial nerve deficits, hydrocephalus, vascular thrombosis, and tissue necrosis. Cerebrospinal fluid evaluation reveals a mononuclear cell predominance, increased protein value, and decreased glucose value.

Disseminated tuberculosis (simultaneous involvement of multiple organs) can be a progressive form of primary disease or a product of reactivating disease. Young children, the elderly, and immunosuppressed persons are most at risk. Chest radiography may show miliary shadows composed of 1- to 2-mm well-defined nodules throughout both lungs. Tuberculin skin testing usually results in no reaction (cutaneous anergy), and the diagnosis of disseminated tuberculosis can be difficult. Extrapulmonary tuberculosis is adequately treated with the same regimens as those for pulmonary tuberculosis, with a few exceptions: an extended course of therapy is recommended for vertebral, central nervous system-meningeal, and disseminated tuberculosis. Adjunctive corticosteroids may be indicated in the management of meningeal and pericardial tuberculosis.

- Unlike in children, more than 90% of cases of mycobacterial lymphadenitis in adults are due to *M. tuberculosis*.
- Adjunctive corticosteroids are beneficial in the management of meningeal and pericardial tuberculosis.
- A prolonged course of therapy is recommended for vertebral, central nervous system, and disseminated tuberculosis.

Screening for Tuberculosis

Current guidelines for detection of latent tuberculosis infection emphasize a "targeted" screening approach toward patients at risk for tuberculosis. Only persons at high risk for recent infection or with clinical conditions that increase the risk for tuberculosis should be screened. Criteria to identify persons with latent tuberculosis infection or high-risk contacts are listed in Table 14-3. Tuberculin skin test (TST) conversion is defined as an increase of 10 mm or more in induration within a 2-year period, regardless of age. All persons with a positive TST test require chest radiography and evaluation to exclude clinical disease. For patients with chest radiographic findings consistent with prior or untreated tuberculosis, an evaluation for active disease, including sputum sample collection, should be performed before therapy is started. If chest radiography or clinical evaluation raises the suspicion for active disease, then combination chemotherapy should be initiated while culture results are awaited. Contacts of persons with infectious cases of tuberculosis should have a baseline TST. If the result is negative, a repeat TST is done 10 to 12 weeks later (a delayed-type hypersensitivity skin test response to *M. tuberculosis* is generally detectable 2 to 12 weeks after infection). Healthy immunocompetent adults may be observed without initiating medical therapy unless the initial TST result is 5 mm or more; however, immunosuppressed adults, HIV-infected persons, and children should start preventive therapy regardless of the initial TST. Treatment can be discontinued in children if repeat skin testing at 12 weeks is negative.

- Only persons at high risk for latent tuberculosis infection or with clinical conditions that increase the risk for tuberculosis should be screened, regardless of age.

Table 14-3 Candidates for Treatment of Latent Tuberculosis Infection or Special Contacts,* by Diameter of Induration Produced by Tuberculin Skin Testing

<5 mm	≥5 mm	≥10 mm	≥15 mm
Child <5 y old and recent close contact	HIV-infected persons	Recent tuberculin skin test converters (within past 2 y)	No risk factors (tuberculin skin test not recommended)
HIV infection and recent close contact	Persons with organ transplants and other immunosuppressed patients (receiving the equivalent of ≥15 mg/day of prednisone for ≥1 mo)	Injection drug users who are HIV-negative	
Immunosuppressed and recent close contact	Recent contact with infectious tuberculosis Fibrotic changes on chest radiograph consistent with prior tuberculosis (if patient not previously fully treated)	High-risk medical conditions† Residents and employees of high-risk congregate settings‡	
		Recent immigrants (within past 5 y) from areas where tuberculosis is common§ Health care workers, depending on individual risk factors Children <4 y old Children or adolescents exposed to adults at high risk	

HIV, human immunodeficiency virus.

*Recent contacts who are initially negative on tuberculin skin testing should have a repeat test 10 to 12 weeks after last exposure to tuberculosis. Treatment can be discontinued if repeat result is negative.

†Gastrectomy, hematologic malignancies, reticuloendothelial diseases, renal failure, other malignancies, diabetes (insulin-dependent), silicosis, jejunoileal bypass.

‡Nursing homes, long-term care facilities, prisons or jails, homeless shelters.

§Asia, Africa, Latin America.

- Tuberculin skin test (TST) conversion is defined as an increase of 10 mm or more in induration within a 2-year period, regardless of age.
- All persons with a positive TST test require chest radiography and evaluation to exclude clinical disease.

Delayed-type hypersensitivity may wane over time in some individuals infected with *M. tuberculosis*. A TST many years after infection in these people may be nonreactive; however, it can stimulate or "boost" hypersensitivity to subsequent skin tests and be misinterpreted as new infection. Two-step testing is designed to identify and distinguish between boosted reactions ("booster effect"), signifying previous infection, and reactions due to new or recent infection. If the first test result is positive, consider the patient to be infected (recent or remote). If the initial TST is negative, a positive repeat skin test 1 to 3 weeks later indicates previous rather than new infection. One should remember that a negative TST *never* excludes tuberculosis. Although less common in otherwise healthy individuals, the TST result may be falsely negative in 20% to 25% of patients with active tuberculosis. In persons infected with both HIV and tuberculosis, the percentage of false-negative skin tests variably ranges between 30% and 80%, depending on the magnitude of cell-mediated immunity damage. Therefore, clinical judgment is always required when screening for tuberculosis.

- Two-step testing may help distinguish boosted reactions from new infection.
- If the first test result is positive, consider the patient to be infected (recent or remote).
- If the first test is negative and the repeat skin test 1-3 weeks later is positive (booster effect), the result most likely represents previous infection.

Outside the United States, the bacille Calmette-Guérin (BCG) vaccine is commonly administered to children and infants and can serve as a source of confusion in TST interpretation. Reactivity to the BCG vaccine by tuberculin skin testing generally decreases with time, and previous BCG vaccination generally should be disregarded in TST interpretation. Unless BCG vaccine was recently administered (i.e., within the past year), significant TST reactions should not be attributable to BCG vaccine and probably indicate infection with *M. tuberculosis*.

Treatment of Latent Tuberculosis Infection

Isoniazid therapy for 9 months is preferred for treatment of latent tuberculosis infection for all patients, including those with HIV infection, chest radiographic lesions suggestive of prior inactive disease, and children and adolescents. Alternative short-course regimens include rifampin plus pyrazinamide for 2 months or rifampin for 4 months. The toxicity with these latter two regimens is considerably higher than with isoniazid alone. Completion of therapy is defined by the total number of doses administered and not on duration of therapy alone. Therefore, the 9-month daily isoniazid regimen should consist of at least 270 doses administered within 12 months, whereas the twice-weekly isoniazid regimen should consist of at least 76 doses administered within 12 months. Baseline and routine laboratory monitoring during treatment are generally not indicated except for patients at increased risk of drug toxicity. Active hepatitis and end-stage liver disease are relative contraindications to use of isoniazid or pyrazinamide for treatment of latent tuberculosis infection. Contrary to the urgency for treatment of active tuberculosis in pregnant women, the need to treat latent tuberculosis infection during pregnancy is more controversial. Although some authorities may delay treatment until after delivery, recently infected women and those with HIV co-infection should most likely be treated (preferably with isoniazid) and monitored closely.

- Isoniazid for 9 months is the preferred treatment for latent tuberculosis infection for all patients, including those with HIV infection, chest radiographic lesions suggestive of prior inactive disease, and children and adolescents.
- Baseline and routine laboratory monitoring during treatment of latent tuberculosis infection is generally not indicated except for certain patients at increased risk of drug toxicity.

Diseases Other Than Tuberculosis Which Are Due to Mycobacteria

Mycobacterium marinum causes swimming pool granuloma and may occur after cleaning an aquarium. It presents with a chronic indurated nodule on the finger or hand. *M. marinum* responds to therapy with rifampin plus ethambutol, doxycycline, or trimethoprim-sulfamethoxazole.

- *M. marinum* causes swimming pool granuloma.

Mycobacterium kansasii produces a pulmonary disease resembling that caused by *M. tuberculosis*. *M. kansasii* is more resistant to isoniazid than is *M. tuberculosis*. Standard treatment regimens include isoniazid, rifampin, and ethambutol and continue for 12 to 24 months.

- *M. kansasii* pulmonary disease resembles tuberculosis.

Mycobacterium avium-intracellulare (MAC) is an important cause of infection in advanced AIDS, in which disseminated disease is common. Although usually only a respiratory tract colonizer, MAC also may cause chronic pulmonary infections. There are four characteristic chest radiographic appearances for MAC pulmonary disease: multiple discrete nodules (71% of patients), bronchiectasis, upper lobe infiltrates, and diffuse infiltrates. The newer macrolides (clarithromycin and azithromycin) are the most active drugs against MAC.

- Chest radiographic findings with MAC pulmonary disease include multiple discrete nodules (71% of patients), bronchiectasis, upper lobe infiltrates, and diffuse infiltrates.

Rapid-growing mycobacteria include *Mycobacterium fortuitum* and *Mycobacterium chelonei*. Typically they cause indolent subcutaneous infections of an extremity. They also are associated with osteomyelitis and nosocomial infection (sternal osteomyelitis after cardiac operation, intramuscular injection). Treatment often requires surgical excision of the lesions. Although resistant to antituberculosis drugs, the rapid growers are usually susceptible to clarithromycin.

SPIROCHETES

Leptospirosis

Leptospira interrogans infection is acquired by contact with urine from infected animals (rats, dogs), and it causes a biphasic disease. The infections occur more often after a rainy season.

The organism can enter directly through the skin from contaminated water that contains animal urine. Leptospirosis can be diagnosed in persons exposed to contaminated freshwater and in persons with fever upon returning from traveling. The *leptospiremic phase* is characterized by abrupt-onset headache (98%), fever, chills, conjunctivitis, severe muscle aching, gastrointestinal symptoms (50%), changes in sensorium (25%), rash (7%), and hypotension. This phase lasts 3 to 7 days. Improvement in symptoms coincides with disappearance of *Leptospira* organisms from blood and cerebrospinal fluid. The *second phase* (immune stage) occurs after a relatively asymptomatic period of 1 to 3 days, when fever and generalized symptoms recur. Meningeal symptoms often develop during this period. The second phase is characterized by the appearance of IgM antibodies. Most patients recover after 1 to 3 days. However, in serious cases, hepatic dysfunction and renal failure may develop. Death in patients with leptospirosis usually occurs in the second phase as a result of hepatic and renal failure.

- *L. interrogans* infection is acquired by contact with urine from infected animals (rats, dogs).
- Leptospirosis is a biphasic disease.

The diagnosis of leptospirosis is established on the basis of clinical presentation and of cultures of blood and, rarely, cerebrospinal fluid in the first 7 to 10 days of infection. Urine cultures can remain positive in the second week of illness. Serologic testing by IgM detection with enzyme-linked immunosorbent assay or microscopic agglutination test has a low sensitivity, especially in the acute phase, but it increases to 89% and 63% in the second phase of disease, respectively. The specificity of both tests is high (>94%) in all specimens. Treatment with penicillin G is effective *only* if given within the first 1 to 5 days from onset of symptoms. Oral amoxicillin or doxycycline can be used for mild-moderate illness.

- Treatment of leptospirosis with penicillin G is effective only if given within the first 1-5 days from onset of symptoms.

Lyme Disease

Epidemiology

Lyme disease is the most common vector-borne (*Ixodes* ticks) disease reported in the United States. The incidence of disease is highest in the spring and summer, when exposure to the tick vector is most common. Experimental evidence suggests that ticks must be attached for more than 24 hours to transmit infection. Although Lyme disease has been reported from most states, it is most common in coastal New England and New York, the mid-Atlantic states, Oregon, northern California, and the Upper Midwest. The white-footed mouse and the white-tailed deer serve as zoonotic reservoirs for the etiologic agent *Borrelia burgdorferi*. Coinfections with *Babesia* or *Ehrlichia* species can occur in up to 15% and may increase the severity of symptoms.

- *B. burgdorferi* is the etiologic agent of Lyme disease.

Clinical Syndromes

Stage 1 (early) occurs from 3 to 32 days after the tick bite. Erythema migrans (solitary or multiple lesions) is the hallmark of Lyme disease and occurs in 80% or more of infected persons. It can be associated with fever, lymphadenopathy, and meningismus. The rash of erythema migrans usually enlarges and resolves over 3 to 4 weeks. *B. burgdorferi* disseminates hematogenously early in the course of the illness.

- Erythema migrans develops in 80% or more of patients with Lyme disease.

Stage 2 occurs weeks to months after stage 1. In 10% to 15% of cases, neurologic abnormalities develop (facial nerve palsy, lymphocytic meningitis, encephalitis, chorea, myelitis, radiculitis, and peripheral neuropathy). Carditis (reversible atrioventricular block) occurs in 5% to 10% of patients. Conduction abnormalities are mostly reversible, and permanent heart block is rare. Temporary pacing may be necessary in approximately 30% of patients. Dilated cardiomyopathy has been reported, and conjunctivitis and iritis also occur.

- During stage 2, 10%-15% of patients have neurologic abnormalities.
- Carditis occurs in 5%-10% of patients.

Stage 3, although uncommon, can develop months to years after initial infection. Monarticular or oligoarticular arthritis occurs in 50% of patients who do not receive effective therapy. It becomes chronic in 10% to 20%. Chronic arthritis is more common in those with HLA-DR2 and HLA-DR4. Other manifestations are acrodermatitis chronica atrophicans (primarily with European strains), progressive, chronic encephalitis, and dementia (rare). Most patients will have detectable serum antibodies against *B. burgdorferi*. Magnetic resonance imaging may show demyelination.

Diagnosis

Anti-*B. burgdorferi* antibodies can be detected by enzyme-linked immunosorbent assay after the first 2 to 6 weeks of illness. Response may be diminished by antimicrobial therapy early in the course. Antibody testing is not standardized. False-positive results occur with infectious mononucleosis, rheumatoid arthritis, systemic lupus erythematosus, echovirus infection, and other spirochetal disease. The Western blot test is an adjunct in diagnosis when antibody response is equivocal or when a false-positive result is suspected. It is particularly useful in the first few months of illness.

Treatment

For stage 1 (early) Lyme disease in the absence of neurologic involvement or complete heart block, doxycycline (100 mg twice a day for 10-21 days), amoxicillin (500 mg 3 times a day for 10-21 days), and cefuroxime axetil (500 mg twice a day for 10-21 days) are effective therapeutic agents. Azithromycin, clarithromycin, or erythromycin is less effective than doxycycline or amoxicillin but can be used in penicillin-allergic patients. Because of the risk of vertical transmission, all pregnant women with active Lyme disease should be treated.

In Lyme carditis, the outcome is usually favorable. If first- or second-degree atrioventricular block is present, it should be treated with oral agents, whereas third-degree heart block should be treated with ceftriaxone, 2 g a day for 14 to 21 days, or penicillin G, 20 million units a day for 14 to 21 days. Lyme meningitis, radiculopathy, or encephalitis should be treated parenterally.

● In Lyme carditis, the outcome is usually favorable.

The outcome in patients with facial palsy is also usually favorable. In one series, 105 of 122 affected patients completely recovered. Corticosteroids have no role. If only facial nerve palsy is present (no symptoms of meningitis, radiculoneuritis), oral therapy with doxycycline or amoxicillin is used. The therapy used if other neurologic manifestations are present is described below.

● The outcome in patients with facial palsy due to Lyme disease is usually favorable.

If Lyme meningitis is present, ceftriaxone, 2 g a day for 14 to 28 days, or penicillin G, 20 million units a day for 14 to 28 days, should be given. Radiculoneuritis and peripheral neuropathy may have a greater tendency for chronicity and often occur with meningitis. Treatment is the same as that for Lyme-associated meningitis. The regimens for encephalopathy and encephalomyelitis are identical to those for meningitis.

● Radiculoneuritis and peripheral neuropathy may have a greater tendency for chronicity and often occur with meningitis.

Optimal regimens for Lyme arthritis (oral vs. intravenous) are not established. Intra-articular corticosteroids may cause treatment failures. Joint rest and aspiration of reaccumulated joint fluid are often needed. Response to antibiotics may be delayed. If no neurologic disease is present, doxycycline is given (100 mg orally twice a day for 28 days). An alternative regimen is amoxicillin and probenecid (500 mg each, 4 times a day for 28 days) or ceftriaxone (2 g per day intravenously for 14-28 days).

Prevention

Prophylactic antibiotic therapy after a tick bite is not recommended. Use of single-dose doxycycline is controversial but may be useful in prolonged, engorged nymphal tick attachment. In the vast majority of tick bites, disease is not transmitted. Appropriate use of repellents and protective clothing are recommended.

● Prophylactic antibiotic therapy after a tick bite is not recommended.

NOCARDIOSIS

Nocardia organisms are aerobic, gram-positive, filamentous, and branching and are visualized with a modified acid-fast stain. *Nocardia asteroides* is the cause of most human infections in the United States (Plate 14-3). *Nocardia brasiliensis* and *Nocardia madurae* cause mycetomas. Infections are most often opportunistic, occurring in immunosuppressed patients, including those with HIV or AIDS, but infections can occur in normal hosts also.

● *Nocardia* infections are most often opportunistic, occurring in immunosuppressed patients.

The respiratory tract is the usual portal of entry for *Nocardia* infection. Chronic pneumonitis and lung abscess are the most common findings. Hematogenous spread to the brain is relatively common. Spread also can occur to the skin (12%) and joints (3%). In patients with chronic pneumonia who have neurologic symptoms or signs, *Nocardia* brain abscess should be considered.

● In patients with chronic pneumonia who have neurologic symptoms, *Nocardia* brain abscess should be considered.

Nocardiosis is not diagnosed until autopsy in up to 40% of cases. Antemortem diagnosis depends on obtaining appropriate stains and cultures (the organism will grow on fungal media). Because sputum culture is relatively insensitive, bronchoscopically obtained specimens or open lung biopsy may be needed to confirm the diagnosis. The disease must be differentiated from other causes of chronic pneumonia (such as bacterial, actinomycotic, tuberculosis, fungal infections).

Therapy involves drainage of abscesses and high doses of sulfonamide drugs (trimethoprim-sulfamethoxazole is the current drug of choice). Some species of *Nocardia* show evidence of sulfonamide resistance. Other antimicrobial agents used for nocardiosis include imipenem, amikacin, minocycline, and cephalosporins. Therapy depends on antimicrobial susceptibility patterns. Newer drugs such as linezolid have activity against *Nocardia* species.

- Nocardiosis is diagnosed at autopsy in up to 40% of cases.
- Trimethoprim-sulfamethoxazole is the current treatment of choice.

RICKETTSIAL INFECTIONS

All rickettsial infections are transmitted by an insect vector except Q fever (respiratory spread). All are associated with a rash except Q fever and ehrlichiosis. The rash of Rocky Mountain spotted fever (RMSF) may be indistinguishable from that of meningococcemia. RMSF rash begins on the extremities and moves centrally. The rash of typhus (both murine and endemic typhus) begins centrally and moves toward the extremities. RMSF is most common in the mid-Atlantic states and Oklahoma, not the Rocky Mountain states. The pathophysiology of all rickettsial infections includes vasculitis and disseminated intravascular coagulation. Rickettsial pox is a common, although usually unrecognized, disease in urban areas of the United States. It is the only rickettsial disease characterized by vesicular rash. The mouse mite is the vector for rickettsial pox. A small eschar is present at the site of inoculation in 95% of patients.

- All rickettsial infections have an insect vector except Q fever.
- All are associated with a rash except Q fever and ehrlichiosis.
- RMSF rash begins on the extremities and moves centrally.
- RMSF is most common in the Mid-Atlantic states and Oklahoma, not the Rocky Mountain states.

Coxiella burnetii, the cause of Q fever, is acquired by inhalation of contaminated aerosol particles of dust, earth, or feces or after exposure to animal products, especially infected placentas. Sheep are common sources, but other animals, including cats, can harbor the disease (for example, a small outbreak occurred in a group of poker players after a cat gave birth beneath their card table). Disease manifests most commonly as an isolated febrile illness, most of those cases presenting with pneumonitis; 15% of patients have hepatitis (granulomatous), 1% have endocarditis, and some also present with central nervous system manifestations. Q fever is one of the causes of culture-negative endocarditis. It usually is diagnosed with serologic testing. Treatment is with tetracyclines or chloramphenicol.

- Among persons with Q fever, most have pneumonitis, and 15% have hepatitis.
- Q fever is one of the causes of culture-negative endocarditis.

Ehrlichia species are gram-negative intracellular bacteria that resemble rickettsial organisms and preferentially infect lymphocytes, monocytes, and neutrophils. The species that cause human ehrlichiosis are *Ehrlichia chaffeensis* (which infects monocytes) and *Ehrlichia equi* and *phagocytophila* (which cause human granulocytic ehrlichiosis, or HGE).

The disease is seasonal; the peak incidence is from May through July. The vectors are the common dog tick (*Dermacentor variabilis*), the lone star tick (*Amblyomma americanum*) for *E. chaffeensis*, and *Ixodes* ticks for the agent of HGE. The incubation period is approximately 7 days, followed by fever, chills, malaise, headache, and myalgia. Less than 50% of patients have a rash. Important laboratory features include leukopenia, thrombocytopenia, and increased levels of hepatic transaminases.

The severity of the disease is variable, but severe complications, including death, can occur. Coinfection with HGE and *B. burgdorferi* (Lyme disease) does occur and can be especially severe. Diagnosis depends on serologic analysis (indirect immunofluorescent assay) or detection by polymerase chain reaction amplification. Treatment is with doxycycline, 100 mg twice a day. Unlike the rickettsial diseases, chloramphenicol is often not effective against *Ehrlichia*.

MYCOPLASMA PNEUMONIAE

This is one of the smallest microorganisms capable of extracellular replication. *Mycoplasma* organisms lack a cell wall. Therefore, cell-wall-active antibiotics such as penicillins are not effective treatment. *Mycoplasma* infection is spread by droplet inhalation. It primarily infects young, previously healthy persons and presents with rapid onset of headache, dry cough, and fever. Results of physical examination are often unremarkable, with the possible exception of bullous myringitis. Chest radiography usually shows bilateral, patchy pneumonitis. The chest radiographic findings are often out of proportion to the physical findings. Pleural effusion is present in 15% to 20% of cases. Neurologic complications include Guillain-Barré syndrome, cerebellar peripheral neuropathy, aseptic meningitis, and mononeuritis multiplex. Hemolytic anemia may occur late in the illness as a result of circulating cold hemagglutinins.

- *M. pneumoniae* infection is spread by droplet inhalation.
- Chest radiography usually shows bilateral, patchy pneumonitis.
- Pleural effusion is present in 15%-20% of cases.
- Neurologic complications include Guillain-Barré syndrome, cerebellar peripheral neuropathy, aseptic meningitis, and mononeuritis multiplex.

The diagnosis is established by specific complement fixation test. Cold agglutinins are nonspecific and unreliable for diagnosing *Mycoplasma* infections. Fluoroquinolones, macrolides, and tetracyclines are effective therapies. Because immunity to *Mycoplasma* infection is transient, reinfection may occur. Clinical relapse of pneumonia occurs in up to 10% of cases of *Mycoplasma* pneumonia.

CHLAMYDIA PNEUMONIAE (TWAR AGENT)

This is a relatively new agent, distinct from *Chlamydia trachomatis* and *Chlamydia psittaci*. In young adults, it causes 10% of cases of pneumonia and 5% of cases of bronchitis. It has been a cause of community outbreaks, and nosocomial transmission has occurred. Fifty percent of adults are seropositive for *C. pneumoniae*. Birds are the source of infection with *C. psittaci* (psittacosis), but there is no reservoir for *C. pneumoniae*. Clinical manifestations of infection are usually mild and may resemble those caused by *M. pneumoniae*. Pharyngitis occurs 1 to 3 weeks before the onset of pulmonary symptoms, and cough may last for weeks. The diagnosis is based on serologic testing. Treatment is with doxycycline or a macrolide.

- In young adults, *C. pneumoniae* causes 10% of cases of pneumonia and 5% of cases of bronchitis.

FUNGAL INFECTIONS

Coccidioidomycosis

Coccidioides immitis is a dimorphic fungus: in tissue it exists as a spherule, and in culture at room temperature it is mycelial (filamentous). It forms arthrospores that are highly infectious. *C. immitis* is endemic in the southwestern United States, especially the San Joaquin Valley of California and central Arizona. Disseminated disease is most likely to occur in males (especially Filipino and black), pregnant females, and immunocompromised hosts regardless of sex. Nonpregnant white females seem to be more resistant to disseminated disease than white males.

- *C. immitis* is endemic in the southwestern United States.

- Disseminated disease is most likely to occur in males (especially Filipino and black), pregnant females, and immunocompromised hosts.

Half to two-thirds (~60%) of primary infections with *C. immitis* are subclinical. The most common clinical manifestation is pneumonitis that is usually self-limited. Common manifestations are dry cough and fever (valley fever) that may resemble influenza. Associated findings include hilar adenopathy, pleural effusion (12%), thin-walled cavities (5%), and solid "coin" lesions. Disseminated infection predominantly affects the central nervous system, skin, bones, and joints.

- Primary infection with *C. immitis* causes pneumonitis that is usually self-limited.

Coccidioidomycosis is one of the causes of erythema nodosum. When present, it usually indicates an active immune response that will control the infection. Erythema nodosum is more common in females and is often associated with arthralgias, especially of the knees and ankles.

- Coccidioidomycosis is one of the causes of erythema nodosum.

The diagnosis of coccidioidomycosis is based on detecting the organism by culture or biopsy with silver stains. A *C. immitis* serologic (complement fixation) titer more than 1:4 is suggestive of infection. Skin testing is of epidemiologic value only. Detection of cerebrospinal fluid anticoccidioidal antibodies is the usual means for diagnosing coccidioidomycosis meningitis. Laboratory abnormalities may include eosinophilia and hypercalcemia.

Fluconazole and amphotericin B are effective for therapy of coccidioidomycosis. The acute pulmonary form is usually self-limited and observation may be adequate. However, therapy is indicated if a patient is pregnant, is immunocompromised (patients with AIDS or receiving immunosuppressive regimens for organ transplantation or other medical reasons), or has worsening infection without therapy. Amphotericin B is the drug of choice for severe manifestations and for pregnant women with coccidioidomycosis. An alternative to fluconazole is itraconazole (200 mg twice daily). For meningitis, therapy with high-dose fluconazole is preferred and has largely replaced intrathecal amphotericin B. Because of the high relapse rate of *C. immitis* meningitis, chronic suppressive therapy is necessary, usually with fluconazole. *Coccidioides* meningitis may be complicated by adhesive arachnoiditis. Newer antifungal medications include voriconazole, which is active in vitro but clinical studies are not available, and caspofungin, which has limited in vitro activity against coccidioidomycosis.

Histoplasmosis

Histoplasma capsulatum is also a dimorphic fungus that grows as a small (3 mm in diameter) yeast in tissue. Culture at room temperature produces the mycelial form. Although present in many areas of the world, histoplasmosis is especially prevalent in the Ohio and Mississippi river valleys. Outbreaks have been associated with large construction projects and exposure to bird droppings. Histoplasmosis is acquired by inhalation of spores and also can be transmitted by organ transplantation from an infected donor. The risk of acquisition is increased with certain activities, including caving and bridge or other construction. Although healthy individuals may acquire histoplasmosis, patients with AIDS are particularly susceptible. *H. capsulatum* infection is one of the causes of caseating granulomata.

- Outbreaks of histoplasmosis have been associated with large construction projects and exposure to bird droppings.
- Although healthy individuals may acquire histoplasmosis, patients with AIDS are particularly susceptible.

Primary (acute) histoplasmosis may be clinically indistinguishable from influenza or other upper respiratory tract infections. After resolution, multiple small, calcified granulomas may be seen on subsequent chest radiography. The progressive (disseminated) form of histoplasmosis is uncommon but serious. The disseminated form and reactivation of prior disease are most likely to occur in infants, elderly men, and immunosuppressed persons, including those with HIV or AIDS and those receiving therapy with tumor necrosis factor-α inhibitor. Manifestations may resemble those of lymphoma, with weight loss, fever, anemia, increased erythrocyte sedimentation rate, and splenomegaly. Mucosal surface lesions, especially in the mouth, are not infrequent. As with tuberculosis, the adrenal glands may be infected, with resulting adrenal insufficiency. Chronic cavitary pulmonary disease due to *Histoplasma* may resemble tuberculosis.

- Primary (acute) histoplasmosis may be indistinguishable from influenza or other upper respiratory tract infections.
- As with tuberculosis, the adrenal glands may be infected by *H. capsulatum*, with resulting adrenal insufficiency.

Serologic testing is of limited sensitivity and specificity and plays little role in the diagnosis of active infection unless increasing or markedly increased titers are detected. Biopsy, silver staining, and cultures of infected tissues are the best means of diagnosis. Bone marrow stains and cultures and fungal blood cultures are frequently helpful. Biopsy specimens of mouth lesions can be diagnostic. Detection of *Histoplasma* antigen in urine or serum is promising as a diagnostic test but is not yet widely available.

The mild, acute forms of histoplasmosis are usually self-limited and do not require therapy. Amphotericin B in a total dose of 35 mg/kg is the drug of choice for all severe, life-threatening cases. Itraconazole is effective for most nonmeningeal, non–life-threatening cases and has largely replaced ketoconazole. The dosage is 200 to 400 mg per day (guided by serum drug concentrations) for 6 to 12 months. Patients with AIDS require chronic maintenance therapy.

Blastomycosis

Yet another dimorphic fungal pathogen is *Blastomyces dermatitidis*. In tissue, the yeast forms are thick-walled and have broad-based buds (±10 μm in diameter) (Plate 14-4). In culture at room temperature, a mycelial form is found. Blastomycosis is endemic in the southeastern and upper midwestern United States. Primary pulmonary blastomycosis may be asymptomatic and may disseminate hematogenously to bone, skin, or prostate. Granulomas occur, but calcification is less frequent than with histoplasmosis or tuberculosis.

Blastomycosis affects lung, skin, bone (especially the vertebrae), male genitalia (prostate, epididymis, testis), and the central nervous system. The pulmonary form has no characteristic findings: pleural effusion is rare, hilar adenopathy develops occasionally, and cavitation is infrequent. It often mimics carcinoma of the lung. Cutaneous involvement with blastomycosis is common. Lesions, especially on the face, are characteristically painless and nonpruritic and have a sharp, spreading border. Chronic crusty lesions may occur.

- Blastomycosis affects lungs, skin, bone (especially the vertebrae), and male genitalia (prostate, epididymis, testis).
- The most common clinical forms of blastomycosis are pulmonary and cutaneous.

The diagnosis of blastomycosis is based on the results of biopsy, stains, and cultures. Serologic and skin testing are rarely helpful.

Amphotericin B (total dose is 20-25 mg/kg) or itraconazole (200-400 mg per day for 6 months) is effective as therapy for blastomycosis. Amphotericin B is reserved primarily for life-threatening infections. Mild-to-moderate nonmeningeal blastomycosis can be treated with itraconazole (200-400 mg/day) for 6 months.

Sporotrichosis

A fourth dimorphic fungal pathogen, *Sporothrix schenckii*, in tissue is a round, cigar-shaped yeast. In culture at room temperature it is mycelial. Sporotrichosis is transmitted by cutaneous inoculation (rose-gardener's disease) and, rarely, through inhalation. It manifests as a suppurative and granulomatous reaction.

Cutaneous infection produces characteristic crusty lesions ascending the lymphatics of the extremities from the initial site of infection. Similar lesions may be produced by infection with *M. marinum*, *Nocardia*, or cutaneous leishmaniasis. Joint spaces rarely are involved. Sporotrichosis occasionally may cause chronic pneumonitis (with cavitation and empyema) or meningitis.

- Cutaneous sporotrichosis produces characteristic crusty lesions ascending the lymphatics of the extremities from the initial site of infection.
- Sporotrichosis occasionally may cause chronic pneumonitis (with cavitation and empyema) or meningitis.

The diagnosis of sporotrichosis may be difficult and depends on clinical recognition of the cutaneous lesions in most instances. Biopsy, culture, or serologic testing may aid in the diagnosis.

For the lymphocutaneous or cutaneous form, itraconazole is the therapy of choice. An effective alternative is supersaturated solution of potassium iodide. Amphotericin B is recommended for disseminated disease (pulmonary, joint), although it may respond poorly to therapy.

Aspergillosis

Aspergillus is an opportunistic pathogen that causes infection in immunocompromised persons. Although any species of *Aspergillus* can cause disease, *Aspergillus fumigatus* is the most common pathogenic species. The organisms have large, septated hyphae (phycomycetes are nonseptated) branching at 45° angles (Plate 14-5). Especially in neutropenic hosts, they may invade blood vessels, producing a striking thrombotic angiitis similar to phycomycosis. Metastatic foci may cause suppurative abscess formation.

- *Aspergillus* organisms may invade blood vessels, producing a striking thrombotic angiitis.

The form of disease produced by aspergillosis primarily is determined by the nature of the immunologic deficit in the infected individual. Neutropenia predisposes to rapidly invasive bronchopulmonary disease with early dissemination to the brain and other tissues. The longer the duration of neutropenia, the higher the risk for invasive aspergillosis. Prompt therapy with high doses of amphotericin B and resolution of the neutropenia are necessary to control the disease. Diagnosis should be suspected when *Aspergillus* is isolated from any source in a susceptible individual.

T-cell deficiencies (primarily from corticosteroids) predispose to somewhat more indolent, although no less dangerous, forms of aspergillosis. Progressive pulmonary infiltrates,

necrotic skin lesions, wound infections, and brain abscesses may result. Sinus infections with *Aspergillus* may be localized or invasive in these patients.

Serologic testing is not helpful for diagnosing invasive *Aspergillus* in the compromised host.

- Neutropenia predisposes to rapidly invasive bronchopulmonary disease with early dissemination to the brain and other tissues.

Aspergillus also can cause localized disease in persons with normal immunologic function. Chronic necrotizing pulmonary aspergillosis occurs in patients with pulmonary emphysema. The chronic, progressive infiltrates of this condition often require tissue sampling for diagnosis. Treatment with surgical resection and systemic antifungal therapy is sometimes curative.

Aspergillus may produce a "fungus ball" in preexisting lung bullae (such as from ankylosing spondylitis, previous tuberculosis, or emphysema). Hemoptysis is the main symptom. Surgical excision may be necessary to prevent lethal hemorrhage.

Localized colonization with *Aspergillus* is common and usually does not produce disease. However, otitis externa (swimmer's ear) and allergic bronchopulmonary aspergillosis are exceptions. The symptoms of allergic bronchopulmonary aspergillosis resemble those of asthma. It is characterized by migratory pulmonary infiltrates, thick, brown, tenacious mucous plugs in the sputum, eosinophilia, and high titers of anti-*Aspergillus* antibodies. Endophthalmitis due to *Aspergillus* may develop after ocular operation or trauma.

Aspergillus frequently colonizes the respiratory tract. Isolating the organism from the sputum of a noncompromised host usually does not indicate disease and does not require treatment.

- Chronic necrotizing pulmonary aspergillosis occurs in patients with pulmonary emphysema.
- *Aspergillus* may produce a "fungus ball" in preexisting lung bullae (such as from ankylosing spondylitis, previous tuberculosis, or emphysema).

Aspergillus infections may respond poorly to currently available antifungal medications. Amphotericin B products are very effective, but they must be given in high doses. Lipid-based formulations of amphotericin B are advised for patients in whom nephrotoxicity develops with deoxycholate amphotericin B. Itraconazole was the first oral agent with substantial activity against *Aspergillus*. However, recently approved newer drugs such as voriconazole and caspofungin have potent in vitro and in vivo activity against *Aspergillus*. Intravenous voriconazole should be avoided in patients with severe renal insufficiency (glomerular filtration rate, <50 mL/min). Caspofungin is approved by the U.S. Food and Drug Administration for refractory invasive aspergillosis. This has been used alone or in combination with amphotericin B products. Surgical debridement of infected tissues is often necessary for cure. Allergic bronchopulmonary aspergillosis responds to corticosteroid therapy, and itraconazole may be an important adjunctive therapy in decreasing or sparing the use of corticosteroids.

- Typical clinical scenario of *Aspergillus* infection: Fever and lung infiltrates in a patient with prolonged neutropenia.

Cryptococcosis

Cryptococcus neoformans is the only species of *Cryptococcus* that is pathogenic for humans. It is a yeast in both tissue and culture, is 4 to 7 μm in diameter, and has thin-walled buds and a capsule (Plate 14-6). It is an opportunistic pathogen infecting persons with T-cell deficiencies or dysfunction (patients with Hodgkin disease, hematologic malignancy, organ transplantation, exogenous corticosteroids, chronic liver disease, and AIDS). The respiratory tract is the probable portal of entry. Cryptococcosis does not incite much inflammatory reaction, and calcification is rare.

- *C. neoformans* is an opportunistic pathogen.
- *Cryptococcus* primarily infects persons with T-cell deficiencies or dysfunction (Hodgkin disease, hematologic malignancy, organ transplantation, exogenous corticosteroids, chronic liver disease, and AIDS).

C. neoformans is acquired by inhalation. From the lungs it disseminates widely and easily crosses into the central nervous system. Pneumonia and meningitis are the most common forms of cryptococcosis. Meningitis may be insidious, with headache as the only symptom. Cranial nerve involvement may develop (including blindness with involvement of the optic nerve). *Cryptococcus* also may cause an indolent form of cellulitis.

- Pneumonia and meningitis are the most common forms of *C. neoformans* infection.

Cryptococcal infection can be diagnosed with fungal culture (cerebrospinal fluid, blood, sputum, urine), silver staining of biopsy tissue, or detection of *Cryptococcus* antigen in body fluids. The cryptococcal antigen test is the most helpful of all fungal serologic tests. It measures capsular antigen, whereas most other fungal serologic tests measure antibody response. Remember that *Cryptococcus* very commonly spreads to the central nervous system. Therefore, if *C. neoformans* is isolated

from any source (such as sputum, urine, blood) in a susceptible patient, simultaneous meningitis should be suspected. India ink preparation largely has been replaced by antigen detection assay.

Cryptococcal infections respond to treatment with amphotericin B or fluconazole. Choice of therapy depends on extent of disease and host immune function. Mild-to-moderate noncentral nervous system cryptococcosis can be treated with fluconazole for 6 to 12 months. However, severe presentation, immunocompromised hosts, and central nervous system involvement should be treated with amphotericin B. Combining oral flucytosine (100-150 mg/kg per day) with amphotericin B for 6 weeks allows a lower dose of amphotericin to be used. Unfortunately, relapse rates are high regardless of the treatment regimen given. In a recent study comparing fluconazole (200 mg/day) with amphotericin B for 10 weeks, fluconazole was as effective as amphotericin B ("effective" is defined as clinical improvement or resolution of symptoms with negative results for culture of cerebrospinal fluid). However, mortality in the first 2 weeks of therapy was higher with fluconazole (15% vs. 8%).

Cryptococcosis in patients with AIDS is virtually impossible to cure. The goal of therapy is to control the infection and then suppress it with long-term antifungal agents. A common approach is to initiate therapy with amphotericin B (with or without flucytosine). Amphotericin therapy is continued until cerebrospinal fluid cultures are negative or there is unacceptable toxicity from the drug. Oral fluconazole (200-400 mg/day) is then given indefinitely. Disappointingly, relapse remains frequent even with maintenance therapy. The newly approved caspofungin does not have any activity against *C. neoformans*.

Candidiasis

Candida is a normal part of the human microflora. It grows as both yeast and hyphal forms simultaneously. Although *Candida albicans* is the most common species, numerous other species can cause human disease. *Candida* causes mucosal and cutaneous infections in both normal and immunocompromised hosts. Invasive disease primarily occurs in neutropenic hosts and as a nosocomial bloodstream infection.

Examples of candidiasis in the normal host include diaper rash and intertrigo, in which *Candida* growth on moist skin surfaces produces irritation. Vulvovaginal candidiasis is common, especially after a woman takes a course of antibiotics for an unrelated infection. Treatment with topical antifungal agents or a single dose of oral fluconazole is usually curative. Diabetes, corticosteroids, oral contraceptives, obesity, and HIV infection predispose to recurrent vulvovaginal candidiasis. Oral thrush may result from the same conditions.

Candida species cause 5% to 10% of nosocomial blood-stream infections. Candidemia most often occurs in critically ill patients receiving broad-spectrum antibiotics and parenteral nutrition. Neutropenia is another predisposing factor. Current blood culture techniques usually detect *Candida*, but culture results may be delayed. All intravenous catheters should always be removed or replaced when bloodstream infection with *Candida* is discovered. Metastatic abscesses can occur in any site after an episode of candidemia. *Candida* osteomyelitis or joint infections can occur as complications after an episode of line-related fungemia. Endophthalmitis may occur as long as 1 month after initial fungemia. For central venous catheter-related candidemias, catheter removal followed by amphotericin B (250-500 mg) or fluconazole is indicated.

Candida tropicalis, *Candida parapsilosis*, *Candida glabrata*, and multiple other species cause nosocomial illness, especially in immunocompromised patients. Note that these non-*albicans* species of *Candida* are more often resistant to fluconazole therapy.

Injection drug use is a risk factor for *Candida* endocarditis (and joint space infections, especially of the sternoclavicular joint). It is often caused by species other than *C. albicans*.

- Fungemia develops from infected intravenous catheters, especially in the immunosuppressed host.
- Risk factors for *Candida* bloodstream infection include previous antibacterial therapy, cytotoxic or corticosteroid therapy, and parenteral nutrition.
- *Candida* endocarditis occurs most often in injection drug users.
- Diabetes, corticosteroids, oral contraceptives, obesity, and HIV infection predispose to recurrent vulvovaginal candidiasis.

Candida urinary tract infection is common in patients with urinary catheters and those receiving antibacterial drugs. Removal of the catheter is the primary therapy. If necessary, treatment with fluconazole or bladder irrigation with dilute amphotericin B may be curative, though recurrence is common.

Hepatosplenic candidiasis, also called chronic disseminated candidiasis, occurs in patients after prolonged chemotherapy-induced neutropenia. Symptoms of fever and increasing liver enzyme values manifest as the leukocyte count recovers. Typical "bull's-eye lesions" can be seen with ultrasonography, computed tomography, or magnetic resonance imaging of the infected liver. The preferred treatment is with at least 2 g of intravenous amphotericin B, but fluconazole or lipid complex amphotericin B also may be effective.

Candida esophagitis is a common cause of odynophagia in immunosuppressed patients, especially those with AIDS. Endoscopy is necessary to prove the diagnosis. *Candida* esophagitis is clinically indistinguishable from, and may coexist with, cytomegalovirus and herpes simplex virus esophagitis. Fluconazole is effective therapy for oral or esophageal candidiasis. Caspofungin is also active and is approved by the U.S. Food and Drug Administration against *Candida* species, including those that are resistant to azoles such as fluconazole. Caspofungin is available only as an intravenous drug.

- Hepatosplenic candidiasis typically develops as chemotherapy-induced neutropenia resolves.
- *Candida* esophagitis is clinically indistinguishable from, and may coexist with, cytomegalovirus and herpes simplex virus esophagitis.
- Typical clinical scenario for *hepatosplenic candidiasis*: A patient recovering from prolonged chemotherapy-induced neutropenia has fever and increasing liver enzyme values. The diagnosis is made with ultrasonography or computed tomography showing characteristic bull's-eye lesions.
- Typical clinical scenario for *Candida* esophagitis: Odynophagia in immunocompromised patients. Differential diagnosis is herpes simplex virus esophagitis. Diagnosis is made with endoscopy and culture.

Mucormycosis (*Rhizopus* Species, Zygomycetes)

Mucormycosis is another disease of immunocompromised hosts. Pulmonary, nasal, and sinus infections are the most common. Rhinocerebral mucormycosis results from direct extension into the brain. Diabetic ketoacidosis, neutropenia, renal failure, and deferoxamine therapy are all risk factors for this dreaded infection. The diagnosis of mucormycosis depends on finding the typical black necrotic lesions (usually in the nose or on the palate) and is confirmed by biopsy. Treatment involves reversing the predisposing condition as much as possible, surgical debridement of necrotic tissue, and amphotericin B.

- The diagnosis of mucormycosis depends on finding the typical black necrotic lesions (usually in the nose or on the palate) and is confirmed by biopsy.
- Diabetic ketoacidosis, neutropenia, renal failure, and deferoxamine therapy are all risk factors for mucormycosis.

VIRAL DISEASES

Herpesviruses

There are now eight known herpesviruses: *herpes simplex virus* (HSV) *types 1 and 2, Epstein-Barr virus* (EBV), *cytomegalovirus* (CMV), *varicella-zoster virus* (VZV), *human herpesvirus 6* (HHV-6), *HHV-7* (not yet known to be associated with clinical disease), and *HHV-8*. All herpesviruses are DNA viruses that share the characteristic of establishing latency after primary infection, whether or not symptomatic.

Serologic evidence of infection is common by adulthood: HSV 1, 87%; HSV 2, 5%; EBV, 95%; CMV, 50%; and VZV, 90%. The rate of infection increases in populations of lower socioeconomic status.

Herpes Simplex Virus

Primary infection with HSV results from exposure of skin or mucous membranes to intact viral particles. Latent infection is then established in sensory nerve ganglia. Genital HSV infection is caused by HSV type 2 in 80% of cases and by HSV type 1 in the remaining 20%. The reverse is true for oral HSV. Genital HSV is more likely to recur when caused by HSV type 2. Recurrence rates can be decreased by 80% with chronic use of antiviral drugs. In normal hosts, this does not promote emergence of acyclovir-resistant strains.

Herpes simplex encephalitis (HSE) is a nonseasonal, life-threatening illness usually caused by HSV type 1. HSE causes confusion, fever, and, frequently, seizures. Simultaneous herpes labialis is present in 10% to 15% of cases. Antemortem diagnosis may be difficult. Although a definitive diagnosis traditionally requires a brain biopsy, new techniques such as magnetic resonance imaging of the temporal lobes and amplification of HSV DNA from cerebrospinal fluid are often helpful. Detecting periodic lateralized epileptiform discharges with electroencephalography is suggestive of HSE. Poor neurologic status, age older than 30 years, and encephalitis of more than 4 days in duration before initiation of therapy are associated with a poor outcome.

Neonatal HSV infection is acquired at the time of vaginal delivery. The mortality rate is high (20%) despite antiviral therapy. In neonates who survive, neurologic sequelae and recurrent HSV lesions are common. Cesarean section is recommended if a woman has active herpetic lesions at the time of delivery.

Acyclovir, famciclovir, valacyclovir, ganciclovir, foscarnet, and vidarabine inhibit replication of both HSV types 1 and 2. Acyclovir resistance may develop in patients with AIDS who are treated with multiple courses of acyclovir. Resistance usually is conferred by a mutation in the thymidine kinase gene, preventing phosphorylation of acyclovir to its active form.

- Recurrence rates of oral HSV can be decreased 80% with chronic suppressive therapy with acyclovir.
- HSE can be diagnosed with magnetic resonance imaging and polymerase chain reaction amplification of HSV DNA from cerebrospinal fluid.
- Delivery by cesarean section is recommended if active genital lesions are present at the end of pregnancy.

HSV pneumonia is rare and usually occurs in immunosuppressed patients. When HSV is isolated from a respiratory source, it most commonly represents shedding from the oral mucosa rather than the lungs. HSV also is associated with visceral disease (such as esophagitis). Biopsy is required to reliably distinguish HSV from CMV or *Candida* esophagitis. *Eczema herpeticum* (Kaposi varicelliform eruption) occurs in areas of eczema. Large areas of skin are involved. *Herpetic whitlow* is a painful HSV infection of a finger, often caused by inoculation with a contaminated needle. Although nosocomial transmission of HSV is rare, recent reports stress the importance of mucous membrane precautions when treating all patients with HSV, particularly those with respiratory infection who undergo invasive procedures.

- *Herpetic whitlow* is a painful HSV infection of a finger, often caused by inoculation with a contaminated needle.

HSV can cause outbreaks among participants in contact sports (in wrestlers it is called *herpes gladiatorum*). The infection is transmitted by skin-to-skin contact. Lesions appear on the head (78%), trunk (28%), and extremities (42%). The rash may be atypical. Large, ulcerative perianal lesions can develop in patients with AIDS. Some of the lesions are mistaken for decubitus ulcers.

- HSV can cause outbreaks among participants in contact sports.
- Large, ulcerative perianal lesions can develop in patients with AIDS.

Epstein-Barr Virus

Most acute EBV infections are asymptomatic. Symptomatic *infectious mononucleosis* causes the clinical triad of fever, pharyngitis (80%), and adenopathy. Splenomegaly occurs in 50% of cases. One of the most serious complications of mononucleosis is splenic rupture. Other complications include hemolytic anemia, airway obstruction, encephalitis, and transverse myelitis. Associated laboratory abnormalities include atypical lymphocytosis, thrombocytopenia, and mild increases in liver enzyme values. Corticosteroids may be beneficial for treatment of hemolytic anemia and acute airway obstruction. Ampicillin or amoxicillin given during infectious mononucleosis commonly causes a diffuse macular rash.

Table 14-4 differentiates EBV from other causes of mononucleosis. The diagnosis of infectious mononucleosis depends on detection of heterophile antibodies (monospot test) or specific EBV IgM antibodies. False-negative results of the monospot test are more likely with increasing age.

- Infectious mononucleosis has the clinical triad of fever, pharyngitis, and adenopathy.

Table 14-4 Infectious Mononucleosis-like Syndromes

Disease	Pharyngitis	Adenopathy	Splenomegaly	Atypical lymphocytes	Heterophile	Other test
Infectious mononucleosis	++++	++++	+++	+++	+	Specific EBV antibody + (VCA IgM)
CMV	-	-	+++	++	-	CMV IgM
Toxoplasmosis	-	++++	+++	++		Toxoplasmosis serology

-, absent; +, ++, +++, and ++++, present to varying degrees; CMV, cytomegalovirus; EBV, Epstein-Barr virus; VCA, viral capsid antigen.

- Splenomegaly occurs in 50% of cases.
- One of the most serious complications is splenic rupture.
- If ampicillin is given, a rash often develops.

Uncomplicated cases require symptomatic care only. The patient should not participate in contact sports for several months because of the risk for splenic rupture. Corticosteroids are not indicated for uncomplicated infection. Acyclovir and other antiviral drug therapy is not effective.

Chronic fatigue syndrome is a syndrome characterized by various nonspecific symptoms. Studies have definitively shown that EBV does not cause chronic fatigue syndrome.

- No therapy is indicated for uncomplicated cases of infectious mononucleosis.
- EBV does not cause chronic fatigue syndrome.

EBV infection in males with X-linked lymphoproliferative syndrome is a rare disorder of young boys in whom fulminant EBV infections develop and is associated with a 57% mortality rate. Complications include severe EBV hepatitis with liver failure and hemophagocytic syndrome with bleeding. In survivors, hypogammaglobulinemia, malignant lymphoma, aplastic anemia, and opportunistic infections develop. Death occurs by age 40 years in all cases. Acyclovir and corticosteroids do not seem to be beneficial.

In *EBV-associated Burkitt lymphoma and nasopharyngeal carcinoma*, patients have high titers of IgA antibodies to EBV. *Polyclonal and monoclonal B-cell lymphoproliferative syndromes* have been associated with EBV in patients who have had organ transplantation and in patients with AIDS. Oral hairy leukoplakia in patients with AIDS is associated with EBV infection and responds to acyclovir therapy. EBV recently has been associated with leiomyosarcomas in transplant recipients.

- Polyclonal and monoclonal B-cell lymphoproliferative syndromes have been associated with EBV.

Cytomegalovirus

Primary CMV infection is usually asymptomatic in immunocompetent patients, but it can cause a heterophile-negative mononucleosis syndrome. It is a significant cause of neonatal disease. Perinatal infection can occur in utero, intra partum, or post partum and can cause congenital malformations. Primary infection of the mother during pregnancy results in a 15% chance of fetal cytomegalic inclusion disease. Young children in day-care centers commonly shed CMV in their urine and saliva. Their parents are at risk of acquiring primary infection from an asymptomatic child.

CMV can be transmitted by leukocytes in blood transfusions. Use of leukocyte-poor packed red blood cells or blood from CMV-seronegative donors decreases the risk of transmission via this route. Symptomatic infection develops about 4 weeks after transfusion and manifests as fever with atypical lymphocytes in the peripheral blood smear. Serologic testing confirms the diagnosis. Viral cultures are rarely helpful in diagnosing CMV disease in the noncompromised patient.

- CMV can cause heterophile-negative mononucleosis syndrome.
- CMV can be transmitted by blood transfusion.
- Fever and infectious mononucleosis-like picture on peripheral smear are characteristics in postoperative patients who have received blood transfusions.

In persons with impaired cellular immunity (such as those with AIDS or organ and bone marrow transplant recipients), CMV causes serious infections (CMV syndrome, retinitis, pneumonia, gastrointestinal ulcerations, encephalitis, adrenalitis). The diagnosis most often is established by isolation of CMV from blood or from culture, by histopathologic evidence of CMV infection in involved tissue (such as liver, lung, gastrointestinal tract), or from clinical findings alone (CMV retinitis).

● CMV causes serious infections (retinitis, pneumonia, gastrointestinal ulcerations, encephalitis, adrenalitis) in patients who have AIDS or take immunosuppressive medications.

The manifestations of CMV disease in persons with advanced AIDS are protean. Disease is almost always caused by reactivation of latent infection in this setting. Finding CMV in the blood or urine of patients with AIDS is common and has a low predictive value for symptomatic CMV disease. CMV retinitis occurs in 20% to 30% of patients with advanced AIDS. Diagnosis is based on ophthalmologic examination. The relapse rate for CMV retinitis in AIDS is very high, even with chronic antiviral therapy.

Solid organ and bone marrow transplant recipients are another group of patients at risk for CMV disease. It is the most common infection after solid organ transplantation (occurring primarily in the first 6 months after transplantation). Those at highest risk are CMV seronegative before transplantation and receive an organ from a seropositive donor. Latent virus is present in almost all tissues and begins replicating shortly after transplantation. Symptomatic disease (CMV syndrome) usually develops in the first 4 to 8 weeks after a solid organ transplantation and causes fever, leukopenia, increases in liver enzyme values, and end-organ involvement. CMV serum antigen testing or CMV detected in blood culture helps confirm the diagnosis. Patients who have had bone marrow transplantation are especially at risk for CMV pneumonia. The mortality rate approaches 50% despite therapy. Prophylactic ganciclovir and, possibly, CMV immune globulin may decrease or delay posttransplantation CMV disease.

● CMV retinitis occurs in 20%-30% of patients with advanced AIDS.
● CMV is the most common infectious complication of organ transplantation.

Ganciclovir is the treatment of choice for most CMV infections in immunocompromised hosts. A randomized, placebo-controlled trial found that foscarnet and ganciclovir are equally efficacious for halting the progression of CMV retinitis in patients with AIDS but that patients taking foscarnet lived longer (12 vs. 8 months). Both drugs are now approved for this indication. Full-dose induction therapy is given for 2 to 3 weeks, followed by chronic suppressive therapy indefinitely (usually as once-daily dosing). Transplant recipients usually do not require suppressive medication after an episode of CMV disease. In patients with CMV pneumonia after bone marrow transplantation, combining ganciclovir with intravenous immune globulin is more effective than ganciclovir alone. Non-immunocompromised patients with CMV do not require treatment.

● Ganciclovir or foscarnet is the treatment of choice for most CMV infections.

Varicella-Zoster Virus

Primary infection with VZV usually occurs in childhood and causes chickenpox. Illness with chickenpox is more likely to be severe in adults and immunocompromised hosts. Varicella pneumonia occurs in 5% to 50% of cases. Pregnant women are especially vulnerable. They should be treated with high-dose acyclovir (10 mg/kg every 8 hours). Acyclovir is not associated with toxicity to the fetus. Pneumonia develops within 1 to 6 days after the onset of illness and usually recedes as the rash does. Encephalomyelitis is another serious complication of varicella infection, occurring predominantly in children. Onset is 3 to 14 days after the appearance of rash.

● Varicella pneumonia occurs in 5% to 50% of adults with chickenpox.
● Pneumonia begins to improve with disappearance of rash.

After primary infection, VZV DNA persists in a latent state in sensory neuron ganglia. Reactivated infection causes zoster (shingles), which manifests as a painful vesicular rash in a dermatomal distribution. Involvement of the fifth cranial nerve, especially the ophthalmic branch, may be sight-threatening. In non-immune persons exposed to zoster, primary VZV infection may develop. Neurologic complications of herpes zoster include motor paralysis (localized to the dermatomal distribution of rash), encephalitis, and myelitis.

● Herpes zoster infection often involves the fifth cranial nerve, especially the ophthalmic branch.

Varicella immune globulin can prevent primary VZV infection, especially when given within 96 hours of exposure. It is indicated for 1) VZV-seronegative immunocompromised hosts who have had close contact with a person with chickenpox and 2) newborns of mothers with varicella infection that occurs 5 days before or 2 days after delivery.

Ten percent of mothers with active varicella will transmit the infection to the fetus. Infection during the first trimester may result in limb hypoplasia, cortical atrophy, and chorioretinitis. During the third trimester, multiple visceral abnormalities can occur, including pneumonia. The fetal and neonatal mortality rate is 31%.

● Among mothers with active varicella, 10% will transmit the infection to the fetus.

Treatment for varicella (*primary varicella-zoster*) infection is based on whether the patient is immunocompetent. Two recent randomized clinical trials showed that oral acyclovir (800 mg 5 times a day or equivalent) reduced the duration of skin lesions and viral shedding in adults and children. Its efficacy for reducing visceral complications (pneumonia) remains unknown. Early treatment (<24 hours) is necessary. The cost of therapy may limit its usefulness, but it is advocated by some to decrease the duration of illness. Acyclovir may reduce the risk of dissemination and of complications in immunocompromised patients. Treatment of zoster ophthalmicus reduces the incidence of uveitis and keratitis. For immunocompetent patients with zoster, three antiviral drugs (acyclovir, famciclovir, and valacyclovir) speed healing and reduce pain. Preliminary data suggest that the new antiviral agent famciclovir might decrease the duration of postherpetic neuralgia. Corticosteroids do not prevent postherpetic neuralgia. For disseminated infections (encephalitis, cranial neuritis), a recent controlled trial showed that high-dose intravenous acyclovir decreases the duration of hospitalization. Acyclovir-resistant VZV infection (which can occur in patients with AIDS) can be treated with intravenous foscarnet.

An effective live virus vaccine for VZV is now available. It is recommended for children and VZV-seronegative adolescent and adult populations. It is contraindicated in pregnancy and in patients with impaired cellular immunity such as AIDS, leukemias, lymphoma, chemotherapy, transplantation, chronic steroid therapy, or other cellular immunodeficiency states. Such immunocompromised patients should avoid contact with persons who have received the vaccine in the past month.

Human Herpesvirus 6

HHV-6 is a recently discovered lymphotropic virus. It causes the mild childhood infectious exanthem known as roseola infantum. Like CMV, reactivation of infection occurs after organ transplantation. HHV-6 has been associated with pneumonitis after bone marrow transplantation.

Human Herpesvirus 8

HHV-8 is also known as Kaposi sarcoma-associated virus. As the name implies, it is thought to be the causative agent of Kaposi sarcoma. It is related to EBV. Most recently, HHV-8 has been linked to body cavity-based lymphomas in patients with AIDS and Castleman disease.

Influenza

Type A is the most common. Epidemics occur every 2 to 4 years; pandemics occur every 20 to 30 years. Epidemics and pandemics are a result of a major antigenic shift in the influenza virus. About 80% to 90% of deaths due to influenza occur in persons older than 65 years. Complications include 1) primary influenza pneumonia (interstitial desquamative

pneumonia) and 2) secondary bacterial infection, which usually is caused by *Streptococcus pneumoniae*, *Haemophilus*, or *Staphylococcus aureus*. Rare cases of toxic shock syndrome have been reported when *S. aureus* pneumonia complicates influenza.

- About 80%-90% of deaths due to influenza occur in persons older than 65 years.
- Secondary infection usually is caused by *Streptococcus pneumoniae* or *Staphylococcus aureus*.
- Typical clinical scenario: An elderly patient, often with chronic obstructive lung disease, develops influenza, which may or may not improve; then, the severity of symptoms increases substantially, with high fever, marked leukocytosis, and often respiratory failure.

Amantadine and rimantadine are effective against only influenza A virus, not influenza B. Therapy is most beneficial if begun within 48 hours of onset of symptoms. Vaccine, together with amantadine, can give about 95% protection against influenza A infection. Newer drugs called neuraminidase inhibitors (oseltamivir and zanamivir) are effective against uncomplicated disease caused by both influenza A and B. Both reduce the duration of symptoms by 1 day when started within 48 hours after onset of symptoms.

A live attenuated intranasal vaccine and an inactivated influenza vaccine are approved by the U.S. Food and Drug Administration for the prevention of influenza. The live attenuated vaccine is approved only for healthy immunocompetent persons between the ages of 5 and 49 years. Adverse reactions to both vaccines include fever, myalgias, and hypersensitivity. Target groups are persons older than 50 years, residents of chronic care facilities, persons with cardiopulmonary disorders, children 6 months to 18 years old receiving long-term aspirin therapy (to prevent Reye syndrome), health care personnel, employees of chronic care facilities, providers of home health care, and those sharing the same household as high-risk persons. Amantadine also is used prophylactically at a dose of 200 mg/day; if the person is older than 65 years, only 100 mg/day is given to decrease the risk of side effects. The decreased dosage also is used for patients with impaired renal function or seizure disorders. Toxicity manifests as dizziness, restlessness, and insomnia. Rimantadine and oseltamivir are also approved by the U.S. Food and Drug Administration and are effective for prophylactic use after exposure to a patient with influenza. High-risk individuals who have not received the vaccine during the influenza season should be considered for chemoprophylaxis.

- Target groups for influenza vaccine are persons older than 50 years, residents of chronic care facilities, persons with cardiopulmonary disorders, health care personnel, employees of chronic care facilities, providers of home health care, and household members of high-risk persons.

Hantavirus Infection, *Hantavirus* Pulmonary Syndrome

In May 1993, an outbreak of an acute illness consisting of fever, rapidly progressive respiratory failure, and death was reported in the four-state area of New Mexico, Arizona, Colorado, and Utah. Most of the initial cases occurred in young Navajo Indians. The causative agent is a virus belonging to the genus *Hantavirus* (family Bunyaviridae) and is now called the Sin Nombre virus. Infection is transmitted through inhalation of aerosolized secretions from the common deer mouse (*Peromyscus maniculatus*).

Since the early reports, cases also have been identified in most other states and Canada. The disease begins with a nonspecific prodrome (fever and generalized myalgia) followed in 4 to 5 days by respiratory symptoms (cough, dyspnea, and tachypnea). This progresses rapidly to an adult respiratory distress syndrome. Diagnosis is possible with serologic studies (such as enzyme-linked immunosorbent assay for antivirus IgM and IgG antibodies). Treatment is mainly supportive. Ribavirin, a guanosine analog, has been used effectively for treating hemorrhagic fever with renal syndrome caused by other related types of *Hantavirus*, but its efficacy in *Hantavirus* pulmonary syndrome is not yet established.

Poliovirus

Although wild-type polio has been eliminated from the Western Hemisphere, it remains endemic in parts of Asia and Africa. Disease still can be imported from these areas. There was a recent outbreak in the Netherlands among members of religious groups who were not vaccinated. Remember that polio is most often an asymptomatic infection. The virus affects the nuclei of cranial nerves and anterior motor neurons of the spinal cord, causing a flaccid paralysis. When paralysis develops, it is usually asymmetric. Vaccine-related polio, although rare, can occur with the live virus vaccine. In July 2000, a vaccine-strain polio outbreak occurred in the Dominican Republic and Haiti. Patients traveling to these countries are advised to receive an injectable inactivated polio vaccine booster.

Rabies

Rabies is difficult to diagnose ante mortem. Manifestations are hydrophobia and copious salivation. It should be considered in any case of encephalitis or myelitis of unknown cause, especially in persons who have recently traveled outside the United States. The virus spreads along peripheral nerves to the central nervous system. The most common sources of exposure are dogs, cats, skunks, foxes, raccoons (Florida, Connecticut), wolves, and bats. Spread by other animals is *very rare*. Rodents rarely, if ever, transmit rabies. From 1980 to 1989, 9 of 13 cases in the United States were due to exposure to rabid animals outside the country. Rabies also has been reported to occur in patients after corneal transplantation. Aerosol spread is possible; it is most often due to exposure to bats during spelunking or in medical laboratories. The risk of nosocomial transmission is low. Definitive diagnosis is established by finding Negri bodies on biopsy of the hippocampus. Serum and cerebrospinal fluid can be tested for rabies antibodies when trying to diagnose the disease. Direct fluorescent antibody testing of a skin biopsy specimen from the nape of the neck is used to detect rabies antigen.

- Rabies should be considered in any case of encephalitis or myelitis of unknown cause.
- Most common sources of exposure are dogs, cats, skunks, foxes, raccoons, wolves, and bats.
- Definitive diagnosis is established by the presence of Negri bodies on biopsy of the hippocampus.

Human diploid vaccine is more effective and less toxic than the older duck embryo vaccine. Human rabies immunoglobulin is now widely available, mitigating the need to use horse serum immune globulin. Human rabies immunoglobulin and vaccine are not of benefit after onset of clinical disease. Preexposure rabies vaccination is advised for patients likely to be in situations that put them at high risk for rabies, such as prolonged travel to rabies-endemic countries. Pre-exposure vaccination mitigates the need for rabies immunoglobulin and decreases the post-exposure doses to only 2 (days 0 and 3 after bite).

Slow Viruses and Prion-Associated Central Nervous System Diseases

Progressive Multifocal Leukoencephalopathy (PML)

PML is associated with AIDS, leukemia, lymphoma, and immunosuppression for organ transplantation. It is caused by a papovavirus (JC virus). PML can cause either diffuse or focal central nervous system abnormalities. Despite its name, PML usually causes solitary brain lesions, as seen on computed tomography or magnetic resonance imaging. Cerebrospinal fluid is normal in most cases. The diagnosis is based on brain biopsy, although detection of JC virus DNA in the cerebrospinal fluid is suggestive of PML. There is no proven effective therapy.

- PML is associated with AIDS, leukemia, lymphoma, and immunosuppression for organ transplantation.
- PML is caused by a papovavirus (JC virus).

Subacute Sclerosing Panencephalitis (Inclusion Body Encephalitis)

This is a progressively fatal disease of children and adolescents. It is thought to be due to rubeola (measles) virus. Patients are younger than 11 years in 80% of cases. Onset is insidious, with progressive mental deterioration. Later, myoclonic jerks and diffuse abnormalities occur. Measles antibody levels in sera and cerebrospinal fluid are markedly increased. Brain biopsy is necessary for diagnosis (inclusion body encephalitis). There is no treatment. The disease is uniformly fatal.

Creutzfeldt-Jakob Disease

This is a rare, fatal, degenerative disease of the central nervous system. It occurs equally in both sexes, usually at older ages. There are both familial and sporadic forms of the disease. Creutzfeldt-Jakob disease usually presents as rapidly evolving dementia with myoclonic seizures. Prions (small proteinaceous infectious particles without nucleic acid) have been proposed as the cause of this disease. Nosocomial transmission of Creutzfeldt-Jakob disease can occur via corneal transplant recipients and exposure to cerebrospinal fluid. Several recent cases in Great Britain were linked to consumption of beef from cattle that had bovine spongiform encephalopathy. There is no treatment.

- Creutzfeldt-Jakob disease presents as rapidly evolving dementia with myoclonic seizures.

Measles (Rubeola)

There was a substantial increase in measles cases in the late 1980s and early 1990s in unvaccinated preschool children and vaccinated high school and college students (1990: 27,786 cases). Prodromal upper respiratory tract symptoms are prominent. Oral lesions (Koplik spots) precede the rash. Both measles infection and measles vaccine cause temporary cutaneous anergy (false-negative purified protein derivative test). Infection may cause more significant immunologic suppression, as exemplified by cases of reactivated tuberculosis in persons with measles.

- In measles, oral Koplik spots precede the rash.
- Measles vaccine may cause temporary cutaneous anergy.

Complications of measles include encephalitis and pneumonia. Encephalitis is often severe. It usually occurs after a period of apparent improvement of measles infection. In primary measles pneumonia, large, multinucleated cells (Warthin-Finkeldey cells) are found on lung biopsy. Secondary bacterial infection is more common than primary measles pneumonia. *S. aureus* and *Haemophilus influenzae* are the most common bacterial pathogens.

- Complications of measles include encephalitis.
- Secondary bacterial infection is more common than primary measles pneumonia.

Atypical measles occurs in patients vaccinated before 1968. After exposure to measles, atypical rash, fever, arthralgias, and headache (aseptic meningitis) may develop. The presence of a high titer of measles antibody in serum helps confirm the diagnosis.

Rubella

The prodromal symptoms of rubella are mild (unlike those of rubeola). Posterior cervical lymphadenopathy, arthralgia (70% in adults), transient erythematous rash, and fever are characteristic. Infection is subclinical in many cases. Central nervous system complications and thrombocytopenia are rare.

- Characteristics of rubella: posterior cervical lymphadenopathy, arthralgia (70% in adults), transient erythematous rash, and fever.

The greatest danger from rubella is to the fetus. When a pregnant female is exposed to rubella, rubella serologic testing should be done. If the titer indicates immunity, there is no danger and no further testing is indicated. If the titer indicates non-immunity, the patient should be followed for evidence of clinical rubella. The serum titer should be checked again in 2 to 3 weeks to evaluate for evidence of asymptomatic infection. If the titer is not increased and there is no evidence of clinical rubella, then no intervention is indicated. If clinical rubella develops or seroconversion is demonstrated, there is a high risk of congenital abnormalities or spontaneous abortion. The risk varies from 40% to 60% if infection occurs during the first 2 months of gestation to 10% by the 4th month. Intravenous gamma globulin may mask symptoms of rubella, but it does not protect the fetus.

- Gamma globulin does not protect the fetus after exposure to rubella.

From 6% to 11% of young adults remain susceptible to rubella after receiving rubella vaccine. A pregnant female should not be given rubella vaccine because it can cause congenital abnormalities. Females of childbearing age should be warned not to become pregnant within 2 to 3 months from the time of immunization. Transient arthralgias develop in 25% of immunized women. Fever, rash, and lymphadenopathy also may develop. Symptoms may occur as long as 2 months after vaccination. They may be confused with other forms of arthritis.

Viral Meningoencephalitis

Etiologic agents of viral meningitis include mumps, enteroviruses, herpes simplex, and, in summer months, the equine encephalitis viruses. Lymphocytic choriomeningitis is acquired by exposure to rodent urine. Lactate levels in cerebrospinal fluid are normal in viral meningitis. The lactate level usually is increased in bacterial meningitis.

Mumps

Mumps virus commonly affects glandular tissue. Parotitis, pancreatitis, and orchitis are characteristic manifestations. Orchitis occurs in 20% of males with mumps. It is unilateral in approximately 75%. Orchitis often is associated with recrudescence of malaise and chills, fever, headache, nausea, vomiting, and testicular pain. Sterility is uncommon, even after bilateral infection.

Mumps meningoencephalitis is one of the most common nonseasonal viral meningitides. It can cause low glucose values in the cerebrospinal fluid, mimicking bacterial meningitis. Deafness is a rare complication of mumps.

- Mumps meningoencephalitis is one of the most common nonseasonal viral meningitides.

Mumps polyarthritis is most common in men between the ages of 20 and 30 years. Joint symptoms begin 1 to 2 weeks after subsidence of parotitis, and large joints are involved. The condition lasts approximately 6 weeks, and complete recovery is usual. This condition may be confused with other forms of arthritis.

- Mumps polyarthritis is most common in men between the ages of 20 and 30 years.

Parvovirus B19

Parvovirus is a single-stranded DNA virus that infects the erythrocyte precursors in bone marrow, with resulting reticulocytopenia. It is the cause of erythema infectiosum (fifth disease) in children, transient arthritis in adults, and aplastic crisis in persons with hemolytic anemias. Infection during pregnancy results in a 5% chance of hydrops fetalis or fetal death. Serologic testing is the preferred diagnostic method in immunologically competent persons.

Parvovirus B19 infection may persist in immunosuppressed patients, resulting in red blood cell aplasia. Diagnosis is established by demonstration of giant pronormoblasts in bone marrow or identification of viral DNA in bone marrow or peripheral blood. Most patients respond to administration of commercial immune globulin infusions for 5 to 10 days. No treatment is recommended for parvovirus infections in the noncompromised host.

- Parvovirus B19 is the cause of erythema infectiosum (fifth disease) and transient arthritis.
- B19 virus can cause red blood cell aplasia in patients with AIDS.

Human T-Cell Lymphotropic Viruses (HTLV)

HTLV-I and -II are non-HIV human retroviruses. HTLV-I is endemic in parts of Japan, the Caribbean basin, South America, and Africa. It may be transmitted by sexual contact, infected cellular blood products (not clotting factor concentrates), and injection drug use. Vertical transmission (breast-feeding, transplacental) also occurs. HTLV-I is associated with human T-cell leukemia/lymphoma and tropical spastic paraparesis (also known as HTLV-I–associated myelopathy). However, clinical disease never develops in 96% of persons infected with HTLV-I. HTLV-II causes no known clinical disease. The seroprevalence of HTLV-I or -II is as high as 18% in certain high-risk groups (injection drug users, patients attending sexually transmitted disease clinics) (HTLV-II is 2.5 times more prevalent than HTLV-I). Among voluntary blood donors, the seroprevalence in the United States is estimated at 0.016%. With current screening practices, the risk of transmission of HTLV-I or -II through blood transfusion is estimated to be 0.0014% (1/70,000 units).

- HTLV-I may be transmitted by sexual contact, infected blood products, and injection drug use.
- HTLV-I infection is usually asymptomatic but is associated with human T-cell leukemia and chronic myelopathy.

PARASITIC DISEASES

Helminths

Neurocysticercosis is an infection of the central nervous system with a larval stage of the pork tapeworm (*Taenia solium*). It is acquired by ingesting tapeworm eggs from fecally contaminated food. It is endemic in Latin America, Asia, and Africa. Recent cases have been reported among household contacts of foreign-born persons (working as domestic employees). The infected persons had not traveled to an affected area. The most common presentation is seizures. Brain imaging reveals cystic or calcified brain lesions. Serum or cerebrospinal fluid serologic testing can aid in the diagnosis. Treatment with praziquantel or albendazole may be beneficial. The coadministration of corticosteroids often is used to decrease cerebral inflammation associated with therapy.

- Neurocysticercosis is acquired by ingesting tapeworm eggs from fecally contaminated food.
- Seizures are the most common symptom of neurocysticercosis.

Strongyloides stercoralis is unique among the intestinal nematode infections. Unlike the other helminths, the larvae of this organism can mature in the human host (auto-infection). In immunocompromised hosts (neutropenia, steroids, AIDS), a superinfection can develop with larval migration throughout the body. Gram-negative bacteremia is a common coinfection, resulting from disruption of the intestinal mucosa by the invasive larvae.

Trichinosis is acquired from eating undercooked meat, especially pork or bear. Features include muscle pain (especially diaphragm, chest, and tongue), eosinophilia, and periorbital edema.

Hookworm (*Necator americanus*) causes anemia. It is found mainly in tropical and subtropical regions. The larval form penetrates the skin. Walking barefoot is a risk factor.

Ascariasis infection may cause intestinal obstruction or pancreatitis (worm migrates up the pancreatic duct).

Schistosomiasis is a tropical disease that causes hepatic cirrhosis, hematuria, and carcinoma of the bladder. Transverse myelitis may develop as a result of schistosomiasis. It is acquired by direct penetration of the *Schistosoma* cercariae from contaminated water (lakes, rivers).

- Trichinosis is acquired from eating undercooked meat, especially pork or bear.
- Transverse myelitis may develop as a result of schistosomiasis.

Protozoan Parasites

Acanthamoeba, a free-living ameba, causes amebic keratitis in persons swimming in fresh water while wearing soft contact lenses. The diagnosis is based on microscopic examination of scrapings of the cornea. Treatment is with topical antifungal agents. Patients often respond poorly to therapy and have progressive corneal destruction.

Symptomatic infection with *Entamoeba histolytica* (amebiasis) may cause diarrhea (often bloody), abdominal pain, and fever. Metronidazole, followed by a lumenocidal agent such as iodoquinol or paromomycin, is the preferred therapy (metronidazole does not kill amebae in the intestinal lumen). Asymptomatic carriage of amebic cysts should be treated with one of the lumenocidal agents.

- Metronidazole, followed by a lumenocidal agent such as iodoquinol or paromomycin, is the preferred therapy for symptomatic amebiasis.

Invasive amebiasis may lead to distant abscesses (primarily the liver, but other organs can be involved). An amebic liver abscess usually is single and is commonly located in the posterior portion of the right lobe of the liver. The anatomical location, the fact that it is usually a single abscess, and the absence of other signs of bacterial infection help to distinguish amebic hepatic abscess from bacterial abscess. Serologic tests (complement fixation) are positive in more than 90% of patients with amebic abscess. Hepatic abscess may rupture through the diaphragm into the right pleural cavity.

- Amebic liver abscess may rupture through the diaphragm into the right pleural cavity.

Giardia lamblia is the parasite most frequently detected in state parasitology laboratories. Infection characteristically produces sudden onset of watery diarrhea with malabsorption, bloating, and flatulence. Prolonged disease that is refractory to standard therapy may occur in patients with IgA deficiency. The organism may be detected in stool specimens, but examination of duodenal aspirates is more sensitive. Treatment with metronidazole usually cures giardiasis.

- *G. lamblia* is the parasite most frequently detected in state parasitology laboratories.
- Giardiasis causes sudden onset of watery diarrhea and malabsorption, bloating, and flatulence. Prolonged disease is particularly common in patients with IgA deficiency.

Toxoplasma gondii is acquired from eating undercooked meat or exposure to cat feces. Primary toxoplasmosis is usually asymptomatic. In immunocompetent persons it may cause a heterophile-negative mononucleosis-like syndrome. Toxoplasmosis causes brain lesions and pneumonia in patients with AIDS. Immunocompromised patients with toxoplasmosis can be treated effectively with pyrimethamine in combination with either sulfadiazine or clindamycin.

- Toxoplasmosis is acquired from eating undercooked meat or exposure to cat feces.
- Toxoplasmosis may cause an infectious mononucleosis-like syndrome.

Malaria is endemic and spreading in many parts of the world. Spiking fevers, rigors, and headache are the hallmark of malaria. With falciparum malaria, the fevers may be irregular or continuous. *Plasmodium vivax* and *Plasmodium malariae* infections cause regular episodic fevers (malarial paroxysms). Malaria is diagnosed by examination of thick and thin blood smears (Plate 14-7).

- Diagnosis of malaria is based on examination of thick and thin blood smears.

Prophylaxis for malaria is increasingly difficult because of drug-resistant *Plasmodium falciparum*. Personal protection should always be used (such as mosquito nets, insect repellents containing DEET [*N,N*-diethyl-3-methylbenzamide]). For travelers to chloroquine-sensitive areas (Central America [north of Panama], Mexico, Haiti, the Dominican Republic, and the Middle East), chloroquine phosphate is still effective. In chloroquine-resistant areas, mefloquine, doxycycline, or an atovaquone-proguanil hydrochloride combination tablet (Malarone) is suggested. Sulfadoxine-pyrimethamine (Fansidar) or a combination of chloroquine with proguanil is not recommended for prophylaxis for chloroquine-resistant falciparum malaria. Travelers to the mefloquine-resistant areas of the Thai-Myanmar and Thai-Cambodian borders should use doxycycline or atovaquone-proguanil hydrochloride. Mefloquine should be avoided in patients with cardiac conduction abnormalities, depression or other psychiatric disorder, or seizure disorder. No regimen guarantees 100% prophylaxis. While receiving mefloquine, patients should be advised not to take halofantrine for a febrile illness because of the risk of fatal cardiac arrhythmias. All patients should be advised to seek medical attention if fever develops within 1 year after return from an endemic area.

Chloroquine is the preferred treatment of infection caused by *P. vivax*, *P. malariae*, and known chloroquine-susceptible strains of *P. falciparum*. Chloroquine-resistant strains may respond to quinine and doxycycline, atovaquone-proguanil hydrochloride, mefloquine, or artemether (this agent is not available in the United States). For severe *P. falciparum* infections, intravenous quinidine or quinine is effective. In the United States, only parenteral quinidine is available for severe malaria. Primaquine is used to eradicate the exoerythrocytic phase of *Plasmodium ovale* and *P. vivax* infections, preventing later relapses. Be aware that primaquine can cause hemolysis in persons with glucose-6-phosphate dehydrogenase deficiency. Exchange transfusion may be beneficial as treatment for cases with overwhelming parasitemia.

Cryptosporidium parvum is an important cause of diarrhea, especially in persons with AIDS. Cryptosporidiosis is also a cause of self-limited diarrhea in otherwise healthy persons. Waterborne outbreaks (Georgia; Milwaukee, Wisconsin) have been reported. They occur most often in late summer or fall. Thirty-five percent of patients have another pathogen simultaneously, most often *Giardia*. The diagnosis may be missed on standard stool examination for ova and parasites. There is no effective therapy for *Cryptosporidium*, except paromomycin, which shows some efficacy.

- Cryptosporidiosis is an important cause of diarrhea in AIDS.

Cyclospora cayetanensis is a recently described cause of persistent diarrhea, fever, and profound fatigue. First described in travelers to tropical areas of the world, disease due to *Cyclospora* also has been linked to consumption of contaminated food in the United States (raspberries from Guatemala). Like *Cryptosporidium*, the organism may not be detected on routine stool examinations. The illness can be effectively treated with trimethoprim-sulfamethoxazole.

- Infection with *C. cayetanensis* causes persistent diarrhea, fever, and profound fatigue.

Leishmaniasis is a protozoan disease transmitted by the sand fly bite. Visceral leishmaniasis (kala-azar, caused by *Leishmania donovani*) causes fever, hepatosplenomegaly, hypergammaglobulinemia, cachexia, and pancytopenia. It has been reported in patients with AIDS in Spain. Bone marrow examination (Giemsa stain) is often diagnostic. Cutaneous leishmaniasis (caused by *L. tropica*, *L. major*, *L. braziliensis*, and *L. mexicana*) may be self-limited. However, South and Central American forms of cutaneous leishmaniasis are often destructive and should be treated. Treatment is with antimony compounds or with amphotericin B or its liposomal formulations.

Babesia microti is a tick-borne (same vector as Lyme disease, *Ixodes dammini*) parasite that infects erythrocytes and causes fever, myalgias, and hemolytic anemia. Often asymptomatic in normal hosts, severe disease may develop in asplenic individuals. Babesiosis is endemic in the northeastern United States, especially around Nantucket and Cape Cod. Cases of transfusion-transmitted babesiosis have been documented. The diagnosis is established with examination of peripheral blood smear or polymerase chain reaction amplification of *Babesia* DNA from peripheral blood. Treatment is with clindamycin and quinine. Simultaneous infection with babesiosis and Lyme disease may be especially severe.

- Babesiosis infects erythrocytes and causes fever, myalgias, and hemolytic anemia.

PART II
Gregory D. Hart, M.D.

CLINICAL SYNDROMES

INFECTIVE ENDOCARDITIS

Native Valve Infective Endocarditis

Native valve infective endocarditis is more common in males and patients older than 65 years. The age- and sex-adjusted incidence rate of infective endocarditis is 4.9 cases per 100,000 person-years. In 60% to 80% of cases, there is a predisposing cardiac lesion. The mitral and aortic valves are most commonly involved. Congenital heart disease is present in 10% to 20% of cases, and rheumatic heart disease is present in less than 15% of cases. The risk of infective endocarditis from mitral valve prolapse is low, but the prevalence of mitral valve prolapse makes it the most common underlying cardiac condition. Infective endocarditis may present with acute or subacute manifestations, depending on the virulence of the infecting organism. The diagnosis of infective endocarditis is often difficult and is based on clinical, microbiologic, and echocardiographic findings. Diagnostic criteria have been developed to aid the clinician in the diagnosis of infective endocarditis (Tables 14-5 and 14-6).

- The risk of infective endocarditis from mitral valve prolapse is low, but the prevalence of mitral valve prolapse makes it the most common underlying cardiac condition.
- Diagnostic criteria have been developed to aid in the diagnosis of infective endocarditis.

Microorganisms causing native valve infective endocarditis include viridans group streptococci (i.e., *Streptococcus sanguis*, *S. mutans*, and *S. mitis*), 30% to 40% of cases; enterococci (i.e., *Enterococcus faecalis* and *E. faecium*), 5% to 18%; other streptococci (i.e., *Streptococcus bovis* and *S. pneumoniae*), 15% to 25%; *Staphylococcus aureus*, 10% to 27%; coagulase-negative staphylococci, 1% to 3%; gram-negative bacilli, 1.5% to 13%; fungi, 2% to 4%; miscellaneous bacteria, less than 5%; mixed infections, 1% to 2%; and "culture-negative," less than 5% to 24%.

- The organisms most commonly involved in native valve infective endocarditis are viridans group streptococci.

Treatment of native valve infective endocarditis includes an emphasis on short-course therapy in patients with uncomplicated left-sided native valve infective endocarditis caused by penicillin-susceptible viridans group streptococci. For enterococcal endocarditis, combination therapy with penicillin G or ampicillin in addition to gentamicin is recommended. Testing for high-level aminoglycoside resistance (gentamicin, >500 μg/mL; streptomycin, >2,000 μg/mL) and penicillin and vancomycin resistance is mandatory.

Table 14-7 lists the recommended treatment regimens for native valve infective endocarditis.

Prosthetic Valve Infective Endocarditis

Prosthetic valve infective endocarditis occurs in up to 3% to 6% of patients with a prosthetic cardiac valve. Some studies suggest that the aortic valve is affected more often than the mitral valve. Early-onset endocarditis is defined as infection occurring 2 months or less after implantation, and late-onset endocarditis is infection occurring more than 2 months postoperatively. Early infection tends to have a more acute presentation. Microorganisms that cause prosthetic valve endocarditis are outlined in Table 14-8. Treatment regimens for prosthetic valve infective endocarditis are given in Table 14-9.

Additional Information About Infective Endocarditis

- Transthoracic echocardiography (TTE) and transesophageal echocardiography (TEE) visualize vegetations in approximately 60% and 90% of patients, respectively. TEE is superior to TTE for diagnosing complications of infective endocarditis such as cardiac abscesses and perivalvular extension.
- Infective endocarditis in injection drug users is caused by *S. aureus* (60%), streptococci (16%), gram-negative bacilli (13.5%), polymicrobial infection (8.1%), and *Corynebacterium JK* (1.4%). *Candida* spp. endocarditis also occurs in this patient population. Tricuspid valve involvement is common. Short-course (2 weeks) therapy with a penicillinase-resistant penicillin with or without an aminoglycoside or 4-week oral regimens with a fluoroquinolone and rifampin may be as effective as longer courses of therapy in uncomplicated right-sided endocarditis due to methicillin-susceptible *S. aureus* in injection drug users, irrespective of whether the patient has human immunodeficiency virus (HIV).
- "Culture-negative" endocarditis may be the result of previous use of antibiotics (most common) and endocarditis due to the following organisms: HACEK organisms,

Table 14-5   Duke Criteria for the Diagnosis of Infective Endocarditis

Definite infective endocarditis
  Pathologic criteria
    Microorganisms: demonstrated by culture *or* histology in vegetation, *or* in vegetation that has embolized, *or* in an
      intracardiac abscess, *or*
    Pathologic lesions: vegetation or intracardiac abscess present, confirmed by histology showing active endocarditis
  Clinical criteria, using specific definitions listed in Table 14-6
    2 major criteria, *or*
    1 major and 3 minor criteria, *or*
    5 minor criteria

Possible infective endocarditis
  Findings consistent with infective endocarditis that fall short of "definite," but not "rejected"

Rejected
  Firm alternative diagnosis for manifestations of endocarditis, *or*
  Resolution of manifestations of endocarditis, with antibiotic therapy for 4 days or less, *or*
  No pathologic evidence of infective endocarditis at surgery or autopsy, after antibiotic therapy for 4 days or less

From Durack DT, Lukes AS, Bright DK, et al: New criteria for diagnosis of infective endocarditis: utilization of specific echocardiographic findings. Am
J Med 1994;96:200-209. By permission of Excerpta Medica.

Table 14-6   Definitions of Terminology Used in the Proposed New Criteria

Major criteria
  1. Positive blood culture for infective endocarditis
     a. Typical microorganism for infective endocarditis from two separate blood cultures
        1) Viridans group streptococci,* *Streptococcus bovis*, HACEK[†] group, *or*
        2) Community-acquired *Staphylococcus aureus* or enterococci, in the absence of a primary focus, *or*
     b. Persistently positive blood cultures, defined as recovery of a microorganism consistent with infective endocarditis from:
        1) Blood cultures drawn more than 12 hours apart, *or*
        2) All of three or a majority of four or more separate blood cultures, with first and last drawn at least 1 hour apart
  2. Evidence of endocardial involvement
     a. Positive echocardiogram for infective endocarditis
        1) Oscillating intracardiac mass, on valve or supporting structures, *or* in the path of regurgitant jets, *or* on implanted
           material, in the absence of an alternative anatomical explanation, *or*
        2) Abscess, *or*
        3) New partial dehiscence of prosthetic valve, *or*
     b. New valvular regurgitation (increase or change in preexisting murmur not sufficient)

Minor criteria
  1. Predisposition: predisposing heart condition *or* intravenous drug use
  2. Fever: 38.0°C (100.4°F)
  3. Vascular phenomena: major arterial emboli, septic pulmonary infarcts, mycotic aneurysm, intracranial hemorrhage,
     conjunctival hemorrhages, Janeway lesions
  4. Immunologic phenomena: glomerulonephritis, Osler nodes, Roth spots, rheumatoid factor
  5. Microbiologic evidence: positive blood culture but not meeting major criteria as noted previously[‡] *or* serologic evidence of
     active infection with organisms consistent with infective endocarditis
  6. Echocardiogram: consistent with infective endocarditis but not meeting major criteria as noted previously

*Including nutritionally variant strains.
[†]HACEK, *Haemophilus* spp., *Actinobacillus actinomycetemcomitans, Cardiobacterium hominis, Eikenella* spp., and *Kingella kingae.*
[‡]Excluding single positive cultures for coagulase-negative staphylococci and organisms that do not cause endocarditis.
From Durack DT, Lukes AS, Bright DK, et al: New criteria for diagnosis of infective endocarditis: utilization of specific echocardiographic findings. Am
J Med 1994;96:200-209. By permission of Excerpta Medica.

nutritionally variant streptococci (i.e., *Abiotrophia* spp.), *Neisseria* spp., *Listeria monocytogenes*, *Brucella* spp., fungi, mycobacteria, *Legionella* spp., *Coxiella burnetii*, *Chlamydia* spp., *Mycoplasma* spp., *Nocardia* spp., *Rothia dentocariosa*, and *Bartonella* spp.

Surgical Therapy

If cardiac valve replacement is needed, it should not be delayed to allow additional days of antimicrobial therapy. Surgical treatment is often indicated in cases of congestive heart failure refractory to medical management. Other generally accepted indications for cardiac valve replacement include evidence of more than one serious systemic embolic episode, uncontrolled bacteremia despite effective antimicrobial therapy, and inadequate antimicrobial therapy. Other indications include invasive perivalvular infection as manifested by abscess or fistula on echocardiography, new or persistent electrocardiographic changes, persistent unexplained fever, fungal endocarditis, and relapse of appropriately treated prosthetic valve endocarditis due to penicillin-sensitive streptococci.

- Surgical treatment is indicated in cases of congestive heart failure refractory to medical management.
- Intractable congestive heart failure is the most common indication for cardiac valve replacement.

Prevention

Most cases of infective endocarditis are not due to invasive procedures. The incidence of endocarditis after invasive procedures is low, and the reported efficacy, in large retrospective studies, of antimicrobial prophylaxis in preventing infective endocarditis is approximately 50%. The lowest-risk group for which antibiotic prophylaxis is currently recommended is patients with mitral valve prolapse with a cardiac murmur or echocardiographic evidence of regurgitation or thickened leaflets. American Heart Association guidelines for the prevention of bacterial endocarditis after invasive dental and medical procedures have been published (JAMA 1997;277:1794-1801). Significant changes from prior guidelines include the following for oral or dental procedures that require prophylaxis: the initial dose of amoxicillin has been reduced to 2.0 g, a follow-up antibiotic dose is not recommended, and erythromycin is not recommended for penicillin-allergic persons (Table 14-10 and 14-11).

- Significant changes from prior guidelines include the following for oral or dental procedures that require prophylaxis: the initial dose of amoxicillin has been reduced to 2.0 g, a follow-up antibiotic dose is not recommended, and erythromycin is not recommended for penicillin-allergic persons.

MENINGITIS

Bacterial Meningitis

The incidence of bacterial meningitis is estimated to be 3.0 cases per 100,000 person-years. The overall case fatality rate was 25% in a report of 443 cases of bacterial meningitis in adults between 1962 and 1988. Forty percent of cases were nosocomial. Common predisposing conditions for community-acquired meningitis include acute otitis media, altered immune states, alcoholism, pneumonia, diabetes mellitus, sinusitis, and a cerebrospinal fluid leak. Risk factors for death among adults with community-acquired meningitis include age 60 years or older, obtundation on admission, and occurrence of seizures within 24 hours of symptom onset. In 66% of patients, fever, nuchal rigidity, and altered mental status are present (N Engl J Med 1993;328:21-28).

Typical initial cerebrospinal fluid characteristics include a cell count of 1,000 to 5,000/μL (range, <100-10,000) and a glucose value less than 40 mg/dL or a cerebrospinal fluid–serum glucose ratio less than 0.31. The leukocyte differential is more likely to show a predominance of polymorphonuclear neutrophils. The Gram stain is positive in 60% to 90% of cases. Countercurrent immunoelectrophoresis or latex agglutination tests are useful for the detection of *Haemophilus influenzae* type B, *S. pneumoniae*, and *Neisseria meningitidis* types A, B, C, and Y, *Escherichia coli* K1, and group B streptococci. Cerebrospinal fluid cultures are positive in 70% to 85% of cases. Blood cultures often are positive. Polymerase chain reaction has been used to diagnose meningitis due to *L. monocytogenes* and *N. meningitidis*.

Organisms most commonly causing community-acquired meningitis in adults are *S. pneumoniae* (38%), *N. meningitidis* (14%), *L. monocytogenes* (11%), streptococci (7%), *S. aureus* (5%), *H. influenzae* (4%), and gram-negative bacilli (4%).

In some studies, dexamethasone has decreased the incidence of neurologic sequelae or sensorineural hearing loss in children with bacterial meningitis due to *H. influenzae*. A prospective, randomized, double-blind, multicenter trial showed that adjunctive treatment with dexamethasone, administered 15 to 20 minutes before or with the first dose of antibiotic, reduced the risk of an unfavorable outcome and death in adults with acute bacterial meningitis. The beneficial effect was most notable among patients with pneumococcal meningitis.

- Risk factors for death in bacterial meningitis: age 60 years or older, decreased mental status at admission, seizures within 24 hours of symptom onset.
- Gram stains of cerebrospinal fluid are positive in 60%-90% of cases.
- Organisms most commonly causing community-acquired infection in adults: *S. pneumoniae*, *N. meningitidis*, *H. influenzae*, and *L. monocytogenes*.

Table 14-7 Treatment of Native Valve Infective Endocarditis

Microorganisms	Therapy*	Alternative therapy*
Penicillin-sensitive viridans group streptococci and *Streptococcus bovis* (MIC, ≤0.1 µg/mL)	Aqueous crystalline penicillin G, 12-18 × 10⁶ U/24 h IV either continuously or in six equally divided doses for 4 wk *Or* Ceftriaxone sodium 2 g IV or IM for 4 wk‡ *Or* Aqueous penicillin G, 12-18 × 10⁶ U/24 h IV either continuously or in six equally divided doses for 2 wk *Plus* Gentamicin sulfate,§ 1 mg/kg IV or IM every 8 h for 2 wk	Vancomycin,† 30 mg/kg IV in two equally divided doses, not to exceed 2 g/24 h unless serum levels are monitored for 4 wk Vancomycin therapy is recommended for patients allergic to β-lactams (immediate-type hypersensitivity); serum concentration of vancomycin should be obtained 1 h after completion of the infusion and should be in the range of 30-45 µg/mL for twice-daily dosing
Relatively penicillin-resistant viridans group streptococci (MIC, >0.1 µg/mL and <0.5 µg/mL)	Aqueous crystalline penicillin G, 18 × 10⁶ U/24 h IV either continuously or in six equally divided doses for 4 wk *Plus* Gentamicin sulfate,§ 1 mg/kg IV or IM every 8 h for 2 wk	Vancomycin,† 30 mg/kg IV in two equally divided doses, not to exceed 2 g/24 h unless serum levels are monitored for 4 wk Vancomycin therapy is recommended for patients allergic to β-lactams (immediate-type hypersensitivity); serum concentration of vancomycin should be obtained 1 h after completion of the infusion and should be in the range of 30-45 µg/mL for twice-daily dosing
Enterococci (gentamicin- or vancomycin-susceptible) or viridans group streptococci with MIC ≥0.5 µg/mL or nutritionally variant streptococci (All enterococci causing endocarditis must be tested for antimicrobial susceptibility in order to select optimal therapy)	Aqueous crystalline penicillin G, 18-30 × 10⁶ U/24 h IV either continuously or in six equally divided doses for 4-6 wk *Or* Ampicillin sodium 12 g/24 h IV either continuously or in six equally divided doses *Plus* Gentamicin sulfate,§ 1 mg/kg IV or IM every 8 h for 4-6 wk (4-wk therapy recommended for patients with symptoms ≤3 mo in duration; 6-wk therapy recommended for patients with symptoms >3 mo in duration)	Vancomycin,† 30 mg/kg IV in two equally divided doses, not to exceed 2 g/24 h unless serum levels are monitored for 4-6 wk *Plus* Gentamicin,§ 1 mg/kg IV or IM every 8 h for 4-6 wk Vancomycin therapy is recommended for patients allergic to β-lactams (immediate-type hypersensitivity); serum concentration of vancomycin should be obtained 1 h after completion of the infusion and should be in the range of 30-45 µg/mL for twice-daily dosing Cephalosporins are not acceptable alternatives for patients allergic to penicillin
Staphylococcus aureus‖ Methicillin-sensitive	Nafcillin sodium or oxacillin sodium, 2.0 g IV every 4 h for 4-6 wk *Plus* Gentamicin sulfate (optional),§ 1 mg/kg every 8 h IV or IM for first 3-5 days. Benefit of additional aminoglycoside has not been established	Cefazolin (or other first-generation cephalosporins in equivalent dosages), 2 g IV every 8 h for 4-6 wk *Plus* Gentamicin (optional),§ 1 mg/kg every 8 h IV or IM for first 3-5 days Cephalosporins should be avoided in patients with immediate-type hypersensitivity to penicillin Vancomycin,† 30 mg/kg IV in two equally divided doses, not to exceed 2 g/24 h unless serum levels are monitored for 4-6 wk Vancomycin therapy is recommended for patients allergic to β-lactams (immediate-type hypersensitivity); serum concentration of vancomycin should be obtained 1 h after

Table 14-7 continued

Microorganisms	Therapy*	Alternative therapy*
		completion of the infusion and should be in the range of 30-45 µg/mL for twice-daily dosing
Methicillin-resistant	Vancomycin,[†] 30 mg/kg IV in two equally divided doses, not to exceed 2 g/24 h unless serum levels are monitored for 4-6 wk	Consult infectious diseases specialist
HACEK group	Ceftriaxone sodium, 2 g IV or IM for 4 wk[†] *Or* Ampicillin,[¶] 12 g/24 h IV either continuously or in six divided doses for 4 wk *Plus* Gentamicin sulfate,[§] 1 mg/kg IV or IM every 8 h for 4 wk Cefotaxime sodium or other third-generation cephalosporins may be substituted	Consult infectious diseases specialist
Neisseria gonorrhoeae	Ceftriaxone, 1-2 g every 24 h for ≥4 wk	Aqueous crystalline penicillin G, 20×10^6 U/24 h IV either continuously or in six equally divided doses for 4 wk, for penicillin-susceptible isolates
Gram-negative bacilli	Most effective single drug or combination of drugs IV for 4-6 wk	
Urgent empiric treatment for culture-negative endocarditis	Vancomycin,[†] 30 mg/kg IV in two equally divided doses, not to exceed 2 g/24 h unless serum levels are monitored for 6 wk *Plus* Gentamicin sulfate,[‡] 1.0 mg/kg IV every 8 h for 6 wk	
Fungal endocarditis	Amphotericin B *Plus* Flucytosine (optional) *Plus* Cardiac valve replacement (flucytosine levels should be monitored)	

HACEK, *Haemophilus* spp., *Actinobacillus actinomycetemcomitans, Cardiobacterium hominis, Eikenella* spp., and *Kingella kingae*; IM, intramuscularly; IV, intravenously; MIC, minimal inhibitory concentration.

*Dosages recommended are for patients with normal renal function.

[†]Vancomycin dosage should be reduced in patients with impaired renal function. Vancomycin given on an mg/kg basis produces higher serum concentrations in obese patients than in lean patients. Therefore, in obese patients, dosing should be based on ideal body weight. Each dose of vancomycin should be infused over at least 1 h to reduce the risk of the histamine-release "red man" syndrome.

[‡]Patients should be notified that IM injection of ceftriaxone is painful.

[§]Dosing of gentamicin on an mg/kg basis produces higher serum concentrations in obese patients than in lean patients. Therefore, in obese patients, dosing should be based on ideal body weight. (Ideal body weight for men is 50 kg + 2.3 kg per inch over 5 feet, and ideal body weight for women is 45.5 kg + 2.3 kg per inch over 5 feet.) Relative contraindications to the use of gentamicin are age older than 65 years, renal impairment, or impairment of the eighth nerve. Other potentially nephrotoxic agents (such as nonsteroidal anti-inflammatory drugs) should be used cautiously in patients receiving gentamicin.

[||]For treatment of endocarditis due to penicillin-susceptible staphylococci (MIC, <0.1 µg/mL), aqueous crystalline penicillin G, $12\text{-}18 \times 10^6$ U/24 h IV either continuously or in six equally divided doses for 4-6 wk can be used instead of nafcillin or oxacillin. Shorter antibiotic courses have been effective in some injection drug users with right-sided endocarditis due to *S. aureus*. The routine use of rifampin is not recommended for the treatment of native valve staphylococcal endocarditis.

[¶]Ampicillin should not be used if laboratory tests show β-lactamase production.

Data from Wilson WR, Karchmer AW, Dajani AS, et al: Antibiotic treatment of adults with infective endocarditis due to streptococci, enterococci, staphylococci and HACEK microorganisms. JAMA 1995;274:1706-1713; and Modified from Steckelberg JM, Giuliani ER, Wilson WR: Infective endocarditis. *In* Cardiology: Fundamentals and Practice. Vol. 2. Second edition. Edited by ER Giuliani, V Fuster, BJ Gersh, et al. St. Louis, Mosby Year Book, 1991, pp 1739-1772. By permission of Mayo Foundation.

Table 14-8   Organisms That Cause Prosthetic Valve Endocarditis

Organism	Time of onset postoperatively, %		
	≤2 mo	>2-12 mo	>12 mo
Coagulase-negative staphylococci	31	34	11
Staphylococcus aureus	23	13	18
Enterococci	9	13	11
Streptococci	1.5	10	31
Gram-negative bacilli	14	3	6
Diphtheroids	7	0	3
Fastidious gram-negative bacilli*	0	0	6
Fungi	9	6	1
Culture negative	3	13	8
Miscellaneous	3	6	5

Haemophilus spp., *Cardiobacterium hominis, Actinobacillus actinomycetemcomitans.*
From Karchmer AW: Infections of prosthetic valves and intravascular devices. *In* Principles and Practice of Infectious Diseases. Vol. 1. Fifth edition. Edited by GL Mandell, JE Bennett, R Dolin. Philadelphia, Churchill Livingstone, 2000, pp 903-917. By permission of Elsevier.

Table 14-9   Treatment of Prosthetic Valve Infective Endocarditis

Organism	Therapy*	Alternative therapy/comments
Staphylococcus aureus or coagulase-negative staphylococci: methicillin-resistant	Vancomycin,[†] 30 mg/kg IV in two equally divided doses, not to exceed 2 g/24 h unless serum levels are monitored for ≥6 wk *Plus* Rifampin,[‡] 300 mg PO every 8 h for ≥6 wk *Plus* Gentamicin sulfate,[§] 1 mg/kg IV or IM every 8 h for first 2 wk of therapy. (If organism is not susceptible to gentamicin, ciprofloxacin may be substituted if the organism is susceptible in vitro)	Rifampin increases the amount of warfarin sodium required for antithrombotic therapy
Staphylococcus aureus or coagulase-negative staphylococci: methicillin-susceptible	Nafcillin sodium or oxacillin sodium, 2 g IV every 4 h for ≥6 wk *Plus* Rifampin,[‡] 300 mg orally every 8 h for ≥6 wk *Plus* Gentamicin sulfate,[§] 1 mg/kg IV or IM every 8 h for first 2 wk of therapy. (If organism is not susceptible to gentamicin, ciprofloxacin may be substituted if the organism is susceptible in vitro)	Rifampin increases the amount of warfarin sodium required for antithrombotic therapy First-generation cephalosporins or vancomycin should be used in patients allergic to β-lactams Cephalosporins should be avoided in patients with immediate-type hypersensitivity to penicillin or to methicillin-resistant staphylococci

Table 14-9   continued

Organism	Therapy*	Alternative therapy/comments
Enterococci (gentamicin- or vancomycin-susceptible) or viridans group streptococci or nutritionally variant streptococci or *Streptococcus bovis* (All streptococci causing endocarditis must be tested for antimicrobial susceptibility in order to select optimal therapy)	Aqueous crystalline penicillin G, $18\text{-}30 \times 10^6$ U/24 h IV either continuously or in six equally divided doses for 6 wk *Or* Ampicillin sodium, 12 g/24 h IV either continuously or in six equally divided doses *Plus* Gentamicin sulfate,[§] 1 mg/kg IV or IM every 8 h for 6 wk	Vancomycin,[†] 30 mg/kg IV in two equally divided doses, not to exceed 2 g/24 h unless serum levels are monitored for 4-6 wk *Plus* Gentamicin sulfate,[§] 1 mg/kg IV or IM every 8 h for 4-6 wk Vancomycin therapy is recommended for patients allergic to β-lactams (immediate-type hypersensitivity); serum concentration of vancomycin should be obtained 1 h after completion of the infusion and should be in the range of 30-45 μg/mL for twice-daily dosing Cephalosporins are not acceptable alternatives for patients allergic to penicillin

IM, intramuscularly; IV, intravenously; PO, orally.

*Dosages recommended are for patients with normal renal function.

[†]Vancomycin dosage should be reduced in patients with impaired renal function. Vancomycin given on an mg/kg basis produces higher serum concentrations in obese patients than in lean patients. Therefore, in obese patients, dosing should be based on ideal body weight. Each dose of vancomycin should be infused over at least 1 h to reduce the risk of the histamine-release "red man" syndrome.

[‡]Rifampin plays a unique role in the eradication of staphylococcal infection involving prosthetic material; combination therapy is essential to prevent emergence of rifampin resistance.

[§]Dosing of gentamicin on an mg/kg basis will produce higher serum concentrations in obese patients than in lean patients. Therefore, in obese patients, dosing should be based on ideal body weight. (Ideal body weight for men is 50 kg + 2.3 kg per inch over 5 feet, and ideal body weight for women is 45.5 kg + 2.3 kg per inch over 5 feet.) Relative contraindications to the use of gentamicin are age older than 65 years, renal impairment, or impairment of the eighth nerve. Other potentially nephrotoxic agents (such as nonsteroidal anti-inflammatory drugs) should be used cautiously in patients receiving gentamicin.

Data from Wilson MR, Karchmer AW, Dajani AS, et al: Antibiotic treatment of adults with infective endocarditis due to streptococci, enterococci, staphylococci, and HACEK microorganisms. JAMA 1995;274:1706-1713.

The causative organisms, affected age groups, and predisposing factors in bacterial meningitis are shown in Table 14-12, and empiric treatment in various age and patient groups is outlined in Table 14-13. Immunocompromised hosts, pregnant women, and elderly patients should receive an empiric antibiotic regimen that includes coverage for *L. monocytogenes*. High-dose ampicillin is the treatment of choice. An aminoglycoside can be added to ampicillin if *L. monocytogenes* meningitis is confirmed. High-dose intravenous trimethoprim-sulfamethoxazole can be used in patients with a penicillin allergy. *L. monocytogenes* can be mistakenly reported as a diphtheroid on cerebrospinal fluid culture and labeled a contaminant.

● Immunocompromised hosts, pregnant women, and the elderly should receive an empiric antibiotic program that includes high-dose ampicillin to cover *L. monocytogenes*.

Meningococcal Meningitis

Meningitis often occurs in patients who are carriers of meningococci in the nasopharynx. Terminal component complement deficiencies predispose to repeated episodes of infection. Serotypes B, C, and Y cause most of the endemic disease in the United States. Many patients have a petechial rash. The pathogenesis of Waterhouse-Friderichsen syndrome (i.e., acute hemorrhagic necrosis of the adrenal glands causing primary adrenocortical insufficiency) is related to disseminated

Table 14-10 American Heart Association Prophylactic Regimens to Prevent Infective Endocarditis After Dental, Oral, Respiratory Tract, or Esophageal Procedures in Adults

Situation	Agent	Regimen
Standard general prophylaxis	Amoxicillin	2.0 g PO 1 h before procedure
Unable to take oral medications	Ampicillin	2.0 g IM or IV within 30 min before procedure
Allergic to penicillin	Clindamycin	600 mg PO 1 h before procedure
	or	
	Cephalexin or cefadroxil*	2.0 g PO 1 h before procedure
	or	
	Azithromycin	500 mg PO 1 h before procedure
	or	
	Clarithromycin	
Allergic to penicillin and unable to take oral medications	Clindamycin	600 mg IV within 30 min before procedure
	or	
	Cefazolin*	1.0 g IM or IV within 30 min before procedure

IM, intramuscularly; IV, intravenously; PO, orally.
*Cephalosporins should not be used in persons with immediate-type hypersensitivity reaction (urticaria, angioedema, anaphylaxis) to penicillins.
From Osmon DR: Antimicrobial prophylaxis in adults. Mayo Clin Proc 2000;75:98-109. By permission of Mayo Foundation for Medical Education and Research.

Table 14-11 American Heart Association Prophylactic Regimens to Prevent Infective Endocarditis After Genitourinary or Gastrointestinal (Excluding Esophageal) Procedures in Adults

Situation	Agent	Regimen*
High-risk patients[†]	Ampicillin plus gentamicin	Ampicillin 2.0 g IM or IV plus gentamicin 1.5 mg/kg (not to exceed 120 mg) within 30 min of starting procedure; 6 h later, ampicillin 1 g IM or IV or amoxicillin 1 g PO
High-risk patients allergic to ampicillin/ amoxicillin	Vancomycin plus gentamicin	Vancomycin 1.0 g IV over 1-2 h plus gentamicin 1.5 mg/kg IM or IV (not to exceed 120 mg); complete injection/infusion within 30 min of starting procedure
Moderate-risk patients[‡]	Amoxicillin or ampicillin	Amoxicillin 2.0 g PO 1 h before procedure, or ampicillin 2.0 g IM or IV within 30 min of starting procedure
Moderate-risk patients allergic to ampicillin/ amoxicillin	Vancomycin	Vancomycin 1.0 g IV over 1-2 h; complete infusion within 30 min of starting procedure

IM, intramuscularly; IV, intravenously; PO, orally.
*No second dose of vancomycin or gentamicin is recommended.
[†]High-risk patients: prosthetic cardiac valves, including bioprosthetic and homograft valves; previous bacterial endocarditis; complex cyanotic congenital heart disease (e.g., single ventricle states, transposition of great arteries, tetralogy of Fallot); surgically constructed systemic pulmonary shunts or conduits.
[‡]Moderate-risk patients: selected congenital cardiac malformations, acquired valvular dysfunction (e.g., rheumatic heart disease), hypertrophic cardiomyopathy, mitral valve prolapse with regurgitation or thickened leaflets or both.
From Osmon DR: Antimicrobial prophylaxis in adults. Mayo Clin Proc 2000;75:98-109. By permission of Mayo Foundation for Medical Education and Research.

intravascular coagulation. Treatment is with penicillin G. If a patient is allergic to penicillin, high-dose ceftriaxone or cefotaxime can be used. If the risk of the carrier state is high (close contacts of the index case, hospital workers with substantial respiratory exposure), chemoprophylaxis should be given. Rifampin, ceftriaxone, and ciprofloxacin (use only in patients 18 years or older) have been used. The carrier state is not eliminated by penicillin. Immunization of certain populations (e.g., military recruits, college students living in dormitories, Hajj pilgrims, patients with terminal complement component deficiencies or asplenia) is also of benefit. The meningococcal vaccine contains polysaccharides of groups A, C, Y, and W-135.

- In meningococcal meningitis, terminal component complement deficiencies predispose to repeated episodes of infection.
- If the risk of the carrier state is high (household contacts), rifampin or ciprofloxacin should be used for prophylaxis.

Aseptic Meningitis

This is a syndrome characterized by an acute onset of meningeal symptoms, fever, cerebrospinal fluid pleocytosis (usually lymphocytes), and negative bacterial cultures from the cerebrospinal fluid. Noninfectious causes of aseptic meningitis include medications, such as nonsteroidal anti-inflammatory drugs and trimethoprim-sulfamethoxazole; chemical meningitis; and neoplastic meningitis. Aseptic meningitis is most often caused by viruses. Common causes include enteroviruses (most common in summer; cause 85%-95% of cases in which a pathogen is identified), mumps virus (most common in winter and spring; decreased incidence with use of vaccine), and others, including arboviruses, lymphocytic choriomeningitis virus (contact with rodents), herpes simplex virus types 1 and 2 (often recurrent), human herpesviruses, cytomegalovirus, HIV (acute retroviral syndrome), varicella-zoster virus, Epstein-Barr virus, and Colorado tick fever virus.

- Characteristics of aseptic meningitis: meningeal symptoms, fever, cerebrospinal fluid pleocytosis, negative bacterial cultures.
- The cause is most often viral.

SEXUALLY TRANSMITTED DISEASES

Neisseria gonorrhoeae

Common uncomplicated infections include urethritis and cervicitis. Symptoms are indistinguishable from those of

Table 14-12 Organisms Involved, Affected Age Groups, and Predisposing Factors in Bacterial Meningitis

Organism	Age group	Comment	Predisposing factors
Streptococcus pneumoniae	Any age, but often elderly	Most common cause of recurrent meningitis in adults	Cerebrospinal fluid leak, alcoholism, splenectomy, functional asplenia, multiple myeloma, hypogammaglobulinemia, Hodgkin disease, HIV
Neisseria meningitidis	Infants to 40 y	Petechial rash is common Epidemics occur in closed populations	Terminal component complement deficiency
Haemophilus influenzae type B	>Neonate to 6 y	Significant decrease in incidence since licensure of H. influenzae B vaccine	Hypogammaglobulinemia in adults, HIV,* splenectomy, functional asplenia
Escherichia coli, group B streptococci	Neonates		Maternal colonization
Gram-negative bacilli	Any age	Staphylococcus aureus and coagulase-negative staphylococci also common after neuro-surgical procedure	Neurosurgical procedures, bacteremia due to urinary tract infection, pneumonia, etc., Strongyloides hyperinfection syndrome
Listeria monocytogenes	Neonates; immuno-suppressed		

HIV, human immunodeficiency virus.

Table 14-13   Empiric Therapy for Bacterial Meningitis

Age group/patient group	Common pathogens	Antimicrobial therapy
0-4 wk	Group B streptococci, *Escherichia coli*, *Listeria monocytogenes*, *Klebsiella pneumoniae*, *Enterococcus* spp., *Salmonella* spp.	Ampicillin plus cefotaxime or ampicillin plus an aminoglycoside
4-12 wk	Group B streptococci, *E. coli*, *L. monocytogenes*, *Haemophilus influenzae*, *Streptococcus pneumoniae*, *Neisseria meningitidis*	Ampicillin plus cefotaxime or ceftriaxone
3 months-18 y	*H. influenzae*, *N. meningitidis*, *S. pneumoniae*	Cefotaxime or ceftriaxone or ampicillin plus chloramphenicol
18-50 y*	*H. influenzae*, *S. pneumoniae*	Cefotaxime or ceftriaxone ± ampicillin
Immunocompromised host	*S. pneumoniae*, *N. meningitidis*, *L. monocytogenes*, aerobic gram-negative bacilli (including *Pseudomonas aeruginosa*)	Vancomycin plus ampicillin plus ceftazidime
Basilar skull fracture	*S. pneumoniae*, *H. influenzae*, group A β-hemolytic streptococci	Cefotaxime or ceftriaxone
Post-neurosurgery	Coagulase-negative staphylococci, *Staphylococcus aureus*, aerobic gram-negative bacilli (including *P. aeruginosa*)	Vancomycin plus ceftazidime

*Vancomycin should be added to empiric therapeutic regimens when highly penicillin-resistant or cephalosporin-resistant strains of *S. pneumoniae* are suspected.
Modified from Tunkel AR, Scheld WM: Central nervous system infections. *In* A Practical Approach to Infectious Diseases. Fourth edition. Edited by RE Reese, RF Betts. Boston, Little Brown, 1996, pp 133-183. By permission of the editors and the publisher.

nongonococcal disease. Gram stain and culture or molecular detection formats are required for diagnosis. The asymptomatic carrier state occurs in both males and females, but it is more common in females. Asymptomatic carriers are primarily responsible for continued transmission of the infection. In females, concomitant proctitis is common (rectal cultures should be done in all women). Gonococcal pharyngitis is often asymptomatic. Coexistence of chlamydial infection is common (both conditions should be treated). For diagnosis in males, a Gram stain of urethral exudate showing intracellular gram-negative diplococci has high sensitivity and specificity. Gram staining of cervical exudate has a sensitivity of only 50%, but the specificity is high. Definitive diagnosis requires culture on modified Thayer-Martin medium.

● *N. gonorrhoeae* commonly causes urethritis, cervicitis, pharyngitis, and proctitis.
● Asymptomatic carrier state occurs in both males and females, but it is more common in females.

The prevalence of multiply resistant gonococcal strains is increasing. Resistance to penicillin and tetracycline is frequent. Quinolone-resistant *N. gonorrhoeae* is common in parts of Asia and the Pacific Rim. Quinolones are no longer recommended for the treatment of gonorrhea in Hawaii, and the use of quinolones in California is inadvisable. Primary treatment is ceftriaxone (125 mg intramuscularly), ciprofloxacin (500 mg orally in a single dose), or ofloxacin (400 mg orally in a single dose) plus doxycycline (100 mg orally twice a day for 7 days) or azithromycin (a single 1-g dose). The latest guidelines from the Centers for Disease Control and Prevention list cefixime 400 mg orally in a single dose as a recommended regimen. Unfortunately, the manufacturer stopped making cefixime in July 2002 and it is no longer available. Alternative drugs include spectinomycin 2 g in a single intramuscular dose, ceftizoxime 500 mg in a single intramuscular dose, cefoxitin 2 g in a single intramuscular dose with probenecid 1 g orally, cefotaxime 500 mg in a single intramuscular dose, gatifloxacin 400 mg orally in a single dose, norfloxacin 800 mg orally in a single dose, and lomefloxacin 400 mg orally in a single dose. Pharyngeal infection is best treated with ceftriaxone, ciprofloxacin, or ofloxacin. Spectinomycin, ciprofloxacin, and ofloxacin may not be active against incubating syphilis. Therapy in pregnant patients involves ceftriaxone (125 mg intramuscularly) plus erythromycin base (500 mg orally four times a day for 7 days). Erythromycin estolate is contraindicated during pregnancy because of drug-related hepatotoxicity. Follow-up gonococcal cultures need to be performed only if nonstandard regimens are used. All patients with sexually transmitted diseases should be considered at risk for HIV infection, and testing should be offered. Sexual partners should be offered evaluation and treatment.

- Primary treatment of *N. gonorrhoeae*: ceftriaxone (125 mg intramuscularly) plus doxycycline (100 mg orally twice a day for 7 days) or azithromycin as a single 1-g dose.

Disseminated gonococcemia occurs in 1% to 3% of infected patients and is most likely to occur in females during menstruation (sloughing of endometrium allows access to blood supply, enhanced growth of gonococci due to necrotic tissue, and change in pH). There are two distinct phases. The bacteremic phase may manifest as tenosynovitis (often around the wrists or ankles), skin lesions (usually less than 30 in number), and polyarthralgia. Results of synovial fluid testing are usually negative. The nonbacteremic phase follows in approximately 1 week and may present as monarticular arthritis of the knee, wrist, and ankle; results of joint culture are positive in about 50%. Culture specimens should be obtained from the urethra, cervix, rectum, and pharynx.

- Disseminated gonococcemia is most likely to occur in females during menstruation.
- A bacteremic phase may manifest as tenosynovitis, skin lesions, and arthralgias; joint cultures are usually negative.
- A nonbacteremic phase may present as monarticular arthritis of the knee, wrist, ankle; results of joint cultures are positive in ±50%.

Treatment is with ceftriaxone (1 g intravenously daily for 7-10 days); alternatives include ceftriaxone (for 3 or 4 days or until improvement is noted) followed by ciprofloxacin to complete a course of 7 to 10 days. If the strain is tested and found to be penicillin-susceptible, treatment includes penicillin G (10 million units intravenously daily) for 7 to 10 days or it is given for 3 or 4 days and then oral amoxicillin is used to finish a 7- to 10-day course. If the patient is allergic to cephalosporins, spectinomycin, ciprofloxacin, or ofloxacin can be given. Chlamydial infection can coexist with gonococcal infection and should be treated. For meningitis, treatment includes ceftriaxone (1-2 g intravenously every 12 hours for at least 10-14 days). Alternative drugs are penicillin, if the strain is susceptible, or chloramphenicol. For endocarditis, ceftriaxone or penicillin is used for at least 28 days.

- Treatment of disseminated gonococcal infection: ceftriaxone (1 g intravenously daily for 7-10 days).
- Chlamydial infections can coexist with gonococcal infection and should be treated.

Nongonococcal Urethritis and Cervicitis

The most common etiologic agent is *Chlamydia trachomatis*. Infection is often asymptomatic. Diagnosis can be made with culture, antigen detection, or molecular detection formats. Doxycycline (100 mg twice a day for 7 days) or azithromycin as a single 1-g dose is standard treatment. Women with *C. trachomatis* cervicitis should be rescreened 3 to 4 months after treatment. *Ureaplasma urealyticum, Trichomonas vaginalis, Mycoplasma genitalium,* and herpes simplex virus are less common causes of nongonococcal urethritis. If urethritis does not resolve and reinfection or relapse of a chlamydial infection has been excluded, consider *Trichomonas* or tetracycline-resistant *Ureaplasma* infection, among others. Treatment consists of metronidazole (2 g orally in a single dose) plus erythromycin base (500 mg orally four times a day for 7 days) or erythromycin ethylsuccinate (800 mg orally four times a day for 7 days).

- Nongonococcal urethritis and cervicitis are most commonly caused by *C. trachomatis*.

Herpes Genitalis

Seventy percent to 90% of cases are caused by herpes simplex virus type 2. For the first episode, therapy with acyclovir (400 mg orally three times a day or 200 mg orally five times a day for 7-10 days) or famciclovir (250 mg orally three times a day or valacyclovir 1 g orally twice a day) shortens the duration of pain, viral shedding, and systemic symptoms. If symptoms are severe, acyclovir at a dosage of 5 mg/kg intravenously every 8 hours for 5 to 7 days is used. Topical acyclovir has marginal benefit for decreasing viral shedding and has no effect on symptoms or healing time. For recurrent episodes with severe symptoms, therapy can be started at prodrome or within 1 day of the onset of symptoms (acyclovir, 400 mg orally three times a day, 200 mg orally five times a day, or 800 mg orally twice a day, or famciclovir, 125 mg orally twice a day, or valacyclovir, 500 mg orally twice a day, all for 5 days). Recurrence after therapy is usually not related to the development of in vitro resistance of herpes simplex to acyclovir. For suppression, in selected patients with more than six recurrences a year, acyclovir (400 mg twice a day), famciclovir (250 mg orally twice a day), or valacyclovir (250 mg, 500 mg, or 1 g orally twice a day) is used for up to 1 year. (The recommended dosages for HIV-infected patients are different than the doses listed above.)

Syphilis

The etiologic agent of syphilis is *Treponema pallidum*. It is estimated that half of the cases are not reported. The incidence of syphilis is increased in large cities among sexually active persons, particularly among inner city minority populations and homosexuals.

The fluorescent treponemal antibody absorption (FTA-ABS) test is the most helpful serologic test for the diagnosis of syphilis (Table 14-14). Results of this test are positive before those on VDRL testing, and thus they may be positive without a positive VDRL result in primary syphilis. VDRL results may be negative in 30% of patients with primary syphilis.

- FTA-ABS is the most helpful serologic test for the diagnosis of syphilis.
- VDRL results may be negative in 30% of patients with primary syphilis.

A chancre (clean, indurated ulcer) is the main manifestation of *primary syphilis*. It occurs at the site of inoculation and is usually painless. The incubation period is 3 to 90 days. It should be distinguished from herpes simplex virus and chancroid (painful exudative ulcer, *Haemophilus ducreyi*). Diagnosis is made by darkfield examination.

The manifestations of *secondary syphilis* result from hematogenous dissemination and usually occur 2 to 8 weeks after appearance of the chancre. Constitutional symptoms occur, in addition to rash, mucocutaneous lesions, alopecia, condylomata lata (i.e., a broad and flat verrucous syphilitic lesion located in warm, moist intertriginous areas, especially about the anus and genitals), lymphadenopathy, and various other symptoms and signs. The diagnosis is based on the clinical picture and serologic testing. The condition resolves spontaneously without treatment.

Table 14-14 Laboratory Diagnosis of Syphilis

Syphilis	Test, % positive		
	VDRL	FTA-ABS	MHA-TP
Primary	70	85	50-60
Secondary	99	100	100
Tertiary	70	98	98

*VDRL, Venereal Disease Research Laboratories; FTA-ABS, fluorescent treponemal antibody absorption; MHA-TP, microhemagglutination assay for *Treponema pallidum*.

From Hook EW III: Syphilis. *In* Cecil Textbook of Internal Medicine. Twentieth edition. Edited by JE Bennett, F Plum. Philadelphia, WB Saunders, 1996, pp 1705-1714. By permission of the publisher.

Latent syphilis is the asymptomatic stage after symptoms of secondary syphilis subside. Those that occur after 1 year are classified as late. The diagnosis is based on serologic testing. A cerebrospinal fluid examination before treatment in patients with latent syphilis is indicated in those with neurologic or ophthalmologic abnormalities, in patients with other evidence of active syphilis, at baseline in patients treated with a non-penicillin regimen, before re-treatment of relapses, and in patients with HIV infection.

Tertiary syphilis can involve all body systems (cardiovascular—aortitis involving the ascending aorta, which can cause aneurysms and aortic regurgitation; gummatous osteomyelitis; hepatitis). However, neurosyphilis is the most common manifestation in the United States.

Neurosyphilis is often asymptomatic. Symptomatic disease is divided into several clinical syndromes that may overlap and occur at any time after primary infection. The diagnosis is made from cerebrospinal fluid examination; abnormalities include mononuclear pleocytosis and an increased protein value. VDRL testing of cerebrospinal fluid is only 30% to 70% sensitive. The FTA-ABS test on cerebrospinal fluid is highly sensitive but not specific. Any cerebrospinal fluid abnormality in a patient who is seropositive for syphilis must be investigated. Syndromes include 1) meningovascular syphilis (occurs 4-7 years after infection and presents with focal central nervous system deficits such as stroke or cranial nerve abnormalities) and 2) parenchymatous syphilis (general paresis or tabes dorsalis). Parenchymatous syphilis occurs decades after infection and may present as general paresis (chronic progressive dementia) or as tabes dorsalis (sensory ataxia, lightning pains, autonomic dysfunction, and optic atrophy).

- Neurosyphilis is the most common manifestation in tertiary disease in the United States.
- The diagnosis is made from cerebrospinal fluid examination.
- VDRL testing of cerebrospinal fluid is only 30%-70% sensitive.

Treatment of syphilis is based on whether the disease is early or late. For early syphilis (primary, secondary, or early latent [<1 year]), benzathine penicillin is used—2.4 million units intramuscularly; follow-up serologic testing is done. (Some experts recommend completing three weekly 2.4 million-unit intramuscular doses in patients with HIV infection.) Alternatives are doxycycline (100 mg twice a day for 14 days) or tetracycline (500 mg orally four times a day for 14 days). Erythromycin (500 mg orally four times a day) is less effective.

Treatment for late disease (>1 year in duration, cardiovascular disease, gumma, late latent syphilis) is with benzathine penicillin, 2.4 million units intramuscularly weekly for 3 weeks. Alternatives are doxycycline (100 mg orally twice a day) or tetracycline (500 mg orally four times a day) for 4 weeks.

Treatment for neurosyphilis is with aqueous penicillin G (12-24 million units intravenously per day) for 10 to 14 days or procaine penicillin (2.4 million units intramuscularly per day) plus probenecid (500 mg four times a day) for 10 to 14 days.

Pregnant patients should receive a penicillin-based regimen for treatment of all stages of syphilis. If a pregnant patient has a penicillin allergy, she should be desensitized to penicillin.

For early and secondary syphilis, follow-up clinical and serologic testing should be performed at 6 and 12 months. Re-treatment with three weekly injections of 2.4 million units of benzathine penicillin G should be given to patients with signs or symptoms that persist or whose VDRL result has a sustained fourfold increase in titer. HIV testing should be performed if not done previously. If the VDRL titer does not decrease fourfold by 6 months, consideration also should be given to re-treatment.

Patients with latent syphilis should have a follow-up examination at 6, 12, and 24 months. If the VDRL result increases fourfold, if a high titer (>1:32) fails to decrease fourfold within 12 to 24 months, or if signs or symptoms attributable to syphilis occur, the patient should be examined for neurosyphilis and re-treated.

Follow-up in cases of neurosyphilis should include testing of cerebrospinal fluid every 6 months if cerebrospinal fluid pleocytosis was present initially; this testing is done until results are normal. If the cell count is not decreased at 6 months or if the cerebrospinal fluid is not entirely normal at 2 years, re-treatment should be considered.

Pelvic Inflammatory Disease

In this condition, proximal spread of infection from the endocervix causes endometritis, salpingitis, tubo-ovarian abscess, or pelvic peritonitis in various combinations. Organisms responsible are *N. gonorrhoeae*, *C. trachomatis*, *Mycoplasma hominis*, and various aerobic gram-negative rods and anaerobes. Fitz-Hugh-Curtis syndrome is an acute perihepatitis caused by direct extension of *N. gonorrhoeae* or *C. trachomatis* to the liver capsule. Occasionally, a friction rub can be auscultated over the liver and "violin string" adhesions between the liver capsule and parietal peritoneum can be observed with laparoscopy. *Actinomyces israelii* can be a pathogen in patients with an intrauterine device. Tuberculosis in older women, including postmenopausal women, should be considered. Clinical signs and symptoms include lower abdominal tenderness, adnexal tenderness, cervical motion tenderness, oral temperature more than 38.3°C, abnormal cervical discharge, increased erythrocyte sedimentation rate, and evidence of *N. gonorrhoeae* or *C. trachomatis* infection. Laboratory evidence includes laparoscopic or ultrasound documentation. The emphasis on early diagnosis is meant to decrease the incidence of infertility as a complication of pelvic inflammatory disease.

- In pelvic inflammatory disease, responsible organisms are *N. gonorrhoeae*, *C. trachomatis*, and anaerobes.
- Fitz-Hugh-Curtis syndrome is an acute perihepatitis caused by direct extension of *N. gonorrhoeae* or *C. trachomatis* to the liver capsule.
- The emphasis on early diagnosis is meant to decrease the incidence of infertility as a complication of pelvic inflammatory disease.

Treatment for inpatients includes cefoxitin (2 g intravenously every 6 hours) or cefotetan (2 g intravenously every 12 hours) or clindamycin and gentamicin plus doxycycline (100 mg intravenously every 12 hours) followed by doxycycline (100 mg orally twice a day) for 14 days. For outpatients, treatment is with ofloxacin (400 mg orally twice a day) plus metronidazole (500 mg orally twice a day) or ceftriaxone (250 mg intramuscularly once) or cefoxitin (2 g intramuscularly plus probenecid, 1 g orally as a single dose, or another third-generation cephalosporin) plus doxycycline (100 mg orally twice a day) for 14 days.

Hospitalization is indicated when the outpatient therapy is precluded by severe nausea and vomiting, the diagnosis is uncertain, pelvic abscess or peritonitis is present, the patient is pregnant, the patient is an adolescent, HIV infection is present, or noncompliance is suspected.

Tubo-ovarian abscess may be characterized by an adnexal mass on physical examination or radiographic examination or by failure of antimicrobial therapy. Medical treatment is successful in 50% of cases. Careful follow-up is required.

- Tubo-ovarian abscess is characterized by an adnexal mass on physical examination or radiographic examination or by failure of antimicrobial therapy.

Trichomonas vaginalis

Infection with this organism produces a yellow, purulent discharge in 5% to 40% of cases. Dysuria and dyspareunia occur in 30% to 50% of cases. Petechial lesions on the cervix are noted with colposcopy (strawberry cervix) in 50% of cases. The vaginal pH is usually more than 4.5. The diagnosis is established with wet mount preparation of vaginal secretion (80% sensitive). Culture is done in difficult cases. Treatment is with metronidazole (2 g as a single dose or 500 mg twice a day for 7 days). All partners should be examined and treated if necessary.

- *T. vaginalis* infection often is characterized by yellow, purulent discharge.
- Diagnosis is established with wet mount of vaginal secretion.
- Treatment: metronidazole orally.

Gardnerella vaginalis (Bacterial Vaginosis)

This condition is characterized by a malodorous "fishy" smell and a grayish white discharge that is homogeneous and coats the vaginal walls. Dysuria and pain are relatively uncommon. Organisms associated with the syndrome are *Mobiluncus* spp., *M. hominis*, *G. vaginalis*, and *Prevotella* spp. The diagnosis is determined by excluding *Candida* and *Trichomonas* infections and other sexually transmitted diseases. The following are characteristics of the vaginal secretion: "clue" cells on wet mount examination, pH more than 4.5 and often more than 6.0, and a "fishy" smell when secretion is mixed with KOH (positive "whiff" test). Recommended treatment regimens include metronidazole (500 mg orally twice a day for 7 days) or topical clindamycin cream or metronidazole gel (the clindamycin cream appears less efficacious than the metronidazole regimens). A single 2-g dose of metronidazole or clindamycin, 300 mg orally twice a day for 7 days, is an alternative. Bacterial vaginosis has been associated with adverse pregnancy outcomes. All symptomatic pregnant women should be treated. In pregnant patients, systemic therapy with metronidazole (250 mg orally three times a day for 7 days) or clindamycin (300 mg orally twice a day for 7 days) is recommended rather than topical agents in order to treat organisms in the upper genital tract. Treatment of asymptomatic nonpregnant carriers is not recommended. Some experts recommend treatment of asymptomatic pregnant women at high risk for preterm delivery. Routine treatment of sex partners is not recommended.

- Diagnosis of *G. vaginalis* is established by excluding *Candida* and *Trichomonas* infections and other sexually transmitted diseases.
- Vaginal discharge has "clue" cells, a "fishy" smell when mixed with 10% KOH (positive "whiff" test), and a pH more than 4.5.
- Routine treatment of sex partners is not recommended.

Vulvovaginal Candidiasis

The predominant symptom of this condition is pruritus. It is typically caused by *Candida albicans*. Seventy-five percent of women will have one episode and 40% to 45%, two or more episodes. Usually there is no odor, and discharge is scant, watery, and white. "Cottage cheese curds" may adhere to the vaginal wall. The diagnosis is made by the addition of 10% KOH to the discharge to demonstrate pseudohyphae. Culture may detect an asymptomatic carrier. Treatment is with various topical agents from 1 to 7 days, depending on the dose and agent. Single-dose fluconazole therapy also is available, although the cost and potential toxicities of the oral azoles must be considered. Multiple-dose oral azole therapy also is used for severe, refractory cases. In severe or recurrent cases, consider HIV infection or drug-resistant candidal species.

- In vulvovaginal candidiasis, "cottage cheese curds" may adhere to the vaginal wall.
- In severe or recurrent cases, consider HIV infection.

Epididymitis

This condition usually is unilateral. It should be distinguished from testicular torsion. In young, sexually active men, *C. trachomatis* and *N. gonorrhoeae* are the common pathogens. In older men, aerobic gram-negative rods and enterococci predominate. Urologic abnormality is more common in this population than in younger men. Doxycycline, 100 mg orally twice a day for 7 days, plus ceftriaxone, 250 mg intramuscularly, is the treatment of choice in young males. In older men, treatment is individualized on the basis of results of urine Gram stain, results of culture, local susceptibility patterns, and presence of recent instrumentation.

- Epididymitis is usually unilateral; it should be distinguished from testicular torsion.
- In young, sexually active men, *C. trachomatis* and *N. gonorrhoeae* are the common pathogens.

GASTROINTESTINAL INFECTION

Bacterial Diarrhea

The principal causes of toxigenic diarrhea are listed in Table 14-15, and those of invasive diarrhea are listed in Table 14-16. Fecal leukocytes usually are absent in toxigenic diarrhea. In invasive diarrhea, fecal leukocytes usually are present. The travel history is often important.

Campylobacter jejuni is being recognized with increasing frequency as a common cause of bacterial diarrhea. Approximately 10% to 30% of cases of Guillain-Barré syndrome are preceded by *C. jejuni* infection. Outbreaks are associated with consumption of unpasteurized dairy products and undercooked poultry. The incidence of disease peaks in summer and early fall. Diarrhea may be bloody. Fever usually is present. The diagnosis is established by isolation of the organism from stool; a special medium is required. Treatment is with erythromycin. Alternatives are ciprofloxacin and norfloxacin (emergence of resistance to fluoroquinolones has been reported). Supportive care also is needed.

Table 14-15   Bacterial Diarrhea: Toxigenic

Organism	Onset after ingestion, h	Preformed toxin	Fever present	Vomiting predominates
Staphylococcus aureus	2-6	Yes	No	Yes
Clostridium perfringens	8-16	No	No	No
Escherichia coli	12	No	No	No
Vibrio cholerae	12	No	Due to dehydration	No
Bacillus cereus				
a.	1-6	Yes	No	Yes
b.	8-16	No	No	No

- Outbreaks of bacterial diarrhea caused by *C. jejuni* are associated with consumption of unpasteurized milk and undercooked poultry.
- Approximately 10%-30% of cases of Guillain-Barré syndrome are preceded by *C. jejuni* infection.

In bacterial diarrhea caused by *S. aureus*, preformed toxin is ingested in contaminated food. Onset is abrupt, with severe vomiting (often predominates), diarrhea, and abdominal cramps. The duration of infection is 8 to 24 hours. Diagnosis is based on rapid onset, absence of fever, and history. Treatment is supportive.

- Bacterial diarrhea due to *S. aureus* is caused by ingestion of preformed toxin in contaminated food.

Bacterial diarrhea caused by *Clostridium perfringens* is associated with ingestion of bacteria that produce toxin in vivo, often in improperly prepared or stored precooked foods (meat and poultry products). Food is precooked and toxin is destroyed but spores survive; when food is rewarmed, spores germinate. When food is ingested, toxin is produced. Diarrhea is worse than vomiting, and abdominal cramping is prominent. Onset of symptoms is later than with *S. aureus* infection. Duration of illness is 24 hours. The diagnosis is based on the later onset of symptoms, a typical history, and Gram staining or culture of incriminated foods. Treatment is supportive.

- In diarrhea caused by *C. perfringens*, ingested bacteria produce toxin in vivo in precooked food.
- Diarrhea is worse than vomiting; abdominal cramping is prominent.

Two types of food poisoning are associated with *Bacillus cereus* infection. Profuse vomiting follows a short incubation period (1-6 hours); this is associated with the ingestion of a preformed toxin (usually in fried rice). A disease with a longer incubation occurs 8 to 16 hours after consumption; profound diarrhea develops and usually is associated with eating meat or vegetables. The diagnosis is confirmed by isolation of the organism from contaminated food. The illness is self-limited and treatment is supportive.

Diarrhea caused by *E. coli* can be either enterotoxigenic or enterohemorrhagic. Enterotoxigenic *E. coli* is the most

Table 14-16   Bacterial Diarrhea: Invasive

Organism	Fever present	Bloody diarrhea present	Antibiotics effective
Shigella species	Yes	Yes	Yes
Salmonella (non-*typhi*)	Yes	No	No
Vibrio parahaemolyticus	Yes	Yes (occasional)	No
Escherichia coli O157:H7	Yes	Yes	No
Campylobacter	Yes	Yes	Yes
Yersinia	Yes	Yes (occasional)	±

common etiologic agent in traveler's diarrhea. Treatment consists of fluid and electrolyte replacement along with loperamide plus trimethoprim-sulfamethoxazole, ciprofloxacin, or norfloxacin. Medical evaluation should be sought if fever and bloody diarrhea occur. For prophylaxis, water, fruits, and vegetables need to be chosen carefully. Routine prophylactic use of trimethoprim-sulfamethoxazole, ciprofloxacin, and doxycycline is not recommended because the risks outweigh the benefits in most travelers. Bismuth subsalicylate reduces the incidence of enterotoxigenic *E. coli*-associated diarrhea by up to 60%.

- Enterotoxigenic *E. coli* is the most common etiologic agent in traveler's diarrhea.

E. coli O157:H7 causes a relatively uncommon form of bloody diarrhea. This agent has been identified as the cause of waterborne illness, outbreaks in nursing homes and child care centers, and sporadic cases. It also has been transmitted by eating undercooked beef. Bloody diarrhea, severe abdominal cramps, fever, and profound toxicity characterize this enterohemorrhagic illness. It may resemble ischemic colitis. At extremes of age (old and young), the infection may produce hemolytic-uremic syndrome and death. This organism should be considered in all patients with hemolytic-uremic syndrome. Antibiotics are not known to be effective and may increase the likelihood of hemolytic-uremic syndrome.

- *E. coli* O157:H7 has been identified as the cause of waterborne illness, outbreaks in nursing homes and child care centers, and sporadic cases.
- Eating undercooked beef also transmits *E. coli* O157:H7.
- Bloody diarrhea, severe abdominal cramps, and profound toxicity characterize *E. coli* O157:H7 infection; it may resemble ischemic colitis.
- Infection should be considered in all patients with hemolytic-uremic syndrome.
- Antibiotic therapy is not recommended.

Vibrio cholerae causes the only toxigenic bacterial diarrheal disease in which antibiotics (tetracycline) clearly shorten the duration of disease. However, fluid replacement therapy is the mainstay of management. It is associated with consumption of undercooked shellfish.

Diarrhea caused by *Shigella* species is often acquired outside the United States. It often is spread by person-to-person transmission but also has been associated with eating contaminated food or water. Bloody diarrhea is characteristic, bacteremia may occur, and fever is present. The diagnosis is based on results of stool culture and blood culture (occasionally positive). Treatment is with ampicillin (ampicillin-resistant strains

are common), trimethoprim-sulfamethoxazole (in some countries, increasing resistance is being reported), norfloxacin, or ciprofloxacin. The illness may precede the onset of Reiter syndrome. Neurotoxin may cause seizures in pediatric patients.

- Diarrhea caused by *Shigella* species is associated with person-to-person transmission and the consumption of contaminated food or water.
- Bloody diarrhea is characteristic, bacteremia may occur, and fever is present.
- Illness may precede the onset of Reiter syndrome.

Salmonella (nontyphi)-associated illness most commonly is caused by *Salmonella enteritidis* and *Salmonella typhimurium* in the United States. It is associated with consumption of contaminated foods or with exposure to pet turtles, ducklings, and iguanas. *Salmonella* infection is a common cause of severe diarrhea and may cause septicemia in patients with sickle cell anemia or acquired immunodeficiency syndrome (AIDS). *Salmonella* bacteremia can lead to the seeding of abdominal aortic plaques resulting in mycotic aneurysms. In *Salmonella* enteritis, fever is usually present, and bloody diarrhea is often absent (a characteristic distinguishing it from *Shigella* infection). The diagnosis is based on stool culture. Treatment is supportive. Antibiotics only prolong the carrier state and do not affect the course of the disease. Antibiotics are used if results of blood culture are positive. Reactive arthritis may be a complication of this illness.

- *Salmonella* infection is a common cause of severe diarrhea.
- *Salmonella* infection may cause septicemia in patients with sickle cell anemia or AIDS.
- Bloody diarrhea is often absent (a feature distinguishing it from *Shigella* infection).

Vibrio parahaemolyticus infection is acquired by eating undercooked shellfish. It is a common bacterial cause of acute food-borne illness in Japan and is appearing with increasing frequency in the United States (Atlantic Gulf Coast and on cruise ships). Acute onset of explosive, watery diarrhea and fever are characteristic. The diagnosis is determined with stool culture. Antibiotic therapy is not required.

- Typical clinical scenario of *V. parahaemolyticus* infection: acute onset of watery diarrhea and fever after eating undercooked shellfish.
- Antibiotic therapy is not required.

Clinical syndromes associated with *Vibrio vulnificus* include bacteremia, gastroenteritis, and cellulitis. Most patients with bacteremia have distinctive bullous skin lesions and underlying hepatic disease (cirrhosis). The condition is associated with consumption of raw oysters. The mortality rate is high. Wound infections occur in patients who have had contact with seawater, such as with fishing injuries or contamination of a wound with seawater. Affected patients have intense pain and cellulitis in the extremities. Gastrointestinal illness is associated with consumption of raw oysters. The incubation period is approximately 18 hours. Vomiting, diarrhea, and severe abdominal cramps are features of this illness. Treatment of uncomplicated gastroenteritis is supportive. Bacteremia or cellulitis is treated with tetracycline, cefotaxime, or ciprofloxacin. *V. vulnificus* is not uniformly susceptible to the aminoglycosides.

- *V. vulnificus* bacteremia can cause distinctive bullous skin lesions and occurs in patients who are immunocompromised or have cirrhosis.
- It is associated with consumption of raw oysters or seawater contact.

Yersinia enterocolitica is the etiologic agent of several major clinical syndromes: enterocolitis, mesenteric adenitis, erythema nodosum, polyarthritis, Reiter syndrome, and bacteremia associated with contaminated blood products. Approximately 20% of infected patients have sore throat. Infection with *Y. enterocolitica* causing mesenteric adenitis can mimic acute appendicitis. Acquisition of infection is thought to be associated with eating contaminated food products. The organism has been cultured from chocolate milk, meat, mussels, poultry, oysters, and cheese.

- In adults with *Y. enterocolitica* infection, erythema nodosum, polyarthritis, and Reiter syndrome can develop.
- Infection with *Y. enterocolitica* causing mesenteric adenitis can mimic acute appendicitis.

Colitis caused by *Clostridium difficile* should be distinguished from other forms of antibiotic-associated diarrhea (watery stools, no systemic symptoms, and negative tests for *C. difficile* toxin). Symptoms often occur 2 to 4 weeks after stopping use of antibiotics. The illness is associated with antibiotic exposure in 99% of cases (any antibiotic can cause it). Nosocomial spread has been documented. Typical features are profuse, watery stools; crampy abdominal pain; constitutional illness; the presence of fecal leukocytes; and a positive *C. difficile* toxin. In toxin-negative disease, proctoscopy or flexible sigmoidoscopy can be used to look for pseudomembranes. Disease can be localized to the cecum (postoperative patient with ileus) and can present as fever of unknown origin. Treatment consists of vancomycin (125 mg orally four times a day for 7-10 days) or metronidazole (250-500 mg orally three or four times a day for 7-10 days). The emergence of vancomycin-resistant enterococci and cost differences favor the use of metronidazole as a first-line agent in most circumstances. Antiperistalsis drugs should not be used. If a patient is unable to take drugs orally, intravenous metronidazole (not vancomycin) or vancomycin enemas can be used. Relapse is frequent (about 15% of cases) and necessitates re-treatment. Treatment of asymptomatic carriers to decrease the nosocomial spread of infection or to reduce the risk of pseudomembranous colitis is not recommended.

- Colitis caused by *C. difficile* often occurs 2-4 weeks after stopping use of antibiotics.
- Illness is associated with antibiotic exposure in 99% of cases (any antibiotic can cause it).
- Features: profuse, watery stools; crampy abdominal pain; constitutional illness; fecal leukocytes; and a positive *C. difficile* toxin.
- Treatment: vancomycin (125 mg orally four times a day for 7-10 days) or metronidazole (250-500 mg orally three or four times a day for 7-10 days).
- Relapse is frequent (about 15% of cases).

Viral Diarrhea

Rotavirus infection is the most common cause of sporadic mild diarrhea in children. It may be spread from children to adults. It usually occurs during the winter. Vomiting is a more common early manifestation than watery diarrhea. Hospitalization for dehydration is common in young children. Diagnosis is made by detection of antigen in stool. Treatment is symptomatic. A vaccine was available but was withdrawn from the market because of a temporal association between the use of the vaccine and the development of intussusception.

Norwalk virus is a common cause of epidemic diarrhea and "winter vomiting disease" in older children and adults. It occurs in families, communities, and institutions. Outbreaks have been associated with eating shellfish, undercooked fish, cake frosting, and salads and with drinking contaminated water. It is the cause of up to 10% of gastroenteritis outbreaks. Recently, Norwalk virus has caused several outbreaks of gastroenteritis on cruise ships. Nausea, vomiting, and watery diarrhea characterize this illness. It is a mild, self-limited (<36 hours) illness. Currently, no commercial diagnostic test is available. Treatment is symptomatic.

- Outbreaks of Norwalk virus are associated with eating shellfish, undercooked fish, cake frosting, and salads and with drinking contaminated water.
- Illness is mild and self-limited (<36 hours).

BACTEREMIA, SEPSIS, AND SEPTIC SHOCK

Bacteremia, or bloodstream infection in general, is defined as the presence of living bacteria or other organisms in the blood and is established by a positive blood culture or other microbiologic techniques. The systemic inflammatory response syndrome (SIRS) is characterized by a group of physiologic responses due to several infectious and noninfectious causes. If SIRS is caused by an infection, then sepsis is said to be present. Some of the common manifestations of SIRS or sepsis include tachypnea, tachycardia, irritability, lethargy, fever or hypothermia, hypoxemia, and leukocytosis. Septic shock is sepsis with hypotension (blood pressure <90 mm Hg or a reduction of 40 mm Hg from baseline) despite adequate fluid replacement.

Severe sepsis and septic shock are characterized by impaired tissue perfusion, hypotension, and multiorgan dysfunction in the setting of infection (blood cultures positive in 50%-60% of cases). Endotoxin activates endogenous mediators of inflammation with catastrophic consequences. The result can be increased vascular permeability, a decrease in peripheral vascular resistance, profound hypotension with progressive lactic acidosis, and death.

Common causative organisms of community-acquired bloodstream infections include *E. coli*, *S. aureus*, and *S. pneumoniae*. Nosocomial infections most often are due to gram-negative aerobic bacilli, coagulase-negative staphylococci, *S. aureus*, enterococci, and *Candida* spp. The frequency of any one organism depends on the host (i.e., neutropenia is associated with *Pseudomonas aeruginosa*, central lines are associated with coagulase-negative staphylococci, *S. aureus*, and *Candida* spp.). The overall mortality rate is 20% to 30%. Management involves maintaining intravascular volume, administering appropriate bactericidal antimicrobials, and correcting any problems that lead to infection (such as draining abscesses). Adjunctive corticosteroids are of no proven benefit. Recombinant human activated protein C (drotrecogin alfa) has been approved by the U.S. Food and Drug Administration for treatment of adults with septic shock.

- In septic shock, blood cultures are positive in 50%-60% of cases.
- Most frequent blood isolates: *E. coli*, *S. aureus*, *S. pneumoniae*.
- Endotoxin activates endogenous mediators of inflammation with catastrophic consequences.

NEUTROPENIA

This condition is characterized by an absolute polymorphonuclear neutrophil value less than 0.5×10^9/L, most often in the setting of chemotherapy for malignancy. Bacteremia is documented in approximately 20% of neutropenic fever episodes. If ecthyma gangrenosum is present, *Pseudomonas* infection should be considered. Other gram-negative aerobic rods (such as *E. coli*) also cause bacteremia. The frequency of bacteremia due to aerobic gram-positive organisms is increasing. Bloodstream infection with these organisms (*S. aureus*, coagulase-negative staphylococci, enterococci, viridans streptococci, and *Corynebacterium jeikeium*) often is associated with central venous catheters or quinolone antibacterial prophylaxis. *Candida* species should be considered in cases associated with nodular skin lesions, fluffy white chorioretinal exudates, and fever unresponsive to empiric antibacterial agents. Anaerobic organisms are uncommon, except in cases of perirectal abscess and gingivitis. Empiric antimicrobial therapy after an attempt to identify the source of the infection is required for fever of 38.3°C or higher. Monotherapy with ceftazidime, cefepime, or imipenem alone is the preferred initial empiric antibacterial regimen. Alternative therapy with antipseudomonal penicillin plus an aminoglycoside is also acceptable. Vancomycin can be added to the initial regimen if there is severe mucositis, quinolone prophylaxis has been utilized, the patient is known to be colonized with methicillin-resistant *S. aureus* or penicillin-resistant *S. pneumoniae*, an obvious catheter-related infection is present, or the patient is hypotensive. If subsequent cultures show the presence of aerobic gram-positive organisms, vancomycin therapy can be continued. If there is no response after 5 to 7 days of treatment and the patient remains neutropenic, empiric therapy with an antifungal agent such as amphotericin B should be considered.

URINARY TRACT INFECTION

Females

Because urethritis or cystitis can occur with low colony counts of bacteria (10^3 colony-forming units), routine urine cultures in young women with dysuria are not recommended. Urinalysis should be done with or without a Gram stain. If pyuria and uncomplicated urinary tract infection (UTI) are present, short-course treatment should be initiated. Only if occult upper urinary tract disease, a complicated UTI, or sexually transmitted disease is suspected should appropriate culture and sensitivity testing be performed. Risk factors for occult infection and complications include emergency room presentation, low socioeconomic status, hospital-acquired infection, pregnancy, use of Foley catheter, recent instrumentation, known urologic abnormality, previous relapse, UTI at age less than 12 years, acute pyelonephritis or three or more UTIs in 1 year, symptoms for more than 7 days, recent antibiotic use, diabetes mellitus, and immunosuppression. Causative organisms include *E. coli* and *Staphylococcus saprophyticus* (susceptible to ampicillin and trimethoprim-sulfamethoxazole), *Proteus mirabilis*, or *Klebsiella pneumoniae*. *S. saprophyticus* may be reported on urine culture as "coagulase-negative staphylococcus."

- Routine urine cultures are not recommended in young women with dysuria.
- Associated organisms: *E. coli*, *S. saprophyticus* (susceptible to ampicillin and trimethoprim-sulfamethoxazole), *P. mirabilis*, or *K. pneumoniae*.

For the first episode of cystitis or urethritis, treatment is given but no investigation is needed. Trimethoprim-sulfamethoxazole or an oral fluoroquinolone is more effective than ampicillin. Short-course treatment (single-dose) has fewer side effects than standard (7-10 days) therapy, but the risk of relapse (due to retention of viable organisms in the vaginal or perivaginal area) is higher. Three-day therapy may be associated with relapse rates equal to those with treatment for 7 to 10 days and with less toxicity. If recurrence develops after 3-day therapy, subclinical pyelonephritis is likely and treatment is then given for 14 days. Urologic evaluation is usually not necessary. It should be performed in patients with multiple relapses, painless hematuria, a history of childhood UTI, renal lithiasis, and recurrent pyelonephritis.

- For first episode of cystitis or urethritis, trimethoprim-sulfamethoxazole or an oral fluoroquinolone is more effective than ampicillin.
- Short-course treatment (3 days) has fewer side effects than standard (7-10 days) therapy, and risk of relapse of infection may be the same.
- Urologic evaluation should be pursued in patients with multiple relapses, painless hematuria, history of childhood UTI, renal lithiasis, and recurrent pyelonephritis.

For acute pyelonephritis, 2 weeks of therapy is equal in efficacy to 6 weeks of therapy. Recent data suggest that 1 week of treatment with a fluoroquinolone may be sufficient for uncomplicated pyelonephritis due to susceptible organisms in women. Most patients are sufficiently ill to require hospitalization. Many are bacteremic. Unless gram-positive cocci are seen on Gram stain (suggesting enterococci), a third-generation cephalosporin, trimethoprim-sulfamethoxazole, or a fluoroquinolone can be used as empiric therapy. If enterococci are suspected, use ampicillin or piperacillin with or without gentamicin. Enterococci are resistant to cephalosporins. Enterococci appear susceptible to trimethoprim-sulfamethoxazole in vitro (and may be reported as such on a susceptibility report), but trimethoprim-sulfamethoxazole fails in the therapy of enterococcal infections because the organism is able to circumvent

the block of folate synthesis by using exogenous folinic acid, dihydrofolate, and tetrahydrofolate from the in vivo environment. Oral regimens can be substituted quickly as the patient improves. A urine culture is recommended 1 to 2 weeks after completion of therapy. If relapse occurs, treatment is given for 6 weeks and a urologic evaluation is done. For recurrent lower UTI (more than two episodes per year), single-dose therapy, 3-day therapy, or 6-week therapy is used. For treatment failure, chronic suppressive therapy may be used; however, the risk of resistant organisms must be weighed. Asymptomatic bacteriuria ($>10^5$ colony-forming units/mL) in a midstream urine specimen should be treated only in pregnant women, diabetic patients, and immunocompromised adults.

- For acute pyelonephritis, 2 weeks of therapy is equal in efficacy to 6 weeks of therapy.
- A follow-up urine culture is recommended.
- Cephalosporins and trimethoprim-sulfamethoxazole should not be used to treat enterococcal UTI.

Males

UTI is less common in males than females. Urologic abnormalities (such as benign prostatic hyperplasia) are common. Symptoms are unreliable for localization. Physical examination should include prostate examination, retraction of the foreskin to look for discharge, and palpation of the testicles and epididymides. When a UTI is suspected, urine culture and sensitivity testing should always be done. Causative organisms include *E. coli* in 50% of cases, other gram-negative organisms in 25%, enterococci in 20%, and others in 5%. If signs and symptoms of epididymitis, acute prostatitis, and pyelonephritis are present, treat accordingly. If uncomplicated lower UTI is present, treat for 10 to 14 days. If symptoms persist or relapse, repeat the urine culture. If results are positive, treat for a minimum of 6 weeks. If culture results are negative, consider chronic prostatitis or nonbacterial or noninfectious diseases and treat accordingly.

- Causes of UTI in males: *E. coli* in 50%, other gram-negative organisms in 25%, enterococci in 20%, others in 5%.

SOFT TISSUE INFECTION

Cellulitis is a skin infection that involves the dermis and subcutaneous fat. The most common causes are β-hemolytic streptococci and *S. aureus*. Patients with lymphedema, patients who have had saphenous vein harvesting for coronary artery bypass grafting, or patients who have tinea pedis are predisposed to cellulitis caused by these organisms. Treatment is typically with an antistaphylococcal penicillin or first-generation cephalosporin. Unusual causes of soft tissue infection are: *Eikenella corrodens* and oral anaerobes after human bites, *Pasteurella multocida* and *Capnocytophaga canimorsus* after animal bites, *Aeromonas hydrophila* after freshwater exposure or exposure to leeches, *Vibrio vulnificus* after saltwater exposure, *Erysipelothrix rhusiopathiae* and *Streptococcus iniae* after fish exposure, and *Pseudomonas aeruginosa* after hot tub exposure.

BONE AND JOINT INFECTIONS

Acute Bacterial Arthritis (Nongonococcal)

This is most commonly due to hematogenous spread of bacteria. The hip and knee joints are commonly involved. Bacteria involved are gram-positive aerobic cocci (about 75% of cases): *S. aureus* (most common) and β-hemolytic streptococci. Gram-negative aerobic bacilli also can cause infection (about 20% of cases); *P. aeruginosa* is a common cause in injection drug users. Anaerobes, fungi, and mycobacteria are unusual. Clinical features include involvement usually of monarticular, large joints. Fever, pain, swelling, and restriction of motion are the most frequent signs and symptoms. The synovial fluid is usually turbid, and the leukocyte count generally exceeds 40,000 cells/mm^3 (=75% polymorphonuclear neutrophils). The condition may overlap and be confused with other inflammatory arthropathies. Gram stain is 50% to 95% sensitive. Culture results are positive unless antibiotics have been used previously or the pathogen is unusual. Blood culture results are often positive. Radiographs are not helpful in routine cases because destructive changes have not had time to occur. Specific antimicrobial therapy is based on results of Gram stain, culture, and sensitivity testing. The duration of therapy is dependent on individual circumstances, such as the presence of complicating osteomyelitis. Usually, treatment is given for 2 to 4 weeks. Empiric therapy should include agents directed against *S. aureus* and gram-negative bacilli. Drainage is essential. Percutaneous, arthroscopic, or open procedures are used. Hip, shoulder, and sternoclavicular joint involvement, development of loculations, and persistently positive culture results (not due to resistant organisms) are the usual indications for arthroscopy or open debridement.

- Acute bacterial arthritis (nongonococcal) is most commonly due to hematogenous spread of bacteria.
- Bacteria most commonly involved are gram-positive aerobic cocci (about 75% of cases): *S. aureus* is most common.
- Monarticular, large joints usually are involved.
- Fever, pain, swelling, and restriction of motion are frequent.
- Synovial fluid is turbid; leukocyte count generally exceeds 40,000 cells/mm^3.

- Blood culture results are often positive.
- Drainage is essential.

Viral Arthritis

This is usually transient, self-limited polyarthritis. It may be caused by rubella (also may occur after vaccination), hepatitis B, mumps, coxsackievirus, adenovirus, parvovirus B19, and HIV, among others.

Chronic Monarticular Arthritis

Organisms involved include Mycobacteria (*Mycobacterium tuberculosis* is more common than *Mycobacterium avium-intracellulare*, *Mycobacterium kansasii*, *Mycobacterium marinum*), fungi (*Coccidioides immitis* and *Sporothrix schenckii* are more common than *Histoplasma capsulatum*, *Blastomyces dermatitidis*–acute, and *Candida* spp.–acute), and others (*Brucella*, *Nocardia*).

- *M. tuberculosis*, *C. immitis*, and *S. schenckii* often are involved in chronic monarticular arthritis.

Osteomyelitis

Acute *hematogenous osteomyelitis* is more common in infants and children than in adults. The metaphysis of long bones (femur, tibia) most commonly is affected. *S. aureus* is the most common organism. Acute onset of pain and fever are typical features. The illness can present with pain only. Compatible radiographic changes and bone biopsy for culture and pathologic examination are used to establish the diagnosis. Results of blood culture may be positive. Specific parenteral antibiotic therapy is used for 3 to 6 weeks on the basis of culture and sensitivity test results. Debridement is usually not necessary unless a sequestrum is present.

- *S. aureus* is the most common organism in acute hematogenous osteomyelitis.
- Acute onset of pain and fever are typical features.

Chronic osteomyelitis is more common in adults. It results from direct inoculation caused by trauma or adjacent soft tissue infection, for example. Open fractures and diabetic foot ulcers are common predisposing factors. *S. aureus* is the most common organism. Coagulase-negative staphylococci are often pathogens if a foreign body (such as plate, screws) is present. Often, osteomyelitis complicating a foot ulcer is polymicrobial, including aerobic gram-positive and gram-negative organisms and anaerobes. Local pain, tenderness, erythema, and draining sinuses are common. Fever is atypical unless there is concurrent cellulitis. The condition can present with pain only. Compatible radiographic changes (often vague) and bone biopsy for culture and pathologic examination are used to establish the diagnosis. Results of blood culture are rarely positive. Adequate debridement, removal of dead space, soft tissue coverage, and fixation of infected fractures are essential. Specific parenteral antibiotic therapy is given for 4 to 6 weeks on the basis of culture and sensitivity test results.

- *S. aureus* is the most common organism in chronic osteomyelitis.
- Coagulase-negative staphylococci are common pathogens if a foreign body is present.
- Local pain, tenderness, erythema, and draining sinuses are common.
- Specific parenteral antibiotic therapy is given for 4-6 weeks.

Vertebral Osteomyelitis

This condition often results from hematogenous dissemination from a focal source of infection (such as urinary tract, pneumonia). *S. aureus* and gram-negative bacilli are the major pathogens. Only 10% of cases have positive results of blood culture. Symptoms include pain and local tenderness. Fever may be present. The leukocyte count may be normal or increased. The sedimentation rate often is increased. Plain radiographs do not show destruction early in the course of disease. Gallium scanning is approximately 80% sensitive. Magnetic resonance imaging is the diagnostic test of choice because it is sensitive and specific and shows anatomical detail (coexistent epidural abscess). Percutaneous needle biopsy (computed tomography-guided) or open biopsy of bone or disk tissue is usually needed to define the microbiology of the infection. Treatment includes appropriate parenteral antimicrobial therapy for 4 to 6 weeks. Drainage may be necessary if a concomitant epidural abscess is present.

- In vertebral osteomyelitis, *S. aureus* and gram-negative bacilli are major pathogens.
- Gallium scanning is about 80% sensitive; magnetic resonance imaging is the diagnostic test of choice.

SINUSITIS IN ADULTS

The physician's overall impression as to the presence or absence of sinusitis is the best clinical predictor of sinusitis. Independent clinical predictors of disease are maxillary toothache, poor transillumination, poor response to decongestants, and a history or examination finding of purulent discharge. Limited computed tomography scanning of the sinuses is the radiographic method of choice. Organisms that are usually involved are *H. influenzae*, *S. pneumoniae*, and oral anaerobes. Treatment is with oral trimethoprim-sulfamethoxazole, amoxicillin, amoxicillin-clavulanate, and levofloxacin, among other options.

- Organisms involved in sinusitis in adults are *H. influenzae*, *S. pneumoniae*, and oral anaerobes.

HEPATIC (BACTERIAL) ABSCESS

Mechanisms of bacterial abscess include portal vein bacteremia resulting from, for example, appendicitis and diverticulitis, bacteremia caused by a primary focus elsewhere in the body, ascending cholangitis, direct extension (subphrenic abscess), or trauma. Fever is common. Right upper quadrant pain, tenderness on percussion, and increased values on liver function tests may or may not be present. Computed tomography and ultrasonography are very helpful in diagnosis. Bacteriology depends on the mechanism of abscess formation. Infection is often polymicrobial and is due to aerobic gram-negative rods, anaerobic streptococci, and *Bacteroides* species. Treatment is individualized and depends on suspected and isolated organisms. Empiric therapy with clindamycin or metronidazole plus a third-generation cephalosporin or aminoglycoside, a β-lactam/β-lactamase inhibitor combination, or a carbapenem is appropriate. If the hematogenous route is suspected, an agent should be used in the regimen that is active against staphylococci. Drainage (surgical or percutaneous) is of primary importance.

TOXIC SHOCK SYNDROME

This syndrome is caused by the establishment or growth of a toxin-producing strain of *S. aureus* in a non-immune person. Clinical scenarios associated with this syndrome include young menstruating women with prolonged, continuous use of tampons, postoperative and nonoperative wound infections, localized abscesses, and *S. aureus* pneumonia developing after influenza. It is a multisystem disease. Clinical criteria include fever, hypotension, erythroderma (often leads to desquamation, particularly on palms and soles), and involvement in three or more organ systems. Onset is acute; blood culture results are usually negative. The condition is caused by production of staphylococcal toxin (TSST-1). Treatment is supportive; subsequent episodes are treated with a β-lactam antibiotic, which decreases the frequency and severity of subsequent attacks. The relapse rate may be as high as 30% to 40% (menstruation-related disease). The mortality rate is 5% to 10%.

- Toxic shock syndrome is caused by a toxin-producing strain of *S. aureus* in a non-immune person.
- Multisystem disease: fever, hypotension, erythroderma (often leads to desquamation, particularly on palms and soles).
- Onset is acute; results of blood culture are usually negative.
- Toxic shock syndrome is caused by production of staphylococcal toxin (TSST-1).

STREPTOCOCCAL TOXIC SHOCK SYNDROME

This syndrome is similar to staphylococcal toxic shock syndrome. Patients have invasive group A streptococcal infections with associated hypotension and two of the following: renal impairment, coagulopathy, liver impairment, adult respiratory distress syndrome, rash (may desquamate), or soft tissue necrosis. Symptoms are caused by production of streptococcal toxin (pyrogenic exotoxin A). Most patients have skin or soft tissue infection, are younger than 50 years, and are otherwise healthy compared with patients with invasive group A streptococcal infections without the toxic streptococcal syndrome. Most patients are bacteremic (different from toxic shock syndrome due to *S. aureus*). Treatment is with appropriate antibiotics, supportive care, and surgical debridement in some cases. The case-fatality rate is 30%.

- Symptoms of toxic streptococcal syndrome are caused by production of streptococcal toxin.
- Most patients are bacteremic (different from toxic shock syndrome due to *S. aureus*).

INFECTIONS IN SOLID ORGAN TRANSPLANTATION AND IMMUNODEFICIENCY STATES

The spectrum of potential pathogens in patients after solid organ transplantation is diverse. The individual risk of specific infection can be classified according to the following: symptoms and signs of illness at presentation (i.e., meningitis vs. pneumonia), posttransplantation time course, serologic status of recipient and donor for certain infections (such as cytomegalovirus, toxoplasmosis), type of organ transplantation, type and duration of immunosuppression, type of antimicrobial prophylaxis patient has received, and travel history and previous exposure to pathogens (such as tuberculosis, coccidioidomycosis). The majority of infections in the first month after transplantation are not opportunistic infections but instead are common nosocomial infections such as wound infections, UTIs, and line infections. Cytomegalovirus is an important pathogen in patients who have had transplantation. Presentations can include febrile illness with viremia, hepatitis, colitis, gastritis, retinitis, myocarditis, and pneumonitis. Cytomegalovirus-seronegative recipients of organs from a seropositive donor are at highest risk for cytomegalovirus disease. The time of occurrence of opportunistic infections after solid organ transplantation is given in Table 14-17. Pathogens associated with various immunodeficiency states are shown in Table 14-18.

- The majority of infections in the first month after transplantation are not opportunistic infections but instead are common nosocomial infections such as wound infections, UTIs, and line infections.
- Cytomegalovirus is an important pathogen in patients who have had transplantation. Presentations can include febrile illness with viremia, hepatitis, colitis, gastritis, retinitis, myocarditis, and pneumonitis. Cytomegalovirus-seronegative recipients of organs from a seropositive donor are at highest risk for cytomegalovirus disease.

BIOTERRORISM

After the September 11, 2001, terrorist attacks and the subsequent deaths from anthrax sent in the mail, it is imperative for physicians to be familiar with likely bioterrorism agents. The Centers for Disease Control and Prevention classified the following diseases as category A, high-priority diseases that pose a risk to national security: smallpox, anthrax, botulism, plague, tularemia, and viral hemorrhagic fevers.

The incubation period, lethality, chemotherapy, and chemoprophylaxis for each agent are described in Table 14-19. These agents cause high mortality rates, can be easily disseminated or transmitted from person to person, and have the potential to have a major public health impact.

SEVERE ACUTE RESPIRATORY SYNDROME

Severe acute respiratory syndrome (SARS) is a rapidly progressive pneumonia that first developed in the Guangdong province of southern China in November 2002. The number of worldwide cases topped 8,000 by July 2003. The infection is caused by a novel coronavirus named SARS-associated coronavirus (SARS-CoV). Symptoms include fever often associated with myalgia, headache, dry cough, and dyspnea.

Table 14-17 Opportunistic Infections in Solid Organ Transplantation

Month	Type of infection after transplantation
1	Bacterial infections (related to wound, intravenous lines, urinary tract), herpes simplex virus, hepatitis B
1-4	Cytomegalovirus, *Pneumocystis carinii*, *Listeria monocytogenes*, *Mycobacterium tuberculosis*, *Aspergillus*, *Nocardia*, *Toxoplasma*, hepatitis B, *Legionella*
2-6	Epstein-Barr virus, varicella-zoster virus, hepatitis C, *Legionella*
>6	*Cryptococcus neoformans*, *Legionella*

Table 14-18 Pathogens Associated With Immunodeficiency

Immunodeficiency	Usual conditions	Pathogens
Neutropenia (<500/mL)	Cancer chemotherapy, adverse drug reaction, leukemia	**Bacteria:** Aerobic gram-negative bacilli (coliforms and pseudomonads, *S. aureus, S. viridans, S. epidermidis*) **Fungi:** *Aspergillus, Candida* spp.
Cell-mediated immunity	Organ transplantation, human immunodeficiency virus infection, lymphoma (especially Hodgkin disease), corticosteroid therapy	**Bacteria:** *Listeria, Salmonella, Nocardia, Mycobacteria* (*M. tuberculosis* and *M. avium*), *Legionella* **Viruses:** CMV, *H. simplex*, varicella-zoster, JC virus **Parasites:** *Pneumocystis carinii, Toxoplasma, Strongyloides stercoralis, Cryptosporidium* **Fungi:** *Candida, Cryptococcus, Histoplasma, Coccidioides*
Hypogammaglobulinemia or dysgammaglobulinemia	Multiple myeloma, congenital or acquired deficiency, chronic lymphocytic leukemia	**Bacteria:** *S. pneumoniae, H. influenzae* (type B) **Parasites:** *Giardia* **Viruses:** Enteroviruses
Complement deficiencies C2, 3 C5 C6-8 Alternative pathway	Congenital	**Bacteria:** *S. pneumoniae, H. influenzae, S. aureus*, Enterobacteriaceae *Neisseria meningitidis, S. pneumoniae, H. influenzae, Salmonella*
Hyposplenism	Splenectomy, hemolytic anemia	*S. pneumoniae, H. influenzae*, DF-2
Defective chemotaxis	Diabetes, alcoholism, renal failure, lazy leukocyte syndrome, trauma, SLE	*S. aureus*, streptococci, *Candida*
Defective neutrophilic killing	Chronic granulomatous disease, myeloperoxidase deficiency	Catalase-positive bacteria: *S. aureus, E. coli, Candida* spp.

CMV, cytomegalovirus; SLE, systemic lupus erythematosus.
From Bartlett JG: Pocket Book of Infectious Disease Therapy. Baltimore, Williams & Wilkins, 1998, p 236. By permission of the publisher.

Table 14-19 Treatment for Infections Potentially Caused by Bioterrorism

Disease	Incubation	Lethality	Chemotherapy	Chemoprophylaxis
			Category A agents	
Smallpox	7-17 d	High to moderate	Cidofovir (in vitro)	Vaccinia immune globulin 0.6 mL/kg IM (within 3 d of exposure)
Anthrax	1-6 d	Very high	Ciprofloxacin 400 mg IV every 8-12 h *Or* Doxycycline 200 mg IV, then 100 mg IV every 8-12 h *Or* Penicillin 2 million U IV every 2 h *Plus* Streptomycin or gentamicin	Ciprofloxacin 500 mg twice daily Levofloxacin 500 mg once daily Doxycycline 100 mg twice daily
Botulism	1-5 d	High without respiratory support	DOD heptavalent equine despeciated antitoxin for serotypes A-G (IND): 1 vial 10 mL IV CDC trivalent equine antitoxin for serotypes A, B, E (licensed)	NA
Plague	2-3 d	High without treatment	Streptomycin 10 mg/kg per day in divided doses × 10 d (or gentamicin) *Or* Doxycycline 200 mg IV then 100 mg IV twice daily × 10-14 d *Or* Chloramphenicol 1 g IV four times daily × 10-14 d	Doxycycline 100 mg PO twice daily × 7 d or duration of exposure Tetracycline 500 mg PO four times daily × 7 d Ciprofloxacin 500 mg PO twice daily × 7 d
Tularemia	1-21 d	Moderate if untreated	Streptomycin 30 mg/kg IM daily × 10-14 d Gentamicin 3-5 mg/kg per day IV × 10-14 d	Doxycycline 100 mg PO twice daily × 14 d Tetracycline 500 mg PO every 8 h × 14 d
Viral hemorrhagic fevers	4-21 d	High	Ribavirin (CCHF/arenaviruses) 30 mg/kg IV initial dose then 15 mg/kg every 6 h × 4 d Passive antibody for AHF, BHF, Lassa, and CCHF	NA

IM, intramuscularly; IV, intravenously; PO, orally; AHF, Argentine hemorrhagic fever (Junin virus); BHF, Bolivian hemorrhagic fever; CCHF, Congo-Crimean hemorrhagic fever; CDC, Centers for Disease Control and Prevention; DOD, Department of Defense; IND, investigational drug.
From Woods CW, Ashford D: Identifying and managing casualties of biological terrorism. *In* UpToDate. Edited by BD Rose. Wellesley, MA, UpToDate, 2004. (http://www.uptodate.com). By permission of the publisher.

The infection can progress to respiratory failure and death; the case fatality ratio is almost 10%.

The infection is suspected in a patient who has documented fever (>38°C) and lower respiratory tract symptoms and has had contact with a person believed to have had SARS or a history of travel to an area of documented transmission. Serum antibody tests and reverse-transcription polymerase chain reaction tests have been developed. The infection is highly contagious, and health care workers are particularly at risk of exposure. Infected patients must be isolated. Infection control precautions for hospitalized patients include standard precautions of good hand hygiene together with airborne isolation and the use of gowns, gloves, and eye protection. No specific treatment recommendations are available.

- SARS is a highly contagious, rapidly progressive respiratory infection caused by a novel coronavirus, SARS-associated coronavirus (SARS-CoV).
- No specific treatment is recommended, although infection control precautions need to be observed to minimize transmission.

PART III
John W. Wilson, M.D.
Lynn L. Estes, Pharm.D.

ANTIMICROBIALS

The mechanisms of action, spectrum of activity, clinical uses, route of excretion, and toxic effects of various antimicrobial agents are emphasized. Some of this information is given in Tables 14-20 through 14-31.

SPECIFIC ANTIBACTERIAL AGENTS

Penicillins

Natural Penicillins

Agents include penicillin G (intravenous, IV), penicillin V (oral), procaine penicillin (intramuscular, IM), and benzathine penicillin (IM, repository formulation).

Their **spectrum of activity** includes non–penicillinase-producing staphylococci (rare); β-hemolytic streptococci (group A, B, C, G); susceptible viridans streptococci; group D streptococci; penicillin-susceptible *Streptococcus pneumoniae* (incidence of penicillin resistance is increasing); most *Neisseria meningitidis*; non–penicillinase-producing *Neisseria gonorrhoeae*; and susceptible anaerobes (*Clostridium* species, most oral *Bacteroides* and *Fusobacterium* species, and *Peptostreptococcus*). Susceptible enterococci are inhibited but not killed by the natural penicillins. Other microbes that these agents are active against include *Erysipelothrix*, *Listeria monocytogenes*, *Pasteurella multocida*, *Streptobacillus*, *Spirillum*, *Treponema pallidum*, *Borrelia burgdorferi*, and *Actinomyces israelii*. Most staphylococci and gram-negative organisms produce β-lactamase that inactivates the natural penicillins.

Pharmacokinetics: These agents have short half-lives necessitating frequent administration or continuous infusions (except long-acting IM formulations such as benzathine and procaine penicillin). They are renally eliminated and require dosage adjustment with renal dysfunction. IV penicillin penetrates the central nervous system when inflammation is present. Oral penicillin V is preferred to penicillin G because it is more acid-stable and attains higher systemic concentrations (but considerably lower than with IV penicillin).

Clinical uses of the natural penicillins include treatment of infections caused by group A streptococci, including streptococcal pharyngitis and skin or soft tissue infections (when staphylococci are not suspected). Additionally, these agents can be used to treat susceptible *S. pneumoniae* infections (e.g., respiratory tract infections) and susceptible enterococcal infections, often with an aminoglycoside if bactericidal activity is needed. Penicillin (benzathine or IV) is the drug of choice for all stages of syphilis. Less common uses of natural penicillins include treatment of Lyme disease (*Borrelia*) and IV penicillin for treatment of meningitis caused by *N. meningitidis*, susceptible *S. pneumoniae*, and *Listeria*. Table 14-22 lists the pathogens for which a penicillin is the drug of choice.

- Natural penicillins are effective treatment of infections caused by susceptible *S. pneumoniae*, group A streptococci, and susceptible *Enterococcus*.

Aminopenicillins

Agents are ampicillin (IV and oral) and amoxicillin (oral). The advantages of amoxicillin over oral ampicillin are increased gastrointestinal absorption, decreased incidence of diarrhea, and dosing three times a day instead of four.

Table 14-20 Routes of Excretion of Antimicrobial Agents

Antimicrobial	Major route of excretion
Abacavir	Liver
Acyclovir, valacyclovir, famciclovir	Renal
Amantadine	Renal
Aminoglycosides	Renal
Azithromycin	Liver
Aztreonam	Renal
Carbapenems (imipenem, meropenem, ertapenem)	Renal
Caspofungin	Liver
Cephalosporins*	Renal
Chloramphenicol	Liver
Clarithromycin	Liver/renal
Clindamycin	Liver
Cotrimoxazole (sulfamethoxazole-trimethoprim)	Renal
Cytomegalovirus agents: foscarnet, ganciclovir, valganciclovir, cidofovir	Renal
Didanosine	Liver/renal
Doxycycline	Liver/intestine
Erythromycin, dirithromycin	Liver
Fluconazole	Renal
Flucytosine	Renal
Fluoroquinolones†	Renal
Itraconazole, ketoconazole, voriconazole	Liver
Linezolid	Liver
Metronidazole	Liver
Nonnucleoside reverse transcriptase inhibitors (nevirapine, delaviridine, efavirenz)	Liver
Oseltamivir	Liver
Penicillins‡	Renal
Protease inhibitors	Liver
Quinupristin/dalfopristin (Synercid)	Liver
Rifamycins (rifampin, rifabutin, rifapentine)	Liver
Rimantadine	Liver
Tetracycline	Renal
Vancomycin	Renal
Zalcitabine, stavudine, lamivudine	Renal
Zidovudine	Liver/renal

*Ceftriaxone has renal and biliary excretion; cefoperazone is excreted primarily in the bile.
†Moxifloxacin and sparfloxacin have liver metabolism; ciprofloxacin and enoxacin have hepatic and renal elimination.
‡Nafcillin and oxacillin are excreted by the liver.

Their **spectrum of activity** extends the antibacterial spectrum of the natural penicillins to include certain strains of *Escherichia coli*, *Proteus mirabilis*, *Salmonella*, *Shigella* (amoxicillin less active than ampicillin), β-lactamase–negative *Haemophilus influenzae* (60%-70%), and β-lactamase–negative *Moraxella catarrhalis* (<20%). Production of β-lactamase by the organism or alterations in binding to the penicillin-binding proteins has resulted in increasing resistance by some of these organisms.

Pharmacokinetics are similar to those of natural penicillins. These agents have short half-lives and are renally excreted.

Clinical uses of aminopenicillins include otitis media caused by *S. pneumoniae* or β-lactamase–negative *Haemophilus*, infections caused by susceptible enterococci, endocarditis prophylaxis for gastrointestinal or genitourinary procedures, and *Listeria* meningitis (IV ampicillin). Aminopenicillins also can be used to treat susceptible *E. coli* infections. However, resistance to this organism has increased to the extent that these agents are no longer empiric drugs of choice for the treatment of urinary tract infections.

- Aminopenicillins are front-line agents for treatment of otitis media, susceptible enterococcal infections, and *Listeria* meningitis.

Penicillinase-Resistant Penicillins

Agents include methicillin (IV), oxacillin (IV), nafcillin (IV), dicloxacillin (oral), and cloxacillin (oral).

The **spectrum of activity** is narrow and includes methicillin-susceptible *Staphylococcus aureus* and group A streptococci. Penicillinase-resistant penicillins have no gram-negative, enterococcal, or anaerobic activity.

Pharmacokinetics: These are the only penicillins that are not cleared renally. The penicillinase-resistant penicillins have hepatobiliary elimination and do not require dosage adjustment for renal function. Similar to the natural penicillins, they have short half-lives and require frequent administration or continuous infusions. The intravenous agents penetrate the central nervous system in the presence of inflammation.

Clinical uses include treatment of skin or soft tissue infections because of good activity for group A streptococci and methicillin-susceptible staphylococci. In addition, these are the drugs of choice for treatment of serious infections (e.g., bacteremia, endocarditis) caused by methicillin-susceptible staphylococci. They are more active than vancomycin in this setting.

- Penicillinase-resistant penicillins primarily are used for treatment of infections caused by group A streptococcus and methicillin-susceptible *S. aureus*. Thus, they are useful

Table 14-21 Mechanisms of Action of Antimicrobials

Cell wall	Protein synthesis	Cell membrane	Cell synthesis	RNA synthesis
Penicillins	Macrolides	Amphotericin	Nalidixic acid	Rifampin
Cephalosporins	Aminoglycosides	Azoles*	Fluoroquinolones	Rifabutin
Carbapenems	Tetracyclines		Flucytosine	Rifapentine
Vancomycin	Chloramphenicol			
Aztreonam	Metronidazole			
Glucan synthesis	Linezolid			
inhibitors (i.e.,	Quinupristin/			
caspofungin)	dalfopristin			

*Ketoconazole, fluconazole, itraconazole, voriconazole.

agents for skin or soft tissue infections caused by these organisms and also are used for treatment of serious methicillin-susceptible staphylococcal infections (e.g., endocarditis).

- These agents are the only penicillins that are not cleared renally. Elimination is hepatobiliary.

Carboxypenicillins

Agents include carbenicillin and ticarcillin.

The carboxypenicillins have a broader gram-negative **spectrum of activity** than ampicillin. When used as antipseudomonal agents, they generally should be used in combination with an aminoglycoside or ciprofloxacin because resistance to these agents can develop. They lack good activity against staphylococci and streptococci and have little or no activity against enterococci or *Klebsiella* species.

Novel **side effects** for the carboxypenicillins compared with other penicillins include sodium overload, hypokalemia, and platelet dysfunction. Because ticarcillin has more (2 to 4 times) antipseudomonal activity in vitro, it is more effective in smaller quantities than carbenicillin against *Pseudomonas aeruginosa*; thus, the adverse effects of large quantities of carbenicillin can be avoided.

- Carboxypenicillins have improved gram-negative activity compared with the natural penicillins or aminopenicillins. However, they lack good activity against staphylococci and streptococci and have little or no activity against enterococci or *Klebsiella* species.

Ureidopenicillins

Agents include piperacillin, azlocillin, and mezlocillin (no longer available).

These agents have a wide **spectrum of activity** against gram-negative bacteria. Compared with penicillin G and ampicillin, they are slightly less active against streptococci and enterococci (except mezlocillin), but they are more active against *H. influenzae* and *M. catarrhalis*. They are more active than carbenicillin and ticarcillin against Enterobacteriaceae, including most strains of *Klebsiella*. In addition, they are more active than ticarcillin against *Bacteroides fragilis*. Against *P. aeruginosa*, piperacillin is the most active of this group, followed by mezlocillin and then azlocillin. Similar to the carboxypenicillins, combination therapy with the ureidopenicillins and an aminoglycoside or ciprofloxacin is suggested for serious infections caused by *Pseudomonas* and *Enterobacter* species because of the frequent emergence of resistance.

Clinical uses of ureidopenicillins include hepatobiliary infections and nosocomial gram-negative infections.

Toxic effects: The ureidopenicillins have a lower sodium content per gram than ticarcillin or carbenicillin, and adverse effects such as hypernatremia, hypokalemia, and bleeding are less common.

- Ureidopenicillins have good gram-negative activity that includes *Klebsiella* and *Pseudomonas*, some gram-positive activity (less than natural or aminopenicillins), and some anaerobic activity against *B. fragilis*.

β-Lactam/β-Lactamase Inhibitors

Agents in this group are amoxicillin-clavulanate (Augmentin), ampicillin-sulbactam (Unasyn), ticarcillin-clavulanate (Timentin), and piperacillin-tazobactam (Zosyn).

The **spectrum of activity** of the parent drug is increased by the addition of β-lactamase inhibitors. This results in enhanced activity against β-lactamase–producing organisms such as *S. aureus* (methicillin-susceptible), *B. fragilis*, most *Klebsiella pneumoniae*, *H. influenzae*, and *M. catarrhalis*. Similar to other β-lactam agents, they are not active against methicillin-resistant *S. aureus*. The addition of the β-lactamase inhibitor usually does not change the activity of the parent compound against most strains of *Pseudomonas* or *Enterobacter*.

Table 14-22   Microorganisms for Which a Penicillin Is the Drug of Choice

Microorganism	Penicillin
Gram-positive cocci	
Enterococcus faecalis (non-penicillinase strains)	Ampicillin or penicillin G (often with an aminoglycoside*)
E. faecium	Ampicillin or penicillin G (often with an aminoglycoside*)
Staphylococcus aureus	
Non-penicillinase strain (rare)	Penicillin G or V
Penicillinase strain	Nafcillin, oxacillin[†]
S. epidermidis[‡]	
Non-penicillinase strain	Penicillin G or V
Penicillinase strain	Nafcillin, oxacillin
Streptococcus pyogenes (group A, B, C, G)	Penicillin G or V
Viridans streptococci	Penicillin G[§]
Streptococcus bovis	Penicillin G
Anaerobic streptococci or peptostreptococci	Penicillin G
Streptococcus pneumoniae (pneumococcus), "penicillin susceptible"	Penicillin G[§]
Gram-negative cocci	
Neisseria meningitidis	Penicillin G[//]
Gram-positive bacilli	
Bacillus anthracis (anthrax)	Penicillin G
Clostridium perfringens	Penicillin G
Clostridium tetani	Penicillin G
Erysipelothrix rhusiopathiae	Penicillin G
Listeria monocytogenes	Ampicillin plus an aminoglycoside
Gram-negative bacilli	
Proteus mirabilis	Ampicillin
Eikenella corrodens	Ampicillin
Fusobacterium spp.	Penicillin G
Leptotrichia buccalis	Penicillin G
Pasteurella multocida	Penicillin G
Pseudomonas aeruginosa	Ureidopenicillin (high dose) plus an aminoglycoside
Spirillum minus	Penicillin G
Streptobacillus moniliformis	Penicillin G
Other	
Actinomyces israelii	Penicillin G
Borrelia burgdorferi (Lyme disease)	Amoxicillin[¶]
Leptospira spp.	Penicillin G
Treponema pallidum (syphilis)	Penicillin G
T. pallidum subsp. *pertenue* (yaws)	Penicillin G

*Aminoglycoside used in combination with penicillin for treatment of enterococcal endocarditis and other serious enterococcal bacteremias.
[†]Penicillins (and other β-lactams) are not active against methicillin-resistant *S. aureus*.
[‡]Between 70% and 80% of *S. epidermidis* organisms are methicillin-resistant (and resistant to other β-lactams).
[§]Resistance to penicillin is increasing.
[//]Resistance to penicillin is uncommon but has been found (especially outside the United States).
[¶]Oral doxycycline or intravenous ceftriaxone also can be used as first-line therapy against Lyme disease.
From Wright AJ. The penicillins. Mayo Clin Proc 1999;74:290-307. By permission of Mayo Foundation for Medical Education and Research.

Clinical uses of amoxicillin-clavulanate and ampicillin-sulbactam include treatment of community-acquired respiratory tract infections (improved activity over the parent compounds for β-lactamase–producing *H. influenzae* and *M. catarrhalis*) and urinary tract infections. Because they have good activity against methicillin-susceptible staphylococci and group A streptococci, they often are used for skin or soft tissue infections. Their enhanced anaerobic activity over the parent compounds also provides coverage for community-acquired intra-abdominal infections and for head, neck, and aspiration pneumonia infections.

Clinical uses of piperacillin-tazobactam and ticarcillin-clavulanate include coverage for mixed gram-negative, anaerobic infections (including intra-abdominal, diabetic skin or soft tissue infections, and nosocomial respiratory tract infections) and empiric broad-spectrum therapy for polymicrobial infections. Their activity against *Enterobacter*, *Pseudomonas*, and other gram-negative organisms provides enhanced coverage over ampicillin-sulbactam or amoxicillin-clavulanate for nosocomial infections.

Toxic effects are similar to those of the parent compounds. Clavulanate may cause diarrhea and rarely hepatitis.

- β-Lactamase inhibitors have good activity against β-lactamase–producing strains of *S. aureus*, *B. fragilis*, *K. pneumoniae*, *H. influenzae*, and *M. catarrhalis*. Thus, their good gram-positive, gram-negative, and anaerobic activity provides good coverage for polymicrobial infections.
- The addition of the β-lactamase inhibitor usually does not change the activity of the parent compound against most strains of *Pseudomonas* or *Enterobacter*. Thus, piperacillin-tazobactam and ticarcillin-clavulanate have activity similar to that of piperacillin and ticarcillin, respectively. Ampicillin-sulbactam and amoxicillin-clavulanate do not have significant activity for these pathogens.
- β-Lactamase inhibitors are not active against methicillin-resistant staphylococci. No currently available β-lactam/β-lactamase inhibitor is active against these organisms.

Adverse Reactions to Penicillins

Hypersensitivity reactions are fairly common (3%-10% of cases). These reactions include maculopapular rash, urticaria, angioedema, serum sickness, and anaphylaxis. True anaphylaxis occurs in 0.004% to 0.015% of patients receiving penicillin. Skin testing in difficult cases can be used to predict subsequent severe (type I) penicillin allergy but will not predict maculopapular drug eruptions. Patients allergic to one penicillin agent should be considered allergic to all penicillins. Furthermore, there is a cross-allergenicity rate of 3% to 7% with cephalosporin compounds, and cross-allergenicity also may occur with the carbapenems. Cephalosporins and

carbapenems should be avoided when possible in patients who have had a severe, immediate penicillin allergy (type I anaphylaxis or urticarial eruption). Rash is common when aminopenicillins (ampicillin and amoxicillin) are given to patients with infectious mononucleosis—this is usually not a true allergy.

Gastrointestinal side effects to penicillins include nausea, vomiting, and diarrhea—including *Clostridium difficile* colitis. Rare hematologic side effects include neutropenia, platelet dysfunction, and hemolytic anemia. Drug fever also can occur with penicillin therapy. Electrolyte disturbances, especially hyperkalemia, can occur when high doses of penicillin potassium are used in patients with renal dysfunction. Central nervous system side effects with penicillin G, when given in high doses, may include tremors, lowered seizure threshold, and neuromuscular irritability.

With penicillinase-resistant penicillins, nephritis (methicillin), phlebitis (nafcillin), hepatitis (oxacillin), and transient neutropenia can occur with prolonged use.

Additional side effects for the carboxypenicillins include sodium overload, hypokalemia, and platelet dysfunction. These are more pronounced for carbenicillin than ticarcillin.

- A person who is allergic to one penicillin agent should be considered allergic to all penicillins. Additionally, there is a cross-allergenicity rate of 3%-7% with cephalosporin compounds and some cross-allergenicity with carbapenems.
- Transient neutropenia with prolonged use can occur with penicillinase-resistant penicillins (e.g., nafcillin).
- Additional side effects for the carboxypenicillins (carbenicillin and ticarcillin) include sodium overload, hypokalemia, and platelet dysfunction. These occur less commonly with ureidopenicillins (piperacillin, mezlocillin, azlocillin).

Cephalosporins

Cephalosporins have been divided into four generations according to spectrum of activity (Table 14-23). In general, first-generation agents have good gram-positive activity; second-generation agents have better gram-negative and somewhat less gram-positive activity; third-generation agents have improved gram-negative activity and variable gram-positive activity; and fourth-generation agents have good gram-negative and fairly good gram-positive activity.

First-Generation Cephalosporins

Representative agents include the injectable agents cefazolin (long serum half-life allows dosing every 8 hours) and cephalothin and the oral agents cephalexin and cefadroxil.

The **spectrum of activity** of the first-generation agents includes good activity against methicillin-susceptible staphylococci, β-hemolytic streptococci, and many strains of

Table 14-23   The Cephalosporins

1st Generation	2nd Generation	3rd Generation	4th Generation
Cefazolin	Cefaclor	Cefotaxime	Cefepime
Cephalexin	Cefamandole	Ceftriaxone	
Cefadroxil	Cefmetazole	Ceftazidime	
Cephalothin	Cefonicid	Cefoperazone	
Cephradine	Cefotetan	Cefixime	
	Cefuroxime	Cefpodoxime	
	Cefprozil	Moxalactam	
	Loracarbef	Ceftizoxime	
	Cefoxitin	Ceftibuten	
		Cefdinir	

P. mirabilis, *E. coli*, and *Klebsiella* species. Similar to all cephalosporins, the first-generation agents are not active against methicillin-resistant staphylococci, enterococci, *L. monocytogenes*, *Legionella* species, *Chlamydia pneumoniae*, *Mycoplasma pneumoniae*, and *C. difficile*. These agents have fairly minimal gram-negative anaerobic activity.

Pharmacokinetics: The first-generation cephalosporins are renally eliminated and require dosage adjustment for renal dysfunction. They do not penetrate the blood-brain barrier and should not be used to treat meningitis or other central nervous system infections.

Clinical uses: The first-generation agents offer activity for treatment of skin or soft tissue infections caused by most streptococci or methicillin-susceptible staphylococci. Similar to nafcillin, cefazolin is often used to treat serious infections caused by methicillin-susceptible staphylococci, including bacteremias and endocarditis. They are also commonly used for surgical prophylaxis and for community-acquired urinary tract infections caused by susceptible organisms. Cephalosporins are not active against methicillin-resistant staphylococci or enterococci.

- First-generation cephalosporins are active against methicillin-susceptible staphylococci and most streptococci.
- Cephalosporins are not active against methicillin-resistant staphylococci or enterococci.

Second-Generation Cephalosporins

Representative IV agents include cefamandole, cefoxitin, cefuroxime, cefmetazole, cefonicid, and cefotetan. Oral second-generation agents include cefuroxime, cefprozil, cefaclor, and loracarbef.

Spectrum of activity: In general, the second-generation agents have improved gram-negative activity but slightly less gram-positive activity than the first-generation agents. Of the

second-generation agents, cefuroxime has the best activity against *S. aureus* and β-lactamase–producing *H. influenzae* and *M. catarrhalis*.

Cefamandole has limited advantage over cefazolin. It has some increase in activity against *E. coli*, *Klebsiella*, indole-positive *Proteus*, *Enterobacter*, and non-β-lactamase–producing *H. influenzae*. It contains the methylthiotetrazole (MTT) side chain, which can produce hypoprothrombinemia (increased international normalized ratio), resulting in bleeding problems and a disulfiram-like reaction when ethanol is consumed. Cephalosporins possessing an MTT side group are listed in Table 14-24.

Cefoxitin has some increase in activity over first-generation agents against *E. coli*, *Klebsiella*, indole-positive *Proteus*, and *Serratia*. It is less active against *S. aureus* and streptococci than first-generation cephalosporins. It is active against most strains of *B. fragilis*.

The activity of cefotetan is fairly similar to that of cefoxitin. It has somewhat better activity than cefoxitin against aerobic gram-negative rods. It also has a longer half-life so

Table 14-24   Cephalosporins With Methylthiotetrazole (MTT) Side Group

Agents:	Cefoperazone	Cefamandole
	Cefotetan	Cefmetazole
	Moxalactam (also decreased platelet aggregation)	

Interactions: 1. Hypoprothrombinemia (↑INR) via competitive inhibition by MTT side group
2. Disulfiram-like reaction (with ethanol consumption)

INR, international normalized ratio.

can be given less frequently than cefoxitin (every 12 hours, compared with every 6). It has the MTT side chain with the associated toxicities described for cefamandole.

The oral second-generation agents have improved gram-negative activity over first-generation agents. Their activity generally includes β-lactamase–producing *H. influenzae* and *M. catarrhalis*, penicillin-sensitive streptococci, and many community-acquired strains of *E. coli*, *Klebsiella*, and *P. mirabilis*. Cefprozil and cefuroxime have the greatest gram-positive activity of the oral second-generation agents.

Pharmacokinetics: The second-generation cephalosporins are renally eliminated. Cefuroxime penetrates the central nervous system with inflammation but has been shown to be less effective for meningitis treatment than ceftriaxone or cefotaxime (slower activity and more long-term sequelae).

Clinical uses: The most common uses of cefuroxime, cefamandole, loracarbef, and cefonicid are for community-acquired respiratory tract infections and urinary tract infections. Cefotetan and cefoxitin have somewhat improved anaerobic activity and are used for community-acquired intra-abdominal infections, pelvic inflammatory infections (usually in combination with doxycycline), and surgical prophylaxis for obstetric and gynecologic procedures.

- Cefuroxime and the oral second-generation cephalosporins often are used for community-acquired respiratory tract infections.
- Cefoxitin and cefotetan have enhanced anaerobic and gram-negative activity. They are used for community-acquired intra-abdominal or pelvic inflammatory infections and surgical prophylaxis for gynecologic procedures.
- Cefotetan and cefamandole have the MTT side chain, which is associated with hypoprothrombinemia (increased international normalized ratio), resulting in bleeding problems and a disulfiram-like reaction when ethanol is consumed.

Third-Generation Cephalosporins

Representative agents are IV cefotaxime, ceftizoxime, ceftriaxone, cefoperazone, and ceftazidime and oral cefixime, cefpodoxime, ceftibuten, and cefdinir.

Spectrum of activity: The third-generation cephalosporins have improved gram-negative activity versus the first- and second-generation agents. The gram-positive activity varies, as described below.

Some organisms, most notably *Enterobacter*, have developed an inducible resistance to these agents. Because resistance can occur during therapy, these agents generally should not be used alone for treatment of *Enterobacter* infections, even if shown to be susceptible initially. Extended-spectrum β-lactamases also have been found in some strains of *Klebsiella* and *E. coli* and can cause resistance to ceftazidime and the other cephalosporins.

Widespread use of ceftazidime may be more likely to select for these resistant organisms. Some hospitals have had success in reducing resistance rates by restricting use of this agent.

Ceftazidime is less active against staphylococci and streptococci than most other third-generation cephalosporins. However, it has the best gram-negative activity of this group, and its spectrum includes *P. aeruginosa*.

Cefotaxime, ceftriaxone, and ceftizoxime have very similar spectra. The primary difference among these agents is their pharmacokinetics. These agents have enhanced gram-negative activity compared with the second-generation agents but are less active against *Pseudomonas* than ceftazidime or cefoperazone. However, they have better activity against methicillin-susceptible staphylococci and streptococci (including *S. pneumoniae* organisms, which are intermediately resistant to penicillin and viridans streptococci) than ceftazidime and cefoperazone. Cefotaxime and ceftriaxone have good cerebrospinal fluid penetration in the presence of inflammation and are commonly used for treatment of community-acquired bacterial meningitis and other central nervous system infections.

Cefoperazone also has some activity against *Pseudomonas* but less than ceftazidime. Penetration into cerebrospinal fluid is less than that of other available third-generation cephalosporins, and it has the MTT side chain with the associated potential toxic effects. Thus, this agent is rarely used.

Oral agents in this class include cefpodoxime proxetil, cefdinir, cefixime, and ceftibuten. They have improved gram-negative activity over the second-generation oral cephalosporins, but they are not as active as the injectable third-generation agents against nosocomial gram-negative infections. None of the oral agents are effective against *Pseudomonas*. Cefixime and ceftibuten have the best gram-negative activity of any oral cephalosporins. However, neither is very active against staphylococci, and ceftibuten has poor streptococcal activity. Cefpodoxime proxetil and cefdinir have better gram-positive activity than the other oral third-generation cephalosporins, particularly against staphylococci and streptococci. Although they have somewhat less gram-negative activity than cefixime or ceftibuten, they are active against *H. influenzae*, *M. catarrhalis*, *N. gonorrhoeae*, and many other gram-negative organisms.

Pharmacokinetics: These agents are renally eliminated except ceftriaxone, which has dual renal and hepatobiliary elimination, and cefoperazone, which is primarily excreted in the bile. Cefotaxime, ceftazidime, and ceftizoxime are usually given every 8 hours, whereas the long half-life of ceftriaxone allows for dosing every 24 hours in most circumstances. Cefotaxime, ceftriaxone, and ceftazidime cross the blood-brain barrier in the presence of inflammation.

Clinical uses: Cefotaxime, ceftriaxone, and ceftizoxime are commonly used for community-acquired respiratory tract infections, urinary tract infections, and pyelonephritis. Cefotaxime and ceftriaxone are used for the treatment of community-acquired meningitis and other central nervous system infections. Additionally, ceftriaxone is used for the treatment of susceptible viridans streptococcal endocarditis. The long half-life of ceftriaxone permits convenient treatment of susceptible outpatient infections that necessitate IV antibiotics.

The enhanced gram-negative activity of ceftazidime (and less commonly cefoperazone) makes this agent useful for the treatment of nosocomial gram-negative infections. Ceftazidime is useful for the treatment of pseudomonal infections—often in combination with another agent such as an aminoglycoside. Ceftazidime also has been used for the treatment of febrile neutropenia.

Third-generation cephalosporins can be used for nosocomial gram-negative infections or in combination with an anti-anaerobic agent (e.g., metronidazole) for polymicrobial infections.

- Ceftazidime is more active than any other third-generation cephalosporin against *Pseudomonas* and is often used for nosocomial infections or treatment of febrile neutropenia.
- Cefotaxime, cefuroxime, ceftizoxime, and the oral third-generation agents provide good coverage of community-acquired respiratory and urinary tract pathogens.
- Third-generation cephalosporins can be used in combination with anti-anaerobic agents such as metronidazole for intra-abdominal and other polymicrobial infections.
- Inducible resistance to ceftazidime and other cephalosporins can develop in *Enterobacter* organisms, and extended-spectrum β-lactamase–producing *E. coli* and *Klebsiella* are an increasing problem.

Fourth-Generation Cephalosporins

Cefepime is the first of the fourth-generation cephalosporins. Its **spectrum of activity** includes gram-positive activity (methicillin-susceptible *S. aureus* and *Streptococcus*) similar to that of cefotaxime. Its gram-negative activity (including *Pseudomonas aeruginosa*) is similar to or better than that of ceftazidime. In addition, cefepime has a lower potential for inducing resistance and may have more durable activity against some gram-negative organisms, such as *Enterobacter*, that may become resistant to third-generation agents. However, cefepime and other cephalosporin agents should not be used against extended-spectrum β-lactamase–producing gram-negative bacilli.

Pharmacokinetics: Cefepime is renally cleared and does penetrate into the cerebrospinal fluid in the presence of inflammation.

Clinical uses: Cefepime has gained widespread popularity because of a broadened spectrum of activity and decreased potential for development of resistance compared with third-generation agents. It is useful for the treatment of nosocomial infections, including respiratory tract, urinary tract, bloodstream, soft tissue, and intra-abdominal infections, in combination with an anaerobic agent. It is also a preferred agent for treatment of febrile neutropenia.

- Cefepime has gram-positive activity similar to cefotaxime and gram-negative activity similar to or better than ceftazidime. Its spectrum includes *Pseudomonas* and *Enterobacter* spp.

Adverse Reactions to Cephalosporins

Cephalosporins usually are well tolerated. The most common **toxic effects** include adverse reactions related to the gastrointestinal tract (such as nausea, vomiting, diarrhea). Hypersensitivity reactions, primarily rashes, occur in 1% to 3% of patients taking cephalosporins. Anaphylaxis is rare. Cross-allergenicity may occur with penicillins. Other adverse reactions associated with cephalosporins include drug fever and *C. difficile* colitis.

The MTT side chain can produce hypoprothrombinemia (increased international normalized ratio), resulting in bleeding problems and a disulfiram-like reaction when ethanol is consumed. Cephalosporins possessing an MTT side group are listed in Table 14-24.

Ceftriaxone has been reported to cause pseudocholelithiasis, cholelithiasis, biliary colic, and cholecystitis as a result of biliary precipitation of ceftriaxone as the calcium salt in up to 2% of cases, especially in children. This effect usually resolves with discontinuation of therapy.

Carbapenems

Imipenem, Meropenem, and Ertapenem

The carbapenems are very broad-spectrum β-lactams. Their mechanism of action is similar to that of other β-lactam antibiotics (inhibition of cell wall synthesis). Unfortunately, bacterial resistance, particularly among *P. aeruginosa*, is increasing and mediated by various mechanisms.

Spectrum of activity: The carbapenems have the broadest antibacterial activity of any antibiotics currently available. The gram-positive spectrum includes β-hemolytic streptococci, pneumococci, and methicillin-susceptible *S. aureus*. Imipenem and, to a lesser extent, meropenem provide coverage for susceptible *Enterococcus* spp. (inhibited only). However, ertapenem has less enterococcal activity than the other carbapenems. They are more active than ceftriaxone or cefotaxime against pneumococci, have intermediate resistance to penicillin (minimal inhibitory concentration, 0.1-1.0 µg/mL), and retain some activity against strains with high-level penicillin resistance (minimal inhibitory concentration, >2.0 µg/mL).

Regarding gram-negative organisms, the carbapenems have good coverage for Enterobacteriaceae, *H. influenzae*, *M. catarrhalis*, and *Nocardia*. The carbapenems remain active against most extended-spectrum β-lactamase–producing *Klebsiella* spp. and *E. coli*. Meropenem and imipenem cover most strains of *P. aeruginosa* and *Acinetobacter* spp.; however, ertapenem lacks good coverage of these organisms.

The spectrum of each of these agents also includes excellent activity against anaerobes, including *Bacteroides* spp., *Clostridium* spp., *Eubacterium* spp., *Fusobacterium* spp., *Peptostreptococcus* spp., *Porphyromonas* spp., and Prevotella spp.

Organisms to which carbapenems are *not* active include methicillin-resistant *Staphylococcus*, *Legionella*, *Chlamydia* spp., *Mycoplasma* spp., *Pseudomonas cepacia*, and *Stenotrophomonas maltophilia*.

Differences in spectra between imipenem and meropenem include slightly better gram-positive activity for imipenem (probably only clinically significant for *Enterococcus faecalis*) and slightly better gram-negative activity for meropenem (including *P. aeruginosa*). In contrast to imipenem and meropenem, ertapenem lacks good coverage for *Enterococcus*, *P. aeruginosa*, and *Acinetobacter*.

Pharmacokinetics: Imipenem is administered intravenously and is hydrolyzed in the kidney by a peptidase located in the brush border of renal tubular cells. Administration with cilastatin, a dehydropeptidase inhibitor, solves this problem and allows imipenem to have activity in the urine. Meropenem and ertapenem do not require the addition of cilastatin. These agents are renally eliminated and require dosage adjustment for renal dysfunction. Ertapenem has a longer half-life than the other carbapenems and can be given once daily, which may be beneficial for outpatient therapy.

Clinical Uses: Carbapenems are commonly used when broad-spectrum empiric therapy is needed in patients with sepsis and for treatment of polymicrobial infections, including intra-abdominal, pelvic, pulmonary, and necrotizing soft tissue infections. Additionally, carbapenems often can be used for the treatment of aerobic gram-negative bacilli that are resistant to the other β-lactam agents (including *Enterobacter* and extended-spectrum β-lactamase–producing Enterobacteriaceae). Imipenem and meropenem also are used for febrile neutropenia, especially when anaerobic activity is needed. Ertapenem is considerably less costly than the other carbapenems and provides cost-effective therapy for mixed infections, for example, intra-abdominal, complicated respiratory tract, and complicated skin or soft tissue infections when *Pseudomonas*, *Acinetobacter*, or *Enterococcus* are not likely to be serious pathogens. (For mixed intra-abdominal infections, it is often not necessary to cover Enterococcus.)

Toxic effects of carbapenems include nausea and vomiting, diarrhea, hypersensitivity, drug fever, and overgrowth of resistant organisms (yeast, *Stenotrophomonas maltophilia*, *C. difficile*). Seizures occur rarely with these agents; affected patients are those with a history of previous seizures, renal insufficiency, or structural central nervous system defects.

- The carbapenems have the broadest spectrum of activity of any antibiotic, including gram-positive, gram-negative, and anaerobic organisms. They commonly are used as broad-spectrum empiric therapy, but the spectrum often can be narrowed when results of cultures and sensitivities are known.
- Ertapenem is considerably less costly than the other carbapenems yet still provides a broad spectrum of activity. However, it does not provide good coverage of *Enterococcus*, *Pseudomonas*, or *Acinetobacter*.

Aztreonam

Aztreonam is the only commercially available monobactam and is a derivative of naturally occurring monocyclic β-lactam compounds. The mechanism of action of aztreonam, like that of β-lactam antimicrobial agents, is the inhibition of cell wall synthesis. Aztreonam is administered intravenously and is excreted by the kidneys. Unlike other β-lactams, cross-reactivity with aztreonam in patients with a penicillin or cephalosporin allergy is rare. However, because of a similar side chain, there may be some cross-allergenicity with ceftazidime.

Its **spectrum of activity** includes most aerobic gram-negative bacteria, including *P. aeruginosa*. However, it has no activity against gram-positive aerobic or anaerobic bacteria, and it is not synergistic with penicillins against the enterococci (in contrast to gentamicin and streptomycin). The **toxic effects** of aztreonam are similar to those of other β-lactams.

Clinical uses of aztreonam include the treatment (as an alternative agent) of aerobic gram-negative infections, especially in penicillin-allergic patients. It may be used in combination with other agents in the treatment of mixed polymicrobial infections.

- Aztreonam is active only against gram-negative aerobes.
- Aztreonam may be useful in cases of penicillin or cephalosporin allergy because cross-reactivity is uncommon.

Aminoglycosides

Agents in this group are gentamicin, tobramycin, amikacin, netilmicin, streptomycin, kanamycin, and neomycin.

The **spectrum of activity** of these agents includes most aerobic gram-negative bacilli, mycobacteria (*Mycobacterium tuberculosis*, streptomycin; *Mycobacterium avium-intracellulare*, amikacin; *Mycobacterium chelonei*, amikacin), *Brucella* (streptomycin), *Nocardia* (amikacin), *Francisella* *tularensis* (streptomycin), and *Yersinia pestis* (streptomycin). They are synergistic with certain β-lactams and vancomycin in the treatment of serious infections due to susceptible enterococci (gentamicin, streptomycin), staphylococci, and several aerobic gram-negative species.

Pharmacokinetics: The aminoglycosides are not absorbed orally and are sometimes used for oral bowel decontamination. They are available as IM or IV preparations; additionally, tobramycin is available as an inhalation formulation for local distribution to the lungs. They are renally eliminated through glomerular filtration, and the half-life in patients with normal renal function is 1.5 to 4 hours. These agents have minimal protein binding and are distributed to extracellular fluid. They do not achieve good penetration to the central nervous system, lungs, eyes, or prostate. In addition, they are less active in a low pH environment (e.g., abscess).

The major **adverse reactions** to aminoglycosides include nephrotoxicity and auditory or vestibular toxicity. Neuromuscular blockade, drug fever, and hypersensitivity reactions are much less common. The risk of nephrotoxicity varies among the different aminoglycosides; neomycin is the most nephrotoxic, and streptomycin is the least nephrotoxic. Gentamicin, tobramycin, and amikacin have intermediate nephrotoxicity. Risk factors include increased serum trough levels, total cumulative dose, advanced age, hypotension, concomitant use of other nephrotoxic drugs, and liver disease. Aminoglycoside nephrotoxicity is almost always reversible with discontinuation of the drug therapy, and it can be minimized if dosages are adjusted to achieve desired serum concentrations and if renal function is carefully monitored. Nephrotoxicity may be delayed or decreased when the entire daily dose is administered at once (single daily dosing of aminoglycosides). Other nephrotoxic drugs such as cisplatin, amphotericin B, vancomycin, and cyclosporine may potentiate nephrotoxicity.

Unlike nephrotoxicity, ototoxicity caused by aminoglycosides is almost always irreversible. Streptomycin, gentamicin, and tobramycin are preferentially toxic to the vestibular system, whereas amikacin and neomycin are primarily toxic to the auditory nerve. Advanced age and concomitant use of ethacrynic acid or furosemide seem to be risk factors for ototoxicity. Because of the imprecision of bedside testing for auditory and vestibular toxicity, routine audiologic and vestibular function evaluation should be considered when prolonged administration is anticipated and in patients predisposed to ototoxicity. Patients also should be routinely questioned about symptoms of ototoxicity.

Single daily dosing (also known as pulse dosing) is a simplified, efficacious, and cost-effective method of aminoglycoside administration. For most infections with gram-negative bacteria, single daily dosing is as effective as the more traditional multiple daily dosing format and may lower the risk of nephrotoxicity. Single daily dosing takes advantage of three basic principles: 1) aminoglycosides display concentration-dependent bactericidal action—that is, higher doses and serum concentrations result in more rapid bacterial killing; 2) aminoglycosides exhibit a long post-antibiotic effect, resulting in persistent bacterial suppression even after serum concentrations decline below the minimal inhibitory concentration (allowing for less frequent drug administration); and 3) large, single daily doses result in periods with negligible serum concentrations, reducing renal cortical and auditory accumulation of the drug. Single daily dosing should not be used for enterococcal endocarditis and requires further evaluation in select patient groups, including pregnant women, children, and persons with cystic fibrosis, severe renal insufficiency, and neutropenic fever.

Although the **clinical uses** of aminoglycosides against gram-negative infections have largely been replaced with alternative, less toxic agents, the aminoglycosides continue to play an important role for some infections. They commonly are used in combination with other agents for the treatment of endocarditis caused by *Enterococcus* spp., *Staphylococcus*, or viridans streptococci. In addition, they may be used in combination for serious pseudomonal and other gram-negative infections, mycobacterial infections, nocardiosis, and brucellosis. Additionally, the aminoglycosides are first-line drugs to treat tularemia and *Yersinia* infections.

- Aminoglycosides are active against most aerobic gram-negative bacilli and are synergistic with β-lactams or vancomycin against susceptible enterococci and staphylococci.
- Major adverse reactions to aminoglycosides are nephrotoxicity and auditory or vestibular toxicity.
- Aminoglycoside nephrotoxicity is almost always reversible with discontinuation of the drug therapy.
- Ototoxicity is almost always irreversible.
- Single daily dosing is a cost-effective, efficacious, and potentially less toxic form of administration than traditional multiple daily dosing.

Tetracyclines

Agents are short-acting (tetracycline, chlortetracycline, oxytetracycline), intermediate-acting (demeclocycline, methacycline), and long-acting (doxycycline, minocycline).

In regard to **spectrum of activity**, these agents are drugs of choice for *Rickettsia*, *Chlamydia* species (including pelvic inflammatory disease), *M. pneumoniae*, *Vibrio cholerae*, *Vibrio vulnificus*, *Brucella* species (with streptomycin or rifampin), *Borrelia burgdorferi* (early stages), and *Borrelia recurrentis*. These agents are also effective therapy or alternatives for *Actinomyces*, anthrax, *Campylobacter*, *P. multocida*, *Spirillum minus*, *Streptobacillus moniliformis*, *Treponema pallidum*, *F.*

tularensis, Whipple disease, *Y. pestis*, *Nocardia* (minocycline), and *Mycobacterium marinum*. Minocycline also may be active against methicillin-resistant staphylococci (for mild disease in patients who cannot tolerate vancomycin) and *Stenotrophomonas*. The tetracyclines also may be used for the treatment of *Helicobacter pylori* infection (as part of combination therapy) and for respiratory tract infections with susceptible *S. pneumoniae*. Although the tetracyclines are active in vitro against many other aerobic gram-positive and gram-negative organisms as well as some anaerobes, they are usually not the drugs of choice to treat the infections caused by these organisms because of the presence or emergence of resistant strains. Further information on the clinical indications for tetracyclines is given in Table 14-25.

Toxic effects include gastrointestinal upset, rash, and photosensitivity. Uremia is increased in patients with renal failure. Other, more rare side effects include acute fatty liver of pregnancy, Fanconi syndrome (old tetracycline), or pseudotumor cerebri. The tetracyclines are not used in pregnant females or in children because they impair bone growth of the fetus and stain the teeth of children. Coadministration of milk, antacids, iron, calcium, or calcium-, magnesium-, or aluminum-containing compounds substantially decreases the enteric absorption of the tetracycline.

In addition to its **clinical use** in treating respiratory, genital, soft tissue, and systemic infections with the aforementioned organisms, the tetracyclines have certain non-antimicrobial therapeutic roles. Demeclocycline inhibits antidiuretic hormone-induced water reabsorption in the renal tubule and collecting duct and therefore is used in treatment of the syndrome of inappropriate antidiuretic hormone. The tetracyclines also are a useful sclerosing agent for the treatment of refractory or malignant pleural effusions.

● The tetracyclines should not be used during pregnancy or in children because they impair bone growth of the fetus and stain the teeth of children.

Chloramphenicol

The **spectrum of activity** of this agent is broad and includes inhibition of most strains of clinically important aerobic and anaerobic bacteria. Exceptions are methicillin-resistant *S. aureus*, many *Klebsiella* isolates, *Enterobacter*, *Serratia*, indole-positive *Proteus*, and *P. aeruginosa*. It is active against *H. influenzae*, *N. meningitidis*, *N. gonorrhoeae*, *Salmonella typhi*, *Brucella* spp., and *Bordetella pertussis*. In addition, chloramphenicol is also active against *Rickettsia*, *Chlamydia*, *Mycoplasma*, and spirochetes.

Toxic effects include two types of hematologic manifestations: idiosyncratic aplastic anemia (not dose-related; severe, often fatal; incidence approximately 1/24,000 to 1/40,000) and

Table 14-25 Major Clinical Indications for Use of Tetracyclines

Genital infections or sexually transmitted diseases
  Chlamydia trachomatis (nongonococcal urethritis, pelvic inflammatory disease, epididymitis, prostatitis, LGV)
  Granuloma inguinale (donovanosis)
  Alternative agent for *Ureaplasma urealyticum*, *Treponema pallidum* (syphilis)
"Atypical" respiratory tract pathogens
  Mycoplasma pneumoniae
  Chlamydia pneumoniae
  Chlamydia psittaci (psittacosis)
  Alternative agent for *Legionella pneumophila*
Systemic infections
  Rickettsia spp. (Rocky Mountain spotted fever, endemic and epidemic typhus, Q fever)
  Brucellosis (in combination with rifampin or streptomycin)
  Ehrlichiosis (HME, HGE)
  Early Lyme disease
  Vibrio infections
Other indications
  Tularemia (*Francisella tularensis*)
  Bacillary angiomatosis (*Bartonella* spp.)
  Leptospirosis
  Helicobacter pylori (in combination therapy)
  Mycobacterium marinum
  Pasteurella multocida (in patients allergic to β-lactam agents)
  As prophylaxis against mefloquine-resistant *Plasmodium falciparum* malaria

HGE, human granulocytic ehrlichiosis; HME, human monocytic ehrlichiosis; LGV, lymphogranuloma venereum.

dose-related, reversible bone marrow suppression (much more common with a dose >4 g/day or increased serum levels). Gray baby syndrome (abdominal distention, cyanosis, vasomotor collapse) can occur in premature infants and possibly in patients with profound liver failure who cannot conjugate chloramphenicol and who have high serum levels. Rare toxic effects are hemolytic anemia, retrobulbar neuritis, peripheral neuritis, and potentiation of oral hypoglycemic agents.

The **clinical use** of chloramphenicol has largely been curbed by the availability of potent, less toxic alternative agents. Although chloramphenicol is no longer the drug of choice for any specific infection, it still remains widely used for typhoid fever in parts of the world where cost and availability limit other drug options. Chloramphenicol remains a useful alternative agent for central nervous system infections and rickettsial infections in patients allergic to β-lactams and tetracyclines, respectively.

- Toxicities with chloramphenicol include two main types of hematologic manifestations: idiosyncratic aplastic anemia (very rare and usually fatal) and dose-related bone marrow suppression.

Clindamycin

Clindamycin has good anaerobic **activity**, including *Actinomyces* spp.; however, 10% to 20% of *B. fragilis* organisms, 10% to 20% of *Clostridium* spp. (non-*C. perfringens*), and 10% of *Peptostreptococcus* spp. are resistant to clindamycin. Clindamycin also is active against many strains of staphylococci and streptococci, but emergence of resistance by staphylococci is common during treatment. Gram-negative aerobic bacteria and enterococci are resistant to clindamycin. Clindamycin does not penetrate well into the central nervous system.

Toxic effects most commonly include rash and gastrointestinal side effects. Antibiotic-associated diarrhea can occur in up to 20% of patients, and *C. difficile* colitis occurs in 1% to 10%. Minor increases of transaminase levels, reversible neutropenia, thrombocytopenia, and neuromuscular blockade are much less common.

The **clinical uses** of clindamycin encompass the treatment of anaerobic infections and infections outside the central nervous system. Examples include anaerobic and mixed pulmonary, intra-abdominal, and pelvic infections. For the treatment of polymicrobial intra-abdominal and pelvic infections, clindamycin is usually combined with a gram-negative active agent. Clindamycin is a useful alternative to penicillin in the treatment of *Clostridium perfringens* soft tissue infections. Clindamycin may reduce pyogenic toxin production, and the combination of clindamycin and penicillin for necrotizing group A streptococcal or clostridial infections may be superior to either drug alone.

- Clindamycin has activity against anaerobic and gram-positive organisms. However, emergence of resistance to clindamycin by staphylococci is common during treatment.
- About 10% to 20% of *B. fragilis* organisms are resistant to clindamycin.
- Antibiotic-associated diarrhea can occur in up to 20% of patients, including *C. difficile* colitis in 1% to 10% of patients.

Metronidazole

Metronidazole has very good antimicrobial **activity** against most anaerobic microorganisms, including *B. fragilis*. The exceptions include some anaerobic gram-positive non-spore–forming bacilli and *Peptostreptococcus*, *Actinomyces*, and *Propionibacterium acnes*. The agent is also effective against infections due to *Entamoeba histolytica*, *Giardia lamblia*, and *Gardnerella vaginalis*. This agent is cleared hepatically.

Toxic effects include nausea, vomiting, reversible neutropenia, metallic taste, a disulfiram reaction when coadministered with alcohol, and potentiation of the effects of oral anticoagulants. Major adverse reactions are rare and usually include central nervous system effects (seizures, cerebellar ataxia, peripheral neuropathy).

In regard to **clinical uses**, the excellent penetration of metronidazole into all tissues (including the central nervous system) and its bactericidal activity make metronidazole an effective drug for the treatment of serious anaerobic infections, including intra-abdominal infections, central nervous system abscesses, skin and soft tissue infections, and even endocarditis with susceptible organisms. Oral metronidazole is the treatment of choice for pseudomembranous colitis from *C. difficile*, giardiasis, amebiasis (followed by a luminal agent), bacterial vaginosis, and trichomoniasis. For polymicrobial infections, additional agents may be necessary for better coverage of aerobes and certain gram-positive anaerobes.

- Metronidazole is quite active against most anaerobic bacteria. It is often used in combination with agents active against aerobes for mixed infections including intra-abdominal infections.
- Oral metronidazole is the treatment of choice for pseudomembranous colitis from *C. difficile*, giardiasis, amebiasis (followed by a luminal agent), bacterial vaginosis, and trichomoniasis.

Macrolides

Erythromycin

Erythromycin is **active** against group A β-hemolytic streptococci, most other β-hemolytic streptococci (including groups B, C, F, and G), and *S. pneumoniae* (although resistance is increasing). Most methicillin-sensitive *S. aureus* isolates are also sensitive to erythromycin, but resistance can develop. Additionally, erythromycin is active against *B. pertussis*, *Campylobacter jejuni*, *T. pallidum*, *Ureaplasma urealyticum*, *Mycoplasma pneumoniae*, *Legionella pneumophila*, *Chlamydia* spp., and some strains of *Rickettsia*.

Toxic effects include gastrointestinal upset (dose-related), cholestatic jaundice (especially the erythromycin estolate compound), and transitory deafness (especially with large doses, such as 4 g/day). Erythromycin is hepatically cleared and can increase the serum levels of several drugs that are metabolized through the P-450 system, including theophylline, carbamazepine, and cyclosporine. High doses (usually of the IV formulation) can prolong the QT interval.

Clinical uses: Erythromycin is a drug of choice for *M. pneumoniae* infections, diphtheria, pertussis, *C. jejuni* gastroenteritis, and bacillary angiomatosis. It remains an active drug for pneumonia caused by *Chlamydia* and *Legionella* spp. Erythromycin is an alternative agent for patients allergic to β-lactams for treatment of mild-to-moderate soft tissue infections caused by susceptible staphylococcal and nonenterococcal streptococcal infections. Additionally, erythromycin can treat and eradicate the carrier state of *Corynebacterium diphtheriae* and shorten the duration of *B. pertussis* disease (whooping cough). Erythromycin is safe during pregnancy and can be used in combination therapy to treat pelvic inflammatory disease. Although it has been previously recommended by the American Heart Association as an alternative to penicillin for endocarditis prophylaxis preceding dental, oral, esophageal, and certain respiratory procedures, updated guidelines have replaced erythromycin with clindamycin, cephalosporins, and the newer macrolides (clarithromycin and azithromycin) because of erythromycin-associated gastrointestinal intolerance.

- Erythromycin can increase the serum levels of several drugs that are metabolized through the hepatic P-450 system.
- Clinical uses include treatment of atypical respiratory pathogens (such as *Mycoplasma*, *Chlamydia*, and *Legionella*), pertussis, diptheria, and *Campylobacter* gastroenteritis.

Clarithromycin

This agent provides good **activity** against most *S. pneumoniae* (resistance is increasing), β-hemolytic streptococci, viridans streptococci, methicillin-sensitive *S. aureus*, *M. catarrhalis*, *L. pneumophila*, *M. pneumoniae*, *C. pneumoniae*, *Chlamydia trachomatis*, *B. burgdorferi*, *M. avium-intracellulare*, and *M. chelonei*. It is superior to erythromycin for *S. pneumoniae* and β-hemolytic streptococci. It is moderately effective against *H. influenzae* and *N. gonorrhoeae*.

In regard to **pharmacokinetics**, excellent concentrations are achieved in many body fluids. The drug penetrates macrophages and polymorphonuclear neutrophils. Food has no effect on absorption. The half-life is 4 to 6 hours, which allows twice-daily dosing. An extended-release, once-daily formulation (clarithromycin XL) is also available. Excretion is through the liver and kidneys.

Adverse effects include nausea (3%) and other gastrointestinal complaints (less often than erythromycin). As with erythromycin, reversible hearing loss may occur at high dosages. Drug interactions (less severe than erythromycin) with theophylline and carbamazepine may occur with concomitant use of clarithromycin.

Clinical uses of clarithromycin include the treatment of mild-to-moderate upper and lower respiratory tract infections, including sinusitis, pharyngitis, acute and chronic bronchitis, and community-acquired pneumonia. Other indications include *M. avium-intracellulare* complex and other atypical mycobacterial infections, in combination with other active agents.

Azithromycin

The **spectrum of activity** is similar to that of clarithromycin. It is twofold to fourfold less active against streptococci, including *S. pneumoniae*, than erythromycin. It is more active against *H. influenzae* than clarithromycin. Azithromycin is the most active macrolide against *Legionella* species and remains active against *M. pneumoniae* and *C. pneumoniae*. *C. trachomatis* and *U. urealyticum* are also highly susceptible to azithromycin.

Pharmacokinetics: Oral bioavailability is approximately 37%. Azithromycin achieves excellent concentrations in many body fluids. The agent penetrates macrophages and polymorphonuclear neutrophils. Food decreases absorption of the capsules but not the tablets or suspension. Its half-life is 68 hours, which allows once-daily dosing. In addition, for many mild to moderate infections, a 5-day course of oral azithromycin is as effective as a 10-day course with an alternative drug. Azithromycin is hepatically metabolized.

Adverse effects are similar to those for clarithromycin. Intravenous azithromycin can cause pain at the injection site. Unlike erythromycin and clarithromycin, azithromycin has minimal interaction issues via the P-450 metabolic pathway.

Clinical uses of azithromycin include oral azithromycin for treatment of community-acquired mild-to-moderate upper and lower respiratory tract infections and skin and soft tissue infections. Because of activity against *Mycoplasma* spp., *Chlamydia* spp., and *Legionella* spp. and the availability in an intravenous form, azithromycin IV also is commonly used with a β-lactam agent as empiric therapy for severe community-acquired pneumonia. Some studies have shown improved survival when a macrolide–β-lactam combination is used, and it is theorized that there may be beneficial anti-inflammatory activity of macrolides.

Azithromycin is a first-line sexually transmitted disease agent against *C. trachomatis* and chancroid, and it can be used in high doses for *N. gonorrhoeae*. It is also first-line prophylaxis (in patients with human immunodeficiency virus [HIV]) against *M. avium* complex and is used as alternative treatment in combination therapy against *M. avium* complex, other atypical *Mycobacteria*, and *Toxoplasma gondii* infections.

Vancomycin

IV vancomycin, a glycopeptide antibiotic, has a **spectrum of activity** against most aerobic and anaerobic gram-positive organisms. However, it is not active against certain strains of *Lactobacillus, Leuconostoc, Actinomyces*, and vancomycin-resistant *Enterococcus* spp. Vancomycin is the drug of choice for infections caused by methicillin-resistant *S. aureus*, methicillin-resistant coagulase-negative staphylococci, highly penicillin-resistant *S. pneumoniae, Bacillus* spp., *Rhodococcus equi*, and other multiply resistant gram-positive organisms such as *Corynebacterium jeikeium*. It is also an alternative agent for infections caused by methicillin-sensitive staphylococci, enterococci (synergistic with aminoglycosides), or streptococci in patients intolerant of β-lactam antimicrobials. Although vancomycin is an active agent, it is less effective than antistaphylococcal β-lactams for treatment of methicillin-susceptible *S. aureus* infections and is not the drug of choice in this setting.

Oral vancomycin is not systemically absorbed and is used for treatment of *Clostridium difficile* colitis after failure, or due to intolerance, of metronidazole.

Vancomycin-resistant strains of *Enterococcus* species are becoming a serious problem. Additionally, vancomycin-resistant staphylococci have now been reported. The widespread use of vancomycin poses a substantial risk for the development of vancomycin-resistant organisms, and the Centers for Disease Control and Prevention has developed guidelines designed to limit the unnecessary use of this drug (Table 14-26).

Pharmacokinetics: Vancomycin is renally eliminated and has a half-life of 4 to 6 hours in patients with normal renal function. Dosing nomograms are available for empiric dosage adjustment for renal function, and serum levels often are monitored for further adjustments. This agent is not orally absorbed, and oral vancomycin is used only for local treatment of *C. difficile* gastroenteritis. Vancomycin has been used for treatment of central nervous system infections, but its penetration is less than that of β-lactam agents.

Adverse effects: Although rare, ototoxicity is the major toxic effect with vancomycin. This side effect is more common in the elderly and when vancomycin and aminoglycosides are administered concurrently. Infusion-related pruritus and the production of an erythematous rash or flushing reaction involving the face, neck, and upper body ("red man" or "red neck" syndrome) are due to a non–immunologic-related release of histamine. Its frequency can be reduced by slowing the rate of infusion and by the administration of antihistamines before vancomycin infusion.

In its early years, vancomycin contained impurities that were nephrotoxic and sometimes was called "Mississippi Mud." However, with the current preparation, nephrotoxicity is rare, except when vancomycin and aminoglycosides (or other nephrotoxic agents) are administered concurrently. With appropriate monitoring, it can be used in patients with underlying renal impairment or those receiving dialysis. Chemical thrombophlebitis (13%) and reversible neutropenia (2%) are also known side effects.

The **clinical uses** for vancomycin outlined by the Centers for Disease Control and Prevention are listed in Table 14-27.

Table 14-26 Situations in Which the Use of Vancomycin Should Be Discouraged

- Routine surgical prophylaxis
- Empiric antimicrobial therapy for a febrile neutropenic patient without high likelihood that infection is due to gram-positive organisms
- Treatment in response to a single blood culture positive for coagulase-negative *Staphylococcus* (i.e., if contamination of the culture is likely)
- Continued empiric use for presumed infections in patients whose cultures are negative for β-lactam–resistant gram-positive microorganisms
- Prophylaxis for infection or colonization of vascular catheters
- Selective decontamination of the digestive tract
- Eradication of methicillin-resistant *Staphylococcus aureus* colonization
- Primary treatment of *Clostridium difficile* colitis (should use metronidazole)
- Routine prophylaxis for infants with very low birth weight
- Routine prophylaxis for patients receiving continuous ambulatory peritoneal dialysis
- Treatment (chosen for convenience) of infections caused by β-lactam–susceptible gram-positive microorganisms in patients with renal dysfunction
- Use of vancomycin for topical application or irrigation

Data from Centers for Disease Control and Prevention: Preventing the spread of vancomycin resistance. Fed Register 1994;59:25758-25763.

Table 14-27   Therapeutic Indications for Vancomycin

- Serious infections caused by methicillin-resistant strains of *Staphylococcus aureus*, coagulase-negative staphylococci, and enterococci (resistant to penicillin/ampicillin)*
- Serious infections caused by *Staphylococcus aureus*, enterococci, or streptococci in patients intolerant of β-lactam antibiotics
- Infections caused by multiply resistant gram-positive organisms (e.g., *Corynebacterium jeikeium* and resistant strains of *Streptococcus pneumoniae*)
- *Clostridium difficile* colitis (oral administration) only if metronidazole therapy fails or in seriously ill patients
- Endocarditis prophylaxis for selected genitourinary or gastrointestinal procedures in penicillin-intolerant patients
- Surgical prophylaxis for major procedures involving implantation of prosthetic materials at institutions with high incidence of methicillin-resistant *Staphylococcus aureus* or methicillin-resistant *Staphylococcus epidermidis*

*Vancomycin may be less rapidly bactericidal than β-lactam agents for β-lactam–susceptible staphylococci.
Data from Centers for Disease Control and Prevention: Preventing the spread of vancomycin resistance. Fed Register 1994;59:25758-25763.

- Vancomycin is bactericidal against most aerobic and anaerobic gram-positive organisms.
- Vancomycin is the drug of choice for infections caused by methicillin-resistant *S. aureus*, methicillin-resistant coagulase-negative staphylococci, ampicillin-resistant enterococci, highly penicillin-resistant *S. pneumoniae*, and *Bacillus* species.
- Oral vancomycin is not absorbed and should not be used to treat systemic infections.
- The major toxic effect is ototoxicity. Nephrotoxicity can occur when vancomycin is coadministered with other nephrotoxic agents.
- "Red man" syndrome is due to non–immunologic-related release of histamine. This is not a true allergy.

Cotrimoxazole (Trimethoprim-Sulfamethoxazole)

Cotrimoxazole consists of two separate antimicrobials, trimethoprim and sulfamethoxazole, combined in a fixed (1:5) ratio. Both trimethoprim and sulfamethoxazole inhibit microbial folic acid synthesis and act synergistically when used in combination.

The **spectrum of activity** of cotrimoxazole includes a wide variety of aerobic gram-positive cocci and gram-negative bacilli, including *S. aureus* (moderate activity), many coagulase-negative staphylococci, most *S. pneumoniae*, *H. influenzae*, *M. catarrhalis*, *L. monocytogenes*, and many Enterobacteriaceae. It is active against *Pneumocystis carinii*, *S. maltophilia*, and *Nocardia asteroides*. Cotrimoxazole is also active against *Shigella* spp. (although resistant strains are reported), *Isospora belli*, and *Cyclospora cayetanensis*. It is not active against anaerobic bacteria and many strains of *Citrobacter freundii*, *Proteus vulgaris*, and *Providencia*. It is inactive against *P. aeruginosa* and enterococci.

Toxic effects with cotrimoxazole commonly include nausea and vomiting (3.2%) and rash (3.4%). Hypersensitivity reactions are more common in patients with acquired immunodeficiency syndrome (AIDS), but desensitization often can be done effectively for mild hypersensitivity. Diarrhea, nephrotoxicity, neutropenia, drug fever, and cholestatic hepatitis are less frequent. Caution or avoidance should be considered during the last trimester of pregnancy (to minimize risk of fetal kernicterus) and in patients with known glucose-6-phosphatase dehydrogenase deficiency. In some patients treated for *Pneumocystis carinii* pneumonia, hyperkalemia due to the trimethoprim component may occur. Cotrimoxazole has several known drug interactions, including increasing the activity of oral anticoagulants, increasing plasma phenytoin concentrations, enhancing hypoglycemia in patients taking oral hypoglycemics, and contributing to pancytopenia when coadministered with immunosuppressive agents.

Clinical uses of cotrimoxazole include the treatment of selected respiratory tract infections, urinary tract infections, prostatitis, and gastrointestinal bacterial infections with susceptible organisms. It is the drug of choice for treatment of *P. carinii* pneumonia, nocardiosis, and infections caused by *Stenotrophomonas*. It is also the drug of choice for prophylaxis against *P. carinii* pneumonia and toxoplasmosis in HIV-infected patients. It is an alternative in penicillin-allergic patients with *Listeria* meningitis.

- The spectrum of activity of cotrimoxazole includes a wide variety of gram-positive and gram-negative aerobic organisms.
- It is the drug of choice for treatment of *P. carinii* pneumonia, nocardiosis, and *Stenotrophomonas* infections and for prophylaxis against *P. carinii* pneumonia and toxoplasmosis in HIV-infected patients.
- With cotrimoxazole, hypersensitivity reactions are common in patients with AIDS.

Fluoroquinolones

Agents include norfloxacin, ciprofloxacin, ofloxacin, lomefloxacin, enoxacin, levofloxacin, sparfloxacin, grepafloxacin, gatifloxacin, and moxifloxacin.

Fluoroquinolones are derivatives of nalidixic acid, the first quinolone. They are bactericidal against a wide variety of microorganisms because of their ability to inhibit DNA gyrase (topoisomerase II) or topoisomerase IV. These enzymes are responsible for maintaining or restoring conformational structure of DNA during the replication process.

The **spectrum of activity** of fluoroquinolones varies from drug to drug. In general, they are active against most aerobic gram-negative bacilli, including the Enterobacteriaceae, *H. influenzae*, and some staphylococci. Gram-positive and anaerobic activity varies. Of concern is that bacterial resistance to fluoroquinolones is increasing, particularly among *P. aeruginosa* and staphylococci.

The fluoroquinolone agents have been somewhat arbitrarily divided into "generations" on the basis of spectra and drug age. These vary slightly according to the reference source but are somewhat helpful for discussing the differences in spectra among the various agents.

The first-generation agent, nalidixic acid, is no longer used. Second-generation agents include ciprofloxacin, ofloxacin, lomefloxacin, and norfloxacin (enoxacin is no longer available). Of these, ciprofloxacin is the primary agent used systemically. These agents achieve good tissue and fluid concentrations and can be used for infections at numerous sites. Ciprofloxacin has the best gram-negative activity (including *Pseudomonas* spp.) of the currently available fluoroquinolones. Ciprofloxacin does not have good activity against *S. pneumoniae*, and clinical failures have been reported. Thus, it should not be used empirically for treatment of community-acquired pneumonia.

The third-generation agent is levofloxacin (sparfloxacin and grepafloxacin are no longer available). Levofloxacin has improved activity against *S. pneumoniae* and other gram-positive organisms. It also retains good gram-negative coverage, but it is somewhat less than that of ciprofloxacin for *P. aeruginosa*. It has good activity against atypical pneumonia pathogens such as *C. pneumoniae*, *M. pneumoniae*, and *Legionella*.

The currently available fourth-generation agents include gatifloxacin and moxifloxacin (trovafloxacin is available only under restricted use). These agents have appreciable activity against anaerobes, including *B. fragilis*, and enhanced activity against gram-positive organisms, such as *S. pneumoniae*, *Staphylococcus*, and *Enterococcus*. These agents also remain quite active against aerobic gram-negative bacilli and have enhanced activity against atypical pneumonia organisms (e.g., *C. pneumoniae*, *M. pneumoniae*, and *Legionella*). However,

they are less active than ciprofloxacin against *P. aeruginosa*.

Intravenous formulations of ciprofloxacin, ofloxacin, levofloxacin, moxifloxacin, and gatifloxacin are currently available. In general, oral formulations should be used whenever possible because they attain plasma levels similar to the IV formulations and are much less costly.

Clinical uses: Fluoroquinolones are useful for treatment of gram-negative aerobic infections such as complicated urinary tract infections (not moxifloxacin because it does not achieve optimal urinary concentrations), prostatitis (good penetration), and many resistant gram-negative organisms (e.g., nosocomial pneumonia). Ciprofloxacin is active against *Pseudomonas* and is often used in combination with other antibiotics for serious infections.

The newer agents, moxifloxacin and gatifloxacin, are particularly well suited to treatment of community-acquired respiratory tract infections. Levofloxacin also has been used successfully for respiratory tract infections. Other uses of fluoroquinolones include infectious diarrhea, osteomyelitis, complicated skin infections, and mycobacterial infections (second-line). Agents with anaerobic activity (e.g., moxifloxacin) may be used in treatment of polymicrobial or mixed infections.

Pharmacokinetics: Fluoroquinolones are very well absorbed; thus, oral therapy often can be used in place of IV therapy. Norfloxacin, ofloxacin, levofloxacin, ciprofloxacin, and gatifloxacin are renally eliminated; doses should be adjusted for renal function. Moxifloxacin and trovafloxacin are primarily metabolized (and do not attain good urinary levels). The fluoroquinolones generally penetrate well into most tissues and fluids.

Fluoroquinolones are generally fairly well tolerated. The more common **toxic effects** are gastrointestinal and include nausea, vomiting, abdominal pain, and diarrhea. *C. difficile* colitis is rare.

Central nervous system effects are rare (incidence is somewhat variable among the agents) but can include headache, dizziness, light-headedness, confusion, hallucinations, restlessness, tremors, and seizures. Seizures are uncommon and usually are associated with an underlying seizure disorder or central nervous system structural defect.

Hypersensitivity reactions, nephrotoxicity, and serum sickness can occur but are uncommon. Phototoxicity can occur with some fluoroquinolones, and its frequency varies among the various agents (uncommon with currently available agents).

Fluoroquinolones can cause erosions in cartilage in animals and thus are not recommended in pregnant women or in patients younger than 18 years (exceptions exist). Tendinitis and tendon rupture are rare complications of fluoroquinolones.

Sparfloxacin and grepafloxacin have been withdrawn because of adverse events associated with prolongation of the QT interval. Levofloxacin, gatifloxacin, and moxifloxacin all now have warnings about QT interval prolongation in their package inserts and generally should be avoided in patients at increased risk of arrhythmias. Trovafloxacin carries a warning about possible serious hepatotoxicity. Gatifloxacin can cause disturbances in glucose homeostasis in some patients, resulting in hyperglycemia or hypoglycemia.

There are several important **drug interactions** with fluoroquinolones. Gastrointestinal absorption of the fluoroquinolones is decreased by coadministration of divalent or trivalent cations, which are found in aluminum- and magnesium-containing antacids, multivitamin preparations that include zinc, oral iron preparations, and calcium supplements. Concurrent administration of sucralfate also inhibits their absorption. Spacing the administration of the fluoroquinolone and interacting drug by several hours can minimize these absorption interactions. Some fluoroquinolones, particularly ciprofloxacin and to a lesser extent, ofloxacin (and previously enoxacin and grepafloxacin) increase serum theophylline and caffeine concentrations.

- The fluoroquinolones should be avoided in pregnant women and used with caution in patients younger than 18 years.
- Coadministration of aluminum-, calcium-, and magnesium-containing antacids, oral iron preparations, sucralfate, and multivitamin preparations with minerals decreases gastrointestinal absorption of the fluoroquinolones.
- Several quinolones have been associated with prolongation of the QT interval and arrhythmias in patients also receiving other drugs that prolong QT intervals and in patients at increased risk of arrhythmias.
- Ciprofloxacin has the best activity against *Pseudomonas*, whereas gatifloxacin and moxifloxacin have enhanced activity against community-acquired respiratory pathogens.

Other Antibacterial Agents

Linezolid is an oxalodinone that possesses activity against gram-positive bacteria, including methicillin-resistant *S. aureus*, methicillin-resistant *Staphylococcus epidermidis*, vancomycin-resistant enterococci (some resistance reported), and penicillin-resistant *S. pneumoniae*. Additionally, it has activity against some mycobacteria species, including *M. tuberculosis* and *M. avium* complex. Linezolid is not active against the Enterobacteriaceae and other gram-negative bacteria.

Pharmacokinetics: Linezolid can be administered either orally or intravenously. Linezolid is rapidly and extensively absorbed after oral dosing, its bioavailability approaching nearly 100%. Thus, oral administration is the preferred route whenever possible. It is well distributed throughout the body and penetrates into the cerebrospinal fluid. It is hepatically metabolized with predominantly inactive metabolites excreted through the kidneys.

The more serious **adverse effect** is myelosuppression (as well as anemia and thrombocytopenia). Headache, diarrhea, and peripheral neuropathy also can occur. Linezolid is also a weak monoamine oxidase inhibitor that can interact with foods containing high tyrosine content and potentially with some medications, such as selective serotonin reuptake inhibitor antidepressants.

Clinical uses of linezolid include the treatment of soft tissue, respiratory, and bloodstream infections with resistant gram-positive bacteria. Many clinicians advise cautious use of this agent so as not to enhance the incidence of resistance, especially to vancomycin-resistant enterococci for which limited treatment options are available. It is an alternative agent for the treatment of susceptible gram-positive infections in patients intolerant to first-line agents.

Dalfopristin-quinupristin (**Synercid**), derived from the streptogramin pristinamycin, acts synergistically to produce good activity against gram-positive cocci, including vancomycin-resistant *E. faecium*; however, activity against *E. faecalis* is substantially decreased. This agent is also active against staphylococci, including methicillin-resistant strains.

Pharmacokinetics: It is available only for intravenous administration and is hepatically metabolized.

Adverse reactions include inflammation and irritation at the infusion site, arthralgias, myalgias, and hyperbilirubinemia.

Anti-tuberculosis Agents

First- and second-line drugs are summarized in Tables 14-28 and 14-29.

For the past 50 years, **isoniazid** (INH) has been the cornerstone of combination drug therapy against *M. tuberculosis* and for treatment of latent tuberculosis infections. INH exerts bactericidal activity most likely through the inhibition of mycolic acid synthesis, an important component of mycobacterial cell walls. It is rapidly absorbed and readily diffuses across all body fluids and tissues. It penetrates into the cerebrospinal fluid and is effective for treatment of central nervous system disease. INH is metabolized by the liver and excreted in the urine, mostly as inactive metabolites. Although the rate of metabolism is determined by genetic acetylation phenotype, the acetylation status of an individual has not been shown to influence the outcome with daily therapy. INH is safe during pregnancy. Hepatitis is uncommon but is the most notable INH-related toxicity. When it occurs, it usually develops during the first 4 to 8 weeks of therapy. A clue to INH-related hepatitis is a rapid improvement in serum transaminase levels after use of the drug is stopped. INH can increase the elimination of pyridoxine (vitamin B_6), resulting in peripheral neuropathy. Malnutrition, alcoholism, diabetes, pregnancy, and uremia increase the risk

Table 14-28   First-Line Antituberculosis Medications

Variable	Isoniazid	Rifampin*	Pyrazinamide	Ethambutol	Streptomycin
Dosage,† daily	5 mg/kg (300 mg)	10 mg/kg (600 mg)	15-30 mg/kg (2 g)	15-25 mg/kg	15 mg/kg (1 g)
Dosage thrice weekly	15 mg/kg (900 mg)	10 mg/kg (600 mg)	50-70 mg/kg (3 g)	25-30 mg/kg	25-30 mg/kg (1.5 g)
Dosage twice weekly	15 mg/kg (900 mg)	10 mg/kg (600 mg)	50-70 mg/kg (4 g)	50 mg/kg	25-30 mg/kg (1.5 g)
Major toxic effects	Hepatitis Peripheral neuropathy Hypersensitivity reactions (+ANA 25%; lupus-like reaction 10%) Mild CNS effects	Drug interactions Hepatitis Cytopenias (↓ WBC, ↓ platelets) Orange discoloration of body fluids (can permanently stain soft contact lenses) Bleeding problems Light-chain proteinuria Hypersensitivity reactions Rash	Hepatitis Hyperuricemia (gout is rare) Arthalgias	Optic neuritis (↓ red-green color discrimination; ↓ visual acuity & fields)	Vestibular toxicity Auditory toxicity (high-frequency range) Nephrotoxicity
Monitoring	Baseline hepatic enzymes Repeat measurements if: baseline results abnormal, patient at high risk for adverse reactions, patient has symptoms of adverse reaction	Baseline CBC Platelets and hepatic enzymes Repeat measurements if: baseline measurements abnormal, patient has symptoms of adverse reaction	Baseline hepatic enzymes and uric acid Repeat measurements if: baseline measurements abnormal, patient has symptoms of adverse reactions, uric acid can be used as marker of compliance	Baseline and monthly testing of visual acuity and color vision	Baseline renal function, audiography and vestibular testing Regular creatinine measurements Repeat audiography and vestibular testing as needed
CNS penetration	20%-100% (good)	5%-20% (fair)	50%-100% (good)	5%-65% (variable)	20%-40% (variable)
Pregnancy	Safe	Safe	Avoid	Safe	Avoid
Elimination	Hepatic metabolism; renal excretion of inactive metabolites	Hepatic metabolism; biliary excretion	Hepatic metabolism; renal excretion of metabolites	Renal excretion	Renal excretion

ANA, antinuclear antibody; CBC, complete blood count; CNS, central nervous system; WBC, white blood cell.

*Alternative rifamycins include rifabutin 300 mg daily (dose adjustment may be needed with some antiretroviral agents) and rifapentine 600 mg weekly.

†Dosing (daily and intermittent) is listed for adults only; maximum recommended doses in parentheses.

Table 14-29 Second-Line Antituberculosis Medications

Variable	Drug								
	Amikacin	Kanamycin	Capreomycin	Levofloxacin	Ciprofloxacin	Moxifloxacin	Ethionamide	Cycloserine	PAS
Major toxic effects	Auditory toxicity Vestibular toxicity Nephrotoxicity	Auditory toxicity Vestibular toxicity Nephrotoxicity	Vestibular toxicity Auditory toxicity Nephrotoxicity	GI upset Dizziness	GI upset Dizziness	GI upset Prolonged QT interval	GI intolerance Hepatotoxicity Hypothyroidism	Psychosis Convulsion Depression	GI intolerance Rash Hepatitis
Elimination	Renal	Renal	Renal	Renal	Renal	Hepatic	Hepatic & renal	Renal	Hepatic & renal
Pregnancy	Avoid	Avoid	Avoid	Avoid	Avoid	Avoid	Avoid	Avoid	Safe

GI, gastrointestinal; PAS, para-aminosalicylic acid.

of peripheral neuropathy. It usually develops in a "stocking-glove" fashion and can be prevented by adding supplemental pyridoxine 5 to 50 mg/day. Hypersensitivity reactions, positive antinuclear antibody titers, and lupus-like reactions can also occur with INH therapy.

- Hepatotoxicity is the most serious adverse effect of INH.
- Peripheral neuropathy can be prevented with the coadministration of pyridoxine.
- Hypersensitivity reactions, positive antinuclear antibody titers, and lupus-like reactions can occur with INH.

Rifampin is a potent antimycobacterial agent and a vital component in 6- and 9-month combination treatment regimens for active infection. Its bactericidal activity acts by binding to DNA-dependent RNA polymerase to block RNA synthesis. It is rapidly absorbed and widely distributed throughout the body and achieves moderate cerebrospinal fluid penetration. It is predominantly hepatically metabolized with enterohepatic circulation; lesser amounts are excreted in the urine. It is safe in pregnancy. Hepatitis with an increase in transaminase value can occur with rifampin; however, increased bilirubin and alkaline phosphatase levels are more characteristic. Leukopenia, thrombocytopenia, orange discoloration of body fluids (including permanent staining of soft contact lenses), light-chain proteinuria, and hypersensitivity reactions can occur with rifampin. Rifampin will induce the hepatic cytochrome P-450 metabolic pathway, causing a substantial decrease in the serum concentration of drugs metabolized by this pathway (Table 14-30). These drug-to-drug interactions should be kept in mind when prescribing rifampin.

Rifabutin has activity similar to that of rifampin against *M. tuberculosis*. Rifabutin induces the hepatic cytochrome P-450 pathway to a lesser extent than rifampin. This allows for rifabutin use by HIV-coinfected patients taking certain protease inhibitors. Rifabutin has a side effect profile similar to that of rifampin and may additionally produce uveitis, arthritis or arthralgias, and bronze skin pigmentation. Of note, *M. tuberculosis* isolates resistant to rifampin are usually resistant to rifabutin. Both rifampin and rifabutin have activity against *M. avium* complex.

Rifapentine is another rifamycin antibacterial agent like rifampin and rifabutin but has a much longer half-life. This allows for less frequent dosing, reduced total number of doses to complete treatment, and easier administration of directly observed therapy. Once-weekly rifapentine and INH may be used in the continuation phase of therapy for select patients.

Fixed-dose combination drugs should be considered for directly observed therapy and are strongly recommended if such therapy is not possible. Two fixed-dose combination drugs are currently available in the United States for the treatment of tuberculosis: INH plus rifampin (**Rifamate**) and INH plus rifampin plus pyrazinamide (**Rifater**). Typical daily doses are 2 tablets of Rifamate (300 mg INH, 600 mg rifampin) or 6 tablets of Rifater (300 mg INH, 720 mg rifampin, 1,800 mg pyrazinamide); however, individualized dosing adjustments may be needed.

- Increased bilirubin and alkaline phosphatase values may occur with rifampin.
- Rifampin and (to a lesser extent) rifabutin induce the hepatic cytochrome P-450 system, decreasing the serum concentration of many coadministered drugs.
- Rifabutin may cause uveitis, arthritis or arthralgias, and bronze skin pigmentation.

Table 14-30   Drugs With Substantially Reduced Serum Concentrations in the Presence of Rifampin*

Azathioprine	Digoxin	Propranolol
Azole antifungals	Haloperidol	Protease inhibitors
Calcium channel blockers	Imidazoles	Quinidine
Corticosteroids	Opioids/methadone	Theophylline
Cyclosporine	Oral contraceptives	Tolbutamide
Dapsone	Oral hypoglycemic agents	Warfarin
Diazepam	Phenytoin	

*The list is not all-inclusive; review drug interactions thoroughly when prescribing.

Pyrazinamide (PZA) is more active in an acidic environment and exerts potent bactericidal activity within cavitary or suppurative disease. PZA is an essential initial component of a 6-month combination drug regimen; the benefit of PZA is less clear beyond the first 2 months of therapy. PZA is readily absorbed and diffuses throughout all body fluids and tissues. It achieves good cerebrospinal fluid penetration for the treatment of central nervous system disease. Because data are insufficient regarding the potential teratogenicity of PZA, the Centers for Disease Control and Prevention recommends it should generally be avoided during pregnancy. As with INH and rifampin, hepatitis also can occur with PZA. A prolonged recovery of increased transaminase levels is a clue toward PZA toxicity. Hyperuricemia is common, although clinical gout is rare.

- PZA is most active during the first 2 months of therapy and within an acidic medium.
- Hepatitis and hyperuricemia may occur with PZA, but clinical gout is rare.
- PZA is an important initial component of a 6-month combination treatment program for active disease.

Ethambutol is bacteriostatic in low concentrations and bactericidal as the dosage is increased. It is readily absorbed, with variable cerebrospinal fluid penetration. It is predominantly excreted in the urine and is safe in pregnancy. Retrobulbar or optic neuritis is the most noteworthy toxic effect of ethambutol. It usually manifests as a decrease in red-green color discrimination, visual acuity, and visual field. Caution must be used in young children because visual testing may be unreliable.

Streptomycin is one of the oldest antituberculosis and aminoglycoside agents in use today. However, because of increased global resistance, streptomycin is no longer considered a first-line agent. It requires IV or IM injection and is renally excreted. Notable toxic effects are vestibular, auditory, and renal. Appropriate drug dosing should be based on serum drug concentrations. Vestibular, auditory, and renal function should be closely monitored.

- Retrobulbar or optic neuritis is the most noteworthy toxic effect of ethambutol.
- Vestibular, auditory, and renal toxicity can occur with streptomycin.

Drug intolerance and microbial resistance are common in the management of tuberculosis and may require the addition of one or more "second-line" antituberculosis agents (Table 14-29). The widespread use of these agents for mycobacterial disease is curbed by reduced activity or increased toxicity or both. **Amikacin**, **kanamycin**, and **capreomycin** are injectable agents with moderate antituberculosis activity. Auditory (high-frequency hearing loss), vestibular, and renal dysfunction are the most common toxic effects. Amikacin and kanamycin are aminoglycosides, whereas capreomycin is a polypeptide antibiotic. **Ethionamide** is highly absorbed and penetrates well into the cerebrospinal fluid. Its use is usually limited by gastrointestinal intolerance (nausea, vomiting, and dysgeusia). Additional side effects include arthralgias and certain endocrine disorders (hypothyroidism, glucose abnormalities, sexual and menstrual abnormalities). **Para-aminosalicylic acid** (PAS) has been in use for the past 50 years and is formulated in delayed-release granules with an acid-resistant outer coating (Paser granules). Rash is common with PAS use, as are gastrointestinal intolerance (nausea, vomiting, and abdominal discomfort), hepatitis, and hypothyroidism. **Levofloxacin**, **ofloxacin**, and **ciprofloxacin** are fluoroquinolones commonly used as second-line agents. They have moderate antituberculosis activity and are usually better tolerated. **Cycloserine** is not as commonly used because of its high side-effect profile, but it has a role against multidrug-resistant tuberculosis. Notable side effects include psychosis, confusion, depression, and headaches. Coadministration of pyridoxine may help decrease the incidence of central nervous system-related side effects.

- Amikacin, kanamycin, capreomycin, levofloxacin, ofloxacin, ciprofloxacin, ethionamide, cycloserine, and PAS are second-line antituberculosis agents.
- They usually have reduced activity and increased toxicity.

ANTIFUNGAL THERAPY

Azole Antifungal Agents

The azole antifungal agents produce their fungistatic effect by interfering with the synthesis and permeability of fungal cell membranes. They do this through inhibition of the fungal cytochrome P-450 enzyme responsible for conversion of lanosterol to ergosterol, which is a major constituent of fungal cell membranes. The azole antifungal agents are less toxic alternatives to amphotericin for many types of fungal infections.

Selected pharmacologic properties of azole antifungal agents are listed in Table 14-31.

Fluconazole

Spectrum of activity: Fluconazole has good activity against most Candida spp. (less activity for C. glabrata and C. krusei), Cryptococcus, Coccidioides, Histoplasma, Blastomyces, and Paracoccidioides infections.

Pharmacokinetics: Because of the long half-life of fluconazole, it can be administered in a once-per-day dose. It is available in oral tablet, oral suspension, and IV formulations. Because of its excellent oral absorption and the considerably higher expense of IV therapy, fluconazole should be given orally whenever possible. Fluconazole achieves good penetration into the cerebrospinal fluid and is primarily renally eliminated.

Clinical uses include treatment of many types of susceptible candidal infections. The drug also may be used for prophylaxis of candidal infection in neutropenic patients, patients undergoing bone marrow transplantation, and AIDS patients with chronic, recurrent mucocutaneous candidiasis. A concern is emergence of resistant fungi, such as C. krusei, resistant C. glabrata, and, more rarely, resistant Candida albicans (especially in HIV). In serious infections, speciation and susceptibility testing of candidal organisms should be considered.

Fluconazole is also used for treatment of cryptococcal meningitis. For this infection, most experts recommend initial therapy for serious infections with amphotericin B and flucytosine, followed by maintenance therapy with fluconazole. Additionally, fluconazole has been used successfully for treatment of Coccidioides meningitis. It is second-line therapy for non–life-threatening cases of histoplasmosis and blastomycosis (after itraconazole and amphotericin).

Adverse effects: This agent is generally well tolerated, and discontinuation of therapy is rarely necessary. The most common effects are gastrointestinal symptoms, rash, and headache. Mild increases in liver function values are occasionally found, but fatal hepatic necrosis is rare. There is no interference with adrenocortical function or synthesis of testosterone, which can occur with ketoconazole.

Table 14-31 Selected Pharmacologic Properties of Azole Antifungal Agents

Factor	Antifungal agent			
	Fluconazole	Itraconazole	Voriconazole	Ketoconazole
Route of administration	Oral, IV	Oral, IV	Oral, IV	Oral
Requires gastric acidity for absorption	No	Yes for oral capsules	No	Yes
Protein binding, %	12	99	60	91-99
Cerebrospinal fluid concentrations	High	Minimal (but some clinical efficacy noted)	High	Minimal
Half-life, h	25-30	24-64	6	8
Clearance route	Renal	Hepatic	Hepatic	Hepatic
Urinary levels of active drug	High	Low	Low	Low
Dose reduction for renal dysfunction	Yes	No for oral*	No for oral*	No

IV, intravenous.

*The manufacturer warns against use of intravenous itraconazole in patients with creatinine clearance <30 mL/min and of voriconazole with creatinine clearance <50 mL/min because of the possible accumulation of the vehicle.

Drug interactions: Although to a lesser degree than other azoles, fluconazole inhibits metabolism of several drugs through inhibition of the cytochrome P-450 isoenzyme 3A4. It can increase serum levels of phenytoin, oral hypoglycemic agents, carbamazepine, cyclosporine, tacrolimus, dihydropyridine calcium channel blockers, and warfarin. It also can increase concentrations of rifabutin, leading to potential uveitis. Coadministration with rifampin or INH decreases serum concentrations of fluconazole.

Itraconazole

Spectrum of activity: A major advantage of itraconazole over fluconazole is its greater activity against *Aspergillus*, *Sporothrix schenckii*, *Histoplasma capsulatum*, and *Blastomycosis dermatitidis*. It also has activity against *Coccidioides immitis* and *Candida* (cross-resistance can occur).

Pharmacokinetics: Itraconazole is available in capsule and oral solution formulations and an IV preparation. The two oral formulations are not bioequivalent; the oral solution produces considerably higher serum concentrations and higher area under the curve. For optimal absorption, the capsule should be taken with food, and the liquid on an empty stomach. Because oral absorption (especially with the capsule formulation) is erratic, serum levels should be checked to document adequate systemic levels when itraconazole is used for serious infections. The IV formulation produces higher systemic levels than equivalent doses of oral itraconazole. Itraconazole is extensively metabolized and has an active metabolite, hydroxyitraconazole.

The IV formulation contains the excipient hydroxypropyl-(β)-cyclodextrin, which produced pancreatic adenocarcinomas in a rat carcinogenicity study. The clinical significance in humans is unknown. Because the excipient is renally eliminated and can accumulate with renal dysfunction, caution should be used in prescribing IV itraconazole in patients with renal insufficiency (i.e., creatinine clearance <30 mL/min).

Clinical uses include histoplasmosis, in which it is used for chronic cavitary pulmonary disease and disseminated, non–life-threatening nonmeningeal disease. Itraconazole also is effective maintenance therapy of histoplasmosis and blastomycosis in patients with AIDS. Itraconazole is now the drug of choice for pulmonary and nonpulmonary (bone, joint, skin) blastomycosis. It also can be used for nonmeningeal coccidioidomycosis (pulmonary, bone, and joint). In a small number of patients, coccidioidal meningitis also has been effectively treated with itraconazole. Itraconazole is an alternative for treatment of many *Candida* species (often cross-resistant with fluconazole), and it is commonly used for treatment of onychomycosis. When used for sporotrichosis, itraconazole is effective in lymphocutaneous and bone and joint diseases, although relapse may occur in disseminated disease. As therapy for *Aspergillus*, success rates of 44% to 77% have been reported for

invasive pulmonary and sinus disease. Amphotericin B or voriconazole are drugs of choice, at least for initial use, for most cases of invasive aspergillosis. Itraconazole also has been studied as a corticosteroid-sparing agent in allergic bronchopulmonary aspergillosis.

The most common **side effects** involve the gastrointestinal tract and rash. Similar to fluconazole, hepatitis can occur but is rare. At lower doses, there is typically little or no effect on glucocorticoid or testosterone synthesis (as can be seen with ketoconazole). With higher doses or systemic levels, edema, hypokalemia, nausea, and vomiting can occur. Congestive heart failure has rarely been reported in patients with cardiac disease.

Drug interactions: Itraconazole inhibits metabolism and increases serum levels of many drugs, such as cyclosporine, tacrolimus, digoxin, midazolam, triazolam, and cisapride. Cyclosporine, tacrolimus, and digoxin levels should be monitored if concomitant therapy is used. Coadministration with rifampin, isoniazid, phenytoin, and carbamazepine can decrease itraconazole levels. Like ketoconazole, itraconazole capsules require gastric acid for absorption; thus, absorption is decreased with concomitant use of histamine$_2$ blockers, antacids, proton pump inhibitors, and didanosine chewable tablets (contain an antacid buffer). These gastric pH interactions are not substantial with the oral liquid formulation of itraconazole.

Voriconazole

Voriconazole is a derivative of fluconazole and has enhanced activity against *Aspergillus* and *Scedosporium apiospermum* (*Pseudallescheria boydii*). It also may have increased activity against *Candida* (including some fluconazole-resistant strains), *Fusarium* spp., and *Cryptococcus*. It has in vitro activity against histoplasmosis, blastomycosis, *Trichophyton* spp., *Microsporum*, and *Coccidiodes*. It does not have activity against Zygomycetes.

Pharmacokinetics: Voriconazole is well absorbed and penetrates tissues well (including central nervous system penetration with inflammation). It undergoes hepatic metabolism via P-450 enzymes. It inhibits the cytochrome P-450 3A4 enzyme and thus interacts with drugs metabolized through this pathway. In patients with creatinine clearance less than 50 mL/min, IV voriconazole should be used only if the benefit outweighs the risk because of potential accumulation of the intravenous vehicle (sulfobutyl ether β-cyclodextrin sodium) (clinical significance unknown).

Clinical uses: Voriconazole has good activity against *Aspergillus* and *Candida* and is a welcome addition to the antifungal agents for immunocompromised patients. Voriconazole is not approved by the U.S. Food and Drug Administration for the empiric treatment of neutropenic fever; however, its performance and measured outcomes were closely similar to those of amphotericin. Its activity against *Scedosporium*, *Fusarium*, and *Candida* spp. less susceptible to fluconazole (e.g., *C. glabrata*) also makes this agent a useful alternative in treating infections caused by these pathogens.

Toxic effects include transient visual disturbances, which have been reported in up to 10% of patients. Similar to other azoles, voriconazole can cause increased liver enzyme values and, rarely, hepatotoxicity.

- Voriconazole has good activity against *Aspergillus* and has become a drug of choice for this infection.
- Voriconazole frequently causes transient visual disturbances, including blurred vision, changes in color vision, photophobia, and other visual perception changes. These are generally mild and typically do not cause discontinuation of therapy.

Ketoconazole

Ketoconazole was the first of the azole antifungals. It has a broad **spectrum of activity**; however, because of its toxicities and the improved pharmacologic characteristics of newer agents, ketoconazole is typically no longer an antifungal drug of choice.

Ketoconazole is available only as an oral agent and requires gastric acid for absorption. It has numerous drug interactions via inhibition of the P-450 cytochrome system. The most common **toxic effect** of ketoconazole is dose-related gastrointestinal upset. Decreased synthesis of adrenal corticosteroids, most notably androgenic corticosteroids, is a dose-related effect that may occur with ketoconazole. This may lead to gynecomastia, menstrual irregularities, and loss of libido with impotence. It also can interfere with cortisol response, and long-term therapy can cause a hypermineralocorticoid effect. Arterial hypertension, edema, and hypokalemia have been reported. Acute hepatitis, which can be fatal, occurs rarely.

- Ketoconazole requires gastric acid for absorption and has serious drug interactions with medications that are metabolized through the P-450 isoenzyme CYP3A4.
- Because of anti-androgenic effects, gynecomastia, menstrual effects, and loss of libido are fairly common side effects.

Polyenes

Amphotericin B Products

Amphotericin B is a fungicidal antifungal agent whose **mode of action** is binding of ergosterol in cell walls and increasing cell wall permeability, which leads to cell death. Its spectrum of activity is the broadest of currently available agents and includes yeasts, *Aspergillus*, *Zygomyces*, dimorphic fungi, and most dematiaceous molds. It is commonly used for serious or life-threatening fungal infections, especially in immunocompromised patients. Organisms that might exhibit resistance include *P. boydii*, *Candida lusitaniae*, *Candida guillermondii*, *Fusarium* species, *Trichosporon* species, some of the species that cause chromoblastomycosis and phaeohyphomycosis, and rare isolates of *C. albicans*, *C. krusei*, *C. glabrata*, and *Aspergillus* species.

Toxic effects include infusion-related reactions such as fever, chills or rigors, nausea, and vomiting. Pretreatment options (such as diphenhydramine, acetaminophen, and meperidine) may lessen these adverse reactions if a patient experiences problems. Nephrotoxicity (usually reversible) is the other major side effect of amphotericin B. This can be lessened by sodium loading, every-other-day dosing, or using a lipid formulation of amphotericin B. Nephrotoxicity is increased with concomitant use of cyclosporine or other nephrotoxic agents. Other adverse effects include hypokalemia, hypomagnesemia, reversible anemia, and phlebitis. More rarely, changes in blood pressure, bradycardia, neurologic effects, and pulmonary decompensation can occur.

Three lipid formulations of amphotericin B are available: amphotericin B lipid complex (Abelcet), amphotericin B cholesteryl sulfate (Amphotec), and liposomal amphotericin (AmBisome). These agents have considerably less renal toxic effect than amphotericin B. The incidence of infusion-related adverse effects varies among the agents; liposomal amphotericin (AmBisome) seems to have the least adverse effects. Unfortunately, these newer agents are very expensive and should be used judiciously.

Clinical uses of amphotericin include the treatment of deep-seated or life-threatening fungal infections. It is often used for serious candidal infections, fever not responding to antimicrobials in neutropenic patients, invasive *Aspergillus* infections, initial treatment of cryptococcal meningitis (often in combination with flucytosine), and life-threatening or disseminated histoplasmosis, blastomycosis, and coccidioidomycosis.

Glucan Synthesis Inhibitors

Caspofungin

Caspofungin is the first agent available in the glucan synthesis inhibitor class of antifungal agents. These agents inhibit the synthesis of β-(1,3)-D-glucan, an integral part of the fungal cell wall.

Spectrum of activity: Caspofungin is fungicidal and has good activity against *Aspergillus* and *Candida*, including most azole-resistant strains. However, it has reduced activity against *Cryptococcus* (not active), *Fusarium*, Zygomycetes, *Histoplasma*, *Blastomyces*, and possibly *Candida parapsilosis* (unclear). Caspofungin is available only in an IV formulation and currently is not approved for use in patients younger than 18 years.

Pharmacokinetics: Caspofungin is slowly metabolized by acetylation and hydrolysis and also undergoes spontaneous chemical degradation. Only a small amount is excreted unchanged in the urine, and dose adjustment is not necessary for renal impairment.

Clinical uses: Caspofungin is a first-line antifungal agent for treatment of serious *Candida* infections and has activity at least equal to amphotericin. It is an alternative agent for treatment of *Aspergillus* infections and for neutropenic fever (not yet approved for this indication).

Adverse effects: Caspofungin is generally well tolerated. Possible histamine-mediated effects such as rash, facial swelling, a sensation of warmth, increased eosinophils, and, rarely, anaphylaxis have been reported. Other adverse effects that have uncommonly been reported include fever, phlebitis, gastrointestinal effects, flushing, increased liver function values, and hypokalemia. An increase in liver function values has been noted during concomitant cyclosporine therapy, and caution is advised when using this combination until further studies are conducted.

● Caspofungin is useful for serious candidal infections and is an alternative for treatment of aspergillosis and neutropenic fever.

Other Antifungal Agents

Flucytosine

The **modes of action** of this agent involve conversion to 5-fluorouracil triphosphate, intracellularly, which causes miscoding of fungal RNA, and the conversion to 5-fluorodeoxyuridine monophosphate, which inhibits DNA synthesis. Resistance develops rapidly when it is used alone, and thus it is typically used in combination with other antifungal agents (most commonly amphotericin). It has **activity** against *Cryptococcus*, *Candida* species, and chromoblastomycosis.

Toxicity is often associated with high serum levels (>100 μg/mL). Side effects include neutropenia, thrombocytopenia, diarrhea, nausea, gastrointestinal upset, and reversible increases in liver function values. Because flucytosine is eliminated renally, renal dysfunction or concomitant use with nephrotoxic drugs without appropriate dosage adjustment can increase toxicity. Serum levels should be monitored and appropriate dose adjustments made to minimize toxicity.

Clinical uses include combination therapy for cryptococcal meningitis (usually used in combination with amphotericin B), *Candida* meningitis, and disseminated candidal infections (usually in combination with amphotericin). Generally, flucytosine should not be used as monotherapy because of rapid development of resistance. However, flucytosine has been used successfully for *Candida* cystitis (urinary levels are high) and chromoblastomycosis, but relapse and resistance can occur.

ANTIVIRAL AGENTS

Current agents are virustatic and have no activity against nonreplicating or latent viruses. Antiretroviral agents are discussed in the chapter on HIV infection, and agents used in treatment of hepatitis are discussed in the gastroenterology chapter. Other antiviral agents are discussed below.

Acyclovir

Acyclovir is a nucleoside analogue of guanosine. It is phosphorylated by virus-specific thymidine kinase to monophosphate and further phosphorylated to the triphosphate form by cellular enzymes. Acyclovir triphosphate inhibits viral DNA polymerase and also acts as a DNA chain terminator.

Acyclovir has good **activity** against herpes simplex viruses 1 and 2 and varicella-zoster virus. It has considerably less activity against Epstein-Barr virus and cytomegalovirus. Resistance to acyclovir can develop through mutations of either viral thymidine kinase or DNA polymerase.

Oral acyclovir is poorly absorbed (bioavailability of 15%-30%). Thus, patients with severe disease or who are immunocompromised should receive IV therapy. Acyclovir generally is well tolerated.

Toxic effects include gastrointestinal distress, headaches, and phlebitis (IV form). Reversible renal dysfunction resulting from crystalline nephropathy can occur with high-dose IV therapy. The risk can be decreased by saline hydration and appropriate dose adjustment for renal function. Confusion, delirium, lethargy, and seizures can occur with high-dose IV therapy in patients with high serum concentrations.

Clinical uses for acyclovir include herpes simplex virus infections (noncurative). It is effective for treatment of primary and recurrent episodes of herpes genitalis and for chronic suppression in patients with frequent recurrences. Topical acyclovir is less effective than oral therapy in genital herpes simplex virus infection. IV therapy should be considered in serious disease. In immunocompromised patients, oral or IV acyclovir is effective in the suppression and treatment of oral-labial disease. IV acyclovir (in high doses of 10 mg/kg every 8 h with normal renal function) is the drug of choice for herpes simplex virus encephalitis.

Acyclovir also is used for varicella-zoster virus. In immunocompetent patients with primary varicella, it can shorten the healing time (about 1 day) and decrease the number of lesions if given early (within 24 hours). IV acyclovir in immunocompromised patients can halt progression and prevent dissemination of varicella-zoster. Varicella-zoster in an immunocompetent host responds to oral acyclovir 800 mg 5 times a day, and this leads to decreased viral shedding and time to healing. It is effective only if given within 72 hours of the onset of symptoms. Early administration may decrease postherpetic neuralgia.

- Crystalline nephropathy can occur with high-dose IV therapy. Its incidence can be reduced by saline hydration and appropriate dose adjustment for renal function.
- IV acyclovir is the drug of choice for herpes simplex encephalitis.

Valacyclovir

Valacyclovir is an oral prodrug of acyclovir that is converted extensively and almost completely to acyclovir and L-valine. Acyclovir is the active drug that inhibits viral DNA synthesis. Approximately 54% to 60% of the valacyclovir dose is available as active acyclovir, representing a twofold to fivefold increase in bioavailability over that achieved after administration of oral acyclovir. The higher bioavailability of valacyclovir also allows for less frequent administration than with oral acyclovir. Like acyclovir, valacyclovir generally is well tolerated.

Toxic effects with valacyclovir are very similar to those with acyclovir (see above). However, when valacyclovir was studied in very high doses (8 g/day) in immunosuppressed patients (patients who had transplantation and patients with HIV), thrombotic thrombocytopenic purpura and hemolytic-uremic syndrome were reported.

Clinical uses of valacyclovir include the treatment of varicella-zoster infections and the treatment and suppression of recurrent genital herpes (noncurative). Some studies have suggested that valacyclovir may be more effective than acyclovir for varicella-zoster. Like acyclovir, valacyclovir may decrease postherpetic neuralgia.

- Valacyclovir is an oral prodrug of acyclovir that increases bioavailability twofold to fivefold. For most indications it can be given less frequently than oral acyclovir.

Famciclovir

Famciclovir is available only as an oral drug. Famciclovir is a prodrug that is converted to its active form, penciclovir, through tissue and hepatic enzymatic processes. A prolonged intracellular half-life allows for dosing three times daily. It has good bioavailability and is well tolerated.

Clinical uses are similar to those of valacyclovir (see above). It is useful for herpes simplex and varicella-zoster virus infections. It may reduce the duration of postherpetic neuralgia when given early in varicella-zoster infections.

Ganciclovir

This agent inhibits DNA polymerase and is dependent on phosphorylation by viral thymidine kinase. Like acyclovir, it is active against herpes simplex viruses and varicella-zoster. However, it is about 10 times more potent than acyclovir against cytomegalovirus and Epstein-Barr virus and also has activity against human herpesvirus 6. It is available as oral, IV, and ocular preparations. The oral formulation is poorly absorbed, and thus IV therapy is needed for serious disease. Valganciclovir (see below) is an oral prodrug of ganciclovir that achieves significantly higher levels than oral ganciclovir.

Toxic effects include neutropenia and thrombocytopenia. The incidence of neutropenia may be increased when ganciclovir is used in combination with other immunosuppressive drugs. Cytopenias are reversible after use of the drug is stopped. It is teratogenic, carcinogenic, and mutagenic in animals. Less common side effects include fever, rash, anemia, and increased values on liver function tests. Like acyclovir, it is renally eliminated and close monitoring of renal function is required. Dosage adjustment for IV ganciclovir is needed even in the presence of mild renal impairment.

Clinical uses for ganciclovir include treatment of cytomegalovirus retinitis in patients with AIDS. Studies also have shown beneficial results in other cytomegalovirus infections (colitis, esophagitis, gastritis, and pneumonia) in patients with AIDS and in other immunocompromised hosts. In patients with AIDS, maintenance therapy may be necessary to prevent relapse. Used in combination with hyperimmune globulin, ganciclovir reduces mortality from cytomegalovirus pneumonitis in patients who have had allogeneic bone marrow transplantation. Oral and IV ganciclovir therapy may be given to at-risk patients before transplantation to prevent cytomegalovirus infection.

Although in vitro activity is seen for Epstein-Barr virus and human herpesvirus 6, clinical efficacy remains unclear.

Oral ganciclovir is an alternative to IV maintenance therapy for cytomegalovirus retinitis in patients who have only peripheral cytomegalovirus lesions. Unfortunately, the oral formulation has poor bioavailability, but the prodrug valganciclovir achieves higher levels.

Ganciclovir ocular implants provide the drug directly to the site of the infection in patients with cytomegalovirus retinitis. Vitrasert implants are surgically implanted into the pars plana and deliver a slow release of drug over 7 to 8 months. Possible disadvantages include the spread of infection to the contralateral eye, a low incidence of endophthalmitis, and the need to replace the inserts.

- Ganciclovir is used for cytomegalovirus infections in immunocompromised patients.
- Bone marrow suppression is the most serious adverse effect. The incidence may be increased when ganciclovir is used in combination with other immunosuppressive drugs.

Valganciclovir

Valganciclovir is an oral prodrug of ganciclovir with 60% bioavailability. Once absorbed, it is rapidly converted to ganciclovir and achieves a similar area under the curve as IV ganciclovir. It is not a substitute on a "one-for-one" basis with ganciclovir (IV or oral) because valganciclovir has its own dosing platform. Its toxicity profile is similar to that of ganciclovir.

Clinical uses are directed against cytomegalovirus infection. It is approved for treatment of cytomegalovirus retinitis in HIV-infected patients, and the efficacy of valganciclovir has been shown to be similar to that of IV ganciclovir for induction therapy. Oral valganciclovir also has been used for treatment of cytomegalovirus disease in transplant and other immunocompromised patients.

Foscarnet

Foscarnet is a noncompetitive inhibitor of viral DNA polymerase and reverse transcriptase. It does not require phosphorylation and may be active against acyclovir-resistant and ganciclovir-resistant strains. It has in vitro activity against all human herpesviruses, HIV, and hepatitis B.

Toxic effects include nephrotoxicity, which usually develops during the second week and is reversible. Substantial renal impairment develops in about a third of patients. The risk of nephrotoxicity is increased with concurrent use of nephrotoxic drugs (e.g., amphotericin B, aminoglycosides, and cyclosporine). Saline hydration may decrease the risk of nephrotoxicity.

Foscarnet is renally eliminated, and close renal monitoring is required to reduce adverse effects. Like IV ganciclovir, foscarnet requires dose adjustment with mild renal impairment.

Electrolyte disturbances, such as hypocalcemia, hyperphosphatemia, hypophosphatemia, hypokalemia, and hypomagnesemia, also commonly occur. The risk of hypocalcemia is increased with concomitant use of IV pentamidine. Central nervous system side effects, fever, nausea, vomiting, anemia, fatigue, headache, leukopenia, pancreatitis, and genital ulceration also have been reported.

Clinical uses of foscarnet include cytomegalovirus retinitis, including disease that is due to ganciclovir-resistant strains. It also may be effective in gastrointestinal cytomegalovirus disease in patients with AIDS. Foscarnet may be active against acyclovir-resistant strains of herpes simplex virus or varicella-zoster virus and against most ganciclovir-resistant strains of cytomegalovirus. However, it is more expensive and less well tolerated than ganciclovir. It requires controlled rates of infusions and large volumes of fluid. Controlled trials in patients with AIDS and cytomegalovirus retinitis showed no difference in the progression of the retinitis between foscarnet-treated and ganciclovir-treated patients. However, there was an unexplained decrease in mortality in the foscarnet group (which may be related to antiretroviral activity). Foscarnet therapy had to be discontinued more often than ganciclovir because of side effects.

- Foscarnet is effective for cytomegalovirus infections, including most strains that are resistant to ganciclovir.
- Nephrotoxicity is the major dose-limiting side effect. It usually develops during the second week and is reversible.

Cidofovir

Cidofovir is a nucleotide analogue with activity against herpesviruses, including cytomegalovirus, herpes simplex virus, varicella-zoster virus, and Epstein-Barr virus. Its Food and Drug Administration indication is for the treatment of cytomegalovirus retinitis in patients with AIDS. Unlike ganciclovir and acyclovir, which require activation by viral-encoded enzymes, conversion of cidofovir to its active intracellular metabolite is performed by host (rather than viral) cellular enzymes. Thus, cidofovir may retain activity against many ganciclovir-resistant strains of cytomegalovirus. The long intracellular half-life of cidofovir-active metabolites allows for weekly intravenous dosing during induction therapy and every-other-week IV administration during maintenance therapy.

The dose-limiting **toxic effect** of cidofovir is nephrotoxicity. Administration with probenecid and saline hydration decreases the incidence and severity of nephrotoxicity. Cidofovir is contraindicated in patients with preexisting renal dysfunction (serum creatinine >1.5 mg/dL, estimated creatinine clearance <55 mL/min, or urine protein ≥100 mg/dL), and renal function must be monitored closely during therapy. Optimally, it should not be given with other nephrotoxic drugs. Neutropenia also has been reported in up to 20% of patients. More rare adverse reactions include ocular hypotony and metabolic acidosis. Adverse effects to probenecid are also fairly common.

Amantadine and Rimantadine

Amantadine and rimantadine inhibit the activity of influenza A virus. They do not have activity against influenza B virus. Most current influenza A viruses are susceptible to these agents, but resistance can develop. Cross-resistance is shared between amantadine and rimantadine.

Pharmacokinetics: Amantadine is well absorbed after oral administration. It is given twice daily in healthy young adults, but the dose must be decreased in elderly patients and in patients with renal dysfunction. It is eliminated unchanged in the urine. Rimantadine is well absorbed and is also usually given twice daily. In contrast to amantadine, it undergoes substantial hepatic metabolism.

Central nervous system side effects are the most important **adverse effects** with these agents. They are more considerable with amantadine (particularly if the dose has not been appropriately adjusted for age or renal function) than rimantadine. Central nervous system effects most commonly include nervousness, anxiety, impaired concentration, insomnia, and light-headedness. Psychotic episodes, seizures, tremor, and even coma have been reported less commonly (typically with very high concentrations of amantadine). Gastrointestinal side effects and rash have occurred with both agents, and anticholinergic effects can occur with amantadine.

Clinical uses for these agents include the prevention and treatment of influenza A infections. Treatment is effective only if given early (within 1-2 days) after the onset of symptoms. Disease severity and duration may be reduced by 1 to 2 days. For prevention, amantadine and rimantadine can be an important adjunct to immunization during influenza outbreaks. They can be used until the vaccine takes full effect or to augment the vaccine (particularly in immunocompromised patients who may not have optimal vaccine response). They also may be useful in patients in whom the vaccine is contraindicated.

Oseltamivir and Zanamivir

These agents are selective inhibitors of viral neuraminidase. Unlike amantadine and rimantadine, the newer agents—oseltamivir and zanamivir—have activity against both influenza A and influenza B viruses. Resistance is also much more difficult to induce with the newer agents than with amantadine or rimantadine.

Pharmacokinetics: Oseltamivir is available as oral tablets and is dosed twice daily. It is eliminated renally, and dose adjustment is necessary in patients with renal impairment. Zanamivir is available as an inhaled preparation and is dosed as 2 puffs given twice daily. Four percent to 17% of the drug is systemically absorbed and then excreted renally. It is dispensed with a special inhalation device called a Diskhaler. Demonstration of the use of this device needs to be provided to patients when this agent is prescribed. Some elderly patients or patients without good manual dexterity may find it difficult to use the device.

Oseltamivir is generally well tolerated. The primary **adverse effects** are nausea and vomiting. These occur in about 10% of patients and are usually not severe. Zanamivir is also generally well tolerated. However, it should not be prescribed for patients with underlying airway disease because they may experience bronchospasm or serious breathing problems. In addition, the drug has not been proved efficacious in this patient population. Elderly patients or patients with poor dexterity may have difficulty with the manipulation required for zanamivir inhalation.

Clinical uses for zanamivir and oseltamivir include the treatment and prophylaxis of influenza A virus and influenza B virus. They are considerably more expensive than amantadine or rimantadine. However, in comparison with the older agents, zanamivir and oseltamivir have the advantages of providing coverage against influenza B (which is less common than influenza A) and of having less resistance induction potential (clinical implications unclear). No studies have been done to compare these newer antiviral agents with the older agents. With both oseltamivir and zanamivir, treatment needs to be started very early after onset of symptoms (within 24-48 hours). These agents can reduce the severity and duration of symptoms (usually by about 1 day). They have not been highly tested in critically ill patients.

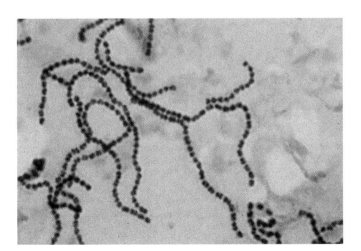

Plate 14-1. Chaining of β-hemolytic *Streptococcus* in a blood culture. (Gram stain.)

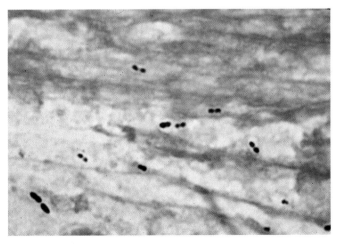

Plate 14-2. *Streptococcus pneumoniae* in sputum. (Gram stain.)

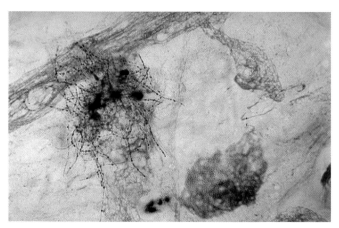

Plate 14-3. *Nocardia asteroides.* (Modified acid-fast stain; ×450.)

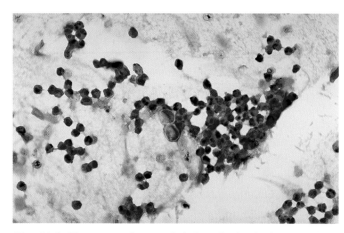

Plate 14-4. *Blastomyces dermatitidis* in bronchoalveolar lavage. (Silver stain; ×450.)

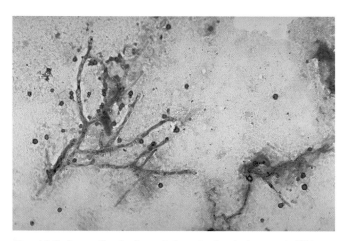

Plate 14-5. *Aspergillus fumigatus* in bronchoalveolar lavage. (×450.)

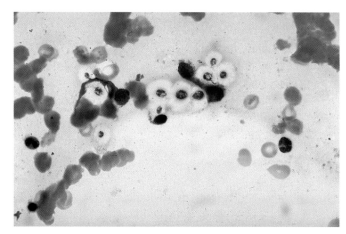

Plate 14-6. *Cryptococcus neoformans* in cerebrospinal fluid. (×450.)

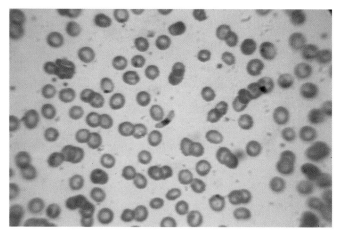

Plate 14-7. Thin blood smear showing banana-shaped gametocyte of *Plasmodium falciparum.*

Infectious Diseases Pharmacy Review
Carrie A. Krieger, PharmD, Lisa K. Buss, PharmD

Drug	Primary toxic/adverse effects	Primary drug interactions*
Penicillins	Hypersensitivity reactions, GI effects (nausea, vomiting, diarrhea), interstitial nephritis, hematologic effects (anemia, neutropenia, thrombocytopenia, platelet dysfunction), neurologic effects (confusion, seizures, neuromuscular irritability)	Probenecid
Natural penicillins		
Penicillin G		
Penicillin V		
Aminopenicillins		
Amoxicillin		
Ampicillin	Higher incidence of diarrhea than with amoxicillin	Allopurinol
Penicillinase-resistant penicillins		
Cloxacillin		
Dicloxacillin		
Methicillin	Not used clinically	
Nafcillin	Thrombophlebitis, hepatitis, neutropenia	
Oxacillin	Neutropenia, thrombophlebitis, hepatitis	
Carboxypenicillins	Sodium overload, hypokalemia, thrombocytopenia, platelet dysfunction	
Carbenicillin		
Ticarcillin		
Ureidopenicillins		
Mezlocillin		
Piperacillin	Neutropenia, thrombocytopenia	
β-Lactam/β-lactamase inhibitors	Refer to individual agents above	
Amoxicillin-clavulanate	Clavulanate may cause diarrhea	
Ampicillin-sulbactam		
Piperacillin-tazobactam		
Ticarcillin-clavulanate	Clavulanate may cause diarrhea	
Cephalosporins	Hypersensitivity reactions, GI effects (including nausea, vomiting, diarrhea), hematologic effects, interstitial nephritis, neurotoxicity (seizures); cephalosporins with MTT side chains can cause hypo-prothrombinemia and disulfiram-like reactions with alcohol	Anticoagulants, probenecid
First-generation		
Cefadroxil		
Cefazolin		
Cephalexin		
Cephalothin		
Cephapirin		
Cephradine		

Infectious Diseases Pharmacy Review (continued)

Drug	Primary toxic/adverse effects	Primary drug interactions*
Cephalosporins (continued)		
Second-generation		
Cefaclor		
Cefamandole	MTT side chain	Alcohol
Cefmetazole	MTT side chain	Alcohol
Cefonicid		
Cefotetan	MTT side chain	Alcohol
Cefoxitin		
Cefprozil		
Cefuroxime		
Loracarbef		
Third-generation		
Cefdinir		
Cefixime		
Cefoperazone	MTT side chain	Alcohol
Cefotaxime		
Cefpodoxime		
Ceftazidime		
Ceftibuten		
Ceftizoxime		
Ceftriaxone	Biliary sludge, gallstones	
Moxalactam	MTT side chain	Alcohol
Fourth-generation		
Cefepime		
Carbapenems	Nausea, vomiting, diarrhea, rash, hematologic effects, hypersensitivity reactions, seizures (rare)	Probenecid
Ertapenem		
Imipenem-cilastatin		
Meropenem		
Aztreonam	Rash, diarrhea, nausea, vomiting	
Aminoglycosides	Nephrotoxicity, auditory toxicity, vestibular toxicity, neuromuscular blockade	Other nephrotoxic drugs, loop diuretics
Amikacin		
Gentamicin		
Kanamycin		
Neomycin		
Netilmicin		
Streptomycin		
Tobramycin		

Infectious Diseases Pharmacy Review (continued)

Drug	Primary toxic/adverse effects	Primary drug interactions*
Tetracyclines	Photosensitivity, permanent staining of developing teeth, GI upset, rash, increased incidence of uremia in renal impairment	Antacids, anticoagulants, digoxin
Demeclocycline Doxycycline Minocycline Oxytetracycline Tetracycline	Vestibular toxicity	
Chloramphenicol	Aplastic anemia, bone marrow suppression, gray baby syndrome, optic and peripheral neuritis	Anticoagulants, phenytoin
Clindamycin	Diarrhea, *Clostridium difficile* colitis, nausea, vomiting	Neuromuscular blockers
Metronidazole	Nausea, diarrhea, disulfiram-like reaction, metallic taste, reversible neutropenia	Alcohol, anticoagulants
Macrolides		
Erythromycin	Abdominal pain, nausea, diarrhea, cholestatic jaundice, transient hearing loss, ventricular arrhythmias, allergic reaction	Benzodiazepines, carbamazepine, cyclosporine, theophylline, warfarin, others
Clarithromycin	Nausea, diarrhea, metallic taste	Similar to erythromycin but to a lesser extent
Azithromycin	Diarrhea, nausea, pain at injection site	May interact with warfarin
Vancomycin	Ototoxicity, red man (red neck) syndrome, nephrotoxicity, chemical thrombophlebitis, reversible neutropenia	Aminoglycosides and other nephrotoxic or ototoxic drugs
Trimethoprim-sulfamethoxazole (cotrimoxazole)	Nausea, vomiting, hypersensitivity reactions (especially common in patients with AIDS), hematologic effects	Antihyperglycemics, methotrexate, phenytoin, warfarin
Fluoroquinolones	GI effects (nausea, vomiting, abdominal pain, diarrhea), CNS effects (headache, dizziness, seizures), photosensitivity, arthropathy, tendon rupture	Antacids, calcium, iron, warfarin, sucralfate
Second-generation Ciprofloxacin Lomefloxacin Norfloxacin Ofloxacin		Theophylline

Theophylline |

Infectious Diseases Pharmacy Review (continued)

Drug	Primary toxic/adverse effects	Primary drug interactions*
Fluoroquinolones (continued)		
Third-generation		
Levofloxacin	QT interval prolongation	Antiarrhythmic agents
Fourth-generation		
Gatifloxacin	QT interval prolongation, hyperglycemia, hypoglycemia	Antiarrhythmic agents
Moxifloxacin	QT interval prolongation	Antiarrhythmic agents
Trovafloxacin	Limited to inpatient use because of risk of hepatotoxicity	
Linezolid	Thrombocytopenia, headache, diarrhea, nausea, rash, peripheral neuropathy	MAO inhibitors, pseudoephedrine, tyramine-containing foods
Quinupristin/Dalfopristin	Pain or inflammation at infusion site, arthralgia, myalgia, hyperbili-rubinemia	Carbamazepine, cyclosporine, delavirdine, diazepam, diltiazem, docetaxel, HMG-CoA reductase inhibitors, indinavir, methyl-prednisolone, midazolam, nevirapine, nifedipine, paclitaxel, ritonavir, tacrolimus, verapamil
Antituberculosis agents		
Isoniazid	Hepatitis, hypersensitivity reactions, lupus-like reactions, peripheral neuropathy	Carbamazepine, cycloserine, phenytoin, levodopa, prednisone, rifampin, theophylline, warfarin
Rifampin and rifapentine	Orange discoloration of body fluids, leukopenia, thrombocytopenia, protein-uria, hypersensitivity reactions, hepatitis	Anticoagulants, azole antifungals, barbiturates, benzodiazepines, corticosteroids, cyclosporine, delavirdine, digoxin, estrogens, haloperidol, hydantoins, macrolides, progestins, protease inhibitors, quinine, tacrolimus, theophylline, thyroid replacements, and others
Rifabutin	Neutropenia, body fluid discoloration, GI intolerance, rash, uveitis, increased liver enzymes	Anticoagulants, azole antifungals, cyclosporine, delavirdine, hydantoins, macrolides, methadone, nelfinavir, quinine, theophylline, and others
Pyrazinamide	Hepatitis, hyperuricemia, nausea, anorexia, polyarthralgia	Ethionamide, probenecid
Ethambutol	Optic neuritis, hyperuricemia	Aluminum salts

Infectious Diseases Pharmacy Review (continued)

Drug	Primary toxic/adverse effects	Primary drug interactions*
Antituberculosis agents (continued)		
Ethionamide	Anorexia, nausea, vomiting, gynecomastia, postural hypotension, drowsiness, asthenia, hepatitis and difficulty managing diabetes in diabetic patients, hypothyroidism	
Para-aminosalicylic acid	Rash, GI intolerance, hypersensitivity	
Cycloserine	CNS toxic effects (somnolence, headache, tremor, psychosis, seizures)	
Antifungal agents		
Amphotericin B	Infusion-related reactions (fever, chills, rigors, nausea, vomiting, headache, hypertension, hypotension), nephrotoxicity, hypokalemia, hypomagnesemia, reversible anemia	Nephrotoxic agents such as aminoglycosides, cyclosporine
Flucytosine	Bone marrow suppression, GI effects (nausea, diarrhea, colitis), increased liver enzymes	
Azole antifungals	GI upset (especially ketoconazole), rash, pruritus, increased liver enzymes	Carbamazepine, cyclosporine, dihydropyridine calcium channel blockers, phenobarbital, phenytoin, midazolam, triazolam, alprazolam, rifampin, tacrolimus, warfarin, or rifabutin
Ketoconazole	Gynecomastia, diminished libido, impotence, menstrual irregularities, adrenal suppression, hypokalemia, edema	Antacids, corticosteroids, didanosine, H_2-receptor blockers, HMG-CoA reductase inhibitors, proton pump inhibitors, sucralfate
Fluconazole	Headache	Antihyperglycemics, theophylline
Itraconazole	Headache, dizziness, hypokalemia, hypertension, edema, congestive heart failure	Antacids, antihyperglycemics, corticosteroids, didanosine, digoxin, H_2-receptor blockers, HMG-CoA reductase inhibitors, proton pump inhibitors, sucralfate
Voriconazole	Visual disturbances (transient)	Cyclosporine, sirolimus, tacrolimus, HMG-CoA reductase inhibitors, vinca alkaloids, and oral hypoglycemics (possible)
Caspofungin	Rash, facial swelling, sensation of warmth, increased eosinophils	Cyclosporine, tacrolimus
Antiviral agents		
Acyclovir	Malaise, nausea, vomiting, diarrhea, phlebitis (IV), drug precipitate in renal tubules (IV)	
Famciclovir	Headache, dizziness, nausea, diarrhea, fatigue	Probenecid
Ganciclovir	Diarrhea, nausea, anorexia, vomiting, leukopenia, neutropenia, rash, anemia, fever	

Infectious Diseases Pharmacy Review (continued)

Drug	Primary toxic/adverse effects	Primary drug interactions*
Antiviral agents (continued)		
Valacyclovir	Nausea, headache, diarrhea, dizziness	
Amantadine	Nausea, dizziness, light-headedness, insomnia, delirium	
Rimantadine	Insomnia, dizziness, nervousness, nausea, vomiting	
Foscarnet	Renal impairment, leukopenia, electrolyte disturbances, seizures, fever, anemia, headache, nausea, vomiting	Nephrotoxic drugs
Cidofovir	Renal impairment, neutropenia, ocular hypotonia, headache, asthenia, alopecia, rash, GI distress	Nephrotoxic drugs
Oseltamivir	Nausea, vomiting, diarrhea, bronchitis, abdominal pain, dizziness	
Zanamivir	Nausea, diarrhea, nasal signs and symptoms, bronchospasm	

AIDS, acquired immunodeficiency syndrome; CNS, central nervous system; GI, gastrointestinal; H_2, histamine$_2$; HMG-CoA, 3-hydroxy-3-methylglutaryl coenzyme-A reductase; IV, intravenous; MAO, monoamine oxidase; MTT, methylthiotetrazole.

*Many antibiotics have the potential to reduce the effectiveness of oral contraceptives.

QUESTIONS

Multiple Choice (choose the one best answer)

1. An acute febrile illness develops in a 20-year-old woman. She complains of pain in both knees and her left wrist. On examination, the symptomatic joints are swollen and warm. A loud mitral regurgitation murmur and an S_3 gallop are found on cardiac examination. The patient recalls having a sore throat about 4 weeks previously, from which she recovered. Which of the following laboratory tests will be most useful for confirming your diagnosis?
   a. Culture of blood for bacteria
   b. Serologic testing for Lyme disease
   c. Antistreptolysin O and anti-DNAse B titers
   d. Serologic testing for human immunodeficiency virus
   e. Synovial biopsy for histologic study and culture for mycobacteria

2. A 57-year-old man presents to the emergency department with septic shock. Four days previously, a dog had bitten his right forearm. Emergency intubation, intravenous fluids, and a dopamine infusion are provided before transfer to the intensive care unit. On examination, multiple purpuric lesions are seen on his extremities. The site of the dog bite is gangrenous. Laboratory studies show evidence of disseminated intravascular coagulation. Despite broad-spectrum intravenous antibiotics and aggressive supportive measures, the patient dies. What is the most likely underlying immunologic deficiency that explains the fulminant course of this patient's infection?
   a. Asplenia
   b. Hypogammaglobulinemia
   c. Common variable immunodeficiency
   d. Terminal complement deficiency
   e. Chédiak-Higashi syndrome

3. A 50-year-old man complains of fever, headache, and a nonhealing lesion on his thumb. On examination, there is a 2×3-cm ulcerating lesion on his left thumb and epitrochlear lymph node enlargement. The patient was previously in good health. There is no travel history, but he frequently hunts and fishes. He relates that he injured the thumb with his knife while skinning a rabbit. A course of therapy with which of the following antibiotics is most likely to resolve this infection?
   a. Amoxicillin
   b. Streptomycin
   c. Ceftriaxone
   d. Trimethoprim-sulfamethoxazole
   e. Amoxicillin-clavulanate

4. The public health department reports an outbreak of *Salmonella* enteritis among diners at a local restaurant. The outbreak is caused by a strain of *Salmonella enteritidis* that is resistant to ampicillin. One of your patients, a 65-year-old woman with hypertension and insulin-dependent diabetes mellitus, comes to your office concerned because she recently ate at the implicated establishment. She reports several episodes of loose stools in the past week; otherwise, she is feeling well. On examination, she is afebrile and has no focal findings. Stool cultures obtained shortly thereafter are reported as growing *S. enteritidis*. You correctly do which of the following?
   a. Begin a 10-day course of therapy with amoxicillin-clavulanate
   b. Begin a 7-day course of therapy with levofloxacin
   c. Perform two more stool cultures to assess for persistence of infection
   d. No further diagnostic testing and no antibiotic therapy
   e. Perform blood culture and ultrasonography of the abdominal aorta to look for an infected aneurysm

5. A 19-year-old female nursing assistant is referred to you because of a reactive tuberculin skin test. The test was obtained as part of new-employee screening at the local hospital. The nursing assistant was originally from western Africa and immigrated to the United States 2 years ago. She does not recall ever receiving bacille Calmette-Guérin vaccine or a previous tuberculin skin test, and she has never had a diagnosis of or been treated for tuberculosis. She is asymptomatic. Examination is unremarkable. Chest radiography shows thickening of the left apical pleura but is otherwise negative. You repeat the tuberculin skin test and observe a reaction with 12 mm of induration. You do which of the following?
   a. Initiate therapy with isoniazid 300 mg daily for 9 months
   b. Initiate therapy with isoniazid 300 mg daily, rifampin 600 mg daily, and ethambutol 1,200 mg daily for 6 months
   c. Arrange for annual repeat tuberculin skin testing
   d. Advise screening all household contacts of the nursing assistant for possible tuberculosis
   e. Advise no intervention because the diameter of induration is less than 15 mm

6. A 47-year-old woman with non-Hodgkin lymphoma is about to receive a course of chemotherapy through a tunneled central venous catheter. Before initiation of the chemotherapy, fever develops. Blood culture specimens obtained both through the catheter and peripherally grow *Staphylococcus aureus*. Susceptibility testing shows the blood isolate is resistant to penicillin but susceptible to

oxacillin. She is given 1 g of cefazolin intravenously every 8 hours. However, after 4 days of therapy she is still febrile and blood cultures are again growing *S. aureus*. On examination, she appears acutely ill. The catheter insertion site is red and the tract is swollen and tender. There are no other important findings. Which of the following interventions will most likely resolve her staphylococcal bacteremia?

a. Change antibiotic therapy from cefazolin to oxacillin
b. Change antibiotic therapy from cefazolin to vancomycin
c. Remove the tunneled catheter
d. Add aztreonam and metronidazole to the cefazolin therapy
e. Obtain an indium-labeled leukocyte scan to look for evidence of focal infection

7. Two months ago, a 72-year-old man underwent transsphenoidal resection of a pituitary tumor. The procedure was uncomplicated, but since then he has noted persistent drainage of clear fluid from his nose. Now he presents to the emergency department with a 12-hour history of fever, headache, and confusion. CT of the head shows postoperative changes in the sella but no evidence for abscess or hemorrhage. Infection with which of the following bacteria is the most likely cause of his symptoms?

a. *Pseudomonas aeruginosa*
b. *Staphylococcus aureus*
c. *Staphylococcus epidermidis*
d. *Streptococcus pneumoniae*
e. *Bacteroides fragilis*

8. A 45-year-old previously healthy man presents with his third episode of diarrhea in the past 9 months. During the two previous episodes, stool bacterial culture showed *Giardia lamblia*. Treatment with metronidazole was successful for both giardiasis episodes. He has been compliant with metronidazole therapy for 2 weeks, but diarrhea has persisted and all the stool tests are still positive for *G. lamblia* only. What test should you order now?

a. Flexible sigmoidoscopy
b. CT of the abdomen and pelvis
c. Colonoscopy
d. Skin test for delayed hypersensitivity
e. Serum immunoglobulin tests

9. A 61-year-old woman with a history of right radical mastectomy and lymph node dissection for breast carcinoma presents with a 2-week history of painful, nonpruritic, multiple, small, raised, red skin lesions on her right hand and forearm. She has had low-grade fever but otherwise no other accompanying symptoms. A course of cephalexin

failed. She denies any animal exposure or insect bites. She gives a history of trauma to her right finger while cleaning in the barn. A tissue culture shows gram-positive bacteria that are beaded with branching filaments that are acid-fast. What drug should you empirically prescribe before final culture results are available?

a. Trimethoprim-sulfamethaxazole
b. Amphotericin B
c. Erythromycin
d. Metronidazole
e. Clindamycin

10. A 19-year-old previously healthy African-American male Navy recruit presents with a 3-week history of fever, nonproductive cough, and shortness of breath. He was treated with levofloxacin for 10 days and had little response. He has no other symptoms. Tests are negative for human immunodeficiency virus and purified protein derivative. He has been at a training camp in San Diego for the past 5 months doing mainly outdoor running and military training. Chest radiography shows a right upper lobe infiltrate. Which one of the following tests is most likely to yield the correct diagnosis?

a. Serologic test for *Legionella* antibodies
b. Fungal serologic test
c. Urine antigen test
d. Test of sputum specimen for acid-fast organisms
e. Sputum Gram stain

11. A 32-year-old woman presents to the emergency department with a 3-month history of low-grade fever and progressive confusion. On examination, she is disoriented and unable to follow any commands. She has an erythematous, nodular, ulcerated lesion on her forearm and crepitations in the right lung base. Chest radiography shows a hazy infiltrate in the right lower lobe of the lung. MRI of the head shows leptomeningeal enhancement. Cerebrospinal fluid examination shows 3,000 total nucleated cells, mostly lymphocytes; protein value is 187 mg/dL, and glucose value is 20 mg/dL. The erythrocyte sedimentation rate is 80 mm in 1 hour. Tests for human immunodeficiency virus and purified protein derivative were negative. According to her family, she had been healthy. Six months ago, she helped build a dock on the Mississippi River. A biopsy of her meninges shows granulomatous inflammation, and special stains show broad-based budding organisms. Cerebrospinal fluid and biopsy culture results are pending. What drug is best for treatment in this patient?

a. Amphotericin B
b. Penicillin G

c. Acyclovir

d. Ganciclovir

e. Itraconazole

12. A 45-year-old woman with a history of acute myelogenous leukemia has been in the hospital for the past 5 weeks undergoing chemotherapy. Persistent fever, chills, rigors, and a mild nonproductive cough have now developed. On examination, she appears ill and is febrile and slightly short of breath. She has some fine crackles in the lungs bilaterally on chest auscultation. The Hickman catheter site is normal. The total leukocyte count is 0.4×10^9/L, and the absolute neutrophil count is 0.1×10^9/L. All blood cultures are negative. She has been neutropenic for the past 3 weeks. Ceftazidime and vancomycin have been used for the past 8 days, and amphotericin B therapy was started 2 days ago. Chest CT shows numerous scattered, small nodules, the largest 2 cm. What is the most likely diagnosis in this patient?

a. Pneumococcal pneumonia

b. Herpes simplex pneumonia

c. Respiratory syncytial virus pneumonia

d. Pulmonary aspergillosis

e. Septic pulmonary emboli

13. You are the physician on a cruise liner to Alaska, and in the past 2 days influenza B has developed in a few of the passengers. No influenza A activity has been reported thus far. Which of the following medications can you provide to protect against influenza B for the unvaccinated patients on the ship?

a. Amantadine

b. Rimantadine

c. Oseltamivir

d. Acyclovir

e. Nelfinavir

14. In July, you are evaluating your friend, a 55-year old, previously healthy male physician, who presents with a 2-day history of fever, malaise, nausea and anorexia, headache, severe myalgias, and arthralgias. On examination, he is ill-appearing but no localizing abnormalities are found. His temperature is 39.2°C, blood pressure 130/80, and pulse 110 beats/min. His leukocyte count is 2.1, and the platelet value is 80/dL. His creatinine level is normal. The aspartate aminotransferase value is 190 U/L (normal, 12-31), and the alanine aminotransferase value is 170 U/L (normal, 10-45); values for bilirubin, alkaline phosphatase, and prothrombin time are normal. He has no exposure to children. He has a dog. He recently attended a meeting in Maryland, where he also hiked and

played golf. Which of the following statements is true about this illness?

a. This disease is transmitted by the deer tick

b. Intracytoplasmic vacuoles are diagnostic in patients with this disease

c. Petechial rash is present in 90% of cases

d. Ceftriaxone is the drug of choice for this illness

e. Blood polymerase chain reaction is not useful for diagnosis of this disease

15. A 20-year-old male sailor stationed at the naval station in Pearl Harbor, Honolulu, Hawaii, presents for evaluation of urethral discharge. One week ago he had sexual intercourse with a prostitute in Honolulu. A Gram stain of the urethral exudate shows intracellular gram-negative diplococci. A nucleic amplification assay confirms the diagnosis. Each of the following treatments would be satisfactory in this patient *except*:

a. Ceftizoxime 500 mg intramuscularly in a single dose plus azithromycin 1 g orally in a single dose

b. Ceftriaxone 125 mg intramuscularly in a single dose plus azithromycin 1 g orally in a single dose

c. Ciprofloxacin 500 mg orally in a single dose plus azithromycin orally in a single dose

d. Spectinomycin 2 g intramuscularly in a single dose plus doxycycline 100 mg orally twice a day for 7 days

e. All of the above treatments would be acceptable in this patient

16. A 28-year-old woman presents for evaluation of a painless genital ulcer. The ulcer has been present for 1 week. The patient is 20 weeks pregnant. A Darkfield examination reveals *Treponema pallidum* spirochetes. The patient has a history of an anaphylactic reaction when she received penicillin as a child. According to the recommendations of the Centers for Disease Control and Prevention, which of the following antibiotics would be an acceptable treatment regimen in this patient?

a. Doxycycline

b. Tetracycline

c. Erythromycin

d. Ceftriaxone

e. Penicillin desensitization followed by intramuscular benzathine penicillin G

17. A 65-year-old man with hypertrophic obstructive cardiomyopathy (HOCM) is admitted to the hospital for evaluation of painless hematuria. The patient has a penicillin allergy. Cystoscopy is scheduled. According to the recommendations of the American Heart Association (AHA),

which of the following is a *true* statement concerning antibiotic prophylaxis in this patient?

a. HOCM is classified as a low-risk condition. Antibiotic prophylaxis is not recommended

b. Cystoscopy is classified as a negligible-risk procedure. Antibiotic prophylaxis is not recommended

c. HOCM is classified as a moderate-risk condition. Endocarditis prophylaxis with vancomycin is recommended

d. HOCM is classified as a moderate-risk condition. Endocarditis prophylaxis with gentamicin is recommended.

e. HOCM is classified as a high-risk condition. Endocarditis prophylaxis with vancomycin and gentamicin is recommended

18. A 72-year-old woman with corticosteroid-dependent chronic obstructive pulmonary disease presents for evaluation of headache, photophobia, fever, and seizure. Physical examination includes a temperature of 39°C, nuchal rigidity, and altered mentation. A funduscopic examination is attempted but it is difficult and the optic discs cannot be visualized. The patient does not answer questions and cannot cooperate with a complete neurologic examination; however, deep tendon reflexes are asymmetric. Significant β-lactam resistance has been reported among local *Streptococcus pneumoniae* isolates. Which answer describes the most appropriate treatment plan?

a. Obtain blood for cultures and immediately obtain a CT scan of the head to exclude a mass lesion. If the CT scan is normal, then perform a lumbar puncture. After a lumbar puncture with cultures is obtained, administer high-dose ceftriaxone before culture results are known

b. Obtain blood for cultures and administer high-dose ceftriaxone before a CT scan of the head is obtained to exclude a mass lesion. Perform a lumbar puncture for cultures if not contraindicated by the CT results

c. Obtain blood for cultures and administer high-dose ceftriaxone and vancomycin before a CT scan of the head is obtained to exclude a mass lesion. Perform a lumbar puncture if not contraindicated by the CT results

d. Obtain blood for cultures and administer high-dose ceftriaxone, vancomycin, and ampicillin before obtaining a CT scan of the head to exclude a mass lesion. Perform a lumbar puncture for cultures if not contraindicated by the CT results

e. Obtain blood for cultures and administer high-dose ceftriaxone and vancomycin before obtaining a CT scan of the head to exclude a mass lesion. Perform a lumbar puncture for cultures if not contraindicated by the CT results. Administer dexamethasone if bacterial cultures grow *S. pneumoniae*

19. A 65-year-old man with cirrhosis from hemochromatosis presents for evaluation of left lower extremity cellulitis, fever, chills, and malaise. Yesterday, the patient sustained a laceration to his left lower extremity while wading to launch his fishing boat in Chesapeake Bay. On physical examination, he has a temperature of 39°C, blood pressure of 80/60 mm Hg, and a pulse of 130 beats per minute. His left lower extremity has several large hemorrhagic bullae. An aspirate of one of the bullous lesions shows gram-negative bacilli on Gram stain. Each of the following antibiotics would be appropriate as empiric therapy for this organism *except*:

a. Tetracycline

b. Gentamicin

c. Cefotaxime

d. Ciprofloxacin

e. All of the antibiotics mentioned above would be appropriate as empiric therapy for this organism

20. A 55-year-old man with neurogenic bladder presents with complaints of urinary frequency, urinary urgency, and dysuria. On urinalysis, the leukocyte value was increased. A urine culture grows more than 100,000 colony-forming units per milliliter of *Enterococcus faecalis*. In vitro susceptibilities report that the isolate is sensitive to penicillin, ampicillin, vancomycin, trimethoprim-sulfamethoxazole, nitrofurantoin, and linezolid. All of the following antibiotics would likely be effective in vivo in treating this isolate *except*:

a. Oral amoxicillin

b. Intravenous ampicillin

c. Intravenous vancomycin

d. Oral trimethoprim-sulfamethoxazole

e. Oral nitrofurantoin

21. A 37-year-old male veterinarian presents for evaluation of fever and pain of his right hand. Yesterday, he was bitten on the hand by an injured dog. The patient required a splenectomy 1 year ago because of a ruptured spleen sustained in a motor vehicle accident. The patient's temperature is 39.2°C, blood pressure is 90/50 mm Hg, and pulse is 140 beats/minute. His hand is red, swollen, warm, and tender. What organism most likely is causing this patient's infection?

a. *Erysipelothrix rhusiopathiae*

b. *Capnocytophaga canimorsus*

c. *Aeromonas hydrophila*

d. *Streptococcus iniae*

e. *Mycobacterium marinum*

22. A previously healthy 41-year-old man with a recently diagnosed sinus infection comes to the emergency department complaining of severe headache and fever of recent onset. There are no focal neurologic findings on examination, but there is considerable nuchal rigidity. He appears quite ill. Which is the most appropriate next step in his management?
    a. Obtain an emergency CT scan of the head to exclude a mass lesion or increased intracranial pressure before performing a lumbar puncture
    b. Start cefazolin and ciprofloxacin therapy; perform lumbar puncture
    c. Start erythromycin and clindamycin therapy; perform lumbar puncture
    d. Start ampicillin and clarithromycin therapy; perform lumbar puncture
    e. Start ceftriaxone and vancomycin therapy; perform lumbar puncture

23. A 58-year-old woman with a history of diabetes-associated nephropathy has been receiving dialysis for the past 4 years. She has been hospitalized for management of cellulitis involving the left lower leg. Which antimicrobial agent does *not* require dose adjustment in the presence of renal dysfunction?
    a. Imipenem
    b. Cefazolin
    c. Clindamycin
    d. Vancomycin
    e. Levofloxacin

24. A 24-year-old woman who has human immunodeficiency virus (HIV) presents to your office with mild fever and symptoms of an upper respiratory tract infection. She is currently in her 26th week of pregnancy and has a recent positive tuberculin skin test conversion of 22-mm induration. Additionally, she has genital ulcerative lesions that test positive for herpes simplex virus. In prescribing antimicrobial therapy for this patient, you should avoid which agent?
    a. Acyclovir
    b. Amoxicillin
    c. Tetracycline
    d. Erythromycin
    e. Isoniazid

25. A 41-year-old man complains of a productive cough that has been present for the past 2 days with general malaise and fever up to 38.3°C. His chest radiograph shows a right mid lung infiltrate. Gram stain of a sputum sample shows many leukocytes, no epithelial cells, and many gram-positive diplococci. The culture results are pending. The patient states that he had a reaction to penicillin 4 years ago, which consisted of laryngeal edema, wheezing, and breathing problems that necessitated emergency medical treatment. Of the agents listed, which is the most appropriate outpatient antimicrobial agent for this patient?
    a. Cefuroxime axetil
    b. Amoxicillin-clavulanate
    c. Meropenem
    d. Ciprofloxacin
    e. Doxycycline

26. A few days ago, you admitted a 26-year-old pharmacology student to the hospital with complicated appendicitis. He recently has been reviewing the mechanism of action of various antibiotics and asks numerous questions about the current regimen that he is receiving. Impressed with your knowledge of antibiotics, he further asks how specific antibiotics function. All the following antimicrobial agents inhibit bacterial wall synthesis *except*:
    a. Nafcillin
    b. Ceftriaxone
    c. Imipenem
    d. Vancomycin
    e. Levofloxacin

27. A 57-year-old woman complains of fever, dysuria, and right-sided flank pain that have been present for 3 days. On further questioning, she describes previous urinary tract infections with similar symptoms and a history of calcium oxalate renal stones discovered in the right kidney and ureteral tract. Her most recent urinary tract infection was approximately 2 weeks ago, for which she received an antibiotic for 3 days. Her previous urine culture grew more than 10^5 colony-forming units/mL *Enterococcus faecalis*. You are concerned that *Enterococcus* is again the most likely urinary pathogen. All the following drugs are active against *E. faecalis except*:
    a. Vancomycin
    b. Cefazolin
    c. Ampicillin
    d. Piperacillin-tazobactam
    e. Linezolid

28. A 35-year-old Somali woman with diabetes presents with a 4-week history of cough and fatigue. Her chest radiograph shows a fibronodular infiltrate in the right upper lobe with a small cavitary lesion. Sputum samples show the presence of acid-fast bacilli on smear. The patient is given a clinical diagnosis of pulmonary tuberculosis and, while culture results are pending, therapy with isoniazid,

rifampin, pyrazinamide, and ethambutol is started. After 1.5 months of therapy, numbness and tingling involving both feet and lower legs develop, and these conditions later become painful. What is the most likely cause of this patient's symptoms?

a. Isoniazid
b. Rifampin
c. Pyrazinamide
d. Ethambutol
e. Spinal cord compression

29. After the second month of therapy, the patient described in question 28 missed her menstrual period. She is married and is sexually active with her husband of 6 years.

You order a pregnancy test, which is positive. A pregnancy test taken at the onset of her antituberculosis treatment was negative. She has been taking all her tuberculosis medications on a daily basis and the oral contraceptive ethinyl estradiol and norethindrone (Ortho-Novum 1/35). She reports no dietary changes and has not started taking any additional medications during the past month. Which one of the following is the most likely cause of the failure of her oral contraceptive?

a. Isoniazid
b. Rifampin
c. Pyrazinamide
d. Ethambutol
e. Noncompliance with taking the birth control pills

ANSWERS

1. Answer c.

The history and symptoms are suggestive of acute rheumatic fever. By Jones criteria, the patient has evidence of two major manifestations (polyarthritis and carditis) and one minor (fever). The history of pharyngitis suggests a recent streptococcal infection. Anti-streptococcal titers provide supporting laboratory evidence for the diagnosis of acute rheumatic fever.

2. Answer a.

Capnocytophaga canimorsus is a common cause of infection after dog bites or scratches. Localized wound infections can develop in anyone. Fulminant disease most commonly develops in persons compromised by splenectomy, alcoholism, or corticosteroid use. Hypogammaglobulinemia and common variable immunodeficiency predispose to respiratory tract infections predominantly. Terminal complement deficiency increases the risk for fulminant or recurrent infections due to encapsulated organisms (e.g., *Streptococcus pneumoniae*, *Neisseria meningitidis*, or *Haemophilus influenzae*). Chédiak-Higashi syndrome is a congenital disorder of neutrophil function that results in recurrent cutaneous and respiratory infections.

3. Answer b.

This is a classic description of ulceroglandular tularemia, also known as rabbit fever. A 7- to 14-day course of intramuscular streptomycin is the most effective therapy. Doxycycline is also effective, although clinical relapse is more common than with streptomycin. The other listed antibiotics are not effective for treating tularemia.

4. Answer d.

Most infections caused by *Salmonella* species are self-limited. Treatment of mild cases of enteritis with antibiotics may actually prolong the carriage of the organism in the gut without changing the clinical outcome. Therefore, antibiotic therapy is indicated only for invasive, severe, or protracted infections. Likewise, further testing is not likely to be beneficial in this patient, who is feeling well and has no signs of invasive disease.

5. Answer a.

This patient has a reactive tuberculin skin test but no evidence of active tuberculosis. Induration of 15 mm is the cutoff for intervention for most persons. However, induration of more than 10 mm is significant for persons from high-risk areas such as Africa. Therefore, she should receive isoniazid therapy for latent tuberculosis infection to prevent subsequent disease. Combination therapy is not indicated because there is no evidence of active disease. Likewise, no contact screening is indicated. Repeat annual skin testing is unhelpful once a skin test is reactive.

6. Answer c.

The patient has evidence of an infected central venous catheter. Although simple line-related bacteremia often is successfully treated with antibiotics alone, the examination findings strongly suggest a tunnel infection. As such, the catheter should be removed to help resolve the infection. Staphylococci that are susceptible to oxacillin also are susceptible to cefazolin. Because drug resistance is not an issue, vancomycin is not indicated. Aztreonam and metronidazole have no antistaphylococcal activity. Indium or other scans are unnecessary because the examination findings already show evidence of a catheter tunnel infection.

7. Answer d.

The patient describes a postoperative cerebrospinal fluid leak. This leak is a risk factor for development of bacterial meningitis. *S. pneumoniae* (pneumococcus) is by far the most common cause of meningitis in this setting.

8. Answer e.

This patient has prolonged giardiasis that is associated with IgA deficiency. Serum immunoglobulin electrophoresis is appropriate in such cases. The other tests listed would not help in identifying the cause of persistent infection in this patient.

9. Answer a.

The patient has cutaneous *Nocardia* infection caused by trauma to the hand. *Nocardia* species are most commonly isolated from respiratory secretions, skin biopsy specimens, or aspirate from deep collections. Direct smears from these specimens show gram-positive, beaded, branching filaments that are usually acid-fast. Sulfonamide therapy remains the treatment of choice in patients with nocardiosis. Other drugs such as amikacin, imipenem, or ceftriaxone also can be used, alone or in combination. The other listed drugs do not have adequate activity against *Nocardia* species.

10. Answer b.

This patient has *Coccidioides immitis* pneumonitis. Common manifestations are dry cough and fever (valley fever) that may resemble influenza. Associated findings include hilar adenopathy, pleural effusion (12%), thin-walled cavities (5%), and solid "coin" lesions. Disseminated infection predominantly affects the central nervous system, skin, bones, and joints. The diagnosis can be made with coccidioidal serologic testing. Other tests would not help in definitive diagnosis.

11. Answer a.

Blastomycosis affects lung, skin, bone (especially the vertebrae), and the central nervous system. Although central nervous system involvement is more common in patients with underlying immunocompromise, it also can occur in patients with normal immune function. Treatment of disseminated blastomycosis, especially that involving the central nervous system, should be with amphotericin B.

12. Answer d.

The most likely diagnosis in this patient with prolonged neutropenia is pulmonary aspergillosis. Neutropenia predisposes to rapidly invasive bronchopulmonary disease with early dissemination to the brain and other tissues. The longer the duration of neutropenia, the higher the risk for invasive aspergillosis. Prompt therapy with high doses of amphotericin B and resolution of the neutropenia are necessary to control the disease. The diagnosis should be suspected when a persistently neutropenic patient has persistent fever with new pulmonary infiltrates. The fact that therapy with amphotericin B was just started does not exclude aspergillosis as the most likely cause in this situation. Other diseases can cause a similar clinical picture; however, aspergillosis is the most likely initially.

13. Answer c.

Amantadine and rimantadine are effective against only influenza A virus, not influenza B. Therapy is most beneficial if begun within 48 hours of onset of symptoms. Vaccine, together with amantadine, can give about 95% protection against influenza A infection. Newer drugs called neuraminidase inhibitors (oseltamivir and zanamavir) are effective against uncomplicated disease caused by both influenza A and B. Both reduce the duration of symptoms by 1 day when given within 48 hours after onset of symptoms. Acyclovir and nelfinavir have no known anti-influenza antiviral activity.

14. Answer b.

The patient's history and exposure are compatible with ehrlichiosis, which infects monocytes. In the mid-Atlantic region, *Ehrlichia chaffeensis* is more common and is transmitted by the Lone Star tick and not the deer tick or *Ixodes* species. Unlike the situation in human granulocytic ehrlichiosis, in which morulae in circulating mononuclear cells are identified in peripheral blood neutrophils in 20% to 80% of patients, ehrlichial morulae are rare in human monocytic ehrlichiosis. However, when present, they are diagnostic. The peak incidence is from May through July. Treatment is with doxycycline. Ceftriaxone is not active against ehrlichiosis. Values on liver function tests are increased in approximately 80% of patients with ehrlichiosis, leukopenia occurs in 67%, and thrombocytopenia occurs in 57%.

15. Answer c.

Because of the high rates of quinolone-resistant *Neisseria gonorrhoeae*, quinolones should not be used for infections in Asia or the Pacific Rim, including Hawaii. The use of quinolones is probably inadvisable for treating *N. gonorrhoeae* acquired in California or other areas with an increased prevalence of quinolone resistance.

16. Answer e.

No alternatives to penicillin have been proved effective for the treatment of syphilis during pregnancy. Pregnant women who have a history of an allergy to penicillin should be desensitized and then receive a penicillin regimen appropriate for the stage of syphilis.

17. Answer c.

HOCM is classified as a moderate-risk condition. Endocarditis antibiotic prophylaxis is recommended before cystoscopy for patients with moderate or high-risk cardiac conditions. For patients with moderate-risk cardiac conditions, antibiotic prophylaxis with oral amoxicillin or intravenous or intramuscular ampicillin is recommended before cystoscopy. Vancomycin is recommended if the patient has a penicillin allergy. A patient with a high-risk cardiac condition requires ampicillin and gentamicin for prophylaxis before a cystoscopy. A patient with a high-risk cardiac condition and a penicillin allergy requires vancomycin and gentamicin. AHA endocarditis recommendations are summarized in Tables 14-10 and 14-11 (JAMA 1997;277:1794-1801).

18. Answer d.

The clinical scenario is consistent with probable meningitis in an elderly, immunocompromised host. The most appropriate empiric antibiotic regimen for this patient includes high-dose ceftriaxone, vancomycin, and ampicillin. Ceftriaxone offers coverage for *Haemophilus influenzae*, *Neisseria meningitidis*, and most isolates of *S. pneumoniae*. Vancomycin should be added in this case because of significant local β-lactam resistance. Ampicillin should be included in the empiric meningitis antibiotic regimen of newborns, pregnant women, elderly patients, and immunocompromised hosts in order to offer coverage for *Listeria monocytogenes*. CT of the head before lumbar puncture is indicated in this patient because she has clinical features predictive of abnormal results of head imaging, including age older than 60 years, immunocompromise, seizure at presentation, focal neurologic examination, and aphasia (N Engl J Med 2001;345:1727-1733). In cases of suspected meningitis in which CT of the head is indicated, the patient should receive antibiotics before the imaging and subsequent lumbar puncture in order to prevent a costly delay in instituting effective treatment. Some evidence suggests a beneficial effect of dexamethasone on meningitis outcomes, especially among patients with pneumococcal meningitis; however, if a decision is made to administer dexamethasone, this therapy should be started 15 minutes before the first dose of antibiotics.

19. Answer b.

Vibrio vulnificus is a gram-negative bacillus found in seawater which has been described as causing a bullous cellulitis with sepsis in immunocompromised hosts, especially those with liver disease or iron overload. Mortality from this infection is considerable. The organism frequently contaminates shellfish from Chesapeake Bay and the Gulf of Mexico and can cause gastroenteritis. Antibiotic therapy for cellulitis or bacteremia includes tetracycline, cefotaxime, or ciprofloxacin. Often a tetracycline is used in combination with a third-generation cephalosporin. Although aminoglycosides are often used as empiric therapy in gram-negative sepsis, *V. vulnificus* is not uniformly susceptible to the aminoglycosides and, therefore, gentamicin monotherapy would not be an appropriate choice for empiric antibiotic therapy in this case.

20. Answer d.

Enterococci appear susceptible to trimethoprim-sulfamethoxazole in vitro, but trimethoprim-sulfamethoxazole fails in the therapy of enterococcal infections because the organism is able to circumvent the block of folate metabolism in vivo by using exogenous folinic acid, dihydrofolate, and tetrahydrofolate.

21. Answer b.

Capnocytophaga canimorsus (Latin for "dog bite"), formerly known as CDC group DF2, is a facultative anaerobic gram-negative bacillus that colonizes the mouths of dogs. The organism can cause soft tissue infections after dog bite and has been reported to cause sepsis in splenectomized patients. *Capnocytophaga cynodegmi* (Greek for "dog bite") also can cause soft tissue infection after dog bite. *Aeromonas hydrophila* causes soft tissue infections after exposure to freshwater or leeches. *Erysipelothrix rhusiopathiae* causes soft tissue infections on the hands of fishermen and butchers. *Streptococcus iniae* soft tissue infections have been described after exposure to the freshwater fish tilapia. *Mycobacterium marinum* causes "fishtank granuloma."

22. Answer e.

This question addresses three important issues. First, if there is a clinical suspicion of bacterial meningitis, there should be no delay in starting antimicrobial therapy. If CT of the head is needed, appropriate empiric therapy with antimicrobial agents should be started *before* the patient has the test. In the absence of focal neurologic findings, seizures, or papilledema, a cerebrospinal fluid examination can be done safely without CT of the head. Second, before starting antimicrobial therapy, the physician needs to consider the most likely bacterial pathogens in an otherwise healthy 41-year-old patient, namely, *Streptococcus pneumoniae* and *Neisseria meningitidis*. The recently diagnosed sinus infection is a clue that *S. pneumoniae* may be the pathogen. Although *Listeria monocytogenes* is frequent in neonates, the elderly, and immunocompromised patients, it is less likely in this patient. It would be prudent, however, to include ampicillin for empiric therapy in these high-risk patients. Third, the physician needs to prescribe antimicrobial agents that adequately penetrate the central nervous system blood-brain barrier to sterilize the cerebrospinal fluid. Of the listed agents, ceftriaxone, ampicillin, vancomycin, and ciprofloxacin penetrate the cerebrospinal fluid with concentrations high enough to sterilize it. Ciprofloxacin variably penetrates the cerebrospinal fluid and does not provide reliable activity against *S. pneumoniae*. Ampicillin is suitable for *Listeria* meningitis (with the addition of gentamicin), but clarithromycin does not adequately penetrate into the cerebrospinal fluid. Ceftriaxone (2 g every 12 hours) and vancomycin provide a suitable initial antimicrobial program for this patient until culture results and drug susceptibilities are available.

23. Answer c.

Clindamycin is hepatically metabolized and requires no dose adjustment for renal insufficiency. Imipenem, cefazolin, vancomycin, and levofloxacin are all renally cleared and require dose adjustments with renal impairment.

24. Answer c.

Acyclovir, amoxicillin, erythromycin, and isoniazid are all safe during pregnancy. There have been no adverse or teratogenic effects reported when they are administered to pregnant women. Tetracyclines have an affinity for developing teeth and bone. They can inhibit fetal bone development and produce tooth discoloration in infants and children. Additionally, acute hepatotoxicity with fatty necrosis has been reported in pregnant women taking tetracyclines. For these reasons, tetracyclines should be avoided in pregnant women, nursing mothers, and children younger than 8 years.

25. Answer e.

This patient has had a previous severe reaction to penicillin. Therefore, he should not receive another member of the penicillin class of antimicrobial agents. Because this reaction is an anaphylactoid reaction and can be life-threatening, it would be prudent to avoid all β-lactam antimicrobial agents because cross-reactions can and do occur. The β-lactams include all the penicillins, cephalosporins, and carbapenems. The quinolones, macrolides, and tetracyclines are acceptable alternatives. Ciprofloxacin is not an optimal choice for outpatient treatment of community-acquired pneumonia because it is not overly active against *S. pneumoniae*. Of agents listed, doxycycline is the most suitable choice. Levofloxacin (third-generation fluoroquinolone),

gatifloxacin or moxifloxacin (both fourth-generation fluoroquinolones), or a macrolide would be appropriate choices in this clinical setting, but these were not listed as options.

26. Answer e.

The β-lactam class of antibiotics (which includes the penicillins, cephalosporins, and carbapenems) and vancomycin exert their antibacterial effect by inhibiting bacterial cell wall formation. Levofloxacin, like all fluoroquinolones, inhibits bacterial DNA replication and repair through the inhibition of topoisomerases (DNA gyrase). DNA gyrase is an enzyme required for DNA replication, repair, and supercoiling.

27. Answer b.

Ampicillin, piperacillin-tazobactam, linezolid, and vancomycin all provide excellent anti-enterococcal activity. The cephalosporins are not active against enterococci. Additionally, the quinolones are not reliably active against enterococci.

28. Answer a.

Peripheral neuropathy has been described in patients taking isoniazid 6 mg/kg per day, but it is less common in patients taking the standard daily dose of 300 mg. Malnutrition, alcoholism, diabetes mellitus, uremia, and slow acetylators of isoniazid increase the risk of neuropathy. Isoniazid promotes the excretion of pyridoxine (vitamin B_6), and supplemental administration of pyridoxine 6 to 50 mg/day (for patients with increased risk of neuropathy) can prevent this complication. Other side effects of isoniazid include hepatotoxicity, positive antinuclear antibody, lupus-like reaction, and drowsiness.

29. Answer b.

Rifampin induces hepatic microsomal cytochrome P-450–mediated enzyme activity, which can profoundly decrease the serum levels of other drugs metabolized by this pathway. Rifampin interaction with more than 100 drugs, including oral contraceptive agents, has been described. Additionally, rifampin may alter intestinal flora that, in turn, alter the enterohepatic circulation of oral contraceptives. In the treatment of HIV and tuberculosis coinfection, rifampin will induce the metabolism of protease inhibitors, reducing their antiviral activity. Other side effects of rifampin include hepatotoxicity, cytopenias (decreased leukocyte and platelet counts), orange discoloration of body fluids, and hypersensitivity reactions.

CHAPTER 15

MEDICAL ETHICS

C. Christopher Hook, M.D.

Medicine is first and foremost a relationship. It is the coming together of one individual, the patient, who is ill or has specific needs and a second individual, the physician, whose goal is to help the patient. Because medicine is fundamentally a relationship, it is at heart an ethical endeavor. Physicians have a long history of creating codes or oaths to provide the ethical norms and framework to support and protect the underlying relationship. Medical ethics is a set of principles that attempts to guide physicians in their relationships with patients and others. These principles are based on moral values shared by both the lay society (may vary from culture to culture) and the medical profession.

- Medical ethics is a set of principles that guide physicians in their relationships with patients and others.

Historically, the Hippocratic Oath has served as the foundation on which much of Western medical ethics has been built. Its principles form the framework for many of our current ethical standards, including beneficence, nonmaleficence, confidentiality, and the prohibition of active euthanasia. In recent times, there have been many other articulations of these core principles, including the Declaration of Geneva (1983), World Medical Association International Code of Medical Ethics (1983), The American College of Physicians Ethics Manual (1989), and The American Medical Association Code of Medical Ethics (1997).

ETHICAL DILEMMAS

Ethical issues in medicine are as dynamic as scientific and technical progress in medicine. In fact, the relentless advances in medical science are greatly responsible for the dynamism in medical ethics. These factors are partly responsible for ethical dilemmas. Furthermore, changes in societal mores and laws also have an impact on the ethical issues in medicine. An ethical dilemma can be defined as a predicament in which there is no clear course to resolve the problem of conflicting

moral principles because of credible evidence both for and against a certain action. Increasing emphasis is being placed on medical ethics in the certifying and licensing examinations for physicians.

- Ethical dilemma: predicament in which there is no clear course to resolve the problem of conflicting moral principles because of credible evidence both for and against a certain action.
- Ethical issues in medicine are dynamic and will continue to change.

PRINCIPLES OF MEDICAL ETHICS

Today, many schools are competing to provide a philosophical framework for deriving the rules or particulars of medical ethics. Historically and foundationally the foremost ethical principle of medicine has been beneficence and its corollary, nonmaleficence, from which we understand our duty in medicine is to do good for the patient and in the process to avoid harm. One of the major contemporary approaches has been labeled principalism. Proposed by Beauchamp and Childress, principalism, although not necessarily providing bedside guidance for each ethical dilemma, provides a useful delineation of overall principles in which to consider many or most of the ethical concerns in the physician-patient relationship. The four major principles that they list are: 1) autonomy, 2) beneficence, 3) nonmaleficence, and 4) justice.

- Four tenets of medical ethics: autonomy, beneficence, nonmaleficence, and justice.

Autonomy

Autonomy derives from two Greek words: *autos* ("self") and *nomes* ("rule"). The principle of autonomy is the articulation that all individuals have the right to determine their individual values and goals and have the right to self-determination. For autonomy to have expression, however, two requirements need to be present. First, the patient must have "agency," that is, the patient must be able to establish his or her own values and goals and be able to make appropriate decisions based on those values. From the requirement of agency, we have the clinically important concept of decision-making capacity. Decision-making capacity often is confused with the legal term "competence." Capacity is the physician's clinical determination of the patient's ability to understand his or her situation and make appropriate decisions for treatment, and competence is the legal determination that an individual has the right to make life-affecting decisions. The judges' or courts' assessment of competence is based in significant part on the clinical assessment of decision-making capacity.

- Autonomy: respecting the patient's right to self-determination and pursuit of one's own life plan.
- Autonomy implies "decision-making" capacity (the right to refuse medical therapy, even at the risk of death).
- Competence is the legal determination that an individual has the right to make life-affecting decisions.

In clinical practice, the lack of decisional capability should be proved and not presumed. Clinical evidence of confusion, disorientation, and psychosis resulting from organic diseases, metabolic disturbances, and iatrogenic interference can adversely affect decision-making ability. Decisionally capable patients have the right to refuse medical therapy, even at the risk of death. If a previously decisionally capable patient had indicated, clearly and convincingly, whether life-sustaining therapy should be administered or withheld in the event of permanent unconsciousness, that wish should be respected (see below, Living Will), unless it was subsequently clearly rescinded.

- The lack of decisional capability should be proved and not presumed.

Several clinical standards are used to assess decision-making capacity: 1) the patient can make and communicate a choice; 2) the patient understands the medical situation and prognosis, the nature of the recommended care, available alternative options, and the risks, benefits, and consequences of each; 3) the patient's decisions are stable over time; 4) the decision is consistent with the patient's values and goals; and 5) the decision is not due to delusions.

The second major element required in autonomy is liberty; that is, the patient must be free to influence the course of his or her life and medical treatment. Many recent court decisions, from the *Quinlan* case in 1976 to the *Cruzan* decision in 1990, along with strong support from the bioethical community, have established the right of patients to refuse any form of medical treatment, even if such refusal will lead to the patient's death.

- Liberty: the patient is free to influence the course of his or her life and medical treatment.

The principle of autonomy, particularly as it affects the right of an individual to die, has been reaffirmed in the recent writings of ethicists and in legal judgments (see Table 15-2). Nevertheless, a survey of physicians published in 1995 reported that 34% of physicians had, at least once in the preceding 12 months, declined to withdraw life-sustaining mechanical ventilation despite being requested to do so by a capable patient or by the family of a patient lacking decision-making capacity. Nearly 20% of physicians engaged in this practice because of the fear of malpractice litigation. Unfortunately, a significant number of physicians in the United States have either a poor or no understanding of the laws of states regarding the principle of autonomy. The 1995 survey revealed that 46% of the respondents from New York incorrectly believed that withdrawal of mechanical ventilation was illegal.

- A significant number of physicians have a poor understanding of the principle of autonomy.

Preservation of the Patient's Autonomy

Can a patient who now is unconscious or lacks decision-making capacity prevent unwanted treatment? Another way of asking this question is, who speaks for the patient when he or she is no longer able to articulate? Because autonomy is based on a respect for persons, caregivers should endeavor to continue treatment in accordance with what the patient would have desired if he or she were still able to interact capably with the caregivers. To preserve the patient's autonomy, patients may communicate through two means to express their wishes: advance directives and surrogate decision makers.

- The patient's autonomy is preserved by 1) advance directives and 2) surrogate decision makers.

Advance Directive

An advance directive is a document in which a person either states choices for medical treatment or designates an individual who should make treatment choices if the person should lose decision-making capacity. The term also can apply to oral statements from the patient to the caregivers, given at a time when the patient was decisionally capable. Advance directives can take several forms: 1) the living will, 2) the durable power of attorney for health care, 3) a document appointing a health care surrogate (in jurisdictions that do not formally recognize a durable power of attorney for health care), and the advance medical care directive.

- Advance directive: a document in which a person either states choices for medical treatment or designates an individual for this purpose.

Living Will

A living will requires that two conditions be present before it takes effect: 1) the patient must be terminally ill, and 2) the patient must lack decision-making capacity. The determination of "terminal" varies from jurisdiction to jurisdiction, as do the laws concerning advance directives. It is therefore advised that each physician be familiar with the local statutes concerning advance directives. Because of the requirement that the patient must be terminally ill, the living will is restricted in its use and may not be useful in many circumstances in which the patient lacks decision-making capacity but cannot necessarily be described as terminally ill. When activated, the living will provides guidance to the caregivers about what treatments the patient does or does not desire. It is, however, ineffective if vaguely written or applied to patients with uncertain prognoses.

- The living will requires that a patient be terminally ill before it takes effect.
- Legal reliability of the living will may vary from state to state.

Durable Power of Attorney for Health Care

The durable power of attorney for health care (DPAHC) is a document that designates a surrogate decision maker should the patient lose decision-making capacity. It does not require that the patient be terminally ill, and therefore it is an advance directive that is more generally useful. Within the DPAHC, the patient can make specific directives concerning different types of treatments such as cardiopulmonary resuscitation (CPR), artificial nutrition, and hydration. The major value, however, is in providing an individual who can dynamically interact with the health care team regarding the great breadth of medical decisions.

- DPAHC designates a surrogate decision maker should the patient lose decision-making capacity.

Surrogate

The surrogate represents the patient's interests and previously expressed wishes in the context of the medical issues. The surrogate is optimally designated by the patient before critical illness. One type of surrogate is the durable power of attorney for health care, in which a legally binding proxy

directive authorizes a designated individual to speak on behalf of the patient. The second type of surrogate is the patient's family or the court. The third type is a moral surrogate (usually a family member) who best knows the patient and has the patient's interests at heart. Difficulties may arise when the moral surrogate is not the legal surrogate. Dialogue between the physician and surrogate is important.

- A surrogate represents the patient's interests and previously expressed wishes in the context of the medical issues.
- Optimally, a surrogate is designated by the patient before critical illness.

Standards of surrogate decision making are characterized as follows. How should the surrogate make decisions for the patient's health care decisions? If the patient has issued explicit directives, the surrogate should follow those instructions, unless it clearly can be demonstrated that the patient did not understand the nature of the information or choices made in that explicit directive. This situation unfortunately occurs when advance directives are completed without discussing the nature of the questions addressed with a health care provider. In the absence of such directives, the surrogate should use "substituted judgment," that is, the surrogate should decide to the best of his or her ability, based on the beliefs and values of the patient, what the choices would be if the patient were able to speak for himself or herself. In some circumstances the surrogate has not had enough communication about health care and life issues to be able to project how the patient would decide. There simply is not enough information to be able to specifically "substitute" for the patient. In these circumstances, the surrogate's obligation is to try to decide the best interests of the patient given the clinical situation.

- A surrogate decision maker represents the patient's interests.
- In the absence of specific advance directives, the surrogate should use "substituted judgment."

Several studies have shown that surrogate decision makers often choose courses that are not what patients would have chosen for themselves in specific circumstances. Because of this, physicians should strongly stress the importance of having patients discuss their values and health care goals with their family members or surrogates. It is also the duty of each physician to discuss these issues with her or his patients personally. This practice allows physicians to understand their patients' values to ensure that their choices are not made on misinformation.

- Each physician should discuss specific advance directives with her or his patients.

It is always helpful when the patient has a specific advance directive appointing a surrogate decision maker. What if there is no advance directive? Who speaks for the patient? The underlying principle is to find a person, or persons, who most likely can share with the caregivers the patient's values and how the patient would most likely choose if he or she could speak for himself or herself. Different jurisdictions may create a specific list of ranking, but a practical approach would be the following list, in descending order of authority: 1) the spouse, 2) an adult child or the majority of adult children, 3) a parent or parents, 4) an adult sibling or the majority of adult siblings, 5) an adult relative who has exhibited special care and concern, and 6) if no relative can be located, a close friend.

● A surrogate decision maker is helpful for directing or enforcing a specific advance directive.

Conflicts

Inescapably, situations arise in which a surrogate's instructions conflict with the patient's previously expressed directive or with those of other family members. Because the primary responsibility of the physician is to the patient, the physician should determine as best as possible what the patient would choose for himself or herself. In these circumstances, it may be helpful to involve an independent third-party arbitrator, such as an ethics consultant or committee or legal counsel, to help work through the issues. This option is useful only if the physician is unable, for whatever reason, to resolve the conflict. In reality, every physician must learn to be a medical ethicist in dealing with her or his own patients. Once it has been established what the patient would want, it is the obligation of the treating physician(s) to comply with those wishes, even in the face of significant disagreement from family members. Only if clear evidence can be provided that the advance directive does not reflect what the patient really desired (for instance, proof that the patient misunderstood what certain procedures involved or what key terms meant) can the directive be overruled.

● The primary responsibility of the physician is to serve the patient's interest.

Advance Medical Care Directive

In some instances, patients have specific desires never to receive certain forms of therapy. For instance, a member of the Jehovah's Witness faith wishes to refuse the administration of blood or blood products in any and all circumstances. Other individuals may refuse dialysis or some other intervention regardless of the circumstance. The advance medical care directive is a document that states this categorical refusal for

a specific treatment. It may take the form of a no-transfusion card or a MedicAlert statement, for example.

● Adults who refuse life-saving measures (such as a blood transfusion) should be allowed to maintain their religious practices.

The Patient Self-Determination Act of 1990

In response to the *Cruzan* decision, the U.S. Congress passed the Patient Self-Determination Act (PSDA) to ensure that patients were informed of their rights to accept or refuse medical care and to create and execute an advance directive. The PSDA requires that hospitals, nursing homes, hospices, managed care organizations, and home health care agencies provide this information to patients at the time of admission or enrollment. The organizations are required to 1) document whether patients have advance directives, 2) establish policies to implement the advance directives, and 3) educate their staff and community about advance directives and these policies.

● The PSDA requires that all health care providers, at the time of admission, dispense information to patients about their rights to accept or refuse care and to create an advance directive.

Informed Consent

A derivative of the principles of autonomy and nonmaleficence, informed consent is the voluntary acceptance of physician recommendations for treatment or research investigations by decisionally capable patients or surrogates who have been furnished with ample truthful information regarding the risks, benefits, and alternatives of the proposed intervention. Informed consent has two preconditions on the part of the patient: 1) decision-making capacity and 2) voluntariness (essentially the same as the agency and liberty associated with the principle of autonomy). Beyond these preconditions are the informational requirements of informed consent. Patients should receive accurate, truthful information sufficient to make a reasoned decision. The amount of information shared with the patient should not be guided only by what the physician believes is adequate (Professional Practice Standard) but that which the average prudent person would need to have in order to make an appropriate decision (Reasonable Person Standard). Included within this information is a discussion of available alternatives to the proposed treatment. For example, a patient with a cancer amenable to surgical resection, chemotherapy, or radiation therapy, all associated with a similar long-term outcome, should receive a thorough discussion of each of the options and their potential complications and side effects, even if the physician may be biased toward one of the three treatments. It is the duty of the physician to set aside personal bias and provide detailed information on each treatment to allow the patient to make a well-informed personal decision. The patient can then take the information and assess it within the context of her or his own life's goals and quality-of-life considerations. Many informed-consent forms do not meet the Reasonable Person Standard and are therefore of no value morally or legally.

- Informed consent requires decision-making capacity and voluntariness.
- Reasonable Person Standard: amount of information needed by a patient is that which the average prudent person would need to have in order to make a decision.
- Many informed-consent forms do not meet the Reasonable Person Standard and are therefore of no value morally or legally.

After a discussion of the available alternatives, the physician should present the patient with a single recommendation that the patient can accept or reject. Patients come to their physicians expecting the caregivers to use their knowledge and experience in providing them with a recommendation. Simply laying out a series of choices before the patient may lead to confusion or the perception by the patient that the physician is unconcerned with his or her welfare. If the patient refuses the recommended treatment and chooses one of the alternatives, the physician should respect the patient's choice. The final plan should reflect an agreement between a well-informed patient and a well-informed, sympathetic, and unbiased physician. In certain circumstances, a patient may require more information than what the average reasonable person might desire. For instance, some religious belief systems may specifically preclude certain forms of medical intervention that might not trouble another individual in the least. It is important to ensure that patients receive sufficient information within the context of their beliefs to help them make an appropriate choice.

- The physician should provide all alternatives, followed by a single recommendation.
- If the patient refuses the recommended treatment, the physician should respect the patient's choice.

Informed consent from surrogates is necessary to perform an autopsy (except in certain instances such as coroners' cases, in which the decision is made by outside authorities) or to practice intubation, placement of intravascular lines, or other procedures on the newly dead. Informed consent is essential when performing new, innovative, nonstandard surgical and research procedures. In rare exceptions, the physician can treat a patient without truly informed consent (e.g.,

in an emotionally unstable patient who requires urgent treatment, informing the patient of the details may produce further problems).

- Informed consent from surrogates is necessary to perform an autopsy.
- Informed consent from surrogates is necessary to perform new, innovative, and nonstandard surgical procedures.

Implied Consent

The principle of implied consent is invoked when true informed consent is not possible because the patient (or surrogate) is unable to express a decision regarding treatment, specifically, in emergency situations in which physicians are compelled to provide medically necessary therapy, without which harm would result. This clarifies that there is a duty to assist a person in urgent need of care. This principle has been legally accepted, and it provides the physician a legal defense against battery (although not negligence).

- Implied consent is invoked when true informed consent is not possible, such as in emergency situations.

Disclosure

Truth-telling on the part of the physician is an integral aspect of autonomy. To make the principle of autonomy function, the physician must provide decisionally capable patients with adequate and truthful information on which to base medical decisions. Without the receipt of sufficient truthful information, patients cannot make truly autonomous decisions about their life plans. Occasionally, however, the physician may withhold part or all of the truth if it is believed that telling the truth is likely to cause significant injury. This is the principle of therapeutic privilege. For example, if it can be well ascertained that a patient will attempt harm to himself or herself or others if certain information is received, such as the diagnosis of cancer, then the information may be withheld. However, there is a high burden of proof on the withholding physician to establish the likelihood of injury, and this decision for intentional nondisclosure must be fully and carefully recorded in the medical record.

- Truth-telling on the part of the physician is an integral aspect of the patient's autonomy.

Justifiable Parentalism

Rarely, it may be necessary for the physician to withhold part or all of the truth if telling the whole truth is likely to cause more harm than good. Making such decisions that would bypass or override the patient's autonomous decision making has been described as paternalistic or parentalistic. Parentalistic behavior may be justified in certain circumstances. The following criteria should be met in these circumstances: 1) the patient is at risk of significant, preventable harm; 2) the parentalistic action probably will prevent the harm; 3) the projected benefits outweigh the risks to the patient; and 4) the least autonomy-restrictive alternative that will secure the benefits and reduce the risks is to be used.

- Parentalistic or paternalistic action: withholding information from a patient to prevent potential harm to the patient which may result if the patient knows the information.

Confidentiality

Privacy is an integral part of the protection of an individual's autonomy. Confidentiality respects that right to privacy and provides the patient the right to keep medical information solely within the realm of the physician-patient relationship. The physician is ethically and legally obliged to maintain a patient's medical information in strict confidence, a tradition dating back to the Hippocratic Oath. However, the obligation to safeguard patient confidences is subject to certain exceptions that are justified because of overriding ethical and social concerns. When a patient threatens to inflict serious bodily harm on another individual, and there is reasonable probability that the patient will carry out the threat, the physician is obligated to take reasonable precautions for the protection of the intended victim, including notification of law enforcement authorities if necessary (American Medical Association Council on Ethical and Judicial Affairs, June 1994). Also, in some exceptions, a patient's data must be shared with public health care agencies, such as in the case of human immunodeficiency virus (HIV), *Mycobacterium tuberculosis*, and other infectious diseases. A growing area of concern regards heritable genetic traits. This concern is undergoing significant ethical and legal scrutiny at the present time. A common example that challenges the principle of confidentiality is a patient with HIV who refuses to inform third parties who may not yet be infected but certainly will have future contact with the individual. A functional solution is the following: 1) attempt to persuade the infected patient to cease endangering the third party or to notify the third party of the risk; 2) if persuasion fails, notify an authority who can intervene; 3) if the authority takes no action or is not available, notify the endangered party of the risk (American Medical Association Council on Ethical and Judicial Affairs, 1988). It must be clearly stated that this approach still may be open to legal liabilities and is based on the medical profession's obligation to prevent harm. Public policy trends have been moving toward stronger protection of patient confidentiality.

- A physician is obliged to maintain medical information in strict confidence.

- Exceptions include instances when data not released to appropriate agencies may cause greater societal harm (e.g., positive results of HIV test, sputum culture for *Mycobacterium tuberculosis*).

Futility

It has been clearly established, both ethically and legally, that patients have the right to refuse any and all medical therapies. But does the principle of autonomy give patients, or their surrogates, the right to demand treatments? This question particularly arises when patients or families request that cardiopulmonary resuscitation, mechanical ventilation, and other aggressive treatment be performed on patients with little chance of recovery or survival to dismissal. Can physicians unilaterally withhold or withdraw medical interventions if, in their opinion, the intervention is futile? The conflict seemingly is between the autonomy of the patients and the moral autonomy and integrity of the caregivers. Physicians are moral agents, just as much as patients, and should not be forced to violate their ethical beliefs and principles.

- Patients have the right to refuse any and all medical therapies.
- Futility: unilateral decision by the physician to withhold or withdraw medical interventions, based on predictable futile outcome.

The definition of futility states that something is futile if it is "leaky, hence untrustworthy, vain, failing of the desired end through intrinsic defect" (*Oxford English Dictionary*). Therefore, a futile intervention is one that cannot achieve the goals of intervention no matter how many times it is repeated. From this definition, it can clearly be stated that physicians are not required to provide treatments that have no pathophysiologic rationale, have already failed in a given patient in the past, or will not achieve the goals of care already agreed on by the physician and patient or surrogate. *Physiologic futility* is determined by the physician, who needs to decide whether a treatment can achieve its physiologic goal. However, most futility conflicts arise in clinical situations in which an intervention is "unlikely" to benefit the patient or there is a conflict about the goals of treatment (such as maintaining physiologic life versus restoration of independent functioning or survival to dismissal). Many have tried to create functional definitions of futility that would cover these circumstances, but all have the flaw of establishing arbitrary thresholds that are value-laden in themselves.

- Physiologic futility is determined by the physician.

When cases of futility conflicts arise in clinical situations in which an intervention is "unlikely" to benefit the patient or there is a conflict about the goals of treatment (such as maintaining physiologic life versus restoration of independent functioning or survival to dismissal), the solution should be one of "due process." The American Medical Association Council on Ethical and Judicial Affairs endorsed such a program ("Houston Policy," JAMA 1996;276:571-574), which requires the following:

1. Earnest attempts to deliberate over and negotiate prior understanding among patient, surrogate, and physician about what constitutes "futile" care for the patient and what falls within acceptable limits for those involved. Many times the disagreement is based on inappropriate expectations of the patient or surrogate. When appropriate data about outcomes are shared, many requests for treatments such as cardiopulmonary resuscitation decrease.
2. Joint decision making should occur to the maximal extent possible.
3. Attempts should be made to negotiate and resolve disagreements (such as through ethics consultation).
4. If disagreements are irresolvable, a consultant or end-of-life decisions committee should become involved.
5. If the committee agrees with the patient and the physician remains unpersuaded, intra- or interinstitutional transfer may be arranged.
6. If the committee agrees with the physician and the patient or surrogate remains unpersuaded, intra- or interinstitutional transfer may be arranged.
7. If transfer is not possible, the intervention need not be offered.

- Cases of futility conflicts should be resolved by due process (see above).

Beneficence

Beneficence is acting to benefit patients by preserving life, restoring health, relieving suffering, and restoring or maintaining function. The physician (acting in good faith) is obligated to help patients attain their own interests and goals as determined by the patient, *not* the physician.

When we think of benefitting the patient, we must remember that there are several levels of defining benefit for a given situation, some objective and some subjective. The first level concerns the biomedical or physiologic benefit of a proposed intervention. This is usually the least controversial area and the one that requires the most physician input. As physicians we often tend to stop at this first level, but the next two patient-defined levels are often of great importance to how a patient defines "benefit." The second level is personal benefit: how the patient interprets the situation in the context of her values and goals. This level may sometimes seem in conflict with the biomedical benefit. For example, a patient with end-stage cancer and ventilator-dependent respiratory failure will not

derive any long-term biomedical benefit from continuing the intensive care. However, that patient may have the goal of living for another 48 hours in order to say good-bye to a child who is going to be arriving from a great distance. That specific goal enables the intervention to be understood as benefitting the patient. The third level has been described as "ultimate" benefit, but it refers to the patient's belief system and world view. Does the patient's faith make claims as to the obligation to preserve life to the last breath? Here the patient's ultimate framework of beliefs may have a specific impact on the definition of benefit. As the patient's advocate, we must consider all three levels as we define benefit.

- Beneficence: preservation of life, restoration of health, relief of suffering, and restoration or maintenance of function.

Nonmaleficence

Nonmaleficence requires that one should not do evil or harm. This principle is based on "do no harm, prevent harm, and remove harm." This tenet also addresses unprofessional behavior: verbal, physical, and sexual abuse of patients, and uninformed and undisclosed experimentation on patients with drugs and procedures that have the potential to cause harmful side effects. Breach of physician-patient confidentiality which results in harm to the patient is another example of maleficence.

- Nonmaleficence: "do no harm, prevent harm, and remove harm."

Nonabandonment

Abandonment connotes leaving the patient (for whom the physician has provided health care in the past) without providing for immediate or future medical care. This action has been "universally condemned as a serious and punishable infraction of both the legal and ethical obligations that physicians owe patients" (Ann Intern Med 1995;122:377-378). In contrast, nonabandonment denotes a requisite ethical obligation of physicians to provide ongoing medical care once the patient and physician mutually concur to enter into an alliance. Nonabandonment is closely related to the principles of beneficence and nonmaleficence and is fundamental to the long-term physician-patient relationship. This tenet has several drawbacks and limitations. The degree of physician involvement in the relationship cannot be measured as to its quantity or quality. Furthermore, the extent of the relationship is dictated by the underlying medical condition. For instance, an annual examination may require a single visit to the physician, whereas a complicated disease process may bring the physician and patient closer to each other over a long period. It would be improper for the physician to force a patient to maintain a long-term physician-patient relationship if the latter is unwilling, for whatever reason. Noncompliance, in terms of taking medications or following a physician's instructions, by the patient is not grounds for abandonment. Physicians should strive to respond to the needs of their patients over time, but they should not trespass their own values in the process.

● Nonabandonment: a requisite ethical obligation of physicians to provide ongoing care once the patient and physician mutually concur to enter into an alliance.

Conflict of Interest

The principle of beneficence requires that the physician not engage in activities that are not in the patient's best interest. This is considered to be a significant problem in the United States and other countries. Some studies have suggested that physicians' prescribing practices are influenced by financial and other significant rewards from drug companies. If the physician does not ardently avoid areas of potential conflict of interest (because of the principle of beneficence), the result may be maleficence. Authorship of scientific papers and editorials to promote drugs and appliances solely for immediate or future personal financial gains also constitutes conflict of interest (Ann Intern Med 1997;126:986-988).

● Conflict of interest is contrary to the tenet of beneficence.

The Impaired Physician

According to the American Medical Association, the impaired physician is one who is "unable to practice medicine with reasonable skill and safety to patients because of physical or mental illness, including deteriorations through the aging process, or loss of motor skill, or excessive use or abuse of drugs including alcohol." Impairment is distinct from competence, which specifically concerns the physician's knowledge and skills to adequately perform his or her duties as a physician. Impairment and incompetence both may seriously compromise patient care and safety. Under the obligation to protect patients from harm, physicians must protect patients from impaired and incompetent colleagues. Physicians have a moral and legal obligation to report impaired and incompetent colleagues to the appropriate authority. Different states vary in the specifics of reporting, but all have a reporting requirement. Typical authorities to contact include the institutional chief of staff or impairment program, local or state medical society impairment programs, or the state licensing body. It is important that reporting the behavior of a colleague be based on objective evidence rather than supposition.

● Physicians have an obligation to report impaired behavior in colleagues.

The Principle of Double Effect (Beneficence vs. Nonmaleficence)

In the medical management of patients, sometimes the pursuit of a beneficent outcome risks the potential for serious injury or death. Consequently, the moral obligations for beneficence and nonmaleficence conflict. The classic example of such a situation is the terminally ill patient who may require high doses of narcotics for adequate analgesia, but such doses also have the potential for respiratory depression and an earlier death. The rule or principle of double effect is a means of trying to resolve the conflict. This principle states that 1) the act itself must be good or morally neutral, 2) the actor or agent intends only the good effect, 3) the bad effect must not be a means to the good effect (e.g., death is the only way to achieve the desired outcome), and 4) the good effect must outweigh the bad effect. By the reasoning of double effect, and the high requirement of beneficence to address the suffering of patients, adequate analgesia for the relief of suffering should always be given even if death is hastened. The analgesics are to be given, however, in such a way as to relieve the pain and not specifically to hasten the death of patients, even terminally ill patients.

● Adequate analgesia, particularly in patients with incurable disease, is the responsibility of the physician.
● The physician has not performed immorally if death in a terminally ill patient is a result of respiratory depression from analgesic therapy; euthanasia is not the goal.

Incurable Disease and Death

Probably the most distressing aspect of medical practice is the encounter with a patient who has an incurable disease and in whom premature death is inevitable. The physician and patient (or surrogate) must formulate appropriate goals of therapy, choose what measures should be taken to maintain life, and decide how aggressive these measures ought to be. It is important to remind oneself that the patient is under enormous mental anguish and physical stress and that the ability to make solid decisions may be clouded. Furthermore, the decision(s) made by the patient may be guided by his or her understanding (whether adequate or not) of the medical condition and prognosis, religious beliefs, financial status, and other personal wishes. The patient may seek counsel from family, friends, and clergy as well as the attending physician.

● In incurable disease, recognize that the patient is under enormous mental anguish and physical stress.
● The ability of the patient to make solid decisions may be clouded.

The following guidelines are suggested in dealing with incurable disease and death. The patient and family (if the patient so desires) must be provided ample opportunity to talk with the physician and ask questions. An unhurried openness and willing-to-listen attitude on the part of the physician are critical for a positive outcome. Patients often find it easier to share their feelings about death with their physician, who is likely to be more objective and less emotional, than with family and friends. Nevertheless, the physician should not remain or "appear" completely detached from the patient's feelings and emotions. Even an attempt on the part of the physician to enter the "inner" feelings of the patient will have a soothing, if not therapeutic, effect.

- The patient and family must be provided every opportunity to talk with the physician and ask questions.
- An unhurried openness and willing-to-listen attitude on the part of the physician are critical for a positive outcome.

The physician should assume the responsibility to furnish or arrange for physical, emotional, and spiritual support. Adequate control of pain, respect for human dignity, and close contact with the family are crucial. The emotional and spiritual support available through local clergy (as appropriate, given the patient's personal beliefs) should not be underestimated. At no other time in life is the reality of human mortality so real as in the terminal phases of disease. It is always preferable to allay the anxiety of the dying patient through adequate emotional and spiritual support rather than by sedation. The physician should constantly remind herself or himself that despite all the medical technology that surrounds the patient, the patient must not be dehumanized.

- Adequate pain control, respect for human dignity, and close contact with the family are crucial.
- It is better to allay the anxiety of the dying patient through adequate emotional and spiritual support rather than by sedation.

Justice

Every patient deserves and must be provided optimal care as warranted by the underlying medical condition. Allocation of medical resources fairly and according to medical need is the basis for this principle. The decision to provide optimal medical care should be based on the medical need of each patient and the perceived medical benefit to the patient. The patient's social status, ability to pay, or perceived social worth should not dictate the quality or quantity of medical care. The physician's clear-cut responsibility is to the patient's well-being (beneficence). Physicians should not make decisions about individual care of their patients based on larger societal needs. The bedside is not the place to make general policy decisions.

- Justice: allocation of medical resources fairly and according to medical need.
- Physicians should not make decisions about individual care of patients based on larger societal needs.

PHYSICIAN-ASSISTED SUICIDE AND EUTHANASIA

All four tenets of medical ethics have an impact on the issue of physician-assisted death, that is, physician-assisted suicide and euthanasia. Historically, the medical profession has taken a strong stand against physicians directly killing patients, but this prohibition has been challenged on the basis of patient autonomy, beneficence or compassion, and other grounds. Numerous opinion polls have shown that significant portions of the general population and the medical community now favor some legalization of physician-assisted suicide, if not euthanasia. The American Medical Association and other large professional medical groups have maintained their stance against these practices.

In 1997, the Supreme Court of the United States ruled that states may maintain laws prohibiting euthanasia and assisted suicide but may also pass laws allowing these practices. The Court, however, emphasized the patient's right to adequate, aggressive pain control even if it might shorten the patient's life. In the election of 1997, the people of the state of Oregon reiterated their support for physician-assisted suicide by reapproving a referendum first passed in 1994 legalizing assisted suicide but still prohibiting euthanasia. The Oregon law requires that the patient 1) be terminal, 2) be decisionally capable, 3) have initiated two verbal requests and one written request for a prescription for a lethal overdose, 4) undergo a second-opinion consultation, 5) receive appropriate psychiatric intervention if perceived to be depressed, and 6) undergo a 15-day waiting period after the request has been made to allow the patient to change his or her mind. At this time, assisted suicide and euthanasia remain illegal in the other 49 states.

- Euthanasia and physician-assisted suicide are legally prohibited in the United States with the exception of the state of Oregon, which permits physician-assisted suicide.

Regardless of one's final position on this difficult issue, physicians are obligated to address the underlying concerns that lead patients and physicians to believe that assisted suicide and euthanasia are necessary (the New York State Task Force on Life and the Law, 1994). Physicians should be acquainted with appropriate means of pain management and palliative care and be willing to be aggressive in the relief of a patient's symptoms. Physicians also are obligated to recognize and appropriately treat depression. Furthermore, physicians should strive to address the other issues that may lead patients to desire assisted death, such as fear of abandonment and loss of control.

"DO NOT RESUSCITATE" (DNR)

DNR orders affect administration of CPR only; other therapeutic options should not be influenced by the DNR order. Every person whose medical history is unclear or unavailable should receive CPR in the event of cardiopulmonary arrest. CPR is not recommended when it merely prolongs life in a patient with terminal illness or when the fatal outcome is clinically evident (Table 15-1).

Of paramount importance are the patient's knowledge of the extent of disease and the prognosis, the physician's estimate of the potential efficacy of CPR, and the wishes of the patient (or surrogate) regarding CPR as a therapeutic tool. The DNR order should be reviewed frequently because clinical circumstances may dictate other measures (e.g., a patient with terminal cardiomyopathy who had initially turned down heart transplantation and wanted to be considered a "DNR candidate" may change her or his mind and now opt for the transplantation). Physicians should discuss the appropriateness of CPR or DNR with patients at high risk for cardiopulmonary arrest and with the terminally ill. The discussion should optimally take place in the outpatient setting, during the initial period of hospitalization, and periodically during hospitalization, if appropriate. DNR orders (and rationale) should be entered in the patient's medical records.

- DNR orders affect CPR only.
- Other therapeutic options should not be influenced by the DNR order.
- Every patient should be considered a candidate for CPR unless clear indications exist otherwise.

- CPR is not recommended when it merely prolongs life in a patient with a terminal illness.
- DNR orders should be reviewed frequently.
- DNR orders (and rationale) should be entered in the patient's medical records.

WITHHOLDING AND WITHDRAWING LIFE SUPPORT

This decision may be compatible with beneficence, nonmaleficence, and autonomy. The right of a decisionally capable person to refuse lifesaving hydration and nutrition was upheld by the U.S. Supreme Court (Table 15-2), but a surrogate decision maker's right to refuse treatment for decisionally incapable persons can be restricted by states. Currently, the states of New York, Missouri, and Florida required "clear and convincing evidence" that withdrawing and withholding of life-supporting treatment would be the patient's desire. Other states have lesser evidentiary standards for surrogates to withhold or withdraw life support. Brain death is not a necessary requirement for withdrawing or withholding life support. The value of each medical therapy (risk:benefit ratio) should be assessed for each patient. When appropriate, the withholding or withdrawal of life support is best accomplished with input from more than one experienced clinician.

- Withholding or withdrawing life support does not conflict with the principles of beneficence, nonmaleficence, and autonomy.
- Brain death is not a necessary requirement for withdrawing or withholding life support.

PERSISTENT VEGETATIVE STATE

This is a chronic state of unconsciousness (loss of self-awareness) lasting for more than a few weeks, characterized by the

Table 15-1 Clinical Situations in Which Cardiopulmonary Resuscitation Is Unlikely to Prolong Life

---

Advanced, progressive, ultimately lethal illness
    Bedfast with metastatic cancer
    Child class C cirrhosis
    Infection by human immunodeficiency virus (with ≥2 episodes of pneumonia caused by *Pneumocystis carinii*)
    Dementia requiring long-term care
Acute, near-fatal illness without evidence of improvement after admission to the intensive-care unit
    Coma (traumatic or nontraumatic) lasting ≥48 hours
    Multiple organ system failure with no improvement after 3 consecutive days in the intensive-care unit
Unsuccessful out-of-hospital cardiopulmonary resuscitation

From Murphy DJ, Finucane TE: New do-not-resuscitate policies: a first step in cost control. Arch Intern Med 1993;153:1641-1648. By permission of the American Medical Association.

Table 15-2 Pertinent Legal Rulings

Case, yr	Legal issue	Court	Decision
Salgo, 1957	Informed consent	California Court of Appeals	First used term "informed consent"
Brooks, 1965	Jehovah's Witness refusal of blood	Illinois District Court	Patients have right to personal treatment on religious grounds
Canterbury, 1972	Degree of disclosure required for adequate informed consent	U.S. District Court	Established "prudent patient test"
Quinlan, 1976	PVS—discontinuation of mechanical ventilation, previously articulated directive	New Jersey Supreme Court	Discontinuation (based on right to privacy)
Brophy, 1986	PVS—discontinuation of gastrostomy feedings, previously articulated directive	Massachusetts Supreme Court	Discontinue feedings (based on autonomy)
Bouvia, 1986	Severely impaired, refusal of nasogastric tube feedings by a decisionally capable patient	California Court of Appeals	Removal of nasogastric tube (based on autonomy)
Corbett, 1986	PVS—discontinuation of nasogastric tube feedings, no predefined directive(s)	Florida Court of Appeals	Discontinue feedings (based on right to privacy)
Cruzan, 1990	PVS—state of Missouri required "clear and convincing" evidence of individual's wishes before allowing withdrawal of life support	U.S. Supreme Court	States have right to restrict exercise of right to refuse treatment by surrogates; decisionally capable patients may refuse life-sustaining therapy, including hydration, nutrition, and mechanical ventilation
Wanglie, 1991	PVS—family wished continued support despite objections to continued life-sustaining therapy by the physicians and institution	Minnesota District Court	Continuation (based on autonomy, substituted judgment)
Lee, 1997	Assisted suicide	U.S. Supreme Court	States have the right to make laws prohibiting or allowing physician-assisted suicide and euthanasia

PVS, persistent vegetative state.

presence of wake/sleep cycles, but without behavioral or cerebral metabolic evidence of possessing cognitive function or of being able to respond in a learned manner to external events or stimuli. The body retains functions necessary to sustain vegetative survival if provided nutritional and other supportive measures—note that the U.S. Supreme Court has ruled that there is no distinction between artificial feeding and hydration versus mechanical ventilation (Table 15-2).

- Persistent vegetative state: unconsciousness (loss of self-awareness) lasting for more than a few weeks.
- U.S. Supreme Court ruling states that there is no distinction between artificial feeding and hydration versus mechanical ventilation.

DEFINITION OF DEATH

Death is irreversible cessation of circulatory and respiratory function or irreversible cessation of all functions of the entire brain, including the brain stem. Clinical criteria (at times substantiated by electroencephalographic testing or assessment of cerebral perfusion) permit the reliable diagnosis of "cerebral death."

The family should be informed of the brain death but should not be asked to decide whether further medical therapy should be continued. One exception is when the patient's surrogate (or the patient, via an advance directive) permits certain decisions, such as organ donation, in the case of brain death.

Once it is ascertained that the patient is "brain dead" and that no further therapy can be offered, the primary physician, preferably after consultation with another physician involved in the care of the patient, may withdraw supportive measures. This is true in general throughout the United States, with the exception of the states of New Jersey and New York, which have modified their definition of death statutes to allow a religious exemption for groups (such as Orthodox Jews) that do not accept brain death as a valid criterion for death. In these states, continued care may be requested of the caregivers until circulatory and respiratory function collapse.

The imminent possibility of harvesting organs for transplantation should in no way affect any of the above-outlined decisions. When organ donation is possible after the determination of brain death, the family should be approached, preferably before cessation of cardiac function, regarding organ donation.

- Death: irreversible cessation of circulatory and respiratory function or irreversible cessation of all functions of the entire brain, including the brain stem.
- Electroencephalography is not necessary to establish death.

AUTHOR'S NOTE

Laws concerning ethical issues in medicine continue to evolve, reflecting changing attitudes of society. Certainly, legal decisions will continue to influence the practice of medicine. Many states have no directly applicable statutes or court cases relating to difficult ethical issues in medical practice. This review is meant as a guide; the individual practitioner is referred to the appropriate state medical society for further information regarding state-specific mandates.

QUESTIONS

Multiple Choice (choose the one best answer)

1. For 6 years, you have been caring for a 54-year-old single man. He has bipolar disease but has been faithful in taking his medication. He is intelligent and works as a computer programmer. He has not had an episode of significant mania or depression for the past 4 years. He is a former smoker; he quit smoking once his bipolar disease was adequately treated. Recently, he presented with the complaint of a new cough without other symptoms of upper respiratory tract infection, and he reported that on a couple of occasions he coughed up blood in his sputum. Chest radiography, followed by CT, showed that he had a solitary lung mass on the right side. Sputum confirmed the presence of adenocarcinoma. His evaluation suggested that the lesion was stage I and therefore there was a high probability that he might be cured by resection (~85% 5-year survival). When you share the diagnosis and recommendations for operation with him, he declines the procedure. In fact, he wants no treatment at all. He acknowledges that he will probably die of this cancer if he does not pursue treatment but indicates that he accepts this as his fate. He is oriented and does not appear to be manic or depressed. What would you do next?
   a. Comply with his refusal and schedule regular appointments to pursue palliative care
   b. Advise psychiatric consultation to assess capacity because of his history of bipolar disease
   c. Declare the patient incompetent because of his irrational choice and seek a court-appointed guardian
   d. Contact his parents and coworkers and enlist them to convince the patient to pursue treatment
   e. Schedule another appointment in 1 week to discuss the issues again after he has had a chance to think about his situation.

2. A 55-year-old man with widely metastatic cancer, unresponsive to chemotherapy, is hospitalized for pain control. On admission, cardiopulmonary resuscitation (CPR) and do-not-resuscitate (DNR) issues were discussed with the patient and his wife. It was learned that he has no advance directive and that the patient and spouse want him to receive full resuscitation efforts in the case of cardiac arrest. He still has much "to do." On the third day of hospitalization, he has arrest and a code is called by his primary nurse. You are the team leader for the advanced cardiac life support (ACLS) team. Which one of the following responses is correct?
   a. Refuse to perform CPR and ACLS because they are physiologically futile

   b. Provide a limited code procedure for a few moments to appease the family
   c. Call the ethics consultation service while resuscitation is being conducted
   d. Have a nurse or colleague discuss the futility of the effort with the wife and try to get her to change her mind
   e. Provide CPR and ACLS according to protocol

3. A 16-year-old boy is brought to the emergency department after a motorcycle accident. Severe, continuous hemorrhage has reduced the patient's hemoglobin value to 4.5 g/dL. His blood pressure is 70 mm Hg systolic. The patient is unconscious. His parents arrive soon after the ambulance and indicate refusal for their son to receive any blood products, in keeping with their religious beliefs. They want to take him home, where they and their neighbors can pray for the boy. You would:
   a. Contact the legal department to get a court order for transfusions and operation
   b. Avoid transfusion and manage with crystalloid
   c. Dismiss the patient to the family against medical advice
   d. Start transfusions immediately and prepare for operation to stop the bleeding
   e. Request that the hospital chaplain reason with the parents

4. A 63-year-old man had a permanent pacemaker placed a year ago for symptomatic complete heart block. He has now had a massive myocardial infarction and is responsive only to deep pain. His ejection fraction is estimated at 12%, and recovery of additional myocardial function is not expected. The patient has a living will stating that he would not want life-sustaining treatments initiated or continued if his chances of recovery from a serious illness were small. Aggressive treatments are being withheld according to the family's request in compliance with the living will. The family now comes to the physician requesting that the pacemaker be deprogrammed. The physician should:
   a. Comply with the request and deprogram the pacemaker
   b. Give the family the deprogrammer and ask them to deprogram the pacemaker
   c. Request an ethics consultation
   d. Refuse to comply with the request because it would constitute actively taking the patient's life, and euthanasia and assisted suicide are illegal in your state
   e. Refuse to comply with the request because the living will is invalid in this circumstance

5. A 73-year-old woman presented with an acute bowel obstruction. Fourteen months earlier, she had had a left hemicolectomy for a stage B2 adenocarcinoma of the

colon. At exploratory operation performed for the current bowel obstruction, the obstruction is found to be due to an adhesion. However, your surgical colleague, who has called you from the operating room to give you an update, also reports that there is a 2-cm lesion in the liver that is metastatic colon cancer. Later that afternoon, you visit the patient's daughter, who has been waiting in her mother's room for the patient's return after the procedure. The daughter, who is an attorney, demands that you not reveal the finding of cancer to her mother, claiming that this information would totally devastate the patient emotionally and cause her to give up hope and die sooner. She states that she will give you a formal document allowing you to withhold the information, absolving you of legal intervention. The next day on rounds, the patient is awake, alert, and specifically asks you, "Did they find any cancer?" You would:

a. Tell the patient that the obstruction was benign, but add no more
b. Tell the patient no cancer was found
c. Stall and tell the patient that you are awaiting the final pathology report
d. Tell the patient that a lesion of metastatic colon cancer was found and removed
e. Tell the patient that she should not worry about such things now, but that she needs to focus on recovering from the operation

6. An 85-year-old woman is admitted to the hospital with end-stage metastatic breast cancer, with metastases involving the brain, lung, liver, kidneys, and multiple areas of the skeleton. She is obtunded and confused as a result of hypercalcemia and cerebral edema from the metastases. She previously had received four different programs of chemotherapy, but her disease progressed through the last two with no response. The patient has a living will on record stating that she does not want CPR or aggressive treatments once she has entered into the terminal phase of her disease, requesting instead comfort measures only. She is being evaluated for an inpatient hospice program because she lives alone. A DNR order has been entered into her chart and orders. At this point a daughter, with whom the patient has not had close contact for several years, arrives at the hospital and demands that her mother be treated aggressively, that the DNR order be rescinded, and that the patient be given more chemotherapy. She accuses the staff of deliberately letting her mother die and indicates that if her demands are not immediately complied with, she will bring suit against the care team and hospital. In fact, she hands then the card of a particularly well-known and aggressive attorney she has already retained, "just in case."

While the physician and daughter are having a discussion on these issues just outside the patient's room, the patient has a cardiac arrest. The physician should:

a. Tell the daughter she needs psychiatric evaluation
b. Call a code and legal counsel
c. Call a code and pursue full resuscitation measures for a minimum of 30 minutes
d. Perform a "slow code" for 10 minutes, hoping to appease the daughter
e. Evaluate the patient and pronounce her dead

7. A 72-year-old man is admitted to the hospital after his third round of chemotherapy for diffuse large-cell non-Hodgkin lymphoma with the acute onset of severe bilateral pneumonia. He is in respiratory failure and consents to intubation. After intubation, he requires chemical paralysis to tolerate mechanical ventilation. Cultures and bronchoalveolar lavage fail to identify an infectious cause, and steroids are added to broad-spectrum antibiotic therapy in the thought that this could be cyclophosphamide-induced pneumonitis. After 1 week of treatment, a little progress is observed, although attempts to wean the patient from chemical paralysis have failed. At this point, the patient's wife and three children demand to meet with the treating physicians. The wife and eldest son demand that use of the ventilator be discontinued and the patient be allowed to die. They claim that he would not want this therapy and that it is torture for him. When queried, they indicate that there is no known advance directive and that neither of them has ever overtly discussed these sorts of issues with the patient. At this point, the youngest son dissents and states that his father is a fighter and would want the ventilator therapy to continue in the hopes that he could improve. He states that his father was always an aggressive businessman and had overcome two previous cancers, lung cancer and prostate cancer. The middle child, a daughter, is very confused and does not know what to think or what her father would want. All again reiterate that none of them have ever discussed issues such as life-sustaining treatment or goals of therapy with the patient. At this point, the physician should:

a. Negotiate a time-limited period of continued aggressive intervention with the family, and encourage them to come to a consensus
b. Stop use of the ventilator as requested by the patient's rightful surrogate, the wife
c. Refuse to withdraw any treatment at any point because there is no advance directive
d. Request an ethics consultation
e. Tell the family they must obtain a court order before use of the ventilator can be stopped

ANSWERS

1. Answer e.

From all appearances, the patient is decisionally capable. Answer "a" is not completely inappropriate. Given that this is the first time the patient is confronting a horrible diagnosis, he may need to take some time to process the information and could change his mind. Answer "b" goes to a very important issue—the patient's capacity in light of his significant psychiatric history. Ultimately, psychiatric consultation might be an important step, but it is probably not the best first response. He has just received horrible news and it might not be the best time to remind him of his psychiatric issues. Rather, it is best to allow him some time to reflect and continue the conversation in the near future. Answer "d" is not appropriate because such action would violate patient confidentiality unless you received specific consent from the patient to make such contacts.

2. Answer e.

Although it is highly unlikely that the patient will survive, or if he survives that he will leave the hospital alive, there is a small chance he will survive the arrest, and, as such, physiologic futility cannot be claimed. Emergency circumstances are not the time to be calling for an ethics consultation. If there were concerns, the consultation should have been obtained soon after admission. It is also inappropriate to try to coerce surrogates to change their minds in such situations or to provide less than a full resuscitation effort. Rather, the patient was "full code" and therefore should receive a legitimate resuscitation effort.

3. Answer d.

The patient is a minor and therefore, under presumed consent, life-sustaining interventions are to be pursued even in the face of parental refusal. Although surrogates can refuse life-sustaining therapy for adults for whatever reason, parents have not been allowed to refuse appropriate medical treatment, especially life-sustaining treatment, of minors for religious convictions. In such cases, physicians are obligated to obtain a court order appointing a guardian and permitting the life-sustaining treatment. In this case, there is not time to have the order in hand before intervening, so it is most appropriate to pursue the life-saving treatment while the legal issues are sorted out.

4. Answer a.

Although an ethics consultation is not unreasonable, it is not really necessary. The living will is valid because the patient's chances of recovery are minuscule to nonexistent. Patients may refuse any form of medical intervention, and that includes pacemaker activity. Although the patient may die rapidly after the deprogramming, the cause of death is the underlying disease, not the physician. Therefore, this approach would not constitute a case of euthanasia or assisted suicide.

5. Answer d.

The patient should always be our guide to how much information to share or not share. In some cultures, patients are protected from "bad news," and they accept and expect that. However, when a patient wants to know the medical information, it is the physician's duty to share it honestly and to the extent the patient wants. The patient clearly wanted to know, because she directly asked the question, and she deserves a truthful answer regardless of what the daughter has requested or promised. The only exception to this approach is when it can be clearly demonstrated that a patient is psychologically or emotionally unstable to the point of engaging in attempts to harm himself or herself if certain information is learned. That is the principle of therapeutic privilege, but it requires a high burden of proof as to the likelihood of harm.

6. Answer e.

Our first obligation is to the patient and his or her directives. The patient has made her choices clear, and they should be respected.

7. Answer a.

It is not at all clear what the patient would want at this point. The last directive from the patient was that he wanted treatment. At the same time, the patient may indeed be in an irreversible situation in which eventual withdrawal of use of the ventilator would be appropriate. The goals are to try to do what is best for the patient and to demonstrate a good-faith commitment to work with the family. A reasonable time limit on the aggressive treatment can accomplish both and allow the family members to resolve the differences among themselves.

CHAPTER 16
NEPHROLOGY

Fernando C. Fervenza, M.D., Ph.D.
Thomas R. Schwab, M.D.
Amy W. Williams, M.D.
Robert C. Albright, Jr., D.O.
Steven B. Erickson, M.D.

PART I
Fernando C. Fervenza, M.D., Ph.D.
Thomas R. Schwab, M.D.

CLINICAL MANIFESTATIONS OF GLOMERULAR INJURY

The glomerular basement membrane is an important size barrier (molecular weight, 70,000) and negative charge barrier, repulsing albumin and immunoglobulins. There is also tubular reabsorption of protein in the range of 500 to 1,500 mg/24 hours by the proximal tubule. Damage to glomeruli is manifested as isolated hematuria, proteinuria, or both, with specific glomerular diseases characteristically tending to present as nephritic or nephrotic syndromes.

Orthostatic proteinuria is usually benign and remits spontaneously. The diagnosis can be made by obtaining two 12-hour urine collections for protein: one supine and one upright. "Normoalbuminuria" is defined as urinary albumin excretion less than 30 mg/24 hours, "microalbuminuria" as "urinary albumin" of 30 to 300 mg/24 hours, and "proteinuria" as more than 300 mg/24 hours. Tubulointerstitial disease is sometimes associated with proteinuria, but it is usually less than 1,500 mg/24 hours. Overflow low-molecular-weight proteinuria is due to increased excretion of light chain or lysozyme without nephrosis.

Renal biopsy is often required in patients with an active urinary sediment (dysmorphic red blood cells, red blood cell casts, and white blood cell casts), proteinuria greater than 1 g/24 hours, or renal insufficiency, in which the diagnosis cannot be determined or the prognosis adequately predicted with a less invasive diagnostic procedure. Other indications for biopsy include acute renal failure lasting longer than 3 to 4 weeks, an atypical course of diabetes mellitus, and systemic diseases in which the differential diagnosis includes amyloidosis, systemic

lupus erythematosus, and systemic vasculitis. Percutaneous renal biopsy is contraindicated if uncontrolled hypertension, acute pyelonephritis or perinephric abscess, or renal neoplasm is present or the patient is uncooperative. Patients with bleeding disorders, including severe thrombocytopenia, should be considered for renal biopsy through a transjugular approach, with the use of fresh frozen plasma and platelet transfusion if indicated. A solitary kidney is not an absolute contraindication to biopsy. Complications include gross hematuria (<10%), arteriovenous fistula (<1%), need for nephrectomy (0.1%), and death (0.001%).

- Renal biopsy: to determine the diagnosis and prognosis for patients with active urinary sediment, proteinuria >1 g/24 hours, or unexplained renal failure.
- Other indications: acute renal failure lasting >3-4 weeks, atypical course of diabetes mellitus, and undiagnosed systemic disease.
- Contraindications to percutaneous renal biopsy: bleeding disorders, uncontrolled hypertension, acute pyelonephritis, renal neoplasm, and uncooperative patient.

Nephrotic Syndrome

"Nephrotic syndrome" is defined by urinary protein greater than 3.5 g/1.73 m^2 per 24 hours, hypoalbuminemia (<3.0 g/dL), peripheral edema, hypercholesterolemia, and lipiduria. Urinalysis demonstrates waxy casts, free fat, oval fat bodies, and lipiduria ("Maltese crosses"). Complications of nephrotic syndrome include hypogammaglobulinemia (increases the risk of infection), vitamin D deficiency from the loss of vitamin

D–binding protein, and iron deficiency anemia due to hypo-transferrinemia. Thrombotic complications are common, for example, renal vein thrombosis, and occur because of an increased thromboembolic tendency (increase in factors V and VIII, fibrinogen, and platelets and a decrease in antithrombin III and antiplasmin). Patients at increased risk include those with proteinuria greater than 10 g/24 hours and serum albumin less than 2 g/dL. Management includes controlling blood pressure and limiting protein (0.8 g/kg daily), sodium, and lipid intake. Anticoagulation should be considered for patients at increased risk, especially if the nephrotic syndrome is due to membranous nephropathy or amyloidosis.

- Nephrotic syndrome: urinary protein >3.5 g/1.73 m² per 24 hours.
- Other features: hypoalbuminemia, peripheral edema, hyperlipidemia, and lipiduria.

Nephritic Syndrome

Nephritic syndrome is characterized by oliguria, edema, hypertension, proteinuria (usually <3.5 g/1.73 m² per 24 hours), and the presence of active urinary sediment (dysmorphic red blood cells or red blood cell casts or both). Because of the formation of methemoglobin in acid urine, the urine has a "Coca-Cola" or smoky appearance.

- Nephritic syndrome: active urinary sediment (dysmorphic red blood cells and/or red blood cell casts). Other features: oliguria, hypertension, edema, and proteinuria (usually <3.5 g/24 hours).

GLOMERULAR DISEASE THAT PRESENTS WITH A NEPHRITIC SYNDROME

Poststreptococcal Glomerulonephritis

Poststreptococcal glomerulonephritis (PSGN) is an acute glomerulonephritis that develops 1 to 4 weeks after pharyngitis or skin infection with specific ("nephritogenic") strains of group A β-hemolytic streptococci. The latent period is 6 to 21 days (type 12 pharyngeal infection) or 14 to 28 days (type 49 skin infection). The typical presentation is an abrupt onset of nephritic syndrome. An active urinary sediment is present in almost all cases. Proteinuria is usually less than 3 g/24 hours, but it may be in the nephrotic range in some cases. Cultures are usually negative, but the antibody titer to streptolysin O (ASO), antistreptokinase, antihyaluronidase, and antideoxyribonuclease may provide evidence of recent streptococcal infection. ASO titers increase 10 to 14 days after infection, peak at 3 to 4 weeks, and then decrease. Total hemolytic (CH50) complement and C3 levels are usually

reduced (activation of the alternative complement pathway), but C4 levels are normal.

Light microscopy shows diffuse hypercellularity of the glomerular tuffs, with mesangial and endothelial cell proliferation and infiltration by polymorphonuclear leukocytes (thus, the name "exudative"), monocytes or macrophages, and plasma cells. All glomeruli are affected in a homogeneous pattern. Early in the disease process, characteristic subepithelial "humps" can be detected with a silver stain. Cellular crescents are uncommon and indicative of severe disease. Immunofluorescence shows the deposition of IgG, C3, and occasionally IgM, which are distributed in the three well-described patterns of "starry sky," "mesangial," and "garland." With electron microscopy, small immune deposits are seen in the mesangial and subendothelial areas. Almost pathognomonic of PSGN is the presence of large "humps," which are dome-shaped subepithelial deposits in the glomerular basement membrane.

The treatment of PSGN is supportive. Appropriate antibiotic therapy is indicated for persistent infection and for contacts to prevent new cases. Sodium restriction and the use of loop diuretics reduce the risk of fluid overload and help to control hypertension. For children, the prognosis is excellent, with most patients recovering renal function within 1 to 2 months after diagnosis. In a few patients, especially adults, microscopic hematuria, proteinuria, hypertension, and renal dysfunction may persist for many years. Patients presenting with a crescentic nephritis have a poorer prognosis, with approximately 50% developing end-stage renal disease (ESRD). Other forms of postinfectious glomerulonephritis include bacterial endocarditis and infected ventriculoatrial shunts.

- PSGN: usually due to group A β-hemolytic streptococcal infections.
- Active urine sediment, with proteinuria <3 g/24 hours.
- Total and C3 complements are low.
- Light microscopy: diffuse hypercellularity of the glomerular tuffs, with mesangial and endothelial cell proliferation and infiltration by polymorphonuclear leukocytes.
- Immunofluorescence: granular deposition of IgG and C3 in a "starry-sky," "mesangial," or "garland" pattern.

IgA Nephropathy

"IgA nephropathy," or Berger disease, is defined as a mesangial proliferative glomerulonephritis characterized by diffuse deposition of IgA in the mesangium. It is the most common glomerulopathy worldwide, with an incidence approaching 1:100 in some countries. The typical presentation is episodic macroscopic hematuria usually accompanying an intercurrent upper respiratory tract infection. This clinical pattern occurs most frequently in the second and third decades of life. Other patients are asymptomatic and may be identified when microscopic hematuria, with or without proteinuria, is found on routine urinalysis. Proteinuria is common, but nephrotic syndrome occurs in less than 10% of all cases. Patients with nephrotic syndrome may have minimal change disease superimposed on IgA nephropathy or other glomerulopathy. The pathogenesis has been linked to abnormal integrity of the intestinal mucosa, resulting in overexposure to ubiquitous environmental antigens. This leads to an exaggerated production of galactose-deficient (GD) IgA1 by bone marrow–derived B cells. Underglycosylation of IgA1 molecules reduces the affinity of the clearance receptors on the Kupffer cells in the liver. This results in an increase in circulating GD-IgA1, the formation of anti–GD-IgA1 autoantibodies, deposition of IgG or IgA anti–GD-IgA1 immune complexes in the mesangium, and activation of complement and cytokine cascades. Secondary causes include advanced chronic liver disease, celiac disease, dermatitis herpetiformis, and ankylosing spondylitis. With light microscopy, glomeruli may look normal or show mesangial expansion. Immunofluorescence studies are diagnostic and demonstrate strong IgA staining within the mesangium. Electron microscopy shows electron-dense deposits in the mesangium that colocalize with the immune deposits.

The disease generally has a benign course, with patients maintaining a proteinuria less than 500 mg/24 hours and having preserved renal function. However, in 20% to 40% of patients, the disease progresses to ESRD within 10 to 25 years. Proteinuria greater than 1 g/24 hours, hypertension, impaired renal function at diagnosis, and glomerular or interstitial fibrosis seen in renal biopsy specimens are the most important predictors of a poor outcome. IgA nephropathy recurs in about 50% of patients after renal transplantation, but loss of the allograft from recurrent disease is uncommon. Progression to ESRD in patients at high risk has been shown to be slowed by angiotensin II converting enzyme blockade, administration of high doses of corticosteroids, and fish oil capsules containing omega-3 fatty acids. Mycophenolate mofetil is a new immunosuppressive agent currently being studied in clinical trials of patients with IgA nephropathy, but the results are not available. Patients with IgA nephropathy and concomitant minimal change disease respond fully to corticosteroid therapy. For patients with rapidly progressive renal failure due to crescentic IgA nephropathy, a regimen of corticosteroids and cyclophosphamide, with the addition of plasma exchange or pulse methylprednisolone, has been tried with variable results.

- IgA nephropathy: the most common glomerulopathy worldwide.
- Presents with synpharyngitic hematuria, often with red blood cell casts.

- Secondary causes: advanced chronic liver disease, celiac disease, dermatitis herpetiformis, and ankylosing spondylitis.
- Prognosis: generally good for patients who are normotensive, with proteinuria <1 g/24 hours, and serum creatinine <1.5 mg/dL.
- Treatment with angiotensin-converting enzyme inhibitors (ACEIs), high-dose corticosteroids, and fish oil capsules containing omega-3 fatty acids slows the progression of the disease.

Henoch-Schönlein Purpura

Henoch-Schönlein purpura represents the systemic form of IgA nephropathy. Patients usually present with microscopic or gross hematuria (or both) along with red blood cell casts, purpura, and abdominal pain. Renal biopsy findings are similar to those of IgA nephropathy with or without vasculitis. The prognosis generally is good for children and variable for adults. In patients with normal renal function, treatment is supportive only. Patients with progressive renal failure should be considered for treatment with high-dose corticosteroids with or without cytotoxic medication.

Membranoproliferative Glomerulonephritis

Membranoproliferative glomerulonephritis (MPGN) is defined by the diffuse proliferation of the mesangium and thickening of the glomerular capillary walls, as seen with light microscopy. MPGN type I affects mainly children of both sexes between the ages of 8 and 16 years. Type II MPGN is a rare disease (<1% of all renal biopsies). Secondary forms of MPGN tend to predominate in adults. The major cause of secondary MPGN is cryoglobulinemia in a patient with hepatitis C virus infection. Other secondary causes include chronic infections, "shunt nephritis," malaria, systemic lupus erythematosus, congenital complement deficiency (C2, C3), sickle cell disease, partial lipodystrophy (only type II), and alpha$_1$-antitrypsin deficiency. The clinical presentations of all forms of MPGN are variable and include nephrotic and nephritic features. Approximately one-third of the patients present with a combination of asymptomatic hematuria and proteinuria. Another third present with nephrotic syndrome and preserved renal function. Some patients (10%-20%) present with a nephritic syndrome. Hypertension is common (50%-80% of patients). In MPGN type I, and in cryoglobulinemic MPGN, the levels of C3, C4, and CH50 are persistently low, reflecting activation of both complement pathways. In MPGN type II, the alternative pathway is activated, with patients having a persistently low level of C3 but a normal level of C4. A C3 nephritic factor is present in many cases. The C3 nephritic factor is an autoantibody to alternative pathway C3 convertase, resulting in persistent C3 breakdown.

In type I MPGN, renal biopsy specimens show diffuse global thickening of capillary walls and endocapillary hypercellularity, giving the glomeruli a lobular appearance. The interposition of mesangium between the glomerular basement membrane and the endothelium triggers the production of neomembrane by the endothelial cells and results in glomerular capillaries developing a double contour, or "tram-track" aspect, best seen with silver staining. Immunofluorescence shows the granular deposition of IgG and C3 in the mesangium and outlines the lobular contours. Electron microscopy demonstrates immune deposits in the subendothelial space and mesangium. In type II MPGN, also known as "dense deposit disease," electron-dense deposits replace the lamina densa and produce a smooth ribbonlike thickening. Immunofluorescence shows intense capillary wall staining for C3.

- MPGN: about one-third of patients present with hematuria and proteinuria; about one-third present with nephrotic syndrome and preserved renal function. Nephritic syndrome is present in 10%-20%.
- Complement values are persistently low.
- C3 nephritic factor is often present.
- Secondary causes: hepatitis B and C, chronic infections, "shunt nephritis," systemic lupus erythematosus, and sickle cell disease.

In children, long-term corticosteroid therapy has been helpful. Dipyridamole (225 mg daily) and aspirin (975 mg daily) may temporarily slow the rate of progression of type I MPGN, but results are not lasting. Treatment in adults is unknown. MPGN type I usually has a slowly progressive course, with 40% to 50% of patients reaching ESRD in 10 years. Patients with MPGN type II have a worse prognosis, and clinical remission rates are less than 5%. Predictors of poor outcome include impaired renal function at presentation, nephrotic-range proteinuria, hypertension, the number of crescents (>50%), and the degree of tubulointerstitial damage. This disorder tends to recur in transplants (type I, 30%; type II, 90%).

- Prognosis: worse with hypertension, poor renal function, proteinuria >3 g/24 hours.

RAPIDLY PROGRESSIVE GLOMERULO-NEPHRITIS—CRESCENTIC GLOMERULONEPHRITIS

"Rapidly progressive glomerulonephritis" (RPGN) is defined as an acute, rapidly progressive (days to weeks to months) deterioration of renal function associated with an active urinary sediment and a focal necrotizing crescentic glomerulonephritis seen on light microscopic examination of renal biopsy specimens. A pulmonary-renal syndrome is frequent, and oliguria is not uncommon. Immunofluorescence demonstrates three patterns: type I, linear IgG deposition (e.g., Goodpasture disease or anti–glomerular basement membrane [GBM]-mediated); type II, granular immune complexes (e.g., systemic lupus erythematosus); and type III, pauci-immune (negative or weak immunofluorescence) (e.g., antineutrophil cytoplasmic antibody [ANCA] vasculitis) (Fig. 16-1). "Goodpasture syndrome" indicates a pulmonary-renal syndrome and can be due to several conditions, including Goodpasture disease, ANCA vasculitis (microscopic polyangiitis, Wegener granulomatosis), systemic lupus erythematosus, cryoglobulinemia, and pulmonary edema.

- RPGN: acute (days to weeks to months) deterioration of renal function.
- Focal necrotizing crescentic glomerulonephritis seen in renal biopsy specimens.
- Pulmonary-renal syndrome (Goodpasture syndrome) is common and can be due to Goodpasture disease, ANCA vasculitis (microscopic polyangiitis, Wegener granulomatosis), systemic lupus erythematosus, cryoglobulinemia, pulmonary edema, and other conditions.

ANCA Vasculitides

In the Chapel Hill classification, systemic vasculitis is classified according to the different size of the vessels involved (Table 16-1). Of particular importance to nephrology are the ANCA vasculitides: microscopic polyangiitis, Wegener granulomatosis, and Churg-Strauss syndrome. This group is

Table 16-1 Chapel Hill Consensus on the Nomenclature of Systemic Vasculitis

Large-vessel vasculitis
Giant cell (temporal) arteritis
Takayasu arteritis
Medium-sized vessel vasculitis
Classic polyarteritis nodosa
Kawasaki disease
Small-vessel vasculitis
Microscopic polyangiitis*
Wegener granulomatosis*
Churg-Strauss syndrome*
Henoch-Schönlein purpura
Essential cryoglobulinemic vasculitis
Cutaneous leukocytoclastic vasculitis

*Strongly associated with antineutrophilic cytoplasmic antibody (ANCA).

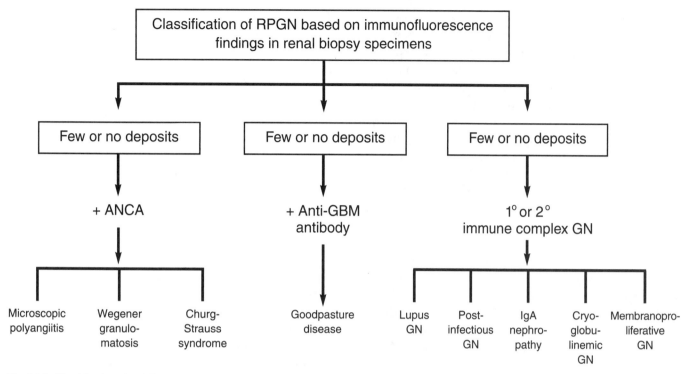

Fig. 16-1. Classification of rapidly progressive glomerulonephritis (RPGN) according to immunofluorescence microscopy findings in renal biopsy specimens. ANCA, antineutrophil cytoplasmic antibody; GBM, glomerular basement membrane; GN, glomerulonephritis.

characterized by inflammation and necrosis of small blood vessels of the kidney and other organs that occur in association with autoantibodies against antigens present in lysosomal granules in the cytoplasm of neutrophils (ANCA). These antigens are myeloperoxidase (MPO) and proteinase-3 (PR3). On ethanol-fixed leukocytes examined with indirect immunofluorescence, anti-MPO antibodies frequently produce a perinuclear pattern (p-ANCA) and antibodies against PR3 form a cytoplasmic pattern (c-ANCA). Because nonspecific antibodies against other cytoplasmic antigens (e.g., enolase, elastase, lactoferrin, and catalase) can also give a positive ANCA pattern on immunofluorescence, confirmation of antibody specificity by enzyme-linked immunosorbent assay (ELISA) is required. Patients with ANCA vasculitis have a wide range of signs and symptoms (Table 16-2).

Microscopic Polyangiitis

Microscopic polyangiitis is a necrotizing vasculitis with few or no immune deposits (pauci-immune) on immunofluorescence that affects small vessels (i.e., capillaries, venules, or arterioles). A necrotizing arteritis involving small- and medium-sized arteries may be present. Necrotizing glomerulonephritis, with crescents, is common, and pulmonary capillaritis often occurs. Fifty percent of patients are MPO-ANCA–positive, 40% are PR3-ANCA–positive, and a few are ANCA-negative.

Wegener Granulomatosis

Wegener granulomatosis is a granulomatous inflammation involving the respiratory tract and necrotizing vasculitis affecting small- to medium-sized vessels (e.g., capillaries, venules, arterioles, and arteries). Similar to microscopic polyangiitis, a necrotizing glomerulonephritis is common. Of patients with Wegener granulomatosis, 75% are PR3-ANCA–positive, and 20% are MPO-ANCA–positive.

Churg-Strauss Syndrome

This syndrome is characterized by peripheral blood eosinophilia, asthma or other form of atopy, an eosinophil-rich

Table 16-2 Signs and Symptoms of ANCA Vasculitis

Cutaneous purpura, nodules, and ulcerations
Peripheral neuropathy (mononeuritis multiplex)
Abdominal pain and blood in stools
Hematuria, proteinuria, and renal failure
Hemoptysis and pulmonary infiltrates or nodules
Necrotizing (hemorrhagic) sinusitis
Myalgias and arthralgias
Muscle and pancreatic enzymes in blood

ANCA, antineutrophilic cytoplasmic antibody.

granulomatous inflammation involving the respiratory tract, and a necrotizing vasculitis affecting small- to medium-sized vessels. Sixty percent of patients are MPO-ANCA–positive.

ANCA vasculitis should be treated with a combination of high-dose corticosteroids and cyclophosphamide (3-6 months). Patients with pulmonary hemorrhage or severe renal failure (serum creatinine >5.5 mg/dL or on dialysis) or both should also receive plasma exchange. The prognosis in ANCA vasculitis is quite variable. According to recent reviews, the mortality rate after the diagnosis is 25% and the ESRD rate is 21%. However, with aggressive treatment up to 75% of patients may recover renal function, even if dialysis therapy was required at the start of treatment. ANCA vasculitides are associated with a high relapse rate (30%-50% within the first 5 years). Long-term treatment with low-dose corticosteroids in combination with azathioprine is beneficial in decreasing the frequency of relapses. Patients with Wegener granulomatosis who are nasal carriers for *Staphylococcus aureus* benefit from long-term treatment with trimethoprim-sulfamethoxazole. The use of serial ANCA testing as a predictor of relapses has variable degrees of success. For making a therapeutic decision, the results of this test should not be considered in isolation but in the context of the patient's clinical history. Several medications (propylthiouracil, hydralazine, and penicillamine) and heavy silica exposure have been associated with the induction of ANCA and necrotizing glomerulonephritis.

Polyarteritis Nodosa

Polyarteritis nodosa is characterized by necrotizing inflammation of medium-sized or small arteries without glomerulonephritis or vasculitis in arterioles, capillaries, or venules. It is ANCA-negative and associated with hepatitis B infection. The diagnosis is made by finding aneurysms on angiography.

- ANCA vasculitis: microscopic polyangiitis, Wegener granulomatosis, Churg-Strauss syndrome.
- ANCA vasculitis: the most common cause of RPGN in patients older than 60.
- Renal biopsy: focal segmental necrotizing glomerulonephritis with crescents.
- Polyarteritis nodosa: ANCA-negative, associated with hepatitis B, normal glomeruli.
- Drug-induced ANCA vasculitis: propylthiouracil, hydralazine, and penicillamine.
- Treatment: high-dose corticosteroids and cyclophosphamide.
- Plasmapheresis is also indicated for patients with ANCA vasculitis who have evidence of pulmonary hemorrhage or severe renal failure (serum creatinine >5.5 mg/dL or on dialysis).

Goodpasture Disease: Anti–GBM Antibody-Mediated Glomerulonephritis

Goodpasture disease is defined by a pulmonary-renal syndrome caused by circulating anti–GBM antibody and linear staining seen along the glomerular and alveolar basement membrane on immunofluorescence. The antibody is directed against the α3 chain of type IV collagen. Pulmonary hemorrhage may be absent or not clinically apparent. Other autoantibodies may coexist with anti-GBM antibodies (~25%-30% of patients are also ANCA-positive). The treatment of Goodpasture disease is with high-dose corticosteroids (prednisone 1 mg/kg daily up to 80 mg daily or pulse methylprednisolone sodium succinate [Solu-Medrol] 1 g for 3 days) in combination with oral cyclophosphamide (2-3 mg/kg daily up to 200 mg daily; decrease the dose by 25% for patients older than 55 or if the creatinine level is >5 mg/dL) and plasma exchange. The prognosis for patients with Goodpasture disease depends on the percentage of circumferential crescents in the renal biopsy specimen, the presence of oliguria, and the need for dialysis. Patients with a serum level of creatinine of 5.7 mg/dL at start of treatment have a greater than 90% probability of renal survival at 5 years. Patients who have 100% circumferential crescents and are receiving dialysis do not recover renal function and should not be treated with the immunosuppressive regimen outlined above, except in the presence of pulmonary hemorrhage. Goodpasture disease is a "single-hit disease" and rarely recurs. Patients with ESRD are candidates for renal transplantation after the antibody has disappeared.

- Goodpasture disease: pulmonary-renal syndrome, positive anti-GBM antibody, and linear staining of the GBM.

GLOMERULAR DISEASE THAT USUALLY PRESENTS AS NEPHROTIC SYNDROME

Minimal Change Nephropathy

Minimal change nephropathy is defined by the absence of structural glomerular abnormalities, except for the fusion of epithelial cell foot processes seen on electron microscopy, in a patient with nephrotic syndrome. Minimal change nephropathy is the most common cause of nephrotic syndrome in children.

- Minimal change nephropathy: 70%-90% of cases of nephrotic syndrome in children younger than 10, although it rarely occurs before the first year of life.
- 50% of cases of nephrotic syndrome in adolescents and young adults.
- Less than 20% of cases of primary nephrotic syndrome in adults.

The pathogenesis of minimal change nephropathy is unknown. The association with Hodgkin lymphoma suggests that minimal change nephropathy may be a consequence of T-lymphocyte abnormalities, with T cells producing a lymphokine that is toxic to glomerular epithelial cells. This results in the fusion of foot processes and detachment of podocytes, the loss of the heparin sulfate negative-charge barrier of the basement membrane, and the increased glomerular permeability to protein. There is a clear association with drugs, allergy, and malignancy. In children, the disease presents with abrupt onset of nephrotic syndrome. The presence of hematuria, hypertension, or impaired renal function is unusual in children. In adults, hypertension and renal insufficiency may be present. In children, the presence of nephrotic syndrome in a patient with normal urinalysis results *is* minimal change nephropathy until proven otherwise. If a child does not have a response to corticosteroid therapy, renal biopsy is justified. In adults, minimal change nephropathy accounts for less than 20% of the cases of patients presenting with a nephrotic syndrome, and renal biopsy is required to establish the diagnosis. The most important differential diagnosis is focal segmental glomerulosclerosis (FSGS). In some patients, minimal change nephropathy may have a secondary cause, as outlined below.

The most common secondary causes of minimal change nephropathy include the following:

- Viral infections—mononucleosis, human immunodeficiency virus (HIV).
- Drugs: nonsteroidal anti-inflammatory drugs (NSAIDs) (with interstitial nephritis).
- Tumors—Hodgkin lymphoma, leukemia.
- Allergies—food, bee sting, poison ivy.

On light microscopic and immunofluorescence examination, the glomeruli are normal. Tubules may accumulate lipid droplets from absorbed lipoproteins. Occasionally, the findings are consistent with acute tubular necrosis. Electron microscopy shows effacement of the foot processes; however, this is a nonspecific finding that is also seen in heavy proteinuria due to other glomerulopathies. In children, high-dose corticosteroid therapy is the cornerstone of treatment, with more than 90% of children achieving complete remission after 4 to 6 weeks of treatment. In adolescents and adults, the response to therapy is also high (>80%), but the response is slower and some patients may require up to 16 weeks of treatment to achieve remission. Generally, therapy is continued for 4 to 8 weeks after remission. Of the patients who have a response to corticosteroid therapy, 25% have a long-term remission. The others have at least one relapse. For patients who have frequent relapses, are steroid-dependent, or are resistant to steroids, alternative therapy includes cyclophosphamide, chlorambucil,

and cyclosporine. Overall, the prognosis is excellent, with patients maintaining renal function long-term. If there is no response to therapy or progressive renal failure develops, an alternative diagnosis must be considered.

- Minimal change nephropathy: abrupt nephrotic syndrome with normal renal function.
- It is the main cause of nephrotic syndrome in children. In adults, it accounts for <20% of cases of nephrotic syndrome.
- Secondary causes: viral, Hodgkin disease, and NSAIDs (with interstitial nephritis).
- Minimal change nephropathy responds to corticosteroid treatment. Failure to respond to this therapy suggests an alternative diagnosis.

Focal Segmental Glomerulosclerosis

Focal segmental glomerulosclerosis (FSGS) accounts for less than 15% of cases of idiopathic nephrotic syndrome in children. In adults, it accounts for approximately 25% of nephropathies. FSGS is the most common form of idiopathic nephrotic syndrome in African Americans. It may be idiopathic or have several different causes (e.g., heroin abuse, HIV infection, sickle cell disease, obesity, vesicoureteral reflux, unilateral renal agenesis, remnant kidneys, and aging). The pathogenesis of idiopathic FSGS is unknown. A circulating permeability factor has been demonstrated in some patients. Glomerular hypertension and hyperfiltration are thought to have a role in secondary causes of FSGS, as in patients with unilateral renal agenesis or remnant kidneys. The presentation is either as asymptomatic proteinuria or full-blown nephrotic syndrome. Hypertension is found in 30% to 50% of patients, with microscopic hematuria in 25% to 75% of them. At presentation, the glomerular filtration rate (GFR) is decreased in 20% to 30% of patients.

The pathologic diagnosis of FSGS is based on the identification in some glomeruli (focal) of areas of capillary obliteration, with increased deposition of mesangial matrix and intracapillary hyalin deposits in parts of the glomerular tufts (segmental lesion). Interstitial fibrosis is a common finding. Immunofluorescence shows IgM and C3 deposition in the areas of glomerular scarring (nonspecific trapping). Electron microscopy demonstrates fusion of epithelial foot processes in the majority of the glomeruli, including those that appear normal on light microscopy. Four histologic variants of FSGS have been described. In the most common pattern, there is a predilection for sclerosis in the perihilar regions. In the collapsing variant, hypertrophy and hyperplasia of the overlying epithelial cells result in global glomerular capillary collapse and sclerosis. The collapsing variant is more common in African Americans and patients with HIV infection.

Prolonged (>4 months) high-dose corticosteroid therapy (prednisone 1 mg/kg daily) has achieved up to a 40% to 60% remission rate of nephrotic syndrome, with preservation of long-term renal function. Alternative therapy includes cytotoxic drugs, either alone or in combination with corticosteroids, and low-dose cyclosporine. For patients who have protein excretion of less than 3 g per day, treatment with an ACEI or angiotensin II receptor antagonist (or both) may be sufficient to reduce proteinuria and improve renal survival. For patients with secondary forms of FSGS, treatment should target the primary cause if possible. In all patients, treatment with an ACEI or an angiotensin II receptor blocker, alone or in combination, may substantially reduce proteinuria and prolong renal survival.

Less than 5% of patients experience spontaneous remission of proteinuria; eventually, ESRD develops in most patients 5 to 20 years after presentation. The degree of proteinuria is a predictor of the long-term clinical outcome. Patients who have a non–nephrotic range proteinuria have the best renal survival (>80% at 10 years). Patients with the collapsing variant have the worst prognosis, with most of them having ESRD within 3 years. Idiopathic FSGS may recur in a transplanted kidney.

- FSGS: accounts for ~25% of cases of adult nephrotic syndrome.
- FSGS is the most common cause of nephrotic syndrome in African Americans.
- Patients present with hypertension, renal insufficiency, proteinuria, and gross or microscopic hematuria.
- Secondary causes: HIV infection, heroin abuse, reflux nephropathy, massive obesity.
- Prolonged high dose corticosteroid therapy: >40% of patients have a response.
- Collapsing variant has the worst prognosis.

HIV-Associated Nephropathy

HIV-associated nephropathy is characterized by progressive renal insufficiency in patients with nephrotic range proteinuria (often massive) but often little edema. Large echogenic kidneys are seen on ultrasonography. Renal biopsy specimens show a collapsing form of FSGS. Tubules are often dilated, forming microcysts. With electron microscopy, numerous tubuloreticular inclusions are seen within the glomerular and vascular endothelial cells. HIV-associated nephropathy is more common, and clinically more severe, in African Americans than in whites. Other types of glomerulonephritis also encountered with some frequency in HIV-infected persons include MPGN, minimal change nephropathy, membranous nephropathy, and postinfectious glomerulonephritis. Thrombotic microangiopathy develops in some patients; it is not related to

E. coli 0157:H7 and carries a high mortality. The optimal treatment for patients with HIV-associated nephropathy is not clear. Suggested therapies include antiretroviral agents, ACEIs to reduce proteinuria, and treatment of underlying infections.

Membranous Nephropathy

Membranous nephropathy is the leading cause of nephrotic syndrome in white adults. It occurs in subjects of all ages and races but is most often diagnosed in middle age, with the incidence peaking during the fourth and fifth decades of life. The male-to-female ratio is 2:1. The pathogenic mechanisms that cause this immune complex localization and the subsequent development of proteinuria and the nephrotic syndrome are not completely understood, but the in situ deposition of cationic antigens in the subepithelial space are thought to be involved. The nature of the antigen involved in the immune complex deposits of membranous nephropathy and its source are not known.

At presentation, proteinuria is greater than 2.0 g per day in more than 80% of patients and more than 10 g per day in as many as 30%. Initially, renal function is preserved in the majority of patients, and hypertension is present in 13% to 55%. A small proportion of patients have microscopic hematuria. Membranous nephropathy is idiopathic (primary) or secondary disease (up to 30% of patients with biopsy-proven membranous nephropathy). Secondary membranous nephropathy is caused by autoimmune diseases (systemic lupus erythematosus and autoimmune thyroiditis), infection (hepatitis B and C), drugs (penicillamine, gold, and NSAIDs), and malignancies (colon cancer and lung cancer). Membranous nephropathy is associated with malignancy in 7% to 15% of patients older than 60 years. Very early in the disease process, the glomeruli may appear normal in light microscopic preparations and the diagnosis can be made only with immunofluorescence or with electron microscopy to detect subepithelial deposits along the GBM. With more advanced lesions, capillary walls are thickened, and the methenamine silver stain shows subepithelial projections ("spikes") along the capillary walls. The spikes represent deposition of new basement membrane material along the subepithelial deposits. Immunofluorescence microscopy shows marked granular deposition of IgG and C3 along the capillary walls.

Therapy for membranous nephropathy is generally supportive. The use of ACEIs and angiotensin receptor blockers is recommended, but their effect in decreasing proteinuria is modest (~40% at most). Therapies other than supportive care include corticosteroids, the combination of corticosteroids and cytotoxic agents, and cyclosporine. Mycophenolate mofetil has been tried with success in some patients. Thrombotic complications (e.g., renal vein thrombosis) are frequent, and anticoagulation should be considered for patients with proteinuria greater than 10 g per day and serum albumin less than 2 g/dL. Without treatment, almost 25% of patients have a spontaneous complete remission and 50% have partial remission. The probability of renal survival is more than 80% at 5 years and 60% at 15 years. The prognosis is worse for patients with nephrosis. In 10% to 15% of patients, the disease has an accelerated course, with ESRD occurring within 1 year after the diagnosis.

- Membranous nephropathy: the primary cause of idiopathic nephrotic syndrome in white adults.
- The peak incidence occurs during the fourth and fifth decades of life.
- Renal vein thrombosis causes sudden loss of renal function in 25%-50% of patients.
- Secondary causes: infections, multisystem disease, neoplasms, and medications.
- Complete remission in 25% of patients and partial remission in 50%.

OTHER GLOMERULAR DISORDERS

Diabetic Nephropathy

Diabetic nephropathy is the commonest cause of ESRD in the United States (>40% of patients on dialysis; 80% or more have type 2 diabetes). Diabetic neuropathy occurs in both type 1 (30%-40% of cases) and type 2 (20%-30% of cases) diabetes mellitus. In diabetes mellitus type 1, the peak onset of nephropathy is between 10 and 15 years after the initial presentation of diabetes. Patients who do not have proteinuria after 25 years of diabetes are unlikely to develop diabetic nephropathy. A similar natural history is likely for patients with diabetes mellitus type 2. The main risk factors for developing diabetic nephropathy are a positive family history for the nephropathy, hypertension, and poor glycemic control. The risk may be greater in some racial groups (e.g., Pima Indians and African Americans). The pathogenesis is secondary to increased glycosylation of proteins, with the accumulation of advanced glycosylation end products that cross-link with collagen, in combination with glomerular hyperfiltration and hypertension.

Diabetic nephropathy is manifested first by the onset of microalbuminuria (defined as urinary albumin excretion ranging from 20 to 200 μg/min or 30-300 mg/24 hours). With time, microalbuminuria evolves into overt proteinuria (>300 mg/24 hours) and subsequent full-blown nephrotic syndrome. The presence of microalbuminuria is the primary predictor of renal disease (in 30%-45% of patients, the microalbuminuria will progress to proteinuria after 10 years), with the degree of proteinuria correlating roughly with the renal prognosis. After overt proteinuria has developed, the progress toward ESRD is

relentless, although rates of decline vary among patients (5-15 years). In patients with type 1 diabetes, there is a great correlation (95%) between the development of nephropathy and other signs of diabetic microvascular compromise such as diabetic retinopathy and diabetic neuropathy. The correlation is not so close for patients with type 2 diabetes, and up to 1/3 of these patients develop nephropathy without evidence of diabetic retinopathy. Hypertension occurs in about 75% of patients with proteinuria. Other renal manifestations of diabetes include frequent urinary tract infections, which may be complicated by the development of acute pyelonephritis and perinephric abscess, and papillary necrosis. A functional obstruction caused by neurogenic bladder may also occur. Because of the accelerated rate of atherosclerosis, patients with diabetes also have a high incidence of cardiovascular disease, including renal artery stenosis. The stages of diabetic nephropathy are listed in Table 16-3.

- Diabetic nephropathy occurs in 30%-40% of patients with diabetes mellitus type 1 and in 20%-30% of those with diabetes mellitus type 2.
- Diabetic nephropathy is the single most common cause of end-stage renal disease in the United States.
- Microalbuminuria is the primary predictor of renal disease.
- Other renal manifestations of diabetes are hypertension, recurrent urinary tract infections, acute pyelonephritis, perinephric abscess, papillary necrosis, and neurogenic bladder.

In the earliest stage of the disease, renal biopsy specimens show glomerular hypertrophy and thickening of the GBM. As the disease progresses, arteriolar hyalinosis and arteriosclerosis develop. This is followed by progressive mesangial expansion (diffuse diabetic glomerulosclerosis) and nodular

Table 16-3 Stages of Diabetic Nephropathy

Stage I	Hyperfiltration, glomerular filtration rate is 20%-50% above normal, microalbuminuria (>300 mg/24 hours)
Stage II	Normalization of glomerular filtration rate with early structural damage
Stage III	Early hypertension
Stage IV	Progression to proteinuria >0.5 g/d, hypertension, declining glomerular filtration rate (lasts 10-15 years)
Stage V	Progression to ESRD (5-7 years), heavy proteinuria persists even to ESRD

ESRD, end-stage renal disease.

formations (Kimmelstiel-Wilson nodules, which are pathognomonic of diabetic nephropathy). Both the diffuse and nodular mesangial expansions are composed of extracellular mesangial matrix and stain positive with silver and the periodic acid-Schiff (PAS) reaction. Capsular drop lesions and fibrin cap lesions are also pathognomonic findings. Late in the disease, tubular atrophy and interstitial fibrosis occur. For patients with long-term diabetes, especially if retinopathy is present and other causes of proteinuria are excluded, renal biopsy may not be necessary. However, renal biopsy is indicated for patients with an atypical course of the disease (e.g., nephrotic range proteinuria within the first 10 years in type 1 diabetes or if loss of renal function is rapidly progressive). The progression of diabetic nephropathy can be retarded by tight glycemic control (glycated hemoglobin <7.5%) and the use of ACEIs or angiotensin receptor blockers (target systolic blood pressure <125 mm Hg). Patients with diabetes who develop microalbuminuria should start ACEI or angiotensin receptor blocker therapy even if they are normotensive. Patients with ESRD due to diabetes mellitus are candidates for a solitary kidney or a combined kidney-pancreas transplant. Hemodialysis and continuous ambulatory peritoneal dialysis are alternatives. Pancreatic islet cell transplantation is a promising new therapy.

- Kimmelstiel-Wilson nodules are pathognomonic for diabetic nephropathy.
- Aggressive glucose and blood pressure control slows progression.
- Diabetes mellitus is the most common cause of type IV renal tubular acidosis.

Systemic Lupus Erythematosus Nephritis

Lupus nephritis is a major cause of morbidity and mortality in patients with systemic lupus erythematosus. Approximately 25% of patients with systemic lupus erythematosus develop substantial renal involvement. If renal involvement occurs with systemic lupus erythematosus, it is usually early in the course of the disease, but rarely is renal involvement the sole manifestation of systemic lupus erythematosus. Lupus nephritis is more severe in children and in African Americans. The World Health Organization (WHO) divides lupus nephritis into six morphologic classes of renal involvement (Table 16-4). These patterns of lupus nephritis are not static and may show a transition from one class to another either spontaneously or after treatment. A few patients may develop a necrotizing glomerulonephritis with crescents. Immunofluorescence shows glomerular deposition of IgG, IgM, IgA, C1q, and C4 (full house). As seen with electron microscopy, immune deposits are localized to the glomerular capillary subendothelium (wire-loop) and a fingerprint-like pattern of tuloreticular inclusions is common within glomerular and vascular endothelial cells. The type of renal lesion strongly influences the management of systemic lupus erythematosus, and kidney biopsy is indicated in patients with proteinuria, active urinary sediment, and with or without decreased glomerular function to define the morphologic class. The histopathologic features correlate with the prognosis, with class III and IV having the worst prognosis (5-year survival is about 80%). Immunosuppressive treatment is indicated for class III or IV lupus nephritis. For patients with severe lupus nephritis, the combination of high-dose corticosteroid (either orally or "pulse" intravenous methylprednisolone) and intravenous cyclophosphamide has produced the most effective therapeutic results, with improvement of serologic and clinical abnormalities. Recent studies have suggested that the combination of mycophenolate mofetil and oral prednisone is as effective as cyclophosphamide plus prednisone. Membranous lupus nephritis is characerized by proteinuria, weakly positive or negative antinuclear antibody, and no erythrocyte casts. Therapy is supportive only, although some patients may benefit from treatment with cyclosporine.

- SLE: 25% of patients have severe renal involvement.
- Proliferative lupus nephritis: requires aggressive treatment with high-dose corticosteroids plus cyclophosphamide.
- Membranous lupus nephritis (without proliferation) usually is not treatable with immunosuppressive agents.

Other manifestations of SLE include acute and chronic tubulointerstitial nephritis and glomerular capillary thrombi in patients with antiphospholipid antibodies. Drug-induced

Table 16-4 The Six WHO Classes of Renal Diseases in Systemic Lupus Erythematosus

Morphologic class	Renal manifestation
I. Normal/minimal glomerular abnormality	Normal urinary sediment
II. Mesangial nephropathy	Low-grade hematuria/ proteinuria
	Normal renal function
III. Focal proliferative lupus nephritis	Active sediment, proteinuria <3 g/24 h
IV. Diffuse proliferative lupus nephritis	Nephritic and nephrotic syndromes
	Hypertension, progressive renal failure
V. Membranous nephropathy	Nephrotic syndrome
VI. Sclerosing nephropathy	Inactive urinary sediment
	Chronic renal failure

WHO, World Health Organization.

SLE rarely involves the kidney. SLE tends to flare during pregnancy, and pregnancy should be delayed until after SLE has been inactive for at least 1 year. SLE "burns out" with ESRD and generally does not recur in transplant recipients.

- Drug-induced SLE rarely involves the kidney.
- Pregnancy should be delayed until after SLE has been inactive.
- SLE "burns out" with ESRD and rarely (2%-4%) recurs in renal transplant recipients.

MONOCLONAL GAMMOPATHIES

Multiple Myeloma

The renal manifestation of multiple myeloma may be acute renal failure or a chronic progressive disease that may occur at any time during the course of the disease. Virtually all patients with multiple myeloma have monoclonal immunoglobulins or light chains in the serum and urine. Acute renal failure may occur as a result of intraluminal precipitation of multiple proteinaceous casts ("cast nephropathy") and the resulting acute noninflammatory interstitial nephritis (myeloma kidney). The casts are usually acellular, with multiple fracture lines (broken casts), seen mainly in the distal nephron, and are the result of aggregates of light chains and Tamm-Horsfall glycoprotein. Coaggregation of Tamm-Horsfall glycoprotein with light chains is facilitated by increasing the concentration of calcium, sodium, and chloride (such as after the use of a loop diuretic) in the urine, by conditions that reduce flow rates (such as intravascular depletion and the use of NSAIDs), or by the use of radiocontrast agents. Other renal manifestations include pseudohyponatremia, low anion gap, and type 2 renal tubular acidosis with Fanconi syndrome (low phosphorus, urate, potassium; glycosuria; aminoaciduria). Ultrasonography shows normal- or large-sized kidneys. Treatment of cast nephropathy includes vigorous hydration, correction of hypercalcemia, and avoidance of nephrotoxic or precipitating agents. Alkalinizing the urine to keep the pH more than 7 may be beneficial in some patients. Plasmapheresis can quickly remove light chains from the circulation and should be considered in patients with acute renal failure or hyperviscosity syndrome. Treatment with melphalan and prednisone decreases the circulating levels of light chains and stabilizes or improves renal function in two-thirds of patients with renal failure. Other therapeutic options include myeloablative therapy followed by bone marrow transplant, but the mortality rate is high.

Amyloidosis

Amyloidosis is due to the systemic extracellular deposition of antiparallel, β-pleated sheet, nonbranching, 8- to 12-nm fibrils that stain positive with Congo red or thioflavin T. In primary amyloidosis, patients are typically older than 50 years, and the kidney is affected in 50% of patients. Common renal manifestations include proteinuria, nephrotic syndrome (25% of patients), and renal failure. Immunofluorescence generally demonstrates λ light chains in the glomeruli (75% of patients). The prognosis is poor, with median survival being less than 2 years. Treatment with prednisone and melphalan can be beneficial in some patients. In selected cases, high-dose melphalan followed by a bone marrow transplant has led to resolution of the disease. Secondary amyloidosis (AA) is most common in patients with rheumatoid arthritis, inflammatory bowel disease, chronic infection, or familial Mediterranean fever and in subcutaneous drug users (heroin). The treatment of AA amyloidosis is directed at the underlying inflammatory process. Colchicine is helpful in patients with familial Mediterranean fever.

Light Chain Deposition Disease

In light chain deposition disease (LCDD), light chain is deposited along the GBM. LCDD is strongly associated with the development of myeloma, lymphoma, and Waldenström macroglobulinemia. Renal involvement is similar to that of amyloidosis, with proteinuria, nephrotic syndrome, and renal insufficiency. Renal biopsy specimens demonstrate acellular, eosinophilic mesangial nodules that are strongly PAS-positive, often mimicking diabetes mellitus. The deposited monoclonal proteins do not form fibrils and do not bind Congo red. Immunofluorescence microscopic findings are diagnostic, that is, diffuse linear Ig light chain deposition (κ in 80% of cases) along the GBM and tubular basement membranes and in the nodules. As in amyloidosis, treatment with melphalan and prednisone has led to stabilization or improved renal function in some patients. At 5 years, the survival rate is 50% to 70%, with renal survival ranging from 20% to 35%. Similar to AL amyloidosis, the disease recurs in transplants.

GLOMERULONEPHRITIS ASSOCIATED WITH HEPATITIS C VIRUS INFECTION

Cryoglobulinemic Glomerulonephritis

Type II or mixed essential cryglobulins (Table 16-5) are commonly found in patients with hepatitis C virus (HCV) infection and contain HCV RNA and anti-HCV IgG. Once they have precipitated in the glomeruli, they bind complement, activate a cytokine cascade, and trigger an inflammatory response. The renal disease may present with proteinuria, microscopic hematuria, nephrotic syndrome, or renal impairment. Hypertension is common and may be severe, particularly in the presence of acute nephritic syndrome. Cryoglobulinemia is usually associated with low levels of C3 and C4. The cryocrits correlate poorly with disease activity (at least 30%-40%

Table 16-5 Cryoglobulins and Associated Diseases

Cryoglobulin type	Immunoglobulin class	Associated disease
I. Monoclonal immunoglobulins	M>G>A>BJP	Myeloma, Waldenström macroglobulinemia
II. Mixed cryoglobulins with monoclonal immunoglobulins	M/G>>G/G	Sjögren syndrome, Waldenström macroglobulinemia, lymphoma, essential cryoglobulinemia
III. Mixed polyclonal immunoglobulins	M/G	Infection, SLE, vasculitis, neoplasia, essential cryoglobulinemia

SLE, systemic lupus erythematosus.

of the patients do not have detectable cryoglobulins). On light microscopy, renal biopsy specimens show a membranoproliferative type I pattern of injury, with massive exudation of cells, mainly monocytic, and a double-contoured appearance of the GBM. Eosinophilic thrombi are often found in the capillary lumen and consist of cryoprecipitated immunoglobulins. On electron microscopy, diffuse dense subendothelial deposits are seen occluding the glomerular capillary; some have a peculiar microtubular or crystalline appearance consisting of parallel fibrils. In some cases, a vasculitis affecting small to medium-sized arteries may be seen. Combination treatment with interferon alfa and ribavirin is effective in clearing the virus from circulation and results in improvement of proteinuria and renal function. However, relapses after discontinuation of antiviral therapy are common. Treatment with prednisone, cytotoxic agents, and plasmapheresis is indicated in patients with acute nephritis. The renal prognosis is usually good, with few patients progressing to ESRD.

HEMOLYTIC UREMIC SYNDROME AND THROMBOCYTOPENIC PURPURA

The two forms of hemolytic uremic syndrome (HUS), a sporadic or diarrhea-associated form (D+HUS) and a non–diarrhea-associated form (D-HUS). D+HUS is strongly linked to ingestion of meat contaminated with *E. coli* O157:H7. These bacteria produce a Shiga-like toxin that binds to a glycolipid receptor on renal endothelial cells and triggers endothelial damage. D-HUS occurs in association with the use of oral contraceptives, cyclosporine, tacrolimus, mitomycin C, bleomycin, ticlopidine, quinine, antiphospholipid-antibody syndrome (in the context of pregnancy), underlying malignancy, and radiotherapy. A familial recurrent form of D-HUS has also been described.

Thrombocytopenic purpura (TTP) can present as an acute form or a chronic (relapsing) form. It also occurs in association with some systemic diseases (systemic lupus erythematosus, scleroderma, or malignancy), drugs (cocaine, quinidine, or ticlopidine), and HIV infection. TTP occurs in the context of

a deficiency of the von Willebrand factor (vWF)–cleaving protease (chronic form) or the development of an autoantibody against vWF-cleaving protease. Both HUS and TTP present with a microangiopathic hemolytic anemia and thrombocytopenia, with HUS more commonly causing acute renal failure and TTP more commonly associated with fever, neurologic signs, and purpura. Markers of hemolysis are present and include low haptoglobin levels, increased levels of lactate dehydrogenase and unconjugated bilirubin, and a high reticulocyte count. Schistocytes are present in peripheral blood smears. In D+HUS, renal biopsy specimens show mainly capillary thrombosis, whereas in D-HUS there is predominant involvement of small arteries, with intimal mucoid proliferation and arterioles with onion-skinning and thrombosis.

Therapy for HUS is supportive. Plasma infusions, plasma exchange, and anticoagulation are ineffective. However, fresh frozen plasma infusions and plasma exchange are effective treatments for TTP. The transfusion of platelets should be avoided because of the risk of accelerating the process. Children with D+HUS have a good prognosis (90% recover renal function), but an increased mortality rate and unfavorable long-term renal survival are seen in older patients.

- D+HUS: Shiga-like toxin production by *E. coli* O157:H7.
- HUS and TTP presentation: microangiopathic hemolytic anemia and thrombocytopenia.
- Therapy: HUS—supportive; TTP—fresh frozen plasma infusion and plasmapheresis.
- D+HUS: good prognosis in children.

DISEASES WITH GBM ABNORMALITIES: ALPORT SYNDROME AND THIN GBM DISEASE

Alport Syndrome

Alport syndrome is an inherited disorder of basement membranes. In more than half of the patients, the disease results from a mutation in the gene (*COL4A5*) that codes for the α5 chain of type IV collagen α5(IV). The syndrome is characterized by a progressive nephritis manifested by persistent or intermittent hematuria and frequently associated with sensorineural hearing loss and ocular abnormalities. Most patients have mild proteinuria, which progresses with age, becoming nephrotic in approximately one-third of patients. The disease is X-linked in at least 80% of patients, but autosomal recessive and autosomal dominant patterns of inheritance have been described. In virtually all male patients, the syndrome progresses to ESRD, often by age 16 to 35. The disease is usually mild in heterozygous females, but some develop end-stage renal failure, usually after age 50. The rate of progression to end-stage renal failure is fairly constant among affected males within individual families, but it varies markedly from family to family. On light microscopy, the glomerular changes are nonspecific. Diagnostic features are usually seen on electron microscopy. At an early stage, thinning of the GBM may be the only visible abnormality and may suggest thin basement membrane disease. With time, the GBM thickens and the lamina densa splits into several irregular layers that may branch and rejoin, producing a characteristic "basket weave" appearance. Immunohistochemistry studies of type IV collagen show the absence of α3(IV), α4(IV), and α5(IV) chains from the GBM and distal tubular basement membrane. This abnormality occurs only in patients with Alport syndrome and is diagnostic. In families with a previously defined mutation, molecular diagnosis of affected males or gene-carrying females is possible. For families in which mutations have not been defined, genetic linkage analysis can determine whether an at-risk person carries the mutant gene provided that at least two other affected members are available for testing. No specific treatment is available for Alport syndrome. Tight control of blood pressure and moderate protein restriction are recommended to retard the progression of renal disease, but the benefit is unproven. Peritoneal dialysis, hemodialysis, and renal transplantation are used successfully. Transplant recipients have a 5% to 10% risk of Goodpasture disease developing (because of the presence of Goodpasture antigen in the transplanted kidney).

Thin GBM Disease

Thin GBM disease, or thin basement membrane nephropathy, is a relatively common condition characterized by isolated glomerular hematuria associated with the renal biopsy finding of excessively thin GBM. The pathogenesis is unclear. In contrast to patients with Alport syndrome, immunohistochemical studies of type IV collagen in the GBM of patients with thin GBM disease do not show abnormality in the distribution on any of the six chains. The clinical presentation is persistent hematuria first detected in childhood. In some patients, hematuria is intermittent and may not be manifested until adulthood. Macroscopic hematuria is not uncommon and may occur in association with an upper respiratory tract infection. When first detected in young adults, 60% have a proteinuria less than 500 mg per day. The glomeruli appear normal in light and immunofluorescence microscopic preparations of renal biopsy specimens. Electron microscopy shows diffuse thinning of the GBM. In adults, a GBM thickness of 250 nm is considered strongly suggestive of thin GBM disease. The condition is usually benign and requires no specific treatment. For the majority of patients, the prognosis is excellent, with renal function preserved for a long time. However, a small proportion of patients have progressive renal disease that leads to end-stage renal failure.

CLINICAL MANIFESTATIONS OF TUBULOINTERSTITIAL RENAL DISEASE

Acute and chronic interstitial disease preferentially involves renal tubules. Some of the patterns of renal tubular injury are 1) tubular proteinuria (<1.5-2 g daily), 2) proximal tubule dysfunction (hypokalemia, hypouricemia, hypophosphatemia, acidosis, glycosuria, aminoaciduria), 3) distal tubule dysfunction (hyperchloremic acidosis, hyperkalemia or hypokalemia, salt wasting), 4) medullary concentration dysfunction, nephrogenic diabetes insipidus with decreased urine-concentrating ability, 5) urine sediment (pyuria, leukocyte casts, eosinophiluria, hematuria), and 6) azotemia, renal insufficiency.

- Tubular proteinuria: <1.5-2 g daily.
- Proximal tubule dysfunction and distal tubule dysfunction.
- Medullary concentration dysfunction.

ACUTE INTERSTITIAL NEPHRITIS

Acute interstitial nephritis is an acute, usually reversible, inflammatory disease characterized by a mononuclear cellular infiltrate within the renal interstitium. It is relatively common (about 10%-15% of cases of acute renal failure) and occurs in any age group, but is rare in children. Acute interstitial nephritis is most frequently associated with drugs, particularly antibiotics and NSAIDs (Table 16-6). Infections are the second most common cause. Acute interstitial nephritis also occurs in association with selected autoimmune systemic diseases and malignancies. In 10% to 20% of patients, it is said to be idiopathic. The presentation is acute, with approximately 40% of patients having oliguria. In patients with drug-induced acute interstitial nephritis, the systemic manifestations of a hypersensitivity reaction include fever (>50% of patients), maculopapular rash (40%), and arthralgias (25%). Flank pain

Table 16-6 Common Causes of Acute Interstitial Nephritis

Drugs

Antibiotics—penicillin, methicillin (anti-tubular basement membrane antibodies), ampicillin, rifampin, sulfa drugs, ciprofloxacin, pentamidine

NSAIDs—interstitial nephritis with nephrotic syndrome and renal insufficiency may have a latent period, not dose-dependent, recurs, possibly T-cell–mediated, allergic signs and symptoms are absent

Diuretics—thiazides, furosemide, bumetanide (sulfa derivatives)

Cimetidine

Allopurinol, phenytoin, phenindione

Cyclosporine

Infections

Bacteria—*Legionella, Brucella, Streptococcus, Staphylococcus, Pneumococcus*

Virus—Epstein-Barr, CMV, *Hantavirus*, HIV, hepatitis B, *Polyomavirus*

Fungus—*Candida, Histoplasma*

Parasites—*Plasmodium, Toxoplasma, Schistosoma, Leishmania*

Systemic disease

Systemic lupus erythematosus

Sjögren syndrome

Sarcoidosis

Lymphoma, leukemic infiltration

Renal transplant rejection

Idiopathic

CMV, cytomegalovirus.

is caused by distention of the renal capsule and occurs in approximately 50% of patients. Renal impairment can vary from a mild increase in the serum level of creatinine to severe acute renal failure requiring dialysis. Tubular damage can impair the urinary concentration mechanism and result in the development of polyuria. Eosinophilia is common (40% of patients). Urinalysis demonstrates pyuria and hematuria in nearly 100% of patients, but macroscopic hematuria is unusual. Rarely, red blood cell casts are seen in the urinary sediment. The presence of eosinophiluria (>1% of patients) is suggestive of acute interstitial nephritis but is also seen in other unrelated renal diseases. The absence of eosinophiluria does not exclude the diagnosis. Proteinuria is generally mild (<1 g/24 hours). The predictive value of gallium scanning is limited. Diagnosis sometimes requires renal biopsy. Therapy is primarily supportive. The likely inciting factor or factors need to be identified and eliminated. Treatment with prednisone (60 mg every

other day) for 2 to 4 weeks may hasten the recovery of renal function and may be of benefit in patients who do not regain renal function within 1 week after the offending agent has been stopped. Corticosteroids are not indicated for infection-related acute interstitial nephritis. Historically, drug-induced acute interstitial nephritis has been considered a reversible process, with renal function returning to baseline in the majority of patients. However, recent studies have shown that impaired renal function can persist long-term in up to 40% of patients.

- Acute interstitial nephritis: ~100% of patients have pyuria, >50% have fever, 60% have renal insufficiency, 50% have eosinophilia, and 25% have arthralgias.
- NSAIDs: interstitial nephritis with nephrotic syndrome and renal insufficiency.

ANALGESIC CHRONIC INTERSTITIAL NEPHRITIS

Analgesic nephropathy is a typical example of slowly progressive chronic interstitial nephritis due to the chronic consumption of mixed analgesic preparations, frequently complicated by papillary necrosis, and resulting in bilateral renal atrophy. It accounts for approximately 3% to 10% of patients reaching ESRD. There are major regional differences in its incidence, reflecting perhaps differences in consumption behavior, availability of phenacetin-containing analgesic mixtures, and medical awareness of the condition. Most of the initial cases of analgesic nephropathy were identified in patients who consumed large amounts of phenacetin, a fact that led to the removal of phenacetin from most markets around the world. More recently, it has been recognized that acetaminophen in combination with acetylsalicylic acid can cause renal damage. Also, chronic use of NSAIDs can result in the development of analgesic nephropathy. The condition is five to seven times more frequent in females than males. Patients usually have a history of chronic pain with the consumption of large amounts of analgesic mixtures over the years, but this can be difficult to ascertain in all patients, partly because of resistance to admitting to analgesic abuse. The frequency of the diagnosis increases with age and is rare in patients younger than 30 years.

The early stages of the disease reflect abnormalities in tubular function, with impaired ability to acidify and concentrate the urine (polyuria). Fifty percent of patients have hypertension, frequently in association with renal artery stenosis. Papillary necroses themselves usually do not cause symptoms. Renal colic and outflow obstruction can result from a sloughed papilla. Occasionally, the obstruction can be bilateral and patients may present with acute renal failure. Anemia is common and may be out of proportion to the degree of renal failure. Urinalysis shows sterile hematuria, pyuria, and mild proteinuria (<3 g/24 hours). Computed tomography without radiocontrast has become the standard method for making the diagnosis of analgesic nephropathy. The demonstration of a bilateral decrease in kidney size in combination with irregular ("bumpy") renal contours and especially papillary calcifications (92% positive predictive value) is considered diagnostic of analgesic nephropathy.

- Analgesic nephropathy: responsible for 20% of cases of chronic tubulointerstitial nephritis (3%-10% of patients have ESRD).
- It is five to seven times more frequent in females than males.
- Characteristics include chronic pain, headaches, arthritis and muscle aches, and history of peptic ulcer.
- Patients generally do not admit to analgesic abuse.
- Computed tomography without contrast: small kidneys bilaterally, irregular ("bumpy") renal contours, and papillary calcifications are diagnostic of analgesic nephropathy.

Potential pathogenic mechanisms include direct drug toxicity to the renal papilla, hemodynamic factors, and genetic predisposition. The metabolism of phenacetin and acetaminophen results in increased concentration of highly reactive oxygen species in the renal papilla. These reactive radicals are normally "detoxified" by glutathione. Depletion of medullary glutathione results in the binding of free reactive intermediates to lipids in the cell membranes and lipid peroxidation. Ultimately, a chain of oxidative damage results in cell death. Aspirin potentiates the toxicity of phenacetin and acetaminophen by depleting renal glutathione. NSAIDs contribute to the renal damage by inhibiting prostaglandin synthesis, which in turn leads to a decrease in renal papillary blood flow and papillary ischemia. The amount necessary to cause analgesic nephropathy is a total intake of 3 kg of phenacetin or 1 g daily for 3 years. There is no specific form of treatment. Chronic consumption of analgesic medications, especially analgesic mixtures, must be discontinued, and if this is not possible, the regimen needs to be switched to single analgesic preparations. Other therapeutic maneuvers are similar to those for other forms of chronic renal failure. The prognosis depends on whether analgesic misuse is stopped. Patients with analgesic nephropathy are at increased risk for uroepithelial tumors, particularly transitional cell carcinomas (renal pelvis, ureter, bladder, and proximal urethra). Tumors frequently occur simultaneously at different sites of the urinary tract, and close follow-up with regular urinary cytologic examination is recommended. These patients are also at increased risk for premature atherosclerosis and coronary artery disease.

- Phenacetin and its metabolites are concentrated in the renal papillae.

- Increased risk for uroepithelial tumors.
- Increased risk for premature atherosclerosis and coronary artery disease.

Other causes of papillary necrosis can be remembered by the mnemonic POSTCARD (pyelonephritis, obstruction, sickle cell disease or trait, tuberculosis, chronic alcoholism with cirrhosis, analgesics, renal vein thrombosis, and diabetes mellitus).

ELECTROLYTE- AND TOXIN-INDUCED INTERSTITIAL NEPHRITIS

Acute uric acid nephropathy is associated with the tumor lysis syndrome that develops after chemotherapy, myeloproliferative disorders, heat stroke, status epilepticus, and Lesch-Nyhan syndrome. In acute uric acid nephropathy, intraluminal crystals cause intrarenal obstruction, the serum level of uric acid is often more than 15 mg, and 24-hour urinary uric acid is more than 1,000 mg. The spot urinary uric acid value divided by spot urinary creatinine value is often greater than 1.0. Prevention requires alkaline diuresis, allopurinol, and, sometimes, hemodialysis. This disorder generally is completetly reversible. Chronic uric acid nephropathy from saturnine gout (lead from "moonshine" or paint) or chronic tophaceous gout is due to interstitial crystal formation, that is, microtophi present in the renal parenchyma. It has only limited reversibility. In renal failure, de novo gout is rare; in this setting, it should be assumed that the patient has lead nephropathy until proved otherwise.

- Acute uric acid nephropathy associated with tumor lysis syndrome and myeloproliferative disorders.
- Serum uric acid is >15 mg, and 24-hour urinary uric acid is >1,000 mg.
- The urine uric acid–to–urine creatinine ratio is >1.
- Prevention: alkaline diuresis and allopurinol.

Early on, hypercalcemia results in mitochondrial deposits of calcium in the proximal and distal tubules as well as in the collecting duct. Later, tubular degeneration with calcium deposition and obstruction occurs. Calcium inhibits sodium transport, induces nephrogenic diabetes insipidus, and causes intrarenal vasoconstriction. It also stimulates the release of renin and catecholamines, increasing blood pressure.

Hypokalemia has been associated with vascularization of the proximal and distal tubules and, possibly, chronic interstitial fibrosis. Nephrogenic diabetes insipidus is also associated with chronic hypokalemia.

Oxalate deposition from primary hyperoxaluria causes renal and extrarenal oxalate deposition. Extrarenal sites include the eyes, heart, bones, joints, and vascular system. Secondary causes of oxalate deposition include ethylene glycol, methoxy-flurane, high doses of ascorbic acid, vitamin B_6 deficiency, and enteric hyperoxaluria.

Lithium induces nephrogenic diabetes insipidus and micro-cystic changes in the renal tubules. Interstitial fibrosis may be present.

Heavy metals such as cadmium, pigments, glass, plastic, metal alloys, electrical equipment manufacturing, and some cigarettes induce proximal renal tubular acidosis and tubu-lointerstitial nephritis. Lead intoxication can cause lead nephropathy, as mentioned above. The organic salt of mer-cury can induce chronic tubulointerstitial nephritis and mem-branous nephritis or acute tubular necrosis.

CYSTIC RENAL DISEASE

Autosomal Dominant Polycystic Kidney Disease

Autosomal dominant polycystic kidney disease (ADPKD) is the most common hereditary kidney disease, with an inci-dence of 1:1,000 to 1:400. It is responsible for about 10% of all patients who reach end-stage renal failure. In approx-imately 50% of patients, end-stage renal failure occurs by the age of 55 to 75 years. The disease is characterized by multiple, bilateral renal cysts in association with cysts in other organs such as the liver and pancreas. Both males and females are affected. Mutations in at least two genes give rise to the disease. The *PKD1* gene is localized to the short arm of chro-mosome 16 and is responsible for 85% to 90% of cases of ADPKD. The *PKD2* gene maps to the long arm of chromo-some 4. *PKD1* and *PKD2* encode for two distinct proteins named, respectively, "polycystin 1" and "polycystin 2." The molecular structure of polycystin 1 suggests it may function as a cell membrane receptor involved in cell-cell or cell-matrix interactions, whereas polycystin 2 has similarities to a volt-age-activated calcium channel.

Manifestations of renal involvement include pain, hema-turia, hypertension, and renal insufficiency. Acute flank pain may occur as a result of cyst hemorrhage, infection, or stone. Macroscopic hematuria occurs in more than 40% of patients with ADPKD and may be the presenting symptom. Cyst hem-orrhage is frequent. It can present as macroscopic hematuria or with pain and fever simulating infection of the cyst. Urinary tract infection may present as cystitis, pyelonephritis, cyst infec-tion, or a perinephric abscess. If cyst infection is suspected, aspiration of the cyst under ultrasonographic or computed tomo-graphic guidance may be needed to confirm the diagnosis and to guide the selection of appropriate antimicrobial therapy. Lipid-soluble antibiotics tend to penetrate the cysts well. Renal stones occur in approximately 20% of patients with ADPKD. In the majority of patients, the stones are composed of uric acid

or calcium oxalate (or both). The diagnosis of renal stones can be difficult because of the distorted renal anatomy and the pres-ence of calcifications in the cyst walls and parenchyma. Computed tomography is the procedure of choice to detect radiolucent stones and to differentiate stones from tumor or clots. The most common extrarenal manifestation of ADPKD is polycystic liver disease. Multiple cysts result in hepatomegaly. Females are more affected than men. Other complications include cyst hemorrhage, infection, and rarely cyst rupture. Intracranial aneurysms are another important extrarenal man-ifestation of ADPKD. The incidence of the aneurysms varies between 5% and 22% depending on a negative or positive fam-ily history. The risk of rupture depends on the size of the aneurysm: minimal risk for aneurysms less than 5 mm in diam-eter but high risk for those more than 10 mm in diameter.

If the patient has a family history of ADPKD, the diagno-sis can be established by using the following renal ultra-sonography criteria: two cysts arising unilaterally or bilaterally for persons younger than 30 years, two cysts in each kidney for those 30 to 59 years old, and at least four cysts in each kid-ney for those older than 60. Presymptomatic screening with ultrasonography before age 20 is not recommended because the results may not be conclusive. Linkage genetic analysis can establish the diagnosis at the molecular level but requires other family members to be available for testing. It can also be used for prenatal diagnosis. Direct mutation analysis is possible in most families with *PKD2*. In patients with *PKD1*, direct muta-tion analysis is difficult because of the larger size of the gene and because a large part of the gene is duplicated on chromo-some 16. Therapy is directed at controlling hypertension and the renal and extrarenal complications of the disease. Lower urinary tract infection or asymptomatic bacteriuria should be treated to prevent retrograde infection of the kidney. Infected cysts may require percutaneous or surgical drainage. Screening for intracranial aneurysms is not routinely indi-cated. Transplantation is the treatment of choice for patients who develop ESRD.

- Autosomal dominant polycystic kidney disease: cause of 10% of cases of end-stage renal failure.
- By age 25, cysts are usually seen with ultrasonography or computed tomography.
- Other cysts occur in the liver, spleen, and pancreas.
- Other associations: diverticulosis, cardiac valve myxomatous degeneration, intracranial aneurysms, and hypertension.

Medullary Sponge Kidney and Acquired Renal Cystic Disease

Medullary sponge kidney is characterized by dilated medullary and papillary collecting ducts. As a result, the renal medulla develops a "spongy" appearance on excretory urography. The disorder may be unilateral or bilateral or involve a single papilla. There is no known pattern of inheritance of this disorder. Medullary sponge kidney is clinically asymptomatic except for the development of nephrolithiasis, hematuria, and recurrent urinary tract infections.

Acquired renal cystic disease can affect up to 50% of long-term dialysis patients and may present with hematuria and an increasing hematocrit. Although these cysts sometimes have neoplastic potential, they rarely metastasize. The disease regresses after transplantation.

PART II
Amy W. Williams, M.D.

ACUTE RENAL FAILURE

Introduction

Acute renal failure is characterized by a rapid decline in renal function accompanied by retention of nitrogenous waste products and electrolyte disorders. Early recognition of acute renal failure, identification of the cause, and initiation of treatment are essential to avoid patient morbidity and irreversible renal dysfunction. The first step in evaluation of acute renal failure is to determine if the increase in creatinine truly reflects a decrease in glomerular filtration rate (GFR) and if the decrease is recent or chronic. A chronically increased level of creatinine usually represents irreversible renal impairment. Drugs such as amiloride and trimethoprim interfere with creatinine secretion in the tubules, resulting in an increased serum level of creatinine without a decrease in GFR. Blood urea nitrogen (BUN), a marker for nitrogenous waste retention, can be increased despite a normal GFR in patients with gastrointestinal tract bleeding, a catabolic state, excessive protein intake, or decreased urinary flow. Another indicator of acute renal failure is a change in urine flow. Oliguria (<400 mL per day), anuria (<50 mL per day), and polyuria (>3,000 mL per day) are all clues to the cause of renal dysfunction and help guide evaluation and treatment. Decreased kidney size indicates a chronic irreversible component to the overall decrease in renal function. Currently, acute renal failure is broadly classified into "prerenal," "renal," and "postrenal" causes. This classification facilitates the clinical evaluation and discovery of the cause from more than 100 potential causes.

- Causes of increased creatinine levels independent of GFR: ketoacidosis (acetoacetate), cefoxitin, cimetidine, trimethoprim, flucytosine, rhabdomyolysis, and large consumption of meat.
- Causes of an increase in BUN independent of GFR: gastrointestinal tract bleeding, tissue trauma, glucocorticoids, tetracycline.

- Anuria <50 mL per day: complete urinary obstruction, rapidly progressive glomerulonephritis, cortical necrosis, and bilateral renal artery occlusion.
- A chronically increased level of creatinine usually represents irreversible renal impairment.
- Decreased kidney size indicates a chronic irreversible component to the overall decrease in renal function.

Prerenal Failure

Prerenal causes of acute renal failure are due to a decrease in renal blood flow that leads to a decrease in GFR. If identified and treated, prerenal failure is usually reversible. Prerenal failure accounts for more than 50% of cases of renal failure in hospitalized patients. Decreased cardiac output (as in congestive heart failure); decreased effective circulating volume due to hemorrhage, gastrointestinal blood losses, use of diuretics, burns and third spacing of fluid (pancreatitis, sepsis, crush injuries, or advanced cirrhosis); and renovascular disease leading to renal artery obstruction and arteriolar obstruction all decrease renal blood flow.

- Prerenal causes of acute renal failure are due to a decrease in blood flow that leads to a decrease in GFR.
- Prerenal failure usually is reversible.

Many vasoactive drugs can cause a decrease in renal blood flow without a decrease in effective circulating volume. Cyclosporine, an immunosuppressive drug used in transplant regimens and to treat immune-mediated diseases, causes renovasal constriction. In the setting of other renal or circulatory insults, cyclosporine can induce acute renal failure. Nonsteroidal anti-inflammatory drugs (NSAIDs) decrease vasodilatory prostaglandin production by inhibiting cyclooxygenase. When renal blood flow is compromised, these vasodilatory prostaglandins maintain the GFR by inducing afferent arteriolar dilatation. Patients with underlying renal insufficiency, volume depletion, and advanced liver disease who take NSAIDs are at risk for acute renal failure.

- Patients with underlying renal insufficiency, volume depletion, and advanced liver disease who take NSAIDs are at risk for acute renal failure.

The intrarenal formation and action of angiotensin II also maintains the GFR when renal perfusion is decreased. Angiotensin II increases efferent arteriolar tone, which increases the intraglomerular hydrostatic pressure, thus preserving the GFR. Medications that interfere with the action of angiotensin can induce acute renal failure when renal blood flow is decreased. Angiotensin-converting enzyme inhibitors (ACEIs) or angiotensin receptor blockers put patients who have compromised intravascular volume, congestive heart failure, and renal artery stenosis at risk for an acute decline in GFR. Another prerenal cause of acute renal failure is obstruction of the renal arteries or of several intrarenal arteries. Chronic renal artery stenosis can cause chronic ischemia and a gradual loss of renal mass and function. These patients usually have hypertension and laboratory findings consistent with prerenal azotemia. A rapid decline in renal function occurs with acute occlusion of the arteries supplying blood to the kidneys (thrombosis, stenosis, emboli, or vasculitis of the main renal arteries or several intrarenal arteries).

- Medications that interfere with the action of angiotensin can induce acute renal failure when renal blood flow is decreased.
- Another prerenal cause of acute renal failure is obstruction of the renal arteries or several intrarenal arteries.
- Rapid decline in renal function: thrombosis, stenosis, emboli, or vasculitis of the main renal arteries or several intrarenal arteries.

Prerenal Failure Due to Liver Disease

Hepatorenal syndrome is characterized by severe liver disease associated with acute renal failure. The pathophysiologic mechanism is not completely understood but splanchnic vasodilatation, an increase in cardiac output, a decrease in systemic resistance, and profound renovascular constriction occur without structural lesions within the vasculature. Mediators proposed to have a role in the severe vasoconstriction include endothelin, vasoconstrictive prostaglandins, and an active renal sympathetic nervous system. Patients with severe liver disease associated with ascites, portal hypertension, jaundice, thrombocytopenia, hepatic encephalopathy, and an increased prothrombin time are at risk for hepatic renal syndrome. Hyponatremia, hypokalemia, and hypoalbuminemia usually accompany the syndrome.

- Hepatorenal syndrome: severe liver disease associated with acute renal failure.

- Hyponatremia, hypokalemia, and hypoalbuminemia usually accompany the syndrome.

The diagnosis of hepatorenal syndrome is one of exclusion. Volume depletion needs to be ruled out. This is often difficult in the setting of severe liver disease associated with ascites, total body sodium, water overload, and oliguria. Urinalysis is often suggestive of acute tubular necrosis, but urinary sediment is benign. Urinary sodium less than 10 mOsm/L, urine osmolality greater than 500 mOsm/L, and a low fractional excretion of sodium are consistent with a prerenal cause. Often, a fluid challenge or central hemodynamic monitoring is used to determine intravascular volume status. The treatment of hepatorenal syndrome includes spironolactone and supportive measures until a liver transplant is available. Many other drugs have been used, with variable success, in an attempt to improve renal function: albumin and terlipressin (an antidiuretic hormone analogue), albumin and misoprostol, and acetylcysteine. The initial results of studies of the α_1-adrenergic agent midodrine and octreotide, a somatostatin analogue, have been promising. This therapy may prove to be effective in stabilizing the condition of the patient until liver transplantation.

- Urinalysis is often suggestive of acute tubular necrosis.
- The treatment of hepatorenal syndrome includes spironolactone, possibly midodrine and octreotide, and supportive measures until a liver transplant is available.

Many disease states that present like hepatorenal syndrome need to be ruled out. Any condition that leads to a decrease in renal blood flow and is associated with liver dysfunction can present as a pseudohepatorenal syndrome (sepsis, hypotension, congestive heart failure). Leptospirosis, acute Wilson syndrome, and immune-mediated diseases such as systemic lupus erythematosus (SLE), polyarteritis, and cryoglobulinemia can involve both liver and kidney. Ingestion of and exposure to toxins (e.g., methoxyflurane) that cause both liver and kidney dysfunction also need to be considered.

Any patient with end-stage liver disease is at risk for acute prerenal failure due to severe systemic vasodilatation and intrarenal vasoconstriction. Endotoxins released systemically from the portal circulation, nitric oxide, and prostacycline have all been implicated as mediators of systemic vasodilatation in these patients. Mediators of the intrarenal vasoconstriction observed under these conditions are thromboxane, F(2)-isoprostanes, vasopressin, endothelin, angiotensin II, and an increase in the stimulation of the renal sympathetic nervous system. All these mechanisms can lead to a decrease in renal blood flow and prerenal failure, especially when diuretics are added to the regimen, attenuating the already decreased renal blood flow by decreasing intravascular volume. In patients with cirrhosis and severe liver disease who present with acute renal failure, the intravascular volume status should be assessed to identify and treat any reversible prerenal component.

- In patients with cirrhosis and severe liver disease who present with acute renal failure, the intravascular volume status should be assessed to identify and treat any reversible prerenal component.

Intrinsic Acute Renal Failure

Intrinsic or structural damage to the kidney that leads to acute renal failure can be divided into three categories: acute tubular necrosis, acute interstitial nephritis, and rapidly progressive glomerulonephritis. (Rapidly progressive glomerulonephritis is discussed in another section of this chapter.) Acute tubular necrosis injury can occur from a decrease in oxygen delivery to the kidney or from nephrotoxic injury. Most likely, there is a continuum, starting with the acute reversible decline in renal function seen in prerenal failure to the irreversible ischemic renal injury due to a prolonged deficiency in oxygen delivery. Between these two extremes is an ischemic injury that is reversible if the contributing factors are readily recognized and corrected. The incidence of acute tubular necrosis in the hospital is 5%. It occurs in 50% of patients undergoing emergency abdominal aortic aneurysm repair, in 10% undergoing elective abdominal aortic aneurysm repair, and in 20% undergoing cardiac surgery or operations related to trauma.

- Acute tubular necrosis injury can occur from a decrease in oxygen delivery to the kidney or from nephrotoxic injury.

Many toxins, both endotoxins (hemoglobinuria, myoglobinuria, calcium, uric acid, bilirubin, and bile salt) and exotoxins (antibiotics, contrast dye, cyclosporine, acyclovir, and chemotherapeutic agents) can cause tubular damage. Retained bilirubin and bile salts as well as altered abdominal hemodynamics may contribute to the increased risk of acute tubular necrosis in patients undergoing biliary tract surgery. The length of time on cardiopulmonary bypass is related directly to the incidence of acute tubular necrosis. Hemoglobinuria and

decreased renal blood flow may have a role in the development of acute tubular necrosis in these patients. Heme pigments (myoglobin and hemoglobin) cause intrarenal vasoconstriction and tubular obstruction that lead to acute renal failure (Table 16-7).

- Many toxins, both endotoxins and exotoxins, can cause tubular damage.
- The length of time on cardiopulmonary bypass is related directly to the incidence of acute tubular necrosis.

In severely ill patients, the cause of acute tubular necrosis is usually multifactorial, and for the recovery of the patient and kidney, it is important that all causes are identified and corrected.

The typical course of acute renal failure due to acute tubular necrosis begins with a rapid increase in the serum level of creatinine, accompanied by a decrease in urine output. The oliguric phase lasts from 7 to 14 days if the initial insult is corrected and no further renal insult (e.g., sepsis or hypotension) occurs. If the oliguric phase lasts longer than 4 weeks, other causes of acute renal failure should be considered. Renal biopsy may be required for further evaluation. The oliguric phase is followed by a diuretic phase, during which urine output increases, followed by delayed improvement in serum creatinine levels and GFR. The last phase occurs over 3 to 12 months as the GFR gradually improves. If the patient is oliguric for more than 16 days, renal function most likely will not return to baseline.

- The typical course of acute renal failure due to acute tubular necrosis begins with a rapid increase in the serum level of creatinine, accompanied by a decrease in urine output.
- The oliguric phase is followed by a diuretic phase.

Another cause of acute intrinsic renal failure is acute interstitial nephritis. This can be mediated by immunologic, infectious, or allergic reactions. The most common cause in the hospital setting is an allergic reaction to a drug. Drugs associated with acute interstitial nephritis include β-lactam antibiotics, diuretics, allopurinol, NSAIDs, cimetidine, sulfonamides, rifampin, and phenytoin.

Table 16-7 Comparison of Heme Pigments

	Serum color	Haptoglobin	CPK	Heme dipstick	Urine benzidine
Hemoglobin	Red	Decreased	Normal	Positive	Negative
Myoglobin	Clear	Normal	Increased	Positive	Positive

CPK, creatine phosphokinase.

- Another cause of acute intrinsic renal failure is acute interstitial nephritis.
- The most common cause in a hospital setting is an allergic reaction to a drug.

Aminoglycoside renal toxicity occurs after 5 to 7 days of therapy and correlates with the cumulative dose received. Its effect on the tubules is reflected by the potassium and magnesium wasting observed in these patients. Despite an increase in creatinine, patients usually are nonoliguric. Aminoglycosides are freely filtered at the glomerulus and partially absorbed in the proximal tubule. The more amino groups on the aminoglycosides, the more toxic the agent (streptomycin is more toxic than gentamicin, which is more toxic than tobramycin). Once-a-day dosing regimens have been shown to decrease nephrotoxicity. Aminoglycoside levels should be monitored to reduce ototoxicity and nephrotoxicity.

- Aminoglycoside renal toxicity occurs after 5-7 days of therapy and correlates with the cumulative dose received.
- Aminoglycoside levels should be monitored to reduce ototoxicity and nephrotoxicity.

Amphotericin B is associated with distal tubule dysfunction. Findings include evidence of a nephrogenic diabetes insipidus (nonoliguric) and type IV renal tubular acidosis. Toxicity occurs after a 2- to 3-g dose. Amphotericin B in liposomes may decrease its toxicity.

- Amphotericin B is associated with distal tubule dysfunction.

Cisplatin is associated with acute renal failure and tubular dysfunction (hypomagnesemia and hypokalemia), with a cumulative dose of 50 to 75 mg/m^2. Forced diuresis while ensuring adequate hydration can prevent renal toxicity.

- Cisplatin is associated with acute renal failure and tubular dysfunction.

NSAIDs can cause acute renal failure by different mechanisms. They block the production of vasodilatory prostaglandins, causing intrarenal vasoconstriction and, when renal blood flow is compromised, reversible acute renal failure. NSAIDs are also associated with an acute tubulointerstitial nephritis (without eosinophils), acute nephrotic syndrome, hyperkalemia, hyponatremia, and an exacerbation of hypertension.

- NSAIDs can cause acute renal failure by different mechanisms.

Contrast-induced acute renal failure is due to the multiple nephrotoxic effects of the contrast dye. Renal vasoconstriction, tubular obstruction, and direct tubular toxicity all negatively affect the GFR. Patients with diabetes mellitus and severe renal dysfunction and those who receive a large dose of dye are at risk for pronounced dye toxicity. Patients become oliguric 24 to 48 hours after the dye load and should recover within 7 days. Nephrotomograms and a low fractional excretion of sodium are clues to the diagnosis. The following may be helpful in preventing toxicity in high-risk patients: normal saline forced diuresis, low ionic contrast agents with lower osmolality, limiting the dose of the agent, administration of acetylcysteine, and spacing repeated dye loads to allow for renal recovery.

Cholesterol atheroembolic-induced renal failure is a cause of acute irreversible intrinsic renal failure. A history of atherosclerotic vascular disease, smoking, hyperlipidemia, hypertension, and diabetes increases the risk for developing acute renal failure due to atheroemboli. It generally occurs in elderly patients, either spontaneously or after an invasive procedure. Clinical findings may include livedo reticularis of the back, flank, abdomen, and extremities; emboli on funduscopic examination; and evidence of microemboli of the digits. Laboratory studies demonstrate an increased erythrocyte sedimentation rate, leukocytosis, eosinophiluria, thrombocytopenia, and a low complement level. Recovery of renal function is rare, and if it does occur, it is gradual and incomplete. No treatment is known to reverse the microvascular occlusion and resulting inflammation. Patients often need support with renal replacement therapy.

- Cholesterol atheroembolic-induced renal failure is a cause of acute irreversible intrinsic renal failure.
- No treatment is known to reverse the microvascular occlusion and resulting inflammation.

Postrenal Failure

Urine flow can be obstructed anywhere along the urinary tract. Crystals can cause obstruction of the collecting system, leading to acute renal failure. Uric acid crystals are the culprits in tumor lysis syndrome and other disease states in which the serum concentration of uric acid is excessive (>15-20 mg/dL). Methotrexate and intravenous acyclovir can precipitate in the tubules and cause acute renal failure. Prevention includes hydrating the patients when these medications are administered.

- Obstruction to urine flow can occur anywhere along the urinary tract.

Ureteral obstruction can occur from stone material, necrosed papillae, blood clots, or tumor. External compression and ureteral obstruction can occur from retroperitoneal fibrosis (idiopathic or due to methysergide) or genitourinary tumors. Surgical ligation is an infrequent cause of acute renal failure but needs to be considered in patients who have had retroperitoneal or genitourinary operations. Bladder outlet obstruction due to prostatic hypertrophy or cancer is a common cause of postrenal acute renal failure in men and genitourinary cancers are a common cause in women. Urine flow patterns and symptom patterns may help distinguish between partial and complete obstruction. Wide fluctuations in urine volume may represent partial obstruction, whereas oliguria or anuria can occur with complete obstruction. Pain is more frequent with complete obstruction because of distention of the renal capsule, collecting system, or bladder. The location of the pain is a clue to the site of obstruction. A normal anion gap (hyperchloremia) acidosis can be seen in cases of urinary obstruction. The creatinine level is usually increased in bilateral or complete obstruction but can be normal or only slightly increased in partial or unilateral obstruction. Despite the normal creatinine level and urine output in partial obstruction, it is important to discover the cause and to correct it to avoid chronic tubular injury and irreversible renal injury.

- The pathogenesis of obstructive uropathy involves early vasoconstriction, followed by vasodilatation.
- A normal anion gap acidosis can be seen in cases of urinary obstruction.

Diagnosis of Acute Renal Failure

Often, the differential diagnosis of the cause of acute renal failure can be determined and narrowed considerably by obtaining a complete past medical history and history of present illness and by understanding the patient's risk factors for the different causes of acute renal failure. Assessment of fluid balance is essential to distinguish between prerenal and intrinsic or postrenal causes. The presence of microinfarction and livedo reticularis suggests atheroemboli as the cause. A palpable bladder or flank tenderness is a clue that the cause is postrenal.

Laboratory studies are also critical for differentiating among causes of acute renal failure. Findings on urinalysis can help to distinguish among prerenal, intrinsic renal, and postrenal causes. Urinary osmolality is increased early in the course of prerenal azotemia and the sediment is usually benign, with only hyaline and occasional granular casts. Acute tubular necrosis is characterized by urine that is isosmotic with the serum and urine sediment that may contain tubular epithelial cells, granular cells, and amorphous material. Urine eosinophils and leukocytes are seen with acute interstitial nephritis. Erythrocyte casts indicate a rapidly progressive or acute glomerulonephritis. A normal urine sediment with a dipstick positive for blood is characteristic of acute renal failure induced

by heme pigments. In postrenal failure, urinalysis findings are often unremarkable. Crystalluria may be present in patients with urolithiasis, and hematuria may be a clue to a genitourinary cancer or to an obstructing lesion or a stone.

- Laboratory studies are also critical for distinguishing among the causes of acute renal failure.
- Findings on urinalysis can easily distinguish among prerenal, intrinsic renal, and postrenal causes.

Urinary chemistry tests or urinary indices can also help distinguish among the three main categories of acute renal failure (Table 16-8). During episodes of decreased renal blood flow (renal artery stenosis, decreased intravascular volume, congestive heart failure, advanced cirrhosis), functional renal tubules reabsorb sodium in an attempt to restore renal perfusion. Under these circumstances, urinary sodium excretion is low (<20 mEq/L) and the fractional excretion of sodium is less than 1%. Initially, in the continuum of prerenal failure, the fractional excretion of sodium is low, but as tubules are damaged by decreased oxygen delivery and acute tubular necrosis develops, the fractional excretion of sodium increases (>3%). Toxins (myoglobins, hemoglobin, contrast media) and medications (ACEIs, angiotensin receptor blockers, cyclosporine, and NSAIDs) that are vasoconstrictive, decreasing renal blood flow, are also associated with a low fractional excretion of sodium. Hepatorenal syndrome, early obstruction, and acute glomerulonephritis are other causes of intrinsic renal failure that affect renal blood flow and are associated with a low fractional excretion of sodium.

- Urinary chemistry tests or urinary indices also can help distinguish among the three main categories of acute renal failure.

Table 16-8 Comparison of Urinary Indices in Prerenal Failure and Acute Tubular Necrosis

Urinary indices	Prerenal failure	Acute tubular necrosis
Urine osmolality, mOsm/L	≥500	≤350
Urine/plasma creatinine ratio	≥40	≤20
Plasma BUN/creatinine ratio	>20	<15
FeNa,* %	<1	>3

BUN, blood urea nitrogen; FeNa, fractional excretion of sodium.

$$*FeNa = \frac{(urinary\ Na) \times (plasma\ creatinine)}{(plasma\ Na) \times (urinary\ creatinine)} \times 100.$$

Postrenal failure due to obstruction can be determined with ultrasonography. Of these studies, however, 2% can be false-negative because of acute obstruction or retroperitoneal fibrosis and 26% are false-positive. A combination of ultrasonography and computed tomography without contrast is 100% diagnostic for obstruction and can determine the cause for obstruction in 84% of cases.

● Postrenal failure due to obstruction can be determined with ultrasonography.
● A combination of ultrasonography and computed tomography without contrast is 100% diagnostic for obstruction and can determine the cause of obstruction in 84% of cases.

Management of Acute Renal Failure

Prevention of acute renal failure begins by determining and managing the risk factors. Avoiding intravascular volume depletion, maximizing cardiac function, and avoiding nephrotoxic medications and intravenous contrast loads are all essential in preventing an acute decline in renal function. Patients with known preexisting renal dysfunction are at risk for losing 10% to 50% of the GFR if they are exposed to these factors.

● Prevention of acute renal failure begins by determining and managing the risk factors.
● Patients with known preexisting renal dysfunction are at risk for losing 10%-50% of the GFR if they are exposed to these factors.

After acute renal failure has occurred, the initial goal is to reverse any ongoing renal insults (restore intravascular volume, discontinue nephrotoxins, improve cardiac function, and relieve urinary obstruction) to prevent ongoing injury. After the obstruction is relieved in patients with obstructive uropathy, there is an initial polyuria. Therapy is aimed at preventing a new prerenal component to the acute renal failure and correcting electrolyte disturbances. Fluid replacement can start with 75 mL/h of 50% normal saline. Patients should be monitored for electrolyte disturbances and volume depletion. In patients with acute tubular necrosis or acute interstitial nephritis, diuretics have been used to maintain urine output.

● The initial goal is to reverse any ongoing renal insult.
● After the obstruction is relieved in patients with obstructive uropathy, replace two-thirds of the postobstructive diuresis volume to prevent adding a new prerenal component to the acute renal failure.

Maintaining the nutritional requirements of patients with acute renal failure is essential. Patients who are seriously ill are usually catabolic and require 35 to 45 kcal/kg daily and 1.5 g/kg of protein daily. Diets must be adjusted to limit potassium, sodium, magnesium, phosphorus, and fluid intake. If serum phosphorus levels increase despite dietary phosphorus restriction, phosphate binders should be added to the regimen.

● Maintaining the nutritional requirements of patients with acute renal failure is essential.

As renal function changes, drug doses need to be adjusted and drug levels monitored. Be cautious prescribing medications that can accumulate and become toxic in patients with declining or low renal function (magnesium, aluminum-containing antacids, digoxin, renally cleared β-blockers, long-acting diltiazem preparations, and benzodiazepines). Treatment with NSAIDs, contrast agents, and other agents known to be nephrotoxic should be avoided.

● As renal function changes, drug doses need to be adjusted and drug levels monitored.

Dialysis

The goals of renal replacement in acute renal failure are to maintain fluid, electrolyte, acid-base, and solute balance; to prevent further insult; to promote healing; and to permit other support measures to be used (intravenous medications and parenteral nutrition). The indications for beginning renal replacement in the acute setting are similar to those for the chronic setting. An increase in BUN indicates the accumulation of uremic toxins. In acutely ill patients, a BUN concentration greater than 100 mg/dL is an indication to begin dialysis even if there are not other signs and symptoms of uremia. In patients who are not receiving adequate protein nutrition or have little muscle mass, the absolute value of BUN can underestimate the degree of renal failure and toxin accumulation. When the estimated GFR is less than 20 mL/min and immediate renal recovery is not anticipated, it is recommended that dialysis be initiated before BUN reaches 100 mg/dL. In acutely or critically ill patients, BUN greater than 60 mg/dL may be an indication to begin dialysis. Hyperkalemia, acidosis, fluid overload not responsive to diuretics, evidence of central nervous system toxicity, pericardial rub, and gastrointestinal tract bleeding believed to be due to uremia are all indications to begin dialysis immediately.

● The goals of renal replacement in acute renal failure are to maintain fluid, electrolyte, acid-base, and solute balance; to prevent further insult; to promote healing; and to permit other support measures to be used.
● Hyperkalemia, acidosis, fluid overload not responsive to diuretics, evidence of central nervous system toxicity, pericardial

rub, and gastrointestinal tract bleeding believed to be due to uremia are all indications to begin dialysis immediately.

The choice of renal replacement must be customized to the needs of the patient. Severe metabolic abnormalities requiring rapid correction (hyperkalemia with electrocardiographic [ECG] changes and severe acidosis) should be treated immediately with short high-flux hemodialysis. Patients with a stable hemodynamic condition able to tolerate rapid fluid and electrolyte shifts can undergo the conventional high-flux intermittent three-times-per-week dialysis. Severely ill catabolic patients requiring intravenous fluids for nutrition, continuous or frequent intravenous administration of medications, and intravenous fluid resuscitation are best dialyzed daily with intermittent dialysis or with continuous dialysis therapy to avoid large fluid gains and to maintain solute homeostasis. Patients with an unstable hemodynamic condition who require renal replacement are best treated with a continuous dialysis modality (CVVHD or CVVHCF). These methods with continuous gentle fluid and solute removal improve hemodynamic stability by decreasing osmolar and solute concentration changes as well as limiting fluid shifts.

CHRONIC RENAL FAILURE

"Chronic renal failure" is defined as a GFR less than 33 mL/min per m^2. As in acute renal failure, the initial steps in evaluating a patient with an increased creatinine level, increased BUN, or decreased GFR are to determine whether it represents a true decrease in GFR, whether the damage is chronic or acute, what the cause is, and if there is a reversible component. The reversible causes of renal insufficiency are listed in Table 16-9.

The diagnosis of chronic renal disease is established by identifying comorbid illnesses known to lead to progressive renal insufficiency and documenting evidence of progressive renal dysfunction (Table 16-10).

Table 16-9 Reversible Causes of Renal Insufficiency

Obstruction
Congestive heart failure
Medications
Hypertension
Infection
Volume loss
Hypothyroidism
Hypoadrenalism
Hypercalcemia
Hyperuricemia

Table 16-10 Causes of Renal Disease

Cause	% of cases
Diabetes mellitus	37
Hypertension	29
Glomerulonephritis	13
Polycystic kidney disease	10

Patients with chronic irreversible renal disease with a GFR less than 33 mL/min usually have atrophic kidneys. Exceptions include patients with renal dysfunction due to amyloidosis, myeloma, diabetes mellitus, or polycystic kidney disease. Chronic renal disease is progressive because of hyperfiltration of the remaining functioning nephrons.

- Patients with chronic renal disease usually have small kidneys.

The goal of identifying and treating chronic renal disease is to prevent progression of the disease, to avoid the morbidity and mortality of end-stage renal disease (ESRD), and to adequately prepare patients for eventual renal replacement. This requires early intervention and adequate follow-up. "End-stage renal disease" is defined as a GFR less than 15 mL/min per m^2, but often patients require renal replacement before the GFR is less than this.

- The goal of identifying and treating chronic renal insufficiency is to prevent progression of the disease, to avoid the morbidity and mortality of ESRD, and to adequately prepare patients for eventual renal replacement.

Strict blood pressure control is essential to slow the progression of any renal disease. Blood pressure should be 130/80 mm Hg or less for those with chronic kidney disease and 125/75 mm Hg or less if proteinuria is present. ACEIs and angiotensin receptor blockers are the first-choice antihypertensive agents. They delay the progression of renal disease by lowering systemic blood pressure and by altering interrenal hemodynamics. Diuretics are also useful in controlling blood pressure. Thiazide diuretics are useful until the GFR is less than 45 mL/min. At that point, loop diuretics should be used. Fluid overload is often an important contributor to hypertension in persons with chronic kidney disease. Electrolyte (hyperkalemia with β-blockers, ACEIs, and angiotensin receptor blockers) and conduction abnormalities (long-acting diltiazem and β-blockers that are renally excreted) need to be monitored.

- Strict blood pressure control is essential to slow the progression of any renal disease.
- ACEIs and angiotensin receptor blockers are the first-choice antihypertensive agents.

Proteinuria is a marker of renal dysfunction and is also a risk factor for progression of chronic renal disease. ACEIs and angiotensin receptor blockers are beneficial in delaying the progression of disease not only by controlling blood pressure but also by decreasing proteinuria. The goal is to decrease proteinuria by 35% to 40%, and blood pressure must be controlled.

- Proteinuria is a risk factor for progression of chronic renal disease.

Dietary adjustments are important for patients with chronic renal failure. As the GFR decreases, the ability of the nephron to handle potassium and phosphorus decreases. Patients should be monitored for hyperkalemia and hyperphosphatemia. Dietary potassium and phosphorus intake should be restricted after the serum levels begin to increase. Hyperkalemia may occur with a GFR greater than 20 mL/min per m^2 if distal tubular function is abnormal (type IV renal tubular acidosis). Hyperphosphatemia, despite adequate compliance with a low phosphorus diet, requires the addition of a phosphate binder. Restriction of dietary protein is recognized to decrease uremic symptoms (decrease acid, sodium, oxalate, and nitrogen loads and nitrogen waste products). The benefits of protein restriction must be balanced against the morbidity and mortality associated with protein malnutrition. If the patient's protein stores are normal, a protein-restricted diet is recommended. After the serum level of albumin decreases, the protein restriction should be liberalized to prevent protein malnutrition.

- Dietary adjustments are important for patients with chronic renal failure.

After the GFR decreases to less than 33 mL/min per m^2, erythropoietin production by the renal parenchyma is not sufficient to prevent anemia. The anemia of chronic renal failure is a normochromic normocytic anemia. Treatment with erythropoietin given subcutaneously should be started for all patients who develop anemia. Also, iron should be given orally to patients without a contraindication for supplemental iron. Resistance to erythropoietin can be caused by iron deficiency, inflammation, malignancy, secondary hyperparathyroidism, hematologic disorders, and increasing uremia. Anemia in patients with chronic kidney disease contributes to the development of left ventricular hypertrophy and progression of the underlying renal disease.

- Treatment with erythropoietin given subcutaneously should be started for all patients who develop anemia.

Uremia

The complications of progressive renal dysfunction and uremia involve all organ systems. Uremic symptoms and signs may occur at different levels of GFR depending on the patient's comorbid diseases and the management of the patient's pre-ESRD.

Anemia of chronic renal failure is multifactorial; decreased erythropoietin production, hemolysis, and blood loss may all contribute to the low hemoglobin concentration. Anemia should be treated with erythropoietin and iron supplementation. Bleeding is common in chronic renal failure because of platelet dysfunction. Treatment with desmopressin is helpful in acutely reversing the bleeding tendency.

- Anemia of chronic renal failure is multifactorial.

The metabolic acidosis in early chronic renal failure is a non–anion gap acidosis due to decreased ammonium secretion. As renal dysfunction progresses and phosphates and sulfates accumulate, the acidosis becomes a high anion gap acidosis.

- The metabolic acidosis in early chronic renal failure is a non–anion gap acidosis.

Cardiovascular disease is a common cause of death in patients with ESRD and advanced renal insufficiency. In this population, hypertension is common and is associated with excess extracellular fluid volume and, in some cases, excess renin production. Hyperlipidemia and accelerated atherosclerosis contribute to the cardiovascular morbidity and mortality. As mentioned above, anemia can lead to left ventricular hypertrophy. Pericarditis may occur in two patterns. Pattern I is a hemorrhagic pericarditis that is treated with hemodialysis. Pattern II can occur in patients who are adequately dialyzed; it may be associated with hemorrhage and tamponade. A viral cause has been implicated, and corticosteroids often need to be given intrapericardially.

- Cardiovascular disease is a common cause of death of patients with ESRD.

Hyperkalemia can occur with a GFR less than 20 mL/min and oliguria, but distal tubular dysfunction (type IV renal tubular acidosis, aldosterone deficiency) and medications (NSAIDs, ACEIs, angiotensin receptor blockers, β-blockers, and potassium-sparing diuretics) that interfere with potassium handling can lead to hyperkalemia with a GFR greater than 20 mL/min.

Hyperkalemia associated with ECG changes should be treated emergently. Acute ECG changes due to hyperkalemia should be treated with an infusion of calcium to protect the myocardium, followed by an infusion of insulin to redistribute the potassium; however, in the setting of ECG changes and a low GFR, dialysis is indicated. Resins and dialysis are used to eliminate potassium. Chronic hyperkalemia can be treated with a scheduled dose of resins, a low potassium diet, and the avoidance of medications that interfere with potassium handling.

● Hyperkalemia can occur with a GFR <20 mL/min and oliguria.

Through a complex feedback system, renal disease leads to phosphorus retention, hypocalcemia, acidosis, decreased 1,25-dihydroxyvitamin D production, and an increase in parathyroid hormone. Relatively early in advancing renal insufficiency (GFR, 30-40 mL/min), the development of hyperphosphatemia and decreased levels of 1,25-dihydroxyvitamin D begin the cascade leading to secondary hyperparathyroidism and the development of osteitis fibrosa cystica. This is the classic form of bone disease in renal failure, with overactive osteoclastic and osteoblastic activity. Osteomalacia (low-turnover bone disease) due to 1,25-dihydroxyvitamin D deficiency is characterized by an increase in osteoid and diminished or absent osteoclastic and osteoblastic activity. Osteoporosis also occurs with ESRD and chronic renal insufficiency. Aluminum bone disease can occur in chronic renal failure and ESRD in patients who ingest aluminum. These patients have low levels of parathyroid hormone and 1,25-dihydroxyvitamin D. They present with a microcytic anemia and frequent bone fractures. Aluminum osteodystrophy is diagnosed with an iliac crest bone biopsy and treated with deferoxamine chelation.

● Through a complex feedback system, renal disease leads to phosphorus retention, hypocalcemia, acidosis, decreased 1,25-dihydroxyvitamin D production, and an increase in parathyroid hormone.
● Osteoporosis also occurs with ESRD and chronic renal insufficiency.

Treatment and prevention of renal osteodystrophy focus on the suppression of parathyroid hormone production by maintaining a normal calcium and phosphorus balance. Treatment begins with a low phosphorus diet. If the serum level of phosphorus remains elevated, enteric phosphate binders are needed. If the serum level of calcium remains low or parathyroid hormone levels remain high (or both), 1,25-dihydroxyvitamin D supplementation is added.

● Treatment and prevention of renal osteodystrophy focus on the suppression of parathyroid hormone production by maintaining a normal calcium and phosphorus balance.

Beta$_2$-microglobulin deposition that occurs in chronic renal failure and ESRD can lead to carpal tunnel syndrome and debilitating arthritis. Pseudogout and periarthritis due to the deposition of hydroxyapatite in joint spaces are other musculoskeletal complications of uremia.

Gastrointestinal complications of uremia include gastritis, colitis, ileitis, peptic ulcer disease, and constipation. Anorexia is a complication that is multifactorial but leads to protein and caloric malnutrition.

● Gastrointestinal complications of uremia include gastritis, colitis, ileitis, peptic ulcer disease, and constipation.

The neurologic complications of uremia range from peripheral neuropathy (sensory fibers affected more than motor fibers) to cognitive impairment and eventual central nervous system irritability associated with asterixis and seizures. Without treatment (dialysis or reversal of the renal failure), eventual coma and death occur.

● Neurologic complications of uremia range from peripheral neuropathy to cognitive impairment and eventual central nervous system irritability associated with asterixis and seizures.

Dialysis

Indications for dialysis include fluid overload, acidosis, hyperkalemia, hypernatremia, and uremic signs and symptoms. The choice of dialysis (hemodialysis or peritoneal dialysis) in chronic nonemergent renal failure depends on many clinical and mechanical factors as well as patient choice. Both types of dialysis can be done in the home. Peritoneal dialysis offers a continuous ultrafiltration and solute clearance, avoiding rapid shifts and hemodynamic instability. Hemodialysis offers more efficient clearance of solutes. Selected patients who have poor hemodialysis access, cardiomyopathy, or a scheduled transplant may be candidates for peritoneal dialysis. Peritoneal dialysis will fail in patients with a history of recurrent abdominal operations or diseases that lead to fibrosis of the peritoneal lining.

● Indications for dialysis include fluid overload, acidosis, hyperkalemia, hypernatremia, and uremic signs and symptoms.

Complications of Dialysis

All patients with ESRD are at increased risk for hepatitis B and C. All of them should receive the vaccine and hepatitis B immunoglobulin.

Hemodialysis—Complications include hemodialysis disequilibrium due to brain edema and osmolar shifts with rapid dialysis and hemodynamic instability due to rapid fluctuations in potassium, calcium, and osmoles and rapid fluid removal.

Infections involving central venous catheters or arteriovenous grafts can occur. Early detection and treatment with antibiotics are essential. If the catheter or graft remains contaminated, removal is required.

Peritoneal dialysis—Complications include infections (peritonitis, exit-site infections, catheter tunnel infection), catheter leak, obesity, protein malnutrition, hyperlipidemia, and hyperglycemia. This form of dialysis is less efficient than high-flux hemodialysis.

Drugs removed with dialysis and those not removed and drugs to be avoided if the patient receives dialysis are listed in Table 16-11.

Table 16-11   Dialysis and Overdoses

Drugs removed with dialysis
  Methanol
  Aspirin
  Ethylene glycol
  Lithium
  Sodium
  Mannitol
  Theophylline

Drugs not removed with dialysis
  Tetracycline
  Benzodiazepines
  Digoxin
  Phenytoin (Dilantin)
  Phenothiazines

Medications to avoid in patients receiving dialysis
  Tetracycline
  Nitrofurantoin
  Probenecid
  Neomycin
  Bacitracin
  Methenamine
  Nalidixic acid
  Clofibrate
  Lovastatin
  Magnesium
  Oral hypoglycemic agents
  Antiplatelet drugs
  Renal-excreted β-blockers

PART III
Robert C. Albright, Jr., D.O.

ELECTROLYTE AND ACID-BASE DISORDERS

DISORDERS OF WATER BALANCE

The most important principle in understanding disorders of water balance is that the serum level of sodium is the clinical index of total body water. However, it is not an index of extracellular volume or total body sodium. Total body sodium can be determined only by physical examination. The serum level of sodium is a useful clinical index for evaluating water balance, not sodium balance. Water balance is regulated by thirst, antidiuretic hormone, and the ability of the renal medulla to concentrate urine.

- The serum level of sodium is not an index of extracellular volume or total body sodium.
- Water balance is regulated by thirst, antidiuretic hormone, and the ability of the renal medulla to concentrate urine.

Hyponatremia

Hyponatremia is the most common electrolyte abnormality in hospitalized patients. Its symptoms are protean and include lethargy, cramps, decreased deep tendon reflexes, and seizures. The diagnosis and management of hyponatremia are shown in Figure 16-2.

Diagnosis

The first step in evaluating patients with hyponatremia is to measure serum osmolality. Isosmotic hyponatremia may be caused by severe hypertriglyceridemia (>1,500 mg/dL, lipemia retinalis is always present), severe hyperproteinemia (>8.0 g/dL, Waldenström macroglobulinemia, myeloma), or isotonic infusions of glucose, mannitol, or glycine. Hyperosmotic hyponatremia may be due to severe hyperglycemia (sodium decreases 1.6 mEq/L for each 100 mg/dL increase in glucose) and to hypertonic infusions of glucose, mannitol, or glycine. The use of ion-selective sodium probes in many clinical chemistry laboratories has markedly decreased the incidence of "pseudohyponatremia."

The second step is to assess the extracellular fluid volume of the hyposmotic hyponatremic patient and to determine whether that patient is hypovolemic, euvolemic, or hypervolemic.

1) Hyposmotic *hypovolemic* hyponatremia: measure urine osmolality and sodium concentration (urinary spot sodium is often <20 mEq/L, fractional excretion of sodium <1%); common causes are severe volume depletion, thiazide diuretics, and adrenal insufficiency.

2) Hyposmotic *hypervolemic* hyponatremia: measure urine osmolality and sodium concentration; edematous states and renal failure are common.

3) Hypotonic *euvolemic* hyponatremia: measure cortisol and thyroid-stimulating hormone levels, urine sodium level, and urine osmolality. Possible diagnoses include hypothyroidism, Addison disease, reset osmostat, psychogenic polydipsia, and the syndrome of inappropriate antidiuresis (SIAD). The term "syndrome of inappropriate antidiuresis" has recently replaced the previous term "syndrome of inappropriate antidiuretic hormone" because up to 20% of patients who fulfill the criteria for SIAD do not have detectable circulating levels of antidiuretic hormone.

SIAD is a diagnosis of exclusion. Patients must meet the following criteria: hypotonic plasma, urine less than maximally dilute (urine osmolality in SIAD is greater than serum osmolality or >100-150 mOsm/kg), urine sodium matches intake, absence of hypoadrenalism and hypothyroidism, and improvement with water restriction. Important clinical clues are low serum levels of uric acid, creatinine, and blood urea nitrogen (BUN).

Acute hyponatremia has been described in several special clinical settings. Hyponatremia may occur in up to 5% of patients after surgery and anesthesia. Plasma vasopressin concentrations are increased because of nonosmolar stimuli such as pain, nausea, and the use of narcotics. Rarely, profound hyponatremia may occur. During transurethral prostatic resection, isotonic or hypotonic fluids containing glycine can be absorbed and depress the serum level of sodium. Schizophrenic patients with severe compulsive water drinking (>14 L daily) occasionally have acute hyponatremia. Also, infusions of oxytocin and cyclophosphamide may induce acute hyponatremia.

Chronic hyponatremia may be induced by the use of thiazides, chlorpropamide, carbamazepine, and nonsteroidal anti-inflammatory drugs (NSAIDs).

- The physical examination, osmolality of plasma and urine, and urine sodium concentration provide important information for diagnosis.
- SIAD: serum levels of uric acid, creatinine, and BUN are low.

Therapy for Hyponatremia

A general tenet of therapy for hyponatremia is that the correction should occur at the rate at which it developed.

Hypovolemic Hyponatremia

This syndrome most often reflects volume depletion. The total sodium deficit can be calculated as follows: sodium deficit

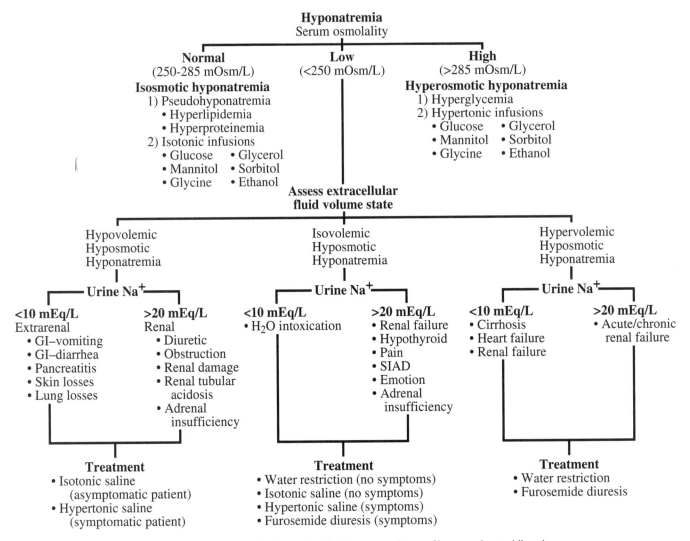

Fig. 16-2. Diagnosis and management of hyponatremia. GI, gastrointestinal; SIAD, syndrome of inappropriate antidiuresis.

= total body water (body weight in kg × 0.5) × desired serum sodium (mEq/L) − current serum sodium (mEq/L).

Euvolemic Hyponatremia

As pointed out above, hyponatremia should be reversed cautiously at a rate similar to that at which it developed, to avoid central pontine myelinolysis. However, the rate of onset often is unknown. Therefore, therapy is directed primarily by signs and symptoms. The treatment for patients with euvolemic hyponatremia who are asymptomatic should be water restriction only. Patients with acute euvolemic hyponatremia who have neurologic symptoms require prompt therapy designed to facilitate the excretion of free water. Options include the infusion of hypertonic saline or the simultaneous infusion of isotonic saline and a loop diuretic. The amount of hypertonic saline required to increase the serum concentration of sodium to appropriate levels can be estimated roughly by calculating free water excess.

However, these calculations assume steady-state urinary concentration, which may not occur as therapy is administered. Therefore, intense monitoring is needed, including hourly measurements of serum sodium and urine sodium and osmolality. Patients with chronic SIAD may benefit from treatment with demeclocycline.

Hypervolemic Hyponatremia

Therapy involves diuretics and correction or treatment of the underlying pathophysiologic state, which often involves liver, heart, or kidney disorders.

Hypernatremia

As in hyponatremia, the symptoms of hypernatremia are often protean, with irritability, hyperreflexia, ataxia, and seizures. Because all forms of hypernatremia are associated with hypertonicity, there is no pseudohypernatremia. Hypernatremia is categorized as "hypovolemic," "hypervolemic," and "euvolemic." The diagnosis and management of hypernatremia are outlined in Figure 16-3.

Hypovolemic hypernatremia often responds to saline, followed by a hypotonic solution. Hypervolemic hypernatremia responds to diuretics; rarely, dialysis may be needed. Euvolemic patients should receive free water, either orally or intravenously, to correct the serum level of sodium, generally no faster than 0.5 mEq/h.

A total free water deficit may be calculated as total body water (0.5 × lean body weight in kg) × [(serum sodium concentration in mEq/L ÷ desired serum sodium in mEq/L) – 1]. Additionally, obligate losses of free water (estimated to be 13 mL/kg daily) need to be considered in these calculations.

- Hypovolemic hypernatremia: check urine sodium; the cause may be osmotic diuresis, excessive sweating, and diarrhea.
- Hypervolemic hypernatremia: may be caused by sodium poisoning.

- Euvolemic hypernatremia: loss of water, extrarenal (skin, lung) vs. renal, diabetes insipidus, central vs. nephrogenic water deprivation test.

DIABETES INSIPIDUS

Polyuria
"Polyuria" is defined as urinary output of more than 3 L per day. This may represent a solute or a water diuresis. The normal daily required osmolar secretion is approximately 10 mOsm/kg. Therefore, water or solute diuresis may be distinguished by measuring urine osmolality and determining the total daily solute excretion. If osmotic diuresis is excluded, polyuria is often due to primary polydipsia or diabetes insipidus.

Central Diabetes Insipidus
An absence of circulating vasopressin (partial or complete) is due to destruction of the pituitary or it is congenital, "familial

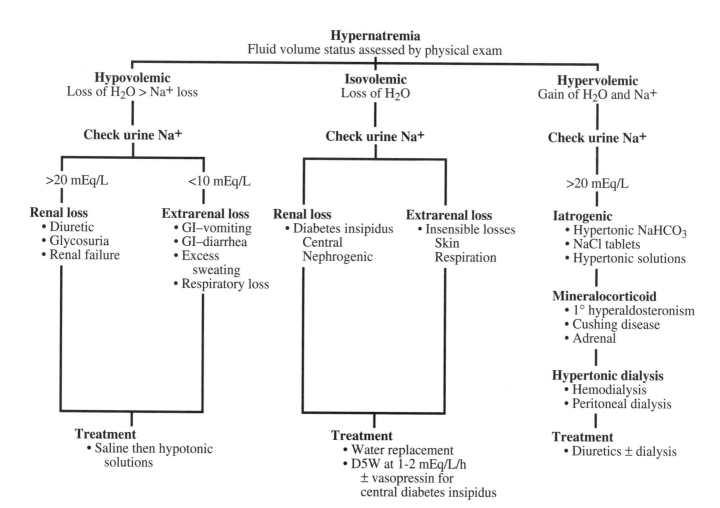

Fig. 16-3. Diagnosis and management of hypernatremia. D5W, 5% dextrose in water; GI, gastrointestinal.

autosomal dominant central diabetes insipidus." This is a result of mutations in the prearginine-proarginine-vasopressin-neurophysin II gene.

Nephrogenic Diabetes Insipidus

A complete or partial resistance of the renal collecting duct cell to the actions of vasopressin may be the result of a familial X-linked disorder or, more commonly, an acquired lesion. Nephrogenic diabetes insipidus may be induced by lithium, demeclocycline, or amphotericin B ("drug-induced nephrogenic diabetes insipidus"). Occasionally, the concentrating defect seen with lithium is not reversible. Renal diseases such as amyloidosis, sickle cell disease, light chain nephropathy, Sjögren syndrome, obstructive uropathy, and renal failure are common causes of nephrogenic diabetes insipidus.

Because of high placenta-derived levels of vasopressinase, a water diuresis may be noted in pregnancy, but technically this is not nephrogenic diabetes insipidus because the women have a normal response to supplemental desmopressin, which is resistant to vasopressinase.

Hypercalcemia and hypokalemia also induce nephrogenic diabetes insipidus via multiple impaired intracellular pathways.

Patients with diabetes insipidus are symptomatic only if access to free water is restricted. This occurs primarily in very elderly, very young, or hospitalized patients or in institutional situations. Differentiating these polyuric states may be challenging. A detailed history of familial issues and use of medications is extremely important. Abrupt onset of polyuria is characteristic of acquired diabetes insipidus. A water deprivation test (or infusion of 5% saline) under closely supervised conditions often allows various polyuric states to be distinguished. The differentiation of diabetes insipidus from primary polydipsia with available laboratory tests is outlined in Table 16-12.

The serum concentration of sodium is often high-normal or increased in diabetes insipidus, whereas it is usually low-normal or low in primary polydipsia.

- Polyuria is defined as urine output >3 L/d.
- Polyuric states are due to either water or solute diuresis.
- A closely supervised water deprivation test will differentiate most polyuric states.

DISORDERS OF SODIUM BALANCE

Disorders of sodium balance can be determined only by clinical examination. Orthostatism implies volume depletion and sodium deficiency. Edema implies volume excess and sodium excess.

Cerebral salt wasting has rarely been documented in situations of severe central nervous system injury. Differentiating this from SIAD may be difficult. A negative sodium balance that causes contraction of the extracellular fluid volume must be documented for cerebral salt wasting to be diagnosed. Often, the "sodium wasting" is physiologic in situations of severe central nervous system injury (such as subarachnoid hemorrhage), because high-volume therapy in the form of albumin and saline is often administered to prevent cerebral vasospasm. Hence, the apparently excess urinary sodium levels are physiologic.

Table 16-12 Comparison of Diabetes Insipidus (DI) With Primary Polydipsia

Test	Normal	Complete CDI	Partial CDI	Nephrogenic DI	Primary polydipsia
Urine osmolality with H$_2$O deprivation,* mOsm/kg H$_2$O	>800	<300	300-800	<300-500	>500
Increase urinary osmolality with exogenous AVP,† mOsm/kg H$_2$O	300	Dramatic	10% increase	0	0
Plasma AVP levels after dehydration, pg/mL	>2	Undetectable	<1.5	>5	<5

AVP, arginine vasopressin; CDI, central diabetes insipidus; DI, diabetes insipidus.
*Water restricted until patient loses 3.5% of body weight or urine osmolality does not change >10% over 2 hours.
†Aqueous AVP (5 U subcutaneous) is given, and urine osmolality is reversed in 60 minutes.

DISORDERS OF POTASSIUM BALANCE

Potassium is predominantly an intracellular cation. Total body potassium is approximately equal to 4,200 mEq, with only 60 mEq in the total volume of extracellular fluid. Gastric fluid contains 5 to 10 mEq of potassium/L and diarrheal fluid, 10 to 100 mEq/L. The internal balance of potassium is regulated by endogenous factors such as acidemia, sodium, potassium, adenosine triphosphatase, insulin, catecholamines, and aldosterone. The external balance is regulated primarily by potassium excretion, which is regulated by urinary flow rate, aldosterone, antidiuretic hormone, and sodium delivery to the distal tubule.

Hypokalemia

Symptoms of hypokalemia include weakness, ileus, polyuria, and, sometimes, rhabdomyolysis. Hypokalemia also aggravates digoxin toxicity. A stepwise approach to the diagnosis of hypokalemia is given in Table 16-13 and outlined in Figure 16-4.

● Hypokalemia symptoms: weakness, ileus, and polyuria.

Therapy—If the serum level of potassium is less than 2 mEq/L, the total potassium deficit is equal to 1,000 mEq; if the serum level of potassium is between 2 and 4 mEq/L, a decrease of 0.3 is equivalent to a 100- to 500-mEq deficit, usually potassium chloride (diabetic ketoacidosis, potassium phosphate, potassium citrate, severe acidosis). Do not exceed 10

mEq of potassium chloride per hour intravenously without use of a central catheter and electrocardiographic monitoring. Dietary sodium restriction decreases the potassium-losing effects of diuretics.

Hyperkalemia

A stepwise approach to the diagnosis of hyperkalemia is given in Table 16-14 and outlined in Figure 16-5.

Therapy—Antagonize the membrane effects and redistribute (treat, in the following order, with calcium, sodium bicarbonate, insulin, resins, and finally dialysis). For chronic therapy, use loop diuretics, sodium bicarbonate, resins, fludrocortisone, or dialysis.

ACID-BASE DISORDERS

Clinically, it is absolutely critical that a stepwise approach to acid-base disorders be followed. The six steps listed in Table 16-15 should always be followed while interpreting an acid-base disorder.

Metabolic Acidosis

"Metabolic acidosis" is defined as a primary disturbance in which the retention of acid consumes endogenous alkali stores. This is reflected by a decrease in bicarbonate. The secondary response is increased ventilation, with a decrease in the partial pressure of carbon dioxide ($PaCO_2$). Metabolic acidosis can be caused by the overproduction of endogenous acid (diabetic ketoacidosis), loss of alkali stores (diarrhea or renal tubular acidosis), or failure of renal acid secretion or base resynthesis (renal failure).

● Metabolic acidosis: the primary disturbance is retention of acid or loss of bicarbonate.
● Secondary response: increased ventilation with decreased $PaCO_2$.

Some of the signs and symptoms of metabolic acidosis include fatigue, dyspnea, abdominal pain, vomiting, Kussmaul

---

Table 16-13 Stepwise Approach to the Diagnosis of Hypokalemia

1. Exclude redistribution—β-agonists (albuterol and terbutaline for asthma and ritodrine for labor), acute alkalosis, vitamin B_{12} therapy for pernicious anemia (especially if thrombocytopenic), barium carbonate
2. Determine whether potassium losses are renal or extrarenal—check urine potassium level on high sodium diet, is potassium > or < 20 mEq/d
3. If loss is extrarenal, determine cause (laxative screen)—usually diarrhea, enemas, laxative abuse, villous adenomas, ureterocolostomy
4. If loss is renal, determine if hypertensive or normotensive (diuretic screen)
5. If hypertensive, check plasma renin and aldosterone levels, includes primary aldosteronism or hyperplasia (glycyrrhizic acid in licorice, chewing tobacco), adrenal abnormalities
6. If normotensive, check plasma HCO_3 levels and urine chloride; the differential diagnosis includes renal tubular acidosis, vomiting, diuretic abuse, Bartter syndrome, magnesium deficiency

---

Table 16-14 Stepwise Approach to the Diagnosis of Hyperkalemia

1. Exclude pseudohyperkalemia—electrocardiogram is normal, heparinized plasma potassium is normal
   Hemolysis of clotted blood (0.3 increase), tourniquet ischemia, severe leukocytosis or thrombocytosis
2. Determine cause based on redistribution or excess total body potassium (see Fig. 16-5)

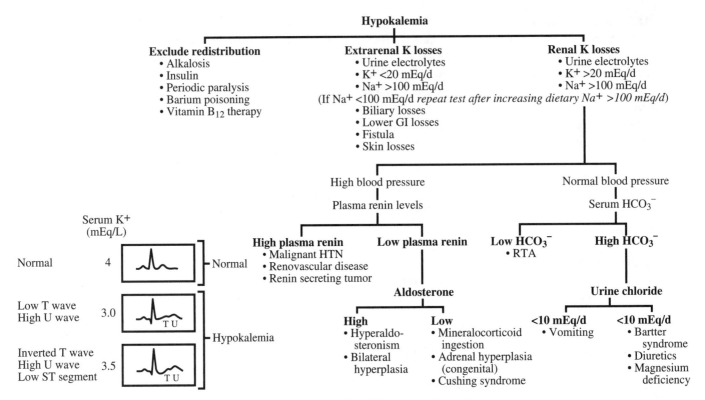

Fig. 16-4. Diagnosis of hypokalemia. GI, gastrointestinal; HTN, hypertension; RTA, renal tubular acidosis.

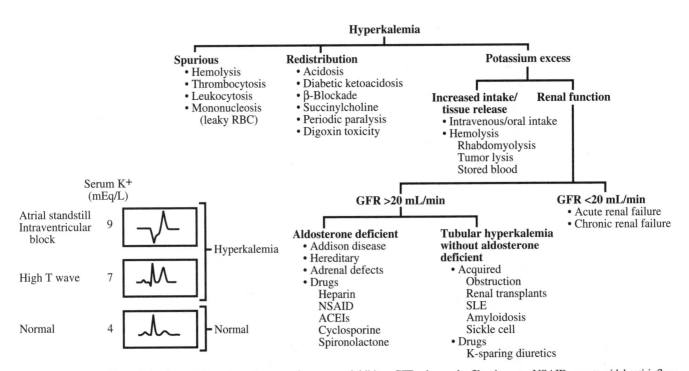

Fig. 16-5. Diagnosis of hyperkalemia. ACEI, angiotensin-converting enzyme inhibitor; GFR, glomerular filtration rate; NSAID, nonsteroidal anti-inflammatory drug; RBC, red blood cell; SLE, systemic lupus erythematosus.

Table 16-15 Six Steps for Interpreting Acid-Base Disorders

1. Note the clinical presentation
2. Always check the anion (hidden acidosis) and osmolar gaps if possible

 Normal anion gap Na − (HCO$_3$ + Cl) = 8 to 12

  Cations = Na, gammaglobulins, Ca, Mg, K

  Anions = Cl, HCO$_3$, albumin, PO$_4$, SO$_4$, organic compounds

 High anion gap >12—MUDPILES (see text)

 Low anion gap <8—bromism, paraproteinemia, hypercalcemia/magnesemia, lithium toxicity, severe hypernatremia, severe hypoalbuminemia

 Osmolar gap >10 "-ols"—meth**ol**, ethan**ol**, ethylene glyc**ol**, isopropyl alcoh**ol**, mannit**ol**

3. Use the Henderson equation to check the validity of the arterial blood gas values:

$$H^+ \ (nEq/L) = \frac{24 \times lungs \ (P_{CO_2})}{kidneys \ (HCO_3)}$$

pH	7.00	7.10	7.20	7.30	7.40	7.50	7.60	7.70
H$^+$	100	79	63	50	40	32	25	20

4. Is the pH high or low?
5. Is the primary disturbance metabolic (HCO$_3$) or respiratory (P$_{CO_2}$)?
6. Is it simple or mixed?

respiration, myocardial depression, hyperkalemia, leukemoid reaction, insulin resistance, and, when the pH is less than 7.1, arteriolar dilatation and hypotension.

Formulas for the predicted compensation of pure metabolic acidosis (which may take up to 24 hours) are listed in Table 16-16.

Metabolic acidoses are classified as either "normal anion gap" or "high anion gap." Normal anion gap acidosis (hyperchloremic metabolic acidosis) may be the result of excess bicarbonate losses from either gastrointestinal or renal sources. These may be discriminated by calculating a urinary net charge (or urine anion gap). The appropriate titration of acidity involves the excretion of excess hydrogen ions as ammonium ions. Electroneutrality is preserved by coupling ammonium ion to chloride, forming ammonium chloride. Hence, appropriate titration of renal acidity should result in high levels of urinary chloride. The urinary net charge (urinary anion gap) is calculated as follows:

Urinary net charge = [Na$^+$ (mEq/L) + K$^+$ (mEq/L)] − Cl$^-$ (mEq/L) (performed on random spot sample)

Urinary net charge (urine anion gap) should result in values of −8 or more negative values in situations of hyperchloremic metabolic acidosis with appropriate renal titration. A positive value or a result less negative than −8 suggests renal tubular disorders (renal tubular acidosis).

Also, normal anion gap metabolic acidosis may be defined in terms of the serum concentration of potassium.

Hypokalemic normal anion gap metabolic acidosis can be associated with diarrhea, ureteral diversion, or the use of carbonic anhydrase inhibitors such as acetazolamide. Renal tubular acidosis type I, or classic renal tubular acidosis, is also a cause. This is associated with nephrocalcinosis and osteomalacia. The causes of type I renal tubular acidosis include glue sniffing (toluene effect), amphotericin B, lithium, Sjögren syndrome, hypergammaglobulinemia, and sickle cell disease. Type II renal tubular acidosis is also a hypokalemic anion gap metabolic acidosis. In adults, it is often associated with other proximal tubule defects, including glycosuria, uricosuria, phosphaturia, and aminoaciduria (Fanconi syndrome). Causes of type II renal tubular acidosis include myeloma, cystinosis (*not* cystinuria), lead, tetracycline, and acetazolamide.

The causes of hyperkalemic normal anion gap metabolic acidosis include acid loads such as ammonium chloride, arginine chloride, lysine chloride, cholestyramine, total parenteral nutrition, hydrogen chloride, oral calcium chloride, obstructive uropathy, hypoaldosteronism (Addison disease), 21-hydroxylase deficiency, sulfur toxicity, and type IV renal tubular acidosis. Type IV renal tubular acidosis is associated with hyporenin and hypoaldosteronism, and it may be caused by diabetes mellitus, interstitial nephritis, spironolactone, amiloride, triamterene, or cyclosporine.

Patients in an intensive care unit often have normal anion gap acidosis because of "dilutional acidosis," which is due to large-volume saline resuscitation. The correction for hypoalbuminemia is necessary if the serum level of albumin is decreased. In this case, a correction factor of roughly 1.3 per gram of albumin below normal needs to be added to the anion gap calculation. Hence, in the intensive care unit or in cases of severe hypoalbuminemia, patients in whom hyperchloremic metabolic acidosis is suspected have high anion gap acidosis.

High anion gap metabolic acidosis has several causes. A common mnemonic is MUDPILES (**m**ethanol, **u**remia, **d**iabetic ketoacidosis, **p**araldehyde, **i**soniazid, **i**ron, **l**actic acidosis, **e**thanol, **e**thylene glycol, **s**alicylates). An anion gap should prompt calculation of an osmolar gap: measured osmolar gap − calculated osmolar gap (normally, the result is <10).

Calculated osmolar gap = Na$^+$ (mEq/L) × 2 + glucose/18 × BUN/2.8

Table 16-16 Formulas for the Predicted Compensation of Metabolic Acidosis and Alkalosis and Respiratory Acidosis and Alkalosis

---

Metabolic acidosis compensation

Pa_{CO_2} = last digits of pH

Pa_{CO_2} decreases by 1-1.3 mm Hg for each mEq decrease in bicarbonate

The Winter formula (favored formula)

$$Pa_{CO_2} = (1.5 \times HCO_3^-) + 8 \pm 2$$

Metabolic alkalosis compensation

$Pa_{CO_2} = 0.9 (HCO_3^-) + 15 \pm 5$

$Pa_{CO_2} = (HCO_3^-) + 15$

Pa_{CO_2} increases 6 mm Hg for each 10 mEq/L increase in HCO_3^-

Respiratory acidosis compensation

HCO_3^- increases by 1 mEq/L for each 10-mm Hg increase in Pa_{CO_2} (acute)

increases by 3 mEq/L for each 10-mm Hg increase in Pa_{CO_2} (chronic)

Increase* in H^+ concentration = $0.75 \times$ increase in Pa_{CO_2} (mm Hg) from normal (acute)

= $0.3 \times$ increase in Pa_{CO_2} (mm Hg) from normal (chronic)

Respiratory alkalosis compensation

HCO_3^- decreases by 2 mEq/L for each 10-mm Hg decrease in Pa_{CO_2} (acute)

decreases by 4 mEq/L for each 10-mm Hg decrease in Pa_{CO_2} (chronic)

Decrease† in H^+ concentration = $0.75 \times$ decrease in Pa_{CO_2} (mm Hg) from normal (acute)

= $0.2 \times$ decrease in Pa_{CO_2} (mm Hg) from normal (chronic)

---

*Delta 0.01 pH = delta 1 nEq [H^+].

†pH 7.40 = 40 nEq [H^+].

In chronic renal failure, the anion gap is usually less than 25. If the anion gap is greater than 25, one should think immediately of ingestion of a poison (generally a toxic alcohol: methanol, ethanol, ethylene glycol, and acetone). Isopropyl alcohol increases the osmolar gap but not the anion gap (acetone is not an anion).

- Dilutional acidosis often occurs in the intensive care unit.
- The anion gap needs to be corrected for hypoalbuminemia.
- In chronic renal failure, the anion gap usually is <25.
- An anion gap >25 should suggest ingestion of a poison.

Metabolic acidosis is generally corrected by treating the underlying disorder, but the bicarbonate deficit can be determined by the following formula:

Bicarbonate deficit = $0.2 \times$ body weight (kg) $\times$ (normal HCO_3 [i.e., 24] – measured HCO_3)

Therapy for ingestion of toxic alcohol (methanol or ethylene glycol) involves inhibiting the metabolism of the relatively nontoxic parent compound to its toxic metabolite. Alcohol dehydrogenase has a much higher affinity for ethanol than for ethylene glycol or methanol. If alcohol dehydrogenase can be occupied by ethanol or another steric

inhibitor (4-methylpyrazole), the ingested substance can be excreted or cleared in its native form, thereby preventing toxicity. This is the rationale for administering either ethanol or 4-methylpyrazole after the ingestion of ethylene glycol or methanol. Clinically, patients who have ingested these compounds often present with very high anion gaps with osmolar gaps (a sign that inhibition of alcohol dehydrogenase is still worthwhile) and complex acid-base disorders. After ensuring that metabolism has been blocked, it is necessary to facilitate the removal of these compounds. Although hemodialysis efficiently removes these compounds, supplemental ethanol is required during dialysis because this will be cleared also.

Aggressive supplementation of bicarbonate is rarely warranted except for cases of severe hemodynamic instability or pH levels less than 7.10. Treatment with bicarbonate may induce hypervolemia by the obligate infusion of sodium along with the bicarbonate (1 ampule of sodium bicarbonate = 50 mEq sodium and 50 mEq bicarbonate) and ultimately requires increased minute ventilation for appropriate buffering.

Metabolic Alkalosis

"Metabolic alkalosis" is defined as a primary disturbance in which plasma bicarbonate is increased. This can be caused by exogenous alkali, acid loss through the gastrointestinal tract or kidney, or loss of nonbicarbonate fluid causing contraction of remaining fluid around unchanged total body bicarbonate. The kidney must also be stimulated to sustain the high level of plasma bicarbonate. This can occur by contraction of extracellular fluid volume, hypercapnia, potassium depletion, steroid excess, hypercalcemia, or hypoparathyroidism. The secondary response is decreased ventilation with an increase in $PaCO_2$. The signs and symptoms of metabolic alkalosis include weakness, muscle cramps, hyperreflexia, alveolar hypoventilation, and arrhythmias.

- Metabolic alkalosis: the primary disturbance is increased plasma bicarbonate.
- The kidney must be stimulated to sustain the high level of plasma bicarbonate.
- Secondary response: decreased ventilation with increased $PaCO_2$.

The predicted compensation for pure renal metabolic alkalosis (which will take up to 24 hours) is presented in Table 16-16.

Metabolic alkalosis can then be classified in terms of the spot urine chloride and spot urinary potassium (Fig. 16-6).

Respiratory Acidosis

The ventilatory system is responsible for maintaining $PaCO_2$ within normal levels by adjustment of minute ventilation. Minute ventilation is controlled by tidal volume and respiratory rate. Normally, minute ventilation matches the production of carbon dioxide. When either carbon dioxide production exceeds the capacity of minute ventilation or respiratory physiology is deranged, carbon dioxide accumulates, causing respiratory acidosis.

Pathophysiologic derangements may be divided into two basic components: 1) the respiratory pump, which generates the forces necessary for airflow, and 2) the loads opposing such forces.

- Respiratory acidosis: the primary disturbance is increased $PaCO_2$.
- Compensation: renal retention of bicarbonate.
- Disorders caused by either a defect in the respiratory pump or an increase in the opposing load.

Abnormalities of the respiratory pump include acute and chronic depressed central drive (medications, anatomical lesions, inflammatory or infectious conditions, and metabolic derangements such as hypothyroidism); abnormal neuromuscular transmission (medications such as succinylcholine and aminoglycosides and metabolic causes [e.g., hypokalemia]); lesions of the nervous system (Guillain-Barré syndrome, myotonic dystrophy, multiple sclerosis, amyotrophic lateral sclerosis); and muscle dysfunction (fatigue, hypokalemia, hypophosphatemia, hyperkalemia, malnutrition, and myopathic disease such as polymyositis).

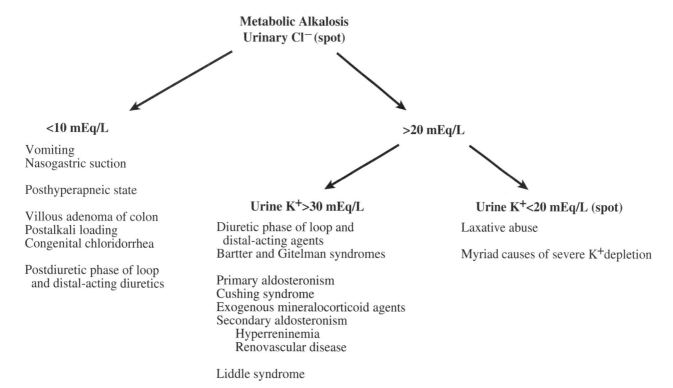

Fig. 16-6. Metabolic alkalosis classified according to spot urine chloride and spot urinary potassium.

Abnormalities of opposing forces (increased load) may be divided into lung stiffness (pneumonia, pulmonary edema, and acute respiratory distress syndrome), chest wall stiffness (flail chest, severe kyphoscoliosis, hemothorax, pneumothorax, obesity, peritoneal insufflation, peritoneal dialysis), increased ventilatory demand (pulmonary embolism, sepsis, overfeeding with carbohydrates), and high airflow resistance (upper and lower airway obstruction, laryngospasm, aspiration, bronchospasm, edema, secretions, chronic obstructive pulmonary disease).

Evaluation of suspected respiratory acidosis first requires determining simultaneously arterial blood gas and electrolyte panel values. Immediate steps should focus on securing a patent airway and providing adequate oxygenation. Historical clues, physical examination findings, assessment of hemodynamics and gas exchange, and radiologic studies help to identify the cause.

Expected compensation for both acute and chronic respiratory acidosis is shown in Table 16-16.

Respiratory Alkalosis

Respiratory alkalosis (primary hypocapnia) results from either increased minute ventilation or decreased carbon dioxide production or both.

- Respiratory alkalosis: the primary disturbance is a decrease in arterial $PaCO_2$.
- Compensation: renal excretion of bicarbonate (over a period of days).

Broadly, disorders that cause primary respiratory alkalosis include hypoxemia, stimulation of ventilatory centers in the central nervous system, various drugs, pregnancy, and sepsis (Table 16-17).

Therapy is directed at correcting the primary cause. Often, sedation or a rebreathing apparatus may be required while the primary disorder is being treated. Occasionally, it may be necessary to consider augmenting the renal excretion of bicarbonate. This can be achieved with acetazolamide (250-500 mg intravenously daily or every 12 hours). Rarely, supplemental hydrochloric acid may be needed in the form of 0.1 N hydrochloric acid. Expected metabolic compensation is indicated in Table 16-16.

- The primary causes of respiratory alkalosis include hypoxemia, stimulation of ventilatory centers in the central nervous system, pregnancy, sepsis, and liver failure.

Mixed Acid-Base Disorders

The coexistence of two primary acid-base disturbances (i.e., metabolic acidosis and metabolic alkalosis) or two disturbances separated by time (i.e., superimposed acute and chronic respiratory acidosis) or the presence of two forms of

Table 16-17   Disorders That Cause Primary Respiratory Alkalosis

Hypoxemia	Stimulation of chest receptors
Decreased FIO_2	Pneumonia
High altitude	Asthma
Laryngospasm	Pneumothorax
Cyanotic heart disease	ARDS
Severe circulatory failure	Pulmonary edema
Pneumonia	Pulmonary fibrosis
Pulmonary edema, embolism	Pulmonary embolism
CNS stimulation	Other
Anxiety	Mechanical ventilation (iatrogenic)
Pain	Pregnancy
Fever	Septicemia
Subarachnoid hemorrhage	Liver failure
Stroke	
Encephalitis	
Tumor	
Drugs or hormones	
Salicylates	
Xanthines	
Angiotensin II	
Catecholamines	
Progesterone	
Nicotine	

ARDS, acute respiratory distress syndrome; CNS, central nervous system; FIO_2, fraction of inspired oxygen.

primary disorder (i.e., metabolic acidosis with high anion gap and normal anion gap concomitantly) is commonly encountered in an acute care setting. These disorders can be differentiated and classified appropriately by applying the compensation formula, as guided by the medical history and physical examination findings. A cardinal tenet is that the pH deviates from normal toward the side of the primary acid-base derangement.

Delta Gap

In the presence of a high anion gap acidosis, the coexistence of nonanion gap acidosis or metabolic alkalosis may be detected by applying the delta gap formula. The premise of the delta gap is based on the accumulation of each excess anion above the normal anion gap accounting for the titration of one bicarbonate (mEq/L). Hence, a patient with an anion gap of 20 has an excess anion gap (assuming a normal anion gap of 12) of 8. Therefore, the expected bicarbonate level measured in the patient's serum should be 16 mEq/L. A bicarbonate level less than this would suggest a coexisting nonanion gap metabolic acidosis (additional loss of bicarbonate). A serum bicarbonate level that is considerably higher than 16 mEq/L suggests a preexisting metabolic alkalosis (previous excess levels of bicarbonate).

The delta gap is calculated as follows:

(Current anion gap − normal anion gap) + serum bicarbonate level (mEq/L) = 24

The delta gap should be calculated in all cases of increased anion gap metabolic acidosis.

Common complex mixed-acid base disorders include the following: 1) salicylate intoxication (high anion gap metabolic acidosis plus respiratory alkalosis), 2) chronic obstructive pulmonary disease with pneumonia (acute-on-chronic respiratory acidosis), 3) hyperemesis gravidarum (metabolic alkalosis superimposed on chronic respiratory alkalosis), 4) sepsis with liver failure (metabolic acidosis with respiratory alkalosis), and 5) metabolic acidosis, respiratory acidosis, metabolic alkalosis (acute ingestion of toxic alcohol, aspiration pneumonia, chronic vomiting).

- Bicarbonate <15 is usually caused partly by a metabolic acidosis.
- Bicarbonate >45 is usually caused partly by a metabolic alkalosis.
- Arterial blood gas values may be normal, but a high anion gap indicates a mixed metabolic alkalosis and acidosis.
- In metabolic acidosis and respiratory alkalosis, PCO_2 is lower than predicted for the acidosis.
- In metabolic alkalosis and respiratory acidosis, bicarbonate is higher than predicted for acidosis.
- In mixed metabolic and respiratory alkalosis, bicarbonate is higher and PCO_2 is lower than expected.
- Triple disorders: diabetic/alcoholic (vomiting) + (ketoacidosis/lactic acidosis) + (pneumonia).
- Calculating the delta gap will allow coexisting metabolic acid-base derangements to be differentiated.

PART IV
Stephen B. Erickson, M.D.

UROLITHIASIS

Epidemiology

The prevalence of urolithiasis in the United States is about 5%. The annual incidence is about 0.1%. Of patients with untreated urolithiasis, 30% to 75% have recurrence within 10 years. Urolithiasis is strongly familial and related to diet and urine volume. Many patients have a metabolic disorder that can be demonstrated with further testing, but conservative treatment with diet and increased fluid intake eliminates the stone-forming tendency in 70% of patients. For those in whom conservative therapy fails, medications are curative in another 25% (Fig. 16-7 and 16-8).

- Prevalence of urolithiasis in the United States: about 5%.
- It is strongly familial and related to diet and urine volume.

Risk Factors

Urine pH is important in the pathogenesis of some renal stones. Struvite and calcium phosphate stones tend to form in alkaline urine; uric acid and cystine stones form in acid urine. Some anatomical factors that predispose to urolithiasis include medullary sponge kidney, polycystic kidney disease, and chronic obstruction. Historic factors include fluid intake, dietary intake, history of urinary tract infection, drugs, family history, and other illnesses. Laboratory studies should include reviewing earlier radiographic findings; radiography of the kidneys, ureters, and bladder (KUB), and stone protocol computed tomography (CT) or excretory urography; stone analysis, serum calcium and phosphorus, urinalysis, urine culture, and 24-hour urinary volume; and calcium, potassium, phosphorus, citrate, creatinine, oxalate, sodium, magnesium, uric acid, and cystine analysis with the usual

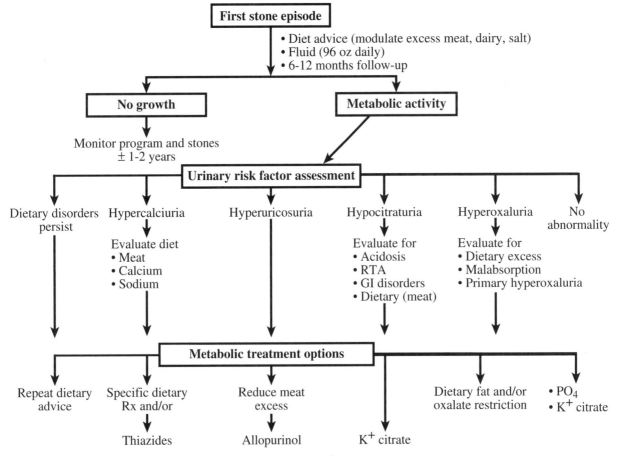

Fig. 16-7. Approach to therapy for idiopathic urolithiasis. GI, gastrointestinal; K^+, potassium; PO_4, phosphate; RTA, renal tubular acidosis; Rx, therapy. (Modified from MKSAP in the Subspecialty of Nephrology and Hypertension. Book 1 Syllabus and Questions, 1994. American College of Physicians. By permission.)

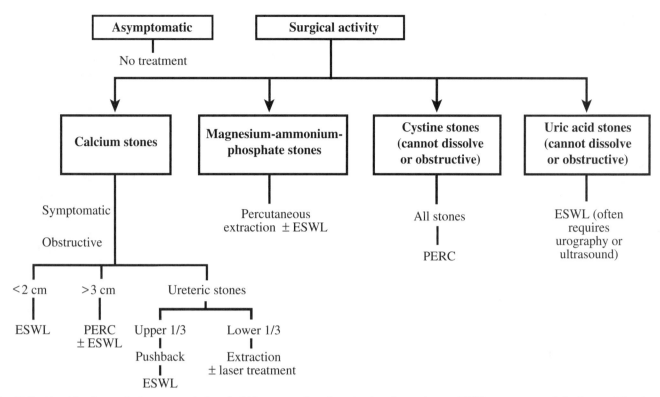

Fig. 16-8. Algorithm for surgical treatment choices for kidney stones based on size, location, and type. ESWL, extracorporeal shock-wave lithotripsy; PERC, percutaneous lithotripsy. (Modified from MKSAP in the Subspecialty of Nephrology and Hypertension. Book 1 Syllabus and Questions, 1994. American College of Physicians. By permission.)

diet. The characteristics of kidney stones are outlined in Table 16-18.

- Struvite and calcium phosphate stones form in alkaline urine.
- Uric acid and cystine stones form in acid urine.

Metabolic Activity

An evaluation of the disease activity to assess surgical activity and metabolic activity of patients who have urolithiasis is important because it dictates treatment. Surgical activity is manifested by unrelieved hydronephrosis, unrelieved pain, or infection (stones <5 mm should pass); metabolic activity is manifested by the formation of a new stone, growth of an existing stone, or passage of stones that did not previously exist within 1 year (Table 16-19).

Calcium Oxalate Stones

About 70% of all kidney stones are predominantly calcium oxalate. The risk factors for calcium oxalate stones are listed

Table 16-18   Kidney Stone Characteristics

Type of stone	Color	Shape	Frequency, %	Male:female	Urine pH
Calcium	White, tan, brown, black	Irregular	80	4:1	Oxalate—no effect Phosphate—relatively alkaline
Uric acid	Orange	Irregular or staghorn	10	10:1	Acid
Struvite	White, tan	Staghorn or irregular	10	1:10	Relatively alkaline
Cystine	Honey	Irregular or staghorn	1	1:1	Acid

From Year 1 Renal Systems Syllabus for Mayo Clinic College of Medicine 2003 and 2004.

Table 16-19 Stone Activity

Metabolic
 New stones, growth of old stones, or passage of
  previously unseen stones in the past year
Surgical
 Unrelenting pain, unrelenting obstruction, or
  infection-related stones

---

in Table 16-20. Causes include idiopathic hypercalciuria, other hypercalciuric states, hyperuricosuria, hyperoxaluria, and decreased excretion of inhibitors of crystallization. Conservative treatment includes correcting dietary stresses and increasing urine volume to more than 2.5 L per day. Medications include potassium citrate for hypocitraturia, neutral phosphates for idiopathic calcium urolithiasis (but not in cases of urinary tract infection or renal insufficiency), thiazides for hypercalciuria (sodium must be restricted for urine calcium to decrease 50%), and allopurinol for hyperuricosuria.

Primary hyperoxaluria is the most aggressive stone disease. Treatment includes fluids, pyridoxine (alters glycine metabolism, an oxalate precursor), neutral phosphates, or liver transplantation.

● Calcium oxalate stones are the most common type.
● Calcium oxalate stones have diverse causes, including various metabolic abnormalities and dietary habits.

Calcium Phosphate Stones

Stones that are predominantly calcium phosphate comprise approximately 10% of kidney stones. The formation of calcium phosphate stones indicates a relatively alkaline urine pH.

Table 16-20 Risk Factors for Calcium Oxalate Stone

Family history
Male gender
Hypercalciuria
Hyperoxaluria
Hyperuricosuria
Hypocitraturia
Low urine volume
Diet
 Low fluids
 Salt
 Protein
 Sugar

Patients who have primary hyperparathyroidism typically have predominantly calcium phosphate stones. Generally, parathyroid adenomas should be resected.

Renal tubular disorders associated with urolithiasis include distal renal tubular acidosis (type I). These patients can often make pure calcium phosphate stones. They may also have nephrocalcinosis, a urine pH that is always greater than 5.3, and a hyperchloremic hypokalemic normal anion gap acidosis with decreased urinary citrate (a stone inhibitor) and a high level of urinary calcium. The primary treatment is to correct the acidosis with alkali and to monitor urinary citrate excretion.

Other conditions associated with predominantly calcium phosphate stones are medullary sponge kidney and the use of absorbable alkalis such as Tums, Rolaids, Alka Seltzer, and baking soda.

● Calcium phosphate stones imply a relatively alkaline urine pH.

Uric Acid Stones

Uric acid stones account for about 10% of all cases of nephrolithiasis. Three-fourths of the patients with uric acid urolithiasis have normal levels of uric acid in the serum and urine. The urine is often very acidic. Of patients with primary gout, 25% form renal stones. An excess of dietary protein also can predispose to uric acid stones, as can any cause of chronic diarrhea because of decreased urine volume and hyperacidity. Uric acid urolithiasis is treated with preventive measures such as increased intake of fluid and decreased intake of protein. Alkalizing the urine to pH 6.5 not only helps prevent uric acid urolithiasis by treating the hyperaciduria, but it may also dissolve renal stones. Although allopurinol usually is not as effective as alkalizing very acidic urine, it may be helpful in patients with hyperuricosuria and in dissolving stones.

● 75% of uric acid stone formers have a persistently low urine pH.
● Renal stones form in 25% of patients with primary gout.
● Colectomy and ileostomy predispose to stones because the urine volume decreases and urine acidity increases.

Struvite Stones

Struvite stones comprise about 10% of all kidney stones. All patients who have magnesium ammonium phosphate stones are infected with urease-producing bacteria, which can include *Proteus*, *Staphylococcus*, *Klebsiella*, *Enterobacter*, and *Pseudomonas*, but only rarely *E. coli*. The urine pH of these patients is alkaline, sometimes greater than the maximum physiologically achievable pH of approximately 8.0. Also, many of these patients have an underlying stone-forming tendency. Staghorn stones are not uncommon, and 50% are bilateral. Treatment includes antibiotics given preoperatively and surgical removal of all stone material, followed by an attempt to identify the underlying stone-forming tendency, and treatment of this followed by bactericidal antibiotics for 6 to 12 months for suppression.

- All patients with magnesium ammonium phosphate stones are infected with urease-producing bacteria.
- Urine pH is very alkaline.
- 50% of staghorn stones are bilateral.
- Treatment: surgical removal, followed by bactericidal antibiotics for 6-12 months for suppression.

Cystine Stones

Only about 1% of kidney stone formers make cystine stones. Cystinuria is an autosomal recessive disorder in which homozygotes develop urolithiasis. Cystine crystalluria in routine urinalysis is diagnostic, as are positive findings on the nitroprusside test. These patients have a defect in the renal and intestinal absorption of cystine, ornithine, lysine, and arginine ("COLA"). The stones can be dissolved with urinary alkalization, cystine chelators such as tiopronin or penicillamine, and a high intake of fluid; however, urinary alkalization must be very intense, with urine pH maintained above 7.0. Adverse effects of penicillamine therapy include blood dyscrasias, gastrointestinal tract upset, membranous glomerulopathy, and a Goodpasture-like syndrome. Patients who have cystinuria often receive pyridoxine (25 mg daily) when taking penicillamine because cystine chelators indiscriminantly bind pyridoxine.

Inhibitors of Crystallization

Multiple inhibitors of calcium crystal formation and aggregation have been discovered. For the most part, they are not routinely measured except for citrate and magnesium. Others include Tamm-Horsfall protein, nephrocalcin, osteopontin, pyrophosphate, and glycosaminoglycans (GAGs). Calcium stone formers who have no metabolic abnormality may be treated successfully with potassium citrate, phosphate, or magnesium salts to prevent further stones.

Drug-Induced Stone Disease

Medications that increase the tendency for stone formation include those listed in Table 16-21.

Urolithiasis and Bowel Disease

Hyperoxaluria: patients must have an intact colon to absorb free oxalate. Free oxalate is overabsorbed when free fatty acids complex calcium and magnesium (the usual oxalate complexers). Fatty acids and bile acids also increase colonic permeability to oxalate. Other factors that increase oxalate

Table 16-21 Medications Increasing the Tendency for Stone Formation

Acetazolamide (calcium phosphate stones)
Calcium carbonate
Allopurinol (xanthine or oxypurinol stones)
Triamterene
Vitamin C (oxalate)
Vitamin D, nonthiazide diuretics, steroids (hypercalciuria)
Chemotherapy (increased urate load)
Indinavir/acyclovir
Topiramate
Ephedra/guaifenesin
Sulfonamides

supersaturation include decreased water absorption, decreased bicarbonate absorption, and decreased absorption of magnesium, phosphate, and pyrophosphate (inhibitors of crystallization). Treatment of this disorder includes correcting the underlying problem, increasing dietary calcium, decreasing dietary oxalate and fat, considering cholestyramine to bind bile acids, and increasing urine pH and inhibitors.

- The absorption of free oxalate requires an intact colon.

Patients with bowel disease, especially those without a colon, may also develop uric acid urolithiasis. Ileostomy patients are frequently susceptible to these stones because of the loss of alkali and water. Treatment includes alkali, fluids, and allopurinol.

- Patients with colectomies preferentially form uric acid stones.

TRANSPLANTATION

Transplantation is the treatment of choice for eligible patients who have end-stage renal disease (ESRD). More than 100,000 renal transplants have been performed; 11,000 are performed annually (8,000 cadaveric and 3,000 living-related). More than 35,000 potential recipients are awaiting a kidney transplant, and this number increases annually. The main limitation is the small number of donor kidneys. Lifetime immunosuppression is required. Recipients range in age from younger than 1 year to older than 50 years. The recipients must not have cancer. Infections (including those of the teeth, sinuses, and bladder) need to be eradicated, and cholecystectomy for gallstones should be performed. Living donors must be older than 18 years and without systemic or renal disease. Cadaveric donors must be older than 6 months and be without infection or malignancy (except for non-metastasizing brain cancer).

- Transplantation is the treatment of choice for eligible patients with ESRD.
- Lifetime immunosuppression is required.

Recurrent Allograft Renal Disease

Causes of recurrent allograft renal disease include membranoproliferative glomerulonephritis, membranous nephropathy, focal segmental glomerulosclerosis, diabetes mellitus, primary hyperoxaluria, hemolytic-uremic syndrome, and IgA (usually not clinically important).

Immunosuppression

Immunosuppressive agents include prednisone, which blocks the production of interleukin-1 by macrophages and the production of cytokine (complications include cataracts, psychoses, peptic ulcer disease, infection, diverticulitis, and aseptic necrosis); azathioprine, which inhibits the proliferation of activated T cells (bone marrow suppression, cholestasis, and infection; never treat with allopurinol); and cyclosporine, which inhibits the activation of helper T cells and the production of interleukin-2, -3, -4, and -5; it is hydrophobic and lipophilic, requiring bile acids for absorption (Fig. 16-9).

Cyclosporine levels are increased by ketoconazole, cimetidine, ranitidine, verapamil, diltiazem, and erythromycin. Cyclosporine levels are decreased by phenytoin, phenobarbital, ethambutol, sulfamethoxazole, ethanol, and cholestyramine.

The adverse effects of cyclosporine include gum hyperplasia, hyperkalemia, hypertension, hemolytic-uremic syndrome, and thrombotic thrombocytopenic purpura.

Graft Failure (Most Commonly Chronic Rejection)

Graft failure is commonly due to chronic rejection. Acute tubular necrosis occurs after transplantation in 20% to 50% of patients. The stages of rejection are hyperacute (hours), acute (days to years), and chronic (months to years). Recurrent disease occurs in 1% of patients. Surgical complications include renal artery stenosis, ureteral obstruction or leak, and lymphocele.

The medical complications of renal transplantation are diverse and complex. Opportunistic infections are the most common cause of death, and the next most common cause is cardiovascular problems. Other complications are hyperlipidemia, malignancy (1%, including skin cancer, sarcomas, lymphomas [Epstein-Barr virus-associated], and solid tumors), polycythemia, proximal/distal renal tubular acidosis, and kidney stones (1%).

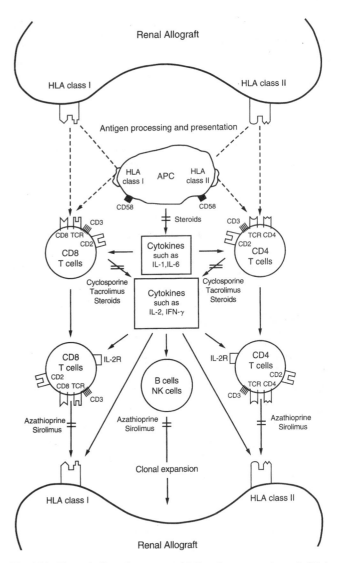

Fig. 16-9. The anti-allograft response. APC, antigen-presenting cell; HLA, human leukocyte antigen; IFN, interferon; IL, interleukin; IL-2R, IL-2 receptor; NK, natural killer; TCR, T-cell receptor. (From Suthanthiran M, Strom T: Renal transplantation. N Engl J Med 1994;331:365-376. By permission of Massachusetts Medical Society.)

PREGNANCY AND THE KIDNEY

Anatomical changes associated with pregnancy are renal enlargement (1 cm) and dilatation of the calyces, renal pelvis, and ureters. Physiologic changes include a 30% to 50% increase in glomerular filtration rate (GFR) and renal blood flow; a mean creatinine level of 0.5 μg/dL and a mean urea of 18 mg/dL (limits: creatinine 0.8 and urea 26); intermittent glycosuria independent of plasma glucose (<1 g per day); proteinuria but less than 300 mg per day (sometimes postural); aminoaciduria less than 2 g per day (most but not all amino acids); increased uric acid excretion; increased total body water (6-8 L) with osmostat resetting; 50% increase in plasma volume and cardiac output; and increased ureteral peristalsis. Bacterial growth in urine is promoted by the intermittent glycosuria and aminoaciduria. Hormonal effects include increased levels of renin, angiotensin II, aldosterone, cortisol, estrogens, prostaglandins (E_2, I_2), and progesterone; insensitivity to the pressor effects of norepinephrine and angiotensin II; and progesterone counteracting the kaliuretic effects of aldosterone.

Urinary Tract Infections

The prevalence of asymptomatic bacteriuria among pregnant women is similar to that among nonpregnant women, except it is higher in those with diabetes mellitus and sickle cell trait. Asymptomatic urinary tract infections progress to pyelonephritis or cystitis in 40% of pregnant women. Recommendations include screening for asymptomatic bacteriuria monthly and treatment of asymptomatic bacteriuria (10 to 14 days). Symptomatic urinary tract infections frequently relapse and reinfect. Pyelonephritis occurs in 1% to 2% of patients. Symptomatic urinary tract infections should be treated aggressively with antibiotics (ampicillin or cephalosporins) for 6 weeks. Follow-up cultures are recommended every 2 weeks. Sulfa drugs near term and tetracyclines (because of fetal bone and teeth development and maternal liver failure) are contraindicated.

Acute Renal Failure in Pregnancy

Conditions that predispose to acute renal failure in pregnancy are sepsis, severe preeclampsia (HELLP [hemolysis, elevated liver enzymes, and low platelet count] syndrome), abruptio placentae, intrauterine fetal death, uterine hemorrhage, and nephrotoxins. Cortical necrosis occurs in 10% to 30% of cases of gestational acute renal failure. Patients become anuric. Although patients may have partial recovery, they may have progression to ESRD years later. Postpartum hemolytic-uremic syndrome (exclude retained placenta) presents at 3 to 6 weeks post partum. This is characterized by acute oliguria, uremia, severe hypertension, and microangiopathic hemolytic anemia. There is disseminated intravascular coagulation and Schwartzman reaction, as in thrombotic thrombocytopenic purpura. Therapy includes dilatation and curettage, support, perhaps antiplatelet therapy (although the evidence is not strong), and plasma infusion. Acute renal failure and acute fatty liver of pregnancy (similar to hepatorenal syndrome) are caused by tetracyclines and possibly disseminated intravascular coagulation. Progressive hepatic failure has a mortality rate of 75%.

Parenchymal Renal Disease in Pregnancy

The outcome of lupus erythematosus depends on the clinical status prepartum. If the disease is quiescent 6 months before birth, 90% of the women have live births. If the disease is active prepartum, 50% have exacerbation and 35%

have fetal loss. If the disease is stable prepartum, 30% of the women have reversible exacerbations. Congenital heart block may occur in the newborn. Glucocorticoids and cytotoxic agents have been used without causing teratogenic effects.

Diabetes mellitus is associated with increased asymptomatic and symptomatic bacteriuria and increased preeclampsia. Proteinuria and hypertension may worsen, but renal function usually is stable.

Renal transplant recipients should postpone pregnancy for 2 years after transplantation. Increased preeclampsia, infection, and adrenal insufficiency have been reported. Pregnancy is usually uncomplicated if the creatinine level is less than 1.5 µg/dL, blood pressure is normal, and the woman is receiving low-dose immunosuppressive therapy. Preeclampsia occurs in 25% of women, prematurity in 7%, and loss of renal function in 7%. Nonobstetrical abdominal pain indicates allograft stone or infection.

EVALUATION OF KIDNEY FUNCTION

Urinalysis

The causes of urine discoloration are listed in Table 16-22.

Dysmorphic erythrocytes (>80%) in the urinary sediment indicate upper urinary tract bleeding. The Hansel stain identifies urine eosinophils.

Table 16-22 Causes of Urine Discoloration

Color	Cause
Dark yellow, brown	Bilirubin
Brown-black	Homogentisic acid (ochronosis)
	Melanin (melanoma)
	Metronidazole
	Methyldopa/levodopa
	Phenothiazine
Red	Beets
	Rifampin
	Porphyria
	Hemoglobinuria/myoglobinuria
	Phenazopyridine hydrochloride (Pyridium)
	Urates
Blue-green	Indomethacin
	Amitriptyline
Turbid white	Pyuria
	Chylous fistula
	Crystalluria

Normal urine osmolality is 40 to 1,200 mOsm/kg and the pH is 4 to 7.5. A pH less than 5.5 excludes renal tubular acidosis type I. A pH greater than 7 suggests infection. Acid urine is indicative of a high protein diet, acidosis, and potassium depletion. Alkaline urine is associated with a vegetarian diet, alkalosis (unless potassium-depleted), and urease-producing bacteria.

Glycosuria in the absence of hyperglycemia suggests proximal tubule dysfunction. Clearance of p-aminohippurate is a measure of renal blood flow. Orthoiodohippurate is used in renal scans. The clearance rates of inulin, iothalamate, diethylenetriamine pentaacetic acid (DTPA), and creatinine are measures of the GFR. The Cockgroft-Gault estimate formula for males is

$$GFR = \frac{(140 - age\ in\ years) \times (lean\ body\ weight\ in\ kg)}{S_{Cr} \times 72}$$

in which S_{Cr} is the serum level of creatinine. For females, the formula is males $\times 0.85$. Creatinine levels are increased independently of the GFR with ketoacidosis (acetoacetate), cefoxitin, cimetidine, trimethoprim, flucytosine, massive rhabdomyolysis, high intake of meat, and probenecid. Urea (blood urea nitrogen) levels are increased independently of the GFR with gastrointestinal tract bleeding, tissue trauma, glucocorticoids, and tetracyclines.

Renal Imaging

KUB-plain films magnify the kidneys 30%. Normal renal size is $3.5 \times$ the height of vertebra L2 (>11 cm). The left kidney is up to 1.5 cm longer than the right one. An enlarged kidney indicates obstruction, infiltration (amyloidosis, leukemia, diabetes mellitus), acute glomerulonephritis, acute tubulointerstitial nephropathy, renal vein thrombosis, or polycystic kidney disease. Calcifications are associated with stone, tuberculosis, aneurysms, and necrosis of the papillary tips.

Excretory urography provides a detailed definition of the collecting system and can be used to assess renal size and contour and to detect and locate calculi. It is also used to assess renal function qualitatively. Rapid sequence excretory urography is a poor screening test for renovascular hypertension. Complications include a large osmotic load (congestive heart failure) and reactions (5%). An iodine load may occur and is a consideration if the patient has hyperthyroidism.

Ultrasonography is used to measure renal size (>9 cm) and to screen for obstruction, but the results may be negative early in the course of obstruction. Ultrasonography can be used to characterize mass lesions (angiomyolipoma and solid vs. cystic) and to screen for polycystic kidney disease. Ultrasonography may be used to assess for renal vein thrombosis, that is, the presence or absence of blood flow. Ultrasonography is not a screening test for renal artery stenosis.

CT demonstrates calcification patterns. It is used to stage neoplasms and as an adjunct to determine the cause of obstruction (no contrast). CT assesses cysts, abscesses, and hematomas.

Magnetic resonance imaging may be used to identify adrenal hemorrhage and to assess a mass in patients sensitive to contrast dyes. Magnetic resonance angiography is a promising screening method for renal artery stenosis.

Arteriography and venography are used to evaluate arterial stenosis, aneurysm, fistulae, vasculitis, and mass lesions and to assess living-related donor transplants.

Gallium and indium scans are used to evaluate acute interstitial nephritis, abscess, pyelonephritis, lymphoma, and leukemia.

DTPA and hippuran renal scanning are useful in assessing a post-transplant kidney, obstruction (pre- and post-furosemide), and infarct (presence or absence of blood flow).

Nephrology Pharmacy Review
Michael A. Schwarz, PharmD

Drug (trade name)	Toxic/adverse effects	Comments
Hematopoietic agent		
Epoetin alfa (Epogen, Procrit)	Hypertension, local pain, iron deficiency, clotted IV access, headache	Administration, SQ or IV
	Rare seizures, CVA	
	Maximize iron stores before & during erythropoietin therapy	
Darbepoetin alfa (Aranesp)	Same as above	Long-acting erythropoietin SQ or IV once weekly
Iron products		
Ferric gluconate (Ferrlecit)	Hypersensitivity reaction, hypotension, flushing, cramps	Less incidence of anaphylaxis than with iron dextran
	Increased hypotension & flushing with rapid infusion	IV infusion route only
		Test dose recommended but not required
Iron dextran (InFeD, Dexferrum)	Hypersensitivity reaction/anaphylaxis, bronchospasm, local pain, tissue staining, arthralgias, flushing, hypotension, rare seizures	Administered by slow IV to avoid tissue discoloration or IM as a "z track"
	Risk decreased with dilution and slow infusion rate	Requires test dose before administration (0.25-0.5 mL slow IV or deep IM)
Iron sucrose (Venofer)	Hypotension, leg cramps, headache, nausea/vomiting, diarrhea, low risk of hypersensitivity reaction	Administration only by slow IV push or injection
		No test dose needed before administration
Oral iron products	GI upset, constipation, nausea/vomiting, dark stools	Typically not adequate to replete iron stores in hemodialysis patient
Ferrous fumarate (33% elemental)		Iron absorption decreased with co-administration of antacids, calcium products, phosphorus binders
Ferrous sulfate (20% elemental)		
Ferrous gluconate (11.6% elemental)		Absorption of quinolone antibiotics decreased with coadministration of iron
Phosphorus-binding agents		
Aluminum carbonate (Basaljel)	Risk of aluminum accumulation/toxicity: encephalopathy, microcytic anemia, osteomalacia, seizures, dementia	Best for short-term use
Aluminum hydroxide (Amphojel, ALternaGEL)		Does not cause hypercalcemia
		Aluminum absorption increased with coadministration of citrate salts (i.e., effervescent tablets), resulting in increased risk of toxicity
		Absorption of quinolone antibiotics & oral iron decrease

Nephrology Pharmacy Review (continued)

Drug (trade name)	Toxic/adverse effects	Comments
Phosphorus-binding agents (continued)		
Calcium acetate (PhosLo)	Hypercalcemia, GI upset, constipation	More potent phosphorus binder than calcium carbonate
		Absorption of quinolone antibiotics & oral iron decreased with coadministration of calcium products
		Absorption of digoxin may be decreased
Calcium carbonate (Tums, Os-Cal)	Same as above	Highest elemental calcium content
		Absorption of quinolone antibiotics & oral iron decreased with coadministration of calcium products
		Absorption of digoxin may be decreased
Sevelamer HCl (Renagel)	Nausea, vomiting, diarrhea, constipation, dyspepsia, hypertension, hypotension	Does not cause hypercalcemia or aluminum toxicity
		May decrease LDL & total serum cholesterol levels
		Absorption of other medications may be decreased with coadministration of sevelamer
Vitamin D analogues		
Calcitriol (Calcijex [IV], Rocaltrol [PO])	Hypercalcemia, hyperphosphatemia, constipation, nausea/vomiting, headache, confusion, somnolence, dry mouth, myalgia	Increases calcium & phosphorus absorption
		Suppresses PTH secretion
Paricalcitol (Zemplar)	Same as above	Less calcium & phosphorus absorption than calcitriol
Miscellaneous		
Vitamins (Nephrocaps, Nephro-Vite)	No important ones documented	Water-soluble vitamin replacement
Quinine sulfate (several)	Hypoglycemia, pancytopenia, tinnitus, nausea/vomiting, visual disturbances, headache, photosensitivity, rare DIC	Prevention or treatment of leg cramps
		Absorption of quinine may be decreased with coadministration of aluminum antacids
		Coadministration with digoxin may lead to increased digoxin levels
		Coadministration with warfarin may potentiate warfarin effects

CVA, cerebrovascular accident; DIC, disseminated intravascular coagulation; GI, gastrointestinal; IM, intramuscular; IV, intravenous; LDL, low-density lipoprotein; PO, by mouth; PTH, parathyroid hormone; SQ, subcutaneous.

Nephrology Pharmacy Review (continued)

Drugs Associated With Acid-Base Disorders

Metabolic acidosis	**Metabolic alkalosis**
Acetaminophen OD	Bicarbonate
Acetazolamide	Citrate salts (esp. with
Alcohol	abnormal renal function)
Amphetamine OD	Diuretics (loop and thiazides)
Cocaine	Phenolphthalein (laxative
Colchicine	abuse)
Cotrimoxazole	**Respiratory acidosis**
Ethylene glycol	Baclofen OD
Iron OD	Barbiturates
Isoniazid OD	Benzodiazepines
Mafenide	Opioids
Metformin	**Respiratory alkalosis**
Methanol	Salicylate OD (early)
Paraldehyde	
Propofol	
Salicylate OD (late)	
Spironolactone	

OD, overdose.

QUESTIONS

Multiple Choice (choose the one best answer)

1. A 65-year-old man loses weight and develops arthralgias and edema. Previously, the serum creatinine level was normal, but now it is 2.5 mg/dL, and urinalysis demonstrates marked proteinuria and red blood cell casts. Which diagnostic test is most likely to establish the diagnosis?
   a. Antinuclear antibody (ANA) cascade
   b. Antineutrophil cytoplasmic antibody (ANCA) serology
   c. Urine eosinophils
   d. Renal arteriography
   e. Erythrocyte sedimentation rate

2. A 25-year-old normotensive woman has had a history of type 1 diabetes mellitus since she was 20 years old. She had abrupt onset of proteinuria and edema 6 weeks ago. The serum creatinine level is 1 mg/dL, and 24-hour urine protein is 16 g. What is the most appropriate next step in the evaluation or management of this patient?
   a. Begin angiotensin-converting enzyme inhibitor (ACEI) therapy
   b. Limit dietary protein intake
   c. Perform renal biopsy
   d. Request serum protein electrophoresis
   e. Obtain an excretory urogram (intravenous pyelography)

3. A 55-year-old man presents to the emergency department with a history of acute hemoptysis and acute renal failure, with a serum creatinine level of 3.9 mg/dL. Urinalysis demonstrates proteinuria with red blood cell casts. Serum anti-GBM (glomerular basement membrane) antibodies are positive. Which therapy is most likely to improve this patient's clinical course?
   a. Plasmapheresis
   b. Oral prednisone and oral cyclophosphamide
   c. Intravenous corticosteroids
   d. Intravenous cyclophosphamide
   e. Plasmapheresis, intravenous corticosteroids, and oral cyclophosphamide

4. A 20-year-old man with progressive hearing loss presents for his college entrance physical examination and is found to have a mild increase in the serum level of creatinine to 2.0 mg/dL. The 24-hour urine protein is 2 g. What is the most likely diagnosis?
   a. Amyloidosis
   b. Poststreptococcal glomerulonephritis
   c. Alport syndrome

d. Interstitial nephritis
e. Familial IgA nephropathy

5. Within the last month, three local high school students have presented to your office with an increase in serum creatinine levels and active urine sediments with proteinuria and red blood cell casts. You clinically diagnose poststreptococcal glomerulonephritis and have detected increased antistreptolysin-O (ASO) titers associated with low serum total and C3 complements in each patient. What is the best choice for diagnosis and treatment of this patient?
   a. Short course of corticosteroids to limit the nephritis
   b. Confirmatory renal biopsy, followed by corticosteroid treatment
   c. Begin penicillin to limit the proteinuria and shorten the clinical course
   d. Supportive therapies to control edema, and begin penicillin to prevent new cases in the community
   e. None of the above

6. IgA nephropathy was diagnosed in a 31-year-old woman. She had presented with recurrent episodes of macroscopic hematuria and a blood pressure of 160/90 mm Hg. The serum creatinine level was 2.0 mg/dL and the 24-hour urine protein was 1.8 g. Which of the following is an unfavorable prognostic indicator in this patient with IgA nephropathy?
   a. Hypertension
   b. Serum creatinine >1.5 mg/dL
   c. Proteinuria >1 g
   d. Macroscopic hematuria
   e. a + b + c are correct

7. A 50-year-old man presents with anemia (hemoglobin 8.0 g/dL) and a serum creatinine of 1.8 mg/dL. Renal ultrasonography shows normal-size kidneys. Routine urinalysis shows 1-3 erythrocytes, 1-3 leukocytes, and 1+ protein. Renal biopsy specimen shows acute interstitial infiltrates with many broken casts in the tubules. Which one of the following is the most likely cause of this patient's condition?
   a. Acute interstitial nephritis
   b. Monoclonal gammopathy
   c. Use of nonsteroidal anti-inflammatory drugs (NSAIDs)
   d. Pyelonephritis
   e. Systemic vasculitis

8. A 65-year-old man who had an abdominal aortic aneurysm repair 48 hours earlier has had minimal urine output. His fluid balance is positive. Six hours ago, the surgical service

gave him 240 mg of furosemide intravenously but without a response. They have asked you to evaluate the patient's oliguria. *Previous medical history*: no known history of renal disease; status post femoral popliteal bypass and coronary artery bypass graft; history of hypertension for more than 5 years; and a history of smoking. *Physical examination*: blood pressure 110/52 mm Hg; pulse rate 62 beats/min; intubated and ventilated; lungs clear; cardiovascular grade: I/VI systolic ejection murmur; abdomen—wound and livedo reticularis of abdomen and flanks; extremities—2+ edema, cool lower extremities, livedo reticularis, and mottled toes bilaterally. *Laboratory values*: sodium 133 mEq/L (normal, 135-145), potassium 4.2 mEq/L (3.6-4.8), phosphorus 5.0 mg/dL (2.5-4.5), creatinine 2.4 mg/dL (0.8-1.2), and blood urea nitrogen (BUN) 48 mg/dL (6-21). *Urinalysis*: osmolality 300 mOsm/kg (300-800), pH 5.5, glucose 30 mg/dL (<20), protein 90 mg/dL, and protein/osmolality 3.11 (<0.12). *Urine microanalysis*: erythrocytes 21-30, leukocytes 11-20, epithelial cells 1-3, granular casts occasional, epithelial casts occasional, and eosinophils >5%. What is the most likely cause of the patient's acute renal failure?

a. Obstruction
b. Prerenal azotemia
c. Acute renal artery occlusion
d. Cholesterol emboli
e. Acute tubular necrosis from clamping the aorta during the surgical procedure

9. Eighteen hours later, the patient in question 8 is still oliguric. Now, the laboratory values are as follows: sodium 132 mEq/L (normal, 135-145), bicarbonate 17 mEq/L (22-29), potassium 6.2 mEq/L (3.6-4.8), creatinine 2.9 mg/dL (6-21), BUN 60 mg/dL (6-21), and phosphorus 5.8 mg/dL. Electrocardiography: normal sinus rhythm and peaked T waves. You recommend which of the following:

a. 1 Ampule of bicarbonate
b. Insulin infusion until a dialysis catheter is placed and hemodialysis can be initiated
c. Oral sodium polystyrene sulfonate (Kayexalate) and initiate urgent hemodialysis
d. Intravenous furosemide 250 mg and metolazone (Zaroxolyn) 5 mg
e. Sodium polystyrene sulfonate (Kayexalate) enema

10. A 68-year-old woman with a 15-year history of diabetes mellitus and a 10-year history of hypertension is evaluated for a 3-day history of persistent nausea, vomiting, and diarrhea. Two months ago, her treatment was changed

from a calcium channel blocker to an ACEI. At that time, her creatinine level was 1.2 mg/dL (normal, 0.6-0.8 mg/dL). Her current medications include atenolol 25 mg twice daily, enalapril (Vasotec) 10 mg twice daily, furosemide 20 mg daily, insulin 30 units NPH every morning, ibuprofen 1 every 6 hours, and calcium 1,000 mg per day. *Physical examination*: blood pressure 120/60 mm Hg; pulse rate 102 beats/min; lungs clear; cardiovascular grade: I/VI systolic ejection murmur; abdomen, obese; and extremities, 2+ edema. *Laboratory values*: glucose 182 mg/dL (normal, 70-100), sodium 137 mEq/L (135-145), potassium 5.0 mEq/L (3.6-4.8), bicarbonate 20 mEq/L (22-29), creatinine 3.8 mg/dL (0.6-0.8), BUN 87 mg/dL (6-21). *Urinalysis*: osmolality 520, pH 5.3, glucose 65 mg/dL (<25), protein/osmolality 2.83 (<0.12). *Microanalysis*: erythrocytes occasional <1, hyaline casts occasional, oval fat bodies occasional. The cause of the patient's acute renal failure is:

a. Prerenal azotemia
b. Diabetic nephropathy
c. Acute allergic interstitial nephritis
d. Hypertensive nephrosclerosis
e. Acute tubular necrosis

11. For the patient in question 10, the fractional excretion of sodium (FeNa) is <0.1% and urinary sodium is 9 mEq/specimen. Which of the following can cause a low FeNa?

a. Furosemide (Lasix) taken 2 hours before urinary sodium and serum sodium are determined
b. β-Blocker
c. Diabetic nephropathy
d. Proteinuria
e. ACEI

12. A 44-year-old man with known cirrhosis due to ethanol use is admitted to the intensive care unit after being found unconscious in his home. His toxicology screen is positive for ethanol. He is now oliguric and his creatinine level is increasing. *Physical examination*: blood pressure 90/50 mm Hg; pulse rate 88 beats/min; lungs clear; cardiovascular findings unremarkable; abdomen, ascites; and extremities, no edema. Which tests would best help differentiate between hepatorenal syndrome and intravascular volume depletion as the cause of his acute renal failure?

a. Urine output in response to intravenous fluid bolus
b. Spot urinary sodium
c. Serum sodium determination
d. Fractional excretion of sodium
e. Urinary sediment

13. An 80-year-old woman underwent coronary angiography 48 hours earlier. You are asked to evaluate her because of an acute decline in renal function.

Laboratory test	Before angiography	After angiography
Creatinine	1.0	2.0
BUN	20	40
Hemoglobin, g/dL	13.1 (12.2-14.8)	12.9
White blood cells, $\times 10^9$/L	6.2 (4.1-8.9)	7.0
% Eosinophils	0.09 (0-0.5) $\times 10^9$/L	0.09
Platelets, $\times 10^9$/L	320	150-450

Urine sediment was unremarkable. Physical examination demonstrates well-controlled blood pressure and normal fluid status. As you examine the patient, her family enters the room. They are anxious about her declining renal function and ask if her kidneys will recover. Your response is:
a. She has a 50% chance of needing short-term hemodialysis
b. Renal function will improve but not return to baseline
c. Renal function will return to normal
d. The increase in creatinine and BUN does not correlate with a decrease in the actual glomerular filtration rate (GFR)
e. Renal function will continue to deteriorate

14. A 72-year-old man is admitted to the hospital with a diagnosis of acute renal failure. He has a very complicated medical history that includes hypertension, poorly controlled benign prostatic hypertrophy, peripheral vascular disease, a left-sided stroke, and recurrent gastrointestinal tract bleeding. He reports decreased appetite, pruritus, restless legs, and fatigue. Laboratory tests performed in the emergency department are as follows: creatinine 4.8 mg/dL (normal, 0.8-1.2), BUN 89 mg/dL (6-21), sodium 130 mEq/L (135-145), potassium 4.0 mEq/L (3.6-4.8), bicarbonate 18 mEq/L (135-145), hemoglobin 9.2 g/dL (13.5-17.6), and phosphorus 5.8 mg/dL (2.5-4.5). You do not have access to previous creatinine levels or physician notes, but you are suspicious that this represents chronic kidney disease. Which test can confirm that the patient's renal dysfunction is not reversible?
a. FeNa
b. Urinalysis
c. Renal ultrasonography
d. Creatinine clearance
e. Parathyroid hormone

15. A 78-year-old woman is admitted from the skilled nursing facility for evaluation of profound mental status changes. According to the staff, she has been eating and drinking little and has had diarrhea. She has a history of frequent urinary tract infections. She takes hydrochlorothiazide for hypertension. Her blood pressure is 90/60 mm Hg, with a supine pulse of 102 beats/min. Her mucous membranes are dry. The laboratory values are as follows: sodium 112 mEq/L, potassium 4 mEq/L, chloride 99 mEq/L, bicarbonate 29 mEq/L, BUN 50 mg/dL, creatinine 1.9 mg/dL, and glucose 99 mg/dL. Serum osmolality is 250 mOsm/L, sensitive thyroid-stimulating hormone (sTSH) is normal, as is serum cortisol. Urine sodium is 18 mg/dL, and urine osmolality is 495 mOsm/L. What is the best treatment?
a. Free water restricted to less than 1.5 L per day
b. Calculate free water excess and infuse hypertonic saline to achieve this
c. Check serum lipids and serum protein electrophoresis
d. Calculate sodium deficit and infuse saline to appropriately correct the deficit
e. Order computed tomography of the chest to exclude malignancy

16. An 20-year-old thin, normotensive nursing student presents with weakness. The physical examination findings are normal except for calluses over her knuckles and severe dental caries. Electrolyte values are as follows: sodium 143 mEq/L, potassium 2.6 mEq/L, chloride 98 mEq/L, bicarbonate 34 mEq/L, BUN 20 mg/dL, and creatinine 0.7 mg/dL. Glucose is normal. Urine studies show an osmolality of 670 mOsm/L, with urinary sodium <10 mEq/L. What is the next step?
a. Diuretic screen
b. Check random renin and aldosterone levels
c. Schedule a captopril renal scan
d. Check urinary anion gap
e. Discuss your concerns about her eating habits and consider psychiatric evaluation

17. A 56-year-old man starts receiving an HMG-CoA (3-hydroxy-3-methylglutaryl coenzyme A) reductase inhibitor in addition to a bile acid sequestrant for severe hyperlipidemia. He has diabetic nephropathy and chronic renal failure. Approximately 1 week after initiation of treatment with the HMB-CoA reductase inhibitor, severe myalgias develop, as well as dyspnea and palpitations. The serum level of potassium is 7.6 mEq/L in the emergency department. What is the next best step?
a. Request that laboratory tests be repeated

b. Immediately administer 1 g calcium gluconate intravenously, followed by an infusion of insulin and dextrose, and consider infusing sodium bicarbonate

c. Immediately check the digoxin level

d. Determine the serum level of potassium

e. Consult nephrology

18. A 34-year-old man is discovered unconscious in his apartment by his neighbors. A jug containing yellowish liquid is found in his room. The following laboratory values were obtained in the emergency department: sodium 140 mEq/L, potassium 4.5 mEq/L, chloride 110 mEq/L, bicarbonate 8 mEq/L, BUN 38 mg/dL, and creatinine 1.9 mg/dL. Glucose is 100 mg/dL, pH 7.22, $PaCO_2$ 22 mm Hg, PaO_2 89 mm Hg. Plasma osmolality is 340 mOsm/L. The laboratory alerts you about the urinalysis result, namely the presence of crystals. The next intervention is:

a. Infuse an alcohol dehydrogenase competitive inhibitor

b. Begin preparation for emergent dialysis

c. Infuse isotonic bicarbonate

d. Order a toxin screen

e. Administer activated charcoal

19. A 28-year-old woman presents for evaluation of malaise, fatigue, and weakness. She also notes that she is always thirsty and her eyes are "gritty." The serum levels of electrolytes are as follows: sodium 135 mEq/L, potassium 1.2 mEq/L, chloride 118 mEq/L, bicarbonate 10 mEq/L, BUN 12 mg/dL, and creatinine 1.2 mg/dL. Arterial blood gases: pH 7.28 and $PaCO_2$ 25 mm Hg. Urinalysis shows pH 6.6, urinary sodium 35 mEq/L, potassium 20 mEq/L, and chloride 50 mEq/L. What should be your next recommendation?

a. Order diuretic screen

b. Order psychiatric consult

c. Order stool electrolytes

d. Begin sodium bicarbonate 450-mEq tablets, 2 taken orally 4 times daily

e. Initiate potassium repletion, followed by potassium citrate

20. A 69-year-old man hospitalized for cervical spine fusion has a long history of deforming rheumatoid arthritis. Postoperatively, his serum level of sodium is 122 mEq/L. Serum osmolality is 256 mOsm/L. Cortisol and sTSH are normal. He is asymptomatic and, postoperatively, has been receiving isotonic saline as resuscitation fluid. A urine sample has been sent for urinalysis. On the basis of which of the following urinalysis results would you recommend free water restriction alone?

a. Urine osmolality of 700 mOsm/L, with a spot urinary sodium of 15 mEq/L

b. Urine osmolality of 306 mOsm/L, with a spot urinary sodium of 100 mEq/L

c. Urine osmolality of 50 mOsm/L, with a spot urinary sodium <10 mEq/L

d. Urine osmolality of 800 mOsm/L, with a spot urinary sodium of 180 mEq/L

e. Urine osmolality of 399 mOsm/L, with a spot urinary sodium of 15 mEq/L

21. A 78-year-old woman who suffers from myriad complications of her diabetes has a long-standing history of severe degenerative joint disease treated with "arthritis pills." She comes to your office with her daugher, who feels that her mother has been more short of breath lately. The patient is reluctant to provide much history but states that she does not have dyspnea, although physical examination discloses tachypnea. The patient is troubled by a "funny noise in her ears." The electrolyte values are sodium 133 mEq/L, potassium 4.0 mEq/L, chloride 100 mEq/L, bicarbonate 16 mEq/L, BUN 55 mg/dL, and creatinine 2.0 mg/dL. Glucose is 135 mg/dL. The arterial blood gas values obtained the same morning at the hospital document pH 7.35, $PaCO_2$ 24 mm Hg, and PaO_2 98 mm Hg. What is your next intervention?

a. Order a toxin screen

b. Check urine for crystals

c. Consult nephrology for uremia

d. Request magnetic resonance imaging of the brain

e. Admit for forced diuresis and perhaps dialysis

22. A 42-year-old male commercial airline pilot comes to your office for advice. One of his copilots has been grounded indefinitely because of kidney stones. The pilot has a strong family history of kidney stones but does not know any details about his family members' stones. At this time, what is the best preventive treatment for your patient to avoid future kidney stones?

a. Allopurinol

b. Antibiotics

c. Citrate

d. Thiazides

e. Water

23. A 44-year-old man comes to your office for consultation about recurrent kidney stones. Pertinent history includes bariatric surgery 10 years ago. The kidney stones "began with a vengence" 2 years ago and have recurred on multiple occasions. However, no stone analysis has been performed. The patient's only medication is a multiple vitamin with extra vitamin C. Pertinent laboratory data include a 24-hour urine specimen with a volume of 2.0 L,

calcium 95 mg (normal, 25-300), citrate undetectable (>400 mg), oxalate 1.08 mmol (0.11-0.46), and uric acid 1,331 mg (<750). What is the root cause of this patient's stone formation?

a. Calcium hyperabsorption
b. Citrate deficiency
c. Oxalate hyperabsorption
d. Uric acid overexcretion
e. Urine volume deficit

24. A 46-year-old white woman comes for treatment of recurrent kidney stones. The patient has made 5 stones over the past 20 years, all of which had to be removed surgically. The first stone resulted in stenosis of the right ureter. Other possible risk factors include a strongly positive family history for kidney stones and recurrent urinary tract infections. Pertinent 24-hour urine data include undetectable urine citrate (normal, >400 mg), urine calcium 238 mg (100-250), urine oxalate 0.25 mmol (0.11-0.46), uric acid 473 mg (<750), and a sterile urine culture. In addition to dilating the ureteral stricture, what would be the most appropriate treatment to prevent further stone formation?

a. Allopurinol
b. Antibiotics
c. Citrate
d. Phosphates
e. Thiazides

25. A 59-year-old woman seeks consultation for a history of recurrent kidney stones. Pertinent history includes previous bariatric surgery, which has resulted in chronic diarrhea. She has recently been hospitalized for bilateral ureteral obstruction with sepsis. However, a kidney, ureter, and bladder (KUB) film taken at that time showed no evidence of stones. What type of kidney stone does this patient most likely make?

a. Calcium
b. Cystine
c. Oxalate
d. Struvite
e. Uric acid

26. A 22-year-old woman comes to your office shortly after being discharged from the hospital where she passed her first kidney stone. The history you elicit does not indicate any risk factors for stone formation. A 24-hour urine collection with the patient following her usual diet shows a urine volume of 653 mL, citrate excretion 803 mg (normal, >400), oxalate excretion 0.15 mmol (0.11-0.46), urine sodium excretion 109 mEq (40-200), calcium excretion 232 mg (100-250), and uric acid excretion 364 mg (<750). A KUB film shows no remaining stones. At this point, what is the best preventive treatment you can advise?

a. Allopurinol
b. Antibiotics
c. Citrate
d. Thiazides
e. Water

27. A 46-year-old man noted the onset of gross intermittent hematuria and intermittent right flank pain 8 months ago. He delayed medical treatment, fearing the discovery of a life-threatening illness. As the episodes of pain become more frequent and intense, he comes to your office for a diagnostic evaluation. A thorough evaluation discloses only a 2-cm radiopaque stone in the right renal pelvis. How would you classify this patient's kidney stone activity?

a. Metabolically active
b. Metabolically indeterminate
c. Metabolically inactive
d. Surgically indeterminate
e. Surgically inactive

28. A 56-year-old woman is evaluated for recurrent uric acid stones. Her brother has gout. According to previous medical records, multiple urinalyses over the years confirm she has a persistently low urine pH. A current 24-hour urine collection with the patient following her usual diet shows a volume of 1.1 L and uric acid excretion of 261 mg (normal, <750). What is the most appropriate treatment to prevent future stone recurrences?

a. Alkalization
b. Allopurinol
c. Antibiotics
d. Penicillamine
e. Thiazides

ANSWERS

1. Answer b.

This elderly patient presents with acute nephritis, and vasculitis is among the top diagnostic considerations. Although ANA serologic testing may be helpful in narrowing the diagnosis, the diagnostic test most likely to establish the correct diagnosis for eventual treatment is ANCA studies.

2. Answer c.

This 25-year-old insulin-dependent diabetic patient has had a short history of diabetes mellitus, and with the clinical course and abrupt onset of renal dysfunction, it is unlikely that diabetes mellitus is the principal cause of the nephrotic range proteinuria. Because of the atypical presentation of nephrotic syndrome in this diabetic woman, the most useful diagnostic step is to perform renal biopsy.

3. Answer e.

The patient presents with Goodpasture syndrome. Evidence clearly demonstrates that patients are most likely to have a response with the intravenous administration of corticosteroids, followed by cyclophosphamide taken orally, and a course of plasmapheresis. Plasmapheresis is most useful in limiting the pulmonary hemorrhage and its sequelae.

4. Answer c.

The most likely diagnosis is Alport syndrome, an X-linked dominantly inherited form of renal disease, in which there is high-frequency hearing loss and often slow progression to end-stage renal disease. The other forms of renal disease listed do not fit as well as Alport syndrome does with the patient's presentation.

5. Answer d.

Poststreptococcal glomerulonephritis generally is treated with supportive therapy alone to control blood pressure and edema. Penicillin therapy is helpful in preventing new cases, particularly in the setting of potential epidemics of these nephritogenic strains of infection.

6. Answer e.

Patients with IgA nephropathy who have hypertension, proteinuria >1 g/24 hours, and impaired renal function at presentation have a worse long-term prognosis than those who are normotensive, have proteinuria <1 g/24 hours, and have normal renal function. The presence or absence of macroscopic hematuria does not seem to be a reliable prognostic factor.

7. Answer b.

Interstitial cell infiltrates together with "broken casts" in the tubules are the classic renal biopsy finding in myeloma kidney.

Also, the degree of anemia is disproportional to the degree of renal failure and suggests suppression of erythropoiesis due to other causes than renal failure. NSAIDs can cause interstitial nephritis but not cast nephropathy.

8. Answer d.

Clues to an embolic event include the livedo reticularis on the patient's back and the mottled, ischemic-appearing toes. The urinalysis findings are consistent with a possible embolic event. In acute prerenal azotemia, urine osmolality would be higher and the BUN-to-creatinine ratio would be elevated. The physical examination results are not consistent with intravascular volume depletion. Prolonged ischemia during aortic clamping is a potential cause of acute tubular necrosis, and this would be the second best answer, but the livedo reticularis and mottled toes are evidence of a shower of cholesterol emboli. Peripheral eosinophilia is associated with cholesterol embolic events to the kidney. Often, urine eosinophils are noted.

9. Answer b.

This patient's acute renal failure has progressed. He now has hyperkalemia, with electrocardiographic changes necessitating immediate therapy. To prepare for hemodialysis, a dialysis central catheter needs to be inserted. While waiting for the initiation of hemodialysis, an infusion of insulin will help shift potassium and decrease serum potassium levels. Once dialysis has begun, the infusion of insulin can be discontinued. In this patient, diuretics would not help eliminate potassium because of his oligoanuria. A sodium polystyrene sulfonate enema does not have an immediate effect and may cause problems with fluid overload because of the sodium-potassium exchange. Bicarbonate should not be used in this case.

10. Answer a.

Diabetic nephropathy and hypertensive nephrosclerosis do not alone cause acute renal failure. They are more a chronic process. The urinalysis findings are not consistent with acute tubular necrosis because the kidney is unable to concentrate the urine. Urine osmolality is 520, and urine sediment only shows oval fat bodies and hyaline casts. Hyaline casts are seen in prerenal conditions and with either low urine volumes or concentrated urine. There are no epithelial cells. Also, the BUN-to-creatinine ratio is greater than 20. All these findings are consistent with a prerenal condition. Clinically, the patient's blood pressure is normal, but it may be on the low side considering that she has a long history of hypertension. Also, her pulse rate is increased despite treatment with a β-blocker. The urinalysis findings in acute allergic interstitial nephritis are quite different from those of this patient's urinalysis. Usually, there are leukocytes, erythrocytes, granular casts, and eosinophils.

Of note, with NSAIDs, an acute interstitial nephritis can occur without eosinophils being found in the urine.

11. Answer e.

The ACEI and NSAID can both cause a decrease in renal blood flow and an increased FeNa. Also, cholesterol emboli acutely can cause a decreased fractional excretion of sodium. A loop diuretic taken 2 hours before a determination of the FeNa even in a prerenal state will usually cause a high FeNa because of sodium wasting in the tubules. β-Blockers do not change renal blood flow. Chronic proteinuria does not cause an FeNa.

12. Answer a.

Hepatorenal syndrome presents with measures that are consistent with a prerenal state. The FeNa is less than 1% and spot urinary sodium is low. Urinary sediment is often benign or can be consistent with an acute tubular necrosis–type condition. Serum sodium can be low if the patient's total body fluid is overloaded. One of the best ways to distinguish between hepatorenal syndrome and intravascular volume depletion is an intravenous fluid bolus. If the patient's urine output increases, suspect intravascular volume depletion as the cause of the acute renal failure. In hepatorenal syndrome, fluid challenges do not result in an increase in urine output.

13. Answer c.

The patient has contrast-induced acute renal failure, which is usually reversible. Her creatinine before angiography was slightly increased, which does increase her risk of acute renal failure from the contrast dye load. The physical examination did not show evidence of cholesterol emboli. The urine sediment is not consistent with acute tubular necrosis or with cholesterol emboli because there are no urine eosinophils. Also, the patient did not have an increase in peripheral eosinophils, which is seen with cholesterol emboli. The syndrome of cholesterol embolic showers to the kidney involves a progressive worsening of renal failure and minimal to no renal recovery. The patient appears to have uncomplicated contrast-induced acute renal failure, and renal function should recover within 7 days. Often, these patients acutely have a low FeNa. To prevent toxicity, an infusion of normal saline using a low ionic contrast agent, limiting the dose of the contrast agent, and the use of acetylcysteine will prevent the toxicity.

14. Answer c.

In this case, renal ultrasonography can distinguish between reversible acute and irreversible chronic renal disease. The finding of atrophic kidneys on renal ultrasonography is consistent with a chronic disease process and minimal to no improvement in renal function. In these patients, urinalysis findings may be abnormal but would not help determine whether the condition was reversible. The FeNa, if low, would indicate a possible reversible component. In this patient, the FeNa would most likely be greater than 1% and it would not distinguish between acute intrinsic renal disease and chronic renal disease. Creatinine clearance would estimate the GFR, but would not reveal whether the GFR could be improved. Parathyroid hormone is not helpful in determining whether a decline in renal function is reversible.

15. Answer d.

This patient has a history and physical examination and laboratory findings consistent with volume contraction (sodium deficit). The calculation of sodium deficit is total body water (TBW) × (current serum sodium − desired serum sodium). TBW is calculated as 0.5 × weight in kilograms for females and 0.6 for males. Correction should not exceed 12 mEq/L per day.

16. Answer e.

This patient has bulemia. The physical findings are a hallmark of this disorder. The urinary studies do not suggest a diuretic effect. Occasionally, determination of urinary electrolyte values may need to be repeated if the patient is intermittently abusing diuretics.

17. Answer b.

He has rhabdomyolysis, from the combination of antihyperlipidemic agents, and severe hyperkalemia. This is an emergency situation and stabilizing cardiac conduction takes priority. In ambiguous situations of hyperkalemia, electrocardiography will often assist in determining the severity of the disorder.

18. Answer a.

This patient has ingested ethylene glycol, as evidenced by the high anion gap metabolic acidosis, the osmolar gap, and the crystalluria (calcium oxalate). The initial step is antagonism of further metabolism of the ethylene glycol to its toxic metabolite, glycolic acid. After forced diuresis, consider initiating dialysis.

19. Answer e.

The patient has sicca complex and renal tubular acidosis, likely due to Sjögren syndrome. This is shown by the inappropriate positive urinary net charge (urine anion gap). The urinary net charge is calculated by the addition of the urinary spot potassium and sodium minus the chloride. The urinary chloride should be in great abundance in the case of a normally functioning nephron due to the acid titration of hydrogen ions as ammonium ions. Because ammonium has a positive charge, ammonium is accompanied into the urine by chloride for electroneutrality. Repletion of potassium is foremost in these situations because a potential disastrous exacerbation of this patient's hypokalemia may occur with base supplementation alone. Note that diuretic abuse often leads to hypokalemia but not metabolic acidosis (except in the case of ingestion of a carbonic anhydrase inhibitor).

20. Answer b.

The criteria for syndrome of inappropriate antidiuresis are met in a euvolemic patient without thyroid or adrenal insufficiency and with urine that is less than maximally dilute in the appropriate clinical situation. Note that the urinary sodium only reflects intake in a euvolemic patient; this patient is euvolemic and receiving isotonic saline (0.9% "normal" saline), which contains 154 mEq of sodium per liter. A low urinary sodium should prompt an investigation for a possible depletion of the effective circulating volume, which may not always be clinically obvious.

21. Answer e.

The patient had a large salicylic acid bezoar in her gastric pyloris which was likely caused by her diabetic gastroparesis. A high anion gap metabolic acidosis with a respiratory alkalosis is noted on review of her laboratory values. The Winter formula [$PaCO_2 = (1.5 \times$ serum bicarbonate) $+ 8 \pm 2$], which is used in metabolic acidosis, demonstrates a respiratory alkalosis in this patient. The tinnitus is another clue to aspirin toxicity. Therapy is directed at discontinuation of aspirin exposure (esophagogastroduodenoscopy and removal in this patient) and forced diuresis or dialysis if signs of mental status changes are noted (with severely elevated aspirin levels).

22. Answer e.

It is inappropriate to advise a life-long medication for a person who may never form kidney stones, particularly when you do not know the type of stone you are trying to prevent. Water, however, is safe, inexpensive, readily available, and reasonably effective when ingested in large quantity for preventing all types of kidney stones.

23. Answer c.

Although the 24-hour urine specimen shows the absence of citrate and excessive uric acid, the extreme hyperoxaluria in the presence of bariatric surgery strongly suggests enteric hyperoxaluria. Thus, the root cause is oxalate hyperabsorption.

24. Answer c.

The most obvious treatable risk factor for stone formation in this case is "c," citrate therapy for the patient's undetectable urinary citrate excretion. The sterile urine culture suggests that the patient does not have chronically infected stones. Her normal excretion of calcium and uric acid should discourage the use of allopurinol and thiazides. Phosphate treatment is appropriate only in the absence of metabolic risk factors.

25. Answer e.

Chronic diarrheal illnesses tend to produce either calcium oxalate or uric acid stones. However, the failure of a KUB film to visualize the obstructing ureteral stones at the time ultrasonography showed bilateral obstruction strongly suggests that these stones were not calcium oxalate and must therefore have been uric acid, which is radiolucent on plain abdominal films.

26. Answer e.

The metabolic activity of this patient's stone formation is indeterminate. Additionally, it is her first stone. You have no definable risk factors to treat other than a low urine volume. In this situation, water is the appropriate recommendation.

27. Answer b.

The severe and recurrent right flank pain in combination with the large size of this stone describes surgical activity. However, this answer is not one of your options. The metabolic activity in this case is indeterminate without previous radiographs to compare whether the right renal stone is actively growing or not.

28. Answer a.

Alkalization is the most appropriate therapy because of the patient's long history of low urine pH. Although allopurinol would reduce the excretion of uric acid, it is already at the low end of the normal range and allopurinol would be minimally helpful.

CHAPTER 17

NEUROLOGY

Eduardo E. Benarroch, M.D.
Robert D. Brown, Jr., M.D.
Frank A. Rubino, M.D.

PART I—GENERAL PRINCIPLES FOR INTERPRETING NEUROLOGIC SYMPTOMS

INTRODUCTION

Neurologic disorders are commonly encountered in general clinical practice. Because of the increasing number of older people throughout the world, cerebrovascular disorders, dementias, and Parkinson disease are becoming more prevalent. Understanding a patient with neurologic disease depends on localizing the problem on the basis of the medical history and examination findings, considering a differential diagnosis, and correlating the clinical findings with abnormalities found on diagnostic testing.

- About 10% of patients of primary care physicians in the United States have neurologic disorders.
- About 25% of inpatients have a neurologic disorder as a primary or secondary problem.
- Primary care physicians should have a good working knowledge of common and emergency neurologic problems.

NEUROLOGIC SIGNS AND SYMPTOMS

General Categories

Neurologic signs and symptoms can be subdivided into four general categories.

- Ill-defined, nonspecific, nonanatomical, and nonphysiologic regional or generalized symptoms.
- Diffuse cerebral symptoms.
- Positive focal symptoms (hyperactivity).
- Negative focal symptoms (loss of function).

Ill-Defined Symptoms

These include such things as ill-defined dizziness, diffuse or unusual regional pain, diffuse and unusual numbness, vague memory problems, and unusual gait. Generally, no serious underlying problem is identified, especially if the symptoms are long-standing. Many patients have a serious underlying psychopathologic disorder, but often the patient either does not recognize this or denies it. However, remember that a psychiatric diagnosis should be made on the basis of positive psychologic factors and not because the physical examination and laboratory findings are normal.

- With ill-defined symptoms, no serious underlying problem is identified in most patients.
- Many of these patients have an underlying psychopathologic condition.
- Establish a psychiatric diagnosis on the basis of positive psychologic factors, not because the physical examination and laboratory findings are normal.

Diffuse Cerebral Symptoms

Diffuse cognitive problems occur in dementia and acute confusional states. However, a common diffuse symptom is syncope or presyncope, which usually implies diffuse and not focal cerebral ischemia. Vasovagal syncope is the major culprit, especially in the young. Syncope is not a transient ischemic attack (TIA). Most causes of syncope are systemic, not neurologic, problems. With primary autonomic dysfunction, other neurologic signs and symptoms usually help make the diagnosis (e.g., multiple system atrophy, diabetic or amyloid autonomic neuropathy).

- Syncope or presyncope implies diffuse, not focal, cerebral ischemia.
- Syncope is not a TIA.
- Systemic, not neurologic, problems usually cause syncope.

Positive Phenomena

An example of a positive sensory phenomenon is marching paresthesia, and an example of a positive motor phenomenon is tonic or clonic movement. Lights, flashes, sparkles, and formed images are examples of positive visual phenomena. An example of a positive language phenomenon is unusual vocalization. Positive central phenomena usually indicate seizures or migraine accompaniments. Positive peripheral phenomena occur with nerve damage and repair.

Negative Phenomena

Negative phenomena usually indicate damage to a specific central or peripheral area. TIAs and strokes usually produce negative phenomena; if there is more than one symptom, all the symptoms tend to appear at the same time. Migraine syndromes may have positive and negative phenomena; if there is more than one symptom, the symptoms tend to come on one after another and "build up."

- TIAs and strokes produce negative phenomena.
- Migraine syndromes have positive and negative phenomena.

Localization

The examination findings may be combined with the neurologic history to clarify the localization of the disorder to the following four levels: supratentorial (cerebral cortex and subcortical regions, including the basal ganglia, hypothalamus, and thalamus); posterior fossa (cerebellum, brainstem, and cranial nerves); spinal cord (including extramedullary, intramedullary, cauda equina, and conus medullaris lesions); and peripheral. Peripheral lesions may be localized further from proximal to distal: radiculopathy, plexopathy, peripheral neuropathy, neuromuscular junction, and muscle. However, many disorders are multifocal. After the level has been determined, it should be considered on the basis of the signs and symptoms whether the lesion is on the right side or the left side or whether it is bilateral. It then is possible to consider a differential diagnosis for the lesion and to outline the diagnostic procedures, therapeutic options, and patient education.

Findings in the Elderly

Examination of healthy elderly persons may show signs that cannot be considered pathologic when present in isolation:

- Decreased acuity of the special senses—olfaction, audition, and vision.
- Decrease in upward gaze, visual pursuit, and saccadic function.
- Abnormal gait with reduced arm swinging, shorter steps, and slow walking speed.
- Difficulty with balance, with wider base and unsteady turns.
- Decreased vibratory sensation in the legs.
- Decreased pupillary response to light.
- Atrophy of the small muscles of the hand.
- Decreased ankle reflexes.

In addition, some neurodiagnostic studies may appear abnormal in most healthy elderly people, including spondylitic abnormalities visible on plain cervical and lumbar radiographs and on magnetic resonance imaging (MRI) and computed tomography (CT) of the same areas, white matter changes on MRI, mild focal slowing on electroencephalography (EEG), and slowing of nerve conduction velocities on electrophysiologic testing.

- Most healthy elderly people have spondylitic abnormalities visible on plain cervical and lumbar radiographs and on MRI of the same areas.

GENERAL PRINCIPLES OF NEUROLOGIC DIAGNOSTIC TESTING

CT and MRI

Vascular Diseases

CT is a good initial test for evaluating suspected TIA or stroke and is superior to MRI for identifying acute hemorrhage in brain parenchyma or the subarachnoid space (Table 17-1). However, gradient echo MRI is now capable of identifying acute blood as well as old hemosiderin. Subacute and chronic intracerebral hemorrhages are better defined by MRI, which is usually the first neuroimaging test to show abnormalities during the evolution of an ischemic cerebral infarct. CT (even with contrast enhancement) often gives equivocal or negative results in the first 24 to 48 hours after an ischemic cerebral infarct. In subacute and chronic stages of an ischemic cerebral infarct, MRI and CT provide equivalent information. Vasculitic lesions or microinfarcts, as in systemic lupus erythematosus, are often seen on MRI but missed on CT.

Table 17-1 Comparison of Computed Tomography (CT) and Magnetic Resonance Imaging (MRI) for Neurologic Imaging

CT preferred	MRI preferred
Evaluation of suspected acute hemorrhage	Evaluation of subacute and chronic hemorrhage
Evaluation of skull fractures	Evaluation of ischemic stroke
Evaluation of meningiomas	Evaluation of posterior fossa and brainstem tumors and lesions
	Diagnosis of multiple sclerosis
	Evaluation of the spinal cord

Magnetic resonance angiography (MRA) is not invasive and has replaced standard angiography for many indications. It is quite sensitive in defining the degree of stenosis in the carotid or vertebrobasilar system. However, MRA does not adequately evaluate more distal intracranial arteries, and arteriography is required for this indication. MRA is also used as a screening study for aneurysms. Arteriography is needed to examine the anatomical details of aneurysms or vascular malformations. With diffusion and perfusion MRI scanning, cerebral infarction or ischemia can be delineated early after the onset of symptoms, usually before CT shows any abnormality.

- For evaluating acute hemorrhage in the brain and subarachnoid space, CT is better than standard MRI. However, gradient echo MRI is now capable of identifying acute blood.
- During an evolving ischemic cerebral infarct, MRI is better than CT.
- CT with contrast is not useful during the first 24-48 hours after an ischemic cerebral infarct.
- For evaluating subacute and chronic stages of an ischemic cerebral infarct, CT and MRI are equivalent.

Trauma

MRI is competitive with but not comparable to CT for assessing the brain after craniocerebral trauma. During the first 1 to 3 days after injury, CT is preferable because the examination time is shorter and hemorrhage at this time is demonstrated more reliably by CT. Standard radiographic examination or CT is necessary to evaluate skull fractures because bone cortex is not visualized with MRI.

CT is highly dependable for demonstrating subdural hematomas, which are also visualized with MRI. Coronal MRI sections are usually best for visualizing the size, shape, location, and extent of subdural hematomas.

- For the first 1-3 days after trauma, CT is best because it is more reliable for demonstrating hemorrhage.
- Radiography or CT is needed to evaluate skull fractures.
- CT is dependable for showing subdural hematomas.

Intracranial Tumors

A wide spectrum of intracranial tumors is visualized with MRI and CT. MRI often shows more extensive involvement than CT, especially in low-grade gliomas or metastasis. CT with contrast and MRI with gadolinium are both excellent for detecting meningiomas. MRI is far superior to CT for identifying all types of posterior fossa tumors. It is the study of choice for identifying brainstem gliomas.

- MRI is superior to CT for identifying posterior fossa tumors and brainstem gliomas.

White Matter Lesions

MRI is superior to CT in detecting abnormalities of the white matter. MRI is far superior to CT for identifying multiple sclerosis lesions and for assessing patients who have isolated optic neuritis. MRI shows that Binswanger disease may be a common cause of adult-onset dementia (along with multi-infarct dementia). However, white matter changes in the elderly must be interpreted carefully because MRI shows changes in the white matter of most normal elderly persons.

- MRI shows changes in the white matter of most normal elderly persons.

Cervical Cord

A wide spectrum of lesions at the cervicomedullary junction and in the cervical spinal cord can be seen clearly with MRI because direct sagittal and coronal sections can be made with this imaging method. Thus, MRI is the study of choice for assessing the cervicomedullary junction and cervical spinal cord. Generally, MRI is better than CT for identifying intramedullary and extramedullary lesions of the spinal cord.

- MRI is better than CT for assessing the cervicomedullary junction and cervical spinal cord and intra- and extramedullary cord tumors.

Dementia

In assessing dementia, either CT or MRI can demonstrate remedial lesions. MRI shows more lesions than CT in multi-infarct dementia.

Disk Disease

Protruding disks are well visualized on MRI sagittal sections, which show the relation of the disk to the spine and nerve roots. MRI is equal to CT myelography for evaluating herniated disks at cervical and thoracic levels, but at the lumbar level, MRI is better than CT myelography. In spinal stenosis, MRI and CT are roughly equivalent and less invasive than myelography.

- MRI sagittal sections show protruding disks.
- For cervical and thoracic herniated disks, MRI is equal to CT myelography, but better at the lumbar level.

Electromyographic Nerve Conduction Velocity Studies

Electromyographic (EMG) studies should be performed by experts familiar with the intricacies of the procedure and who know its value and limitations. EMG tests are excellent for eliciting motor unit problems and, thus, are valuable for identifying diseases of the anterior horn cell, nerve root, peripheral nerve, neuromuscular junction, and muscle. By helping to localize and to better define further diagnostic studies, EMG tests are an extension of the neurologic examination.

- EMG should be performed by experts.
- EMG is valuable for identifying motor unit problems—anterior horn cell, nerve root, neuromuscular junction, and muscle.

EEG

EEG is used mainly to study seizure disorders, but the EEG is specific in only a few forms of epilepsy, such as typical absence epilepsy. Seizure disorder is a clinical diagnosis and not an EEG diagnosis, and a normal EEG does *not* rule out a seizure disorder. EEG has many nonspecific patterns that should not be overinterpreted.

Ambulatory EEG is available for detecting frequent unusual spells. EEG telemetry with videomonitoring is helpful in defining epileptic surgical candidates, nonepileptic spells (pseudoseizures), and unusual seizures. EEG is imperative in diagnosing nonconvulsive status epilepticus.

- The EEG is specific in only a few forms of epilepsy, including typical absence epilepsy.
- Seizure disorder is a clinical, not an EEG, diagnosis.
- A normal EEG does not rule out seizure disorder.
- EEG telemetry is helpful in defining epileptic surgical candidates, nonepileptic spells, and unusual seizures.

EEG is valuable for evaluating various encephalopathies. Many drugs cause an unusual fast pattern, and most metabolic encephalopathies cause a diffuse slow or triphasic pattern. Diffuse slow patterns are seen also in diffuse cerebral disease (Alzheimer disease). Unusual high-amplitude sharp wave activity helps define Creutzfeldt-Jakob disease and subacute sclerosing panencephalitis. EEG is often valuable in diagnosing infectious encephalopathies (herpes simplex encephalitis).

EEG is essential for diagnosing various sleep disorders and is an *adjuvant* tool for diagnosing brain death. Recall that brain death is a clinical diagnosis. EEG may be used as a monitoring device in surgery (e.g., during carotid endarterectomy).

At 6 hours or more after a hypoxic insult, the EEG indicates the likelihood of neurologic recovery. Poor outcome is seen with "alpha" coma, burst suppression, periodic patterns, and electrocerebral silence.

- EEG is valuable in diagnosing infectious encephalopathies (herpes simplex encephalitis).
- EEG is an adjuvant tool for diagnosing brain death.
- Brain death is a clinical diagnosis.

Evoked Potentials

Evoked potentials indicate the intactness of various pathways: visual evoked potentials, somatosensory evoked potentials, brainstem auditory evoked potentials, and motor evoked potentials. These tests generally are not practical clinical tools. They are excellent monitoring devices for spinal surgery and posterior fossa surgery (monitoring cranial nerve function intraoperatively), and they may be useful for substantiating nonorganic disease, for example, hysterical paraplegia or hysterical blindness.

- Evoked potentials may be useful for substantiating nonorganic disease (hysterical paraplegia, hysterical blindness).

Lumbar Puncture and Cerebrospinal Fluid Analysis

Perform lumbar puncture only after a thorough clinical evaluation and after serious consideration of the potential value versus the hazards of the procedure.

Indications for Lumbar Puncture

Urgent lumbar puncture is performed for suspected acute meningitis, encephalitis, or subarachnoid hemorrhage (unless preceding CT findings indicate otherwise) and for fever (even without meningeal signs) in infancy, acute confusional states, and neurologic manifestations in immunocompromised patients. Another indication for lumbar puncture is unexplained dementia.

Multiple sclerosis is an indication for lumbar puncture. If the cerebrospinal fluid (CSF) cell count is greater than 100, look for another disease (e.g., sarcoidosis). Although IgG synthesis is increased in multiple sclerosis, this finding is nonspecific. The demonstration of oligoclonal bands is useful, but they also occur in other inflammatory diseases of the central nervous system (CNS).

Lumbar puncture is used to assess CSF pressure. High pressure occurs with pseudotumor cerebri and low pressure with positional headache and CSF leak.

Lumbar puncture is indicated in cases of infectious disease, including acquired immunodeficiency syndrome (AIDS), Lyme disease, and any suspected acute, subacute, or chronic infection (viral, bacterial, or fungal). It also is indicated in cases of paraneoplastic syndromes: Hu and Yo antibodies to cerebellar Purkinje cells in paraneoplastic cerebellar degeneration, neuronal antinuclear antibodies in subacute sensory neuronopathy and sensory neuropathy, and retinal antibodies in paraneoplastic retinopathy.

Other indications for lumbar puncture are meningeal carcinomatosis, non-Hodgkin lymphoma, certain neuropathies (Guillain-Barré syndrome, acute inflammatory demyelinating polyneuropathy, and chronic inflammatory demyelinating polyradiculopathy [CIDP]), and gliomatosis cerebri.

There is no difference in headache frequency after immediate mobilization or after 4 hours of bed rest following lumbar puncture. Spinal headache depends on the size of the needle used and the leakage of CSF through a dural rent.

Contraindications for Lumbar Puncture

Suppuration in the skin and deeper tissues overlying the spinal canal and anticoagulation therapy or bleeding diathesis are contraindications for lumbar puncture. A minimum of 1 or 2 hours should elapse between lumbar puncture and initiation of heparin therapy. If the platelet count is less than 20×10^9/L, transfuse platelets before performing a lumbar puncture.

Increased intracranial pressure is a contraindication. Lumbar puncture is dangerous when papilledema is due to an intracranial mass, but it is safe (and has been used therapeutically) in pseudotumor cerebri. In complete spinal block, lumbar puncture may aggravate the signs of spinal cord disease.

- Perform lumbar puncture only after a thorough clinical evaluation.
- Increased IgG synthesis in the CSF is a nonspecific finding.
- CSF pressure is high in pseudotumor cerebri (idiopathic intracranial hypertension).
- CSF pressure is low in positional headache and CSF leak.
- Lumbar puncture is dangerous when an intracranial mass is present, with or without papilledema.
- Lumbar puncture is safe in and therapeutic for pseudotumor cerebri.
- Lumbar puncture aggravates the signs of spinal cord disease in complete spinal block.

PART II—GENERAL PRINCIPLES FROM THE LEVEL OF THE CEREBRAL CORTEX THROUGH THE NEURAXIS TO MUSCLE

SUPRATENTORIAL LEVEL: SYMPTOMS AND CLINICAL CORRELATIONS

The supratentorial region is large and includes all levels of the nervous system inside the skull and above the tentorium cerebelli. Symptoms and signs related to disorders of the cerebral cortex may lead to alterations in cognition and consciousness. Focal neurologic symptoms involving a single limb and a single neurologic symptom (such as numbness [sensory system] or weakness [motor system]) commonly localize to the cerebral cortex. Abnormalities of speech and language are localized to the dominant cerebral hemisphere, whereas abnormalities of the nondominant hemisphere may lead to visuospatial deficits, confusion, or neglect of the contralateral side of the body. Abnormalities in the subcortical

region may lead to weakness or numbness; they typically involve more than one limb. Abnormalities in the basal ganglia may lead to movement disorders, including tremor, bradykinesia (as in Parkinson disease), and chorea (as in Huntington disease). Disorders of the thalamus, another subcortical structure, typically cause unilateral sensory abnormalities. The hypothalamus is important in many functions that affect everyday steady-state conditions, including temperature, hunger, water regulation, sleep, endocrine functions, cardiovascular functions, and regulation of the autonomic nervous system. Cortical and subcortical abnormalities may also lead to visual system deficits, usually homonymous visual field deficits.

Disorders of Consciousness

Consciousness has two dimensions: arousal and cognitive content. "Arousal" is a vegetative function maintained by the brainstem and medial diencephalic structures. "Cognitive content"—learning, memory, self-awareness, and adaptive behavior—depends on the functional integrity of the cerebral cortex and associated subcortical nuclei.

Coma or unconsciousness results from either bilateral dysfunction of the cerebral cortex or dysfunction of the reticular activating system in the upper brainstem (above the middle level of the pons). Unconsciousness implies global or total unawareness; coma implies the lack of both wakefulness and awareness.

- "Brain death" is the absence of function of the cerebral cortex and brainstem.
- Coma implies the lack of both wakefulness and awareness.
- "Persistent vegetative state" is the absence of cerebral cortex function with normal brainstem function (deafferentated state). The patient has no detectable awareness but, unlike a patient in a coma, is wakeful and has sleep-wake cycles.
- "Locked-in syndrome" is normal cerebral cortex function with absence of brainstem function. The lesion usually is in the pons and causes quadriplegia and the inability to speak, swallow, and move the eyes horizontally, that is, the de-efferentated state. The patient is wakeful and aware but is unable to communicate because of the neurologic deficits.
- "Acute confusional state" is malfunction of the cerebral cortex and reticular activating system.
- "Dementia" is chronic malfunction of the cerebral cortex but normal function of the brainstem.

Stupor and Coma

For a person to stay awake, the cerebral hemispheres and reticular activating system must be intact. Patients with dysfunction of only one cerebral hemisphere have a focal neurologic deficit but are awake. The most common, important, potentially reversible causes of stupor and coma are toxic, metabolic, and infectious problems that affect both cerebral hemispheres diffusely. Thus, most patients in stupor or coma have an underlying systemic problem. In adults and children with traumatic brain injury, recovery from unconsciousness is unlikely after 12 months. Recovery is rare after 3 months in adults and children with nontraumatic brain injury.

- The most common reversible causes of stupor and coma are toxic, metabolic, and infectious problems.

Patients with systemic encephalopathies have changes in mental status and awareness before going into stupor or coma, but they have no focal signs. Corneal reflexes are lost early in the disease, but pupillary reflexes remain. Ocular motility tested by the doll's eye maneuver (oculocephalic reflexes) and the cold caloric response (oculovestibular reflex) are fully intact, at least early in the disease.

- Patients with systemic encephalopathies have no focal signs.
- Corneal reflexes are lost early in the disease, but pupillary reflexes remain.

Patients with a large unilateral cerebral lesion may go into stupor or coma if the lesion causes shifting and pressure changes in other parts of the brain, such as the opposite hemisphere or brainstem. These patients have focal neurologic signs. Patients with brainstem lesions that directly affect the ascending reticular activating system are in coma but have focal signs. Persons who feign coma have no focal signs, no abnormal reflexes, normal caloric responses, and a normal EEG. They account for a small percentage of patients with stupor and coma.

- Large unilateral cerebral lesions that cause a shift and pressure changes in the other hemisphere or brainstem produce focal neurologic signs together with coma.
- Brainstem lesions that cause coma also produce focal signs.
- Persons who feign coma have no focal signs, no abnormal reflexes, normal caloric responses, and a normal EEG.

Acute Confusional States

Acute confusional states are abrupt, of recent onset, and often associated with fluctuations in the state of awareness and cognition. They are manifested by confusion, inattention, disorientation, and delirium. Thus, patients may be inattentive, dazed, stuporous, restless, agitated, or excited and may have marked autonomic dysfunction and visual and tactile hallucinations. Abnormal motor manifestations are common, including paratonia, asterixis, tremor, and myoclonus. The usual etiologic factors of acute confusional states are toxic, metabolic, traumatic, infectious, organ failure of any sort, or ictal or postictal encephalopathies. Three large

categories of general causes are systemic, neurologic, and psychophysiologic. Withdrawal states from alcohol, benzodiazepines, and barbiturates are also important causes of acute confusion or delirium.

- Three large categories of causes of acute confusional states are systemic, neurologic, and psychophysiologic.

Dementia

Dementia is a clinical state characterized by a marked loss of function in multiple cognitive domains not due to an impaired level of arousal. The presence of dementia does not necessarily imply irreversibility, a progressive course, or any specific disease. Dementia is not a disease but an entity with various causes (Table 17-2).

Table 17-2 Differential Diagnosis of Dementia

Potentially treatable dementias
  Metabolic-toxic disorders
    Vitamin B_{12} deficiency
    Hypothyroidism
    Alcoholism
  Structural lesions
    Normal-pressure hydrocephalus
    Subdural hematoma
    Neoplasm
    Vascular dementia
  Infections
    Chronic meningitis
    Neurosyphilis
    HIV dementia
    Whipple disease
  Inflammatory/immune disorders
    Vasculitis
    Limbic encephalitis
    Hashimoto encephalopathy
    Multiple sclerosis

Degenerative dementias
  Alzheimer disease
  Diffuse Lewy body disease
  Frontotemporal dementia (including Pick disease)
  Huntington disease
  Progressive supranuclear palsy

Prion-related disorders
  Creutzfeldt-Jakob disease

HIV, human immunodeficiency virus.

A small percentage of patients have reversible causes of dementia. These include medication-induced encephalopathy, depression, thyroid disease, CNS infections, vitamin deficiencies, and structural brain lesions (neoplasms, subdural hematomas, and symptomatic hydrocephalus).

● Dementia is not a disease.

Alzheimer disease is the most common cause of dementia. It occurs in both young and old persons and is no longer subcategorized into "presenile" and "senile" types. Generally, patients present first with difficulties of memory, but eventually difficulties develop in several cognitive areas, including aphasia, apraxia, or agnosia. The patients also have various behavioral and psychiatric manifestations, and some may have myoclonus or akinesia. Alzheimer disease is not simply diffuse atrophy of the brain but a regionally specific illness that first affects hippocampal structures.

Mild cognitive impairment (MCI) consists of memory loss that is clearly evident at bedside testing but does not interfere with everyday function. MCI may represent a very early stage of dementia. In about 50% of patients, MCI may progress to Alzheimer disease over a 4-year period. MRI, with focus in the temporal lobes, may detect atrophy early in the mesial temporal lobe of patients with MCI at risk for developing Alzheimer disease. The *APOE* ε 4 genotype also predicts a higher likelihood of Alzheimer disease. Additional study is needed to clarify the association of the subtypes and the power of prediction of a specific finding.

Some symptoms of Alzheimer disease are thought to be due to partial depletion of acetylcholine in the brain. Currently available centrally active noncompetitive reversible cholinesterase inhibitors, including donepezil, rivastigmine, and galantamine, may improve symptoms slightly and slow the decline of cognitive function in a small proportion of patients. Donepezil can be given once daily, whereas rivastigmine and galantamine are taken twice daily after meals. Tacrine, the first anticholinesterase agent used for the treatment of Alzheimer disease, may cause hepatotoxicity and is now rarely prescribed. The main side effects of these drugs are nausea, vomiting, and diarrhea. Donepezil is administered at bedtime but may cause vivid dreams, requiring that the dose be taken in the morning. Treatment with these drugs is continued until dementia reaches severe stages. The drugs should not be discontinued abruptly because it may cause abrupt cognitive deterioration. Vitamin E is also commonly used in Alzheimer disease, although its efficacy in slowing the rate of progression is not clearly defined.

Another common degenerative dementia is dementia with Lewy bodies. These patients typically exhibit parkinsonism, fluctuations of cognitive function, visual hallucinations, and rapid eye movement (REM) sleep behavior disorder. Antipsychotic medications may trigger a neuroleptic malignant-type syndrome in these patients. Cholinesterase inhibitors may improve hallucinations and other symptoms. Patients with a frontotemporal dementia such as Pick disease exhibit difficulties with executive function, inappropriate behavior, and aphasia.

A typical diagnostic work-up for dementia may include a complete blood count, electrolyte survey (including calcium, glucose, blood urea nitrogen, and creatinine), liver function tests, thyroid function tests, serum level of vitamin B_{12}, and serologic testing for syphilis. In selected patients, erythrocyte sedimentation rate, human immunodeficiency virus (HIV) testing, paraneoplastic antibody screening, chest radiography, urine collection for heavy metals, and toxicology screens should be performed. Neuroimaging should be considered for all persons with dementia. Neuropsychometric testing may also be considered. Lumbar puncture is indicated for persons who have had recent onset of symptoms, persons younger than 55 years who have dementia, and those with immunosuppression, possible CNS infection, reactive serum syphilis serologic findings, or metastatic cancer without findings on an imaging study. EEG may be useful in evaluating for Creutzfeldt-Jakob disease. In these patients, fluid-attenuated inversion recovery (FLAIR) MRI techniques can detect abnormalities in the cerebral cortex, basal ganglia, or thalamus when the findings of a standard MRI study are negative. The presence of increased levels of 14-3-3 protein in the CSF, although a nonspecific finding, strongly supports the diagnosis of Creutzfeldt-Jakob disease.

Typical Clinical Scenarios
● Alzheimer disease: a 70-year-old patient has had progressive loss of recent memory over the last 2 years. The results of neurologic examination, laboratory tests, and CSF examination are normal. The EEG is diffusely slow. MRI shows moderate cerebral atrophy but no specific lesions.
● Multi-infarct dementia: an elderly patient with known coronary artery disease and hypertension has progressive memory loss and difficulty walking. Deep tendon reflexes of the lower limb are brisk. The results of routine laboratory tests and CSF examination are normal. MRI shows multiple infarcts in both cerebral hemispheres.
● Creutzfeldt-Jakob disease: a 60-year-old patient has had rapidly progressive dementia and myoclonic jerks over several months. The EEG shows unusual high-amplitude sharp waves. FLAIR MRI shows increased signal intensity in the cerebral cortex and basal ganglia. The results of routine laboratory tests and CSF examination are normal, except for an increased level of 14-3-3 protein, which is highly supportive of the diagnosis.

Seizure Disorders

"Seizures" refer to electroclinical events, and "epilepsy" indicates a tendency for recurrent seizures. A classification of seizures is given in Table 17-3.

The proper treatment of epilepsy includes accurate diagnosis of the seizure type, identification of the cause (if possible), and management of psychosocial problems. The EEG can be important in deciding whether to treat a first unprovoked seizure. The risk of recurrent seizures is high if the initial EEG shows epileptiform activity and low if two EEGs (one of them sleep-deprived) are normal.

Causes

Seizures occur at any age, but 70% to 90% of all patients with epilepsy have their first seizure before age 20. Both the cause and the type of epilepsy are related to age at onset. However, the cause may not be found in many patients. Neonatal seizures are often due to congenital defects or prenatal injury, and head trauma is often the cause of focal seizures in young adults. Brain tumors and vascular disease are major known causes of seizures in later life. Seizures often occur during withdrawal from alcohol, barbiturates, or benzodiazepines in young and old adults. Seizures also occur with the use of such drugs as cocaine, usually in young adults. Metabolic derangements (e.g., hypoglycemia, hypocalcemia, hyponatremia, and hypernatremia) can occur at any age, as can infections (e.g., meningitis and encephalitis). Metabolic abnormalities usually cause primary generalized tonic-clonic seizures and rarely focal or multifocal seizures. CNS infections usually cause partial and secondary generalized tonic-clonic seizures.

Pseudoseizures (psychogenic, nonepileptic) are sudden changes in behavior or mentation not associated with any physiologic cause or abnormal paroxysmal discharge of electrical activity from the brain. They are often the cause of so-called intractable seizures. Effective treatment is elusive. A favorable outcome may be associated with an independent lifestyle, the absence of coexisting epilepsy, and a formal psychologic approach to therapy.

Anticonvulsant Therapy

Drugs used to treat seizures are listed in Table 17-4. Monotherapy is the treatment of choice. The dose of the drug may be increased as high as necessary and as much as can be tolerated. The coadministration of antiepileptic drugs has not been shown to have more antiseizure efficacy than the administration of only one drug without concurrently increasing toxicity. In studies of a large population, one particular drug may be shown more efficacious and less toxic, but for a given patient, an alternate drug may be more effective or have fewer side effects. The classic antiepileptic drugs are phenobarbital, phenytoin, carbamazepine, valproic acid, benzodiazepines, and ethosuximide. Simple and complex partial seizures are most likely to be controlled with phenytoin and carbamazepine, whereas secondary generalized tonic-clonic seizures respond equally well to carbamazepine, phenytoin, or valproic acid. Phenobarbital is equally efficacious but less well tolerated because of sedative side effects. Idiopathic generalized epilepsy with absence seizures is well controlled with ethosuximide. Valproic acid controls all forms of generalized seizures. Extended-release formulations are available for carbamazepine and valproic acid, and a rectal formulation is available for diazepam.

The new anticonvulsant drugs include gabapentin, tiagabine, lamotrigine, topiramate, felbamate, zonisamide, oxcarbazepine, and levetiracetam. These agents generally have less potential for drug interactions and fewer side effects than the older drugs. They are indicated as add-on therapy for partial seizures. Felbamate and oxcarbazepine are also used as single-drug therapy for partial seizures. Felbamate, lamotrigine, and topiramate are also used as monotherapy for generalized seizures. Because the efficacy, high cost, and dosing schedule (twice daily) are similar for most of these new anticonvulsants,

Table 17-3 Classification of Seizures

Partial (focal) seizures
    Simple partial seizures
        Partial simple sensory
        Partial simple motor
        Partial simple special sensory (unusual smells or tastes)
        Speech arrest or unusual vocalizations
    Complex partial seizures
        Consciousness impaired at onset
        Simple partial onset followed by impaired
          consciousness
    Evolving to generalized tonic-clonic convulsions
    (secondary generalized tonic-clonic seizures)
        Simple evolving to generalized tonic-clonic
        Complex evolving to generalized tonic-clonic
        (including those with simple partial onset)
    True auras—are actually simple partial seizures
Generalized seizures—convulsive or nonconvulsive (primary generalized seizures—generalized from onset)
    Absence and atypical absence
    Myoclonic
    Clonic
    Tonic
    Tonic-clonic
    Atonic
Unclassified epileptic seizures (includes some neonatal seizures)

Table 17-4 Guidance for Use of Antiepileptic Drugs

Criteria	Possibilities	Drug
Type of seizures	GTCSs	PHT, CBZ, VPA, lamotrigine, topiramate
	Partial seizures with or without secondary GTCSs	PHT, CBZ, VPA, PB, lamotrigine, topiramate, zonisamide, levetiracetam
	Absence seizures	Ethosuximide, VPA, lamotrigine
	Myoclonic seizure	VPA, clonazepam, lamotrigine
	Atonic, akinetic, or mixed	VPA, felbamate, topiramate, lamotrigine
Use of other drugs metabolized in the liver	Use drugs that do not affect metabolism of other drugs	Gabapentin, tiagabine, lamotrigine, zonisamide, levetiracetam
Avoid oral contraceptive pill failure	Use drugs with no or minimal effect on contraceptive metabolism	VPA, clonazepam, gabapentin, tiagabine, lamotrigine, zonisamide, levetiracetam

CBZ, carbamazepine; GTCS, generalized tonic-clonic seizure; PB, phenobarbital; PHT, phenytoin; VPA, valproic acid.

tolerability is frequently the major determinant in choosing a particular drug.

Anticonvulsants have both neurologic and systemic side effects. Dose-initiation side effects such as fatigue, dizziness, incoordination, and mental slowing are common in most patients and can be prevented with slow introduction of the drug. Dose-related side effects may limit the use of a particular drug in a given patient. A dose-related side effect common to most drugs is cognitive impairment. Other neurologic side effects include cerebellar ataxia (phenytoin), diplopia (carbamazepine), tremor (valproic acid), and chorea or myoclonus (phenytoin and carbamazepine). Idiosyncratic side effects are rare, unpredictable, severe, and sometimes life-threatening. Idiosyncratic and systemic side effects are listed in Table 17-5.

Many antiepileptic drugs are metabolized in the liver and are responsible for important drug interactions. Liver enzyme inducers such as carbamazepine, phenobarbital, phenytoin, primidone, oxcarbazepine, felbamate, and topiramate increase metabolism and decrease the efficacy of oral contraceptives in preventing pregnancy. Valproic acid and felbamate are enzyme inhibitors and increase the levels of other anticonvulsants. Gabapentin has the advantage of fewer drug interactions because it is eliminated primarily by renal excretion. It may be safer than other anticonvulsants in the management of seizures in patients with porphyria.

Special issues must be considered when managing epilepsy in pregnancy. Seizure control is attempted first with monotherapy, with the lowest possible dose of anticonvulsant and monitoring of drug levels. There is risk of fetal hemorrhage if the mother is taking phenytoin, phenobarbital, or carbamazepine. This risk can be minimized by administering vitamin K to the mother before delivery and to the fetus at delivery. Offspring of women with epilepsy are at increased risk for intrauterine growth retardation, minor abnormalities (digit hypoplasia and craniofacial abnormalities), major malformations (neural tube defects and cardiac malformations), microcephaly, cognitive dysfunction, and infant mortality. Various combinations of these findings, referred to as "fetal anticonvulsant syndrome," have been described with virtually all anticonvulsants. Multiple drugs at high doses generally are associated with a greater frequency of anomalies. Valproic acid and carbamazepine are selectively associated with increased risk of neural tube defects. All women with epilepsy and childbearing potential should receive folate supplementation of at least 0.4 mg daily. Prenatal screening should be offered to all women with epilepsy to detect any fetal malformation.

When to Start and When to Stop Anticonvulsant Therapy

The decision to begin anticonvulsant therapy after a first seizure should be individualized for each patient. It depends on the risk of additional seizures, risk of seizure-related injury, loss of employment or driving privileges, or other psychosocial factors. An important decision is whether a single generalized tonic seizure is provoked, for example, by sleep deprivation, alcohol, or concurrent illness. After the first seizure, the risk of recurrence ranges from 30% to 60%, with higher risks for patients with an abnormal EEG and a remote symptomatic cause. After a second seizure, the risk of recurrence increases to 80% to 90%.

For many patients who have been seizure-free for 2 to 5 years, anticonvulsant therapy can be withdrawn. The benefit of discontinuing the drugs should be weighed against the

Table 17-5   Systemic Side Effects of Antiepileptic Drugs

Side effect	Drug most commonly involved
Skin rash and Stevens-Johnson syndrome	10% risk with lamotrigine, CBZ, or PHT 5% risk with other AEDs, least with VPA Topiramate and zonisamide contraindicated for patients with allergy to sulfa drugs
Liver failure	Highest risk with VPA and felbamate Risk increased in infants with mental retardation & receiving polytherapy, with underlying metabolic disease or poor nutritional status
Bone marrow suppression	Highest risk with felbamate and CBZ
Gum hypertrophy, hirsutism, acne, osteoporosis	Phenytoin
Weight gain, hair loss, tremor	VPA
Weight loss	Felbamate, topiramate
Headache, insomnia	Felbamate
Behavioral and cognitive disturbances	Barbiturates, benzodiazepines, topiramate
Kidney stones	Topiramate, zonisamide
Hyponatremia	CBZ or oxcarbazepine
Atrioventricular conduction defect	CBZ, PHT
Neural tube defect	VPA, CBZ, but all AEDs are potentially teratogenic

AED, antiepileptic drug; CBZ, carbamazepine; PHT, phenytoin; VPA, valproic acid.

possibility of seizure recurrence and its potential adverse consequences. In adults, relapse occurs in 26% to 63% of patients within 1 to 2 years after the withdrawal of medication. Predictors of relapse are an abnormal EEG before or during medication withdrawal, abnormal findings on neurologic examination, frequent seizures before entering remission, or mental retardation. To lessen the chance of seizures after the withdrawal of medication, withdrawal should not proceed faster than a 20% reduction in dose every 5 half-lives.

Typical Clinical Scenarios
- Absence seizures: a child has abrupt episodes of staring and unresponsiveness that last less than 10 seconds and are associated with complete recovery and no postictal abnormalities. These episodes occur several times a day, but otherwise the child appears normal. The diagnosis is absence seizure, for which ethosuximide or valproic acid is effective.
- Seizure due to an intracranial neoplasm: an elderly patient with a history of recent headaches has a generalized seizure. He has a 50-pack-year history of smoking, but no previous history of a seizure disorder. Chest radiography shows a 2-cm mass in the left upper lobe of the lung. Brain metastases should be included in the differential diagnosis. Neuroimaging is indicated to establish the diagnosis.
- Drug-induced agranulocytosis: a neutropenic fever develops a month after a patient starts taking carbamazepine for a seizure disorder. The absolute neutrophil count is 100. Treatment is discontinuation of carbamazepine and use of an alternative antiseizure agent. The neutropenic fever should be managed with antibiotics.
- Interaction with oral contraceptives: a young woman with a chronic seizure disorder that has been well controlled with phenytoin for several years indicates that she has become pregnant despite taking birth control pills. The oral contraceptives have been rendered ineffective because of induction of liver microenzymes by phenytoin. Valproic acid does not induce liver enzymes and would be a good choice for women with a seizure disorder who take oral contraceptives.

Anticonvulsant Blood Levels
Anticonvulsant blood levels are readily available and help attain the best control of seizures. It is extremely important to

remember that therapeutic levels represent an average bell-shaped curve and that patients with well-controlled seizures are included under the bell-shaped curve. Seizures are well controlled in many patients who have anticonvulsant blood levels below or above the therapeutic range. The anticonvulsant dose should *never* be changed on the basis of blood levels alone. Remember, toxicity is a clinical, *not* a laboratory, phenomenon.

- Therapeutic levels represent an average bell-shaped curve.
- The dose of anticonvulsant should never be changed on the basis of blood levels alone.
- Toxicity is a clinical, not a laboratory, phenomenon.
- From 70% to 90% of patients with epilepsy have their first seizure before age 20.
- The cause and type of epilepsy are related to age at onset.
- Head trauma is a major cause of focal seizures in young adults.
- Brain tumors and vascular disease are major causes of seizures in older persons.
- Seizures occur with withdrawal from alcohol, barbiturates, and benzodiazepines.
- Seizures occur during the use of cocaine (young adults).
- Pseudoseizures are often the basis of so-called intractable seizures.

If a patient with epilepsy under treatment has breakthrough seizures, several things need to be considered. These include compliance issues; excessive use of alcohol or other recreational drugs; psychologic and physiologic stress (lack of sleep or anxiety); a combination of the preceding; systemic disease of any type, organ failure of any type, or systemic infection; a new cause of seizures (neoplasm); newly prescribed medication, including other anticonvulsants (polypharmacy) and over-the-counter drugs; toxic levels of anticonvulsants (with definite clinical toxicity); pseudoseizures; progressive CNS lesion not identified previously with neuroimaging or lumbar puncture; or no cause found. If no cause is found, anticonvulsant doses must be readjusted or the drug replaced with another one.

- The treatment of choice is monotherapy.
- Essentially all anticonvulsant drugs have the potential to cause developmental abnormalities.
- Valproic acid and carbamazepine may cause neural tube defects.

Surgery for Epilepsy

With improved technology, the anatomical site of seizure origin can be identified more accurately. Also, technical advances have made surgical management safer. Of the 150,000 patients in whom epilepsy develops each year, 10% to 20% have "medically intractable epilepsy." Seizures that are medically refractory may respond to stimulation of the left vagus nerve with a permanent stimulator.

Brain surgery is an alternative therapy if treatment with antiepileptic drugs fails. However, before seizures are deemed intractable, ascertain that the correct drugs have been given in the correct amounts. Anterior temporal lobe operations and other cortical resections involve removal of the epileptic focus. These operations are performed for complex partial seizures. Corpus callosotomy (the severing of connections between the right and left cerebral hemispheres) is performed for some types of generalized epilepsy.

- If treatment with antiepileptic drugs fails, vagal nerve stimulation and brain surgery are alternatives.
- Anterior temporal lobe operations and other cortical resections remove the epileptic focus.
- Resection operations are performed for complex partial seizures.
- Corpus callosotomy severs the connections between the left and right sides of the brain and is performed for generalized epilepsy.

Status Epilepticus

Status epilepticus is a medical emergency and a life-threatening condition. The seizure is prolonged, lasting more than 15 to 30 minutes, or there are repetitive seizures, without recovery between seizures. The most common causes of status epilepticus include withdrawal of an anticonvulsant agent or alcohol, recreational drug toxicity, and CNS infection. The management of status epilepticus is summarized in Figure 17-1.

Nonconvulsive status epilepticus may cause an acute confusional state or stupor and coma, especially in the elderly. EEG is a valuable diagnostic tool in these cases because nonconvulsive status epilepticus must be treated as quickly and vigorously as convulsive status epilepticus.

- Status epilepticus is life-threatening and a medical emergency.
- The seizure lasts >15-30 minutes or there are repetitive seizures without recovery.
- Administer 50 mL of 50% dextrose with 100 mg thiamine intravenously.
- Slowly administer diazepam or lorazepam intravenously.
- Treatment can begin with a loading dose of fosphenytoin.
- Cardiorespiratory monitoring is required if fosphenytoin or phenytoin is infused rapidly.

Headache and Facial Pain

Headache may indicate intracranial or systemic disease, a personality or situational problem, or a combination of these.

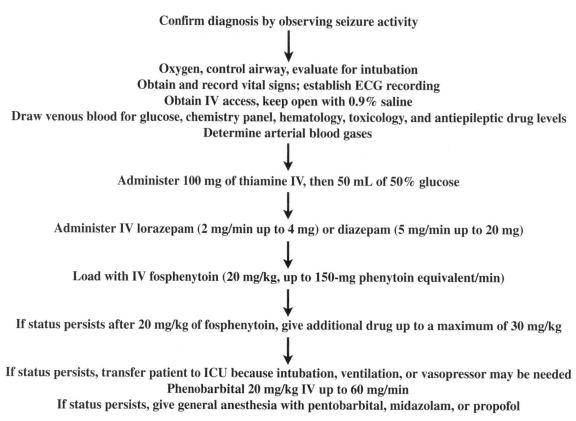

Confirm diagnosis by observing seizure activity

↓

Oxygen, control airway, evaluate for intubation
Obtain and record vital signs; establish ECG recording
Obtain IV access, keep open with 0.9% saline
Draw venous blood for glucose, chemistry panel, hematology, toxicology, and antiepileptic drug levels
Determine arterial blood gases

↓

Administer 100 mg of thiamine IV, then 50 mL of 50% glucose

↓

Administer IV lorazepam (2 mg/min up to 4 mg) or diazepam (5 mg/min up to 20 mg)

↓

Load with IV fosphenytoin (20 mg/kg, up to 150-mg phenytoin equivalent/min)

↓

If status persists after 20 mg/kg of fosphenytoin, give additional drug up to a maximum of 30 mg/kg

↓

If status persists, transfer patient to ICU because intubation, ventilation, or vasopressor may be needed
Phenobarbital 20 mg/kg IV up to 60 mg/min
If status persists, give general anesthesia with pentobarbital, midazolam, or propofol

Fig. 17-1. Algorithm for the management of status epilepticus. ECG, electrocardiography; ICU, intensive care unit; IV, intravenous.

Some headaches have a readily identified organic cause. Classic migraine and cluster headaches form distinctive, easily recognized clinical entities, but their pathophysiologic mechanism is not understood. The major challenge is that often neither the location nor the intensity of the pain is a reliable clue to the nature of the problem. Episodic tension headache and migraine can be difficult to distinguish.

- Neither location nor intensity of headache pain is a reliable clue to the nature of the problem.

Conditions alerting physicians that a headache may have a serious cause are listed in Table 17-6. Chronic recurrent headaches are rarely, if ever, caused by eye strain, chronic sinusitis, dental problems, food allergies, high blood pressure, or temporal mandibular joint syndrome. Headache without other neurologic signs or symptoms is rarely caused by a brain tumor. Serious causes of headache in which neuroimaging findings may be normal and lead to a false sense of security are listed in Table 17-7.

- "Worst or first headache of my life" is serious.
- Headache with abnormal neurologic findings, papilledema, obscuration of vision, or diplopia is serious.

- Most of the signs and symptoms in Table 17-6 can occur with chronic benign headache (tension-migraine headache).
- Headache without other neurologic signs or symptoms is rarely caused by a brain tumor.

Migraine and Tension Headache

Psychologic and physical therapy and pharmacotherapy are components of a systemic approach to treating headache.

Abortive headache medications may range from simple analgesics to anxiolytics, nonsteroidal anti-inflammatory drugs, ergots, and corticosteroids to major tranquilizers and narcotics. Dihydroergotamine (DHE 45) as well as sumatriptan and related serotonin 1B/1D receptor agonists (zolmitriptan, naratriptan, rizatriptan, almotriptan, eletriptan, and frovatriptan) are effective in aborting acute migraine attacks. Dihydroergotamine and sumatriptan can be administered parenterally or intranasally to patients who have severe nausea or vomiting. Sumatriptan and other vasoconstrictor drugs are contraindicated in patients with migraine associated with a focal neurologic deficit and in patients with coronary artery disease.

Prophylactic medication should not be given when the attacks occur no more than 2 or 3 times a month unless they are incapacitating, associated with focal neurologic signs, or of

Table 17-6   Conditions Indicating That a Headache May Have a Serious Cause

"Worst or first headache of my life"

Headache in a person not prone to headache, especially a middle-aged or elderly patient

Headache associated with abnormal neurologic findings, papilledema, obscurations of vision, or diplopia

Headache that changes with different positions or increases with exertion, coughing, or sneezing

Changes in headache patterns—character, frequency, severity—in someone who has had chronic recurring headaches previously

Headache that awakens one from sound sleep

Headache associated with trauma

Headache associated with systemic symptoms, e.g., fever, malaise, weight loss

Most of the above signs and symptoms may occur in chronic benign headache (e.g., tension-migraine)

Table 17-7   Serious Causes of Headache in Which Neuroimaging Findings May Be Normal

Cranial arteritis

Glaucoma

Trigeminal or glossopharyngeal neuralgia

Lesions around sella turcica

Warning leak of aneurysm

Inflammation, infection, or neoplastic invasion of leptomeninges

Cervical spondylosis

Pseudotumor cerebri

Low intracranial pressure syndromes (cerebrospinal fluid leaks)

prolonged duration. When prophylactic medication is indicated, the following should be observed:

- Begin with a low dose and increase it slowly.
- Perform an adequate trial of medication (1-2 months).
- Confirm that the patient is not taking drugs that may interact with the headache agent (vasodilator, estrogens, oral contraceptives).
- Determine that a female patient is not pregnant and she is using effective contraception.
- Attempt to taper and discontinue prophylactic medication after the headaches are well-controlled.
- Avoid polypharmacy.
- Establish a strong doctor-patient partnership; emphasize that management of headache is often a team effort, with the patient having a role equal to that of the physician.
- The best medication is *no* medication.

Drugs used for prophylaxis include β-blockers, calcium channel blockers, amitriptyline, valproic acid, and other anticonvulsants. The most widely used β-blocker is propranolol; others are atenolol, metoprolol, and timolol. Valproic acid is an excellent preventive agent, but its use may be limited because of weight gain and hair loss. Amitriptyline is particularly useful in patients with migraine and chronic-type tension headache. Verapamil is a good alternative to β-blockers in athletes and is recommended for patients with suspected vasospasm as a cause of migrainous infarction. There is some evidence that gabapentin, lamotrigine, and topiramate potentially have a role in preventing migraine.

Naproxen and other nonsteroidal anti-inflammatory drugs produce analgesia through alternate pathways that do not appear to induce dependence. They may be useful for the following headaches: migraine, both for acute attacks and prophylaxis; menstrual migraine (especially naproxen); benign exertional migraine and sex-induced headache (especially indomethacin); cluster variants (chronic paroxysmal hemicrania, episodic paroxysmal hemicrania, and hemicrania continua); idiopathic stabbing headache, jabs-and-jolts, needle-in-the-eye, and ice-pick headaches (indomethacin is often effective); muscle contraction headaches; mixed headaches; and ergotamine-induced headache.

Cluster Headache

Cluster headache, unlike migraine, predominantly affects men. The onset is usually in the late 20s but may occur at any age. Its main feature is periodicity. On average, the cluster period lasts 2 to 3 months and typically occurs every 1 or 2 years between clusters. Attacks occur at a frequency of 1 to 3 times daily and tend to be nocturnal in more than 50% of patients. The average period of remission is about 2 years between clusters. Cluster is not associated with an aura. The pain reaches a peak in about 10 to 15 minutes and lasts 45 to 60 minutes. It is excruciating, penetrating, usually nonthrobbing, and maximal behind the eye and in the region of the supraorbital nerve and temples. Attacks of pain typically are unilateral. The autonomic features are both sympathetic paresis and parasympathetic overreaction. They may include 1) ipsilateral lacrimation, injection of the conjunctiva, and nasal stuffiness or rhinorrhea, and 2) ptosis and miosis (ptosis may become permanent), periorbital swelling, and bradycardia. The scalp, face, and carotid artery may be tender.

- Cluster headache affects men, with onset in the 20s.
- Periodicity is the main feature.

- The cluster period lasts 2-3 months.
- Cluster headache is not associated with an aura.
- The pain peaks in 10-15 minutes and lasts 45-60 minutes.
- The pain typically is unilateral, excruciating, penetrating, nonthrobbing, and maximal behind the eye.
- In >50% of patients, the pain is nocturnal.
- Autonomic features are present.

Abortive therapy includes oxygen inhalation, 5 to 8 L/min for 10 minutes; sumatriptan, a serotonin 1B/1D agonist; dihydroergotamine; ergotamine, especially inhalation or suppositories; corticosteroids (e.g., 8 mg dexamethasone); local anesthesia (intranasal 4% lidocaine); and capsaicin in the ipsilateral nostril. Sumatriptan is the drug of choice for management of an acute attack of cluster headache. Surgical intervention may be indicated under certain circumstances for chronic cluster headache but never for episodic headache.

Prophylactic treatment is the mainstay of cluster headache treatment. Calcium channel blockers (verapamil) are widely used. The usual dose of lithium is 600 to 900 mg in divided doses. Its effectiveness is known within 1 week. Methysergide is most effective in the early course of the disease and least effective in later years. Ergotamine at bedtime is particularly beneficial for nocturnal attacks. Corticosteroids are helpful for short-term treatment, especially for patients resistant to the above drugs or to a combination of the above. The usual dose is 40 mg prednisone tapered over 3 weeks. The most effective treatment for chronic cluster headache is the combination of verapamil and lithium. Valproic acid may also be useful.

- Prophylaxis of cluster headaches is the mainstay of treatment.
- Calcium channel blockers are widely used.
- Methysergide is effective early in the disease.
- Ergotamine is effective for nocturnal attacks.
- Corticosteroids are helpful short-term.
- The combination of verapamil and lithium is best for prophylaxis of chronic cluster headache.

Typical Clinical Scenarios

- Migraine: a young patient with recurrent, episodic (once a week or so), and severe headache. Often, the headache is unilateral and associated with nausea and vomiting. CSF and MRI findings are normal.
- Tension headache: a young patient has a 3-year history of headaches, which occur almost every month and last several days. They are bilateral and are not associated with any neurologic deficit, nausea, or vomiting.
- Cluster headache: a 27-year-old man has a 1-month history of severe, excruciating headaches that occur daily and last for approximately 1 hour. He had a similar episode 1 year ago, in which the headache lasted 3 months and then resolved

completely. The pain is unilateral and worse behind the right eye. The right eye becomes red and teary during the headache.

Medication-Overuse Headache

Chronic daily headache (intractable headache) may occur de novo, probably as a form of tension headache or, more important, it may be part of an evolution from periodic migraine or tension headache. Chronic daily headache is often accompanied by sleep disturbances, depression, anxiety, and overuse of analgesics; 90% of patients with this disorder have a family history of headache. Episodic migraine and other episodic benign headaches can evolve into a daily refractory, intense headache. This syndrome is usually due to the overuse (>2 days a week) of ergotamine tartrate, analgesics (especially analgesics combined with barbiturates), narcotics, and perhaps even benzodiazepines. To control the headache, the use of these medications has to be discontinued. Two points have to be stressed: the overuse of these medications causes daily headache, and the daily use of these medications prevents other useful medications from working effectively.

The treatment of daily refractory headaches usually requires hospitalization and withdrawal of the overused medication, with repetitive intravenous administration of dihydroergotamine together with an antiemetic drug such as metoclopramide or prochlorperazine.

Nonsteroidal anti-inflammatory drugs, β-blockers, calcium channel blockers, and tricyclic antidepressants do not cause transformation/withdrawal syndrome. Also, patients who do not have headache but who take large amounts of analgesics for other conditions, for example, arthritis, do not develop analgesic or rebound headache. Simple withdrawal from analgesics produces marked improvement in patients with chronic daily headache. A nonprescription medication can be withdrawn abruptly. However, prescription medications (ergotamine tartrate, narcotics, barbiturates) have to be withdrawn gradually. When narcotics or compounds containing codeine and ergotamine tartrate are withdrawn, clonidine may be helpful in repressing withdrawal symptoms. Some think even simple analgesics (aspirin, acetaminophen [Tylenol]) taken more than 2 days a week can cause daily headache syndrome. The overuse (more than 3 days a week for 2 weeks or more) of "triptan" drugs is now becoming a common cause of medication-overuse syndrome.

- Chronic daily headache is often accompanied by sleep disturbances, depression, anxiety, and analgesic overuse.
- 90% of patients with chronic daily headache have a family history of headache.
- Migraine and other headaches can become a refractory intense headache.
- Overuse of medications causes daily headache and prevents the effective action of other drugs.

- Hospitalization and withdrawal of overused drugs are usually required.
- Nonsteroidal anti-inflammatory drugs, β-blockers, calcium channel blockers, and tricyclic antidepressants do not cause transformation/withdrawal syndrome.
- There is marked improvement after withdrawal of analgesics.

Temporal Arteritis

In an elderly person, temporal arteritis (also called "cranial arteritis" or "giant cell arteritis") should be in the differential diagnosis of any new temporal headache of mild to moderate severity. About 50% of persons with this diagnosis have headache or tender temporal arteries. Common additional symptoms include low-grade fever, jaw claudication, weight loss, anorexia, and other systemic symptoms. The erythrocyte sedimentation rate is consistently increased. If vision loss has already occurred, emergent therapy with high doses of corticosteroids is needed. To prevent vision loss in those who have no visual problem, prednisone therapy should be initiated immediately after the diagnosis has been made. Temporal artery biopsy is used to confirm the diagnosis before long-term treatment with prednisone is prescribed. However, if the biopsy cannot be performed immediately, prednisone therapy may be initiated until biopsy results are available. The erythrocyte sedimentation rate may be followed to help gauge the response to treatment. The prednisone dose can be tapered slowly after several months of therapy, although longer term treatment with prednisone may be needed.

Polymyalgia rheumatica is another rheumatologic syndrome that is sometimes associated with cranial arteritis. It affects elderly patients and is associated with aching or pain and stiffness in the neck, upper back, shoulders, upper arms, and hip girdle. Systemic symptoms include various degrees of fever, anorexia, weight loss, apathy, and depression. True muscle weakness is not present except when attributed to pain.

Trigeminal Neuralgia

Characteristically, patients with trigeminal neuralgia always have symptoms on the same side and usually in the second or third division of the trigeminal nerve. The idiopathic variety occurs in middle-aged and elderly patients and is heralded by a sharp, lancinating pain that usually can be triggered. Chewing often precipitates the pain of trigeminal neuralgia, and swallowing often precipitates the pain of glossopharyngeal neuralgia.

In the elderly, trigeminal neuralgia may be caused by an enlarged artery (rarely a vein) that compresses the trigeminal nerve. Importantly, in idiopathic trigeminal neuralgia, sensory and motor functions of the trigeminal nerve are normal when the patient is examined during an asymptomatic period. If there are signs or symptoms other than pain, evaluate for other compressive lesions, for example, neoplasm. Consider

the possibility of multiple sclerosis if trigeminal neuralgia occurs in a young person. Treatment options include carbamazepine, phenytoin, baclofen, gabapentin, clonazepam, and surgical management.

- Chewing often precipitates pain in trigeminal neuralgia, as does swallowing in glossopharyngeal neuralgia.
- In idiopathic trigeminal neuralgia, there should be no other neurologic signs or symptoms when the patient is examined during an asymptomatic period.
- Consider multiple sclerosis if trigeminal neuralgia occurs in a young person.

Glossopharyngeal Neuralgia

The pain in glossopharyngeal neuralgia is similar to that in trigeminal neuralgia, but it occurs in the throat and neck and often radiates to the ear. Glossopharyngeal neuralgia may cause hypotension and syncope. It is usually idiopathic but has been reported with leptomeningeal metastasis or jugular foramen syndrome (head and neck malignancies). The treatment is the same as for trigeminal neuralgia, that is, carbamazepine and, occasionally, surgical management.

- Glossopharyngeal pain occurs in the throat and neck and radiates to the ear.

Intracranial Lesions

Leptomeningeal Lesions

Inflammation, infection, or neoplastic invasion of the leptomeninges may present with similar signs and symptoms, as follows:

- Cerebral—headache, seizures, focal neurologic signs.
- Cranial nerve—any cranial nerve (CN) can be affected, especially CN III, IV, VI, and VII (the latter is often affected in Lyme disease).
- Radicular (radiculoneuropathy or radiculomyelopathy)—neck and back pain as well as radicular pain and spinal cord signs.

Parasagittal Lesions

Because the cortical leg area and cortical area for control of the urinary bladder are located on the medial surface of each hemisphere, parasagittal lesions can cause spastic paraparesis with urinary problems. Meningioma is a common lesion in this location and may also cause seizures and headache.

- Parasagittal lesions may cause paraparesis with urinary problems.
- Meningioma may also cause seizures and headache.

Cortical Lesions

Cortical lesions produce focal signs. If the lesions are in the dominant hemisphere, they cause language dysfunction, including problems of reading, writing, and speaking. Cortical lesions can also impair higher intellectual function, producing apraxias, agnosias, and denial of illness or body parts, and they often impair cortical sensation (e.g., stereognosis). A dense loss of primary sensation (e.g., pinprick and touch) occurs with thalamic lesions.

● Cortical lesions may produce apraxia and agnosia.
● Thalamic lesions cause loss of primary sensation (e.g., touch).

Ventricular System

Hydrocephalus

A combination of signs and symptoms—impaired mental status, gait disturbance, urinary problems—suggests hydrocephalus. If it is the obstructive type, signs of increased intracranial pressure may be present, including lethargy, nausea, vomiting, and headache; obscurations of vision are often associated with changes in position.

The following are types of hydrocephalus:
1. Communicating hydrocephalus
   a. Hydrocephalus ex vacuo—due to the loss of parenchyma, either gray or white matter, and not associated with the signs listed above (if the hydrocephalus is due to aging, the findings on neurologic examination are normal; if it is due to Alzheimer disease, clinical examination shows signs of dementia).
   b. Normal-pressure hydrocephalus—due to decreased reabsorption of CSF.
   c. Hydrocephalus due to overproduction of CSF—rare and controversial; supposedly occurs with choroid plexus lesions.
2. Obstructive (noncommunicating) hydrocephalus—due to an obstructive lesion anywhere in the ventricular system.

● Normal-pressure hydrocephalus is due to decreased reabsorption of CSF and may be associated with urinary symptoms, gait disturbance, and memory dysfunction.

POSTERIOR FOSSA LEVEL: SYMPTOMS AND CLINICAL CORRELATIONS

Brainstem Lesions

Brainstem lesions can produce crossed neurologic syndromes; cranial nerve signs are ipsilateral to the lesion, but long-tract signs are usually contralateral (crossed syndrome). Other symptoms associated with brainstem lesions include impairment of ocular motility; medial longitudinal fasciculus syndrome (internuclear ophthalmoplegia); rotary, horizontal, and vertical nystagmus (downbeat nystagmus is highly suggestive of a lesion at the cervicomedullary junction); ataxia; dysarthria; diplopia; vertigo; and dysphagia.

● Downbeat nystagmus is highly suggestive of a lesion at the cervicomedullary junction.
● Cranial nerve signs are ipsilateral to the brainstem lesion.
● Long-tract signs are usually contralateral to the brainstem lesion.

Cerebellar Lesions

Problems with equilibrium and coordination suggest a cerebellar lesion. Lesions of the cerebellar hemisphere usually produce ipsilateral ataxia of the arm and leg. Lesions restricted to the anterior superior vermis, as in alcoholism, usually cause ataxia of gait, that is, a wide-based gait and heel-to-shin ataxia, with relative sparing of the arms, speech, and ocular motility. Lesions of the flocculonodular lobe cause marked difficulty with equilibrium and walking but not much difficulty with finger-to-nose and heel-to-shin tests if the patient is lying down.

Vertigo and Dizziness

Accurate visual, vestibular, proprioceptive, tactile, and auditory perceptions are necessary for normal spatial orientation. These inputs are integrated in the brainstem and cerebral hemispheres. The outputs are the cortical, brainstem, and cerebellar motor systems. The impairment of any of these functions or their input, integration, or output causes a complaint of "dizziness" (a sensation of altered orientation or space). Dizziness, vertigo, and dysequilibrium are common complaints. The results of diagnostic tests are often normal. Diagnosis depends mainly on the medical history, with physical examination findings in some cases. Vestibular tests rarely provide an exact diagnosis. The types of dizziness are listed in Table 17-8.

Vertigo

"Vertigo" is an illusion of movement (usually that of rotation) and the feeling of vertical or horizontal rotation of either the person or the environment around the person. Most patients report this as "spinning" or "rotational" feelings. Others experience mainly a sensation of staggering. In contrast to vertigo, "dysequilibrium" is a feeling of unsteadiness or insecurity about the environment, without a rotatory sensation. Vertigo occurs when there is imbalance, especially acute, between the left and right vestibular systems. The sudden unilateral loss of vestibular function is dramatic; the patient complains of severe vertigo and nausea and vomiting and is pale and diaphoretic. With

Table 17-8 Types of Dizziness

Vertigo
    Peripheral
    Central
Presyncopal light-headedness
    Orthostatic hypotension
    Vasovagal attacks
    Impaired cardiac output
    Hyperventilation
Psychophysiologic dizziness
    Acute anxiety
    Agoraphobia (fear and avoidance of being in public
      places)
    Chronic anxiety
Disequilibrium
    Lesions of basal ganglia, frontal lobes, and white matter
    Hydrocephalus
    Cerebellar dysfunction
Ocular dizziness
    High magnification and lens implant
    Imbalance in extraocular muscles
    Oscillopsia
Multisensory dizziness
Physiologic dizziness
    Motion sickness
    Space sickness
    Height vertigo

acute vertigo, the patient also has problems with equilibrium and vision, often described as "blurred vision," or diplopia. Autonomic symptoms are common—sweating, pallor, nausea, vomiting—and occasionally can cause vasovagal syncope.

Fluctuating hearing loss and tinnitus are characteristic of Meniere syndrome. Abrupt complete unilateral deafness and vertigo occur with viral involvement of the labyrinth or CN VIII (or both) and with vascular occlusion of the inner ear. Patients who slowly lose vestibular function bilaterally, as with ototoxic drugs, often do not complain of vertigo but have oscillopsia with head movements and instability with walking. Even with unilateral vestibular loss, if it is a slow process (acoustic neuroma), patients usually do not complain of vertigo; they typically present with unilateral hearing loss and tinnitus. Vertigo invariably occurs in episodes. Common vestibular disorders with a genetic predisposition include migraine, Meniere syndrome, otosclerosis, neurofibromatosis, and spinocerebellar degeneration.

Benign positional vertigo is the most common cause of vertigo. Symptoms include brief episodes of vertigo that usually last less than 30 seconds with positional change, for example, turning over in bed, getting in or out of bed, bending over and straightening up, and extending the neck to look up. No cause is found in about half of the patients. For the other half, the most common causes are post-traumatic and postviral neurolabyrinthitis.

Typically, bouts of benign positional vertigo are intermixed with variable periods of remission. Periods of vertigo rarely last longer than 1 minute, although after a flurry of episodes, patients may complain of more prolonged nonspecific dizziness that lasts hours to days (light-headedness, swimming sensation associated with nausea). Management includes reassurance, positional exercises (vestibular exercises), and the canalith repositioning maneuver. Drugs are not very useful, but meclizine and promethazine may help with the nausea and nonspecific dizziness. Rarely, in intractable cases, surgical treatment (section of the ampullary nerve) may be undertaken.

Vertigo of CNS origin is caused by acute cerebellar lesions (hemorrhages or infarcts) or acute brainstem lesions (especially the lateral medullary [Wallenberg] syndrome). Vertebrobasilar arterial disease is also a cause, but vertigo by itself is never a TIA. Other symptoms are necessary to make the diagnosis of vertebrobasilar insufficiency, such as dysarthria, dysphagia, diplopia, facial numbness, crossed syndromes, hemiparesis or alternating hemiparesis, ataxia, and visual field defects.

Presyncopal Light-Headedness

This is best described as the "sensation of impending faint." It results from pancerebral ischemia. Presyncopal light-headedness is not a symptom of focal occlusive cerebrovascular disease, but it may indicate orthostatic hypotension, usually due to decreased blood volume, chronic use of hypotensive drugs, or autonomic dysfunction. Symptoms of vasovagal attacks are induced when such emotions as fear and anxiety activate medullary vasodepressor centers. Vasodepressor episodes can also be precipitated by acute visceral pain or sudden severe attacks of vertigo. Impaired cardiac output causes presyncopal light-headedness, as does hyperventilation. Chronic anxiety with associated hyperventilation is the most common cause of persistent presyncopal light-headedness in young patients. In most subjects, only a moderate increase in respiratory rate can decrease the $PaCO_2$ level to 25 mm Hg or less in a few minutes.

Five types of syncopal attacks especially common in the elderly are the following:

1. Orthostatic—multiple causes
2. Autonomic dysfunction due to peripheral (postganglionic) or central (preganglionic) involvement

3. Reflex—such as carotid sinus syncope or cough or micturition syncope

4. Vasovagal syncope—occurs less frequently in the elderly than in the young; however, the prognosis is worse in the elderly, with about 16% of them having major morbidity and mortality in the following 6 months compared with less than 1% of patients younger than 30 years; common precipitating events in the elderly include emotional stress, prolonged bed rest, prolonged standing, and painful stimuli

5. Cardiac syncope

- Presyncopal light-headedness is the sensation of impending faint.
- It is not an isolated symptom of occlusive cerebrovascular disease.
- Vasovagal attacks occur less frequently in the elderly.
- In the young, a common cause of persistent presyncopal light-headedness is chronic anxiety with hyperventilation.
- The prognosis of vasovagal syncope is worse for the elderly; 16% have major morbidity or mortality within 6 months.
- In the elderly, vasovagal syncope may be precipitated by emotional stress, bed rest, prolonged standing, or pain.

Psychophysiologic Dizziness

Patients usually describe psychophysiologic dizziness as "floating," "swimming," or "giddiness." They also may report a feeling of imbalance, a rocking or falling sensation, or a spinning inside the head. The symptoms are not associated with an illusion of movement or movement of the environment or with nystagmus. Commonly associated symptoms include tension headache, heart palpitations, gastric distress, urinary frequency, backache, and generalized feeling of weakness and fatigue. Psychophysiologic dizziness can also be associated with panic attacks.

Disequilibrium

Patients who slowly lose vestibular function on one side, as with an acoustic neuroma, usually do not have vertigo but often describe a vague feeling of imbalance and unsteadiness on their feet. Disequilibrium may be a presenting symptom of lesions involving motor centers of the basal ganglia and frontal lobe, for example, Parkinson disease, hydrocephalus, and multiple lacunar infarction syndrome. The broad-based ataxic gait of cerebellar disorders is readily distinguished from milder gait disorders seen with vestibular or sensory loss or with senile gait.

- Disequilibrium may be a presenting symptom of basal ganglia or frontal lobe lesions.

Multisensory Dizziness

This is common in the elderly and especially in patients with systemic disorders such as diabetes mellitus. A typical combination includes, for example, mild peripheral neuropathy that causes diminished touch and proprioceptive input, decreased visual acuity, impaired hearing, and decreased baroreceptor function. In these patients, an added vestibular impairment, as from an ototoxic drug, can be devastating.

The resulting sensation of dizziness is usually present only when the patient walks or moves and not when supine or seated. There is a feeling of insecurity of gait and motion. The patient is usually helped by walking close to a wall, using a cane, or by holding on to another person. Drugs should *not* be prescribed for this disorder. Instead, the use of a cane or walker is important to improve support and to increase somatosensory signals.

- Multisensory dizziness is common in elderly diabetic patients.
- Added vestibular impairment can be devastating.
- Do not prescribe drugs for this disorder.

SPINAL LEVEL: SYMPTOMS AND CLINICAL CORRELATIONS

Sensory levels, signs of anterior horn cell involvement (atrophy and fasciculations), and long-tract signs in the posterior columns, corticospinal tract, and spinothalamic tract suggest a spinal cord lesion. Extramedullary cord lesions are usually heralded by radicular pain. Intramedullary cord lesions are usually painless but may have an ill-described nonlocalizable pain, sensory dissociation, and sacral sparing. Conus medullaris lesions are often indicated by "saddle anesthesia" and early involvement of the urinary bladder.

- Extramedullary lesions are heralded by radicular pain.
- Intramedullary lesions are usually painless.
- Conus medullaris lesions are indicated by saddle anesthesia and early bladder involvement.

Spinal Cord Disease-Related Weakness

A compressive or noncompressive spinal cord lesion may cause muscle weakness, which typically occurs in the arm and leg if the lesion is at the cervical level or only in the leg if the lesion is below the lower cervical level. The weakness is often bilateral. Bowel and bladder difficulties and numbness are frequently noted. The findings on examination include limb weakness, spasticity, and increased muscle stretch reflexes below the level of the lesion. Extensor plantar reflexes may also be elicited. Sensory findings are often noted.

The most common noncompressive lesion is transverse myelitis, usually of unknown cause. Some patients have a history of vaccination or symptoms suggestive of viral disease that usually precede the neurologic symptoms by a few days to 1 or 2 weeks.

Compressive myelopathy is commonly due to metastatic epidural neoplasm. These patients usually present with local vertebral column pain at the level of the spinal cord lesion. This symptom is present for weeks to months before the gross neurologic deficits occur, although occasionally bony pain may antedate other symptoms by only a few hours.

- Muscle weakness may be associated with a compressive or noncompressive spinal cord lesion.
- Transverse myelitis is the most common noncompressive lesion.

Anterior Horn Cell Disease

Degenerative disorders that affect the motor neurons in the cerebral cortex and the anterior horn cells are called "motor neuron diseases." The most common one is amyotrophic lateral sclerosis (ALS). This disorder is one of the causes of weakness. It typically presents with bilateral weakness that usually begins distally and is associated with cramps and fasciculations. Bowel and bladder difficulties are very uncommon, and sensory abnormalities are not noted. Findings on examination include weakness, severe atrophy, fasciculations, and decreased or increased muscle stretch reflexes and extensor plantar responses.

A mutation in the oxygen radical detoxifying enzyme superoxide dismutase can cause a familial form of ALS. However, no drug has been found to be effective in altering the progressive course of this disease. Recently, some beneficial effect has been noted with riluzole, especially in patients with bulbar onset of the disease. However, treating ALS with immunosuppression such as irradiation, corticosteroids, cyclophosphamide, or intravenous immunoglobulin (IVIG) is at best futile and at worst, costly and harmful. However, treatment for multifocal motor neuropathy with cyclophosphamide or perhaps IVIG can be effective. "Multifocal motor neuropathy" is a syndrome of purely lower motor neuron disease. It is often distal and asymmetrical, accompanied by motor conduction block on EMG, and associated with high titers of serum antibodies to GM_1 gangliosides. However, antibody determinations are costly and have no therapeutic implication. Therefore, patients with purely lower motor neuron disease accompanied by the presence of conduction block on EMG should receive treatment with cyclophosphamide or IVIG.

Radiculopathy

Nerve root lesions usually are indicated by pain that is often sharp and lancinating, follows a dermatomal pattern, and is increased by increasing intraspinal pressure (e.g., sneezing and coughing) or by stretching of the nerve root. Pain often follows a myotomal (e.g., C5 and C6 root pain in the deltoid and biceps muscles) rather than a dermatomal pattern, with paresthesias occurring in the dermatomal pattern. Findings are in the root distribution and include weakness, sensory impairment, and decreased muscle stretch reflexes. Radiculopathies have many causes, including compressive lesions (osteophytes, ruptured disks, and neoplasms) and noncompressive lesions (postinfectious and inflammatory radiculopathies and metabolic radiculopathies, as in diabetes).

- Nerve root lesions are indicated by sharp, lancinating pain with a dermatomal pattern.
- Pain is increased by sneezing and coughing.
- Pain often has a myotomal rather than a dermatomal pattern.
- Findings are weakness, sensory impairment, and decreased muscle stretch reflexes.
- Radiculopathies have many causes.

Degenerative Disease of the Spine

Cervical Spondylosis

MRI in combination with plain radiographs is the preferred approach for evaluating patients who have cervical spondylosis. Surgical results for the relief of symptoms of cervical radiculopathy are better when the cause is a soft disk herniation than when spondylitic radiculopathy and myelopathy are present. In fact, surgical treatment of cervical radiculopathy due to the herniation of a soft disk is so successful that most patients and doctors prefer surgical therapy to prolonged conservative treatment. However, surgical treatment for cervical spondylitic myelopathy is much less successful, with fewer than two-thirds of patients having improvement. Cervical spondylitic myelopathy is a condition in which the spinal cord is damaged either directly by traumatic compression or indirectly by arterial deprivation or venous stasis as a consequence of proliferative bony changes in the cervical spine.

Lumbar Spine Disease

Bulging disks after the age of 30 years should be considered normal and are unlikely to cause nerve root compression. Bulging disks appear round and symmetrical compared with herniated disks, which appear angular and asymmetrical and extend outside the disk space. The criteria for surgical treatment of lumbar disk herniations include the presence of disk herniation on anatomical imaging; dermatome-specific reflex, sensory, or motor deficits; and failure of 6 to 8 weeks of conservative treatment.

The lateral recess syndrome (facet syndrome) is characterized by the following: it produces radicular pain; it is usually caused by an osteophyte on the superior articular facet; the symptoms are unilateral or bilateral pain or paresthesias in the distribution of L5 or S1; the pain is provoked by standing and walking and is relieved by sitting; and the results of the straight leg raising test are usually negative.

Lumbar stenosis is characterized by the following: most patients are older than 50 years; neurogenic intermittent claudication (pseudoclaudication) occurs; the symptoms are usually bilateral but can be asymmetrical or unilateral; the pain usually has a dull, aching quality; the whole lower extremity is generally involved; the pain is provoked while walking or standing; sitting or leaning forward provides relief; and there is often a "dead" feeling in the legs. Decompressive operations for lumbar stenosis can be performed with low morbidity despite the advanced age of most patients. A very high initial success rate can be expected, although about 25% of patients become symptomatic again within 5 years. On reoperation, three-fourths of the patients ultimately have a successful outcome; failures result from progression of stenosis at levels not previously decompressed or restenosis at levels previously decompressed.

Musculoskeletal low back pain is treated best with a formal program of physical therapy and exercise, weight reduction, and education on postural principles.

PERIPHERAL LEVEL: SYMPTOMS AND CLINICAL CORRELATIONS

Neuropathy

Peripheral neuropathies are usually characterized by distal weakness and distal sensory changes. They are usually symmetrical, occur more often in the legs than in the arms, and are often accompanied by impaired or absent distal muscle stretch reflexes. Weakness related to peripheral nerve disorders is typically worse distally, with footdrop and clumsy gait often associated with distal numbness and paresthesias. Examination findings include distal weakness, sensory loss, atrophy, and, sometimes, fasciculations. Muscle stretch reflexes usually are decreased. If a single plexus (lumbosacral or brachial) is involved, the weakness may be isolated to a single limb. However, the findings still are consistent with a "lower motor neuron" lesion, with decreased reflexes, weakness, atrophy, and sensory loss. Neuropathy has many causes, and the pattern of the neuropathy might suggest its cause (Table 17-9). The evaluation of peripheral neuropathy is summarized in Table 17-10. An extensive search usually uncovers the cause in 70% to 80% of cases. A high percentage of the cases of "idiopathic neuropathy" referred to specialty centers are in fact hereditary neuropathies.

Table 17-9 Main Clinical Features and Differential Diagnosis of Peripheral Neuropathies

Pattern of neuropathy	Common or important causes
Mononeuropathy	Compressive neuropathy
	Tumor
	Trauma
	Diabetes mellitus
Mononeuropathy multiplex	Diabetes mellitus
	Vasculitis
	Lyme disease
	HIV neuropathy
	Sarcoidosis
	Leprosy
	Multifocal motor neuropathy
	Hereditary predisposition to pressure palsies
Acute motor polyradiculoneuropathy	AIDP (Gullain-Barré syndrome)
	Lyme disease
	HIV neuropathy
	Porphyria
	Toxins (arsenic, thallium)
	Carcinomatous or lymphomatous meningitis

Table 17-9 Continued

Pattern of neuropathy	Common or important causes
Chronic motor or sensorimotor polyradiculopathy	CIDP
	Paraproteinemia (e.g., osteosclerotic myeloma)
	Hereditary neuropathy (Charcot-Marie-Tooth disease)
	Lead toxicity
	Diabetes mellitus
Distal (stocking-and-glove) sensorimotor neuropathy	Diabetes mellitus
	Alcoholism
	Uremia
	Toxins (hexacarbons)
	Hereditary neuropathy
Sensory ataxic neuropathy	Diabetes mellitus
	Paraneoplastic disorder
	Sjögren syndrome
	Paraproteinemia
	Vitamin B_{12} deficiency
	HIV infection
	Cisplatin
	Vitamin B_6 excess
	Hereditary neuropathy
Painful peripheral neuropathy	Diabetes mellitus
	Vasculitis
	Toxins (arsenic, thallium)
	Hepatitis C
	Cryoglobulinemia
	HIV neuropathy
	CMV polyradiculoneuropathy in HIV-positive patients
	Alcoholism
	Fabry disease
Neuropathy with prominent autonomic involvement	Acute or subacute
	Guillain-Barré syndrome
	Subacute pandysautonomia
	Paraneoplastic pandysautonomia
	Porphyria
	Vincristine neuropathy
	Botulism
	Chronic
	Diabetes mellitus
	Amyloidosis
	Sjögren syndrome

AIDP, acute inflammatory demyelinating polyradiculopathy; CIDP, chronic inflammatory demyelinating polyradiculoneuropathy; CMV, cytomegalovirus; HIV, human immunodeficiency virus.

Table 17-10 Evaluation of Peripheral Neuropathy

Basic laboratory investigations	Special investigations	Investigations in selected cases
CBC with platelets	Thyroid function test	Autonomic function tests
Erythrocyte sedimentation rate	Vitamin B_{12}	Cerebrospinal fluid analysis
Fasting blood glucose	Vitamin E	Sural nerve biopsy
Serum electrolytes	Cholesterol and triglycerides	Investigation for inborn errors of metabolism
Serum creatinine	HIV serology	Genetic studies
Liver function tests	Lyme serology	
Serum and urine electrophoresis and immunoelectrophoresis	Hepatitis serology	
	Cryoglobulins	
Urinalysis	Antineutrophil cytoplasmic antibodies	
Chest radiography	Antibodies against extractable nuclear antigens	
Electromyography	Antineuronal nuclear (anti-Hu) antibodies	
	GM_1 antibodies	
	MAG antibodies	
	Porphyrins	
	Heavy metal screen	

CBC, complete blood count; HIV, human immunodeficiency virus; MAG, myelin-associated glycoprotein.

- Peripheral neuropathy: distal weakness and sensory changes more in the legs than in the arms, usually symmetrical, and with distal muscle stretch reflexes impaired or absent.
- The cause of peripheral neuropathy is usually found in 70%-80% of cases.

Mononeuropathy

Mononeuropathy is characterized by sensory and motor impairment in a single nerve. The usual cause is compression, as in compressive ulnar neuropathy at the elbow, compressive median neuropathy in the carpal tunnel, and compression of the peroneal nerve as it winds around the fibula.

Mononeuropathy Multiplex

Mononeuropathy multiplex consists of asymmetrical involvement of several nerves either simultaneously or sequentially. It suggests such causes as trauma or compression, diabetes mellitus, vasculitis, Lyme disease, HIV neuropathy, sarcoidosis, leprosy, tumor infiltration, multifocal motor neuropathies, or hereditary predisposition to pressure palsies.

Acute Motor Neuropathy

A progressive motor neuropathy of rapid onset that affects both distal and proximal muscles suggests acute inflammatory demyelinating polyneuropathy (AIDP), or Guillain-Barré

syndrome. This may be associated with respiratory muscle weakness, cranial neuropathy (particularly facial palsy, which can be bilateral), and autonomic manifestations. Typically, it is associated with an increased CSF protein concentration but no pleocytosis. About 50% of patients have a mild respiratory or gastrointestinal tract infection 1 to 3 weeks before the neurologic symptoms appear. In the other patients, the syndrome may be preceded by surgery, viral exanthems, or vaccinations. Also, the syndrome may develop in patients who have autoimmune disease or a lymphoreticular malignancy. This syndrome has no particular seasonal, age, or sex predilection. Plasma exchange or IVIG is the treatment for AIDP.

- In Guillain-Barré syndrome, 50% of patients have a mild respiratory or gastrointestinal tract infection 1-3 weeks before neurologic symptoms appear.
- Surgery, viral exanthems, or vaccinations may precede Guillain-Barré syndrome.

Typical Clinical Scenarios

- Guillain-Barré syndrome: a 35-year-old patient has a fairly acute, 1-week history of weakness in both legs that is progressively worsening. The patient does not have any constitutional symptoms, and the results of routine laboratory testing are unremarkable. The patient has some tingling sensation in both feet. Neurologic examination shows mild sensory loss over the toes and generalized loss of deep tendon reflexes. The Babinski sign is not elicited. CSF analysis shows a high concentration of protein but no increase in cell count. Treatment includes plasma exchange or IVIG.

- Amyotrophic lateral sclerosis ("motor neuron disease"): a 50-year-old patient has a 6-month history of slowly progressive muscle weakness. Weakness involves all four extremities. It started distally and now also involves proximal muscles. Physical examination demonstrates muscle wasting and fasciculations. The upper limb reflexes are absent, lower limb reflexes are brisk, and the Babinski sign is elicited. No sensory abnormalities are detected on examination.

- Other causes of subacute, predominantly motor neuropathy are Lyme disease, HIV-related polyradiculopathy, porphyria, organophosphate poisoning, hypoglycemia, toxins (arsenic, thallium), and malignancy. "Acute intermittent porphyria" produces a severe, rapidly progressive, symmetrical polyneuropathy with or without psychosis, delirium, confusion, and convulsions. In most patients, weakness is most pronounced in the proximal muscles. "Tick paralysis" is a rapid, progressive ascending motor weakness caused by neurotoxin injected by the female wood tick. It occurs endemically in the southeastern and northwestern United States. After an asymptomatic period (about 1 week), symptoms develop, usually with leg weakness.

Chronic Predominantly Motor Neuropathies

Chronic, predominantly motor or sensorimotor neuropathies include CIDP, paraproteinemic neuropathies (e.g., associated with osteosclerotic myeloma), hereditary neuropathies, lead toxicity, and diabetes mellitus. Most neuropathies are distal, but occasionally there is predominant proximal weakness, which suggests AIDP, CIDP, porphyria, diabetic proximal motor neuropathy, or idiopathic acute brachial plexopathy. In sharp contrast to AIDP, the argument for corticosteroid treatment of CIDP is strong; plasma exchange is also effective, and corticosteroids alone or in combination with plasma exchange remain the treatment of choice. IVIG may be beneficial for some patients.

Sensory Ataxic Neuropathy

Sensory ataxic neuropathies are characterized by severe proprioceptive sensory loss, ataxia, and areflexia. Some neuropathies are due to peripheral nerve demyelination and others to involvement of large dorsal root ganglion neurons. A predominantly sensory polyneuropathy suggests diabetes mellitus, paraneoplastic disorder, Sjögren syndrome, paraproteinemias, HIV infection, vitamin B_{12} deficiency, cisplatin toxicity, vitamin B_6 excess, or hereditary neuropathy. More than 60% of neuropathies associated with monoclonal gammopathy of undetermined significance (MGUS) are idiopathic, but some are associated with multiple myeloma, amyloidosis, lymphoma, or leukemia. The patients usually are older than 50 years and present early with symmetrical sensory radiculoneuropathy. Later, a motor polyradiculoneuropathy develops, involving mostly the legs. The CSF protein concentration is usually increased; IgM is more common than IgG or IgA. Plasma exchange can be effective therapy for patients with IgG or IgA neuropathy. They have a better response than those with IgM neuropathy. Other immunosuppressive therapy such as IVIG may also be effective.

Painful Neuropathy

Some peripheral neuropathies affect predominantly the small-diameter nociceptive fibers or dorsal root ganglion neurons and are characterized by severe burning pain distally in the extremities. The examination findings are normal except for the distal loss of pain and temperature sensation. Typical causes are diabetes mellitus, vasculitis, toxins, hepatitis C, cryoglobulinemia, some HIV-associated neuropathies, and alcoholism.

Autonomic Neuropathy

Neuropathy with autonomic dysfunction (e.g., orthostatic hypotension, urinary bladder and bowel dysfunction, and impotence) suggests Guillain-Barré syndrome, acute pandysautonomia, paraneoplastic dysautonomia, porphyria, diabetes mellitus, amyloidosis, or familial neuropathy.

Acute pandysautonomia is a heterogeneous, monophasic, usually self-limiting disease that involves both the sympathetic and parasympathetic nervous systems. It may produce orthostatic hypotension, anhidrosis, diarrhea, constipation, urinary bladder atony, and impotence. The syndrome usually evolves over a few days to a few months, with recovery generally being prolonged and partial. This may be an immunologic disorder, but it is indistinguishable from paraneoplastic autonomic neuropathy. Some of the patients may have antibodies against the ganglion-type nicotinic acetylcholine receptor. IVIG treatment limits the duration and reduces the long-term disability of patients with acute pandysautonomia.

- The pattern of neuropathy suggests its cause.
- Mononeuropathy multiplex: diabetes, vasculitis, leprosy, sarcoidosis, Lyme disease.
- Neuropathy with autonomic dysfunction: amyloidosis, diabetes, Guillain-Barré syndrome, porphyria, familial neuropathy.
- Motor polyneuropathy: inflammatory demyelinating polyneuropathy, hereditary neuropathy, osteosclerotic myeloma, porphyria, lead poisoning, organophosphate toxicity, hypoglycemia.

- Sensory polyneuropathy: diabetes, cancer, Sjögren syndrome, dysproteinemias, HIV infection, vitamin B_{12} deficiency, cisplatin toxicity, vitamin B_6 excess, hereditary neuropathy.

Diabetic Neuropathy

Diabetes mellitus may cause CN III neuropathy, usually presenting with sudden diplopia, eye pain, impairment of the muscles supplied by CN III, and relative sparing of the pupil. With compressive CN III lesions, the pupil usually is involved early. Painful diabetic neuropathies include CN III neuropathy, acute thoracoabdominal neuropathy (truncal), acute distal sensory neuropathy, acute lumbar radiculoplexopathy, and chronic distal small-fiber neuropathy.

- Diabetes may cause CN III neuropathy.
- The pupil is involved early in compression of CN III.

Acute or subacute muscle weakness can occur in various forms of diabetic neuropathy. Weakness, atrophy, and pain affect the pelvic girdle and thigh muscles (asymmetrical or unilateral—diabetic amyotrophy). In the second form, elderly patients with diabetes have bilateral proximal and pelvic girdle weakness, wasting, weight loss, and autonomic dysfunction.

Neuromuscular Transmission Disorders

Neuromuscular transmission disorders often are missed clinically. They present as fluctuating weakness, with fatigable weakness in the limbs, eyelids (ptosis), tongue and palate (dysarthria and dysphagia), and extraocular muscles (diplopia). Sensation, muscle tone, and reflexes usually are normal except in myasthenic syndrome, in which the weakness is more constant and reflexes are diminished. Drugs may cause problems at neuromuscular junctions, for example, penicillamine can cause a syndrome that appears similar to myasthenia gravis. Three major clinical syndromes of the neuromuscular junction are myasthenia gravis, myasthenic syndrome, and botulism. Several drugs adversely affect neuromuscular transmission and may exacerbate weakness in these disorders. They include aminoglycoside antibiotics, quinine, quinidine, procainamide, propranolol, calcium channel blockers, and iodinated radiocontrast agents.

Myasthenia Gravis

This usually occurs in young women and older men and is often heralded by such cranial nerve findings as diplopia, dysarthria, dysphagia, and dyspnea. The deficits are usually fatigable, worsening with repetition or late in the day. However, muscle stretch reflexes, sensation, mentation, and sphincter function are normal. Because of remissions and exacerbations in this disease, patients often are considered "hysterical." The diagnosis of myasthenia gravis is based on the detection of nicotinic acetylcholine receptor antibodies and the presence of decremental responses to repetitive electrical stimulation of motor nerves. Acetylcholine receptor antibodies are rare in conditions other than myasthenia gravis (they do not occur in patients with congenital myasthenia gravis and in only about 50% of those with purely ocular myasthenia gravis). Striational antibodies are highly associated with thymoma and sometimes occur in Lambert-Eaton myasthenic syndrome or small cell lung carcinoma. They can occur in penicillamine recipients, bone marrow allografts, and autoimmune liver disorders.

Treatment strategies for myasthenia gravis include anticholinesterase and immunomodulatory agents. Cholinesterase inhibitors, such as pyridostigmine bromide, are often given as initial therapy for myasthenia gravis. This therapy provides symptomatic improvement for most patients for a period of time. Thymectomy is indicated for selected patients younger than 60 years with generalized weakness and for all patients with thymoma. Prednisone is the most commonly used immunomodulatory agent, but initial administration of high doses may exacerbate the weakness. Plasma exchange is an effective short-term therapy for patients with severe weakness and is particularly useful for a recent exacerbation, for preparation for surgery, or during the initiation of corticosteroid therapy. Other immunomodulatory agents include azathioprine, cyclophosphamide, cyclosporine, mycophenolate mofetil, and IVIG (IgG). Older patients receive the most benefit from azathioprine, especially when used as a steroid-sparing drug.

Myasthenic Syndrome (Lambert-Eaton Syndrome)

Patients with myasthenic syndrome often have proximal weakness in the legs and absent or decreased muscle stretch reflexes (sometimes reflexes are elicited after brief exercise). This syndrome usually is diagnosed in middle-aged men who often have vague complaints such as diplopia, impotence, urinary dysfunction, paresthesias, mouth dryness, and other autonomic dysfunctions (orthostatic hypotension). Lambert-Eaton syndrome is due to the presence of antibodies directed against presynaptic voltage-gated P/Q-type calcium channels. It often is associated with small cell lung carcinoma.

Botulism

Botulism should be suspected when more than one person has a syndrome that resembles myasthenia gravis or when one person has abdominal and gastrointestinal symptoms that precede a syndrome that resembles myasthenia gravis. Botulism occurs after the ingestion of improperly canned vegetables, fruit, meat, or fish contaminated by exotoxin of *Clostridium botulinum*. There is increased concern about the potential use of this toxin as a biologic weapon. Paralysis is caused by toxin-mediated inhibition of acetylcholine release from axon terminals at the neuromuscular junction. Although an antitoxin is available, treatment is mainly supportive, especially respiratory but also psychologic, because the signs and symptoms are reversible.

- Often, lesions of the neuromuscular junction are missed clinically.
- Botulism: suspect it if more than one person has a syndrome that resembles myasthenia gravis.
- Onset of myasthenia gravis: diplopia, dysarthria, dysphagia, dyspnea, fatigability, often in young women and older men.
- Myasthenic syndrome: proximal weakness of the legs and decreased or absent muscle stretch reflexes.
- Myasthenic syndrome occurs in middle-aged men who have vague complaints of diplopia, impotence, urinary dysfunction, and dry mouth.
- Myasthenic syndrome is often associated with small cell lung carcinoma.
- Ingestion of the exotoxin of *C. botulinum* causes botulism.
- In botulism, the release of acetylcholine is inhibited at the neuromuscular junction.

Organophosphate Toxicity

This causes the characteristic combination of miosis, excessive bodily secretions, and fasciculations. A key pathophysiologic factor is decreased acetylcholinesterase activity that causes excessive acetylcholine at the neuromuscular junction. The onset of symptoms varies from 5 minutes to 12 hours after exposure. Treatment is with atropine.

- In organophosphate toxicity, decreased acetylcholinesterase activity causes excessive acetylcholine at the neuromuscular junction.
- Atropine is the treatment for organophosphate toxicity.

Muscle Disease

Muscle disease is usually indicated by symmetrical proximal weakness (legs more than arms) and weakness of neck flexors and, occasionally, of smooth muscle and cardiac muscle. Other neurologic findings are normal. Muscle stretch reflexes are usually normal early in muscle disease. Muscle disease presents as proximal weakness greater than distal weakness, with the person having difficulty arising from a chair or raising the arms over the head.

Muscle disease may be acquired disease or progressive hereditary disease. "Myopathy" is a general term for muscle disease. If the disease is progressive and familial, it is called "dystrophy." A classification of myopathies is given in Table 17-11. The diagnosis of myopathy is based on the history and physical examination, increased levels of creatine kinase, and EMG and muscle biopsy results.

Table 17-11   Classification of Myopathies

Dystrophies
Nonprogressive or relatively nonprogressive congenital myopathies
Inflammatory myopathies
   Infectious and viral—toxoplasmosis, trichinosis
   Granulomatous—sarcoidosis
   Idiopathic—polymyositis, dermatomyositis
   With collagen vascular disease
Metabolic myopathies
   Glycogenoses
   Mitochondrial disorders
   Endocrine
   Periodic paralysis
   Toxic—emetine, chloroquine, vincristine, HMG-CoA reductase inhibitors
   Paroxysmal rhabdomyolysis
Miscellaneous

HMG-CoA, hydroxymethylglutaryl coenzyme A.

Two exceptions to proximal weakness in myopathy are the following:

1. Unusual distal myopathy, called "distal myopathy," occurs mainly in residents of Scandinavian countries.
2. Myotonic dystrophy is more common and occurs everywhere. Atrophy and weakness begin distally and in the face and especially in the sternocleidomastoid muscles. An interesting feature of this dystrophy is myotonia, which is normal contraction of muscle with slow relaxation. Test for myotonia by striking the thenar eminence with a reflex hammer and also by shaking the patient's hand and noting that he or she cannot let go quickly.

Inflammatory Myopathy

Inflammatory myopathies include polymyositis, dermatomyositis, and inclusion body myositis. In evaluating acquired myopathies such as inflammatory myopathy, look for the underlying cause. The incidence of occult carcinoma is probably increased in patients with dermatomyositis. Inclusion body myositis occurs mainly in men older than 60 years; they have symmetrical weakness of proximal and distal muscles. At times, there is asymmetrical weakness, and at other times, there is greater predominance of distal muscle involvement. Early in the course of muscle disease, muscle stretch reflexes are normal. Inclusion body myositis is not associated with collagen vascular disease or neoplasms, and the creatine kinase level may be normal or slightly increased. The diagnosis of an inflammatory myopathy, although suggested by the history and examination findings, increased serum levels of creatine kinase, and EMG results, should be confirmed with muscle biopsy.

Prednisone is the cornerstone for treatment of polymyositis and dermatomyositis. The most common pitfall in treating these conditions is not treating with high enough doses of prednisone for sufficient time. The main difference between polymyositis and dermatomyositis is dermatomyositis responds to IVIG (IgG). In both disorders, other immunomodulatory agents, including azathioprine, methotrexate, cyclosporine, cyclophosphamide, chlorambucil, and mycophenolate mofetil, are indicated if relapse occurs during prednisone taper, unacceptable side effects develop from prednisone, or there is no response to prednisone or the response is slow. Plasma exchange is ineffective for both polymyositis and dermatomyositis. There is no convincing evidence that inclusion body myositis responds to immunosuppression.

- "Myopathy" is muscle disease.
- If the disease is progressive and familial, it is called "dystrophy."
- Distal myopathy is unusual and occurs mainly in Scandinavia.
- Myotonic dystrophy: atrophy and weakness in the face and sternocleidomastoid muscles.
- Myotonia (normal contraction, slow relaxation) is a feature of myotonic dystrophy.
- With myotonia, the patient cannot let go quickly after a handshake.
- Acquired myopathy: no underlying cause is found in most adults.
- Patients with dermatomyositis: increased incidence of occult carcinoma.
- Causes of myopathies: collagen vascular disease, endocrinopathy, sarcoidosis, and remote nonmetastatic effects of cancer.

Acute Alcoholic Myopathy

Patients have acute pain, swelling, tenderness, and weakness of mainly proximal muscles. Gross myoglobinuria may cause renal failure.

- Gross myoglobinuria often occurs in acute alcoholic myopathy.

Toxic Myopathies

"Statin" drugs (HMG-CoA inhibitors) may produce an acute necrotizing myopathy characterized by myalgia, weakness, myoglobinuria, and a marked increase in creatine kinase. This toxic effect is potentiated by fibric acid–derivative drugs and cyclosporine.

Electrolyte Imbalance

Severe hypokalemia (<2.5 mEq/L) and hyperkalemia (>7 mEq/L) produce muscle weakness, as do hypercalcemia, hypocalcemia, and hypophosphatemia. Familial periodic paralysis of hypokalemic-, hyperkalemic-, or normokalemic-type consists of episodes of acute paralysis that last 2 to 24 hours and can be precipitated by a large carbohydrate meal or strenuous exercise; cranial or respiratory muscle paralysis is rare.

Endocrine Diseases

Hyperthyroidism and hypothyroidism, hyperadrenalism and hypoadrenalism, acromegaly, and primary and secondary hyperparathyroidism cause muscle weakness.

Acute Muscle Weakness

Physicians may overlook serious underlying diseases in patients whose chief or only complaint is weakness, especially if there are few or no obvious clinical signs. Delayed or missed diagnosis can lead to life-threatening complications such as respiratory failure, irreversible spinal cord dysfunction, and acute renal failure. Respiratory muscles may be affected, although strength in the extremities is relatively normal. Patients with early Guillain-Barré syndrome may have distal paresthesias and increased respiratory effort and be given the diagnosis of hysterical hyperventilation.

- Missed diagnosis can lead to life-threatening complications: respiratory failure, irreversible spinal cord dysfunction, and acute renal failure.
- Early Guillain-Barré syndrome may be misdiagnosed as hysterical hyperventilation.

Acute muscle weakness can be classified into four groups according to the anatomical location of the disorder: disease of the spinal cord, peripheral nerve, neuromuscular junction, or muscle. Causes of acute muscle weakness are summarized in Table 17-12.

PART III—DISORDERS BY MECHANISM

CEREBROVASCULAR DISEASE

Ischemic Cerebrovascular Disease

Pathophysiologic Mechanisms

The causes of ischemic cerebrovascular disorders, including TIA and cerebral infarction, can be classified on the basis of the site of the source for the arterial blockage (embolus from a proximal site or thrombosis in situ from distal causes) within the vascular system starting from most proximal to distal. First, a cardiac source as the most proximal site includes both arrhythmias and structural disorders such as valve disease, dilated

Table 17-12 Important Causes of Acute Muscle Weakness

Spinal cord disease
    Transverse myelitis
    Epidural abscess
    Extradural tumor
    Epidural hematoma
    Herniated intervertebral disk
    Spinal cord tumor
Peripheral nerve disease
    Guillain-Barré syndrome
    Acute intermittent porphyria
    Arsenic poisoning
    Toxic neuropathies
    Tick paralysis
Neuromuscular junction disease
    Myasthenia gravis
    Botulism
    Organophosphate poisoning
Muscle disease
    Polymyositis
    Rhabdomyolysis-myoglobinuria
    Acute alcoholic myopathy
    Electrolyte imbalances
    Endocrine disease

From Karkal SS: Rapid accurate appraisal of acute muscular weakness. Updates Neurology 1991, pp 31-39. By permission of American Health Consultants.

cardiomyopathy, recent myocardial infarction, and other cardiac structural disorders. Also, paradoxical emboli with a right-to-left shunt must be considered. Another potential proximal site of emboli is the aorta. The second site includes large-vessel disorders, with the most common cause being atherosclerosis or dissection in the carotid or vertebrobasilar system. The third site involves small-vessel occlusive disease caused by either inflammatory or noninflammatory arteriopathies (hypertension-induced disease, isolated CNS angiitis, systemic lupus erythematosus) and hematologic disorders, including polycythemia, sickle cell anemia, thrombocytosis, severe leukocytosis, protein C deficiency, protein S deficiency, anticardiolipin antibody syndrome, lupus anticoagulant positivity, and hypercoagulable states caused by carcinoma. Illicit drug use is a common cause of stroke in young persons and results in arrhythmia, inflammatory arteriopathies, and a relative hypercoagulable state.

Pathophysiologic mechanisms of ischemic cerebrovascular disease include artery-to-artery emboli (e.g., extracranial carotid bifurcation to a branch of the middle cerebral artery), cardiac embolic stroke, and lacunar infarction (small-vessel

disease). Other causes are hematologic disorders and states of altered coagulability (polycythemia; sickle cell anemia; thrombocytosis; severe leukocytosis; abnormalities of the cellular constituents of blood such as serologic factors like homocystinuria; deficiencies of antithrombin III, protein C, and protein S; anticardiolipin antibodies; lupus anticoagulant; and mucin produced by adenocarcinomas that can cause a hypercoagulable state). Still other causes are nonarteriosclerotic vasculopathies (fibromuscular hyperplasia, granulomatous angiitis, congophilic angiopathy, systemic lupus erythematosus), dissection of the carotid or vertebral arteries, hemodynamic crisis with impaired distal flow, mechanical compression of arteries, steal syndromes, and AIDS. Recreational drugs are a major risk factor for stroke in young adults.

- Pathophysiologic mechanisms of ischemic cardiovascular disease include a cardiac source, large-vessel disorders, small-vessel disorders, and hematologic causes.
- In young adults, recreational drugs are a major risk factor for stroke.

Risk Factors

Risk factors for atherosclerotic occlusive disease are similar to those predisposing to coronary artery disease: hypertension, male sex, advanced age, cigarette smoking, diabetes mellitus, and hypercholesterolemia. Emboli from intracardiac mural thrombi are also an important cause of TIA and cerebral infarction. Major cardiac risk factors include left-sided chamber enlargement or aneurysm, congestive heart failure, atrial fibrillation, transmural myocardial infarction, mitral valve disease, septic emboli, paradoxical emboli, and atrial myxoma.

Hypertension is the most powerful modifiable risk factor for stroke, but other modifiable risk factors include cigarette smoking, alcohol consumption, physical activity, and cholesterol level. Although low levels of alcohol consumption appear to have a protective effect for ischemic stroke, heavy alcohol consumption increases the risk of all types of stroke, particularly intracerebral and subarachnoid hemorrhage.

Transient Ischemic Attacks

TIAs place patients at high risk for subsequent cerebral infarctions; estimates are from 4% to 10% within 1 year to 33% within the patient's lifetime. Most TIAs are short-lived, usually lasting less than 10 to 15 minutes; 88% resolve within 1 hour. Infarcts, hemorrhages, and mass lesions can present like TIAs.

"Amaurosis fugax" is defined as temporary, partial, or complete monocular blindness and is a classic symptom of a carotid artery TIA. It can be mimicked by glaucoma, vitreous hemorrhage, retinal detachment, papilledema, migrainous aura, temporal arteritis, and even ectopic floaters.

The long-term prognosis for patients who have a TIA generally follows the rule of 3s: 1/3 go on to have cerebral infarction, 1/3 have at least one more TIA, and 1/3 have no more TIAs.

- With TIAs, the risk for subsequent cerebral infarction is high.
- The rule of 3s for patients with TIA: 1/3 will have cerebral infarction, 1/3 will have at least one more TIA, 1/3 will have no more TIAs.
- Most TIAs last less than 10-15 minutes.
- Infarcts, hemorrhages, and mass lesions can present with symptoms like those of a TIA.
- Amaurosis fugax is a classic symptom of a carotid artery TIA.

Carotid Endarterectomy

Carotid endarterectomy markedly decreases the risk of stroke and death of *symptomatic* patients who have a 70% to 99% stenosis of the carotid artery, as seen on angiography. For a 50% to 60% stenosis, carotid endarterectomy is moderately efficacious in selected symptomatic patients. Medical treatment alone is better than carotid endarterectomy for patients with a 0% to 49% stenosis. Symptoms must be those of a carotid territory TIA or minor stroke and must be of recent onset (<4 months). The benefits of carotid endarterectomy require a low perioperative complication rate (4%-6%). Carotid angioplasty with stent placement may be used as an alternative to carotid endarterectomy, particularly for higher risk patients such as those who previously had carotid endarterectomy, radiotherapy to the neck, or neck dissection; those with a stenosis high in the internal carotid artery; or those otherwise deemed at high risk for the operation. The safety and durability of the endovascular approach in comparison with those of carotid endarterectomy are not well defined.

According to the report of the Asymptomatic Carotid Atherosclerosis Study (ACAS), selected patients with asymptomatic carotid stenosis of at least 60% benefit from carotid endarterectomy in terms of future risk for an ipsilateral stroke or death. In ACAS, medical patients were treated with aspirin and risk-factor reduction. The risk for stroke was low for patients treated surgically and for those treated medically (5-year risk of ipsilateral stroke or death was 11% for those treated medically and 6% for those treated surgically). This amounted to approximately a 1% difference per year. No trend was noted on the basis of the various degrees of stenosis, but the number of events was small in each stenosis subdivision. Importantly, surgeons and hospitals were particularly chosen for having reported perioperative complication rates of less than 3% in asymptomatic patients. However, most conservative neurologists advise caution in accepting the premise that patients

with asymptomatic carotid stenosis less than 79% will benefit from surgical endarterectomy.

Patients with asymptomatic carotid occlusive disease who require an operation for some other reason (e.g., coronary artery bypass graft or abdominal aortic aneurysm repair) usually can have that procedure performed without prophylactic carotid endarterectomy, because in this context the risk of stroke in asymptomatic persons is quite low. If a patient has recently had symptoms in the distribution of the carotid stenosis, the decision is more complicated. Generally, if a patient with an asymptomatic carotid stenosis is experiencing cardiac symptoms such as angina, coronary artery bypass graft is performed first and carotid endarterectomy may be considered later if the patient is otherwise an excellent surgical candidate.

The role of carotid angioplasty with stent placement for extracranial carotid occlusive disease has not been entirely clarified. Because the comparative risks and long-term durability of the angioplasty-with-stent procedure are unclear, many consider carotid angioplasty a reasonable alternative, especially if carotid endarterectomy poses a high risk for the patient.

Antiplatelet Agents

Aspirin, ticlopidine, and clopidogrel are all effective for secondary prevention of stroke. The optimal dose of aspirin is uncertain, with ranges recommended from 30 to 1,300 mg daily. Clopidogrel is given as a single dose, 75 mg daily. The dose of ticlopidine is 250 mg twice daily. Ticlopidine is now rarely given because of the associated neutropenia (thus, a complete blood count must be monitored every 2 weeks for the first 3 months of treatment) and thrombotic thrombocytopenic purpura, which also has rarely been reported with clopidogrel. A combination of low-dose aspirin and extended-release dipyridamole is well tolerated and provides another useful alternative to aspirin for prevention of stroke.

Management of Acute Cerebral Infarction

If a patient has an important neurologic deficit caused by an acute cerebral infarction, the immediate decision in the emergency department is whether the patient is a candidate for thrombolytic therapy (tissue plasminogen activator [TPA]). The initial therapeutic approach to ischemic infarction depends greatly on the time from the onset of symptoms to the presentation for emergency medical care. If the onset of symptoms was less than 3 hours before the evaluation, emergent thrombolytic therapy should be considered. If a patient awakens from sleep with the deficit, thrombolytic therapy should not be considered unless the duration of the deficit is clearly less than 3 hours.

The CT findings are important in selecting patients for TPA. CT should not show any evidence of intracranial hemorrhage, mass effect, or midline shift. Patients who may be excluded by clinical criteria are those with rapidly improving deficit, obtunded or comatose status or presentation with seizure, history of intracranial hemorrhage or bleeding diathesis, blood pressure elevation persistently greater than 185/110 mm Hg, gastrointestinal tract hemorrhage or urinary tract hemorrhage within the previous 21 days, a large ischemic stroke within the previous 14 days or a small ischemic stroke within the previous 4 days, or mild deficit. Eligible patients should have marked weakness in at least one limb or severe aphasia. Laboratory abnormalities that may preclude treatment are heparin use within the previous 48 hours with an increased activated partial thromboplastin time, prothrombin time greater than 15 seconds, or blood glucose concentration less than 50 mg/dL or greater than 400 mg/dL.

In a treatment trial of intravenous TPA, the efficacy in improving neurologic status at 3 months was defined for TPA compared with placebo, with the agent administered within 3 hours after the onset of symptoms. Although there was a greater proportion (12% greater) of subjects with minimal or no deficit in the TPA group at 3 months after the event, there was no increase in the proportion of persons with severe deficits or disability. This is particularly important because there was an increased occurrence of symptomatic hemorrhage in the TPA group.

Intravenous TPA should be given in a 0.9-mg/kg dose (maximum, 90 mg), with 10% given as a bolus and the rest over 60 minutes.

- Intravenous TPA should be considered for patients evaluated within 3 hours after the onset of symptoms of severe cerebral infarction.
- Do not treat with TPA if CT shows hemorrhage, mass effect, or midline shift.

Stroke Risks With Nonvalvular Atrial Fibrillation

Atrial fibrillation is associated with up to 24% of ischemic strokes and 50% of embolic strokes. The stroke rate for the entire cohort of patients with chronic atrial fibrillation is generally about 5% per year. However, patients younger than 60 with "lone atrial fibrillation" have a lower risk of stroke than other patients with atrial fibrillation. Stroke risk factors with atrial fibrillation include a history of hypertension, recent congestive heart failure, previous thromboembolism (including TIAs), left ventricular dysfunction identified on two-dimensional echocardiography, and increased size of the left atrium identified on M-mode echocardiography. Patients with atrial fibrillation who have one or more risk factors generally should receive anticoagulation with warfarin (international normalized ratio [INR] 2.0-3.0) and those at low risk should receive aspirin.

For patients receiving anticoagulant therapy, the dominant risk factor for intracranial hemorrhage is the INR. Age is another risk factor for subdural hemorrhage. An INR of 2.0 to 3.0 is probably an adequate level of anticoagulation for nearly all warfarin indications except for preventing embolization from mechanical heart valves. Generally, the lowest effective intensity of anticoagulant therapy should be given.

- Atrial fibrillation is associated with 24% of ischemic strokes and 50% of embolic strokes.
- The stroke rate is about 5% per year.
- Patients with "lone atrial fibrillation" have a lower risk of stroke.

HEMORRHAGIC CEREBROVASCULAR DISEASE

Intracerebral Hemorrhage

Hypertension commonly affects deep penetrating cerebral vessels, especially ones supplying the basal ganglia, cerebral white matter, thalamus, pons, and cerebellum. The following are common misconceptions of intracerebral hemorrhage: the onset is generally sudden and catastrophic, hypertension is invariably severe, headache is always present, reduced consciousness or frank coma is usually present, the CSF is always bloody, and the prognosis is poor and mortality is high. None of these may be present, and the prognosis depends on the size and location of the hemorrhage. Amyloid angiopathy is the second most common cause of intracerebral hemorrhage in older persons and often causes recurrent lobar hemorrhages.

- Intracerebral hemorrhage: the prognosis depends on the size and site of the hemorrhage.

Surgical evacuation of intracerebral hematomas may be necessary for patients who have signs of increased intracranial pressure or for those whose condition is worsening.

Cerebellar Hemorrhage

It is important to recognize cerebellar hemorrhage because drainage may be lifesaving. The important clinical findings are vomiting and inability to walk. Long-tract signs usually are not present. Patients may have ipsilateral gaze palsy, ipsilateral CN VI palsy, or ipsilateral nuclear-type CN VII palsy. They may or may not have headache, vertigo, and lethargy. Cerebellar hemorrhage may cause obstructive hydrocephalus.

- Vomiting and the inability to walk are important findings in cerebellar hemorrhage.
- Long-tract signs usually are not present.
- Cerebellar hemorrhage may cause obstructive hydrocephalus.

Subarachnoid Hemorrhage

Subarachnoid hemorrhage accounts for about 5% of strokes, including about half of those in patients younger than 45, with a peak age range between 35 and 65 years. In up to 50% of cases, an alert patient with an aneurysm may have a small sentinel bleed with a warning headache, or the expansion of an aneurysm may cause focal neurologic signs or symptoms, for example, an incomplete CN III palsy. The prognosis is related directly to the state of consciousness at the time of intervention. The headache is characteristically sudden in onset, and although one-third of subarachnoid hemorrhages occur during exertion, one-third occur during rest and one-third during sleep. The peak incidence of vasospasm associated with subarachnoid hemorrhage occurs between days 4 and 12 after the initial hemorrhage. Other complications include 1) hemorrhagic infiltration into the brain, ventricles, and even subdural space, which requires evacuation; 2) hyponatremia associated with diabetes insipidus or the syndrome of inappropriate secretion of antidiuretic hormone; and 3) communicating hydrocephalus.

In addition to the initial hemorrhage, vasospasm and rehemorrhaging are the leading causes of morbidity and mortality of patients who have a subarachnoid hemorrhage.

The outpouring of catecholamines may cause myocardial damage, with accompanying electrocardiographic abnormalities, pulmonary edema, and arrhythmias. Arrhythmias can be both supraventricular and ventricular and are most likely to occur during the initial hours or days after a moderate-to-severe subarachnoid hemorrhage.

- About 5% of strokes are a subarachnoid hemorrhage.
- In 50% of cases, an alert patient with an aneurysm may have a small sentinel bleed.
- The prognosis is related directly to the state of consciousness at the time of intervention.
- Characteristically, the headache has a sudden onset.

The differential diagnosis of subtypes of hemorrhagic cerebrovascular disease is outlined in Table 17-13.

Table 17-13 Differential Diagnosis of Subtypes of Hemorrhagic Cerebrovascular Disease

Hemorrhage into parenchyma
    Hypertension
    Amyloid angiopathy
    Aneurysm
    Vascular malformation
        Arteriovenous malformation
        Cavernous malformation
        Venous malformation (rare cause of hemorrhage)
    Trauma—primarily frontal and temporal
    Hemorrhagic infarction
    Secondary to brain tumors (primary and secondary neoplasms)
    Inflammatory diseases of vasculature
    Disorders of blood-forming organs (blood dyscrasia, especially leukemia and thrombocytopenic purpura)
    Anticoagulant or thrombolytic therapy
    Increased intracranial pressure (brainstem) (Duret hemorrhages)
    Illicit drug use
    Postsurgical
    Fat embolism (petechial)
    Hemorrhagic encephalitis (petechial)
    Undetermined cause (normal blood pressure, no other recognizable disorder)
Hemorrhage into subarachnoid space (subarachnoid hemorrhage)
    Trauma
    Aneurysm
        Saccular ("berry," "congenital")
        Fusiform (arteriosclerotic)—rarely causes hemorrhage
        Mycotic
    Arteriovenous malformation
    Many of the same causes as for parenchyma above
Subdural and epidural hemorrhage (hematoma)
    Mainly traumatic
    Many of the same causes as for parenchyma above
Hemorrhage into pituitary (pituitary apoplexy)

NEOPLASTIC DISEASE

The most common neurologic symptoms of patients with systemic cancer are back pain, altered mental status, and headache. However, the most common neurologic complication of systemic cancer is metastatic disease, of which cerebral metastasis is most frequent. In patients with cancer and back pain, epidural metastasis and direct vertebral metastasis are common, but no malignant cause is found in about 15% to 20% of patients. Nonstructural causes are the most common reasons for headache. Some identified causes include fever, side effects of therapy, lumbar puncture headache, metastasis (cerebral, leptomeningeal, base of skull), and intracranial hemorrhage (thrombocytopenia, hemorrhage due to intracranial metastasis). The most common cause of altered mental status is metabolic encephalopathy, which is also the most common nonmetastatic manifestation of systemic cancer. Less common causes include intracranial metastatic disease (parenchymal and meningeal), intracranial hemorrhage, primary dementia, cerebral infarction, psychiatric disorder, known primary brain tumor, bacterial meningitis, and transient global amnesia.

Neoplasms that commonly cause neurologic problems are those of the lung and breast, leukemia, lymphoma, and colorectal cancer. Breast, lung, and prostate cancer are commonly associated with bony metastasis and epidural metastasis. The most common brain metastasis is from the lung. Meningeal metastases are common in lung and breast cancer, melanoma, leukemia, and lymphoma. Colorectal cancer causes local pelvic metastasis and is the most frequent cause of tumor plexopathy. Head cancer and neck cancer are the most frequent sources of metastasis to the base of the skull. Melanoma produces a disproportionate number of metastases in the CNS. Gastrointestinal tract tumors (stomach, esophagus, pancreas) have the least number of neurologic complications.

Many neurologic problems in patients with cancer can be diagnosed on the basis of the medical history and findings on neurologic examination and require knowledge of both nonmetastatic- and noncancer-related neurologic illness. Neurologic complications of systemic cancer can be divided generally into the following categories:

Metastatic—parenchymal, leptomeningeal, epidural, subdural, brachial and lumbosacral plexuses, and nerve infiltration; this is common

Infectious—unusual CNS infections because of immunosuppression

Complications of systemic metastases—hepatic encephalopathy

Vascular complications—cerebral infarction from hypercoagulable states, nonbacterial thrombotic endocarditis, and radiation damage to carotid arteries; cerebral hemorrhage from such entities as thrombocytopenia and hemorrhagic metastases

Systemic encephalopathies—usually from multiple causes, hypercalcemia, syndrome of inappropriate secretion of antidiuretic hormone, medications, and systemic infections

Complications of treatment—irradiation, chemotherapy, surgery: radiation necrosis of the brain, radiation myelopathy, radiation plexopathy, fibrosis of the carotid arteries, neuropathies, encephalopathies, and cerebellar ataxia

Nonmetastatic "remote" effect—syndromes have been described from the cerebral cortex through the central and peripheral neuraxes to muscle; they are rare

Miscellaneous—various systemic and neurologic illnesses having nothing to do with cancer

- Cerebral metastasis is the most common neurologic complication of systemic cancer.
- Metabolic encephalopathy is the most common nonmetastatic manifestation of cancer.
- Cancers commonly causing neurologic problems are lung, breast, and colorectal cancers, leukemia, and lymphoma.

- The most common source of brain metastasis is from lung and breast cancer, melanoma, leukemia, and lymphoma.
- The most frequent cause of tumor plexopathy is colorectal cancer.
- Melanoma produces a disproportionate number of metastases in the CNS.
- Common metastatic sites are the parenchyma of the cerebral hemispheres and cerebellum, leptomeninges, epidural and subdural spaces, brachial and lumbosacral plexuses, and nerve.

Radiosurgery (gamma knife and the LINAC-based systems) has been used to treat vascular malformations, acoustic neuromas, pituitary adenomas, and meningeal and (recently) metastatic tumors.

Primary CNS lymphoma is becoming more common in both AIDS and immunocompetent patients. Median survival has been increased with the combination of radiotherapy and chemotherapy, including hydroxyurea, procarbazine, lomustine (CCNU), vincristine, cytosine arabinoside, and intrathecal methotrexate.

MOVEMENT DISORDERS

Tremor

Tremor is an oscillatory rhythmical movement disorder. A simple classification of tremor is rest tremor, postural tremor, and kinetic tremor.

"Rest tremor" is observed with the arms lying in the patient's lap while he or she is sitting or with the arms at the patient's side while walking. Rest tremor occurs in Parkinson disease. "Postural tremor" is seen mainly with the arms outstretched, although there is often a kinetic component as well. Postural tremor is seen in physiologic tremor, but it is also noted pathologically in essential tremor. Drugs such as methylxanthines, β-adrenergic agonists, lithium, and amiodarone may produce postural tremor. "Kinetic tremor" is seen mainly in action, as in finger-to-nose testing. This type of tremor occurs with cerebellar disease and diseases of the cerebellar connections in the brainstem.

Essential Tremor

Essential tremor is the most common movement disorder. It is often misdiagnosed and inappropriately treated. It is a monosymptomatic condition that is manifested as rhythmic oscillations of various parts of the body. Middle-aged and older persons are most commonly affected, and there is often a genetic component. The hands are affected most, with the tremor present in postural position and often having a kinetic component. The head and voice are often affected. Head tremor can be either horizontal ("no-no") or vertical ("yes-yes"). Head tremor almost never occurs in Parkinson disease, but parkinsonian patients may have tremor of the mouth, lips, tongue, and jaw. The legs and trunk (orthostatic tremor) are affected less frequently in essential tremor. Essential tremor is a slowly progressive condition; its pathophysiologic mechanism is not known.

The agent most effective in decreasing essential tremor is alcohol. Alcoholic drinks substantially reduce the tremor for 45 to 60 minutes. However, the rate of alcoholism among patients with essential tremor is no different from that of the general population. Propranolol (80-320 mg daily), other β-blockers, and primidone (25-250 mg at bedtime) are effective. Other drugs that have been prescribed are benzodiazepines, especially clonazepam and lorazepam; methazolamide has also been effective in some patients, especially for head tremor. Botulinum toxin has been used recently. Stereotactic thalamotomy can be effective for patients with severe functional disability whose tremor is unresponsive to drug therapy; surgery probably is underused. Thalamic stimulation (deep brain stimulation) is effective for all types of tremor.

- Movement disorders occur mostly in middle-aged and older persons.
- There is often a genetic component.
- The hands are affected most.
- Head tremor is almost never seen in Parkinson disease.

Parkinson Disease

Patients with Parkinson disease present with tremor (the initial symptom in 50%-70%, but 15% never have tremor), rigidity, and bradykinesia. Also, gait is unsteady—a slow, shuffling gait. Decreased blinking rate, lack of change in facial expression, small handwriting, and asymptomatic orthostatic hypotension are also common. Although dementia is more frequent among patients with Parkinson disease, it is noted in only about 25% of those in whom the disease develops after age 60. The detection of cerebellar findings (ataxia), corticospinal signs (increased deep tendon reflexes, spasticity, extensor plantar response), lower motor neuron findings (decreased reflexes, flaccidity, or fasciculations) should all suggest a disorder other than Parkinson disease as a cause for parkinsonism.

- Tremor does not occur in 15% of those with Parkinson disease.
- If ataxia, increased reflexes, spasticity, extensor plantar responses, or lower motor neuron findings are present, consider other diagnoses.

The treatment for Parkinson disease is summarized in Table 17-14.

Initial treatment options for Parkinson disease include a combination of levodopa and carbidopa (Sinemet), anticholinergic agents, amantadine, or dopaminergic agonists. Anticholinergic agents should not be given to patients older than 65 because of the high incidence of such side effects as memory loss, delirium, urinary hesitancy, and blurred vision. When given to a patient with newly diagnosed Parkinson disease, selegiline (a monoamine oxidase type B inhibitor) may delay the initiation of levodopa therapy as well as give mild symptomatic relief. Initial doses of a combination of levodopa and carbidopa include a 25/100 tablet three times daily. Common side effects include hallucinations, confusion, dyskinesias, and orthostatic hypotension. Long-term high-dose levodopa monotherapy leads to dyskinesias and motor fluctuations. Management strategies include the use of smaller and more frequent doses of levodopa, long-acting levodopa preparations, dopaminergic agonists, and inhibitors of catechol *O*-methyltransferase. Unpredictable off periods may also be helped with the use of a protein restriction diet.

Dopaminergic agonists include the ergot derivatives bromocriptine and pergolide and the nonergot derivatives pramipexole and ropinirole. Although monotherapy with dopamine agonists does not cause the delayed motor complications associated with long-term levodopa therapy, these agents are less efficacious than levodopa. The use of dopaminergic agonists rather than levodopa for early treatment of Parkinson disease has been proposed. The rationale is that this will delay the potential toxic effects of dopamine metabolites in the brain. However, this point is controversial. Like levodopa, dopaminergic agonists may cause hallucinations, postural hypotension, and edema. An important side effect of all these agents is the development of unpredictable episodes of daytime sleepiness. Bromocriptine has been associated with pulmonary and retroperitoneal fibrosis. Reportedly, pergolide is associated potentially with valvular heart disease. New generation antipsychotic drugs, such as clozapine, olanzapine, and quetiapine, can be used to manage drug-induced psychosis because they have a lower risk of exacerbating parkinsonism in these patients. Stereotactic pallidotomy and subthalamic nucleus stimulation are performed in patients with predominantly unilateral symptoms. These treatments are particularly effective for tremor and drug-induced dyskinesia.

Many patients with parkinsonism develop orthostatic hypotension, bladder dysfunction, and other autonomic manifestations. In these patients, Parkinson disease should be distinguished from multiple system atrophy. Findings suggestive of multiple system atrophy include lack of a predictable response to levodopa, the presence of cerebellar or pyramidal signs, severe orthostatic hypotension and urinary incontinence, sleep apnea, and laryngeal stridor. The management of orthostatic hypotension includes eliminating potentially offending

Table 17-14   Treatment of Parkinson Disease

Treatment	Indications	Caveats/problems
Anticholinergic agent (e.g., trihexyphenidyl)	Tremor predominant in young patients	Anticholinergic and cognitive side effects in patients >65 years
Amantadine	Early disease, adjuvant treatment for patients with dyskinesia	Dizziness, livedo reticularis, edema
Levodopa-carbidopa Sinemet 25/100 Sinemet CR 50/200	Most efficacious treatment, give early in disease to patients with marked impairment	Nausea, vomiting, orthostatic hypotension, hallucinations, motor fluctuations with chronic treatment
Dopaminergic agonists Bromocriptine Pergolide Pramipexole Ropinirole	Motor fluctuations while taking Sinemet Some recommend use of these agonists early in course of disease	As with Sinemet (except fluctuations), pleuro-pulmonary reaction and retroperitoneal fibrosis with ergots; patients may fall asleep while driving
COMT inhibitors Entacapone	Prolong duration of action of levodopa in patients with "wearing-off" effect	As with levodopa, diarrhea
MAO-B inhibitors Selegiline	Delay the need to start levodopa therapy, potential (not proven) neuroprotective effect	Insomnia
Atypical antipsychotics Clozapine Olanzapine Quetiapine	Hallucinations, try to avoid extra-pyramidal side effects, may improve akathisia and dyskinesia	Risk of myelosuppression and orthostatic hypotension with clozapine
Surgical treatment Pallidotomy Subthalamic nucleus stimulation	Prominent unilateral symptoms, particularly when associated with dyskinesia	Does not help axial problems/gait instability; risk of optic tract damage with pallidotomy; risk of paresis; speech or swallowing disturbances, particularly with bilateral pallidotomy

COMT, catechol *O*-methyltransferase; MAO, monoamine oxidase.

drugs (vasodilators, diuretics, dopaminergic agonists, clozapine), increasing sodium and water intake, performing postural maneuvers, elevating the head of the bed, and wearing support stockings. Drug treatment includes fludrocortisone (0.1-1.0 mg daily) and vasoconstrictors such as midodrine (10-40 mg daily).

Other Movement Disorders: Botulinum Toxin Therapy

Botulinum toxin, which blocks the neuromuscular junction, is effective therapy for cervical dystonia, blepharospasm, hemifacial spasm, spasmodic dysphonia, jaw-closing oromandibular dystonia, and limb dystonia, including occupational dystonias.

INFLAMMATORY AND IMMUNE DISORDERS

Demyelinating Diseases

Idiopathic inflammatory demyelinating diseases of the CNS are as follows:

Multiple sclerosis

Isolated demyelinating syndromes—optic neuritis and transverse myelitis

Primary progressive demyelinating diseases—chronic progressive myelopathy and progressive cerebellar syndrome

Asymptomatic demyelinating diseases (noted on MRI or autopsy)

Multiple sclerosis is a common, disabling neurologic demyelinating disorder of young adults 20 to 50 years old. It affects women twice as often as men. Multiple sclerosis has a variable prognosis and an unpredictable course. Polygenetic and environmental (possibly viral) factors probably have a substantial effect on susceptibility to multiple sclerosis. The disease involves central white matter of the cerebral hemispheres, brainstem, cerebellum, spinal cord, and optic nerve. From 80% to 85% of patients present with relapsing-remitting symptoms. In about 15% of patients, the disease is progressive from onset (primary progressive). Over time, 70% of patients with the relapsing-remitting form will develop secondary progressive multiple sclerosis. Thus, symptoms reflect multiple central white matter lesions "disseminated in space and time" and include spastic weakness of the limbs, ataxia, diplopia, sensory disturbances, loss of vison, and urinary bladder and bowel dysfunction. Other important symptoms include fatigue, subtle memory and cognitive dysfunction, and depression.

The diagnosis is based on established clinical criteria and supportive laboratory data. Abnormalities on MRI are most helpful and include multifocal lesions of various ages in the periventricular white matter, corpus callosum, brainstem, cerebellum, and spinal cord. Gadolinium-enhanced lesions are presumed to be active lesions of inflammatory demyelination. CSF findings include oligoclonal bands, increased IgG synthesis, and moderate lymphocytic pleocytosis (<50 mononuclear cells). Visual and somatosensory evoked potential studies are less helpful.

Predictors associated with a more favorable long-term course of multiple sclerosis include age younger than 40 at onset, female sex, optic neuritis or isolated sensory symptoms as the first clinical manifestation, and relatively infrequent attacks. Prognostic factors associated with a poor outcome include age older than 40 at onset, male sex, cerebellar or pyramidal tract findings at initial presentation, relatively frequent attacks during the first 2 years, incomplete remissions, and a chronically progressive course. However, no single clinical variable is sufficient to predict the course or outcome of this disease. Acute transverse myelopathy is usually a monophasic disorder and is rarely the first sign of multiple sclerosis. Abnormal MRI findings at the time of presentation of a clinically isolated syndrome suggestive of multiple sclerosis (isolated involvement of the optic nerve, brainstem, or spinal cord) are a strong predictor of the eventual clinical diagnosis of multiple sclerosis in the next 5 years. Interferon beta-1b, interferon beta-1a, and glatiramer acetate decrease the relapse rate and the intensity of relapse in patients with the relapsing-remitting type of multiple sclerosis.

A study of corticosteroid therapy for optic neuritis found that oral prednisone therapy was ineffective. The recommendation is for either a 3-day course of a high dose of intravenous methylprednisolone followed by an 11-day course of oral prednisone taper or no treatment at all.

Several drugs are used to treat specific symptoms of multiple sclerosis. Trigeminal neuralgia, flexor spasms, and other paroxysmal symptoms respond to carbamazepine, and spasticity responds to baclofen and tizanidine. Fatigue, a disabling symptom of multiple sclerosis, occasionally responds to amantadine.

- Typical clinical scenario for multiple sclerosis: A 35-year-old woman has a history of rapid loss of vision in the right eye, with pain on eye movement. A similar episode occurred 2 years ago and involved the same eye, and recovery was complete. She also has noticed weakness and paresthesias of both legs in the last 6 months. CSF analysis shows increased protein levels and oligoclonal bands on electrophoresis. Multiple hypodense areas consistent with demyelination are seen on MRI.

Paraneoplastic Disorders

The paraneoplastic disorders are associated with increased circulating antibodies against membrane (e.g., ion channels) or cytoplasmic components of neoplastic cells. The most common underlying malignancies are small cell lung carcinoma and breast cancer. Others include ovarian or testicular carcinoma, thymoma, Hodgkin disease, and parotid tumors. Paraneoplastic autoimmunity occurs with various neurologic syndromes, including limbic encephalitis (characterized by behavioral and memory abnormalities), brainstem encephalitis, opsoclonus-myoclonus, cerebellar ataxia, myelopathy, motor neuron disease, stiff-man–like syndrome (with axial and limb rigidity), sensory ganglionopathies, Lambert-Eaton myasthenic syndrome, dermatomyositis, and retinopathy. These syndromes are characterized by an acute or subacute onset and increased levels of one or multiple antibodies. Neither the neurologic syndrome nor the antibody is pathognomonic for a particular neoplasm, and many neurologic syndromes and antibodies may coexist in the same patient.

Of patients with Lambert-Eaton myasthenic syndrome, 80% who have primary lung cancer (small cell, squamous cell, adenocarcinoma) and 36% who have no evidence of cancer, are found to have anti-calcium channel antibodies. Those with Lambert-Eaton syndrome who have cancer other than lung cancer usually are negative for these antibodies. Antineuronal nuclear antibodies (ANNA) type I (anti-Hu) are a marker of various neurologic disorders that occur with small cell lung cancer, and the ANNA type II (anti-Ri) antibodies occur in a spectrum of neurologic disorders associated with breast cancer, including cerebellar ataxia, myelopathy, opsoclonus, and other brainstem disorders. Purkinje cell antibodies (sometimes called "anti-Yo" antibodies) are detected in women with paraneoplastic cerebellar degeneration and are associated with ovarian, fallopian tube, endometrial, surface papillary, and breast carcinomas and occasionally with lymphoma. They are not found in men with paraneoplastic cerebellar degeneration or in women with gynecologic cancer without a neurologic syndrome. In a woman who does not have clinically known or laboratory-proven cancer but is positive for these antibodies, exploratory laparotomy probably is warranted. Amphiphysin antibodies occur in patients who have rigidity, peripheral neuropathy, and other neurologic syndromes generally associated with breast cancer.

NEUROLOGIC INFECTIOUS DISEASES

Infectious diseases of the nervous system are manifested in various combinations of meningitis, encephalitis, brain abscess, granulomas, and vasculitis. The typical clinical and CSF findings and common causes of these diseases are summarized in Table 17-15. The most common causes and empiric treatment of bacterial meningitis are summarized in Table 17-16.

Lyme Disease—Multisystem Disorder

Stage I Lyme disease begins with the bite of an infected tick. Any body area may be bitten, but the thigh, groin, and axilla are common sites. Often, patients cannot recall the tick bite.

Stage II disease begins weeks to months after the initial infection and is characterized by neurologic, cardiac, and ophthalmic involvement. About 15% of the patients in the United States have neurologic involvement, usually meningoencephalitis, cranial neuritis, or radiculoneuropathy. Cranial neuropathies are common, most frequently CN VII (bilaterally in one-third of patients). Thus, bilateral CN VII palsy in a patient from an endemic area is almost diagnostic of Lyme disease. Peripheral nervous system involvement can include the spinal roots, plexuses, and peripheral nerves.

Stage III disease marks the chronic phase and begins months to years after the initial infection. This stage is heralded by arthritic and neurologic symptoms. Any CNS symptom is possible, and there may be psychiatric symptoms and cognitive impairment. Severe fatigue is a particularly prominent feature. Rarely, a multiple sclerosis–like demyelinating illness featuring gait disturbance, urinary bladder dysfunction, spastic paraparesis, and dysarthria may develop. These symptoms may have exacerbations and remissions; MRI and CT show multifocal white matter lesions.

- Lyme disease is a multisystem disorder.
- Patients often do not recall the tick bite.
- In the United States, 15% of patients have neurologic involvement.

- Cranial neuropathies, especially CN VII, are common.
- Bilateral CN VII palsy in an endemic area is almost diagnostic of Lyme disease.
- In stage III disease, severe fatigue is prominent.

The longer the duration of symptoms before diagnosis and effective antibiotic treatment, the greater the risk that serious symptoms will outlast the period of acute infection. Laboratory diagnosis can be difficult; an enzyme-linked immunosorbent assay can be undependable both in identifying new cases and in distinguishing acute from remote healed infection. Asymptomatic tick bites have a less than 1% chance of Lyme infection, and treating such patients for Lyme disease is not cost-effective. However, typical erythema migrans accompanying either a tick bite or other typical symptoms is sufficiently diagnostic to warrant treatment after exposure in an endemic area, even without abnormal serologic findings.

Neurologic Complications of AIDS

The nervous system is affected clinically in up to 40% of patients with HIV infection, and pathologic changes in the nervous system are found at autopsy in up to 90%. Neurologic features may be the presenting manifestation of the illness in 5% to 10% of patients. HIV infection is associated with various central and peripheral nervous system disorders, and multiple levels of the nervous system can be affected simultaneously. Therapy is available for many of these syndromes. HIV dementia is treated with a high dose of zidovudine (AZT). Cytomegalovirus encephalitis is treated with ganciclovir. A syndrome of lumbosacral polyradiculomyelopathy presenting as or manifested by progressive lumbosacral radicular symptoms (with weakness, areflexia, and sensory loss in the legs) is often due to cytomegalovirus and, thus, treated with ganciclovir. Cryptococcal meningitis is treated with amphotericin B (also with flucytosine or fluconazole). CNS lymphoma in AIDS patients is treated the same way as CNS lymphoma in immunocompetent patients, that is, with radiotherapy and chemotherapy. The acute inflammatory demyelinating polyradiculoneuropathy responds well to plasma exchange or prednisone. Zidovudine-induced myopathy responds to dose reduction or withdrawal of the medication. Polymyositis is treated the same as it is in other patients, that is, with corticosteroid therapy.

The major HIV-related neurologic conditions include dementia, toxoplasmic encephalitis, CNS lymphoma, progressive multifocal leukoencephalopathy, cytomegalovirus encephalitis, cryptococcal meningitis, neurosyphilis, vacuolar myelopathy, distal symmetrical polyneuropathy, inflammatory demyelinating polyradiculoneuropathy, mononeuropathy multiplex, progressive polyradiculopathy, and myopathy.

Table 17-15   Infectious Syndromes in the Central Nervous System

Syndrome	Clinical features	CSF and other findings	Common or important causes
Aseptic meningitis	Headache, fever, neck stiffness <4 wk duration	Mild-to-moderate mononuclear pleocytosis, normal glucose levels	Infectious—enteroviruses, arboviruses, HSV-2 and 6, HIV, mumps, *Borrelia burgdorferi*, *Treponema pallidum*, *Mycoplasma* Noninfectious—autoimmune disease, drug-induced
Septic meningitis	Headache, fever, neck stiffness <4 wk duration	Moderate-to-marked polynuclear pleocytosis, low glucose levels	*Streptococcus pneumoniae*, *Neisseria meningitidis*, *Listeria monocytogenes*, *Haemophilus influenzae*
Recurrent meningitis	Multiple acute episodes, <4 wk duration	Mild-to-moderate mixed pleocytosis, variable glucose levels	Anatomical defects (*Streptococcus pneumoniae*), HSV-2-autoimmune disease Chemical meningitis
Chronic meningitis	Chronic headache & cognitive, cranial nerve, or other focal symptoms >4 wk duration	Mild-to-moderate mononuclear pleocytosis, low glucose levels, meningeal enhancement and/or hydrocephalus on MRI	Infectious—*Mycobacterium tuberculosis*, fungal (e.g., *Cryptococcus neoformans*) Noninfectious—sarcoidosis, neoplastic disease, vasculitis, autoimmune disorders
Acute encephalitis	Headache, fever, altered state of consciousness; frequently associated with seizures & focal or multifocal neurologic deficits	Mononuclear (occasionally polynuclear) pleocytosis, normal (occasionally low) glucose levels, abnormal EEG, high T_2 signal lesions on MRI	HSV-1, La Crosse encephalitis, St. Louis encephalitis, Rocky Mountain spotted fever VZV, EBV, CMV, HHV-6, and enteroviruses in immunosuppressed patients
Postinfectious encephalomyelitis	Fever, multifocal neurologic signs, altered consciousness	Multiple areas of hyperintense T_2 signal consistent with multifocal demyelinating disease, lymphocytic pleocytosis	Postviral (varicella, mumps, measles, URTI), postimmunization

CMV, cytomegalovirus; CSF, cerebrospinal fluid; EBV, Epstein-Barr virus; EEG, electroencephalography; HHV, human herpesvirus; HIV, human immunodeficiency virus; HSV, herpes simplex virus; MRI, magnetic resonance imaging; URTI, upper respiratory tract infection; VZV, varicella-zoster virus.

Toxoplasmic encephalitis is a common opportunistic infection in AIDS patients. Treatment for this infection is with either pyrimethamine plus sulfadiazine or pyrimethamine plus clindamycin. However, CNS lymphoma and toxoplasmic encephalitis can be difficult to differentiate because they have similar clinical manifestations and CT and MRI characteristics. Therefore, patients with AIDS who present with a contrast-enhancing CNS mass lesion are treated empirically for toxoplasmic encephalitis, and they have follow-up CT or MRI

scans to determine whether the lesion decreases in size. Patients whose lesions do not respond to medical treatment should have a stereotactic biopsy to exclude other causes, including lymphoma.

Patients with AIDS dementia complex have an increased concentration of CSF beta$_2$-microglobulin, which may be a valuable marker for the severity of the dementia and response to treatment. Treatment with zidovudine markedly decreases the concentration of beta$_2$-microglobulin.

Table 17-16 Causes and Management of Bacterial Meningitis by Age

Age	Major pathogens	Empiric antibiotic regimen	Pathogen	Specific therapy
3 mo-18 y	*Neisseria meningitidis, Streptococcus pneumoniae, Haemophilus influenzae*	Ceftriaxone (or cefotaxime), add vancomycin in areas with >2% incidence of highly drug-resistant *S. pneumoniae*	*N. meningitidis* *H. influenzae*	Penicillin G or ampicillin for 7-10 d Ceftriaxone for 7-10 d
18-50 y	*S. pneumoniae, N. meningitidis*	Ceftriaxone (or cefotaxime), add vancomycin in areas with >2% incidence of highly drug-resistant *S. pneumoniae*	*S. pneumoniae* (MIC <0-0.1) *S. pneumoniae* (MIC >0-0.1)	Ceftriaxone (or cefotaxime) for 10-14 d Vancomycin plus ceftriaxone for 10-14 d
>50 y	*S. pneumoniae, Listeria monocytogenes,* gram-negative bacilli	Ampicillin plus ceftriaxone (or cefotaxime), add vancomycin in areas if drug-resistant *S. pneumoniae* is suspected	*L. monocytogenes*	Ampicillin plus gentamicin for 14-21 d (for patients with major penicillin allergy, TMP-SMX may be substituted for ampicillin)

MIC, minimal inhibitory concentration; TMP-SMX, trimethoprim-sulfamethoxazole.

Neurology of Sepsis

The nervous system is commonly affected in sepsis syndrome. The neurologic conditions encountered are septic encephalopathy, critical-illness polyneuropathy, septic myopathy, cachexia, and panfascicular muscle necrosis. Neurologic complications also occur in an intensive care unit for critical medical illness. These complications include metabolic encephalopathy, seizures, hypoxic-ischemic encephalopathy, and stroke.

Septic Encephalopathy

Septic encephalopathy is brain dysfunction in association with systemic infection *without* overt infection of the brain or meninges. Early encephalopathy often begins before failure of other organs and is not due to single or multiple organ failure. Endotoxin does not cross the blood-brain barrier and so probably does not directly affect adult brains. Cytokines, important components of sepsis syndrome, may contribute to encephalopathy. Gegenhalten or paratonic rigidity occurs in more than 50% of patients, and tremor, asterixis, and multifocal myoclonus occur in about 25%. Seizures and focal neurologic signs are rare.

EEG is a sensitive indicator of encephalopathy. The mildest abnormality is diffuse excessive theta low-voltage activity (4-7 Hz). The next level of severity is intermittent rhythmic delta activity (<4 Hz). As the condition worsens, delta activity becomes arrhythmic and continuous. Typical triphasic waves occur in severe cases.

Adult respiratory distress syndrome is common in severe but not in mild cases of encephalopathy.

- Brain dysfunction is associated with systemic infection.
- Encephalopathy precedes failure of other organs.
- Cytokines are an important part of sepsis syndrome.
- More than 50% of patients have paratonic rigidity.
- 25% of patients have tremor, asterixis, and multifocal myoclonus.
- EEG is a sensitive indicator of encephalopathy.

Critical Illness Polyneuropathy

This occurs in 70% of the patients with sepsis and multiple organ failure. There is often unexplained difficulty in weaning from mechanical ventilation. Nerve biopsy specimens show primary axonal degeneration of motor and sensory fibers without inflammation. Recovery from polyneuropathy is satisfactory if the patient survives sepsis and multiple organ failure.

- Nerve biopsy specimens show primary axonal degeneration of motor and sensory fibers without inflammation.
- Recovery from polyneuropathy is satisfactory.

Neurologic Complications of Organ Transplantation

Because almost all organ transplant recipients require some degree of chronic, life-long immunosuppressive therapy, the major neurologic complications of organ transplantation are due to immunosuppression. These include the direct neurotoxic side effects of immunosuppressive drugs, infections, and the development of de novo malignancies. Direct neurologic side effects include the following:

Cyclosporine—Tremor is the most common side effect of cyclosporine, which also may produce various motor syndromes such as hemiparesis, paraparesis, and quadriparesis. Cyclosporine may cause encephalopathy and, less commonly, neuralgia and neuropathy; it is epileptogenic.

Corticosteroids—The side effects of corticosteroids include myopathy, steroid psychosis, withdrawal (myalgias, arthralgias, headache, lethargy, nausea), and spinal cord or cauda equina compression due to epidural lipomatosis.

Azathioprine—It has no direct neurotoxic side effects.

CNS Infections

Infection of the CNS in immunosuppressed patients is relatively frequent and life-threatening. The three organisms that cause more than 80% of CNS infections are *Listeria monocytogenes*, *Cryptococcus neoformans*, and *Aspergillus fumigatus*. The greatest risk factor for CNS infection is the magnitude and duration of immunosuppression. Severe and advanced CNS infections may present with little or no clinical evidence of infection. The period of the risk of infection is mainly from 1 to 6 months after transplantation. Specific infections include 1) acute meningitis, most often due to *Listeria*; 2) subacute or chronic meningitis, generally due to *Cryptococcus*; 3) slowly progressive dementia, frequently due to progressive multifocal leukoencephalopathy; and 4) focal brain disease due to infection usually caused by *Aspergillus*, *Toxoplasma*, *Listeria*, or *Nocardia*.

CNS Involvement by de Novo Lymphoproliferative Diseases

There is an increase in non-Hodgkin lymphoma, especially primary CNS lymphomas. These lymphomas may be linked to infection with Epstein-Barr virus.

Other Neurologic Complications

Other complications affecting the nervous system can be classified as follows:

Complications arising from the underlying diseases
Problems resulting from the transplant procedure
Side effects of immunosuppression
Post-transplantation disorder peculiar to the specific type of transplant

The complications include compressive neuropathies, plexopathies, and radiculopathies; encephalopathy (especially with kidney, liver, and heart transplants); and cerebral infarctions (with bone marrow and heart transplants). Chronic graft-versus-host disease (especially with bone marrow transplant) involves the peripheral nervous system (but not the CNS), for example, polymyositis, myasthenia gravis, and peripheral neuropathy, including CIDP. A complication associated with liver transplantation is central pontine myelinolysis, which is manifested as altered mental status or coma, pseudobulbar palsy, and quadriplegia.

Neurology Pharmacy Review
Kelly K. Wix, PharmD

Drug (trade name)	Toxic/adverse effects	Drug interactions	Comments
		Parkinson disease	
Dopamine precursor			
Levodopa-carbidopa (Sinemet, Sinemet CR)	Contraindicated: narrow-angle glaucoma, MAO inhibitors used within previous 2 wk Dyskinesias, psychiatric disturbances, nausea/vomiting, orthostatic hypotension	Decreased levodopa effect: antipsychotics, iron, pyridoxine (vitamin B_6), phenytoin, TCAs Increased levodopa effect: antacids, tolcapone Affected by levodopa: antihypertensives, MAO-A inhibitors	Carbidopa prevents dopa-decarboxylase activity peripherally Regular release product *without* food; CR product *with* food Wearing off & on/off phenomena require adjustments in dose and administration schedule Taper dose over 2-3 d for discontinuation
Dopamine agonist			
Pramipexole (Mirapex)	Dyskinesias, psychiatric disturbances, nausea, constipation, orthostatic hypotension, syncope, confusion, hallucinations, sedation/ sleep attacks	Increased pramipexole effect: cimetidine Decreased pramipexole effect: DA antagonists*	Weekly titration to target dose Short-term efficacy without concomitant levodopa therapy Reduce pramipexole dose in renal failure Take with food to decrease nausea/vomiting
Ropinirole (Requip)	Same as for pramipexole, more syncope, fewer hallucinations	Increased ropinirole effect: ciprofloxacin, estrogen Decreased ropinirole effect: smoking, DA antagonists*	Short-term efficacy without concomitant levodopa therapy
Pergolide (Permax)	Same as for pramipexole except sleep attacks; in addition, pleuropulmonary reaction, retroperitoneal fibrosis, erythromelalgia, pedal edema	Decreased pergolide effect: DA antagonists*	If pleuropulmonary reaction, retroperitoneal fibrosis, or erythromelalgia occurs, must discontinue drug Take with food to decrease nausea/vomiting
Bromocriptine (Parlodel)	Same as for pergolide	Increased bromocriptine effect: erythromycin Increased effect by bromocriptine: cyclosporine, sirolimus, tacrolimus	Same as for pergolide

Neurology Pharmacy Review (continued)

Drug (trade name)	Toxic/adverse effects	Drug interactions	Comments
MAO-B inhibitor			
Selegiline (Eldepryl)	Contraindicated: meperidine, sibutramine Exacerbates levodopa side effects, agitation, insomnia	Increased effect by selegiline: meperidine, sibutramine, SSRIs, TCAs, bupropion, oral contraceptives, tramadol, amphetamine, sumatriptan, dextromethorphan	Last dose given with lunch Hypertensive crises with tyramine foods not a concern because selegiline does not inhibit MAO-A in doses <20 mg daily
Anticholinergic			
Benztropine (Cogentin) Trihexyphenidyl (Artane)	Confusion, dry mouth, blurred vision, constipation, urinary retention	Decreased effect by anticholinergics: phenothiazines	Use with caution in the elderly and in narrow-angle glaucoma Only effective in about 25% of patients
COMT inhibitor			
Entacapone (Comtan)	Diarrhea, nausea, anorexia, orthostatic hypotension, dyskinesias, psychiatric disturbances, orange urine	Increased effect by entacapone: COMT substrates (Epi, NE, dobutamine), nonselective MAO inhibitors, probenecid, cholestyramine, ampicillin, erythromycin	COMT inhibitors are for adjunctive therapy to levodopa only Do not administer with nonselective MAO inhibitors
Tolcapone (Tasmar)	Same as for entacapone Acute fulminant hepatic failure	Increased effect by tolcapone: levodopa, warfarin (possible)	Requires written informed consent from patient Monitor LFTs q 2 wk × 1 y; then q 4 wk × 6 mo; then q 8 wk thereafter
Miscellaneous			
Amantadine (Symmetrel)	Dizziness, confusion, nausea, ankle edema, livedo reticularis	Increased effect by amantadine: medications with anticholinergic properties Increased amantadine effect: triamterene, trimethoprim-sulfamethoxazole	Not for use in renal failure Tolerance develops in 6-12 wk Need to taper dose for discontinuation

Neurology Pharmacy Review (continued)

Drug (trade name)	Toxic/adverse effects	Drug interactions	Comments
		Alzheimer disease	
		[See Drug Class Note†]	
Donepezil (Aricept)	Nausea/vomiting, diarrhea, headache	Possible increased donepezil effect: ketoconazole Possible decreased donepezil effect: phenytoin, phenobarbital, carbamazepine, rifampin, dexamethasone	Fewer side effects than tacrine because works only in CNS
Rivastigmine (Exelon)	Nausea/vomiting, diarrhea, dizziness, headache, anorexia/weight loss	None known	Take with food
Galantamine (Reminyl)	Nausea/vomiting, diarrhea, anorexia/weight loss	Increased effect by galantamine: ketoconazole, erythromycin, cimetidine, fluoxetine, paroxetine, fluvoxamine	Because of marked GI adverse reactions, start dose at 1.5 mg twice daily and titrate to maintenance dose If treatment is interrupted more than several days, start again with lowest daily dose Take with food Dose reduction in renal or hepatic failure
Tacrine (Cognex)	Nausea/vomiting, diarrhea, dizziness, elevated LFTs	Increased effect by tacrine: theophylline Increased tacrine effect: cimetidine, estradiol, fluvoxamine, riluzole	Monitor LFTs every other week for weeks 4-16, then q 3 mo Dose adjustments indicated if LFTs >2 × ULN Discontinue if jaundice, total bilirubin >3 mg/dL, and/or signs/symptoms or hypersensitivity in association with ALT elevation

Neurology Pharmacy Review (continued)

Drug (trade name)	Toxic/adverse effects	Drug interactions	Comments
Multiple sclerosis			
Interferon beta-1a (Avonex, Rebif)	Contraindicated: pregnancy Depression, anxiety, injection site reaction, influenza-like symptoms, photosensitivity, increased LFT & leukopenia (Rebif)	Increased effect by interferon beta-1a: zidovudine, live vaccines	Avonex, weekly IM dosing; Rebif, 3 times weekly dosing Both interferon beta-1a and 1b decrease number of exacerbations, but only interferon beta-1a has retarded disease progression in clinical studies For both interferon beta-1a and 1b, caution patients to immediately report depression or any thoughts of suicide, caution in preexisting seizure disorder Avonex, Rebif: use with caution if preexisting seizure disorder Rebif: stop if jaundice/ symptoms of liver dysfunction
Interferon beta-1b (Betaseron)	Same as for interferon beta-1a, side effects generally more severe with interferon beta-1b	Increased effect by interferon beta-1b: live vaccines	Every other day SQ dosing Must enroll in program to prescribe Also monitor WBCs, Plt, LFTs periodically
Glatiramer acetate (Copaxone)	Injection site reaction, flushing, palpitations, chest tightness, dyspnea	Not known	Daily SQ dosing at bedtime

*Common DA antagonists include phenothiazines, droperidol, metoclopramide, atypical antipsychotics.
†Antagonistic effects with anticholinergics; additive effects with cholinergics or other cholinesterase inhibitors.
ALT, alanine aminotransferase; CNS, central nervous system; COMT, catechol O-methyltransferase; CR, continuous release; DA, dopamine; Epi, epinephrine; GI, gastrointestinal; IM, intramuscular; LFT, liver function test; MAO, monoamine oxidase; NE, norepinephrine; Plt, platelets; q, every; SQ, subcutaneous; SSRI, selective serotonin reuptake inhibitor; TCA, tricyclic antidepressant; ULN, upper limit of normal; WBC, white blood cell.

Neurology Pharmacy Review (continued)

Review of Headache Drugs

Drug (trade name)	Toxic/adverse effects	Drug interactions	Comments
Acute treatment			
Ergots			
Ergotamine tartrate (Ergostat) Ergotamine/caffeine (Cafergot, Ercaf) Dihydroergotamine (DHE 45, Migranal)	Contraindicated: pregnancy, PVD, CAD, sepsis, liver or renal disease, severe HTN N/V, CNS, rebound headache, dependence, numbness/tingling of extremities Diarrhea with DHE 45	Protease inhibitors, macrolides, NNRT inhibitors decrease ergot metabolism Triptans add to vasospastic effects, avoid use within 24 h of ergots Sibutramine: could lead to serotonin syndrome β-Blockers: unopposed ergot action may lead to peripheral ischemia Nitrates: decreased ergot metabolism, decreased antianginal effects of nitrates	Avoid prolonged administration or excessive dose because of danger of gangrene Caffeine enhances intestinal absorption of ergotamine Most effective if given early in headache course DHE 45: used IM, IV, or SC; pretreat with antiemetic
Triptans			
Sumatriptan (Imitrex) Naratriptan (Amerge) Rizatriptan (Maxalt, Maxalt-MLT) Zolmitriptan (Zomig) Almotriptan (Axert) Frovatriptan (Frova) Eletriptan (Relpax)	Contraindicated: IHD, Prinzmetal angina, uncontrolled HTN, use with or within 24 h of ergots or other serotonin agonist, use with or within 2 wk of MAO inhibitors, hemiplegic or basilar migraine CNS, chest pain, GI, photo-sensitivity, headache recurrence	MAO-A inhibitors (but not MAO-B inhibitors) decrease metabolism of triptans. Naratriptan is not metabolized by MAO-A & is less likely to interact with MAO inhibitors Ergots (see above) SSRIs, sibutramine: possible serotonin syndrome Propranolol increases rizatriptan by 70% and frovatriptan (in males) by 60% Almotriptan & eletriptan have important interactions with CYP3A4 inhibitors	Do not exceed recommended dose, each agent has specific requirements for daily maximum Do not give Imitrex injectable product IV Headache recurrence rate may be lower with naratriptan and frovatriptan (longer half-life)
Analgesics Acetaminophen (Tylenol) NSAIDs Butorphanol nasal spray (Stadol)	Somnolence, dizziness, nasal congestion; may precipitate withdrawal in the opioid-dependent		Drugs of choice for menstrual migraine prophylaxis Ketorolac: given IV/IM for acute headache treatment Poor tolerance is often limiting factor for routine use

Neurology Pharmacy Review (continued)

Review of Headache Drugs (continued)

Drug (trade name)	Toxic/adverse effects	Drug interactions	Comments
Midrin (isometheptene [sympathomimetic], dichloralphenazone [mild sedative], acetaminophen)	Contraindicated: glaucoma, severe renal disease, HTN, organic heart disease, liver disease, MAO inhibitor therapy CNS, agranulocytosis (dichloralphenazone)	MAO inhibitors with isometheptene may cause hypertensive crisis May potentiate effects of warfarin	Max 5 caps/24 h
Acute treatment			
Analgesics Meperidine (Demerol)	Contraindicated: concurrent MAO inhibitor, respiratory depression CNS, dependence	MAO inhibitor: hypertensive crisis Ritonavir inhibits meperidine metabolism Sibutramine: possible serotonin syndrome	Give SC/IM for acute headache treatment Metabolized to normeperidine, which accumulates with chronic dosing and renal dysfunction to cause CNS SEs
Butalbital products (Fiorinal, Fioricet)	Contraindicated: porphyria CNS, respiratory depression, tolerance/dependence, depression	Butalbital may increase metabolism of warfarin Avoid ethanol with butalbital	Fiorinal: butalbital + caffeine + aspirin Fioricet: butalbital + caffeine + acetaminophen
Corticosteroids Dexamethasone (Decadron)	Contraindicated: systemic fungal infection Peptic ulceration, immunosuppression, psychosis, HPA-axis suppression, fluid retention, osteoporosis	Anticholinesterases: steroids antagonize ACHE effects Rifamycins: increased metabolism of steroids	Give IV/IM for acute headache treatment Pretreat with antiemetic Limit to 1 dose
Prophylactic treatment*			
β-Blockers Propranolol (Inderal) Timolol (Blocadren) Metoprolol (Lopressor)	Contraindicated: asthma or bronchospasm, sinus bradycardia, 2nd/3rd-degree heart block Fatigue, depression, blunting of hypoglycemic/hyperthyroid reactions Abrupt withdrawal may precipitate angina or MI	Clonidine plus β-blocker: discontinue gradually and remove β-blocker first Epinephrine: initial hypertensive episode followed by bradycardia Verapamil: effects of both drugs are enhanced Ergots (see above)	Drugs of choice for migraine prophylaxis Avoid agents with ISA activity Failure of 1 agent does not preclude trial of another
Tricyclic antidepressants Amitriptyline (Elavil) Nortriptyline (Pamelor)	Contraindicated: avoid in acute recovery stage after MI Anticholinergic SE, cardiac abnormalities, decreased seizure threshold, CNS, photosensitivity	Clonidine: hypertensive crisis Sparfloxacin, grepafloxacin: risk of torsades de pointes MAO inhibitors: hypertensive crisis	Very toxic in overdose

Neurology Pharmacy Review (continued)

Review of Headache Drugs (continued)

Drug (trade name)	Toxic/adverse effects	Drug interactions	Comments
Prophylactic treatment* (continued)			
Miscellaneous			
Verapamil (Calan, Isoptin)	Contraindicated: advanced heart failure, 2nd/3rd-degree AV block, LV dysfunction, sick sinus syndrome	β-Blockers: increased effects of both drugs	
	Arrhythmias, constipation	Digoxin: increased digoxin levels	
		Use with dofetilide is contra-indicated	
		Prolongs half-life of quinidine	
Divalproex sodium (Depakote ER)	See table for antiepileptic agents (valproic acid derivatives)	See table for antiepileptic agents (valproic acid derivatives)	
Methysergide (Sansert)	Same as for ergots	Same as for ergots	Requires 3-4-wk drug holiday between each 6-mo treatment course
	Retroperitoneal, pleuro-pulmonary, & cardiac fibrosis		Last-line agent because of severe SEs

ACHE, acetylcholinesterase; AV, atrioventricular; CAD, coronary artery disease; CNS, central nervous system; GI, gastrointestinal; HPA, hypothalamo-pituitary-adrenocortical; HTN, hypertension; IHD, ischemic heart disease; IM, intramuscular; ISA, intrinsic sympathomimetic activity; IV, intravenous; LV, left ventricular; MAO, monoamine oxidase; MI, myocardial infarction; NNRT, nonnucleoside reverse transcriptase; NSAID, nonsteroidal anti-inflammatory drug; N/V, nausea and vomiting; PVD, peripheral vascular disease; SC, subcutaneous; SE, side effect; SSRI, selective serotonin reuptake inhibitor.
*Prophylaxis is indicated for patients with 1) prolonged aura, 2) >2 or 3 attacks per month where abortive agents are ineffective or contraindicated, 3) headache requiring daily symptomatic therapy.

Neurology Pharmacy Review (continued)

Review of Antiepileptic Drugs

Drug (trade name)	Toxic/adverse effects	Drug interactions	Comments
Traditional AEDs*			
Phenytoin (Dilantin)	Contraindicated: sinus brady-cardia, SA block, 2nd/3rd-degree AV block or Adams-Stokes syndrome Increased LFTs, nystagmus, gingival hyperplasia, folic acid deficiency, blood dyscrasias, hirsutism, metabolic bone disease, coarsening facial features, hyperglycemia Monitor ECG & BP during IV administration	IV administration of phenytoin during dopamine infusions may cause severe hypotension and cardiac arrest Liver enzyme inducer: causes increased metabolism of many other drugs (cyclosporine, tacrolimus, theophyllines, oral contraceptives, itraconazole, antiarrhythmics, steroids, other AEDs) Rifampin, chemotherapy agents, theophyllines, steroids decrease phenytoin levels Phenytoin interacts with tube feedings, separate phenytoin and tube feeding by 2 h Cimetidine, fluconazole, sulfas, SSRIs, felbamate, topiramate increase phenytoin concentration	IV phenytoin precipitates in solution: give IV push Max rate 50 mg/min, avoid IM use Metabolism is capacity-limited & shows saturability: avoid large dose changes Highly protein bound to albumin: may choose to check free phenytoin levels in hypoalbuminemic states Avoid frequent dose changes: steady state reached in 10-14 d
Fosphenytoin (Cerebyx)	Same as for phenytoin Groin paresthesia with IV administration	As for phenytoin	Antiepileptic activity is due to phenytoin (fosphenytoin = prodrug) Dose is expressed as PE IM product must be diluted before administration IV Max rate of IV infusion = 150 mg PE/min Continuous monitoring of ECG, BP, & RR is essential during IV administration and for 10-20 min after end of infusion Avoid IM for treatment of status epilepticus

Neurology Pharmacy Review (continued)

Review of Antiepileptic Drugs (continued)

Drug (trade name)	Toxic/adverse effects	Drug interactions	Comments
Traditional AEDs (continued)			
Carbamazepine (Tegretol, Tegretol XR, Carbatrol)	Contraindicated: bone marrow suppression, with or within 14 d of MAO inhibitors Blood dyscrasias: leukopenia (10%), aplastic anemia (rare), thrombocytopenia Hyponatremia Cholestatic jaundice	Liver enzyme inducer: causes increased metabolism of other drugs (warfarin, oral contraceptives, cyclosporine, TCAs, bupropion, other AEDs) Metabolized by CYP3A4 Macrolides, azole antifungals, grapefruit, fluoxetine, cimetidine, verapamil, propoxyphene, isoniazid increase carbamazepine concentrations Valproic acid increases carbamazepine epoxide (active metabolite) by 45% Felbamate, phenobarbital, phenytoin, rifampin decrease carbamazepine concentrations	Monitor CBC/DC at baseline, monthly ×2 mo, then every 12-24 mo (discontinue if WBC $<3\times10^9$/L or ANC $<1.5\times10^9$/L), LFTs baseline and periodically, serum sodium periodically Structurally related to TCAs Carbamazepine induces its own metabolism, so true steady state may not be seen for 30 d even though half-life is short
Valproic acid derivatives (Depakote, Depakote Sprinkles, Depakote ER, Depakene, Depacon)	Contraindicated: liver disease/dysfunction Pancreatitis, rare fatal hepatotoxicity (risk greatest if age <2 y), GI, platelet aggregation inhibition, alopecia, thrombocytopenia (dose related), weight gain, hyperammonemia	Liver enzyme inhibitor: causes decreased metabolism of lamotrigine, phenobarbital, phenytoin, diazepam, & ethosuximide & increased levels of carbamazepine-epoxide Use caution in patients taking other agents affecting platelet function Carbamazepine, phenytoin, phenobarbital, rifampin decrease valproic acid concentrations Felbamate, salicylates, erythromycin increase valproic acid concentrations	Do not give injectable product IM. Typical max infusion rate = 20 mg/min (some evidence that faster rate over 5-10 min is safe) Depakote tablets are not bioequivalent to Depakote ER tablets, do not crush any Depakote product
Phenobarbital	Contraindicated: respiratory disease when dyspnea or obstruction is present, porphyria Tolerance/dependence, hyperactivity in children, cognitive impairment, metabolic bone disease	Liver enzyme inducer: causes increased metabolism of other drugs (warfarin, metronidazole, theophyllines, oral contraceptives, steroids, β-blockers) Felbamate, valproic acid, chloramphenicol decrease metabolism of phenobarbital	Max infusion rate = 60 mg/min, avoid intraarticular or SC injection

Neurology Pharmacy Review (continued)

Review of Antiepileptic Drugs (continued)

Drug (trade name)	Toxic/adverse effects	Drug interactions	Comments
Traditional AEDs (continued)			
Primidone (Mysoline)	As for phenobarbital	As for phenobarbital Phenytoin causes increased serum concentration of phenobarbital component	Metabolized by liver to phenylethyl-malonamide (active) and phenobarbital
Felbamate (Felbatol)	Contraindicated: history of blood dyscrasias, liver dysfunction Aplastic anemia, hepatotoxicity, photosensitivity	Inducers (phenytoin, carbamazepine, phenobarbital) decrease felbamate concentrations Felbamate increases phenytoin, valproic acid, phenobarbital, carbamazepine-epoxide concentrations	Monitoring: CBC/DC at baseline and every 2-4 wk LFTs and bilirubin every 1-2 wk Recommended for use *only* in severe epilepsy refractory to all other treatment
Newer AEDs†			
Lamotrigine (Lamictal)	Photosensitivity Risk of severe, potentially life-threatening rash increases if age <16 y Risk *may* increase if lamotrigine is given concurrently with VA, dose exceeds recommended dose, or dose is escalated faster than recommended	Valproic acid increases lamotrigine concentrations Lamotrigine decreases valproic acid concentrations Inducers (phenytoin, carbamazepine, phenobarbital) decrease lamotrigine concentrations Lamotrigine inhibits dihydrofolate reductase, be aware if administering other inhibitors of folate metabolism	*Must* use smaller doses of lamotrigine in combination with valproic acid Discontinue lamotrigine at the first sign of rash
Tiagabine (Gabitril)	GI (give with food) Weakness	Inducers (phenytoin, carbamazepine, phenobarbital) decrease tiagabine concentration by 60% Metabolized by CYP3A	Decrease dose and/or increase interval in hepatic insufficiency
Gabapentin (Neurontin)	GI	Separate aluminum/magnesium antacids and gabapentin by 2 h	Renally eliminated, not metabolized, must be adjusted for renal insufficiency
Topiramate (Topamax, Topamax Sprinkles)	Nephrolithiasis Paresthesias	Inducers (phenytoin, carbamazepine, phenobarbital) may decrease topiramate concentrations Topiramate has additive effect with carbonic anhydrase inhibitors Topiramate decreases efficacy of estrogen component of oral contraceptives	70% of dose excreted unchanged in urine: use 1/2 normal dose in patients with renal impairment Encourage hydration to avoid nephrolithiasis

Neurology Pharmacy Review (continued)

Review of Antiepileptic Drugs (continued)

Drug (trade name)	Toxic/adverse effects	Drug interactions	Comments
Newer AEDs†(continued)			
Zonisamide (Zonegran)	Contraindicated: hypersensitivity to sulfa Do not use in renal failure (creatinine clearance <50 mL/min) Urolithiasis	Inducers (phenytoin, carbamazepine, phenobarbital) may decrease zonisamide concentration Concurrent drugs that induce or inhibit CYP3A4 would be expected to alter zonisamide concentrations Zonisamide is not expected to interfere with metabolism of other drugs metabolized by CYT P450	Long half-life, may take up to 2 wk to reach steady state Encourage fluid intake to avoid urolithiasis
Newest AEDs			
Oxcarbazepine (Trileptal)	Hyponatremia 25%-30% of patients with hypersensitivity to carbamazepine have hypersensitivity to oxcarbazepine	Oxcarbazepine inhibits CYP2C19, induces CYP3A4/5 Inducers (phenytoin, carbamazepine, phenobarbital) decrease 10-monohydroxy-carbazepine (active metabolite) levels Oxcarbazepine increases metabolism of oral contraceptives, felodipine	Initiate at 1/2 normal dose if creatinine clearance <30 mL/min
Levetiracetam (Keppra)	Decreased erythrocytes, hemoglobin, hematocrit Infection	Per clinical trials, levetiracetam does not appear to affect or be affected by other AEDs, but cases of increased phenytoin concentrations have been reported	2/3 of dose excreted unchanged in urine Must be adjusted for renal dysfunction

AED, antiepileptic drug; ANC, absolute neutrophil count; AV, atrioventricular; BP, blood pressure; CBC, complete blood count; CNS, central nervous system; DC, differential count; ECG, electrocardiography; GI, gastrointestinal; IM, intramuscular; IV, intravenous; LFT, liver function test; LTG, lamotrigine; MAO, monoamine oxidase; PE, phenytoin equivalents; RR, respiratory rate; SA, sinoatrial; SC, subcutaneous; SE, side effect; SSRI, selective serotonin reuptake inhibitor; TCA, tricyclic antidepressant; WBC, white blood cell.

*For all AEDs, the most common SEs are CNS effects (drowsiness, dizziness, ataxia). With chronic administration, tolerance usually develops to these SEs. The general rule for dosing AEDs is "start low and go slow." Do not discontinue AEDs abruptly.

†Generally, the newer/newest AEDs tend to have fewer side effects than older agents, to have fewer drug interactions than older AEDs, and are approved as adjunctive agents to older AEDs. The value of blood level monitoring is undefined for newer/newest AEDs.

QUESTIONS

Multiple Choice (choose the one best answer)

1. A 65-year-old man is evaluated for progressive memory decline, shuffling gait, visual hallucinations, and sleep disorder. Neurologic examination revealed impaired attention and recall and parkinsonism. A sleep study indicates that the patient has rapid eye movement (REM) sleep behavior disorder. Which of the following drugs is indicated for management of hallucinations and cognitive symptoms?
   a. Levodopa
   b. Amitriptyline
   c. Haloperidol
   d. Donepezil
   e. Carbamazepine

2. A 55-year-old man is evaluated for a 6-month history of progressive cognitive deterioration and recent onset of muscle twitches. Neurologic examination revealed severe impairment in attention and visuospatial tasks, parkinsonism, and abrupt jerky limb movements indicative of myoclonus. An electroencephalogram showed periodic sharp wave, and a fluid-attenuated inversion recovery (FLAIR) magnetic resonance imaging (MRI) study showed increased signal in the cortex and basal ganglia. Which of the following cerebrospinal fluid (CSF) findings is most likely to confirm the presumptive diagnosis?
   a. Mononuclear pleocytosis
   b. Increased IgG index
   c. Elevated 14-3-3 protein
   d. Positive polymerase chain reaction for herpes simplex virus
   e. Positive syphilis serology

3. A 55-year-old woman has been taking phenytoin, 300 mg daily, after two episodes of generalized tonic-clonic seizures as a consequence of a stroke 2 months ago. She has been seizure-free since that time. She is also taking warfarin for atrial fibrillation and prednisone for rheumatoid arthritis. Her serum phenytoin level is 6 µg/mL (therapeutic range, 10-20 µg/mL). Which of the following is the most appropriate approach?
   a. Obtain a free phenytoin level
   b. Increase the phenytoin dose to 400 mg daily
   c. Maintain the current dose of phenytoin
   d. Substitute carbamazepine for phenytoin to avoid drug interactions
   e. Monitor the phenytoin level frequently to assess compliance

4. A 23-year-old woman has had recent onset of generalized tonic-clonic seizures. The findings on neurologic examination and magnetic resonance imaging are normal. She is taking oral contraceptives and is concerned about the loss of their efficacy as a consequence of starting antiepileptic drug therapy. On counseling the patient, you should mention that loss of contraceptive efficacy is least likely to occur with which of the following drugs?
   a. Phenytoin
   b. Valproic acid
   c. Carbamazepine
   d. Oxcarbazepine
   e. Phenobarbital

5. A 73-year-old woman complained of headache and malaise for 1 week and an episode of transient monocular blindness in the right eye a few hours before evaluation. Which of the following would be the most appropriate next step in her evaluation?
   a. Carotid ultrasonography
   b. Lumbar puncture
   c. CT of the head
   d. Erythrocyte sedimentation rate (ESR)
   e. Magnetic resonance (MR) angiography

6. A 26-year-old presents with a severe headache involving the retrobulbar region. The headaches have occurred in groups over the last 6 months. Which of the following would be *incorrect* about the likely cause of these headaches?
   a. They are most common in men
   b. They occur at night
   c. They last 30 to 60 minutes
   d. They are preceded by warning symptoms
   e. They are associated with sympathetic paresis

7. A 67-year-old man has a 2-month history of varying diplopia and alternating ptosis; over the next several weeks, he develops flaccid dysarthria, bifacial weakness, mild proximal arm and leg weakness, and marked weakness of neck flexion. Cognition, sensation, and reflexes are normal. Which of the following tests is most likely to establish an accurate diagnosis?
   a. MRI of the head
   b. Lyme polymerase chain reaction of the CSF
   c. Paraneoplastic antibody panel
   d. Electromyography (EMG) with repetitive stimulation
   e. Muscle and nerve biopsy

8. A 55-year-old woman has a 3- to 4-week history of progressive asymmetrical, mainly proximal weakness of the

legs, with pain in the low back, buttocks, and thighs. The weakness is greater in the left leg and is most marked in the iliopsoas muscle, followed by the quadriceps and hamstrings. Distal strength is mildly reduced. The knee reflexes are absent and the ankle reflexes are reduced, with flexor toe signs. The most likely diagnosis is:

a. Inflammatory polyradiculopathy
b. Spinal cord tumor
c. Inflammatory myopathy
d. Spinal stenosis
e. Paraneoplastic myasthenic syndrome

9. A 50-year-old woman has a subacute course of progressive symmetrical proximal weakness of the limbs, the legs greater than the arms. No systemic signs or symptoms are present. Reflexes, mentation, and cranial nerve function are normal. The most effective initial therapy after appropriate diagnostic studies would be:

a. Intravenous immunoglobulin
b. High-dose oral corticosteroids
c. Plasma exchange
d. Intravenous pulse cyclophosphamide
e. Oral 3,4-diaminopyridine

10. A 45-year-old man initially complained of tingling of the feet and fingers; over the next 1 to 2 weeks he had progressive symmetrical weakness of the legs and then the arms, both proximally and distally, accompanied by pain in the low back and legs. Reflexes are absent and toe signs are flexor. Which of the following would be the most appropriate treatment?

a. High-dose intravenous corticosteroids
b. Intravenous immunoglobulins
c. Epidural corticosteroids
d. Intravenous patient-controlled analgesia
e. Neurosurgical intervention

11. A 42-year-old woman presents with acute onset of headache, vertigo, nausea, and vomiting. Neurologic examination reveals left nystagmus, left Horner syndrome, absent left gag reflex, left appendicular ataxia, and anesthesia to pinprick in the left face and right upper extremity. Which of the following is the most likely diagnosis?

a. Complicated migraine
b. Vertebral artery dissection
c. Subarachnoid hemorrhage
d. Acute multiple sclerosis
e. Transverse sinus thrombosis

12. A 69-year-old person with hypertension presents with sudden vertigo accompanied by staggering, nausea, and vomiting but no headache or altered consciousness. On examination, the patient is unable to stand and to walk but has no weakness except mild right facial weakness involving the forehead, eye closure, and lower face. Which of the following is the most likely diagnosis?

a. Lateral medullary syndrome (Wallenberg syndrome)
b. Acute multiple cranial neuropathy (cranial nerves VII and VIII)
c. Acute Bell palsy with functional overlay (astasia-abasia)
d. Spontaneous intracerebellar hemorrhage
e. Pontine infarction

13. A 65-year-old man with Parkinson disease has been taking levodopa-carbidopa for 1 year, with good response of the motor symptoms. However, he has developed disturbing visual hallucinations that have persisted despite attempts to decrease the dose of levodopa. Which of the following is the most appropriate approach?

a. Substitute pramipexole for levodopa
b. Add haloperidol
c. Increase the dose of carbidopa
d. Add an anticholinergic agent
e. Add quetiapine

14. A 58-year-old woman presents with subacute onset of ataxia that has been slowly worsening. The neurologic examination demonstrates marked gait and appendicular ataxia. MRI of the head does not show any abnormality. What would be the most appropriate next diagnostic step?

a. Cerebral arteriography
b. Cerebellar cortical biopsy
c. Anti-Purkinje cell (anti-Yo) antibodies
d. Laparoscopy
e. Acetylcholine receptor antibodies

ANSWERS

1. Answer d.

The combination of dementia, parkinsonism, fluctuating cognitive function, visual hallucinations, and REM sleep behavior disorder is highly suggestive of dementia with Lewy bodies, also referred to as "Lewy body disease." Cholinesterase inhibitors such as donepezil may improve the hallucinations and cognitive symptoms. Antipsychotic medications such as haloperidol may trigger a neuroleptic malignant-type syndrome in these patients. Levodopa may worsen hallucinations; amitriptyline, because of its anticholinergic effect, may worsen memory and other cognitive function and contribute to the hallucinations. Carbamazepine, although useful for management of agitation, does not have an antihallucinatory effect and may predispose the patient to hyponatremia.

2. Answer c.

Rapidly progressive dementia and myoclonic jerks over several months should raise the suspicion of Creutzfeldt-Jakob disease. The clinical manifestations may include visual agnosia or cortical blindness, parkinsonism, or ataxia. Electroencephalography (EEG) shows unusual high-amplitude sharp waves. FLAIR MRI typically shows increased signal in the cerebral cortex and basal ganglia. Findings on CSF examination are normal except for an increased level of 14-3-3 protein, which is highly supportive of the diagnosis. This prion-related disorder typically is not accompanied by CSF pleocytosis or evidence of intrathecal immunoglobulin synthesis, as in inflammatory diseases. Neurosyphilis is a chronic disorder and is not associated with periodic sharp waves on the EEG. Herpes simplex encephalitis is an acute disorder that affects predominantly the temporal lobes and may produce focal deficits and seizures, but typically no myoclonus. An important differential diagnosis of Creutzfeldt-Jakob disease is immune encephalopathy associated with elevated thyroperoxidase antibodies, commonly referred to as "Hashimoto encephalopathy."

3. Answer c.

Seizures may be well controlled in many patients who have anticonvulsant blood levels below or above the therapeutic range. The anticonvulsant dose should *never* be changed on the basis of blood levels alone. Toxicity is a clinical, *not* a laboratory, phenomenon. Routine monitoring of anticonvulsant levels is rarely useful, particularly in patients taking other medications such as warfarin or corticosteroids that may affect hepatic drug metabolism. Levels should be checked at the beginning of antiepileptic drug therapy, when other potentially interacting drugs are added, when symptoms suggest toxicity, or when seizures are poorly controlled, particularly to assess compliance.

4. Answer b.

Hepatic enzyme inducers (carbamazepine, phenobarbital, phenytoin, primidone, oxcarbazepine, felbamate, and topiramate) increase metabolism and decrease the efficacy of oral contraceptives in preventing pregnancy. Valproic acid, gabapentin, tiagabine, lamotrigine, and levetiracetam do not induce clinically important liver enzyme induction and have not been associated with decreased efficacy of oral contraceptives. Special issues must be considered when managing epilepsy in pregnancy, and counseling in this regard is also necessary. Although essentially all anticonvulsants may produce teratogenic effects, valproic acid and carbamazepine are selectively associated with an increased risk of neural tube defects. All women with epilepsy and childbearing potential should receive folate supplementation of at least 0.4 mg daily. Prenatal screening should be offered to all women with epilepsy to detect any fetal malformation.

5. Answer d.

The combination of headache preceding transient monocular loss of vision in an older person must suggest temporal arteritis until proven otherwise. Although headache and malaise are nonspecific, if the potential diagnosis of temporal arteritis is not considered and the condition is left untreated, then permanent loss of vision could occur quickly. The ESR should be determined urgently and appropriate medical management with prednisone be initiated. If the ESR result is negative, additional evaluation of the carotid artery with carotid ultrasonography or MR angiography would be appropriate. CT of the head is not clearly indicated. Lumbar puncture would not be part of the urgent evaluation.

6. Answer d.

The recurrent severe headaches occurring in groups suggest the diagnosis of cluster headache. As opposed to migraine, these headaches predominantly affect men. They occur in clusters of 2 to 3 months with periods of several months to 1 to 2 years between clusters. They often occur at night. Clinically, the headache is a severe, nonthrobbing pain, typically maximally behind the eye and without any warning. The attacks are usually unilateral. Each episode reaches a peak in about 10 minutes and lasts 45 to 60 minutes. The headache often is associated with sympathetic paresis, including ptosis and miosis, and the patient may also have ipsilateral lacrimation, injection of the conjunctiva, and periorbital swelling.

7. Answer d.

The history of fluctuating weakness and fatigability involving extraocular, bulbar, or limb muscles in any combination should raise the suspicion of a defect in neuromuscular transmission such as myasthenia gravis. This diagnosis may be supported by a positive result on the Tensilon test, but it has to be confirmed with electrophysiologic and immune studies. The most important test is EMG with repetitive stimulation. Laboratory tests include acetylcholine receptor antibodies and, if a presynaptic defect is suggested by the EMG findings, paraneoplastic P/Q antibodies to diagnose Lambert-Eaton myasthenic syndrome. Although diplopia, facial weakness, dysarthria, and limb weakness may occur in brainstem lesions that can be detected on MRI or in inflammatory polyradiculopathy such as Lyme disease, the fluctuation of symptoms, normal sensation, and normal reflexes in this patient would not be consistent with either possibility. The clinical features are atypical for Lambert-Eaton myasthenic syndrome or other paraneoplastic disorders. The fluctuation of symptoms is atypical for myopathy or neuropathy.

8. Answer a.

The history of subacute to chronic, asymmetrical weakness with reduced deep tendon reflexes should raise the possibility of an inflammatory polyradiculopathy. Although spinal stenosis may affect multiple nerve roots, its course is chronic and rarely produces fixed weakness. Spinal cord neoplasms frequently affect the pyramidal tract, leading to areflexia and extensor plantar responses, unlike in this patient. In general, inflammatory myopathies produce symmetrical weakness and are not associated with the loss of muscle stretch reflexes. Myasthenic syndrome also produces symmetrical weakness and is not associated with low back pain.

9. Answer b.

The pattern of subacute, progressive proximal and symmetrical limb muscle weakness, without involvement of the cranial nerves and preservation of sensation and reflexes, should raise the possibility of polymyositis. The diagnosis is supported by an increase in the serum level of creatine kinase and EMG findings and is confirmed by muscle biopsy findings. The treatment of choice is high-dose oral corticosteroids. There is no evidence that plasma exchange or intravenous immunoglobulin is helpful in this condition. Cyclophosphamide could be one of several options for patients who do not have a response to corticosteroid therapy, but it is rarely used. Oral 3,4-diaminopyrimidine is efficacious in treating Lambert-Eaton myasthenic syndrome, but normal reflexes would be an unusual finding in this condition.

10. Answer b.

The pattern of subacute, progressive severe weakness and loss of muscle stretch reflexes frequently associated with distal sensory symptoms and low back pain and leg pain should raise the suspicion of acute inflammatory demyelinating polyradiculoneuropathy, or Guillain-Barré syndrome. The

presence of a high protein level in the CSF, with minimal or no pleocytosis, and the slow conduction velocities or conduction block demonstrated on EMG confirm the diagnosis. Treatment includes intravenous immunoglobulin or plasma exchange. There is no evidence that intravenous or epidural corticosteroid therapy is of benefit. The history of this patient does not suggest structural spinal lesions, including cervical myelopathy or spinal stenosis.

11. Answer b.

The clinical findings, with nystagmus, Horner syndrome, cerebellar abnormalities, and crossed sensory loss, suggest a brainstem and cerebellar localization. The acute onset of the deficit is most consistent with an ischemic or hemorrhagic process. Migraine is a very unusual cause of cerebral infarction and is more cortically based when it does occur. Subarachnoid hemorrhage usually does not cause acute onset of focal findings in the brainstem. Although multiple sclerosis can develop acutely, a subacute onset is more typical and is not associated with headache. Transverse sinus thrombosis can cause cerebral infarction but not infarction of the brainstem. The abrupt onset of pain in combination with a focal neurologic process would be more consistent with an arterial dissection with resultant cerebral infarction.

12. Answer d.

The abrupt onset of vertigo with unsteadiness in combination with the examination findings of ataxia and facial weakness suggests a disorder involving the cerebellum or cerebellar tracts and a compressive effect on cranial nerve VII. The lack of other pontine findings argues against a brainstem process. Facial weakness involving the upper and lower part of the face suggests a "peripheral" cranial nerve VII process rather than a "central" cause of the facial weakness. (A central process, as in the frontal lobe, causes weakness that is greater in the lower than upper part of the face.) The abrupt onset suggests a vascular process, and infarction or hemorrhage would be possible. A hemorrhagic process would be more likely because the process involves the peripheral aspect of cranial nerve VII, implying that a mass lesion from the cerebellum is compressing this cranial nerve. A spontaneous intracerebellar hemorrhage would be a key concern. This may represent a neurosurgical emergency because a compressive effect of the hemorrhage on the fourth ventricle can cause acute hydrocephalus and rapid deterioration. Should this patient become drowsy in the early period, emergency repeat imaging and neurosurgical consultation are indicated. There are no other lateral medullary findings such as a crossed sensory loss (loss of ipsilateral facial and contralateral body pain and temperature sensation), decreased gag or difficulty swallowing, or Horner syndrome. Acute multiple cranial neuropathies would be unusual, and the ataxia implies a cerebellar process.

13. Answer e.

Hallucinations are a relatively common side effect of dopaminergic drugs, including levodopa-carbidopa, and dopamine agonists such as pramipexole or ropinirole. Hallucinations may be exacerbated by the concomitant use of anticholinergic drugs. Classic antipsychotic drugs such as haloperidol pose a high risk of exacerbation of parkinsonian symptoms. In contrast, newer antipsychotic agents such as quetiapine and olanzapine are efficacious in treating hallucinations in Parkinson disease at doses that do not usually exacerbate parkinsonism.

14. Answer c.

Subacute onset of ataxia in a woman in conjunction with normal MRI findings should suggest a paraneoplastic disorder. Cerebral angiography is unlikely to be useful if the MRI results are negative. A biopsy would not be indicated. Acetylcholine receptor antibodies evaluate for the presence of myasthenia gravis, and the clinical findings would not be consistent with that diagnosis. Purkinje cell antibodies (anti-Yo antibodies) occur with ovarian, fallopian tube, endometrial, surface papillary, and breast carcinomas and occasionally with lymphoma. They cause paraneoplastic cerebellar degeneration with subacute ataxia. The specificity of the paraneoplastic antibodies is extremely high, and exploratory laparoscopy should be performed if the appropriate paraneoplastic antibodies are present and the imaging studies of the abdomen and pelvis are negative.

CHAPTER 18

ONCOLOGY

Scott H. Okuno, M.D.

BREAST CANCER

Magnitude of the Problem

In the United States, 211,000 new cases of breast cancer are diagnosed annually. Breast cancer will develop in approximately 1 in 8 women who achieve a normal life expectancy. Breast cancer is the second most common cause of cancer death among women in the United States (lung cancer is the most common). The incidence is increasing largely due to screening.

- Breast cancer will develop in 1 in 8 American women.
- Incidence is increasing (largely due to screening).
- Breast cancer is the second most common cause of cancer death in American women.

Risk Factors

The risk factors for breast cancer are outlined in Table 18-1. In addition, women with breast cancer-associated genes (*BRCA1* and *BRCA2*) have up to an 80% chance for breast cancer developing in their lifetime. Less than 25% of women with breast cancer have known high-risk factors.

- Less than 25% of women with breast cancer have known high-risk factors.

Screening

The use of screening mammography in the age group 50 years or older has decreased mortality by 20% to 30%. The use of screening mammography in the age group 40 to 50 years is controversial. There is general consensus that women 50 years or older should be screened with annual clinical examination and mammography. For women deemed at high risk for breast cancer, screening should be instituted at an appropriate earlier age, generally taken as 5 to 10 years before the earliest diagnosis of breast cancer in the family. Currently, mammography misses about 10% of breast cancers detectable on physical examination. Thus, a biopsy specimen should be obtained of any suspicious palpable lump despite a negative mammogram.

- Screening for breast cancer can reduce mortality.
- Women 50 years or older need annual examinations and mammography.
- There is controversy about screening normal women who are 40 to 50 years old.
- Ten percent of breast cancers found on physical examination are missed by mammography.
- Biopsy is recommended for a suspicious palpable lump, even if mammography is negative.

Table 18-1 Risk Factors for Breast Cancer

High risk: relative risk >4.0	Moderate risk: relative risk 2-4	Low risk: relative risk 1-2
Older age	Any first-degree relative with breast cancer	Menarche before age 12 y
Personal history of breast cancer		Menopause after age 55 y
Family history of premenopausal bilateral breast cancer or familial cancer syndrome	Personal history of ovarian or endometrial cancer	Caucasian race
		Moderate alcohol intake
Breast biopsy showing proliferative disease with atypia	Age at first full-term pregnancy >30 y	Long-duration (≥15 y) estrogen replacement therapy
	Nulliparous	
	Obesity in postmenopausal women	
	Upper socioeconomic class	

Pathology

Breast cancers are classified as ductal or lobular, corresponding to the ducts and lobules of the normal breast (Fig. 18-1). Invasive, or infiltrating, breast cancer has the potential for systemic spread, as opposed to carcinoma in situ, which does not have the metastatic potential because by definition it has not invaded through the basement membrane. Ductal carcinoma in situ is noninvasive, does not have the potential for systemic spread, and is treated with local therapy only. Infiltrating ductal carcinoma is the most common histologic type (70% of breast cancers), and lobular cancer is more frequently multifocal and bilateral.

- Infiltrating ductal carcinoma is the most common histologic type of breast cancer.
- Lobular disease is more frequently multifocal and bilateral.
- Ductal carcinoma in situ is noninvasive, does not have the potential for systemic spread, and is treated with local therapy only.

Staging

The staging system of the American Joint Committee on Cancer is shown in Table 18-2.

Natural History and Prognostic Factors

Nodal Status

The number of involved axillary nodes remains the single best predictor of outcome (Fig. 18-2).

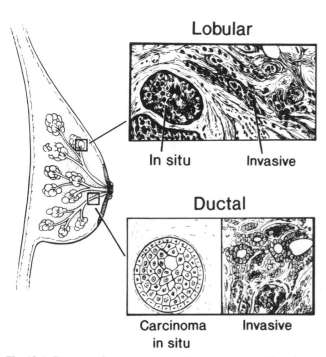

Fig. 18-1. Breast carcinomas: ductal and lobular, in situ and invasive.

Tumor Size

After nodal status, tumor size is generally the most important prognostic factor (Table 18-3).

Table 18-2   Staging of Breast Cancer

Primary tumor (T)
TIS	Carcinoma in situ
T1	T = ≤2 cm
T2	T = 2.1-5 cm
T3	T = >5 cm
T4	T of any size with direct extension to chest wall or skin

Regional nodes (N)
N0	No involved nodes
N1	Movable ipsilateral axillary nodes
N2	Matted or fixed nodes, or in clinically apparent ipsilateral internal mammary nodes in the absence of clinically evident axillary lymph node metastasis
N3	Metastasis in ipsilateral infraclavicular lymph nodes

Distant metastasis (M)
M0	None detected
M1	Distant metastasis present (includes ipsilateral supraclavicular nodes)

Stage grouping

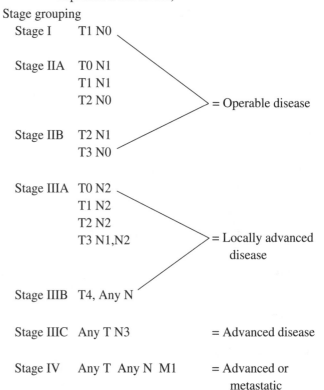

Data from Singletary SE, Allred C, Ashley P, et al: Revision of the American Joint Committee on Cancer Staging System for Breast Cancer. J Clin Oncol 2002;20:3628-3636.

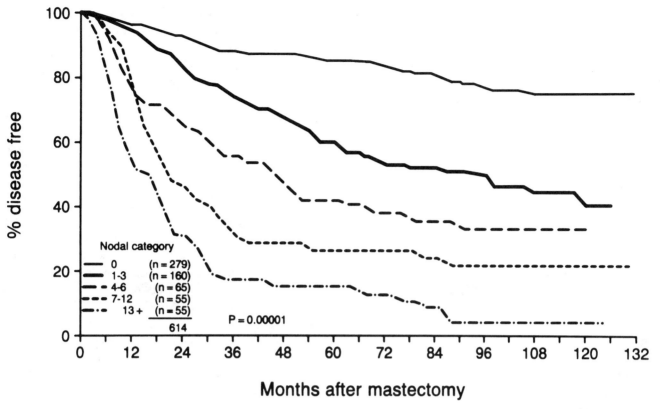

Fig. 18-2. Relation of disease-free survival to numbers of nodal metastases in more than 600 women with breast cancer treated with radical mastectomy alone in the early 1970s. (From Fisher ER, Sass R, Fisher B, et al: Pathologic findings from the National Surgical Adjuvant Project for Breast Cancers [protocol no. 4]. X. Discriminants for tenth year treatment failure. Cancer 1984;53:712-723. By permission of American Cancer Society.)

Hormone Receptor Status

In general, patients with estrogen-receptor–positive tumors have a better prognosis. However, the difference in recurrence rates at 5 years is only 8% to 10%.

Grade

Most breast cancers are high-grade. Patients with low-grade tumors have fewer recurrences and longer survival.

- The number of involved axillary nodes is the best predictor of outcome.
- After nodal status, tumor size is the most important prognostic factor.
- Patients with receptor-positive tumors have a better prognosis.
- Patients with low-grade tumors have a better prognosis.

Treatment

Primary or Local-Regional Therapy

Primary local treatment for invasive breast cancer is either breast conservation (lumpectomy with axillary lymph node dissection and breast radiation) or mastectomy. Several randomized controlled clinical trials have shown therapeutic equivalence for breast conservation and mastectomy. The outcome for women with invasive breast cancer depends on the presence of distant microscopic metastatic disease rather than on the treatment of local disease.

- Breast conservation and mastectomy have therapeutic equivalence.

Table 18-3   Long-Term Results[*] in Patients With Node-Negative Breast Cancer Treated Surgically

Tumor size, cm	No. of patients	% free of recurrence	% dead of disease
<1	171	88	10
1.1-2.0	303	74	24
2.1-3.0	188	72	24
3.1-5.0	105	61	36

[*]Median duration of follow-up was 18 years.
Data from Rosen PP, Groshen S, Kinne DW: Survival and prognostic factors in node-negative breast cancer: results of long-term follow-up studies. Monogr Natl Cancer Inst 1992;11:159-162.

Adjuvant Treatment

After primary treatment of the breast, additional systemic treatment (adjuvant) may be offered to women to help eradicate the microscopic metastatic disease and ultimately improve overall survival. The number of involved axillary lymph nodes is the single best predictor of outcome. All women with metastatically involved axillary lymph nodes should be offered adjuvant treatment (Table 18-4). Women with negative lymph nodes have only a 25% chance of microscopic metastatic disease, and their risk of recurrence can be further estimated according to the data in Table 18-5. Adjuvant systemic treatment should be offered to women in the intermediate- and high-risk groups.

- Women with node-positive disease are at high risk of systemic disease and should be offered adjuvant treatment.
- Women with node-negative disease have only a 25% chance of systemic disease, and adjuvant treatment should be given to women in the intermediate- and high-risk groups.

Treatment of Advanced Disease

We currently lack curative therapy for recurrent or metastatic breast cancer. The median duration of survival for recurrent disease is 2.5 years. Survival is longer with bone or soft tissue recurrence than with visceral recurrence. Because treatment is not curative, the initial systemic treatment for patients with estrogen-receptor–positive advanced disease is usually hormonal. Chemotherapy is used once women have progressed on hormonal therapy or in women with estrogen-receptor–negative breast cancer.

- There is no curative therapy for recurrent or metastatic breast cancer.
- The average survival with recurrent breast cancer is 2.5 years.

Chemotherapy

Active drugs against breast cancer include doxorubicin (Adriamycin, A), cyclophosphamide (C), methotrexate (M), 5-fluorouracil (F), paclitaxel (Taxol), docetaxel (Taxotere), capecitabine (Xeloda), vinorelbine (Navelbine), vincristine, vinblastine, mitomycin-C, etoposide, and cisplatin. Common combination regimens are CMF, CAF, and AC. The side effects of chemotherapy include reversible lowering of the blood counts and reversible hair loss. After 20 years of follow-up, there has been no increased risk of second malignancies for women who received adjuvant chemotherapy.

Hormonal Agents

Tamoxifen is the most widely used hormonal agent in the treatment of patients with breast cancer. Tamoxifen is a nonsteroidal compound that on selected tissue acts like an antiestrogen (breast tissue) but on other tissue acts like an estrogen (bones, lipids, uterus). Its beneficial effects include 1) antitumor effects on breast cancer cells, 2) decreased risk (by 40%) of contralateral breast cancer for women taking adjuvant tamoxifen, 3) improved bone density, and 4) favorable effects on lipid profiles. Tamoxifen also has some side effects, including 1) vaginal dryness and hot flashes, 2) thromboembolic risk (1%-2%), and 3) increased risk of endometrial cancer.

- Tamoxifen has both antiestrogen and estrogen-like activity.
- Beneficial effects of tamoxifen: antitumor effects, increased bone density, improved lipid profile, and decreased risk of contralateral breast cancer.
- Side effects of tamoxifen: hot flashes, vaginal dryness, thromboembolic risk, and increased risk of endometrial cancer.

Other hormonal agents include megestrol acetate (Megace), a progestational agent; fluoxymesterone (Halotestin), an androgen; the nonsteroidal aromatase inhibitors anastrozole (Arimidex) and letrozole (Femara); the steroidal aromatase inactivator exemestane (Aromasin); and the estrogen receptor antagonist fulvestrant (Falsodex).

Table 18-4 Adjuvant Therapy: Node-Positive Breast Cancer

	Estrogen-receptor status	
	Positive	Negative
Premenopausal	Chemo + Tam	Chemo
Postmenopausal	Chemo + Tam	Chemo

Chemo, combination chemotherapy; Tam, tamoxifen.

Table 18-5 Adjuvant Therapy: Node-Negative Breast Cancer[*]

	Risk		
	Low	Intermediate	High
Tumor size, cm	<1	1-2	>2
ER or PR	+	+	–
Grade	1	1-2	2-3

ER, estrogen receptor; PR, progesterone receptor.
[*]Most oncologists would not treat tumors less than 1 cm.

Other Agents

Herceptin

About 25% of breast cancers overexpress the growth factor HER2. A monoclonal antibody directed against HER2 (herceptin) has been shown to have activity against refractory breast cancer, is synergistic with certain chemotherapy agents, and can cause heart failure when used in conjunction with doxorubicin.

Zoledronic Acid (Zometa) and Pamidronate (Aredia)

The use of the bisphosphonates can reduce the need for palliative radiation, bone fixation, and pain medicine in women with lytic bone metastases.

Typical Clinical Scenarios

Localized node-positive breast cancer: A 40-year-old woman has a 3-cm mass in the right breast and two lymph nodes involved in the axilla. Biopsy reveals adenocarcinoma that is hormone-receptor–negative. The diagnosis is node-positive adenocarcinoma of the right breast. Treatment is local therapy (modified radical mastectomy or lumpectomy plus radiation) followed by adjuvant chemotherapy.

Metastatic breast carcinoma: A 65-year-old patient has a history of breast carcinoma treated 10 years earlier with operation and chemotherapy. The patient presents with back pain, and bone scanning shows multiple areas of increased uptake throughout the skeleton. There is no evidence of metastatic disease elsewhere. The diagnosis is metastatic breast carcinoma. Initial therapy is usually hormonal and use of bisphosphonates.

CERVICAL CANCER

Background

The incidence of and mortality from cervical cancer have decreased by 30% to 40% in recent decades, attributed to widespread use of Papanicolaou smear screening. Currently, 12,200 new cases of cervical cancer are diagnosed in U.S. women each year, and there are 4,100 deaths annually. In addition, more than 50,000 cases of carcinoma in situ of the cervix are diagnosed annually. Risk factors for cervical cancer include first intercourse at an early age, a greater number of sexual partners, smoking, history of sexually transmitted disease, especially herpesvirus or human papillomavirus lesions, and lower socioeconomic class. It is now understood that human papillomavirus is an etiologic agent for cervical carcinogenesis.

If a cytologic smear shows dysplasia or malignant cells, colposcopy with directed biopsy should be done. The Papanicolaou smear has limited sensitivity; false-negative rates of 20% frequently are quoted. The American Cancer Society recommends that asymptomatic, low-risk women 20 years of age or older, and those younger than 20 years who are sexually active, have a Papanicolaou smear annually for 2 consecutive years and, if those are negative, at least one every 3 years.

Treatment

Treatment for carcinoma in situ of the cervix is usually total hysterectomy. If additional childbearing is desired, a more conservative approach, such as a therapeutic conization, is another option. Early invasive carcinoma of the cervix is usually treated with total hysterectomy. For patients with higher-stage disease, a combination of chemotherapy (cisplatin-based) and radiation therapy is recommended.

COLORECTAL CANCER

Background

Colorectal cancer is diagnosed in approximately 148,000 Americans each year and causes 57,000 deaths. Colorectal cancer is most common in North America and Europe. It is associated with high fat, low fiber diets. Population screening with fecal occult blood testing remains problematic. Although one study showed a reduction in mortality from colorectal cancer with fecal occult blood screening (N Engl J Med 1993;328:1365-1371), it should be noted that any participants who had positive results went on to have colonoscopy. Another study showed that fecal occult blood tests failed to detect 70% of colorectal cancers and 80% of large ($\geq$2 cm) polyps (JAMA 1993;269:1262-1267). Although specific screening recommendations vary, some form of screening process should be initiated by age 50 years regardless of risk. For high-risk patients, such as those with a family history of colorectal cancer or a prior colorectal cancer, structural studies of the entire large bowel, such as colonoscopy or proctoscopy plus barium enema, should be performed at appropriate intervals (such as every 1-3 years).

- Colorectal cancer is associated with high fat, low fiber diets.
- Although specific screening recommendations vary, some form of screening process should be initiated by age 50 years regardless of risk.
- For high-risk patients, the entire large bowel should be studied at appropriate intervals.

Risk Factors

High-risk groups include persons with 1) familial polyposis syndromes (familial adenomatous polyposis—gene recently identified on chromosome 5—and Gardner syndrome—gut polyps plus desmoid tumors, lipomas, sebaceous cysts, and other abnormalities), 2) familial cancer syndromes without polyps (hereditary nonpolyposis colorectal cancer or Lynch syndromes, which are marked by colon cancer with or without endometrial, breast, and other cancers), and 3) inflammatory bowel disease (incidence 12% after 25 years).

● High-risk factors for colorectal cancer are familial polyposis syndromes, including familial adenomatous polyposis and Gardner syndrome, both inherited as an autosomal dominant trait; select familial cancer syndromes without polyps; and inflammatory bowel disease.

Treatment

Surgery

Surgical resection is the preferred method of curative treatment for carcinomas of the colon or rectum. Surgical exploration and resection allows for pathologic determination of tumor depth of penetration through the bowel wall and assessment of regional lymph nodes. Prognosis is directly related to the stage of disease (Table 18-6), although rectal tumors tend to have a worse prognosis than colon carcinomas. Five-year survival rates for locoregional disease have improved in recent decades as a result of many factors, including improvements in preoperative staging, surgical technique, and adjuvant therapy.

● Surgical resection is the preferred treatment for colorectal cancer.
● Prognosis is directly related to the stage of disease.
● Five-year survival rates are improving.

Adjuvant Therapy

For colon cancers, adjuvant 5-fluorouracil (5-FU) and leucovorin, given for 6 months, are recommended for node-positive (stage III) disease. Controversy exists on standard recommendations for deeply invasive (stage II) colon carcinomas. For *rectal cancers*, a combination of chemotherapy (5-FU–based) and pelvic irradiation is standard for stage II and III disease.

● For stage III colon cancers, adjuvant chemotherapy includes 5-FU and leucovorin.

● For rectal cancer, a combination of chemotherapy (5-FU–based) and radiotherapy is the standard recommendation.

Metastatic Disease

Certain patients with locally recurrent or advanced colorectal cancer may be candidates for an attempt at curative resection. Of carefully selected patients with limited metastatic disease to the liver or lung, approximately 25% survive beyond 5 years without further evidence of disease recurrence (Ann Intern Med 1998;129:27-35).

Palliative chemotherapy is the only option for the vast majority of patients with advanced metastatic colorectal cancer. The median survival for patients treated with chemotherapy is about 18 months. The combination of oxaliplatin (Eloxatin), 5-FU, and leucovorin is the standard chemotherapy for metastatic disease. Other agents that have activity against colorectal cancer include capecitabine (Xeloda) and irinotecan (Camptosar). Bevacizumab (Avastin) was approved by the U.S. Food and Drug Administration in 2004 for patients with metastatic colon cancer as first-line therapy in combination with any 5-FU regimen. In addition, cetuximab (Erbitux) was approved in 2004 as combination treatment with intravenous irinotecan (or alone if irinotecan is not tolerated) for metastatic colon cancer.

● Surgical resection of metastatic disease can result in long-term disease-free survival.
● Palliative chemotherapy options for advanced colorectal carcinoma include oxaliplatin, 5-FU, leucovorin, capecitabine, and irinotecan.
● Bevacizumab in combination with 5-FU is approved first-line therapy for metastatic colon cancer.
● Cetuximab in combination with intravenous irinotecan is approved therapy for metastatic colon cancer.

Carcinoembryonic Antigen (CEA)

Proponents of CEA monitoring after operation for colorectal cancer argue that early recurrences, curable surgically, can be detected. However, CEA monitoring lacks sensitivity and specificity. It is estimated that cancer cures attributable to CEA monitoring occur in less than 1% of patients monitored (JAMA 1993;270:943-947).

Table 18-6   Staging of Colorectal Cancer and Survival

Dukes stage	AJCC stage	Depth of penetration	Nodal status	5-Year survival, %
A	I	Submucosa or muscularis	Negative	90
B	II	Through muscularis or to other organs	Negative	60-80
C	III	Any	Positive	30-60

AJCC, American Joint Committee on Cancer.

Typical Clinical Scenarios

Node-positive colon cancer: A 60-year-old patient has a history of altered bowel habits over 3 months. Colonoscopy shows adenocarcinoma in the descending colon. The patient undergoes left hemicolectomy. Regional lymph nodes are found to be involved. In view of the positive lymph nodes, adjuvant chemotherapy with 5-FU and leucovorin is warranted.

Metastatic colon carcinoma: A 70-year-old patient with a history of colon carcinoma resected 10 years previously presents with increasing abdominal girth and jaundice. Computed tomography shows multiple nodules in the liver. The diagnosis is metastatic colon carcinoma, and therapy consists of palliative chemotherapy with oxaliplatin, 5-FU, and leucovorin.

Localized ascending colon carcinoma: A 50-year-old patient has a new diagnosis of iron deficiency anemia. A mass in the ascending colon is found on a work-up for iron deficiency. The diagnosis is adenocarcinoma of the ascending colon.

LUNG CANCER

Magnitude of the Problem

Approximately 172,000 new cases of lung cancer are diagnosed in the United States annually, resulting in approximately 157,000 deaths. Thus, only approximately 10% of patients with lung cancer survive the disease. Lung cancer is the leading cause of cancer mortality in American men and women.

Risk Factors

About 95% of lung cancers in men and about 80% of lung cancers in women result from cigarette smoking. Men who smoke 1 to 2 packs per day have up to a 25-fold increase in lung cancer compared with those who have never smoked. The risk of lung cancer in an ex-smoker declines with time. Passive smoking is associated with an increased risk of lung cancer. Certain occupations (smelter workers, iron workers), chemicals (arsenic, methyl ethyl ether), and exposure to radioactive agents (radon, uranium) and asbestos have been associated with increased risks for development of lung cancer.

- 95% of lung cancers in men and 80% in women result from cigarette smoking.
- Men who smoke 1 to 2 packs a day have a 25-fold increase in lung cancer compared with those who have never smoked.
- Passive smoking is associated with an increased risk of lung cancer.

Screening

Several large, randomized trials have tested the utility of chest radiography and sputum cytology in screening for lung cancer. None of these studies have shown that either sputum cytology or regular chest radiography improves survival from lung cancer. Thus, screening is not standard at the present time. However, there are recognized methodologic problems with these studies, and some believe that there is benefit to screening for this disease (Chest 1995;107 Suppl:270S-279S).

- Randomized trials have not shown an advantage to screening for lung cancer.

Histologic Types and Characteristics

Lung cancer is divided into small-cell and non–small-cell types. Small-cell lung cancer occurs almost exclusively in smokers. The primary tumors are often small but are associated with bulky mediastinal adenopathy. They may be associated with paraneoplastic syndromes, including the syndrome of inappropriate secretion of antidiuretic hormone, and various neurologic abnormalities. Non–small-cell lung cancers can be divided into squamous, adenocarcinoma, and large-cell types. Squamous cell carcinomas may be associated with hypercalcemia due to the secretion of a parathyroid hormone-like peptide. Squamous carcinomas tend to occur centrally, whereas large-cell and adenocarcinoma types tend to be more peripheral. Adenocarcinoma is the most frequent histologic subtype in nonsmokers. Bronchoalveolar carcinoma is a low-grade non–small-cell carcinoma that frequently presents as a patchy infiltrate. It may be multifocal.

Staging

The classic *T*umor-*N*ode-*M*etastasis system is simplified in Table 18-7.

Natural History

The natural history of surgically treated lung cancer, by stage, is shown in Figure 18-3.

Treatment

Non–Small-Cell Lung Cancer (NSCLC)

Operation is the treatment of choice for clinical stages I, II, and selected IIIA disease. The use of adjuvant chemotherapy recently was shown to improve survival by about 5% compared with operation alone. The use of adjuvant radiation does not improve survival in resected stage II and III disease, but it is able to decrease the likelihood of local recurrence. In patients with locally advanced unresectable NSCLC, the use of chemotherapy before radiation therapy improves the long-term survival compared with radiation alone. Although patients with metastatic disease are not cured, the use of chemotherapy has improved the overall survival and the quality of life compared with best supportive care.

Table 18-7 Staging of Lung Cancer

Non–small-cell type	
Stage I	Primary tumor >2 cm from carina; node negative
Stage II	Primary tumor >2 cm from carina; hilar nodes positive
Stage IIIA	Tumor <2 cm from carina, or invading a resectable structure, or ipsilateral mediastinal nodes positive
Stage IIIB	Tumor invading an unresectable structure, supraclavicular or contralateral mediastinal nodes positive or cytologically positive pleural effusion
Stage IV	Metastatic disease
Small-cell type	
Limited	Limited to one hemithorax less supraclavicular lymph nodes. Can be encompassed within a tolerable radiation port
Extensive	All other disease (metastatic disease)

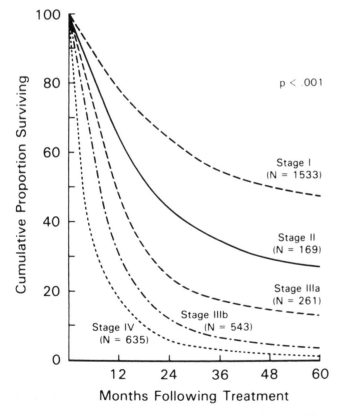

Fig. 18-3. Survival curves for patients with lung cancer by stage. (From Mountain CF: A new international staging system for lung cancer. Chest 1986;89:225S-233S. By permission of American College of Chest Physicians.)

- Operation is the treatment of choice for stages I and II and selected IIIA NSCLC.
- There is some improvement in survival with adjuvant chemotherapy.
- Chemotherapy is not curative for metastatic NSCLC.
- Chemotherapy improves the overall survival and quality of life for patients with metastatic NSCLC.

Chemotherapy for NSCLC

Active chemotherapy agents for NSCLC include etoposide, cisplatin, carboplatin, cyclophosphamide, mitomycin-C, ifosfamide, gemcitabine, irinotecan, docetaxel, and paclitaxel.

Small-Cell Lung Cancer

Treatment of limited-stage small-cell lung cancer consists of both chemotherapy and chest irradiation. Surgical resection has not been shown to improve survival. For patients who have a complete response to chemotherapy and chest radiation therapy, prophylactic cranial irradiation is used to decrease the frequency of failure in the central nervous system and improve overall survival. Unfortunately, it is associated with the risk of a delayed leukoencephalopathy, but this risk can be reduced by the administration of radiation in small-dose fractions without concomitant chemotherapy. For limited-stage small-cell disease, the median duration of survival is approximately 18 months; 30% to 40% of patients survive 2 years, and 10% to 20% survive 5 years.

- For small-cell lung cancer, treatment of limited-stage disease consists of both chemotherapy and chest irradiation.
- Prophylactic cranial irradiation decreases the frequency of failure in the central nervous system and improves overall survival.
- Median survival is 18 months with limited-stage disease.

Chemotherapy is used for the treatment of extensive stage (stage IV) small-cell lung cancer. Combination chemotherapy is favored over single-agent therapy. Active drugs include etoposide, cisplatin, cyclophosphamide, doxorubicin, and vincristine. High-dose chemotherapy with or without autologous bone marrow transplantation or marrow colony-stimulating factors has not yet been proved superior to standard chemotherapy. The median duration of survival is approximately 9 months; about 10% of patients survive 2 years, and 1% or less survive 5 years.

- For extensive stage small-cell lung cancer, treatment is chemotherapy.
- High-dose chemotherapy has not yet been proved superior to standard chemotherapy.
- Median survival is 9 months.

Typical Clinical Scenarios

Localized lung cancer: A 60-year-old smoker presents with cough. Chest radiography and computed tomography reveal a 2-cm nodule in the right upper aspect of the chest without evidence of lymph node or metastatic disease. After the diagnosis of non–small-cell lung carcinoma is confirmed, therapy is surgical resection.

Small-cell lung carcinoma: This patient is similar to the one described above, but biopsy reveals small-cell lung carcinoma. Treatment consists of systemic chemotherapy.

MELANOMA

Background

Malignant melanoma is increasing at a rapid rate. If current trends continue, the lifetime risk for malignant melanoma to develop in an American will be 1 in 75. Fortunately, the 5-year survival rate has doubled from approximately 40% in the 1940s to approximately 80% now, a change attributed to earlier detection. Melanoma is more common among fair-skinned people, persons with multiple atypical nevi, patients with freckling tendency, and certain families (first-degree relatives or persons with familial atypical mole/melanoma [FAMM] syndrome, formerly called the dysplastic nevus syndrome).

- The incidence of malignant melanoma is increasing rapidly.
- The 5-year survival rate has improved as a result of earlier detection.
- High-risk populations are identifiable.

Diagnosis ("ABCD") and Prognosis

Keys to the early diagnosis of malignant melanoma include the following:
- A: Asymmetry, especially a changing lesion
- B: Borders are irregular
- C: Color is variable, especially with blues, blacks, and tans dispersed throughout the lesion
- D: Diameter 6 mm or more

The Breslow microstaging method measures the thickness (i.e., depth of penetration of the tumor from the epidermis into the dermis/subcutis) of a malignant melanoma and is the best independent predictor of survival (Table 18-8).

Management

Surgical excision to achieve a 1- to 3-cm margin around the lesion remains the principal treatment for primary malignant melanoma. In the absence of palpable adenopathy, an elective lymph node dissection is not routinely performed. With clinically palpable regional nodes, a node dissection is

Table 18-8 Ten-Year Survival in Melanoma, by Depth of Tumor

Depth, mm	% alive
<0.85	96
0.85-1.69	87
1.7-3.6	66.5
>3.6	46

Data from Friedman RJ, Rigel DS, Silverman MK, et al: Malignant melanoma in the 1990s: the continued importance of early detection and the role of physician examination and self-examination of the skin. CA Cancer J Clin 1991 July/Aug;41:201-226.

performed for curative intent and to achieve maximal local tumor control. For patients at high risk for recurrence (deep primary tumor more than 4.0 mm or resected node-positive disease), recent clinical trials demonstrate conflicting results, and therefore adjuvant therapy remains controversial.

Treatment for metastatic melanoma is primarily palliative. Surgical resection in selected patients (those with a long disease-free interval and limited disease at recurrence) can be considered. Systemic treatments commonly include immunotherapy (interleukin-2 or interferon), chemotherapy (dacarbazine or nitrosoureas), or various combinations.

Typical Clinical Scenario

Malignant melanoma: A 60-year-old patient presents with a mole on the right leg that has been increasing in size during the past 3 months. Resection reveals malignant melanoma with a depth of invasion of 0.75 mm. Definitive therapy is reexcision to obtain a 1- to 3-cm margin around the lesion. No adjuvant therapy is recommended.

OVARIAN CANCER

This disease is diagnosed annually in approximately 25,400 American women. It is the leading cause of death due to gynecologic cancer, resulting in 14,300 deaths annually. There are no early warning signs; most patients present with vague gastrointestinal complaints such as bloating. Most patients (75%) present with advanced disease (i.e., stages III and IV, disease spread beyond the pelvis). The term "ovarian cancer" refers to tumors derived from the ovarian surface epithelium, not germ cell tumors.

- Ovarian cancer is the leading cause of death due to gynecologic cancer.
- There are no early warning signs.
- Most patients (75%) present with advanced disease.

Staging

Stage I is confined to the ovary, stage II is confined to the pelvis, stage III includes spread to the upper abdomen, and stage IV includes spread to distant sites.

CA 125

Cancer antigen 125 (CA 125) is expressed by approximately 85% of epithelial ovarian tumors and released into the circulation. However, it is detectable in only 50% of patients with stage I disease. The highest serum levels of CA 125 are found in patients with ovarian cancer, but the serum CA 125 level also may be increased in other malignancies, as well as in pregnancy, endometriosis, and menstruation. CA 125 is clearly of value for monitoring the course of ovarian cancer.

- CA 125 is expressed by about 85% of epithelial ovarian tumors.
- The CA 125 level also may be increased in other malignancies and in pregnancy, endometriosis, and menstruation.
- CA 125 is useful for monitoring the course of ovarian cancer.

Screening

The tools evaluated thus far, namely, pelvic ultrasonography and determination of the serum CA 125 value, are inadequate for screening the general female population. Screening for this disease is difficult for several reasons. The incidence of ovarian cancer is relatively low, and there are no recognized pre-invasive lesions. Moreover, pelvic ultrasonography and CA 125 lack sufficient sensitivity and specificity. However, it seems reasonable to apply these techniques on a periodic basis to women at particularly high risk of ovarian cancer, for example, those with a strong family history of the disease (two or more affected relatives). The cause of epithelial ovarian cancer is unknown. A small subset of patients (<5%) has an inherited predisposition to this disease. Generally, this occurs in families with both breast and ovarian cancer.

- Population screening for ovarian cancer is not recommended.
- Pelvic ultrasonography and CA 125 testing lack sufficient sensitivity and specificity.
- A small subset of patients (<5%) has an inherited predisposition to ovarian cancer and should be screened.

Treatment

The initial management of patients with epithelial ovarian cancer includes a thorough surgical staging and debulking procedure. Outcome in this disease depends on the amount of tumor tissue removed at initial operation. Subsequently, patients are treated with six cycles of platinum- and paclitaxel-based chemotherapy.

- Management of ovarian cancer includes thorough surgical staging and debulking followed by chemotherapy.
- The outcome depends on the amount of tumor tissue removed at initial operation.
- Subsequent chemotherapy consists of a platinum compound and paclitaxel.

Outcome

Outcome depends on the stage of disease. Ninety percent of patients with stage I disease are alive at 5 years, versus 80% for stage II disease. Unfortunately, survival with advanced disease is poor: 15% to 20% of patients with stage III disease are alive at 5 years and only 5% of patients with stage IV disease are alive.

Typical Clinical Scenario

Ovarian cancer: A 50-year-old patient presents with ascites. Evaluation reveals a mass in the right ovary. Therapy consists of surgical debulking followed by chemotherapy.

PROSTATE CANCER

Background

There are approximately 220,900 new cases of prostate cancer annually in the United States. It is the most common cancer in men in the United States and is the second leading cause of death from cancer in men in the United States (29,000 deaths annually). Identified risk factors for the development of prostatic cancer include older age, race (African American), family history (first-degree relative), and possibly dietary fat. The American Cancer Society recommends a digital rectal examination in men 40 years or older and determination of the prostate-specific antigen (PSA) value in men 50 years or older. Use of the PSA value for prostate cancer screening is a controversial issue and has not been shown to reduce mortality.

- Prostate cancer is the most common cancer among U.S. men and the second leading cause of death from cancer in men.
- Risk factors include older age, race (African American), family history, and a high fat diet.

Prostate-Specific Antigen

PSA is a serine protease produced by normal and neoplastic prostatic ductal epithelium. Its concentration is proportional to the total prostatic mass. The inability to differentiate benign prostatic hyperplasia from carcinoma on the basis of the PSA level renders it inadequate as the sole screening method for prostate cancer. PSA is useful for monitoring response to therapy in cases of known prostate cancer, particularly after radical prostatectomy, when PSA should be undetectable.

- The concentration of PSA is proportional to the total prostatic mass.
- The PSA test is inadequate as the sole screening test for prostate cancer.
- PSA is useful for monitoring response to therapy.

Prognostic factors for prostate cancer include stage of disease, grade of tumor, and pretreatment PSA level. Table 18-9 simplifies the staging of prostate cancer, including the TNM classification. Grading of tumors is performed by the pathologist with the Gleason scoring system. The surgical specimen is graded by the most predominant pattern of differentiation added to the secondary architectural pattern (e.g., $3 + 5 = 8$). Gleason grades 2 through 6 are associated with a better prognosis. Recent retrospective results indicate that the pretreatment PSA value is a strong predictor of disease outcome after operation or radiotherapy.

Table 18-9 Staging of Prostate Cancer

Whitmore	TNM*	Criteria
A1	T1A	Incidental focus of tumor in ≤5% of resected tissue
A2	T1B	Incidental tumor in >5% of resected tissue
B0	T1C	Tumor identified by needle biopsy (performed on basis of increased PSA value)
B1	T2A	Tumor ≤1/2 of one lobe
B2	T2B	Tumor >1/2 of one lobe but not both lobes
	T2C	Tumor involvement of both lobes
C	T3 or T4	Extracapsular local disease or local invasion
D1	N1	Pelvic node involvement
D2	M1	Distant disease

*Tumor-Node-Metastasis system.

- Prognostic factors for the outcome of prostate cancer include tumor stage, grade, and pretreatment PSA value.
- Gleason grades 2 through 6 have a better prognosis.

Management

Management of Specific Stages

Significant controversy surrounds the primary treatment of prostate cancer in nearly all stages of the disease. In general, patients with T1A prostate tumors are observed without treatment. For organ-confined prostate cancer (T1B, T1C, and T2 tumors), both radiation therapy and radical prostatectomy are equally viable options. Recently, some investigators have proposed observation alone and treatment with hormonal agents at the time of progression because the rate of death from prostate cancer is low for well-differentiated early-stage disease. A large trial is currently under way in the United States to test the value of operation compared with observation for organ-confined prostate cancer.

For stage C (T3 or T4) disease (locally advanced), radiotherapy is generally used. A trial combining androgen deprivation with local radiation therapy showed improved local control and overall survival in this patient cohort (N Engl J Med 1997;337:295-300). Some centers use androgen deprivation to downstage tumors before an aggressive surgical approach.

For stage D1 disease (positive pelvic nodes), the management is controversial. Divergent approaches include androgen deprivation alone, x-ray therapy with or without androgen deprivation, close observation with androgen deprivation at progression, or, infrequently, prostatectomy with androgen deprivation. For advanced (D2) disease, androgen deprivation is the treatment of choice.

Prostatectomy

This is reserved for patients with localized disease. The 15-year disease-specific survival rate after prostatectomy is 85% to 90% for stage A2 or B disease. Impotence occurs in most patients, especially older individuals. Total urinary incontinence is rare (<2% of patients).

- Prostatectomy is used for localized disease.
- The 15-year survival rate is 85%-90% for stage A2 or B disease.

Radiation Therapy

External beam radiotherapy is considered the equivalent of prostatectomy. It is preferred for stage C disease at most centers. Impotence can occur, but less often than with prostatectomy. A concern related to radiotherapy is that repeat biopsies after treatment have shown apparently viable tumor in more than 35% of patients. The clinical importance of this residual tumor is unclear, but there may be a correlation with the subsequent appearance of distant metastasis, especially with a persistent, palpable abnormality in the gland.

- External beam radiotherapy is considered the equivalent of prostatectomy at most centers.
- Impotence is less frequent with radiotherapy than prostatectomy.

Androgen Deprivation

For advanced (D2) disease, bone is the most frequent site of metastatic disease. Hormonal therapy, although it is very effective and produces a response in most patients, is noncurative. The average duration of response to initial hormonal maneuver is 18 months. The average duration of survival is 2 to 3 years. Once the disease progresses after the initial hormonal maneuver, it is typically very refractory to secondary treatment attempts (such as hormonal or chemotherapy).

- Bone is the most frequent site of metastatic disease from the prostate.
- Hormonal therapy is effective and produces a response, but it is noncurative.
- The average duration of survival with advanced prostatic cancer is 2-3 years.

The two sources of androgens in men are the testes (testosterone, 95%) and adrenal glands (5%). Androgen deprivation can be accomplished surgically with orchiectomy or medically. Potential agents include luteinizing hormone-releasing hormone (LHRH) agonists such as leuprolide, buserelin, and goserelin. They decrease androgen levels through continuous binding of the LHRH receptor and subsequent decrease of LH and thus testosterone. They are administered as a monthly injection of a depot preparation. A 3- or 4-month depot preparation is also available. LHRH agonists, on initial binding of the LHRH receptor, transiently stimulate LH release and thus cause an initial increase in the testosterone level. This explains the transient flare of prostate cancer that can occur in men with advanced disease when therapy with an LHRH agonist is initiated. This possibility must be considered in patients with impending spinal cord compression or urinary obstruction.

- Androgen deprivation is accomplished with orchiectomy or medically.
- LHRH agonists decrease androgen levels.
- These agonists initially stimulate a transient release of LH and testosterone.

Antiandrogens compete with androgens at the receptor level. These include flutamide, nilutamide, and bicalutamide. To effect total androgen blockade, an antiandrogen is added to therapy in patients who have had orchiectomy or who are receiving an LHRH agonist (these block testicular testosterone production but not adrenal androgen production). A prospective U.S. study in which a combination of an LHRH analogue with flutamide was compared with placebo suggested an advantage for the addition of flutamide. However, other studies of total blockade have failed to show an advantage. A recent clinical trial comparing orchiectomy alone with orchiectomy plus flutamide failed to show a survival advantage for total androgen blockade. The antiandrogens may also block the "flare" induced by LHRH agonists.

- The use of an antiandrogen in combination with orchiectomy or an LHRH agonist to treat advanced prostate cancer remains controversial.
- Antiandrogens block the "flare" induced by LHRH agonists.

Chemotherapy

Chemotherapy for prostate cancer is palliative and has limited impact on overall survival. The judicious use of chemotherapy can improve the symptoms of prostate cancer with manageable side effects.

Bisphosphonates

The use of bisphosphonates in men with bone metastasis can delay skeletal complications but does not improve overall survival.

- Chemotherapy and bisphosphonates can be used for palliative effects in men with prostate cancer.

Typical Clinical Scenario

Prostate cancer: A 70-year-old patient presents with back pain. The PSA value is markedly increased and the prostate is enlarged. Prostatic biopsy reveals prostatic carcinoma. Radiography and bone scanning reveal multiple areas of increased uptake throughout the skeleton, consistent with metastatic disease. Therapy consists of hormonal manipulation, with either orchiectomy or LHRH agonists.

TESTICULAR CANCER

Background

This cancer is diagnosed in 7,600 men annually. It is the most common carcinoma in males 15 to 35 years old. It is highly curable, even when metastatic. At high risk are males with cryptorchid testes (40-fold relative risk) or Klinefelter syndrome (also increased risk of breast cancer). Two broad categories are seminomas (40%) and nonseminomas. Types of nonseminomas include embryonal carcinoma, mature and immature teratoma, choriocarcinoma, yolk sac tumor, and endodermal sinus tumor. There is often an admixture of several cell types within nonseminomas. Any nonseminomatous component plus seminoma is treated as a nonseminoma.

- Testicular cancer is the most common carcinoma in males 15-35 years old.
- Testicular cancer is highly curable, even when metastatic.
- High-risk factors: cryptorchid testes, Klinefelter syndrome.
- Two categories: seminomas (40%) and nonseminomas.

Evaluation includes determination of β-human chorionic gonadotropin (hCG) and α-fetoprotein values and computed tomography of the abdomen (retroperitoneal nodes) and chest (mediastinal nodes or pulmonary nodules).

Staging

Stage I disease is confined to the testis, stage II includes infradiaphragmatic nodal metastases, and stage III is spread beyond retroperitoneal nodes. About 85% of nonseminomas are associated with an increased β-hCG or α-fetoprotein value. Approximately 10% of seminomas are associated with an increased β-hCG level. The α-fetoprotein value is never increased in pure seminoma; if it is increased, the tumor is not seminoma and should be treated as such.

- 85% of nonseminomas are associated with an increased β-hCG or α-fetoprotein value.
- 10% of seminomas are associated with an increased β-hCG value.
- The α-fetoprotein value is never increased in pure seminoma.

Management

Radical (inguinal) orchiectomy is the definitive procedure for both pathologic diagnosis and local control. Scrotal orchiectomy or biopsy is associated with a high incidence of local recurrence or spread to inguinal nodes. After orchiectomy, management depends on cell type (Table 18-10). Seminomas are radiosensitive. For stage I and nonbulky stage II seminoma, infradiaphragmatic lymphatic irradiation is used. The 5-year disease-free survival rate is more than 95%. For bulky stage II disease and stage III, platinum-based chemotherapy is used. Approximately 85% of patients are cured. For stage I nonseminoma, close follow-up is often used rather than immediate retroperitoneal node dissection (a controversial issue). For stages II and III, platinum-based chemotherapy is given. Cure rates are more than 95% for minimal metastatic disease, 90% for moderate bulk disease, and about

Table 18-10 Management of Testicular Cancer

| Stage | Treatment, by cell type | |
	Seminoma	Nonseminoma
I	XRT	? Observe
II	XRT	Chemo
III	Chemo	Chemo

Chemo, chemotherapy; XRT, x-ray therapy.

50% for bulky disease (multiple pulmonary metastases, bulky abdominal masses, liver, bone, or central nervous system metastases).

- Radical orchiectomy is the definitive initial procedure for testicular cancer.
- Early-stage seminoma is treated with radiation.
- Stage I nonseminoma may require no treatment after orchiectomy.
- Platinum-based chemotherapy is used for all other patients and results in high cure rates.

Extragonadal Germ Cell Tumor

This is uncommon. Patients present with increased β-hCG or α-fetoprotein values with midline mass lesions (retroperitoneum, mediastinum, or pineal gland). No gonadal primary tumor is identifiable on examination or ultrasonography. Cisplatin-based chemotherapy is frequently effective.

UNKNOWN PRIMARY LESION

Background

Patients presenting with metastatic carcinoma with an unknown primary lesion make up 5% to 10% of general oncologic practice. The first principle of management is to establish the diagnosis with a sufficient histologic specimen. In general, open biopsy is preferable to fine-needle aspiration, because a larger specimen allows optimal histologic and immunohistochemical analysis. All patients should have a careful history and complete physical examination, including pelvic and rectal examinations. Most patients, approximately 60%, have an adenocarcinoma. In 35% of patients, a diagnosis of poorly differentiated carcinoma will be made. Once a pathologic diagnosis is established, additional evaluation should be tailored according to the patient's symptoms and signs, sites of metastasis, and the histologic diagnosis. Special consideration should be given to rule out possible treatable malignancies, such as germ cell tumors, breast or ovarian carcinoma, or prostate cancer. Women presenting with axillary adenocarcinomas, with no clear breast primary lesion, should receive treatment for breast cancer. Women with peritoneal carcinomatosis generally have exploratory laparotomy with surgical cytoreduction, as for ovarian carcinoma. Men presenting with bone metastases, particularly osteoblastic metastases, should have a PSA test and their tumor material stained for PSA expression.

Treatment

If a potentially treatable neoplasm is ruled out, most patients with metastatic cancer of an unknown primary lesion have a very poor prognosis, with expected survival of 4 to 6 months. Some may benefit from palliative treatment (radiation or chemotherapy); many are managed best with supportive care.

PARANEOPLASTIC SYNDROMES

General

These conditions are the effects of a cancer occurring at a distance from the tumor; they are called "remote effects." They do not indicate metastatic disease. Common paraneoplastic syndromes and associated tumor types are listed in Table 18-11.

Carcinoid Syndrome

This is caused by peptide mediators secreted by carcinoid tumors of the small intestine which have metastasized extensively to the liver. It is less frequent with primary carcinoid tumors arising from other sites such as lung, thymus, or ovary. The most common symptoms are episodic flushing and diarrhea; bronchospasm may occur. Flushing and diarrhea may occur

Table 18-11 Classification of Paraneoplastic Syndromes

Syndrome	Mediator	Tumor type
Endocrine		
Cushing syndrome[*]	ACTH	Small-cell lung cancer
SIADH[*]	ADH	Lung, especially small cell
Hypercalcemia[*]	PTH-like peptide	Lung, especially squamous; breast; myeloma
Carcinoid syndrome	? Serotonin	Gut neuroendocrine tumors
	? Substance P	
Hypoglycemia	Insulin	Gut neuroendocrine tumors; other
	Insulin-like growth factors	
Neuromuscular		
Cerebellar degeneration	Anti-Purkinje cell antibodies	Lung, especially small cell; ovarian; breast
Dementia	?	Lung
Peripheral neuropathy[*]	Autoantibodies	Lung, gastrointestinal, breast
Lambert-Eaton	Antibodies to cholinergic receptor	Small-cell lung cancer
Dermatomyositis	?	Lung, breast
Skin		
Dermatomyositis	?	Lung, breast
Acanthosis nigricans	? TGF-α	Intra-abdominal cancer, usually gastric
Hematologic		
Venous thrombosis[*]	Activators of clotting cascade and platelets	Various adenocarcinomas, especially pancreatic and gastric
Nonbacterial thrombotic endocarditis	Activators of clotting cascade and platelets	Various adenocarcinomas, especially pancreatic and gastric

ACTH, adrenocorticotropic hormone; ADH, antidiuretic hormone; PTH, parathyroid hormone; SIADH, syndrome of inappropriate secretion of antidiuretic hormone; TGF-α, transforming growth factor-α.
[*]Most common types.

spontaneously or be precipitated by emotional factors or ingestion of food or alcohol. Carcinoid heart disease (right-sided valvular disease) is a potential late complication.

Lambert-Eaton Syndrome

This consists of muscle weakness (proximal) and gait disturbance. Strength is increased with exercise. It is associated with small-cell lung cancer.

Dermatomyositis

The female:male ratio is 2:1. Findings include muscle weakness (proximal), inflammatory myopathy, and increased creatine kinase values. Skin changes are variable and include heliotrope rash, periorbital edema, and Gottron papules. An underlying malignancy (lung, breast, gastrointestinal) is common in patients older than 50 years.

CHEMOTHERAPY

Basic Concepts

Currently, approximately 40 cytotoxic agents are available for use in North America. Taken generally, chemotherapeutic agents impair the process of cell division. Their selectivity for tumor cells is based primarily on a higher replicative rate in neoplastic cells. This selectivity for rapidly dividing cells explains the typical patterns of toxicity that occur with chemotherapy (that is, bone marrow, gastrointestinal mucosa, and hair follicles). The general classes and mechanisms of chemotherapeutic agents are shown in Figure 18-4 and the Oncology Pharmacy Review.

Applications

Chemotherapy can be used in the following settings: 1) advanced disease, 2) as adjuvant therapy after definitive local treatment, and 3) as primary or neoadjuvant therapy. The last application refers to situations in which patients present with a locally advanced malignancy and initial tumor reduction is needed before a primary treatment (such as operation or radiation) can be applied.

Solid Tumors Sensitive to Chemotherapy

Germ cell tumors of the testis and ovary, choriocarcinomas, breast cancer, ovarian cancer, and small-cell lung cancer are sensitive to chemotherapy. In recent years, combination chemotherapy regimens also have produced impressive tumor reductions in transitional cell carcinomas of the bladder, head and neck cancer, and cervical cancer.

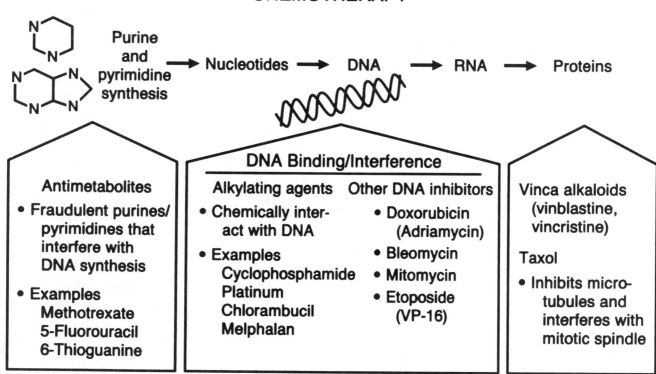

Fig. 18-4. General classes of chemotherapeutic agents.

Why Chemotherapy Fails to Cure Most Advanced Solid Tumors

The reasons for failure are 1) tumor cell heterogeneity, including populations of cells resistant to cytotoxic agents; 2) large numbers of noncycling or resting cells; and 3) pharmacologic sanctuaries—blood-tissue barriers and blood supply-tumor barriers.

Side Effects

The most common side effects of various chemotherapeutic agents are outlined in the Oncology Pharmacy Review.

Mechanisms of Tumor Cell Drug Resistance

Mechanisms include decreased drug uptake, increased drug efflux, decreased drug activation, increased drug inactivation, and increased production of a target enzyme.

Tumor cells may be resistant to a specific drug or they can have broad cross-resistance to structurally dissimilar drugs. This latter phenomenon is referred to as "multidrug resistance." This seems to be mediated by a large plasma membrane glycoprotein, termed the "p-glycoprotein," that functions as an energy-dependent drug-efflux pump.

- Tumor cells may be resistant to structurally dissimilar chemotherapy drugs ("multidrug resistance").

Colony-Stimulating Factors

In recent years, bone marrow colony-stimulating factors have been isolated and are now available for clinical use. These naturally occurring glycoproteins stimulate the proliferation, differentiation, and function of specific cells in the bone marrow. They may act at the level of the earliest stem cell or at later mature functional cells. They differ in their specificity.

Granulocyte colony-stimulating factor (G-CSF), for example, acts fairly specifically to stimulate production of mature neutrophils; granulocyte-macrophage CSF (GM-CSF) acts more generally, stimulating several cell lineages, including monocytes, eosinophils, and neutrophils. Both CSFs have been used to stimulate leukocyte recovery after chemotherapy-induced myelosuppression. As a general rule, CSFs do not affect the depth of the leukocyte nadir but shorten the duration of neutropenia. Unfortunately, no currently available CSF reliably protects against thrombocytopenia. To be effective, a CSF should be initiated shortly after completion of chemotherapy (1-2 days) and delivered through the expected neutrophil nadir. Placebo-controlled studies examining the efficacy of G-CSF initiated at the start of a documented chemotherapy-induced neutropenia have failed to show clinical benefit in patients who are not at high risk.

ONCOLOGIC COMPLICATIONS AND EMERGENCIES

Hypercalcemia

The most common underlying causes are malignancies and primary hyperparathyroidism. Patients with primary hyperparathyroidism have increased serum parathyroid hormone (PTH) values, but PTH is suppressed in cancer-associated hypercalcemia. Cancer-related hypercalcemia is often mediated by a PTH-related protein secreted by the tumor. This PTH-related protein can be detected with current assays. Tumors also can cause hypercalcemia by secreting other bone-resorbing substances or by enhancing conversion of 25-hydroxy-vitamin D to 1,25-dihydroxyvitamin D. Another mechanism is due to the local effects of osteolytic bone metastases.

Effects on bone and kidney contribute to hypercalcemia. Accelerated bone resorption is due to activation of osteoclasts by various mediators, primarily the PTH-like peptide. The same factors that induce osteoclast-mediated bone resorption also stimulate renal tubular resorption of calcium. The hypercalcemic state interferes with renal resorption of sodium and water, leading to polyuria and eventual depletion of extracellular fluid volume. This reduces the glomerular filtration rate, further increasing the serum calcium level. Immobilization tips the balance toward bone resorption, worsening the hypercalcemia.

- PTH is suppressed in cancer-associated hypercalcemia.
- Malignancy-associated hypercalcemia is often mediated by PTH-related protein secreted by a tumor.
- Bone and kidney pathophysiologic effects lead to an increased calcium level.

Symptoms of hypercalcemia include gastrointestinal (anorexia, nausea, vomiting, constipation), renal (polyuria, polydipsia, dehydration), central nervous system (cognitive difficulties, apathy, somnolence, or even coma), and cardiovascular (hypertension, shortened QT interval, enhanced sensitivity to digitalis).

Cancers associated with hypercalcemia include lung (squamous cell), renal, myeloma, lymphoma, breast, and head and neck. Patients with breast cancer and those with myeloma are more likely to have bony involvement with their disease.

For treatment of hypercalcemia, the magnitude of the hypercalcemia and the degree of symptoms are key considerations. Generally, patients with a serum calcium value more than 14 mg/dL should be hospitalized for immediate treatment. The serum calcium value should be adjusted if the serum albumin value is abnormal. The conversion formula is 0.8 mg/dL of serum total calcium for every 1 g of serum albumin more or less than 4 g/dL. If the serum albumin value is increased (as with dehydration), the total calcium value should be adjusted downward; if the serum albumin value is reduced (as in chronic illness), the total calcium value should be adjusted upward.

For hydration, intravenously administered normal saline (200-400 mL/h) is initially given. Loop diuretics are used *after* volume expansion. Furosemide facilitates urinary excretion of calcium by inhibiting calcium resorption in the thick ascending loop of Henle. A loop diuretic will help correct for volume overload once the patient has been rehydrated.

Bisphosphonates (pamidronate or zoledronic acid) are given intravenously (gastrointestinal absorption is poor). They bind to hydroxyapatite and inhibit osteoclasts. In addition to fluids, bisphosphonates have become the mainstay of treatment for hypercalcemia.

Gallium nitrate (200 mg/m^2 per day) is administered as continuous intravenous infusion for 5 days (unless normocalcemia is achieved earlier). It is a highly effective inhibitor of bone resorption. Renal impairment limits its usefulness.

Mithramycin (25 µg/kg) is given intravenously over 4 hours; this treatment can be repeated if necessary. Maximal hypocalcemic effect is reached at 48 to 72 hours. It is associated with hepatic and renal side effects and thrombocytopenia.

Glucocorticoids have an antitumor effect on neoplastic lymphoid tissue.

Calcitonin is given subcutaneously or intramuscularly. It has a rapid onset of action; thus, it is useful in immediate life-threatening situations. Calcitonin is a relatively weak agent with short-lived effect. Allergic reactions to salmon calcitonin are unusual, but an initial skin test with 1 unit is recommended before a full dose is given.

- Volume expansion must precede administration of furosemide.
- Furosemide inhibits calcium resorption in the thick ascending loop of Henle.
- Bisphosphonates bind to hydroxyapatite and inhibit osteoclasts.
- Mithramycin has hepatic and renal side effects.
- Calcitonin is a relatively weak agent with a rapid, short-lived effect.

Tumor Lysis Syndrome

This syndrome occurs as a result of the overwhelming release of tumor cell contents into the bloodstream such that concentrations of certain substances become life-threatening. It most commonly occurs in cancers with large tumor burdens and high proliferation rates which are exquisitely sensitive to chemotherapy. Examples include high-grade lymphomas, leukemia, and, much less commonly, solid tumors. The syndrome is characterized by an increased uric acid value, which leads to renal complications; acidosis; an increased potassium value, which can cause lethal cardiac arrhythmias; an increased phosphate value,

which leads to acute renal failure; and a decreased calcium value, which causes muscle cramps, cardiac arrhythmias, and tetany. The syndrome can be prevented with adequate hydration, alkalinization, and administration of allopurinol before chemotherapy.

- Tumor lysis syndrome is a result of the overwhelming release of tumor cell contents into the bloodstream.
- It is most common in cancers with large tumor burdens and high proliferation rates which are exquisitely sensitive to chemotherapy.
- It is characterized by increased uric acid, increased potassium, increased phosphate, acidosis, and decreased calcium.

Febrile Neutropenia

This is defined as a temperature of 38.5°C or more on one occasion or three episodes of 38°C or more plus an absolute neutrophil count of 500×10^9/L or less (or leukocyte count of $1,000 \times 10^9$/L or less). Management generally involves hospitalization and institution of parenteral broad-spectrum antibiotics. Patients usually have no infection documented, but appropriate specimens for culture should be rapidly obtained before antibiotics are given. Use of colony-stimulating factors at the time of documentation of febrile neutropenia has not been shown to have clinical utility.

Spinal Cord Compression

Acute cord compression is a neurologic emergency. It results most commonly from epidural compression by metastatic tumor (lung, breast, prostate, myeloma, kidney). Occasionally, compression can occur from neighboring nodal involvement and tumor infiltration through intervertebral foramina (lymphoma). The locations are cervical in 10% of cases, thoracic in 70%, and lumbar in 20%. Multiple noncontiguous levels are involved in 10% to 40%.

More than 90% of patients present with pain. Cervical pain may radiate down the arm. Thoracic pain radiates around the rib cage or abdominal wall; it may be described as a compressing band bilaterally around the chest or abdomen. Lumbar pain may radiate into the groin or down the leg. Pain may be aggravated by coughing, sneezing, or straight-leg raising. Focal neurologic signs depend on the level affected. Paresthesias (tingling, numbness), weakness, and altered reflexes also can be present (Table 18-12). Tenderness over the spine may help localize the level. Autonomic changes of urinary or fecal retention or incontinence may be present.

Imaging studies include bone scanning or plain radiography, which reveal vertebral metastases in approximately 85% of patients with epidural compression. Myelography or magnetic resonance imaging of the entire spine is generally recommended.

Treatment usually includes an initial bolus of 10 to 100 mg of dexamethasone intravenously, depending on the severity of

Table 18-12 Reflexes and Their Corresponding Roots and Muscles

Reflex	Root(s)	Muscle
Biceps	C5-6	Biceps
Triceps	C7-8	Triceps
Knee jerk	L2-4	Quadriceps
Ankle jerk	S1	Gastrocnemius

block. Thereafter, dexamethasone is given (4 mg four times a day), although some physicians favor higher doses for a few days followed by a rapid taper. Radiation therapy is applied to the involved area(s). Surgical procedures are used in select circumstances, including no previous diagnosis of malignancy, spine instability, prior radiation to cord tolerance, and progressive neurologic decline despite radiation therapy. The outcome depends on the patient's neurologic function at presentation (Table 18-13).

PALLIATIVE CARE

Background

More than 70% of patients with cancer have significant pain during the course of their disease. Multiple studies have shown that patients with cancer-related pain are not given adequate analgesic therapy (42% of patients are not given adequate pain relief). Primary barriers to optimal management of cancer pain include inadequate pain assessment by health care professionals; physician reluctance to prescribe opioids; and patient reluctance to take opioids. Physician reluctance to prescribe opioids stems from concern about addiction, lack of familiarity with the agents, and problems with management of side effects of opioids. Of note, psychological addiction to opioids in cancer patients is very rare, occurring in less than 1%.

Evaluation

Evaluation should include 1) a history regarding onset, quality, severity, and location of pain; exacerbating and relieving

Table 18-13 Outcome of Patients With Spinal Cord Compression, by Neurologic Status

Status at presentation	% ambulatory after radiation
Ambulatory	>80
Paraparetic	<50
Paraplegic	<10

factors; associated symptoms, and 2) physical examination, which should include a complete neurologic examination. Diagnostic studies are determined by the results of the history and physical examination.

Treatment

Three-Tiered Approach

Step 1: For mild pain, administer acetaminophen or a nonsteroidal anti-inflammatory drug around the clock. Of note, studies of nonsteroidal anti-inflammatory drugs for cancer pain have shown that these agents are only 1.5 to 2 times more effective than placebo.

Step 2: When step 1 fails to provide adequate analgesia, or for moderate pain, add codeine or oxycodone.

Step 3: For severe pain or inadequate pain relief with steps 1 and 2, agents include morphine, hydromorphone, oxycodone, methadone, and fentanyl (see the Oncology Pharmacy Review).

General Principles

For most cancer pain, opioids are the main treatment approach. Orally administered immediate-release morphine is the usual first-line drug selected for severe pain from cancer. The average starting oral dosage is 10 to 30 mg every 4 hours. There is no "standard dosage." This should be increased until analgesia is achieved. Around-the-clock dosing, not as-needed, is necessary. When the patient's total daily morphine requirements are defined, convert that total daily dose to a long-acting morphine product that can be given every 8 or every 12 hours. Provide rescue doses of immediate-release morphine (usually 5%-10% of the total daily dose should be available every 1-2 hours as needed). Adverse effects of opioids include sedation, nausea, constipation, respiratory depression, and myoclonus. Tolerance to opioid-induced sedation and nausea usually develops within a few days. For opioid-induced constipation, initiate the use of docusate sodium and senna with opioids. Respiratory depression typically follows sedation; if a patient is somnolent, doses should be held. No narcotic is more or less likely to result in a particular side-effect profile. However, one narcotic may produce an adverse effect in a patient whereas another will not. Thus, sequential trials of different opioids may be needed to determine the one best suited for a patient. The fentanyl patch (a transdermal formulation) delivers drug continuously over 72 hours. It is especially useful for patients with poor tolerance of orally administered opioids or those unable to take medications orally.

ACKNOWLEDGMENT

We gratefully acknowledge Lynn Hartmann, M.D., for her extensive work on this chapter in previous editions.

Oncology Pharmacy Review — Part I: General Classes of Agents
Robert C. Wolf, PharmD, Darryl C. Grendahl, RPh

A. Alkylating Agents

Drug	Toxic/adverse effects	Comments
Carboplatin	Myelosuppression (especially thrombocytopenia)	Commonly dosed with the Calvert formula
Carmustine	Myelosuppression (delayed) Renal dysfunction Pulmonary fibrosis	Crosses blood-brain barrier Pain with infusion
Cisplatin	Nephrotoxicity Peripheral neuropathy Ototoxicity Anemia	Magnesium or potassium wasting is common Dose adjustment is needed for renal insufficiency Minimize concomitant nephrotoxins
Cyclophosphamide	Myelosuppression Hemorrhagic cystitis SIADH (high dose) Cardiomyopathy (high dose)	
Dacarbazine	Myelosuppression Flu-like symptoms Photosensitivity	Pain with infusion
Ifosfamide	Myelosuppression Hemorrhagic cystitis CNS toxicity	Mesna is used to prevent hemorrhagic cystitis Lethargy, confusion, seizures
Mechlorethamine	Myelosuppression Thrombosis Thrombophlebitis Vomiting	Nitrogen mustard
Oxaliplatin	Peripheral neuropathy Hypersensitivity Myelosuppression Diarrhea	Acute, transient, cold-exacerbated dysesthesia or delayed-onset, cumulative paresthesias
Streptozocin	Nephrotoxicity	Dose adjustment is needed for renal insufficiency Vesicant
Temozolomide	Myelosuppression Lethargy Ataxia Increased LFTs	

CNS, central nervous system; LFTs, liver function test results; SIADH, syndrome of inappropriate secretion of antidiuretic hormone.

Oncology Pharmacy Review — Part I (continued)

B. Antimetabolites

Drug	Toxic/adverse effects	Comments
Capecitabine	Hand-foot syndrome Diarrhea Mucositis Fatigue	Oral prodrug of 5-fluorouracil Dose adjustment is needed for renal insufficiency Contraindicated in severe renal impairment

Fluorouracil	Diarrhea
	Mucositis
	Myelosuppression
	Ocular irritation
	Skin toxicity
	Myocardial ischemia
		Toxicity profile is dependent on administration schedule
		  • Bolus—myelosuppression
		  • Continuous infusion—GI toxicity
		Leucovorin is concomitantly used to enhance enzyme inhibition

Gemcitabine	Myelosuppression (especially thrombocytopenia) Increased LFTs Peripheral edema Flu-like symptoms Rash Anal pruritus Hemolytic uremic syndrome	
Methotrexate	Myelosuppression Mucositis Nephrotoxicity (high dose) CNS toxicity (high dose or IT) Hepatotoxicity Pulmonary fibrosis	Leucovorin rescue for doses >100 mg/m^2 with serum level monitoring Urinary alkalinization for high dose Distributes in "third-space" fluids, leading to prolonged elimination and toxicity Drug interactions—NSAIDs, probenecid

CNS, central nervous system; GI, gastrointestinal; IT, intrathecal; LFTs, liver function test results; NSAIDs, nonsteroidal anti-inflammatory drugs.

Oncology Pharmacy Review — Part I (continued)

C. Plant Derivatives

Drug	Toxic/adverse effects	Comments
Vincristine	Neurotoxicity (peripheral, autonomic, cranial) SIADH	Dose reduction for biliary dysfunction Vesicant
Vinblastine	Myelosuppression Neuromuscular (myalgias)	Dose reduction for biliary dysfunction Vesicant
Etoposide	Myelosuppression Alopecia Mucositis (high dose) Hypotension Secondary leukemia	Renal & hepatic elimination
Paclitaxel	Myelosuppression Peripheral neuropathy Alopecia Hypersensitivity Myalgias Bradycardia	Vesicant Dose adjustment for liver dysfunction Premedicate with dexamethasone & antihistamine (H1 and H2) Drug interaction (administer before cisplatin)
Docetaxel	Myelosuppression Fluid retention Peripheral neuropathy Skin reactions Hand-foot syndrome Hypersensitivity	Dose adjustment is needed for liver dysfunction Prevent fluid retention with dexamethasone 4 mg twice daily for 5 days (begin 1 day before docetaxel)
Irinotecan	Diarrhea (acute & delayed) Myelosuppression Abdominal cramping/pain	Dose adjustment is needed for liver dysfunction Loperamide ($\leq$24 mg/day) is used for delayed diarrhea
Topotecan	Myelosuppression Alopecia Mucositis (high dose)	Dose adjustment is needed for renal insufficiency

SIADH, syndrome of inappropriate secretion of antidiuretic hormone.

Oncology Pharmacy Review — Part I (continued)

D. Antitumor Antibiotics

Drug	Toxic/adverse effects	Comments
Bleomycin	Pulmonary fibrosis (chronic) (>400 units) Febrile reaction Hyperpigmentation Mucositis	Dose adjustment is needed for severe renal insufficiency
Doxorubicin	Myelosuppression Cardiomyopathy (chronic) (>550 mg/m^2) Mucositis Alopecia Red-orange urine Secondary leukemia	Dose reduction is needed for biliary dysfunction Dexrazoxane may be used as cardioprotectant Vesicant Venous flare reaction on injection Radiation recall
Epirubicin	Myelosuppression Cardiomyopathy Mucositis Red-orange urine	Vesicant
Mitomycin	Myelosuppression (delayed) Blue-green urine Hemolytic uremic syndrome Pulmonary toxicity	Vesicant
Mitoxantrone	Myelosuppression Blue-green urine Cardiomyopathy	Vesicant

Oncology Pharmacy Review — Part I (continued)

E. Immunotherapy

Drug	Toxic/adverse effects	Comments
Aldesleukin (IL-2)	Capillary leak syndrome (fever, fluid retention, respiratory distress, hypotension) Myelosuppression Erythema	Concurrent corticosteroids may limit efficacy
Interferon-α	Flu-like symptoms Fatigue Myelosuppression Increased LFTs	

LFTs, liver function test results.

F. Targeted Therapy

Drug	Toxic/adverse effects	Comments
Bevacizumab	Bleeding Wound healing complications	Recombinant monoclonal antibody that inhibits vascular endothelial growth factor
Cetuximab (IMC-225)	Folliculitis	Monoclonal antibody against epidermal growth factor
Gefitinib	Diarrhea Rash (acne) Interstitial lung disease Ocular irritation	Inhibits the epidermal growth factor receptor tyrosine kinase
Herceptin	Fever Chills or rigors Cardiac dysfunction Diarrhea	Cardiac dysfunction most common when used in combination with doxorubicin

Oncology Pharmacy Review — Part I (continued)

G. Endocrine Therapy

Drug	Toxic/adverse effects	Comments
Tamoxifen	Hot flashes Vaginal dryness Endometrial cancer Thromboembolism	Antiestrogen
Anastrozole Letrozole Exemestane	Nausea (mild) Peripheral edema Diarrhea Asthenia Hot flashes	Aromatase inhibitors
Megestrol	Fluid retention Weight gain Thromboembolism	Progestin
Leuprolide Goserelin	Decreased libido Impotence Hot flashes Tumor flare	LHRH agonists
Flutamide Bicalutamide Nilutamide	Gynecomastia Diarrhea Increased LFTs Impaired adaptation to dark (nilutamide) Pulmonary fibrosis (nilutamide)	Antiandrogens

LFTs, liver function test results; LHRH, luteinizing hormone-releasing hormone.

H. Emetogenic Potential of Select Oncology Agents

High (level 5)	Moderately high (level 4)	Moderate (level 3)	Mild (level 2)	Low (level 1)
Cisplatin	Carboplatin	Ifosfamide	Fluorouracil	Temozolomide
Carmustine	Cyclophosphamide	Gemcitabine	Methotrexate	Capecitabine
Mechlorethamine	Methotrexate*	Irinotecan	Etoposide	Vincristine
Dacarbazine	Doxorubicin	Epirubicin	Paclitaxel	Vinblastine
Streptozocin		Mitoxantrone	Docetaxel	Bleomycin
		Mitomycin	Topotecan	

*High-dose.

Oncology Pharmacy Review — Part II: Analgesics
Lisa G. Hall, PharmD, Robert C. Wolf, PharmD

A. Dosage Information: Common Opioid Agonists

Agonist	Dosage form	Onset, min	Duration, h	Approximate equianalgesic dose, mg	
				Parenteral	Oral
Morphine	Tablet/capsule	15-60	3-12	10	30-60
	Solution	15-60	3-12		
	Suppository	15-60	3-12		
	Injection	IV: <5	3-12		
Oxycodone	Tablet/capsule	15-30	4-12	Not	20-30
	Solution	15-30	4-12	applicable	
Fentanyl	Transdermal patch	12-18 h	48-72	0.1	Patch: ~17 μg/h
	Transmucosal lozenge	TM: 5-15			
	Injection	IV: 1-5	IV: 1-2		
Hydromorphone	Tablet	15-30	4-5	1.5	7.5
	Solution	15-30	4-5		
	Suppository	15-30	4-5		
	Injection	IV: <5	4-5		
Methadone	Tablet	30-60	4-12	5-10	5-10
	Solution	30-60	4-12		
	Injection	IV: <5	4-12		
Codeine	Tablet	30-60	4-6	120	200
	Solution	30-60	4-6		
	Injection	IV: 10-30	4-6		
Hydrocodone	Tablet/capsule	60	2-6	Not	30
	Solution			applicable	
Meperidine	Tablet	10-15	2-4	75	300
	Solution	10-15	2-4		
	Injection	IV: <5	2-4		

IV, intravenous; TM, transmucosal.

Oncology Pharmacy Review — Part II (continued)

B. Dosage Information: Common Nonopioid Analgesics

Analgesic	Dosage form	Onset, min	Duration, h
Miscellaneous			
Acetaminophen	Tablet	10-30	4-6
	Solution		
	Suppository		
Aspirin	Tablet	30	3-6
	Suppository		
Tramadol	Tablet	30-60	6-8
Nonsteroidal anti-inflammatory drugs			
Ibuprofen	Tablet	30	4-6
	Suspension		
Naproxen	Tablet	60	6-12
	Suspension		
Ketorolac	Tablet	30	4-6
	Injection	IV: 10	IV: 6
Cyclooxygenase-2 inhibitors			
Celecoxib	Capsule	45-60	4-8
Rofecoxib	Tablet	30-60	6
	Suspension		
Adjuvant analgesics			
Gabapentin	Tablet/capsule	1-5 days	6-8
Amitriptyline	Tablet	3-14 days	12-24
	Injection		
Carbamazepine	Tablet	3-14 days	8-12
	Suspension		

IV, intravenous.

Oncology Pharmacy Review — Part II (continued)

C. Effects and Other Considerations for Common Opioid Agonists and Nonopioid Analgesics

Drug	Toxic/adverse effects	Comments
Common opioid agonists		
Morphine	Sedation	Morphine: orthostatic hypotension, use cautiously with hemodynamic instability
Oxycodone	Respiratory depression	
Fentanyl	Nausea or vomiting	Fentanyl: delayed onset with the transdermal patch
Hydromorphone	Constipation	Hydromorphone: neuroexcitation leading to seizures (rare)
Methadone	Euphoria	Methadone: longer duration of effect with chronic use
Codeine	Delirium	Codeine: ceiling effect
Hydrocodone	Hallucinations, dry mouth,	Meperidine: neuroexcitatory active metabolites accumulate
Meperidine	urinary retention, itching, physical dependence	with renal insufficiency; *not* recommended for chronic pain states; drug-drug interaction with MAO inhibitors
		There are many combination products that contain both an opioid agonist and nonopioid analgesic. The cumulative dose of the nonopioid analgesic generally limits the ability to increase doses
Common nonopioid analgesics		
Miscellaneous analgesics		
Acetaminophen	Hepatic dysfunction with higher doses or chronic use	Maximal dose = 4,000 mg/day
	Renal tubular necrosis	Higher doses inhibit warfarin metabolism, which may prolong the INR
Aspirin	GI ulceration, inhibits platelet aggregation, renal insufficiency, tinnitus	Maximal dose = 3,600 mg/day
Tramadol	Dizziness, sedation, constipation, nausea or vomiting	Maximal dose = 400 mg/day (300 mg/day in elderly)
		Higher doses increase seizure potential
Nonsteroidal anti-inflammatory drugs/cyclooxygenase-2 inhibitors		
Ibuprofen	Dyspepsia	Ketorolac: maximal duration of use is 5 days because of risk of GI or renal side effects
Naproxen	GI ulceration	
Ketorolac	Salt and water retention	Use cautiously with other nephrotoxic agents
Celecoxib	Renal insufficiency	Celecoxib and rofecoxib have fewer GI side effects than traditional nonsteroidal anti-inflammatory agents and do not inhibit platelet aggregation
Rofecoxib	Inhibition of platelet aggregation	
Adjuvant analgesics		
Gabapentin	Sedation	Usual effective dose: 1,200-1,800 mg/day in divided doses (maximal, 3,600 mg/day)
	Dizziness	
	Fatigue	Dose reduction is necessary with renal insufficiency
		Initiate bedtime dosing and titrate to effective dose
Amitriptyline	Sedation, dizziness, dry mouth, confusion, constipation, blurred vision, urinary retention, orthostatic hypotension	Usual effective dose: 50-150 mg/day
		Other tricyclic antidepressants are also effective
Carbamazepine	Dizziness, sedation, nausea or vomiting, mild leukopenia, agranulocytosis (rare)	Usual effective dose: 400-800 mg/day
		Erythromycin, clarithromycin, and propoxyphene inhibit carbamazepine metabolism

GI, gastrointestinal; INR, International Normalized Ratio; MAO, monoamine oxidase.

QUESTIONS

Multiple Choice (choose the one best answer)

1. A 65-year-old man with a 25 pack-year history of smoking and a family history of colon cancer presents with hemoptysis. Chest radiography and CT of the chest show a mass in the right lung. Bronchoscopy with biopsy of the mass is positive for non–small-cell lung carcinoma. He undergoes resection of this lung mass, and two mediastinal lymph nodes are metastatically involved. The pathologic stage is T2 N2 M0 (stage IIIA). The most appropriate statement is:
   a. Postoperative radiation therapy will improve survival
   b. Postoperative chemotherapy will improve overall survival
   c. Postoperative radiation therapy will improve local failure rate
   d. Combined chemotherapy and radiation therapy is indicated and has been shown to improve overall survival
   e. CT of the brain is necessary to exclude brain metastasis

2. A 72-year-old woman with a 45 pack-year history of smoking presents with unsteady gait and weight loss of 15 lb. MRI of the head is negative for metastasis. A lumbar puncture and cytologic analysis are negative for malignancy. Chest radiography is negative, but CT of the chest shows evidence of a mediastinal mass, which on mediastinoscopy is positive for small-cell lung carcinoma. Anti-Purkinje cell antibodies are positive in the serum. CT of the abdomen and pelvis shows a solitary liver metastasis, which on biopsy is positive for small-cell carcinoma. The rest of the imaging studies were otherwise negative. What is the next appropriate treatment?
   a. Whole brain radiation therapy
   b. Resection of the liver metastasis
   c. Combination chemotherapy
   d. Intrathecal methotrexate
   e. Radiation therapy to the chest

3. A 50-year-old male lawyer with a 50 pack-year history of smoking presents with cough. He has evidence of bilateral pulmonary nodules on chest radiography. This is confirmed with CT of the chest. CT of the abdomen confirms three liver lesions and an enlarged adrenal gland. A biopsy of the liver lesion is positive for non–small-cell lung carcinoma. He has not lost any weight and he is otherwise in good performance status (Eastern Cooperative Oncology Group performance status 0). A bone scan is negative. Which of the following recommendations is appropriate?
   a. Supportive care is as good as chemotherapy

   b. Chemotherapy will improve overall survival and improve quality of life
   c. Chemotherapy is curative
   d. Prophylactic cranial radiation therapy is indicated
   e. Bisphosphonates are needed to improve the complication rates of bony metastasis

4. A 45-year-old anxious white woman comes to your office because she found a new mass in her breast while performing breast self-examination. There is no family history of breast carcinoma or ovarian cancer. She took birth control pills from ages 20 to 40 years and discontinued their use when bilateral deep venous thrombosis and symptomatic pulmonary embolism developed at age 40 years. The examination confirms a 2-cm, firm lump in the left outer quadrant. No other adenopathy or organomegaly is noted. Mammography is negative. Ultrasonography shows a solid mass. What is the next recommendation?
   a. Reassure the patient that the lump is benign because the mammogram is negative
   b. Reassure the patient that the lump is benign because there is no family history of breast carcinoma
   c. Recommend genetic screening for *BCR2*
   d. Begin tamoxifen therapy
   e. Recommend a biopsy

5. A 52-year-old postmenopausal woman undergoes a lumpectomy and sentinel lymph node biopsy for lobular breast carcinoma. The lesion measured 2 cm, and a sentinel node was positive. An axillary node dissection is performed, and 10 of 10 lymph nodes are metastatically involved. The tumor is estrogen-receptor–negative, progesterone-receptor–negative, and HER2 markedly positive. The examination and laboratory data are otherwise negative. What is the next recommendation?
   a. Tamoxifen
   b. Anastrozole
   c. Chemotherapy followed by breast radiation therapy
   d. Breast radiation therapy alone
   e. Herceptin alone

6. A 72-year-old woman with a history of breast carcinoma 2 years ago presents with nausea, vomiting, dehydration, and diffuse bone pain. Examination shows a right modified radical mastectomy scar and palpable liver 5 cm below the right costal margin. She has tenderness in the lumbar spine, and neurologically she has weakness in the right lower extremity. Her calcium value is increased (12 mg/dL), and her creatinine value is 2.5 mg/dL. MRI of the lumbar spine shows an epidural mass at L3-5. Ultrasonography of the liver confirms multiple liver

metastases, which on biopsy are positive for adenocarcinoma consistent with a breast primary lesion that is estrogen-receptor– and progesterone-receptor–positive. Which one of the following recommendations is appropriate at this time?
a. Therapy with intravenous fluids and corticosteroids
b. Tamoxifen therapy
c. Cytotoxic chemotherapy
d. Intravenous bisphosphonate therapy
e. Radiofrequency ablation of the liver lesions

7. A 75-year-old woman, otherwise healthy, presents with fullness in the abdomen and increasing abdominal girth. A right pelvic mass and ascites are found on examination. CT confirms a right-sided pelvic mass. The level of cancer antigen 125 (CA 125) is 5 times increased. She undergoes maximal debulking of her ovarian carcinoma, and the pathologic stage is III. Postoperatively, her CA 125 returns to normal. What is the next recommendation?
a. Six cycles of postoperative chemotherapy
b. Estrogen therapy
c. No adjuvant therapy because her CA 125 level has returned to normal
d. Herceptin
e. Tamoxifen

8. A 55-year-old man was found to have a 3-cm transverse colon mass that, on biopsy, was invasive adenocarcinoma. He underwent surgical resection, and three regional lymph nodes were metastatically involved. This was pathologically staged as stage III. He had no family history of colon cancer and recovered well from the operation. You should also recommend:
a. Radiation
b. Interarterial chemotherapy to the liver
c. Genetic p53 analysis
d. Six cycles of 5-fluorouracil and leucovorin-based chemotherapy
e. Serial fecal occult blood testing every month

9. A 65-year-old man presents with a 2-month history of rectal bleeding and bloating with nausea and vomiting and a 25-lb weight loss. He is thin and cachetic and is not jaundiced. His liver is enlarged 6 cm below the right costal margin. On rectal examination, there is a firm mass that is bloody. Imaging studies confirm metastatic disease in the liver. A biopsy of the liver is consistent with metastatic rectal cancer. What is the next appropriate treatment?
a. Radiofrequency ablation of the liver metastasis
b. Chemotherapy
c. Radiation with concurrent chemotherapy
d. Surgical consultation for diverting colostomy
e. Hepatic infusion of floxuridine

10. A 27-year-old man presents with a left testicular mass. Physical examination confirms a solitary mass in the left testicle. Ultrasonography confirms the solitary mass, and CT of the chest, abdomen, and pelvis is negative. He undergoes a left radical orchiectomy, and the pathologic diagnosis is seminoma. Which one of the following laboratory reports would be inconsistent with the diagnosis?
a. The β-human chorionic gonadotropin and α-fetoprotein levels are increased
b. The α-fetoprotein value is normal
c. The β-human chorionic gonadotropin value is increased
d. The lactate dehydrogenase value is increased
e. The testosterone level is normal

11. A 76-year-old man with a history of coronary artery disease and left deep venous thrombosis was referred to the emergency department because of back pain and lower extremity weakness. He has a history of localized prostate carcinoma treated 2 years ago with primary radiation. On physical examination, the patient is somewhat anxious and has weakness of the left lower extremity with good sphincter control. His prostate-specific antigen level is increased at 400 ng/mL. Previously, after radiation therapy, this value was normal. MRI shows epidural extension at L2. After dexamethasone therapy, he is improved and pain-free. What is your next step?
a. Combination cytotoxic chemotherapy
b. Diethylstilbestrol (estrogen)
c. Orchiectomy
d. Luteinizing hormone-releasing hormone alone
e. Bisphosphonates

12. A 36-year-old female medical resident presents with an enlarging right axillary lump. She has no fevers or chills. On examination, a 4-cm mobile lump is found in her right axilla. The breast examination is negative. There is a changing mole on the right forearm. On biopsy of the mole, malignant melanoma is found. What is the next treatment?
a. Combination chemotherapy
b. Radiation therapy to the mole and lymph node
c. Wide local excision and axillary lymph node dissection
d. Interferon therapy
e. Tumor necrosis factor

13. A new compound is developed from the snail of the Black Sea. It works by inhibiting and binding DNA. Your project

manager wants you to combine this new agent with agents that work on microtubules. Which chemotherapy would you use?

a. Paclitaxel
b. Cisplatin
c. 5-Fluorouracil
d. Methotrexate
e. Bleomycin

14. An 80-year-old man with history of hormone-refractory prostate carcinoma presents with lumbar pain. It is not responsive to over-the-counter pain medicines. MRI shows extensive bony metastasis with no cord compression. His bowel and bladder function are otherwise preserved. On examination, he is a weak, elderly man with a performance status of 3. Prior radiation therapy, corticosteroid therapy, and radionucleotide therapy have failed. He wants hospice care. What is the next appropriate step?

a. Avoid opioids because of fear of addiction and constipation
b. Recommend that the patient not have hospice care because there are proven treatments that could substantially improve his overall survival
c. Prescribe meperidine shots every 6 hours
d. Initiate therapy with a narcotic for pain control as needed and begin a bowel and bladder regimen
e. Initiate a plan to use scheduled narcotics to control the pain and then convert to a long-acting pain regimen

15. A 72-year-old male smoker with a 42 pack-year history of smoking presents with anorexia and cough. Chest radiography shows a right-sided mass, which on bronchoscopy is positive for squamous cell carcinoma. On physical examination, the patient is thin, cachectic, and dehydrated. The calcium value is increased at 15 mg/dL, and the creatinine value at 2.5 mg/dL. Bone scan shows multiple bony metastases. What should be the initial treatment?

a. Cisplatin-based chemotherapy
b. Radiation to the lung
c. Intravenous fluids
d. Bisphosphonates
e. Mithramycin

ANSWERS

1. Answer c.

Postoperative radiation therapy will improve local control but has not been shown to improve overall survival. The addition of chemotherapy to radiation therapy has not been shown to increase overall survival. Without central nervous system symptoms, routine imaging of the brain for non–small-cell lung carcinoma is not required for staging.

2. Answer c.

Patients with small-cell lung carcinoma may have paraneoplastic syndrome with cerebellar degeneration due to anti-Purkinje cell antibodies. The treatment for a neurologic disease is treatment of the systemic disease (small-cell lung carcinoma). Initial treatment is combination chemotherapy. Because small-cell lung carcinoma is a systemic disease, isolated metastasectomy for metastatic disease is not generally indicated.

3. Answer b.

Chemotherapy will improve overall survival and quality of life but is not curative. Studies have shown that chemotherapy compared with best supportive care does improve survival. Prophylactic cranial radiation is indicated only in small-cell lung carcinoma in patients who achieve a complete regression. This patient has non–small-cell lung carcinoma and therefore would not be a candidate for prophylactic cranial radiation therapy. Bisphosphonates are helpful for bony complications when they are present. It has not been a practice to use bisphosphonates to prevent bony metastasis.

4. Answer e.

Mammography is normal in about 10% of breast cancers. All lumps in the breast need further evaluation regardless of family history. The use of tamoxifen is contraindicated in someone with significant thrombotic risks.

5. Answer c.

Adjuvant chemotherapy and postoperative breast radiation therapy are indicated. Because the tumor is estrogen-receptor– and progesterone-receptor–negative, hormonal manipulation is not indicated. The value of herceptin is its synergy with systemic chemotherapy. Its use at this point on an adjuvant basis alone is not recommended.

6. Answer a.

Spinal cord compression is a medical emergency, as is hypercalcemia. Both should respond to treatment with intravenous fluids and corticosteroids. Systemic treatment with chemotherapy or hormonal therapy might take several days to be effective and several weeks to show maximal benefit.

Appropriate fluid and corticosteroid therapy is all that might be needed to help control the calcium level. If it still remains increased after this therapy, bisphosphonates would be the next option.

7. Answer a.

Standard of care is the addition of chemotherapy after undergoing maximal debulking. Normalization of the CA 125 level postoperatively is a favorable sign but still does not indicate the absence of persistent disease in the abdomen and pelvis.

8. Answer d.

Adjuvant chemotherapy with 5-fluorouracil and leucovorin is the standard of care after resection of stage III colon cancer. Radiation therapy is indicated for rectal cancer to improve local control. The use of genetic testing or fecal occult blood testing is not recommended.

9. Answer d.

This patient has metastatic rectal cancer, and treatment is not curative. Chemotherapy options are palliative. If he is to undergo systemic treatment, he will need to improve his nutritional status and relieve the rectal obstruction. If operation is not recommended, other options include a rectal stent. If he is not a good candidate after these procedures, symptomatic supportive care is reasonable.

10. Answer a.

Pure seminomas do not produce any α-fetoprotein. Some β-human chorionic gonadotropin is produced by seminomas. The testosterone value is normal and the lactate dehydrogenase value frequently is increased in patients with germ cell tumors.

11. Answer c.

Improvement of metastatic prostate carcinoma with corticosteroids is temporary. Additional treatments for the localized disease are indicated. Because prostate cancer is a hormone-responsive disease (he has not had previous hormonal manipulation), it is reasonable to expect some long-term benefit with orchiectomy. The use of diethylstilbestrol (estrogen) is contraindicated in someone with coronary artery disease and left deep venous thrombosis. Luteinizing hormone-releasing hormone will cause a temporary flare; it can actually cause worsening neurologic symptoms and should be used after blockade with bicalutamide or flutamide.

12. Answer c.

Local treatment is still curative in its intent. Melanomas do tend to metastasize to the regional lymph nodes. Chemotherapy and radiation therapy is palliative, as is cytokine therapy.

13. Answer a.

Paclitaxel works by stabilizing microtubule formation. Cisplatin and bleomycin inhibit DNA-binding interface interactions. Methotrexate and 5-fluorouracil are antimetabolites.

14. Answer e.

Pain is very common in palliative medicine. It is important to remember the need for a bowel regimen to prevent constipation. The fear of addiction to narcotics and of constipation is moot in this situation. It is better to try to control the pain before it becomes intolerable, and scheduled pain medicine is recommended.

15. Answer c.

Patients need intravenous fluids and hydration before any treatment with a platinum-base therapy. Cisplatin causes renal insufficiency and is contraindicated with renal insufficiency. Given the patient's marginal performance status, it is unclear whether he should receive chemotherapy. If, after appropriate intravenous fluid resuscitation, he still remains hypercalcemic, the addition of bisphosphonates would be recommended. Mithramycin is not recommended in renal insufficiency.

CHAPTER 19

PREVENTIVE MEDICINE

Sally J. Trippel, M.D., M.P.H.

DEFINITIONS

"Preventive medicine" is the practice of medicine that detects and alters or ameliorates host susceptibility in a premorbid state (e.g., immunization), risk factors for disease in a predisease state (e.g., increased cholesterol level), and disease in the presymptomatic state (e.g., in situ cervical cancer). Not all disease is preventable because not all risk factors (or all individuals at risk) are known, the cost of screening everyone is not feasible, barriers to medical access exist, interval disease occurs, characteristics of the target disease vary, and screening tests and treatments are imperfect.

"Primary prevention" is the prevention of disease occurrence (e.g., immunization to prevent infection and blood pressure control to prevent stroke). "Secondary prevention" is the detection and amelioration of disease in a presymptomatic or preclinical stage (e.g., mammography detects small foci of cancer and Pap smear detects in situ cancer). "Tertiary prevention" is the prevention of future negative health effects of existing clinical disease (e.g., use of aspirin and β-blockers after myocardial infarction to prevent recurrence).

"Efficacy" is the potential or maximal benefit derived from applying a test or procedure under ideal circumstances (e.g., research studies with compliant patients, with ideal testing conditions and techniques). "Effectiveness" is the actual benefit that is derived from a test or procedure that is applied under usual—less than ideal—circumstances. Randomized trials in which results are analyzed by the "intention-to-treat" principle (that is, all members of a group are included in the analysis whether they complied or not) give a measure of effectiveness in a population. "Cost-effectiveness" is the unit of cost incurred to achieve a given level of effectiveness. It is often expressed as the dollars spent per year of life saved. Often, the most cost-effective method of testing is not the most effective. For example, performing Pap smears every 5 or 10 years is more cost-effective, but performing them every year is more effective.

- Cost-effectiveness: cost incurred to achieve a given level of effectiveness.

- The most cost-effective test may not be the most effective test.

"Years of potential life lost" is one measure of the relative impact of a disease on society. This term usually refers to the years lost because of death from a disease before age 65 years (or sometimes 70). For example, colon cancer kills approximately 57,000 men and women annually and breast cancer kills approximately 40,000 women. However, on average, breast cancer kills at a younger age and so has nearly 3× as many years of potential life lost.

- Years of potential life lost: the years lost because of death from a disease before age 65 (or sometimes 70) years.

"Incidence (rate)" refers to the number of new events (deaths, diagnoses) that occur in a population in a given time (e.g., 170 cancer deaths per 100,000 people in the United States annually). "Prevalence" refers to the number of cases of a condition existing at a point in time in a population (e.g., currently, 800,000 to 900,000 people in the United States are infected with the human immunodeficiency virus [HIV]).

PRINCIPLES OF SCREENING FOR DISEASE

The term "mass screening" is generally applied to the relatively indiscriminate testing of a population with the intent to improve the aggregate health of the population but not necessarily of every person in the population. An example is blood pressure or cholesterol testing in a public setting such as a shopping mall.

- Mass screening: indiscriminate testing of a population to improve the aggregate health of the population.

"Case finding" is the technical term often used for screening conducted in the office setting. The intent is to detect asymptomatic disease and to improve the health of the person.

In testing asymptomatic persons, it is important to bear in mind the dictum "first do no harm."

- Case finding: screening conducted in the office setting to detect asymptomatic disease and to improve the health of a person.

Desirable Screening Characteristics

1. Disease characteristics: the diseases screened should be common, cause substantial morbidity and mortality, have a long preclinical phase (during which disease is curable or modifiable), have an effective treatment that is available to those screened, and have an acceptable treatment (i.e., one that is not excessively painful or disfiguring).

2. Test characteristics: the tests should be inexpensive, safe, acceptable, easy to administer, technically easy to perform, highly sensitive, and have a complementary, highly specific confirmatory test.

3. Host characteristics: the person should be at risk, have access to testing, be likely to comply with follow-up testing, and have adequate overall life expectancy or functional life expectancy.

Burden of United States Disease

Diseases that cause the most morbidity and mortality in the United States may or may not be amenable to screening or case finding. Heart disease and cancer are clearly the leading causes of death in the United States (Tables 19-1 and 19-2). The most recent year for which all actual statistics exist is 2000.

Table 19-1 Leading Causes of Death in the United States, 2000

	No. of deaths	Death rate (per 100,000 population)	% of total deaths
Heart disease	710,760	257.5	29.6
Cancer	553,091	199.6	23.0
Cerebrovascular disease	167,661	60.8	7.0
Chronic lower respiratory tract disease	122,009	44.2	5.1
Accidents (unintentional injuries)	97,900	34.9	4.1

From Jemal A, Murray T, Samuels A, et al: Cancer Statistics, 2003. CA Cancer J Clin 2003;53:5-26. By permission of Lippincott Williams & Wilkins.

Table 19-2 Cancer Mortality for Women and Men, 2000 (U.S. Vital Statistics)

Age, y					
40-59		60-79		80+	
Women					
Breast	11,937	Lung & bronchus	39,311	Lung & bronchus	14,693
Lung & bronchus	10,613	Breast	17,842	Colon & rectum	12,379
Colon & rectum	3,619	Colon & rectum	12,612	Breast	10,648
Ovary	3,033	Pancreas	7,825	Pancreas	5,319
Pancreas	1,871	Ovary	7,217	Non-Hodgkin lymphoma	4,039
Men					
Lung & bronchus	15,827	Lung & bronchus	57,470	Lung & bronchus	16,626
Colon & rectum	4,801	Colon & rectum	15,420	Prostate	15,630
Pancreas	2,929	Prostate	14,428	Colon & rectum	7,821
Esophagus	2,345	Pancreas	8,179	Urinary bladder	3,222
Liver	2,308	Non-Hodgkin lymphoma	6,107	Leukemia	3,187

Data from Jemal A, Murray T, Samuels A, et al: Cancer statistics, 2003. CA Cancer J Clin 2003;53:5-26.

Cancer Screening

Lung Cancer

Lung cancer is a highly lethal form of cancer (it kills most of the people it afflicts) and is the leading cause of cancer death for men and women. Burden of disease (2003 estimates from the American Cancer Society): 171,900 new cases and 157,200 deaths. The peak incidence occurs in 60- to 79-year-old men and women. Risk factors include 1) smoking—10× increased risk over nonsmoker; 2) age—70 years, 10× greater risk than for 40 years old; 3) sex—male-to-female ratio (lung cancer deaths) is 1.78:1 and is related primarily to duration and intensity of smoking; 4) environmental, industrial, and occupational carcinogen exposure—radon, asbestos, hydrocarbons, and uranium. Screening tests include chest radiography and sputum cytology. Screening probably is not effective. Although the Mayo Clinic Lung Project detected more cases of cancer, mortality was not altered in approximately 12 years of follow-up study. This may have been because of "overdiagnosis" of clinically irrelevant lesions or lead-time bias. Annual chest radiography (or sputum cytology) solely to look for treatable-stage lung cancer should not be performed.

Studies are under way to evaluate newer imaging modalities as well as cytologic and molecular evaluation of sputum for lung cancer screening. On the basis of these studies, low-dose radiation computed tomography (CT) of the chest appears to be better than chest radiography for detecting small lung cancers. Large population-based screening studies of chest CT have not been completed, so currently it is uncertain whether this technology will be effective in screening for lung cancer.

Smoking is the leading preventable cause of cancer in the United States and a leading cause of heart disease and stroke. Physician advice to quit smoking and referral to smoking cessation programs are the most cost-effective preventive measures available.

- Lung cancer: the leading cause of cancer death for men and women.
- Risk factors for lung cancer: smoking, age, sex (male > female), and environmental exposure.
- Annual chest radiography or sputum cytology solely to look for treatable stage lung cancer should not be performed.
- Smoking is the leading preventable cause of cancer in the United States.

Breast Cancer

Breast cancer is the second leading cause of cancer death for women. The lifetime risk is estimated at 1 in 8 women. Burden of disease (2003 estimates from the American Cancer Society): 212,600 new cases and 40,200 deaths. Thus, breast cancer is moderately lethal (it kills many but not most of the people it afflicts). The risk factors include 1) age—the risk increases throughout life, and the risk for an 80-year-old woman is 12× that for a 30-year-old woman; 2) family history—one first-degree relative with breast cancer, 2×-3× risk, and two first-degree relatives, 4×-6× risk; 3) socioeconomic status—high, increases risk 2×; 4) nulliparity or age at first full-term pregnancy older than 30 years, risk is increased 2×; 5) history of proliferative breast disease, history of breast cancer, and high-dose radiation exposure all increase risk approximately 2×.

- Breast cancer: the second leading cause of cancer death for women.
- Lifetime risk: 1 in 8 women.
- One first-degree relative with breast cancer, 2×-3× risk; two first-degree relatives, 4×-6× risk.

Screening procedures include the following:

1. Breast self-examination—No demonstrated effectiveness.
2. Clinical breast examination—Sensitivity of about 50% to 70% and specificity greater than 90%.
3. Mammography—Sensitivity of 75% to 95% for women 50 or older. Sensitivity is lower for women who are younger than 50, have dense breast tissue, or take hormone replacement therapy. The specificity is 95% to 99%. Positive predictive values (PPVs) are about 5% to 10%, with 20% to 50% of biopsy examinations finding cancer, depending on age (higher percentages in older women).
4. Randomized controlled trials worldwide have examined the effectiveness of mammography. They showed an approximate 30% decrease in mortality, but only two trials showed statistical significance. Data are conflicting or inconclusive in women younger than 50 or older than 70 years.

- Breast physical examination has a sensitivity of 50%-70% and a specificity >90%.
- Mammography has a sensitivity of 75%-95% and a specificity of 95%-99%.
- Studies are inconclusive about the benefit of mammography for women younger than 50 or older than 70.

Screening risks—Radiation is estimated to produce 80 additional radiation-induced breast cancer deaths among 1,000,000 women screened annually for 10 years, compared with over 90,000 breast cancers expected to be detected. The Breast Cancer Detection and Demonstration Project showed that 2% of women were referred for surgical evaluation or aspiration, and of the 50- to 65-year-old women referred for biopsy, half were found to have cancer. About 3% of women 40 to 49 years old were referred for biopsy, with a smaller percentage yielding cancer.

- Radiation: 80 additional cases of breast cancer among 1,000,000 women screened.
- Approximately 2% of screened women 50-65 years old will have biopsy, as will 3% of women 40-49 years old.

Cost-effectiveness—If 25% of women 40 to 75 years old in the United States were screened annually, 11,000,000 per year would be screened at a cost of $1.3 billion annually for physical examination and mammography. The cost of screening and the work-up would be 100× as expensive as the cost saved by reduced treatment. Cost per year of life saved ranges from about $9,000 to $12,000, with lower costs in the 50- to 69-year-old group and higher costs in both younger and older age groups.

- The cost of screening and work-up would be 100× as expensive as the cost saved by reduced treatment.
- The cost per year of life saved is $9,000-$12,000.

Recommendations:
1. General agreement—Clinical breast examination and mammography every 1 to 2 years for women 50 to 69 years old. Otherwise, recommendations vary.
2. American Cancer Society and several other groups—Screening with mammography and clinical breast examination beginning at age 40. Organizations differ in recommendations for screening interval.
3. United States Preventive Services Task Force (USPSTF)—Screening mammography alone or clinical breast examination and mammography every 1 to 2 years for women 40 and older.

Colorectal Cancer
Colorectal cancer is the second leading cause of cancer death in the United States. Burden of disease (2003 estimates from the American Cancer Society): 105,500 new cases of colorectal cancer and 57,100 deaths due to colorectal cancer. The lifetime risk of developing this cancer is approximately 5% to 6%. Less than 2% of these cancers occur in people younger than 40 and 90% occur in those older than 50. The risk of developing colorectal cancer is approximately 2× greater than the risk of dying of it (which reflects potential survivability of colorectal cancer and the age of the population involved, i.e., there are competing causes of mortality). Colorectal cancer is now the second cancer for which randomized controlled trial evidence has demonstrated decreased mortality because of screening.

- Colorectal cancer is the second leading cause of cancer death.
- Lifetime risk is 5%-6%.

- Of colorectal cancers, 90% occur in patients older than 50.

Natural history: Cancer may develop de novo in the colon, but most tumors probably develop from adenomatous polyps. The risk of a polyp becoming malignant appears to be related to time and size. Clinically significant polyps are ones larger than 7 mm. The average time from formation to malignant transformation for a polyp is 7 to 10 years. Ten-year survival for Dukes stage A or B cancer is 74%, 36% for Dukes stage C, and 5% for Dukes stage D.

- The risk of a polyp becoming malignant appears to be related to time and size.
- Clinically significant polyps: ones >7 mm.
- The time from polyp formation to malignant transformation is 7-10 years.

Risk factors: Age—risk doubles every 7 years over age 50. Family history—if a first-degree relative has disease, the risk increases 2×-3×. Previous adenomatous polyps increase risk 2×-4×. A history of endometrial, ovarian, or breast cancer increases risk 2×. Familial polyposis (Gardner syndrome)—the risk is approximately 100% by age 40. Ulcerative colitis—approximately a 50% risk with a 30-year history of disease. Cancer family syndrome (adenocarcinoma at various locations at an early age in multiple siblings)—approximately a 50% risk.

- Risk for colorectal cancer doubles every 7 years over age 50.
- If a first-degree relative has colorectal cancer, the risk increases 2×-4×.
- Previous adenomatous polyps, risk increases 2×-3×.
- History of endometrial, ovarian, or breast cancer, risk increases 2×.
- Familial polyposis (Gardner syndrome), risk is nearly 100% by age 40.
- Ulcerative colitis, about a 50% risk with a 30-year history of disease.

Tests: Fecal occult blood test (FOBT) is 26% to 92% sensitive and does not detect polyps well. Proctoscopy is more than 90% sensitive for the area of the colon visualized and could detect about 30% of cancers. Flexible sigmoidoscopy is also more than 90% sensitive for the area of the colon visualized and could detect about 60% of cancers. Barium enema and colonoscopy usually visualize the entire colon and are 85% to 95% sensitive.

- FOBT is 26%-92% sensitive.
- Proctoscopy and flexible sigmoidoscopy are >90% sensitive for the area of colon visualized.

- Barium enema and colonoscopy visualize the entire colon and are 85%-95% sensitive.

Recommendations: The available randomized controlled trial data show about a 30% decrease in mortality for persons older than 50 with annual FOBT. There is little consensus about how to screen for colorectal cancer. Mathematical modeling suggests that annual screening with barium enema or colonoscopy might reduce mortality by 85%, but the cost would be prohibitive.

For persons with average risk, the American Cancer Society recommends screening starting at age 50 with FOBT annually, flexible sigmoidoscopy every 5 years, or a combination of these tests. Alternative options include double-contrast barium enema every 5 years or colonoscopy every 10 years.

The USPSTF strongly recommends colorectal cancer screening for men and women 50 years and older. Screening options include FOBT, flexible sigmoidoscopy, colonoscopy, and double-contrast barium enema. There is insufficient evidence for determining the optimal screening strategy and interval. The guidelines also recommend that persons with a family history of hereditary syndromes associated with a high risk for colon cancer should be referred for diagnosis and management.

- FOBT screening annually decreases mortality by 30% for persons older than 50.
- Annual screening with barium enema or colonoscopy might reduce mortality by 85%, but the cost would be prohibitive.

Prostate Cancer

For the purposes of screening, prostate cancer is a troublesome disease, primarily because of the great difference between the "burden" of prevalent disease and the "burden" of clinical disease. The 2003 estimates from the American Cancer Society are 220,900 new cases of prostate cancer and 28,900 deaths. Pathology studies show that a small focus of prostate cancer can be found in 30% to 40% of 60-year-old men. Prostate cancer will be diagnosed in only 8% to 9% of the men, with many cases diagnosed incidentally at transurethral resection of the prostate. Currently, 80% of diagnoses are made in men older than 65. Relatively few men with prostate cancer die of the disease, only 3% to 4% of men in the United States.

- 8%-9% of U.S. males will have the diagnosis of prostate cancer in their lifetime.
- 3%-4% of U.S. males die of prostate cancer.
- 80% of the diagnoses are made in men older than 65 years.

Natural history: Prostate cancer is a hormonally induced cancer that is generally slow growing. In most host males, it does not alter the life span or lifestyle. Growth of a tiny nidus of cancerous cells into a clinically important cancer takes 10 to 15 years. In elderly hosts, this process is usually halted by intervening causes of mortality. Aggressiveness and morbidity are related to size, grade, and ploidy.

- Prostate cancer is a hormonally induced cancer.
- It does not alter the life span or lifestyle of most host males.
- Growth into a clinically important cancer takes 10-15 years.

Risk factors: Age—the risk increases exponentially after age 50. Race—in the United States, African-American men have 2× the risk of whites, and whites have 2× the risk of Asians. Family history—a first-degree relative increases the risk 3×, a brother with cancer before age 63 increases the risk 4×, and a sister with breast cancer increases the risk 2×.

- For prostate cancer in the United States, African-American men have twice the risk of whites, who have twice the risk of Asians.

Tests: A digital rectal examination has a PPV of 6% to 33%. Transrectal ultrasonography has a PPV of about 10% to 20% (values vary depending on population and previous screening). The prostate-specific antigen (PSA) test has a PPV of 10% to 35% (values vary depending on population and prior screening). Because there is much undetected disease, PPV values do not have the usual meaning.

Recommendations: No good data are available from randomized controlled trials on the effect of early detection and treatment on survival. There is little agreement on recommendations for screening. Aggressive screening for prostate cancer will uncover many new cases (causing a surge in incidence) and result in many additional treatments. However, because of the natural history of the disease, screening may have minimal effect in decreasing mortality, the desired benefit. The American Cancer Society recommends that a digital rectal examination and the PSA test be offered annually to men older than 50 who have a life expectancy of at least 10 years. The USPSTF guidelines conclude that there is insufficient evidence to recommend for or against routine screening with a digital rectal examination or PSA test for prostate cancer.

- There is little agreement on recommendations for prostate cancer screening.

Some authorities have recommended *against* any form of screening—rectal examination, ultrasonography, or PSA—primarily because of concern that the effect on survival will be minimal and that the costs in detection and follow-up treatment and in deaths due to treatment (perioperative deaths) will be substantial. There is a risk that the harm outweighs the good from detection of early-stage disease. Screening, if performed, should be done in men likely to have a 10-year survival.

Cervical Cancer

The 2003 estimates from the American Cancer Society are 12,200 new cases of cervical cancer and 4,100 deaths. Cervical cancer has a bimodal risk curve divided between in situ carcinoma and invasive carcinoma. This cancer has a long preclinical phase, and progression from dysplasia to invasive cancer may take 10 to 15 years or more. A strong association exists between human papillomavirus (HPV) infection (types 16, 18, and others) and cervical cancer. Cervical cancer is largely a sexually transmitted disease.

- Cervical cancer: bimodal risk curve divided between in situ carcinoma and invasive carcinoma.
- It has a long preclinical phase.
- Cervical cancer is strongly associated with human papillomavirus infection.

Risk factors: 1) Age—the risk of invasive carcinoma increases throughout life; 2) sexual activity—early age at onset; 3) multiple sexual partners; 4) a history of sexually transmitted disease, especially HIV infection; and 5) smoking.

- Cervical cancer risk factors: early age at onset of sexual activity, multiple sexual partners, a history of sexually transmitted disease, and smoking.

Test: The Pap smear has a sensitivity of 55% to 80% and a specificity of 90% to 99%. Experienced cytologists and pathologists as well as clinician sampling technique are important to test effectiveness. The USPSTF has concluded that the evidence is insufficient to recommend for or against routine use of new technology (liquid-based cytology, computerized rescreening, and algorithm-based screening) to screen for cervical cancer. No current guidelines recommend using HPV testing for cervical cancer screening.

- Pap smear: 55%-80% sensitivity and 90%-99% specificity.

Screening effectiveness: No randomized controlled trial of screening has been conducted in a general population. However, evidence from case-control studies and observational studies suggests effectiveness. Estimated overall effect of Pap smear: every 10 years, 64% reduction in invasive cancer; every 5 years, 84% reduction; every 3 years, 91% reduction; every 2 years, 92.5% reduction; and every year, 93.5% reduction.

Recommendations: There is general agreement on screening starting at the onset of sexual activity and every 1 to 3 years thereafter, depending on risk. The USPSTF guidelines recommend routine screening for all women who have been sexually active and who have a cervix. Screening should begin with the onset of sexual activity and should be repeated at least every 3 years. The American Cancer Society recommends that cervical cancer screening start 3 years after onset of sexual activity, but no later than age 21. Also, it recommends annual screening with a conventional Pap test, or every 2 years if liquid-based cytology is used, until age 30. The recommendation permits less frequent testing after age 30 (every 2-3 years) based on past screening results and risk factors. The recommendation suggests offering women the option to discontinue screening after age 65 to 70 if there is evidence of adequate past screening.

- General recommendation: screen at the onset of sexual activity and every 1-3 years thereafter, depending on risk.

Ovarian Cancer

Ovarian cancer is the fifth leading cause of cancer death in women. Burden of disease (2003 estimates from the American Cancer Society): 25,400 new cases of ovarian cancer and 14,300 deaths. Ovarian cancer is the leading cause of gynecologic cancer death. Age-adjusted death rates have been increasing slowly in the last 25 years.

- Ovarian cancer is the fifth leading cause of cancer death in women.
- Age-adjusted death rates have been increasing slowly.

Risk factors: Lower risk—history of at least one term pregnancy has a relative risk of 0.6 to 0.8. The use of oral contraceptives for 3 to 6 months has a relative risk of 0.6; if used more than 10 years, the relative risk is 0.2. Higher risk—family history as a risk is not well quantified, but it is an important factor if a first-degree relative had disease (only 1%-5% of ovarian cancers are familial). High fat diet and long duration of ovulatory years (i.e., early menarche or late menopause) are possible risk factors.

- 1%-5% of ovarian cancers are familial.

Screening tests: Bimanual examination is insensitive. Ultrasonography, transvaginal or transabdominal, is more sensitive than bimanual examination but has a poor PPV. CA 125 (blood test) is more sensitive than bimanual examination but also has a poor PPV. Ultrasonography and CA 125 have a significant false-positive rate. It is estimated that 10 to 60 abdominal operations would have to be performed for every one cancer detected, at a cost of more than $13 billion annually to screen the 43 million women older than 45. An adequate study of efficacy, even with a highly sensitive and specific test, would require tens of thousands of participants.

- For ovarian cancer, bimanual examination is insensitive.
- Ultrasonography and CA 125 are more sensitive than bimanual examination, but both have a poor PPV.
- For every one ovarian cancer detected, 10-60 abdominal operations would have to be performed.

Recommendations: USPSTF guidelines recommend against screening for ovarian cancer. The American Cancer Society recommends regular pelvic examination, including adnexal palpation, as part of cervical cancer screening.

A 1994 National Institutes of Health (NIH) Consensus Conference recommended that women with presumed hereditary cancer syndrome should have a pelvic examination, CA 125 test, and transvaginal ultrasonography annually until childbearing is completed or at age 35, at which time prophylactic bilateral oophorectomy is recommended.

Tuberculosis Prevention

Burden of disease: In 1997, the worldwide prevalence of tuberculosis (TB) infection (latent or active) was estimated to be 1.86 billion cases, with an annual incidence rate of about 8 million. Approximately 2,000,000 people worldwide die annually of TB. The U.S. incidence is approximately 15,000 cases per year, with fewer than 1,000 deaths per year. The incidence decreased from 1953 to 1985, and then TB made a resurgence because of immigration from endemic areas, HIV infection, and increased use of immunosuppressive drugs. Since 1993, the incidence has consistently decreased.

- TB: the U.S. incidence is approximately 15,000 cases and fewer than 1,000 deaths annually.

Natural history: Infection occurs through inhalation of *Mycobacterium tuberculosis*-bearing droplets. After being infected, healthy persons are usually asymptomatic. However, it is believed that the tubercle bacillus remains viable in granulomata for many years. The risk of reactivation after asymptomatic infection (purified protein derivative [PPD] conversion) is 5% for the first 1 or 2 years after infection. Another 5% will develop disease sometime later in life.

- The tubercle bacillus remains viable in granulomata for many years.
- The risk of reactivation (after PPD conversion) is 5% for the first 1-2 years after infection.
- Another 5% develop disease later in life.

Persons at higher risk for TB infection include those with close contact with a person with active TB, foreign-born persons from areas of high prevalence, residents and employees of high-risk congregate settings (e.g., nursing homes and prisons), health care workers, medically underserved low-income populations, high-risk racial or ethnic minority populations, and persons who inject illicit drugs.

Persons at higher risk for developing active TB after infection include HIV-infected persons (7%-10% risk each year), persons recently infected with TB (5% risk for first 1 or 2 years after infection), persons with certain medical conditions (e.g., diabetes mellitus and end-stage renal disease), persons who inject illicit drugs, and persons with a history of inadequately treated TB.

- Persons infected with both *M. tuberculosis* and HIV have a 7%-10% risk of developing active TB each year.

Test: The PPD (Mantoux) skin test—5-tuberculin-unit intradermal skin test. Measure the area of induration (not erythema) at 48 to 72 hours. Targeted skin testing is recommended for high-risk groups. In low-risk persons, consider the reaction positive if it is larger than 15 mm. A 10-mm reaction is considered positive for the following groups: recent arrivals from countries of high prevalence, persons who inject illicit drugs, residents and employees of high-risk congregate settings, mycobacteriology laboratory personnel, and persons with medical conditions that increase the risk for TB.

A 5-mm reaction is considered positive for HIV-positive persons, recent contacts of a person with active TB, persons with fibrotic changes on chest radiographs consistent with old healed TB, and immunosuppressed patients.

Persons exposed in the past may be relatively anergic, but the response can be boosted by repeating the test (two-step PPD testing procedure). Previous bacille Calmette-Guérin (BCG) vaccination may produce skin reactivity, but positive reactors should be considered to have true infection and be given appropriate follow-up care. Recent measles-mumps-rubella (MMR) and oral polio vaccine (OPV) vaccination (within 6 weeks) may diminish skin reactivity, and testing should be avoided during this interval. Chest radiography and sputum are not useful screening tests for conversion but may detect active disease in high-risk persons.

- Chest radiography and sputum are not useful screening tests for TB.

All persons with a positive PPD test should have chest radiography and clinical evaluation for active TB.

Preventive measures: Primary prevention is with BCG vaccine, an attenuated species of *Mycobacterium bovis*. It may be up to 80% effective when used properly. It is appropriate in high-risk areas because it is inexpensive, requires a single dose, and has a low risk (only 100 fatalities in 2 billion administrations). BCG vaccine is not indicated in areas of low prevalence because it confuses interpretation of the PPD response. Currently, BCG vaccination is not recommended for any adult in the United States. Another primary preventive measure is environmental controls, especially in a health care environment, with respiratory isolation, high-efficiency filter masks, and special venting of rooms and wards with TB cases.

● BCG vaccine may be 80% effective when used properly.
● Its use is not indicated in low-prevalence areas.

Secondary prevention is with isoniazid (INH) treatment. Its use is indicated for recent converters (<2 years), contacts of infected persons with a 5-mm or more PPD, history of TB with inadequate treatment, positive skin test with abnormal but stable chest radiographic findings, and positive PPD (of any duration). The dosage is 5 to 10 mg/kg daily, up to a maximum of 300 mg daily (the usual adult dose) given as a single oral dose. Treatment should continue for 9 months. Primary side effects are liver toxicity and peripheral neuropathy. Peak toxicity is in persons older than 50 years (2%-3%). Monitoring for side effects is generally through symptoms only. Baseline laboratory testing and periodic monitoring of liver transaminase (aspartate aminotransferase [AST] or alanine aminotransferase [ALT]) levels is not routinely recommended. Testing should be considered for pregnant or postpartum women, persons with liver disease or other chronic medical condition, and those taking other medications.

Alternative treatment regimens for latent TB infection include rifampin and pyrazinamide daily for 2 months or rifampin alone for 4 months.

● Isoniazid: 5-10 mg/kg daily up to a maximum of 300 mg daily.
● Treatment should continue for 9 months.
● Peak toxicity is in persons older than 50 (2%-3%).

IMMUNIZATIONS

One of the greatest successes of modern medicine for preventing disease and extending life has been immunization. Adults have continuing immunization needs throughout life. Physicians who administer vaccines are required by law to keep permanent vaccine records (National Childhood Vaccine Act of 1986) and to report adverse events through the Vaccine Adverse Event Reporting System (VAERS). Service in the U.S. military may be considered verification of vaccination for measles, rubella, tetanus, diphtheria, and polio. Providers are now required to give patients "vaccine information pamphlets" before vaccination as a mechanism for informed consent.

Immunity may be of two types. Passive immunity—preformed antibodies are provided in large quantities to prevent or to diminish the impact of infection or associated toxins (e.g., tetanus immune globulin [TIG] and hepatitis B immune globulin [HBIG]). Passive immunity lasts for several months only. Active immunity—an antigen is presented to the host immune system that in turn develops antibodies (e.g., hepatitis or tetanus) or specific immune cells (e.g., BCG). Active immunity generally lasts from years to a lifetime. Active immunity may be induced by live virus vaccines (e.g., measles), killed virus vaccines (e.g., influenza), or refined antigen vaccines (e.g., pneumococcal).

Live virus vaccines are contraindicated in some persons. In general, pregnant women, people with immunodeficiency diseases, leukemia, lymphoma, generalized malignancy, or those who are immune-suppressed because of therapy with corticosteroids, alkylating drugs, antimetabolites, or radiation should *not* be given live virus vaccines. HIV-infected persons who are immunocompetent and leukemia patients who have been in remission for 3 or more months after chemotherapy generally may be vaccinated with *some* live virus vaccines. Live virus vaccines include measles, mumps, rubella, smallpox, varicella, yellow fever, and OPV.

Inactivated virus vaccines include enhanced inactivated polio (eIPV), hepatitis A, hepatitis B, influenza, and rabies. Inactivated bacterial vaccines include cholera, typhoid, meningococcal, plague, and pneumococcal.

An adult immunization schedule has been developed and endorsed by several groups (Fig. 19-1).

Specific Vaccines and Chemoprophylaxis

Diphtheria
Diphtheria is a rare disease primarily because of vaccination. However, up to 40% of adults lack protective antibody levels. Recommendation: vaccination in combination with tetanus toxoid (see below, Tetanus), as Td. The diphtheria-tetanus-pertussis (DTP) preparation recommended for children should not be used for adults.

Tetanus
Approximately 50 cases of tetanus are reported each year. Most cases occur in adults who are either unvaccinated or inadequately vaccinated. Vaccination is nearly 100% effective. Recommendation: The primary series, a three-dose series, should be completed before adulthood, usually in early childhood. The primary series consists of Td (DTP in childhood). The last childhood dose is usually a booster at age 15. For adults who have had a primary series, vaccinate every 10 years (e.g., mid-decade is easy to remember; if last childhood dose

Age group (y)

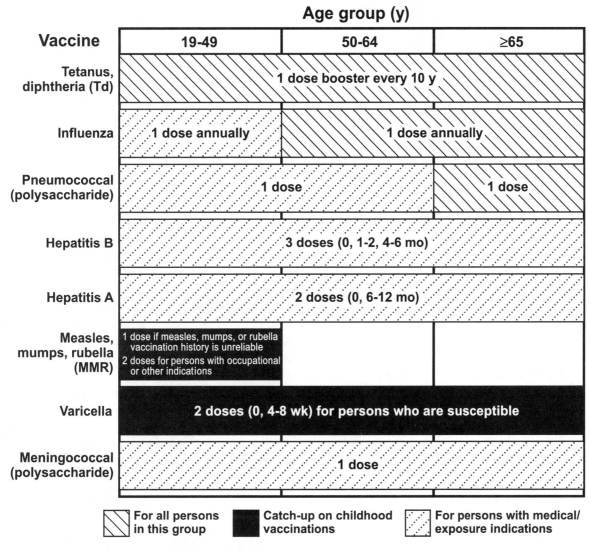

Vaccine	19-49	50-64	≥65
Tetanus, diphtheria (Td)	1 dose booster every 10 y		
Influenza	1 dose annually	1 dose annually	
Pneumococcal (polysaccharide)	1 dose		1 dose
Hepatitis B	3 doses (0, 1-2, 4-6 mo)		
Hepatitis A	2 doses (0, 6-12 mo)		
Measles, mumps, rubella (MMR)	1 dose if measles, mumps, or rubella vaccination history is unreliable / 2 doses for persons with occupational or other indications		
Varicella	2 doses (0, 4-8 wk) for persons who are susceptible		
Meningococcal (polysaccharide)	1 dose		

Legend:
- For all persons in this group
- Catch-up on childhood vaccinations
- For persons with medical/exposure indications

Fig. 19-1. Recommended adult immunization schedule, United States, 2003-2004, by age group. (From The Advisory Committee on Immunization Practices. Summary of Recommendations. Atlanta, Center for Disease Control and Prevention.)

was at 15, vaccinate at ages 25, 35, 45, etc.). Clean, minor wounds received in the 10-year interval require no further vaccination. However, for a contaminated wound, the patient should get a Td booster if it has been more than 5 years since the last booster. If immune status is unknown or lacking (specifically, no primary series), both toxoid (Td) and TIG (250 U intramuscularly) should be given. Td is the preferred toxoid in an emergency setting as well as for routine vaccination. Td and TIG when given in the emergency setting should be given in separate syringes at separate locations, but they may be given at the same time.

- Tetanus vaccination: the primary series is a three-dose series.
- Adults who have had a primary series should receive a booster every 10 years.

- For a contaminated wound, the patient should get a booster if it has been more than 5 years since the last booster.

Side effects: Td may be given in pregnancy, although it is desirable to wait until the second trimester. Maternal antibodies are passed to the infant transplacentally and confer passive immunity for several months after birth.

- Maternal antibodies are passed to the infant transplacentally.

A history of neurologic reaction, urticaria, anaphylaxis, or other severe hypersensitivity reaction is a contraindication to the readministration of toxoids. Skin testing may be performed if necessary. In the emergency setting, TIG may be used when T or Td is contraindicated if other than a clean minor wound is sustained. Arthus-type hypersensitivity, a severe local reaction starting 2 to 8 hours after injection, often with fever and malaise, may occur in persons who have received multiple boosters. These people have very high levels of antitoxin and do not need boosters, even in the emergency setting, more frequently than every 10 years.

Measles

Vaccination reduced the number of cases of measles from 500,000 yearly (with 500 deaths) to 3,500 yearly in the mid-1980s. A disease resurgence occurred in 1989-1991, with a peak incidence of more than 27,000 cases in 1990. Since 1993, fewer than 500 cases have been reported in most years. Measles is no longer considered to be endemic in the United States. All cases appear to be the result of importation, with limited spread among U.S. residents. The risk of encephalitis with measles infection in an adult is approximately 1 in 1,000. Infection during pregnancy may result in spontaneous abortion or premature labor and low birth weight. Malformation does not appear to be as much of a problem as with rubella.

● The risk of encephalitis with measles infection in an adult is approximately 1 in 1,000.

Target: Adults born after 1956 who have no medical contraindication and who have no dated documentation of at least one dose of live measles vaccine on or after their first birthday, physician-documented disease, or documented immune titer should receive vaccination. Persons with expected exposure to measles should consider revaccination or titer measurement because up to 10% of persons born before 1957 may not be immune. Persons at risk include travelers to endemic areas, those in school settings, and health care workers. They should have two doses of measles vaccine documented on or after their first birthday. MMR is the preferred vaccine. If they have never been vaccinated, they should receive two doses given at least 1 month apart.

Exposure precautions: If an exposed person is unvaccinated, vaccinate within 72 hours if possible or give immune globulin (up to 6 days after exposure) if the person is not a vaccine candidate (0.25-0.5 mL/kg body weight, up to 15 mL—the dose depends on immunocompetence). Health care workers should remain away from work for 5 to 21 days after exposure if they are not immune.

Side effects include fever with a temperature higher than 103°F (usually occurs on day 5 to 12) in 5% to 15% of those vaccinated and a rash in 5%. Encephalitis is rare (1 case per 1 million immunizations). No apparent increase in side effects occurs with a second vaccination. Contraindications are immune globulin or blood products given within the previous 3 months, pregnancy, egg or neomycin allergy, and others as noted above for live virus vaccines.

Mumps

A highly effective vaccination program has decreased the number of cases of mumps from approximately 200,000 yearly to less than 1,000 yearly during the 1990s. Vaccine side effects of fever, rash, pruritus, and purpura are uncommon, and central nervous system problems and parotitis are rare. There is no increased risk with revaccination. The contraindications are the same as for measles.

Rubella

Infection with rubella in the first trimester results in congenital rubella syndrome in up to 85% of infected fetuses. The goal of vaccination is to prevent the occurrence of this disease. Vaccination is highly effective, and there is no evidence of transmission of vaccine virus to close household contacts. The target population includes all women of childbearing age, all health care workers, and travelers to endemic areas. The side effects include arthralgias in 25% and transient arthritis in 10%, usually 1 to 3 weeks after vaccination. Vaccination rarely causes chronic joint problems, certainly much less frequently than natural infection. Contraindications are immune globulin given within the previous 3 months (but not blood products, e.g., Rho(D) immune globulin [RhoGAM]), pregnant women or women likely to become pregnant within 3 months (although there are no documented cases of congenital rubella syndrome in vaccinated pregnant women), and allergy to neomycin but not to egg (as prepared in a diploid cell culture).

Influenza

During the 20th century, influenza pandemics occurred in 1918, 1957, and 1968, and each one resulted in a large number of deaths worldwide. Epidemics of influenza occur in the United States almost annually and are caused primarily by influenza A viruses and occasionally by influenza B viruses or both. Incidence peaks occur in mid to late winter, earlier in recent years. Influenza A is classified by two surface antigens: hemagglutinin (subtypes H1, H2, H3) and neuraminidase (subtypes N1, N2). Because of differing subtypes and antigenic drift, infection or vaccination more than 1 year previously may not give protection the following year. Influenza B is antigenically more stable but still has moderate drift. Control of both influenza A and B is with vaccination or chemoprophylaxis or both.

The vaccine is an inactivated (killed) virus vaccine (virus grown in egg culture). Each year it contains three viruses: two A-type viruses and one B-type virus. Vaccines may contain whole virus or split virus (subvirion). Split-virus vaccines are used in children to decrease febrile reaction. All forms may be used in adults. Ideally, vaccination should be given in October and November.

The side effects include local soreness; fever, malaise, myalgia (occur 6-12 hours after vaccination and may last 1-2 days); and anaphylactic reaction (probably due to egg protein). The target populations include persons 65 and older, especially those who reside in a nursing home or chronic care facility; persons with chronic pulmonary or cardiovascular disease, including asthma, chronic metabolic disease such as diabetes mellitus, renal dysfunction, or immunosuppression; health care workers; and women in the second or third trimester of pregnancy during influenza season (November-March). Consideration may be given to persons in vital roles, to those in institutional settings, and to travelers. Contraindications are the first trimester of pregnancy, except for those at high risk because of underlying disease, and egg allergy.

Chemoprophylaxis for type A influenza has been available for many years, with either amantadine hydrochloride or rimantadine hydrochloride. These drugs interfere with the replication cycle of influenza A. In healthy populations, they are 70% to 90% effective if given daily throughout an epidemic. For treatment of disease, they decrease fever and other symptoms if given within 48 hours of disease onset. These agents are used to control influenza outbreaks, usually in institutions, and are given to all unvaccinated workers and residents. They may be given regardless of vaccination status to persons at high risk. Workers should continue taking the medication until 2 weeks after vaccination or indefinitely during the period of risk if the vaccine is contraindicated. Drug dosage (100-200 mg daily) varies with age.

- Amantadine and rimantadine are used for influenza A only.
- They are 70%-90% effective.
- They are used to control influenza outbreaks, usually in institutions, and are given to all unvaccinated workers and residents.

The side effects are usually minor, occurring in 5% to 10% of recipients, and may abate with continued use. Rimantadine has less frequent central nervous system side effects than amantadine. Central nervous system side effects are nervousness, anxiety, insomnia, and decreased concentration, and those of the gastrointestinal system include anorexia and nausea. Serious side effects are seizure and confusion, usually seen in the elderly or in those with kidney or liver disease. In these groups, the dose should be decreased in accordance with the recommendations made in the package inserts.

Chemoprophylaxis using the neuramidase inhibitor oseltamivir has been shown to be effective in preventing both influenza A and B. When given in a dosage of 75 mg daily for up to 6 weeks during an influenza outbreak, the medication has a protective efficacy of 74%. The most common side effects of oseltamivir are nausea and vomiting.

Hepatitis A

In the United States, the rate of hepatitis A infection tends to vary from year to year. In 2001, the infection rate was 4 per 100,000 population. More than 70% of infected older children and adults develop clinical disease. Also, more than 10,000 infected persons are hospitalized yearly, and approximately 80 deaths are due to fulminant hepatitis. Signs and symptoms usually last less than 2 months. However, 10% to 15% of patients have prolonged or relapsing illness, which may last up to 6 months.

Spread of hepatitis A virus (HAV) occurs by the fecal-oral route, most commonly within households. Common-source outbreaks due to contaminated food and water supplies have occurred. Blood-borne transmission is uncommon but can occur through blood transfusion and contaminated blood products and from needles shared with an infected viremic person. Sexual transmission has also been reported.

Hepatitis A vaccination provides an opportunity to lower disease incidence and ultimately to eradicate infection because humans are the only natural reservoir of the virus. A single dose of hepatitis A vaccine induces a protective antibody level within 4 weeks after vaccination. A second dose of vaccine 6 to 12 months later induces long-lasting immunity. Target groups for immunization include persons traveling to or working in countries that have high or intermediate HAV endemicity; homosexual males; illicit drug users; persons who have an occupational risk for infection (those who work with HAV-infected primates or with HAV in a research laboratory), chronic liver disease, or clotting-factor disorders; and some food handlers. Hepatitis A vaccination of children has been used effectively to control outbreaks in communities that have high rates of hepatitis A.

Travelers who are allergic to a vaccine component or who elect not to receive vaccine should be encouraged to get immune globulin (0.02-0.06 mL/kg provides protection for 3-5 months). Immune globulin should also be given to travelers leaving on short notice, and it can be given concomitantly with vaccine, using separate sites and syringes.

Prevaccination serologic testing may be cost-effective for adults who were born or lived for extended periods in areas of high HAV endemicity and homosexual males. Postvaccination testing is not necessary because of the high rate of vaccine response.

Hepatitis B

The lifetime risk of acquiring hepatitis B is 5% for the general population; 150,000 cases occur annually in the United States, resulting in 8,000 hospitalizations and 200 deaths. Of the patients affected, 90% are 20 or older; 5% to 10% become carriers, and one-fourth of these develop chronic active hepatitis. Annually, 4,000 persons die of hepatitis B virus-related cirrhosis and 1,500 die of hepatitis B virus-related liver cancer.

- The lifetime risk of acquiring hepatitis B is 5% for the general population.

- 5%-10% become carriers.
- Annually, 4,000 persons die of hepatitis B virus-related cirrhosis and 1,500 die of hepatitis B virus-related liver cancer.

The current vaccine is yeast recombinant, developed from the insertion of a plasmid into *Saccharomyces cerevisiae*, which produces the copies of the surface antigen. Human-plasma–derived vaccine is no longer made. The target population includes adults at increased risk, that is, homosexual males, intravenous drug users, heterosexual persons with multiple sexual partners, and those with a history of other sexually transmitted diseases; household and sexual contacts of hepatitis B virus carriers; workers in health-related and public safety occupations involving exposure to blood or body fluids; hemodialysis patients; recipients of concentrates of clotting factors VIII and IX; morticians and their assistants; and travelers who will be living for extended periods in high-prevalence areas or who are likely to have sexual contacts or contact with blood in the endemic areas (especially in eastern Asia and sub-Saharan Africa).

Vaccination—Normally, vaccination consists of three doses at 0, 1 month, and 6 months. An alternative dosing schedule to induce immunity more rapidly, for example, after exposure, involves 4 doses, the first three given 1 month apart and a fourth dose at 12 months. Postexposure prophylaxis consists of HBIG given in a single dose of 0.06 mL/kg or 5 mL for adults. It should be administered along with the vaccine in separate syringes at separate sites, but they may be administered at the same time. Current evidence suggests that for most vaccinees the vaccination has a duration of 7 or more years. Currently, revaccination is not routinely recommended. For persons who received the vaccine in the buttock or whose management depends on knowledge of immune status (e.g., surgeons or venipuncturists), periodic serologic testing may be valuable. Those with antibody to hepatitis B surface antigen (anti-HBsAg) titers less than 10 mIU/mL should be revaccinated. Revaccination with a single dose is usually effective.

- Currently, revaccination for hepatitis B is not routinely recommended.

The most common side effect of hepatitis B vaccination is localized soreness. Guillain-Barré syndrome (0.5 per 100,000) has been associated with human-plasma–derived hepatitis B vaccine. Comparable information is not available for the recombinant vaccines. Vaccination during pregnancy is considered advisable for women who are at risk for hepatitis B infection. The risk of hepatitis B virus infection in pregnancy far outweighs the risk of vaccine-associated problems.

- Guillain-Barré syndrome (0.5 per 100,000) has been associated with human-plasma–derived hepatitis B vaccine.

Pneumococcal Disease

Pneumococcal pneumonia is an important cause of death of older persons. The overall case fatality rate is 5% to 10%, but it is higher (20%-40%) among persons with underlying disease or alcoholism. The risk of bacteremia for persons 65 years or older with *Streptococcus pneumoniae* infection is 50 per 100,000. Two-thirds of persons with serious pneumococcal disease have been hospitalized in the previous 5 years, which represents a missed opportunity for vaccination.

The current adult vaccine contains purified capsular polysaccharide of 23 pneumococcal serotypes that cause approximately 90% of bacteremic pneumococcal infections in the United States. Following a single dose of vaccine, the titers persist for 5 or more years in healthy adults. Side effects of vaccination include localized erythema and pain, which occur in about 50% of all vaccinees. Other side effects, which occur in less than 1% of persons vaccinated, include fever, myalgia, and severe local reactions. A total of 5 per 1,000,000 of those vaccinated develop anaphylaxis. Revaccination within approximately 1 year is associated with increased local reactions. The target population for vaccination includes persons 65 or older, adults with chronic cardiovascular or pulmonary disease, diabetics, and persons at higher risk for pneumococcal infection because of, for example, alcoholism or cerebrospinal fluid leak. The target population also includes immunocompromised persons (e.g., those who are asplenic) and patients with Hodgkin disease, lymphoma, multiple myeloma, chronic renal failure, nephrotic syndrome, HIV infection, or organ transplant.

It is not necessary to revaccinate persons who received the original 14-valent pneumococcal vaccine. However, persons at highest risk for pneumococcal infections, especially immunocompromised persons, should be revaccinated with the 23-valent vaccine. Revaccination once after 5 years should be considered for adults with conditions associated with rapid antibody decline after initial immunization, especially those with nephrotic syndrome, renal failure, and renal transplantation. Anyone 65 or older should be given a second dose of vaccine if they received an original dose more than 5 years previously and were younger than 65 at the time of primary immunization.

- The target population is persons ≥65 years old or adults with chronic disease.

Smallpox (Vaccinia)

The World Health Organization declared the world free of smallpox in May 1980. Smallpox vaccination subsequently was given only to laboratory personnel working directly with orthopoxviruses. During 2002 preparations began for use of smallpox vaccine for bioterrorism preparedness. Vaccination of health care workers started in 2003. The Advisory Committee on Immunization Practices of the Centers for Disease Control and Prevention has released detailed recommendations for preexposure vaccination and for use of smallpox vaccine in the event of a smallpox emergency. The live virus smallpox vaccine is highly effective in inducing immunity that lasts for up to 5 years after primary vaccination. Additional doses may confer long-term immunity, possibly for a decade or more. Side effects include fever, skin rash, eczema vaccinatum, generalized vaccinia, and postvaccinal encephalitis. Inadvertent inoculation at other sites may occur. Transmission of vaccine virus to close contacts has been documented. Contraindications include pregnancy, history or presence of eczema, HIV infection, altered immunocompetence, and known allergy to vaccine component. Vaccinia immune globulin can be given to persons with complications of vaccination.

Polio

Polio has now been eradicated from the entire Western Hemisphere. The few cases that occur in the Western Hemisphere are due to the oral vaccine virus strain. There are OPV (live virus) and eIPV (killed virus) vaccines. A primary series with either one has more than 95% effectiveness. Polio vaccination is not recommended for persons older than 18 unless they plan to travel to an endemic area and have no history of a previous primary series. For these persons, eIPV is recommended because of the lower risk of paralysis. The primary series consists of three doses of eIPV given at 0, 1, and 6 to 12 months. If it is less than 4 weeks before travel, give a single dose of eIPV. If the primary series is incomplete, complete it despite the interval since the last dose. If the person previously received OPV, give one dose of eIPV. For OPV, the risk of paralysis is approximately 1 in 1,000,000 after the first dose, and for susceptible household contacts, it is approximately 1 in 2,000,000.

- Polio vaccination is not recommended for persons older than 18 unless they plan to travel to an endemic area.

Rabies

Preexposure prophylactic vaccination is recommended for animal handlers, laboratory workers, persons traveling to hyperendemic areas for more than 1 month, or those with vocations or avocations with exposure to skunks, raccoons, and bats, as well as other animals. In the United States, the reservoir of infection includes carnivorous animals, particularly skunks, raccoons, foxes, and bats. Except for woodchucks, rodents are rarely infected. Preexposure vaccination consists of 3 doses of rabies vaccine given on days 0, 7, and 21 or 28.

Ideally, preexposure vaccination should be completed at least 1 month before travel or potential exposure.

Following a potential or known rabies exposure (e.g., animal bite or bat contact), a person who has had preexposure vaccination needs only two doses of rabies vaccine: one immediately and another 3 days later. Appropriate postexposure treatment for unimmunized persons includes administration of rabies immune globulin (part of it infiltrated in and around the bite and the rest given intramuscularly) and five doses of rabies vaccine. The first dose of vaccine should be given as soon as possible after exposure and additional doses on days 3, 7, 14, and 28 to 35 after the first dose.

Varicella

Primary infection with varicella zoster virus (VZV) results in chickenpox, and recurrent infection produces herpes zoster or shingles. Factors associated with recurrent disease include aging, immunosuppression, and intrauterine exposure to VZV and varicella at a young age (<18 months).

Complications of VZV infection, which occur more commonly in older children and adults, include bacterial infection of lesions, viral or secondary bacterial pneumonia, central nervous system manifestations (aseptic meningitis and encephalitis), hospitalization, and death.

Varicella vaccination is recommended for all children between 12 and 18 months old. It is also recommended for nonimmune adolescents and adults who are at highest risk for exposure and those most likely to transmit varicella to others. These groups include health care workers, family members of immunocompromised persons, teachers of young children, women of childbearing age, military personnel, persons working in institutional settings, and international travelers.

Persons older than 13 should receive two doses of varicella vaccine separated by 4 to 8 weeks. Vaccine contraindications include severe allergy to neomycin, moderate or severe illness, immunosuppression, pregnancy, and recent receipt of a blood product. Adverse events following vaccination include injection site lesions, swelling, or pain; generalized varicella-like rash; and systemic reaction with fever. There is a risk of transmission of vaccine virus from a vaccinated person, especially with vaccine-associated rash, to a susceptible contact. However, this potential risk is low, and the benefits of vaccinating susceptible health care workers are thought to outweigh this risk.

Prevaccination serologic testing of adolescents and adults is probably cost-effective. Postvaccination testing is not necessary because of the high rate of seropositivity after two doses of vaccine (>99%).

QUESTIONS

Multiple Choice (choose the one best answer)

1. A 42-year-old woman presents in November for a pre-employment medical evaluation. She will start working as a venipuncture technician. She is currently 5 months pregnant and in very good health. She was born and raised in the United States and has never traveled outside the United States. She believes that she received all recommended childhood vaccinations but has no documentation of vaccination dates. She is certain that she has not received any vaccinations for many years, probably since high school, when she thinks she had a tetanus booster. A serologic test for hepatitis B is negative. She cannot recall having had chickenpox during childhood. You recommend all the following *except*:
   a. Tetanus diphtheria booster (Td)
   b. Influenza vaccination
   c. First dose of hepatitis B vaccine
   d. MMR vaccination
   e. Varicella serology

2. A 60-year-old Somali man comes to your office for a refugee health assessment. A tuberculin (PPD) skin test shows 9 mm of induration after 48 hours. He is not aware of exposure to anyone with active pulmonary tuberculosis (TB). He denies TB symptoms. Physical examination demonstrates mildly elevated blood pressure, but the findings are otherwise unremarkable. You recommend:
   a. Repeat PPD skin test in 2 weeks
   b. Chest radiography
   c. Isoniazid (INH) 300 mg daily for 9 months
   d. BCG vaccination
   e. No further evaluation or treatment

3. A 79-year-old woman presents for a periodic medical evaluation during early winter. She has known valvular heart disease and moderately severe asthma with documented chronic obstructive pulmonary disease. She is allergic to sulfa and eggs. In the past, she has had swelling of the lips and mouth as well as a skin rash after ingesting eggs. She developed a skin rash on her hands after handling chicken. She received a pneumococcal vaccination at age 63 when her valvular heart disease was diagnosed. She had a Td booster 4 years ago. Influenza B has just recently been reported in a few schoolchildren in the community. You recommend:
   a. Pneumococcal and influenza vaccinations
   b. Influenza vaccination
   c. Pneumococcal vaccination and rimantadine (100 mg daily)

   d. Pneumococcal vaccination and oseltamivir (75 mg daily)
   e. Pneumococcal vaccination, influenza vaccination, and oseltamivir (75 mg daily)

4. A 35-year-old physician is evaluated before starting a fellowship in gastrointestinal medicine. He mentions that he was bitten by an unknown dog on his buttock while jogging some distance from his home 7 days ago. He is sure that the bite punctured his skin because his shorts were torn and there was blood on them. He has no other health concerns. His past medical history is unremarkable. He received his last Td booster 4 years ago. He received rabies preexposure vaccine series (three doses of unknown vaccine) before serving in the Peace Corps in central Africa during his early 20s. Physical examination findings are normal except for a small, mostly healed superficial laceration on his right buttock. You recommend:
   a. Rabies immune globulin
   b. Two doses of rabies vaccine (first dose as soon as possible, then an additional dose 3 days later)
   c. Rabies immune globulin and five doses of rabies vaccine (first dose as soon as possible, then additional doses on days 3, 7, 14, and 28-35)
   d. That he find the dog and observe it for 10 days for signs of rabies
   e. No additional treatment because the attack was likely provoked by his jogging

5. A 48-year-old man requests recheck of chronic hepatitis B infection. He was first found to be a hepatitis B surface antigen carrier approximately 20 years ago at the time of blood donation. The serum levels of transaminases (aspartate [AST] and alanine aminotransferase) have been mildly elevated over the past 10 years. He currently has no symptoms suggesting liver disease. He feels good and has no complaints. He is homosexual and has had a single partner for the past 8 years. Before that, he was sexually active with multiple male partners. He is negative for human immunodeficiency virus. He has smoked one pack of cigarettes per day for 30 years and drinks one or two glasses of wine every day with dinner. His father was found to have prostate cancer at age 68. There is no other family history of cancer. The physical examination findings are unremarkable, and the serum level of AST is now 100 U/L (normal 12-32 U/L). You recommend all the following *except*:
   a. Smoking cessation
   b. Abstaining from alcohol
   c. Hepatitis A serology
   d. Digital rectal examination of the prostate and serum prostate-specific antigen (PSA) test
   e. Alpha-fetoprotein and ultrasonography of the liver

6. A 53-year-old woman presents for a periodic medical evaluation. Her last evaluation was 5 years ago. She has smoked one pack of cigarettes daily for 33 years. She has two to three alcoholic drinks daily. She feels well and has no specific complaints. Her menses stopped 13 years ago. She had a few "hot flashes" then but none in recent years. Physical examination findings are unremarkable. You recommend all the following *except*:

a. Smoking cessation
b. Chest radiography
c. Screening mammography
d. Fecal occult blood test (FOBT) × 3 days
e. Spine and hip bone mineral density

7. A 60-year-old man presents for a periodic medical evaluation. He has asymptomatic coronary artery disease (CAD), for which he takes low-dose aspirin therapy and metoprolol. He has taken omeprazole for the past 3 years, with good control of his symptoms of gastroesophageal reflux disease. He smoked one pack of cigarettes daily for 40 years and quit smoking 5 years ago when CAD was diagnosed. His father and an older brother had prostate cancer in their late 60s. There is no other family history of cancer. He has never had any cancer screening. Randomized controlled trial data would support screening this patient for which of the following cancers:

a. Lung, with chest radiography with or without sputum cytology
b. Prostate, with digital rectal examination of the prostate and serum PSA test
c. Colon, with FOBT × 3 days
d. Bladder, with urine cytology
e. Esophageal, with esophagogastroduodenoscopy (EGD)

ANSWERS

1. Answer d.

A second dose of MMR vaccine is recommended for persons born after 1956 who are beginning employment in a health care facility. However, MMR is a live virus vaccine that is contraindicated during pregnancy. It would be appropriate to perform a measles serologic test. In the event of a possible measles exposure, she could safely be given immune globulin prophylaxis (for up to 6 days after exposure) if the test result is negative. She is due for a Td booster, which can safely be given during the second or third trimester of pregnancy. Influenza vaccination is also indicated because she will be in the second and third trimesters of pregnancy during the influenza season (November-March). Influenza vaccination would not be appropriate if she were in her first trimester, unless she had a high-risk condition such as valvular heart disease, which places her at higher risk for decompensation in the event of severe influenza. Hepatitis B vaccination is also appropriate because she is starting employment that places her at risk for hepatitis B exposure. This can safely be given during pregnancy, when the risks associated with disease are thought to outweigh risks associated with vaccination. Finally, varicella serologic testing would also be appropriate. If the result is negative, she is not a candidate for the live-virus varicella vaccine during pregnancy, but she could be given varicella zoster immune globulin following a high-risk exposure.

2. Answer a.

A tuberculin (PPD) skin test reaction of 10 mm or more at 48-72 hours is considered positive for recent arrivals from countries of high TB prevalence. Therefore, this patient's initial skin test is negative. He may have been exposed to TB in the past and may be relatively anergic; therefore, "boosting" reactivity by repeating the test (two-step PPD testing procedure) would be appropriate. A chest radiograph would be appropriate if you anticipate that the patient will not return for follow-up skin testing. A negative chest radiograph would rule out active pulmonary TB but not rule out extrapulmonary TB, which is more common among some refugee populations. Therefore, repeat PPD skin testing would be the preferred clinical management. Isoniazid treatment would be appropriate only if a positive PPD skin test is confirmed on repeat testing and subsequent evaluation did not reveal physical findings to suggest active TB and the chest radiograph is negative. Currently, there is no indication for BCG vaccination of adults in the United States, which is a low prevalence area for TB.

3. Answer d.

Influenza vaccination is contraindicated in this patient because of known significant egg allergy. Repeat pneumococcal vaccination would be indicated because she received an original dose more than 5 years earlier and was younger than 65 at the time of primary immunization. Antiviral prophylaxis with oseltamivir (75 mg daily) would be appropriate for preventing both influenza A and B. Oseltamivir has been shown to be effective for up to 6 weeks in preventing influenza A and B, with a protective efficacy of 74%. Rimantadine and amantadine are not effective against type B influenza.

4. Answer b.

The patient has had an unprovoked attack by an unknown dog with uncertain rabies vaccination status. Rabies postexposure prophylaxis is indicated in this setting. Because the patient's wound is mostly healed, thorough wound cleansing is no longer necessary. He has had a rabies preexposure vaccination series in the past. Therefore, he needs only two doses of rabies vaccine for postexposure prophylaxis, with the first dose given as soon as possible and another dose 3 days later. After a severe potential rabies exposure (e.g., head bites), it would be appropriate to give a third dose 7 days later. Rabies immune globulin is not necessary for postexposure prophylaxis if the person has had a previous full course of antirabies immunization or after preexposure immunization in the past. State public health laws require an immediate report of potential or known rabies exposure. Therefore, the health care practitioner must report this event to a local public health official who is responsible for trying to identify the animal involved. In the event that the dog was a known neighborhood pet or captured soon after the incident, postexposure prophylaxis could be delayed during a 10-day observation period. Because this is an unknown (e.g., escaped) animal, it is necessary to start postexposure prophylaxis immediately.

5. Answer d.

Currently, no confirmatory data are available from randomized controlled trials on the effect of early detection and treatment of prostate cancer on survival. Also, there is little agreement on recommendations for prostate cancer screening. The American Cancer Society recommends that digital rectal examination plus a serum PSA test be offered annually to men 50 years or older who have a life expectancy of at least 10 years. This patient is not yet 50 years old and, furthermore, his life expectancy is likely to be decreased because of his (probable) chronic active hepatitis B. Chronic active hepatitis B increases his risk of developing cirrhosis of the liver and hepatocellular carcinoma. Alcohol consumption is a known risk factor for developing hepatocellular carcinoma. Therefore, it would be appropriate to counsel him to abstain from alcohol. There is some evidence of an association between smoking and hepatocellular carcinoma, although this is equivocal. It would be appropriate to counsel this patient about smoking cessation to decrease his risk of developing lung and many other cancers (possibly hepatocellular carcinoma) and cardiovascular disease. Hepatitis A infection is more common among homosexual males. Therefore, it would be appropriate to perform a hepatitis A serologic test. If the test result is negative, hepatitis A vaccination would be appropriate to decrease his risk of contracting hepatitis A, which may result in further liver damage. Screening studies in the Native American population in Alaska and in China have demonstrated the effectiveness of alpha-fetoprotein measurement and liver ultrasonography in detecting asymptomatic early-stage hepatocellular carcinoma.

6. Answer b.

Studies completed in the past have failed to show benefit, in terms of mortality reduction, with the use of chest radiography (with or without sputum cytology) for lung cancer screening. Smoking is the leading preventable cause of cancer in the United States and a leading cause of heart disease and stroke. Physician advice to quit smoking and/or referral to a smoking cessation program has been shown to be effective in getting patients to quit smoking. Randomized controlled trial data in the United States have demonstrated an approximate 30% decrease in mortality associated with mammography screening for breast cancer and FOBT for colon cancer. This patient had menopause prematurely at approximately age 40, which places her at increased risk for developing osteoporosis. In addition, heavy alcohol use is a known risk factor for developing osteoporosis. Therefore, screening for osteoporosis with lumbar spine and hip bone mineral density would be appropriate because there are interventions known to prevent further bone loss and bone fracture.

7. Answer c.

Randomized controlled trial data have shown a 30% decrease in mortality for persons older than 50 with annual FOBT for colon cancer screening. Lung cancer screening studies using chest radiography with or without sputum cytology completed in the past have failed to show mortality reduction associated with this screening. Currently, there are no data available from randomized controlled trials that prostate cancer screening with a digital rectal examination of the prostate or serum PSA test is effective in decreasing mortality. Cytologic examination of the urine and testing for asymptomatic hematuria have been investigated as screening methods for bladder cancer. However, both tests have low sensitivity, so repeat testing is necessary. In addition, the prevalence of preclinical bladder cancer is fairly low in the general population, so large-scale screening programs would be costly. Currently, no population-based data document the effectiveness of screening for bladder cancer with either urine cytology or testing for asymptomatic hematuria. This patient has had gastroesophageal reflux disease symptoms for the past 3 years. His symptoms are well controlled with proton pump inhibitor therapy. Therefore, EGD to check for Barrett esophagus (and dysphagia) is not necessary. A history of symptoms of long duration or dysphagia in spite of appropriate acid-reducing therapy would be an appropriate indication for EGD.

CHAPTER 20

PSYCHIATRY

Marcia J. Slattery, M.D.
Lois E. Krahn, M.D.

A comprehensive psychiatric evaluation is essential because many psychiatric symptoms are nonspecific. This situation is analogous to a patient presenting in general internal medicine with fever or nausea. The presence of a single symptom, for example, depressed mood, is never pathognomonic of a specific disorder. All psychiatric disorders are based on a set of inclusion and exclusion criteria outlined in *The Diagnostic and Statistical Manual of the American Psychiatric Association (DSM)*, which is periodically updated by the American Psychiatric Association. The edition currently in use is the DSM-IV, which was published in 1994 and is expected to be revised in 2006-2007. For patients with psychiatric symptoms, the biopsychosocial model is widely used. With this approach, the biologic, psychologic, and social factors contributing to the patient's clinical presentation are evaluated. Some psychiatric symptoms indicate severe problems, whereas others are much less important to the extent that they may not be clinically relevant. A key concept is whether the symptom interferes with a patient's functioning or causes distress. For example, a patient may have a fear of heights. If this acrophobia never causes an alteration in activity, then intervention likely is not necessary. However, if a patient hesitates to visit offices on higher floors of an office building, the distress during the visits or avoidance of these situations warrants intervention.

The common psychiatric disorders confronting general physicians in outpatient settings are anxiety disorders, mood disorders, substance abuse, and somatoform functional disorders. In the general hospital setting, the common psychiatric conditions are mood disorders, adjustment disorders, substance abuse, delirium, and dementia. Psychiatric disorders are difficult to identify and manage because frequently two or more specific conditions coexist. For example, comorbid alcohol or substance abuse or dependence, delirium, or dementia can complicate the presentation, course, and treatment response of major depression. Suicide, a leading cause of death in the United States, has been reported to occur in all psychiatric conditions.

- Common psychiatric disorders confronting general physicians in an outpatient setting: anxiety disorders, mood disorders, substance abuse, somatoform (functional) disorders, and adjustment disorders.
- Common psychiatric groups in a general hospital setting: mood disorders, adjustment disorders, substance abuse, delirium, and dementia.

THE SUICIDAL PATIENT

Suicide presents as a complication of psychiatric disorders. Emergency medicine physicians are often the first to deal with patients who have suicidal ideation or who have attempted or completed suicide. The recognition of risk factors for suicide, a thorough assessment of the psychiatric and medical factors, and urgent intervention are critically important. Although the patient who overdoses with a benzodiazepine may be very serious about the intent to die, the person who overdoses with acetaminophen is more at risk for serious medical complications.

Recognition of a suicidal gesture is essential in evaluating a patient in an emergency department. Although drug overdoses are the commonest form, alcohol intoxication, single-vehicle accidents, and falls from heights may merit further investigation. Many suicidal patients see a physician the week before the attempt. Some of the risk factors to be aware of include recent psychiatric hospitalization, an older divorced or widowed man, unemployment, poor physical health, past suicide attempts, family history of suicide (especially if a parent), psychosis, alcoholism, drug abuse, chronic pain syndrome, sudden life changes, loneliness, and anniversary of significant loss. Almost without exception, patients come to an emergency department with intense suicidal ideation or gestures. These patients should not be sent home alone.

- In evaluating patients in an emergency department, it is important to recognize a suicidal gesture.
- Many patients see a physician the week before they attempt suicide.

823

- Patients who come to an emergency department with intense suicidal ideation or gestures should not be sent home alone.
- Typical clinical scenario: A 68-year-old, lonely, divorced man has a sudden life change.

MOOD DISORDERS

The prevalence of mood disorders in the general population of the United States is estimated to be 5% to 8%. However, in the general medical setting, the rate may be as high as 5% to 15%.

The essential feature of this group of disorders is a disturbance of mood (depressed or manic), which is in the context of related cognitive, psychomotor, vegetative (e.g., sleep and appetite), and interpersonal difficulties. Mood fluctuation or swings are a normal occurrence. A mood disorder is diagnosed only when the frequency or intensity (or both) of these changes is extreme and accompanied by the other features. Mood disorders range in severity from mild to severe.

- Mood disorders: the essential feature is disturbance of mood in a constellation of other symptoms.
- Mood disorders are accompanied by related cognitive, psychomotor, vegetative, and interpersonal difficulties.
- Mood disorders may also be related to a general medical condition or be substance-induced.

Major Depression

Major depression is a serious psychiatric disorder that must be distinguished from an adjustment disorder and dysthymia by the severity of the mood and cognitive disturbances and potentially by the presence of major physical somatic complaints. The primary symptoms of major depression include depressed mood, diminished interest or pleasure in many activities, notable weight loss or weight gain (>5% of body weight in a month), decrease or increase in appetite, insomnia or hypersomnia, psychomotor agitation or retardation, fatigue or loss of energy, feelings of worthlessness or of excessive or inappropriate guilt, diminished ability to concentrate, recurrent thoughts of death or suicidal ideation, or a suicide attempt. These must be present for at least 2 weeks. This time frame helps in differentiating major depression from acute changes in mood seen in delirium or medical processes, for example, acute blood loss.

If delusions or hallucinations are also present, they are less prominent than in a primary psychotic disorder, and the disorder is referred to as "major depression with psychotic features." The presence of psychotic symptoms increases the likelihood of treatment resistance. Another major depression, the melancholic type, is a severe subtype of depression. In addition to the symptoms listed above, this form is characterized

by the lack of reactivity to pleasurable stimuli (does not feel better even temporarily if involved in what is usually a pleasurable activity), diurnal mood variation (depression regularly worse in the morning), and early morning awakening (at least 2 hours before the usual time of awakening).

- Major depression: symptoms include depressed mood, diminished interest or pleasure in all or almost all activities, and notable weight loss or weight gain.
- Major depression with psychotic features: presence of hallucinations or delusions, which are often subtle.
- Major depression, melancholic type: characterized by lack of reactivity to pleasurable stimuli, diurnal mood variation, and early morning awakening.
- Typical clinical scenario: A 43-year-old woman who has lost weight and has fatigue and feelings of worthlessness and excessive guilt is much less interested in many things that used to attract her. Her ability to concentrate has decreased.

Every year about 10 million Americans have a depressive episode, but about only 20% usually seek treatment. The prevalence of depression in women is twice as high as in men. The peak age at onset of depression in women is 33 to 45 years and in men, more than 55 years. Of those who seek treatment from a physician, the diagnosis is not made in as many as one-third or sometimes it is a misdiagnosis because patients often present primarily with physical or somatic complaints. As the population ages and more elderly patients seek medical care, diagnosing and treating their mood disorders become more complicated because many of these patients often have overlapping medical and neurologic problems. Patients occasionally present with the combination of a dementing process and depression. When the depressive symptoms are treated effectively in these patients, cognitive performance may also improve.

- Of persons seeking treatment for major depression, the diagnosis is not made in as many as one-third or it is a misdiagnosis.
- In elderly patients, diagnosing and treating mood disorders become more complicated because of possible comorbid psychiatric and medical conditions.
- The prevalence of depression among women is twice as high as among men.

Seasonal Affective Disorder

Seasonal affective disorder is a subtype of depression usually characterized by the onset of depression in the autumn or winter. It is twice as common in women as in men and is associated with psychomotor retardation, hypersomnia, overeating (carbohydrate craving), and weight gain. To establish the diagnosis, winter episodes of depression must recur for 3 or more consecutive years. These episodes must resolve during the spring and summer months. Treatment has relied primarily on phototherapy, using a full-spectrum light source of 10,000 lux sources, which must be used for a minimum of 30 minutes a day. Antidepressant agents that selectively block serotonin reuptake are also of benefit in treating this disorder.

- Seasonal affective disorder: onset of depression in the autumn and winter; it resolves in the spring.
- It is twice as common among women as among men.
- It is associated with psychomotor retardation, hypersomnia, and overeating.
- Treatment: phototherapy and antidepressant agents.
- Typical clinical scenario: A 45-year-old woman has had recurrent depression in the winter for three consecutive winters.

Because depressive disorders are heterogeneous in clinical presentation, the cause is expected to be multifactorial. There probably is no single etiologic agent. According to current theories, depression appears to be related to alterations of several neurotransmitter systems and neuropeptides, effects on presynaptic and postsynaptic receptors, neurohormonal alterations, and, in general, an alteration in the overall balance of these systems, which are interdependent on one another. Adverse life events (marital discord, bankruptcy, professional setbacks, and failure) can initiate or perpetuate a depressive episode by overwhelming a person's coping mechanisms.

Dysthymia

Dysthymia is chronic depression that is milder in severity than major depression. It may have either an early or a late onset, as defined by onset before or after age 21 years. It can be disabling for the person because the depressed mood is present most of the time during at least a 2-year period. Many patients have one or two associated vegetative signs, such as disturbance of sleep and appetite. Also, patients often feel inadequate, have low self-esteem, and struggle with interpersonal relationships. If onset is in late adolescence, the dysthymia may become intertwined with the person's personality, behavior, and general attitude toward life. Treatment is usually a combination of psychotherapy (cognitive or interpersonal) and pharmacotherapy. Psychopharmacotherapy may be particularly useful for patients with a family history of mood disorders or for those who have the early onset form of dysthymia. In patients with dysthymia, superimposed major depressive episodes may develop. Also, some are prone to turn to alcohol or other substance abuse to "treat" their dysphoria.

- Dysthymia: a form of chronic depression.
- Depressed mood is present most of the time during at least a 2-year period.
- Treatment is usually a combination of psychotherapy and pharmacotherapy.
- Major depressive episodes may develop in patients with dysthymia.
- Typical clinical scenario: A 25-year-old woman has had disturbed sleep, appetite changes, low self-esteem, and issues with interpersonal relationships for 3 years.

Adjustment Disorder With Depressed Mood

Adjustment disorder with depressed mood is a reaction that develops in response to an identifiable psychosocial stressor, for example, divorce, job loss, or family or marital problems. The severity of the adjustment disorder (degree of impairment) does not always parallel the intensity of the precipitating event. The critical factor appears to be the relevance of the event or stressor to the individual and his or her ability to cope with the stress. In general, these reactions are relatively transient. Although patients generally can be managed by an empathic primary care physician, the development of extreme withdrawal, suicidal ideation, or failure to improve as the circumstances improve may prompt psychiatric referral. Treatment includes supportive psychotherapy, psychosocial interventions, and, sometimes, use of antidepressant agents.

Treatment of Depression

There are four major groups of treatment modalities for depression: psychotherapy, pharmacotherapy, electroconvulsive therapy (ECT), and circadian rhythm manipulation such as sleep deprivation or phototherapy. Generally, these therapeutic modalities are used in some combination.

Psychotherapy

There are multiple forms of psychotherapy, many of which can be used in the treatment of depression. However, the two forms that have been used extensively for treating depression are cognitive therapy and interpersonal therapy. Cognitive therapy strives to help patients have a better integration of cognition (thoughts), emotion, and behavior. This therapy is based on the premise that thoughts have a profound effect on emotions, which have an effect on behavior. For example, if a patient repeatedly thinks that he or she is failing professionally because of striving for unrealistic, perfectionist goals, then over time that person's emotions and behavior will be affected. If patients can perceive themselves in more realistic or adaptive ways, their general outlook will be expected to improve. Ultimately, they may experience an increase in a sense of worth and self-esteem. Interpersonal therapy focuses on current interpersonal functioning. It is based on the concept that depression is associated with impaired social relationships that either precipitate or perpetuate the disorder.

- Cognitive therapy: helps patients achieve a better integration of cognition (thoughts), emotion, and behavior.
- Interpersonal therapy: focuses on current interpersonal functioning.

Pharmacotherapy

The selection of medication is based on the side-effect profile of the medication and the clinical profile of the patient. Research is under way to select or avoid particular medications according to an individual patient's cytochrome P450 polymorphisms, but this has not been incorporated into clinical practice. For the dose, begin slowly and titrate to a therapeutic dose based on clinical assessment. Blood levels of a drug are used less often than previously because they are meaningful only for tricyclic antidepressants. The duration of treatment is usually a minimum of 6 months, counting from the time the patient attained noticeable improvement. Often, patients may benefit from extended use of antidepressant agents, especially if they have had multiple episodes of depression. Generally, antidepressant agents should be tapered rather than stopped abruptly when treatment is discontinued. If the response to the first antidepressant agent is minimal, reevaluate the diagnosis, change to a different class of drug, or treat with ECT, which is still probably the most consistently effective treatment for severe depression. ECT is especially valuable if psychotic symptoms complicate the major depression.

Mania and Bipolar Disorder

The essential features of a manic episode are the presence of an abnormally euphoric, expansive, or irritable mood associated with some of the following features: inflated self-esteem or grandiosity, decreased need for sleep, pressured speech, flight of ideas, distractibility, increase in goal-directed activity or psychomotor agitation, and excessive involvement in pleasurable activities that have a high potential for painful consequences (e.g., unrestrained buying sprees, sexual indiscretions, or inappropriate financial investments). These episodes must last a minimum of 1 week (unless the course is altered by treatment). To establish the diagnosis of bipolar disorder, the patient must have had at least one episode of mania. Most bipolar patients have had recurrent depressive episodes in addition to manic episodes, although rare patients exclusively have mania. Some patients do not experience a fully developed manic episode but have fewer symptoms. The term "hypomania" has been introduced to describe this form of bipolar disorder (type II), which generally is challenging to clinicians because its more subtle features make it more difficult to recognize.

- Mania: the essential feature is an abnormally euphoric, expansive, or irritable mood.
- The prevalence of bipolar disorder is estimated to be about 1%.
- Bipolar disorder occurs about as frequently in women as in men.
- The usual age at onset is from the teens to age 30.
- A family history of bipolar or other mood disorder is more common for patients with bipolar disorder than for other mood disorders.
- Typical clinical scenario: For more than 1 week, a 25-year-old man has had a euphoric mood, flight of ideas, decreased need for sleep, and unrestrained buying sprees.

Treatment is aimed at mood stabilization and improved social and occupational functioning. The traditional pharmacologic treatment is lithium carbonate. In recent years, valproic acid has replaced lithium as the first-line agent for treatment of bipolar disorder. Other helpful agents include carbamazepine and newer anticonvulsants, including gabapentin. All these mood stabilizers may take up to 10 days to be effective. During this waiting period, the judicious use of antipsychotic agents or clonazepam is helpful in controlling the acute symptoms. Bipolar patients should not receive monotherapy with an antidepressant because antidepressants can trigger a hypomanic or manic episode. For bipolar patients with a depressive episode, a mood-stabilizing medication should be given simultaneously with an antidepressant to reduce the risk of triggering a hypomanic or manic episode.

- Treatment of mania and bipolar disorder: aimed at stabilizing mood and improving social and occupational functioning.
- Primary pharmacologic treatment: valproic acid, lithium carbonate, newer anticonvulsants.

Mood Disorders Caused by a General Medical Condition

The essential feature of mood disorders caused by a general medical condition is depression or mania that is attributable to the physiologic effects of a specific medical condition. The full criteria for one of these episodes regarding the number of symptoms and time course need not be met. Medical conditions that may cause mood symptoms include endocrinopathies (Cushing syndrome, Addison disease, hyperthyroidism, hypothyroidism, hyperparathyroidism, and hypoparathyroidism), certain malignancies (lymphomas, pancreatic carcinoma, and astrocytomas), neurologic conditions (Parkinson disease and Huntington disease), autoimmune conditions (systemic lupus erythematosus), and infections (chronic hepatitis

C, encephalitis, mononucleosis, and human immunodeficiency virus [HIV]).

- In mood disorders due to a general medical condition, the essential feature is a disturbance of mood attributable to the physiologic effects of a specific medical condition.
- Many medical conditions may induce mood changes, so the clinical interview needs to identify coexisting symptoms such as excessive guilt, social withdrawal, or suicidal ideation, which are more specific for a depressive disorder.
- Some potential depressive symptoms such as energy, sleep, and appetite changes may be due to the medical condition in the absence of a depressive disorder.

Substance-Induced Mood Disorders

The essential feature of a substance-induced mood disorder is a disturbance of mood, either depressed or manic, that is judged to be due to the direct physiologic effects of a substance. Many substances can induce mood changes, including medications, toxins, and drugs of abuse. The mood symptoms may occur during the use of or exposure to the substance or during withdrawal from the substance. Medications that have been implicated in inducing mood disturbances include corticosteroids, interferon, reserpine, methyldopa, carbonic anhydrase inhibitors, stimulants, sedative-hypnotics, benzodiazepines, and narcotics as well as the long-term use or abuse of alcohol or hallucinogens. Recent studies have demonstrated that β-adrenergic agents are less likely to cause depressive disorders than previously thought.

- In substance-induced mood disorders, the essential feature is a disturbance of mood due to the physiologic effects of a substance.
- Many medications and drugs of abuse may induce mood changes.

PSYCHOTIC DISORDERS

"Psychosis" is a generic term used to describe altered thought and behavior in which the patient is incapable of interpreting his or her situation rationally and accurately. Psychotic symptoms can occur in various medical, neurologic, and psychiatric disorders. Many psychotic reactions seen in medical settings are associated with the use of recreational or prescription drugs (Table 20-1). Some of these drug-induced psychotic reactions are nearly indistinguishable from schizophrenia in terms of hallucinations and paranoid delusions (e.g., amphetamine and phencyclidine [PCP] psychoses). Many brain regions may be involved with the production of psychotic symptoms, but abnormalities in the frontal, temporal, and limbic regions are more likely than others to produce psychotic features.

- Psychosis: a generic term describing altered thought and behavior in which the patient is incapable of interpreting his or her situation rationally and accurately.
- Many psychotic reactions may be associated with the use of recreational or prescription drugs.
- Some drug-induced psychotic reactions have symptoms similar to those found in schizophrenia.

There are disorders throughout the life span that may be associated with schizophrenia-like psychoses. These include genetic abnormalities (e.g., a microdeletion of chromosome 22, the velocardiofacial syndrome), childhood neurologic disorders (autism and epilepsy), adult neurologic disorders (narcolepsy), medical and metabolic diseases (infections, inflammatory disorders, endocrinopathies, nutritional deficiencies, uremia, and hepatic encephalopathy), drug abuse, and psychologic stressors.

Schizophrenia may have multifactorial causes. Symptoms have been subdivided into positive (delusions and hallucinations) and negative (apathy and amotivation) symptoms. Current diagnostic criteria are divided into inclusion and exclusion criteria. Inclusion criteria include the presence of delusions and hallucinations; marked decrement in functional level in areas such as work, school, social relations, and self-care; and continuous signs of the disturbance for at least 6 months. Exclusion criteria include consistent mood disorder component and evidence of an organic factor that produces the symptoms. The five subtypes of schizophrenia are catatonic, disorganized, paranoid, undifferentiated, and residual. These subtypes are not used extensively in clinical practice because of diagnostic overlap over the course of an individual patient's illness.

- Schizophrenia may be a neurodevelopmental disorder resulting from possible environmental or genetic factors occurring before birth.

Table 20-1   Classes of Drugs That Can Produce Psychotic Symptoms

Stimulants
Hallucinogens
Phencyclidine (PCP)
Catecholaminergic drugs
Anticholinergic drugs
Central nervous system depressants
Glucocorticoids
Heavy metals (lead, mercury, manganese, arsenic, thallium)
Others (digitalis, disulfiram, cimetidine, bromide, tacrolimus)

- The psychotic symptoms and altered interpersonal skills typically become evident initially in the teenage years.

ANXIETY DISORDERS

This group of disorders is encountered most frequently in the outpatient setting. Anxiety symptoms may be misinterpreted as those of medical illness because many of the symptoms overlap, for example, tachycardia, diaphoresis, tremor, shortness of breath, nausea, abdominal pain, and chest pain. Autonomic arousal and anxious agitation in a medically ill patient can also be attributed quickly to stress or anxiety when it may represent pulmonary embolus or cardiac arrhythmia. Common sources of anxiety in the medical setting are related to fears of death, abandonment, loss of function, pain, dependency, and loss of control. When to treat or to seek psychiatric consultation depends on the assessment of the degree of anxiety. Is the patient able to function in his or her role without distress or avoidance?

- Anxiety symptoms may be misinterpreted as those of medical illness.
- Common sources of anxiety in the medical setting are related to fears of death, abandonment, loss of function, and pain.

Panic Disorder With or Without Agoraphobia

Panic disorder is recurrent, discrete episodes of extreme anxiety accompanied by various somatic symptoms such as dyspnea, unsteady feelings, palpitations, paresthesias, hyperventilation, trembling, diaphoresis, chest pain or discomfort, or abdominal distress. Agoraphobia refers to extreme fear of being in places or situations from which escape may be difficult or embarrassing. This may lead to avoidance of such situations as driving, travel in general, being in a crowded place, and many other situations, ultimately causing severe limitations in daily functioning for the patient. Panic disorder is more common in women (prevalence, 2%-3%) than in men (prevalence, 0.5%-1.5%). The usual age at onset is from the late teens to the early thirties. A history of childhood separation anxiety is reported in 20% to 50% of patients. The incidence is higher in first- and second-degree relatives. Most patients describe their first panic attack as spontaneous. They generally go to an emergency department after the first attack, believing they are having a heart attack or some severe medical problem.

- Panic disorder: recurrent, discrete episodes of extreme anxiety accompanied by various somatic symptoms.
- Agoraphobia: extreme fear of being in places or situations from which escape may be difficult.
- Agoraphobia is more common in women than in men.
- Patients generally go to an emergency department after their first panic attack, believing they are having a heart attack or some severe medical problem.

The differential diagnosis of panic disorder includes several medical disorders, for example, endocrine disturbances (hyperthyroidism, pheochromocytoma, and hypoglycemia), gastrointestinal disturbances (colitis and irritable bowel syndrome), cardiopulmonary disturbances (pulmonary embolism, exacerbation of chronic obstructive pulmonary disease, and acute allergic reactions), and neurologic conditions (especially conditions like seizures that are episodic or are associated with paresthesias, faintness, or dizziness).

Patients with panic attacks may also be prone to major episodes of depression. Alcohol use may temporarily reduce some of the distress of the panic attack and the interim anticipatory anxiety but symptoms may soon rebound, potentially leading to alcohol abuse. Benzodiazepines may similarly be abused.

- Patients with panic attacks may be prone to episodes of major depression.
- Alcohol and benzodiazepines may reduce the distress of panic attacks, but symptoms may rebound, potentially leading to the abuse of these substances.

Post-Traumatic Stress Disorder

Post-traumatic stress disorder can be a brief reaction that follows an extremely traumatic, overwhelming, or catastrophic experience or it may be a chronic condition that produces severe disability. The syndrome is characterized by intrusive memories, flashbacks, nightmares, avoidance of reminders of the event, and often a restricted range of affect. It may occur in adults or children. There is increased comorbidity with substance abuse, depression, and other anxiety disorders. Patients may be more prone to impulsivity, including suicide. As for other anxiety disorders, treatment is usually a combination of behavioral, psychotherapeutic, and, if necessary, pharmacologic interventions.

- Post-traumatic stress disorder may be a brief reaction or a chronic condition that produces severe disability.
- Patients may be prone to impulsivity, including suicide.
- Typical clinical scenario: A 30-year-old man who is a military veteran has flashbacks, nightmares, and depression.

Generalized Anxiety Disorder

Generalized anxiety disorder is characterized by chronic excessive anxiety and apprehension about life circumstances accompanied by somatic symptoms of anxiety, such as trembling, restlessness, autonomic hyperactivity, and hypervigilance. Treatment is usually a mixture of behavioral, progressive muscle relaxation, psychotherapeutic, and adjunctive psychopharmacologic modalities.

Obsessive-Compulsive Disorder

Obsessive-compulsive disorder is characterized by recurrent obsessions or compulsions that are severe enough to disrupt daily life. The obsessions are distressing thoughts, ideas, or impulses experienced as unwanted. Compulsions are repetitive, intentional behaviors usually performed in response to an obsession. The obsessions cause marked anxiety or distress, and the compulsions serve to neutralize the anxiety. Prevalence rates are about 2% to 3% and are about equal in men and women. The onset of this disorder is usually in adolescence or early adulthood. Obsessive traits are often present before onset of the disorder. The predominant neurobiologic theory for the cause of obsessive-compulsive disorder involves dysfunction of brain serotonin systems. Pharmacologic treatment of this disorder is with antidepressants that are more selective for effects on the serotonin transmission system. These include clomipramine, selective serotonin reuptake inhibitors (SSRIs) (fluvoxamine, fluoxetine, paroxetine, and sertraline), and, occasionally, lithium augmentation of any of the preceding agents. In extremely severe, debilitating cases for which other treatments have failed, neurosurgical procedures such as cingulotomy, stereotactic limbic leukotomy, or anterior capsulotomy may be of some benefit. The effectiveness of these procedures is thought to be related to disruption of the efferent pathways from the frontal cortex to the basal ganglia. Behavioral therapies and some forms of psychotherapy can also be helpful adjunctive therapies. As with the treatment of many psychiatric disorders, a combination of treatments is most often used. With obsessive-compulsive disorder, the pharmacologic treatments are generally not as effective as with major depressive episodes. Also, higher doses of antidepressants may be needed for longer trial periods to see effectiveness in reducing symptoms of obsessive-compulsive disorder.

- Obsessive-compulsive disorder is characterized by recurrent obsessions (distressing thoughts) and compulsions (repetitive behaviors) that are recognized as unreasonable but irresistible.
- Treatment consists primarily of antidepressants with serotonergic activity and behavioral therapy.

Adjustment Disorder With Anxious Mood

Adjustment disorder with anxious mood is a maladaptive reaction to an identifiable environmental or psychosocial stress accompanied primarily by symptoms of anxiety that interfere with the patient's usual functioning. Treatment may include supportive counseling and help with identifying the stressor. However, in some cases, the anxiety may be so severe as to require short-term use of anxiolytic agents. However, these should be used with caution to avoid problems of long-term use and possible dependence.

- Adjustment disorder with anxious mood is characterized by a maladaptive reaction to an identifiable environmental or psychosocial stress accompanied by symptoms of anxiety.
- This disorder may require short-term use of anxiolytic agents.

SOMATOFORM DISORDERS, FACTITIOUS DISORDERS, AND MALINGERING

Each of these disorders represents medical symptoms that are excessive for the degree of objective disease. These conditions differ with regard to whether the symptoms and motivations for their persistence are conscious or unconscious.

Somatoform Disorders

This category includes somatization disorder, conversion disorder, hypochondriasis, chronic pain disorder, and body dysmorphic disorder. In all these conditions, the patient experiences physical complaints because of an effort to satisfy unconscious needs. These patients are not deliberately seeking to appear ill.

Somatization Disorder

Somatization disorder is a heterogeneous disorder that begins in early life and is characterized by recurrent multiple somatic complaints. It mostly affects women. It is often best managed by collaborative work with an empathic primary care physician and mental health professional. Regularly scheduled appointments with the primary care physician are a cost-effective strategy that lessens "doctor shopping" and frequent visits to an emergency department.

- Somatization disorder begins in early life and is characterized by recurrent multiple physical complaints.
- It mostly affects women.
- It is associated with high utilization of health care.

Conversion Disorder

Conversion disorder is a loss or alteration of physical functioning suggestive of a medical or neurologic disorder that cannot be explained on the basis of known physiologic mechanisms. The disorder is not limited to pain or sexual dysfunction. It is seen most often in the outpatient setting. Patients frequently respond to any of several therapeutic modalities that suggest hope of a cure. When conversion disorder becomes chronic, it carries a poorer prognosis and is difficult to treat. Treatment focuses on management of the symptoms rather than cure, much as in somatization or chronic pain disorder.

- Conversion disorder is characterized by a loss or alteration of physical functioning.

- It cannot be explained by known physiologic mechanisms.
- It is usually seen in the outpatient setting.
- Treatment focuses on management of the symptoms and encouraging the patient to resume normal functioning.

Chronic Pain Disorder

Chronic pain somatoform disorder (somatoform, chronic pain syndromes) may occur at any age but most often develops in the 30s or 40s. It is diagnosed twice as often in women as in men and is characterized by preoccupation with pain for at least 6 months. No organic lesion is found to account for the pain, or if there is a related organic lesion, the complaint of pain or resulting interference with usual life activities is in excess of what would be expected from the physical findings. A thorough assessment is essential before this diagnosis can be established. Treatment is usually multidisciplinary and focused on helping the patient manage or live with the pain rather than continuing with the expectation of "cure." Avoidance of long-term dependence on addictive substances is an important goal.

- Chronic pain disorder: occurs at any age but usually develops in the 30s or 40s.
- It is diagnosed twice as often in women as in men.
- It is characterized by preoccupation with pain for at least 6 months.
- Treatment: usually multidisciplinary, ideally with involvement of primary care, psychiatry, psychology, and physiatry.
- Typical clinical scenario: A 33-year-old woman has been preoccupied with pain for 8 months, and this has interfered with normal function. An extensive medical evaluation has not found any organic lesion.

Hypochondriasis

Hypochondriasis is an intense preoccupation with the fear of having or the belief that one has a serious disease despite the lack of physical evidence to support the concern. It tends to be a chronic problem for the patient. The differential diagnosis includes obsessive-compulsive disorder (somatic presentation) and delusional disorder (somatic type). Patients with hypochondriasis and obsessive-compulsive disorder tend to have fleeting insight into their excessive concern for their health, unlike patients with delusional thinking. The treatment of hypochondriasis, similar to that of obsessive-compulsive disorder, depends on a combination of serotonergic antidepressants and cognitive-behavioral psychotherapy.

Factitious Disorders

Factitious disorders are characterized by the deliberate production of signs or symptoms of disease. The diagnosis of these disorders requires that the physician maintain a high index of suspicion and look for objective data at variance with the patient's history (e.g., surgical scars are inconsistent with past surgical history). The more common form of factitious disorder generally occurs among socially conforming young women of a higher socioeconomic class who are intelligent, educated, and frequently work in a medically related field. The possibility of a coexisting medical disorder or intercurrent illness needs to be appreciated in the diagnostic and therapeutic management of these difficult cases. Factitious disorders are often found in patients with a history of childhood emotional traumas. These patients, through their illness, may be seeking to compensate for childhood traumas and secondarily to escape from and make up for stressful life situations. The most extreme form of the disorder is Munchausen syndrome, which is characterized by the triad of simulating disease, pathologic lying, and wandering. This syndrome has been recognized primarily in men of lower socioeconomic class who have a lifelong pattern of poor social adjustment. The subtype of Munchausen disorder is not included in DSM-IV, which instead uses the more inclusive category "factitial disorder."

- Factitious disorder: the voluntary production of signs or symptoms of disease to assume the sick role.
- Common form: occurs among socially conforming young women of a higher socioeconomic class.
- Munchausen syndrome is the most extreme form of factitious disorder, with the characteristic triad of simulating disease, pathologic lying, and wandering.
- Factitious disorders often occur in patients with a history of childhood emotional traumas.
- Typical clinical scenario: A 32-year-old woman who is a registered nurse has recurrent fevers but no presenting signs or symptoms with a documented double-organism bacteremia due to self-injection.

Malingering

The essential feature of malingering is the intentional production of false or exaggerated physical or psychologic symptoms. It is motivated by external incentives such as avoiding military service or work, obtaining financial compensation or drugs, evading criminal prosecution, or securing better living conditions. Malingering should be suspected in cases in which a medicolegal context overshadows the clinical presentation, a marked discrepancy exists between the person's claimed stress or disability and the objective findings, there is lack of cooperation during the diagnostic evaluation and in compliance with prescribed treatments, and there is presence of an antisocial personality disorder. The person who is malingering is much less likely to present his or her symptoms in the context of emotional conflict, and the presenting symptoms are less likely to be related symbolically to an underlying emotional conflict.

- Malingering is the intentional production of false or exaggerated physical or psychologic symptoms.
- It is motivated by external incentives such as disability payments, housing, release from jail, or avoiding court appearances.

DELIRIUM AND DEMENTIA

The primary distinguishing feature between delirium and dementia is the retention and stability of alertness in dementia.

Delirium

Delirium is characterized by a fluctuating course of an altered state of awareness and consciousness. Although the onset typically is abrupt, the symptoms of this disorder may occasionally be insidious. It may be accompanied by hallucinations (tactile, auditory, visual, or olfactory), illusions (misperceptions of sensory stimuli), delusions, emotional lability, paranoia, alterations in the sleep-wake cycle, and psychomotor slowing or hyperactivity. The symptoms can be dramatic and mimic primary psychotic disorders. Delirium is usually reversible with correction of the underlying cause. It often is related to an external toxic agent, medication side effect, metabolic abnormality, central nervous system abnormality, or withdrawal of a medication or drug. Delirium is relatively common (range, 10%-30%) in medical or surgical inpatients older than 65 years. The diagnosis is made primarily by clinical assessment and changes in the results of a patient's mental status examination. Patients may present with either agitation or withdrawal, the latter being more difficult to recognize. High-risk groups include elderly patients with medical illness (especially congestive heart failure, urinary tract infection, renal insufficiency, hyponatremia, dehydration, or stroke), postcardiotomy patients, patients with dementia, patients in drug withdrawal, patients with severe burns, and patients with acquired immunodeficiency syndrome (AIDS).

- Delirium is characterized by a fluctuating course of inattention and altered level of consciousness.
- Delirium usually is reversible with correction of the underlying cause.
- It often is related to an external toxic agent, medication side effect, metabolic abnormality, central nervous system abnormality, or withdrawal of a medication or drug.
- Delirium is relatively common in medical or surgical patients older than 65 years.

The most common cause of delirium in the elderly probably is intoxication with psychotropic drugs, especially drugs with sedative and anticholinergic side effects. The first step in management is determining whether a specific cause can be identified. Comprehensive medical investigations are frequently warranted. After the cause of the delirium has been recognized, a treatment is selected that can reverse the disease process. If the cause is unknown and the patient's behavior interferes with safety and medical care, several categories of intervention can be considered. Management aspects include monitoring vital signs, electrolytes, and fluid balance and giving neuroleptic agents such as haloperidol intravenously. Environmental supports aid orientation; these include calendars, clocks, windows, and family and other persons. Also, psychosocial support, including family or other care providers, is helpful. Severely agitated patients may require physical restraints to prevent injury to themselves or others if medications are not yet effective. Restraints should be avoided whenever possible.

- The most common cause of delirium in the elderly is intoxication with psychotropic drugs.
- Typical clinical scenario: A 70-year-old man hospitalized for renal insufficiency and hyponatremia has abrupt onset of visual hallucinations and paranoia accompanied by alternation of his sleep-wake cycle.

Dementia

Dementia is a syndrome of acquired persistent impairment of mental function involving at least three of the following five domains: memory, language, visuospatial skills, personality or mood, and cognition (including abstraction, judgment, calculations, and executive function). The most common form of cortical dementia is Alzheimer disease. The lifetime prevalence for patients reaching age 65 is estimated at 5% to 10% and for those over age 85, 15% to 20%. Dementia with Lewy bodies is a progressive neurodegenerative disorder that typically has a faster rate of decline than Alzheimer disease. Autopsy findings in this disorder include eosinophilic inclusion bodies in the cerebral cortex and brainstem. Patients have prominent visual hallucinations and extrapyramidal symptoms. Another common type of dementia is multi-infarct dementia, which represents 15% of cases of dementia in a pure form and an additional 10% in a mixed form.

Subcortical dementia is another important subtype. Patients with this type of dementia often have other focal neurologic signs, including an associated gait disturbance. They also may have normal-pressure hydrocephalus, Huntington disease, or Parkinson disease.

Dementia may be associated with HIV infection, multiple sclerosis, amyotrophic lateral sclerosis, vitamin B_{12} deficiency, hypothyroidism, and Wilson disease. Other rare types of dementia include Pick disease and Creutzfeldt-Jakob disease.

- Cortical dementia: the common form is Alzheimer disease.
- Subcortical dementia: focal neurologic signs, including

gait disturbance, other than cognitive dysfunction are often present.

Dementia is differentiated from delirium by appropriate levels of arousal, more preserved attention, and persistence of the cognitive changes. Some forms may be reversible, as in dementia related to hypothyroidism, and some may be "treatable" without reversing the intellectual deficits, for example, preventing further ischemic injury in patients with vascular dementia. Dementia may be a chronic progressive form in which treatment is generally related to improved control of the behavioral disturbances.

PSYCHOLOGIC ASPECTS OF AIDS

From the early to the terminal phases of AIDS and its sequelae, many psychiatric symptoms and complications are possible. The organic mental disorders associated with this process can be primary (i.e., directly induced by HIV infection), secondary (i.e., related to the effects of the HIV infection leading to immunodeficiency and opportunistic infections or tumors systemically or within the central nervous system), or iatrogenic (i.e., resulting from the treatment of HIV or its sequelae). The delirium of AIDS often has a multifactorial cause, similar to delirium in general, namely, electrolyte imbalance, encephalopathy from intracranial or systemic infections, hypoxemia, or medication side effects. HIV itself can cause encephalopathy. The dementia of AIDS can result from the chronic sequelae of most of the causes of delirium. However, direct cerebral infection with HIV probably causes much of the dementia. Other psychiatric symptoms are more nonspecific, such as anger, depression, mania, psychosis, and the general problems of dealing with a terminal illness. Also, all these might be complicated by undiagnosed and, thus, untreated alcohol or drug dependence, especially in the early phases of the disease. A patient who contracted HIV infection through intravenous drug abuse may need chemical dependency treatment as well as thoughtful management of pain complaints.

- AIDS has many possible psychiatric symptoms and complications.
- Organic mental disorders can be primary (due to HIV infection), secondary (due to immunodeficiency and opportunistic infections), or iatrogenic.
- Delirium in AIDS is multifactorial.
- Dementia in AIDS can result from the chronic sequelae of most of the causes of delirium.

EATING DISORDERS

The two common eating disorders are anorexia nervosa and bulimia. Both are markedly more prevalent among women than men. Onset is usually in the teenage or young adult years; although it can start prepubertally, this is rare. Eating disorders are increasingly found across all income, racial, and ethnic groups. Both disorders have a primary symptom of preoccupation with weight and distortion of body image. For example, the patient perceives herself to look less attractive than an observer would. The disorders are not mutually exclusive, and about 50% of patients with anorexia nervosa also have bulimia. Many patients with bulimia previously had at least a subclinical case of anorexia nervosa.

- The two common eating disorders are anorexia nervosa and bulimia.
- They are markedly more prevalent among women than men.
- Primary symptom: preoccupation with weight and a desire to be thinner.

Anorexia Nervosa

To meet the diagnostic criteria of anorexia nervosa, weight must be 15% below that expected for age and height. However, weight of 30% to 40% below normal is not uncommon and leads to the medical complications of starvation, such as depletion of fat, muscle wasting, bradycardia, arrhythmias, ventricular tachycardia and sudden death, constipation, abdominal pain, leukopenia, hypercortisolemia, and osteoporosis. In extreme cases, patients develop lanugo (fine hair of the body) and metabolic alterations to conserve energy. Thyroid effects include low levels of triiodothyronine (T_3), cold intolerance, and difficulty maintaining core body temperature. Reproductive effects included a pronounced decrease or cessation of the secretion of luteinizing hormone and follicle-stimulating hormone, resulting in secondary amenorrhea.

Bulimia

Patients with bulimia frequently lose control and consume large quantities of food. Many patients may have a concurrent depressive or anxiety disorder. Physical complications of the binge-purge cycle may include fluid and electrolyte abnormalities, hypochloremic-hypokalemic metabolic alkalosis, esophageal and gastric irritation and bleeding, colonic abnormalities from laxative abuse, marked erosion of dental enamel with associated decay, parotid and salivary gland hypertrophy, and amylase levels 25% to 40% higher than normal. If bulimia is untreated, it often becomes chronic. Some patients have a gradual spontaneous remission of some symptoms.

- Patients with bulimia may have a concurrent depressive or anxiety disorder.
- The binge-purge cycle causes physical complications.

ALCOHOLISM AND SUBSTANCE ABUSE DISORDERS

Alcoholism and substance abuse disorders are a major concern in all age groups and across all ethnic, socioeconomic, and racial groups. Despite national and international efforts to curb the problem and to make treatment more readily available, the condition is not diagnosed in many persons and fewer than 10% of persons with addiction are involved in some form of treatment, either self-help groups or with professional supervision. The lifetime incidence of alcohol and drug abuse approaches 20% of the population. These disorders have devastating effects on families and other persons and contribute to social problems such as motor vehicle accidents and fatalities, domestic violence, suicide, and increased health care costs. Untreated alcoholics have been estimated to generate twice the general health care costs of nonalcoholics. Persons with addictive disorders are a heterogeneous group and may present in many different ways. Recognizing addictive disorders is critically important. The current definition of alcoholism approved by the National Council on Alcoholism and Drug Dependence may also be applicable to other drugs of abuse: alcohol abuse and dependence are primary, chronic diseases with genetic, psychosocial, and environmental factors influencing their development and manifestations. The disease is often progressive and fatal. It is characterized by continuous or periodic impaired control over drinking, preoccupation with the drug alcohol, the use of alcohol despite adverse consequences, and distortions in thinking, most notably denial.

- Fewer than 10% of persons with addiction receive some form of treatment.
- Persons with addictive disorders are a heterogeneous group.
- The lifetime incidence of alcohol and drug abuse approaches 20% of the population.
- Untreated alcoholics generate twice the general health care costs of nonalcoholics.

The adverse consequences of alcohol and substance abuse disorders cross over into several domains. Physical health issues include alcohol withdrawal syndromes, liver disease, gastritis, anemia, and neurologic disorders. Psychologic functioning issues include impaired cognition and changes in mood and behavior. Interpersonal functioning issues include marital problems, child abuse, and impaired social relationships. Occupational functioning issues include academic, scholastic, or job problems. Legal, financial, and spiritual problems also occur.

Substance abuse disorders are divided by the substance involved into 10 major groups: alcohol, amphetamines, cannabis, cocaine, hallucinogens, inhalants, nicotine, opioids, PCP, and benzodiazepines, sedative-hypnotics, and anxiolytics.

Some characteristics are specific to each of these groups, but what may be unexpected is that they probably have more similarities than differences when it comes to diagnosing a problem of abuse or dependence (or both). These drugs are grouped according to their perceived effects in Table 20-2. The descriptive titles of the groups give an idea of the physiologic and psychologic activity of the drug when taken. Within the group of central nervous system depressants ("downers"), there is considerable potential for crossover addictions (barbiturates and alcohol).

- Within the group of central nervous system depressants, there is considerable potential for crossover addictions.

Alcoholism

Medical data from physical examination and laboratory tests can be helpful. However, most of the pertinent findings are not apparent until after several years (often up to 5 years) of notable alcohol use and, thus, do not reflect the earliest stages of the disease. Two of the earlier detectable signs are increases in serum γ-glutamyltransferase level and mean corpuscular volume. In both men and women, the combination of increased γ-glutamyltransferase level and mean corpuscular volume can identify up to 90% of alcoholics. Carbohydrate-deficient transferrin is the most sensitive screening test. Other abnormal laboratory findings include increased levels of alkaline phosphatase, bilirubin, uric acid, and triglycerides. However, because of the number of false-negative results, it is not practical to rely on laboratory data alone to establish the diagnosis of alcoholism. The CAGE questions (attempts to cut down on alcohol use, other persons expressing annoyance, experiencing guilt, early morning drinking) have excellent sensitivity and specificity. Alcohol withdrawal can range from mild to quite severe, with the occurrence of withdrawal seizures or delirium tremens (or both). The medical complications of alcoholism can affect nearly every organ system, but the liver, gastrointestinal tract, pancreas, and central nervous system are particularly susceptible to the effects of alcohol.

Table 20-2 Drugs Grouped According to Their Perceived Effects

Uppers	Downers	Multiple effects
Cocaine	Alcohol	Cannabis
Amphetamines	Opioids	Hallucinogens
Caffeine	Benzodiazepines	Inhalants
Nicotine	Sedative-hypnotics	Phencyclidine
	Barbiturates	(PCP)

- Increased γ-glutamyltransferase level and mean corpuscular volume can identify up to 90% of alcoholics.
- It is not practical to rely on laboratory data alone to diagnose alcoholism.
- Medical complications of alcoholism can affect nearly every organ system.

Benzodiazepines, Sedative-Hypnotics, and Anxiolytics

Benzodiazepines, sedative-hypnotics, and anxiolytics are widely prescribed in many areas of medicine, so abuse and dependence are often iatrogenic. However, five characteristics may help distinguish medical use from nonmedical use. Intent—What is the purpose of the use? Effect—What is the effect on the user's life? Control—Is the use controlled by the user only or does a physician share in the control? Legality—Is the use of the drug legal or illegal? Medical drug use is legal. Pattern—In what settings is the drug used?

These same characteristics may also be used to distinguish between the medical and nonmedical use of opioids. Withdrawal from use of benzodiazepines and barbiturates, in particular, may be serious because of the increased risk of withdrawal seizures.

- Withdrawal of the use of benzodiazepines and barbiturates, in particular, can be serious because of the increased risk of withdrawal seizures.

PSYCHOPHARMACOLOGY

The use of a pharmacologic treatment for a psychiatric disorder or the use of psychoactive medications in other disorders is a decision that generally is made after considering multiple factors in the case. Medication alone is rarely the sole treatment for a psychiatric disorder but rather a component of a comprehensive treatment plan. Because psychoactive medications are used in various circumstances for many different indications, the major groups of these medications—antidepressants, antipsychotics, antimanic agents, anxiolytics, and sedative drugs—are discussed below in general terms rather than for treatment of specific disorders. The choice of a medication usually is based on its side-effect profile and the clinical profile of the patient. There are many effective drugs in each of the major groups, but they differ in terms of pharmacokinetics, side effects, and available routes of administration.

- Medication alone is rarely the sole treatment for a psychiatric disorder.
- The choice of a medication generally is based on its side-effect profile and the clinical profile of the patient.

Antidepressants

In the United States, more than 30 antidepressants are available to treat depression, and several others have been approved by the U.S. Food and Drug Administration exclusively for certain indications, such as obsessive-compulsive disorder (clomipramine and fluvoxamine) and attention-deficit/hyperactivity disorder (atomoxetine). First-generation antidepressants include tricyclic agents and monoamine oxidase inhibitors. Newer generation antidepressants are not easily grouped by their chemical structure or function; they are instead a diverse group of compounds. Currently, the most widely used of this group of agents are SSRIs.

Although older generation antidepressants were effective in treating depression, they were associated with important side effects that limited their use in certain groups of patients, especially those with other medical problems. In particular, tricyclic agents are associated with orthostatic hypotension, anticholinergic side effects, and cardiac conduction defects. Monoamine oxidase inhibitors are effective antidepressants but require special dietary restrictions and attention to interactions with other medications. Because the newer generation antidepressants have fewer potential side effects and drug interactions than older agents, they are prescribed more widely, but they are not optimal for all patients.

- Tricyclics—tertiary amines (including amitriptyline, doxepin, imipramine, and trimipramine), and secondary amines (including desipramine, nortriptyline, and protriptyline).
- Monoamine oxidase inhibitors—pargyline, phenelzine, and tranylcypromine.
- SSRIs—citalopram, fluoxetine, fluvoxamine, paroxetine, and sertraline.
- Norepinephrine reuptake inhibitors—atomoxetine.
- Newer generation antidepressants—bupropion, nefazodone, trazodone, and venlafaxine.
- Isolated enantiomer of an SSRI—escitaolpram (S-enantiomer [single isomer] of citalopram)

The mechanism of action of virtually all antidepressants is their effect, to varying degrees, on the noradrenergic and serotonergic systems of the central nervous system. Various antidepressant agents block the reuptake of norepinephrine or serotonin (or both), thus increasing the amount of these neurotransmitters at the synapse. Bupropion, an example of an antidepressant with insignificant serotonergic action, instead works through dopaminergic and not adrenergic systems. The ability of this agent to increase levels of dopamine in the synaptic cleft likely underlies its unique efficacy in nicotine dependence.

Monoamine oxidase inhibitors block the catabolism of several biogenic amines (norepinephrine, serotonin, tyramine, phenylephrine, and dopamine), thereby increasing the amount of these neurotransmitters available for synaptic release.

- Antidepressants affect the noradenergic and serotonergic systems of the central nervous system.
- Bupropion acts on dopamine and norepinephrine neurotransmission and not serotonin
- Monoamine oxidase inhibitors block the catabolism of several biogenic amines.

Antidepressants have been approved primarily for use in the treatment of depression. However, they are useful in several other disorders, including panic disorder, obsessive-compulsive disorder, generalized anxiety disorder, social anxiety disorder, post-traumatic stress disorder, enuresis, bulimia, and attention-deficit/hyperactivity disorder. Noradrenergic antidepressants such as tricyclic agents and venlafaxine can be beneficial for the treatment of chronic pain and migraines. Theoretically, SSRIs have potential for these conditions as well but as yet have not been tested extensively.

Because antidepressants are widely used, familiarity with the basic facts of their use, side effects, and drug interactions may be helpful. The choice of which antidepressant to use is often made on the basis of the side-effect profile of the drug and the clinical presentation of the patient. The side effects of the major groups of antidepressant agents are listed in Table 20-3. A complete trial of antidepressant medication consists of 6 weeks of therapeutic doses before considering refractoriness. If improvement has occurred with the initial trial of the

Table 20-3 Side Effects of the Major Groups of Antidepressants

---

Orthostatic hypotension—The cardiovascular side effect that most commonly results in serious morbidity, especially in the elderly

Anticholinergic effects—Dry mouth, blurred vision, urinary retention; beware of these side effects in patients with prostatic hypertrophy and narrow-angle glaucoma. Drugs with more anticholinergic side effects also seem to be the more sedating, e.g., tertiary amine tricyclics

Cardiac conduction effects—Most of the tricyclics prolong PR and QRS intervals. Thus, these drugs need to be used with caution in patients with preexisting heart block, such as second-degree heart block or markedly prolonged QRS and QT intervals. The tricyclics are potent antiarrhythmic agents because of their quinidine-like effect. Newer generation antidepressants have considerably fewer cardiac interactions

Sedating types—Tertiary amine tricyclics and trazodone

Potentially more stimulating types—Secondary amine tricyclics, bupropion, fluoxetine, sertraline, and paroxetine

---

medication but the patient's condition has not returned to baseline, it may be worthwhile augmenting therapy with lithium carbonate before changing the medication to another class of antidepressant. After clinical improvement has been noted, the medication may need to be maintained for an extended period. A complete trial of antidepressant medication consists of 6 weeks of therapeutic doses. Another option is to switch to an antidepressant with a different mechanism of action that interacts with different neurochemical pathways.

Monoamine Oxidase Inhibitors

This group of medications is now seldom used because of concerns about drug-drug and drug-food interactions. The mechanism of action is to inhibit irreversibly the enzyme monoamine oxidase A or B, which degrades catecholamines, serotonin, and the neurotransmitter amino acid precursor tyramine. Most clinical concerns about the use of monoamine oxidase inhibitors are related to reactions from the ingestion of tyramine, which is not metabolized because of the inhibition of intestinal monoamine oxidase. Tyramine may act as a false transmitter and displace norepinephrine from synaptic vesicles. Patients should be instructed in a tyramine-restricted diet, especially to avoid aged cheeses, smoked meats, pickled herring, beer, red wine, yeast extracts, fava beans, and overripe bananas and avocadoes. Certain general anesthetics and drugs with sympathomimetic activity should be avoided; patients should beware especially of over-the-counter cough and cold preparations, decongestants, and appetite suppressants. Meperidine (Demerol) is absolutely contraindicated because of its potentially lethal interaction with monoamine oxidase inhibitors.

- Clinical concerns about monoamine oxidase inhibitors: reactions due to ingestion of tyramine, which is not metabolized.
- Tyramine is a false neurotransmitter that displaces norepinephrine from synaptic vesicles.
- Meperidine (Demerol) is absolutely contraindicated because of its potentially lethal interaction with monoamine oxidase inhibitors.

Treatment of hypertensive reactions relies on administering drugs with α-adrenergic blocking properties, such as intravenous administration of phentolamine.

Antipsychotic Agents

Clinically, "atypical" antipsychotic agents are now used widely and are replacing "standard antipsychotics" such as chlorpromazine and haloperidol. The currently available newer generation antipsychotics include aripiprazole, clozapine, olanzapine, quetiapine, risperidone, and ziprasidone.

The choice of medication is based on the patient's clinical situation, side-effect profile of the chosen agent, history of previous response, and issues related to compliance. The prevailing theory about the mechanism of action of these agents is that they cause blockade of postsynaptic dopamine receptors. This is related to both the antipsychotic activity and other side effects, depending on which dopamine pathways in the brain are affected and which of the several types of dopamine receptor is preferentially affected. If the nigrostriatal dopaminergic system (involved with motor activity) is affected, extrapyramidal symptoms may result. Blockade of the dopamine pathways in the pituitary and hypothalamus causes increased release of prolactin and changes in appetite and temperature regulation. The effects of these drugs on the limbic system, midbrain tegmentum, septal nuclei, and mesocortical dopaminergic projections are thought to be responsible for their antipsychotic action. Atypical antipsychotic medications combine dopaminergic and serotonergic antagonism, which appears to minimize extrapyramidal side effects.

- The theory about the mechanism of action of antipsychotic agents is that they cause blockade of postsynaptic dopamine receptors.
- The antipsychotic effects of these agents are due to their actions on the limbic system, midbrain tegmentum, septal nuclei, and mesocortical dopaminergic projections.

Side Effects: Extrapyramidal Reactions

Atypical antipsychotic agents have a lower rate of extrapyramidal side effects. Yet, because these events are still reported occasionally, it is important to recognize these possible complications of therapy. Acute dystonic reactions occur within hours or days after treatment is initiated with antipsychotic drugs. These reactions are characterized by uncontrollable tightening of the face and neck muscles with spasms. The effect on the eyes may cause an oculogyric crisis, and the effect on the laryngeal muscles may cause respiratory or ventilatory difficulties. Treatment is usually with intravenous or intramuscular administration of an anticholinergic agent, followed by the use of an oral anticholinergic agent for a few days.

- Acute dystonic reactions occur within hours or days after treatment is initiated with antipsychotic drugs.
- Reactions include uncontrollable tightening of the face and neck muscles with spasms.
- Treatment: intravenous or intramuscular administration of an anticholinergic agent.

Parkinsonian syndrome has a more gradual onset and can be treated with oral anticholinergic agents or decreased doses of the antipsychotic agent (or both). "Akathisia" is an unpleasant feeling of restlessness and the inability to sit still. It often occurs within days after treatment is initiated with an antipsychotic agent. Akathisia is sometimes mistaken for exacerbation of the psychosis. Treatment, if possible, is to decrease the dose of the antipsychotic agent or to try using a β-adrenergic blocking agent such as propranolol, if not contraindicated.

Tardive dyskinesia has an incidence of 3% to 5% annually and consists of involuntary movements of the face, trunk, or extremities. The most consistent risk factors for its development are long-term use (>6 months) of typical antipsychotics and older age. Prevention is the most important aspect of management because no reliable treatment is available. It is best if treatment with the antipsychotic agent can be discontinued because the dyskinesia is sometimes reversible, although the involuntary movements may increase temporarily.

- Tardive dyskinesia is involuntary movements of the face, trunk, or extremities.
- Prevention is the most important aspect of management.

Neuroleptic malignant syndrome is a potentially life-threatening disorder that may occur after the use of any antipsychotic agent, although it is more common with rapid increases in dosage of high-potency antipsychotic agents. Its clinical presentation is characterized by severe rigidity, fever, leukocytosis, tachycardia, tachypnea, diaphoresis, blood pressure fluctuations, and marked increase in creatine kinase levels because of muscle breakdown. Treatment consists of discontinuing the use of the antipsychotic agent and providing life-support measures (ventilation and cooling). Pharmacologic interventions may include the use of one or both of the following: dantrolene sodium, which is a direct-acting muscle relaxant, or bromocriptine, which is a centrally acting dopamine agonist. Often, one of the most effective treatments is ECT, which likely increases presynaptic dopamine release markedly and this reverses the extreme degree of dopamine receptor blockade present in neuroleptic malignant syndrome.

- Neuroleptic malignant syndrome is potentially life-threatening.
- It may occur after the use of any antipsychotic agent.
- Characteristics include severe rigidity, fever, leukocytosis, tachycardia, tachypnea, diaphoresis, blood pressure fluctuations, and marked increase in creatine kinase levels (from muscle breakdown).

Side effects of antipsychotic agents other than extrapyramidal effects are listed in Table 20-4.

Newer ("Atypical") Antipsychotic Agents

The atypical antipsychotic agents are different from their predecessors in terms of potential mechanisms of action and

Table 20-4   Side Effects of Antipsychotic Agents Aside From Extrapyramidal Effects

---

Anticholinergic

Orthostatic hypotension—related to α-adrenergic receptor blockade

Hyperprolactinemia—gynecomastia possible in men and women, galactorrhea (rare), amenorrhea, weight gain, breast tenderness, decreased libido

Sexual dysfunction

Dermatologic—pigmentary changes in the skin, photosensitivity

Decreased seizure threshold

---

side-effect profiles. They are less likely to cause bothersome extrapyramidal side effects, and their potential for causing tardive dyskinesia may be less. The evidence for the latter will take time to establish because the onset of the symptoms is delayed and the drugs have not been widely used long enough to determine the risk of tardive dyskinesia. Neuroleptic malignant syndrome has been reported to occur with clozapine and risperidone. Clozapine has a 1% to 2% risk of producing agranulocytosis, which is reversible if use of the medication is withdrawn immediately. Because of this serious potential side effect, a specific requirement is that blood cell counts be made regularly (weekly for the first 6-18 months and then every 2 weeks). Similar to their predecessors, increased levels of prolactin are associated with risperidone and notable weight gain may occur with olanzapine. These newer generation antipsychotic agents are also considerably more expensive than their predecessors. Currently, they are not available in parenteral form, which makes them less versatile in the case of psychiatric emergencies.

Antianxiety Medications

These drugs are used most appropriately to treat time-limited anxiety or insomnia related to an identifiable stress or change in sleep cycle. If used long term (>2-3 months), benzodiazepines and related substances should be tapered rather than be discontinued abruptly to avoid any of the three "discontinuation syndromes," which include relapse, rebound, and withdrawal.

"Relapse" is the return of the original anxiety symptoms, often after weeks to months. "Rebound" is the intensification of the original symptoms that usually lasts several days and appears within hours to days after abrupt cessation of drug use. "Withdrawal" may be mild to severe and includes autonomic and central nervous system symptoms that are different from the original presenting symptoms of the disorder.

Benzodiazepines are well-absorbed orally but have unpredictable availability with intramuscular use, except for lorazepam. There is great variability in the pharmacokinetics of benzodiazepines. Several of these drugs have metabolites with a long half-life. Therefore, much smaller doses need to be used in the elderly, in patients with cognitive dysfunction, and in children. All these patient groups are prone to paradoxical reactions (anxiety, irritability, aggression, agitation, insomnia), especially patients with known brain damage.

- Benzodiazepines have great variability in their half-life, which directly determines the duration of action and side effects.

Buspirone is a non-benzodiazepine anxiolytic drug whose mechanism of action is well understood. However, the drug has effects on many neurotransmitter systems, especially the serotonergic and dopaminergic systems. Cross-tolerance does not exist between benzodiazepines and buspirone. It generally takes 2 to 3 weeks for the drug to become effective. Patient compliance can be an issue because of the long latency to effectiveness and the need for divided doses daily.

- Buspirone is a non-benzodiazepine anxiolytic drug.
- It takes 2-3 weeks for the drug to become effective.

LITHIUM

For many years, lithium carbonate was the drug of choice for treating bipolar disorders. It may also be effective in patients with recurrent unipolar depression and as an adjunct for maintenance of remission of depression after ECT. Acute manic symptoms usually respond to treatment with lithium within 7 to 10 days. While waiting for this effect, the adjunctive use of antipsychotic agents and benzodiazepines may be helpful. Lithium is well absorbed from the gastrointestinal tract, with peak levels in 1 to 2 hours. Its half-life is about 24 hours. Levels are generally checked 10 to 12 hours after the last dose. Relatively common side effects include resting tremor, diarrhea, polyuria, polydipsia, thirst, and nausea, which is often improved by taking the medication on a full stomach. Lithium is contraindicated in the first trimester of pregnancy because of its potential for causing defects in the developing cardiac system. Renal effects generally can be reversed with discontinuation of lithium therapy. The most noticeable renal effect is the vasopressin-resistant effect leading to impaired concentrating ability and nephrogenic diabetes insipidus with polyuria and polydipsia. Most patients who take lithium develop some polyuria but not all develop more severe manifestations of nephrogenic diabetes insipidus. Renal function should be followed in all patients receiving maintenance lithium therapy. However, whether lithium has severe nephrotoxic effects is a matter of controversy. A hematologic side effect is benign leukocytosis. Hypothyroidism may occur in as many as 20% of patients taking lithium because of the direct inhibitory effects on thyroid hormone production or increased antithyroid antibodies.

- Lithium carbonate: the common side effects are hand tremor, diarrhea, polyuria, polydipsia, thirst, and nausea.
- Renal effects generally can be reversed with discontinuation of lithium therapy.
- The most noticeable renal effect is impaired concentrating ability.
- Hypothyroidism occurs in as many as 20% of patients taking lithium.

Because the range between the therapeutic and toxic levels of lithium in the plasma is narrow, patients and physicians should be familiar with conditions that may increase or decrease lithium levels and with the signs and symptoms of lithium toxicity so it can be recognized and treated promptly (Tables 20-5 and 20-6).

Other Mood Stabilizers

The anticonvulsant valproic acid is effective in the treatment of acute manic episodes and for prophylactic maintenance therapy of bipolar disorders. Because of fewer side effects and a wider therapeutic index (reducing potential toxicity), valproic acid is now the most commonly prescribed mood stabilizer. The mechanism of action for its mood-stabilizing effects is not clear. The side effect of most concern with valproic acid is hepatotoxicity, which has occurred mostly in children receiving treatment with multiple anticonvulsants. Carbamazepine has also been used in this context, and because

Table 20-5   Conditions That Increase or Decrease Lithium Levels in the Plasma

Increase levels	Decrease levels
Dehydration	Increased caffeine consumption
Overheating and increased perspiration with exercise and/or hot weather	Theophylline
Nonsteroidal anti-inflammatory drugs	
Thiazide diuretics	
Angiotensin-converting enzyme inhibitors	
Certain antibiotics—tetracycline, spectinomycin, and metronidazole	

Table 20-6   Signs and Symptoms of Lithium Toxicity

Mild-to-moderate toxicity (plasma level, 1.5-2.0 mEq/L)	Moderate-to-severe toxicity (plasma level, 2.0-2.5 mEq/L)	Severe toxicity (plasma level, >2.5 mEq/L)
Vomiting	Persistent nausea and vomiting	Generalized seizures
Abdominal pain	Anorexia	Oliguria and renal failure
Dry mouth	Blurred vision	Death
Ataxia	Muscle fasciculations	
Slurred speech	Hyperactive deep tendon reflexes	
Nystagmus	Delirium	
Muscle weakness	Convulsions	
	Electroencephalographic changes	
	Stupor and coma	
	Circulatory system failure	
	Decreased blood pressure	
	Cardiac arrhythmias	
	Conduction abnormalities	

Modified from Silver JM, Hales RE, Yudofsky SC: Biological therapies for mental disorders. *In* Clinical Psychiatry for Medical Students. Edited by A Stoudemire. Philadelphia, JB Lippincott Company, 1990, pp 459-496. By permission of publisher.

its chemical structure is similar to that of tricyclic antidepressants, it has a quinidine-like effect. Other anticonvulsants such as gabapentin and lamotrigine are also being investigated as mood-stabilizing agents.

- Valproic acid is effective for the treatment of acute mania and maintenance therapy of bipolar disorders.

ELECTROCONVULSIVE THERAPY

ECT is the most effective treatment for severely depressed patients, especially those with psychotic features. It is also helpful in treating catatonia and mania and may be used in children and adults. Also, ECT can be administered safely to pregnant women, provided fetal monitoring is available. It may be effective in patients with overlapping depression and Parkinson disease or dementia. ECT is administered with the patient under barbiturate anesthesia, with succinylcholine or a similar muscle relaxant to minimize peripheral manifestations of the seizure. An anticholinergic agent such as atropine is generally given to decrease secretions and to prevent bradycardia caused by central stimulation of the vagus nerve. A usual course of treatment is 6 to 12 sessions given over 2 to 4 weeks. Therapy is often initiated with unilateral, nondominant electrode placement to minimize memory loss. If satisfactory results cannot be obtained with this method, bilateral electrode placement is used.

- ECT is the most effective treatment for severely depressed patients, especially those with psychotic features.

- It is also helpful in treating catatonia and mania.
- ECT can be administered to pregnant women.
- It may be helpful in cases of overlapping depression and Parkinson disease or dementia.
- Mechanism of action—ECT induces rapid changes in several transmitter-receptor systems simultaneously, particularly acetylcholine, norepinephrine, dopamine, and serotonin.

ECT no longer has any absolute contraindications, although it has several relative contraindications. Previously, the only absolute contraindication was the presence of an intracranial space-occupying lesion and increased intracranial pressure. Serious complications or mortality is generally reported as less than 1 per 10,000, which makes this therapy one of the safest interventions that uses general anesthesia. Morbidity and mortality usually are due to cardiovascular complications, such as arrhythmia, myocardial infarction, or hypotension. The major risks are those associated with the brief general anesthesia. Medical evaluations performed before ECT is administered should pay particular attention to cardiovascular function, pulmonary function, electrolyte balance, neurologic disorder (epilepsy), and the patient's previous experiences with anesthesia.

- ECT no longer has any absolute contraindications.
- It has several relative contraindications.
- Morbidity and mortality are usually due to cardiovascular complications.

Psychiatry Pharmacy Review
Carrie A. Krieger, PharmD

Review of Antipsychotic Agents

Drug	Toxic/adverse effects	Comments

Typical antipsychotic agents
Phenothiazines
Chlorpromazine
Fluphenazine
Mesoridazine
Perphenazine
Thioridazine
Trifluoperazine
Nonphenothiazines
Haloperidol
Loxapine
Molindone
Thiothixene
Atypical antipsychotic agents
Aripiprazole
Clozapine
Olanzapine
Quetiapine
Risperidone
Ziprasidone
	Extrapyramidal side effects—dystonia, pseudoparkinsonism, akathisia, tardive dyskinesia
	Neuroleptic malignant syndrome
	Sedation—most frequent with clozapine
	Anticholinergic effects
	Orthostatic hypotension—more frequent with thioridazine and clozapine
	ECG changes—thioridazine, clozapine, risperidone, ziprasidone
	Galactorrhea, amenorrhea, gynecomastia, weight gain, sexual dysfunction
	Seizures—higher risk with clozapine (dose-related)
	Photosensitivity—more common with phenothiazines, haloperidol, thiothixene, risperidone
	Hypersalivation—clozapine
	Pigmentary retinopathy—thioridazine
		Drug interactions—generally minor, usually involve additive CNS or sedative effects, common to all the following:
		  Anticholinergics
		  Anticonvulsants (carbamazepine, phenobarbital, phenytoin)
		  Antidepressants (selective serotonin reuptake inhibitors, tricyclic antidepressants)
		  β-Blockers
		  Cimetidine
		  Ethanol
		  Quinolone antibiotics
		  Smoking
		Thioridazine—contraindicated for patients with QT interval >450 ms & coadministration of other drugs that cause QT-interval prolongation
		Clozapine—requires strict leukocyte monitoring because of risk of agranulocytosis
		Quetiapine—recommend slit-lamp exam at baseline & 6-month intervals because of increased risk of cataracts
		Ziprasidone—contraindicated for patients with QT-interval prolongation, recent acute MI, or uncompensated heart failure

CNS, central nervous system; ECG, electrocardiographic; MI, myocardial infarction.

Psychiatry Pharmacy Review (continued)
Julie L. Cunningham, PharmD

Review of Antidepressants*†

Drug	Toxic/adverse effects	Comments
Bupropion (Wellbutrin)	Can cause agitation, insomnia, psychosis, confusion, weight loss	Contraindicated for patients with seizure or history of anorexia, bulimia, MAOIs Low incidence of sexual dysfunction and minimal drug interactions Available as SR and XL formulations

MAOIs
  Phenelzine (Nardil)
  Tranylcypromine
    (Parnate)
	Associated with weight gain, orthostatic hypotension, sexual dysfunction
	Hypertensive crisis may occur with tyramine-containing foods
		Limited use because of drug/food interactions
		Contraindicated with use of other antidepressants, ethanol, meperidine, general anesthesia

Mirtazapine (Remeron)	Low risk of sexual dysfunction May cause weight gain & increase serum cholesterol & triglycerides Can lower seizure threshold Incidence of agranulocytosis	Avoid with use of MAOIs, clozapine, carbamazepine Unique mechanism of action & may be beneficial for resistant cases Lower doses more sedating than higher doses
Nefazodone (Serzone)	Low risk of sexual dysfunction Some sedative, orthostatic hypotensive & anticholinergic effects	May improve symptoms of anxiety & insomnia Contraindicated with use of triazolam, alprazolam, MAOIs, & cisapride because nefazadone inhibits their metabolism

SSRIs
  Citalopram (Celexa)
  Fluoxetine (Prozac)
  Paroxetine (Paxil)
  Sertraline (Zoloft)
  Escitalopram
    (Lexapro)
	Can exacerbate insomnia, GI upset, headache
	Can cause sexual dysfunction, tremors, & rare extrapyramidal symptoms
	Hyponatremia/SIADH
	May impair platelet aggregation
		No significant anticholinergic effects, minimal weight gain, relatively safe in overdose
		Avoid with use of MAOIs & migraine agents (may cause serotonin syndrome)
		Fluoxetine—long half-life & active metabolites, available in weekly formulation
		Paroxetine—also available in CR formulation

Tricyclic antidepressants
  Tertiary amines
    Amitriptyline
     (Elavil)
    Imipramine
     (Tofranil)
    Doxepin
     (Sinequan)
  Secondary amines
    Nortriptyline
     (Pamelor)
    Desipramine
     (Norpramin)
	Potentially fatal in overdose
	Increased risk of seizures, conduction abnormalities, hyponatremia/SIADH
	May cause anticholinergic effects, weight gain, sedation, sexual dysfunction, orthostatic hypotension
		Secondary amines generally have milder side effects
		Blood levels are useful for monitoring
		Contraindicated with use of MAOIs & for patients with recent MI
		SSRIs may inhibit metabolism & cause toxicity

Psychiatry Pharmacy Review (continued)

Review of Antidepressants*† (continued)

Drug	Toxic/adverse effects	Comments
Venlafaxine (Effexor)	Can cause insomnia, GI upset, headache, sexual dysfunction, sustained increase in blood pressure (especially higher doses) Minimal weight gain	No significant anticholinergic effects May be beneficial for resistant cases (higher doses) Avoid with use of MAOIs
Mood stabilizer Lithium (Lithobid, Eskalith)	Hand tremor, nausea, polyuria, polydipsia, diarrhea, weight gain, hypothyroidism	Adjust for kidney function Monitor trough levels Use cautiously with drugs that affect sodium—diuretics, NSAIDs, ACEIs (lithium toxicity) Caffeine may decrease lithium level Contraindicated in severe cardiovascular or kidney disease, dehydration, sodium depletion

ACEI, angiotensin-converting enzyme inhibitor; CR, continuous release; GI, gastrointestinal; MAOI, monoamine oxidase inhibitor; MI, myocardial infarction; NSAID, nonsteroidal anti-inflammatory drug; SIADH, syndrome of inappropriate antidiuretic hormone; SR, sustained release; SSRI, selective serotonin reuptake inhibitor; XL, extended release.

*Avoid abrupt discontinuation because all antidepressants may have withdrawal effects.

†All antidepressants have the potential to cause switch to mania in patients with bipolar disorder.

Psychiatry Pharmacy Review (continued)
  Kari L. Beierman, PharmD

Review of Anxiolytics

Drug	Toxic/adverse effects	Drug interactions	Comments
Benzodiazepines	Tachycardia, chest pain CNS effects—drowsiness, fatigue, light-headedness, insomnia, headache Rash Decreased libido GI effects—nausea, vomiting, diarrhea, increased/decreased appetite, decreased salivation Blurred vision	Mild, usually involve additive CNS effects Alcohol Sedative-hypnotics Cimetidine MAOIs Carbamazepine & rifampin may enhance metabolism of benzodiazepines	Benzodiazepines with active metabolites need to be dosed carefully, especially in the elderly Doses of all benzodiazepines may need adjusting for hepatic failure Avoid abrupt discontinuation if used long-term Grapefruit juice may increase serum levels & adverse effects
Buspirone (BuSpar)	CNS effects—dizziness, drowsiness, light-headedness, restlessness Nausea	SSRIs & trazodone may cause serotonin syndrome MAOIs—increased blood pressure Erythromycin, clarithromycin, ketoconazole, itraconazole—increased concentration of buspirone	Non-benzodiazepine anxiolytic Adjust dosage for hepatic/renal failure

CNS, central nervous system; GI, gastrointestinal; MAOI, monoamine oxidase inhibitor; SSRI, selective serotonin reuptake inhibitor.

Review of Benzodiazepines

Drug	Metabolite (active/inactive)	Comments
Alprazolam	Inactive	Used commonly to treat panic attacks
Chlordiazepoxide	Active	Also used for alcohol withdrawal symptoms
Clonazepam	Inactive	Used mainly for seizure control
Clorazepate	Active	Also used as an anticonvulsant
Diazepam	Active (very long half-life)	Also used for sedation, as a muscle relaxant, for treatment of status epilepticus
Estazolam	Inactive	Hypnotic, good choice for elderly patients because of lack of active metabolites
Flurazepam	Active	Short-term treatment of insomnia
Lorazepam	Inactive	May be given intramuscularly
Midazolam	Inactive	Given intravenously only, used mainly for sedation before procedures
Oxazepam	Inactive	May also be used as an anticonvulsant
Quazepam	Active	Long-acting, treats insomnia
Temazepam	Inactive	Most often used to treat panic attacks, insomnia, sleep latency
Triazolam	Inactive	Short-term treatment of insomnia, short onset of action

QUESTIONS

Multiple Choice (choose the one best answer)

1. A 32-year-old woman has a 4-year history of frequent and severe tension headaches. She has no other depression or medical problems. Periodically, she goes to the emergency department and receives an injection of meperidine. Which medication is best suited for her needs?
   a. Fluoxetine
   b. Nefazodone
   c. Nortriptyline
   d. Phenelzine
   e. Sertraline

2. A 55-year-old man has been depressed for 13 years. He describes ongoing sadness with a sense of helplessness about his career. He states that he does not have problems with sleep, appetite, or energy level. Many years ago, he completed his training as an architect. He has been hired numerous times but has been unable to keep any job for longer than 3 months. Typically, he has been asked to leave because of estranged relationships with coworkers. He denies any drug or alcohol problems. The preferred management plan would include:
   a. Electroconvulsive therapy
   b. Returning to school
   c. Methylphenidate
   d. Psychotherapy
   e. Lithium

3. A 19-year-old college student is brought in by the police. He has been found yelling obscenities outside his dormitory. He is agitated and describes hearing voices. He expects he will be harmed in some way. His parents report no previous episodes of this type of behavior. On laboratory testing, the most likely abnormality is:
   a. Positive phencyclidine screen
   b. Positive lorazepam screen
   c. Positive opioid screen
   d. Positive zolpidem screen
   e. Positive γ-hydroxybutyrate screen

4. A 32-year-old woman has a history of multiple drug overdoses. She reports that for the past 2 months she has been having depressed mood, excessive sleep, binge eating, frequent fights with her boyfriend, self-critical attitude, and suicidal ideation. The optimal treatment plan is psychotherapy in combination with:
   a. Sertraline
   b. Diazepam

   c. Desipramine
   d. Phenelzine
   e. Lithium

5. A 45-year-old unmarried man is very meticulous in hoarding many possessions. He has not thrown out any mail, newspapers, or periodicals for more than 7 years. He lives alone and his house is filled with stacks of material. He keeps this on hand in case he needs to refer to it and obtain some information. He recognizes that his house is now filled with piles of paper, but he finds that he cannot toss any away. His concern is that if he discards any particular item, he would then regret it because he would not be able to access the valuable information when needed. His neighbors are beginning to complain because some of the stacks of material are now visible from outside the house. The best treatment would include:
   a. Behavioral therapy and bupropion
   b. Insight-oriented psychotherapy and fluoxetine
   c. Electroconvulsive therapy
   d. Behavioral therapy and fluoxetine
   e. Social skills training and nortriptyline

6. A 75-year-old woman presents with a 1-week history of severe insomnia, hyperactivity, pressured speech, flight of ideas, and grandiose delusions. On bedside examination, she demonstrates moderate cognitive impairment. She has congestive heart failure, for which she takes a thiazide, diuretic, and potassium. Her past psychiatric history is remarkable for multiple psychiatric hospitalizations. The preferred medication for this condition is:
   a. Lithium
   b. Carbamazepine
   c. Valporic acid
   d. Electroconvulsive therapy
   e. Donepezil

7. A 34-year-old woman has a long history of medical complaints that include virtually every organ system. She describes herself as being ill since adolescence. She takes a total of 25 prescription and over-the-counter medications, including prednisone and multiple pain medications. A comprehensive assessment provides little evidence of objective disease. Which one of the following interventions should you pursue?
   a. Transfer her care to a psychiatrist
   b. Request that she see your partner
   c. Admit her to the hospital
   d. Recommend that she visit the emergency department as needed
   e. Schedule monthly visits to the office

ANSWERS

1. Answer c.

Antidepressants that increase the level of norepinephrine in the brain have been shown to be useful in patients who have chronic pain. Although most of the research studies have examined amitriptyline, nortriptyline, and desipramine, newer studies have investigated the antidepressant venlafaxine. Generally, medications that selectively increase serotonin levels, such as selective serotonin reuptake inhibitors, are not as useful for chronic pain. The issue to consider is whether the patient appears to have clear depressive symptoms—pain being one of these. In this situation, any antidepressant probably would be effective for treating the depressive symptoms, although medications that selectively increase norepinephrine levels have been shown to be most effective in treating pain syndromes. A monoamine oxidase inhibitor such as phenelzine should absolutely be avoided if there is any possibility that the patient may receive meperidine, because of the serotonin syndrome caused by a probable drug-drug interaction.

2. Answer d.

The patient's depressed mood has lasted longer than 2 years. He has interpersonal difficulties that have led to his having difficulties succeeding professionally. Currently, no other depressive symptoms suggest a major depressive episode. This scenario is most consistent with a patient who has dysthymia, a chronic milder form of depression. Dysthymia can coexist with episodes of major depression, but in these cases more symptoms suggesting poor sleep, poor appetite, or other issues would be present. The preferred treatment is psychotherapy to help the patient examine his perception of himself and others. Sometimes antidepressants can be beneficial, especially if the patient has a history of major depressive episodes, a family history of mood disorders, or the early-onset form of dysthymia. Psychostimulants such as methylphenidate are used occasionally to treat attention-deficit/hyperactivity disorder. Although this may be a reason for a patient to have persisting vocational problems, there is not enough information in this case vignette to support the use of these medications, which may lead to physical dependence because they are amphetamine-like compounds.

3. Answer a.

When patients present with a first episode of markedly disturbed thoughts and behavior, a thorough diagnostic assessment should be made. Many psychotic episodes seen in medical settings are associated with the use of recreational or prescription drugs. The symptoms of drug-induced psychotic reactions can be very similar to those seen in chronic psychotic disorders. This college student has a positive phencyclidine screen, and this drug can cause agitation, hallucinations, and delusions. The other drugs listed (lorazepam, opiods, and zolpidem) are all central nervous system depressants and would not cause agitation or psychosis when patients are in an intoxicated state. If these drug levels were negative, it could indicate drug withdrawal, in which case agitation and psychosis could be expected. γ-Hydroxybutyrate is a newer recreational drug that typically causes sedation with intoxication rather than agitation; currently, it is not easily detected with blood or urine screening tests.

4. Answer a.

This patient appears to have an atypical depression. The most appropriate therapy would be sertraline, a selective serotonin reuptake inhibitor, which is relatively safe even in overdose because of its lack of effect on cardiac conduction and seizure threshold. Optimal treatment would be a combination of medication and psychotherapy. Outpatient psychotherapy alone is not sufficient for this severely ill patient. Hospitalization or partial hospitalization may be a reasonable consideration when the patient is in crisis.

5. Answer d.

Both behavioral therapy and antidepressants that increase serotonin levels in the central nervous system are effective in treating obsessive-compulsive disorder. Electroconvulsive therapy, insight-oriented psychotherapy, and antidepressants that act primarily on neurotransmitters other than serotonin have not been shown to be as therapeutic for this condition.

6. Answer c.

The diagnosis of bipolar mood disorder appears clear even in the setting of a possible cognitive disorder. This patient needs long-term therapy with a mood-stabilizing medication. With the patient's need for diuretics, potential fluid and nutrition shifts, and possible medication errors because of memory problems, valproic acid is the preferred mood stabilizer. It has a wider therapeutic index than either lithium or carbamazepine. Electroconvulsive therapy could be effective in the short term but is difficult to administer long term for maintaining normal mood.

7. Answer e.

Although choices a and b may be attractive, they are likely unacceptable to a patient with somatization disorder (and to the physician's partner). Hospital or emergency department care will reinforce the patient's identity as a medically ill person, deflect attention from her suspected underlying emotional needs, and not be cost-effective. Scheduled monthly office visits have been demonstrated to be most reassuring to the patient and to reduce polypharmacy, minimize repetitive diagnostic testing, and overall to be more cost-effective. Ideally, a consulting psychiatrist will assist in managing a patient with this difficult disorder in an outpatient setting. Most patients with this disorder refuse to see a psychiatrist in place of their primary care or specialty care provider.

CHAPTER 21

PULMONARY DISEASES

John G. Park, M.D.
Timothy R. Aksamit, M.D.
Karen L. Swanson, D.O.
Charles F. Thomas, Jr., M.D.

PART I
John G. Park, M.D.

SYMPTOMS AND SIGNS

Cough

"Cough" is an explosive expiration that clears and protects the airways. It is one of the most common presenting complaints encountered in an outpatient practice. The coughing act is under both voluntary and involuntary control. The latter is the cough reflex, which has five components: cough receptors, afferent nerves, cough center (medulla), efferent nerves, and effector organs. The afferent limb of the cough reflex includes the sensory branches of the trigeminal, glossopharyngeal, and vagus nerves. Inflammatory, mechanical, chemical, or thermal stimulation of the receptors and sensory pathways can trigger cough. The efferent limb includes the recurrent laryngeal and spinal nerves that innervate the expiratory and laryngotracheobronchial musculature. Lesions in the nose, ears, pharynx, larynx, bronchi, lungs, pleura, or abdominal viscera can cause cough.

- Cough is one of the most common symptoms in an outpatient practice.
- Lesions in the nose, ears, pharynx, larynx, bronchi, lungs, pleura, or abdominal viscera can cause cough.
- Cough can be the presenting manifestation or the only manifestation of asthma.

"Chronic cough" is cough that lasts 3 weeks or longer without an obvious cause such as cigarette smoking. The most common causes of chronic cough are postinfectious (viral, *Mycoplasma*, *Chlamydia pneumoniae* TWAR, or *Bordetella pertussis*), postnasal drip, asthma, and gastroesophageal reflux. Connective tissue diseases such as giant cell arteritis, rheumatoid

bronchiolitis, and Sjögren syndrome may also present with cough. Cough is a complication in up to 10% of patients who take angiotensin-converting enzyme inhibitors (ACEIs). Angiotensin-converting enzyme (ACE) receptor blockers are much less likely to produce cough. About one-half of the patients with persistent cough may have more than one cause for the cough. Initial diagnostic testing may include computed tomography (CT) of the sinuses and ear-nose-throat (ENT) consultation, sputum analysis, methacholine inhalation challenge, 24-hour esophageal pH monitoring, or esophagography. If no chest radiographic (CXR) abnormalities are detected, bronchoscopy has a low (4%) diagnostic yield. In cough syncope, a hard cough produces increased intrathoracic pressure, which decreases cardiac output and cerebral perfusion.

- Postnasal drip, asthma, reflux, chronic obstructive pulmonary disease, and recent infection account for 80%-90% of cases of chronic cough.
- ACEIs cause cough in 6%-10% of patients.
- Up to 50% of patients may have more than one cause for chronic cough.
- Bronchoscopy: low diagnostic yield if CXR is normal.
- Complications of cough: cough syncope, rib fracture, pneumothorax.

Sputum

Purulent sputum is found in bronchiectasis and lung abscess. The sputum is frothy pink in pulmonary edema. Expectoration of bronchial casts, mucous plugs, or thin strings occurs in asthma, bronchopulmonary aspergillosis, and mucoid impaction syndrome. Plastic bronchitis is the formation of thick bronchial casts in asthma, bronchopulmonary aspergillosis, and other conditions. Bronchorrhea (expectoration of thin serous fluid >100 mL daily) occurs in 20% of patients with diffuse alveolar cell carcinoma.

- Bronchorrhea is uncommon in diffuse alveolar cell carcinoma.
- The most common cause of broncholithiasis: histoplasmosis.
- Sputum analysis may identify eosinophils, Charcot-Leyden crystals, and Curschmann spirals in patients with asthma.

Hemoptysis

"Hemoptysis" is the expectoration of blood or blood-streaked sputum that originates below the level of the larynx. "Pseudohemoptysis" is expectoration of blood previously aspirated into the airways or lungs from the gastrointestinal tract, nose, or supraglottic areas. Bronchial arterial bleeding occurs in chronic bronchitis, bronchiectasis, malignancies, and broncholithiasis and with the presence of foreign bodies. Pulmonary arterial bleeding occurs in pulmonary arteriovenous malformations, fungus ball, tumors, vasculitis, pulmonary hypertension, and lung abscess. Pulmonary capillary bleeding occurs in mitral stenosis, left ventricular failure, pulmonary infarction, vasculitis, Goodpasture syndrome, and idiopathic pulmonary hemosiderosis. Airway-vessel fistula (e.g., tracheoinnominate) can cause massive hemoptysis (>200 mL/24 hours).

- History, examination, and CXR findings are important in the diagnosis of hemoptysis.
- Common cause of streaky hemoptysis: acute exacerbation of chronic bronchitis.
- The cause of death in massive hemoptysis is asphyxiation, not exsanguination.

Dyspnea

"Dyspnea" is the subjective awareness of breathlessness. It usually is the result of increased work of breathing. Other mechanisms include abnormal activation of respiratory centers, voluntary hyperventilation, and Cheyne-Stokes breathing. Dyspnea may be due to cardiopulmonary disease or disorders of the skeletal (e.g., kyphoscoliosis), endocrine, metabolic, neurologic, or hematologic systems. Other causes are physiologic dyspnea of pregnancy, drugs, psychogenic, deconditioning, and obesity. The grades of severity are based on the New York Heart Association classification: grade 0, no dyspnea except with strenuous exercise; grade 1, slight dyspnea on hurrying on a level surface or walking up a hill; grade 2, dyspnea while walking on a level surface and being unable to keep up with peers and having to stop to catch breath; grade 3, dyspnea on walking 100 yards or after a few minutes and the need to stop for breath; grade 4, dyspnea on dressing or undressing

or minimal exertion; and grade 5, dyspnea at rest. Recent studies have suggested that an increased serum level of brain natriuretic peptide (>100 pg/mL) differentiates dyspnea due to congestive heart failure from that due to pulmonary dysfunction.

- Disease in any organ can cause dyspnea, but the most common cause is cardiopulmonary dysfunction.
- The grades of dyspnea are defined according to the New York Heart Association classification.

A medical history, physical examination, CXR, electrocardiography (ECG), complete blood count, and pulmonary function tests (PFTs) are required for most patients. Arterial blood gases and cardiopulmonary physiologic testing may also be required. "Tachypnea" is more than 20 breaths/min, and "bradypnea" is fewer than 10 breaths/min. "Orthopnea" is dyspnea in the supine posture, as in congestive heart failure, bilateral diaphragmatic paralysis, severe chronic obstructive pulmonary disease (COPD), asthma, sleep apnea, or severe reflux. "Trepopnea" is dyspnea in the lateral decubitus position, as in tumors of the main bronchi, unilateral pleural effusion, or after pneumonectomy. "Platypnea" is dyspnea in the upright posture and is due to an increased right-to-left shunt in lung bases; it is seen in liver disease, severe lung fibrosis, or after pneumonectomy. "Paroxysmal nocturnal dyspnea" is nocturnal episodes of dyspnea, resulting in frequent waking up (associated with pulmonary edema and asthma).

Chest Pain

Pulmonary causes of chest pain are often difficult to distinguish from cardiac and other causes. Tightness of the chest and dyspnea are also described as "chest pain" by patients. Pleuritic pain is encountered in pleuritis, pleuropericarditis, pericarditis, pneumothorax, pleural effusion, mediastinitis, pulmonary embolism, pulmonary infarction, esophageal disease, aortic dissection, and chest wall trauma. Subdiaphragmatic diseases that produce chest pain include pancreatitis, cholecystitis, and colonic distention.

Cyanosis

Cyanosis, the bluish discoloration of the skin and mucous membranes that appears when the capillary content of reduced hemoglobin is greater than 5 g/dL, may be difficult to detect clinically. The causes of central cyanosis are severe hypoxia (PaO_2 is usually <55 mm Hg), anatomical right-to-left shunt, mild hypoxia with polycythemia, shock, and abnormal hemoglobin. Methemoglobinemia and sulfhemoglobinemia, argyria (from silver nitrate), and hemochromatosis cause pseudocyanosis. Anemia does not cause cyanosis. Peripheral cyanosis results from decreased peripheral perfusion with increased oxygen extraction.

- Cyanosis occurs when reduced hemoglobin is >5 g/dL.
- Central cyanosis should be distinguished from peripheral cyanosis.
- Polycythemia vera causes "red cyanosis."
- Methemoglobinemia and hemochromatosis: "pseudocyanosis."
- Cherry-red flush (not cyanosis) is caused by carboxyhemoglobinemia.

Clubbing

"Clubbing" is the bulbous enlargement of the distal segment of a digit (fingers or toes) caused by increased soft tissue mass. Its mechanisms are neurogenic, humoral/hormonal, hereditary, and idiopathic. Common causes for CLUBBING include: **C** (cyanotic heart diseases, cystic fibrosis), **L** (lung cancer, lung abscess), **U** (ulcerative colitis), **B** (bronchiectasis), **B** (benign mesothelioma), **I** (infective endocarditis, idiopathic pulmonary fibrosis, idiopathic, inherited), **N** (neurogenic tumors), and **G** (gastrointestinal diseases, e.g., cirrhosis and regional enteritis). Clubbing can be the presenting manifestation of any of the above entities.

- Clubbing may precede other clinical features of lung cancer.
- Common causes: pulmonary fibrosis, congenital heart disease with right-to-left shunt, cystic fibrosis, and idiopathic.

Hypertrophic Pulmonary Osteoarthropathy

Hypertrophic pulmonary osteoarthropathy (HPO) is characterized by clubbing, painful periosteal hypertrophy of long bones, and symmetrical arthralgias of large joints (usually knees, elbows, and wrists). Other features include gynecomastia, fever, and an increased erythrocyte sedimentation rate (ESR). The mechanisms of HPO are neurogenic (vagal afferents), hormonal, and idiopathic. The most common cause is bronchogenic carcinoma, usually adenocarcinoma or large cell carcinoma. HPO is an early sign of pulmonary metastasis from nasopharyngeal carcinoma. Clubbing is present in 30% of patients with non–small cell lung cancer; it is more common in women than in men (40% vs. 19%). Radiographs of long bones show thickened and raised periosteum. Bone scans show increased uptake of radionuclide by the affected periosteum. If HPO does not resolve after tumor resection, treatment options include the administration of a somatostatin analogue or ipsilateral vagotomy.

- Common causes of HPO: idiopathic and adenocarcinoma or large cell carcinoma of the lung.
- Radionuclide bone scans show characteristic changes.
- Therapy: resection of the tumor, somatostatin analogue, or ipsilateral vagotomy.

- Typical clinical scenario: An adult with clubbing, pain in the long bones, symmetrical arthralgias of large joints, increased ESR, and fever.

Horner Syndrome

Horner syndrome consists of ipsilateral miosis, anhidrosis, and ptosis on the side of the lesion. It is a complication of a superior sulcus tumor (Pancoast tumor) of the lung.

- Horner syndrome: ipsilateral miosis, anhidrosis, and ptosis.
- Superior sulcus tumor (Pancoast tumor).

Other Signs and Symptoms of Pulmonary Disease

Conjunctival suffusion is seen in severe hypercarbia, superior vena cava syndrome, and conjunctival sarcoidosis. Asterixis is seen in severe acute or subacute hypercarbia. Telangiectasia of the skin and mucous membranes occurs in patients with pulmonary arteriovenous malformation. Skin lesions of various types occur in patients with pulmonary involvement by Langerhans cell granuloma (eosinophilic granuloma or histiocytosis X), tuberous sclerosis, sarcoidosis, or lung cancer.

- Asterixis is seen in severe acute or subacute hypercarbia.
- Mental obtundation is seen with hypercarbia.

HISTORY AND EXAMINATION

An approach to the history and physical examination of patients with pulmonary disease is outlined in Table 21-1. Percussion and auscultation findings associated with various pulmonary conditions are also listed in Table 21-1.

DIAGNOSTIC TESTS

Radiology

Plain CXR, CT, magnetic resonance imaging (MRI), bronchography, pulmonary angiography, and bronchial angiography are among the tests performed in the diagnosis of chest diseases.

Plain Chest Radiography

Internists should become familiar with the interpretation of common abnormalities on a plain CXR. Even normal CXRs should be viewed so that reading CXRs becomes routine. Many of the "radiographic" diagnoses such as pneumothorax, pleural effusion, and lung nodule can be established by CXR. It is essential to correlate clinical and other laboratory data with CXR findings.

It is important to compare the present film with previous films, particularly in assessing the seriousness of a "newly" identified abnormality. A lateral CXR is of most help in identifying retrocardiac and retrodiaphragmatic abnormalities.

- Develop the habit of reading CXRs.
- Obtain earlier CXRs for comparison.

- Lateral CXRs are important in identifying retrocardiac and retrodiaphragmatic abnormalities.

The ability to identify normal radiographic anatomy is essential. A "routine" step-by-step method of interpretation should be developed so that subtle abnormalities are not

Table 21-1 History and Physical Examination of Patients With Pulmonary Disease

History
  Smoking
  Occupational exposure
  Exposure to infected persons or animals
  Hobbies and pets
  Family history of diseases of lung and other organs
  Past malignancy
  Systemic (nonpulmonary) diseases
  Immune status (corticosteroid therapy, chemotherapy,
    cancer)
  History of trauma
  Previous chest radiography
Examination
  Inspection
    Respiratory rate, hoarseness of voice
    Respiratory rhythm (abnormal breathing pattern)
    Accessory muscles in action (FEV_1 <30%)
    Postural dyspnea (orthopnea, platypnea, trepopnea)
    Intercostal retraction
    Paradoxical motions of abdomen/diaphragm
    Cough (type, sputum, blood)
    Wheeze (audible with or without stethoscope)
    Pursed lip breathing/glottic wheeze (patients with
      chronic obstructive pulmonary disease)
    Cyanosis (central vs. peripheral)
    Conjunctival suffusion (CO_2 retention)
    Clubbing
    Thoracic cage (e.g., anteroposterior diameter,
      kyphoscoliosis, pectus)
    Trachea, deviation
    Superior vena cava syndrome

    Asterixis, central nervous system status
    Cardiac impulse, jugular venous pressure, pedal edema
      (signs of cor pulmonale)
  Palpation
    Clubbing
    Lymphadenopathy
    Tibial tenderness (hypertrophic pulmonary
      osteoarthropathy)
    Motion of thoracic cage (hand or tape measure)
    Chest wall tenderness (costochondritis, rib fracture,
      pulmonary embolism)
    Tracheal deviation, tenderness
    Tactile (vocal) fremitus
    Subcutaneous emphysema
    Succussion splash (effusion, air-fluid level in thorax)
  Percussion
    Thoracic cage (dullness, resonance)
    Diaphragmatic motion (normal, 5-7 cm)
    Upper abdomen (liver)
  Auscultation
    Tracheal auscultation
    Normal breath sounds
    Bronchial breath sounds
    Expiratory slowing
    Crackles
    Wheezes
    Pleural rub
    Mediastinal noises (mediastinal crunch)
    Heart sounds
    Miscellaneous (muscle tremor, etc.; see Other
      Signs and Symptoms of Pulmonary Disease)

Percussion/auscultation finding	Chest expansion	Fremitus	Resonance	Breath sounds	Egophony	Bronchophony
Pleural effusion	Decreased	Decreased	Decreased	Decreased	Absent>>present	Absent>>present
Consolidation	Decreased	Increased	Decreased	Bronchial	Present	Present
Atelectasis	Decreased	Decreased	Decreased	Decreased	Absent>present	Absent>present
Pneumothorax	Variable	Decreased	Increased	Decreased	Absent	Absent

Note: The trachea is shifted ipsilaterally in atelectasis and contralaterally in effusion. Whispered pectoriloquy is present in consolidation. FEV_1, forced expiratory volume in 1 second.

missed. Initially, the CXR should be "eyeballed," without focusing on any one area or abnormality. This is to ensure that the technical aspects are adequate and the patient identification markers and the orientation of the CXR (identification of the left and right sides) are correct. Next, the extrapulmonary structures are viewed. For instance, destructive arthritis of a shoulder joint seen on a CXR may be the result of rheumatoid arthritis and may prompt the CXR reader to look for pulmonary manifestations of this disease. The absence of a breast shadow on the CXR of a female suggests the need to look for signs of pulmonary metastases. The visualization of a tracheostomy stoma or cannula on the CXR may indicate previous laryngeal cancer, suggesting the possibility of complications such as aspiration pneumonia and lung metastases. Infradiaphragmatic abnormalities such as calcifications in the spleen, displacement of the gastric bubble and colon, and signs of upper abdominal surgery (metal sutures, feeding tubes) may indicate the cause of a pleuropulmonary process.

- Initially look at the entire CXR as a single picture.
- Look for the absence of a breast shadow, infradiaphragmatic abnormalities, and extrapulmonary skeletal abnormalities.

The skeletal thorax should be viewed to exclude rib fracture, osteolytic and other lesions of the ribs, rib notching, missing ribs, and vertebral abnormalities. Changes due to a previous thoracic surgical procedure such as coronary artery bypass, thoracotomy, lung resection, or esophageal surgery may provide clues to the pulmonary disease. Next, the intrathoracic but extrapulmonary structures such as the mediastinum (great vessels, esophagus, heart, lymph nodes, and thymus) should be assessed. The superior mediastinum should be viewed to see whether the thyroid gland extends into the thoracic cage. A calcified mass in the region of the thyroid almost always indicates a goiter. The esophagus can produce important abnormalities in the CXR. A large esophagus, as in achalasia, may mimic a mass, and a large hiatal hernia with an air-fluid level may mimic a lung abscess. The aortopulmonary window (a notch below the aortic knob on the left, just above the pulmonary artery), if obliterated, may indicate a tumor or lymphadenopathy. Right paratracheal and paramediastinal lymphadenopathy can be subtle. Hilar regions are difficult to interpret because lymphadenopathy, vascular prominence, or tumor may make the hila appear larger. The retrocardiac region may show hiatal hernia with an air-fluid level; this may be helpful in the diagnosis of reflux or aspiration. A lateral CXR is important to assess the retrocardiac and retrodiaphragmatic recesses.

- Rib lesions: osteolytic, expansile, notching, or absence of a rib.
- Note changes due to previous surgical procedures.
- Assess the mediastinum: the esophagus, thyroid, thymus, and great vessels.

The pleural regions should be examined for pleural effusion, pleural thickening (particularly in the apices), blunting of costophrenic angles, pleural-based lesions such as pleural plaques or masses, and pneumothorax. A lateral decubitus film may be necessary to confirm the presence of free fluid in the pleural space. An air bronchogram depicting the major airways may indicate a large tumor (cut-off of air bronchogram), deviation of airways, signs of compression or stenosis, and the relation of major airways to the esophagus. Finally, the lung parenchyma should be evaluated. Nearly 15% of the pulmonary parenchyma is located behind the heart and diaphragm; a lateral CXR is helpful in examining this region. It is important *not* to overinterpret increased interstitial lung markings. Oligemia of the lung fields is difficult to assess because the clarity of the film depends on the duration of the exposure of the film. Generally, bronchovascular markings should be visible throughout the lung parenchyma. The complete absence of any markings within the lung parenchyma should suggest a bulla or an air-containing cyst. Apical areas should be evaluated carefully for the presence of pleural thickening, pneumothorax, small nodules, and subtle infiltrates. If the apices cannot be visualized properly with a standard CXR, a lordotic view should be obtained.

- Look for small pneumothorax, nodules, and large airway lesions.
- Examine the apices for thickening, pneumothorax, nodules, and subtle infiltrates.
- Examine the lung parenchyma behind the heart and diaphragm.

Some of the common CXR abnormalities are depicted in Figures 21-1 to 21-26.

Fluoroscopy

Fluoroscopy is useful in localizing lesions during biopsy and aspiration procedures. It also is valuable in assessing diaphragmatic motion and in diagnosing diaphragmatic paralysis by the sniff test. Paradoxic motion of the diaphragm suggests diaphragmatic paralysis.

- Up to 6% of normal subjects exhibit paradoxic diaphragmatic motion.

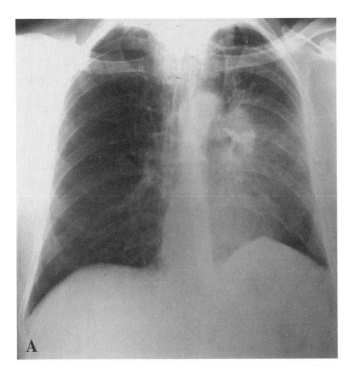

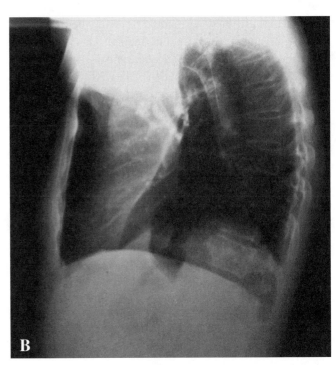

Fig. 21-1. Collapsed left upper lobe. *A*, PA CXR and, *B*, lateral CXR. The ground-glass haze over the left hemithorax is typical of a partially collapsed left upper lobe. In more than 50% of patients with collapsed lobes, loss of volume is evidenced by left hemidiaphragmatic elevation; the mediastinum is shifted to the left and the left hilus is pulled cranially. Also, left main bronchus deviates cranially. Calcification in the left hilar mass represents an unrelated old granulomatous infection. In *B*, the density from the left hilus down toward the anterior portion of the chest represents the partially collapsed left upper lobe. The radiolucency substernally is the right lung.

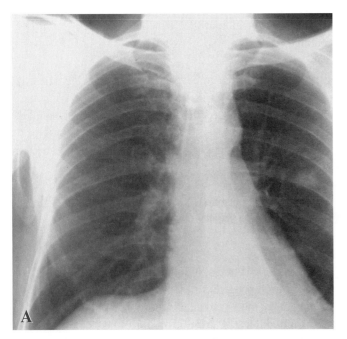

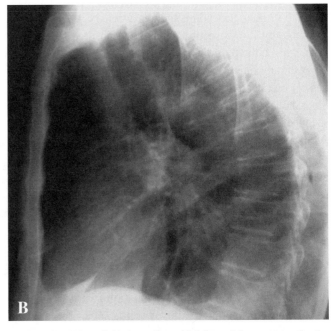

Fig. 21-2. Collapsed left lower lobe. *A*, PA CXR and, *B*, lateral CXR. Note nodule in left mid lung field plus collapsed left lower lobe, seen as a density behind the heart. This entity represents two separate primary lung cancers: synchronous bronchogenic carcinomas. Do not stop with the first evident abnormality, such as the nodule in the mid lung field, without looking carefully at all other areas. *B* demonstrates an increased density over the lower thoracic vertebrae without any obvious wedge-shaped infiltrate. Over the anterior portion of the hemidiaphragm, the small wedge-shaped infiltrate is not fluid in the left major fissure because the left major fissure is pulled away posteriorly. Instead, it is an incidental normal variant of fat pushed up into the right major fissure.

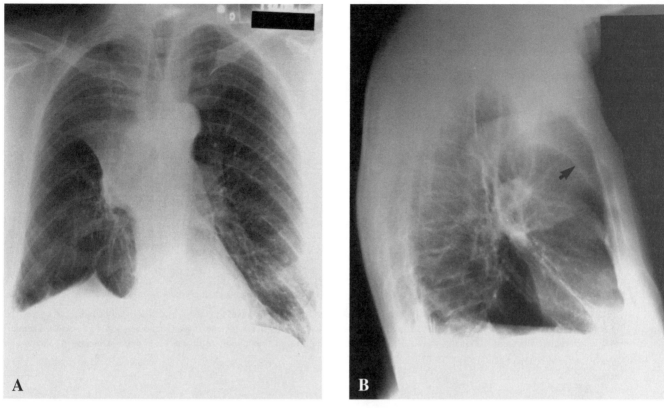

Fig. 21-3. Collapsed right upper lobe. *A*, PA CXR and, *B*, lateral CXR. *A*, This is a classic "reversed S" mass in the right hilus with partial collapse of the right upper lobe. Loss of volume is evident with the elevation of the right hemidiaphragm. In *B*, the partially collapsed right upper lobe is faintly seen in the upper anterior portion of the hemithorax (*arrow*).

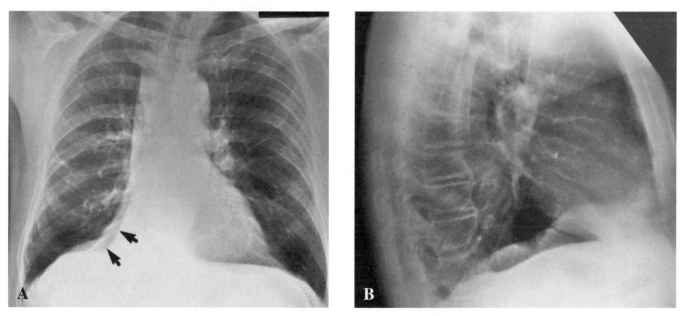

Fig. 21-4. Collapsed right lower lobe. *A*, PA CXR and, *B*, lateral CXR. *A*, This 75-year-old smoker had hemoptysis for 1.5 years; his CXR had been read as "normal" on several occasions. Note the linear density (*arrows*) projecting downward and laterally along the right border of the heart. It projects below the diaphragm and is not a normal line. Also, the right hilus is not evident; it has been pulled centrally and downward because of carcinoma obstructing the bronchus of the right lower lobe. Note the very slight shift in the mediastinum to the right, indicative of some loss of volume. *B*, In the lateral view, in spite of notable collapse of the right lower lobe, only a subtle increased density over lower thoracic vertebrae represents this collapse.

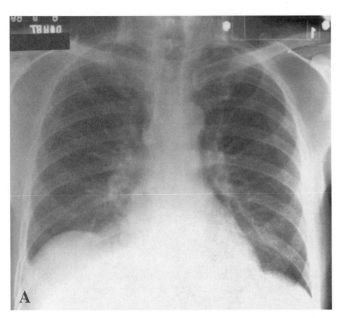

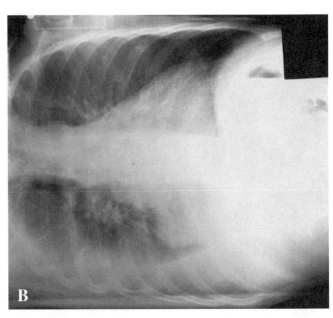

Fig. 21-5. *A*, PA CXR and, *B*, decubitus CXR. *A*, "Elevated right hemidiaphragm" that is really an infrapulmonic effusion, or subpulmonic, as seen on the decubitus film. *B*, For unknown reasons, a meniscus is not formed in some people with infrapulmonic pleural effusion. Thus, any seemingly elevated hemidiaphragm should be examined with the suspicion that it could be an infrapulmonic effusion. Subpulmonic effusions occur more frequently in patients with nephrotic syndrome. Decubitus CXR or ultrasonography would disclose the free fluid.

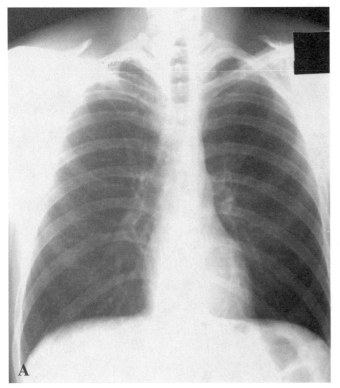

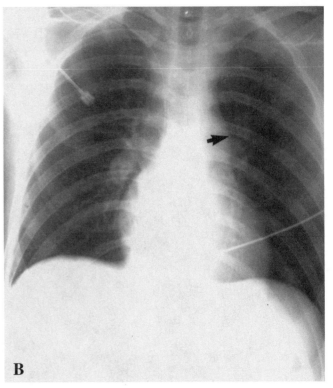

Fig. 21-6. *A*, Normal, prepulmonary embolism on PA CXR; *B*, pulmonary embolism. The CXR is read as normal in up to 30% of patients with angiographically proven pulmonary embolism. In comparison with *A*, *B* shows a subtle elevation of the right hemidiaphragm. In *A*, the right and left hemidiaphragms are equal. In some series, an elevated hemidiaphragm is the most common finding with acute pulmonary embolism. Also, note the plumpness of the right pulmonary artery, prominent pulmonary outflow tract on the left (*arrow*), and subtle change in cardiac diameter. At the time of CXR, this 28-year-old man was in shock from massive pulmonary emboli as a result of major soft tissue trauma produced by a motorcycle accident 7 days earlier.

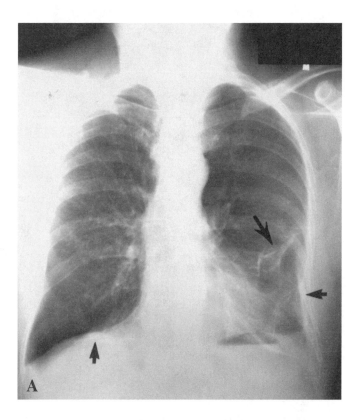

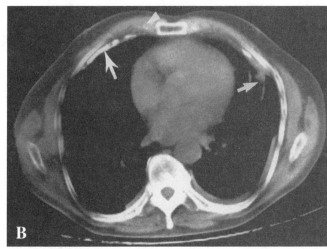

Fig. 21-7. Abnormal CXR, *A*, in a 68-year-old asymptomatic man. *Small arrows* indicate areas of pleural calcification, particularly on the right hemidiaphragm. This is a tip-off to previous asbestos exposure. The process in the left mid lung was worrisome (*large arrow*), perhaps indicating a new process such as bronchogenic carcinoma in this smoker. However, CT, *B*, disclosed rounded atelectasis (*small arrow*). The "comma" extending from this mass is characteristic of rounded atelectasis, which is the result of subacute-to-chronic pleural effusion resolving and trapping some lung as it heals. Also note pleural calcification in *B* (*large arrow*).

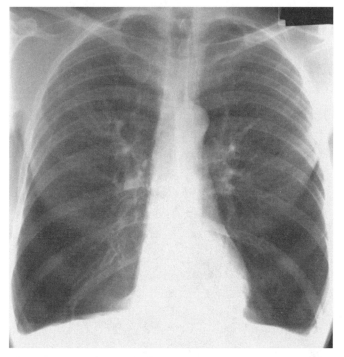

Fig. 21-8. Panlobular emphysema at the bases consistent with the diagnosis of alpha$_1$-antitrypsin deficiency. Emphysema should not be read into a CXR because all it usually represents is hyperinflation that can occur with severe asthma as well. However, in this setting, there are markedly diminished interstitial markings at the bases, with radiolucency. Also, blood flow is increased to the upper lobes because that is where most of the viable lung tissue is. Note the flattening of the hemidiaphragms from hyperinflation.

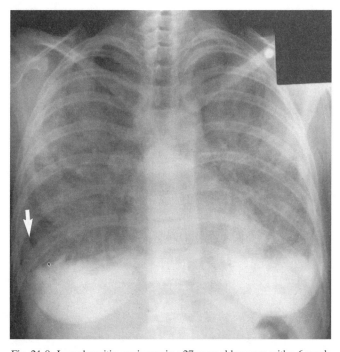

Fig. 21-9. Lymphangitic carcinoma in a 27-year-old woman with a 6-week history of progressive dyspnea and weight loss. Because of her young age, neoplasm may not be considered initially. However, the CXR features suggest it, viz., bilateral pleural effusions, Kerley B lines as evident in the right base (*arrow*), and mediastinal and hilar lymphadenopathy in addition to diffuse parenchymal infiltrate.

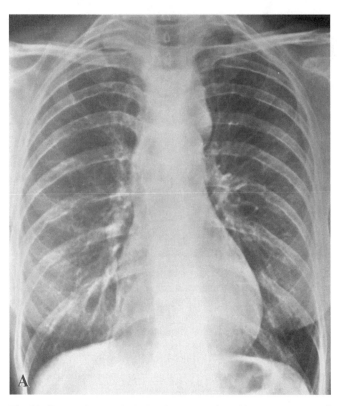

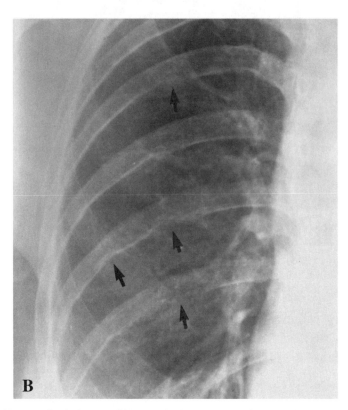

Fig. 21-10. *A* and *B*, PA CXR showing coarctation with a tortuous aorta mimicking a mediastinal mass. This occurs in about one-third of patients with coarctation. Rib notching is indicated by the *arrows* in *B*.

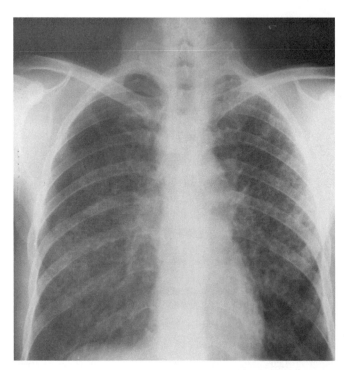

Fig. 21-11. Histiocytosis X, or eosinophilic granuloma, shows extensive change but predominantly in the upper two-thirds of the lung fields. Eventually 25% of these patients have pneumothorax, as seen on this CXR. The honeycombing, also described as microcysts, is characteristic of advanced histiocytosis X.

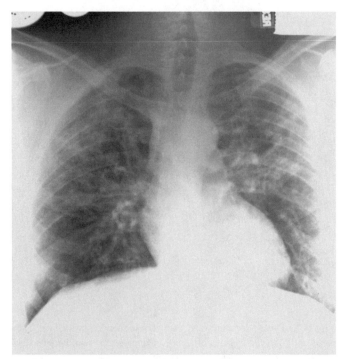

Fig. 21-12. Sarcoidosis in a 35-year-old patient. This CXR shows the predominant upper two-thirds parenchymal pattern seen in many patients with stage II or III sarcoidosis. The pattern can be interstitial, alveolar (which this one is predominantly), or a combination. There probably is some residual adenopathy in the hila and right paratracheal area.

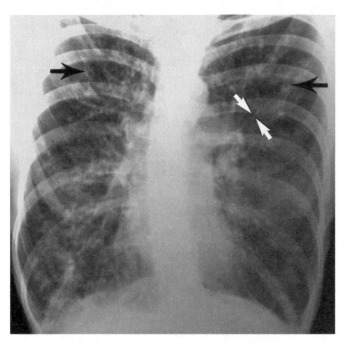

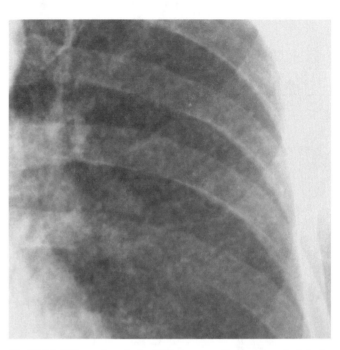

Fig. 21-13. Advanced cystic fibrosis showing hyperinflation with low-lying hemidiaphragms, bronchiectasis (*white arrows* pointing to parallel lines), and microabscesses (*black arrows*) representing small areas of pneumonitis distal to the mucous plug that has been coughed out. Cystic fibrosis almost always begins in the upper lobes.

Fig. 21-14. Miliary tuberculosis. CXR shows a miliary pattern of relatively discrete micronodules, with little interstitial (linear or reticular) markings. Disseminated fungal disease has a similar appearance, as does bronchoalveolar cell carcinoma; however, these patients do not usually have the systemic manifestations of miliary tuberculosis. Other, less common differential diagnoses include lymphoma, lymphocytic interstitial pneumonitis, and pulmonary edema. *Pneumocystis carinii* pneumonia usually has a more interstitial reaction.

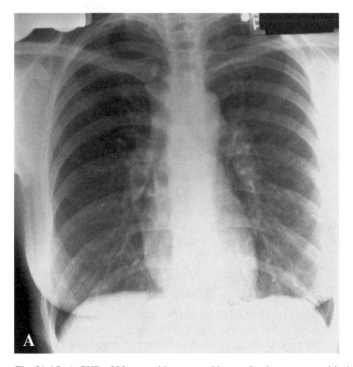

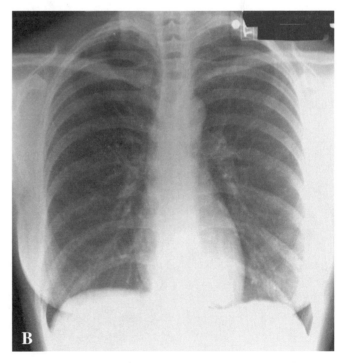

Fig. 21-15. *A*, CXR of 30-year-old woman with stage I pulmonary sarcoidosis with subtle bilateral hilar and mediastinal adenopathy, particularly right paratracheal and left infra-aortic adenopathy. *B*, CXR 1 year later, after spontaneous regression of sarcoidosis.

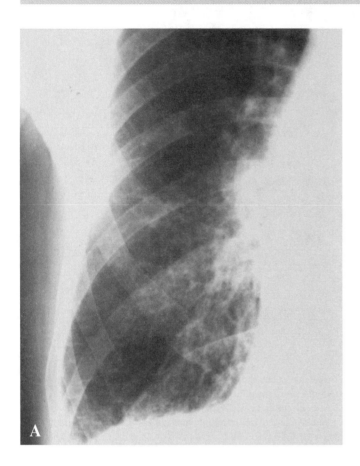

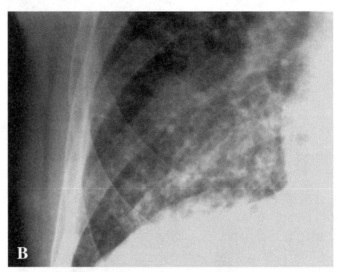

Fig. 21-16. *A* and *B*, Two examples of Kerley B lines that can be helpful in interpreting CXRs. *A*, Kerley B lines in a 75-year-old man with colon cancer. *B*, Kerley B lines are from metastatic adenocarcinoma of the colon and were a tip-off that the parenchymal process in this patient was due to metastatic carcinoma and not to a primary pulmonary process such as pulmonary fibrosis, which was the working diagnosis.

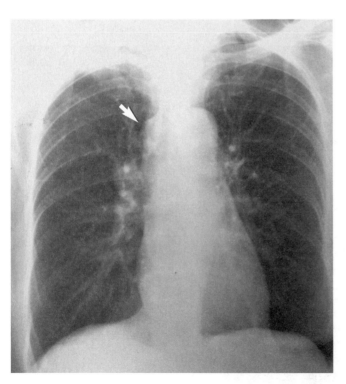

Fig. 21-17. CXR of a 55-year-old woman who had had a right mastectomy for breast carcinoma now shows subtle but definite right paratracheal (*arrow*) and right hilar adenopathy from metastatic carcinoma of the breast.

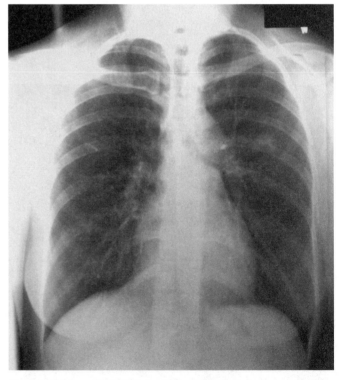

Fig. 21-18. The nodule in the left mid lung field is technically not a "solitary pulmonary nodule" because of another abnormality in the thorax that might be related to it, left infra-aortic adenopathy. The differential diagnosis would be bronchogenic carcinoma with hilar nodal metastasis or, as in this case, acute primary pulmonary histoplasmosis. Had this patient been in an area with coccidioidomycosis, it would also be included in the differential diagnosis.

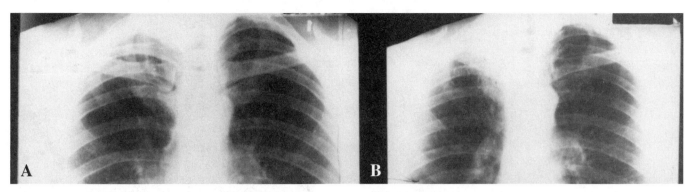

Fig. 21-19. Pancoast tumor. *A*, Subtle asymmetry at the apex of the right lung was more obvious 3.5 years later, *B*, at the time the Pancoast lesion (primary bronchogenic carcinoma) was diagnosed. The patient was symptomatic at the time of the initial CXR, with the symptoms attributed to a cervical disk.

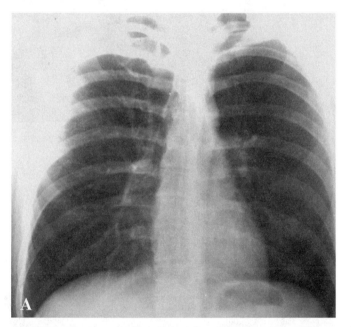

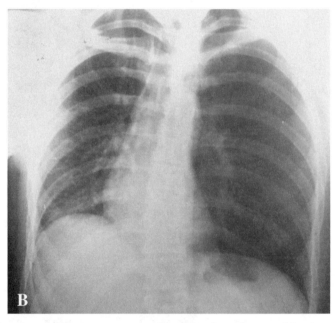

Fig. 21-20. The adage that "not all that wheezes is asthma" should be remembered every time you encounter a patient with asthma whose condition does not seem to improve. In the case shown here, *A*, wheezes were predominant over the left hemithorax. A forced expiration film, *B*, showed air trapping in the left lung. Bronchial carcinoid of the left main bronchus was diagnosed at bronchoscopy.

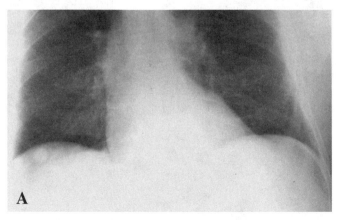

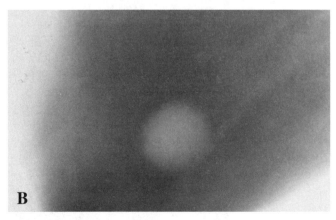

Fig. 21-21. *A*, A solitary pulmonary nodule is evident below the right hemidiaphragm, where at least 15% of the lung is obscured. *B*, Tomography shows that the nodule has a discrete border but is noncalcified. It was not present 18 months earlier. This is an adenocarcinoma.

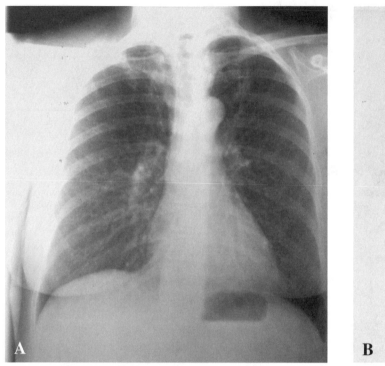

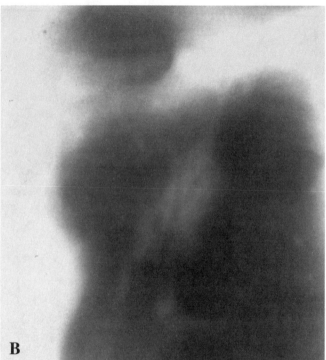

Fig. 21-22. *A*, Solitary infiltrate in the left upper lobe with air bronchogram, as evident on tomography or CT. *B*, Air bronchogram should be considered a sign of bronchoalveolar cell carcinoma or lymphoma until proved otherwise.

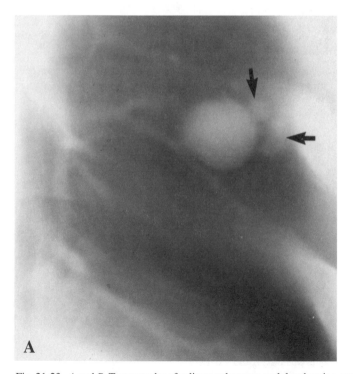

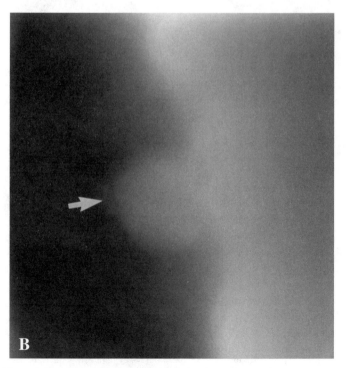

Fig. 21-23. *A* and *B*, Tomography of solitary pulmonary nodules showing satellite nodules (*arrows*). This is characteristic of granulomas.

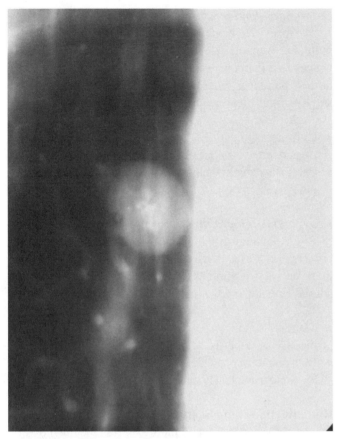

Fig. 21-24. Popcorn calcification of hamartoma. This can be seen also in granuloma and represents a benign process.

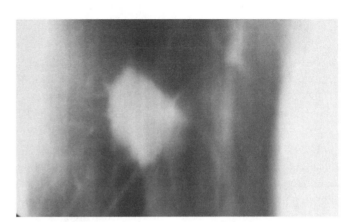

Fig. 21-25. Tomography of a solitary nodule showing spiculation, or sunburst effect, characteristic of primary bronchogenic carcinoma. Spicules represent extension of the tumor into septa. CT showed a similar appearance.

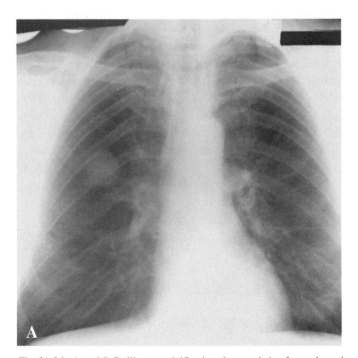

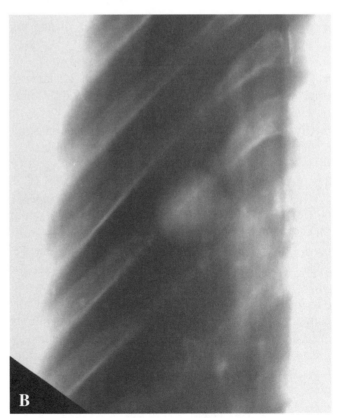

Fig. 21-26. A and B, Bull's-eye calcification characteristic of granuloma in a solitary pulmonary nodule. They occasionally enlarge but even then almost never warrant removal.

Computed Tomography

Standard CT is useful in the staging of lung cancer and in assessing mediastinal and hilar lesions, diffuse lung disease, and pleural processes. High-resolution CT (HRCT) demonstrates characteristic findings in pulmonary bronchiectasis, Langerhans cell granulomatosis (nodular-cystic spaces in the upper lung fields), lymphangitic carcinomatosis (nodular interlobular septal thickening), lymphangioleiomyomatosis (well-defined cystic spaces in lung parenchyma), and idiopathic pulmonary fibrosis (subpleural honeycombing). HRCT findings in pulmonary fibrotic diseases are more than 90% accurate; honeycombing may be seen in up to 90% of patients, as compared with 30% with traditional CXR. HRCT is also helpful in diagnosing certain granulomatous lung diseases (sarcoidosis and mycobacterial infections), asbestosis, pulmonary alveolar phospholipoproteinosis, chronic eosinophilic pneumonia, and bronchiolitis obliterans. Ultrafast CT is better than a ventilation-perfusion (V/Q) scan in detecting pulmonary emboli in the main and lobar arteries. The role of CT in the diagnosis of peripheral pulmonary emboli has not been established.

- HRCT demonstrates characteristic features in pulmonary Langerhans cell granulomatosis, lymphangioleiomyomatosis, idiopathic pulmonary fibrosis, and lymphangitic pulmonary metastasis.
- HRCT has replaced bronchography for diagnosing bronchiectasis.
- CT is helpful in the staging of lung cancer.
- CT is useful in evaluating the presence of solitary pulmonary nodule, multiple lung nodules (metastatic), and calcification in the nodule(s).
- Ultrafast CT is better than a V/Q scan for diagnosing pulmonary emboli.

Magnetic Resonance Imaging

MRI is recommended for the initial evaluation of superior sulcus tumors (Pancoast tumor), lesions of the brachial plexus, and paraspinal masses that on CXR appear most consistent with neurogenic tumors. MRI is superior to CT in the evaluation of chest wall masses and in the search for small occult mediastinal neoplasms (e.g., ectopic parathyroid adenoma). MRI is useful when CT with contrast media is contraindicated for patients with renal failure or contrast allergy. MRI may be superior to CT in evaluating pulmonary sequestration, arteriovenous malformation, vascular structures, and tumor recurrence in patients with total pneumonectomy.

- MRI: useful for the evaluation of superior sulcus tumors and neurogenic tumors.

Pulmonary Angiography

The main indication for pulmonary angiography is to detect pulmonary emboli. However, small peripheral emboli may not be seen. Pulmonary angiography is also useful in the diagnosis of pulmonary arteriovenous fistulas and malformations, and it is usually a prerequisite if embolotherapy is planned.

- Common indications: pulmonary embolism and pulmonary arteriovenous malformations and fistulas.
- Pulmonary angiography may not detect a peripheral or tiny pulmonary embolism.

Bronchial Angiography

Bronchial angiography is used to determine whether the bronchial arteries are the cause of massive pulmonary hemorrhage or massive hemoptysis. It is a prerequisite if bronchial arterial embolotherapy is planned.

- Main indication: suspected bronchial arterial bleeding in massive hemoptysis.
- Both pulmonary and bronchial angiography may be needed for some patients who have massive hemoptysis.

Radionuclide Lung Scans

The V/Q scan is still commonly used in the diagnosis of pulmonary embolism, although CT angiography is assuming an increasingly larger diagnostic role. The likelihood of pulmonary embolism in a V/Q scan that shows "high probability" and a scan that shows "low probability" is greater than 90% and less than 5%, respectively. An "intermediate probability" scan usually is an indication for HRCT or pulmonary angiography. However, clinical suspicion of pulmonary embolism should guide the decision. The quantitative V/Q scan is used to assess unilateral and regional pulmonary function by measuring V/Q relationships in different regions of the lungs. It is indicated for patients who are poor surgical candidates for lung resection because of underlying pulmonary dysfunction. If the lung region to be resected shows minimal or no lung function on a quantitative V/Q scan, the resection is unlikely to impair further the patient's pulmonary reserve. The gallium scan is of minimal or no use in the diagnosis of diffuse lung diseases. The technetium 99m scan is useful in detecting diffuse pulmonary calcification associated with chronic hemodialysis.

- Quantitative V/Q scan is used to assess unilateral or regional pulmonary function.
- The gallium scan has no role in the diagnosis of diffuse lung disease.
- The technetium 99m lung scan detects diffuse pulmonary calcification.

Sputum Microscopy

Simple microscopy with a "wet" slide preparation of sputum is helpful in assessing the degree of sputum eosinophilia and detecting the presence of Charcot-Leyden crystals. Gram staining of sputum should be used to evaluate suspected bacterial infections. However, routine examination with Gram stain is not necessary for all patients with COPD who present with acute exacerbations. Induced sputum is helpful in identifying mycobacteria, fungi, *Pneumocystis carinii*, and malignant cells. Gastric washings are used to identify mycobacteria and fungi. Hemosiderin-laden macrophages in sputum do not always indicate alveolar hemorrhage; smokers can have a large number of hemosiderin-laden macrophages in their sputum.

- A sputum "wet prep" detects eosinophilia and Charcot-Leyden crystals.
- Induced sputum is excellent for identifying *P. carinii*.

Pulmonary Function Tests

The major indication for PFTs is dyspnea. PFTs do not diagnose lung disease. They assess the mechanical function of the respiratory system and quantify the loss of lung function. PFTs can separate obstructive from restrictive phenomena. Bronchoprovocation testing with agents such as methacholine is useful in detecting airway hyperresponsiveness. Results of previous PFTs are helpful in following the course of lung disease.

- Obstructive dysfunction: indicates airflow limitation, as in asthma, bronchitis, and emphysema.
- An increase (>20%) in flow rates after bronchodilator therapy suggests reversible component airway disease, although the absence of response does not preclude a clinical trial with inhaled bronchodilator medications.
- Restrictive dysfunction: limitation to full expansion of the lungs because of a large pleural effusion or disease in the lung parenchyma, chest wall, or diaphragm; volumes are diminished.
- A combination of obstructive and restrictive patterns is also possible (e.g., COPD with pulmonary fibrosis).

Provocation Inhalational Challenge

This test is useful when the diagnosis of asthma or hyperreactive airway disease is uncertain. The test uses agents that elicit a bronchospastic response, for example, methacholine, carbachol, histamine, industrial irritants, exercise, isocapneic hyperventilation, and cold air. A 20% decrease in forced expiratory volume in 1 second (FEV_1) from baseline is considered a positive test result. Normal subjects exhibit a positive response to provocation challenge without symptoms of asthma.

- A 20% decrease in FEV_1 from baseline is considered positive.
- Up to 10% of normal subjects exhibit a positive response to an inhalational challenge.

Interpretation of Pulmonary Function Tests

A simplified step-by-step approach is as follows:

1. Evaluate volumes and flows separately.
2. Total lung capacity (TLC), functional residual capacity (FRC), and residual volume (RV) indicate volumes. TLC = VC (vital capacity) + RV. Increases in TLC and RV suggest hyperinflation (asthma, COPD). If TLC and VC are decreased, consider restrictive lung disease (fibrosis) or loss of lung volume (surgery, diaphragmatic paralysis, skeletal problems).
3. VC measured during a slow (not forced) expiration is not affected by airway collapse in COPD. Forced VC may be low with forced expiration because of airway collapse. In normal subjects, VC equals forced VC (i.e., VC = FVC).
4. FEV_1 and forced expiratory flow between 25% and 75% of VC (FEF_{25-75}) indicate flow rates. Flow rates are diminished in COPD, but smaller decreases can be seen if lung volumes are low. Decreased FEV_1/FVC (<70%) indicates obstruction to airflow.
5. The maximal voluntary ventilation (MVV) test requires rapid inspiratory and expiratory maneuvers and, thus, tests airflow through major airways and muscle strength. Disproportionately reduced MVV may be from poor effort, variable extrathoracic obstruction, and respiratory muscle weakness.

- MVV is decreased in obstructive disease (i.e., MVV = FEV_1 × 33).
- Respiratory muscle weakness can be assessed by maximum inspiratory pressure (PI_{max}) and maximum expiratory pressure (PE_{max}).
- Clinical features should be correlated with the results of PFTs.

6. Diffusing capacity (DLCO) is dependent on the thickness of the alveolocapillary membrane (DM), hemoglobin level (θ), and pulmonary capillary volume (Vc). DLCO is represented by $\left(\frac{1}{DLCO} = \frac{1}{DM} + \frac{1}{\theta Vc}\right)$. DLCO is low in anatomical emphysema ($\downarrow$Vc), anemia ($\downarrow\theta$), restrictive lung diseases ($\uparrow$DM), pneumonectomy ($\downarrow$Vc), pulmonary hypertension, and recurrent pulmonary emboli ($\downarrow$Vc). DLCO is increased in the supine posture ($\uparrow$Vc), after exercise ($\uparrow$Vc), in polycythemia ($\uparrow\theta$), obesity ($\uparrow$Vc), left-to-right shunt ($\uparrow$Vc), and in some patients with asthma. Isolated low DLCO (with normal results on

PFTs) is seen in pulmonary hypertension, multiple pulmonary emboli, and anemia.

- DLCO is decreased in anatomical emphysema.
- An isolated decrease in DLCO (normal volumes and flows) may occur in pulmonary hypertension, multiple pulmonary emboli, and severe anemia.
- A decrease in hemoglobin by 1 g diminishes DLCO by 7%.
- Flow-volume curves are helpful to distinguish between intrathoracic and extrathoracic major airway obstructions.

Explanation of Table 21-2

Patient 1. Typical features of hyperinflation (high TLC and RV). VC is low because of high RV ($TLC - RV = VC$). Flow rates are very low, and MVV is moderately reduced. The very low DLCO suggests parenchymal damage. Without inhalational challenge, it is not possible to discern a bronchospastic component. Clinical diagnosis: moderately severe obstructive disease with severe anatomical emphysema.

Patient 2. Young nonsmoker with hyperinflation (high TLC and RV). Flow rates and MVV are also severely decreased. These suggest obstructive lung disease. The low DLCO suggests parenchymal damage (emphysema). Clinical diagnosis: severe emphysema caused by familial deficiency of alpha$_1$-antitrypsin.

Patient 3. Flow rates and lung volumes are decreased only slightly but are within normal limits. MVV is severely decreased. In this patient, PImax and PEmax are severely decreased, suggesting muscle weakness. Clinical diagnosis: severe thyrotoxicosis with proximal muscle weakness (thyrotoxic myopathy). This pattern of results on PFTs can also occur in neuromuscular diseases such as amyotrophic lateral sclerosis and myasthenia gravis.

Patient 4. Slightly increased but normal TLC and slightly diminished VC. Flow rates are moderately decreased. This patient has a mild-to-moderate obstructive phenomenon. Normal DLCO excludes anatomical emphysema or other parenchymal problems. Bronchodilator testing elicited improvement in lung volumes and flow rates. Clinical diagnosis: typical asthma.

Patient 5. Mild hyperinflation (increased TLC and RV). Because these are within normal limits (80%-120% of predicted), true hyperinflation is not present. Flow rates are slightly reduced, and MVV and DLCO are normal. Bronchodilator inhalation showed no improvement. Note the slightly diminished FEV_1/FVC ratio. This together with a slightly diminished FEF_{25-75} suggests a mild obstructive lung disease of a nonasthmatic type. Because of normal DLCO, marked anatomical emphysema can be excluded. Clinical diagnosis: nonasthmatic bronchitis.

Patient 6. Normal lung volumes and flow rates (80%-120% of predicted normal). A former "superathlete," he recently noted cough and chest tightness after exertion. Previous PFTs were unavailable. Important points: 1) In a young, otherwise healthy patient, the lung volumes and flow rates are usually above normal, more so in an athlete. 2) This patient may have

Table 21-2 Try to Interpret These Results of Pulmonary Function Tests Before Reading the Explanations*

Patient	1	2	3	4	5	6	7	8	9	10
Age, y, and sex	73 M	43 M	53 F	43 M	50 M	20 M	58 F	40 M	28 F	44 M
Weight, kg	52	53	50	63	73	80	59	75	52	148
Tobacco	63PY	NS	NS	NS	20PY	NS	NS	NS	NS	NS
Total lung capacity, %	140	128	84	118	110	100	56	68	108	90
Vital capacity, %	52	75	86	78	82	95	62	58	106	86
Residual volume, %	160	140	90	110	112	90	65	80	98	90
FEV_1, %	35	38	82	48	80	90	85	42	112	96
FEV_1/FVC, %	40	34	80	40	60	85	88	50	85	78
FEF_{25-75}	18	14	80	35	75	88	82	24	102	88
Maximal voluntary ventilation, %	62	48	40	60	105	120	108	62	88	90
Diffusing capacity	9	10	20	28	26	32	8	8	6	40
(normal)	(22)	(28)	(20)	(28)	(27)	(34)	(26)	(28)	(32)	(28)

FEF_{25-75}, forced expiratory flow between 25% and 75% of vital capacity; FEV_1, forced expiratory volume in 1 second; FVC, forced vital capacity; NS, nonsmoker; PY, pack-years of smoking.

*Values of 80%-120% of predicted are considered normal.

had very high volumes and flow rates in the past, but without previous PFTs, no comparison can be made (if earlier PFT results were available, the new results might represent a severe decrease in pulmonary function). 3) The history suggests the possibility of exercise-induced asthma; spirometry after an exercise test showed a 28% reduction in flow rates 5 to 10 minutes after termination of exercise. 4) Note the relatively high DLCO in this patient, a phenomenon seen in patients with asthma. Clinical diagnosis: exercise-induced asthma.

Patient 7. Moderately severe decrease in lung volumes and normal flow rates. MVV is normal, but DLCO is severely diminished. These suggest severe restrictive lung disease. The slightly diminished flow rates are the result of decreased lung volumes. Clinical diagnosis: biopsy-proven idiopathic pulmonary fibrosis. Patients who have had lung resection also have low lung volumes and decreased DLCO.

Patient 8. Moderately decreased lung volumes. Flow rates are also diminished more than expected from the decreases in lung volumes. Reduction in the FEV_1/FVC ratio suggests the presence of obstructive dysfunction. MVV is also reduced, and DLCO is severely decreased. Compared with patient 7, this patient has obstructive disease plus severe restrictive lung disease. A very low DLCO suggests parenchymal disease. CXR showed bilaterally diffuse nodular interstitial changes, especially in the upper two-thirds of the lungs. Biopsy specimens of the bronchial mucosa and lung showed extensive endobronchial sarcoidosis. Clinical diagnosis: severe restrictive lung disease from parenchymal sarcoidosis and obstructive dysfunction caused by endobronchial sarcoidosis.

Patient 9. Normal lung volumes and flow rates. MVV is slightly reduced but within normal limits. DLCO is very low. PaO_2 is 56 mm Hg. Clinical diagnosis: primary pulmonary hypertension.

Patient 10. Normal lung volumes and flow rates. Previous PFT results were not available. DLCO is abnormally high. This patient was extremely obese, and all the abnormal results on PFTs can be explained on the basis of this. Obese patients show diminished lung volumes because of poor effort made during testing. Abnormally high DLCO is reported to be a result of increased Vc. Clinical diagnosis: obesity-related pulmonary dysfunction.

Preoperative Evaluation of Lung Functions

If patients scheduled to undergo lung resection have suspected or documented lung disease, PFTs should be performed preoperatively. A patient can tolerate pneumonectomy if the values are more than 50% of predicted for FEV_1, MVV, RV/TLC, and DLCO. If the values are less than 50% of predicted, a quantitative V/Q scan will help assess regional lung functions. Preoperative bronchodilators, chest physiotherapy, incentive spirometry, and physical conditioning decrease the risk of postoperative pulmonary complications. Increased morbidity and mortality are associated with severe COPD and $PaCO_2$ greater than 45 mm Hg (hypoxemia is not a reliable indicator). Upper abdominal operations (gallbladder and abdominal aortic aneurysm repair) have higher rates of pulmonary complications than lower abdominal procedures.

Exercise Testing

Exercise testing can assess cardiopulmonary function. Indications for exercise testing include unexplained dyspnea or effort intolerance, ability-disability evaluation, quantification of severity of pulmonary dysfunction, differentiation of cardiac from pulmonary causes of disability, evaluation of progression of a disease process, estimation of operative risks before cardiopulmonary surgery (lung resection or heart-lung or lung transplantation), rehabilitation, and evaluation of need for supplemental oxygen. Special equipment and expertise are required to perform an optimal exercise study.

Blood Gases and Oximetry

The interpretation of blood gas abnormalities is discussed in Chapter 4, Critical Care Medicine.

Bronchoscopy

Common diagnostic indications for bronchoscopy include persistent cough, hemoptysis, suspected cancer, lung nodule, atelectasis, diffuse lung disease, and lung infections. Therapeutic indications include atelectasis, retained secretions, tracheobronchial foreign bodies, airway stenosis (dilatation), and obstructive lesions (laser therapy, stent placement). Bronchoscopy is valuable in the staging of lung cancer. Complications from bronchoscopy are minimal and include bleeding from mucosal or lung biopsy, pneumothorax (from lung biopsy), and hypoxemia.

- Bronchoscopy: low diagnostic yield in pleural effusion.
- Useful in the diagnosis and staging of lung cancer.

Bronchoalveolar Lavage

Bronchoalveolar lavage (BAL) is performed by instilling 100 to 150 mL of normal saline into the diseased segment(s) of the lung. The instilled saline is aspirated back via the bronchoscope. The aspirated effluent can be analyzed for cells, chemical constituents, and cultures for infectious agents. BAL in normal subjects shows alveolar macrophages (93%±3%) and lymphocytes (7%±1%). Other types of leukocytes (neutrophils <1%) are rarely found in normal subjects.

- BAL can quantify and identify cell morphology at the alveolar level.

- Normal subjects: macrophages (93%), lymphocytes (7%), and neutrophils (<1%).

BAL may be helpful in diagnosing alveolar proteinosis, pulmonary Langerhans cell granuloma, and lymphangitic pulmonary metastasis. The CD4/CD8 ratio in BAL effluent is reversed in patients with acquired immunodeficiency syndrome (AIDS) complicated by lymphocytic interstitial pneumonitis and in many patients with hypersensitivity pneumonitis. BAL is extremely helpful in the diagnosis of infections in immunocompromised hosts, *P. carinii* infection, tuberculosis, mycoses, and other infections.

- BAL is helpful in diagnosing opportunistic lung infections.
- BAL has a limited role in the diagnosis of sarcoidosis and idiopathic pulmonary fibrosis.
- BAL is diagnostic in >60% of patients with pulmonary lymphangitic carcinomatosis.

Lung Biopsy

Lung biopsy can be performed via bronchoscopy, thoracoscopy, or thoracotomy. The indications for lung biopsy in diffuse lung disease should be based on the clinical features, treatment planned, and risks from biopsy and from treatment without a pathologic diagnosis. Bronchoscopic lung biopsy can provide up to an 80% to 90% diagnostic yield in sarcoidosis, pulmonary Langerhans cell granuloma, eosinophilic pneumonitis, lymphangioleiomyomatosis, infections, pulmonary alveolar proteinosis, lymphangitic carcinomatosis, drug-induced lung disease, and hypersensitivity pneumonitis, especially when performed in combination with special stains. The major complications after bronchoscopic lung biopsy are pneumothorax (<2%) and hemorrhage (<3%).

OBSTRUCTIVE LUNG DISEASES

A common pathophysiologic feature of obstructive lung diseases is the obstruction to flow of air. Obstructive lung diseases include emphysema, bronchitis, asthma, bronchiectasis, cystic fibrosis, bronchiolitis, bullous lung disease, and airway stenosis. The three most prevalent obstructive lung diseases are emphysema, chronic bronchitis, and asthma; they affect at least 25 to 30 million people in the United States. The salient features of these diseases are compared in Table 21-3.

COPD represents the fourth leading cause of chronic morbidity and mortality in the United States. The current working definition of COPD is a disease state characterized by airflow limitation that is not fully reversible. This implies that asthma, which is considered fully reversible (at least in its early stages), is separate from COPD. Although there is airway inflammation

Table 21-3 Salient Differential Features of Bronchial Asthma, Chronic Bronchitis, and Emphysema*

Differential feature	Bronchial asthma	Chronic bronchitis	Emphysema
Onset	70% <30 y old	≥50 y old	≥60 y old
Cigarette smoking	0	++++	++++
Pattern	Paroxysmal	Chronic, progressive	Chronic, progressive
Dyspnea	0 to ++++	+ to ++++	+++ to ++++
Cough	0 to +++	++ to ++++	+ to +++
Sputum	0 to ++	+++	+ to ++
Atopy	50% (adult)	15%	15%
Infections	↑ Symptoms	↑↑↑ Symptoms	↑ Symptoms
Chest radiograph	Usually normal	↑ Marking	Hyperinflation
$Paco_2$	Normal or ↓ in attack	Increased	Normal or increased
Pao_2	Normal or ↓ in attack	Low	Low
DLCO	Normal	Normal or slight decrease	Decreased
FEV_1, %	↓↓ in attack or normal	↓↓	↓↓
Total lung capacity	Normal or ↑ in attack	Normal or slight ↑	↑↑↑
Residual volume	Normal or ↑ in attack	Normal or slight ↑	↑↑↑
Cor pulmonale	Rare	Common	Rare
Hematocrit	Normal	Normal or increased	Normal or increased

*↑ indicates increase; ↓, decrease; ↑↑, increased more; ↓↓, decreased more; ↑↑↑, increased greatly; ↓↓↓, decreased greatly; +, present; ++, bothersome; +++, major problem; ++++, significant problem; DLCO, diffusion capacity:total lung capacity ratio; and FEV_1, %, percentage of vital capacity expired in 1 second.
From Kaliner M, Lemanske R: Rhinitis and asthma. JAMA 1992;268:2807-2829. By permission of the American Medical Association.

in both diseases, the inflammation characteristics of COPD appear to be different from those of asthma. In some instances, however, the two diseases can coexist. A classification of the severity of COPD has been proposed and should guide management at various stages of the disease (Table 21-4).

Etiology

Tobacco smoking is the major cause of COPD. Nearly 10% to 20% of smokers exhibit an accelerated rate of decrease in FEV_1. This decrease is proportional to the number of pack years of smoking. Smokers have 10 times the risk of nonsmokers of dying of chronic bronchitis and emphysema. Pipe and cigar smokers have between 1.5 and 3 times the risk of nonsmokers. Smoking increases the risk of developing COPD in persons who have alpha$_1$-antitrypsin deficiency. Smokers have an increased incidence of COPD, atherosclerosis, abdominal aortic aneurysm, and carcinoma of the lung, larynx, esophagus, and bladder. Diseases associated with or aggravated by smoking include asthma, lung fibrosis, calcification of pleural plaques in asbestosis, pulmonary alveolar phospholipoproteinosis, pulmonary Langerhans cell granuloma, and lung hemorrhage in Goodpasture syndrome. Sidestream tobacco exposure ("second-hand smoke") is also carcinogenic. Other increased risks (particularly in children) include infections of the lower respiratory tract, fluid collection in the middle ear, decreased lung function, increased severity of preexistent asthma, and increased risk of developing asthma.

- Nearly 15%-20% of smokers exhibit an accelerated rate of decrease in FEV_1.
- Pulmonary Langerhans cell granuloma and pulmonary alveolar proteinosis are more common in smokers.
- Sidestream smoke is also carcinogenic.

Air pollution caused by oxidants, oxides of nitrogen, hydrocarbons, and sulphur dioxide has an important role in exacerbating COPD. Occupational exposures, heredity (alpha$_1$-antitrypsin deficiency), infections, allergy (in asthma), and other factors are also involved in the etiology of COPD.

Pathology

Obstruction to airflow in COPD can result from damage of lung tissue by mucus hypersecretion and hypertrophy, airway narrowing (bronchospasm) and fibrosis, destruction of lung parenchyma, and pulmonary vascular changes. The premature collapse of airways leads to air-trapping and hyperinflation of the lungs (barrel chest). Bronchospasm in susceptible persons occurs from increased bronchomotor tone in the smooth muscles of the airways. Bronchospasm can occur as a result of many underlying complex mechanisms mediated by the vagus nerve, extrinsic allergens, release of intrinsic chemicals, external physical and chemical injury, hypothermia of airways, and other factors. Mucous gland hypertrophy occurs in chronic bronchitis, asthma, and other airway diseases as a result of direct or indirect stimulation of mucous glands. Increased bronchomotor tone can be elicited by the provocation inhalational challenge (see above). Histologically, centrilobular emphysema is the most common type of COPD and usually starts in the upper lobes. The panlobular type usually starts in the lower lobes and is often seen in COPD associated with alpha$_1$-antitrypsin deficiency.

- Causes of airway obstruction: expiratory collapse of airways, bronchospasm, mucosal inflammation, pulmonary vascular changes, and mucous gland hypertrophy.
- Upper lobe centrilobular emphysema is the most common type of emphysema in susceptible smokers.

Table 21-4 Practical Aspects of Managing Chronic Obstructive Pulmonary Disease (COPD)

Steps in management
  Identify the type of COPD
  Identify pathophysiology
  Assess lung dysfunction
  Eliminate causative/exacerbating factors
  Aim drug therapy at underlying pathophysiology
  Anticipate and treat complications
  Enroll in a rehabilitation program
  Educate patient and family
Stepped care approach
  Mild COPD (FEV_1/FVC <70%, FEV_1 ≥80% of
    predicted)
      Short activity bronchodilators as needed
  Moderate COPD
      IIA (FEV_1/FVC <70%, FEV_1 ≤50%, <80% of
        predicted)
          Scheduled use of bronchodilators with/without
            inhaled steroids if marked symptoms and lung
            function response, rehabilitation
      IIB (FEV_1/FVC <70%, 30% ≤FEV_1, <50% of
        predicted)
          Scheduled use of bronchodilators with/without
            inhaled steroids if repeated exacerbations or
            lung function response, rehabilitation
  Severe COPD (FEV_1/FVC <70%, FEV_1 <30% of
    predicted or presence of respiratory failure or right
    heart failure)
      Regular use of bronchodilators with/without inhaled
        steroids, rehabilitation, long-term oxygen if
        respiratory failure

FEV_1, forced expiratory volume in 1 second; FVC, forced vital capacity.

- Lower lobe panlobular emphysema is the usual pattern in patients with alpha$_1$-antitrypsin deficiency.

Physiology

Decreased flow rates are characteristic of COPD. Lung compliance is increased in emphysema, and elastic recoil of the lung is decreased (the opposite occurs in restrictive lung disease). DLCO is diminished in emphysema (as well as in most restrictive lung diseases). Hyperexpansion is manifested by increased total lung capacity and residual volume. As COPD progresses, continued parenchymal destruction and pulmonary vascular abnormalities result in hypoxemia, which eventually may progress to hypercapnia.

- Lung compliance is increased in emphysema (decreased in restrictive lung disease).

Chronic Bronchitis

"Chronic bronchitis" is defined as cough with sputum for 3 months or more per year for 2 or more consecutive years. Pathologically, the Reid index (i.e., the ratio of bronchial mucous glands to bronchial wall thickness) is increased. Cigarette smoking is the most common cause of chronic bronchitis. Occupational exposure and air pollution also contribute to the exacerbations. Patients exhibit productive cough, have a tendency to retain carbon dioxide, have a lower PaO$_2$, develop polycythemia and cyanosis ("blue bloaters"), and tend to be overweight and deconditioned.

- Patients with chronic bronchitis ("blue bloaters") tend to retain carbon dioxide, cough, be overweight, and develop cor pulmonale.

Emphysema

"Emphysema," a pathology term, is characterized by enlargement of the airspaces distal to the terminal bronchioles and destruction of the alveolar walls. This entity describes only one of several structural abnormalities present in patients with COPD. CT of the lungs is excellent for documenting emphysema and bullous lung disease. Pure anatomical emphysema is less common than chronic bronchitis. Patients with emphysema are typically thin, maintain near normal PaO$_2$ by increasing the work of breathing, and look adequately oxygenated ("pink puffers"). Severe weight loss is a relatively common finding in severe emphysema. Carbon dioxide retention does not occur until late in the disease.

- Patients with emphysema are "pink puffers."

Bullous Lung Disease

Small apical bullae are present in many healthy persons. Bullous lung disease can be congenital or acquired. Lack of communication with bronchi may cause air-trapping. Complications include pneumothorax, COPD, infection and formation of lung abscess, bleeding into a bulla, and compression of adjacent normal lung. Surgical therapy may improve lung function by 5% to 10% in 10% to 15% of patients. The incidence of lung cancer is increased in patients with bullous emphysema.

- Panlobular emphysema may look like a bulla.
- Bullous changes may be seen in Marfan and Ehlers-Danlos syndromes, burned-out sarcoidosis, and cadmium exposure.
- Bullous lung disease is associated with an increased risk of lung cancer.

Alpha$_1$-Antitrypsin Deficiency

The synthesis of alpha$_1$-antitrypsin, a secretory glycoprotein, by hepatocytes is determined by the alpha$_1$-antitrypsin gene on chromosome 14. Alpha$_1$-antitrypsin inhibits many proteolytic enzymes and, thus, protects the lungs from destructive emphysema. Alpha$_1$-antitrypsin deficiency is an autosomal recessive disease; the phenotypes are normal (P$_I$MM), heterozygote (P$_I$MZ), homozygote (P$_I$ZZ), and null (P$_I$Null). Other phenotypes with either no increased risk or a slightly increased risk of disease are P$_I$SS and P$_I$SZ, respectively. The threshold for disease is set at plasma alpha$_1$-antitrypsin level of less than 11 μmol/L (normal, 20-53 μmol/L). The prevalence of P$_I$ZZ in the United States is 1:1,670 to 1:5,097. Up to 10% of patients with P$_I$ZZ alpha$_1$-antitrypsin deficiency do not develop lung disease. Up to 95% of those with the P$_I$ZZ phenotype may have an unrecognized deficiency because they are asymptomatic or the disease is unrecognized. In nonsmoking P$_I$ZZ persons, lung function decreases with increasing age, especially after age 50. Men are at greater risk for deterioration of lung function than women. Smoking hastens the onset of emphysema. Signs and symptoms appear during the 3rd or 4th decade of life. Alpha$_1$-antitrypsin deficiency is associated with neonatal liver disease (hepatitis, cryptogenic cirrhosis, periportal fibrosis) and respiratory distress syndrome. A lack of alpha$_1$-antitrypsin seems to increase the propensity to develop asthma. Alpha$_1$-antitrypsin derived from human plasma has been used as replacement therapy; minimal decreases in the rate of decrease of FEV$_1$ (~27 mL per year) have been observed in patients with severe emphysema.

- In alpha$_1$-antitrypsin deficiency, smoking hastens the onset of emphysema.
- Features of the disease: basal emphysema on CXR, absence of alpha$_1$-globulin on protein electrophoresis, patient with COPD, and family history of COPD.
- Hepatic cirrhosis develops in up to 3% of patients.

- In young patients with clinical features of COPD, consider asthma, alpha$_1$-antitrypsin deficiency, cystic fibrosis, ciliary dyskinesia, and bronchiectasis.
- Replacement therapy for persons with the P$_1$ZZ phenotype should be considered when the serum level of alpha$_1$-antitrypsin is <11 µmol/L.

Asthma

Asthma is characterized by chronic airway inflammation with episodes of reversible bronchospasm. Nocturnal cough or chronic, nonproductive cough can be the only presenting symptom of bronchial asthma. Exercise-induced asthma typically presents as intermittent chest tightness or cough (without wheeze) shortly after the termination of exercise. It occurs in 10% to 50% of recreational and elite athletes. Inhaled corticosteroids are considered the first line of therapy by many physicians, and long-acting bronchodilators and leukotriene modifiers are used as adjunctive agents to control more severe disease. A more detailed discussion of asthma is given in Chapter 2, Allergy.

- All that wheezes is not asthma, and not all persons who have asthma wheeze.
- Drug-induced bronchospasm: β-blockers, prostaglandin inhibitors (acetylsalicylic acid, indomethacin), ultrasonic nebulizers, acetylcysteine, *Ascaris* antigen, and occupational exposures.
- Provocation inhalational challenge is used to detect latent asthma.

Treatment of COPD

The therapeutic approach to COPD consists of reducing risk factors (e.g., smoking cessation), identifying the type of COPD, quantification of pulmonary dysfunction and response to bronchodilator therapy, selection of appropriate bronchodilators, anticipation and appropriate treatment of complications, and initial as well as continued education of the patient and family about long-term therapy. Pulmonary rehabilitation decreases disability and improves the handicap, but PFTs show minimal improvement.

Reducing Risk Factors

Because cigarette smoking represents a major risk factor in the development and progression of COPD, smoking cessation should be discussed and programs offered to those who continue to smoke. Smoking cessation can prevent or delay the onset of symptoms in persons without disease and slow the progression in those with disease. Brief physician intervention can be effective in 5% to 10% of smokers. A formal multidisciplinary program with the use of skills training, problem solving, social support, and medications (nicotine replacement

therapy and/or bupropion) can increase smoking cessation in up to 35% of smokers. Reduction in occupational dusts, gases, and fumes and other pollutants is also important in the management of COPD.

- Smoking cessation is vital in the treatment of COPD.
- Minimize exposure to other occupational and environmental pollutants.
- Formal smoking cessation programs can be effective in up to 35% of smokers.

Bronchodilators

Bronchodilator drugs are administered to reverse bronchoconstriction (bronchospasm). They can be divided into β-adrenergic agonists (β$_2$-selective agonists), anticholinergics (ipratropium), adrenergic agonists (sympathomimetics), phosphodiesterase inhibitors (theophylline), mast cell inhibitors (cromolyn), leukotriene modifiers, antihistamines, anti-inflammatory agents (corticosteroids and methotrexate), and other agents (troleandomycin, gamma globulin, and mucolytics).

Short-Acting β-Adrenergic (β$_2$-Selective) Agonists

These are the most commonly used bronchodilators. They include albuterol, bitolterol, metaproterenol, pirbuterol, and terbutaline. They produce bronchodilatation by stimulating the production of cyclic adenosine monophosphate (cAMP) through activation of adenyl cyclase in the cell membrane. In most patients, single doses of these agents produce clinically important bronchodilatation within 5 minutes, a peak effect 30 to 60 minutes after inhalation, and a beneficial effect that lasts for 3 to 4 hours. Many of these agents are available in inhaled form (metered dose inhalers) as well as in tablet, powder, and syrup form and as injections. The standard dose for inhalation therapy is two inhalations four times daily. It is essential to tailor the dosage on the basis of the clinical features and the potential side effects. Adverse effects include tremor, anxiety, restlessness, tachycardia, palpitations, increased blood pressure, and cardiac arrhythmias. Prostatism may become exacerbated. Side effects are more likely in the elderly and in the presence of cardiovascular, liver, or neurologic disorders and in patients taking other medications for nonpulmonary diseases (e.g., β-blockers for cardiac disease). Normal therapeutic dosages of theophylline and β-agonists taken in combination usually are not associated with serious side effects. Rarely, paradoxic bronchospasm may result from tachyphylaxis (a rapidly decreasing response to a drug after a few doses) or from exposure to preservatives and propellants. A newer single-isomer β-agonist, levalbuterol, binds to β-adrenergic receptors with 100-fold greater affinity than albuterol. Because of the narrow therapeutic window for methylxanthines (i.e., theophylline) and the wide range of toxic effects (e.g., cardiac arrhythmias and grand mal convulsions) and drug interactions, the use of theophylline has decreased. The use of inhaled bronchodilators is preferred.

- β-Adrenergic agonists stimulate cAMP.
- Standard dose: two inhalations four times daily.
- Side effects: tremor, anxiety, tachycardia, palpitations, increased blood pressure, cardiac arrhythmias, exacerbated prostatism.

Long-Acting β-Adrenergic (β₂-Selective) Agonists

These include salmeterol, fenoterol, and formoterol. Currently, only salmeterol is available in the United States. Salmeterol is more β_2-selective than isoproterenol, a short-acting bronchodilator that has approximately equal agonist activity on β_1- and β_2-adrenergic receptors. Albuterol has a β_2- to β_1-adrenergic receptor selectivity ratio of 1:1,400. Salmeterol is at least 50 times more selective for β_2-adrenergic receptors than albuterol. Salmeterol is highly lipophilic (albuterol is hydrophilic), hence the depot effect in tissues. Salmeterol has a prolonged duration of action (10-12 hours) and inhibits the release of proinflammatory and spasmogenic mediators from respiratory cells. It has a persistent effect in inhibiting histamine release for up to 20 hours, as compared with the short duration of action of isoproterenol, albuterol, and formoterol. Salmeterol is also effective in preventing exercise-induced asthma, methacholine-induced bronchospasm, and allergen challenge. The dosage of salmeterol is two inhalations (100 µg) twice daily. The longer duration of action may aid in the management of nocturnal asthma. The side effects are similar to those of other β-adrenergic agents. However, tachyphylaxis is distinctly uncommon. Salmeterol and other β-adrenergic bronchodilators may potentiate the actions of monoamine oxidase inhibitors and tricyclic antidepressants.

- Salmeterol is lipophilic (albuterol is hydrophilic).
- Salmeterol: long-acting bronchodilator (>12 hours).
- Dose: two inhalations (100 µg) twice daily.

Anticholinergic Agents

Anticholinergic agents (e.g., ipratropium and atropine) prevent the increase in intracellular concentration of cyclic guanosine monophosphate (cGMP) caused by the muscarinic receptors in bronchial smooth muscle. They also inhibit vagally mediated reflexes by blocking the effects of acetylcholine. Anticholinergic agents are useful in treating chronic bronchitis or asthmatic bronchitis, but they are not beneficial in pure emphysema. Ipratropium is a synthetic quaternary ammonium congener of atropine. As a single agent, it is not effective in the management of acute or chronic airway disease.

It is efficacious if given with β-adrenergic agents and theophylline in the treatment of mild-to-moderate asthma. Ipratropium prevents bronchoconstriction caused by cholinergic agents such as methacholine and carbachol. It does not protect against bronchoconstriction produced by tobacco smoke, citric acid, sulfur dioxide, or carbon dust. Allergen-induced bronchospasm also responds poorly to ipratropium therapy. Ipratropium has no effect on mucus production, mucus transport, or ciliary activities. The usual dose is two inhalations four times daily. The duration of action is 3 to 5 hours. No more than 12 inhalations should be permitted in 24 hours. Side effects include nervousness, headache, gastrointestinal tract upset, dry mouth, and cough. The drug may aggravate narrow-angle glaucoma, prostatic hypertrophy, and bladder neck obstruction.

- Ipratropium inhibits vagally mediated reflexes by blocking the effects of acetylcholine.
- It has minimal or no benefit in pure emphysema.
- It is not very effective if used alone.

Adrenergic Agonists (Sympathomimetics)

These include epinephrine, isoproterenol, ephedrine, and isoetharine. Epinephrine acts on both α- and β-receptors of effector cells. It is used in the treatment of acute severe asthma or anaphylaxis. For adults, the common dose is 0.1 to 0.3 mg (0.1-0.3 mL of a 1:1,000 dilution) by injection. The maximal dose is three injections (each 15 minutes apart). Isoproterenol has a rapid onset of action (<5 minutes) and a duration of action of 2 hours. Adverse reactions associated with excessive use of adrenergic agonists such as ephedrine include anxiety, headache, palpitations, cardiac arrhythmias, skin flushing, tremor, diaphoresis, and paradoxic bronchospasm.

- Sympathomimetics are used to treat acute severe bronchospasm or anaphylaxis.

Phosphodiesterase Inhibitors

Theophylline (methylxanthine) is the main drug in this group. The proposed mechanisms of action include inhibition of cGMP, augmentation of adrenergic terminal output to airway smooth muscle, adenosine receptor antagonism, and stimulation of endogenous catecholamine. The result is a decrease in free calcium levels in smooth muscle. Overall, the use of theophylline has diminished, with β-agonists being given more often in its place. Theophylline is effective in combination with β_2-agonists in the management of moderate and severe asthma. It increases the contractility of respiratory muscles in a dose-related fashion. The clearance of theophylline is shown in Table 21-5.

Table 21-5 Theophylline Clearance

Increased by	Decreased by
β-Agonists	Allopurinol
Carbamazepine	Antibiotics (macrolides)—
Dilantin	ciprofloxacin, norfloxacin,
Furosemide	isoniazid
Hyperthyroidism	β-Blocker—propranolol
Ketoconazole	Caffeine
Marijuana	Cirrhosis
Phenobarbital	Congestive heart failure
Rifampin	H_2-blocker—cimetidine
Tobacco smoke	Mexiletine
	Oral contraceptives
	Viral infection

- The exact mechanism of action of theophylline is unclear.
- Theophylline is effective in combination with β_2-agonists.

The recommended blood level of theophylline is 10 to 15 µg/mL. The loading dose is 6 mg/kg (range, 5-7 mg); the maintenance dose is 0.5 mg/kg per hour or 1.15 g/24 hours. The normal adult dose is usually less than 1,000 mg daily. Longer acting preparations may be given in a single dose of 300 to 600 mg. The dose should be decreased by 50% if the patient has received theophylline in the preceding 24 hours or has heart failure, severe hypoxemia, hepatic insufficiency, or seizures. Each dose should be increased by 50 to 100 mg if the therapeutic effect is suboptimal and in smokers who can tolerate the increased dose. Each dose should be decreased by 50 to 100 mg if toxic effects develop or if progressive heart or liver failure develops. Tobacco smoking decreases the efficacy (half-life) of theophylline. The main side effects are tremor, aggravation of prostatism, tachycardia, and arrhythmias.

- Tobacco smoking decreases the half-life of theophylline.
- The recommended blood level is 10-15 µg/mL.
- In clinical practice, it is not necessary to measure frequently the serum levels of theophylline.

Mast Cell Inhibitors

Cromolyn and nedocromil (pyranoquinoline) block the release of IgE-mediated mast cell mediators, histamine, and other mediators of bronchoconstriction. Nedocromil is 4 to 10 times more potent than cromolyn. These are "preventive" drugs and should not be administered to reverse a full-blown asthma attack. They are available as powdered inhaler preparations or liquids for aerosolization. They are excellent drugs for exercise-induced asthma and for patients with asthma who have known allergens. The duration of action is 4 to 6 hours.

The dose is two inhalations three or four times daily. For exercise-induced asthma, treatment is given 15 to 20 minutes before exercise. The side effects include irritation of the throat, hoarseness, and dry mouth.

- Mast cell inhibitors: not true bronchodilators (they prevent bronchospasm).
- Mast cell inhibitors should be used to prevent extrinsic asthma.
- They are excellent for exercise-induced and allergen-induced asthma.

Antileukotrienes

Leukotrienes are formed by the breakdown of arachidonic acid (membrane component) via the 5-lipoxygenase pathway. By occupying the receptor sites, leukotrienes cause airway edema, contraction of bronchial smooth muscle, and altered airway cellular activity in patients with asthma. There are several leukotrienes, including LTC_4, LTD_4, and LTE_4. Persons with asthma are up to 100 times more sensitive to the bronchoconstrictor effects of LTD_4 than those without asthma. The leukotriene receptor antagonists available in the United States include zafirlukast and montelukast. Zileuton is an inhibitor of leukotriene synthesis (5-lipoxygenase inhibitor). These agents improve FEV_1 by 8% to 20% but are effective in only 50% to 70% of patients with asthma. Antileukotrienes are not true bronchodilators; they prevent bronchospasm. The standard doses are montelukast orally 10 mg daily, zafirlukast 20 mg orally twice daily, and zileuton 600 mg orally four times daily. The most common side effects associated with zafirlukast are headache in 13% of patients, respiratory infection in 3.5% (in those older than 55 years), nausea in 3%, and diarrhea in 2%. Patients taking warfarin should have the prothrombin time (PT) checked and the dose altered as necessary (mean PT increases by 35% by inhibiting cytochrome P450). The simultaneous use of zafirlukast with theophylline, terfenadine, or erythromycin decreases the mean plasma level of zafirlukast. Aspirin also decreases the mean plasma level of zafirlukast. Zileuton may cause dyspepsia, nausea, myalgia, abdominal discomfort, and increased serum levels of alanine aminotransferase (ALT). Churg-Strauss syndrome has also been reported in several patients taking antileukotrienes, most of them while systemic corticosteroid therapy was being withdrawn. The efficacy of these agents in the treatment of COPD is not known.

- Leukotrienes cause bronchoconstriction in persons with asthma.
- Antileukotrienes can be administered for the prevention and long-term control of asthma.

- The efficacy of antileukotrienes in the treatment of COPD is not known.

Corticosteroids

Corticosteroids are the most effective anti-inflammatory drugs available for the treatment of asthma. The mechanism of action of corticosteroids (inhaled and systemic) is unclear. Because inflammation is a main feature of asthma, inhaled corticosteroid is considered by many to be the first-line drug in the treatment of mild asthma. The doses of oral or injectable corticosteroids depend on the severity and duration of the asthma. Corticosteroids have no bronchodilating effect in patients with emphysema. Patients with bronchitis, however, may benefit from the anti-inflammatory action. Short- or long-term systemic corticosteroid therapy is an important aspect of treating moderate-to-severe asthma. Systemic corticosteroid therapy in nonasthmatic COPD has a limited role; only about 15% of patients have improvement. Inhaled corticosteroids can be given in conjunction with systemic (oral) corticosteroids, especially during the weaning period of long-term or high-dose systemic (oral) corticosteroids. All inhaled corticosteroids, when given at higher doses, are associated with greater side effects and fewer benefits. The most common side effect with aerosolized corticosteroids is oral candidiasis. Inhaled corticosteroids in doses greater than 1.5 mg per day (0.75 mg daily for fluticasone propionate) may lead to slowing of linear growth velocity in children, decrease in bone density (particularly in perimenopausal women), posterior subcapsular cataracts, or glaucoma. The use of corticosteroids, inhaled or oral, in the treatment of COPD is limited. A short course of oral corticosteroids may be tried for COPD, but studies have suggested that, unlike for patients with asthma, the response to a short course of treatment is a poor predictor of a long-term response in patients with COPD. Steroid myopathy in those receiving long-term treatment with oral corticosteroids may lead to worsening respiratory muscle function and eventually to respiratory failure. Several large studies on the use of inhaled corticosteroids have suggested that their regular use may be appropriate for patients who have a documented FEV_1 response to inhaled corticosteriods or for those with moderate-to-severe COPD who have repeated exacerbations requiring oral corticosteroid therapy.

- Corticosteroids are considered by many to be first-line drugs in the treatment of asthma.
- Oropharyngeal candidiasis is a complication of aerosolized corticosteroids.
- Systemic corticosteroid therapy is important in the treatment of refractory asthma.
- The use of corticosteroids in the treatment of COPD is limited.

Nonsteroidal Anti-Inflammatory ("Steroid-Sparing") Agents

The efficacy and safety of methotrexate as a steroid-sparing agent is controversial, and the beneficial responses are not consistent. Therefore, methotrexate should not be considered a standard antiasthma drug. Gold salts have been used as anti-inflammatory agents in treating asthma. The bronchodilator effect may not be apparent until a daily dose of 1,500 mg has been administered for 6 to 12 months. Troleandomycin, a macrolide antibiotic, has shown a steroid-minimizing effect by decreasing the elimination of steroid. It works best with methylprednisolone rather than with prednisone or prednisolone. The normal dose is 250 mg four times daily. Other agents in this group include cyclosporine, hydroxychloroquine, and dapsone. High-dose immunoglobulin therapy has been tried in some refractory cases.

- Steroid-sparing agents have a limited role in the management of asthma.
- Some steroid-sparing agents (methotrexate and gold) can produce lung toxicity.

Antihistamines

Because asthma is provoked in many patients by the release of histamine and histamine analogues, antihistamines have been used to treat asthma. Astemizole (10 mg once daily) and terfenadine (60 mg twice daily) are effective in preventing pollen-induced asthma. Histamine (H_1) antagonists produce bronchodilatation without inducing sedation. These drugs can produce prolongation of the QTc interval, which may lead to ventricular tachycardia. This serious side effect is more likely if the patient has liver or heart disease or is taking ketoconazole or macrolide antibiotics.

- Antihistamines are not standard antiasthma drugs.
- Astemizole: prolongation of the QTc interval.

Adjuvant Therapy

Expectorants and mucolytics (acetylcysteine, guaifenesin, iodinated glycerol, and potassium iodide) are used to treat symptoms rather than the underlying bronchospasm. They are not considered standard drugs for asthma or COPD. Antibiotic therapy is helpful for patients with symptoms suggestive of bacterial infection. Desensitization therapy in patients with proven extrinsic allergies may prevent acute asthma attacks on exposure to known allergens. Maintenance of good oral hydration, avoidance of tobacco smoking and other respiratory irritants, annual influenza vaccination, and prompt treatment of respiratory infections are equally important.

Asthma in a pregnant female should be treated as aggressively as asthma in a nonpregnant female. Fetal growth and development and maternal lung function should be monitored. Therapy for asthma during pregnancy should include a short-acting agent to relieve symptoms (usually an inhaled short-acting β_2-agonist) and long-term daily medication to control intermittent disease.

Oxygen

Nocturnal low-flow oxygen (<2 L/min) therapy is recommended when the PaO_2 is 55 mm Hg or less, PaO_2 is 59 mm Hg or less with polycythemia or clinical evidence of cor pulmonale, or arterial oxygen saturation (SaO_2) is 88% or less. The lack of carbon dioxide retention should be assured before recommending oxygen. Continuous oxygen therapy is more useful than nocturnal-only treatment. Oxygen therapy is indicated for patients who have persistent polycythemia, recurrent episodes of cor pulmonale, severe hypoxemia, or central nervous system symptoms induced by hypoxemia. The need for chronic or indefinite oxygen therapy should be reassessed after 3 months of treatment. For each liter of oxygen administered, the fraction of inhaled oxygen (FIO_2) increases by 3%. Exercise therapy improves exercise tolerance and maximal oxygen uptake but does not improve the results of PFTs.

- Oxygen therapy is recommended if PaO_2 is ≤55 mm Hg and/or SaO_2 is ≤88%.
- FIO_2 increases by 3% for each liter of supplemental oxygen.
- An exercise program does not improve PFT results.

The practical aspects of managing COPD are outlined in Table 21-4.

Complications and Causes for Exacerbation of COPD

The complications and causes for exacerbation of COPD include viral and bacterial respiratory infections (commonly *Haemophilus influenzae*, *Moraxella catarrhalis*, and *Streptococcus pneumoniae*), cor pulmonale, myocardial infarction, cardiac arrhythmias, pneumothorax, pulmonary emboli, bronchogenic carcinoma, environmental exposure, oversedation, neglect of therapy, excessive oxygen use (suppression of hypoxemic drive), and excessive use of β_2-agonist (tachyphylaxis). Nocturnal oxygen desaturation is common in "blue bloaters," as are premature ventricular contractions and episodic pulmonary hypertension. A decrease in SaO_2 correlates with an increase in pulmonary artery pressure. Severe weight loss, sometimes more than 50 kg, is noted in 30% of patients with severe COPD.

- Bacterial infections in COPD are caused by *H. influenzae*, *M. catarrhalis*, and *S. pneumoniae*.

- Nocturnal oxygen desaturation is more common in "blue bloaters."
- A decrease in SaO_2 correlates with an increase in pulmonary artery pressure.
- Severe weight loss is seen in 30% of patients with COPD (emphysema).

Other Topics in COPD

Nicotine gum and patch help maintain nicotine blood levels while a smoker tries to cope with the psychologic and other aspects of nicotine addiction. Nearly 25% of smokers require treatment for more than 12 months to remain tobacco-free. Nicotine from gum is absorbed more slowly from the buccal mucosa and stomach than from the airways with inhaled smoke. Side effects include mucosal burning, light-headedness, nausea, stomachache, and hiccups. The patch causes a rash in a large number of patients. Use of the nicotine patch with continued smoking aggravates heart problems. Bupropion has been shown to be effective either as a single agent or in combination with nicotine replacement therapy in achieving smoking cessation. This medication is contraindicated for persons who have a seizure disorder, anorexia nervosa, or bulimia. The most common side effects of bupropion include insomnia, headache, and dry mouth.

- Nicotine gum and patch are important aspects of a tobacco cessation program.
- The simultaneous use of cigarette and nicotine products aggravates heart problems.
- Bupropion is effective in achieving smoking cessation, but its use is contraindicated for those who have a seizure or eating disorder.

Lung volume reduction surgery (resection of 20%-30% of peripheral lung parenchyma) in patients with emphysema appears to improve pulmonary function at least during short-term follow-up, but multicenter investigations are ongoing. The benefit is thought to be the result of regaining normal or near-normal mechanical function of the thoracic cage that was compromised by the severe hyperinflation of the lungs. However, lung volume reduction surgery is associated with increased mortality for patients whose FEV_1 is less than 20% and who have either a DLCO less than 20% or homogeneous changes on chest CT. Lung transplantation is used to treat various end-stage pulmonary diseases. It does not confer a survival advantage for patients with advanced emphysema, but it does confer a survival advantage for patients with cystic fibrosis or idiopathic pulmonary fibrosis. Regardless of the underlying disease for which a transplant is performed, the procedure improves the quality of life.

- Lung volume reduction surgery is experimental.
- It is associated with increased mortality for those with severe disease.

Cystic Fibrosis

Cystic fibrosis is the most common lethal autosomal recessive disease among whites in the United States. The locus of the responsible gene is on the long arm of chromosome 7. This gene codes for cystic fibrosis transmembrane conductance regulator (CFTR), a protein that regulates the function of epithelial cell chloride channels. The most common genetic mutation is the DeltaF(508) mutation, which results in the omission of a phenylalanine residue at the regulatory site. Cystic fibrosis develops in 1 in 2,000 to 3,500 live births among whites; about 1 in 20 (2%-5%) whites is a heterozygous carrier. There is no sex predominance. Occurrence in African Americans is 1 in 15,300 and 1 in 32,100 in Asian Americans. Both parents of a child with cystic fibrosis must be heterozygotes; siblings of such a child have a 50% to 65% chance of being heterozygotes. The diagnosis is made in 80% of patients before the age of 10 years. Obstruction of exocrine glands, with the exception of sweat glands, by viscous secretions causes almost all the clinical manifestations. Mucociliary clearance is normal in patients with minimal pulmonary dysfunction and is decreased in those with obstructive phenomena.

- Cystic fibrosis: the most common lethal autosomal recessive disease among whites.
- In 10% of patients, the diagnosis is not made until the adolescent years.
- Siblings of children with cystic fibrosis have a 50%-65% chance of being heterozygotes.
- All exocrine glands, except sweat glands, are affected.

Up to 10% of patients with cystic fibrosis and heterozygous carriers demonstrate nonspecific airway hyperreactivity and an increased susceptibility to asthma and atopy. Because of chronic airway obstruction from viscous secretions, bacteria such as *Haemophilus influenzae*, *Staphylococcus aureus*, and *Pseudomonas aeruginosa* often colonize the airways. Also, defective CFTR protein may be responsible for the ineffective clearance of *P. aeruginosa*. There is an increased risk of allergic bronchopulmonary aspergillosis developing in patients with atopic cystic fibrosis. Many patients exhibit type I and type III hypersensitivity reactions to antigens. Positive serologic reactions to *Aspergillus* species and *Candida albicans* occur with higher frequency in patients with cystic fibrosis than in those with asthma. Allergic bronchopulmonary aspergillosis occurs in up to 10% of patients with cystic fibrosis, and up to 57% of patients with cystic fibrosis become colonized with *Aspergillus fumigatus*.

- Up to 10% of patients with cystic fibrosis and carriers exhibit increased airway response.
- Up to 10% of patients show increased susceptibility to asthma and atopy.
- Allergic bronchopulmonary aspergillosis occurs in up to 10% of patients.
- Organisms such as *H. influenzae*, *S. aureus*, *P. aeruginosa*, and *A. fumigatus* often colonize the airways.

There is no evidence for a primary defect in sodium transport. However, the epithelial cells in cystic fibrosis are poorly permeable to chloride ions because of the defect in CFTR protein in most cases. The normally negative potential difference across the cell membrane becomes more negative (because of chloride impermeability) in cystic fibrosis. This leads to defects in intracellular chloride and, secondarily, to sodium homeostasis.

- No evidence for a primary defect in sodium transport.
- Because of a defect in CFTR protein, chloride ion transport is defective.
- There is a marked increase in the electrical potential difference across the nasal and tracheobronchial epithelium compared with that of normal subjects and heterozygote relatives.

Quantitative pilocarpine iontophoresis is helpful in making the diagnosis; abnormal results on at least two tests are necessary for the diagnosis (abnormal sweat chloride: adult, >80 mEq/L; child, >60 mEq/L). Note that normal sweat chloride values do not exclude cystic fibrosis. This test must be performed with extreme care because inaccurate collection is a common source of misdiagnosis. Conditions associated with high levels of sodium and sweat chloride include smoking, chronic bronchitis, malnutrition, hereditary nephrogenic diabetes insipidus, adrenal insufficiency, hypothyroidism, hypoparathyroidism, pancreatitis, hypogammaglobulinema, and ectodermal dysplasia. The concentrations of sodium and sweat chloride increase with age. Heterozygotes may have normal sodium and sweat chloride values. False-negative test results are common in edematous states or in persons receiving corticosteroids. When sweat chloride levels are normal in a patient in whom cystic fibrosis is highly suspected, alternative diagnostic tests (e.g., nasal transepithelial voltage measurements and genotyping) should be considered.

- Diagnosis in adults requires at least three of the following: clinical features of cystic fibrosis, positive family history, sweat chloride >80 mEq/L, and pancreatic insufficiency.
- Respiratory manifestations: sinusitis, nasal polyps, progressive cystic bronchiectasis, purulent sputum, atelectasis, hemoptysis, and pneumothorax.

Cystic fibrosis is the most common cause of COPD and pancreatic deficiency in the first 3 decades of life in the United States. Males constitute 55% of the adult patients. The diagnosis is made after the age of 15 years in 17% to 25% of patients. In adults, COPD is the major cause of morbidity and mortality. Adults with cystic fibrosis have a higher incidence of minor hemoptysis (60% of patients), major hemoptysis (71%), pneumothorax (16%), and sinusitis and nasal polyposis (48%). Pancreatic insufficiency is present in 95% of patients, but it is seldom symptomatic. Intussusception and fecal impaction (similar to meconium ileus) are more frequent (21%) in adults than in children. Hyperinflation of lungs on CXR and lobar atelectasis are both less frequent in adults than in children. The mean age at onset of massive hemoptysis is 19 years, and median survival from the initial episode of hemoptysis is about 3.5 years. The mean age at occurrence of pneumothorax in adults is 22 years. Azoospermia occurs in 95% of male patients.

- COPD is present in 97% of adults with cystic fibrosis; COPD is the major cause of morbidity and mortality.
- Adults with cystic fibrosis: minor hemoptysis (60% of patients), major hemoptysis (71%), pneumothorax (16%), and sinusitis and nasal polyposis (48%).
- Pancreatic insufficiency occurs in 95% of patients; it is seldom symptomatic.

Respiratory therapy of cystic fibrosis includes management of obstructive lung disease, chest physiotherapy, postural drainage, immunization against influenza, and hydration. *P. aeruginosa* is the dominant organism and is impossible to eradicate. The presence of *Burkholderia cepacia* is associated with rapid deterioration in lung function. Inhaled antipseudomonal antibiotic therapy, such as inhaled tobramycin, is an option; it has been associated with an increase in FEV_1 and a decrease in the likelihood of hospitalization. Lung transplantation is an option for advanced disease. The sputum of patients with cystic fibrosis contains high concentrations of extracellular DNA, a viscous material released by leukocytes. Aerosolized recombinant human DNase I (dornase alfa) reduces sputum viscosity by degrading the DNA. Results of DNase I therapy have shown decreased risk of lung infections, improvement in FEV_1, and reduced antibiotic requirement. The usual dose is 2.5 mg once daily via nebulizer; patients older than 21 years may benefit from 2.5 mg twice daily. However, recent studies have suggested that alternate-day dosing may have equivalent clinical outcomes. Serum antibodies to dornase alfa develop in about 2% to 4% of patients, but anaphylaxis has not been noted. Side effects of dornase alfa have included voice alteration, hoarseness, rash, chest pain, pharyngitis, and conjunctivitis. Although systemic glucocorticoids are administered during acute exacerbations or to those with allergic bronchopulmonary

aspergillosis, routine use has been associated with notable side effects and is not recommended. Small studies have shown some benefit with inhaled glucocorticoids, which may be beneficial for patients with airway hyperreactivity. If examination of the sputum does not show nontuberculous mycobacteria, treatment with azithromycin (500 mg three times a week) appears to sustain the improvement in FEV_1 and to decrease the frequency of pulmonary exacerbations. The risk of death from cystic fibrosis is 38% to 56% within 2 years when FEV_1 has reached 20% to 30% of predicted. Patients younger than 18 years have worse survival rates once the deterioration in FEV_1 has occurred. Bilateral lung transplantation is an option for patients with declining lung function. Survival rates are comparable to those of patients who undergo lung transplantation for other reasons. The 5-year survival rate is between 40% and 60%.

- Nearly 50% of patients with cystic fibrosis survive to age 25.
- The overall survival rate for patients older than 17 years is closer to 50%.
- Aggressive chest physical therapy, prompt treatment of upper and lower respiratory tract infections, intensive nutritional support, and conditioning improve survival and quality of life.
- Poor prognostic factors: female sex, residence in a nonnorthern climate, pneumothorax, hemoptysis, recurrent bacterial infections, presence of *B. cepacia*, and systemic complications.
- Bilateral lung transplantation is an option for patients with declining lung function.

Bronchiectasis

"Bronchiectasis" is ectasia, or dilatation, of the bronchi due to irreversible destruction of bronchial walls. Its clinical features are similar to those of COPD. Airway inflammation in bronchiectasis is characterized by tissue neutrophilia, a mononuclear cell infiltrate composed mainly of CD4+ T cells and CD68+ macrophages, and increased interleukin-8 expression. Bronchiectasis is reversible when it results from severe bronchitis, acute pneumonia, or allergic bronchopulmonary aspergillosis. Bronchiectasis most commonly occurs in the lower lung fields. Mild cylindrical bronchiectasis seen in many heavy smokers with chronic bronchitis may be diffuse. Distal bronchial segments (second- to fourth-order bronchi) are involved in most cases of bronchiectasis. An exception is proximal bronchial involvement in allergic bronchopulmonary aspergillosis. Disease is bilateral in 30% of patients.

- Bronchiectasis is reversible in chronic bronchitis, acute pneumonia, and allergic bronchopulmonary aspergillosis.
- Upper lobe involvement in cystic fibrosis and chronic mycotic and mycobacterial infections.

- Central (perihilar) involvement is suggestive of allergic bronchopulmonary aspergillosis.
- Lower lobe predominance is suggestive of idiopathic bronchiectasis.

Most cases are diagnosed on clinical grounds (chronic cough with purulent sputum expectoration). Some patients with "dry bronchiectasis" caused by tuberculosis do not have productive cough, but episodes of severe hemoptysis may develop (this presentation is uncommon). Many mildly symptomatic or asymptomatic patients with atelectatic segments of the right middle lobe (right middle lobe syndrome) and lingular segments of the left upper lobe have minor degrees of bronchiectasis. CXR shows segmental atelectasis, loss of lung volume, dilated and thickened airways (manifested as "tram tracks" or parallel lines), and air-fluid levels (if cystic bronchiectasis is present). HRCT can have a diagnostic sensitivity as high as 97%; it is the preferred test to confirm the presence of bronchiectasis. Findings include signet-ring shadows (a dilated bronchus, with bronchial artery forming the "stone"), bronchial wall thickening, dilated bronchi extending to the periphery (lack of tapering), bronchial obstruction due to inspissated purulent secretions, loss of volume, and air-fluid levels if cystic or saccular changes are present. The HRCT diagnosis of "nodular bronchiectasis" usually indicates peribronchial granulomatous infiltration caused by secondary infection by *Mycobacterium avium* complex. High seroprevalence of *Helicobacter pylori* has been reported in active bronchiectasis, but the clinical implications are unclear.

- Nonpulmonary symptoms: fetor oris, anorexia, weight loss, arthralgia, clubbing, and HPO.
- HRCT of the chest has replaced bronchography in making the diagnosis.
- PFTs usually show obstructive phenomena.
- Typical clinical scenario: A patient has asymptomatic or chronic cough, and HRCT shows signet-ring shadows and bronchial wall thickening.

Causes and Associations of Bronchiectasis

Infections

In adults, many cases of bronchiectasis are related to adenoviral or bacterial infections (measles, influenza, adenovirus, or pertussis) in childhood. Various infections, including *Mycoplasma pneumoniae*, nontuberculous mycobacteria, and anaerobic organisms, have also been associated with bronchiectasis. Tuberculosis is a common cause of bronchiectasis, particularly in the upper lobes. Occasionally, chronic histoplasmosis and coccidioidomycosis can cause bronchiectasis. However, in patients with chronic stable bronchiectasis, *P. aeruginosa* is the predominant organism in respiratory secretions.

- "Dry bronchiectasis" with episodes of marked hemoptysis without sputum is usually due to bronchiectasis in an area of old tuberculous damage.
- Bronchiectasis may result from a chronic infection or be a complication of a previous viral infection.

Ciliary Dyskinesia (Immotile Cilia) Syndrome

Cilia are normally present in many organs, and their absence or abnormality may cause clinical problems (which are listed in parentheses): nasal mucosa (nasal polyps), paranasal sinuses (chronic sinusitis), eustachian tube (inner ear infection, deafness), and tracheobronchial tree (chronic bronchitis, bronchiectasis). Many types of ciliary abnormalities (loss of radial spokes, eccentric tubules, absence of tubules, adhesion of multiple cilia) occur. Although the term "immotile cilia" is commonly used, the cilia do move, but their motion is abnormal; thus, the preferred term is "primary ciliary dyskinesia" (PCD).

- Many forms of ciliary abnormalities can occur.
- Ciliary dyskinesia—not ciliary immotility—is the major abnormality.

Kartagener syndrome, a classic example of PCD, is an autosomal recessive disorder that involves the triad of situs inversus, sinusitis, and bronchiectasis or at least bronchitis. Loss of the dynein arm—the fundamental defect—is an inherited abnormality involving a single protein. The prevalence of Kartagener syndrome is 1 in 40,000 to 60,000 persons, whereas the prevalence of PCD is approximately 1 in 20,000 to 40,000 persons. The loss of the dynein arm results in sinusitis and otitis (less common in adults), nasal polyposis, bronchiectasis (in 75% of adults), situs inversus, and infertility in males. Infertility is not a universal phenomenon, and, in fact, approximately 50% of women with immotile cilia syndrome are often fertile. Kartagener syndrome accounts for 0.5% of the cases of bronchiectasis and 15% of the cases of dextrocardia.

- Kartagener syndrome is an autosomal recessive disorder.
- Loss of the dynein arm is the fundamental defect.
- Typical clinical scenario: A patient presents with situs inversus, sinusitis, and bronchiectasis.

Diagnosis of PCD depends on the clinical features and documentation of ciliary abnormalities by electron microscopic examination of the nasal mucosa, bronchial mucosa, or semen. At least 20 types of axonemal defects have been described. Ciliary defects are not always inherited; acquired forms occur in smokers and patients with bronchitis, viral infections, or other pulmonary diseases. However, these acquired defects are different from those of PCD.

- Ciliary defects are not always inherited but are separate from PCD.
- Acquired ciliary defects occur in smokers, in patients with bronchitis, and after viral infections.

Hypogammaglobulinemia

Congenital (or Bruton X-linked) agammaglobulinemia predisposes to recurrent bacterial infections and bronchiectasis. The bacteria that are isolated include *Haemophilus influenzae*, *Staphylococcus aureus*, and *Streptococcus pneumoniae*. Acquired agammaglobulinemia (common variable) may be manifested as sinopulmonary infections in the 2nd or 3rd decade. Selective IgA deficiency is the most common immunoglobulin deficiency; most of these patients are asymptomatic. IgA deficiency is frequently associated with IgG subclass (IgG2 and IgG4) deficiency. Despite the inability to form antibody, most patients have a normal number of circulating B cells, which fail to dedifferentiate into plasma cells that make immunoglobulins. Pulmonary disease occurs more commonly and is more severe than in patients with X-linked agammaglobulinemia. Infections caused by encapsulated bacteria are more common. Bronchiectasis and obstructive airway disease occur in up to 73% of patients.

Hyperimmunoglobulinemia E (Job syndrome) is a rare disorder characterized by phagocyte dysfunction, high serum levels of IgE and IgD, and normal levels of IgG, IgA, and IgM. Respiratory complications include sinusitis, pneumonia, bronchiectasis, pneumatoceles, and chronic dermatitis.

- The overall incidence of bronchiectasis in hypogammaglobulinemia and agammaglobulinemia can be as high as 73%.
- Typical clinical scenario: Selective IgA deficiency is the most common immunoglobulin deficiency; most of these patients are asymptomatic or minimally symptomatic.

Right Middle Lobe Syndrome

"Right middle lobe syndrome" is recurrent atelectasis associated with localized bronchiectasis of the right middle lobe. Mechanisms include compression of the middle lobe bronchus by lymph nodes, acute angulation of the origin of the bronchus, narrow opening of the bronchus, lengthy bronchus, and lack of collateral ventilation. CXR usually points to the diagnosis, although many patients are asymptomatic.

- Typical clinical scenario for right middle lobe syndrome: An asymptomatic patient has chronic atelectasis and volume loss in the right middle lobe.
- The diagnosis is frequently made as an incidental CXR finding.

Allergic Bronchopulmonary Aspergillosis

Central bronchiectasis is present in 85% of patients with allergic bronchopulmonary aspergillosis at the time of the initial diagnosis and has been used as a diagnostic criterion of the disease.

Yellow Nail Syndrome

This syndrome consists of the triad of yellow to yellow-green discoloration of the nails (with a thickened and curved appearance in all extremities), lymphedema of the lower extremities, and lymphocyte-predominant pleural effusion. Bronchiectasis is noted in about 20% of patients. Some patients have sinusitis. Lymphedema may affect the breasts. Some patients have Raynaud phenomenon. Patients may present with chronic and insidious edema of the extremities. Lymphatic hypoplasia or atresia is a proposed mechanism for this syndrome. Pleural effusions occur in 35% to 40% of patients, and recurrent pleural effusions are noted in about one-third. Pleural effusions may appear years after the nail changes occur and tend to be bilateral and small-to-moderate in amount. Both exudates and transudates have been described.

- Typical clinical scenario: A patient has the triad of yellow discoloration of the nails, lymphedema of the lower extremities, and pleural effusion.

Obstructive Azoospermia (Young Syndrome)

Obstructive azoospermia denotes primary infertility in males who have normal spermatozoa in the epididymis but none in the ejaculate. The reason for the relation between obstructive azoospermia and lung disease is unknown. The following pulmonary abnormalities have been noted: grossly abnormal sinus radiograph (59% of patients), sinusitis (56%), repeated otitis media (32%), chronic bronchitis (35%), abnormal CXR findings (53%), and bronchiectasis (29%).

- Typical clinical scenario: A patient has obstructive azoospermia and bronchiectasis.
- Pulmonary and ENT symptoms occur in 30% of patients.

Unilateral Hyperlucent Lung Syndrome (Swyer-James or Macleod Syndrome)

The diagnosis of this syndrome is usually an incidental CXR finding. Hyperlucency and hyperinflation of the lung (usually left) are found in conjunction with a small pulmonary artery. Bronchiectasis is noted in 25% of patients, but most patients are asymptomatic. The cause is unknown, but congenital atresia of the pulmonary artery or acquired bronchiolitis after a viral or nonviral lower respiratory tract infection, inhalation of toxic fumes, or aspiration of a foreign body soon after birth has been postulated.

- Typical clinical scenario: A CXR shows unilateral hyperlucency of the lung, with a small ipsilateral pulmonary artery.
- Most patients are asymptomatic, and 25% have bronchiectasis.

Miscellaneous Causes and Associations

Nearly 10% of patients with bronchiectasis may have an abnormal alpha$_1$-antitrypsin phenotype, with serum levels less than 66% of normal. Other causes and associations include rheumatoid arthritis (Felty syndrome), toxic chemicals, recurrent aspiration, heroin, inflammatory bowel disease, foreign body, sequestrated lung, relapsing polychondritis, chronic tracheoesophageal fistula, heart-lung transplantation, chronic granulomatous disease of childhood, and postobstructive (tumors, long-standing foreign body, stenosis) status.

- Uncommon causes of bronchiectasis include alpha$_1$-antitrypsin deficiency, Felty syndrome, inflammatory bowel disease, toxic inhalation, and chronic tracheobronchial stenosis.

Complications of Bronchiectasis

Complications include hemoptysis (in 50% of patients), progressive respiratory failure with hypoxemia and cor pulmonale, and secondary infections by fungi and noninfectious mycobacterioses. The presence of these organisms usually represents a saprophytic state, but active infection has to be excluded. The most commonly isolated bacterium in bronchiectasis is *P. aeruginosa*. As in cystic fibrosis, it is impossible to eradicate this bacterium. Patients with bronchiectasis infected by *P. aeruginosa* have more extensive bronchiectasis than those without this infection. Routine culture of respiratory secretions is not warranted for all patients.

- The source of bleeding in bronchiectasis is the bronchial (systemic) circulation; hence, it can be brisk.
- The presence of mycobacteria and fungi may represent saprophytic growth.

Treatment

Treatment of bronchiectasis is aimed at controlling the symptoms and preventing complications. Predisposing conditions should be sought and treated aggressively (gamma globulin injections, removal of foreign body or tumor, control of aspiration, and treatment of infections of paranasal sinuses, gums, and teeth). Postural drainage, chest physiotherapy, humidification, bronchodilators, and cyclic antibiotic therapy are effective in many patients. Surgical treatment is reserved for patients with troublesome symptoms, localized disease, and severe hemoptysis. High-dose inhaled corticosteroid therapy (fluticasone) is reportedly effective in reducing the sputum inflammatory indices in bronchiectasis.

DIFFUSE LUNG DISEASE

"Diffuse lung disease" usually refers to an infiltrative process affecting most of the segments of both lungs. The term generally implies interstitial or alveolar filling defects (or both). It is the result of injury to structures in the alveolar space, interstitial space, or both. The interstitial space is located between the alveolar lining cells and the capillary endothelium. The interstitium contains reticular and elastic fibers, alveolar interstitial cells (alveolar cells and histiocytes), small lymphocytes, arterioles, and a capillary network. Diffuse lung disease has many causes. The following discussion includes the causes not discussed in Part II, Diffuse Lung Disease, of this chapter.

Causes

Acute Eosinophilic Pneumonia

Acute eosinophilic pneumonia, a rare entity, was first described as a cause of acute respiratory failure in 1989. It is considered to affect all ages, but more commonly persons between 20 and 40 years old. Most patients have had a febrile illness lasting fewer than 7 days, with nonproductive cough, dyspnea, myalgia, night sweats, and pleuritic chest pains. Most of the patients are hypoxemic at presentation and require mechanical ventilation. Initially, CXR shows reticular or ground-glass opacities, which are often bilateral and diffuse (unlike the commonly peripheral infiltrates of chronic eosinophilic pneumonia). BAL shows eosinophilia, with eosinophils accounting for more than 25% of the cells. For the diagnosis of acute eosinophilic pneumonia, other causes of eosinophilic pneumonia such as drugs, asthma, or infections need to be excluded. Although spontaneous resolution has been reported, most patients are treated with corticosteroids, with therapy continuing for several weeks after the symptoms and radiographic abnormalities have completely resolved.

- Acute eosinophilic pneumonia often results in acute respiratory failure.
- Features: diffuse, bilateral infiltrates with BAL eosinophilia.
- Treatment is with corticosteroids, although spontaneous resolution has been reported.

Chronic Eosinophilic Pneumonia

Chronic eosinophilic pneumonia is another idiopathic disorder. Its clinical presentation is more of a subacute illness with cough, fever, wheezing, night sweats, and progressive dyspnea that is accompanied by peripheral blood eosinophilia. The pathognomonic finding is bilateral peripheral infiltrates seen on CXR which have been described as "photographic-negative" pulmonary edema. However, this is found in only about 30% of cases. Asthma may accompany or precede the diagnosis in up to 50% of patients. After other causes of peripheral and pulmonary eosinophilia have been excluded, treatment is with corticosteroids for 6 to 9 months because relapse is common.

- Chronic eosinophilic pneumonia is another idiopathic disorder.
- "Photographic-negative" pulmonary edema is pathognomonic, although it is seen in only about 30% of cases.
- Treatment is with corticosteroids.

Allergic Bronchopulmonary Aspergillosis

Allergic bronchopulmonary aspergillosis is often difficult to distinguish from asthma, but the eosinophilia is more severe (30%) and longer lasting. More than 95% of patients have extrinsic asthma, and the disease develops in 10% of those with intrinsic asthma. Indicators of allergic bronchopulmonary aspergillosis are asthma previously under control that becomes refractory to treatment with nonsteroidal bronchodilators, expectoration of brownish mucous plugs, segmental atelectasis, and increasing eosinophilia and serum levels of IgE. Allergic bronchopulmonary aspergillosis also occurs in about 10% of patients with cystic fibrosis. The disease is caused by both IgG- and IgE-mediated immune responses directed at *Aspergillus* species. Type I (bronchospasm), type III (pulmonary-destructive changes), and type IV (parenchymal granuloma and mononuclear cell infiltrates) reactions are involved. The major criteria are asthma, blood eosinophilia greater than 1×10^9/L, immediate skin reactivity (type I reaction—IgE dependent) to *Aspergillus* antigen, IgG antibodies (type III reaction) to *Aspergillus* antigen, high IgE titer (>1,000 ng/mL), transient or fixed pulmonary infiltrates, and central bronchiectasis (noted in 85% of patients). A normal IgE level in a symptomatic patient virtually excludes allergic bronchopulmonary aspergillosis.

Minor criteria include the presence of *Aspergillus* in sputum, expectoration of brownish mucous plugs, and late-phase (Arthus) skin test reactivity to *Aspergillus* antigen. CXR shows fleeting infiltrates ("gloved finger" sign, "tramtrack" line lesions, and "toothpaste shadows") in 85% of patients, mucoid impaction in 15% to 40%, atelectasis, and central bronchiectasis. Although generally associated with *A. fumigatus*, allergic bronchopulmonary mycosis can be caused by *Candida albicans*, *A. terreus*, *Curvularia lunata*, *Helminthosporium* species, and *Stemphylium lanuginosum*. Systemic corticosteroid therapy for more than 6 months is required for most patients.

- Allergic bronchopulmonary aspergillosis: almost always in patients with extrinsic asthma.
- May develop in 10% of patients with cystic fibrosis.
- Types I, III, and IV immune reactions may be involved.
- An increased IgE level is the most useful laboratory finding.

- Presence of *A. fumigatus* is only a minor criterion for the diagnosis.
- Therapy consists of long-term systemic corticosteroids.
- Typical clinical scenario: A patient has refractory asthma, expectoration of brownish mucous plugs, segmental atelectasis, and eosinophilia.

Churg-Strauss Syndrome

Churg-Strauss syndrome, also known as "allergic granulomatous angiitis," may affect multiple organ systems. Patients usually present with symptoms of asthma, allergic rhinitis, and peripheral neuropathy, but any number of organ systems may be affected. According to the American College of Rheumatology, the diagnosis is suggested by the presence of vasculitis in conjunction with four or more of the following: asthma, paranasal sinus abnormality, transient or migratory pulmonary infiltrates, mononeuropathy or polyneuropathy, peripheral eosinophilia (greater than 10%), or extravascular eosinophilic infiltration seen in a vascular biopsy specimen. The patients often have increased IgE levels and ESRs in combination with perinuclear antineutrophil cytoplasmic antibody (pANCA) positivity and, often, a low-titer rheumatoid factor. Treatment is most often with corticosteroids for 2 to 3 months or until the symptoms have resolved. Relapse may occur and may require treatment with other immune modulators.

- Churg-Strauss syndrome is a multisystem disorder.
- It is often responsive to corticosteroids.

Parasitic Infections

Almost all parasitic infections encountered in the tropics are known to cause pulmonary infiltrates with eosinophilia (PIE). PIE syndromes due to parasites are considered distinct from PIE syndromes caused by tropical eosinophilia (see below). In the United States, the most commonly encountered parasites are *Ascaris lumbricoides*, *A. suum*, *Strongyloides stercoralis*, *Necator americanus*, *Entamoeba histolytica*, and *Toxocara canis*. The clinical features of strongyloidiasis include peripheral blood eosinophilia, skin rash, and transient lung infiltrates. Pulmonary infiltrates occur before ova can be detected in the stool. Chronic, recurrent strongyloidiasis can last for several years. Ascariasis produces skin rash, nonproductive cough, chest pain, and, occasionally, hemoptysis. CXR shows bilateral discrete densities several centimeters large in perihilar regions. Respiratory symptoms resolve over 8 to 10 days. *Toxocara* causes visceral larva migrans.

- In the United States: strongyloidiasis, ascariasis, and *Toxocara* infection are common causes of PIE syndrome.
- Typical clinical scenario: A patient has skin rash, eosinophilia, and patchy lung infiltrates.

Drug Reactions

Many drugs can cause PIE syndrome. The important ones include aminosalicylate (para-aminosalicylic acid), aspirin, bleomycin, chlorpromazine, clofibrate, cocaine, cromolyn, desipramine, heroin, ibuprofen, inhaled pentamidine, interleukin 2, iodinated contrast dye, mesalamine, methotrexate, minocycline, nitrofurantoin, penicillin, phenytoin, sulfasalazine, sulindac, tamoxifen, tetracycline, and trazodone.

Neoplasms

Pulmonary neoplasms (adenocarcinoma, lymphoma, and other tumors) are associated with peripheral eosinophilia. The mechanism is unknown, although an eosinophilic chemotactic factor secreted by the tumors is thought to be responsible.

- Pulmonary neoplasms may be associated with peripheral eosinophilia.

Tropical Eosinophilia

The cause of tropical eosinophilia is unclear, although parasitic infestation (filariasis) from *Wuchereria bancrofti* and *Brugia malayi* most likely is responsible. Microfilariae surrounded by eosinophils have been identified in lung sections. Repeated laboratory examinations may be required to rule out parasitic infection as the cause of a PIE syndrome. Symptoms progress gradually and include dry nocturnal cough, dyspnea, wheezing, fever, weight loss, and malaise. An asthma-like illness develops in many patients. Eosinophil counts range from 20% to 50% (usually $>3 \times 10^9$/L). CXR may be normal (in 20%-30% of patients) or show diffuse reticulonodular infiltrates. Diethylcarbamazine citrate (Hetrazan) is the drug of choice.

- Tropical eosinophilia: very high eosinophilia.
- Diethylcarbamazine citrate is the drug of choice.

Hypereosinophilic Syndrome

Idiopathic hypereosinophilic syndrome is a rare and often fatal disease of unknown cause manifested by peripheral eosinophilia greater than 1.5×10^9/L for more than 6 months, absence of obvious reasons for eosinophilia, and signs of end-organ damage related directly to the eosinophilia. Most patients are in their 3rd or 4th decade, and the male-to-female ratio is 7:1. Symptoms include cough, fever, weight loss, night sweats, anorexia, and pruritus. The leukocyte count is usually greater than 10×10^9/L, with eosinophil counts of 30% to 70%. The lung is involved in 40% of patients, and CXR shows interstitial nodular infiltrates, with pleural effusions in 50% of patients. BAL may show more than 70% eosinophils. Pulmonary fibrosis may develop in chronic cases. Other serious complications include endomyocardial fibrosis, restrictive cardiomyopathy, mural thrombus formation, arterial thromboembolic disease, deep venous thrombosis, cerebrovascular lesions, and peripheral neuropathy.

- Typical clinical scenario: Very high eosinophilia in men in the 3rd or 4th decade; 40% of patients have lung involvement, i.e., nodular infiltrates or pleural effusion.

Hypersensitivity Pneumonitis

Hypersensitivity pneumonitis, also known as "extrinsic allergic alveolitis," is an immune-mediated lung disease. Many fungal precipitins and several avian proteins (pigeon breeder's lung), animal proteins, chemicals (isocyanates), and metals (trimellitic anhydride and phthalic anhydride) cause this condition. Studies have shown the presence of viruses (influenza A) in the lower airways of some patients with acute hypersensitivity pneumonitis.

Acute (classic) and chronic forms of hypersensitivity pneumonitis occur. Acute farmer's lung is the prototype of the acute form. *Micropolyspora faeni* and *Thermoactinomyces vulgaris* are usually responsible. Symptoms appear 4 to 6 hours after exposure and include fever, chills, sweats, dry cough, and dyspnea. Examination shows tachypnea and basal crackles without wheezing. Leukocytosis, hyperglobulinemia, and precipitating antibody can be detected. Symptoms resolve rapidly (within 18-24 hours) and recur on reexposure. CXR may show increased bronchovascular markings and fine reticular and nodular defects that are often fleeting. HRCT may be required to confirm the infiltrates because CXR findings are often normal. Biopsy (rarely indicated) may show poorly formed peribronchial noncaseating granulomas.

- Typical clinical scenario: Symptoms start 4-6 hours after exposure to the causative precipitin; respiratory distress of varying intensity; wheezing is not a feature; symptoms resolve within 18-24 hours and recur on reexposure.

Chronic farmer's lung follows repeated exposure to precipitins. Obtaining a good history is important in establishing the diagnosis of chronic hypersensitivity pneumonitis because symptoms are insidious in onset, eventually resulting in progressive fibrosis. A decrease in lung volumes, compliance, and diffusing capacity and exercise-induced hypoxemia are typical in late stages. Clinically, this disease is identical to idiopathic pulmonary fibrosis. BAL may show reversal of the CD4/CD8 ratio. Lung biopsy specimens usually demonstrate a granulomatous reaction with bronchiolitis obliterans (with or without organizing pneumonia), epithelioid cells, septal swelling with lymphocytes and plasma cells, and honeycombing. Hypersensitivity pneumonitis has occurred from exposure to *M. avium* complex contaminating the water in hot tubs.

- Hypersensitivity pneumonitis: most cases are due to fungal precipitins.
- The typical feature is restrictive lung dysfunction.
- Water in hot tubs contaminated by *M. avium* complex can cause hypersensitivity pneumonitis.

The points to remember about occupational lung diseases are summarized in Table 21-6.

The histologic features of pigeon-breeder's lung disease consist of foamy macrophages and interstitial granulomas. Positive serologic findings are not diagnostic because 20% of asymptomatic farmers and 40% of asymptomatic pigeon breeders are positive for precipitins and 10% of symptomatic farmers are negative for precipitins. Digital clubbing is frequent (51% of patients) in pigeon breeder's disease and may help to predict clinical deterioration. The treatment for symptomatic patients is to avoid exposure to the causative precipitins. If the patient is still symptomatic or severely ill, corticosteroids have been shown to improve symptoms dramatically. As long as the causative agent is avoided, maintenance therapy usually is not required.

PLEURAL EFFUSION

The normal volume of pleural fluid is 0.2 to 0.3 mL/kg of body weight. Excess pleural fluid collects in the pleural space when fluid collection exceeds normal removal mechanisms. Hydrostatic, oncotic, and intrapleural pressures regulate fluid movement in the pleural space. Any of the following mechanisms can produce pleural effusion: changes in capillary permeability (inflammation), increased hydrostatic pressure, decreased plasma oncotic pressure, impaired lymphatic drainage, increased negative intrapleural pressure, and movement of fluid (through diaphragmatic pores and lymphatic vessels) from the peritoneum. The principal causes of pleural effusion are listed in Table 21-7. The diagnosis may be suggested by certain characteristics of the effusion. For example, obvious pus suggests empyema; lupus erythematosus cells and a ratio of pleural fluid to serum antinuclear antibody greater than 1 suggests lupus pleuritis; a high salivary amylase level with pleural fluid acidosis suggests esophageal rupture; and a ratio of pleural fluid hematocrit to blood hematocrit greater than

Table 21-6 Pulmonary Diseases: Causes and Associations

Pulmonary disease	Causes and associations
Progressive massive fibrosis	Silicosis, coal, hematite, kaolin, graphite, asbestosis
Autoimmune mechanism	Silicosis, asbestosis, berylliosis
Monday morning sickness	Byssinosis, bagassosis, metal fume fever
Metals and fumes producing asthma	Bakers' asthma, meat wrappers' asthma, printers' asthma, nickel, platinum, toluene diisocyanate, cigarette cutters' asthma
Increased incidence of tuberculosis	Silicosis, hematite lung
Increased incidence of carcinoma	Asbestos, hematite, arsenic, nickel, uranium, chromate
Welder's lung	Siderosis, pulmonary edema, bronchitis, emphysema
Centrilobular emphysema	Coal, hematite
Generalized emphysema	Cadmium
Silo filler's lung	Nitrogen dioxide
Farmer's lung	*Thermoactinomyces, Micropolyspora*
Asbestos exposure	Mesothelioma, bronchogenic cancer, gastrointestinal tract cancer
Eggshell calcification	Silicosis, sarcoid
Sarcoid-like disease	Berylliosis
Diaphragmatic calcification	Asbestosis (also ankylosing spondylitis)
Nonfibrogenic pneumoconioses	Tin, emery, antimony, titanium, barium
Minimal abnormality in lungs	Siderosis, baritosis, stannosis
Bullous emphysema	Bauxite lung
Occupational asthma	Toluene diisocyanate, laboratory animals, grain dust, biologic enzymes, gum acacia, tragacanth, silkworm, anhydrides, wood dust, platinum, nickel, formaldehyde, Freon, drugs

Table 21-7 Principal Causes of Pleural Effusion

Osmotic-hydraulic*
  Congestive heart failure
  Superior vena caval obstruction
  Constrictive pericarditis
  Cirrhosis with ascites
  Hypoalbuminemia
  Salt-retaining syndromes
  Peritoneal dialysis
  Hydronephrosis
  Nephrotic syndrome
Infections[†]
  Parapneumonic (bacterial) effusions
  Bacterial empyema
  Tuberculosis
  Fungi
  Parasites
  Viruses and mycoplasma
Neoplasms[†]
  Primary and metastatic lung tumors
  Lymphoma and leukemia
  Benign and malignant tumors of pleura
  Intra-abdominal tumors with ascites
Vascular disease[†]
  Pulmonary embolism
  Wegener granulomatosis
Intra-abdominal diseases[†]
  Pancreatitis and pancreatic pseudocyst
  Subdiaphragmatic abscess
  Malignancy with ascites
  Meigs syndrome*
  Hepatic cirrhosis with ascites*
Trauma[†]
  Hemothorax
  Chylothorax
  Esophageal rupture
  Intra-abdominal surgery
Miscellaneous
  Drug-induced effusions[†]
  Uremic pleuritis[†]
  Myxedema*
  Yellow nail syndrome[†]
  Dressler syndrome[†]
  Familial Mediterranean fever[†]

*Usually a transudate.
[†]Usually an exudate.

0.5 suggests hemothorax. On the basis of clinical suspicion, testing of the effusion should be selective. Despite thorough testing of pleural fluid, the cause of up to one-third of pleural effusions is unknown.

Transudate Versus Exudate
Traditionally, the effusion is considered an exudate if

- The pleural fluid protein-to-serum protein ratio is >0.5 *or*
- The pleural fluid lactate dehydrogenase (LDH)-to-serum LDH ratio is >0.6 *or*
- Pleural fluid LDH is >2/3 the upper limit of serum LDH.

A recent meta-analysis found that any one of the following findings can also differentiate the fluid as being an exudate:

- Pleural fluid protein >2.9 g/dL.
- Pleural fluid cholesterol >45 mg/dL.
- Pleural fluid LDH >60% of the upper limit of that of normal serum.

An increased level of LDH in the fluid is nonspecific, but it is increased in pulmonary embolism, rheumatoid effusion, lymphoma, and most exudative effusions.

- It is not necessary to perform all the above tests to differentiate a transudate from an exudate.
- Clinically, it is more useful to classify the cause by considering the source (organ system) of the fluid (Table 21-7).
- The classification of pleural fluid into transudates and exudates does not permit the consideration of all causes.
- The most common cause of a transudate is congestive heart failure (pulmonary artery wedge pressure >25 mm Hg).
- The most common cause of an exudate is pneumonia (parapneumonic effusion).

Glucose and pH
Pleural fluid hypoglycemia (<60 mg/dL or fluid/plasma glucose <0.5) is found in rheumatoid effusion, malignant mesothelioma, empyema, systemic lupus erythematosus, esophageal rupture, and tuberculous pleurisy. In some cases of rheumatoid pleurisy and empyema, pleural fluid glucose may not be detectable. The pH of normal pleural fluid, which should be determined with a blood gas machine instead of a pH meter, is approximately 7.60. A pleural fluid pH less than 7.30 is found in empyema, esophageal rupture, rheumatoid effusion, tuberculosis, malignancy, and trauma. If the pH is low (<7.20) and clinical suspicion is high for infection, drainage with a chest tube should be considered. Empyema caused by *Proteus* species produces a pH greater than 7.8 (because of the production of ammonia).

- The pleural fluid glucose concentration and pH usually go together (i.e., if glucose is low, so is pH).
- Glucose levels are low in rheumatoid effusion, malignant mesothelioma, and empyema.

Amylase

The concentration of amylase in the pleural fluid (pleural fluid amylase:serum amylase is >1.0) is increased in pancreatitis, pseudocyst of the pancreas, malignancy (typically a primary tumor in the lung), and rupture of the esophagus or abdominal viscera. The amylase level in the fluid remains higher for longer periods than in the serum. Rare causes include ruptured ectopic pregnancy, hydronephrosis, cirrhosis, and pneumonia.

- The concentration of amylase in the pleural fluid is increased in esophageal rupture because of leakage of salivary amylase.
- In any unexplained left-sided effusion, consider pancreatitis and measure the amylase level in the pleural fluid.

Chylous Effusion

Chylous effusion is suggested by a turbid or milky white appearance of the fluid. However, chylothorax is confirmed by the presence of chylomicrons. Supportive evidence includes a pleural fluid triglyceride concentration greater than 110 mg/dL. A concentration less than 50 mg/dL excludes chylothorax. Chylous effusions can occur in numerous conditions: Kaposi sarcoma with mediastinal adenopathy, after Valsalva maneuver, during childbirth, amyloidosis, esophagectomy, esophageal sclerotherapy, and thrombosis of the superior vena cava or the innominate or subclavian vein. Lymphoma is the most common nontraumatic cause of chylothorax. Cholesterol effusions (fluid cholesterol >250 mg/dL, triglyceride <110 mg/dL, absence of chylomicrons) are not true chylous effusions but are also known as "pseudochylothorax." They are seen in the setting of chronic pleural effusions and in some cases of nephrotic syndrome; the more common causes are old tuberculous effusions and rheumatoid effusions.

- Chylous effusion is seen in the "5 Ts": **T**horacic duct, **T**rauma, **T**umor (lymphoma), **T**uberculosis, and **T**uberous sclerosis (lymphangiomyomatosis).
- True chylous effusions contain chylomicrons.
- Cholesterol effusions are not true chylous effusions.

Complement

Total complement, C3, and C4 components in the pleural fluid are decreased in systemic lupus erythematosus (80% of patients), rheumatoid arthritis (40%-60% of patients), carcinoma, pneumonia, and tuberculosis. Increased pleural fluid antinuclear antibody (>1:160) is strongly suggestive of lupus erythematosus. The presence of lupus erythematosus cells in the pleural fluid is diagnostic of systemic lupus erythematosus. Rheumatoid factor is greater than 1:320 in rheumatoid pleural effusion.

- Low pleural fluid complement: systemic lupus erythematosus (also in the drug-induced form).

Cell Counts

A hemorrhagic effusion (pleural fluid hematocrit >50%) is seen in trauma, tumor, asbestos effusion, pancreatitis, pulmonary embolism with infarctions, and other conditions. Pleural fluid eosinophilia (>10%) is nonspecific and occurs in trauma (air or blood in the pleural space), pulmonary infarction, psittacosis, drug-induced effusion, pulmonary infiltrate with eosinophilia-associated effusions, benign asbestos pleural effusion, and malignancy. Pleural fluid lymphocytosis occurs in tuberculosis, chronic effusions, lymphoma, sarcoidosis, chylothorax, and some collagenoses such as yellow nail syndrome and chronic rheumatoid pleurisy.

- A bloody effusion in lung cancer usually denotes pleural metastasis, even if the cytologic results are negative.

Cytology

Most effusions in adults should be examined cytologically if the clinical features do not suggest an obvious benign cause. Cytologic findings are positive in 60% of all malignant effusions, and pleural biopsy results are positive in fewer than 50%. Cytologic examination and biopsy give a slightly higher yield than either one alone, and repeated cytologic examination from sequential thoracentesis increases the diagnostic yield. Cytologic examination is less helpful in malignant mesothelioma, and an open biopsy is often necessary. Positive fluid cytologic findings in primary lung carcinoma mean unresectability (stage IIIB disease).

- Cytologic examination is an important test in most adults with an "unknown" effusion.
- The overall yield from a cytologic examination is 60%, less in cases of mesothelioma and lymphoma.

Cultures

Tuberculous effusions (fluid alone) yield positive cultures in fewer than 15% of cases. Pleural biopsy (histology and culture) has a higher (>75%) diagnostic yield. Culture is of value if the effusion is due to actinomycosis or *Nocardia* infection but is less helpful in other mycoses. However, if fungal infection of the pleural space is suspected, the pleural fluid should be cultured. Cultures for viruses (influenza A, ornithosis, coxsackievirus B, and mycoplasma) are often negative. Paragonimiasis causes pleural effusion. The diagnosis of tuberculous pleuritis is strongly suggested by a high adenosine deaminase level in the pleural fluid. Another relatively sensitive test for the diagnosis of tuberculous pleuritis is the level of interferon-gamma in the pleural fluid.

- In tuberculosis, it is important to culture pleural biopsy specimens.
- The adenosine deaminase level is increased in tuberculous pleural effusion.
- Poor yield in viral infections.

Pleural Biopsy

Pleural biopsy, now most commonly performed through a thoracoscope, is indicated if tuberculous involvement of the pleural space is suspected. The diagnostic rate from pleural biopsy in tuberculosis is greater than 75%, whereas pleural fluid alone has a much lower yield (<15%). The overall diagnostic yield in malignant pleural effusions is about 50%. Diagnostic rates are low (<30%) in malignant pleural mesothelioma.

- Pleural biopsy is indicated if tuberculous pleural disease is suspected.

Miscellaneous

At least 350 to 400 mL of fluid has to be present to be seen on CXR. It is important to look for subpulmonic effusions, elevated hemidiaphragms, and blunting of the costophrenic angle. When in doubt, obtain a lateral decubitus CXR.

Ultrasonography is helpful in tapping small amounts of fluid and loculated fluid collections. Assess for signs of trauma (rib fracture), abdominal surgery, acute abdomen, pancreatitis, and cirrhosis. Asbestos-induced effusions frequently mimic malignant pleural mesothelioma, with pain, bloody fluid, and recurrence. Mesothelioma should be excluded by repeated thoracentesis, pleural biopsy, or thoracotomy.

- Small effusions are common after abdominal operations and the normal labor of pregnancy; almost all resolve spontaneously.
- Drug-induced pleural effusion: nitrofurantoin, methysergide, drug-induced systemic lupus erythematosus, and busulfan.
- Nearly 30% of all effusions are undiagnosed despite extensive studies, including open pleural biopsy.

Complications

Complications of thoracentesis include pneumothorax (in 3%-20% of patients), hemothorax, pulmonary edema, intrapulmonary hemorrhage, hemoptysis, vagal inhibition, air embolism, subcutaneous emphysema, bronchopleural fistula, empyema, seeding of a needle tract with malignant cells, and puncture of the liver or spleen.

PART II
Timothy R. Aksamit, M.D.

DIFFUSE LUNG DISEASE

"Diffuse lung disease" includes a wide range of parenchymal lung diseases that have infectious, inflammatory, malignant, drug, occupational/environmental, and other causes. Although many identifiable causes are recognized, the cause of most cases of diffuse lung disease in many published series is idiopathic. The clinical course may be acute or prolonged and may progress rapidly to life-threatening respiratory failure with death or it may be indolent over many years. In most instances, a differential diagnosis can readily be formulated by taking the medical history, with emphasis on the nature of the symptoms, duration, and pertinent environmental, occupational, drug, and travel exposures. The physical examination, blood tests, pulmonary function tests (PFTs), chest radiography (CXR) and computed tomography (CT) often provide clues to the diagnosis. The diagnosis may be confirmed on clinical grounds but may also require bronchoscopy with bronchoalveolar lavage (BAL) and transbronchial biopsy or open lung biopsy via video-assisted thoracoscopy (VATS).

This overview of diffuse lung disease emphasizes the differential diagnosis, classification schemes, clinical clues to diagnosis, and available diagnostic tools and summarizes a diagnostic strategy for approaching diffuse lung disease in clinical practice.

Some of the numerous causes of diffuse lung disease and the diseases associated with them are listed in Figure 21-27. The numerous idiopathic causes are listed in Table 21-8. The relative proportions of the causes of diffuse lung disease are given in Table 21-9. In a typical internal medicine practice, approximately three-fourths of the cases of diffuse lung disease represent one of three diagnoses: idiopathic pulmonary fibrosis (IPF) (also called "usual interstitial pneumonitis" [UIP]), sarcoidosis, or collagen vascular disease-associated interstitial lung disease (especially nonspecific interstitial pneumonitis). Many of the causes of diffuse lung disease usually described in textbooks are uncommon in clinical practice.

The abbreviations and clinicopathologic correlates of diffuse lung disease are listed in Tables 21-10 and 21-11, respectively. In most instances, the histopathologic findings alone are not sufficient to establish a specific clinical diagnosis of diffuse lung disease. The pathology findings are common to several diagnostic possibilities and need to be correlated with the clinical history and laboratory test and radiographic results to establish the diagnosis. Similarly, different disease entities have overlapping histopathologic features. The histopathologic features of UIP or nonspecific interstitial pneumonitis may be found separately or together, as in collagen vascular disease-associated interstitial diffuse lung disease. In other instances, the histopathologic features are

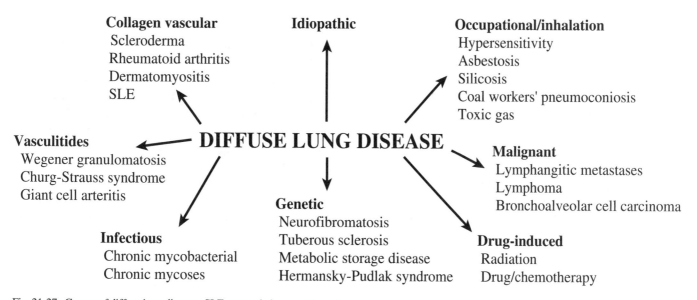

Fig. 21-27. Causes of diffuse lung disease. SLE, systemic lupus erythematosus.

Table 21-8 Idiopathic Diffuse Lung Disease

Idiopathic pulmonary fibrosis (IPF/UIP)
Nonspecific interstitial pneumonitis
Sarcoidosis
Bronchiolitis obliterans with organizing
   pneumonia/cryptogenic organizing pneumonia
Eosinophilic lung diseases
Lymphocytic interstitial pneumonitis
Alveolar microlithiasis
Lymphangioleiomyomatosis
Langerhans cell histiocytosis/eosinophilic granulomatosis
Pulmonary alveolar proteinosis
Acute respiratory distress syndrome/acute lung injury
Others

IPF, idiopathic pulmonary fibrosis; UIP, usual intersitital pneumonitis.

Table 21-9 Epidemiology of Diffuse Lung Disease*†

Diagnosis	%
IPF	12-42
Sarcoidosis	8-41
ILD-CVD	10-17
Hypersensitivity	2-8
Vasculitides	2-8
Histiocytosis	1-11
Drug/radiation	1-10
Pneumoconioses	5-10
BOOP	1-3
LAM	1-2
Lymphangitic cancer	1-2
LIP	1-2

BOOP, bronchiolitis obliterans with organizing pneumonia; CVD, colla-
   gen vascular disease; ILD, interstitial lung disease; IPF, idiopathic pulmonary fibrosis; LAM, lymphangioleiomyomatosis; LIP, lymphocytic
   interstitial pneumonitis.
*Prevalence is 2 to 200 per 100,000 persons.
†Prevalence of IPF is higher among males and the elderly.
Data from American Thoracic Society (ATS), European Respiratory
   Society (ERS): Idiopathic pulmonary fibrosis: diagnosis and treatment.
   International consensus statement. Am J Respir Crit Care Med
   2000;161:646-664; Coultas DB, Zumwalt RE, Black WC, et al: The epidemiology of interstitial lung diseases. Am J Respir Crit Care Med
   1994;150:967-972; Grenier P, Chevret S, Beigelman C, et al: Chronic
   diffuse infiltrative lung disease: determination of the diagnostic value of
   clinical data, chest radiography, and CT and Bayesian analysis. Radiology
   1994;191:383-390.

Table 21-10 Abbreviations for Diffuse Lung Disease

AIP	Acute interstitial pneumonia (Hamman-Rich syndrome)
BOOP/COP	Bronchiolitis obliterans with organizing pneumonia/cryptogenic organizing pneumonia
DAD	Diffuse alveolar damage (acute respiratory distress syndrome)
DIP	Desquamative interstitial pneumonia
GIP	Giant cell pneumonitis
ILD	Interstitial lung disease
IPF	Idiopathic pulmonary fibrosis
NSIP	Nonspecific interstitial pneumonia
RB-ILD	Respiratory bronchiolitis-associated interstitial lung disease
UIP	Usual interstitial pneumonitis

specific for a particular diagnosis, for example, lymphangioleiomyomatosis. The histopathologic features may also
have prognostic and therapeutic implications. For example,
the histopathologic findings of UIP, compared with those of
nonspecific interstitital pneumonia, are consistently correlated with less responsiveness to corticosteroid therapy and
poorer prognosis. In contrast, nonspecific interstitial pneumonia–interstitial diffuse lung disease is more common in
younger persons, is often associated with drug-induced or
collagen vascular disease-associated diffuse lung disease,
and has a more cellular inflammatory process.

Thus, the physician needs to formulate a systematic approach
to diffuse lung disease that involves a complete medical history,
physical examination, PFTs, blood tests, and radiographic
studies before considering bronchoscopy with BAL and transbronchial biopsy or open lung biopsy via VATS. Occasionally,
specific patterns of diagnostic test results provide additional
clues to assist the physician.

In diffuse lung disease, PFTs generally demonstrate restrictive change, with various degrees of gas exchange abnormalities and hypoxemia. A component of obstructive change may
be found in some cases. Specifically, the causes of diffuse
lung disease that demonstrate various degrees of airflow
obstruction on PFTs with or without restrictive change and
gas exchange abnormalities include rheumatoid arthritis,
Langerhans cell histiocytosis, lymphangioleiomyomatosis,
tuberous sclerosis, sarcoidosis, bronchiectasis, cystic fibrosis,
eosinophilic pneumonia, and hypersensitivity pneumonitis.

CXR is the initial radiographic study for virtually all patients
who present with respiratory symptoms attributed to diffuse
lung disease. The findings may include interstitial or alveolar patterns or both. However, the differences between alveolar

Table 21-11   Clinicopathologic Classification of Diffuse Lung Disease

Idiopathic pulmonary fibrosis
Usual interstitial pneumonitis: idiopathic > collagen-vascular disease, others
Nonspecific interstitial pneumonitis: collagen-vascular disease, drugs
DIP/RB-ILD: smokers
Lymphocytic interstitial pneumonitis: Sjögren syndrome, AIDS, lymphoma, dysproteinemia, inflammatory bowel disease/Crohn
  disease, primary biliary cirrhosis, lymphomatoid granulomatosis
Acute interstitial pneumonia: Hamman-Rich syndrome, diffuse alveolar damage-ARDS
BOOP (idiopathic): also drugs, collagen-vascular disease
Hypersensitivity pneumonitis: drugs, avian, mold

AIDS, acquired immunodeficiency syndrome; ARDS, acute respiratory distress syndrome; BOOP, bronchiolitis obliterans with organizing pneumonia; DIP, desquamative interstitial pneumonia; RB-ILD, respiratory bronchiolitis-associated interstitial lung disease.

and interstitial infiltrates can be subtle; also, they are sufficiently nonspecific to be of limited usefulness. Nonetheless, alveolar infiltrates generally predominate in processes of diffuse lung disease that include diffuse alveolar damage (which is the histopathologic diagnosis that corresponds to acute respiratory distress syndrome [ARDS], the clinical diagnosis), pulmonary edema (cardiogenic and noncardiogenic), aspiration pneumonia, alveolar hemorrhage syndromes, pulmonary alveolar proteinosis, bronchoalveolar cell carcinoma, toxic gas exposure, desquamative interstitial pneumonia, infectious pneumonitis, and hematogenous metastases. Infiltrates may be nodular, cavitary, or mixed. An upper versus lower predominance may be suggestive of specific diagnoses. Upper predominance often occurs in diffuse lung disease related to ankylosing spondylitis, silicosis/coal workers' pneumoconiosis, sarcoidosis, Langerhans cell histiocytosis, tuberculosis and mycotic lung disease, cystic fibrosis, and allergic bronchopulmonary aspergillosis. Basilar predominance is common in UIP/IPF, asbestosis, desquamative interstitial pneumonia, lymphocytic interstitial pneumonitis, and hematogenous metastatic disease.

Chest CT, including high-resolution chest CT (HRCT, thin-section CT), is commonly used to evaluate patients who present with diffuse lung disease. In conjunction with a "characteristic" clinical history, physical examination, blood tests, and PFTs, HRCT findings may preclude the need for bronchoscopy or VATS open lung biopsy (or both) to establish the clinical diagnosis, to outline a therapeutic strategy, and to provide prognostic information. Similarly, specific chest CT findings alone may suggest the diagnosis of Langerhans cell histiocytosis, lymphangioleiomyomatosis, UIP, and lymphangitic metastases and, occasionally, sarcoidosis, bronchiolitis obliterans with organizing pneumonia (BOOP), eosinophilic pneumonia, asbestosis, and mycobacterial disease. Ground-glass opacities seen with HRCT are patchy, hazy areas of increased

attenuation with preserved bronchial and vascular margins. They may represent airspace or interstitial abnormalities, although rarely they are seen in nondisease states because of technical limitations. In the case of airspace opacification and interstitial lung disease, ground-glass opacities have been correlated with increased cellularity, as in nonspecific interstitial pneumonitis. In contrast, interlobular septal thickening and subpleural "reticular" honeycombing with traction bronchiectasis reflect a less cellular lesion that is more fibrotic, with scattered fibroblastic foci, and are characteristic of UIP. Both ground-glass opacities and peripheral reticular honeycombing occur in many cases of interstitial diffuse lung disease.

Flexible fiberoptic bronchoscopy has dramatically improved the ability to sample the airway and lung in stabilized outpatients and in inpatients with hypoxemic respiratory failure due to diffuse lung disease. BAL generally can be performed safely in most settings and the findings can be used to quickly identify the cause of diffuse lung disease, especially atypical or typical infectious causes or lymphangitic metastases. BAL is safe for patients who have thrombocytopenia or hypoxemia. Nonetheless, BAL has a limited role in establishing many specific diagnoses of diffuse lung disease, including IPF, sarcoidosis, hypersensitivity pneumonitis, and asbestosis. In many cases, transbronchial biopsy can be performed in combination with BAL, resulting in a diagnostic yield greater than 70% for sarcoidosis, hypersensitivity pneumonitis, Langerhans cell histiocytosis, pulmonary alveolar proteinosis, lymphangitic metastases, diffuse pulmonary lymphoma, bronchoalveolar cell carcinoma, mycobacterial and mycotic lung disease, pneumoconioses, and lung rejection after transplantation. The complication rates of transbronchial biopsy are 1% to 5% for pneumothorax, 1% to 2% for hemorrhage, and less than 0.2% for death. In comparison, the mortality rate for BAL is 0.04%.

In most cases, the results of blood tests provide supportive but not definitive diagnostic information. Results that are often abnormal but nonspecific, and thus not helpful diagnostically, include the leukocyte count, antinuclear antibody titer, rheumatoid factor, and gamma globulins. Moreover, an increase in the angiotensin-converting enzyme (ACE) level is neither specific nor sensitive enough to establish the diagnosis of sarcoidosis. The level may be increased in many other causes of granulomatous lung disease. When the ACE level is increased in sarcoidosis, it may be a marker of disease activity and thus be helpful in follow-up evaluations. In other cases, blood test abnormalities are specific but lack sensitivity; these include fungal serologic tests (e.g., for histoplasmosis, blastomycosis, coccidioidomycosis, and cryptococcal disease), serum precipitins (for hypersensitivity pneumonitis), and specific autoantibody titers in connective tissue diseases or vasculitis. An exception is the test for cytoplasmic antinuclear cytoplasmic antibody (cANCA) which has an estimated overall sensitivity of 81% and a specificity of 98% for Wegener granulomatosis when performed in an experienced laboratory. This antibody is directed specifically against proteinase 3 (PR3). The perinuclear antinuclear cytoplasmic antibody (pANCA) is directed against myeloperoxidase and may also be positive in Wegener granulomatosis as well as in microscopic polyangiitis, Churg-Strauss syndrome, and other vasculitides. Higher sensitivity and specificity rates may be expected during disease activity.

The pretest probability, including medical history and laboratory data, and radiographic findings need to be combined to optimize the diagnostic yield. The diagnostic yield increases from 27% to 53% to 61% when clinical information is added to CXR and HRCT findings, respectively. An algorithm for

diagnosing diffuse lung disease is given in Figure 21-28. With this strategy, including HRCT, the diagnostic yield may approach 90% if the diffuse lung disease is rapidly progressive. The likelihood of establishing a specific diagnosis using this algorithm is greatest for sarcoidosis, Langerhans cell histiocytosis, hypersensitivity pneumonitis, asbestosis, lymphangitic metastases, silicosis, and possibly UIP. VATS open lung biopsy may still be required in up to one-third of patients.

SPECIFIC DIAGNOSES

IPF/UIP

The onset of UIP is insidious and involves a dry progressive cough. It affects persons 50 to 70 years old. Serologic tests are too nonspecific to be helpful diagnostically. Antinuclear antibody, erythrocyte sedimentation rate, rheumatoid factor, and gamma globulins are often mildly abnormal. HRCT findings vary but typically include lower lobe predominance of interlobular septal thickening with subpleural fibrosis and honeycombing with few, if any, ground-glass opacities. In many cases of UIP, peripheral honeycombing and ground-glass opacities are seen together. Classic HRCT findings in combination with a compatible clinical presentation suggest UIP and may obviate the need for bronchoscopy or biopsy. PFTs are expected to demonstrate restrictive abnormalities, with reduced diffusing capacity and abnormal gas exchange with various degrees of hypoxemia. By the time the diffusing capacity is about 50% of predicted or less, hypoxemia with

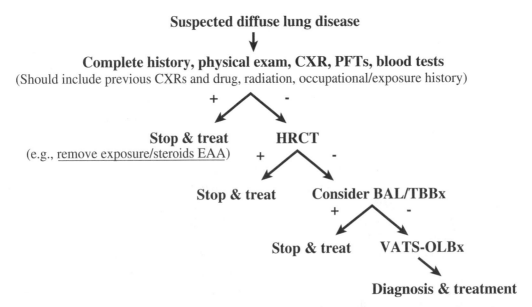

Fig. 21-28. Strategy for diagnosing diffuse lung disease. BAL, bronchoalveolar lavage; CRX, chest radiography; EAA, extrinsic allergic alveolitis; HRCT, high-resolution computed tomography; OLBx, open lung biopsy; PFT, pulmonary function test; TBBx, transbronchial biopsy; VATS, video-assisted thoracoscopy.

exercise is usually present. As a rule, the response to treatment is poor. Corticosteroids, other immunosuppressive agents (e.g., azathioprine and cyclophosphamide), and antifibrotic drugs (e.g., colchicine and penicillamine) have not been shown clearly to be of benefit. Some data suggest that corticosteroids worsen the outcome of IPF/UIP if more than a low dose (prednisone equivalent of ≥10 mg/day) is administered. Whether newer therapies, including gamma interferon and antifibrotic agents, will be effective is not known, but they are being studied in large multicenter trials. The overall prognosis is poor, with 5-year survival from the time of diagnosis estimated to be 20%.

Nonspecific Interstitial Pneumonia

Nonspecific interstitial pneumonia represents a distinct histopathologic type of interstitial lung disease. Its pathologic features often are found in drug-induced or collagen vascular disease-associated interstitial diffuse lung disease. However, in many cases, it appears to be idiopathic. Nonspecific interstitial pneumonia generally occurs in younger patients (≤50 years) and has a female-to-male ratio of 2:1. HRCT often shows ground-glass opacities, in contrast to the basilar subpleural honeycombing, fibrosis, and traction bronchiectasis typical of UIP. The course usually includes various degrees of cough, dyspnea, and fever over weeks or months. The cellularity detected with BAL and the inflammatory components seen in biopsy specimens tend to be greater than those of IPF/UIP. Thus, nonspecific interstitial pneumonia tends to be more responsive to corticosteroid therapy and to have a better prognosis overall, with a 5-year survival rate of approximately 65% to 80%.

Sarcoidosis

Sarcoidosis is a granulomatous disease of patients who generally are younger than 50 years. It may present as lung disease, either as acute inflammatory disease or chronic end-stage diffuse fibrotic lung disease. The development of sarcoidosis has not been linked to tobacco use. Although the lymph nodes and lungs are the most commonly involved organs, the disease can affect virtually any organ, including the heart, liver, spleen, eye, bone, skin, bone marrow, parotid glands, pituitary, reproductive organs, and the nervous system. If the disease is systemic, hypercalcemia, anemia, and increased liver enzyme levels may be noted. Familial clusters of sarcoidosis have been reported. The incidence, clinical course, and prognosis are influenced by ethnic and genetic factors. Stages 0 through IV correlate with the severity of pulmonary disease and the prognosis. Radiographic stage 0 is a normal chest CXR; stage I, hilar adenopathy; stage II, hilar adenopathy with pulmonary infiltrates; stage III, infiltrates without adenopathy; and stage IV, fibrotic lung disease. CXRs may also demonstrate characteristic right paratracheal, bilateral hilar, or mediastinal lymphadenopathy (or a combination of these) with or without eggshell calcification. Chest CT may show small nodules with a bronchovascular and subpleural distribution, thickened intralobular septa, architectural distortion, or conglomerate masses.

A diagnosis of acute sarcoidosis (Löfgren syndrome) can be made on the basis of clinical findings in a young patient who presents with fever, erythema nodosum, polyarthritis, and hilar adenopathy. For the diagnosis in most other cases, granulomatous histopathologic features need to be demonstrated and other causes of granulomatous inflammation need to be excluded, primarily infectious (mycotic and mycobacterial) causes. If hilar adenopathy and parenchymal infiltrates are present, bronchoscopy with biopsy confirms granulomatous changes in more than 90% of cases. Thus, sarcoidosis must be considered a diagnosis of exclusion after other causes of granulomatous disease have been ruled out.

Although rales may be present when acute parenchymal interstitial changes occur, the lung fields typically are clear on auscultation even if parenchymal infiltrates are substantial. The serum levels of ACE are not sufficiently sensitive or specific to be of diagnostic value, but they may be helpful as a marker of disease activity.

Corticosteroids are first-line therapy. However, whether any immunosuppressive therapy, including corticosteroids, alters the natural course of the disease is debated. Other immunosuppressive regimens used as second-line therapy for pulmonary sarcoidosis have included methotrexate, azathioprine, pentoxifylline, and cyclosporine. Treatment is reserved for progressive disease or advanced-stage disease with active granulomatous inflammation. In up to 90% of patients with stage I pulmonary sarcoidosis, the disease is expected to remain stable or to resolve spontaneously with no treatment. Stage III pulmonary sarcoidosis is expected to spontaneously remit in only 10% of patients. Pregnancy does not alter disease activity, although a flare in disease activity may occur post partum. Pulmonary sarcoidosis is expected to progress within the first 2 to 5 years after diagnosis, although increased disease activity can occur at any time. Indefinite long-term follow-up is recommended for patients with stage II or higher pulmonary or extrapulmonary sarcoidosis.

Desquamative Interstitial Pneumonia and Respiratory Bronchiolitis–Associated Interstitial Lung Disease

Desquamative interstitial pneumonia and respiratory bronchiolitis-associated interstitial lung disease likely represent similar entities along a spectrum of disease. Both are diagnosed universally in current or former smokers who present with worsening cough and dyspnea over weeks or months. Crackles may be present. In desquamative interstitial pneumonia, chest CT demonstrates diffuse ground-glass opacities, but in respiratory bronchiolitis-associated interstitital lung disease, it shows a mix of diffuse, fine reticular, or nodular interstitial abnormalities. PFTs may show restrictive, obstructive, or mixed abnormalities, with various degrees of reduced diffusing capacity and hypoxemia. Macrophages are thought to be an integral part of the disease process. Abnormal accumulations of macrophages are seen in the alveoli in desquamative interstitial pneumonia and in the peribronchiolar airway–respiratory bronchioles in respiratory bronchiolitis-associated interstitial lung disease. Mild fibrosis of the peribronchiolar area is more prominent in respiratory bronchiolitis-associated interstitial lung disease than in desquamative interstitial pneumonia, in which little fibrosis is noted. Cellularity, including lymphocytic infiltration, is also more prominent in the airway-oriented lesions of respiratory bronchiolitis-associated interstitial lung disease than the relatively bland macrophage accumulations seen in the alveoli in desquamative interstitial pneumonia. Smoking cessation is the mainstay of therapy, although corticosteroids have been used in some instances. Overall, prognosis is better for both of these conditions than for IPF/UIP. The expected 10-year mortality rate for desquamative interstitial pneumonia is approximately 30%.

Lymphangioleiomyomatosis

This is a disease of women of childbearing age. It is characterized clinically by a history or recurrent pneumothoraces, chylous pleural effusions, diffuse infiltrates with hypoxemia, and airflow obstruction. HRCT typically demonstrates well-defined cysts scattered throughout the lungs, without nodules or interstitial fibrosis. Hemoptysis is common. Pregnancy or exogenous estrogens may worsen the course of the disease. The histopathologic features, similar to those of tuberous sclerosis, include a distinctive proliferation of atypical interstitial smooth muscle and thin-walled cysts within the lung. Extrapulmonary involvement may include uterine leiomyomas and renal angiomyolipomas. The response to treatment with hormonal manipulation has been limited. Currently, lung transplantation is the definitive treatment.

Langerhans Cell Histiocytosis

Langerhans cell histiocytosis is a rare diffuse lung disease of young white smokers. Spontaneous pneumothoraces are common. CXR demonstrates diffuse interstitial infiltrates with classic cystic and nodular changes, predominantly in the upper lobe. The distinctive nodular component with cystic change seen on HRCT differentiates Langerhans cell histiocytosis from lymphangioleiomyomatosis. Airflow obstruction with decreased diffusing capacity and hypoxemia is expected. In the systemic variant of the disease, bone may be involved, especially in children. Pituitary insufficiency with central diabetes insipidus has been described, as it has been for other granulomatous processes, including sarcoidosis. Peripheral blood eosinophilia is not expected, although eosinophilia may be detected on BAL. PFTs often demonstrate restrictive, obstructive, or mixed changes, with reduced diffusing capacity and various degrees of gas exchange abnormality and hypoxemia. Aggregates of Langerhans cells interspersed with normal lung parenchyma are the characteristic histopathologic finding. An increase in the number of Langerhans cells can be detected by staining BAL specimens for OKT6, which is overexpressed in these cells. Absolute cessation from smoking is mandatory. The response to abstinence from all tobacco products varies, with stabilization or improvement noted in as many as two-thirds of patients. Langerhans cell histiocytosis increases the risk of bronchogenic cancer. The success of corticosteroid treatment and chemotherapy has been limited. Transplantation is reserved for advanced, progressive disease.

Hypersensitivity Pneumonitis (Extrinsic Allergic Alveolitis): Farmer's Lung Disease, Hot-Tub Lung, and Bird Fancier's Lung Disease

Hypersensitivity pneumonitis is an uncommon but often discussed form of diffuse lung disease. It respresents an allergic sensitization to a wide variety of antigens, including molds, grain dusts (farmer's lung), pets and birds (bird fancier's lung), and mycobacterial antigens (hot-tub lung). Serum precipitins for specific antigens are inconsistently specific and have poor sensitivity for diagnostic purposes. In many cases, serum precipitins are tested but the results are not helpful diagnostically except for patients who have a clear history of exposure to birds and positive serologic results to testing with an avium panel of antigens. Other blood tests are expected to demonstrate nonspecific and various degrees of leukocytosis and eosinophilia and an increase in the erythrocyte sedimentation rate and rheumatoid factor and a mild increase in antinuclear antibodies. Patients may present with acute inflammatory disease, subacute mixed inflammatory–fibrotic disease, or chronic fibrotic lung disease. The symptoms and clinical course are related temporally to antigen exposure. Acutely, patients may experience dyspnea, cough, fever, chest pain, headache, malaise, fatigue, and flulike illness. Clinically, radiographically, histopathologically, or bronchoscopically, chronic diffuse fibrotic lung disease may be indistinguishable from IPF/UIP.

The histopathologic features of hypersensitivity pneumonitis show a range of bronchiolar-oriented, loosely organized, noncaseating granulomas with lymphocytic-predominant centrilobular infiltrates and various degrees of fibrosis, depending on how long the disease has been present. PFTs show restrictive abnormalities, although an airway component may also be present and result in an obstructive component. Gas exchange abnormalities and hypoxemia may be profound in more severe cases of acute or chronic disease. Bronchodilators may be needed to treat airflow obstruction. CXR generally demonstrates reticulonodular changes, with various amounts of alveolar infiltrates. HRCT findings often include nonspecific nodules and ground-glass opacities, predominantly in the upper lobe. Diffuse fibrotic changes indistinguishable from those of UIP may be seen in chronic disease. Acute symptoms generally improve after the patient is removed from antigen exposure. Severe cases require treatment with corticosteroids.

Asbestos-Related Lung Disease

Asbestos-related lung disease manifests as diffuse interstitial lung disease (asbestosis), but it may also present as benign pleural plaques and effusions, malignant mesothelioma, pulmonary nodules, or rounded atelectasis. The asbestos fibers usually associated with the disease are the amphibole type, of which the crocidolite subtype is the most fibrogenic and carcinogenic. A dose-response relation has been reported consistently between the intensity and duration of exposure to asbestos fibers and the development of asbestosis. A long dormant period between exposure and symptomatic disease is common. The dormant period for interstitial disease, pleural plaques, and malignant mesothelioma is generally longer (20-40 years) than for the development of benign pleural effusions (<15 years). Progressive isolated pleural disease may lead to restrictive pulmonary function without parenchymal change. Asbestos-related interstitial lung disease is characterized by a progressive course of dry cough, dyspnea, and basilar rales in association with restrictive abnormalities detected with PFTs, decreased diffusing capacity, and hypoxemia. Smoking greatly increases the risk of bronchogenic cancer for patients with asbestos-related interstitial disease and may accelerate the rate of progression of parenchymal lung disease. A basilar predominance of interstitial infiltrates seen on CXR resembles that of IPF/UIP. Pleural plaques, when present, may differentiate asbestosis from IPF/UIP. Although HRCT is not needed as often to establish the diagnosis of asbestosis as it is for IPF/UIP, it is able to detect parenchymal changes earlier than CXR and it demonstrates the characteristic subpleural lines, parenchymal bands, thickened interlobular septal lines, and honeycombing. Treatment, including corticosteroids, is not effective.

Silicosis

Silicosis-related diffuse lung disease may result from acute or chronic exposure to silica dust. Generally, the disease affects predominantly the upper lobe, with typical 1- to 3-mm nodular infiltrates. Coalescence may lead to conglomerate masses and fibrosis. Dry cough and dyspnea are typical symptoms. Eggshell calcifications of mediastinal and hilar lymph nodes may be seen, as in sarcoidosis. The antinuclear antibodies are often high titer, but their role in disease progression is unclear. PFTs are usually normal, unless the disease is advanced. Restrictive changes and a decrease in diffusing capacity without obstructive change are expected. Patients with silicosis are at increased risk for *Mycobacterium tuberculosis* infection and should have screening tests for latent tuberculosis infection and active disease. The risk of bronchogenic cancer is less for silicosis than for asbestosis.

BOOP

BOOP is a specific histopathologic entity that can occur with collagen vascular- and drug-induced diffuse lung disease, various infections, radiation injury, and other conditions. Idiopathic BOOP appears to represent a distinct clinical diagnosis, assuming that other secondary causes have been excluded. It generally affects men and women between 50 and 70 years old. The presentation is more acute, occurring over days or weeks, than that of UIP, which occurs over months or years. Approximately 75% of cases of idiopathic BOOP present within 8 weeks after symptoms appear. Most often, the symptoms are cough, dyspnea, fever, fatigue, and flulike illness not responsive to antibiotics. CXR findings include consolidation, interstitial infiltrates, alveolar infiltrates, or mixed infiltrates. Often, the infiltrates are predominantly peripheral, resembling chronic eosinophilic pneumonia. Diagnosis is usually confirmed by transbronchial or VATS open lung biopsy. The response to corticosteroid therapy is generally dramatic. Overall, the prognosis is favorable. Long-term outcome studies do not usually indicate progression.

Diffuse Alveolar Damage, Adult Respiratory Distress Syndrome, and Acute Interstitial Pneumonitis

Diffuse alveolar damage is a specific pathologic diagnosis made on the basis of lung biopsy findings. When diffuse alveolar damage is found in combination with causes of the systemic inflammatory response syndrome, including sepsis, pneumonia, pancreatitis, and trauma, the clinical diagnosis is acute respiratory distress syndrome or, if it is less severe, acute lung injury. If a patient presents with acute or subacute hypoxemic respiratory failure and diffuse lung disease without any identifiable cause and the histopathologic features of diffuse alveolar damage, the diagnosis is acute interstitial pneumonitis. The mortality rate is high (>50%-80%), and the disease is not very responsive to treatment, including high-dose corticosteroids or other aggressive immunosuppressive regimens. Treatment is largely supportive.

Eosinophilic Pneumonia

Acute and chronic eosinophilic pneumonias are two of several forms of eosinophilic lung disease. Acute eosinophilic pneumonia has acute onset (days) of severe dyspnea and cough associated with fulminant hypoxemic respiratory failure and diffuse alveolar and interstitial infiltrates and, usually, pleural effusions. Peripheral blood eosinophilia is not necessarily present, but marked eosinophilia is expected in BAL and pleural fluid specimens. Typically, the response to corticosteroid therapy is complete and without relapse. The long-term prognosis is excellent. In comparison, chronic eosinophilic pneumonia presents with cough, dyspnea, and fever over months or years and, clinically and radiographically, may be essentially indistinguishable from IPF/UIP or chronic BOOP. In the subacute form of the disease, CXR typically shows the negative image of pulmonary edema, which may also be seen in some cases of BOOP and occasionally in sarcoidosis and drug reactions. BAL eosinophilia with peripheral blood eosinophilia (88% of patients) is expected. Usually, long-term corticosteroid therapy is required to prevent disease relapse.

Lymphocytic Interstitial Pneumonitis

This is an unusual form of interstitial diffuse lung disease that is related to several hematologic diseases (e.g., lymphoma), autoimmune disorders (e.g., Sjögren syndrome), dysproteinemia, human immunodeficiency virus infection, and transplant rejection (graft-versus-host disease). The response to treatment is highly variable and depends primarily on the underlying disease process.

Giant Cell Pneumonitis

Another rare form of interstitial diffuse lung disease, giant cell pneumonitis is most often associated with hard-metal (e.g., cobalt) pneumoconioses.

Pulmonary Alveolar Proteinosis

This rare and idiopathic form of diffuse lung disease is characterized by the filling of alveoli with proteinaceous material consisting mostly of phospholipoprotein (dipalmitoyl lecithin). A defect in the signaling of granulocyte-macrophage colony-stimulating factor is thought to contribute to the clinical manifestations. Most patients are smokers younger than 50 years, with a male predominance (male-to-female ratio of 3:1). Symptoms of dyspnea, cough, and low-grade fever are common. Many infectious, occupational, inflammatory, and environmental secondary causes of pulmonary alveolar proteinosis-like presentations have been recognized. Increased predisposition to *Nocardia* infections has been reported. CXR may demonstrate an alveolar filling pattern infiltrate that resembles "bat wings," mimicking pulmonary edema. A nonspecific but characteristic alveolar filling pattern seen with HRCT, described as a "crazy paving" pattern with airspace consolidation and thickened interlobular septa, is suggestive of pulmonary alveolar proteinosis. A milky white return of BAL fluid or lung biopsy findings usually indicate the diagnosis. In addition to smoking cessation, therapy has involved whole lung lavage and, more recently, trials of granulocyte-macrophage colony-stimulating factor.

Alveolar Microlithiasis

Alveolar microlithiasis, a rare form of idiopathic familial (autosomal recessive) diffuse lung disease, is characterized by interstitial infiltrates. Fine miliary nodular changes due to the deposition of microliths occur throughout all lung fields. Most patients are asymptomatic through the third to fourth decades of life. Symptoms of dyspnea may progress to cor pulmonale as the disease advances. No therapy has been shown to be effective.

SUMMARY

In summary, diffuse lung disease represents a wide range of idiopathic and secondary disease processes of the lung that have various presentations and prognoses. A directed, complete medical history and physical examination in combination with judicious use of laboratory data, PFTs, chest imaging, bronchoscopy, and open lung biopsy when needed can considerably narrow the differential diagnosis and provide important therapeutic and prognostic information.

PART III
Karen L. Swanson, D.O.

PULMONARY NEOPLASMS

Solitary Pulmonary Nodule

A "solitary pulmonary nodule" is defined as a solitary lesion seen on plain chest radiography (CXR). It is less than 4 cm in diameter and is round, ovoid, or slightly lobulated. The lesion is located in lung parenchyma, is at least moderately circumscribed, and is uncalcified on plain CXRs. It is not associated with satellite lesions or other abnormalities on plain CXRs. Common causes include carcinoma of the lung (15%-50% of patients), mycoses (5%-50%), tuberculosis, uncalcified granulomas, resolving pneumonia, hamartoma, and metastatic lesions. Uncommon causes include carcinoid tumors, bronchogenic cysts, resolving infarction, rheumatoid and vasculitic nodules, and arteriovenous malformations.

- Granulomas and hamartomas make up 40%-60% of all solitary pulmonary nodules and 90% of nonmalignant solitary pulmonary nodules.
- Hamartomas alone comprise <10% of nonmalignant nodules.

Clinical Evaluation

The following are important in the evaluation of solitary pulmonary nodules: age of patient, availability of previous CXRs, smoking history, previous malignancy, exposure to tuberculosis, travel to areas endemic for mycoses, recent respiratory infection, recent pulmonary embolism (suggestive of infarction), recent trauma to the chest, asthma, mucoid impaction, systemic diseases (congestive heart failure, rheumatoid arthritis), ear-nose-throat symptoms (Wegener vasculitis), exposure to mineral oil or oily nose drops, immune defense mechanisms, and family history (arteriovenous malformation seen in hereditary hemorrhagic telangiectasia).

- History: old CXRs for comparison, age, smoking history, previous malignancy, and exposure history are important.

Diagnosis

Physical examination, routine blood tests, chemistry group, and the exclusion of obvious causes (e.g., congestive heart failure, vasculitis, and rheumatoid arthritis) are important for making the diagnosis. Obtain an earlier CXR for comparison if possible. Generally, sputum cytology, skin tests, serologic studies, and cultures are unrewarding in evaluating asymptomatic patients. Chest computed tomography (CT) is helpful in assessing the location of a solitary pulmonary nodule, calcification, cavitation, satellite lesions, margins, density, and multiple nodules (particularly in evaluating metastatic malignancy) and in the staging of lung cancer. A nodule is more likely to show contrast enhancement on CT if it is malignant. For nodules larger than 1 cm, dynamic positron emission tomography with fluorodeoxyglucose F 18 imaging reportedly differentiates malignant from benign pulmonary lesions more accurately than CT. For asymptomatic patients who have a single lung nodule, extensive studies (gastrointestinal tract series, intravenous pyelography, and scans of bone, brain, liver, bone marrow) are not indicated because of the low diagnostic yield (<3%).

- CT detects 30% more nodules than CXR.
- A nodule is more likely to show contrast enhancement on CT if it is malignant.
- Bronchoscopy has a 60% diagnostic yield in cancer.
- Transthoracic needle aspiration (CT- or fluoroscopy-guided) has an 85% diagnostic yield in cancer but a 20% risk of pneumothorax.

Decision Making

General guidelines for decision making are given in Table 21-12. If a benign cause cannot be firmly established after complete clinical, imaging, culture, and biopsy evaluations, the following clinical decisions advocate surgical resection: 1) the solitary pulmonary nodule is probably malignant because little or no other clinical information is available to indicate a benign diagnosis or 2) the nodule may be benign but must be resected now because the benign nature cannot be established. If the clinical information firmly indicates a benign cause, follow-up CXR is recommended.

- If there is no change in the size or shape of the nodule for more than 2 years, repeat CXR every 6-12 months.
- If the patient is a poor surgical risk, repeat CXR every 3 months (enlargement of the lesion may alter the decision).

Primary Lung Cancer

Lung cancer is the most common malignant disease and the most common cause of cancer death in the United States. The estimated incidence of new lung cancer cases in 2000 was 14% (of all cancers) for both men and women. It was estimated that more than 190,000 new cases would be diagnosed and more than 160,000 deaths would be attributable to lung

Table 21-12 Likelihood of Benign or Malignant Single Pulmonary Nodule According to Clinical and Radiographic Variables

Clinical factor, radiographic result	More likely benign	More likely malignant
Age	<35 y	≥35 y
Sex	Female	Male
Smoking	No	Yes
Symptoms	No	Yes
Exposure to tuberculosis, cocci, etc.	Yes	No
Previous malignancy	No	Yes
Nodule size	<2.0 cm	≥2.0 cm
Nodule age	≥2 y	<2 y
Doubling time	<30 d	≥30 d
Nodule margins	Smooth	Irregular
Calcification	Yes	No
Satellite lesions	Yes	No

cancer. The risk factors include cigarette smoking (25% of cancers may result from passive smoking), other carcinogens, cocarcinogens, radon exposure (uranium mining), arsenic (glass workers, smelters, and pesticides), asbestos (insulation, textile, and asbestos mining), coal dust (coke oven, road work, and roofer), chromium (leather, ceramic, and metal), vinyl chloride (plastic), chloromethyl ether (chemical), and chronic lung injury (idiopathic pulmonary fibrosis and chronic obstructive pulmonary disease [COPD]). Genetic and nutritional factors (perhaps deficiency of vitamin A) have been implicated.

The World Health Organization (WHO) classification of pathologic types of pulmonary neoplasms is given in Table 21-13 and the TNM classification for staging of non–small cell lung carcinoma, in Table 21-14.

Small cell carcinoma is staged as follows:
1. Limited: single hemithorax, mediastinum, ipsilateral supraclavicular nodes
2. Extensive: anything beyond limited stage

Overall Survival

The overall 5-year survival for all stages of lung cancer is 14%. The overall survival rate for patients with occult and in situ cancers is greater than 70%. The overall survival for other stages is as follows: stage I, 50%; stage II, less than 20%; stage III, less than 10%. One-year survival for stage I cancer is greater than 80%. In small cell cancer, the median survival is less than 12 months; the 5-year survival for limited stage cancer is 15% to 20% and for extensive disease, 1% to 5%.

- The overall 5-year survival for all lung cancers is 14%.

Cell Types

Primary lung cancer is broadly divided into non–small cell lung carcinoma (adenocarcinoma, 35%; squamous cell carcinoma, 30%; and large cell carcinoma, 1%-15%), small cell carcinoma (20%-25%), mixed (small and large cell), and others (metastatic lesions).

Clinical Features

Most patients are older than 50 years. Only 5% of patients with lung cancer are asymptomatic. The presentation is highly variable and depends on the cell type, location, rate of growth, paraneoplastic syndromes, systemic symptoms, and other factors. Cough is the most frequent symptom and is more likely in squamous cell carcinoma and small cell lung carcinoma than in other types of lung cancer. Hemoptysis occurs in 35% to 50% of patients and is more common with squamous cell, small cell, carcinoid, and endobronchial metastases than with other types of tumors. Wheezing is due to intraluminal tumor or extrinsic compression. Dyspnea depends on the extensiveness of the tumor, COPD, degree of bronchial obstruction, and other factors. Persistent chest pain may suggest rib metastasis, local extension, or pleural involvement. Superior vena cava syndrome may suggest small cell carcinoma, lymphoma,

Table 21-13 World Health Organization Classification of Pulmonary Neoplasms

Type	Histologic type
I	Squamous cell carcinoma
II	Small cell carcinoma
	Oat cell carcinoma
	Intermediate cell carcinoma
	Combined oat cell carcinoma
III	Adenocarcinoma
	Acinar adenocarcinoma
	Papillary adenocarcinoma
	Bronchoalveolar carcinoma
	Solid carcinoma with mucus formation
IV	Large cell carcinoma
	Giant cell carcinoma
	Clear cell carcinoma
V	Combined cell types
VI	Carcinoid
VII	Bronchial gland tumors
	Cylindroma
	Mucoepidermoid
VIII	Papillary tumors

Table 21-14   Staging of Lung Cancer: TNM Classification

T, primary tumor		
T0	No evidence of primary tumor	
TX	Cancer cells in respiratory secretions; no tumor on chest radiographs or at bronchoscopy	
Tis	Carcinoma in situ	
T1	Tumor ≤3 cm in greatest dimension, surrounded by lung tissue; no bronchoscopic evidence of tumor proximal to lobar bronchus	
T2	Tumor >3 cm in diameter, or tumor of any size that involves visceral pleura, or associated with atelectasis extending to hilum (but not involving entire lung); must be ≥2 cm from main carina	
T3	Tumor involves chest wall, diaphragm, mediastinal pleura, or pericardium, or is <2 cm from main carina (but does not involve it)	
T4	Tumor involves main carina or trachea, or invades mediastinum, heart, great vessels, esophagus, or vertebrae, or malignant pleural effusion	
N, nodal involvement		
NX	Regional lymph nodes cannot be assessed	
N0	No demonstrable lymph node involvement	
N1	Ipsilateral peribronchial or hilar lymph nodes involved	
N2	Metastasis to ipsilateral mediastinal lymph nodes or to subcarinal lymph nodes	
N3	Metastasis to contralateral mediastinal and/or hilar lymph nodes or to scalene and/or supraclavicular lymph nodes	
M, metastasis		
MX	Presence of distant metastasis cannot be assessed	
M0	No known distant metastasis	
M1	Distant metastasis present (specify site or sites)	

Stage Grouping—TNM Subsets[*]

Stage 0	Carcinoma in situ	Stage IIIB	T4 N0 M0
			T4 N1 M0
Stage IA	T1 N0 M0		T4 N2 M0
Stage IB	T2 N0 M0		T1 N3 M0
			T2 N3 M0
Stage IIA	T1 N1 M0		T3 N3 M0
Stage IIB	T2 N1 M0		T4 N3 M0
	T3 N0 M0		
		Stage IV	Any T Any N M1
Stage IIIA	T3 N1 M0		
	T1 N2 M0		
	T2 N2 M0		
	T3 N2 M0		

[*]Staging is not relevant for occult carcinoma, designated TX N0 M0.

squamous cell carcinoma, or Pancoast tumor. Horner syndrome is indicative of Pancoast tumor. Fever, postobstructive pneumonitis, nonthoracic skeletal pain, central nervous system symptoms, abdominal pain or discomfort, and hepatomegaly are indicative of possible distant metastases. During the course of the disease, central nervous system metastasis is found in 15% of patients with squamous cell carcinoma, in 25% with adenocarcinoma, in 28% with large cell carcinoma, and in 30% with small cell carcinoma.

- Cough and hemoptysis are more common in squamous cell carcinoma and carcinoid.
- Chest pain may indicate pleural effusion, pleural metastasis, or rib lesion.

- Nonpulmonary symptoms may indicate distant metastases or paraneoplastic syndromes.
- Central nervous system metastasis is more common with small cell carcinoma.

Squamous Cell Carcinoma

More than 65% of squamous cell carcinomas arise in the proximal tracheobronchial tree (first four subdivisions). They also may arise in the upper airway and esophagus. Symptoms appear early in the course of the disease because of proximal bronchial involvement and consist of cough, hemoptysis, and lobar or segmental (or both) collapse with postobstructive pneumonia. CXR findings include atelectasis (23% of patients), obstructive pneumonitis (13%), hilar adenopathy (38%), and cavitation (5%). One-third of cases present as peripheral masses. Sputum cytology and bronchoscopy are indicated in almost all patients. One-third of squamous cell carcinomas have thick-walled irregular cavities. Treatment is with resection, irradiation, and chemotherapy. Laser bronchoscopy and endobronchial brachytherapy are palliative measures.

- Squamous cell carcinoma: proximal airway disease in 66% of cases, peripheral mass in 33%, and cavitation in 35%.
- Sputum cytology and bronchoscopy are important tests.

Adenocarcinoma

Most adenocarcinomas arise in the periphery and, thus, remain asymptomatic and undetected until they have spread locally or distally. This means that the chance of dissemination to extrapulmonary sites is higher for these tumors. However, incidentally detected peripheral carcinomas tend to be in an early stage. Adenocarcinoma is the most common type of peripheral primary lung cancer. Sputum cytology has a low diagnostic yield. The most common presentation is as a solitary peripheral nodule. A small number cavitate. Clubbing and hypertrophic pulmonary osteoarthropathy are more common than in other kinds of primary lung cancer. The response to radiotherapy and chemotherapy is generally poor.

- Adenocarcinoma: A solitary pulmonary nodule in the periphery of the lung.
- The symptomatic stage usually denotes advanced disease.
- Sputum cytology has a low diagnostic yield.
- Clubbing and hypertrophic pulmonary osteoarthropathy are more common than in squamous cell carcinoma.

Bronchoalveolar Cell Carcinoma

Bronchoalveolar cell carcinoma is thought to arise from alveolar type II pneumocytes or Clara cells (or both). The tumor presents in two forms: as a localized solitary nodular lesion and as a diffuse alveolar process. More than 60% of patients are asymptomatic. The cancer presents as a solitary nodule in the majority of patients and as lobar pneumonitis or a diffuse infiltrate in a minority. The solitary form has the best prognosis of all types of lung cancer, with a 1-year survival rate greater than 80%. The diffuse form has a mean survival of less than 6 months. Bronchorrhea (>100 mL of thin serous mucus secretion in 24 hours) is seen in 20% of patients. CXR shows a solitary nodule, localized infiltrate with vacuoles (on tomography), or pneumonic lesions. Both forms of bronchoalveolar cell carcinoma can mimic ordinary pneumonia. Because of the slow growth, the chronic course of the disease may suggest a benign process; thus, close surveillance is imperative. The treatment for a solitary lesion is resection. The response to radiotherapy and chemotherapy is poor, although bronchorrhea seems to respond to radiotherapy in some patients.

- Bronchoalveolar cell carcinoma: unrelated to tobacco smoking.
- The solitary form grows slowly and may mimic a benign lung nodule.
- The solitary (localized) form has >80% 1-year survival rate after resection.
- The diffuse form has a mean survival of <6 months.
- Bronchorrhea occurs in 20% of patients (usually the diffuse form).

Large Cell Carcinoma

Large cells are seen on histologic examination, and CXR shows large masses. Large cell carcinoma grows more rapidly than adenocarcinoma. Cavitation occurs in 20% to 25% of patients. Clubbing and hypertrophic pulmonary osteoarthropathy are more common than in other tumors except for adenocarcinoma. The treatment is surgical. The response to irradiation and chemotherapy is poor.

- Large cell carcinoma: A large, rapidly growing lung mass, with cavitation in 25% of patients; clubbing and hypertrophic pulmonary osteoarthropathy are common.

Small Cell Carcinoma

Small cell carcinoma (oat cell carcinoma) accounts for 25% of all bronchogenic carcinomas. The tumor originates from neuroendocrine cells and invades the tracheobronchial tree and spreads submucosally. Later, it breaks through the mucosa and produces changes similar to those seen in squamous cell carcinoma. CXR shows a unilateral, rapidly enlarging hilar or perihilar mass or widening of the mediastinum. Less than 20% of these tumors are peripheral. Bronchoscopy may show heaped-up or thickened mucosa. This tumor responds better to radiotherapy and chemotherapy than do other lung tumors. Brain metastasis is common. Prophylactic brain irradiation is standard at many medical centers; this decreases the frequency of brain metastasis but does not prolong survival. Peripheral nodules that are found after resection to be small cell carcinoma should be treated as any small cell carcinoma.

- Small cell carcinoma: Smokers and uranium miners are at high risk; it is associated with many paraneoplastic syndromes, including the syndrome of inappropriate antidiuretic hormone (SIADH), adrenocorticotropic hormone (ACTH) production, and myasthenic syndrome.
- Surgical treatment is not a standard therapeutic option; radiotherapy and chemotherapy are.

Carcinoid

Carcinoid arises from the same cells as small cell carcinoma, but its clinical behavior is different. Typically, carcinoid presents with cough, with or without hemoptysis, in young adults. CXR may show a solitary nodule or segmental atelectasis. Paraneoplastic syndromes develop from hormonal secretion (ACTH and parathyroid hormone [PTH]). Treatment is surgical resection of the tumor without lung resection. The diagnosis of malignant carcinoid is based on the extent of spread noted at resection or clinical behavior.

- Typical clinical scenario for carcinoid: A young adult presents with cough and hemoptysis; symptoms may be related to the production of ACTH (Cushing syndrome, hypertension) and PTH (hypercalcemia).
- Carcinoid "syndrome" is rare, occurring in <1% of patients with bronchial carcinoid.

Bronchial Gland Tumors

Cylindroma (adenoid cystic carcinoma) and mucoepidermoid tumors usually are located centrally and cause cough, hemoptysis, and obstructive pneumonia. Distant metastasis is unusual. Surgical treatment is used for lesions causing major airway obstruction. The response to radiotherapy and chemotherapy is poor.

- Cylindromas arising in salivary glands can metastasize to the lungs after many years.

Mesenchymal Tumors

This group of tumors includes lymphoma, lymphosarcoma, carcinosarcoma, fibrosarcoma, mesothelioma, and soft tissue sarcomas. Many of these present as large peripheral masses, homogeneous densities, and cavitated lesions.

Lymphoma

Patients with Hodgkin or non-Hodgkin lymphoma may have pulmonary involvement. CXR findings include bilateral hilar adenopathy, chylous pleural effusion, segmental atelectasis from endobronchial lesions, a diffuse nodular process, fluffy infiltrates, and diffuse interstitial or alveolar infiltrates (or both). Almost all cases of lymphocytic interstitial pneumonitis represent low-grade lymphomas that originate from the mucosa-associated lymphoid tissue ("maltoma"). They are very responsive to chemotherapy.

- Intrathoracic involvement is common in Hodgkin lymphoma.
- Bilateral hilar lymphadenopathy and chylous pleural effusion may occur.
- Hodgkin lymphoma can produce any type of CXR abnormality.

Diagnostic Tests

Sputum cytology findings are positive in 60% of patients with squamous cell carcinoma, in 21% with small cell carcinoma, in 16% with adenocarcinoma, and in 13% with large cell carcinoma. More tumors are diagnosed with CXR than with sputum cytology, but CXR is not recommended as a surveillance tool for all patients. Bronchoscopy is helpful in diagnosing the cell type, in assessing staging and resectability, in using laser treatment for large airway tumors, and in brachytherapy. Transthoracic needle aspiration has an 85% to 90% yield, but the incidence of pneumothorax is 25%, with most patients requiring chest tube drainage. CT is helpful in assessing the number of nodules in patients with pulmonary metastasis and in examining the hila and mediastinum. Positive results on pleural fluid cytology establish stage IIIB disease. Mediastinoscopy and mediastinotomy (Chamberlain procedure) are staging procedures that are often used before thoracotomy is performed.

- More lung tumors are diagnosed with CXR than with sputum cytology.
- Sputum cytology findings are positive in 60% of patients with squamous cell cancer.
- Routine surveillance of all susceptible persons (heavy smokers) with CXR and sputum cytology is not recommended.

Paraneoplastic Syndromes

As a group, primary lung tumors are the most common cause of paraneoplastic syndromes. The presence of a paraneoplastic syndrome does not indicate metastatic spread of lung cancer. It is more helpful to consider paraneoplastic manifestations based on each organ system (see below).

- Primary lung tumors cause most of the paraneoplastic manifestations.
- A paraneoplastic syndrome does not indicate metastatic spread of lung cancer.

Endocrine

Small cell carcinoma is associated with SIADH and ACTH production. Hypokalemia, muscle weakness, and CXR abnormality should suggest ACTH production. These patients do not survive long enough for the typical Cushing syndrome to develop. The ACTH levels are high and not suppressed by dexamethasone. Hypercalcemia is not associated with small cell carcinoma. The overall frequency of hypercalcemia is 13%, with squamous cell cancer as the cause in 25% of patients, large cell carcinoma in 13%, and adenocarcinoma in 3%. Bony metastasis may also cause hypercalcemia. Hyperpigmentation from melanocyte-stimulating hormone occurs in small cell carcinoma. Calcitonin is secreted in 70% of patients with small cell carcinoma and in adenocarcinoma. SIADH is also seen in some patients with alveolar cell carcinoma and adenocarcinoma. Hypoglycemia with insulin-like polypeptide is found in patients with squamous cell carcinoma and mesothelioma. The human chorionic gonadotropin, luteinizing hormone, and follicle-stimulating hormone secreted by adenocarcinoma and large cell carcinoma may be responsible for gynecomastia.

● Abnormal CXR, hypokalemia, and muscle weakness: small cell carcinoma (ACTH).
● ACTH is also produced by bronchial carcinoid.
● Hypercalcemia: squamous cell carcinoma and carcinoid.

Nervous System

The mechanisms for encephalopathy, myelopathy, sensorimotor neuropathies, and polymyositis are unknown but may include toxic, nutritional, autoimmune, and infectious causes. Cerebellar ataxia is similar to alcohol-induced ataxia and is more common with squamous cell carcinoma. Myasthenic syndrome (Lambert-Eaton syndrome) is closely associated with small cell carcinoma; the proximal muscles are initially weak, but strength returns to normal with repeated stimulation. Focal neurologic signs should suggest central nervous system metastasis. Acute and rapidly progressive lower extremity signs should indicate spinal cord compression by tumor. Antineuronal nuclear antibody (ANNA)-1 is positive in many patients with small cell carcinoma.

● Myasthenic syndrome may precede the clinical detection of small cell carcinoma.
● Cerebellar ataxia (similar to alcohol-induced ataxia) is more common in squamous cell carcinoma.

Skeletal

Hypertrophic pulmonary osteoarthropathy (HPO) indicates periosteal bone formation and is associated with clubbing and symmetrical arthralgias. Other features include fever, gynecomastia, and an increased erythrocyte sedimentation rate (ESR).

The proposed mechanisms include neural (vagal afferents), hormonal, and others. HPO is more common in adenocarcinoma and large cell carcinoma than in squamous cell and small cell lung carcinoma, and it may precede detection of the tumor by months. Clubbing may be the only feature. Removal of the tumor relieves the HPO. Octreotide appears to be effective in treating HPO.

● HPO is more common in adenocarcinoma and large cell carcinoma.
● Tumor resection relieves HPO.
● Treatment: octreotide (somatostatin analogue) or ipsilateral vagotomy if the HPO persists after resection of the tumor.

Others

Other paraneoplastic manifestations include malignant cachexia, marantic endocarditis, increased incidence of thrombophlebitis, fever, erythrocytosis, leukocytosis, lymphocytopenia, eosinophilia, thrombocytosis, leukemoid reaction, disseminated intravascular coagulation, dysproteinemia, fever, acanthosis nigricans (adenocarcinoma), epidermolysis bullosa (squamous cell carcinoma), and nephrotic syndrome.

Pulmonary Metastases

Nearly 30% of all cases of malignant disease from extrapulmonary sites metastasize to the lung. More than 75% present with multiple lesions, and the rest may present as a solitary pulmonary nodule, a diffuse process, lymphangitic spread (breast, stomach, thyroid, pancreas, and the lung itself), and endobronchial metastases (kidney, colon, Hodgkin lymphoma, and breast). Solitary metastases are more common with carcinoma of the colon, kidneys, testes, and breast and with sarcoma and melanoma. The estimated occurrence of pulmonary metastasis by primary tumor is as follows: choriocarcinoma, 80%; osteosarcoma, 75%; kidney, 70%; thyroid, 65%; melanoma, 60%; breast, 55%; prostate, 45%; nasopharyngeal, 20%; gastrointestinal tract, 20%; and gynecologic malignancies, 20%.

VASCULAR DISEASES

Pulmonary Embolism

Pulmonary embolism (PE) is the cause of death of 5% to 15% of patients who die in hospitals in the United States. A multicenter study of PE observed that the mortality rate at 3 months was 15% and important prognostic factors included age older than 70 years, cancer, congestive heart failure, COPD, systolic arterial hypotension, tachypnea, and right ventricular hypokinesis. PE is detected in 25% to 30% of routine autopsies.

Antemortem diagnosis is made in fewer than 30% of cases. Among hospitalized patients, the prevalence of PE is 1%. In about 90% of patients who die of PE, death occurs within 1 to 2 hours. The risk of fatal PE is greater among patients with severe deep venous thrombosis (DVT).

- PE is a common problem; consider PE in all patients who have lung problems.
- Antemortem diagnosis is made in <30% of cases.
- The risk of death from untreated PE is 8%.

Etiology

The factor responsible for most PEs is DVT of the lower extremities. Among patients with fatal PE, DVT has been identified clinically in only 50%. In those with a large angiographically diagnosed PE, DVT is detected in about 35%. About 60% of patients with PE have asymptomatic lower extremity DVT. Approximately 45% of femoral and iliac DVTs embolize to the lungs. Other sources of emboli include thrombi in the upper extremities, right ventricle, and indwelling catheters. In up to 20% of patients, DVTs from the calves propagate to the thigh and iliac veins, and up to 10% of cases of superficial thrombophlebitis are complicated by

DVT. The risk of recurrent DVT is similar among carriers of factor V Leiden and patients without this mutation. The primary and secondary coagulation abnormalities that predispose to the development of DVT and PE are listed in Table 21-15.

- DVT is detected in only 40% of cases of pulmonary embolism.
- Consider factor V Leiden mutation and deficiencies of antithrombin III, protein S, and protein C and the presence of lupus anticoagulant among predisposing factors for DVT and PE.
- In idiopathic, recurrent DVT, look for an occult neoplasm.

The incidence of DVT in various clinical circumstances is listed in Table 21-16. Idiopathic DVT, particularly when recurrent, may indicate the presence of neoplasm in 10% to 20% of patients. The presence of varicose veins does not increase the risk of developing DVT.

- Risk of DVT: thoracic surgery, 25%-60%; hip surgery, 50%-75%; post-myocardial infarction, 20%-40%; congestive heart failure, 70%; and stroke with paralysis, 50%-70%.

Table 21-15   Coagulation Disorders Predisposing to the Development of Deep Venous Thrombosis and Pulmonary Embolism

Primary hypercoagulable states	Secondary hypercoagulable states
Activated protein C resistance* (factor V Leiden carriers)	Cancer
Antithrombin III deficiency†	Postoperative states (stasis)
Protein C deficiency†	Lupus anticoagulant syndrome
Protein S deficiency†	Increased factor VII and fibrinogen
Fibrinolytic abnormalities	Pregnancy
Hypoplasminogenemia	Nephrotic syndrome
Dysplasminogenemia	Myeloproliferative disorders
TPA release deficiency	Disseminated intravascular coagulation
Increased TPA inhibitor	Acute stroke
Dysfibrinogenemia	Hyperlipidemias
Homocystinuria	Diabetes mellitus
Heparin cofactor deficiency	Paroxysmal nocturnal hemoglobinuria
Increased histidine-rich glycoprotein	Behçet disease and vasculitides
	Anticancer drugs (chemotherapy)
	Heparin-induced thrombocytopenia
	Oral contraceptives
	Obesity

TPA, tissue plasminogen activator.

*Prevalence of factor V Leiden in patients with deep venous thrombosis is 16%; presence of factor V Leiden is associated with a 40% risk of recurrent deep venous thrombosis (*N Engl J Med* 336:399-403, 1997).

†Prevalence of these protein deficiencies in patients with deep venous thrombosis is 5% to 10%.

From Prakash UBS: Pulmonary embolism. *In* Mayo Clinic Cardiology Review. 2nd ed. Edited by JG Murphy. Philadelphia, Lippincott Williams & Wilkins, 2000, pp 379-406. By permission of Mayo Foundation for Medical Education and Research.

Table 21-16 Incidence of Deep Venous Thrombosis (DVT) in Various Clinical Circumstances

Clinical circumstance	Incidence of DVT, %
Major abdominal surgery*	14-33
Thoracic surgery	25-60
Gynecologic surgery	
Patients ≤40 years old	<3
Patients >40 years old	10-40
Patients >40 years + other risks	40-70
Urologic surgery	10-40
Hip surgery	50-75
Post-myocardial infarction	20-40
Congestive heart failure	70
Stroke with paralysis	50-70
Post partum	3
Trauma	20-40

*Odds are 1:20 without prophylaxis and 1:50 with prophylaxis.

DVT is diagnosed in only 50% of clinical cases. A diagnosis based on physical examination findings is unreliable. The Homan sign (pain and tenderness on dorsiflexion of the ankle) is elicited in fewer than 40% of cases of DVT, and a false-positive Homan sign occurs in 30% of high-risk patients. Impedance plethysmography (IPG) and duplex ultrasonography together are the most commonly used noninvasive tests and have a diagnostic accuracy of 90% to 95% in detecting iliac and femoral DVTs. They are clinically unreliable in the diagnosis of calf vein thrombosis. Serial (daily) IPG or duplex ultrasonography (or both) is recommended for high-risk patients, because of a 15% detection rate of DVT after an initial negative study. Currently, IPG is performed less often than ultrasonography. Duplex ultrasonography is less accurate for the diagnosis of chronic DVT and less useful in pelvic DVT than in the diagnosis of acute femoral DVT. Venography is considered nearly 100% sensitive and specific. Venography should be performed when other tests are nondiagnostic or cannot be performed. Magnetic resonance imaging (MRI) has a high sensitivity and specificity for the diagnosis of pelvic DVT.

- DVT is diagnosed in only 50% of clinical cases.
- IPG plus duplex ultrasonography is up to 95% accurate for detecting iliac and femoral DVTs.

Clinical Features

PE has no typical clinical symptoms and signs. Tachypnea and tachycardia are observed in nearly all patients. Other symptoms include dyspnea in 80% of patients, pleuritic pain in up to 75%, hemoptysis in fewer than 25%, pleural friction rub in 20%, and wheezing in 15%. The differential diagnosis of PE includes myocardial infarction, pneumonia, congestive heart failure, pericarditis, esophageal spasm, asthma, exacerbation of COPD, intrathoracic malignancy, rib fracture, pneumothorax, pleurisy from any cause, pleurodynia, and nonspecific skeletal pains. Acute cor pulmonale occurs if more than 65% of the pulmonary circulation is obstructed by emboli. PE should be suspected in the setting of syncope or acute hypotension.

- PE has no typical signs or symptoms.
- Acute cor pulmonale occurs when >65% of the pulmonary circulation is obstructed by PE.

Diagnostic Tests

Clinical examination, electrocardiography, CXR, blood gas abnormalities, and increased plasma D-dimer level have low specificity and sensitivity for the diagnosis of PE. Clinical suspicion is the most important factor in steering a clinician toward the appropriate tests to diagnose PE. CXR may show diaphragmatic elevation in 60% of patients, infiltrates in 30%, focal oligemia in 10% to 50%, effusion in 20%, an enlarged pulmonary artery in 20%, and normal findings in 30%. Nonspecific electrocardiographic changes are noted in 80%, ST and T changes in 65%, T inversion in 40%, S_1Q_3 pattern in 15%, right bundle branch block in 12%, and left axis deviation in 12%. In critical patients, echocardiography should be performed early to assess right ventricular hypokinesia or dysfunction. The recommendations of the American Thoracic Society for the diagnosis of PE are listed in Figure 21-29.

- Normal CXR in 30% of patients with PE.
- The classic S_1Q_3 pattern is seen in only 15% of patients.

Both the PaO_2 and $P(A-a)O_2$ gradient may be normal in 15% to 20% of patients. The $P(A-a)O_2$ gradient shows a linear correlation with the severity of the PE. A normal $P(A-a)O_2$ gradient does not exclude PE. Indeed, in the Prospective Investigation of Pulmonary Embolism Diagnosis (PIOPED) study, about 20% of patients with angiographically documented PE had a normal $P(A-a)O_2$ gradient (≤20 mm Hg). Most patients with acute PE demonstrate hypocapnia.

- The $P(A-a)O_2$ gradient correlates linearly with the severity of PE.
- Of patients with PE, 20% have a normal $P(A-a)O_2$ gradient (≤20 mm Hg).

The plasma levels of D-dimer (a specific fibrin degradation product) are increased in DVT and PE. However, high levels themselves have no positive predictive value for PE. A normal level of D-dimer does not exclude PE but makes it unlikely in

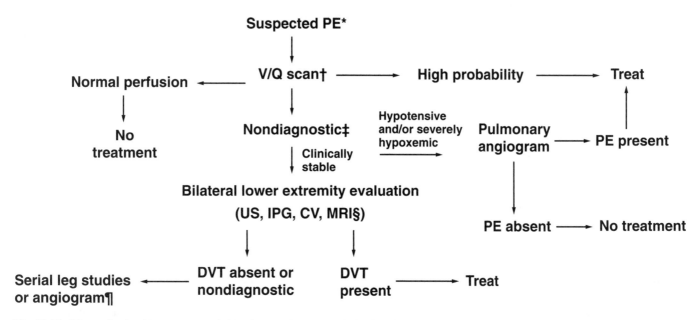

Fig. 21-29. Diagnostic algorithm, recommended by the American Thoracic Society, for patients with symptoms suggesting acute pulmonary embolism (PE). CV, contrast venography; DVT, deep venous thrombosis.

*When PE is suspected and the risk of bleeding is deemed low, it is appropriate to begin anticoagulation while diagnostic testing is under way.

†A perfusion scan alone may suffice. Diagnostic alternatives to the ventilation-perfusion (V/Q) scan include spiral computed tomography (CT) and magnetic resonance imaging (MRI).

‡If clinical suspicion is low and the patient has a low probability V/Q scan, PE is unlikely. Others require further evaluation. There are several options when the V/Q scan (or spiral CT or lung MRI) is nondiagnostic. Pulmonary angiography is the appropriate approach if the patient's condition is unstable. Otherwise, leg studies can be performed. If spiral CT or lung MRI is performed, a negative result should be interpreted together with the level of clinical suspicion. Although these techniques appear to be sensitive, additional studies (pulmonary angiography or leg studies) should be performed as deemed appropriate.

§A positive test is useful. The sensitivity for compression ultrasonography (US) and impedance plethysmography (IPG) is low in asymptomatic patients, and negative or nondiagnostic studies require additional data.

¶Negative serial IPG in this setting has been associated at certain centers with excellent outcome without anticoagulation.

Modified from American Thoracic Society: The diagnostic approach to acute venous thromboembolism. Clinical practice guidelines. Am J Respir Crit Care Med 160:1043-1066, 1999. By permission of American Thoracic Society.

patients with a low pretest probability of PE. Age and pregnancy are associated with increased levels. Levels less than 300 μg/L (by ELISA) or less than 500 μg/L (by latex agglutination) are considered to reliably exclude PE in patients with an abnormal but not high-probability ventilation-perfusion (V/Q) lung scan. A plasma concentration of D-dimer less than 500 μg/L allows the exclusion of PE in fewer than 30% of patients with suspected PE. Currently, the D-dimer test cannot be recommended as a standard part of the PE or DVT diagnostic algorithm.

- Increased D-dimer levels have no positive predictive value for PE.
- Normal (<500 μg/L) D-dimer levels exclude PE in fewer than 30% of cases.

Echocardiography can identify thrombi in the right side of the heart in up to 15% of patients with PE. Dysfunction of the right ventricle, frequently seen in massive as well as recurrent PE, can be detected with echocardiography. Although the echocardiographic findings are abnormal in more than 80% of patients with documented PE, the findings are nonspecific. The presence of associated abnormalities (intracardiac tumors, myxoma) poses a difficulty in distinguishing among the lesions. A highly mobile intracavitary thrombus-in-transit has a 98% risk of acute PE and a 1-week mortality of 50%. Transesophageal echocardiography is reportedly 97% sensitive and 86% specific for the diagnosis of centrally located pulmonary arterial thrombi. Currently, the role of echocardiography in the diagnosis of acute PE is undefined.

The V/Q scan is commonly used in the diagnosis of PE. A "high-probability" lung scan has a sensitivity of 41% and a specificity of 97%. A "low-probability" lung scan excludes the diagnosis of PE in more than 85% of patients. A normal lung scan excludes PE in 100% of cases. An "intermediate- or indeterminate-probability" scan is associated with PE in 21%

to 30% of patients. Therefore, patients with an "intermediate-probability" lung scan usually require pulmonary angiography. A negative or normal perfusion-only scan (excluding ventilation scan) rules out PE with a very high probability.

- High-probability scan = 90% probability of PE.
- Intermediate-probability scan = 30% probability of PE.
- Low-probability scan = 15% probability of PE.
- Normal scan excludes PE in 100% of cases.

CT permits ultrafast scanning of pulmonary arteries during contrast injection. In some institutions, spiral (helical) CT with intravenous contrast (CT angiography) is being used more frequently than V/Q scans to detect PE. Sensitivity and specificity rates greater than 95% have been reported. Spiral CT has the greatest sensitivity in the diagnosis of PE in the main, lobar, or segmental arteries. Lymph node enlargement may result in false-positive studies. MRI may have the advantage of detecting both DVT and PE.

- Spiral CT has the greatest sensitivity in the diagnosis of PE in the main, lobar, or segmental arteries.

Pulmonary angiography is the best diagnostic test. It should be performed within 24 to 48 hours after the diagnosis has been considered. However, it is nondiagnostic in 3% of cases. Major and minor complications following pulmonary angiography occur in 1% and 2% of patients, respectively, and mortality from the procedure is 0.5%. Pulmonary angiography followed by therapy with tissue plasminogen activator (TPA) is associated with a 14% risk of major hemorrhage.

- Major and minor complications from pulmonary angiography are 1% and 2%, respectively.

Treatment

The therapy for uncomplicated DVT is identical to that for PE. For acute disease, treatment can begin simultaneously with both heparin (low-molecular-weight heparin [LMWH] or unfractionated heparin [UFH]) and warfarin unless warfarin is contraindicated. When treatment with both drugs is begun simultaneously, an overlap for 4 to 5 days is recommended. For patients with acute disease, UFH (80 IU/kg) is administered as a bolus, followed by a maintenance dose of 18 IU/kg per hour intravenously. The dose should be adjusted to maintain an activated partial thromboplastin time (APTT) above 1.5 times the control value. The non–weight-based UFH dose in acute DVT and acute PE consists of initial intravenous boluses of 5,000 IU and 15,000 to 20,000 IU, respectively; the maintenance dose is more than 1,200 IU per hour intravenously or 15,000 to 20,000 IU subcutaneously to maintain an APTT

greater than 1.5 times control. With LMWH regimens, suggestions for outpatient therapy include stable proximal DVT or PE, normal vital signs, low risk for bleeding, and availability of appropriate monitoring.

- In acute DVT or PE, heparin (LMWH or UFH) and warfarin treatment can begin simultaneously.
- UFH dose: bolus = 80 IU/kg; maintenance = 18 IU/kg per hour.

Long-term anticoagulant therapy can be maintained with either heparin or warfarin. Heparin is indicated when warfarin is contraindicated or not tolerated. The usual dose of UFH is 5,000 to 10,000 IU subcutaneously twice daily. However, the dose should be adjusted based on the APTT, as noted above. The weight-based UFH dose is not reliable for maintenance therapy by the subcutaneous route. LMWH has been prescribed for patients who have difficulty monitoring the APTT. Warfarin at a dose to achieve an international normalized ratio (INR) of 2.0 to 3.0 is recommended. The loading dose of warfarin usually is 10 mg/daily for 1 or 2 days, followed by adjustment of the dose to maintain an INR of 2.0 to 3.0. Recurrent and complicated cases (e.g., coagulopathies) may require lifelong anticoagulation, maintenance of higher APTT or prothrombin time (PT), and other measures such as plication of the inferior vena cava. The recommended duration of treatment for venous thromboembolic disease is given in Table 21-17.

- APTT in uncomplicated cases: 1.5-2 times normal.
- PT in uncomplicated cases: INR of 2.0-3.0.
- Length of treatment for first episode of idiopathic DVT or PE: 6 months.

Table 21-17 Recommended Duration of Treatment for Venous Thromboembolic Disease

Patient characteristic	Duration of treatment, mo
First event, with a reversible or time-limited risk factor*	≥3
First episode of idiopathic DVT or PE	≥6
Recurrent idiopathic DVT or PE or a continuing risk factor†	≥12

DVT, deep venous thrombosis; PE, pulmonary embolism.
*Surgery, trauma, immobilization, or estrogen use.
†Cancer, antithrombin deficiency, anticardiolipin antibody syndrome.
Modified from Hyers TM, Agnelli G, Hull RD, et al. Antithrombotic therapy for venous thromboembolic disease. Chest 2001;119:176S-193S. By permission of the American College of Chest Physicians.

Thrombolytic agents are administered in cases of massive PE and massive iliofemoral thrombosis. The indications are debated, although these drugs generally are indicated for patients with massive DVT or PE (or both). One-year mortality among those treated with heparin alone and those treated with thrombolytic agents is 19% and 9%, respectively. The rate of recurrent PE in heparin-alone therapy and thrombolytic therapy is 11% and 5.5%, respectively. Ideally, thrombolytic agents should be administered within 24 hours after PE. The doses for different agents are as follows: streptokinase, loading dose of 250,000 IU infused over 30 minutes, followed by a maintenance dose of 100,000 IU per hour for up to 24 hours; urokinase, loading dose of 4,400 IU/kg infused over 10 minutes, followed by continuous infusion of 4,400 IU/kg per hour for 12 hours; and TPA, a total dose of 100 mg given intravenously over a 2-hour period. The adequacy of thrombolytic therapy is monitored with the thrombin time. Heparin infusion is begun or resumed if the APTT is less than 80 seconds after thrombolytic therapy.

- Thrombolytic agents should be administered within 24 hours after PE.
- Heparin therapy is necessary after thrombolytic therapy.

Among patients receiving chronic warfarin therapy, the cumulative incidence of fatal bleeding is 1% at 1 year and 2% at 3 years. A greater risk of major hemorrhage exists when anticoagulation is continued indefinitely. The presence of malignant disease at the initiation of warfarin therapy is significantly associated with major hemorrhage. Patients with PE treated with thrombolytic drugs have about a 1% risk of intracranial bleeding.

- Thrombolytic therapy: 1% risk of intracranial bleeding.

Drugs that prolong the effect of warfarin include, among others, salicylates, heparin, estrogen, antibiotics, clofibrate, quinidine, and cimetidine. Drugs that decrease the effect of warfarin include glutethimide, rifampin, barbiturates, and ethchlorvynol. This is only a partial list of drugs that interfere with warfarin metabolism. Therefore, the physician recommending warfarin therapy should ascertain the drug-drug interaction or consult a pharmacist.

- Knowledge of the interaction of warfarin with other drugs is important.

Inferior Vena Cava Interruption
Inferior vena cava interruption is aimed at preventing PE while maintaining blood flow through the inferior vena cava. It is indicated if anticoagulant therapy is contraindicated,

complications result from anticoagulant therapy, anticoagulant therapy fails, a predisposition to bleeding is present, chronic recurrent PE and secondary pulmonary hypertension occur, or surgical pulmonary thromboendarterectomy has been or is intended to be performed. Inferior vena cava plication does not replace anticoagulant therapy; many patients require both. After the filter has been inserted, anticoagulant therapy is aimed at preventing DVT at the insertion site, inferior vena cava thrombosis, cephalad propagation of a clot from an occluded filter, or propagation or recurrence of lower extremity DVT.

- Inferior vena cava plication does not replace chronic anticoagulant therapy.
- PE occurs in 2.5% of patients despite inferior vena cava interruption.

Prophylaxis
Prophylaxis against DVT and PE includes early ambulation after surgery or immobilization, intermittent pneumatic compression of the lower extremities, active and passive leg exercises, and a low dose of heparin given subcutaneously (10,000-15,000 IU daily). A low dose of heparin decreases the incidence of DVT from 25% to 8%; 5,000 IU are given preoperatively and then every 8 to 12 hours postoperatively. Prophylactic enoxaparin, 40 mg daily subcutaneously, safely reduces the risk of DVT in patients with acute medical illnesses. LMWH has been approved in the United States for prophylaxis against DVT and PE after total hip arthroplasty and total knee arthroplasty. A postoperative, fixed-dose LMWH (enoxaparin, 30 mg subcutaneously every 12 hours) is more effective than adjusted-dose warfarin (INR 2.0-3.0) in preventing DVT after total hip or knee arthroplasty. LMWH has a rapid onset of action, is safe, and is approximately 50% more effective than standard heparin. Because of a more predictable dose response to LMWH, it is not as important to monitor the dose and APTT.

- LMWH has been approved in the United States for DVT and PE prophylaxis after total hip arthroplasty.
- LMWH therapy does not require measuring APTT.
- Heparin-induced thrombocytopenia is reduced with LMWH.

Complications of PE
Pulmonary infarction occurs in fewer than 10% of patients with PE. Pulmonary infarction and hemorrhage occur more frequently in patients with disseminated intravascular coagulation. Complications of pulmonary infarction include secondary infection, cavitation, pneumothorax, and hemothorax. Recurrent PE is a common cause of secondary pulmonary hypertension. Mechanical obstruction of one-half

to two-thirds of the pulmonary vascular bed by emboli is necessary for this complication to develop.

- Pulmonary infarction in <10% of patients.
- Recurrent PE in 8%.
- Secondary pulmonary hypertension in 0.5%.

Pulmonary Vasculitides

The vasculitides are a heterogeneous group of disorders of unknown cause characterized by various degrees of inflammation and necrosis of the arteries and, sometimes, veins. Immunologic factors, the absence or deficiency of certain chemical mediators in the body, and infectious processes caused by mycoses, particularly *Aspergillus* and *Mucor*, are associated with vasculitis. The common vasculitides and their frequency in North America are as follows: giant cell (temporal) arteritis, 26.5%; polyarteritis nodosa, 14.6%; Wegener granulomatosis, 10.5%; Schönlein-Henoch purpura, 10.5%; Takayasu arteritis, 7.8%; and Churg-Strauss syndrome, 2.5%.

Wegener Granulomatosis

Wegener granulomatosis is a systemic vasculitis of arteries and veins characterized by necrotizing granulomatous vasculitis of the upper and lower respiratory tract, glomerulonephritis, and variable degrees of small-vessel vasculitis. The Wegener triad consists of necrotizing granulomas of the upper or lower respiratory tract (or both), generalized focal necrotizing vasculitis of arteries and veins in the lungs, and glomerulonephritis. Bronchiolitis obliterans-organizing pneumonia (BOOP), bronchocentric inflammation, a marked eosinophilic infiltrate, and alveolar hemorrhage are atypical features. Pulmonary capillaritis occurs in up to 40% of patients. Eosinophilic infiltrates are seen in tissue samples, but peripheral blood eosinophilia is *not* a feature of Wegener granulomatosis. The term "limited Wegener granulomatosis" is used to describe the disease involving the lungs only.

- Typical clinical scenario for Wegener granulomatosis: systemic disease with major respiratory manifestations and renal involvement with focal segmental glomerulonephritis.

The cause of Wegener granulomatosis is unknown. Occupational exposure has been suggested as an etiologic factor; a sevenfold risk for development of Wegener granulomatosis was observed in persons with a history of inhalation of silica-containing compounds and grain dust. Heterozygotes for the P_I*Z variant of the α_1-antitrypsin gene are reported to have a sixfold greater risk of developing the disease than the general population. The prevalence of Wegener granulomatosis in the United States is approximately 3 per 100,000 persons. Some have noted associations between disease exacerbations during the winter months and during pregnancy.

The mean age at the onset of symptoms is 45.2 years (the male-to-female ratio is 2:1); 91% of the patients are white. The initial symptoms are nonspecific: fever, malaise, weight loss, arthralgias, and myalgias. The organs affected are the ear-nose-throat (initial complaints in 90% of patients: rhinorrhea, purulent or bloody nasal discharge, sinus pain, nasal mucosal drying and crust formation, epistaxis, and otitis media), the skin (40%-50% of patients), eyes (43%), and central nervous system (25%). Arthralgias occur in 58% of patients and frank arthritis in 28%. Patients older than 60 have a relatively low incidence of upper respiratory tract complaints but a high incidence (4.5-fold) of neurologic involvement.

- Major organs affected: "ELKS," i.e., **E**NT, **l**ungs, **k**idney, and **s**kin.
- Ear-nose-throat symptoms are the initial complaints in 90% of patients.
- Nasal septal perforation and ulceration of the vomer bone are two important signs.
- Differential diagnosis of "saddle-nose" deformity: Wegener granulomatosis, relapsing polychondritis, and leprosy.

Ulcerated lesions of the larynx and trachea occur in 30% of untreated patients and subglottic stenosis in 8% to 18% of treated patients. The pulmonary parenchyma is affected in more than 60% of patients. Symptoms include cough, hemoptysis, and dyspnea. The clinical manifestations can range from subacute to rapidly progressive respiratory failure. Most patients with pulmonary symptoms have associated nodular infiltrates on CXR. Hemoptysis is seen in 98% of patients and CXR abnormalities in 65% (unilateral in 55% and bilateral in 45%), including infiltrates (63%), nodules (31%), infiltrates with cavitation (8%), and nodules with cavitation (10%). CXR shows rounded opacities (from a few millimeters to several centimeters large). The nodules are usually bilateral and one-third cavitate. Solitary nodules occur in 30% to 40% of patients. Pneumonic infiltrates, lobar consolidation, and pleural effusions are also seen. Massive pulmonary alveolar hemorrhage is occasionally a life-threatening emergency. Benign stenoses of the tracheobronchial tree are more likely in chronic cases and in patients whose disease is stable.

- Hemoptysis occurs in almost all patients.
- CXR: multiple nodules or masses with cavitation in 35% of patients.
- Diffuse alveolar infiltrates indicate alveolar hemorrhage.
- Tracheobronchial stenosis occurs in 15% of patients.

Laboratory tests demonstrate mild-to-moderate normochromic normocytic anemia, mild leukocytosis, mild thrombocytosis, positive rheumatoid factor, and elevations of immunoglobulins IgG and IgA and circulating immune complexes. A highly increased ESR (often >100 mm/h) is a consistent finding. Peripheral blood eosinophilia is not a feature. All these abnormalities are nonspecific. Urinalysis is an important test because hematuria, proteinuria, and red cell casts are found in 80% of patients.

- Increased ESR.
- Hematuria, proteinuria, and red cell casts in 80% of patients.

The antineutrophil cytoplasmic antibodies (ANCAs) are used to corroborate the diagnosis of Wegener granulomatosis. The two main patterns of ANCA are cytoplasmic (c-ANCA) and perinuclear (p-ANCA). Almost all c-ANCAs are directed to proteinase 3 (Pr3), whereas myeloperoxidase (mpo) is the major target antigen of p-ANCA. Also, c-ANCA is highly specific and sensitive for Wegener granulomatosis and is present in more than 90% of patients with systemic Wegener granulomatosis. In active disease, the sensitivity and specificity are 91% and 98%, respectively, whereas in inactive disease, the values are 63% and 99.5%. The following points are important: a positive c-ANCA without clinical evidence of disease does not establish the diagnosis; some patients with active disease are negative for c-ANCA; some patients have persistently positive c-ANCA results despite inactive disease or disease in remission; c-ANCA titers may increase without evidence of an increase in disease activity; and c-ANCA is present in other diseases such as hepatitis C virus infection and in some cases of microscopic polyangiitis and ulcerative colitis and as a manifestation of sulfasalazine toxicity.

- c-ANCA is generally considered specific for Wegener granulomatosis.
- Positive c-ANCA without clinical evidence of disease does not establish the diagnosis.
- c-ANCA can be positive in other diseases.

p-ANCA is positive in various diseases, including inflammatory bowel disease, autoimmune liver disease, rheumatoid arthritis, and many other vasculitides. Reportedly, p-ANCA with specificity against mpo is closely associated with microscopic polyangiitis, mononeuritis multiplex, leukocytoclastic vasculitis of the skin, pauci-immune necrotizing-crescentic glomerulonephritis, and other vasculitides affecting small vessels. Some cases of Churg-Strauss syndrome may demonstrate p-ANCA with specificity for mpo.

- p-ANCA has been noted in other vasculitides and collagen diseases.

- p-ANCA with specificity for mpo should suggest small-vessel vasculitis (microscopic polyangiitis).

The combination of corticosteroids and cyclophosphamide produces complete remission in more than 90% of patients. The usual dosage of each drug is up to 2 mg/kg daily orally. In milder cases, corticosteroids alone may be sufficient. Because of immunosuppression, the overall incidence of *Pneumocystis carinii* pneumonia in these patients is approximately 6%. Respiratory infection, particularly from *Staphylococcus aureus*, is more common. The nasal carriage rate for this bacteria is higher in patients with Wegener granulomatosis. Disease relapse usually is associated with viral or bacterial infections. A combination of trimethoprim, 160 mg daily, and sulfamethoxazole, 800 mg daily, is an effective prophylactic regimen to prevent disease relapse; 82% of treated patients remain in remission for 24 months compared with 60% who do not receive prophylaxis. Stenosis of large airways may require bronchoscopic interventions, including dilation by rigid bronchoscope, YAG-laser treatment, and placement of silicone airway stents.

- Cyclophosphamide and corticosteroids are effective.
- Trimethoprim-sulfamethoxazole is effective in preventing relapse.

Giant Cell (Temporal) Arteritis

Giant cell arteritis, also known as "temporal arteritis," "cranial arteritis," and "granulomatous arteritis," is a vasculitis of unknown cause. It usually affects middle-aged or older persons. Pulmonary complications include cough, sore throat, and hoarseness. Nearly 10% of the patients have prominent respiratory symptoms, and respiratory symptoms are the initial manifestation in 4%. Giant cell arteritis should be considered in older patients who have a new cough or throat pain without obvious cause. Pulmonary nodules, interstitial infiltrations, pulmonary artery occlusion, and aneurysms have been described. Virtually all patients have a favorable response to systemic corticosteroid therapy.

- Giant cell arteritis: nearly 10% of patients have prominent respiratory symptoms.
- Cough, sore throat, and hoarseness may be the presenting features.

Churg-Strauss Syndrome

Churg-Strauss syndrome, also called "allergic granulomatosis" and "angiitis," is among the least common of the vasculitides. It is characterized by pulmonary and systemic vasculitis, extravascular granulomas, and eosinophilia, which occur exclusively in patients with asthma or a history of allergy.

Allergic rhinitis, nasal polyps, nasal mucosal crusting, and septal perforation occur in more than 70% of patients. Nasal polyposis is a major clinical finding. The chief pulmonary manifestation is asthma, which is noted in almost all patients. CXR abnormalities are noted in more than 60% of patients: patchy and occasionally diffuse alveolar-interstitial infiltrates in the perihilar area, with a predilection for the upper two-thirds of the lung fields. Up to one-third of patients with Churg-Strauss vasculitis develop pleural effusions. A dramatic response can be expected with high doses of systemic corticosteroids.

● Churg-Strauss syndrome: Refractory asthma, progressive respiratory distress, allergic rhinitis, nasal polyps, nasal mucosal crusting, septal perforation in >70% of patients, tissue and blood hypereosinophilia, and increased IgE.

Behçet Disease

Behçet disease is a chronic relapsing multisystem inflammatory disorder characterized by aphthous stomatitis along with two or more of the following: aphthous orogenital ulcerations (in >65% of patients), uveitis, cutaneous nodules or pustules, synovitis, and meningoencephalitis. Superficial venous thrombosis and DVT of the upper and lower extremities and thrombosis of the inferior and superior venae cavae occur in 7% to 37% of patients. Pulmonary vascular involvement produces major hemoptysis. Severe hemoptysis, initially responsive to therapy with corticosteroids, tends to recur; death is due to hemoptysis in 39% of patients. CXR may show lung infiltrates, pleural effusions, prominent pulmonary arteries, and pulmonary artery aneurysms. Aneurysms of the pulmonary artery communicating with the bronchial tree (bronchovascular anastomosis) should be considered in patients with Behçet disease and massive hemoptysis. Because of the high incidence of DVT of the extremities and the venae cavae, PE commonly occurs in these patients. Corticosteroids and chemotherapeutic agents have been used to treat Behçet disease. The prognosis is poor if marked hemoptysis develops.

● Behçet disease: Aphthous stomatitis, uveitis, cutaneous nodules, and meningoencephalitis.
● Major hemoptysis is the cause of death in 39% of patients.
● A fistula between the airway and vascular structures is common.
● High incidence of DVT and PE.

Takayasu Arteritis

Takayasu arteritis, also known as "pulseless disease," "aortic arch syndrome," and "reversed coarctation," is a chronic inflammatory disease of unknown cause that affects primarily the aorta and its major branches, including the proximal coronary arteries and renal arteries and the elastic pulmonary arteries. The pulmonary arteries are involved in more than 50% of patients, with lesions in medium- and large-size arteries. Early abnormalities occur in the upper lobes, whereas the middle and lower lobes are involved in later stages of the disease. Perfusion lung scans have shown abnormalities in more than 75% of patients; pulmonary angiography has demonstrated arterial occlusions in 86%. Corticosteroid therapy has produced symptomatic remission within days to weeks. Pulmonary involvement signifies a poor prognosis.

● Takayasu arteritis: pulmonary artery involvement in >50% of patients.

Urticarial Vasculitis

Urticarial vasculitis is manifested by urticarial lesions, pruritus, and arthralgias in 60% of patients, arthritis in 28%, abdominal pain in 25%, and glomerulonephritis in 15%. Many of the pulmonary complications described have been in patients with the hypocomplementemic variety of the disease. Pulmonary vasculitis has not been demonstrated in patients with urticarial vasculitis. However, up to 62% of those with hypocomplementemic urticarial vasculitis acquire COPD. Many of these patients have been smokers.

● Higher incidence of COPD among patients who have hypocomplementemic urticarial vasculitis.

Eosinophilia-Myalgia Syndrome

The eosinophilia-myalgia syndrome is a multisystem inflammatory disease with features characteristic of myalgia and eosinophilia. An epidemic of eosinophilia-myalgia syndrome in 1989 was linked to dietary ingestion of L-tryptophan tablets. Clinical manifestations of this syndrome included myalgias, fatigue, muscle weakness, arthralgias, edema of the extremities, skin rash, oral and vaginal ulcers, scleroderma-like changes, ascending neuropathy, and peripheral blood eosinophilia. About 60% of the patients had pulmonary complications: pulmonary infiltrates associated with severe pulmonary distress and progressive hypoxemia, pleural effusion, diffuse bilateral reticulonodular infiltrates, and pulmonary hypertension.

● Eosinophilia-myalgia syndrome: caused by a contaminant in L-tryptophan preparations.
● Pulmonary hypertension, interstitial granulomas, and respiratory distress.
● Similar features were observed in a Spanish toxic oil syndrome.

Mixed Cryoglobulinemia

This disease is characterized by recurrent episodes of purpura, arthralgias, weakness, and multiorgan involvement.

Frequently, cryoglobulin and rheumatoid factor are increased. Biopsy findings in vascular structures are similar to those in leukocytoclastic vasculitis. The most serious complication is glomerulonephritis caused by deposition of immune complexes. Pulmonary insufficiency, Sjögren syndrome-like illness with lung involvement, subclinical T-lymphocytic alveolitis, diffuse pulmonary vasculitis with alveolar hemorrhage, BOOP, and bronchiectasis have been described in isolated cases.

- Mixed cryoglobulinemia: lymphocytic alveolitis, BOOP, alveolar hemorrhage.

Polyarteritis Nodosa

Polyarteritis nodosa is characterized by a necrotizing arteritis of small- and medium-size muscular arteries involving multiple organ systems. Note that this disease seldom affects the lungs. Arteritis affecting bronchial arteries and producing diffuse alveolar damage has been reported. Lung involvement is rare also in Schönlein-Henoch purpura.

- Polyarteritis nodosa and Schönlein-Henoch purpura rarely affect the lungs.

Secondary Vasculitis

Many of the rheumatologic diseases (e.g., systemic lupus erythematosus, rheumatoid arthritis, and scleroderma) demonstrate secondary vasculitic processes in the tissues involved. Certain infectious processes, particularly mycoses, may cause secondary vasculitis. When confronted with vasculitic lesions, the well-known etiologic agents such as drugs and chemicals should be considered.

- Collagen diseases are common causes of secondary vasculitis.

Alveolar Hemorrhage Syndromes

Diffuse hemorrhage into the alveolar spaces is called "alveolar hemorrhage syndrome." Disruption of the pulmonary capillary lining may result from damage caused by different immunologic mechanisms (e.g., Goodpasture syndrome, renal-pulmonary syndromes, glomerulonephritis, and systemic lupus erythematosus), direct chemical or toxic injury (e.g., toxic or chemical inhalation, abciximab, all-*trans*-retinoic acid, trimellitic anhydride, and smoked crack cocaine), physical trauma (pulmonary contusion), and increased vascular pressure within the capillaries (mitral stenosis and severe left ventricular failure). The severity of hemoptysis, anemia, and respiratory distress depends on the extent and rapidity with which bleeding occurs in the alveoli. More than 20% of hemosiderin-laden macrophages among the total alveolar macrophages recovered with bronchoalveolar lavage is reported to indicate alveolar hemorrhage. Pulmonary alveolar hemorrhage is strongly associated with thrombocytopenia (50×10^9/L), other abnormal coagulation variables, renal failure (creatinine, ≥ 2.5 mg/dL), and a history of heavy smoking.

- Alveolar hemorrhage syndrome is caused by different mechanisms.
- Hemoptysis is not a consistent feature.
- Increased risk if platelets 50×10^9/L, other coagulopathy, creatinine ≥ 2.5 mg/dL, and heavy smoking.
- Drugs that cause alveolar hemorrhage: penicillamine, abciximab, all-*trans*-retinoic acid, mitomycin.

Goodpasture Syndrome

Goodpasture syndrome is a classic example of a cytotoxic (type II) disease. The Goodpasture antigen (located in type IV collagen) is the primary target for the autoantibodies. The highest concentration of Goodpasture antigen is in the glomerular basement membrane (GBM). The alveolar basement membrane is affected by cross-reactivity with the GBM. Lung biopsy specimens show diffuse alveolar hemorrhage. Immunofluorescent microscopy shows linear deposition of IgG and complement along basement membranes. Anti-GBM antibody is positive in more than 90% of patients, but it is also present in persons exposed to influenza virus, hydrocarbons, or penicillamine and in some patients with systemic lupus erythematosus, polyarteritis nodosa, or Schönlein-Henoch purpura. The cause of Goodpasture syndrome is unknown, but influenza virus, hydrocarbon exposure, penicillamine, and unknown genetic factors are known to stimulate anti-GBM antibody production. Inadvertent exposure to hydrocarbons has resulted in the exacerbation of Goodpasture syndrome. The treatment of rheumatoid arthritis and other diseases with penicillamine and carbimazole has been associated with Goodpasture syndrome, circulating anti-GBM antibodies, and focal necrotizing glomerulonephritis with crescents. Azathioprine hypersensitivity may mimic pulmonary Goodpasture syndrome.

- Goodpasture syndrome: a classic example of a cytotoxic (type II) disease.
- Anti-GBM antibody is positive in >90% of patients.
- Anti-GBM antibody is also present in persons exposed to influenza virus, hydrocarbons, or penicillamine and in some patients with collagen diseases.
- Exposure to hydrocarbons may exacerbate the disease.

Patients with anti-GBM antibody–mediated nephritis demonstrate two principal patterns of disease: 1) young men presenting in their twenties with Goodpasture syndrome (glomerulonephritis and lung hemorrhage) and 2) elderly patients, especially women, presenting in their sixties with glomerulonephritis alone. In the classic form (in younger patients) of Goodpasture syndrome, men are affected more often than women (the male-to-female ratio, 7:1) and the average age at onset is approximately 27 years. Recurrent hemoptysis, pulmonary insufficiency, renal involvement with hematuria and renal failure, and anemia are the classic features. Pulmonary hemorrhage almost always precedes renal manifestations. Active cigarette smoking increases the risk of alveolar hemorrhage. Frequent initial clinical features include hemoptysis, hematuria, proteinuria, and an increased serum level of creatinine.

- Typical clinical scenario for the classic form: A young man with glomerulonephritis and lung hemorrhage.
- Typical clinical scenario for the atypical form: An elderly patient, especially a woman, with glomerulonephritis alone.
- Pulmonary hemorrhage almost always precedes renal manifestations.
- Active cigarette smoking increases the risk of alveolar hemorrhage.

CXR demonstrates a diffuse alveolar filling process, with sparing of the costophrenic angles. One-third of the patients with anti-GBM disease (Goodpasture syndrome) test positive for p-ANCA–mpo. These patients are more prone to develop fulminant pulmonary hemorrhage than those who are p-ANCA–negative. Plasmapheresis is the treatment of choice for Goodpasture syndrome. Although complete recovery can be expected in most patients treated with systemic corticosteroids, immunosuppressive agents, or plasmapheresis, relapse occurs in up to 7% of them. A previous history of pulmonary hemorrhage markedly decreases the diffusing capacity of the lung for carbon monoxide without affecting other variables of pulmonary function.

- One-third of the patients with anti-GBM disease test positive for p-ANCA–mpo.
- Patients with positive p-ANCA–mpo are more likely to have fulminant pulmonary hemorrhage.
- Plasmapheresis is the treatment of choice.

Glomerulonephritis

Rapidly progressive glomerulonephritis, in the absence of anti-GBM antibody, is a major cause of pulmonary alveolar hemorrhage. Nearly 50% of the patients with alveolar hemorrhage syndromes caused by a renal mechanism do not have anti-GBM antibody. Alveolar hemorrhage is mediated by immune-complex disease. Several vasculitic syndromes, including Wegener granulomatosis and microscopic polyangiitis, belong to this group. ANCAs have been detected in patients with idiopathic crescentic glomerulonephritis and alveolar hemorrhage syndrome. The alveolar hemorrhage syndrome in systemic lupus erythematosus and other vasculitides is discussed elsewhere.

- Glomerulonephritis: a major cause of pulmonary alveolar hemorrhage.
- Alveolar hemorrhage is mediated by immune-complex disease.

Vasculitides

Diffuse alveolar hemorrhage is seen sometimes in patients with vasculitis. Alveolar hemorrhage is rare as an initial symptom of Wegener granulomatosis and is more common in Churg-Strauss syndrome and Schönlein-Henoch purpura. Alveolar hemorrhage is more common in Behçet disease than in other vasculitides. Pulmonary capillaritis is a distinct histologic lesion characterized by extensive neutrophilic infiltration of the alveolar interstitium. Subclinical alveolar hemorrhage may occur in patients with this disease. This lesion can be seen in various vasculitides such as Wegener granulomatosis, microscopic polyarteritis, systemic lupus erythematosus, and other collagen diseases.

Microscopic Polyangiitis

Microscopic polyangiitis is distinct from classic polyarteritis nodosa, which typically affects medium-size arteries. Pulmonary capillaritis is the most common lesion in microscopic polyangiitis but does not occur in classic polyarteritis nodosa. Microscopic polyangiitis is a systemic vasculitis associated with renal involvement in 80% of patients, characterized by rapidly progressive glomerulonephritis. Other features include weight loss (70% of patients), skin involvement (60%), fever (55%), mononeuritis multiplex (58%), arthralgias (50%), myalgias (48%), and hypertension (34%). Males are affected more frequently than females; the median age at onset is 50 years. Pulmonary alveolar hemorrhage is observed in 12% to 29% of patients and is an important contributory factor to morbidity and mortality. ANCA is detected in 75% of patients with microscopic polyangiitis, and the majority are the p-ANCA–mpo type.

- Microscopic polyangiitis: progressive glomerulonephritis is a major feature.
- Pulmonary alveolar hemorrhage is observed in 12%-29% of patients.
- p-ANCA–mpo is positive in 75% of patients.

Mitral Valve Disease

Diffuse alveolar hemorrhage is a well-known feature of mitral stenosis, even though the possibility is rarely considered in clinical practice. Severe mitral insufficiency can also produce alveolar hemorrhage. Hemoptysis can be the presenting feature. It is caused by the rupture of dilated and varicose bronchial veins early in the course of mitral stenosis or it is the result of stress failure of pulmonary capillaries. In patients not treated surgically, recurrent episodes of alveolar hemorrhage may lead to chronic hemosiderosis of the lungs, fibrosis, and punctate calcification or ossification of the lung parenchyma.

● Mitral stenosis is an important cause of alveolar hemorrhage syndrome.

Idiopathic Pulmonary Hemosiderosis

Idiopathic pulmonary hemosiderosis is a rare disorder of unknown cause. The term "idiopathic pulmonary hemorrhage" has been suggested instead of the traditional name. Idiopathic pulmonary hemosiderosis is a diagnosis of exclusion. It manifests as recurrent intra-alveolar hemorrhage, hemoptysis, transient infiltrates on CXR, and secondary iron deficiency anemia. The cause is unknown, but many factors have been implicated: heritable defect, an immunologic mechanism based on the presence of antibodies to cow's milk (Heiner syndrome), cold agglutinins, increased serum IgA, viral infections, a primary disorder of airway epithelial cells, and a structural defect of pulmonary capillaries. Idiopathic pulmonary hemosiderosis has been described in association with idiopathic thrombocytopenic purpura, autoimmune hemolytic anemia, and nontropical sprue (celiac disease). A pediatric form of pulmonary hemosiderosis, presumed to be caused by the toxins of a spore growing in humid basements, has been described.

● Idiopathic pulmonary hemosiderosis: a diagnosis of exclusion.

Most cases begin in childhood. Although this disease is often fatal, a prolonged course is common. In childhood, the male-to-female ratio is 1:1 and in adults, 3:1. Pathologic features include hemosiderin-laden macrophages. No autoimmune phenomena are noted. Some patients have cold agglutinins. The iron content in the lung depends on the duration of the disease. Clinical features are chronic cough with intermittent hemoptysis, iron deficiency anemia, fever, and weight loss. CXR shows transient, blotchy, perihilar alveolar infiltrates in the mid and lower lung fields. Small nodules, fibrosis, and cor pulmonale may also be found. Intrathoracic lymphadenopathy occurs in up to 25% of patients. Treatment is repeated blood transfusions, iron therapy, corticosteroids, and, possibly, cytotoxic agents. A 30% mortality rate within 5 years after disease onset has been reported.

● Generalized lymphadenopathy in 25% of patients, hepatosplenomegaly in 20%, and clubbing in 15%.
● The kidneys are not involved.
● Eosinophilia in 10% of patients.

Toxic Alveolar Hemorrhage

Dust or fumes of trimellitic anhydride (a component of certain plastics, paints, and epoxy resins) cause acute rhinitis and asthma symptoms if exposure is minor. With greater exposure, alveolar hemorrhage occurs. The trimellitic anhydride-hemoptysis anemia syndrome occurs after "high-dose exposure" to fumes. Antibodies to trimellitic anhydride, human proteins, and erythrocytes have been found in these patients. Isocyanates have caused lung hemorrhage. Other toxins known to cause alveolar hemorrhage syndromes are penicillamine and mitomycin C. Lymphangiography has been complicated by pulmonary alveolar hemorrhage. Pulmonary lymphangioleiomyomatosis is an uncommon cause of alveolar hemorrhage syndrome. Alveolar hemorrhage occurs in a large number of patients with pulmonary veno-occlusive disease. Anticardiolipin antibody syndrome is another cause of alveolar hemorrhage.

● Alveolar hemorrhage occurs with penicillamine and mitomycin C.
● Trimellitic anhydride can cause pulmonary hemorrhage-anemia syndrome.
● Alveolar hemorrhage occurs with tumor emboli and after a bone marrow transplant.

PART IV
Charles F. Thomas, Jr., M.D.

PULMONARY INFECTIONS

Viral Infections

The common cold is caused by rhinovirus, parainfluenza virus, adenovirus, respiratory syncytial virus, and coxsackievirus. The temporary interference with mucociliary clearance caused by acute viral infection may increase the risk of other infections. Viral respiratory tract infections constitute 80% of all acute infections. Nearly one-half of the general population has a viral respiratory tract infection in December–February and only 20% in June–August. Respiratory syncytial virus is an important cause of acute lower respiratory tract disease among children and the elderly. Coxsackieviruses are a more frequent cause of viral respiratory tract infections in the summer and autumn.

- Coxsackieviral infections are more frequent in the summer and autumn.
- Typical clinical scenario: Coxsackievirus B causes pleurodynia (Bornholm disease or "devil's grip")—fever, headache, malaise, and severe pleuritic pain lasting from several days to weeks.

Viral Pneumonia

Common causes of viral pneumonia are parainfluenza virus, adenovirus, and influenza viruses A and B. In adults, varicella (chickenpox) pneumonia is a severe illness, the resolution of which may be followed by nodular pulmonary calcification. In adults with chickenpox, cough (25% of patients), profuse rash, fever for more than 1 week, and age older than 34 years are the most important predictors of varicella pneumonia. Early aggressive therapy with intravenous acyclovir is recommended for patients at risk for pneumonia. Corticosteroids reportedly are of value in the treatment of previously well patients with life-threatening varicella pneumonia. Herpes simplex virus may cause pneumonia in an immunocompromised host or in patients with extensive burns. Cytomegalovirus is seen more commonly in immunocompromised patients such as those with acquired immunodeficiency syndrome (AIDS) (also associated with *Pneumocystis carinii* infection) or transplant recipients, in hematologic malignancy, and after multiple blood transfusions and cardiopulmonary bypass. Diffuse, small nodular, or hazy infiltrates are seen on chest radiography (CXR) in 15% of patients with pneumonia caused by cytomegalovirus, but interstitial pneumonia due to cytomegalovirus is seen in 50% of bone marrow graft recipients. Findings of inclusion bodies and high titers of cytomegalovirus may help in making the diagnosis.

- Viral pneumonia in nonimmunocompromised adults is caused by influenza virus and adenovirus.
- Typical clinical scenario for varicella pneumonia: An adult with a characteristic chickenpox rash who has cough and fever lasting more than 1 week; acyclovir is recommended for patients at risk.
- Cytomegalovirus infection is associated with immunocompromised patients, such as those with AIDS (CD4 count <50/μL).
- Isolation of cytomegalovirus from respiratory tract secretions does not always establish that infection is present.

Influenza

Influenza is responsible for more than 50% of cases of viral pneumonia diagnosed in adults. Influenza A pneumonia is a major cause of morbidity and mortality during the winter months in the United States. Influenza B is more endemic than influenza A and is responsible for 20% to 30% of influenza infections. Parainfluenza viruses are responsible for 15% of all cases of viral pneumonia. Nearly all patients with influenza A pneumonia have underlying heart disease, usually rheumatic valvular disease. The clinical features are high temperature, dyspnea, cyanosis, fluffy or nodular infiltrates in the mid-lung fields, and respiratory failure. Annual (in the autumn) influenza vaccination is recommended for high-risk persons (chronic obstructive pulmonary disease [COPD], heart disease, diabetes mellitus, kidney disease, chronic anemia, debilitated condition, age older than 60, and immunocompromised status). Overall protection rates are 70%. Recently, antiviral agents have been approved to shorten the duration of illness from influenza.

- Typical clinical scenario for influenza A pneumonia: A 73-year-old woman presents with fever, dyspnea, cyanosis, mid-lung infiltrates, and underlying valvular heart disease.

Hantavirus Pulmonary Syndrome

Hantavirus pulmonary syndrome, first recognized in the southwestern United States in 1993, is caused by an RNA virus (family, Bunyaviridae; genus, *Hantavirus*). The rodent reservoir for this virus is the deer mouse (*Peromyscus maniculatus*). Infection occurs by inhalation of rodent excreta. No human-to-human transmission has been documented. The syndrome is more common in the southwestern United States. The demographic features are the following: median age of patients, 32 years (range, 12-69 years); males (52%); and Native Americans (55%). The illness is characterized by a short prodrome of fever, myalgia, headache, abdominal pain, nausea or vomiting (or both), and cough, followed by the abrupt onset of respiratory distress. Bilateral pulmonary infiltrates (noncardiogenic pulmonary edema) that occur within 48 hours after the onset of illness have been reported in all patients. Pleural effusions are common and can be transudates or exudates. Hemoconcentration and thrombocytopenia occur in 71% of patients. Autopsy has routinely documented serous pleural effusions and heavy edematous lungs, with interstitial mononuclear cells in the alveolar septa, alveolar edema, focal hyaline membranes, and occasional alveolar hemorrhage. *Hantavirus* antigens are detected with immunohistochemistry. Serologic (*Hantavirus*-specific IgM or increasing titers of IgG), polymerase chain reaction, and other studies are available. For those in shock and who have lactic acidosis, the prognosis is poor. No sequelae have been reported in survivors. The mortality rate has been 50% to 75%.

- The reservoir for *Hantavirus* is the deer mouse.
- Typical clinical scenario for hantavirus pulmonary syndrome: After a prodrome, a Native American male has abrupt onset of respiratory distress, shock, and hypoxemia. CXR demonstrates bilateral pulmonary infiltrates and pleural effusion. Laboratory studies demonstrate a leftshift neutrophilia, hemoconcentration, thrombocytopenia, and circulating immunoblasts.

Severe Acute Respiratory Syndrome

Severe acute respiratory syndrome (SARS) is a viral respiratory infection caused by a novel coronavirus that previously had infected only animals. The majority of patients with SARS have been adults 25 to 70 years old who were previously healthy. Many of the cases have been reported in Asia, particularly Hong Kong, Taiwan, and the People's Republic of China; however, cases have been reported in other countries in Asia as well as in North America and Europe. SARS has an incubation period of 2 to 7 days and as long as 10 days in some patients. The illness begins with fever (>38.0°C) and associated chills and rigors. Other frequent symptoms are headache, malaise, and myalgia. No skin rash or neurologic symptoms are present. Diarrhea may occur in 10% to 20% of patients. Within the first 7 days, a dry nonproductive cough and dyspnea develop, with hypoxemia. This worsens in 20% of patients, who require mechanical ventilation and treatment in an intensive care unit. Currently, the fatality rate is approximately 15%. CXR shows interstitial infiltrates that progress to areas of consolidation. Leukocyte counts generally have been

normal or decreased, with more than 50% of patients having leukopenia and thrombocytopenia. Increased levels of liver aminotransferases and creatine kinase have been noted. Most patients have normal renal function during the illness. It is not known what treatment regimen would be most efficacious. Supportive care is recommended.

- SARS is caused by a coronavirus.
- Typical clinical scenario for SARS: After a febrile prodrome with associated myalgias, a dry nonproductive cough with dyspnea and hypoxemia develop in a 39-year-old traveler from Asia. CXR demonstrates bilateral interstital pulmonary infiltrates. Laboratory studies demonstrate leukopenia, thrombocytopenia, and elevated levels of creatine kinase and liver aminotransferases.

Bacterial Infections

Sinusitis

Most bacterial sinus infections occur after an acute viral infection of the nasal mucosa. Bacteria in acute and chronic sinusitis are listed in Table 21-18. *Moraxella catarrhalis* is also frequently involved. The maxillary sinus is commonly involved, and nearly 10% of the cases of maxillary sinusitis are related to odontogenic infections. Cultures of the nasal secretions from more than 90% of patients with chronic rhinosinusitis are positive for fungi. Computed tomography (CT) of the sinuses is better than traditional radiography for detecting sinusitis.

- Sinus involvement is also seen in asthma, chronic bronchitis, bronchiectasis, cystic fibrosis, Kartagener syndrome, and Wegener granulomatosis.
- Fungal sinusitis is common in chronic rhinosinusitis.

Otitis Media

The relation between otitis media and common viral infections is strong, especially in children. Nearly 10% of children

Table 21-18 Bacteria in Acute and Chronic Sinusitis

Bacteria	Sinusitis, % of patients	
	Acute	Chronic
Pneumococci	20-35	5-15
Haemophilus influenzae	15-30	3-10
Streptococcus, anaerobes and aerobes	5-35	10-25
Staphylococcus aureus	3-6	5-15
No growth	2-25	25-60

with measles have otitis media. Bacteria are isolated from 70% to 80% of patients with otitis media and include pneumococci (25%-75% of patients), *Haemophilus influenzae* (15%-30%), anaerobes, peptococci and propionibacteria (20%-30%), group A streptococci (2%-10%), and *Staphylococcus aureus* (1%-5%). Ampicillin-resistant *H. influenzae* is found in 15% to 40% of patients.

- Otitis media in adults occurs in severe diabetes mellitus and cystic fibrosis.

Pharyngitis

Pharyngitis is caused by group A *Streptococcus pyogenes* (>30% of patients), *Neisseria gonorrhoeae*, *Corynebacterium diphtheriae*, and *Mycoplasma pneumoniae* (5%). Sore throat is also caused by adenovirus, Epstein-Barr virus, and other viruses.

Pneumonia

Streptococcus pneumoniae

S. pneumoniae is responsible for 90% of cases of pneumonia in adults. The incidence peaks in the winter and spring, when carrier rates in the general population may be as high as 70%. It is most common in infants and the elderly and in alcoholic or immunocompromised patients. At high risk are persons with cardiopulmonary disease (especially pulmonary edema), viral respiratory tract infections, or hemoglobinopathy and immunosuppression, including patients with hyposplenism. The incidence of bacteremic pneumonia among hospitalized patients is 25%, and the mortality rate is 20%. Of the elderly with bacteremic pneumonia, 30% do not have fever, 50% have minimal respiratory symptoms, 50% have altered mental state, and 50% have volume depletion. Leukocytosis of 10 to 30×10^9/L is common. Sputum may be blood-streaked or rusty. Early in the disease, CXR findings may be normal, but later, they may show classic lobar pneumonia. Pleurisy or effusion is common, and cavitation is rare.

- *S. pneumoniae*: mortality rate of about 30% among patients older than 50 with bacteremic pneumonia.
- Of the elderly with bacteremic pneumonia, 30% do not have fever and 50% each have minimal respiratory symptoms, altered mental state, and volume depletion.
- Typical clinical scenario for streptococcal pneumonia: A patient with cardiopulmonary disease has a recent viral respiratory tract infection, leukocytosis, and rusty sputum.

The pneumococcal vaccine consists of purified capsular polysaccharide from the 23 pneumococcal types, accounting for at least 90% of pneumococcal pneumonias. It offers as much protection against drug-resistant pneumococci as against drug-sensitive ones. Vaccination decreases serious complications of pneumococcal infection by about one-half and reduces the carrier state among the general population. Pneumococcal vaccination is recommended for elderly persons (older than 65) and for those with diabetes mellitus, heart and lung diseases, renal insufficiency, hepatic insufficiency, sickle cell anemia, asplenia or hyposplenia, hematologic and other malignancies, alcoholism, cerebrospinal fluid leakage, immunodeficiency states, organ transplants, or AIDS. Some recommend pneumococcal vaccination for all adults, especially health care workers. Repeat vaccination guidelines are controversial. Patients with nephrotic syndrome and other protein-losing nephropathies rapidly lose pneumococcal antibody and, thus, should receive pneumovax every 5 or 6 years. Pneumococcal vaccination should be given to pregnant women only if clearly needed.

- The overall efficacy of the pneumococcal vaccine is 60%.
- Efficacy rates for certain diseases vary (diabetes mellitus, 84%; coronary artery disease, 73%; congestive heart failure, 69%; COPD, 65%; and anatomical asplenia, 77%).
- Pneumovax decreases the incidence of pneumonia by 79%-92%.

Staphylococcus aureus

S. aureus may be isolated from the nasal passages of 20% to 40% of normal adults, but pneumonia is uncommon. *S. aureus* pneumonia is more likely to occur in patients with severe diabetes mellitus or an immunocompromised state, in patients receiving dialysis, in drug abusers, and in those with influenza or measles. In drug addicts, it may begin as septic emboli from right-sided endocarditis. It is a nosocomial type of pneumonia. Consolidation, bronchopneumonia, abscess with air-fluid level, pneumatocele, empyema, and a high mortality rate characterize staphylococcal pneumonia.

- Lung abscess and pneumatoceles are more common complications of *S. aureus* pneumonia.
- Associations with *Staphylococcus* pneumonia: diabetes mellitus, immunocompromised host, dialysis patients, influenza or measles infection, or drug abuse.

Pseudomonas aeruginosa

P. aeruginosa is a ubiquitous organism commonly isolated from patients with cystic fibrosis and bronchiectasis. Pneumonia may occur in patients with COPD, congestive heart failure, diabetes mellitus, kidney disease, alcoholism, tracheostomy, or prolonged ventilation. It also may develop postoperatively and in immunocompromised hosts. *Pseudomonas* pneumonia results in microabscess, alveolar hemorrhage, and necrotic areas. CXR may show bilateral patchy infiltrates.

- *P. aeruginosa*: it may be difficult to distinguish between colonization and true infection.
- It is an important pathogenic organism in cystic fibrosis, bronchiectasis, malignant otitis media, immunocompromised state, and ventilator-associated pneumonia.

Klebsiella pneumoniae

Pneumonia due to *K. pneumoniae* is more likely in persons who are alcoholic, have diabetes, or are hospitalized. Also, it is more common in males. Dependent lobes are affected more frequently than nondependent ones. In lobar pneumonia caused by *K. pneumoniae*, CXR may show a "bulging fissure." Complications include abscess and empyema.

- Typical clinical scenario for *K. pneumoniae* pneumonia: A patient is alcoholic, has diabetes, or is hospitalized and has a "bulging fissure" sign on CXR.

Haemophilus influenzae

Unencapsulated strains of *H. influenzae* are present in the sputum of 30% to 60% of normal adults and 58% to 80% of patients with COPD. In contrast, bacteremia is almost always associated with encapsulated strains. Both strains cause pulmonary infections and otitis, sinusitis, epiglottitis, and pneumonia. Most patients with pneumonia have underlying COPD or alcoholism, even though *H. influenzae* pneumonia develops in healthy military recruits. Pneumonia is detected in the lower lobes more often than in the upper lobes. CXR findings are typical for bronchopneumonia or lobar pneumonia. Pleural effusions occur in 30% of patients, and cavitation is rare.

- Typical clinical scenario for *H. influenzae* pneumonia: A patient has COPD or is alcoholic; 30% of patients have pleural effusions, and cavitation is rare.

Moraxella catarrhalis

M. catarrhalis, a gram-negative diplococcus, is part of the normal flora. Colonization is more common in the winter. It causes sinusitis, otitis, and pneumonia. The latter is more likely in patients who are alcoholic or have COPD, diabetes mellitus, or immunocompromised status. Bacteremia is rare. Infection produces segmental patchy bronchopneumonia in the lower lobes. Cavitation and pleural effusion are rare. These bacteria produce β-lactamase, and most are resistant to penicillin and ampicillin.

- Typical clinical scenario for *M. catarrhalis* pneumonia: A patient has COPD or is immunocompromised or alcoholic

and has gram-negative diplococci that are β-lactamase–positive.

Legionella pneumophila

Legionella is a gram-negative bacillus whose natural habitat is water. Infection results from inhalation of aerosolized organisms. Epidemics have occurred from contaminated air-conditioning cooling towers, construction or excavation in contaminated soil, and contaminated hospital showers. Most cases occur in the summer and early autumn. Risk factors include COPD, smoking, cancer, diabetes mellitus, immunosuppression, and chronic heart and kidney diseases. Almost all cases of pneumonia are caused by *L. pneumophila* (85% of patients) and *L. micdadei* (10%). Bacteria can be demonstrated in tissue with the Dieterle and fluorescent antibody stains. The incubation period is 2 to 10 days. Symptoms, in decreasing order of frequency, are abrupt onset of cough (hemoptysis in 30% of patients), chills, dyspnea, headache, myalgia, arthralgia, and diarrhea. Common signs include fever, relative bradycardia, and change in mental status. The diagnosis is established with the fluorescent antibody stain, which is positive in the sputum in 20% of serologically positive patients. Bacteria can be cultured from tissue or other samples. Serologic testing takes from 1 to 3 weeks before a titer of 1:64 is seen; the peak titer is reached in 5 to 6 weeks. A titer of 1:128 is suspicious, and a fourfold increase in titer is diagnostic.

- Typical clinical scenario for *L. pneumophila* pneumonia: A 67-year-old with COPD, diabetes mellitus, and chronic heart failure presents with hyponatremia and hypophosphatemia, lobar consolidations on CXR, leukocytosis (>10 $\times 10^9$/L), proteinuria, and increased serum level of aspartate aminotransferase (AST).
- A false-positive titer can be seen in plague, tularemia, leptospirosis, and adenovirus infections.
- A *Legionella* serology titer of 1:128 is suspicious, and a fourfold increase in titer is diagnostic.

Anaerobic Bacteria

Bacteroides melaninogenicus, Fusobacterium nucleatum, anaerobic cocci, and anaerobic streptococci are responsible for most cases of anaerobic pneumonia. *Bacteroides fragilis* is recovered from 15% to 20% of patients with anaerobic pneumonia. Most of these anaerobes reside in the oropharynx as saprophytes. Common factors responsible for aspiration of anaerobes include altered consciousness, tooth extraction, poor dental hygiene, oropharyngeal infections, and drug overdose. Anaerobic bacterial infections may complicate underlying pulmonary problems (e.g., cancer, bronchiectasis, or foreign body). More than 50% of patients have foul-smelling sputum. Patchy pneumonitis in dependent segments may progress to lung abscess and empyema.

- Typical clinical scenario for anaerobic bacterial pneumonia: Aspiration of anaerobes is facilitated by altered consciousness, tooth extraction, poor dental hygiene, oropharyngeal infections, and drug overdose; the patient has cavitated lung abscesses in dependent lobes.

Community-Acquired "Atypical" Pneumonia

Organisms causing "atypical" community-acquired pneumonia include *Mycoplasma pneumoniae*, *Chlamydia psittaci*, *Chlamydia pneumoniae*, *Coxiella burnetii*, and *Francisella tularensis*. Community-acquired "typical" pneumonias are caused by *Streptococcus pneumoniae* (45% of patients), gram-negative bacilli (15%), and *Haemophilus influenzae* (15%). For patients not admitted to the hospital, the mortality from community-acquired pneumonia is less than 1%. However, the overall mortality for patients admitted to the hospital is 14% and it is 18% for elderly patients and 20% for those with bacteremia. The mortality of patients with community-acquired pneumonia who are admitted to an intensive care unit is 37%.

- Community-acquired "atypical" pneumonia is caused by *Mycoplasma pneumoniae*, *Chlamydia psittaci*, *Chlamydia pneumoniae*, *Coxiella burnetii*, and *Legionella* species.

Mycoplasma

Mycoplasma spp is spread from person to person by droplet nuclei. Infections occur in epidemic and endemic form, and outbreaks occur in closed populations (e.g., military camps and colleges). Epidemics are more common in the summer and autumn. Illness is more common in school-aged children and young adults. The incubation period is 2 to 3 weeks. Clinical features include cough (>95% of patients), fever (85%), pharyngitis (50%), bullous myringitis (20%), coryza, and tracheobronchitis. Rare complications include pleural effusion, hemolytic anemia, erythema multiforme, hepatitis, thrombocytopenia, and Guillain-Barré syndrome. Nearly 20% of all community-acquired pneumonias and 50% of all pneumonias in healthy young adults in close living quarters (e.g., military recruits and dormitory students) may be caused by *Mycoplasma pneumoniae*. Pneumonia occurs in only 3% to 10% of infected persons and is more likely in younger adults (military recruits or children in summer camps); it causes interstitial pneumonia and acute bronchiolitis. CXR shows unilateral bronchopneumonia, lower lobe involvement (65% of patients), and pleural effusion (5%). Cold agglutinins (>1:64 in 50% of patients) appear during the second or third week after the onset of symptoms, and the titer decreases to insignificant levels by 4 to 6 weeks. With complement fixation serologic testing, a fourfold increase in titer is noted in 50% to 80% of patients. The organism can be cultured from respiratory tract secretions, the middle ear, and the cerebrospinal fluid.

- Typical clinical scenario for *Mycoplasma* pneumonia: Cough, fever, pharyngitis, coryza, and tracheobronchitis, with bullous myringitis, hemolytic anemia, erythema multiforme, or Guillain-Barré syndrome; it causes interstitial pneumonia and acute bronchiolitis.
- Cold agglutinins (>1:64 in 50% of patients) appear during the second to third week.

Chlamydia pneumoniae (TWAR Strain)

C. pneumoniae is confined to the human respiratory tract; no reservoirs are known. Person-to-person spread occurs among schoolchildren, family members, and military recruits. The incubation period is 10 to 65 days (mean, 31 days). Reinfection is common, with cycles of disease every few years. *C. pneumoniae* is the cause of at least 10% of all cases of community-acquired pneumonia. About 15% of patients are symptomatic and have clinical features that include pharyngitis (90% of patients), pneumonia (10%), bronchitis (5%), and sinusitis (5%). Pharyngeal erythema and wheezing are common. Among older adults, 40% of community-acquired cases of pneumonia are due to *C. psittaci*. CXR shows unilateral segmental patchy opacity. The complement fixation test is insensitive and nonspecific.

- *C. pneumoniae*: person-to-person spread among schoolchildren, family members, and military recruits.
- Pneumonia in 10% of patients, and bronchitis in 5% of symptomatic patients.
- *C. pneumoniae* is considered an etiologic agent in coronary artery disease.

Chlamydia psittaci

C. psittaci causes psittacosis (ornithosis) in humans. The organism is found in psittacine birds (parrots and lories), turkeys, pigeons, and other birds. Infected birds have anorexia, weight loss, diarrhea, ruffled feathers, conjunctivitis, and rhinitis, and they are not able to fly. In humans, the incubation period is 1 to 6 weeks. Clinical features include myalgias, fever, headache, pharyngitis, lethargy, confusion, delirium, neutropenia (in 25% of patients), and splenomegaly (in 1%-10%). Pulmonary symptoms are late and mild. CXR shows patchy unilateral or bilateral lower lobe pneumonia and an occasional small pleural effusion. Laboratory findings include a normal leukocyte count, increased creatine kinase level, and a fourfold increase in complement fixation over more than 2 weeks.

- Typical clinical scenario for psittacosis: Exposure to sick birds that harbor *C. psittaci*; patients have myalgias, fever, headache, lethargy, confusion, delirium, and splenomegaly.
- Note the differences: *C. pneumoniae* pneumonia (human-to-human transmission), psittacosis (birds-to-human

transmission), and pigeon-breeder's or bird fancier's lung (hypersensitivity pneumonitis caused by immune reaction to avian proteins).

Coxiella burnetii

C. burnetii, a rickettsia shed in the urine, feces, milk, and birth products of sheep, cattle, goats, and cats, is responsible for Q fever. However, epidemiologic factors such as contact with cats or farm animals are found in only 40% of patients. Humans are infected by inhalation of dried aerosolized material. The incubation period is 10 to 30 days. Clinical features include fever, myalgias, chills, chest pain, and cough (late). The leukocyte count is normal, and the erythrocyte sedimentation rate is increased. CXR findings may be normal or show unilateral bronchopneumonia and small pleural effusions. Lobar consolidation is seen in 25% of patients. Hepatitis and endocarditis can occur. Hyponatremia occurs in more than 25% of patients. Liver enzyme levels may increase; the complement fixation serologic test is positive.

- *C. burnetii*: rickettsial illness (Q fever).
- Inhalation of dried inoculum from urine, feces, milk, or birth products of sheep, cattle, goats, or cats.
- Bronchopneumonia and pleural effusion.

Francisella tularensis

F. tularensis is a gram-negative bacillus transmitted to humans from wild animals and by bites of ticks or deer flies. The incubation period is 2 to 5 days. Cutaneous ulcer and lymphadenopathy are common features. Cough, fever, and chest pain are frequent, but many patients are asymptomatic. CXR shows unilateral lower lobe patchy infiltrates (bilateral in 30% of patients) and pleural effusion (30% of patients). The leukocyte count is normal; the organism is not seen with Gram staining of the sputum. Serologic testing (agglutinins) shows a fourfold change (titer >1:160).

- Tularemia: transmitted from wild rabbits, squirrels, and other wild animals.
- Typical clinical scenario for tularemia: Patients may be asymptomatic or have cough and fever, with cutaneous ulcer, lymphadenopathy, bronchopneumonia, and pleural effusion.

Yersinia pestis

Y. pestis is a gram-negative bacillus that causes plague. It is more prevalent in New Mexico, Arizona, Colorado, and California than in other states. It is spread from wild rodents (occasionally cats), either directly or by fleas, usually in May to September. The incubation period is 2 to 7 days. Clinical features include fever, headache, bubo (groin or axilla), cough, and tachypnea.

Pneumonia occurs in 10% to 20% of patients. CXR shows bilateral lower lobe alveolar infiltrates. Pleural effusion is common, and nodules and cavities can occur. The leukocyte count is higher than 15×10^9/L. The organism is seen with Giemsa or direct fluorescent antibody staining and in cultures of blood, lymph node, or sputum. Serologic testing gives positive results.

- Typical clinical scenario for *Y. pestis* pneumonia: A patient from the southwestern United States has alveolar infiltrates and pleural effusion; the leukocyte count is $>15 \times 10^9$/L.

Burkholderia pseudomallei

B. pseudomallei is a gram-negative rod responsible for melioidosis. The disease is most prevalent in parts of Southeast Asia; sporadic cases have been reported in the United States. The organism is widely distributed in water and soil, and infection occurs after direct inoculation through the skin or, less commonly, by inhalation. Although the incubation period can be as short as 3 days, the disease remains latent and may become evident months to years later. Up to 2% of U.S. Army personnel stationed in Vietnam were seropositive for *B. pseudomallei* even though the majority of them were free of clinical disease. Clinical features include acute community-acquired pneumonia, pleurisy, subacute presentation with upper lobe lesions (sometimes with cavitation), or chronic cavitary lung disease that resembles tuberculosis. Diagnosis is by positive findings on culture.

- Melioidosis may resemble chronic cavitary tuberculosis.

Nocardia Pneumonia

Nocardia asteroides, *N. brasiliensis*, and *N. otitidis-caviarum* can cause pneumonia in susceptible persons. *N. asteroides* is a weakly acid-fast saprophytic bacteria present in the soil, dust, plants, and water. Infection is more common in immunosuppressed patients and in those with pulmonary alveolar proteinosis. Primary infection leads to necrotizing pneumonia with abscess formation. No inflammatory response or granuloma formation occurs. Infection may produce pleural effusion. Lymphohematogenous spread is seen in 20% of patients; nearly all such patients develop a brain abscess. The diagnosis is made at autopsy in 40% of cases. Isolation of the organism from respiratory secretions is not diagnostic of infection because the saprophytic state is well recognized.

- Typical clinical scenario for *Nocardia* pneumonia: An immunocompromised patient or patient with pulmonary alveolar proteinosis, necrotizing pneumonia, and lung abscess.
- Brain abscess is common in those with disseminated infection.

Actinomycosis

Actinomycosis is caused by *Actinomyces israelii* or *A. bovis*. The organism is easily isolated from scrapings around the teeth, gums, and tonsils in subjects with poor dental or oral hygiene. It is an opportunistic organism and becomes invasive with severe caries, tissue necrosis, and aspiration. In tissue, the organism grows into a "sulfur granule" caused by mycelial clumps in a matrix of calcium phosphate. The disease is more common in rural areas and has a male-to-female ratio of 2:1. Infection is always mixed with anaerobes. Skin abscesses, ulcers, sinus tracts, and cervicofacial node involvement are found in up to 40% of patients. Pulmonary involvement is seen in 20% of patients, along with cough, fever, pulmonary consolidation, pleurisy with effusion, and, eventually, draining sinuses.

- Typical clinical scenario for actinomycosis: A patient has severe dental caries, tissue necrosis, and aspiration, with cough, fever, pulmonary lesions, pleural effusion, and fistula and sinus tracts.

Hospital-Acquired (Nosocomial) Pneumonia

About 60% of the cases are caused by gram-negative bacilli, 10% by *Staphylococcus aureus*, 10% by *Steptococcus pneumoniae*, and the rest by anaerobes, *Legionella* species, and others. Risk factors include coma, hypotension, shock, acidosis, azotemia, prolonged treatment with antibiotics, major surgical operations, lengthy procedures, mechanical ventilation, and immunosuppressive therapy.

- About 60% of cases of nosocomial pneumonia are caused by gram-negative bacilli, 10% by *Staphylococcus aureus*, and 10% by *Streptococcus pneumoniae*.
- In hospital outbreaks involving a single type of organism, consider contaminated respiratory equipment.

Aspiration Pneumonia

Aspiration pneumonia can be either acute or chronic. The acute type usually results from aspiration of a volume larger than 50 mL, with a pH less than 2.4. It produces classic aspiration pneumonia. Predisposing factors include nasogastric tube, anesthesia, coma, seizures, central nervous system problems, diaphragmatic hernia with reflux, and tracheoesophageal fistula. Nosocomial aspiration pneumonia is caused by *Escherichia coli*, *Staphylococcus aureus*, *Klebsiella pneumoniae*, and *Pseudomonas aeruginosa*. Community-acquired aspiration pneumonias are caused by infections due to anaerobes (*Bacteroides melaninogenicus*, *Fusobacterium nucleatum*, and gram-positive cocci). Preventive measures are important. Chronic aspiration pneumonia results from recurrent aspiration of small volumes. Examples include patients with reflux aspiration who develop mineral oil granuloma. Symptoms include chronic cough, patchy lung infiltrates, and nocturnal wheeze.

- Acute aspiration pneumonia: from the aspiration of a volume >50 mL, with a pH <2.4.
- Chronic aspiration pneumonia: from recurrent aspiration of small volumes.

Lung Abscess

"Lung abscess" is a circumscribed collection of pus in the lung that leads to cavity formation and a CXR finding of an air-fluid level in the cavity. It usually is caused by bacteria, particularly anaerobic bacilli (30%-50% of cases), aerobic gram-positive cocci (25%), and aerobic gram-negative bacilli (5%-12%). Suppuration leading to lung abscess can result from primary, opportunistic, and hematogenous lung infection. Primary lung abscess is caused by oral infection; aspiration accounts for up to 90% of all abscesses. Alcohol abuse and dental caries also contribute. Lung abscesses caused by opportunistic infections are seen in elderly patients with a blood dyscrasia and in patients with cancer of the lung or oropharynx. Hematogenous lung abscesses occur with septicemia, septic embolism, and sterile infarcts (3% of patients). A history of any of these conditions in association with fever, cough with purulent or bloody sputum, weight loss, and leukocytosis suggests the diagnosis. CXR may show cavitated lesions. The abscess may rupture into the pleural space and cause empyema. Bronchoscopy may be necessary to obtain cultures, to drain the abscess, and to exclude obstructing lesions. High rates of morbidity and mortality (20%) are associated with lung abscess despite antibiotic therapy. The prognosis is worse for patients with a large abscess and for those infected with *Staphylococcus aureus*, *Klebsiella pneumoniae*, and *Pseudomonas aeruginosa*. Treatment includes drainage (physiotherapy, postural, and bronchoscopic), antibiotics for 4 to 6 weeks, and surgical treatment if medical therapy fails.

- Typical clinical scenario for primary lung abscess: A 54-year-old alcoholic male presents with fever. CXR demonstrates a cavity with an air-fluid level.
- Hematogenous lung abscess is seen in septicemia and septic embolism.

Mycobacterial Diseases

Mycobacterium tuberculosis

Mycobacterium tuberculosis causes the most common type of human-to-human chronic infection by mycobacteria worldwide. The most common mode of transmission is by inhalation of droplet nuclei from expectorated respiratory secretions.

Of those exposed to *M. tuberculosis*, 30% become infected, and among the latter group, fewer than 5% develop active primary disease and fewer than 5% develop active disease from reactivation. Active infection is diagnosed by documenting the presence of *M. tuberculosis* in respiratory secretions or other body fluids or tissues. Sputum and gastric washings have approximately a 30% diagnostic yield. Bronchoscopy with bronchoalveolar lavage has an approximately 40% diagnostic yield, which increases to almost 95% if biopsy is performed. Culture of pleural fluid alone provides the diagnosis in fewer than 20% of cases, but culture of pleural biopsy specimens has a 70% diagnostic yield. Faster culture results are available with the use of broth culture systems (1.5-2 weeks) and nucleic acid amplification (8 hours). Culture-positive pulmonary tuberculosis with normal CXR findings is not uncommon, and the incidence of this presentation is increasing. "Latent tuberculosis infection" (LTBI) is the current term for a person who does not have active tuberculosis but has a positive purified protein derivative (PPD) skin test. Such a person is infected with mycobacteria but does not have active disease.

- The PPD skin test indicates infection with mycobacteria and not active disease.
- Active infection should be confirmed by the growth of *M. tuberculosis* in respiratory secretions or other body fluids or tissues.
- Bronchoscopically obtained specimens have a higher diagnostic yield.
- CXR findings can be normal in active tuberculosis.

A positive PPD tuberculin skin test is an example of a delayed (T-cell–mediated) hypersensitivity reaction. The PPD is negative in 25% of patients with active tuberculosis. A false-negative PPD is also seen in infections with viruses or bacteria, live virus vaccinations, chronic renal failure, nutritional deficiency, lymphoid malignancies, leukemias, corticosteroid and immunosuppressive drug therapy, newborn or elderly, recent or overwhelming infection with mycobacteria, and acute stress. The annual risk of active tuberculosis for those who are PPD-positive depends on the underlying medical condition (annual risk in parentheses): human immunodeficiency virus (HIV)-positive (8%-10%), recent converters (2%-5%), abnormal CXR (2%-4%), intravenous drug abuse (1%), end-stage renal disease (1%), and diabetes mellitus (0.3%). PPD skin testing should use a 5-tuberculin unit (TU) preparation; the widest induration is read at 48 and 72 hours.

- The PPD reaction is a delayed type of hypersensitivity reaction.
- The PPD skin test can become positive within 4 weeks after exposure to *M. tuberculosis*.

- The PPD skin test is negative in 25% of patients with active tuberculosis.

Targeted tuberculin testing for LTBI identifies persons at high risk for developing tuberculosis who would benefit from treatment of LTBI. Indications for the PPD skin test include persons with signs and symptoms suggestive of current tuberculous infection, recent contacts with known or suspected cases of tuberculosis, abnormal CXR findings compatible with past tuberculosis, patients with diseases that increase the risk of tuberculosis (silicosis, gastrectomy, diabetes mellitus, immune suppression, and HIV infection), and groups at high risk for recent infection with *M. tuberculosis* (immigrants and long-time residents and workers in hospitals, nursing homes, or prisons). The following criteria are used to diagnose LTBI (i.e., a "positive" PPD skin test):

- ≥5 mm: adults and children with HIV infection, close contact with infectious cases, and those with fibrotic lesions on CXR.
- ≥10 mm: other at-risk adults and children, including infants and children <4 years old.
- ≥15 mm: any person without a defined risk factor for tuberculosis.
- Recent PPD skin test converters: ≥10-mm increase within a 2-year period for those <35 years old; ≥15-mm increase for those ≥35 years old; and a ≥10-mm skin reaction for infants and children <4 years old.

Pleural tuberculosis used to be more common in younger (<40 years) patients; now, it is more common among the elderly. In the United States, 4% of all tuberculous patients have pleural involvement, and pleural tuberculosis constitutes 23% of the cases with extrapulmonary tuberculosis. Effusions usually occur 3 to 6 months after the primary infection. Acute presentation (cough, fever, and pleuritic chest pain) is more common in younger patients. Bilateral exudative effusions occur in up to 8% of patients, and the PPD skin test is positive in more than 66%. Low levels of glucose (<50 mg/dL) in the pleural fluid and a low pH occur in 20% of patients. Pleural biopsy specimens show caseous granulomas in up to 80% of patients, and cultures of biopsy specimens are positive in more than 75%. Cultures of pleural fluid are positive in only 15% of patients and the sputum is positive in 40%. Bronchopleural fistula is a complication.

- Pleural tuberculosis is seen in younger (<40 years) patients.
- Effusion occurs 3-6 months after primary infection.

Miliary tuberculosis constitutes 10% of cases of extrapulmonary tuberculosis. It is characterized by the diffuse presence of small (<2 mm) nodules throughout the body. The spleen, liver, and lung are frequently involved. The disease can be acute and fatal or insidious in onset and slowly progressive. CXR shows typical miliary lesions in more than 65% of patients. Mortality is high (30%) even with therapy. Tuberculous lymphadenitis (scrofula) is the most common form of extrapulmonary tuberculosis. It is more common in children and young adults than in older persons. Cervical lymph nodes are affected most commonly; one or more nodes (painless, nontender, and rubbery) may be palpable. Abscess and sinus formation may occur. Skeletal tuberculosis is becoming less common; when seen, it is more common in the young than in older adults. Any bone can be involved, but the vertebrae are involved in 50% of cases. Pott disease is tuberculous spondylitis and may produce severe kyphosis. Tuberculous meningitis is the most common form affecting the nervous system and is localized mainly to the base of the brain. It occurs more commonly in intravenous drug users who are HIV-positive and in immunocompromised patients. Tuberculous meningitis is often insidious in onset. Abdominal tuberculosis frequently affects the peritoneum. Ileocecal tuberculosis can lead to ulcerative enteritis, strictures, and fistulas. Genitourinary tuberculosis is responsible for up to 13% of extrapulmonary disease. It is usually a late manifestation of the infection and is more common in older patients. The renal cortex is affected initially, and the infection can then spread to the renal pelvis, ureter, bladder, and genitalia. Sterile pyuria is an important feature. Laryngeal tuberculosis is usually a complication of pulmonary tuberculosis. Pericardial tuberculosis is usually due to hematogenous spread. Pericardial constriction may begin subacutely and become a chronic problem.

- Miliary tuberculosis is responsible for 10% of cases of extrapulmonary tuberculosis.
- Tuberculous lymphadenitis is the most common form of extrapulmonary tuberculosis.
- Tuberculous meningitis is often insidious in onset.

Tuberculosis is particularly prone to develop in HIV-positive persons. In this group of patients, a CD4 count less than 200/μL and a PPD-positive status increase the risk. Furthermore, there is an increased rate of reactivation, increased rate of progressive primary infection, increased incidence of multidrug resistance, atypical clinical features, and increased progression of HIV disease. Among those who are HIV-positive and are exposed to *M. tuberculosis*, nearly 40% develop primary tuberculosis, and the rate of reactivation is 8% to 10% per year. Tuberculous pleurisy and hilar and mediastinal lymphadenopathy are more common in AIDS than in non-AIDS patients with tuberculosis. Treatment of tuberculosis is identical in HIV-negative and HIV-positive patients. Rifampin-containing regimens are effective in curing tuberculosis in HIV-positive patients. Initiation of HIV protease inhibitor therapy in patients who are HIV-positive or have AIDS increases the symptoms and signs of the underlying mycobacterial infection. Rifampin accelerates the metabolism of protease inhibitors (decreased plasma levels) and leads to HIV resistance. Isoniazid prophylaxis for 12 months decreases the incidence of tuberculosis and increases the life expectancy for HIV-infected patients.

- Tuberculosis is particularly prone to develop in HIV-positive persons.
- The simultaneous presence of HIV and tuberculosis leads to increased severity of both infections.
- HIV protease inhibitor therapy may lead to worsening of the signs and symptoms of tuberculosis.

Definitive therapy is indicated for all patients with culture-positive tuberculosis. Treatment usually should include multiple drug (>2 drugs) therapy for all patients who have active tuberculosis (Tables 21-19–21-21). With rigidly administered 6-month regimens, more than 90% of patients are smear-negative after 2 months of therapy, more than 95% are cured, and fewer than 5% have relapse. A 9-month regimen provides a cure rate higher than 97% and a relapse rate less than 2%. All treatment programs should be recommended and preferably undertaken by physicians and health care workers experienced in the management of mycobacterial diseases.

Extrapulmonary tuberculosis can be treated effectively with either a 6- or 9-month regimen. However, miliary tuberculosis, bone and joint tuberculosis, and tuberculous meningitis in infants and children may require treatment for 12 or more months. Systemic corticosteroid therapy may be useful in the prevention of pleural fibrosis, pericardial constriction, neurologic complications from tuberculous meningitis, tuberculous bronchial stenosis, and adrenal insufficiency caused by tuberculosis. Extrapulmonary tuberculosis confined to lymph nodes has no effect on obstetrical outcomes, but tuberculosis at other sites adversely affects the outcome of pregnancy.

- Miliary, skeletal, and meningeal tuberculosis may require >12 months of therapy.
- Corticosteroids are helpful in treating extrapulmonary tuberculosis.

Drug-resistant tuberculosis is a problem in many large cities; for example, a rate of 30% has been reported in New York City. Drug resistance can develop against a single drug or multiple drugs. Multidrug resistance is usually defined as *M. tuberculosis* resistant to at least isoniazid and rifampin.

Multidrug resistance is more likely in the following settings: nonadherence to treatment guidelines and treatment "errors" by physicians and health care workers, lack of compliance by patients, homelessness, drug addiction, and exposure to multidrug-resistant tuberculosis in high-prevalence countries with inadequate tuberculosis control programs. Multiple-drug resistance occurs rapidly in HIV-infected persons. The American Thoracic Society (ATS) and the Centers for Disease Control and Prevention (CDC) recommend an intensive phase of therapy with four drugs if the local rate of resistance to isoniazid is more than 4%. Even though the mortality from multidrug-resistant tuberculosis is high in HIV-positive and HIV-negative patients, appropriate treatment produces a favorable outcome (>80%).

● Drug-resistant tuberculosis may require multidrug (4-6) therapy.

To prevent drug resistance and to effectively decrease the number of cases of tuberculosis, many health care organizations recommend administration of antituberculous drugs by directly observed therapy (DOT) in which a health care provider monitors each patient as every dose of a 6-month regimen is taken. This approach makes a cure almost certain in those

Table 21-19 Regimen Options for Treatment of Tuberculosis (TB)*[†]

Option	Indication	Total duration, wk	Initial phase		Continuation phase		Comments
			Drugs	Interval and duration	Drugs	Interval and duration	
1	Pulmonary and extrapulmonary TB in adults and children	24	INH, RIF, PZA, and EMB or SM	Daily for 8 wk	INH, RIF	Daily or 2 or 3 times/wk[‡] for 16 wk[§]	EMB or SM should be continued until susceptibility to INH and RIF is demonstrated. In areas where primary INH resistance is <4%, EMB or SM may be unnecessary for patients with no individual risk factors for drug resistance
2	Pulmonary and extrapulmonary TB in adults and children	24	INH, RIF, PZA, and EMB or SM	Daily for 2 wk and then 2 times/wk[‡] for 6 wk	INH, RIF	2 times/wk[‡] for 16 wk[§]	Regimen should be directly observed. After the initial phase, continue EMB or SM until susceptibility to INH and RIF is demonstrated, unless drug resistance is unlikely
3	Pulmonary and extrapulmonary TB in adults and children	24	INH, RIF, PZA, and EMB or SM	3 times/wk[‡] for 6 mo[§]	...	...	Regimen should be directly observed. Continue all 4 drugs for 6 mo.[//] This regimen has been shown to be effective for INH-resistant TB
4	Smear- and culture-negative pulmonary TB in adults	16	INH, RIF, PZA, and EMB or SM	Follow option 1, 2, or 3 for 8 wk	INH, RIF, PZA, and EMB or SM	Daily or 2 or 3 times/wk[‡] for 8 wk	Continue all 4 drugs for 4 mo. If drug resistance is unlikely (primary INH resistance is <4% and patient has no individual risk factors for drug resistance), EMB or SM may be unnecessary, and PZA may be discontinued after 2 mo

Table 21-19 (continued)*†

Option	Indication	Total duration, wk	Initial phase Drugs	Initial phase Interval and duration	Continuation phase Drugs	Continuation phase Interval and duration	Comments
5	Pulmonary and extra-pulmonary TB in adults and children when PZA is contraindicated	36	INH, RIF, and EMB or SM¶	Daily for 4-8 wk	INH, RIF	Daily or 2 times/wk‡ for 24 wk§	EMB or SM should be continued until susceptibility to INH and RIF is demonstrated. In areas where primary INH resistance is <4%, EMB or SM may be unnecessary for patients with no individual risk factors for drug resistance

EMB, ethambutol; INH, isoniazid; PZA, pyrazinamide; RIF, rifampin; SM, streptomycin.

*For all patients, if susceptibility results show resistance to any of the first-line drugs or if the patient remains symptomatic or smear or culture remains positive after 3 mo, consult a TB medical expert.

†INH, RIF, PZA, and EMB are administered orally; SM is administered intramuscularly.

‡Directly observed therapy should be used with all regimens administered 2 or 3 times a week.

§For infants and children with miliary TB, bone and joint TB, or TB meningitis, treatment should be given for at least 12 months. For adults with these types of extrapulmonary TB, response to therapy should be monitored closely. If response is slow or suboptimal, treatment may be prolonged, as judged on a case-by-case basis.

//Some evidence shows that SM may be discontinued after 4 months if the isolate is susceptible to all drugs.

¶Avoid SM in pregnant women because of the risk of ototoxicity to the fetus.

From Centers for Disease Control and Prevention, Division of Tuberculosis Elimination: Core Curriculum on Tuberculosis. 3rd ed. 1994.

with drug-sensitive tuberculosis. The DOT regimen is particularly important for the homeless, chronic alcoholics, intravenous drug abusers, AIDS patients, and prison inmates. Even though fixed-dose combinations of antituberculous drugs (Rifamate and Rifater, Table 21-22) are available and have been strongly recommended by the World Health Organization, CDC, ATS, and the International Union Against Tuberculosis and Lung Disease, less than 25% of rifampin-containing therapies use the fixed-dose regimen. Treatment completion rates for pulmonary tuberculosis are most likely to exceed 90% with DOT. However, DOT may not increase the cure rate in areas where the rate of cure is high (without DOT).

● DOT for 6 months is effective in preventing relapses and emergence of drug-resistant tuberculosis.
● DOT is also useful in the treatment of drug-resistant tuberculosis and tuberculosis in immunocompromised patients.
● A fixed-dose combination should be considered in cases of newly diagnosed disease.

Treatment of LTBI is indicated for persons with a positive PPD skin test who do not have active infection (Table 21-23). If an isoniazid-sensitive organism is suspected to have caused LTBI, the treatment options include isoniazid 300 mg daily or 900 mg biweekly. Rifampin (600 mg daily) is an alternative option. If isoniazid resistance is suspected or known, the options include rifampin (600 mg daily) or rifabutin (300 mg daily). A short course of therapy (4 months) with rifampin and pyrazinamide was an alternative regimen for LTBI, but this is no longer routinely recommended because of the increased frequency of cases of fatal hepatitis. Therapy with this combination should be supervised by a specialist. The recommended duration for LTBI therapy is outlined below:

● Isoniazid for HIV-positive adults and children: 12 months.
● Isoniazid for HIV-negative adults: at least 6 months.
● Isoniazid for HIV-negative children: 9 months.
● Rifampin or rifabutin: 12 months.
● Silicosis or old fibrotic lesion on CXR without active tuberculosis: 4-month therapy with isoniazid and rifampin, although 12 months of isoniazid alone is an acceptable alternative.

In the United States, bacille Calmette-Guérin (BCG) vaccine is recommended for PPD-negative 1) infants and children who are at high risk for intimate and prolonged exposure to persistently untreated or ineffectively treated patients with infectious pulmonary tuberculosis, who cannot be removed from the source of exposure, and who cannot be given long-term

Table 21-20   First-Line Drugs for Tuberculosis (TB)*†

Drug	Dose, mg/kg Daily Children§	Daily Adults	2 times/wk‡ Children§	2 times/wk‡ Adults	3 times/wk‡ Children§	3 times/wk‡ Adults	Adverse reactions	Monitoring
INH// (maximal dose, mg)	10-20 (300)	5 (300)	20-40 (900)	15 (900)	20-40 (900)	15 (900)	Liver enzyme elevation, hepatitis, peripheral neuropathy, mild effects on central nervous system, drug interactions	Baseline measurements of liver enzymes for adults Repeat measurements if baseline results are abnormal, if patient is at high risk for adverse reactions, if patient has symptoms of adverse reactions
RIF¶ (maximal dose, mg)	10-20 (600)	10 (600)	10-20 (600)	10 (600)	10-20 (600)	10 (600)	GI upset, drug interactions, hepatitis, bleeding problems, influenza-like symptoms, rash	Baseline measurements for adults: complete blood cell count, platelets, liver enzymes Repeat measurements if baseline results are abnormal, if patient has symptoms of adverse reactions
PZA# (maximal dose, g)	15-30 (2)	15-30 (2)	50-70 (4)	50-70 (4)	50-70 (3)	50-70 (3)	Hepatitis, rash, GI upset, joint aches, hyperuricemia, gout (rare)	Baseline measurements for adults: uric acid, liver enzymes Repeat measurements if baseline results are abnormal, if patient has symptoms of adverse reactions
EMB**	15-25	15-25	50	50	25-30	25-30	Optic neuritis	Baseline and monthly tests: visual acuity, color vision
SM†† (maximal dose, g)	20-40 (1)	15 (1)	25-30 (1.5)	25-30 (1.5)	25-30 (1.5)	25-30 (1.5)	Ototoxicity (hearing loss or vestibular dysfunction), renal toxicity	Baseline and repeat as needed: hearing, kidney function

EMB, ethambutol; GI, gastrointestinal; INH, isoniazid; PZA, pyrazinamide; RIF, rifampin; SM, streptomycin.
*Adjust weight-based dosages as weight changes.
†INH, RIF, PZA, and EMB are administered orally; SM is administered intramuscularly.
‡Directly observed therapy should be used with all regimens administered 2 or 3 times a week.
§Younger than 12 years.
//Hepatitis risk increases with age and alcohol consumption. Pyridoxine can prevent peripheral neuropathy.
¶Severe interactions with methadone, oral contraceptives, and many other drugs. Drug colors body fluids orange and may permanently discolor soft contact lenses.
#Treat hyperuricemia only if patient has symptoms.
**Not recommended for children too young to be monitored for changes in vision unless TB is drug resistant.
††Avoid or decrease dose in adults older than 60 years.
From Centers for Disease Control and Prevention, Division of Tuberculosis Elimination: Core Curriculum on Tuberculosis. 3rd ed. 1994.

prophylactic therapy and 2) health care workers in settings in which the likelihood of transmission and subsequent infection with *M. tuberculosis* strains resistant to isoniazid and rifampin is high, provided comprehensive tuberculosis infection-control precautions have been implemented in the workplace and have not been successful. BCG is not recommended for HIV-positive children and adults.

• BCG is indicated for children who are at high risk for intimate and prolonged exposure to *M. tuberculosis*.

Table 21-21 Treatment Regimens for Patients With Tuberculosis, According to HIV Status*

| Drug resistance | Patients | | Antiretroviral therapy |
	Without HIV infection	With HIV infection	
None	I,R,P,E for 2 mo, I,R for 4 mo[†]	I,R,P,E for 2 mo, I,R for 4-7 mo[‡]	No protease inhibitors or NNRTIs can be used with rifampin[§]
		or	
		I,P,E plus rifabutin for 2 mo, I plus rifabutin for 4-7 mo	Rifabutin can be used with indinavir or nelfinavir but not with saquinavir, ritonavir, or NNRTIs
Isoniazid	R,P,E for 6 mo	R,P,E for 6-9 mo[¶]	No protease inhibitors or NNRTIs can be used with rifampin
		or	
		Rifabutin plus P,E for 6-9 mo	Rifabutin can be used with indinavir or nelfinavir but not with saquinavir, ritonavir, or NNRTIs
Rifampin	I,P,E for 18-24 mo	I,P,E for 18-24 mo	All antiretroviral drugs can be used
		or	
		I,P,S,E for 2 mo, I,P,S for 7-10 mo	All antiretroviral drugs can be used

E, ethambutol; HIV, human immunodeficiency virus; I, isoniazid; NNRTI, non-nucleoside reverse-transcriptase inhibitor; P, pyrazinamide; R, rifampin; S, streptomycin.

*Recommendations are based on those of the American Thoracic Society, the Centers for Disease Control and Prevention, and expert opinion.

[†]Streptomycin may be substituted for ethambutol. Ethambutol may be omitted only if rates of isoniazid resistance in the community are documented to be less than 4%.

[‡]Therapy should be more prolonged in patients with a slow clinical or bacteriologic response to treatment. A total of 12 months of therapy is recommended for patients who have miliary or skeletal tuberculosis, with or without HIV infection.

[§]Protease inhibitors and NNRTIs should not be given for at least 2 weeks after rifampin has been discontinued, because of persistent induction of cytochrome P450 CYP3A.

[¶]The American Thoracic Society recommends 6 months of therapy; the CDC recommends 6 to 9 months.

- BCG is not recommended for HIV-positive adults or children.

Nontuberculous Mycobacteria

Mycobacteria other than *Mycobacterium tuberculosis* and *M. leprae* are commonly classified as "nontuberculous mycobacteria" (NTM) even though tubercle formation occurs. The types of human disease and the NTM responsible are listed in Table 21-24.

Most NTM have been isolated from natural water and soil. Human-to-human spread has not been documented. Natural waters are the source for most human infections caused by *M. avium* complex; some cases are likely acquired from hospital tap water. *M. kansasii* has not been cultured from soil or natural water even though it has been recovered from tap water. *M. xenopi*, an obligate thermophile, grows in hot water and hot water taps. Colonization or a saprophytic state of NTM is uncommon.

- Human-to-human spread has not been documented.
- NTM disease is not reportable in the United States.

Chronic pulmonary disease is caused most frequently by *M. avium* complex and *M. kansasii*. Pulmonary disease is more common in older adults, those with underlying COPD, smokers, alcohol abusers, and some children with cystic fibrosis. CXR features include thin-walled cavities with minimal surrounding infiltrates and pleural thickening adjacent to areas of lung involvement. Another group of patients who develop pulmonary infection from *M. avium* complex are white women in their 60s who are HIV-negative without preexisting lung disease. Most (>90%) of these patients demonstrate bronchiectasis or small nodules without predilection for any lobe. Nearly 90% of patients with *M. kansasii* and most of those with *M. avium* complex disease show cavitation. High-resolution CT may show associated multifocal bronchiectasis with small (<5 mm) nodular infiltrates. Bilateral nodular or interstitial lung disease (or both) or isolated disease in the right middle lobe or lingular disease is more predominant in elderly nonsmoking women. Hypersensitivity pneumonitis caused by exposure to *M. avium* complex growing in a hot tub has been reported. *M. avium* complex is responsible for 5% of the cases of mycobacterial lymphadenitis in adults and more than 90%

Table 21-22 Antituberculosis Drugs, Dosages, and Major Toxic Effects

Drug (brand name)	Adult dosage (daily)	Pediatric dosage (daily)	Main adverse effects
Isoniazid (INH)*†	300 mg PO, IM	10-20 mg/kg (max. 300 mg)	Liver toxicity, peripheral neuropathy
Rifampin*‡ (Rifadin, Rimactane)	600 mg PO, IV	10-20 mg/kg (max. 600 mg)	Liver toxicity, flulike syndrome
Pyrazinamide§	1.5-2.5 g PO	15-30 mg/kg (max. 2 g)	Arthralgias, hepatic toxicity, hyperuricemia
Ethambutol¶ (Myambutol)	15-25 mg/kg PO	15-25 mg/kg PO	Optic neuritis
Streptomycin//	15 mg/kg IM	20-30 mg/kg	Vestibular toxicity, renal damage
Combinations			
Rifamate (isoniazid 150 mg, rifampin 300 mg)	2 tablets	Not recommended	
Rifater (isoniazid 50 mg, rifampin 120 mg, pyrazinamide 300 mg)	≤44 kg: 4 tablets 45-54 kg: 5 tablets ≥55 kg: 6 tablets	Not recommended	
Second-line drugs			
Capreomycin (Capastat)	15 mg/kg IM	15-30 mg/kg	Auditory and vestibular toxicity, kidney damage
Kanamycin (Kantrex and others)	15 mg/kg IM, IV	15-30 mg/kg	Auditory toxicity, kidney damage
Amikacin (Amikin)	15 mg/kg IM, IV	15-30 mg/kg	Auditory toxicity, kidney damage
Cycloserine# (Seromycin and others)	250-500 mg bid PO	10-20 mg/kg	Psychiatric symptoms, seizures
Ethionamide (Trecator-SC)	250-500 mg bid PO	15-20 mg/kg	Gastrointestinal and liver toxicity, hypothyroidism
Ciprofloxacin (Cipro)	500-750 mg bid PO	Not recommended	Nausea, abdominal pain, restlessness, confusion
Ofloxacin (Floxin)	300-400 mg bid or 600-800 mg/d PO	Not recommended	Nausea, abdominal pain, restlessness, confusion
Aminosalicylic acid (PAS, Teebacin)	4-6 g bid PO	75 mg/kg bid	Gastrointestinal disturbance

bid, twice daily; IM, intramuscularly; IV, intravenously; PO, orally.

*Intravenous preparations of isoniazid and rifampin are available.

†For intermittent use after a few weeks to months of daily therapy, dosage is 15 mg/kg (max. 900 mg) twice/wk for adults. Pyridoxine 10 to 25 mg should be given to prevent neuropathy in malnourished or pregnant patients and in those with human immunodeficiency virus infection, alcoholism, or diabetes mellitus.

‡For intermittent use after a few weeks to months of daily therapy, dosage is 600 mg twice/wk.

§For intermittent use after a few weeks to months of daily therapy, dosage is 2.5 to 3.5 g twice/wk.

¶Usually not recommended for children younger than 6 years because visual acuity cannot be monitored. Some clinicians use 25 mg/kg per day during first 1 to 2 months or longer if organism is isoniazid-resistant. Decrease dosage if renal function is diminished. For intermittent use after a few weeks to months of daily therapy, dosage is 50 mg/kg twice/wk.

//Available from Pfizer (800-254-4445) free of charge to physicians, clinics, or hospitals. When oral drugs are given daily, streptomycin is generally given 5 times/wk (15 mg/kg, or a maximum of 1 g per dose) for an initial 2- to 12-week period, and then (if needed) 2 to 3 times/wk (20-30 mg/kg, or a maximum of 1.5 g per dose). For patients older than 40 years, dosage is reduced to 500 to 750 mg 5 times/wk and 20 mg/kg when given twice/wk. Some clinicians change to lower dosage at 60 rather than 40 years old. Dosage should be decreased if renal function is diminished.

#Some authorities recommend pyridoxine 50 mg for every 250 mg of cycloserine to decrease the incidence of adverse neurologic effects.

From Drugs for Tuberculosis. The Medical Letter 37:67-70, Aug 4, 1995. By permission of The Medical Letter.

of the cases in children. Lymphadenopathy is usually unilateral and nontender. Disseminated disease caused by NTM presents as a fever of unknown origin in immunocompromised patients without AIDS.

- *M. avium* complex infection occurs in bronchiectasis.
- Cavitation occurs in >90% of patients with *M. kansasii* infection.

HIV-infected persons are at high risk for developing NTM infections. More than 95% of NTM disease in HIV-infected persons is caused by *M. avium* complex. In those with AIDS,

disseminated infection occurs in up to 40% and localized infection in 5%; dissemination is more likely in those with a CD4 cell count less than 50/μL. The risk of developing disseminated infection is 20% per year when the CD4 cell count is less than 100/μL. High fever and sweats are common, as are anemia and increased alkaline phosphatase levels. Dissemination is usually documented with positive blood cultures.

- Disseminated *M. avium* complex in AIDS is more likely when the CD4 count is <50/μL.
- A single blood culture in disseminated *M. avium* complex infection has a sensitivity of 90%.

Table 21-23   Targeted Tuberculin Testing for Latent Tuberculous Infection

Prophylactic group description	PPD, mm
Persons with known or suspected HIV infection	≥5
Close contacts of person with infectious TB	≥5
Persons with chest radiographic findings suggestive of previous TB and inadequate or no treatment*	≥5
Persons who inject drugs and are known to be HIV-negative	≥10
Persons with certain medical conditions or factors	≥10
Diabetes mellitus, silicosis, prolonged corticosteroid or other immunosuppressive therapy, cancer of the head and neck, hematologic and reticuloendothelial diseases (e.g., leukemia and Hodgkin disease), end-stage renal disease, intestinal bypass or gastrectomy, chronic malabsorption syndromes, low body weight (≥10% below ideal)	
Persons in whom PPD converted from negative to positive within the past 2 y	†
Age <35 y in the following high-prevalence groups	≥10
Foreign-born persons from areas of the world where TB is common (e.g., Asia, Africa, Caribbean, and Latin America)	
Medically underserved, low-income populations including high-risk racial and ethnic groups (e.g., Asians and Pacific Islanders, African Americans, Hispanics, and American Indians)	
Residents of long-term care facilities (e.g., correctional facilities and nursing homes)	
Children <4 y	
Other groups identified locally as having an increased prevalence of TB (e.g., migrant farm workers or homeless persons)	
Persons <35 y with no known risk factors for TB	≥15
Occupational exposure to TB (e.g., health care workers and staff of nursing homes, drug treatment centers, or correctional facilities)	‡
Close contacts with an initial PPD <5 mm and normal findings on chest radiography	<5
Circumstances suggest a high probability of infection	
Evaluation of other contacts with a similar degree of exposure demonstrates a high prevalence of infection	
Child or adolescent	
Immunosuppressed (e.g., HIV infection)	

HIV, human immunodeficiency virus; PPD, purified protein derivative of tubercle bacillus; TB, tuberculosis.

*Isolated calcified granulomas are excluded.

†10 mm or greater increase if person is younger than 35 years or is a health care worker; 15 mm or greater increase if person is 35 years or older.

‡Appropriate cutoff for defining a positive reaction depends on the employee's individual risk factors for TB and on the prevalence of TB in the facility.

From Van Scoy RE, Wilkowske CJ: Antimicrobial therapy. Mayo Clin Proc 74:1038-1048, 1999. By permission of Mayo Foundation.

Specific skin tests are not available for the diagnosis of NTM. Routine cultures of sputum, blood, or stool are not recommended for asymptomatic patients. All specimens positive for acid-fast bacilli must be considered to indicate *M. tuberculosis* until final culture results are available. Bronchoscopy or open lung biopsy is required for diagnosis in nearly half the cases. Therapy fails in half the patients. More than 80% of patients remain symptomatic, and 60% do not tolerate the initial multidrug regimen. Treatment of infections caused by NTM should be undertaken by a physician who specializes in infections caused by mycobacteria. It should be noted that isoniazid is no longer used in the treatment of infections caused by

Table 21-24 Classification of Nontuberculous Mycobacteria Recovered From Humans

Clinical disease	Common etiologic species	Features of the common species		Unusual etiologic species
		Geography	Morphologic features*	
Pulmonary disease	*M. avium* complex	Worldwide	Usually not pigmented; slow growth (>7 days)	*M simiae*
				M. szulgai
	M. kansasii	U.S., coal mining regions, Europe	Pigmented; often large and beaded on acid-fast stain	*M. fortuitum*
				M. celatum
	M. abscessus	Worldwide, but mostly U.S.	Rapid growth (<7 days); not pigmented	*M. asiaticum*
				M. shimoidei
	M. xenopi	Europe, Canada	Slow growth; pigmented	*M. haemophilum*
	M. malmoense	UK, northern Europe	Slow growth; not pigmented	*M. smegmatis*
Lymphadenitis	*M. avium* complex	Worldwide	Usually not pigmented	*M. fortuitum*
	M. scrofulaceum	Worldwide	Pigmented	*M. chelonei*
	M. malmoense	UK, northern Europe (especially Scandinavia)	Slow growth	*M. abscessus*
				M. kansasii
				M. haemophilum
Cutaneous disease	*M. marinum*	Worldwide	Photochromogen; requires low temperatures (28-30°C) for isolation	*M. avium* complex
				M. kansasii
				M. nonchromogenicum
	M. fortuitum	Worldwide, mostly U.S.	Rapid growth; not pigmented	*M. smegmatis*
	M. chelonae			*M. haemophilum*
	M. abscessus			
	M. ulcerans	Australia, tropics, Africa, SE Asia	Grows slowly; pigmented	
Disseminated disease	*M. avium* complex	Worldwide	Isolates from patients with AIDS; usually pigmented (80%)	*M. abscessus*
				M. xenopi
				M. malmoense
	M. kansasii	U.S.	Photochromogen	*M. genavense*
	M. chelonae	U.S.	Not pigmented	*M. simiae*
	M. haemophilum	U.S., Australia	Not pigmented; requires hemin, often low temperatures, and CO_2 to grow	*M. conspicuum*
				M. marinum
				M. fortuitum

AIDS, acquired immunodeficiency syndrome.

*Photochromogen: isolate is buff-colored in the dark but turns yellow with brief exposure to light.

From American Thoracic Society: Diagnosis and treatment of disease caused by nontuberculous mycobacteria. Am J Respir Crit Care Med 156:S1-S25, 1997. By permission of American Lung Association.

M. avium complex; the macrolides azithromycin and clarithromycin are more important in the treatment of *M. avium* complex.

- Isoniazid is not used to treat infection with *M. avium* complex.
- Macrolides are important in the therapy of infections with *M. avium* complex.

Toxicity From Antituberculous Drugs

When streptomycin is not included in a 6- to 9-month regimen, the incidence of adverse reactions is about 3%. Streptomycin increases the frequency of side effects to 8%. Patient compliance improves, and the risk of monotherapy (emergence of resistant organisms) diminishes when fixed-dose drug combinations are used. In adults, it is important to assess baseline liver function, creatinine level, complete blood count, platelet count, and uric acid (if pyrazinamide is used) and to perform an ophthalmic examination (if ethambutol is used) before antituberculous therapy is begun. All patients should be evaluated periodically for adverse reactions to the drugs (Tables 21-20 and 21-22).

Isoniazid

Hepatitis is the most serious side effect. The incidence of hepatitis is age-dependent: it is rare in patients younger than 20 years, 0.3% for those between 20 and 34 years, 1.2% for those between 35 and 49 years, and 2.3% for those older than 50 years. The overall incidence is less than 1%. Liver dysfunction develops in 46% of patients within the first 2 months, in 36% during the second month, and in 54% after the third month. Middle-aged and black females are at higher risk. Hepatitis is more likely in patients who are "rapid acetylators," and neuritis is more likely in those who are "slow acetylators." Isoniazid also causes skin rash, purpura, drug-induced systemic lupus erythematosus, and arthritis. The addition of pyridoxine is recommended for patients with neuropathy (diabetes mellitus, uremia, alcoholism, and malnutrition), pregnancy, and seizure disorder. Before initiating treatment for LTBI, baseline laboratory testing is indicated in patients with known liver disease or HIV infection, in pregnant women, in women in the immediate postpartum period (within 3 months after delivery), and in persons who drink alcohol regularly. Routine monitoring of liver function during treatment is recommended for patients with abnormal baseline liver function tests or those at risk for liver disease.

- The incidence of isoniazid-induced hepatitis increases with age.
- Isoniazid causes hepatitis and peripheral neuropathy.
- Stop therapy if AST is >5 times normal or 3 times above baseline.

Rifampin

The overall incidence of serious side effects is 1%. Gastrointestinal upset is the most common reaction. A transient increase in serum AST is common; true hepatitis occurs in fewer than 4% of patients. Hepatitis is worse with isoniazid therapy. Larger or intermittent doses (>10 mg/kg) (or both) are associated with thrombocytopenia, flulike syndrome, hemolytic anemia, and cholestatic jaundice. Harmless orange discoloration of body secretions occurs. Rifampin increases the metabolism of contraceptive pills, corticosteroids, warfarin, oral hypoglycemic agents, theophylline, anticonvulsant agents, ketoconazole, cyclosporine, methadone, and antiarrhythmic drugs (digitalis, quinidine, verapamil, and mexiletine); therefore, dosages of these drugs may have to be increased.

- Rifampin: gastrointestinal upset is the most common side effect.
- Hepatitis is worse with isoniazid therapy.
- Rifampin induces liver microsomal enzymes.

Pyrazinamide

The most serious adverse reaction is liver damage. Hyperuricemia is common but gout is not, although arthralgias are reported occasionally. Skin rash and gastrointestinal upset are sometimes encountered.

- Pyrazinamide: liver damage is the most serious adverse reaction.

Ethambutol

Ethambutol in doses greater than 25 mg/kg causes retrobulbar neuritis in fewer than 3% of patients; symptoms usually are observed 2 months after therapy has been initiated. Because ophthalmoscopic findings are normal in these patients, symptoms are important (blurred vision, central scotoma, and red-green color blindness). These symptoms precede changes in visual acuity.

- Ethambutol: retrobulbar neuritis (dose-related) is the most frequent and serious side effect.
- Renal failure prolongs the half-life of the drug and increases the frequency of ocular toxicity.

Streptomycin

Because streptomycin is excreted by the kidneys, the dosage should be decreased in renal insufficiency. The most common adverse side effect is vestibular toxicity, which causes vertigo. Hearing loss may also occur. These side effects are more likely in the elderly. Ototoxicity and nephrotoxicity are related to both the cumulative dose and the peak serum concentration.

- Streptomycin: nephrotoxicity and vestibular toxicity are more common in persons >60 years.
- Streptomycin should be avoided in pregnancy.

Fungal Diseases of the Lung

Serious fungal infections are found at autopsy in 2% of patients overall, in up to 10% of those with solid tumors, and in up to 40% of those dying of leukemia. Renal transplantation patients (15%) have a fungal infection at some time during their post-transplantation course. Almost all fungi produce granulomas. The saprophytic state of fungi is a common problem, particularly with *Aspergillus* species. Pulmonary manifestations are described here. Diagnostic methods and treatment of the mycoses are discussed in Chapter 14.

Histoplasmosis

Histoplasma capsulatum infections are more common in the Mississippi, Ohio, and St. Lawrence River valleys than elsewhere. Infection is by inhalation of fungal spores, which are especially numerous in chicken coops, dusty areas, starling roosts, bat-infested caves, and decayed wood. Clinically, patients may present with asymptomatic infection, acute pneumonia or acute respiratory distress syndrome (ARDS), disseminated infection (AIDS or other immunocompromised hosts), chronic cavitary disease (underlying lung structural defects), or late complications of mediastinal granuloma, mediastinal fibrosis, broncholithiasis, or residual pulmonary nodules seen on CXR. The nodules may be calcified, and hilar adenopathy may be seen.

- Typical clinical scenario for histoplasmosis pneumonitis: Exposure to chicken coops, dusty areas, starling roosts, bat-infested caves, and decayed wood in the Mississippi River Valley, with late complications that include chronic cavitary disease, mediastinal granulomas, calcified hilar adenopathy, and hilar adenopathy.

Coccidioidomycosis

The endemic zone for *Coccidioides immitis* extends from northern California to Argentina. Infections are more common when dry windy conditions exist, with epidemics occurring in the dry hot months after the rainy season, often after the soil has been disturbed. Clinically, patients may be asymptomatic, with CXR showing nodules or thin-walled cavities, or they may have a range of symptomatic disease: "valley fever" (erythema nodosum, erythema multiforme, arthralgia, arthritis, and eosinophilia), acute pneumonia (mildly symptomatic flulike illness in 40% of patients), disseminated disease (more common in Filipinos, African Americans, Mexicans, and immunocompromised patients), and chronic cavitary disease. Infection acquired late during pregnancy is associated with higher maternal and fetal mortality.

- Typical clinical scenario for coccidioidomycosis pneumonitis: A patient from the southwestern United States presents with erythema nodosum, arthalgias/arthritis, acute pneumonia, and chronic cavitary disease.

Blastomycosis

Blastomyces dermatitidis infections occur most commonly in the southern, south central, and Great Lakes states. Persons and animals (canines) in contact with soil are more likely to be infected. Patients with pulmonary infections can be asymptomatic or have acute pneumonia (mimicking an acute bacterial pneumonia), chronic progressive pneumonia, or extrapulmonary dissemination (typically to skin, bone, prostate, or central nervous system). The most characteristic CXR finding is a perihilar mass that mimics carcinoma. Sputum analysis with 10% potassium hydroxide is helpful in diagnosis. Laryngeal blastomycosis can resemble cancer. Serologic testing is unreliable.

- Typical clinical scenario for blastomycosis pneumonitis: A person has contact with the soil, lives in one of the Great Lakes states, and has the CXR finding of a perihilar mass mimicking carcinoma.

Cryptococcosis

Cryptococcus neoformans is a unimorphic fungus that is widely distributed in the soil and excreta of pigeons and other animals. In humans, it may exist as a saprophyte in preexisting lung disease, but one-third to one-half of patients with cryptococcosis are immunosuppressed. The lung is the portal of entry, but the most common clinical presentation is subacute or chronic meningitis (the common cause of death). Diseases that predispose to cryptococcosis include an immunocompromised state, Hodgkin and non-Hodgkin lymphomas, leukemia, sarcoidosis, and diabetes mellitus. The onset of neurologic symptoms, fever, nausea, and anorexia is insidious. Pulmonary features include cough with scant sputum (15% of patients), chest pain (45%), dyspnea (25%), hemoptysis (7%), and night sweats (25%). Nodular infiltrates with cavitation, especially in the lower lobes, occasional hilar adenopathy, and a solitary mass may be found. In non-AIDS patients with pulmonary cryptococcosis, masses and air space consolidation are common and atelectasis, lymphadenopathy, and pleural effusion or empyema are relatively rare. The diagnosis can be established with positive sputum cultures (35% of patients), bronchoscopic specimens (35%), and open lung biopsy (100%). India ink preparations of the cerebrospinal fluid are positive in 30% to 60% of patients. In HIV-infected patients, serum cryptococcal antigen testing is highly sensitive. Serologic testing (detects polysaccharide antigen) of the cerebrospinal fluid is positive in 90% of cases of central nervous system infection and in 30% of cases of non-central nervous system infection. Serologic testing should be performed on blood, cerebrospinal fluid, and urine.

- Typical clinical scenario for *Cryptococcosis neoformans* pneumonitis: An immunocompromised patient or a patient with diabetes who has nodular, cavitary, and patchy infiltrates on CXR, fever, and pulmonary and neurologic symptoms.
- The cerebrospinal fluid should be examined in almost all patients who have organisms in respiratory secretions.

Aspergillosis

Aspergillus fumigatus, *A. flavus*, and *A. niger* are responsible for several pulmonary manifestations. The clinical forms include 1) allergic bronchopulmonary aspergillosis (see above), 2) hypersensitivity pneumonitis in red cedarwood workers, 3) mycetoma or fungus ball in preexisting lung disease, 4) locally invasive (chronic necrotizing) aspergillosis of lung tissue, 5) tracheobronchial form in immunocompromised or HIV-infected persons and lung transplant recipients (at anastomotic site), 6) disseminated, 7) bronchocentric granulomatosis, and 8) saprophytic. The organism frequently colonizes the respiratory tract in patients with lung disease. Invasive aspergillosis in immunosuppressed hosts is the most serious form of infection and occurs mainly in granulocytopenic patients with a hematologic malignancy. The occurrence of life-threatening complications in patients with invasive fungal pneumonia is closely related to rapid granulocyte recovery. *Aspergillus* is isolated at autopsy from 10% of subjects who had acute leukemia. Of all patients with invasive aspergillosis (diagnosed premortem or post mortem), 40% have acute lymphocytic leukemia, 20% have acute myelomonocytic leukemia, 10% have chronic myelogenous leukemia, 5% have Hodgkin disease, and 10% have other hematologic malignancies. The presence of the organism in respiratory secretions is not diagnostic; tissue invasion should be documented.

Aspergilloma is a mass of fungal hyphae in preexisting lung cavities, almost always in the upper lobes. The major symptoms include hemoptysis, cough, low-grade fever, and weight loss. CXR and CT show a meniscus of air around the fungus ball. Because surgical therapy of aspergilloma has a high morbidity and mortality, another therapeutic option is the intracavitary instillation of amphotericin.

- Typical clinical scenario for pulmonary invasive aspergillosis: Fever and pulmonary infiltrates with prolonged neutropenia in acute leukemias and Hodgkin disease.
- Aspergillosis: tissue invasion should be documented.

- Aspergilloma (fungus ball) occurs in previously damaged lung; hemoptysis is a serious complication.

Zygomycosis (Mucormycosis)

Zygomycosis is caused by Mucorales (Phycomycetes) species. Serious infections of the upper respiratory tract, lungs, central nervous system, and skin occur in patients with severe diabetes mellitus, hematologic malignancy, skin or mucosal injury, or immunocompromised status. The organism invades blood vessels in the lungs and causes hemoptysis. CXR may show patchy infiltrates, consolidation, cavitation, and effusions. Bronchial stenosis is a peculiar complication of zygomycosis. The diagnosis must be established by biopsy, although sputum culture may suggest it. No serologic test is available.

- Zygomycosis: immunocompromised and diabetic patients.
- Propensity to invade blood vessels; hemoptysis is common.

Candidiasis

Candida species are present in the oropharynx of 30% of normal persons, in the gastrointestinal tract of 65%, and in the vagina of up to 70% of women. Systemic candidiasis is found at autopsy in as many as 25% of patients with leukemia. Risk factors for developing candidiasis include diabetes mellitus, cancer, cirrhosis, renal failure, blood dyscrasia, cytotoxic therapy, intravenous or urinary catheters, intravenously administered antibiotics, prostheses, cachexia, burns, and HIV infection. Lung involvement is relatively rare, and CXR shows patchy or diffuse infiltrates. *Candida* bronchitis, an occupational disease of tea tasters, is manifested by low-grade fever, cough, and patchy infiltrates.

- Typical clinical scenario for candidiasis: A patient with hematologic malignancy and prolonged granulocytopenia.
- Lung involvement is uncommon; patchy or diffuse lung infiltrates.

Sporotrichosis

Sporothrix schenckii is a dimorphic fungus that exists as a saprophyte in the soil, plants, wood, straw, sphagnum moss, decaying vegetation, cats, dogs, and rodents. Sporotrichosis is an occupational hazard of farmers, florists, gardeners, horticulturists, and forestry workers. Infection is by cutaneous inoculation and inhalation. Cutaneous nodules along lymphatic vessels may appear in 75% of patients. Hematogenous dissemination to the lungs is rare, but inhalation-induced pulmonary disease mimics cavitary tuberculosis.

- Sporotrichosis: occupational hazard of florists, horticulturists, and gardeners.
- Lymphangitis of the skin and subcutaneous nodules.
- Pulmonary infection mimics chronic tuberculosis.

Pneumocystis carinii

Pneumocystis carinii is a fungus with trophic and cyst forms. *P. carinii* infections occur in immunosuppressed patients, especially those with AIDS (CD4 <200/μL) or malignancy, and after organ transplantation. Infection causes alveolar and interstitial inflammation and edema with plasma cell infiltrates. Clinical features in patients with AIDS include the gradual onset of dyspnea, fever, tachypnea, and hypoxia. In patients without AIDS, the onset is more abrupt and progression to respiratory failure occurs quickly. Patients typically have relatively normal findings on lung examination and a patchy or diffuse interstitial or alveolar process on CXR. The typical CT finding is ground-glass attenuation. However, this classic radiographic presentation is less frequent now and is being replaced by cystic lung disease, spontaneous pneumothorax, and an upper lobe distribution of parenchymal opacities. Routine laboratory data are unhelpful. The diagnosis can be made with induced sputum, bronchoalveolar lavage, or lung biopsy. Induced sputum or bronchoalveolar lavage is an excellent method for diagnosis, and the cyst stains best with methenamine silver nitrate. The number of organisms present in immunocompromised patients without AIDS is smaller and overall mortality is greater.

- Typical clinical scenario: AIDS patient with CD4 <200/μL and gradual onset of dyspnea, fever, tachypnea, hypoxia, cyanosis, cough; relatively normal findings on lung examination; and a patchy or diffuse interstitial or alveolar process on CXR.
- An upper lobe process is seen on CXR of patients receiving pentamidine aerosol prophylaxis.

Parasitic Diseases

Parasitic infections of the lung are less common in the United States than in other parts of the world. Travelers to regions that are endemic for parasitic infestations may become infected and, when they return to the United States, present as difficult diagnostic problems. However, dirofilariasis is indigenous to the eastern and southeastern United States. Other parasitic infections, including helminthic infestations, also occur in the United States. Even though the respiratory system may be affected by many parasitic infections, the parasites more likely to cause chronic pulmonary manifestations include *Paragonimus westermani* (paragonimiasis), *Echinococcus granulosus* (echinococcosis or hydatid disease), *Dirofilaria immitis* (dirofilariasis), *Schistosoma japonicum* and *S. mansoni* (schistosomiasis), and *Entamoeba histolytica* (amebiasis). Protozoal infections are more likely in patients whose cellular immunity is suppressed.

Dirofilariasis is caused by the "dog heartworm" and transmitted to humans by mosquitoes. The disease is endemic to the Mississippi River valley, the southeastern United States, and the Gulf Coast. Characteristically, the infection presents in the form of a well-defined solitary lung nodule or multiple lung nodule(s) 1.5 to 2.5 cm in diameter. Eosinophilia occurs in fewer than 15% of patients. Serologic tests may aid in the diagnosis.

Echinococcosis has occurred in Alaska and the southwestern United States. Lung disease presents with the CXR findings of well-defined round or oval cystic or solid lesions up to 15 cm in diameter. Rupture of the cysts can cause anaphylactic shock, hypersensitivity reactions, and seeding of adjacent anatomical areas. Liver involvement (in 40% with lung disease) and positive serologic findings are common.

Paragonimiasis is more likely in immigrants from Southeast Asia, but sporadic cases occur in the United States. It is transmitted typically through consumption of raw or undercooked crabs or crayfish. Respiratory features resemble those of chronic bronchitis, bronchiectasis, or tuberculosis. Profuse brown-colored sputum and hemoptysis can be seen. Pleural effusion is relatively common, and peripheral eosinophilia is common. Ova can be found in pleural fluid, bronchial wash, or sputum.

Schistosomiasis is not acquired in the United States. The infection leads to gradual development of secondary pulmonary hypertension caused by occlusion of the pulmonary arterial tree by the parasite. Cor pulmonale develops in 5% of patients.

Amebiasis may present as lobar pneumonia or lung abscess. Rupture into the bronchial tree (hepatobronchial fistula) may be followed by expectoration of "anchovy paste" or "chocolate" sputum. Rupture of the liver abscess into the pleural space causes empyema along with respiratory distress in many patients. Pericardial involvement can also occur.

Strongyloidiasis involving the lungs can mimic asthma. Risk factors include corticosteroid use, age older than 65, chronic lung disease, and chronic debilitating illness. Pulmonary signs and symptoms include cough, shortness of breath, wheezing, and hemoptysis in more than 90% of patients. ARDS has been observed in 45% of patients and pulmonary infiltrates in 90%. Preexisting chronic lung disease and ARDS are important predictors of a poor prognosis.

- Typical clinical scenario for dirofilariasis: A patient from the Mississippi River valley, southeastern United States, or the Gulf Coast who has exposure to a dog and a solitary lung nodule or multiple nodules.
- Schistosomiasis: pulmonary hypertension.
- Amebiasis: pleuropulmonary complications are almost always right-sided; rupture into the bronchial tree, with "anchovy paste" or "chocolate" sputum.
- Strongyloidosis: mimics asthma with eosinophilia.

Noninfectious Pulmonary Complications in AIDS

Infectious pulmonary complications are discussed in Chapter 14. The noninfectious pulmonary complications in AIDS are discussed below (see Chapter 12).

Nonspecific interstitial pneumonitis is common in patients with AIDS. It represents 30% to 40% of all episodes of lung infiltrates in these patients. More than 25% of patients with this problem have concurrent Kaposi sarcoma, previous experimental treatments, or a history of *Pneumocystis carinii* pneumonia or drug abuse. The clinical features are similar to those of patients with *P. carinii* pneumonia. Histologic examination of the lung may show various degrees of edema, fibrin deposition, and interstitial inflammation with lymphocytes and plasma cells. No specific therapy is known.

- Nonspecific interstitial pneumonitis occurs in up to 40% of patients with AIDS, and *P. carinii* pneumonia should be excluded.

Lymphocytic interstitial pneumonitis is caused by pulmonary infiltration with mature polyclonal B lymphocytes and plasma cells. It occurs in children of mothers at high risk for AIDS and in patients with AIDS. Corticosteroid therapy may produce marked improvement. Pulmonary lymphoid hyperplasia has been reported in 40% of children with AIDS.

- Lymphocytic interstitial pneumonitis is diagnostic of AIDS when it occurs in a child younger than 13 years who is seropositive for HIV.

Cystic lung disease is more common in patients with *P. carinii* infections and in those receiving aerosolized pentamidine therapy. Cystic lesions are more common in the upper and mid lung zones. Chest CT identifies these small- to medium-size cystic lesions.

- Cystic lung disease is more common in patients with *P. carinii* pneumonia receiving aerosolized pentamidine therapy.

Pneumothorax occurs with increasing frequency in patients with *P. carinii* pneumonia and in those receiving pentamidine aerosol therapy. Other causes of pneumothorax include Kaposi sarcoma, tuberculosis, and other infections. Pneumothorax in patients with AIDS has a poor prognosis.

- High incidence of bilateral synchronous pneumothoraces.

Pleural effusion is found in 25% of hospitalized patients with AIDS. Nearly one-third of the pleural effusions are due to noninfectious causes. Hypoalbuminemia is the leading cause of these effusions. Other important noninfectious causes include Kaposi sarcoma and atelectasis. Among the infectious causes, bacterial pneumonias, *P. carinii* pneumonia, and *M. tuberculosis* are important. Fungal infections can also produce pleural effusion. Large effusions are caused by tuberculosis and Kaposi sarcoma.

- Pleural effusion is caused by infections in two-thirds of hospitalized patients with AIDS.
- Kaposi sarcoma and tuberculosis cause large effusions.

Pulmonary hypertension has been found in patients with AIDS. It is more common in those with HLA-DR6 alleles. The mechanism is not clear, but HIV is thought to affect the endothelium directly and to cause vascular changes. The clinical, physiologic, and pathologic features are identical to those of primary pulmonary hypertension.

- Pulmonary hypertension is clinically identical to idiopathic pulmonary hypertension.

Kaposi sarcoma occurs with greater frequency among homosexuals with AIDS than among other patients with AIDS. It is believed to be caused by human herpesvirus 8. The incidence of its occurrence has diminished. Previous or concurrent pulmonary opportunistic infections have been noted in more than 70% of patients with Kaposi sarcoma. Kaposi sarcoma occurs in the lungs of up to 35% of patients who have this tumor. The lung may be the only site in about 15% of patients. In most patients, pulmonary Kaposi sarcoma is established only at autopsy. The diagnostic yield from bronchoscopy is 24% and from lung biopsy, 56%. Hemoptysis is an uncommon complication of Kaposi sarcoma, although endobronchial metastasis develops in 30% of patients. CXR may show typical nodular infiltrates in fewer than 10% of patients. Pleural effusion may be seen.

- Pulmonary Kaposi sarcoma is usually preceded by cutaneous lesions.
- Lung involvement due to Kaposi sarcoma occurs in up to 35% of patients with this neoplasm.
- Clinically, pulmonary Kaposi sarcoma is indistinguishable from *P. carinii* pneumonia or opportunistic pneumonia.
- Multiple, discrete, raised, violaceous, or bright red tracheobronchial lesions can be seen on bronchoscopy.

Non-Hodgkin lymphoma involving the lungs is seen in fewer than 10% of patients with AIDS who develop lymphoma. The lymphoma in these patients is usually extranodal non-Hodgkin B-cell lymphoma. Lung involvement is a late occurrence. Nodules, masses, and infiltrates can be seen on CXR. A 6.5-fold increased incidence of primary lung cancer has been noted among HIV-infected and AIDS patients.

Pulmonary Diseases Pharmacy Review
Todd M. Johnson, PharmD

Drugs for Pulmonary Disease

Drug	Toxic/adverse effects	Drug interactions	Comment
Bronchodilators Levalbuterol (Xopenex) Salmeterol (Serevent) Albuterol (Proventil, Ventolin, Vomax) Bitolterol (Tornalate) Isoetharine Metaproterenol (Alupent) Pirbuterol (Maxair) Terbutaline (Bricanyl) Isoproterenol (Isuprel, Medihaler-Iso) Epinephrine (AsthmaHaler, Primatene)	Palpations, tachycardia, hypertension, arrhythmia, tremor, nervousness, headache, insomnia, gastroesophageal reflux disease, or pharyngitis	β-Blockers may inhibit effect of bronchodilators in asthmatic patients Tricyclic antidepressants & sympathomimetics may cause hypertension Isoproterenol or epinephrine may sensitize the myocardium to the effects of general anesthetic	Bronchodilators must be used with caution in patients with diabetes mellitus, cardiovascular disorders, hyperthyroidism, or seizure Use of β-blockers in asthmatics may precipitate asthma
Ipratropium (Atrovent) Ipratropium & albuterol (Combivent)	Ipatropium may cause blurred vision & dry mouth		
Leukotriene receptor antagonists Montelukast (Singulair) Zafirlukast (Accolate) Zileuton (Zyflo)	Rarely may cause systemic eosinophilia with vasculitis, consistent with Churg-Strauss syndrome	Zafirlukast & zileuton can increase warfarin effects Zileuton can double theophylline concentrations	
Anti-inflammatory inhalant products Beclomethasone (Beclovent, Vanceril, QVAR) Budesonide (Pulmicort) Flunisolide (Aerobid) Fluticasone (Flovent) Fluticasone & salmeterol (Flovent Diskus) Triamcinolone (Azmacort) Cromolyn (Intal) Nedocromil (Tilade)			Corticosteroids, cromolyn, & nedocromil are not effective for the relief of acute bronchospasm When systemic corticosteroids are withdrawn, inhaled corticosteroids do not provide systemic effects necessary to prevent symptoms of adrenal insufficiency

Pulmonary Diseases Pharmacy Review (continued)

Drugs for Pulmonary Tuberculosis

Drug	Toxic/adverse effects	Drug interactions
Isoniazid	Hepatitis, hypersensitivity reactions, lupus-like reactions, peripheral neuropathy	Carbamazepine, cycloserine, phenytoin, levodopa, prednisone, rifampin, theophylline, warfarin
Rifampin	Orange discoloration of body fluids, leukopenia, thrombocytopenia, proteinuria, hypersensitivity	Aminosalicylic acid, anticoagulants, azole antifungals, barbiturates, benzodiazepines, contraceptives (oral), corticosteroids, cyclosporine, delavirdine, digoxin, estrogens, haloperidol, hydantoins, isoniazid, macrolides, progestins, protease inhibitors, quinine, sulfones, tacrolimus, theophylline, thyroid replacement
Rifabutin	Neutropenia, body fluid discoloration, GI intolerance, rash, uveitis, increased liver enzymes	Anticoagulants, azole antifungals, cyclosporine, delavirdine, hydantoins, macrolides, methadone, nelfinavir, quinine, theophylline
Pyrazinamide	Hepatitis, hyperuricemia, nausea, anorexia, poly-arthralgia	Ethionamide, probenecid, zidovudine
Ethambutol	Optic neuritis, hyperuricemia	Aluminum salts
Cycloserine	CNS (somnolence, headache, tremor, psychosis, seizures)	Isoniazid
Para-aminosalicylic acid	Skin rash, GI intolerance, hypersensitivity	
Acyclovir	Malaise, nausea, vomiting, diarrhea, phlebitis (IV)	
Famciclovir	Headache, dizziness, nausea, diarrhea, fatigue	Probenecid
Ganciclovir	Diarrhea, nausea, anorexia, vomiting, leukopenia, neutropenia, rash, anemia, fever, abdominal pain	
Valacyclovir	Nausea, headache, diarrhea, dizziness	
Amantadine	Nausea, dizziness, light-headedness, insomnia	
Rimantadine	Insomnia, dizziness, nervousness, nausea, vomiting	
Foscarnet	Renal impairment, leukopenia, electrolyte disturbances, seizures, fever, anemia, headache, nausea, vomiting	Nephrotoxic drugs
Cidofovir	Renal impairment, neutropenia, ocular hypotony, headache, asthenia, alopecia, rash, GI distress, anemia, infection, fever	Nephrotoxic drugs
Oseltamivir	Nausea, vomiting, diarrhea, bronchitis, abdominal pain, dizziness	
Zanamivir	Nausea, diarrhea, nasal signs & symptoms, bronchitis	

CNS, central nervous system; GI, gastrointestinal; IV, intravenous.

QUESTIONS

Multiple Choice (choose the one best answer)

1. A 45-year-old man with a 45 pack-year smoking history presents with a complaint of right shoulder pain and weakness of the right hand. Physical examination shows atrophy of the right hand muscles, constriction of the right pupil, and drooping of the right eyelid. The next step in the diagnosis would be:
   a. CT of the head
   b. Electromyography of the right arm
   c. CT-guided needle biopsy
   d. Bronchoscopy
   e. Ophthalmology evaluation

2. A 47-year-old woman, current smoker, who is receiving hormone replacement therapy presents with acute onset of pleuritic chest pain and shortness of breath. She was evaluated in the clinic 3 days earlier, when right lower lobe pneumonia was diagnosed on the basis of chest radiographic (CXR) findings. On physical examination, the left calf is tender and swollen, with some erythema. You suspect pulmonary embolism (PE) as the cause of the chest pain and shortness of breath. In this patient, the best diagnostic test for PE would be:
   a. Lower extremity duplex ultrasonography
   b. Spiral CT of the chest with contrast
   c. V/Q scan
   d. Repeat CXR
   e. Echocardiography

3. Chronic obstructive pulmonary disease (COPD) is characterized by:
   a. Alpha$_1$-antitrypsin deficiency
   b. Reduction in FEV_1 in 90% of smokers
   c. Reduction in total lung capacity with a preserved FEV_1/FVC ratio
   d. Airflow limitation that is not fully reversible
   e. Reduction in diffusing capacity (DLCO)

4. A 35-year-old man with a current 3 pack-year smoking history presents with progressive dyspnea on exertion. CXR shows lower lobe emphysema. The next best step in the diagnosis would be:
   a. Measurement of carboxyhemoglobin
   b. CT of the chest
   c. Detailed history of occupational exposure
   d. Microscopic urinalysis
   e. Measurement of alpha$_1$-antitrypsin level

5. In the treatment of COPD, you should:

   a. Offer assistance in smoking cessation
   b. Offer inhaled corticosteroids to all patients to decrease development of fibrosis
   c. Initiate methotrexate therapy if the disease is severe
   d. Offer lung volume reduction surgery if the disease is severe
   e. Have the patient follow peak flowmeter values

6. Cystic fibrosis is:
   a. Most common among Asian Americans
   b. Associated with allergic bronchopulmonary aspergillosis
   c. A disease for which lung transplantation is contraindicated
   d. Rarely associated with *Pseudomonas* colonization
   e. Not diagnosed in persons older than 15 years

7. A pleural effusion is considered an exudate if:
   a. Pleural fluid lactate dehydrogenase (LDH) is >1/3 the upper limit of serum LDH
   b. Pleural fluid protein-to-serum protein ratio is >0.6
   c. Pleural fluid cholesterol is >75 mg/dL
   d. Pleural fluid LDH-to-serum LDH ratio is >0.5
   e. Pleural fluid protein is >2.9 g/dL

8. A 25-year-old woman who is a nonsmoker presents with a 1-week history of mild cough and dyspnea following a flulike illness with fever, arthralgias, and tender erythematous lesions on the anterior aspects of the legs. She has no history of asthma or no notable past medical history. No environmental or occupational high-risk exposures are noted. Physical examination reveals clear lung fields without other abnormality. Chest radiography demonstrates bilateral interstitial infiltrates with prominent bihilar adenopathy. On pulmonary function tests (PFTs), vital capacity is 88% of predicted and the forced expiratory volume in 1 second (FEV_1) is 76% of predicted, with an FEV_1- to-vital capacity ratio of 68%. Diffusing capacity is 83% of predicted. The next most appropriate treatment is:
   a. Systemic corticosteroids
   b. Methotrexate
   c. Cyclosporine
   d. Azathioprine
   e. Nonsteroidal anti-inflammatory drug (NSAID)

9. The patient in question 8 subsequently developed Bell palsy on the right side. The most appropriate therapy would be:
   a. Systemic corticosteroids
   b. Methotrexate
   c. Cyclosporine

d. Azathioprine

e. NSAID

10. A 62-year-old man and previous smoker presents with a 2-year history of progressive dry cough and dyspnea. No occupational or environmental exposures are noted. Findings on examination include bibasilar Velcro rales and clubbing. Chest radiography shows prominent interstitial infiltrates in the middle and lower lung fields. High-resolution CT (HRCT) demonstrates subpleural honeycombing with thickened alveolar septa in the lower lobes and bilateral mediastinal lymph nodes (1.5 cm large) but only minimal ground-glass opacities. On PFTs, vital capacity is 62% of predicted, FEV_1 is 69% of predicted, and the FEV_1-to-vital capacity ratio is 78%, with diffusing capacity 52% of predicted. You start treatment with corticosteroids. What is the *most* likely clinical course?

a. Clinical and radiographic clearing of the lung disease

b. Clinical but not radiographic clearing of the lung disease

c. No improvement likely

d. No improvement; start treatment with immunomodulating agents

11. A 36-year-old man who is a nonsmoker without previous known pulmonary disease or respiratory symptoms presents with a several-hour history of dyspnea, dry cough, fever, chills, malaise, headache, and wheezing. The symptoms began while he was on the job at a plastics manufacturing company. His vital signs are stable. Bilateral crackles and scattered wheezes are detected on physical examination. Chest radiography demonstrates bilateral mixed interstitial and alveolar reticular nodular infiltrates, with apical sparing. Oxygen saturation is 84% on room air at rest. Diffusing capacity is 78% of predicted. Spirometry documents a vital capacity 65% of predicted, FEV_1 58% of predicted along with a forced expiratory flow ($FEF_{25\%-75\%}$) 25% of predicted. After removal from the workplace, this patient's symptoms and physiologic abnormalities are expected to resolve within a few:

a. Seconds

b. Minutes

c. Days

d. Weeks

e. Months

12. A 52-year-old man, a current 75 pack-year smoker, is evaluated for acute dyspnea and right-sided chest pain. He says he does not have fever, chills, sweats, cough, sputum production, or hemoptysis. On physical examination, diminished breath sounds are noted throughout, right more than left. Previous PFTs demonstrated a vital capacity of 4.0 L (72% of predicted) and FEV_1 of 2.5 L (53% of predicted). Chest radiography and CT demonstrate scattered interstitial changes with cystic and nodular abnormalities in addition to a right-sided pneumothorax. The best treatment for this patient's underlying disease is:

a. Systemic corticosteroids

b. Azathioprine

c. Plasmapheresis

d. Smoking cessation

e. Monthly pulse cyclophosphamide

13. A 68-year-old man who is an exsmoker presents with a 6- to 12-month history of dry cough and dyspnea. He says he does not have fever, chest pain, or hemoptysis. No reflux or dysphagia is reported. His past medical history is notable for diabetes, hyperlipidemia, and benign prostatic hypertrophy. No known hobby, travel, or environmental exposures are noted. His past occupational history includes ship refurbishing while in the armed services. Medications include pravastatin, glyburide, and prazosin. His vital signs are stable. He is afebrile. No adenopathy is noted. Bibasilar crackles are present. Heart rhythm is regular. The abdomen is normal, and no edema is noted. Clubbing is present. Blood test results are normal. PFTs demonstrate mild restriction and a low diffusing capacity. Chest radiography and HRCT demonstrate bilateral lower lobe infiltrates, with some honeycombing, pleural thickening, diaphragmatic calcification, and an area of consolidation in the right lower lobe consistent with rounded atelectasis. The next appropriate diagnostic test is:

a. Video-assisted thoracoscopy (VATS)–open lung biopsy

b. Trial of systemic corticosteroids

c. Bronchoscopy with bronchoalveolar lavage, brush biopsy, and transbronchial biopsy

d. Mediastinoscopy

e. Observation

14. A 53-year-old woman who is a nonsmoker has had a several-year history of progressive dyspnea, cough, and chest tightness. No important occupational, travel, environmental, or hobby exposures are noted. She says she does not have any arthralgias, reflux, or dysphagia and is not taking any medication. The past medical history is notable for a left lower extremity deep venous thrombosis and pulmonary embolism following a pregnancy at age 25. Her vital signs are stable. Examination reveals bibasilar crackles. Heart rhythm is regular. No murmurs are present. Joints are normal. No clubbing, cyanosis, or edema is present. Chest radiography demonstrates bibasilar

peripheral interstitial infiltrates. HRCT confirms peripheral honeycombing without marked adenopathy or pleural fluid. Ground-glass opacities are not present. The following were normal on blood tests: complete blood count, manual differential, liver-associated enzymes, and renal function. Urinalysis demonstrates a rare leukocyte and hyaline cast. The antinuclear antibody (ANA) titer is minimally elevated at 1:40. Serum protein electrophoresis demonstrates a polyclonal increase. Rheumatoid factor is also minimally elevated at 1:40. On PFTs, vital capacity is 60% of predicted, FEV_1 is 56% of predicted, total lung capacity is 72% of predicted, residual volume is 75% of predicted, and diffusing capacity is 62% of predicted. The most likely diagnosis is:

a. Nonspecific interstitial pneumonitis (NSIP)–idiopathic pulmonary fibrosis (IPF)
b. Usual interstitial pneumonitis–IPF
c. Rheumatoid arthritis
d. Amyloidosis
e. Bronchiolitis obliterans with organizing pneumonia (BOOP) or cryptogenic organizing pneumonia (COP)

15. A 67-year-old asymptomatic woman with a 50-pack-year cigarette smoking history (still smoking) presents for her annual physical examination. A chest radiograph shows a new 1.3-cm right upper lobe nodule that was not present 3 years previously. The results of physical examination and routine laboratory testing are unremarkable. Spirometry demonstrates mild obstruction. The nodule is found to enhance significantly on chest CT. Which of the following is the next most appropriate step in the management of this patient?

a. Bronchoscopy with transbronchial biopsy
b. Positron emission tomography (PET)
c. Surgical resection
d. Transthoracic needle aspiration
e. Repeat chest CT in 1 year

16. A 50-year-old woman with a 55-pack-year smoking history presents with mild dyspnea, cough, and streaky hemoptysis. On physical examination, temperature is 39.2°C, pulse rate is 100 beats/min, respirations are 24/min, and blood pressure is 168/92 mm Hg. Auscultation of the lungs detects signs of consolidation in the right upper lobe. No adenopathy or clubbing is noted. Laboratory findings include the following: hematocrit 35%, leukocyte count 12×10^9/L (12,000 mm^3), serum creatinine 1.2 mg/dL, and serum calcium 12 mg/dL. Chest radiography shows a 4-cm right hilar mass with partial cavitation. Bronchoscopy demonstrates extensive neoplastic involvement of the right main bronchus, with near occlusion of the right

upper lobe orifice. Biopsy of the hilar mass is most likely to show which one of the following?

a. Small cell carcinoma
b. Adenocarcinoma
c. Non-Hodgkin lymphoma
d. Squamous cell carcinoma
e. Bronchoalveolar carcinoma

17. A 69-year-old man is brought to the emergency department because of increasing confusion, headache, nausea, and vomiting for the last 3 days. On physical examination, the pulse rate is 64 beats/min, blood pressure is 138/72 mm Hg, and temperature is 37.4°C. The patient is lethargic but responds to questions appropriately. Auscultation of the lungs demonstrates diminished breath sounds in the left lower lung fields. Mild peripheral edema is present. Laboratory findings include the following: hemoglobin concentration 12.8 g/dL, leukocyte count 8.6×10^9/L (8,600 mm^3), serum sodium 119 mEq/L, serum potassium 4 mEq/L, serum creatinine 1.1 mg/dL, and serum osmolality 268 mOsm/kg. Urine osmolality is 600 mOsm/kg. Chest radiography shows a left hilar mass and a left pleural effusion. What is the most likely diagnosis in this patient?

a. Small cell carcinoma
b. Adenocarcinoma
c. Non-Hodgkin lymphoma
d. Squamous cell carcinoma
e. Bronchoalveolar carcinoma

18. A 60-year-old man is brought to the emergency department following a syncopal episode. His wife stated that they had just returned from a trip to Europe 2 days earlier. On physical examination, the pulse rate is 140 beats/min, blood pressure is 64/30 mm Hg, and respirations are 30/min. Helical (spiral) CT demonstrates a large near-occlusive thrombus in the main pulmonary artery extending to the right main pulmonary artery and to the orifice of the left main pulmonary artery. Which of the following is the next most appropriate step in the management of this patient?

a. Placement of a vena cava filter
b. Pulmonary thromboendarterectomy
c. Low-molecular-weight heparin
d. Thrombolytic therapy
e. Unfractionated heparin

19. A 45-year-old man complains of progressive dyspnea on exertion and nonproductive cough. Wegener granulomatosis was diagnosed 4 years previously when he presented with sinus pain and epistaxis; the diagnosis was

supported with cytoplasmic-antineutrophil cytoplasmic antibodies (c-ANCA). He was treated conservatively at that time and had done well. Over the last several months, he has developed a persistent cough and progressive dyspnea so that he is not able to play basketball. He states that he does not have hemoptysis. On physical examination, blood pressure is 130/70 mm Hg, pulse rate is 76 beats/min, and respirations are 20/min. There is expiratory wheezing with forced expiration. Chest radiography shows several cavitary pulmonary nodules. The flow-volume loop showed flattening of the expiratory curve consistent with a variable intrathoracic obstruction. Which of the following is the next most appropriate step in the management of this patient?

a. CT of the chest
b. Otorhinolaryngology consultation
c. Bronchoscopy
d. Bronchodilator therapy
e. Immunosuppressive therapy

20. A 45-year-old woman presents for evaluation of fever, arthralgias, and a truncal rash. She has a history of steroid-dependent asthma and nasal polyps diagnosed 5 years previously. One month ago, she started treatment with a steroid inhaler and the corticosteroids were tapered off. On physical examination, blood pressure is 138/84 mm Hg, pulse rate is 92 beats/min, and respirations are 20/min. Physical examination of the nose shows nasal mucosal crusting and bilateral nasal polyps. Auscultation of the chest detects scattered wheezes. Laboratory findings include the following: leukocytes 11×10^9/L (11,000/mm^3) (70% neutrophils, 8% lymphocytes, 18% eosinophils, 5% monocytes) and serum creatinine 1.1 mg/dL. Chest radiography demonstrates bilateral upper lobe infiltrates. Which of the following diagnoses is most likely?

a. Behçet disease
b. Wegener granulomatosis
c. Churg-Strauss syndrome
d. Giant cell arteritis
e. Allergic bronchopulmonary aspergillosis

21. A 25-year-old male smoker is admitted to the hospital because of hemoptysis, shortness of breath, and hypoxemia. His symptoms began 3 days ago while he was recovering from an upper respiratory tract infection. On physical examination, respirations are 24/min, pulse rate is 100 beats/min, blood pressure is 112/64 mm Hg, and oxygen saturation is 87% on 2 L per minute of oxygen. Chest examination demonstrates bilateral crackles. Chest radiography shows bilateral alveolar infiltrates. Laboratory

findings include the following: hemoglobin concentration 8.8 g/dL, leukocytes 9.4×10^9/L (9,400 mm^3), serum creatinine 3.3 mg/dL, c-ANCA negative, and perinuclear-ANCA (p-ANCA) positive, with specificity for myeloperoxidase. The anti-streptococcal O titer is normal. Urinalysis shows many red blood cells and red blood cell casts. Which of the following diagnoses is most likely?

a. Acute poststreptococcal glomerulonephritis
b. Microscopic polyarteritis
c. Wegener granulomatosis
d. Goodpasture syndrome
e. Behçet disease

22. A 36-year-old man with stage IV sarcoidosis presents with hemoptysis. CXR shows an infiltrate in the left upper lobe with associated pleural thickening. CT of the chest demonstrates a cavity with a free-floating density. A mycetoma is suspected. The most common species of fungus that would cause a mycetoma in this patient is:

a. *Histoplasma capsulatum*
b. *Candida albicans*
c. *Aspergillus flavus*
d. *Aspergillus fumigatus*
e. *Candida glabrata*

23. Which of the following patients should have baseline measurements of liver function before beginning treatment for latent tuberculosis infection (LTBI)?

a. 30-year-old man with no medical problems
b. 28-year-old woman who is 3 weeks post partum
c. 55-year-old man with diabetes and renal failure
d. 66-year-old woman with COPD
e. 25-year-old woman with scleroderma

24. Screening for LTBI should be performed in which of the following high-risk persons?

a. 67-year-old man with bronchiectasis and COPD
b. 39-year-old man with cirrhosis
c. 54-year-old man with congestive heart failure
d. 33-year-old woman with inflammatory arthritis
e. 45-year-old woman with end-stage renal disease

25. LTBI is diagnosed in which of the following asymptomatic patients with a PPD skin test of 7 mm?

a. 23-year-old woman medical student
b. 44-year-old man with Hodgkin lymphoma
c. 32-year-old man in whose child active TB was recently diagnosed
d. 22-year-old man emigrating from Nigeria
e. 18-year-old woman with cystic fibrosis

26. A 35-year-old man with human immunodeficiency virus (HIV) infection develops malaise, cough, and fever. CXR shows diffuse interstitial infiltrates. Induced sputum is obtained, and special smears for *Pneumocystis carinii* and an acid-fast bacillus (AFB) smear are negative. Bronchoscopy with bronchoalveolar lavage (BAL) is performed and *Cryptococcus neoformans* is recovered. This patient should receive antifungal treatment for what duration?
   a. Life-long
   b. 2 months
   c. 6 months
   d. 9 months
   e. Until CXR findings are normal

27. A 73-year-old man is hospitalized for community-acquired pneumonia and levofloxacin is given after sputum and blood specimens are cultured. His condition quickly deteriorates, and he has to be transferred to an intensive care unit for mechanical ventilation. CXR demonstrates diffuse patchy areas of bronchopneumonia. All the sputum and blood cultures are negative at 48 hours, but a *Legionella* urinary antigen test is positive. Which of the following should be performed?
   a. Stop levofloxacin and substitute intravenous ciprofloxacin
   b. Continue levofloxacin as monotherapy

   c. Add intravenous aztreonam
   d. Add intravenous gentamicin
   e. Add rifampin

28. A 42-year-old woman is referred for chronic cough, low-grade fevers, and dyspnea. The physical examination findings are normal. The results of CXR are normal, but the pulmonary function tests indicate mild restriction with a low diffusing capacity. High resolution CT of the chest shows 4-mm nodules in both upper lobes and areas of ground-glass attenuation. She has no pets and no history of recent travel and is not taking any medications. She uses her hot tub frequently. Bronchoscopy with a biopsy specimen from the right upper lobe demonstrates granulomatous inflammation. Mycobacterial and fungal stains of the tissue are negative but culture results are pending. Hypersensitivity pneumonitis from *Mycobacterium avium* complex is suspected. Which would be the most appropriate recommendation for this patient?
   a. Treat with isoniazid, rifampin, pyrazinamide, and ethambutol for 9 months
   b. Treat with isoniazid for 6 months
   c. Treat with prednisone for 9-12 months
   d. Treat with isoniazid, rifampin, and clarithromycin for 18 months
   e. Drain the hot tub and stop using it

ANSWERS

1. Answer c.

The presenting signs and symptoms are suggestive of Pancoast tumor. The shoulder and arm weakness is common, and the ipsilateral miosis and ptosis suggest Horner syndrome. Thus, a CT-guided needle biopsy of the superior sulcus tumor would be the best diagnostic test. Although bronchoscopy is a reasonable option, the peripheral location of the lesion would decrease the diagnostic yield.

2. Answer b.

Although a V/Q scan is used in many centers for the diagnosis of PE, the sensitivity of this test decreases if a person has existing radiographic abnormalities. CT with contrast using a PE protocol has been shown to have high sensitivity and specificity for identifying segmental and subsegmental PEs. Echocardiography may show increased right-sided pressures, but this would not be diagnostic of PE. Lower extremity duplex

ultrasonography may show deep venous thrombosis but would not be diagnostic of PE.

3. Answer d.

This is the definition of COPD according to the Global Initiative for Chronic Obstructive Lung Disease (GOLD). A rapid decline in FEV_1 is noted in only 10% to 15% of smokers. A reduction in total lung capacity with a preserved FEV_1/FVC ratio is suggestive of restrictive lung disease. Although a reduction in DLCO can be seen in severe COPD (emphysema), this does not characterize the disease.

4. Answer e.

Emphysematous changes in this relatively young man with a minor smoking history should trigger an evaluation of alpha$_1$-antitrypsin deficiency. Furthermore, lower lobe emphysema is characteristic of alpha$_1$-antitrypsin deficiency. The presence of carboxyhemoglobin would confirm that he is currently smoking, but it would not aid in the diagnosis. CT of the chest may confirm the presence of structural changes, but the findings would not be diagnostic. Because no other signs or symptoms are suggestive of pulmonary-renal diseases, urinalysis would not be helpful.

5. Answer a.

Smoking cessation is vital in the treatment of COPD. The use of inhaled corticosteroids is usually limited to patients with pronounced symptoms or with a lung function response to inhaled steroids. According to the recent results of the National Emphysema Treatment Trial (NETT), the mortality of patients with severe COPD who underwent lung volume reduction surgery was increased compared with those who received medical management.

6. Answer b.

Cystic fibrosis is commonly associated with allergic bronchopulmonary aspergillosis (up to 10% of patients). The disease is most prevalent among whites (1 in 2,000-3,500), compared with 1 in 32,100 Asian Americans. Of the patients in whom cystic fibrosis is diagnosed, up to 25% are older than 15 years. *Pseudomonas* colonization is common in cystic fibrosis. The defective gene may be responsible for ineffective clearance of *Pseudomonas*.

7. Answer e.

Traditionally, pleural fluid is considered an exudate if the pleural fluid protein-to-serum protein ratio is >0.5, the pleural fluid LDH-to-serum LDH ratio is >0.6, or pleural fluid LDH is >2/3 the upper limit of serum LDH. A meta-analysis found that pleural fluid protein >2.9 g/dL or pleural fluid cholesterol >45 mg/dL can differentiate the fluid as an exudate.

8. Answer e.

Sarcoidosis is a granulomatous disease that most often affects the lung and lymph nodes. It can occur after a flulike illness, and it may be diagnosed on the basis of a specific constellation of symptoms and signs of Lofgren syndrome (erythema nodosum, bihilar adenopathy, fever, and polyarthritis) when present. In most other cases, the diagnosis of sarcoidosis requires a compatible history, findings of noncaseating granulomas in a biopsy specimen, and the exclusion of other possible causes of disease. Blood tests may show abnormalities, including hypercalcemia, anemia, and elevated liver enzymes if systemic involvement is present. Angiotensin-converting enzyme (ACE) levels are neither specific nor sensitive to use as a diagnostic tool, but they may be helpful in following disease activity when they are elevated. Bronchoscopy can confirm granulomatous disease in more than 90% of patients with hilar adenopathy and parenchymal lung involvement. Although rales may be present when acute parenchymal interstitial changes occur, the typical examination finding is clear lung fields. The incidence, clinical course, and prognosis of sarcoidosis are also influenced by ethnic and genetic factors. CT findings may demonstrate small nodules with a bronchovascular and subpleural distribution, thickened intralobular septa, architectural distortion, or conglomerate masses. Viruses, mycobacteria, mycoplasma, and other environmental factors are possible etiologic risk factors for developing sarcoidosis. Tobacco use has not been associated with the development of sarcoidosis. Extrapulmonary involvement may include the heart, liver, spleen, eye, bone, skin, bone marrow, parotid gland, pituitary gland, and reproductive organs. This patient's presentation is most consistent with Lofgren syndrome, which should be treated symptomatically with an NSAID. For progressive pulmonary and extrapulmonary disease, corticosteroids or immunosuppressive therapy should be considered.

9. Answer a.

Bell palsy is the most common manifestation of neurosarcoidosis. It occurs in 49% to 67% of patients with neurologic involvement. Treatment of Bell palsy as an isolated manifestation of neurosarcoidosis is controversial, but when therapy is required, the initial treatment of choice is systemic corticosteroids. Neurosarcoidosis, other than Bell palsy, clearly warrants immunosuppressive therapy, including cyclosporine, methotrexate, azathioprine, chlorambucil, or cyclophosphamide for patients who do not have a response to systemic corticosteroid therapy or who cannot tolerate the treatment because of adverse side effects.

10. Answer c.

The combination of lower lung field interstitial lung disease, lack of occupational exposure, duration of symptoms, and peripheral honeycombing make the diagnosis of IPF most likely. Favorable prognostic factors for IPF/usual interstitial fibrosis (UIP) include age younger than 50, female sex, shorter duration of symptoms before presentation, presence of ground-glass opacities on chest CT, and lymphocytic bronchoalveolar lavage. PFTs in IPF are restrictive. No more than 20% to 30% of patients with IPF are expected to have a response to corticosteroid or other immunosuppressive therapy. Oxygen has been shown to extend survival in chronic obstructive pulmonary disease but not in IPF. Familial clusters of IPF suggest a potential genetic predisposition in some cases. Although subjective improvement of patients with IPF/UIP may be expected to be as high as 70%, objective improvement in PFTs occurs in no more than 20% to 30% of patients. Most studies require single parameter improvement of at least 15% to 20% in vital capacity, total lung capacity, or diffusing capacity to be considered a response. Radiographic improvement generally does not occur. Currently, no treatment is available.

11. Answer c.

Symptoms of acute hypersensitivity pneumonitis usually resolve 8 to 12 hours after exposure ceases but are likely to recur if exposure is repeated. Airflow obstruction may occur if occupational asthma and airway disease develop. Corticosteroid therapy is seldom required but may accelerate improvement in symptoms and gas exchange in severe cases. Isocyanates used in plastic manufacturing and automobile body repair can cause both occupational asthma and hypersensitivity pneumonitis. Skin testing, an IgE-mediated reaction, is not usually helpful for the diagnosis of hypersensitivity pneumonitis. In contrast, serum precipitants, with precipitating IgG antibodies, indicate a host response to specific antigens and may be correlated with disease activity in some patients. After removal from the offending antigen, physiologic abnormalities are expected to resolve within a few days for acute hypersensitivity pneumonitis and within a month for chronic hypersensitivity pneumonitis. The prognosis is generally excellent if permanent radiographic or physiologic abnormalities are not present at the onset of acute hypersensitivity pneumonitis.

12. Answer d.

This patient's presentation is most consistent with a course of Langerhans cell histiocytosis. Absolute smoking cessation is the primary form of treatment. Stabilization or improvement (or both) with smoking cessation alone is expected to occur in as many as two-thirds of patients. Other therapies, including systemic corticosteroids and immunosuppressive agents, have been used with limited success. No role has been described for plasmapheresis.

13. Answer e.

Asbestosis, in contrast to all the other choices, typically has a basilar predominance. Rounded atelectasis is suggestive of asbestos exposure. It should be noted that known or remembered histories of occupational asbestos exposure may not always be elicited, although when they are, they can be helpful. Common findings include pleural plaques or diaphragmatic calcifications (or both). Malignant mesothelioma is strongly associated with asbestos exposure but not with smoking. Pleural surfaces are generally abnormal and involved with asbestos-related parenchymal lung disease. However, in some instances, pleural and parenchymal abnormalities may occur independently of each other. Asbestos fibers typically are dormant for decades before pulmonary fibrosis develops. No clinical response is expected to corticosteroid treatment of asbestos-related pulmonary fibrosis. Smoking in the setting of asbestos-related pulmonary fibrosis increases the rate of progression of fibrosis and the risk of developing bronchogenic carcinoma. Tuberculosis is not a common complication of asbestosis. No therapy has been shown to be effective in preventing progressive pulmonary fibrosis due to asbestos exposure.

14. Answer b.

This patient's presentation, medical history, examination findings, laboratory data, and radiographic findings are most consistent with IPF/UIP. Pulmonary function tests are expected to demonstrate decreased vital capacity with a preserved FEV_1-to-vital capacity ratio, decreased lung volumes (including total lung capacity and residual volume), and decreased diffusing capacity. Hypoxemia at rest or with exercise may also be present. Blood tests may demonstrate an elevated ANA, polyclonal gammopathy, elevated rheumatoid factor, or elevated erythrocyte sedimentation rate. Serum precipitants for farmer's lung battery, including thermophilic actinomycetes, are not expected to be positive. The important differentiation is whether this patient has IPF/UIP, a steroid-unresponsive process, or NSIP-IPF, generally a steroid-responsive process. In contrast, had there been historical elements, examination findings, or laboratory data to suggest collagen vascular disease-associated or drug-induced lung disease, the diagnosis of NSIP should be considered. If ground-glass opacities were seen on HRCT and the duration of symptoms was shorter, the possibility of a more steroid-responsive process such as NSIP-IPF would need to be considered in this relatively young female patient. Proceeding with additional diagnostic tests, including bronchoscopy or VATS, would be the next appropriate step.

15. Answer c.

Surgical resection is correct because this is a new pulmonary nodule in a smoker which was not present 3 years previously. The enhancement on chest CT is worrisome for malignancy. Bronchoscopy with transbronchial biopsy has a low diagnostic yield for small peripheral pulmonary nodules. PET would likely show enhancement of the nodule, which is already known to enhance, so it would not be helpful. Although transthoracic needle aspiration could be attempted, the patient would still have surgical resection whether the findings were positive or negative. Repeating chest CT would be reasonable; however, waiting 1 year is too long.

16. Answer d.

Squamous cell carcinoma is the type of lung cancer most likely to be located centrally, to be cavitated, and to be associated with hypercalcemia from the production of parathyroid hormone-related protein secreted by tumor cells. Proximal tracheobronchial involvement occurs in 65% of these malignancies, resulting in the early onset of symptoms such as cough, hemoptysis, and obstructive pneumonitis.

17. Answer a.

This patient has the syndrome of inappropriate antidiuretic hormone (SIADH), which is associated most commonly with small cell carcinoma. It is characterized by hyponatremia in the setting of euvolemia, a low serum osmolality with a high urinary osmolality. Other paraneoplastic syndromes associated with small cell carcinoma include Cushing syndrome, Lambert-Eaton myasthenic syndrome, and cerebellar degeneration.

18. Answer d.

Thrombolytic therapy is indicated in massive pulmonary embolism with hemodynamic instability. Thrombolytic therapy accelerates the resolution of acute embolism and improves right ventricular function. If thrombolytic therapy and subsequent anticoagulation fail, the patient may be a candidate for pulmonary thromboendarterectomy.

19. Answer c.

The flow-volume loop shows a normal inspiratory curve and flattening with plateau of the expiratory curve consistent with a variable intrathoracic obstruction. Bronchoscopy is indicated because tracheobronchial stenosis occurs in 15% of patients with Wegener granulomatosis. Bronchoscopic intervention including dilation by rigid bronchoscopy, YAG-laser treatment, or placement of silicone airway stents may be necessary to relieve the obstruction and the patient's dyspnea.

20. Answer c.

The patient has features of Churg-Strauss syndrome that had previously been controlled with oral corticosteroids. Her presenting symptoms represent a flare of the vasculitis as the oral corticosteroid therapy was tapered. The presentation of difficult-to-control asthma, nasal polyps, infiltrates seen on chest radiography, and peripheral blood eosinophilia all point to Churg-Strauss syndrome as the correct diagnosis. A dramatic response can be expected with high doses of systemic corticosteroids.

21. Answer d.

The most likely diagnosis in a young male smoker presenting with alveolar hemorrhage and glomerulonephritis is Goodpasture syndrome. Active cigarette smoking increases the risk of alveolar hemorrhage, and one-third of patients with Goodpasture syndrome test positive for p-ANCA. The diagnosis is established by finding anti-GBM (glomerular basement membrane) antibody in the blood or, with immunofluorescent microscopy, finding linear deposition of IgG and complement along basement membranes in renal biopsy specimens.

22. Answer d.

A mycetoma, or fungus ball, is a complication in patients with cavitary lung disease. *Aspergillus fumigatus* is the organism most frequently recovered from the lung cavity. *Aspergillus* is a dimorphic fungus with a mycelial phase (which grows at room temperature) and a yeast phase (which grows at body temperature). Typically, the mycelial phase comprises the bulk of the mycetoma. Complications include hemoptysis, malaise, and weight loss.

23. Answer b.

The recommendations for baseline measurements of liver function before beginning treatment for LTBI were modified in 1999. According to recommendations from the American Thoracic Society and the Centers for Disease Control and Prevention, patients whose initial examination suggests liver disease should have baseline liver function measured. Additionally, baseline testing is indicated for patients with HIV infection, pregnant women, and those within the immediate postpartum period (3 months after delivery), persons with known liver disease, and those who drink alcohol regularly. Follow-up examinations need to be performed at least monthly and patients educated about the side effects of these medications.

24. Answer e.

Targeted tuberculin testing is the strategy for identifying patients at high risk for LTBI. The rationale is that a positive PPD skin test should indicate LTBI once active disease is excluded and the patient should receive treatment for LTBI. Of the patients listed, only the one with end-stage renal disease would be considered at high risk, and a PPD skin test induration of 10 mm or more would be positive. The relative risk for active TB developing in this patient compared with a control population is 10 to 25.

25. Answer c.

Persons infected with HIV, persons with recent contacts with a patient with tuberculosis (as in this patient) or fibrotic changes on CXR consistent with previous tuberculosis, and patients with an organ transplant or immunosuppressed status (those receiving the equivalent of ≥15 mg of prednisone for ≥1 month) have a positive PPD skin test indicating LTBI if the induration is more than 5 mm.

26. Answer a.

Cryptococcal disease that develops in a patient with HIV infection requires treatment. Usually fluconazole at 200-400 mg daily is efficacious; however, patients with severe disease may require the addition of flucytosine or treatment with amphotericin B. It is recommended that all HIV-infected patients continue maintenance therapy for life.

27. Answer e.

Legionella pneumonia should be suspected in patients with severe community-acquired pneumonia. Delay in instituting appropriate therapy for *Legionella* pneumonia markedly increases mortality; therefore, empirical therapy for this infection should be included in the treatment of severe community-acquired pneumonia. The *Legionella* urinary antigen test is relatively inexpensive and rapid and detects the antigens of *L. pneumophila* in the urine. Traditionally, macrolides such as erythromycin have been used to treat this infection, but the high doses required have marked side effects. Newer macrolides and quinolones have been shown to be effective. For a patient who is severely ill, rifampin is recommended as part of a combination therapy with a macrolide or a quinolone because it is highly active against *Legionella*.

28. Answer e.

"Hot tub lung" is a form of hypersensitivity pneumonitis due to *Mycobacterium avium* complex and is not considered infectious. If this patient stops using the hot tub, the exposure source will be removed and her symptoms and pulmonary function should recover rapidly. Antimycobacterial therapy is not necessary and corticosteroids are rarely helpful.

CHAPTER 22

RHEUMATOLOGY

Clement J. Michet, Jr., M.D.
Kevin G. Moder, M.D.
William W. Ginsburg, M.D.

PART I
Clement J. Michet, Jr., M.D.
Kevin G. Moder, M.D.

RHEUMATOID ARTHRITIS

Rheumatoid arthritis is a chronic systemic inflammatory disease characterized by joint destruction. It affects 0.03% to 1.5% of the population worldwide. Its incidence peaks between the ages of 35 and 45 years; however, the age-related prevalence continues to increase even after age 65. It occurs 3 times more frequently in women than men. The cause remains unknown. The presentation of an unknown antigen to genetically susceptible persons is believed to trigger rheumatoid arthritis.

There is an immunogenetic predisposition to the development of rheumatoid arthritis. Class II major histocompatibility complex molecules on the surface of antigen-presenting cells are responsible for initiating cellular immune responses and for stimulating the differentiation of B lymphocytes into plasma cells that produce antibody. Most white patients with rheumatoid arthritis have class II major histocompatibility complex type HLA-DR4 or HLA-DR1 or both. HLA-DR4 can be divided into five subtypes, two of which independently promote susceptibility to rheumatoid arthritis ("shared epitope"). The risk of rheumatoid arthritis is increased 3 to 5 times in white Americans with HLA-DR4. The concordance of rheumatoid factor–positive rheumatoid arthritis is increased 6 times among dizygotic twins. The risk of rheumatoid arthritis in a monozygotic twin is increased 30 times when a sibling has the disease.

- Rheumatoid arthritis affects 0.03%-1.5% of the population.
- Most white patients with rheumatoid arthritis have class II major histocompatibility complex type HLA-DR4 or HLA-DR1 or both.

- The concordance of rheumatoid factor–positive rheumatoid arthritis is increased 6 times among dizygotic twins.
- The risk of rheumatoid arthritis in a monozygotic twin is increased 30 times when a sibling has the disease.

Pathogenesis of Rheumatoid Arthritis

The immune reaction begins in the synovial lining of the joint. The earliest pathologic changes in the disease are microvascular injury that increases vascular permeability and the accumulation of inflammatory cells (CD4+ lymphocytes, polymorphonuclear leukocytes, and plasma cells) in the perivascular space. Pro-inflammatory cytokines are released. Mediators of inflammation promote synovial angiogenesis and synovial cell proliferation, the accumulation of neutrophils in synovial fluid, and the maturation of B cells into plasma cells. Plasma cells in the joint locally synthesize rheumatoid factor and other antibodies that promote inflammation. Immune complexes activate the complement system, releasing chemotactic factors and promoting vascular permeability and opsonization. Phagocytosis releases lysosomal enzymes and fosters the digestion of collagen, cartilage matrix, and elastic tissues. The release of oxygen free radicals injures cells. Damaged cell membranes set free phospholipids that fuel the arachidonic acid cascade.

The local inflammatory response becomes self-perpetuating. Cytokines continue to play an important role, including tumor necrosis factor-α, interleukin-1, and interleukin-6. Proliferating synovium of activated macrophages and fibroblasts polarizes into a centripetally invasive pannus, destroying the weakened cartilage and subchondral bone. Chondrocytes, stimulated in the inflammatory milieu, release their own proteases and collagenases. Patients have swelling, pain, and joint stiffness with the onset of vascular injury of the synovial lining, angiogenesis, and cellular proliferation. Joint warmth, swelling, pain, and limitation of motion worsen as the synovial membrane proliferates and the inflammatory reaction builds.

Rheumatoid factor is an immunoglobulin (usually IgM) that binds other immunoglobulins (usually IgG) at their Fc components, forming immune complexes.

- Swelling, pain, and joint stiffness occur with the onset of immune-mediated vascular injury of the synovial lining, angiogenesis, and cellular proliferation.
- Rheumatoid factor is an immunoglobulin (usually IgM) that binds other immunoglobulins (usually IgG) at their Fc components, forming immune complexes.
- Cytokines, in particular tumor necrosis factor-α, and immune complexes, including rheumatoid factor, are important components of the joint inflammatory reaction.

Clinical Features of Rheumatoid Arthritis

The joints most commonly involved (more than 85% of patients) in rheumatoid arthritis are the metacarpophalangeal, proximal interphalangeal, wrist, and metatarsophalangeal joints (Fig. 22-1). The distal interphalangeal joints are typically spared. The distribution of involvement is symmetric and polyarticular (five or more joints); predominantly, small joints are involved. Ultimately, the knees (80% of patients),

ankles (80%), shoulders (60%), elbows (50%), hips (50%), acromioclavicular joints (50%), atlantoaxial joint (50%), and temporomandibular joints (30%) can be involved. The sternoclavicular joints, cricoarytenoid joints, and the ear ossicles are affected infrequently. Joints affected with rheumatoid arthritis are warm and swollen. The joint enlargement feels spongy and occurs with the thickening of the synovium. An associated joint effusion may make the joint feel fluctuant. Patients describe deep aching and soreness in the involved joints, which are aggravated by use and can be present at rest. Prolonged morning joint stiffness and "gelling" throughout the body and recurrence of this stiffness after resting are some of the many constitutional features that complicate rheumatoid arthritis.

- The joints most commonly involved in rheumatoid arthritis are the metacarpophalangeal, proximal interphalangeal, wrist, and metatarsophalangeal joints.
- The distribution of involvement is symmetric and polyarticular; predominantly, small joints are involved.
- Hallmarks of joint inflammation: stiffness, heat, redness, soft tissue swelling, pain, and dysfunction.

Constitutional Features of Rheumatoid Arthritis

Fatigue initially affects up to 40% of patients. Weight loss, muscle pain, excessive sweating, or low-grade fever occurs in 20% of patients presenting with rheumatoid arthritis. Adult seropositive rheumatoid arthritis is not a cause of fever of

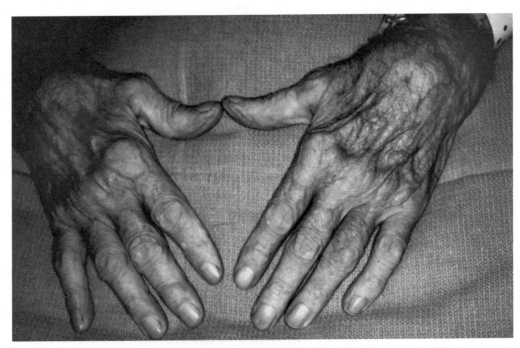

Fig. 22-1. Moderately active seropositive rheumatoid arthritis. The patient has soft tissue swelling across the entire row of metatarsophalangeal joints and proximal interphalangeal joints bilaterally and soft tissue swelling mounding up over the wrists. Note the nearly complete lack of change at the distal interphalangeal joints.

unknown origin because temperatures greater than 101°F cannot be attributed to the disease. A high temperature should raise concern about another problem, such as infection or malignancy. Most patients with *active* arthritis have more than 1 hour of morning stiffness. The musculoskeletal complications of rheumatoid arthritis are listed in Table 22-1.

Musculoskeletal Complications of Rheumatoid Arthritis

Cervical Spine

One-half of all patients with chronic rheumatoid arthritis have radiographic involvement of the atlantoaxial joint. It is diagnosed with cervical flexion and extension radiographs showing subluxation. Alternatively, some patients have subaxial subluxations, typically at two or more levels. The cervical instability is usually asymptomatic; however, patients may have pain and stiffness in the neck and occipital region. Patients may present dramatically with drop attacks or tetraplegia, but more commonly progression can be slow and subtle with symptoms of hand weakness or paresthesias or signs of cervical myelopathy. Interference with blood flow by compression of the anterior spinal artery or vertebral arteries (vertebrobasilar insufficiency) causes the neurologic symptoms. All patients with destructive rheumatoid arthritis should be managed with intubation precautions and the assumption that cervical instability is present. New neurologic symptoms mandate urgent

Table 22-1 Musculoskeletal Complications of Rheumatoid Arthritis

---

Characteristic deformities include

Boutonnière deformity of the finger, with hyperextension of the distal interphalangeal joint and flexion of the proximal interphalangeal joint

Swan-neck deformity of the finger, with hyperextension at the proximal interphalangeal joint and flexion of the distal interphalangeal joint

Ulnar deviation of the metacarpophalangeal joints; it can progress to complete volar subluxation of the proximal phalanx from the metacarpophalangeal head

Compression of the carpal bones and radial deviation at the carpus

Subluxation at the wrist

Valgus of the ankle and hindfoot

Pes planus

Forefoot varus and hallux valgus

Cock-up toes from subluxation at the metatarsophalangeal joints

---

neurologic evaluation, including magnetic resonance imaging of the cervical spine and consideration of surgical intervention. Indications for surgical treatment include neurologic or vascular compromise and intractable pain. In active patients, prophylactic cervical spine stabilization is recommended when there is evidence of extreme (>8 mm) subluxation of C1 over C2. The probability of cervical involvement is predicted by the severity of peripheral arthritis.

- One-half of all patients with chronic rheumatoid arthritis have radiographic involvement of the atlantoaxial joint.
- Patients with cervical spine involvement may present with occipital pain, signs of myelopathy, weakness and paresthesias of the hands, or drop attacks.
- Indications for surgical treatment: neurologic or vascular compromise or intractable pain.
- The probability of cervical involvement is predicted by the severity of peripheral arthritis.

Popliteal Cyst

Flexion of the knee markedly increases the intra-articular pressure of a swollen joint. This pressure produces an outpouching of the posterior components of the joint space, termed a "popliteal" or a "Baker" cyst. Ultrasonographic examination of the popliteal space can be diagnostic. A popliteal cyst should be distinguished from a popliteal artery aneurysm, lymphadenopathy, phlebitis, and (more rarely) a benign or malignant tumor. The cyst can rupture down into the calf or, rarely, superiorly into the posterior thigh. Rupture of the popliteal cyst with dissection into the calf may resemble acute thrombophlebitis and is called "pseudophlebitis." Fever, leukocytosis, and ecchymosis around the ankle (crescent sign) can occur with the rupture. Treatment of an acute cyst rupture includes bed rest, elevation of the leg, ice massage or cryocompression, and an intra-articular injection of corticosteroid. Treatment of the popliteal cyst requires improvement in the knee arthritis.

- Popliteal cyst is also called Baker cyst.
- Rupture of a popliteal cyst may resemble acute thrombophlebitis (pseudophlebitis).
- Ultrasonography can distinguish a cyst from a popliteal artery aneurysm, lymphadenopathy, phlebitis, and tumor.

Tenosynovitis

Tenosynovitis of the finger flexor and extensor tendon sheaths is common. It presents with diffuse swelling between the joints and a palpable grating within the flexor tendon sheaths in the palm with passive movement of the digit. Other tenosynovial syndromes in rheumatoid arthritis include de Quervain and wrist tenosynovitis. Persistent inflammation can produce stenosing tenosynovitis, loss of function, and, ultimately, rupture of tendons. Treatment of acute tenosynovitis includes immobilization, warm soaks, nonsteroidal anti-inflammatory drugs, and local injections of corticosteroid in the tendon sheath.

● Tenosynovitis of the finger flexor and extensor tendon sheaths is common and can lead to tendon rupture.

Carpal Tunnel Syndrome

Rheumatoid arthritis is a common cause of carpal tunnel syndrome (pregnancy is the commonest cause). The sudden appearance of bilateral carpal tunnel syndrome should raise the question of an early inflammatory arthritis. This syndrome is associated with paresthesias of the hand in a typical median nerve distribution. Discomfort may radiate up the forearm or into the upper arm. The symptoms worsen with prolonged flexion of the wrist and at night. Late complications include thenar muscle weakness and atrophy and permanent sensory loss. Treatment includes resting splints, control of inflammation, and local injection of glucocorticosteroid. Surgical release is recommended for persistent symptoms.

● Rheumatoid arthritis is a common cause of carpal tunnel syndrome.
● Carpal tunnel syndrome: paresthesias of the hand in a typical median nerve distribution.

Extra-Articular Complications of Rheumatoid Arthritis

Extra-articular complications of rheumatoid arthritis occur almost exclusively in patients who have high titers of rheumatoid factor. In general, the number and severity of the extra-articular features vary with the duration and severity of disease.

Rheumatoid Nodules

Rheumatoid nodules are the most common extra-articular manifestation of seropositive rheumatoid arthritis. More than 20% of patients have rheumatoid nodules, which occur over extensor surfaces and at pressure points. They are rare in the lungs, heart, sclera, and dura mater. The nodules have characteristic histopathologic features. A collagenous capsule and a perivascular collection of chronic inflammatory cells surround a central area of necrosis encircled by palisading fibroblasts. Breakdown of the skin over rheumatoid nodules, with ulcers and infection, can be a major source of morbidity. The infection can spread to local bursae, infect bone, or spread hematogenously to joints.

● Extra-articular complications in rheumatoid arthritis occur almost exclusively in seropositive rheumatoid arthritis.

● Rheumatoid nodules are the most common extra-articular complication.
● Rheumatoid nodules occur over extensor surfaces and at pressure points and are prone to ulceration and infection.

Rheumatoid Vasculitis

Rheumatoid vasculitis usually occurs in persons with severe, deforming arthritis and a high titer of rheumatoid factor. The vasculitis is mediated by the deposition of circulating immune complexes on the blood vessel wall. At its most benign, it occurs as rheumatoid nodules, with small infarcts over the nodules and at the cuticles. Proliferation of the vascular intima and media causes this obliterative endarteropathy, which has little associated inflammation. It is best managed by controlling the underlying arthritis. Leukocytoclastic or small vessel vasculitis produces palpable purpura or cutaneous ulceration, particularly over the malleoli of the lower extremities. This vasculitis can cause pyoderma gangrenosum or peripheral sensory neuropathy. Secondary polyarteritis, which is clinically and histopathologically identical to polyarteritis nodosa, results in mononeuritis multiplex. Occasionally, the vasculitis appears after the joint disease appears "burned out."

● Rheumatoid vasculitis usually occurs in the setting of severe, deforming arthritis and a high titer of rheumatoid factor.
● Rheumatoid vasculitis is mediated by the deposition of circulating immune complexes on the blood vessel wall.
● Rheumatoid vasculitis comprises a spectrum of vascular disease, including rheumatoid nodules and obliterative endarteropathy, leukocytoclastic or small vessel vasculitis, and secondary polyarteritis (systemic necrotizing vasculitis).

Neurologic Manifestations

Neurologic manifestations of rheumatoid arthritis include mild peripheral sensory neuropathy. Sensory-motor neuropathy (mononeuropathy) suggests vasculitis or nerve entrapment (e.g., carpal tunnel syndrome). Cervical vertebral subluxation can cause myelopathy. Erosive changes may promote basilar invagination of the odontoid process of C2 into the underside of the brain, causing spinal cord compression and death.

Pulmonary Manifestations

Pleural disease has been noted in more than 40% of autopsies in cases of rheumatoid arthritis, but clinically significant pleural disease is less frequent. Characteristically, rheumatoid pleural effusions are asymptomatic until they become large enough to interfere mechanically with respiration. The pleural fluid is an exudate with a concentration of glucose that is low (10-50 mg/dL) because of impaired transport of glucose into the pleural space. Pulmonary nodules appear singly or in clusters. Single nodules have the appearance of a coin lesion. Nodules typically are pleural-based and may cavitate and create a bronchopleural fistula. Pneumoconiosis complicating rheumatoid lung disease, or Caplan syndrome, results in a violent fibroblastic reaction and large nodules.

Acute interstitial pneumonitis is a rare complication that may begin as alveolitis and progress to respiratory insufficiency and death. Interstitial fibrosis is a chronic, slowly progressive process. It has physical findings of diffuse dry crackles on lung auscultation and a reticular nodular radiographic pattern affecting both lung fields, initially in the lung bases. A decrease in the diffusing capacity for carbon dioxide and a restrictive pattern on pulmonary function testing complicate symptomatic interstitial fibrosis. Interstitial disease is highly associated with smoking. Bronchiolitis obliterans with or without organizing pneumonia may occur with rheumatoid arthritis or its treatment. It produces an obstructive picture on pulmonary function testing and typically responds to corticosteroid treatment. High-resolution computed tomography is useful for distinguishing these different interstitial rheumatoid lung syndromes and predicting treatment response. Methotrexate treatment causes a hypersensitivity lung reaction in 1% to 3% of patients. It can present insidiously with a dry cough or with life-threatening pneumonitis.

- Rheumatoid pleural disease is common but asymptomatic until pleural effusions interfere with respiration.
- The exudative pleural fluid is remarkable for low levels of glucose.
- Pleural-based rheumatoid nodules can cause a bronchopleural fistula.
- High-resolution computed tomography distinguishes among rheumatoid-associated interstitial lung diseases, including interstitial pneumonitis, interstitial fibrosis, and bronchiolitis obliterans with or without organizing pneumonia.

Cardiac Complications

Pericarditis has been noted in 50% of autopsies in cases of rheumatoid arthritis. However, patients rarely present with acute pericardial symptoms or cardiac tamponade. Recurrent effusive pericarditis without symptoms may evolve to chronic constrictive pericarditis. Signs of unexplained edema or ascites may be the presenting manifestations. Untreated constrictive pericarditis has a 70% 1-year mortality. Surgical pericardectomy is necessary.

- Patients rarely present with acute pericardial symptoms despite frequent serous pericarditis.
- Rheumatoid pericardial disease frequently presents with edema or ascites due to occult constrictive disease.
- Untreated constrictive pericarditis has a 70% 1-year mortality. Surgery is necessary.

Liver Abnormalities

Patients with rheumatoid arthritis can have increased levels of liver enzymes, particularly alkaline phosphatase. Increased levels of aspartate aminotransferase, γ-glutamyltransferase, and acute-phase proteins and hypoalbuminemia also occur in active rheumatoid arthritis. Liver biopsy shows nonspecific changes of inflammation. Nodular regenerative hyperplasia is rare and causes portal hypertension and hypersplenism. Many medications used to treat rheumatoid arthritis may cause increased levels of the transaminases.

- Increased levels of liver enzymes, particularly alkaline phosphatase, may occur in rheumatoid arthritis.
- Nodular hyperplasia of the liver can complicate rheumatoid arthritis and lead to portal hypertension and hypersplenism.
- Many medications used to treat rheumatoid arthritis increase the levels of transaminases.

Ophthalmic Abnormalities

Keratoconjunctivitis sicca, or secondary Sjögren syndrome, is the most common ophthalmic complication in rheumatoid arthritis. Episcleritis and scleritis also occur independently of the joint inflammation and are usually treated topically. Severe scleritis progressing to scleromalacia perforans causes blindness. Infrequent ocular complications of rheumatoid arthritis include episcleral nodules, palsy of the superior oblique muscle caused by tenosynovitis of its tendon sheath (Brown syndrome), and uveitis. Retinopathy is an infrequent complication of antimalarial drug treatment.

- Keratoconjunctivitis sicca, or secondary Sjögren syndrome, is the most common ophthalmic complication in rheumatoid arthritis.
- Severe scleritis progressing to scleromalacia perforans causes blindness.

Laboratory Findings of Rheumatoid Arthritis

Nonspecific alterations in many laboratory values are common. In very active disease, normocytic anemia (hemoglobin in the range of 10 g/dL), leukocytosis, thrombocytosis, hypoalbuminemia, and hypergammaglobulinemia are common. Rheumatoid factor (IgM) occurs in 90% of patients, but its presence may not be detected for months after the initial joint symptoms occur. Rheumatoid factor is a marker of immune stimulation and occurs in various connective tissue diseases and infections, including primary Sjögren syndrome, lupus erythematosus, Wegener granulomatosis, hepatitis C, subacute bacterial endocarditis, and lymphoproliferative disorders. Diseases in bold type in Table 22-2 are most likely to have high titers of rheumatoid factor. Five percent of the general population has a low titer of rheumatoid factor.

Table 22-2 Diseases That May Have Positive Rheumatoid Factor[*]

Rheumatoid arthritis
Sjögren syndrome
Systemic lupus erythematosus
Scleroderma
Sarcoidosis
Idiopathic pulmonary fibrosis
Mixed cryoglobulinemia
Hypergammaglobulinemic purpura
Asbestosis
Malignancies
Infectious mononucleosis
Influenza
Chronic active hepatitis
Vaccinations
Tuberculosis
Syphilis
Subacute bacterial endocarditis
Brucellosis
Leprosy
Salmonellosis
Malaria
Kala-azar
Schistosomiasis
Filariasis
Trypanosomiasis

[*]Diseases in boldface type are the most likely to have high-titer rheumatoid factor.

Antinuclear antibodies are common in seropositive rheumatoid disease. C-reactive protein correlates with disease activity, but it is not more helpful than the erythrocyte sedimentation rate. Patients with rheumatoid arthritis who have active disease have low iron-binding capacity, low plasma levels of iron, and an increased ferritin value, unless they are iron-deficient.

- Normocytic anemia, leukocytosis, thrombocytosis, and hypoalbuminemia are common in active rheumatoid arthritis.
- Rheumatoid factor is not specific for the diagnosis of rheumatoid arthritis.
- Antinuclear antibodies occur in seropositive rheumatoid arthritis.
- C-reactive protein correlates with disease activity, but it is not more helpful than the erythrocyte sedimentation rate.

Synovial fluid is cloudy and light yellow, has poor viscosity, and typically contains 10,000 to 75,000 leukocytes/μL, predominantly neutrophils.

Radiographic Findings of Rheumatoid Arthritis

The radiographic findings in early rheumatoid arthritis are normal or show soft tissue swelling. Later, the characteristic changes of periarticular osteoporosis, symmetric narrowing of the joint space, and marginal bony erosions become obvious. These signs are most common in radiographs of the hands and forefeet. Radiographic changes at end-stage rheumatoid arthritis include subluxation and other deformities, joint destruction, fibrous ankylosis, and, rarely, bony ankylosis (Fig. 22-2).

- The characteristic radiologic changes in rheumatoid arthritis include periarticular osteoporosis, symmetric narrowing of the joint space, and bony erosions of the joint margin. These occur earliest in the hands and forefeet.

Diagnosis of Rheumatoid Arthritis

Adult rheumatoid arthritis should be considered in a person older than 16 years with inflammatory joint symptoms lasting for more than 6 weeks. The time criterion is important because there are viral arthropathies, such as parvovirus B19 infection, that mimic acute rheumatoid arthritis. Morning stiffness lasting for more than 30 minutes, small joint involvement in the metatarsophalangeal joints (morning metatarsalgia), metacarpophalangeal joints with tenderness and swelling, and more than three joints affected are clues to an early rheumatoid arthritis presentation. Four of the seven criteria of the American Rheumatism Association, listed in Table 22-3, must be satisfied for the diagnosis to be made.

Natural History of Rheumatoid Arthritis

The majority of patients have insidious onset of the joint disease, occurring over weeks to months. However, in a third of patients, the onset is rapid, occurring in days or weeks. Early in the course of the disease, most patients have oligoarthritis. Their disease becomes polyarticular with time. From 10% to 20% of patients have relentlessly progressive arthritis, and 70% to 90% have persistent, chronic, progressive arthritis. The course may be slow, fluctuating, or rapid, but the end point is the same: disabling, destructive arthritis. Seventy percent of patients experience polycyclic disease, with repeated flares interrupted by partial or complete remissions. Spontaneous remissions in the polycyclic or progressive group almost never occur after 2 years of disease. Patients who experience a persisting polyarthritis with increased acute phase reactants and a positive rheumatoid factor are at high risk for early erosive disease within 1 to 2 years of symptom onset and early disability.

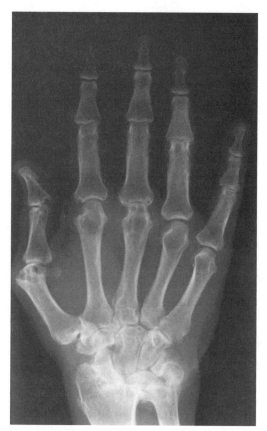

Fig. 22-2. Radiographic features of long-standing rheumatoid arthritis. Periarticular osteoporosis is marked by decreased cortical margins and reduction in trabecular textures in the periarticular areas. There is symmetric narrowing of the joint space at the proximal interphalangeal joints and second and third metacarpophalangeal joints. Marginal erosions are best seen at the thumb interphalangeal and metacarpophalangeal joints and at the second and third metacarpophalangeal joints. Additional destructive changes have nearly obliterated the usual margins of the carpal bones, making it difficult to distinguish them individually.

Table 22-3   American Rheumatism Association Criteria for Making the Diagnosis of Rheumatoid Arthritis[*]

One or more hours of morning stiffness in and around the joints

Arthritis of three or more joint areas involved simultaneously

Arthritis of at least one area in the wrist, metacarpophalangeal or proximal interphalangeal joints

Symmetrical arthritis involving the same joint areas on both sides of the body

Rheumatoid nodules

Serum rheumatoid factor

Radiographic changes typical of rheumatoid arthritis, including periarticular osteoporosis, joint-space narrowing, and marginal erosions

[*]1987 revision.

The relationship between disease duration and inability to work is nearly linear. After 15 years of rheumatoid arthritis, 15% of patients are completely disabled. Life expectancy in seropositive rheumatoid arthritis is shortened, but it may be improving with more aggressive early intervention in the illness. Age, disease severity, comorbid cardiovascular disease, and functional status predict mortality. Educational level and socioeconomic factors also influence mortality.

- In a third of patients, the onset of rheumatoid arthritis is rapid (days or weeks).
- 70%-90% of patients have persistent, chronic, progressive arthritis.
- The relationship between disease duration and inability to work is nearly linear.
- With seropositive rheumatoid arthritis, life expectancy is decreased.

Treatment of Rheumatoid Arthritis

The management of patients with rheumatoid arthritis requires making the correct diagnosis, determining the functional status of the patient, and selecting the goals of management with the patient. Goals of management include relieving inflammation and pain and maintaining function.

The principles emphasized by physical medicine include bed rest or rest periods, improving nonrestorative sleep, and joint protection (including modification of activities of daily life, range-of-motion exercises, orthotics, and splints, if they help the pain). Exercise should begin with range of motion and stretching to overcome contracture. Strengthening and conditioning exercises should be prescribed carefully, depending on the activity of the patient's disease.

Initial treatment is with a nonsteroidal anti-inflammatory drug given at anti-inflammatory doses. If the response is inadequate after 3 or 4 weeks, a trial of a second, chemically unrelated nonsteroidal anti-inflammatory drug is used. Low-dose prednisone (≤7.5 mg daily) may be necessary to reduce symptoms while disease-modifying therapies are initiated. Intra-articular corticosteroids are effective for symptomatic joints not responding to oral anti-inflammatory drugs. A disease-modifying agent of rheumatic disease (DMARD) is also known as a second-line agent, slow-acting antirheumatic drug, or remittive agent. The goal of DMARD therapy is to slow disease progression (erosive damage) and maintain joint function. A goal of disease remission will be possible as new therapies are introduced. Disease-modifying agents include the following:

- Methotrexate
- Hydroxychloroquine
- Sulfasalazine
- Minocycline
- Leflunomide

- Cyclosporine
- Azathioprine
- Anticytokine therapies, including anti-tumor necrosis factor and interleukin-1 inhibitors

DMARD therapy should be started early, once rheumatoid arthritis is diagnosed. The choice of first DMARD is empiric, but usually consists of methotrexate, sulfasalazine, hydroxychloroquine, or minocycline. Uninterrupted treatment with a disease-modifying agent for 3 to 6 months is usually necessary to assess its effect. Traditionally, DMARDs have been used sequentially, although recent studies have shown an enhanced benefit with combination DMARD treatments that include methotrexate. A second disease-modifying drug is substituted or added to the first one when a therapeutic or toxic roadblock is reached. Evidence supporting the pivotal proinflammatory role of tumor necrosis factor-α in rheumatoid arthritis has been exploited clinically with the development of several effective tumor necrosis factor-α antagonists. These generally are reserved for patients not responding to trials of more traditional and less expensive DMARDs.

- Goals of management include relieving inflammation and pain and maintaining function.
- A disease-modifying regimen is started when rheumatoid arthritis is diagnosed.
- Low-dose prednisone may be necessary to preserve function during initiation of DMARD therapy.
- With disease-modifying agents, uninterrupted treatment for 3 to 6 months is needed to assess efficacy. Combination DMARD therapy has become more common.

Surgery in the Treatment of Rheumatoid Arthritis

An orthopedic surgical procedure for resistant rheumatoid arthritis remains the most important therapeutic option for preserving or enhancing function. Synovectomy of the wrist and nearby tendon sheaths is beneficial when medication alone fails to control the synovitis. The operation preserves joint function and prevents the lysis of extensor tendons that can result in a loss of function. Synovectomy of the knee, either open or through an arthroscope, can delay the progression of rheumatoid arthritis from 6 months to 3 years. Removal of nodules and treatment for local nerve entrapment syndromes are also important surgical treatments for rheumatoid arthritis. Arthroplasty is reserved for patients in whom medical management has failed and in whom intractable pain or compromise in function developed because of a destroyed joint. Arthroplasty, arthrodesis (wrist), and synovectomy are important components of well-balanced rheumatology treatment programs. Total joint arthroplasty has a slightly poorer long-term outcome in rheumatoid arthritis than in osteoarthritis.

Nevertheless, joint replacement has had a major impact on reducing patient disability.

- Orthopedic surgery is the most important advance in the treatment of medically resistant rheumatoid arthritis.
- Total joint arthroplasty has a slightly poorer long-term outcome in rheumatoid arthritis than in osteoarthritis.
- Typical clinical scenarios:
  Rheumatoid arthritis—A patient presents with bilateral inflammation of metacarpophalangeal and proximal interphalangeal joints and considerable morning stiffness. The joint involvement is symmetric. Laboratory tests are positive for rheumatoid factor.
  Baker cyst—A patient with a known history of rheumatoid arthritis who is receiving therapy presents with acute pain and swelling in the posterior aspect of the right knee. Mild fever and leukocytosis are present.

CONDITIONS RELATED TO RHEUMATOID ARTHRITIS

Seronegative Rheumatoid Arthritis

Rheumatoid factor-negative (seronegative) rheumatoid arthritis is not associated with extra-articular manifestations. However, the arthritis usually is destructive, deforming, and otherwise indistinguishable from seropositive rheumatoid arthritis.

- Seronegative rheumatoid arthritis is not associated with extra-articular manifestations.

Seronegative Rheumatoid Arthritis of the Elderly

A subgroup of patients older than 60 years with seronegative rheumatoid arthritis may have milder arthritis. In this subgroup, polyarticular inflammation suddenly develops and is controlled best with low doses of prednisone. Minimal destructive changes and deformity occur. An additional group of elderly patients with seronegative arthritis (men in their 70s) present with acute polyarthritis and pitting edema of the hands and feet. They have a prompt and gratifying response to low doses of prednisone.

- Typical clinical scenario: In a patient older than 60 years, rheumatoid factor-negative polyarticular arthritis suddenly develops. It is best controlled initially with low doses of prednisone.

Adult-Onset Still Disease

Systemic *juvenile* rheumatoid arthritis is known as Still disease. It has quotidian (fever spike with return to normal all in

1 day) high-spiking fevers, arthralgia, arthritis, seronegativity (negative rheumatoid factor and antinuclear antibody), leukocytosis, macular evanescent rash, serositis, lymphadenopathy, splenomegaly, and hepatomegaly. Fever, rash, and arthritis are the classic triad of Still disease.

Adult-onset Still disease (AOSD) has a slight female predominance. Its onset commonly occurs between ages 16 and 35. Temperature more than 39°C occurs in a quotidian or double quotidian pattern in 96% of patients. The rash has a typical appearance: a macular salmon-colored eruption on the trunk and extremities. The transient rash is usually noticed at the time of increased temperature. Arthritis occurs in 95% of these patients, and in about a third the joint disease is progressive and destructive. AOSD has a predilection for the wrists, shoulders, hips, and knees. Sixty percent of patients complain of sore throat, which can confuse the diagnosis with rheumatic fever. Weight loss is common. Lymphadenopathy occurs in two-thirds of patients and hepatosplenomegaly in about half. Pleurisy, pneumonitis, and abdominal pain occur in less than a third of patients. The serum ferritin level is markedly increased.

Treatment of AOSD includes high doses of aspirin or indomethacin. Corticosteroids may be needed to control the systemic symptoms. Half of patients require methotrexate to control the systemic and articular features.

- Typical clinical scenario: A patient presents with the classic triad of fever, rash, and arthritis.
- Rheumatoid factor and antinuclear antibodies are absent.
- There is a predilection for the wrists, shoulders, hips, and knees.
- Sore throat occurs in 60% of patients.

Felty Syndrome

Felty syndrome has the classic triad of rheumatoid arthritis, leukopenia, and splenomegaly. (Classic Felty syndrome usually occurs after 12 years or more of rheumatoid arthritis.) It occurs in less than 1% of patients with rheumatoid arthritis. Splenomegaly either may not be clinically apparent or may manifest only after the arthritis and leukopenia have been present for some time. Other features of Felty syndrome are listed in Table 22-4. Patients with this syndrome frequently have bacterial infections, particularly of the skin and lungs. Infection related to the cytopenia is the major cause of mortality. High titers of rheumatoid factor are the rule, and a positive antinuclear antibody occurs in two-thirds of patients. Hypocomplementemia often occurs with active vasculitis. Patients often die of sepsis despite vigorous antibacterial treatment. Treatment can include corticosteroids, methotrexate, granulocyte colony-stimulating factor, and splenectomy.

Table 22-4 Features of Felty Syndrome

Classic triad
Rheumatoid arthritis
Leukopenia
Splenomegaly
Other features
Recurrent fevers with and without infection
Weight loss
Lymphadenopathy
Skin hyperpigmentation
Lower extremity ulcers
Vasculitis
Neuropathy
Keratoconjunctivitis sicca
Xerostomia
Other cytopenias

- Felty syndrome occurs in <1% of patients with rheumatoid arthritis.
- Felty syndrome has the classic triad of rheumatoid arthritis, leukopenia, and splenomegaly.
- High titers of rheumatoid factor are the rule.
- Patients with Felty syndrome frequently die of infection.

Sjögren Syndrome

Sjögren syndrome has a triad of clinical features: keratoconjunctivitis sicca (with or without lacrimal gland enlargement), xerostomia (with or without salivary gland enlargement), and connective tissue disease (usually rheumatoid arthritis). Histologically, CD4 lymphocytic infiltration and destruction of lacrimal salivary glands characterize it. Clinically, it is manifested by dry eyes and dry mouth. Primary Sjögren syndrome is diagnosed predominantly in middle-aged women. Additional features of primary Sjögren syndrome are listed in Table 22-5. Most patients have a polyclonal hypergammaglobulinemia. Autoantibodies typically are present, including rheumatoid factor, antinuclear antibodies, and antibodies to extractable nuclear antigens (SS-A and SS-B).

Patients can present with primary Sjögren syndrome without any additional connective tissue disease. The primary syndrome typically has episodic and nondeforming arthritis. More commonly, rheumatoid arthritis, systemic lupus erythematosus, scleroderma, polyarteritis nodosa, or polymyositis accompanies Sjögren syndrome. There is no perfect definition for Sjögren syndrome, and no test is completely diagnostic. Simple dry eyes of the elderly must be distinguished from Sjögren syndrome. Patients with Sjögren syndrome have an increased risk for development of non-Hodgkin lymphoma.

Table 22-5 Features of Sjögren Syndrome

Classic triad
    Arthritis: typically episodic polyarthritis
    Dry eyes
    Dry mouth (and other dry mucous membranes)
Other features
    Constitutional features: fatigue, malaise, myalgia
    Raynaud phenomenon
    Cutaneous vasculitis
    CNS abnormalities
        Cerebritis, CNS vasculitis
        Stroke
        Multiple sclerosis-like illness
    Peripheral neuropathy
        Sensory
        Autonomic
        Interstitial lung disease
        Pleurisy

CNS, central nervous system.

Treatment of primary Sjögren syndrome is mainly symptomatic. Pilocarpine, 5 mg orally 4 times daily, improves salivary and lacrimal gland function in the majority of patients. Side effects, including flushing and sweating, limit its usefulness. In addition to hydration, systemic therapy is indicated if there is evidence of systemic inflammation. A Sjögren-like syndrome has been described in patients with human immunodeficiency virus (HIV) infection.

- Typical clinical scenario: A patient presents with dry eyes, dry mouth, and a connective tissue disorder (usually rheumatoid arthritis).
- Sjögren syndrome can exist by itself or with another formal connective tissue disease such as rheumatoid arthritis, systemic lupus erythematosus, scleroderma, or myositis.
- Treatment focuses on control of inflammation and symptoms of dryness.
- A Sjögren-like syndrome has been described in patients with HIV infection.

OSTEOARTHRITIS

Osteoarthritis is the failure of articular cartilage and subsequent degenerative changes in subchondral bone, bony joint margins, synovium, and para-articular fibrous and muscular structures. Osteoarthritis is the most common rheumatic disease; 80% of patients have some limitation of their activities, and 25% are unable to perform major activities of daily living. More than 10% of the population older than 60 years has osteoarthritis. Annually, symptomatic hip or knee osteoarthritis develops in half a million new patients.

- Osteoarthritis is the most common rheumatic disease.
- More than 10% of the population older than 60 years has osteoarthritis.

Pathogenesis of Osteoarthritis

Two principal changes associated with osteoarthritis are the progressive focal degeneration of articular cartilage and the formation of new bone in the floor of the cartilage lesion at the joint margins (osteophytes). Not all the mechanisms causing osteoarthritis have been identified. Current theories include 1) mechanical process: cartilage injury, particularly after impact loading, and 2) biochemical process: failure of cartilage repair processes to adequately compensate for injury. A combination of mechanical and biochemical processes likely contributes in most cases of osteoarthritis. It must be emphasized that osteoarthritis is not just the consequence of "wear and tear."

- Osteoarthritis: progressive focal degeneration of articular cartilage, with subsequent degeneration of surrounding soft tissues and proliferation (osteophytosis) of bone.
- Osteoarthritis is not the consequence of normal use ("wear and tear").

Clinical Features of Osteoarthritis

The pain of an osteoarthritic joint is usually described as a deep ache. The pain occurs with use of the joint and is relieved with rest and cessation of weight bearing. As the disease progresses, the involved joint may be symptomatic with minimal activity or even at rest. The pain originates in the structures around the disintegrating cartilage (there are no nerves in cartilage). There may be stiffness in the joint with initial use, but this initial stiffness is not prolonged as it is in inflammatory arthritis, such as rheumatoid arthritis. Although the symptoms are related predominantly to mechanical failure and motion limits, joint debris and the associated repair process promote mild inflammation, accumulation of synovial fluid, and mild hypertrophy of the synovial membrane. Acute inflammation can transiently occur at Heberden nodes (distal interphalangeal joints with prominent osteophytes as a consequence of osteoarthritis) or at the knee with tearing of a degenerative meniscal cartilage.

- Osteoarthritic pain is usually described as a deep ache with joint use, improved with rest.
- The stiffness with initial use of the joint is not prolonged in osteoarthritis as it is in inflammatory arthritis (rheumatoid arthritis).

Physical examination documents joint margin tenderness, fine crepitance, limits to motion, and enlargement of the joint. The enlargement is usually bony (proliferation of cartilage and bone to form osteophytes), but it can include effusions and mild synovial thickening. Deformity is a late consequence of the osteoarthritis and is associated with atrophy or derangement of the local soft tissues, ligaments, and muscles. Radiographic or physical examination evidence of osteoarthritis severity does not reliably predict a patient's symptoms.

Clinical Subsets of Osteoarthritis

Primary Osteoarthritis

Primary osteoarthritis is cartilage failure without a known cause that would predispose to osteoarthritis. It almost never affects the shoulders, elbows, ankles, metacarpophalangeal joints, or ulnar side of the wrist. It is divided into several clinical patterns, as described below.

1. *Generalized osteoarthritis* involves the distal interphalangeal joints, proximal interphalangeal joints, first carpometacarpal joints, hips, knees, and spine (Fig. 22-3). It occurs most frequently in middle-aged postmenopausal women.

2. *Isolated nodal osteoarthritis* is primary osteoarthritis that affects only the distal interphalangeal joints. It occurs predominantly in women and has a familial predisposition.

3. *Isolated hip osteoarthritis* is more common in men than in women. It has no clear association with obesity or activity.

4. *Erosive osteoarthritis* affects only the distal and proximal interphalangeal joints. Patients with erosive osteoarthritis have episodes of local inflammation. Mucous cyst formation at the distal interphalangeal joint is common. Painful flare-up of the disease recurs for years. Symptoms usually begin about the time of menopause. Bony erosions and collapse of the subchondral plate—features not usually seen in primary osteoarthritis—with osteophytes are markers of erosive osteoarthritis. Joint deformity can be severe. In many cases, bony ankylosis develops. Ankylosis is usually associated with relief of pain. The synovium is intensely infiltrated with mononuclear cells. This condition may be confused with rheumatoid arthritis.

5. *Diffuse idiopathic skeletal hyperostosis* is a variant of primary osteoarthritis. It occurs chiefly in men older than 50 years. It is also known as Forestier disease. The diagnosis requires finding characteristic exuberant, flowing osteophytosis that connects four or more vertebrae with preservation of the disk space. Diffuse

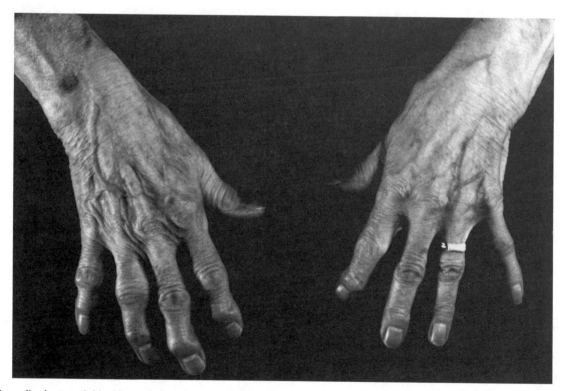

Fig. 22-3. Generalized osteoarthritis. Note prominent bony swelling at the proximal (Bouchard nodes) and distal (Heberden nodes) interphalangeal joints. The metacarpophalangeal joints are spared. Early hypertrophic changes are seen on profile at the first carpometacarpal joint, giving a slight squaring of the hand deformity, appreciated best on the left.

idiopathic skeletal hyperostosis must be distinguished from typical osteoarthritis of the spine with degenerative disk disease and from ankylosing spondylitis. Extraspinal sites of disease involvement include calcification of the pelvic ligaments, exuberant osteophytosis at the site of peripheral osteoarthritis, well-calcified bony spurs at the calcaneus, and heterotopic bone formation after total joint arthroplasty. Patients with diffuse idiopathic skeletal hyperostosis are often obese, and 60% have diabetes mellitus or glucose intolerance. Symptoms include mild back stiffness and, occasionally, back pain. Pathologically and radiologically, diffuse idiopathic skeletal hyperostosis is distinct from other forms of primary osteoarthritis.

- Primary osteoarthritis almost never affects the shoulders, elbows, ankles, metacarpophalangeal joints, or the ulnar side of the wrist.
- Generalized osteoarthritis involves the distal interphalangeal joints, proximal interphalangeal joints, first carpometacarpal joints, hips, knees, and spine.
- Isolated nodal osteoarthritis is primary osteoarthritis affecting only the distal interphalangeal joints.
- Isolated hip osteoarthritis is more common in men than in women.
- Erosive osteoarthritis affects only the distal and proximal interphalangeal joints.
- Diffuse idiopathic skeletal hyperostosis is a variant of primary osteoarthritis and should not be confused for ankylosing spondylitis.

Secondary Osteoarthritis

Secondary osteoarthritis is cartilage failure caused by some known disorder, trauma, or abnormality. Any patient with an unusual distribution of osteoarthritis or widespread chondrocalcinosis should be considered to have secondary osteoarthritis. Secondary osteoarthritis frequently complicates trauma and the damage caused by inflammatory arthritis. Inherited disorders of connective tissue and several metabolic abnormalities, including ochronosis, hemochromatosis, Wilson disease, and acromegaly, are complicated by secondary osteoarthritis. Paget disease of bone, involving the femur or pelvis about the hip joint, can predispose to osteoarthritis.

- Osteoarthritis involving the shoulder, metacarpophalangeal joints, or isolated large joints or with chondrocalcinosis should prompt physicians to consider secondary causes of osteoarthritis.

Trauma. Trauma or injury to a joint and supporting periarticular tissues predisposes persons to the most common type of secondary osteoarthritis. Stress from repeated impact loading could weaken subchondral bone. Internal joint derangement with ligamentous laxity or meniscal damage alters the normal mechanical alignment of the joint. Isolated large joint involvement is a clue to posttraumatic osteoarthritis. Chronic rotator cuff tear with subsequent loss of shoulder joint cartilage (cuff arthropathy) and knee osteoarthritis that develops years after meniscal cartilage damage are examples of secondary osteoarthritis.

Congenital malformations of joints. Congenital hip dysplasia and epiphyseal dysplasia lead to premature osteoarthritis. Other developmental abnormalities, including slipped capital femoral epiphysis and Legg-Calvé-Perthes disease (idiopathic avascular necrosis of the femoral head), may first present as premature osteoarthritis years after they occur. Inherited disorders of connective tissue frequently predispose the afflicted person to premature osteoarthritis. Table 22-6 describes several inherited disorders, including their gene defects and characteristics.

- Injury to a joint or supporting periarticular tissues can predispose to osteoarthritis.
- Posttraumatic osteoarthritis is the most common form of secondary osteoarthritis.
- Isolated large joint involvement is a clue to posttraumatic osteoarthritis.

Alkaptonuria/ochronosis. This is a rare autosomal recessive disorder of tyrosine metabolism. Deficiency of the enzyme homogentisic acid oxidase leads to excretion of large amounts of homogentisic acid in the urine. Black, oxidized, polymerized homogentisic acid pigment collects in connective tissues (ochronosis). The diagnosis may go unrecognized until middle life. The first manifestation can be secondary osteoarthritis. The patient's urine darkens when allowed to stand or with the addition of sodium hydroxide. Ochronotic arthritis affects the large joints (e.g., the hips, knees, and shoulders) and is associated with calcium pyrophosphate crystals in the synovial fluid. The radiographic finding of calcified intervertebral disks at multiple levels is characteristic of ochronosis. Other manifestations include grayish brown scleral pigment and generalized darkening of the ear pinnae.

- Alkaptonuria/ochronosis is a rare autosomal recessive disorder of tyrosine metabolism.
- Ochronosis: black, oxidized, polymerized homogentisic acid pigment collects in connective tissues.
- Ochronotic arthritis affects the large joints: the hips, knees, and shoulders.

Hemochromatosis. Hemochromatosis was formerly considered an unusual autosomal recessive disorder of white

Table 22-6 Inherited Disorders of Connective Tissue

Condition	Gene defect	Characteristics
Marfan syndrome (autosomal dominant)	Fibrillin gene	Hypermobile joints: osteoarthritis, arachnodactyly, kyphoscoliosis Lax skin, striae, ectopic ocular lens Aortic root dilatation (aortic insufficiency), mitral valve prolapse, aneurysms, and aortic dissection
Ehlers-Danlos syndrome (10 subtypes)	Type I and type III collagen gene defects	Joint hypermobility, friable skin, osteoarthritis Type III collagen defects associated with vascular aneurysms
Osteogenesis imperfecta (autosomal dominant and recessive variations; the most common heritable disorder of connective tissue: 1:20,000; 4 subtypes)	Type I collagen gene defects	Brittle bones, blue sclerae, otosclerosis and deafness, joint hypermobility, and tooth malformation
Type II collagenopathies: Achondrogenesis type II Hypochondrogenesis Spondyloepiphyseal dysplasia Spondyloepimetaphyseal dysplasia Kniest dysplasia Stickler syndrome Familial precocious osteoarthropathy	Type II collagen gene defects	Spectrum from lethal (achondrogenesis) to premature osteoarthritis (Stickler syndrome)
Achondroplasia (autosomal dominant)	Fibroblast growth factor III receptor gene defect	Dwarfism, premature osteoarthritis
Pseudoachondroplasia	Cartilage oligomeric matrix protein (COMP) gene defect	Short stature, premature osteoarthritis
Multiple epiphyseal dysplasia (autosomal dominant)		

males. It is now considered the commonest inherited disease. The full clinical spectrum of hemochromatosis includes hepatomegaly, bronze skin pigmentation, diabetes mellitus, the consequences of pituitary insufficiency, and degenerative arthritis. The arthropathy affects up to 50% of patients with hemochromatosis and generally resembles osteoarthritis; however, it involves the metacarpophalangeal joints and shoulders, joints not typically affected by generalized primary osteoarthritis. Attacks of acute pseudogout arthritis may occur in relation to deposition of calcium pyrophosphate dihydrate crystals. Chondrocalcinosis is commonly superimposed on chronic osteoarthritic change in hemochromatosis. The pathogenesis of joint degeneration in hemochromatosis is not clear.

- Arthropathy affects up to 50% of patients with hemochromatosis.

- It involves the metacarpophalangeal joints and shoulders.

Wilson disease. Arthropathy occurs in 50% of adults with Wilson disease, a rare autosomal recessive disorder. This disease is suspected in anyone younger than 40 years with unexplained hepatitis, cirrhosis, or movement disorder. The diagnosis is suggested when the serum level of ceruloplasmin is less than 200 mg/L. Arthropathy is unusual in children with the disease. The radiologic appearance varies somewhat from that of primary osteoarthritis. There are more subchondral cysts, sclerosis, cortical irregularities, and radiodense lesions, which occur centrally and at the joint margins. Focal areas of bone fragmentation occur, but they are not related to neuropathy. Although chondrocalcinosis occurs, calcium pyrophosphate dihydrate crystals have not been observed in the synovial fluid.

- Arthropathy occurs in 50% of adults with Wilson disease.
- Arthropathy is unusual in children.

Apatite microcrystals. They are associated with degenerative arthritis and are found in patients with hypothyroidism, hyperparathyroidism, and acromegaly. They occur without an associated endocrinopathy. The role of microcrystalline disease in the progression of osteoarthritis is not clear, especially in the absence of acute recurrent flares of pseudogout.

Neuroarthropathy (Charcot joint). Neuroarthropathy commonly affects patients with diabetes mellitus. Men and women are equally affected. Patients with diabetic neuroarthropathy have had diabetes an average of 16 years. Frequently, the diabetes is poorly controlled. Diabetic peripheral neuropathy causes blunted pain perception and poor proprioception. Repeated microtrauma, overt trauma, small vessel occlusive disease (diabetes), and neuropathic dystrophic effects on bone contribute to neuroarthropathy.

Patients can present with an acute arthritic condition that includes swelling, erythema, and warmth. The foot, particularly the tarsometatarsal joint, is involved most commonly in diabetics. Patients usually describe milder pain than the condition would suggest, and they walk with an antalgic limp. Callus formation occurs over the weight-bearing site of bony damage, and the callus subsequently blisters and ulcerates. Infection can spread from skin ulcers to the bone. Osteomyelitis frequently complicates diabetic neuroarthropathy. Radiography shows disorganized normal joint architecture. Bone and cartilage fragments later coalesce to form characteristic sclerotic loose bodies. There is an attempt at reconstruction with new bone formation. This periosteal new bone is inhibited by small vessel ischemic change in some diabetics. Diabetic osteopathy is a second form of neuroarthropathy. Osteopenia of para-articular areas, particularly the distal metacarpals and proximal phalanges, results in rapidly progressive osteolysis and juxta-articular cortical defects. This can be associated with osteomyelitis.

Initial treatment in diabetics includes good local foot care, treatment of infection, and protected weight bearing. Involvement of the knee, lumbar spine, and upper extremity is uncommon in diabetics. Classically, hip and spinal neuroarthropathy is caused by tertiary syphilis, and shoulder neuroarthropathy is associated with cervical syringomyelia.

- Neuroarthropathy (Charcot joint) most commonly affects the feet and ankles of patients with diabetes mellitus.
- Neuroarthropathy is a consequence of peripheral neuropathy and local injury.
- Osteomyelitis is caused by skin ulcers extending to the bone and should be suspected when an affected diabetic has sudden worsening of his or her glucose control.

Aseptic necrosis of the bone. Aseptic necrosis of the bone, also known as avascular necrosis of bone, may lead to collapse of the articular surface and subsequent osteoarthritis. It usually occurs in the hip after femoral neck fracture. Systemic corticosteroid therapy increases the risk of aseptic necrosis. Aseptic necrosis of the bone has other causes, including alcoholism, sickle cell disease, and systemic lupus erythematosus (Table 22-7). No underlying cause can be identified in 10% to 25% of patients.

Aseptic necrosis of bone usually affects the hips, shoulders, knees, or ankles. Treatment is conservative, including reduced weight bearing and analgesics. Some investigators have treated patients successfully with vascularized bone grafts in the bed of necrotic trabecular bone, although controlled studies are not available. Core decompression may help with pain but does not influence progression to gonarthritis. When there is evidence of cortical bone collapse, progression to advanced osteoarthritis is inevitable. The most sensitive test for aseptic necrosis is magnetic resonance imaging. Plain radiography is insensitive to early aseptic necrosis.

- Aseptic necrosis usually occurs in the hip after femoral neck fracture and may lead to osteoarthritis.
- Alcoholism and corticosteroid use are other common causes of avascular necrosis.

Hypertrophic osteoarthropathy. Hypertrophic osteoarthropathy is characterized by clubbing of the fingernails and painful distal long bone periostitis. The patient may have a noninflammatory arthritis at the ankles, knees, or wrists. This condition complicates primary and metastatic pulmonary malignancies, chronic pulmonary infections, cystic fibrosis, and hypoxic congenital heart disease. Treatment is usually symptomatic.

Hemophilic arthropathy. Patients with hemophilia and recurrent hemarthroses are at risk for hemophilic arthropathy,

Table 22-7 Mnemonic Device for Causes of Aseptic Necrosis of Bone

A	Alcohol, atherosclerotic vascular disease
S	Steroids, sickle cell anemia, storage disease (Gaucher disease)
E	Emboli (fat, cholesterol)
P	Postradiation necrosis
T	Trauma
I	Idiopathic
C	Connective tissue disease (especially SLE), caisson disease

SLE, systemic lupus erythematosus.

a type of progressive degenerative arthropathy that is more destructive than primary osteoarthritis. Widening of the intercondylar notch of the knees is an early radiographic feature suggesting the diagnosis of this condition.

Radiographic Features of Osteoarthritis

The radiographic features of osteoarthritis do not always predict the extent of symptoms. Common radiographic features include osteophyte formation, asymmetric joint-space narrowing, subchondral bony sclerosis, subchondral cysts, and buttressing of angle joints. Later bony changes include malalignment and deformity (Fig. 22-4). In the spine, the radiographic finding called spondylosis includes anterolateral spinous osteophytes, degenerative disk disease with disk-space

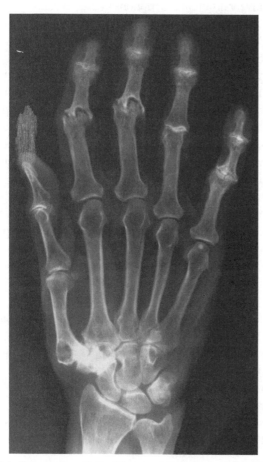

Fig. 22-4. Severe osteoarthritis. Hypertrophic changes, asymmetric joint-space narrowing, and subchondral sclerosis are prominent at the interphalangeal joints and at the first carpometacarpal joint. Note that the metacarpophalangeal joints are completely spared, distinguishing this arthritis from rheumatoid arthritis. Also, there is joint-space narrowing and sclerosis at the base of the thumb at the first carpometacarpal joint and between the trapezium and the scaphoid. Osteoarthritis does not affect equally the entire wrist compartment. The involvement seen here is the most common. An additional interesting feature seen here is central erosions at the second and third proximal interphalangeal joints. This variant occasionally has been called "erosive osteoarthritis."

narrowing, and facet sclerosis. A defect in the bony structure of the posterior neural arch produces spondylolysis. With bilateral spondylolysis, subluxation of one vertebra on another may occur, a condition called spondylolisthesis. The causes of spondylolisthesis are trauma, osteoarthritis, and congenital. No laboratory studies of blood are useful in the diagnosis of osteoarthritis.

- Common radiographic features of osteoarthritis include osteophyte formation, asymmetric joint-space narrowing, subchondral bony sclerosis, subchondral cysts, and buttressing of angle joints.
- No laboratory studies of blood are useful in the diagnosis of osteoarthritis.

Therapy for Osteoarthritis

Therapeutic goals include relieving pain, preserving joint motion and function, and preventing further injury and wear of cartilage. Weight loss (important in knee osteoarthritis), use of canes or crutches, correction of postural abnormalities, and proper shoe support are helpful measures. Isometric or isotonic range-of-motion exercises and muscle strengthening provide para-articular structures with extra support and help reduce symptoms. Relief of muscle spasm with local application of heat or cold to decrease pain can help.

Initial drug therapy should be analgesics, such as acetaminophen (1 g 4 times daily as needed). Nonsteroidal antiinflammatory drugs are beneficial for inflammatory flares of osteoarthritis and usually do not need to be taken in antiinflammatory doses every day. Selective use of opioid analgesics can be considered for disabling pain, especially in persons who are not surgical candidates. Intra-articular corticosteroids offer some temporary relief but should be used only if there is a symptomatic effusion or synovitis. Injections of hyaluronic acid into the knee joint may provide short-term improvement in symptomatic osteoarthritis in selected patients.

Joint arthroplasty may relieve pain, stabilize joints, and improve function. Total joint arthroplasty is very successful at the knee or hip. Table 22-8 describes the indications for total joint arthroplasty in radiographically advanced osteoarthritis. Surgical treatment for osteoarthritis of the shoulder is usually reserved for patients with intractable pain. Tibial osteotomy redistributes knee-joint forces. Arthroscopy removes loose bodies and trims torn menisci to correct lockup or giving way of the joint. Herniated disks or spinal stenosis with radicular symptoms may require decompression.

- Simple analgesics such as acetaminophen are the first choice for treating osteoarthritis.

Table 22-8 Indications for Total Joint Arthroplasty

Radiographically advanced osteoarthritis
Night pain that cannot be modified by changing position
Lockup or giving way of the weight-bearing joint associated
  with falls or near falls
Joint symptoms compromise activities of daily living

ARTHRITIS IN CHRONIC RENAL FAILURE

Up to 75% of patients undergoing chronic renal dialysis have musculoskeletal complaints after 4 years of dialysis. Renal failure arthritis affects the interphalangeal joints, metacarpophalangeal joints, wrists, shoulders, and knees. Symmetric joint-space narrowing and para-articular osteoporosis, subchondral cysts, and erosions have been described. There is no osteophytosis to confuse this condition with osteoarthritis. The synovial fluid is noninflammatory, and the synovitis on biopsy is nonspecific. Possible causes of this arthritis include apatite microcrystal deposition, hyperparathyroidism, and renal failure amyloidosis. Aseptic necrosis occasionally affects large joints.

After 10 years of hemodialysis, 65% of patients have pathologic or radiologic evidence of amyloid deposition (renal failure amyloid arthropathy). The amyloid is composed of β_2-microglobulin, is arthrotropic, and results in complete joint-space loss that occurs over a 3- to 12-month period. Shoulder pain and stiffness syndrome and carpal tunnel syndrome are strongly related to this amyloid deposition. Currently, treatment is aimed at relieving the symptoms.

- Up to 75% of patients undergoing chronic renal dialysis have musculoskeletal complaints after 4 years of dialysis.
- Destructive arthritis, shoulder pain and stiffness syndrome, and carpal tunnel syndrome are strongly related to amyloid deposition.

NONARTICULAR RHEUMATISM

Fibromyalgia

Fibromyalgia is characterized by chronic diffuse musculoskeletal pain. Older synonyms include fibrositis, tension myalgias, generalized nonarticular rheumatism, and psychogenic rheumatism. For the diagnosis, the pain should be present for at least 3 months and should involve areas on both sides of the body above and below the waist and some part of the axial skeleton. Symptoms should not be explainable on the basis of other coexisting diseases or conditions. A high tender point count is an additional obligatory criterion for classification of fibromyalgia. Fibromyalgia affects 2% to 10% of all populations studied and 15% of all general medical patients seen by internists; 75% to 95% of all patients are women. It is unusual for the diagnosis to be made in a person younger than 12 years or after age 65. Of the patients (or their parents), 60% recall childhood growing pains (leg pains). Fibromyalgia is the second most common reason (after the common cold) for lost workdays.

- Fibromyalgia: chronic diffuse musculoskeletal pain.
- Fibromyalgia affects 2%-10% of all populations studied; 75%-95% of patients are women.

Symptoms

Patients typically describe pain all over the body and use qualitatively different descriptions of the pain and discomfort than used by patients with rheumatoid arthritis. Patients localize the pain poorly, referring it to muscle attachment sites or muscles. The discomfort may be worse late in the day after activity. Some patients report morning stiffness, but it is usually not as long or as severe as in patients with inflammatory arthritis. Physical activity or changes in the weather typically aggravate the symptoms. Most patients describe nonrestorative, nonrestful sleep. Anxiety is common. Depression is not uncommonly associated. Other patient complaints can include subjective joint swelling (without objective synovitis on examination), arthralgias, headaches, and paresthesias. About a third of patients have visceral symptoms, including urinary irritability, pelvic pain, temporomandibular joint symptoms, and irritable bowel syndrome. The onset of fibromyalgia can occur after an acute illness, such as a viral syndrome, or after trauma.

- Patients with fibromyalgia typically describe pain all over the body.
- Physical activity or weather changes typically aggravate the symptoms.
- Headaches, paresthesias, numbness, and irritable bowel symptoms are common.
- The onset of fibromyalgia occurs after an acute illness, typically a viral syndrome, in more than half of patients.

Diagnosis

A detailed history and physical examination will exclude most rheumatologic and neurologic diseases. The finding of painful points at muscle attachment sites supports the diagnosis of fibromyalgia. Laboratory evaluation should include a complete blood count, erythrocyte sedimentation rate, thyroid function studies, and baseline chemistry studies of electrolytes, creatinine, calcium, and liver function. In selected cases, if liver transaminase values are increased, then creatine kinase and hepatitis serologic tests may be indicated. Radiographs are helpful for excluding other diseases. There is no diagnostic test for fibromyalgia. If sleep disturbance is prominent, sometimes sleep studies are helpful because some patients with sleep apnea have fibromyalgia symptoms.

- The finding of painful points at muscle attachment sites supports the diagnosis of fibromyalgia.
- No laboratory test confirms the diagnosis of fibromyalgia.

Natural History

Fibromyalgia is a chronic waxing and waning condition. Patients have periods of pain and dysfunction alternating with variable periods of feeling reasonably well. Over a period of years, a patient's symptoms and concerns can shift considerably from musculoskeletal concerns to fatigue or other associated symptoms. There is no increased physical disability in patients who have had fibromyalgia for longer periods in comparison with those for whom the diagnosis is recent. Treatment includes reassurance and education, addressing sleep problems, and establishing an exercise program. NSAIDs, simple analgesics, and medications to help with sleep (such as tricyclic antidepressants) have a role in some patients. Chronic pain management techniques may be helpful for patients with impaired life skills.

- In fibromyalgia, symptoms wax and wane.
- There is no progressive physical disability.

Low Back Pain

One-third of all people older than 50 years have episodes of acute low back pain. Chronic low back pain is the number one compensable work-related injury. The many causes of low back pain include mechanical, neurologic, inflammatory, infectious, neoplastic, and metabolic and referred pain from the viscera. Only 3% of patients presenting with acute low back pain have an organic cause not apparent after the initial interview and physical examination. Clinical suspicion of acute spinal cord compromise, spinal infection, or neoplasm requires immediate evaluation and prompt therapy. More than 90% find relief on their own or with the help of a medical practitioner within the first 6 weeks after symptoms occur.

- Only 3% of patients presenting with acute low back pain have an organic cause not apparent after the initial interview and physical examination.

Diagnosis

The most important consideration during the initial evaluation of acute low back pain is the possibility of severe compromise of the spinal cord or cauda equina. In the absence of evidence for acute spinal cord compromise, spinal infection, or neoplastic involvement, immediate pursuit of a cause for the acute back pain is often not helpful. Objective leg weakness or bladder or bowel dysfunction is an indication for more extensive examination and possible surgical decompression. Substantial weight loss or pain that increases with recumbency suggests a neoplastic or infectious process. Pain that worsens with coughing, straining, or sneezing suggests irritation of the dura mater. Radiating pain, weakness, or numbness in an extremity implicates irritation of a spinal nerve root. Exertional calf or thigh cramping but normal peripheral pulses suggest pseudoclaudication (spinal stenosis). Pseudoclaudication symptoms improve with leaning forward on a shopping cart while walking or with sitting (not standing still). Referred pain from an abdominal, pelvic, or hip area suggests an extra-axial cause. An insidious onset with prominent morning stiffness suggests an inflammatory axial arthropathy.

- Objective leg weakness or bladder or bowel dysfunction is an indication for more extensive examination.
- Substantial weight loss or pain that interferes with sleep suggests a neoplastic or infectious process.
- Exertional calf or thigh cramping but normal peripheral pulses suggest pseudoclaudication.
- An insidious onset with prominent morning stiffness suggests an inflammatory axial arthropathy.

In the absence of specific historical or physical examination findings, laboratory or plain radiographic findings often are unrevealing. The radiographic findings of spondylosis, disk degeneration, facet osteoarthritis, transitional lumbosacral segments, Schmorl nodes, spina bifida occulta, or mild scoliosis are often incidental findings not relevant to a patient's complaints of acute back pain. The routine use of bone scans, electromyography, computed tomography, or magnetic resonance imaging is usually not necessary to evaluate acute low back pain. The indications for spinal radiography in patients with acute low back pain are listed in Table 22-9.

Treatment

The treatment of acute nonspecific low back pain begins with reassuring the patient, because 90% of all patients with acute low back pain have considerable improvement in 6 weeks. Temporary modification of activities by empowering the patient to adjust lifestyle and demands works best. Bed rest should never be prescribed for more than 3 days to treat acute nonspecific low back pain, because longer bed rest has not been shown to be more beneficial. Short-term use of narcotic analgesics or tramadol can supplement the use of acetaminophen, nonsteroidal anti-inflammatory drugs, and muscle relaxants such as cyclobenzaprine. Physical therapy measures include

Table 22-9   Indications for Spinal Radiography in Patients
With Acute Low Back Pain

First episode of acute back pain is after age 50
History of back disease
History of back surgery
History of neoplasm
Acute history of direct trauma to the back
Fever
Weight loss
Severe pain unrelieved in any position
Neurologic symptoms or signs

---

local heat and ice massage. Pelvic traction and transcutaneous electrical nerve stimulation add little to the management of acute nonspecific low back pain. Epidural glucocorticosteroid injections are best suited to acute disk herniation, although their role is controversial. Injections into the facets are helpful occasionally, particularly if the patient describes a locking or catching as part of the pain syndrome.

- In 90% of patients, acute low back pain (local or sciatic presentations) remits within 6 weeks.
- Clinical suspicion of acute spinal cord compromise, spinal infection, or neoplasm requires immediate evaluation and prompt therapy.
- Pelvic traction and transcutaneous electrical nerve stimulation add little to the management of acute nonspecific low back pain.

Bursitis

A bursa is a closed sac containing a small amount of synovial fluid and lined with a membrane similar to that surrounding a diarthrodial joint. Bursae are present in the areas where tendons and muscles move over bony prominences. Additional bursae form in response to irritative stimuli. Trauma or overuse, microcrystalline disease, chronic inflammatory arthritis, and infection cause bursitis. Treatment of aseptic bursitis involves strict immobilization, ice compresses, nonsteroidal anti-inflammatory drugs, bursal aspiration, corticosteroid injections, and, occasionally, physical therapy. Glucocorticosteroids should not be given if there is a clinical suggestion of sepsis.

- Always consider infection or microcrystalline disease in the differential diagnosis of acute bursitis.

Septic bursitis may result from puncture wounds or cellulitis or occur after a local injection. Half of the time, there is no portal of entry for infection in septic superficial bursitis (olecranon and prepatellar bursae). The organisms frequently responsible for infection are staphylococci and streptococci. Patients with septic superficial bursitis present with localized pain and swelling. Warmth about the area of the superficial bursa should raise the possibility of a septic bursa. If there is doubt, the bursa should be aspirated with strict aseptic technique. The needle should enter from the side through uninvolved skin—not at the point of maximal fluctuance—to avoid creating a chronic draining fistula.

When infection is suspected, patients should be treated empirically with antistaphylococcal and antistreptococcal oral antibiotics, pending the microbiologic results. Gram stains are positive in only 40% to 60% of patients. The number of leukocytes in infected bursal fluid can be low compared with that in infected joint fluid. This may be due to the modest blood supply of the bursae compared with that of joints. Patients with more severe infections or with associated cellulitis frequently do not respond to outpatient management. They should be hospitalized and given antibiotics intravenously, and the affected part should be immobilized for 3 or 4 days. Repeated aspirations or percutaneous suction drainage may be necessary until the fluid stops accumulating. In chronic cases, surgical bursectomy may be indicated.

- Septic bursitis frequently occurs without evidence of a portal of entry.
- Bursal warmth is the best predictor of infection.
- Gram stains are positive in only 40%-60% of patients.
- The number of leukocytes in infected bursal fluid can be low.
- Patients with more severe infections should be hospitalized.

Polymyalgia Rheumatica

Polymyalgia rheumatica is a clinical syndrome usually characterized by the onset of aching and morning stiffness in the proximal musculature (hip and shoulder girdles). It is more common in females than males and is usually seen in patients older than 60 years. Patients usually have an increased erythrocyte sedimentation rate; autoantibodies including rheumatoid factor and antinuclear antibody are usually negative or normal. A small number of patients may have a normal sedimentation rate at presentation. The C-reactive protein value is usually increased in these cases. The presence of other specific diseases such as rheumatoid arthritis, chronic infection, inflammatory myositis, or malignancy should be excluded. Patients with polymyalgia rheumatica have prompt (within 24-72 hours) response to small doses of prednisone (10-15 mg daily).

- Typical clinical scenario: An elderly patient presents with aching and morning stiffness in the proximal musculature, increased erythrocyte sedimentation rate, and negative rheumatoid factor and antinuclear antibody tests.

Features and Differential Diagnosis

Patients with polymyalgia rheumatica complain of stiffness and pain. This stiffness is most prominent in the mornings and after prolonged sitting. They also have problems getting comfortable at night to sleep. They occasionally have mild constitutional symptoms, including sweats, fevers, anorexia, and weight loss. Very prominent constitutional features and markedly increased erythrocyte sedimentation rate could suggest associated giant cell arteritis. Extremity edema or oligoarticular synovitis can occur, particularly at the knees, wrists, and shoulders. Radionuclide joint scans in patients with active polymyalgia rheumatica confirm hip and shoulder synovitis. Polyarticular small joint arthritis is not a feature. Table 22-10 summarizes the rheumatic syndromes and other diseases that occasionally present with a polymyalgia rheumatica-like syndrome. Depression should be considered in patients with atypical features. Clinical evaluation and screening laboratory tests usually distinguish polymyalgia rheumatica from these other conditions.

- Polymyalgia rheumatica: stiffness is more prolonged in the mornings and after prolonged sitting.
- Prominent constitutional features and markedly increased erythrocyte sedimentation rate could suggest associated giant cell arteritis.
- Extremity edema or oligoarticular synovitis can occur.

Pathogenesis and Relationship to Giant Cell Arteritis

Polymyalgia rheumatica can begin before, appear simultaneously with, or develop after the symptoms of giant cell arteritis. The pathogenesis of polymyalgia rheumatica is unknown. Clinicians appreciate the close relationship between giant cell arteritis and polymyalgia rheumatica. Up to 15% of patients with polymyalgia rheumatica also have giant cell arteritis. Familial aggregation and increased incidence in patients of northern European background suggest a genetic predisposition. HLA-DR4 is associated with these conditions more commonly than would be expected by chance. Among patients with giant cell arteritis, 40% have symptoms of polymyalgia rheumatica during the course of their disease.

- Up to 15% of patients with polymyalgia rheumatica also have giant cell arteritis.
- Among patients with active giant cell arteritis, 40% have symptoms of polymyalgia rheumatica.
- Polymyalgia rheumatica can begin before, appear simultaneously with, or develop after the symptoms of giant cell arteritis.

Treatment

All patients with polymyalgia rheumatica should respond completely after 3 to 5 days of treatment with prednisone, 10 to 20 mg/day. Sometimes, split-dose (5 mg 3 times daily) prednisone is more effective than a single daily dose of 15 mg. Patients should be followed clinically, and usually the erythrocyte sedimentation rate should be measured monthly to confirm the disease flare. Polymyalgia rheumatica is thought to be a self-limited disease, although relapses occur. Prednisone treatment is discontinued in more than half the patients within 2 years.

- All patients with polymyalgia rheumatica should respond completely after 3-5 days of treatment with prednisone.
- Polymyalgia rheumatica is thought to be a self-limited disease, although relapses occur.

VASCULITIC SYNDROMES

Vasculitis, or angiitis, is an inflammatory disease of blood vessels. It often causes damage to the vessel wall and stenosis or occlusion of the vessel lumen by thrombosis and progressive intimal proliferation of the vessel. Vasculitic symptoms reflect the nonspecific systemic features of inflammation (constitutional features) and the ischemic consequences of vascular occlusion. The distribution of the vascular lesions and the size of the blood vessels involved vary considerably in different vasculitic syndromes and in different patients with the same syndrome. Vasculitis can be transient, chronic, self-limited, or progressive. It can be the primary abnormality or secondary to another systemic process. Histopathologic classification does not distinguish local from systemic illness or secondary from primary insult. The key clinical features suggestive of vasculitis are listed in Table 22-11. Vasculitis "look-alikes," or simulators, are listed in Table 22-12. These diseases and conditions should be considered whenever the patient's condition suggests vasculitis. A scheme for diagnosing vasculitis

Table 22-10 Systemic Illnesses Presenting With a Polymyalgia-Like Syndrome

Rheumatic syndromes	Other systemic illnesses
Systemic vasculitis	Paraneoplastic syndromes
Myositis	Systemic amyloidosis
Systemic lupus erythematosus	Infectious endocarditis
Seronegative rheumatoid arthritis	Hyperthyroidism
Polyarticular osteoarthritis	Hypothyroidism
Fibromyalgia	Hyperparathyroidism
Remitting seronegative, symmetric synovitis and peripheral edema	Osteomalacia
	Depression

Table 22-11 Clinical Features That Suggest Vasculitis

Constitutional features
    Fatigue, fever, weight loss, and anorexia
Skin lesions
    Palpable purpura, necrotic ulcers, livedo reticularis,
      urticaria, nodules, and digital infarcts
Arthralgia or arthritis
Myalgia or prominent fibrositis
    Polymyalgia rheumatica symptoms
Claudication or phlebitis
Headache
Cerebrovascular accident
Neuropathy
    Mononeuritis multiplex
Hypertension
Abnormal renal sediment
Pulmonary abnormalities
    Pulmonary hemorrhage, pulmonary nodules with cavities
Abdominal pain or intestinal hemorrhage
Nonspecific indicators of inflammation
    Anemia, thrombocytosis, low levels of albumin, elevated
      erythrocyte sedimentation rate, increased levels of liver
      enzymes, or eosinophilia

Table 22-12 Syndromes That Mimic Vasculitis

Cardiac myxoma with embolization
Infective endocarditis
Thrombotic thrombocytopenic purpura
Atheroembolism: cholesterol or calcium emboli
Ergotism
Pseudoxanthoma elasticum
Ehlers-Danlos type 4
Neurovasculopathy secondary to antiphospholipid syndrome
Arterial coarctation or dysplasia
Infectious angiitis
    Lyme disease
    Rickettsial infection
    HIV infection

HIV, human immunodeficiency virus.

Table 22-13 The Diagnostic Approach to Vasculitis

Proper clinical suspicion for vasculitis[*]
Consider conditions that mimic vasculitis
Recognize clinical pattern of involvement
Define the extent and severity of disease
Narrow the diagnostic possibilities with laboratory tests
Select the confirmatory study
    Efficient (highest-yield study)
    Safe as possible
Weigh urgency of diagnosis with risk of
    Diagnostics
    Therapeutics

[*]Table 22-11.

is outlined in Table 22-13. The ability to recognize characteristic clinical patterns of involvement is very helpful in making the diagnosis of systemic necrotizing vasculitis (Fig. 22-5).

- Vasculitic symptoms reflect the nonspecific systemic features of inflammation (constitutional features) and the ischemic consequences of vascular occlusion.

Specific Vasculitic Syndromes

Giant Cell Arteritis

Giant cell arteritis, also known as temporal arteritis, predominantly affects persons older than 50 years. The prevalence exceeds 223 cases per 100,000 persons older than 50. It is most common in persons of northern European ancestry. Females outnumber males by 3:1. Polymyalgia rheumatica symptoms may develop in 40% to 50% of all patients with giant cell arteritis. Up to 15% of patients with polymyalgia rheumatica have temporal artery biopsy findings positive for giant cell arteritis. There is considerable morbidity with this disease; however, the rate of blindness is declining. The mortality rate for patients with giant cell arteritis is similar to that for the general population.

- Giant cell arteritis is most common in persons of northern European ancestry.
- Polymyalgia rheumatica develops in 40% of patients with giant cell arteritis.
- Up to 15% of patients with polymyalgia rheumatica have temporal artery biopsy findings positive for giant cell arteritis.

Pathology—Giant cell arteritis involves the primary and secondary branches of the aorta in a segmental or patchy fashion. However, any artery, and occasionally veins, can be affected. It is unusual for intracranial arteries to be involved. Histopathologically, all layers of the vessel wall are extensively disrupted, with intimal thickening and a prominent mononuclear and histiocytic infiltrate. Multinucleated giant cells infiltrate the vessel wall in 50% of cases. Fragmentation

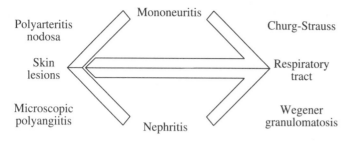

Fig. 22-5. Common organ involvement in systemic vasculitis.

Table 22-14   Classic Clinical Features of Giant Cell Arteritis

Fever, weight loss, fatigue
Polymyalgia rheumatica symptoms
Temporal headache
Jaw or tongue claudication
Ocular symptoms
   Blindness
   Diplopia
   Ptosis
Scalp tenderness
Dry cough
Peripheral large vessel vasculitis (10%)

and disintegration of the internal elastic membrane, the other characteristic features, are closely associated with the accumulation of giant cells and vascular occlusive symptoms.

- Giant cell arteritis affects primary and secondary branches of the aorta in a segmental or patchy fashion.

Clinical features—Early clinical features of giant cell arteritis include temporal headache, polymyalgia rheumatica symptoms, fatigue, and fever. The classic features of this disease are included in Table 22-14. Arteritis of the branches of the ophthalmic or posterior ciliary arteries causes ischemia of the optic nerve (ischemic optic neuritis) and blindness. Less often, retinal arterioles are occluded. Blindness occurs in fewer than 15% of untreated patients. Large peripheral artery involvement in giant cell arteritis occurs in about 10% of patients. Extremity claudication, Raynaud phenomenon, aortic dissection, decreased pulses, and vascular bruits suggest large peripheral artery involvement. Patients with large peripheral artery involvement do not differ from those with more classic giant cell arteritis, either histologically or with regard to laboratory findings. Late features include a markedly increased risk of thoracic aortic aneurysm.

- Typical clinical scenario: A 60-year-old patient presents with temporal headache, polymyalgia rheumatica-like symptoms, fatigue, and fever. Laboratory tests reveal a markedly increased sedimentation rate. Physical examination reveals scalp tenderness.
- Blindness occurs in <15% of untreated patients.

Diagnosis—The temporal artery biopsy specimen should be at least 3 cm long to compensate for patchy involvement. In 15% of patients, the biopsy is positive on the opposite side if that on the initial side is negative. Typical laboratory abnormalities in acute active giant cell arteritis include a markedly increased erythrocyte sedimentation rate, moderate normochromic anemia, and thrombocytosis. A mild increase in liver enzyme values, most typically alkaline phosphatase,

occurs in one-third of patients because of granulomatous hepatitis. The erythrocyte sedimentation rate is rarely normal in patients with active giant cell arteritis. The diagnostic criteria for giant cell arteritis are given in Table 22-15.

- The temporal artery biopsy specimen should be at least 3 cm long to compensate for patchy involvement.
- In 15% of patients, the biopsy is positive on the opposite side if that on the initial side is negative.
- Typical laboratory abnormalities: markedly increased erythrocyte sedimentation rate, moderate normochromic anemia, and thrombocytosis.

Treatment—Treatment is initiated with corticosteroids when the diagnosis of giant cell arteritis is considered and the biopsy is requested. A temporal artery biopsy specimen remains positive for disease even after several weeks of corticosteroid treatment. Initial treatment includes prednisone, typically 40 to 60 mg/day. A higher dose of corticosteroids can be given parenterally in cases of visual or life-threatening symptoms. Most symptoms of giant cell arteritis begin to respond within 24 hours after corticosteroid therapy is initiated. Visual changes

Table 22-15   Diagnostic Criteria for Giant Cell Arteritis

Temporal artery biopsy findings positive for classic giant cell arteritis

or

Four of the five following criteria:
   Tender, swollen temporal artery
   Jaw claudication
   Blindness
   Polymyalgia rheumatica symptoms
   Rapid response to corticosteroids

that are present for more than a few hours are often irreversible. Alternate-day administration of corticosteroids does not control symptoms in at least half of patients.

- Treatment is initiated with corticosteroids when the diagnosis of giant cell arteritis is considered and the biopsy is requested.
- Initial treatment: prednisone, typically 40-60 mg/day.
- Alternate-day administration of corticosteroids does not initially control symptoms in at least half of patients.

Outcome—Giant cell arteritis typically has a self-limited course. In 24 months, half of patients are able to discontinue treatment with corticosteroids. An effective steroid-sparing agent has not been identified, but methotrexate or azathioprine has been used in some patients. The diagnosis of giant cell arteritis does not influence mortality rates. Relapse may occur in a third of patients, and a thoracic or abdominal aneurysm develops in a third.

- Giant cell arteritis typically has a self-limited course over about 2 years, although relapses and late consequences, including aortic aneurysms, occur.

Takayasu Arteritis

Takayasu arteritis is also known as aortic arch syndrome or pulseless disease. Each year, about 2.6 new cases per 1,000,000 population occur. Most patients are between the ages of 15 and 40 years. At least 80% of them are female. This disease is more common in the Orient, Latin America, and Eastern Europe. Its pathologic features cannot be distinguished from those of giant cell arteritis. Takayasu arteritis affects the aorta and its primary branches. The arterial wall is irregularly thickened, with luminal narrowing, dilatations, aneurysms, and distortions. The aortic valve and coronary ostia can be involved.

- Takayasu arteritis: most patients are female, between the ages of 15 and 40 years.
- The aorta and its primary branches are affected.

Clinical and laboratory features—The constitutional features of fever, weight loss, fatigue, and arthralgia can precede symptoms of ischemia to the brain or claudication of the extremities. Renovascular hypertension, pulmonary hypertension, and coronary artery insufficiency can complicate Takayasu arteritis. Cutaneous vasculitis, erythema nodosum, and synovitis occasionally occur in cases of active Takayasu arteritis. Compromise of the cerebral vasculature can lead to dizziness, blurry or fading vision, syncope, and, occasionally, stroke. Physical examination findings confirm vascular bruits, absence of peripheral pulses, and, occasionally, fever. When the disease

is active, abnormal values of laboratory studies reveal increased erythrocyte sedimentation rate, normochromic anemia, and thrombocytosis. The diagnosis can be confirmed by conventional angiography, although magnetic resonance angiography may become the imaging method of choice.

- Typical clinical scenario: A young patient presents with fever, weight loss, fatigue, and arthralgia. Physical examination reveals carotid bruits and absence of peripheral pulses. Laboratory testing reveals increased erythrocyte sedimentation rate.

Treatment and outcome—Corticosteroid therapy alone is usually adequate for controlling the inflammation. Methotrexate or cyclophosphamide treatment is indicated in resistant cases. On average, patients receive corticosteroids for about 2 years. Late stenotic complications are amenable to vascular operation and bypass grafting. Survival is more than 90% at 10 years. Congestive heart failure from previous coronary artery involvement and cerebrovascular accidents are major causes of mortality.

- Renovascular hypertension, pulmonary hypertension, and coronary artery insufficiency can complicate Takayasu arteritis.
- Survival is >90% at 10 years.

Polyarteritis

Polyarteritis is a systemic necrotizing vasculitis that occurs by itself or in association with several diseases (secondary). When it occurs as a primary vasculitis, it is called "polyarteritis nodosa." A necrotizing vasculitis that is indistinguishable from polyarteritis nodosa can occur in association with rheumatoid arthritis, systemic lupus erythematosus, other connective tissue diseases, cryoglobulinemia, hepatitis-B infection, hairy cell leukemia, and other malignant conditions. Polyarteritis occurs in 1 to 3 patients per year per 100,000 population. The peak incidence occurs at ages 40 to 60 years, although all age groups are affected. Males are more commonly affected than females. If untreated, the systemic form of polyarteritis is associated with a less than 15% survival at 5 years.

- Polyarteritis: systemic necrotizing vasculitis that occurs by itself or in association with several diseases.

Pathology—Polyarteritis involves small systemic muscular arteries. Histopathologically, there is a focal transmural inflammation of small muscular arteries marked by fibrinoid necrosis and a pleomorphic, neutrophil-predominant infiltration. Elastic laminae are disrupted, producing a characteristic "blow out" of the vessel wall and microaneurysms. The coexistence of normal, active, and healed areas in the same vessel is unique to polyarteritis.

- Small systemic muscular arteries are involved in polyarteritis.
- The coexistence of normal, active, and healed areas in the same vessel is unique to polyarteritis.

Clinical features—Polyarteritis is usually a systemic illness associated with prominent constitutional features, including fever, fatigue, weight loss, and, occasionally, myalgia or arthralgia along with manifestations of multisystem involvement such as a rash, peripheral neuropathy, and asymmetric polyarthritis. Virtually any organ can be affected eventually. Other features are listed in Table 22-16. Occasionally, polyarteritis is limited to a single organ or found incidentally associated with cancer at the time of operation and cured by surgical removal. Other cases are limited to isolated involvement of the skin or peripheral nerves.

The two primary forms of polyarteritis include classic polyarteritis nodosa (PAN) and microscopic polyangiitis (MPA). Classic PAN is a necrotizing vasculitis of small and medium-sized arteries and is associated with vascular nephropathy (usually without glomerulonephritis), causing multiple renal infarctions, hypertension, and renal failure. Hypertension develops as a result of angiographically demonstrable renal artery compromise or, less commonly, glomerular involvement. Lung involvement is very uncommon. MPA is a necrotizing vasculitis that affects capillaries, venules, and arterioles and most frequently presents with pauci-immune and sometimes rapidly progressive necrotizing glomerulonephritis. Proteinuria is common and, rarely, a nephrotic syndrome may develop. There is an active urinary sediment, with red blood cells and red cell casts characteristic of glomerular involvement. Renal insufficiency is frequently noted at presentation, and glomerulonephritis causes oliguric renal failure in one-third of all patients. Renal angiograms in MPA are usually normal. Hypertension is uncommon. Lung involvement, including pulmonary capillaritis and hemorrhage, may eventually affect up to one-third of patients with MPA.

Clinically distinguishing between classic PAN and MPA is frequently difficult. Their clinical features and natural history frequently overlap. Antineutrophil cytoplasmic antibodies (ANCA) may help distinguish between them because these antibodies occur mostly in patients with the microscopic form of the disease.

Polyarteritis may be a manifestation or complication of other diseases. This secondary polyarteritis complicates hepatitis B infection, rheumatoid arthritis, Sjögren syndrome, mixed cryoglobulinemia, hairy cell leukemia, myelodysplastic syndrome, and other hematologic malignancies. Secondary polyarteritis is suggested by complement consumption and is histopathologically and clinically indistinguishable from the primary forms of polyarteritis. However, some forms of secondary polyarteritis have favored clinical presentations. For instance, systemic rheumatoid vasculitis most commonly manifests with constitutional symptoms, skin lesions, and neuropathy. It uncommonly causes a necrotizing glomerulonephritis.

- Polyarteritis is usually a systemic illness associated with prominent constitutional features, including fever, fatigue, weight loss, and, occasionally, myalgia or arthralgia along with manifestations of multisystem involvement, including kidney disease, lung lesions, rash, and neuropathy.

Table 22-16 Clinical Features of Polyarteritis

Common features	Uncommon features
Fever, fatigue, weight loss	Coronary arteritis
Arthralgia, arthritis	Myocardial infarction
Myalgia	Congestive heart failure
Mononeuritis multiplex	Central nervous system abnormalities
Focal necrotizing glomerulonephritis	Seizures
Abnormal renal sediment	Cerebrovascular accident
Hypertension	Lung (interstitial pneumonitis)
Skin abnormalities	Eye (retinal hemorrhage)
Palpable purpura	Testicular pain
Livedo reticularis	
Cutaneous infarctions	
Abdominal pain/ischemic bowel	
Liver enzyme abnormalities	

- Classic PAN is distinguished from MPA by aneurysms seen on visceral angiography and the absence of glomerulonephritis or a positive ANCA. Classic PAN usually does not involve the lungs.
- Secondary polyarteritis may be a complication of other diseases.

Diagnosis—Abnormal laboratory findings include normocytic anemia, increased erythrocyte sedimentation rate, and thrombocytosis. MPA presents 90% of the time with positive c-ANCA or myeloperoxidase-specific p-ANCA. Complement consumption is not part of primary polyarteritis. Low complement may be evident if immune complexes such as cryoglobulins are part of the pathogenesis of secondary polyarteritis. Hepatitis B infection is found in a small proportion of patients with ANCA-negative (classic) PAN and should always be sought, because treatment is directed against the infection. Hepatitis C is associated with the secondary polyarteritis that complicates some cases of cryoglobulinemia. Evaluation should document the extent and severity of the condition. The confirmatory test typically is angiography or biopsy of involved tissue showing vasculitis. The biopsy should be of accessible symptomatic tissue. Visceral angiography, including views of the renal and mesenteric arteries, shows saccular or fusiform aneurysm formation coupled with smooth, tapered stenosis alternating with normal or dilated blood vessels (Fig. 22-6).

- MPA often presents with positive myeloperoxidase-specific p-ANCA.
- Hepatitis B infection is found in a small proportion of patients with ANCA-negative (classic) PAN and should always be sought, because treatment is directed against the infection.
- Hepatitis C is associated with the secondary polyarteritis that complicates some cases of cryoglobulinemia.
- Confirmatory test: typically, angiography or biopsy of involved tissue showing vasculitis.
- Visceral angiography shows saccular or fusiform aneurysm formation coupled with smooth, tapered stenosis.
- Consider visceral angiography to make the diagnosis when the patient has significant gastrointestinal symptoms or markedly increased liver enzyme values and no tissue or organ system (nerve, skin) is affected or easily sampled by biopsy. Angiography is abnormal in classic PAN and in cases in which classic PAN and MPA overlap.

Treatment—The cornerstone of treatment is early diagnosis and corticosteroid therapy. Cytotoxic and antimetabolite drugs such as cyclophosphamide, chlorambucil, methotrexate, and azathioprine are often used in combination with

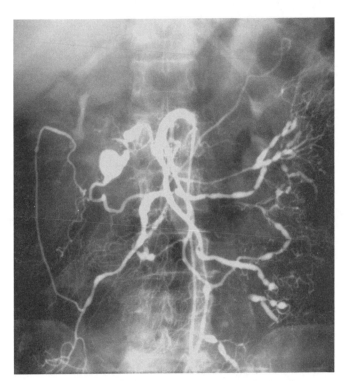

Fig. 22-6. Visceral polyarteritis nodosa. Angiography shows the classic features of smooth tapers followed by normal or dilated vessels. Note the large saccular aneurysm in the hepatic artery. (From Audiovisual Aids Subcommittee of the Education Committee of the American College of Rheumatology: Syllabus: Revised Clinical Slide Collection on the Rheumatic Diseases and 1985, 1988, and 1989 Slide Supplements. Atlanta, Georgia, American College of Rheumatology. By permission.)

corticosteroids. These agents are added when the disease is rapidly progressive, particularly if polyarteritis involves an internal organ such as the kidney, gut, or heart. They also are useful as steroid-sparing agents. When a patient's condition deteriorates in the face of potent treatment, consider possible progression of disease, superimposed infection, or noninflammatory, proliferative, occlusive vasculopathy. Hepatitis-associated polyarteritis is treated best with antiviral drugs.

- Cyclophosphamide, chlorambucil, methotrexate, and azathioprine are often used in conjunction with corticosteroids.

Outcome—In the first year after diagnosis of polyarteritis, deaths are related to the extent of disease activity, particularly gastrointestinal tract ischemia and renal insufficiency. Distinguishing classic PAN from MPA and type of organ involvement may influence treatment, complications, relapse rate, and mortality. After 1 year, complications of treatment, including infections in the immunocompromised patient, contribute most to mortality rates. Survival at 5 years with treatment is between 55% and 60% for MPA and between 75% and 90% for classic PAN.

- In the first year after diagnosis, deaths are related to the extent of disease activity, particularly gastrointestinal tract ischemia and renal insufficiency.
- Complications from treatment affect long-term mortality.
- Typical clinical scenario: A patient presents with fever, fatigue, weight loss, arthralgia, mononeuritis multiplex, and renal failure. Renal angiography shows saccular and fusiform aneurysm formation with smooth, tapered stenosis of the vessels. Laboratory testing shows increased sedimentation rate and negative c- and p-ANCA antibodies. Chest radiography is normal.

Churg-Strauss Vasculitis

Churg-Strauss vasculitis, or Churg-Strauss syndrome, is similar to polyarteritis and usually accounts for 6% to 30% of series that combine polyarteritis and Churg-Strauss syndrome. The median age at onset is about 38 years (range, 15-69 years). Churg-Strauss vasculitis is defined by 1) a history of, or current symptoms of, asthma, 2) peripheral eosinophilia (>1.5×10^9 eosinophils/L), and 3) systemic vasculitis of at least two extrapulmonary organs. There is a slight male predominance. The histopathologic features of the disease include eosinophilic extravascular granulomas and granulomatous or nongranulomatous small vessel necrotizing vasculitis. It typically involves the small arteries, veins, arterioles, and venules.

- Churg-Strauss vasculitis: history of, or current symptoms of, asthma, peripheral eosinophilia (>1.5×10^9 eosinophils/L), and systemic vasculitis of at least two extrapulmonary organs.
- It involves small arteries, veins, arterioles, and venules.

Clinical features—Churg-Strauss syndrome has three clinical stages. Patients need not progress in an orderly manner from one stage to another. There usually is a prodrome of allergic rhinitis, nasal polyposis, or asthma. In the second stage, peripheral blood and tissue eosinophilia develops, suggesting Löffler syndrome. Chronic eosinophilic pneumonia and gastroenteritis may remit or recur over years. The third stage is life-threatening vasculitis. Transient, patchy pulmonary infiltrates or nodules, pleural effusions, pulmonary angiitis and cardiomegaly, eosinophilic gastroenteritis, extravascular necrotizing granulomata of the skin, mononeuritis multiplex, and polyarthritis can complicate Churg-Strauss syndrome. A Churg-Strauss–like syndrome has been reported in some patients treated with the asthma medication zafirlukast (Accolate).

- Churg-Strauss syndrome: prodrome of allergic rhinitis, nasal polyposis, or asthma.
- Peripheral blood and tissue eosinophilia develops.

- Transient, patchy pulmonary infiltrates, extravascular necrotizing granulomata of the skin, and mononeuritis multiplex can complicate Churg-Strauss syndrome.

Treatment and outcome—The 1-year survival with treated Churg-Strauss syndrome is similar to that with polyarteritis. There is more cardiac involvement but fewer renal deaths than in polyarteritis. Treatment includes corticosteroids with or without the addition of cytotoxic agents. The eosinophilia resolves with treatment.

- Churg-Strauss syndrome: more cardiac involvement but fewer renal deaths than in polyarteritis.
- Typical clinical scenario: A patient presents with a history of bronchial asthma with recent worsening of pulmonary symptoms and development of mononeuritis multiplex. There is a history of nasal polyposis. Physical evaluation reveals palpable purpura. Laboratory testing reveals markedly increased eosinophil count.

Buerger Disease

Buerger disease, or thromboangiitis obliterans, occurs almost exclusively in young adult smokers, who typically present with claudication of the instep and loss of digits from ischemic injury. Buerger disease affects the small- and medium-sized arteries and veins of the extremities. Acute vasculitis in Buerger disease is accompanied by characteristic intraluminal thrombus that contains microabscesses. Usually, the disease is arrested when smoking is stopped. In contrast to other forms of vasculitis, Buerger disease is best thought of as a vasculopathy.

- Buerger disease occurs almost exclusively in young adult smokers.
- Patients present with loss of digits from ischemic injury.
- The disease is arrested when smoking is stopped.

Isolated (Primary) Angiitis of the Central Nervous System

Clinical features—Isolated, or primary, angiitis of the central nervous system, once thought to be rare, has a chronic fluctuating and progressive course. The average age of patients presenting with this disease is 45 years. Forty percent of patients have had symptoms for less than 4 weeks at presentation, and another 40% present with symptoms that have been noted for more than 3 months. The most common symptom is headache (mild or severe), often associated with nausea or vomiting. Nonfocal neurologic abnormalities (including confusion, dementia, drowsiness, or coma) may interrupt prolonged periods of apparent remission. Acute stroke-like focal neurologic presentations are increasingly described. Cerebral hemorrhage occurs in fewer than 4% of patients. Focal and nonfocal neurologic abnormalities coexist in half of patients. Systemic features—fever, weight loss, arthralgia, and myalgia—are uncommon and occur in fewer than 20% of patients; seizures occur in about 25%.

- Isolated angiitis of the central nervous system: a chronic fluctuating and progressive course, most commonly without evidence of systemic inflammation.
- Most common symptom is headache.
- Complications include acute strokes, with or without nonfocal neurologic abnormalities (decreased consciousness or cognition).
- Cerebral hemorrhage occurs in <4% of patients.

Diagnosis—There are no reliable noninvasive tests for making the diagnosis. The mainstays of diagnosis are cerebral angiography and biopsy of central nervous system tissues, including the leptomeninges. The cerebrospinal fluid is abnormal in most patients with pathologically documented primary angiitis of the central nervous system. Computed tomography of the head is not specific or sensitive for the condition. Magnetic resonance imaging may be sensitive but does not distinguish this primary angiitis from other vasculopathic or demyelinating lesions of the brain, and it is not useful for following the condition. Patients with a chronic progressive course are more likely to have the diagnosis made pathologically and have abnormal results on examination of the cerebrospinal fluid.

- Mainstays of diagnosis: cerebral angiography and biopsy of central nervous system tissues, including the leptomeninges.

Rheumatologic syndromes that may produce a clinical picture similar to that of primary angiitis of the central nervous system include Cogan syndrome (nonsyphilitic keratitis and vestibular dysfunction), Behçet syndrome (uveitis, oral and genital ulcers, meningitis, and vasculitis), systemic lupus erythematosus, and polyarteritis. Drug-induced vasculopathy (particularly cocaine), demyelinating disease, human immunodeficiency virus (HIV) infection, Lyme disease, syphilis, carcinomatous meningitis, angiocentric immunoproliferative lesions, and antiphospholipid antibody syndrome are also part of the differential diagnosis in patients presenting with a syndrome suggesting primary angiitis of the central nervous system.

Treatment—The treatment for primary angiitis of the central nervous system may be influenced by the clinical subset. Younger patients with acute disease in whom the diagnosis was made with angiography may have a benign course and typically respond well to a short course of treatment with corticosteroids and calcium channel blockers to prevent vasospasm. Patients with a protracted course, abnormal cerebrospinal fluid, and diagnosis made with brain and leptomeningeal biopsy are best treated with combination therapy, including corticosteroids and cytotoxic agents. If untreated, this clinical subset has a high mortality rate.

- The mortality rate is high among patients with histopathologically confirmed or recurrent symptoms treated without cytotoxic agents.

Wegener Granulomatosis

Clinical features—Wegener granulomatosis is a well-recognized pathologic triad of upper and lower respiratory tract necrotizing granulomatous inflammation and focal segmental necrotizing glomerulonephritis. Wegener granulomatosis occurs in less than 1 person annually per 100,000 population. The peak incidence of the disease occurs in the fourth and fifth decades of life. There is a slight male predominance. Eighty-five percent of the patients have generalized disease, including glomerulonephritis; 15% can present with local inflammation involving only the upper respiratory tract or kidneys. The clinical features of this disease are summarized by the mnemonic ELKS: involvement of *e*ar/nose/throat, *l*ung, *k*idney, and *s*kin. Lung involvement most commonly includes thick-walled, centrally cavitating pulmonary nodules. Alveolitis and pulmonary hemorrhage occur in up to 20% of patients. Biopsy in patients with renal involvement shows focal segmental necrotizing glomerulonephritis and, occasionally, granulomatous vasculitis. Skin involvement may include urticaria, petechiae, papules, vesicles, ulcers, pyoderma, and livedo reticularis. Inflammatory arthritis is usually oligoarticular and transient, occurring early in the clinical presentation. Central nervous system involvement includes distal sensory neuropathy, mononeuritis multiplex, and cranial nerve palsies. Conjunctivitis, uveitis, and proptosis are not unusual. Neurosensory hearing loss has been described together with serous otitis and inner ear vasculitis. Wegener granulomatosis-associated subglottic tracheal stenosis due to chondritis should be distinguished from primary polychondritis. Laboratory testing shows a positive c-ANCA test.

- Typical clinical scenario: A 50-year-old patient presents with the triad of upper and lower respiratory tract necrotizing granulomatous inflammation and focal segmental necrotizing glomerulonephritis. Laboratory testing shows a positive c-ANCA test.
- ELKS: involvement of *e*ar/nose/throat, *l*ung, *k*idney, and *s*kin.
- Alveolitis and pulmonary hemorrhage occur in up to 20% of patients.

- Central nervous system involvement: distal sensory neuropathy, mononeuritis multiplex, and cranial nerve palsies.

Pathologic diagnosis—The diagnosis of Wegener granulomatosis may require finding characteristic pathologic features in biopsy specimens. Biopsy of the upper respiratory tract suggests the diagnosis in 55% of patients, but only 20% show granulomata or vasculitis associated with necrosis. An open lung biopsy has a higher diagnostic yield than transbronchial biopsy. Renal biopsies usually document only a focal segmental necrotizing glomerulonephritis. Infrequently, renal biopsy shows vasculitis. Relevant laboratory findings in active Wegener granulomatosis include nonspecific increases in the erythrocyte sedimentation rate and platelet count, normocytic anemia, and low levels of albumin. A positive c-ANCA test in a patient with the clinical features of Wegener granulomatosis may be sufficient for diagnosis, especially if tissue is not easily obtained.

- Laboratory findings: nonspecific increases in erythrocyte sedimentation rate and platelet count, normocytic anemia.
- Diagnosis: positive c-ANCA test and granulomatous inflammation on biopsy.

ANCA—c-ANCA is directed against proteinase 3, a serine protease from azurophilic granules. c-ANCA occurs in more than 90% of active cases of generalized Wegener granulomatosis. Occasionally, it is found in idiopathic crescentic glomerulonephritis, microscopic polyarteritis nodosa, and Churg-Strauss syndrome. The antibody titer tends to correlate with disease activity.

p-ANCA is directed against myeloperoxidase and other neutrophil cytoplasmic constituents. p-ANCA (anti-myeloperoxidase-specific) is found in idiopathic crescentic glomerulonephritis, microscopic polyarteritis nodosa, Churg-Strauss syndrome, Wegener granulomatosis, and other connective tissue diseases. p-ANCA directed against other antigens can occur in patients with inflammatory bowel disease, autoimmune liver disease, other connective tissue diseases, malignancies, and even drug-induced syndromes.

- c-ANCA occurs in >90% of active cases of Wegener granulomatosis.
- p-ANCA is found in many different conditions.

Treatment and outcome—If untreated, generalized Wegener granulomatosis is associated with a mean survival of 5 months and 95% mortality in 1 year. More than 95% of patients eventually have clinical remission with oral cyclophosphamide treatment. Corticosteroids are useful initially, and the dose can be tapered quickly after the disease is controlled. Mortality in the first year of disease is related primarily to the inflammatory process, with pulmonary hemorrhage or renal failure. In subsequent years, drug toxicity may dominate, with opportunistic infection and increasing risk of neoplasm and hemorrhagic cystitis related to the use of cyclophosphamide. Relapses even years after treatment are not uncommon.

- If untreated, generalized Wegener granulomatosis has a mean survival of 5 months.
- Cyclophosphamide has revolutionized the treatment of Wegener granulomatosis and dramatically altered the natural history.
- Corticosteroids are useful initially, and the dose can be tapered quickly after the disease is controlled.

Small Vessel Vasculitis/Cutaneous Vasculitis

Clinical features—Small vessel vasculitis occurs by itself or complicates many infectious, neoplastic, and connective tissue diseases. In the skin, it manifests with urticaria, palpable purpura, livedo reticularis, or skin ulceration. It can be associated with peripheral neuropathy, arthralgia, or synovitis. Mononeuritis multiplex, diffuse pulmonary hemorrhage, and renal vasculitis are complications of systemic small vessel vasculitis as part of the formal primary or secondary vasculitis syndromes already mentioned. Small vessel vasculitis occurs with many illnesses; a partial listing is given in Table 22-17.

- Small vessel vasculitis: occurs by itself or complicates many infectious, neoplastic, and connective tissue diseases.
- In the skin, it manifests with urticaria, palpable purpura, livedo reticularis, or skin ulceration.
- It can complicate most types of primary and secondary systemic vasculitis.

Histopathology—A neutrophilic- or (uncommonly) lymphocytic-predominant infiltrate surrounds small arteries, veins, arterioles, or venules. The histopathologic picture called "leukocytoclastic vasculitis" includes immune complexes deposited in vessel walls, along with fibrin deposition, endothelial cell swelling and necrosis, and a polymorphonuclear leukocytoclasis with scattering of nuclear fragment or nuclear dust. This is a pathologic diagnosis and not a specific clinical condition.

- Classic clinical correlate of leukocytoclastic vasculitis: palpable purpura.

Diagnosis—The clinician must interpret small vessel/cutaneous vasculitis as a clinical finding and not a diagnosis. These various conditions are distinguished clinically and pathologically. For instance, Schönlein-Henoch vasculitis is suggested by the clinical features of abdominal pain or gastrointestinal

Table 22-17 Conditions With Small Vessel Vasculitis

Systemic small vessel vasculitis
  Systemic vasculitis
    Wegener granulomatosis
    Polyarteritis (primary and secondary)
    Churg-Strauss vasculitis
    Takayasu arteritis
    Schönlein-Henoch purpura/vasculitis
  Serum sickness
  Goodpasture syndrome
Nonsystemic small vessel vasculitis
  Hypocomplementemic vasculitis
  Leukocytoclastic vasculitis related to:
    Rheumatoid arthritis
    Sjögren syndrome
    Systemic lupus erythematosus
    Other connective tissue diseases
  Drug-induced and postinfectious angiitis
  Mixed cryoglobulinemia
  Malignancy-associated vasculitis
  Inflammatory bowel disease
  Organ transplant-associated vasculitis
  Hypergammaglobulinemic purpura of Waldenström

hemorrhage in addition to the classic picture of lower extremity purpura, arthritis, and hematuria. Schönlein-Henoch vasculitis has IgA deposition in vessel walls and normal complement levels. Mixed cryoglobulinemia has circulating cryoglobulins and evidence of complement consumption. Complement levels, especially C4, may be low transiently in hypersensitivity vasculitis. Hypersensitivity vasculitis is almost always a nonsystemic small vessel vasculitis temporally related to infection, ingestion of drugs, or, less commonly, malignancy. The results of other laboratory studies are nonspecific. The leukocyte count and platelet count may be increased. Eosinophilia may be present. The erythrocyte sedimentation rate is usually increased.

- Complement levels may be low in mixed cryoglobulinemia and hypersensitivity vasculitis.
- Schönlein-Henoch vasculitis has four classic clinical features: lower extremity purpura, arthritis, gastrointestinal hemorrhage, and nephritis. IgA is noted on biopsy.

Treatment and outcome—The outcome of nonsystemic small vessel vasculitis depends on the underlying condition. Control of the infection or discontinuation of the offending drug may be all that is required. In other cases, corticosteroids

or nonsteroidal anti-inflammatory drugs are beneficial. Hypersensitivity vasculitis is usually self-limited, but it may recur with repeated exposure to the antigen or drug.

- Nonsystemic small vessel vasculitis: the outcome is good.
- Hypersensitivity vasculitis may recur with repeated exposure to the antigen or drug.

Cryoglobulinemia
   Cryoglobulins are immunoglobulins that reversibly precipitate at reduced temperatures. They are grouped into two major categories. *Type I cryoglobulins* are aggregates of a single monoclonal immunoglobulin and are generally associated with multiple myeloma, Waldenström macroglobulinemia, and lymphomas. They are usually found in high concentrations (1-5 g/dL). Patients with type I cryoglobulins are often asymptomatic. Symptoms of type I cryoglobulinemia are usually related to increased viscosity and include headaches, visual disturbances, nosebleeds, Raynaud phenomenon, and ischemic ulceration from occlusion of arterioles and venules by precipitated immune complexes. Vasculitis is rare.

- Type I cryoglobulins are aggregates of a single monoclonal immunoglobulin.
- Patients with type I cryoglobulins are often asymptomatic.
- Symptoms are usually related to increased viscosity.
- Vasculitis is rare.

Type II and type III cryoglobulins consist of more than one class of immunoglobulin (mixed cryoglobulinemia) and can occur alone (essential, primary) or be due to another disease. Type II cryoglobulinemia involves a monoclonal immunoglobulin (usually IgM) with anti-immunoglobulin specificity (rheumatoid factor). Type III cryoglobulinemia involves polyclonal immunoglobulins (usually IgM) directed against other polyclonal immunoglobulins (usually IgG). Not all rheumatoid factors are cryoglobulins. Other components of the immune complexes formed in mixed cryoglobulinemia include hepatitis C antigen, other infectious agents, cellular/nuclear antigens, and complement. These immune complexes precipitate slowly and are present in smaller quantities (50-500 mg/dL) than type I cryoglobulins.

   Type II cryoglobulins are frequently associated with chronic infections (most commonly hepatitis C), autoimmune disorders, and, occasionally, lymphoma. The immune complexes that form precipitate on endothelial cells in peripheral blood vessels and fix complement, promoting vasculitic inflammation. The size of immune complexes, ability to fix complement, persistent IgM production, and many other factors may influence the clinical presentation of mixed cryoglobulinemia. The typical presentation is that of nonsystemic small vessel vasculitis with palpable purpura, urticaria, and cutaneous ulceration. Peripheral neuropathy, arthralgia, and arthritis are common. Less commonly, mixed cryoglobulinemia is complicated by hepatosplenomegaly, pneumonitis or pulmonary hemorrhage, focal segmental necrotizing glomerulonephritis, serositis (pleurisy, pericarditis), and thyroiditis.

- Type II cryoglobulins are frequently associated with chronic infections (most often hepatitis C) and immune disorders.
- Typical presentation: nonsystemic small vessel vasculitis with palpable purpura, urticaria, and cutaneous ulceration.
- Peripheral neuropathy, arthralgia, and arthritis are common.

Laboratory studies—Patients with type II cryoglobulinemia and small vessel vasculitis usually have an increased erythrocyte sedimentation rate, increased immunoglobulin levels, positive rheumatoid factor, and low levels of complement. Evidence of chronic hepatitis infection (particularly hepatitis C) is frequently identified. For cryoglobulin testing, it is important to draw blood into a warmed syringe and to keep it warm until transferred to a cryocrit tube. Cooled specimens must be kept for up to 3 days to identify type II cryoglobulins. Serum protein electrophoresis, immunoelectrophoresis, and quantitative immunoglobulin determinations can be helpful in some cases.

- Immunoglobulin levels and the erythrocyte sedimentation rate are increased, rheumatoid factor is positive, and complement levels are low.
- Evidence of chronic hepatitis infection (particularly hepatitis C) is frequently identified.

Outcome—The clinical course depends on the underlying condition associated and on the organs involved. Progressive renal disease is the most common systemic complication. Pulmonary hemorrhage can be life-threatening.

- Outcome depends on associated conditions and organs involved.
- Progressive renal disease is the most common systemic complication.

Vasculitis Associated With Connective Tissue Diseases

Obliterative endarteropathy—Vascular involvement in rheumatoid arthritis can have various presentations. Vasculitis in patients with rheumatoid arthritis usually occurs only in seropositive (rheumatoid factor-positive) patients. Digital nail fold and nodule infarcts occur in some patients with active rheumatoid arthritis. Histopathologically, this is a bland, obliterative endarteropathy with intimal proliferation. Managing the rheumatoid arthritis itself is all that is needed, because these

vasculopathic changes require no other therapy. A process similar to that of obliterative endarteropathy occurs in scleroderma and systemic lupus erythematosus. A renal arcuate artery vasculopathy is responsible for scleroderma renal crisis.

- Rheumatoid factor is invariably present in patients with rheumatoid arthritis who have vasculitis.

Small and medium-sized vessel vasculitis—Small vessel vasculitis or leukocytoclastic vasculitis with palpable purpura and systemic vasculitis (polyarteritis) can occur with seropositive nodular rheumatoid arthritis. A systemic necrotizing vasculitis, histopathologically indistinguishable from polyarteritis nodosa, complicates some cases of seropositive rheumatoid arthritis. Systemic lupus erythematosus can present with leukocytoclastic vasculitis or a polyarteritis-like picture. Sjögren syndrome uncommonly includes small vessel vasculitis, with either a polymorphonuclear leukocyte or a lymphocyte predominance. Type II cryoglobulins and vasculitis may complicate many different connective tissue diseases. Cryoglobulins should be assayed in any patient with an autoimmune disease in whom vasculitis develops.

- Rheumatoid arthritis, Sjögren syndrome, and systemic lupus erythematosus can present with skin-limited vasculitis or a polyarteritis-like picture.
- Cryoglobulins should be assayed in any patient with an autoimmune disease in whom vasculitis develops.

Large vessel vasculitis—Aortitis, an inflammation of the aortic root with dilatation and aortic insufficiency, occurs in a minority of patients with HLA-B27–associated spondyloarthropathies. Patients present with aortic valve insufficiency.

Atypical Vasculitic Syndromes: Differential Diagnosis

Patients may present with the classic features of one of the vasculitic syndromes described above. When they do not, a diagnostic approach to determine what type of vasculitis is present may prove difficult. Some patterns suggesting vasculitic disease and their differential diagnoses are listed in Tables 22-18 and 22-19 and Figure 22-7.

Skin Lesions Associated With Vasculitis

Palpable purpura suggests leukocytoclastic vasculitis, but this pathologic diagnosis does not define the clinical syndrome. Table 22-19 outlines the differential diagnosis of palpable purpura. Nodules or papules diagnosed as necrotizing granuloma on biopsy occur in Churg-Strauss syndrome, Wegener granulomatosis, rheumatoid arthritis, and, occasionally, systemic

Table 22-18   Acute Pulmonary-Renal Syndrome:
Differential Diagnosis

Common
    Wegener granulomatosis
    Churg-Strauss syndrome
    Goodpasture syndrome
    Systemic small vessel vasculitis
        Systemic lupus erythematosus (SLE)
        Cryoglobulinemic vasculitis
Uncommon
    Schönlein-Henoch purpura/vasculitis
    Connective tissue disease (other than SLE)-associated
        vasculitis
        Rheumatoid arthritis
        Mixed connective tissue disease
        Polychondritis
        Behçet syndrome
    Thrombotic thrombocytopenic purpura
    Thromboembolic disease
    Infectious pneumonia-associated hypersensitivity vasculitis
        Streptococcus
        Mycoplasma
        Legionella

lupus erythematosus. Other nodules or papules without necrotizing granulomata can be the sign of angiocentric lymphoproliferative disorders or sarcoidosis or they may be related to inflammatory bowel disease. Urticarial or pustular lesions complicate hypocomplementemic vasculitis, inflammatory bowel arthritis syndrome, and Behçet syndrome. Livedo reticularis, which is associated with proliferative endarteropathy, occurs in connective tissue diseases and antiphospholipid antibody syndrome and in association with cholesterol emboli and many systemic necrotizing vasculitides.

Table 22-19   Palpable Purpura: Differential Diagnosis

Polyarteritis
Churg-Strauss syndrome
Wegener granulomatosis
Schönlein-Henoch purpura/vasculitis
Cryoglobulinemic vasculitis
Connective tissue disease-associated vasculitis (rheumatoid
    arthritis, Sjögren syndrome, systemic lupus erythematosus)
Hypersensitivity vasculitis
    Drugs, infection, malignancy

- Urticarial or pustular lesions complicate hypocomplementemic vasculitis, inflammatory bowel arthritis syndrome, and Behçet syndrome.
- Livedo reticularis occurs in connective tissue diseases and antiphospholipid antibody syndrome.

Sinusitis and Vasculitis
    Included in the differential diagnosis of sinusitis and presumed vasculitis are Wegener granulomatosis, Churg-Strauss syndrome, relapsing polychondritis, angiocentric lymphoproliferative disorders, sarcoidosis, nasopharyngeal carcinoma, and, occasionally, systemic bacterial or fungal infection.

ANTIRHEUMATIC DRUG THERAPIES
Colchicine and allopurinol treatments are considered in the section on gout.

Nonsteroidal Anti-Inflammatory Drugs (NSAIDs)
    NSAIDs are among the most commonly prescribed medications in the world. There are no clear guidelines for selecting a particular NSAID on the basis of toxicity or efficacy. Patients vary in their responsiveness to different drugs. The various NSAIDs available permit individualization of therapy. All of them are equivalent to aspirin with regard to efficacy. They are all potent cyclooxygenase (COX) inhibitors or prodrugs of COX inhibitors. Clinical studies have not consistently found greater efficacy or tolerance for any one of these medications. NSAIDs are used to treat all types of arthritis and many types of soft tissue rheumatism.

- Patients vary in their responsiveness to different drugs.
- NSAIDs are all potent COX inhibitors or prodrugs of COX inhibitors.

Mechanisms of Action of NSAIDs
    The mechanism of action of NSAIDs is incompletely understood. They decrease prostaglandin synthesis by inhibiting COX conversion of arachidonic acid to prostaglandin precursors. Prostaglandins cause vasodilatation, mediate pain, and potentiate the inflammatory effects of histamines and bradykinin. Furthermore, prostaglandins act as immunomodulators, influencing cellular and humoral immune responses. NSAIDs have potent analgesic effects that are related to their suppression of prostaglandin synthesis. Decreased levels of prostaglandin decrease the sensitivity of peripheral nerve receptors and may affect pain transmission. Acetaminophen is not a potent prostaglandin inhibitor in peripheral tissue. However, it does affect prostaglandin concentrations in neural tissue. This may explain the analgesic effect of acetaminophen.

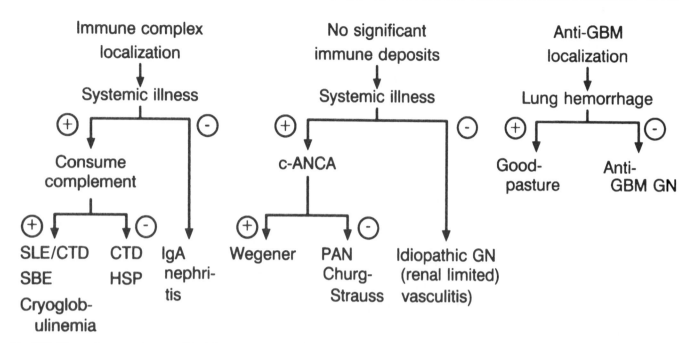

Fig. 22-7. Diagnostic approach to vasculitis. Disease pattern recognition. Focal segmental necrotizing glomerulonephritis (kidney biopsy). c-ANCA, anti-neutrophil cytoplasmic antibody with cytoplasmic staining; CTD, connective tissue disease; GBM, glomerular basement membrane; GN, glomerulonephritis; HSP, Henoch-Schönlein purpura; PAN, polyarteritis nodosa; SBE, subacute bacterial endocarditis; SLE, systemic lupus erythematosus. (Modified from Rosen S, Falk RJ, Jennette JC: Polyarteritis nodosa, including microscopic form and renal vasculitis. *In* Systemic Vasculitides. Edited by A Churg, J Churg. New York, Igaku-Shoin Medical Publishers, 1991, pp 57-77. By permission of publisher.)

Acetaminophen, salicylates, and other NSAIDs are potent antipyretic medications.

- NSAIDs decrease prostaglandin synthesis by inhibiting COX conversion of arachidonic acid to prostaglandin precursors, explaining most of their therapeutic effects.
- Prostaglandins cause vasodilatation, mediate extravasation and pain sensation, potentiate inflammatory mediators, and influence cellular and humoral immunity.
- Acetaminophen is not a potent prostaglandin inhibitor in peripheral tissue.

Mechanisms of Toxicity of NSAIDs

Toxic reactions are due primarily to inhibition of COX-1 and prostaglandin production. Recent investigation has uncovered two forms of COX: COX-1 and COX-2. COX-1 is constitutively expressed in most tissues and produces the prostaglandin precursors needed for "housekeeping function." Prostaglandins protect the gastric mucosal barrier from autodigestion. Patients with renal insufficiency or liver or cardiac disease may have prostaglandin-dependent renal blood flow. NSAIDs interfere with the synthesis of thromboxane via COX-1, which influences vascular tone, platelet aggregation, and hemostasis. COX-2 is not found in resting cells but is rapidly induced in activated fibroblasts, endothelial cells, and smooth muscle cells by cytokines, growth factors, and lipopolysaccharide. Simply

viewed, the acute anti-inflammatory effects of NSAIDs relate to their ability to inhibit COX-2. The side effects of NSAIDs reside mostly with their ability to inhibit COX-1 and the "housekeeping function" associated with the prostaglandins synthesized by COX-1. Selective COX-2 inhibitors have been developed to improve the cost:benefit ratio of NSAID therapy by reducing the risk of gastrointestinal toxicity.

Blocking COX with currently available NSAIDs augments conversion of arachidonic acid to leukotrienes. Leukotrienes (previously known as "slow-reacting substance of anaphylaxis") aggravate asthma, rhinitis, hives, and nasal polyps.

- Acute anti-inflammatory action of NSAIDs is mediated by COX-2 inhibition.
- Toxic reactions are due primarily to inhibition of COX-1.
- Selective COX-2 inhibitors are available to reduce the risk of gastrointestinal toxicity.
- NSAIDs interfere with the synthesis of thromboxane and influence platelet function.
- Leukotrienes aggravate asthma, rhinitis, hives, and nasal polyps. NSAIDs may increase the production of leukotrienes.

NSAIDs are bound extensively to plasma proteins. Protein binding has obvious implications for other medications that are also protein-bound. Indomethacin, diclofenac, and piroxicam decrease lithium excretion. NSAIDs also can influence methotrexate toxicity at high doses (>50 mg/week) by interfering with the renal clearance of methotrexate. At the dose range of methotrexate used in rheumatic diseases, this is not a concern.

Most NSAIDs attenuate the effects of antihypertensive medications. Diuretics, β-blockers, and angiotensin-converting enzyme inhibitors are the drugs affected most by the influence of NSAIDs on renal prostaglandins. Aspirin irreversibly inhibits COX-1. The effect of all the other NSAIDs on COX-1 is reversible. These drugs prolong bleeding time. Aspirin therapy needs to be discontinued for up to 10 days before the bleeding time returns to normal. NSAID therapy should be discontinued at least four drug half-lives before invasive procedures in which bleeding is a concern. NSAIDs with a short half-life are best when an acute effect (e.g., treatment of acute gout) is required. The half-life is proportional to the onset of maximal clinical benefit. The common side effects of NSAIDs are listed in Table 22-20.

● Diuretics, β-blockers, and angiotensin-converting enzyme inhibitors are the drugs affected most by the influence of NSAIDs on renal prostaglandins.
● Aspirin irreversibly inhibits COX-1.
● NSAIDs usually prolong the bleeding time.

Gastrointestinal Side Effects of NSAIDs

Twenty percent of chronic users of NSAIDs have gastric ulcer noted on endoscopy, and 15% to 35% report dyspepsia, but this complaint does not appear to be related to abnormal findings on endoscopy. Nausea and abdominal pain are described in up to 40% of users of NSAIDs. Stomach upset or pain forces discontinuation of therapy with these drugs in more than 10% of patients. Gastrointestinal blood loss related to these drugs is most often occult and can result in iron deficiency anemia. The true incidence of significant gastrointestinal bleeding requiring hospitalization or operation or resulting in death is unknown. However, the elderly, persons with considerable cardiovascular morbidity, and persons with a previous history of NSAID-associated ulcer are at greatest risk for significant gastrointestinal toxicity related to NSAIDs. These patients are the most likely candidates to benefit from the risk reduction of selective COX-2 inhibitors. Alcohol, corticosteroid, or tobacco use also predisposes to the development of gastrointestinal toxicity.

● Of chronic users of NSAIDs, 20% have gastric ulcer and 15%-35% have dyspepsia.
● Stomach upset or pain forces discontinuation of therapy with these drugs in >10% of patients.
● Gastrointestinal blood loss related to these drugs is most often occult.

Table 22-20   Common Side Effects of Nonsteroidal Anti-Inflammatory Drugs

Gastrointestinal
    Nausea
    Abdominal pain
    Constipation or diarrhea
    Occult blood loss and iron deficiency anemia
    Peptic ulcer disease
    Colitis and colonic hemorrhage
Renal
    Reduced renal blood flow
    Reduced glomerular filtration rate
    Increased creatinine clearance
    Pyuria
    Interstitial nephritis
    Papillary necrosis
    Nephrotic syndrome
    Hyperkalemia and type IV renal tubular acidosis
    Fluid retention
Hematologic
    Bone marrow suppression
        Agranulocytosis
        Aplastic anemia
    Iron deficiency anemia
    Platelet-aggregating defect
Neurologic
    Delirium/confusion
    Headache
    Dizziness
    Blurred vision
    Mood swings
    Aseptic meningitis
Dermatologic
    Urticaria
    Erythema multiforme
    Exfoliative syndromes (toxic epidermal necrolysis)
    Oral ulcers
    Dermatitis
Pulmonary
    Pulmonary infiltrates
    Noncardiac pulmonary edema (aspirin toxicity)
    Anaphylaxis and bronchospasm
    Nasal polyps
Drug interactions
    Augment hemostatic effect of warfarin
    Attenuate antihypertensive effect of diuretics, β-blockers, angiotensin-converting enzyme inhibitors
    Influence drug metabolism
        Methotrexate (high doses only)
        Lithium
        Oral hypoglycemic agents

- The elderly, persons with considerable cardiovascular morbidity, and persons with a previous history of NSAID-associated ulcer are especially at risk for significant gastrointestinal toxicity related to NSAIDs. They are candidates for selective COX-2 inhibitors.

Other Toxic Effects of NSAIDs

Central nervous system symptoms such as headaches, dizziness, mood alterations, blurred vision, and confusion are reported most frequently with the use of indomethacin. Ibuprofen, tolmetin, and sulindac have been associated with aseptic meningitis in patients with systemic lupus erythematosus. All the central nervous system effects resolve when the use of NSAIDs is discontinued. Rashes, urticaria, exfoliative dermatitis, erythema multiforme, and scalded skin syndrome or toxic epidermal necrolysis all occur, albeit rarely, with the use of NSAIDs. Easy bruisability is a common complaint of chronic users of these drugs. Dependent petechiae may develop if platelet function is already compromised. Pulmonary infiltrates, bronchospasm, and anaphylaxis may occur with all NSAIDs, including aspirin. Although it is not IgE-mediated, anaphylaxis occurs most commonly in patients who have the classic triad of asthma, nasal polyps, and aspirin sensitivity. Combination therapy with NSAIDs should be avoided. Whereas toxicity is additive, there is no evidence that the therapeutic effect is additive.

- Combination therapy with two different NSAIDs should be avoided.

Nonacetylated Salicylates

Careful studies have not identified significant differences in efficacy of nonacetylated salicylates compared with NSAIDs. Nonacetylated salicylates (e.g., salsalate) minimally inhibit COX-1 and are about half as potent as aspirin for inhibiting COX-2. Although their use decreases the incidence of gastrointestinal bleeding, they can cause many of the gastrointestinal symptoms that influence patient compliance. Tinnitus remains a potential problem. Nonacetylated salicylates do not interfere with renal blood flow, and they do not inhibit platelet function. They usually can be safely prescribed for patients with aspirin allergy.

- Nonacetylated salicylates minimally inhibit COX-1.
- Nonacetylated salicylates do not interfere with renal blood flow, and they do not inhibit platelet function.
- Nonacetylated salicylates can cause stomach upset or tinnitus.

Disease-Modifying Antirheumatic Drugs

Antimalarial Compounds (Hydroxychloroquine)

Open and randomized placebo-controlled studies have confirmed the benefit of hydroxychloroquine in the management of rheumatoid arthritis and systemic lupus erythematosus. The dose typically does not exceed 4.5 mg/kg daily. Retinopathy is the major toxic effect associated with the use of hydroxychloroquine. The risk of irreversible retinopathy is small (<3%) in patients taking less than 4.5 mg/kg daily. The elderly may be at somewhat increased risk. Regular eye examinations can identify the premaculopathy stage of the toxic reaction, which is reversible. Permanent symptomatic retinopathy is preventable when patients have eye examinations every 6 to 12 months.

- Retinopathy is the major toxic effect associated with the use of hydroxychloroquine.
- The risk of irreversible retinopathy is small (<3%) in patients taking <4.5 mg/kg daily.

The clinical response to hydroxychloroquine does not appear before 8 weeks. Improvement may not occur until 6 months of continuous therapy. Approximately 40% to 60% of patients with rheumatoid arthritis may respond (based on established criteria for response). It is used most commonly in combination with NSAIDs or low doses of corticosteroids in patients with early or mild polyarthritis.

- The clinical response to hydroxychloroquine does not appear before 8 weeks and may not occur until 6 months of continuous therapy.

Sulfasalazine

Enteric-coated tablets of sulfasalazine (Azulfidine EN-tabs) have reduced some of the immediate gastrointestinal upset associated with this drug. The metabolites of sulfasalazine include 5-aminosalicylic acid and sulfapyridine. The results of short-term randomized trials indicate significant efficacy in mild-to-moderate rheumatoid arthritis. Rheumatologists also recommend treatment with sulfasalazine for seronegative spondyloarthropathies and psoriatic arthritis; however, peripheral arthritis responds more effectively than axial or spinal inflammation. The benefit of this drug in rheumatoid arthritis is equal to that of intramuscular injections of gold but with fewer toxic effects. Sulfasalazine treatment is usually reserved for milder cases of inflammatory polyarthritis. Although the onset of efficacy occurs as early as 8 weeks, the effect may not be documented for as long as 6 months. The toxic effects include nausea, vomiting, gastric ulcers, and, more rarely, hepatitis or cholestasis. Ten percent of patients complain of headache or sense of fatigue. Recently, a combination of sulfasalazine, hydroxychloroquine, and methotrexate was found to be superior to single-drug therapy for patients with rheumatoid arthritis in whom treatment with at least one DMARD had failed.

- Sulfasalazine treatment is usually reserved for milder cases of inflammatory polyarthritis.
- The benefit of this drug in selected cases of rheumatoid arthritis is equal to that of intramuscular injections of gold.

Methotrexate

Methotrexate is a structural analogue of folic acid and is considered an antimetabolite rather than a cytotoxic agent. It is used extensively in rheumatoid arthritis and also has a place in the treatment of psoriatic arthritis and peripheral arthritis of seronegative spondyloarthropathies. Methotrexate may have a role in the treatment of arthritis in systemic lupus erythematosus and scleroderma. Its mechanism of action includes inhibition of folate metabolism (critical in nucleotide production), inhibition of leukotriene B_4, and increasing intracellular adenosine. It has both immunomodulatory and anti-inflammatory effects. Its strongest effect is on rapidly dividing cells, particularly those in the S phase of the cell cycle. Methotrexate is unique among disease-modifying antirheumatic drugs because its antirheumatic effect occurs within 4 to 6 weeks. Oral, subcutaneous, intramuscular, and intravenous routes are equally effective for low dosages.

- Methotrexate is used extensively in rheumatoid arthritis and has a place in the treatment of psoriatic arthritis, peripheral arthritis of seronegative spondyloarthropathies, and the arthritis in systemic lupus erythematosus and scleroderma.
- The antirheumatic effect occurs within 4-6 weeks.

Of rheumatoid arthritis patients receiving treatment with methotrexate, 80% have substantial improvement within the first year of therapy. At 5 years, it is estimated that at least 35% of patients treated with methotrexate still take it. No other DMARD has this combination of efficacy and tolerability. Most patients with rheumatoid arthritis have a severe flare of their disease within 3 weeks after discontinuation of methotrexate therapy. This drug should not be used in patients with significant renal dysfunction (creatinine >2.0 mg/dL). Coadministration of trimethoprim-sulfamethoxazole and methotrexate increases the risk of hematologic toxicity.

- 80% of rheumatoid arthritis patients taking methotrexate have substantial improvement within the first year of treatment.
- Most patients with rheumatoid arthritis have a severe flare of their disease within 3 weeks after discontinuation of methotrexate therapy.

Gastrointestinal toxic reactions are common side effects of methotrexate. Nausea and vomiting may persist for 24 to 48 hours after ingestion. Stomatitis and diarrhea are insurmountable problems for some patients. Methotrexate treatment should be withheld from patients with significant gastric ulceration until their ulcers have healed. Methotrexate should not be used in patients with significant liver disease. Increased liver enzyme levels suggest a subclinical hepatic toxic effect due to methotrexate. Persistent increase in aspartate aminotransferase levels or decreasing albumin levels are markers for developing hepatic fibrosis and, potentially, cirrhosis. Cryptic cirrhosis may develop without liver enzyme abnormalities being detected. Stomatitis and the less common hematologic abnormalities such as leukopenia, thrombocytopenia, and pancytopenia may respond to folic acid supplementation. Pulmonary toxic side effects include chemical pneumonitis and insidious pulmonary fibrosis, beginning with a dry cough. Acute pneumonitis due to methotrexate may be associated with eosinophilia. Neurologic features such as headache and seizure are uncommon. Methotrexate is teratogenic and should be withheld for 3 months before the patient attempts to conceive.

Supplemental folic acid, 1 mg daily, is provided to patients taking methotrexate. This strategy often reduces mild side effects and may help to prevent cytopenia and liver toxicity.

- Gastrointestinal toxic reactions are common side effects of methotrexate.
- Methotrexate should not be used in patients with significant liver disease.
- Stomatitis and diarrhea are insurmountable problems for some patients.

Leflunomide

Leflunomide (Arava) is an immunoregulatory agent that interferes with pyrimidine synthesis and is approved for the treatment of rheumatoid arthritis. Its efficacy may be comparable to that of methotrexate and is noted within 12 weeks after initiation of therapy. Toxic effects are also comparable to those of methotrexate, although no pulmonary complications have been reported. The most common side effects include gastrointestinal distress, rashes, and alopecia. The monitoring of side effects, including cytopenias and liver toxicity, that is recommended currently is the same as that recommended for methotrexate. This drug is a teratogen and must be avoided in pregnancy. A protocol with cholestyramine is used to accelerate the clearance of leflunomide.

Azathioprine

Azathioprine and its metabolites are purine analogues. It is considered a cytotoxic agent. Azathioprine is metabolized by xanthine oxidase and thiopurine methyltransferase. Allopurinol, an inhibitor of xanthine oxidase, delays the metabolism of azathioprine and can lead to toxic reactions if the dose of azathioprine is not decreased by 50% to 66%. Thiopurine methyltransferase can be assayed; low levels of this enzyme predict the 1 in 300 patients in whom a severe hematologic reaction to azathioprine will develop. Controlled studies have documented the efficacy of azathioprine in the treatment of rheumatoid arthritis and systemic lupus erythematosus.

The most common toxic effects of azathioprine are gastrointestinal effects and cytopenias. An idiosyncratic, acute pancreatitis-like attack is an absolute contraindication to further treatment with this drug. Cholestatic hepatitis is rare, but if it occurs, it generally does so within the first several weeks after drug administration. If tolerated initially, hematologic toxic effects become the most significant concern. In patients who have undergone organ transplant, azathioprine treatment increases the risk of neoplasia, particularly lymphomas, leukemias, and skin and cervical malignancies. Azathioprine does not alter fertility, but it may have some teratogenic potential. For pregnant women, azathioprine should be reserved for those with severe or life-threatening rheumatic diseases.

- Azathioprine is a cytotoxic agent.
- The most common toxic effects of azathioprine are gastrointestinal effects and cytopenias.
- Allopurinol should be avoided in patients taking azathioprine.

Cyclophosphamide

Cyclophosphamide is a potent alkylating agent. It acts on dividing and nondividing cells, interfering with cellular DNA function. It depletes T cells and B cells, causing considerable immunosuppression. Oral cyclophosphamide is well absorbed and completely metabolized within 24 hours, and most of its metabolites are excreted in the urine. Allopurinol increases the risk of leukopenia in patients taking cyclophosphamide. Short-term studies document significant efficacy of this drug in the treatment of rheumatoid arthritis at doses of 1 to 2 mg/kg per day. Unequivocal healing and arrest of erosive change occur. The considerable toxicity associated with chronic administration of cyclophosphamide has raised questions about whether it should be used in rheumatoid arthritis. It is the drug of choice in the treatment of generalized Wegener granulomatosis. Intravenous administration of cyclophosphamide is efficacious in managing systemic necrotizing vasculitis and severe systemic lupus erythematosus, including proliferative glomerulonephritis. Short-term advantages of intravenous pulse of cyclophosphamide may include fewer toxic effects on the bladder and perhaps a lower risk of infection.

- Cyclophosphamide depletes T cells and B cells, causing considerable immunosuppression.

- Cyclophosphamide is efficacious in managing systemic necrotizing vasculitis and severe systemic lupus erythematosus.

Dose-related bone marrow suppression is common in patients receiving cyclophosphamide and requires close laboratory monitoring. Immunosuppression from treatment with cyclophosphamide increases the risk of infection. Herpes zoster infection occurs in most patients receiving the drug orally. Cyclophosphamide directly affects ovarian and testicular function. Premature ovarian failure frequently occurs in premenopausal lupus patients taking the drug. Spermatogenesis also can be affected by this drug, which causes atrophy of seminiferous tubules. Cyclophosphamide has teratogenic potential. Alopecia, stomatitis, cardiomyopathy (with drug doses used to treat cancer), and pulmonary fibrosis may complicate cyclophosphamide therapy. The metabolites of this drug, including acrolein, accumulate in the bladder. Acrolein has direct mucosal toxic effects and causes hemorrhagic cystitis. This complication is potentially life-threatening. The chronic use of cyclophosphamide taken orally is associated with an increased risk of neoplasia, including hematologic and bladder malignancies. The risk of malignancy with intravenous pulse therapy has not been established. All patients who have had cyclophosphamide therapy should have urinalysis and urine cytology performed at regular intervals for life.

- Cyclophosphamide: dose-related bone marrow suppression is common.
- Cyclophosphamide directly affects ovarian and testicular function.
- The chronic use of cyclophosphamide is associated with an increased risk of neoplasia.

Glucocorticosteroids

Glucocorticosteroids modify the inflammatory response dramatically. They are potent inhibitors of neutrophil function. Glucocorticosteroids suppress cellular immune activity and, to a lesser extent, inhibit the humoral response. Low doses of glucocorticosteroids (<10 mg of prednisone per day) are frequently used in the day-to-day management of the articular manifestations of rheumatoid arthritis. At least one-third of all patients with rheumatoid arthritis take glucocorticosteroids chronically. High doses of glucocorticosteroids (1-2 mg of prednisone per kilogram of body weight) may be required for life-threatening or serious inflammatory disorders, including systemic vasculitis and complications of systemic lupus erythematosus. Prednisone doses of more than 30 mg/day are associated with a higher risk of infection, including *Pneumocystis carinii*. This is particularly the case if prednisone is given in addition to cyclophosphamide, azathioprine, or methotrexate.

Many clinicians add one double-strength trimethoprim-sulfamethoxazole tablet twice a week to these immunosuppressive regimens as prophylaxis against *Pneumocystis* infection.

- Glucocorticosteroids are potent inhibitors of neutrophil function.
- They suppress cellular immune activity and, to a lesser extent, inhibit the humoral response.
- One-third of all patients with rheumatoid arthritis take glucocorticosteroids chronically.

These drugs have many side effects, which are not idiosyncratic but actually unwanted effects of the medication. The duration of treatment and the dose used determine how fast an unwanted effect appears. Many patients with rheumatoid arthritis tolerate prednisone doses of 1 to 5 mg/day for years without having serious side effects. Patient concerns about glucocorticosteroids include weight gain from increased appetite, water retention, and hirsutism. Longer-term concerns include thinning of the skin, easy bruising, progressive osteoporosis (unclear if this happens with physiologic doses of prednisone) and compression fractures, high blood pressure, glucose intolerance, cataract formation, and aggravation of glaucoma. Glucocorticosteroids interfere with wound healing and increase the risk of opportunistic infection. Steroid-induced osteoporosis should be anticipated, and patients should be treated with calcium, vitamin D supplementation, and oral bisphosphonates. The psychoactive potential of high doses of glucocorticosteroids is an additional factor in treating older patients. Glucocorticosteroid psychosis can complicate the diagnosis of neuropsychiatric lupus.

- Many patients with rheumatoid arthritis tolerate prednisone doses in the 1-5 mg/day range for years without having serious side effects.
- Long-term concerns: thinning of the skin, progressive osteoporosis and compression fractures, high blood pressure, glucose intolerance, cataract formation, and aggravation of glaucoma.
- Glucocorticosteroid psychosis can complicate the diagnosis of neuropsychiatric lupus.
- Glucocorticosteroids interfere with wound healing and increase the risk of opportunistic infection.
- Bisphosphonates, calcium, and vitamin D are used to reduce the risk of glucocorticoid osteoporosis.

Anti-Cytokine Therapies

Appreciation of the role of tumor necrosis factor-α and interleukin-1 in the inflammatory process in rheumatoid arthritis has led to the development of specific inhibitors of these cytokines. Tumor necrosis factor antagonists include neutralizing antibodies (infliximab and adalimunab) and soluble receptor recombinant fusion protein (etanercept). Anakinra is a recombinant interleukin-1 receptor antagonist. Anti-cytokine therapies are very expensive. Their roles in the management of rheumatoid arthritis are still being defined. Because of evidence that they delay radiographic progression, they are usually added to other therapies such as methotrexate when the disease has not been adequately controlled. The primary risk of these agents, especially the tumor necrosis factor inhibitors, is infection. Reactivation of latent tuberculosis is a major concern, and potential candidates for tumor necrosis factor inhibitors must be evaluated with tuberculin testing before treatment.

PART II
William W. Ginsburg, M.D.

CRYSTALLINE ARTHROPATHIES

Hyperuricemia and Gout

Hyperuricemia has been described in 2% to 18% of normal populations. Hyperuricemia is associated with hypertension, renal insufficiency, obesity, and arteriosclerotic heart disease. The prevalence of clinical gouty arthritis ranges from 0.1% to 0.4%. There is a family history of gout in 20% of patients with gouty arthritis. Genetic studies suggest a multifactorial inheritance pattern. Of patients with hyperuricemia whose uric acid level is more than 9 mg/dL, gout develops in 5 years in approximately 20%.

- Hyperuricemia is associated with hypertension, renal insufficiency, obesity, and arteriosclerotic heart disease.
- The prevalence of gouty arthritis is 0.1%-0.4%.
- 20% of patients with gouty arthritis have a family history of gout.
- In patients with a uric acid level more than 9 mg/dL, gout develops in 20% in 5 years.

Ninety percent of patients with gout have underexcretion of uric acid. They have reduced filtration of uric acid, enhanced tubular reabsorption, or decreased tubular secretion. Overproduction of uric acid is the cause of hyperuricemia in approximately 10% of patients with primary gout. Of these 10%, about 15% have one of the two X-linked inborn errors of purine metabolism: 1) hypoxanthine-guanine phosphoribosyltransferase deficiency (Lesch-Nyhan syndrome) and 2) 5-phosphoribosyl-1-pyrophosphate synthetase overactivity. Of the remaining 85% of patients who have overproduction, most are obese, but the cause of overproduction and the relationship between obesity and overproduction of uric acid remain unknown.

- 10% or less of patients with gout have overproduction of uric acid.

Events leading to initial crystallization of monosodium urate in a joint after many years of asymptomatic hyperuricemia are unknown. Trauma with disruption of microtophi in cartilage may lead to release of urate crystals into synovial fluid. The urate crystals become coated with immunoglobulin and then complement. They are then phagocytosed by leukocytes with subsequent release of chemotactic protein, activation of the kallikrein system, and disruption of the leukocytes, which release lysosomal enzymes into synovial fluid.

Important Enzyme Abnormalities in the Uric Acid Pathway (Fig. 22-8)

Lesch-Nyhan syndrome is a complete deficiency of hypoxanthine-guanine phosphoribosyltransferase. It is characterized by an X-linked disorder in young boys, hyperuricemia, self-mutilation, choreoathetosis, spasticity, growth retardation, and severe gouty arthritis.

Overactivity of 5-phosphoribosyl-1-pyrophosphate synthetase is associated with hyperuricemia, X-linked genetic inheritance, and gouty arthritis.

Adenosine deaminase deficiency is inherited in an autosomal recessive pattern. It causes a combined immunodeficiency state with severe T-cell and mild B-cell dysfunction. There is a buildup of deoxyadenosine triphosphate in lymphocytes, which is toxic to immature lymphocytes. Features of the disorder are hypouricemia, recurrent infection, chondro-osseous dysplasia, and an increased deoxyadenosine level in plasma and urine. Treatment for the disorder is with irradiated frozen red blood cells or marrow transplantation.

Xanthine oxidase deficiency is also inherited in an autosomal recessive pattern. It is characterized by hypouricemia, xanthinuria with xanthine stones, and myopathy associated with deposits of xanthine and hypoxanthine.

Causes of Secondary Hyperuricemia

Secondary hyperuricemia can be attributed to overproduction or underexcretion of uric acid (Table 22-21).

- Important causes of overproduction of uric acid include cancer, psoriasis, and sickle cell anemia.
- Important causes of underexcretion of uric acid include chronic renal insufficiency, lead nephropathy, alcohol, diabetic ketoacidosis, and drugs, notably thiazide diuretics, nicotinic acid, and cyclosporine.

Causes of Hypouricemia

Increased urinary excretion of uric acid contributes to hypouricemia. It can develop in healthy persons with an isolated defect in tubular reabsorption of uric acid. It also can be related to diminished reabsorption of urate, such as in Fanconi syndrome, Fanconi syndrome associated with Wilson disease, carcinoma of the lung, acute myelogenous leukemia, light-chain diseases, and use of outdated tetracycline. Malignant neoplasms, such as carcinoma, Hodgkin disease, and sarcoma, also are associated with increased excretion of uric acid. Hypervolemia caused by inappropriate secretion of antidiuretic hormone also can be a factor. Drugs involved in increased

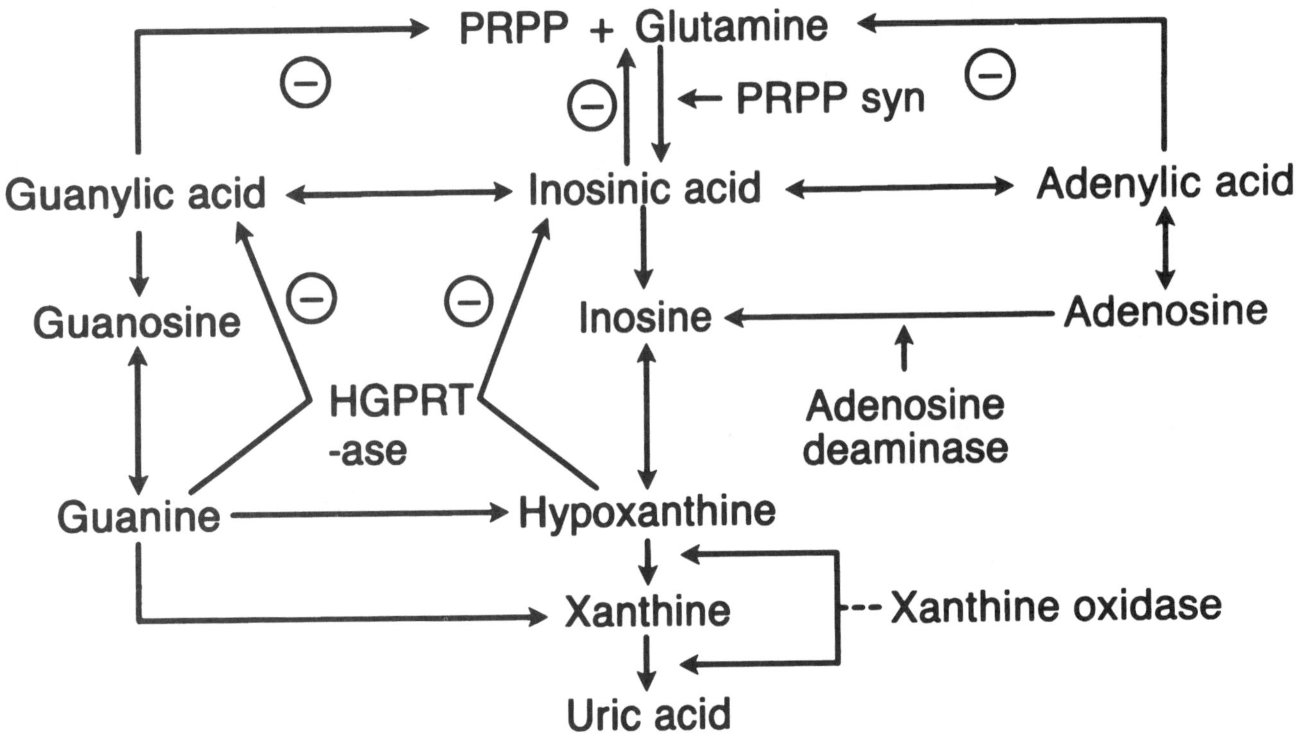

Fig. 22-8. Purine metabolism. HGPRTase, hypoxanthine-guanine phosphoribosyltransferase; PRPP, phosphoribosylpyrophosphate; PRPP syn, phosphoribosylpyrophosphate synthetase; $\ominus$, feedback inhibition.

excretion of uric acid are high-dose aspirin, probenecid and other uricosuric agents, and glyceryl guaiacolate. Radiographic contrast agents that can cause hypouricemia are iopanoic acid (Telopaque), iodipamide meglumine (Cholografin), and diatrizoate sodium (Hypaque). It also can occur in severe liver disease.

Decreased synthesis of uric acid also can cause hypouricemia. The drug allopurinol inhibits the enzyme xanthine oxidase, causing hypouricemia. The decrease also can be caused by congenital deficiencies in enzymes involved in purine biosynthesis: 5-phosphoribosyl-1-pyrophosphate synthetase deficiency, adenosine deaminase deficiency, purine nucleoside phosphorylase deficiency, and xanthine oxidase deficiency (xanthinuria). Acquired deficiency in xanthine oxidase activity (metastatic adenocarcinoma of lung) also can cause decreased synthesis of uric acid, as can acute intermittent porphyria.

Factors Predisposing to Gout and Pseudogout

The following can predispose to an attack of gout or pseudogout: trauma, operation (3 days after), major medical illness (myocardial infarction, cerebrovascular accident, pulmonary embolus), fasting, alcohol use, infection, and acidosis. The attacks are precipitated by changes in the urate equilibrium between the blood and joints.

- Factors that precipitate gout and pseudogout include trauma, operation, alcohol use, and acidosis.

Clinical Manifestations of Acute Gout

In 50% of patients with gout, the metatarsophalangeal joint of the great toe is involved initially (podagra), and this joint is eventually involved in more than 75% of patients. Rapid joint swelling is associated with extreme tenderness. Uric acid crystals, which are needle-shaped and strongly negatively birefringent under polarized light, are always found in the joint during an acute attack. The diagnosis of gout is established by the demonstration of uric acid crystals in the joint aspirate. The joint fluid is usually inflammatory, with between 5 and 75×10^9/L polymorphonuclear neutrophils.

Gout occurs most commonly in middle-aged men, but, after menopause, the incidence of gout in women increases. Although gout is usually monarticular and usually involves the joints in the lower extremity, attacks may become polyarticular over time in some patients.

- Podagra is the initial presentation of gout in 50% of cases.
- Uric acid crystals are negatively birefringent under polarized light microscopy.
- Gout is usually monarticular and most often involves the joints in the lower extremities.

Table 22-21   Causes of Secondary Hyperuricemia

Overproduction
   Myeloproliferative disorders
      Polycythemia, primary or secondary
      Myeloid metaplasia
      Chronic myelocytic leukemia
   Lymphoproliferative disorders
      Chronic lymphocytic leukemia
   Plasma cell proliferative disorders
      Multiple myeloma
   Disseminated carcinoma and sarcoma
   Sickle cell anemia, thalassemia, and other forms of chronic
    hemolytic anemia
   Psoriasis
   Cytotoxic drugs
   Infectious mononucleosis
   Obesity
   Increased purine ingestion
Underexcretion
   Intrinsic renal disease
      Chronic renal insufficiency of diverse cause
      Saturine gout (lead nephropathy)
   Drug-induced
      Thiazide diuretics, furosemide, ethacrynic acid,
        ethambutol, pyrazinamide, low-dose aspirin,
        cyclosporine, nicotinic acid, laxative abuse, levodopa
   Endocrine conditions
      Adrenal insufficiency, nephrogenic diabetes insipidus,
        hyperparathyroidism, hypoparathyroidism,
        pseudohypoparathyroidism, hypothyroidism
   Metabolic conditions
      Diabetic ketoacidosis, lactic acidosis, starvation,
        ethanolism, glycogen storage disease type I, Bartter
        syndrome
   Other
      Sarcoidosis
      Down syndrome
      Beryllium disease

- Typical clinical scenario: Pain, swelling, redness, and tenderness develop over the right metatarsophalangeal joint of the great toe 3 days after myocardial infarction in an elderly patient. Aspiration of the joint reveals needle-like crystals, which are strongly negatively birefringent under polarized light. Joint fluid shows 50×10^9/L polymorphonuclear neutrophils.

Treatment of Acute Gouty Arthritis

Indomethacin or other nonsteroidal anti-inflammatory drugs (NSAIDs) are the drugs of choice for the treatment of acute gouty arthritis and should be used for a 7- to 10-day course. These drugs are relatively contraindicated in patients with congestive heart failure, active peptic ulcer disease, or renal insufficiency. NSAIDs should not be used in patients with nasal polyps and aspirin sensitivity because they may cause bronchospasm.

- NSAIDs are the initial drugs of choice for an acute attack of gouty arthritis.
- Avoid NSAIDs in patients with congestive heart failure, peptic ulcer disease, and renal insufficiency.

Intra-articular or oral corticosteroids and subcutaneous adrenocorticotropic hormone are other treatments, especially in patients who have contraindications to colchicine and NSAIDs. Oral corticosteroids may need to be given for 10 days to avoid relapses. Allopurinol or probenecid should not be administered until the acute attack completely subsides. Because of severe gastrointestinal side effects, high-dose oral colchicine is rarely used for an acute attack. Intravenously administered colchicine in a single dose (1-2 mg) has no gastrointestinal side effects. It has increased toxicity in patients with renal insufficiency, bone marrow depression, sepsis, and immediate prior use of oral colchicine. Repeat dosages should be avoided. It can cause severe skin necrosis if it infiltrates into subcutaneous tissues.

- Colchicine: there is potential for gastrointestinal side effects with the oral form, but there are no gastrointestinal side effects with single-dose intravenous administration.
- Avoid intravenous colchicine in patients with renal insufficiency, bone marrow depression, sepsis, or immediate prior use of oral colchicine.

Treatment During Intercritical Period

Oral colchicine, 0.6 mg twice a day, should be given prophylactically with probenecid or allopurinol for 6 to 12 months to prevent exacerbation of acute gout.

Probenecid inhibits tubular reabsorption of filtered and secreted urate, thereby increasing urinary excretion of uric acid. It should not be used if the patient has a history of kidney stones or if the 24-hour urine uric acid value is more than 1,000 mg (normal, less than 600 mg/day). Probenecid delays the renal excretion of indomethacin and thereby increases its blood level. Probenecid delays the renal excretion of acetylsalicylic acid (ASA), and ASA completely blocks the uricosuric effect of probenecid. ASA also blocks tubular secretion of urates. Do not use probenecid with methotrexate because probenecid increases methotrexate blood levels, increasing toxicity.

- Probenecid inhibits tubular reabsorption of filtered and secreted urate.
- Probenecid should not be used if the patient has a history of kidney stones or if 24-hour uric acid value is more than 1,000 mg.
- Probenecid delays renal excretion of indomethacin and ASA.

Allopurinol is a xanthine oxidase inhibitor. It is the drug of choice to prevent gouty attacks if the patient has a history of renal stones, tophi, or renal insufficiency. Allopurinol also can precipitate gout. Allopurinol and probenecid usually are not used simultaneously unless the patient has extensive tophaceous gout with good renal function. Allopurinol can cause a rash and a severe toxicity syndrome consisting of eosinophilia, fever, hepatitis, decreased renal function, and an erythematous desquamative rash. This syndrome usually occurs in patients with decreased renal function. Allopurinol should be given in the lowest dose possible to keep the uric acid value less than 6 mg/dL. If allopurinol is used in conjunction with 6-mercaptopurine or azathioprine, the dose of 6-mercaptopurine or azathioprine needs to be reduced at least 25% or bone marrow toxicity can occur. Both of these drugs are metabolized by xanthine oxidase, which allopurinol inhibits. Patients who have had transplantation frequently receive both medications.

- Allopurinol is a xanthine oxidase inhibitor.
- Allopurinol can precipitate gout.
- It is the drug of choice if patient has a history of renal stones, tophi, or renal insufficiency.
- It can cause a severe toxicity syndrome: eosinophilia, fever, hepatitis, decreased renal function, erythematous desquamative rash.

The indications for use of allopurinol rather than probenecid for lowering the uric acid level are tophaceous gout, gout complicated by renal insufficiency, uric acid excretion more than 1,000 mg/day, history of uric acid calculi, use of cytotoxic drugs, and allergy to uricosuric agents. Allopurinol should be used before treatment of rapidly proliferating tumors. The nucleic acid liberated with cytolysis is converted to uric acid and can cause renal failure secondary to precipitation of uric acid in collecting ducts and ureters (acute tumor lysis syndrome). Patients also should have adequate hydration and alkalinization of the urine before chemotherapy.

- Indications for allopurinol include tophaceous gout, gout complicated by renal insufficiency, history of uric acid calculi, and use of cytotoxic drugs.

Renal Disease and Uric Acid

Renal function is not necessarily adversely affected by an increased serum urate concentration. The incidence of interstitial renal disease and renal insufficiency is no greater than that in patients of comparable age with similar degrees of hypertension, arteriosclerotic heart disease, diabetes, and primary renal disease. Correction of hyperuricemia (to 10 mg/dL or less) has no apparent effect on renal function.

Most rheumatologists do not treat asymptomatic hyperuricemia if the uric acid level is less than 10.0 mg/dL (normal to 8.0). When hyperuricemia is associated with a urinary uric acid of more than 1,000 mg/24 hours, which increases the risk of uric acid stones, renal function should be monitored closely. Excessive exposure to lead may contribute to the renal disease found in some patients with gout.

- Renal function is not necessarily adversely affected by an increased serum urate concentration.
- Correction of hyperuricemia (to 10 mg/dL or less) has no apparent effect on renal function.

Miscellaneous Points of Importance

- Positive diagnosis of a crystalline arthritis requires identification of crystal by polarization microscopy.
- Do not start allopurinol therapy during an acute attack of gout.
- 30% of patients with chronic tophaceous gout are positive for rheumatoid factor (usually weakly positive).
- 10% of patients with acute gout will be positive for rheumatoid factor (usually weakly positive).
- 5%-10% of patients will have a gout and a pseudogout attack simultaneously.
- 50% of synovial fluids aspirated from first metatarsophalangeal joints of asymptomatic patients with gout have crystals of monosodium urate.
- Up to 20% of patients with acute gout have a normal level of serum uric acid at the time of the acute attack.
- Gout in a premenopausal female is very unusual.
- Sulfinpyrazone is also uricosuric and potentially therapeutic.
- There have been many recent reports of superimposed gout occurring in Heberden and Bouchard nodes in older women taking thiazide diuretics.
- A septic joint can trigger a gout or pseudogout attack in a predisposed person. Synovial fluid should always be analyzed for crystals, Gram stain, and culture.
- The frequency of gout in patients who have had cardiac

transplantation is high (25%). (Both cyclosporine and diuretics cause hyperuricemia.)

Calcium Pyrophosphate Deposition Disease

Etiologic Classification

Calcium pyrophosphate deposition (CPPD) is classified as idiopathic, hereditary, or associated with metabolic disease. The associated diseases include hyperparathyroidism, hemochromatosis-hemosiderosis, hypothyroidism, gout, hypomagnesemia, hypophosphatasia, Wilson disease, and ochronosis.

- CPPD associations include hyperparathyroidism, hemochromatosis-hemosiderosis, hypothyroidism, and hypomagnesemia.

Pseudogout

When CPPD causes an acute inflammatory arthritis, the term "pseudogout" is applied. CPPD crystals are weakly positively birefringent and are rhomboid. Pseudogout rarely involves the first metatarsophalangeal joint. It most commonly affects the knees, but the wrists, elbows, ankles, and intervertebral disks may be involved. It usually occurs in older individuals. Most patients with pseudogout have chondrocalcinosis on radiography. The presence of chondrocalcinosis does not necessarily mean that a patient will have pseudogout or even CPPD.

- Pseudogout is an acute inflammatory arthritis caused by CPPD.
- CPPD crystals are weakly positively birefringent under polarized light microscopy.
- Pseudogout most commonly affects the knees, but the wrists, elbows, ankles, and intervertebral disks can be affected.
- Chondrocalcinosis is found on radiographs in most patients with pseudogout.
- Chondrocalcinosis does not mean that patients will have pseudogout or even CPPD.

Treatment of Pseudogout

For treatment of acute attacks, NSAIDs or injection of a steroid preparation can be used. Intravenously administered colchicine is effective for acute attacks, but oral administration is not consistently effective. Prophylactic oral colchicine (0.6 mg 2-3 times daily) can lead to a decrease in the frequency and severity of pseudogout attacks. In patients with underlying metabolic disease, the frequency of acute attacks of pseudogout does not necessarily decrease with treatment of the underlying disease (such as hypothyroidism or hyperparathyroidism).

- Treatment of acute attacks of pseudogout: NSAIDs, injection of steroid preparation, or colchicine given intravenously.

- Prophylactic oral colchicine can lead to a decrease in the frequency and severity of attacks.
- Typical clinical scenario: An elderly patient presents with acute pain, swelling, and redness over the right knee joint. Radiographic examination reveals chondrocalcinosis. Aspiration of joint fluid reveals rhomboid crystals that are weakly positively birefringent on polarized light examination.

Hydroxyapatite Deposition Disease (Basic Calcium Phosphate Disease)

Presentation

Clinical presentations include 1) acute inflammation, including calcific tendinitis, osteoarthritis with inflammatory episodes, periarthritis or arthritis dialysis syndrome, and calcinotic deposits in scleroderma and 2) chronic inflammation, including severe osteoarthritis and Milwaukee shoulder or knee: advanced glenohumeral and knee osteoarthritis, rotator cuff tear, noninflammatory paste-like joint fluid containing hydroxyapatite.

- Hydroxyapatite deposition disease can present as acute or chronic inflammation.

Diagnosis and Treatment

Individual crystals cannot be seen on routine polarization microscopy (Table 22-22). Small, round (shiny coin) bodies 0.5 to 100 μm are seen. On electron microscopy these represent lumps of needle-shaped crystals. Positive identification requires transmission electron microscopy or elemental analysis. Alizarin red stain showing calcium staining provides a presumptive diagnosis (if CPPD is excluded). Treatment involves NSAIDs and intra-articular steroids.

- Individual crystals are not seen on polarization microscopy.
- Positive identification requires transmission electron microscopy.

Calcium Oxalate Arthropathy

This disorder occurs in patients with primary oxalosis and in patients undergoing chronic hemodialysis. It can cause acute inflammatory arthritis. Crystals are large, bipyramidal, and birefringent. Calcium oxalate can cause chondrocalcinosis or large soft tissue calcifications.

- Calcium oxalate arthropathy occurs in patients with primary oxalosis and patients undergoing chronic hemodialysis.

Other Crystals Implicated in Joint Disease

Cholesterol crystals are a nonspecific finding and have been found in the synovial fluid of patients with various types of chronic inflammatory arthritis. Cryoglobulin crystals are

Table 22-22 Differential Diagnosis According to Results of Synovial Fluid Analysis

Diagnosis	Leukocyte count, ×10^9/L	Differential	Polarization microscopy
Degenerative joint disease	<1	Mononuclear cells	Negative
Rheumatoid arthritis	5-50	PMNs	Negative
Gout	5-100	PMNs	Monosodium urate
Pseudogout	5-100	PMNs	CPPD
Hydroxyapatite	5-100	PMNs	Negative
Septic arthritis	≥100	PMNs	Negative

CPPD, calcium pyrophosphate deposition disease; PMN, polymorphonuclear leukocytes.

found in essential cryoglobulinemia and paraproteinemia. Corticosteroid crystals are found in an arthritis flare after a corticosteroid injection, and Charcot-Leyden crystals have been found in hypereosinophilic syndromes. In patients undergoing hemodialysis, aluminum phosphate crystals can develop.

SPONDYLOARTHROPATHIES

Conditions that form the spondyloarthropathies include ankylosing spondylitis, reactive arthritis, enteropathic spondylitis, and psoriatic arthritis.

Spondyloarthropathies are characterized by involvement of the sacroiliac joints (uncommon in rheumatoid arthritis), peripheral arthritis that is usually asymmetric and oligoarticular, absence of rheumatoid factor, and an association with HLA-B27 in more than 90% of cases. They are enthesopathic disorders.

The HLA region of chromosome 6 contains genes of the human histocompatibility complex. Every person has two of chromosome 6, one inherited from each parent. On each of these there is an HLA-A and HLA-B allele. Therefore, everyone has two HLA-A types and two HLA-B types. With regard to inheritance, an offspring has a 50% chance of acquiring a specific HLA-A or HLA-B antigen from a parent (Fig. 22-9). Siblings have a 25% chance of being identical for all four HLA-A and HLA-B alleles.

The frequency of HLA-B27 in control populations is as follows: whites (United States), 8%; African blacks, 0%; Asians, 1%; Haida (North American Indian), 50%.

The rheumatic diseases associated with HLA-B27 are ankylosing spondylitis (HLA-B27 in more than 90%), reactive arthritis (more than 80%), enteropathic spondylitis (approximately 75%), and psoriatic spondylitis (approximately 50%).

- Ankylosing spondylitis is associated with HLA-B27 in more than 90% of cases.

Many theories have been proposed to explain the association between HLA-B27 and the spondyloarthropathies: B27 may act as a receptor site for an infective agent, may be a marker for an immune response gene that determines susceptibility to an environmental trigger, and may induce tolerance to foreign antigens with which it cross-reacts.

An offspring of a person with HLA-B27 has a 50% chance of carrying the antigen. In randomly selected persons with HLA-B27, the chance of the disease developing is 2%. In B27-positive relatives of B27-positive patients with ankylosing spondylitis, the risk of the disease developing is 20%.

Ankylosing Spondylitis

Ankylosing spondylitis is a chronic systemic inflammatory disease that affects the sacroiliac joints, the spine, and the peripheral joints. Sacroiliac joint involvement defines this disease, and back pain, decreased spinal motion, and reduced chest expansion also are often found.

- Sacroiliac joint involvement defines ankylosing spondylitis, and back pain, decreased spinal motion, and reduced chest expansion also are often found.

Features

Characteristic features of low back pain in ankylosing spondylitis are age at onset usually between 15 and 40 years, insidious onset, duration of more than 3 months, morning stiffness, improvement with exercise, family history, involvement of other systems, and diffuse radiation of back pain.

- Typical clinical scenario: A 20-year-old man has a history of low back pain of insidious onset that improves with exercise. He has diminished chest expansion, iritis, and tenderness over the sacroiliac joints. Laboratory testing shows an increased sedimentation rate. Rheumatoid factor is negative. Radiographic examination reveals sclerosis and erosions of the sacroiliac joints and squaring of the vertebral bodies with the presence of syndesmophytes.

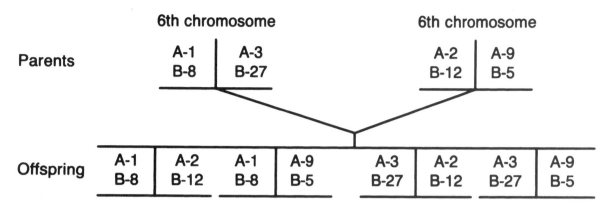

Fig. 22-9. Inheritance of HLA antigens.

Findings of ankylosing spondylitis on physical examination are listed in Table 22-23. Other physical findings in ankylosing spondylitis are listed in Table 22-24.

The radiographic findings in ankylosing spondylitis are 1) sacroiliac involvement with erosions, "pseudo widening" of joint space, sclerosis (both sides of sacroiliac joint; this finding is needed for diagnosis), and fusion and 2) spine involvement with squaring of superior and inferior margins of vertebral body, syndesmophytes, and bamboo spine.

- Radiographic findings in ankylosing spondylitis include sacroiliac sclerosis and possible erosions, spine involvement with squaring of the vertebral bodies, syndesmophytes, and bamboo spine.

Laboratory Findings

The erythrocyte sedimentation rate may be increased, there may be an anemia of chronic disease, rheumatoid factor is absent, and 95% of white patients are positive for HLA-B27.

Extraspinal Involvement

Enthesopathic involvement distinguishes spondyloarthropathies from rheumatoid arthritis and consists of plantar

Table 22-23 Findings in Ankylosing Spondylitis

Characteristic	
Scoliosis	Absent
Decreased range of movement	Symmetric
Tenderness	Diffuse
Hip flexion with straight-leg raising	Normal
Pain with sciatic nerve stretch	Absent
Hip involvement	Frequently present
Neurodeficit	Absent

fasciitis, Achilles tendinitis, and costochondritis. Hip and shoulder involvement are common (up to 50%), but peripheral joints can be affected, usually with asymmetric involvement of the lower extremities. Some patients in whom juvenile rheumatoid arthritis is diagnosed, especially male adolescents, may have juvenile ankylosing spondylitis in which peripheral arthritis preceded the axial involvement.

- Enthesopathic involvement is characteristic of ankylosing spondylitis and the other spondyloarthropathies and consists of plantar fasciitis, Achilles tendinitis, and costochondritis.
- Hip and shoulder involvement are common (up to 50%).

Extraskeletal Involvement

Other findings in active disease include 1) fatigue, 2) weight loss, 3) low-grade fever, and 4) iritis (25% of patients). Iritis is an important clinical clue in the diagnosis of spondyloarthropathies. It is not found in adults with rheumatoid arthritis.

- Iritis is an important clue to the diagnosis of spondyloarthropathies and is not found in adults with rheumatoid arthritis.

Late complications can include 1) traumatic spinal fracture leading to cord compression, 2) cauda equina syndrome (symptoms include neurogenic bladder, fecal incontinence, radicular leg pain), 3) fibrotic changes in upper lung fields, 4) aortic insufficiency in 3% to 5% of patients, 5) complete heart block, and 6) secondary amyloidosis.

- Late complications of ankylosing spondylitis include traumatic spinal fractures leading to cord compression, cauda equina syndrome, fibrotic changes in upper lung fields, and aortic insufficiency.

Table 22-24 Results of Testing in Ankylosing Spondylitis

Test	Method	Results
Schober	Make a mark on the spine at level of L-5 and one at 10 cm directly above with the patient standing erect. Patient then bends forward maximally and the distance between the two marks is measured	An increase of <5 cm indicates early lumbar involvement
Chest expansion	Measure maximal chest expansion at nipple line	Chest expansion of <5 cm is clue to early costovertebral involvement
Sacroiliac compression	Exert direct compression over sacroiliac joints	Tenderness or pain suggests sacroiliac involvement

Ankylosing Spondylitis in Men and Women

Ankylosing spondylitis has been thought to be a disease primarily of men, but it is now recognized that the incidence in women is higher than originally thought, although women have less tendency for spinal ankylosis. The ratio of men to women is approximately 3:1. Women more frequently have osteitis pubis and peripheral joint involvement.

Differential Diagnosis

The differential diagnosis includes diffuse hypertrophic skeletal hyperostosis (DISH), osteitis condensans ilii, fusion of sacroiliac joint seen in paraplegia, osteitis pubis, infection, and degenerative joint disease. The clinical symptoms of DISH are "stiffness" of spine and relatively good preservation of spine motion. It generally affects middle-aged and elderly men. Patients with DISH can have dysphagia related to cervical osteophytes. Criteria for DISH are "flowing" ossification along the anterolateral aspect of at least four contiguous vertebral bodies, preservation of disk height, absence of apophyseal joint involvement, absence of sacroiliac joint involvement, and extraspinal ossifications, including ligamentous calcifications.

Osteitis condensans ilii usually affects young to middle-aged females with normal sacroiliac joints. Radiography shows sclerosis on the iliac side of the sacroiliac joint only.

The sacroiliac joint also can be involved with 1) tuberculosis, 2) metastatic disease, 3) gout, 4) Paget disease, or 5) other infections (*Brucella, Serratia, Staphylococcus*).

- Osteitis condensans ilii usually affects young to middle-aged females; radiography shows sclerosis on the iliac side of the sacroiliac joint only.
- The sacroiliac joint can be involved with metastatic disease, gout, Paget disease, or infection (*Brucella, Serratia, Staphylococcus*).

Treatment

Treatment involves physical therapy (upright posture is very important), exercise (swimming), cessation of smoking, genetic counseling, and drug therapy with NSAIDs such as indomethacin. Sulfasalazine and methotrexate therapy also may provide benefit, especially in patients with peripheral joint involvement.

Reactive Arthritis

This is an aseptic arthritis induced by a host response to an infectious agent rather than direct infection. HLA-B27 is associated in 80% of cases. The condition develops after infections with *Salmonella* organisms, *Shigella flexneri*, *Yersinia enterocolitica*, and *Campylobacter jejuni*, which cause diarrhea, and *Chlamydia* and *Ureaplasma urealyticum*, which cause nonspecific urethritis. Inflammatory eye disease (conjunctivitis or iritis) and mucocutaneous disease (balanitis, oral ulcerations, or keratoderma) also can occur. Keratoderma blennorrhagicum is a characteristic skin disease on the palms and soles which is indistinguishable histologically from psoriasis. Joint predilection is for the toes and asymmetric large joints in the lower extremities. It can cause "sausage" toe, as can psoriatic arthritis. The distal interphalangeal joints in the hands can be affected also. Cardiac conduction disturbances and aortitis can develop. Sacroiliitis (sometimes unilateral) can occur. Long-term studies indicate that the disease remains episodically active in 75% of patients and that disability is a frequent outcome.

- Reactive arthritis: aseptic arthritis induced by a host response to an infectious agent rather than direct infection.
- HLA-B27 is associated in 80% of cases.
- Develops after infections with *Salmonella, Shigella flexneri, Yersinia enterocolitica, Campylobacter jejuni, Chlamydia, Ureaplasma urealyticum*.

Treatment is with NSAIDs (indomethacin). Sulfasalazine and methotrexate are used in patients with chronic disease. Treatment with tetracycline or erythromycin-type antibiotics may decrease the duration and severity of illness in some cases of *Chlamydia*-triggered reactive arthritis.

Arthritis Associated With Inflammatory Bowel Disease

Two distinct types of arthritis are associated with chronic inflammatory bowel disease: 1) a *non*destructive oligoarthritis of the peripheral joints tending to correlate with the activity of the bowel disease and 2) ankylosing spondylitis (enteropathic spondylitis). The spondylitis is not a complication of the bowel disease. It may be diagnosed many years before the onset of bowel symptoms, and its subsequent progress bears little relationship to the bowel disease. Approximately 75% of patients with enteropathic spondylitis and inflammatory bowel disease are HLA-B27–positive. Patients with inflammatory bowel disease alone do not have an increased frequency of HLA-B27 and are not at increased risk for development of spondylitis.

- Patients with inflammatory bowel disease may have a nondestructive oligoarthritis of the peripheral joints which tends to correlate with the activity of the bowel disease.

Psoriatic Arthritis

Psoriatic arthritis develops in 7% or less of patients with psoriasis. Pitting of nails is strongly associated with joint disease. Patients with more severe skin disease are at higher risk for the development of arthritis. A "sausage" finger or toe is characteristic of psoriatic arthritis and is very uncommon in rheumatoid arthritis. Radiographic evidence of involvement of the distal interphalangeal joint with erosions is common in psoriasis and uncommon in rheumatoid arthritis. Psoriatic arthritis also can, in severe cases, cause a characteristic "pencil-in-cup" deformity of the distal interphalangeal and proximal interphalangeal joints on radiography.

- Psoriatic arthritis develops in 7% or less of patients with psoriasis.
- Pitting of nails is strongly associated with joint disease.
- "Sausage" finger or toe is characteristic.
- "Pencil-in-cup" deformity of the distal and proximal interphalangeal joints is found on radiography.

There are five clinical groups of psoriatic arthritis: 1) predominantly distal interphalangeal joint involvement, 2) asymmetric oligoarthritis, 3) symmetric polyarthritis-like rheumatoid arthritis but negative for rheumatoid factor, 4) arthritis mutilans, and 5) psoriatic spondylitis (HLA-B27–positive in 50%-75%

of cases). Treatment is with NSAIDs, methotrexate, and tumor necrosis factor antagonists.

IRITIS AND RHEUMATOLOGIC DISEASES

Various rheumatologic diseases are associated with iritis, particularly the seronegative spondyloarthropathies. Iritis is uncommon in rheumatoid arthritis and systemic lupus erythematosus. Nongranulomatous iritis without any other associated symptoms may be associated with HLA-B27 in almost 50% of patients.

BEHÇET SYNDROME

Behçet syndrome is most common in Middle Eastern countries and Japan. HLA-B51 is associated with the syndrome. In addition to oral and genital ulcerations, uveitis, synovitis, cutaneous vasculitis, and meningoencephalitis may be present. The pathergy reaction (hyperreactivity of the skin in response to superficial trauma) is also seen. Migratory, superficial thrombophlebitis and erythema nodosum also have been associated with this syndrome. The combination of recurrent aphthous dermatitis, similar ulcerations in the genital area, and uveitis is most common. Treatment is with corticosteroids, although more aggressive immunosuppression is often required.

OSTEOID OSTEOMA

Osteoid osteoma is a benign bone tumor. It usually occurs in males and females between the ages of 5 and 30 years. The classic symptom is bone pain at night, which is relieved completely with aspirin or another NSAID. The diagnosis may be made with routine radiography, but often this is negative and a bone scan may be helpful in localizing the tumor. Tomography or computed tomography then can be done for better visualization. Radiography shows a small nidus, usually less than 1 cm, varying from radiolucent to radiopaque, depending on the age of the lesion. There is usually a lucent ring around the nidus and adjacent bone sclerosis. Definitive treatment includes excision, which is curative.

- Osteoid osteoma is a benign bone tumor.
- Bone pain at night is relieved by aspirin or another NSAID.
- Treatment includes excision, which is curative.

BYPASS ARTHRITIS

This occurs in patients who have undergone intestinal bypass operations, including jejunocolic or jejunoileal. The arthritis may be acute or subacute, is usually intermittent, and can last occasionally for short periods, only to recur. The most commonly affected joints are the metacarpophalangeal, proximal interphalangeal, wrists, knees, and ankles. It is commonly associated with a dermatitis, which can be pustular. Circulating immune complexes composed of bacterial antigens have been found in both the circulation and the synovial fluid and are thought to be the cause of this disorder. Treatment consists of NSAIDs and antibiotics such as tetracycline, but reanastomosis may be necessary for complete resolution of symptoms.

- Bypass arthritis occurs in patients who have had intestinal bypass operations.
- Most commonly affected joints: metacarpophalangeal, proximal interphalangeal, wrists, knees, ankles.
- Bypass arthritis is commonly associated with a dermatitis.

SYSTEMIC LUPUS ERYTHEMATOSUS

Systemic lupus erythematosus (SLE) is a chronic inflammatory disease of unknown cause with a wide spectrum of clinical manifestations and variable course characterized by exacerbations and remissions. Antibodies that react with nuclear antigens commonly are found in patients with the disease. Genetic, hormonal, and environmental factors seem to be important in the cause.

- SLE is characterized by exacerbations and remissions.

Diagnosis

At least four of the following findings are needed for the diagnosis of SLE: malar rash; discoid lupus; photosensitivity; oral ulcers; nonerosive arthritis; proteinuria (protein >0.5 g/day) or cellular casts; seizures or psychosis; pleuritis or pericarditis; hemolytic anemia, leukopenia, lymphopenia, or thrombocytopenia; antibody to nDNA, antibody to Sm (Smith), IgG or IgM anticardiolipin antibodies, positive test for lupus anticoagulant, or false-positive results of VDRL test; and positive results of fluorescent antinuclear antibody test.

Epidemiology

The female:male ratio is 8:1 during the reproductive years. The first symptoms usually occur between the second and fourth decades of life. The disease seems to be less severe in the elderly. In SLE with onset at an older age, the female:male ratio is equal. The frequency of SLE is increased in American blacks, Native Americans, and Asians.

- Female:male ratio in SLE is 8:1 during the reproductive years.
- The frequency of SLE is increased in American blacks, Native Americans, and Asians.

Etiology

In human disease, viral-like particles in glomeruli of patients with SLE have been reported; however, attempts to isolate viruses have been unsuccessful. A direct causal relationship between virus and SLE has not yet been established. Patients with SLE have increased antibody titers to a wide range of antigens without much sign of specificity for a particular viral agent.

- In SLE, there are increased antibody titers to a wide range of antigens without much sign of specificity for a particular viral agent.

Genetics

Among relatives of patients with SLE, 20% have a different immunologic disease. Another 25% have antinuclear antibodies, circulating immune complexes, antilymphocyte antibodies, or a false-positive result on VDRL test without clinical disease. Concordance for SLE among monozygotic twins is much greater than among dizygotic twins. Multiple genetic and environmental factors are important in the development of SLE. Immune complex levels are much higher in persons with close contact to SLE patients than in unexposed consanguineous relatives. The frequency of HLA-B8, HLA-DR2, and HLA-DR3 is increased.

- 20% of relatives of patients with SLE have a different immunologic disease.
- In SLE, the frequency of HLA-B8, HLA-DR2, and HLA-DR3 is increased.

Pathogenesis

There is a change in the activity of the cellular immune system with an absolute decrease in T-suppressor cells. There is an increase in the activity of the humoral immune system with B-cell hyperactivity resulting in polyclonal activation and antibody production.

Circulating immune complexes (anti-nDNA) may contribute to glomerulonephritis and skin disease, among other manifestations. Immune complexes bind complement, which initiates the inflammatory process. Organ-specific autoantibodies also contribute to the pathophysiology of the disease and include antibodies that are 1) antierythrocyte, 2) antiplatelet, 3) antileukocyte, 4) antineuronal, and 5) antithyroid.

- Circulating immune complexes (anti-nDNA) are responsible for glomerulonephritis and certain skin manifestations.
- Organ-specific autoantibodies also may contribute to the pathophysiology.

Late complications of SLE are related to vascular damage, sometimes in the relative absence of active immunologic disease. Damage to the intima during active disease may ultimately result in various thrombotic, ischemic, and hypertensive manifestations.

Clinical Manifestations

Fever in SLE usually is caused by the disease, but infection must be ruled out. Shaking chills and leukocytosis strongly suggest infection.

Articular

The arthritis is characteristically inflammatory but nondeforming and nonerosive. Avascular necrosis of bone occurs, and not only in patients taking steroids. The femoral head, navicular bone, and tibial plateau are most commonly affected.

Dermatologic

Discoid lupus involves the face, scalp, and extremities. There is follicular plugging with atrophy leading to scarring. Subacute cutaneous LE is a subset of SLE that primarily has skin involvement with psoriasiform or annular erythematous lesions. Patients may be negative for antinuclear antibodies but frequently are positive for antibodies to the extractable nuclear antigen SS-A (Ro).

Cardiopulmonary

Cardiac involvement in SLE is manifested by pericarditis, myocarditis, valvular involvement, accelerated coronary atherosclerosis, and coronary vasculitis.

Pulmonary involvement in SLE is manifested by any of the following: pleurisy, pleural effusions, pneumonitis, pulmonary hypertension, hemorrhage, and diaphragmatic dysfunction.

Neuropsychiatric

Central nervous system lupus is a most variable and unpredictable phenomenon. Manifestations such as impaired cognitive function, seizures, long tract signs, cranial neuropathies, psychosis, and migraine-like attacks occur with little apparent relationship to each other or to other systemic manifestations. Immune complexes in the choroid plexus are *not* specific for central nervous system disease because they also occur in patients without central nervous system disease. Patients may have increased cerebrospinal fluid protein (IgG), pleocytosis, and antineuronal antibodies.

Results of electroencephalography can be abnormal. Magnetic resonance imaging usually shows areas of increased signal in the periventricular white matter, similar to those found in multiple sclerosis. Magnetic resonance imaging findings are often nonspecific and sometimes can be seen in patients who have SLE without central nervous system manifestations. Pathologic examinations of autopsy specimens usually reveal microinfarcts, nerve cell loss, rarely vasculitis, or no detectable abnormalities.

Proposed pathogenetic mechanisms causing neuropsychiatric manifestations include autoneuronal antibodies, vasculitis, leukoagglutination, antiphospholipid-associated hypercoagulability, and cytokine effect.

Psychosis caused by steroid therapy is probably rarer than previously thought. When in doubt about the cause of the psychosis in patients with SLE, the steroid dose can be increased and the patient observed. Patients rarely can have isolated central nervous system involvement and normal results of cerebrospinal fluid examination and no other organ involvement.

Particularly with neuropsychiatric symptoms or respiratory symptoms, secondary causes must be considered, particularly infection, hypertension, anemia, hypoxia, and fever. Fever should be considered due to infection until proved otherwise.

- Central nervous system lupus is a most variable and unpredictable phenomenon.
- Immune complexes in the choroid plexus are not specific for central nervous system disease.
- Magnetic resonance imaging findings are nonspecific.
- Particularly with neuropsychiatric symptoms or respiratory symptoms, secondary causes must be considered, particularly infection, hypertension, anemia, hypoxia, and fever.
- Fever should be considered due to infection until proved otherwise.

Pregnancy and SLE

Women with SLE who become pregnant have a high prevalence of spontaneous abortion. Because abortion itself may lead to a flare of the disease, therapeutic abortion ordinarily is not recommended after the first trimester. Flares of disease should be treated with steroids, particularly during the postpartum period.

In infants of mothers with SLE, thrombocytopenia and leukopenia can develop from passive transfer of antibodies. They also can have transient cutaneous lesions and transient complete heart block. Mothers usually have anti-SS-A (Ro), which crosses the placenta and is transiently present in the infant. Mothers usually are HLA-B8/DR3-positive, but there is no HLA association in the child.

Renal Involvement

The types of renal disease in SLE are 1) mesangial, 2) focal glomerulonephritis, 3) membranous glomerulonephritis, 4) diffuse proliferative glomerulonephritis, 5) interstitial nephritis with defects in the renal tubular handling of K^+, and 6) renal vein thrombosis with nephrotic syndrome.

Treatment of renal disease depends in part on the results of renal biopsy. Patients with high activity indices on biopsy such as active inflammation, proliferation, necrosis, and crescent formation are considered for aggressive therapy. Patients with high chronicity indices such as tubular atrophy, scarring, and glomerulosclerosis are less likely to respond to aggressive therapy. Patients with mesangial changes alone do not require aggressive therapy. Active diffuse proliferative glomerulonephritis is treated with high-dose steroids and immunosuppressive agents. Immunosuppressive agents lower the incidence of renal failure in patients with diffuse proliferative glomerulonephritis and may improve overall survival. Appropriate treatment for focal proliferative glomerulonephritis and membranous glomerulonephritis is controversial because the prognosis is more favorable.

- Renal biopsies are helpful for directing therapy.
- Patients with mesangial changes alone do not require aggressive therapy.
- Active diffuse proliferative glomerulonephritis is treated with high-dose steroids and immunosuppressive agents.

Laboratory Findings

Anemia of chronic disease and hemolytic anemia (Coombs positive) can occur. Leukopenia usually does not predispose to infection. Antilymphocyte antibodies cause lymphopenia in SLE. Idiopathic thrombocytopenic purpura with the presence of platelet antibodies can be the initial manifestation of SLE. Polyclonal gammopathy due to hyperactivity of the humoral immune system is common. The erythrocyte sedimentation rate usually correlates with disease activity.

Hypocomplementemia (CH_{50}, C3, C4) usually correlates with active disease. Hypocomplementemia with increased anti-nDNA antibodies usually implies renal disease (or skin disease). Complement split products (such as C3a, C5a, Ba/BB) are increased in active disease. A total complement value too low to measure with normal C3 and C4 values suggests a hereditary complement deficiency. Familial C2 deficiency is the most common complement deficiency in SLE, but C1r, C1s, C1q, C4, C5, C7, and C8 deficiencies also have been reported.

Patients with SLE may have false-positive results of the VDRL test as a result of antibody to phospholipid, which cross-reacts with VDRL. Patients with SLE also can have false-positive results of the fluorescent treponemal antibody test, but usually have the "beaded pattern" of fluorescence. LE cells are present in approximately 70% of patients with SLE and are caused by antibody to deoxyribonucleoprotein (DNP). This test is not specific and is no longer performed in many centers. Anti-DNP also is detected by the fluorescent antinuclear antibody test in a homogeneous pattern.

Anti-nDNA levels fluctuate with disease activity, whereas levels of other autoantibodies (ribonucleoprotein, Sm, antinuclear antibody) show *no* consistent relationship to levels of anti-nDNA or disease activity. Methods used to measure anti-nDNA are 1) an immunofluorescent method using *Crithidia lucilia*, an organism with a kinetoplast that contains helical native DNA free of other nuclear antigens—therefore, there is no single-stranded DNA contamination, and 2) radioimmunoassay and enzyme-linked immunosorbent assay, which suffer from the difficulty of maintaining DNA in its native double-stranded state and so are contaminated with single-stranded DNA.

Although all patients with lupus should have positive results of antinuclear antibody tests, a positive result is by no means specific for lupus. Antinuclear antibody patterns are outlined in Table 22-25. Other autoantibodies and disease associations are outlined in Table 22-26.

- Hemolytic anemia (Coombs positive) can occur in SLE.
- Idiopathic thrombocytopenic purpura can be the initial manifestation of SLE.
- Hypocomplementemia (CH_{50}, C3, C4) usually correlates with active disease.
- Hypocomplementemia with increased anti-nDNA antibodies usually implies renal disease (or skin disease).
- Anti-nDNA levels fluctuate with disease activity, but other associated antibodies do not.
- A positive result of an antinuclear antibody test is by no means specific for lupus.

Treatment

Treatment should match the activity of SLE in the individual patient. Serial monitoring of organ function and appropriate laboratory evaluation (anti-nDNA, C3, erythrocyte sedimentation rate) allow rapid recognition and treatment of flares and appropriate tapering of steroid dose during periods of disease

Table 22-25 Antinuclear Antibody Patterns

Fluorescent pattern	Antigen	Disease association
Rim, peripheral, shaggy	nDNA	SLE
Homogeneous	DNP	SLE, others
Speckled	ENA	MCTD, SLE, others
Nucleolar	RNA	Scleroderma

DNP, deoxyribonucleoprotein; ENA, extractable nuclear antigen; MCTD, mixed connective tissue disease; SLE, systemic lupus erythematosus.

Table 22-26 Autoantibodies in Rheumatic Diseases

Antibody	Disease association
Anti-nDNA	SLE, 50%-60%
Anti-Sm (Smith)	SLE, 30%
Anti-RNP (ribonucleoprotein)	MCTD, 100% high titer
	SLE, 30% titer
	Scleroderma, low frequency, low titer
Anti-SS-A	Sjögren, 70%
	SLE, 35%
	Scleroderma + MCTD, low frequency, low titer
Anti-SS-B	Sjögren, 60%
	SLE, 15%
Antihistone	Drug-induced SLE, 95%
	SLE, 60%
	RA, 20%
Anti-Sc1-70 (antitopoisomerase I)	Scleroderma, 25%
Anticentromere	CREST, 70%-90%
	Scleroderma, 10%-15%
Anti-PM1	PM, 50%
Anti-Jo1 (histidyl-tRNA synthetase)	PM/interstitial lung disease, 30%

CREST, syndrome of *c*alcinosis cutis, *R*aynaud phenomenon, *e*sophageal dysmotility, *s*clerodactyly, *t*elangiectasia; MCTD, mixed connective tissue disease; PM, polymyositis; RA, rheumatoid arthritis; SLE, systemic lupus erythematosus.

quiescence. Table 22-27 provides guidelines for treatment, and Table 22-28 outlines the complications of treatment.

Outcome

The 10-year survival rate is 90% in newly diagnosed SLE. Prognosis is worse in blacks and Hispanics than in whites. Prognosis is worse in patients with creatinine values more than 3.0 mg/dL. The major causes of death are 1) renal disease, 2) infection, 3) central nervous system involvement, and 4) vascular disease (such as myocardial infarction).

- The 10-year survival rate is 90% in newly diagnosed SLE.
- The prognosis is worse in blacks and Hispanics.
- Typical clinical scenario: A young woman presents with malar rash and photosensitivity. She has a history of oral ulcers and arthralgias. Laboratory testing reveals significant proteinuria and red blood cell casts in the urine. There is a normochromic normocytic anemia with a positive Coombs test. Antibody to native DNA is present. Results of the VDRL test are positive.

DRUG-INDUCED LUPUS

Many drugs have been implicated in drug-induced lupus. The most common drugs are listed in Table 22-29. One must differentiate between the clinical syndrome of drug-induced lupus and only a positive antinuclear antibody result without clinical symptoms. Many drugs can cause a positive antinuclear antibody result without ever causing the clinical syndrome of drug-induced lupus. Only hydralazine and procainamide have been strongly implicated in drug-induced lupus. A drug-induced lupus syndrome develops in approximately 5% of persons taking hydralazine and in 15% to 25% of those who take procainamide. Virtually all patients taking procainamide for 1 year will have a positive result of the antinuclear antibody test.

- Only hydralazine and procainamide are strongly implicated in drug-induced lupus.
- Virtually all patients taking procainamide for 1 year have a positive result of the antinuclear antibody test.

Clinical Features

The clinical manifestations of drug-induced lupus include arthralgias and polyarthritis, which occur in approximately 80% of cases. Malaise is common, and fever has been reported in up to 40% of cases. Cardiopulmonary involvement is also common, and approximately 30% of patients have pleural-pulmonary manifestations as their presenting symptoms. Pericarditis has been reported in approximately 20% of cases. Diffuse interstitial pneumonitis has been noted. Asymptomatic

Table 22-27 Treatment of Manifestations of Systemic Lupus Erythematosus

Manifestation	Treatment
Arthritis, fever, mild systemic symptoms	ASA, NSAID
Photosensitivity, rash	Avoidance of sun, use of sunscreens
Rash, arthritis	Hydroxychloroquine (Plaquenil)
Significant thrombocytopenia, hemolytic anemia	Steroids
Renal disease, CNS disease, pericarditis, other significant organ involvement	Steroids
Rapidly deteriorating renal function	Cytotoxic agents

ASA, acetylsalicylic acid; CNS, central nervous system; NSAID, nonsteroidal anti-inflammatory drug.

Table 22-28 Complications of Treatment for Systemic Lupus Erythematosus

Treatment	Complication
Ibuprofen	Aseptic meningitis (headache, fever, stiff neck, CSF pleocytosis)
NSAID	Decreased renal blood flow
ASA	Salicylate hepatitis (common), benign
Cyclophosphamide	Hemorrhagic cystitis, alopecia, opportunistic lymphomas, infection, increased incidence of lymphomas (CNS)
Hydroxychloroquine (Plaquenil)	Retinal toxicity

ASA, acetylsalicylic acid; CNS, central nervous system; CSF, cerebrospinal fluid; NSAID, nonsteroidal anti-inflammatory drug.

Table 22-29 Implicated Agents in Drug-Induced Lupus

Definite	Probable
Common	Phenytoin
Procainamide	Carbamazepine
Hydralazine	Ethosuximide
Uncommon	Propylthiouracil
Isoniazid	Penicillamine
Methyldopa	Sulfasalazine
Chlorpromazine	Lithium carbonate
Quinidine	Acebutolol
Minocycline	Lovastatin

- In drug-induced lupus, arthralgias and polyarthritis occur in about 80% of cases.
- Malaise is common, and fever occurs in up to 40% of cases.
- About 30% of patients have pleural-pulmonary manifestations on presentation.
- Pericarditis is reported in about 20% of cases.
- The incidence of renal and central nervous system involvement is low.

SLE is predominantly a disease of premenopausal females, whereas drug-induced disease has an almost equal sex distribution and occurs in an older population. This disparity in age reflects the use of hydralazine and procainamide primarily in an older population.

Laboratory Abnormalities

Virtually all patients with SLE and drug-induced lupus have antinuclear antibodies. Although patients with SLE and drug-induced lupus are serologically similar in many respects, there are notable differences. Antibodies to native DNA are found in only a small percentage of cases of drug-induced lupus but in approximately 60% of cases of SLE. Serum total hemolytic complement, C3, and C4 are usually normal in drug-induced

pleural effusions may be found on routine chest radiography. A few cases of pericardial tamponade have been reported. In contrast to SLE, the incidence of renal and central nervous system involvement is low in drug-induced lupus. Therefore, it is regarded as more benign than SLE. Other clinical differences include a lower incidence of skin manifestations, lymphadenopathy, and myalgias in drug-induced disease.

disease, in contrast to SLE. Antibodies such as anti-Sm, SS-A, SS-B, and RNP are also unusual in drug-induced lupus. The frequency of antihistone antibodies in drug-induced lupus is high (>95% of cases), but these also occur in approximately 60% of cases of SLE. Other, less frequent laboratory abnormalities in drug-induced lupus can include a positive LE preparation, positive Coombs test, positive rheumatoid factor, false-positive result of serologic test for syphilis, circulating anticoagulants, and cryoglobulins.

Metabolism

Drugs involved in drug-induced lupus have different chemical structures, but three of them—isoniazid, procainamide, and hydralazine—contain a primary amine that is acetylated by the hepatic *N*-acetyltransferase system. Persons who are taking one of these drugs and who are *slow* acetylators have a much higher incidence of serologic abnormalities and clinical disease than rapid acetylators. These manifestations also occur over a shorter period in slow acetylators than in rapid acetylators.

- Slow acetylators have a much higher incidence of serologic abnormalities and clinical disease.

Treatment

When possible, patients with drug-induced lupus should stop using the offending drug. Symptoms usually subside within several weeks, although the duration for complete resolution varies depending on the drug. Serologic abnormalities can remain for years after resolution of clinical symptoms. Patients taking procainamide are most likely to have a rapid remission once use of the drug is stopped, but patients taking hydralazine might have prolonged clinical manifestations. Treatment depends on the clinical manifestations and could include NSAIDs or possibly low-dose prednisone if needed.

- Typical clinical scenario: A patient presents with a history of fever, arthralgias, fatigue, and a rash. The patient is taking procainamide for suppression of a ventricular arrhythmia. Laboratory testing reveals a positive antinuclear antibody test and negative anti-native DNA antibody.

OVERLAP SYNDROMES

An overlap syndrome is a disease characterized by features of more than one connective tissue disease. Secondary Sjögren syndrome accompanying another connective tissue disease is not classified as an overlap syndrome.

Mixed Connective Tissue Disease

This is a distinct disease with variable features of SLE, polymyositis, systemic sclerosis, and rheumatoid arthritis. The incidence of renal disease is low. It is serologically characterized by a positive antinuclear antibody and by a high titer of the autoantibody anti-RNP. Anti-nDNA antibodies usually are not present. Raynaud phenomenon is common.

Undifferentiated Connective Tissue Disease

This category includes patients with symptoms that do not fulfill the diagnostic criteria for a definite or specific connective tissue disease. Common symptoms include Raynaud phenomenon, arthralgias, fatigue, and variable joint or soft tissue swelling. The antinuclear antibody may be positive, but other autoantibodies are not present. Patients need to be observed to determine whether progression to a distinct connective tissue disease occurs.

ANTIPHOSPHOLIPID ANTIBODY SYNDROME

The lupus anticoagulant and various phospholipid antibodies have been associated with recurrent arterial and venous thromboses. Antiphospholipid antibodies may be either the IgG or the IgM class and are routinely measured as anticardiolipin antibodies. The hallmark of the antiphospholipid antibody syndrome is prolongation of all phospholipid-dependent coagulation tests. The antibodies prolong the partial thromboplastin time at the level of the prothrombin activator complex of the clotting cascade. The antiphospholipid antibodies are thought to interact with the β_2-glycoprotein-1 that binds to phospholipid, interfering with the calcium-dependent binding of prothrombin factor Xa to the phospholipid. The failure of normal plasma to correct the prolonged clotting time distinguishes the lupus anticoagulant and antiphospholipid antibody clotting factors from clotting factor deficiencies. In the usual coagulation screening tests, the lupus anticoagulant results in prolongation of the activated partial thromboplastin time without prolongation of the prothrombin time (Table 22-30).

- Antiphospholipid antibodies are of either the IgG or the IgM class.

Table 22-30 Coagulation Tests Characterizing the Lupus Anticoagulant

Screening tests
Prothrombin time normal
Partial thromboplastin time (PTT) prolonged
Plasma clot time prolonged
Tests identifying the lupus anticoagulant
Prolonged PTT not corrected by adding normal plasma

- Prolongation of all phospholipid-dependent coagulation tests is the laboratory hallmark of the antiphospholipid antibody syndrome.
- Activated partial thromboplastin time is prolonged and not corrected by adding normal plasma, but it is corrected with the addition of platelet-rich plasma, and this is the laboratory hallmark of a lupus anticoagulant.

Various other tests are reported to be sensitive for detection of lupus anticoagulants, including the plasma clotting time, kaolin clotting time, a platelet neutralization procedure, and modified Russell viper venom time.

Many, but not all, patients with the lupus anticoagulant also have increased IgG or IgM antiphospholipid antibody levels.

The lupus anticoagulant and antiphospholipid antibodies are associated with SLE, but they also have been reported in various other autoimmune, malignant, infectious, and drug-induced diseases. Other associated diseases include Sjögren syndrome, rheumatoid arthritis, idiopathic thrombocytopenic purpura, Behçet syndrome, myasthenia gravis, and mixed connective tissue disease. The antibodies are also found in persons with no apparent disease but in whom recurrent thrombosis develops. This is the primary antiphospholipid antibody syndrome, which represents approximately 50% of cases.

- Lupus anticoagulant and antiphospholipid antibodies also have been reported in various other autoimmune, malignant, infectious, and drug-induced diseases.
- The primary antiphospholipid antibody syndrome represents 50% of cases.

Clinical Features

There is an association between the presence of the lupus anticoagulant and antiphospholipid antibodies and recurrent venous or arterial thrombosis. Thrombotic events described have included stroke, transient ischemic attacks, myocardial infarctions, brachial artery thrombosis, deep venous thrombophlebitis, retinal vein thrombosis, hepatic vein thrombosis resulting in Budd-Chiari syndrome, and pulmonary hypertension. Other manifestations include recurrent fetal loss, thrombocytopenia, positive results of Coombs test, migraines, chorea, epilepsy, chronic leg ulcers, livedo reticularis, and progressive dementia resulting from cerebrovascular accidents. Recently, acquired valvular heart disease, especially aortic insufficiency, has been described. The mechanism or mechanisms by which antiphospholipid antibodies are associated with thromboembolic manifestations remain unclear. Blocking the production of prostacyclin from vascular endothelial cells, inhibition of the prekallikrein activity protein C pathway and fibrinolysis, and decreased plasminogen activator release have all been described.

Although many patients with lupus and other diseases can have a lupus anticoagulant or antiphospholipid antibodies, of either the IgG or the IgM class, thrombosis will not necessarily develop. In general, patients with the highest levels of antiphospholipid antibodies are more prone to thrombosis than those with lower levels. Also, the IgG antiphospholipid antibody is more strongly associated with recurrent thrombosis than is the IgM antiphospholipid antibody. If there is no history of thrombosis, most physicians are reluctant to treat the patient with a lupus anticoagulant or increased antiphospholipid antibodies alone without clinical manifestations.

- There is an association between the presence of the lupus anticoagulant and antiphospholipid antibodies and recurrent venous or arterial thrombosis.
- Other manifestations: recurrent fetal loss, thrombocytopenia, positive Coombs test, migraines, chorea, epilepsy, chronic leg ulcers, livedo reticularis, and progressive dementia from cerebrovascular accidents.
- Acquired valvular heart disease, especially aortic insufficiency, has been described.
- Patients with the highest levels of antiphospholipid antibodies are more prone to thrombosis.
- IgG antiphospholipid antibody is more strongly associated with recurrent thrombosis.

Treatment

For most patients who have recurrent thrombosis and high-titer anticardiolipin antibody, warfarin (Coumadin) is prescribed in doses sufficient to yield international normalized ratio values close to 3 and will need to be taken for life. Low-dose aspirin and subcutaneous heparin have been used in pregnant women to prevent fetal loss. Corticosteroids have not been clearly demonstrated to be efficacious in preventing thrombosis.

- Typical clinical scenario: A young patient presents with recurrent deep vein thrombosis. In the absence of anticoagulant therapy, the activated partial thromboplastin time is prolonged. Laboratory tests show that this prolongation is not corrected by the addition of normal plasma.

RAYNAUD PHENOMENON

This is biphasic or triphasic color changes (pallor, cyanosis, erythema) accompanied by pain and numbness in the hands or feet. Cold is a common precipitating agent. Associated factors are listed in Table 22-31.

- Cold is a common precipitating agent for Raynaud phenomenon.

Table 22-31 Causes of Secondary Raynaud Phenomenon

Chemotherapeutic agents
   Bleomycin
   Vinblastine
Toxins
   Vinyl chloride
Vibration-induced injuries
   Jackhammer use
Vascular occlusive disorders
   Thoracic outlet obstruction
   Atherosclerosis
   Vasculitis
Connective tissue diseases
   Scleroderma, 90%-100%
   Mixed connective tissue disease, 90%-100%
   Systemic lupus erythematosus, 15%
   Rheumatoid arthritis, <10%
   Polymyositis
Miscellaneous
   Cryoglobulinemia
   Cold agglutinins
   Increased blood viscosity

Raynaud phenomenon is related to an abnormality of the microvasculature associated with intimal fibrosis. In male patients with Raynaud phenomenon, a rare occurrence, a connective tissue disease may develop. Although Raynaud phenomenon is common in females, it usually is not associated with a connective tissue disease unless the patient has positive results for antinuclear antibody, which suggest that a connective tissue disease may develop in the future.

Skin capillary microscopy reveals tortuous, dilated capillary loops in systemic sclerosis, mixed connective tissue disease, and polymyositis. They also may be present in patients with Raynaud phenomenon who will go on to have systemic sclerosis, polymyositis, or mixed connective tissue disease.

Treatment involves smoking cessation, wearing gloves, biofeedback, 2% nitrol paste, and antihypertensive agents (prazosin, nifedipine). A stellate ganglion block, digital nerve block, or surgical digital sympathectomy is used if ischemia is severe. β-Adrenergic blockers increase spasm and should be avoided.

To differentiate primary Raynaud phenomenon from the secondary form (resulting from a connective tissue disease), clinical features are considered. In primary Raynaud disease, females are usually affected, the onset is at menarche, usually all digits are involved, and attacks are very frequent. The severity of symptoms is mild to moderate, and they can be precipitated by emotional stress. Digital ulceration and finger edema are rare, as is periungual erythema. Livedo reticularis is frequent.

In persons with Raynaud phenomenon due to a connective tissue disease, both males and females are affected. The onset of Raynaud phenomenon is in the mid-20s or later. It often begins in a single digit, and attacks are usually infrequent (zero to five a day). It is moderate to severe, and the disorder is not precipitated by emotional stress. Digital ulceration, finger edema, and periungual erythema are frequent. Livedo reticularis is uncommon.

SYSTEMIC SCLEROSIS (SCLERODERMA)

For the diagnosis of systemic sclerosis, one major criterion or two or more minor criteria need to be present. The major criterion is symmetric induration of the skin of the fingers and skin proximal to metacarpophalangeal or metatarsophalangeal joints. The minor criteria are sclerodactyly, digital pitting scars or loss of substance from the finger pad, and bibasilar pulmonary fibrosis.

● Systemic sclerosis is characterized by symmetric induration of the skin of the fingers and skin proximal to metacarpophalangeal or metatarsophalangeal joints, sclerodactyly, fingertip pitting or scarring, and bibasilar pulmonary fibrosis.

Clinical Manifestations

Skin

Patients are at risk for the development of rapidly progressive acral and trunk skin thickening and early visceral abnormalities. Skin and visceral changes tend to parallel each other in severity, but not always. Some patients have rapid progression for 2 to 3 years and then arrest of the disorder, allowing for some improvement of the disorder.

Raynaud Phenomenon

Raynaud phenomenon occurs in almost all patients. It usually occurs more than 2 years before skin changes. The vasospasm in the hands can be associated with reduced perfusion to the heart, lungs, kidneys, and gastrointestinal tract. If Raynaud phenomenon is not present but skin findings are suggestive of scleroderma, another disease such as eosinophilic fasciitis should be considered.

Articular

Nondeforming symmetric polyarthritis similar to rheumatoid arthritis may precede cutaneous manifestations by 12 months. Patients can have both articular erosions and nonarticular bony resorptive changes of ribs, mandible, radius, ulna, and distal phalangeal tufts which are unique to systemic sclerosis. Up to 60% of patients have "leathery" crepitation of the tendons of the wrist.

Pulmonary

A considerable decrease in diffusing capacity can be present with a normal chest radiograph. Diffuse interstitial fibrosis occurs in approximately 70% of patients and is the most common pulmonary abnormality. Patients who have active alveolitis demonstrated by 1) bronchopulmonary lavage, 2) high-resolution computed tomography showing ground-glass appearance without honeycombing, or 3) lung biopsy are most likely to respond to prednisone and cyclophosphamide therapy with improvement of pulmonary function. Pleuritis (with effusion) is very rare. Pulmonary hypertension is more common in patients with CREST (calcinosis cutis, Raynaud phenomenon, esophageal dysmotility, sclerodactyly, telangiectasias) variant.

- A considerable decrease in diffusing capacity can be present with a normal chest radiograph.
- Diffuse interstitial fibrosis occurs in approximately 70% of patients and is the most common pulmonary abnormality.
- Pleuritis is very rare.
- Pulmonary hypertension is more common in patients with CREST variant.

Cardiac

Cardiac abnormalities occur in up to 70% of patients. Conduction defects and supraventricular arrhythmias are most common. Pulmonary hypertension with cor pulmonale is the most serious problem.

- Cardiac abnormalities occur in up to 70% of patients. Pulmonary hypertension with cor pulmonale is a serious potential problem.

Gastrointestinal

Esophageal dysfunction is the most frequent gastrointestinal abnormality. It occurs in 90% of patients and often is asymptomatic. Lower esophageal sphincter incompetence with acid reflux may produce esophageal strictures or ulcers. Medications to reduce acid production are important. Reduced esophageal motility may respond to therapy with metoclopramide, cisapride, or erythromycin. Small bowel hypomotility may be associated with pseudo-obstruction, bowel dilatation, bacterial overgrowth, and malabsorption. Treatment with tetracycline may be helpful, but promotility agents are less effective. Colonic dysmotility also occurs and wide-mouthed diverticuli may be seen.

Renal

Renal involvement may result in fulminant hypertension, renal failure, and death if not treated aggressively. Proteinuria, newly diagnosed *mild* hypertension, microangiopathic hemolytic anemia, vascular changes on renal biopsy, and rapid progression of skin thickening may precede overt clinical findings of renal crisis. Renal involvement with hyperreninemia necessitates the use of angiotensin-converting enzyme inhibitors. Aggressive early antihypertensive therapy can extend life expectancy.

Laboratory Findings

Antitopoisomerase I antibody (anti-Scl-70) is found in approximately 25% of patients with scleroderma, and anticentromere antibody occurs in 10% to 20%.

Treatment

No remissive or curative therapy is available. Retrospective studies suggest that D-penicillamine (62.5 mg daily) may decrease skin thickness, prevent or delay internal organ involvement, and perhaps prolong life expectancy, but enthusiasm for this treatment has faded. Aggressive nutritional support, including hyperalimentation, may be required for extensive gastrointestinal disease.

- No remissive or curative therapy is available for systemic sclerosis.

CREST SYNDROME

This is characterized by *c*alcinosis cutis, *R*aynaud phenomenon, *e*sophageal dysmotility, *s*clerodactyly, and *t*elangiectasias. Skin involvement progresses slowly and is limited to the extremities. Development of internal organ involvement occurs but is delayed. Lung involvement occurs in 70% of patients. Diffusing capacity may be low, and pulmonary hypertension can develop. The latter is more common in CREST than in diffuse scleroderma. Onset of Raynaud phenomenon occurs less than 2 years before skin changes. Anticentromere antibody is found in 70% to 90% of patients and antiscleroderma-70 antibody in 10%. The incidence of primary biliary cirrhosis is increased.

- In CREST syndrome, 70% of patients have lung involvement.
- The diffusing capacity may be low, and pulmonary hypertension can develop.
- Anticentromere antibody is present in 70%-90% of patients.
- There is an increased incidence of primary biliary cirrhosis.

The clinical manifestations of limited and systemic scleroderma are listed in Table 22-32.

Table 22-32 Clinical Findings in Limited and Diffuse Scleroderma

Clinical finding	Cutaneous disease	
	Limited	Diffuse
Raynaud phenomenon	Precedes other symptoms by years	Onset associated with other symptoms within 1 year
Nailfold capillaries	Dilated	Dilated with dropout
Skin changes	Distal to elbow	Proximal to elbow with involvement of trunk
Telangiectasia, digital ulcers, calcinosis	Frequent	Rare early, but frequent later in the course
Joint and tendon involvement	Uncommon	Frequent (tendon rubs)
Visceral disease	Pulmonary hypertension	Renal, intestinal, and cardiac disease; pulmonary interstitial fibrosis
Autoantibodies	Anticentromere (70%-90%)	Antitopoisomerase 1 (Scl-70) (25%)
10-year survival	>70%	<70%

SCLERODERMA-LIKE SYNDROMES

Disorders Associated With Occupation or Environment

This group includes polyvinyl chloride disease, organic solvents, jackhammer disease, silicosis, and toxic oil syndrome.

Eosinophilic Fasciitis

Clinical features of this disorder include tight bound-down skin of the extremities, characteristically sparing the hands and feet. Peau d'orange skin changes can develop. Onset after vigorous exercise is common. Raynaud phenomenon does not occur, and there is no visceral involvement. Flexion contractures and carpal tunnel syndrome can develop.

Laboratory findings are peripheral eosinophilia, increased sedimentation rate, and hypergammaglobulinemia. The diagnosis is based on the findings of inflammation and thickening of the fascia on deep fascial biopsy. Treatment is with prednisone (40 mg daily). The response is usually good. Associated conditions are aplastic anemia and thrombocytopenia (both antibody-mediated) as well as leukemia and myeloproliferative diseases.

- Eosinophilic fasciitis is characterized by tight bound-down skin of the extremities, usually sparing the hands and feet.
- Raynaud phenomenon does not occur.
- There is no visceral involvement.
- Laboratory findings include peripheral eosinophilia.
- Treatment with prednisone provides good response.

Metabolic Causes of Scleroderma-Like Syndrome

This group includes porphyria, amyloidosis, carcinoid, and diabetes mellitus (flexion contractures of the tendons in the hands, cheiropathy, can develop).

Other Causes

As a manifestation of *graft-versus-host disease*, skin induration develops in up to 30% of patients who receive bone marrow transplant. *Drug-induced disorders* are caused by carbidopa, bleomycin, and bromocriptine. *Eosinophilic myalgia syndrome* is associated with ingestion of contaminated L-tryptophan. Eosinophilia, myositis, skin induration, fasciitis, and peripheral neuropathy develop. Skin changes are similar to those of eosinophilic fasciitis. There is a poor response to steroids. *Scleredema* frequently occurs after streptococcal upper respiratory tract infection in children. It is usually self-limiting. Swelling of the head and neck is common. In adults, diabetes mellitus often is associated. *Scleromyxedema* is associated with IgG monoclonal protein. Cocaine use and appetite suppressants also cause scleroderma-like illness.

THE INFLAMMATORY MYOPATHIES

Inflammatory myopathies can be classified into several categories, including polymyositis, dermatomyositis, myositis associated with malignancy, childhood-type, and overlap connective tissue disease. Polymyositis is an inflammatory myopathy characterized by proximal muscle weakness. Patients with dermatomyositis have an associated rash that includes a heliotrope hue of the eyelids, a rash on the metacarpophalangeal and proximal interphalangeal joints (Gottron papules), and photosensitivity dermatitis of the face. Most patients have an increased creatine kinase level, a characteristic electromyogram, and a characteristic muscle biopsy.

Electromyography is characteristic but not diagnostic of inflammatory myopathies. It shows decreased amplitude and increased spike frequency, it is polyphasic, and conduction speed is normal. Fibrillation is not specific for inflammatory myopathies, but when present it indicates active disease. Loss of fibrillation usually means the inflammatory myopathy is under control, but if the electromyogram is still myopathic, it suggests an associated steroid myopathy caused by treatment. The muscle biopsy, which is mandatory in all patients with inflammatory myopathy, shows degeneration, necrosis, and regeneration of myofibrils with lymphocytic and monocytic infiltrate in a perivascular or interstitial distribution.

In patients older than 40 years, perhaps 10% of those with dermatomyositis have an associated malignancy. The antibody anti-Jo1 is associated with polymyositis and dermatomyositis in approximately 25% of cases. This antibody is associated with inflammatory arthritis, progressive interstitial lung disease, Raynaud phenomenon, and increased mortality primarily due to respiratory failure. The autoantibody anti-Mi-2 is associated with dermatomyositis in 2% to 20% of patients.

- Polymyositis is an inflammatory myopathy characterized by proximal muscle weakness.
- Dermatomyositis is an inflammatory myopathy plus a rash that includes heliotrope hue of eyelids.
- Electromyography is characteristic but not diagnostic of polymyositis.
- Perhaps 10% of patients older than 40 years with dermatomyositis have associated malignancy.
- Anti-Jo1 is associated with polymyositis and dermatomyositis, pulmonary disease, and increased mortality.
- Typical clinical scenario: A 50-year-old patient presents with bilateral progressive proximal muscle weakness. There is a history of arthralgias. Physical examination reveals a rash over the eyelids bilaterally. Laboratory testing reveals positive anti-Jo1 antibody and increased creatine kinase level.

Treatment of polymyositis includes prednisone (60 mg daily), usually for 1 to 2 months, until the muscle enzyme values normalize. The dosage is slowly reduced thereafter, and the clinical course and creatine kinase values are monitored. In severe or steroid-resistant cases, either azathioprine (1-2 mg/kg per day) or methotrexate can be used.

Aspiration pneumonia can occur as a result of pharyngeal weakness. If so, a liquid diet, feeding tube, or feeding gastrostomy is needed until there is clinical improvement.

Inclusion Body Myositis

Inclusion body myositis needs to be considered in the differential diagnosis of inflammatory myopathies. This usually occurs in the older age group. The onset of weakness is more insidious, occurring over many years. The creatine kinase value often is only minimally to several times increased, and distal and proximal weakness occur. The electromyogram,

besides showing a myopathic picture, also has an associated neuropathic picture. The diagnosis of inclusion body myositis is made from biopsy. Histopathologic findings are indistinguishable from those of polymyositis except for the presence of eosinophilic inclusions and rimmed vacuoles with basophilic enhancement. Inclusion body myositis responds poorly to prednisone and immunosuppressive therapy, and the course is one of slow, progressive weakness.

- Inclusion body myositis usually occurs in the older age group.
- Diagnosis is made from biopsy.
- It responds poorly to prednisone.

DRUG-INDUCED MYOPATHIES

Muscle Disease

Drugs may cause an inflammatory myopathy. The myopathy associated with colchicine mimics polymyositis, and patients have muscle weakness and an increased creatine kinase level. This often occurs in the setting of a patient with gout and renal insufficiency receiving long-term therapy with colchicine. Lipid-lowering drugs such as the statins, other drugs including zidovudine, D-penicillamine, and hydroxychloroquine, and addictive drugs such as heroine or cocaine have all been associated with myopathy. Corticosteroids cause a steroid myopathy with proximal muscle weakness and a normal creatine kinase value.

INFECTIOUS ARTHRITIS

An infectious cause should be ruled out immediately in a patient with acute monarticular arthritis. Approximately 5% to 10% of patients with septic arthritis present with multiple joint involvement.

Bacterial Arthritis

Nongonococcal bacterial arthritis is caused by hematogenous spread of bacteria, direct inoculation (which is usually traumatic), or extension of soft tissue infection with osteomyelitis into the joint space. Large joints are more commonly affected. Patients who are elderly or immunosuppressed are predisposed to septic arthropathy, including patients with cancer, diabetes mellitus, chronic renal failure, liver disease, or sickle cell anemia. Patients with chronic inflammatory and degenerative arthritis are also at increased risk for septic arthritis, and the possibility of septic arthritis should be considered in patients with a preexisting polyarthritis who have a single joint flare that is out of proportion to the rest of their joint symptoms. In any patient with a septic joint, the possibility of infectious endocarditis, other septic joints, or a disk space infection should be considered.

Septic arthritis is a medical emergency. A thorough search for a source of infection is important. Joint aspiration is required. Gram staining of centrifuged synovial fluid and appropriate cultures should be performed. Typically, patients with non-gonococcal septic arthritis have a leukocyte value of more than 50,000/μL in the synovial fluid. Low glucose levels in synovial fluid and high levels of lactic acid are common but not specific for septic arthritis. Blood cultures should be performed when septic arthritis is considered. Radiographs of an involved joint may show an associated osteomyelitis or previous local trauma, but radiographic findings of infection usually lag considerably behind clinical symptoms.

Staphylococcus aureus is the most common pathogen in adult patients with nongonococcal bacterial arthritis. In sickle cell anemia, *Salmonella* is the organism commonly causing septic arthritis. *Pseudomonas* should be considered in the context of cat or dog bites, and an anaerobic infection should be considered in cases of human bites. Intravenous drug users may have bacteremia with unusual organisms, such as *Pseudomonas* or *Serratia*, and this may present with septic arthritis in unusual locations, such as the sternoclavicular or sacroiliac joints. The portal of entry may help predict the infecting organism; for example, gram-negative bacilli, such as *E. coli* and *Klebsiella*, may cause septic arthritis in older patients with gastrointestinal or genitourinary infections or instrumentation.

Broad-spectrum antibiotics should be used until culture results are available. Daily aspiration and lavage of the affected joint should be performed until clinical improvement is obvious. Synovial fluid leukocytes and volume should decrease, or orthopedic arthroscopic or even open drainage should be considered. Such drainage usually is indicated in joints such as the hip, which are not readily accessible. The duration of treatment depends on the virulence of the organisms, but antibiotics usually are given intravenously for at least 2 weeks.

- Nongonococcal bacterial arthritis usually is caused by hematogenous spread of bacteria, direct inoculation (which is usually traumatic), or extension of soft tissue infection or osteomyelitis.
- Synovial fluid Gram stain and culture are essential.
- The portal of entry may predict the organism causing septic arthritis.
- Antibiotic therapy should be initiated even before culture results are available.
- If repeated aspiration and antibiotics do not lead to clinical improvement as well as a decrease in synovial fluid volume and leukocytosis, then arthroscopic or open drainage and debridement may be necessary.

- Typical clinical scenario: A patient presents with acute swelling of the right knee, fever, and constitutional symptoms. The joint is tender and painful.

Gonococcal Arthritis

Disseminated gonococcal infection develops in approximately 0.2% of patients with gonorrhea. The male:female ratio is 3:1. This is the most common form of septic arthritis in younger, sexually active persons who may be asymptomatic carriers of gonococci. When gonococcal infection is suspected, specimens from the pharynx, joints, rectum, blood, and genitourinary tract should be cultured. Females present with gonococcal arthritis commonly during pregnancy or within 1 week after onset of menses, possibly related to the pH of vaginal secretions. The most common form of gonococcal arthritis is the disseminated gonococcal arthritis syndrome with fever, dermatitis, and an inflammatory tenosynovitis. Approximately 50% of these patients present with an inflammatory arthritis, commonly of the knee, wrist, or ankle. Tenosynovitis is more common than large joint effusions. Rash, sometimes with pustules or hemorrhagic vesicles, is common. The second form of gonococcal arthritis commonly begins as a migratory polyarthralgia, which subsequently localizes to one or more joints.

Synovial fluid cultures are positive in only 30% of patients with known disseminated gonococcal infection. Culture of the skin lesion is positive for gonococcus in 40% to 60% of patients with disseminated gonococcal infection. The leukocyte count in the joint fluid may be lower than in the other types of septic arthritis. Joint effusions in patients with disseminated gonococcal infection may be related to a *reactive* postinfectious response rather than to bacterial invasion. Rare patients who have recurrent disseminated gonococcal infection may have an associated terminal complement component deficiency (C5-C9).

Most patients with disseminated gonococcal arthritis are treated as outpatients. Current treatment recommendations suggest a later third-generation cephalosporin, such as ceftriaxone, 1.0 g per day. Treatment involves a minimum 7-day course. Treatment should include an anti-chlamydial antibiotic.

- Gonococcal arthritis develops in 0.2% of patients with gonorrhea.
- In the disseminated gonococcal arthritis syndrome, fever, dermatitis, and tenosynovitis are common.
- In the nonbacteremic form of gonococcal arthritis, migratory polyarthralgias are followed by inflammation localizing to one or more joints.
- Synovial fluid cultures are positive in 30% of patients with known disseminated gonococcal infection.
- Joint fluid leukocyte counts may be lower than in other types of septic arthritis.

- Joint effusions may be related to a reactive or postinfectious arthritis.
- Treatment recommendations are the use of a later third-generation cephalosporin (e.g., ceftriaxone).
- Treatment should include an antichlamydial antibiotic.

Mycobacterial and Fungal Joint Infections

These types of organisms usually cause chronic bone and joint infections. Months are required for radiographic changes to be obvious. A synovial biopsy and culture may be required to document these infections. Tuberculous arthritis is often otherwise asymptomatic and usually is caused by direct extension from adjacent bony infection. Atypical mycobacterial infection may cause an inflammatory arthritis and tenosynovitis frequently involving the hand and wrist. Surgical excision and prolonged treatment with multiple drug regimens are often required. Sporotrichosis and blastomycosis are the fungi most likely to have osteoarticular manifestations.

- Tuberculous arthritis is often otherwise asymptomatic and is caused by direct extension from adjacent bony infection.
- Atypical mycobacterial infection may cause an inflammatory arthritis and tenosynovitis.
- Sporotrichosis and blastomycosis are the fungi most likely to have osteoarticular manifestations.

Spinal Septic Arthritis

This condition should be suspected in patients with acute or chronic, unrelenting back pain associated with fever and marked local tenderness. The thoracolumbar region is most commonly affected. An antecedent infection or procedure predisposing to bacteremia may help suggest this diagnosis. Imaging studies usually have evidence for infection crossing the disk space. In tuberculous spinal septic arthritis (Pott disease), the site of involvement is most commonly T10-L2, and there is usually an associated paraspinal abscess.

Intravertebral disk infection is often a difficult diagnosis to establish because pain patterns may be unusual and localizing signs may be absent. Bone scanning may be helpful, but magnetic resonance imaging may be very helpful, particularly because of the ability to show extension of infection into surrounding tissues.

Infected Joint Prostheses

Infection in joint prostheses occurs in approximately 1% to 5% of all joint replacements. Symptoms and signs of infection may be difficult to detect during the postoperative period. Fever may not be present, and laboratory findings are often unhelpful, although the erythrocyte sedimentation rate may be increased. There may or may not be evidence of loosening of the cement holding the new joint in place, and radiographs may reveal lytic changes around the prosthesis. A negative bone scan is reassuring. Aspiration of fluid from the prosthetic joint is necessary to confirm infection. Prosthetic joint arthritis usually is caused by gram-positive organisms, particularly *Staphylococcus aureus* and *Staphylococcus epidermidis* in the first 6 months after the replacement operation, and by gram-negative and fungal organisms after 6 months. In long-standing prosthetic joints, return of pain and evidence of prosthetic loosening may be the only signs and symptoms. Patients with prosthetic joints do not require antibiotic prophylaxis before invasive dental, gastrointestinal, or genitourinary procedures according to the recent guidelines, unless obvious immunosuppression is present.

- Prosthetic joint arthritis usually is caused by a gram-positive organism within the first 6 months after joint replacement.
- Prosthetic joint infections usually are caused by gram-negative or fungal organisms beyond the initial 6 months after joint replacement.

LYME DISEASE

Lyme disease is a tick-borne spirochetal illness with acute and chronic manifestations primarily affecting the skin, heart, joints, and nervous system. Diagnosis is important because treatment with appropriate antibiotics at an early stage of disease can prevent chronic sequelae. Even some chronic symptoms are treatable. Endemic areas in the United States include Connecticut, Delaware, Maryland, Massachusetts, New Jersey, New York, Pennsylvania, Rhode Island, Minnesota, Wisconsin, California, Nevada, Oregon, and Utah.

- Lyme disease is a tick-borne spirochetal illness.
- Acute and chronic manifestations affect skin, heart, joints, and nervous system.

The Tick

Ticks that transmit Lyme disease include *Ixodes dammini* in the northeastern and midwestern United States and *Ixodes pacificus* in the western United States. *Amblyomma americanum* ("lone star" tick) is a possible vector in the eastern, southern, and western United States. *Ixodes scapularis* is the common deer tick. It has a wide distribution. Humans are accidental hosts.

The Spirochete

Borrelia burgdorferi was an unknown organism until isolated initially from ticks by Burgdorfer in 1983. It is similar to an organism causing relapsing fever. It apparently exists only in the digestive tract of tick vectors.

Clinical Stages

Signs and symptoms occur in stages that may overlap. Later stages may occur without evidence of previous disease.

Stage I

About 50% to 67% of patients experience erythema chronicum migrans. Flu-like symptoms, including fever, headache, malaise, and adenopathy, can occur. They usually occur several days to a month after the tick bite.

- In stage I Lyme disease, 50%-67% of patients experience erythema chronicum migrans.

Stage II

Symptoms begin weeks to months after the initial symptoms in stage I. Disseminated infection develops and can include symptoms of the skin, musculoskeletal system, heart, and nervous system. In approximately 15% of untreated patients, neurologic symptoms develop, including Bell palsy, meningoencephalitis, and sensory and motor radiculoneuritis. Approximately 5% of untreated patients have cardiac abnormalities, including heart block. About 30% to 50% of untreated patients have arthritis. This usually affects large joints, primarily the knees, and joint fluid analysis shows a leukocytosis similar to that in rheumatoid arthritis. Baker cysts may form early and are prone to rupture in patients who have arthritis of the knees.

- In stage II Lyme disease, symptoms begin weeks to months after initial symptoms of stage I.
- Disseminated infection develops.
- 15% of untreated patients have neurologic symptoms.
- 5% of untreated patients have cardiac abnormalities.
- 30%-50% of untreated patients have arthritis.

Stage III

This usually occurs several years after the initial onset of illness. Episodes of arthritis can develop and become chronic. Histologically, the synovium resembles that in rheumatoid arthritis, although a unique feature of Lyme arthritis is the finding of an obliterative endarteritis. Spirochetes occasionally are seen in and around the blood vessels. Patients in whom chronic joint disease develops have increased frequency of HLA-DR4, often in combination with HLA-DR2. Patients with chronic arthritis have a poor response to antibiotics.

- Stage III Lyme disease occurs several years after initial onset of illness.

- Episodes of arthritis can be chronic.
- Synovium resembles that in rheumatoid arthritis.
- A unique feature of Lyme arthritis is obliterative endarteritis in the synovium.
- Patients with chronic joint disease have increased frequency of HLA-DR4, often in combination with HLA-DR2.

Diagnosis

Culturing the organism is difficult and of low yield. Antibody to spirochete can be measured by several techniques. The enzyme-linked immunosorbent assay (ELISA) is most commonly performed, but there is a substantial frequency of false-positive results. Patients with other autoimmune disease can have false-positive results. Also, such results may occur in syphilis, relapsing fever, and Rocky Mountain spotted fever. Up to 25% of patients with lupus and rheumatoid arthritis have false-positive results of Lyme test by ELISA. It is important to remember that test results remain negative for up to 4 to 6 weeks after infection. Also, if patients are treated early with tetracycline or another antibiotic, the results might never be positive, although symptoms of chronic Lyme disease can result. The Western blot assay for Lyme disease is now being used as a confirmatory test if the ELISA test result is positive.

- In Lyme disease, culturing the organism is difficult and of low yield.
- The ELISA assay is commonly performed but there is a substantial frequency of false-positive results.
- False-positive ELISA results may occur in syphilis, relapsing fever, and Rocky Mountain spotted fever.
- Up to 25% of patients with lupus and rheumatoid arthritis have false-positive results of Lyme test by ELISA.
- Patients treated early with tetracycline or other antibiotics may never have positive results.

Treatment

For early treatment of Lyme disease, either oral tetracycline or doxycycline, or amoxicillin in children, for 14-21 days, can prevent later complications. The optimal treatment for patients with neurologic, cardiac, and arthritic symptoms of Lyme disease includes ceftriaxone, 2 g intravenously daily for 28 days. Patients with Lyme disease can experience worsening of symptoms analogous to the Jarisch-Herxheimer reaction and can be treated with acetaminophen.

- Early treatment of Lyme disease is either oral tetracycline or doxycycline (amoxicillin in children) for 14-21 days.
- Treatment for neurologic, cardiac, and arthritic symptoms of Lyme disease includes ceftriaxone for 28 days.

RHEUMATIC FEVER AND POSTSTREPTOCOCCAL REACTIVE ARTHRITIS

Arthritis affects two-thirds of all patients with rheumatic fever. One-third of patients with acute rheumatic fever have no obvious antecedent pharyngitis. In adults, arthritis may be the only clinical feature of acute rheumatic fever and often occurs early. The arthritis usually involves the large joints, particularly the knees, ankles, elbows, and wrists. The arthritis may be migratory, with each joint remaining inflamed for approximately 1 week. The arthritis of rheumatic fever is nonerosive; however, repeated attacks may result in a "Jaccoud deformity," in which the metacarpophalangeal joints are in ulnar deviation as a result of tendon laxity rather than bony damage.

Patients with joint symptoms without carditis may be treated with high-dose salicylates (3-6 g per day). Corticosteroids may be required if patients do not respond to salicylates. Joint symptoms may rebound when anti-inflammatory therapy is discontinued.

- The arthritis in rheumatic fever may be migratory and usually involves the large joints, particularly the knees, ankles, elbows, and wrists.
- Repeated attacks of rheumatic fever may result in "Jaccoud deformity."
- The mainstay treatment for the arthritis of rheumatic fever is high-dose salicylates (3-6 g per day).

VIRAL ARTHRITIS

Viruses associated with arthralgia and arthritis include human immunodeficiency virus (HIV), hepatitis B, rubella, parvovirus, and, less commonly, mumps, adenovirus, herpesvirus, and enterovirus. Most viral-related arthritides have joint symptoms with a semiacute onset, but fortunately they are usually of brief duration. The arthritis is nondestructive.

Although *parvovirus* infection in children is usually mild, in adults associated arthralgias and arthritis are common, and the distribution of involved joints is symmetric and may mimic rheumatoid arthritis. Joint symptoms in adults are usually self-limited, but chronic disease develops in some patients. The diagnosis of parvovirus infection is made by demonstrating the presence of anti-B19 IgM antibodies, but these may be increased in patients for only 2 months after acute infection. Because the joint symptoms usually occur approximately 1 to 3 weeks after the initial infection, the antibodies are usually present at the time of onset of rash or joint symptoms. Treatment is usually conservative and includes anti-inflammatory medications, but in more chronic infections more aggressive treatment such as low-dose corticosteroids may be warranted. Parvovirus infection also has been associated rarely with significant hematologic abnormalities.

Hepatitis B virus infection has been associated with an immune complex-mediated arthritis, which can be dramatic. The arthritis is usually limited to the pre-icteric prodrome, although patients with chronic types of hepatitis may have recurrent arthralgias or arthritis. Polyarteritis nodosa has been associated with chronic hepatitis. *Hepatitis B* and more commonly *C* are associated with mixed cryoglobulinemia. *Rubella* virus infection is frequently associated with joint complaints in adults. In a few patients, the symptoms have persisted for months to years. Joint symptoms may occur just before or after the appearance of the characteristic rash.

- Parvovirus infection in adults may cause a symmetric polyarthritis mimicking rheumatoid arthritis.
- Parvovirus infection can be documented by demonstrating the presence of anti-B19 IgM antibodies.
- Hepatitis B virus infection has been associated with an arthritis limited to the pre-icteric prodrome.
- Hepatitis B and C viremia have been associated with cryoglobulinemia and vasculitis.
- Rubella virus infection frequently is associated with joint complaints in young adults.

RHEUMATOLOGIC MANIFESTATIONS OF HIV INFECTION (TABLE 22-33)

Musculoskeletal complaints can be among the first manifestations of HIV infection. Articular manifestations can be extremely debilitating. Epidemiologic studies have not concluded whether HIV infection predisposes to arthritis or whether other viral or new mechanisms associated with HIV infection have a role in the pathogenesis of arthritis.

Table 22-33 Rheumatologic Manifestations of Human Immunodeficiency Virus (HIV)

Arthralgia
Painful articular syndrome
HIV arthropathy
Reactive arthritis
Psoriatic arthritis
Undifferentiated spondyloarthropathy
Myositis
Vasculitis
Raynaud phenomenon
Sjögren-like syndrome (diffuse infiltrative lymphocytosis syndrome)
Septic arthritis
Fibromyalgia
Serologic abnormalities

Reactive Arthritis and Undifferentiated Spondyloarthropathy

Signs and symptoms of reactive arthritis, psoriatic arthritis, or a nonspecific enthesopathy and related destructive arthritis may occur before or simultaneously with the onset of HIV infection. The prevalence of these conditions in HIV-infected patients varies from 0.5% to 10% in reports. These HIV-associated spondyloarthropathies have a predisposition for patients who are HLA-B27–positive and frequently are associated with severe enthesopathy and dactylitis. Progressive axial involvement is less common in HIV-associated arthritides. The foot and ankle are common sites of enthesopathy in reactive arthritis, which may be severe. Symptoms may be episodic. Most HIV-infected patients with reactive arthritis have skin and mucocutaneous manifestations, including urethritis, keratoderma blennorrhagicum, circinate balanitis, or painless oral ulcers, but conjunctivitis is unusual. In approximately one-third of patients, the onset of HIV-associated reactive arthritis has been linked to a documented infection with specific enteric organisms known to precipitate reactive arthritis. Genitourinary tract infection with *Ureaplasma* or *Chlamydia* is less common.

- Enthesopathy and dactylitis may be severe in HIV-infected patients.
- Mucocutaneous features are common, but conjunctivitis is unusual.

Lupus-Like Illnesses in HIV Infection

Some of the features of systemic lupus erythematosus are similar to those in patients with HIV infection. Fever, lymphadenopathy, mucous membrane lesions, rashes, arthritis, and hematologic abnormalities are common to both lupus and HIV infection. HIV infection also may be associated with polyclonal B-cell activation resulting in autoantibody production, including antinuclear and antiphospholipid antibodies. HIV infection should be considered in the differential diagnosis of systemic lupus erythematosus in any patient who is at risk for HIV. Antinuclear antibodies in high titer have not been observed in HIV infection, and antibodies to double-stranded DNA are absent.

- Although some features of HIV infection may resemble lupus, antinuclear antibodies are present in low titer only, and antibodies to double-stranded DNA are absent.

HIV-Associated Vasculitis

Different types of vasculitic syndromes have been described in association with HIV infection. Primary angiitis of the central nervous system, angiocentric lymphoproliferative lesions related to lymphomatoid granulomatosis, and polyarteritis nodosa have been reported. It has not been established whether the association of vasculitis and HIV infection is coincidental, related to comorbidities such as drugs or other infections, or represents a direct pathogenetic role for the HIV virus. All patients with primary angiitis of the central nervous system and lymphoproliferative angiocentric vasculopathies should be tested for HIV. Any person with known HIV infection who presents with new mononeuritis should be evaluated for vasculitis.

Other HIV-Associated Rheumatic Syndromes

The diffuse, infiltrative lymphocytosis syndrome is manifested by xerostomia, xerophthalmia, and salivary gland swelling mimicking Sjögren syndrome. The glands are infiltrated with CD8 lymphocytes. In contrast to Sjögren syndrome, HIV-positive patients usually do not have antibodies to SS-A or SS-B and are usually rheumatoid factor-negative.

There is an inflammatory articular syndrome associated with HIV infection which is distinct from any resemblance to spondyloarthropathy. This is usually an oligoarthritis affecting joints of the lower extremities and is usually short-lived.

There is an acquired immunodeficiency syndrome-associated myopathy that may be viral. There is also a myopathy due to zidovudine therapy. Fibromyalgia also has been reported in up to 25% of HIV-infected patients.

OTHER TYPES OF INFECTIOUS ARTHRITIS

Whipple disease is a rare cause of arthropathy and usually is associated with constitutional symptoms, fever, neurologic symptoms, malabsorption, lymphadenopathy, and hyperpigmentation. There may be a slow, progressive dementia. The arthritic symptoms may precede the gastrointestinal manifestations. The infectious agent is *Tropheryma whippelii*. Small bowel or synovial biopsy may be necessary to establish the diagnosis. Treatment is usually with doxycycline or trimethoprim-sulfamethoxazole, often required for a year.

Rheumatology Pharmacy Review

Robert B. McMahan, PharmD, MBA, Christopher M. Wittich, PharmD, MD

Drug	Toxic/adverse effects	Drug interactions	Comments
Nonsteroidal anti-inflammatory drugs (NSAIDs), by chemical group			

Acetic acids
    Diclofenac potassium
    Diclofenac sodium
    Etodolac
    Indomethacin
    Ketorolac
    Sulindac
  Propionic acids
    Flurbiprofen
    Ibuprofen
    Ketoprofen
    Naproxen
    Naproxen sodium
  Salicylates
    Aspirin
    Diflunisal
    Salicylate
  Fenamates
    Mefanamic acid
  Oxicams
    Piroxicam
  COX-2 inhibitors
    Celecoxib
    Rofecoxib
	Central nervous system: dizziness, headache, drowsiness
	Gastrointestinal: constipation, dyspepsia, nausea, abdominal pain, gastrointestinal bleeding
	Hematologic: irreversible platelet inhibition (salicylates)
	Renal: decreased renal perfusion and glomerular filtration
		ACE inhibitors: antihypertensive effects may be reduced
		Antacids: antacids may decrease effectiveness of enteric coating
		Anticoagulants: coadministration may increase bleeding risk
		Cyclosporine: coadministration may increase nephrotoxicity
		Digoxin: serum digoxin levels may increase
		Diuretics: decreased effects
		Lithium: serum lithium levels may increase
		Methotrexate: methotrexate clearance may be reduced
		Phenytoin: serum phenytoin levels may increase
			If an NSAID from one chemical group is not effective, one from another chemical group may be more effective
			Use with caution in patients with asthma

Glucocorticosteroids			

Betamethasone
  Dexamethasone
  Methylprednisolone
  Prednisone
	Cardiovascular: fluid retention, hypertension
	Central nervous system: euphoria, depression, insomnia, mania, hallucinations, anxiety, pseudotumor cerebri
	Dermatologic: acneiform eruptions, bruising, atrophy, hirsutism, impaired wound healing, striae, telangiectasia
	Endocrine: hypothalamic-pituitary-adrenal axis suppression, central obesity, moon facies, buffalo hump, growth suppression, hyperglycemia
		Cyclosporine: plasma clearance may be decreased by certain glucocorticoids
		NSAIDs: concomitant use may cause gastrointestinal ulcerations or perforation
		Diuretics: concomitant use may cause increased potassium loss
		Anticholinesterase agents: concomitant use may cause weakness in patients with myasthenia gravis
		Vaccines: glucocorticoids may decrease response to vaccines
		Anticoagulants: concomitant use can increase or decrease anticoagulant effects	

Rheumatology Pharmacy Review (continued)

Drug	Toxic/adverse effects	Drug interactions	Comments
Glucocorticosteroids (continued)			
	Gastrointestinal: candidiasis, perforations, ulcers		
	Hematologic: increased absolute granulocyte count, decreased lymphocyte and monocyte counts		
	Musculoskeletal: myopathy, osteoporosis		
	Ocular: posterior subcapsular cataracts, increased intraocular pressure		
Disease-modifying antirheumatic drugs (DMARDs)			
Hydroxychloroquine	Ocular: macular damage Dermatologic: accumulation in melanin-rich tissues, pruritus	Decreased digoxin levels Gold compounds lead to an increase in dermatologic adverse effects	Initial ophthalmologic exam, then every 6 to 12 mo Periodic CBC Hemolysis possible in G-6-PD–deficient patients
Gold salts	Dermatologic: rash, stomatitis, alopecia Hematologic: blood dyscrasias Gastrointestinal: diarrhea, worse with oral gold Renal: hematuria, proteinuria Special senses: metallic taste, may be a precursor to other reactions	Increased phenytoin levels Use with immunosuppressants, penicillamine, or antimalarials increases risk of blood dyscrasias	Before initiation of therapy: CBC, UA, renal and liver function Before each injection: CBC and UA
D-Penicillamine	Dermatologic: stomatitis, rashes Hematologic: possible induction of autoimmune diseases, myelosuppression Renal: glomerulonephritis, proteinuria Special senses: hypogeusia	Antacids and iron decrease penicillamine absorption Decreased digoxin concentrations Increased gold concentrations	UA and CBC every week for 1 month, then monthly LFT every 6 mo

Rheumatology Pharmacy Review (continued)

Drug	Toxic/adverse effects	Drug interactions	Comments
Disease-modifying antirheumatic drugs (DMARDs) (continued)			
Sulfasalazine	Genitourinary: crystalluria, urine discoloration Gastrointestinal: nausea, vomiting, diarrhea, anorexia Dermatologic: hypersensitivity	Increased effect of warfarin Antibiotics and iron decrease absorption Decreased folic acid absorption Decreased digoxin absorption	CBC w/diff at initiation CBC w/diff and LFT should be done every 2 wk for 3 mo, then every mo for 3 mo, then every 3 mo Can lead to folic acid deficiencies
Methotrexate	Hepatotoxicity: hepatic fibrosis and cirrhosis Hematologic: myelosuppression Gastrointestinal: mucositis, stomatitis Pulmonary: pneumonitis	NSAIDs, salicylates, cisplatin, cyclosporine, and penicillamine delay methotrexate excretion, leading to toxicities	Initial CBC, LFT, and renal function tests CBC monthly LFT and renal function tests every 1 to 2 mo
Leflunomide	Liver: hepatotoxicity Cardiovascular: hypertension Dermatologic: alopecia, rash Pregnancy: teratogen with a long half-life and dangerous blood levels for up to 2 years after therapy	Cytochrome P-450 inhibitor Increased methotrexate concentrations Rifampin increases leflunomide Cholestyramine decreases leflunomide	Initial LFT Baseline LFTs followed by monthly LFTs until the enzyme levels are stable
Azathioprine	Hematologic: myelosuppression Liver: hepatotoxicity Gastrointestinal: nausea, vomiting, diarrhea	Allopurinol increases concentration of azathioprine; reduce the dose of azathioprine by 70% ACE inhibitors and methotrexate increase azathioprine Decreased anticoagulant concentrations	
Cyclophosphamide	Genitourinary: cystitis Hematologic: leukopenia (nadir at 8-15 days) Dermatologic: alopecia Gastrointestinal: nausea, vomiting Cardiovascular: cardiotoxicity	Phenytoin and barbiturates induce liver enzymes, which increase conversion to the active metabolite, leading to cyclophosphamide toxicities Allopurinol and thiazide diuretics can increase cyclophosphamide concentrations Doxorubicin can increase cardiotoxic potential Increased anticoagulant effects Decreased digoxin effects	Initial UA and CBC, then every week for 1 mo, then every 2-4 wk The risk for hemorrhagic cystitis from high-dose cyclophosphamide may be reduced by the coadministration of mesna

Rheumatology Pharmacy Review (continued)

Drug	Toxic/adverse effects	Drug interactions	Comments
Disease-modifying antirheumatic drugs (DMARDS) (continued)			
Cyclosporine	Renal: nephrotoxicity Liver: hepatotoxicity Cardiovascular: hypertension	Carbamazepine, phenytoin, phenobarbital, rifamycin decrease effect Increased toxicities are azoles, macrolides, grapefruit juice, protease inhibitors, immuno-suppressants, calcium channel blockers, and oral contraceptives NSAIDs and aminoglyco-sides increase nephrotoxic potential	Initial monitoring of blood pressure and serum creatinine; then monitor every 2 wk for 3 mo, then monthly
Tumor necrosis factor inhibitors			
Etanercept	Injection site reactions Respiratory tract infections Sepsis Formation of autoimmune antibodies	Do not give live vaccines with etanercept	Monitor for signs of infection
Infliximab	Injection site reactions Respiratory tract infections Sepsis Formation of autoimmune antibodies	Do not give live vaccines with infliximab	Monitor for signs of infection Do not administer using PVC tubing or equipment

ACE, angiotensin-converting enzyme; CBC, complete blood count; COX, cyclooxygenase; exam, examination; LFT, liver function tests; PVC, polyvinyl chloride; UA, urinalysis; w/diff, with differential.

QUESTIONS

Multiple Choice (choose the one best answer)

1. A 37-year-old woman presents with a 4-month history of polyarthralgias, fatigue, and a rash on her legs. She gave a history of intravenous drug use in her 20s. There was no history of pleurisy, photosensitivity, or oral ulcers. No overt joint swelling is found on examination. She has multiple raised, red papules several millimeters in diameter from just below her knees to the feet.

   Laboratory values:

Hemoglobin	13.1 g/dL
Leukocytes	5.6×10^9/L
Erythrocyte sedimentation rate	77 mm/h
Rheumatoid factor	256 IU/mL
	(normal <15)
Antinuclear antibody	1:40
Cryoglobulins	Positive
Anti-nDNA	Negative
C3	Low
Aspartate aminotransferase	65 U/L
	(normal <30)
Creatinine	1.2 mg/dL

   Which one of the following is the most likely diagnosis?
   a. Rheumatoid arthritis
   b. Lupus erythematosus
   c. Hepatitis C
   d. Polyarteritis nodosa
   e. Autoimmune hepatitis

2. A 45-year-old woman with a 3-year history of scleroderma has new-onset hypertension with a blood pressure of 180/100 mm Hg. The creatinine value is 1.5 mg/dL. Which one of the following medications is the best choice at this time?
   a. Diltiazem
   b. Atenolol
   c. Hydrochlorothiazide
   d. Lisinopril
   e. Hydralazine

3. A 35-year-old man has a 2-month history of swollen knees. He gives no history of rash, pleurisy, or Raynaud phenomenon. He is an avid hunter. He had Bell palsy, which resolved 3 months previously. Examination findings include bilateral knee effusions with Baker cysts.

   Laboratory values:

Erythrocyte sedimentation rate	45 mm/h
Rheumatoid factor	Negative
Antinuclear antibody	1:40
Synovial fluid analysis	4.5×10^9/L leukocytes Negative culture

   Which of the following is the most likely diagnosis?
   a. Seronegative rheumatoid arthritis
   b. Lupus
   c. Lyme disease
   d. Osteoarthritis
   e. Reactive arthritis

4. A 33-year-old woman with lupus is positive for both IgG and IgM antiphospholipid antibodies. There is no history of miscarriages or abnormal arterial or venous clotting. Which one of the following would you do?
   a. Begin heparin therapy
   b. Begin warfarin therapy
   c. Begin clopidogrel bisulfate therapy
   d. Begin hydroxycloroquine therapy
   e. Observe

5. A 35-year-old woman presents with Raynaud phenomenon, polyarthralgias, photosensitivity, and mild muscle weakness. She has sclerodactyly on skin examination.

   Laboratory values:

Antinuclear antibody	1:640
Anti-nDNA	Negative
Sm	Negative
Ribonucleoprotein	Positive
Jo1	Negative
Rheumatoid factor	50 IU/mL
	(normal <15)
Erythrocyte sedimentation rate	47 mm/h
Creatine kinase	390 U/L
	(normal ≤200)

   Which of the following is the most likely diagnosis?
   a. Mixed connective tissue disease
   b. Rheumatoid arthritis
   c. Lupus
   d. Scleroderma
   e. Polymyositis

6. An 18-year-old woman presents with polyarthralgias of 3 weeks in duration and a 3-day history of pleurisy. There is no fever. She is receiving minocycline for acne, an oral contraceptive, and sertraline (Zoloft).

   Laboratory values:

Hemoglobin	13.2 g/dL
Leukocytes	4.3×10^9/L
Erythrocyte sedimentation rate	37 mm/h
Creatinine	0.7 mg/dL
Urinalysis	Normal

Antinuclear antibody	1:1,280
Anti-nDNA	Negative
C3	Normal
Rheumatoid factor	Negative
Chest radiograph	Normal

In addition to beginning therapy with nonsteroidal anti-inflammatory drugs, which one of the following should be done next?

a. Begin azathioprine therapy 100 mg daily
b. Begin hydroxychloroquine therapy 200 mg daily
c. Begin cyclophosphamide therapy 100 mg daily
d. Stop minocycline therapy
e. Stop sertraline therapy

7. A 32-year-old woman with a 5-year history of systemic lupus erythematosus manifested by skin and joint disease presents for evaluation of right groin pain with ambulation of 2 weeks in duration. Her lupus erythematosus is well controlled on hydroxychloroquine and 5 mg of prednisone. A radiograph of the hip is normal, as is the sedimentation rate. Deep tendon reflexes and muscle strength in the legs are normal. There is normal range of motion of the hip but pain with movement. Which one of the following is the most likely diagnosis?

a. Avascular necrosis of the hip
b. L2 radiculopathy
c. Femoral neuropathy
d. Stress fracture of the pubic ramus
e. Flare of lupus arthritis

8. An 82-year-old man presents with an acutely swollen right great toe. Joint aspiration shows monosodium urate crystals. He has a history of hypertension treated with diltiazem 240 mg daily. One month previously, therapy had been started with allopurinol 300 mg daily and colchicine 0.6 mg twice daily for recurrent gout attacks.
Laboratory values:

Hemoglobin	12.1 g/dL
Leukocytes	5.1×10^9/L
Creatinine	1.7 mg/dL
Uric acid	8.1 mg/dL (normal ≤8.0)

Which one of the following would be the most appropriate treatment at this time?

a. Indomethacin 50 mg four times daily
b. Celecoxib (Celebrex) 200 mg daily
c. Colchicine 1 g intravenously
d. Increase of allopurinol to 400 mg daily
e. Methylprednisolone dose pak

9. A 45-year-old woman presents with a 2-week history of a swollen left ankle and right knee. There is no history of fever. She has had a 10-lb weight loss and complains of three to five loose bowel movements per day over the past 3 months. Which one of the following tests is most likely to help make a diagnosis?

a. Synovial fluid analysis, including leukocyte count and culture
b. Colonoscopy
c. Stool cultures for ova and parasites
d. HLA-B27 antigen test
e. *Clostridium difficile* antigen test

10. A 65-year-old man presents with a swollen painful right wrist of 2 days in duration. He has a 20-year history of diabetes mellitus and a recent diagnosis of a cardiomyopathy. Radiography of the wrist shows calcification of the triangular fibrocartilage. Joint aspiration shows weakly positive birefringent crystals.
Laboratory values:

Hemoglobin	13.2 g/dL
Leukocytes	4.8×10^9/L, normal differential
Creatinine	1.2 mg/dL
Calcium	10.2 mg/dL (normal ≤10.1)
Aspartate aminotransferase	95 U/L (normal <31)

Which one of the following associated diseases is most likely to be present?

a. Hemochromatosis
b. Ochronosis
c. Hyperparathyroidism
d. Hypomagnesemia
e. Hypothyroidism

11. A 42-year-old man is seen for a general medical evaluation. He is not receiving any medications and considers himself in good health. The uric acid value is 9.1 mg/dL (normal <8.0). He has no history of gout. His blood pressure is 110/70 mm Hg, and the creatinine value is normal. His father does have gout. Besides limiting foods high in purine content, which one of the following would you advise?

a. Allopurinol
b. Colchicine
c. Probenecid
d. Indomethacin
e. Observation

12. A 35-year-old man presents with a 2-week history of a swollen right ankle. He gives a history of iritis 2 years previously and Achilles tendinitis 3 months ago treated successfully with ibuprofen. Which one of the following is the most likely diagnosis?

a. Rheumatoid arthritis
b. Gout
c. Spondyloarthropathy
d. Lyme disease
e. Sarcoid

13. A 39-year-old woman presents for evaluation of a swollen second left toe. She had a previous episode 1 year ago involving the third right toe, for which she took ibuprofen and had improvement. She has a history of hypertension. Medications include hydrochlorothiazide 25 mg and atenolol 50 mg daily. On physical examination, a "sausage-like" (dactylitis) swelling of the second left toe is found. There was a scaly erythematous rash in her scalp in the occipital area.
    Laboratory values:

Hemoglobin	14.2 g/dL
Leukocytes	5.1×10^9/L
Creatinine	0.7 mg/dL
Uric acid	8.3 mg/dL (normal ≤8.0)
Calcium	10.3 mg/dL (normal ≤10.1)
Rheumatoid factor	21 IU/mL (normal ≤20)

Which one of the following is the most likely diagnosis?
a. Pseudogout
b. Gout

c. Reactive arthritis
d. Rheumatoid arthritis
e. Psoriatic arthritis

14. A 23-year-old man presents for evaluation of an acutely swollen left ankle. There is no history of injury. Two weeks previously, he had an episode of severe diarrhea, and stool cultures showed *Salmonella*, which was successfully treated with a 10-day course of amoxicillin, just completed.
    Laboratory values:

Hemoglobin	14.1 g/dL
Leukocytes	6.2×10^9/L
Erythrocyte sedimentation rate	62 mm/h
Rheumatoid factor	22 IU/mL (normal <20)
Uric acid	7.8 mg/dL (normal ≤8.0)

Which one of the following is the most likely diagnosis?
a. Rheumatoid arthritis
b. Gout
c. Pseudogout
d. Reactive arthritis
e. Septic arthritis

ANSWERS

1. Answer c.

Patients with hepatitis C can present with polyarthralgias and cutaneous vasculitis manifested by palpable purpura. This patient also had a positive rheumatoid factor and a low C3 value. Cryoglobulins, which occur in hepatitis C, will cause both of these abnormalities. The increased aspartate aminotransferase value also is in keeping with hepatitis C infection. Although rheumatoid arthritis can be associated with vasculitis, palpable purpura would be very unusual and the associated low complement value and increased aspartate aminotransferase value also would be unlikely. Polyarteritis nodosa and autoimmune hepatitis are not characteristically associated with cryoglobulins, a positive rheumatoid factor, or low complement values. Patients with lupus erythematosus can have low complement values and vasculitis, but cryoglobulins would be unusual.

2. Answer d.

Hyperreninemia is associated with renal involvement of scleroderma and necessitates the use of angiotensin-converting

enzyme inhibitors such as lisinopril. Other antihypertensive medications are not as effective.

3. Answer c.

This patient has a history of Bell palsy, which can occur in Lyme disease and is not associated with the other answers. Also, Lyme disease characteristically involves the knees with Baker cysts. An inflammatory fluid on synovial fluid analysis is compatible with Lyme disease. Synovial fluid cultures are characteristically negative in Lyme disease.

4. Answer e.

Although this patient has both IgG and IgM antiphospholipid antibodies, she gives no history of miscarriages or clotting. Therefore, she does not fit the criteria for an antiphospholipid antibody syndrome, which requires both the presence of antibodies and a history of clotting. Observation is the treatment of choice.

5. Answer a.

This patient has classic mixed connective tissue disease. She has both laboratory and clinical features, including an increased creatine kinase value indicative of a myositis, sclerodactyly indicative of a scleroderma-like picture, and photosensitivity and polyarthralgias, which can occur in lupus erythematosus. In conjunction, she has the characteristic serologic findings of mixed connective tissue disease, including a positive ribonucleoprotein and negative Sm. This serologic combination in conjunction with the clinical picture is needed to make a diagnosis.

6. Answer d.

This woman has drug-induced lupus caused by minocycline. The appropriate treatment would be to stop the minocycline therapy. There is no evidence of renal disease, which would necessitate the use of azathioprine or cyclophosphamide. Symptoms can be treated with nonsteroidal anti-inflammatory drugs, and there is no reason to prescribe hydroxychloroquine unless she has persistence of her symptoms after discontinuation of the minocycline.

7. Answer a.

Patients with systemic lupus erythematosus are more susceptible to avascular necrosis, even without prednisone. The hip radiograph can be normal for several months before changes of avascular necrosis are seen. MRI is much more sensitive. Avascular necrosis also can characteristically occur in the wrist (navicular) and tibial plateau.

8. Answer e.

A methylprednisolone dose pak would give prompt relief of gouty arthritis. The patient has contraindications to the other proposed treatments. He has a history of hypertension and renal insufficiency, which would make indomethacin and celecoxib both relative contraindications. The increased creatinine value and his baseline use of colchicine 0.6 mg twice daily increase the risk of intravenous colchicine toxicity, which can cause pancytopenia. Allopurinol is not used to treat acute gout. He has been receiving allopurinol for 1 month, and there is no reason to increase his dosage to 400 mg daily at this time.

9. Answer b.

Colonoscopy would provide the most useful information for a diagnosis of inflammatory bowel disease. A synovial fluid analysis would show an inflammatory fluid but would give no further information. Parasitic infection of the bowel should not cause inflammatory arthritis. The HLA-B27 antigen does not have a higher increased frequency in patients with inflammatory bowel disease with associated arthritis. Patients with *C. difficile* colitis do not have an inflammatory arthritis.

10. Answer a.

This patient has hemochromatosis, as manifested by diabetes mellitus, pseudogout, and a cardiomyopathy. Ochronosis,

hyperparathyroidism, hypomagnesemia, and hypothyroidism can all be associated with chondrocalcinosis and pseudogout. Only hemochromatosis can also cause both diabetes mellitus and a cardiomyopathy. The increased value of aspartate aminotransferase reflects chronic liver disease from hemochromatosis.

11. Answer e.

This patient can continue to be observed. He has never had an attack of gout. He is at increased risk for gouty attacks in the future, but there is no reason for treatment at this time. An increased uric acid value does not lead to renal disease by itself.

12. Answer c.

This patient has clinical manifestations to suggest a spondyloarthropathy. Besides the inflammatory arthritis, he has a history of iritis and Achilles tendinitis. Spondyloarthropathies characteristically cause an enthesopathy such as Achilles tendinitis. Iritis occurs in up to 25% of patients with a spondyloarthropathy. Rheumatoid arthritis characteristically does not cause iritis or an enthesopathy. Sarcoid can be associated with iritis, but Achilles tendinitis would be unusual. Neither gout nor Lyme disease has this clinical presentation.

13. Answer e.

This patient has a sausage-like swelling of a digit, which is very characteristic of psoriasis. She also had an erythematous rash in her scalp. Many patients are not aware of the rash. Although gout can cause a swollen toe and this patient's uric acid level was slightly increased, she was taking hydrochlorothiazide, and this would explain both the increased uric acid and calcium levels. Gout in a premenopausal woman would be unusual. Rheumatoid arthritis would not characteristically cause a sausage-like swelling of a digit. Also, rheumatoid arthritis usually has polyarticular involvement. Similar to psoriatic arthritis, reactive arthritis can cause a swollen toe, but this patient's history does not suggest a reactive arthritis, and the finding of a scaly erythematous rash would lead to the diagnosis of psoriatic arthritis.

14. Answer d.

This patient has a reactive arthritis, which characteristically occurs several weeks after an episode of bacterial diarrhea. Eighty percent of patients are HLA-B27–positive. Both gout and pseudogout can cause an acutely swollen ankle, but given the history of diarrhea, reactive arthritis would be much more likely. The clinical scenario described is very unusual in rheumatoid arthritis. Although the patient had a *Salmonella* bacterial diarrhea, synovial fluid cultures would be sterile, indicative of a reactive arthritis.

CHAPTER 23
VASCULAR DISEASES

Peter C. Spittell, M.D.

Peripheral vascular diseases are prevalent in current medical practice. Characteristic clinical features, accurate diagnostic techniques, and improved treatment of peripheral vascular disease further emphasize the need for increased awareness of this group of disorders.

DISEASE OF THE AORTA

Aneurysmal Disease

Thoracic Aortic Aneurysm

Thoracic aortic aneurysms are caused most commonly by atherosclerosis, but they also occur in patients with systemic hypertension, inherited disorders of connective tissue (e.g., Marfan syndrome), giant cell arteritis (cranial and Takayasu disease), and infection and as a result of trauma. There is also a familial tendency. Most thoracic aortic aneurysms are asymptomatic and are discovered incidentally on chest radiography (Fig. 23-1).

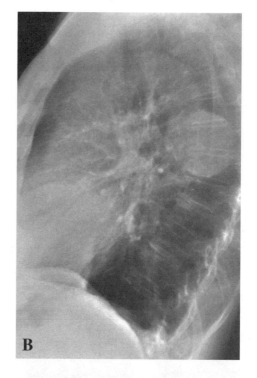

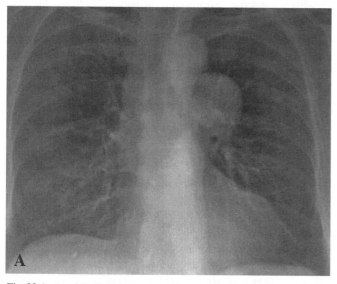

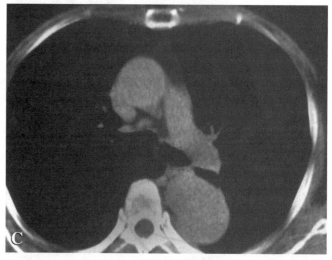

Fig. 23-1. *A* and *B*, Chest radiographs (*A*, anteroposterior; *B*, lateral) show a large mass in the left posterior chest. *C*, Computed tomogram reveals a saccular aneurysm in the mid-descending thoracic aorta.

1013

Symptoms, when present, may include chest or back pain, vocal hoarseness, cough, dyspnea, stridor, and dysphagia. Findings on physical examination may include systemic hypertension, fixed distention of a neck vein(s), aortic regurgitation, a fixed vocal cord, and signs of cerebral or systemic embolism. Complications of thoracic aortic aneurysm include rupture, dissection, embolism, pressure on surrounding structures, infection, and, rarely, thrombosis. Factors that seem to worsen the prognosis include female sex, diastolic hypertension, aneurysm size (critical hinge point for rupture >6 cm ascending aorta and >7 cm descending thoracic aorta), traumatic aneurysm, and associated coronary and carotid artery disease. The overall cumulative risk of rupture after 5 years is 20%, but rupture risk is a function of aneurysm size at recognition (0% for aneurysms less than 4 cm in diameter, 16% for aneurysms 4.0-5.9 cm, and 31% for aneurysms ≥6.0 cm). Computed tomography (CT), magnetic resonance imaging (MRI) (Fig. 23-2), and transesophageal echocardiography (TEE) are all noninvasive techniques that are accurate in the diagnosis of thoracic aortic aneurysms. Medical management of thoracic aortic aneurysm includes control of systemic hypertension (preferably with a β-adrenergic blocking agent), discontinuation of tobacco use, diagnosis and treatment of associated coronary and carotid artery disease, and follow-up combining clinical assessment and noninvasive imaging tests. Indications for surgical resection include the presence of symptoms attributable to the aneurysms, an aneurysm enlarging under observation (particularly if the patient has hypertension), traumatic aneurysm, pseudoaneurysm, mycotic aneurysm, and an aneurysm 6 cm or more in diameter (5.5-6 cm in low-risk patients). In patients with Marfan syndrome, operation is usually indicated when the ascending aortic diameter exceeds 5 cm.

Abdominal Aortic Aneurysm

Approximately three-fourths of all atherosclerotic aneurysms involve the abdominal aorta. Most abdominal aortic aneurysms (AAAs) are infrarenal, and 2% to 5% are suprarenal, usually the result of distal extension of a thoracic aneurysm (thoracoabdominal aneurysm). Men are affected more frequently than women (9:1), and the majority of patients are older than 50 years. There is a familial tendency for development of AAA, and both sex-linked and autosomal patterns of inheritance are involved. Infection and trauma are additional causes of AAA.

The majority of patients with AAA are asymptomatic. The most common physical examination finding is the presence of a pulsatile abdominal mass. The sensitivity of abdominal palpation for the detection of AAA is 43% overall (57% for aneurysms ≥4.0 cm in diameter, 29% for aneurysms <4.0 cm in diameter). A tortuous abdominal aorta, transmitted pulsation from an abdominal mass, or a horseshoe kidney anteriorly displacing the abdominal aorta are conditions that can mimic AAA on physical examination. Because physical examination for the detection of AAA lacks sensitivity, screening tests are indicated in high-risk subsets of patients. Early detection of AAA can reduce mortality. Furthermore, single screening ultrasonography for men older than 65 years can identify the majority of AAAs. Current recommendations for screening for AAA include initial ultrasonography of the general population at age 60 to 65 years and screening of siblings and first-degree relatives of patients with aneurysm at age 50 years.

When AAAs are symptomatic without rupture, the most common complaint is abdominal pain. New low back pain can occur and may be due to dissection within the aneurysm or retroperitoneal hematoma. Abdominal pain radiating to the flank, groin, or testes also may occur. Livedo reticularis, blue toes with palpable pulses, hypertension, renal insufficiency, increased erythrocyte sedimentation rate, and transient eosinophilia characterize atheroembolism in association with AAA (Fig. 23-3).

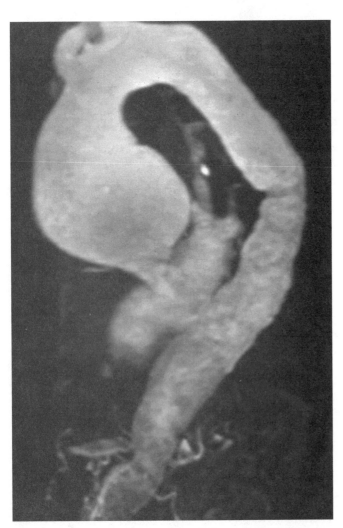

Fig. 23-2. Magnetic resonance angiograph (longitudinal view) shows a large ascending aortic aneurysm and moderate aortic regurgitation.

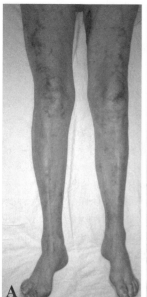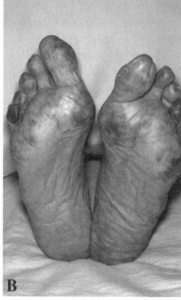

Fig. 23-3. *A* and *B*, Patient with atheroembolism, characterized by livedo reticularis (upper thighs, plantar surface of feet) and multiple blue toes.

Atheroembolism can occur spontaneously or as a result of anti-coagulants (warfarin or thrombolytic therapy) or angiographic or surgical procedures. Treatment of choice is surgical resection of the symptomatic AAA if feasible.

The most frequent complication of AAA is rupture, which is related to aneurysm size: 1-year incidence of rupture for AAA diameter 5.5 to 5.9 cm is 9.4%; diameter 6.0 to 6.9 cm, 10.2%; diameter 7.0 cm or more, 32.5%. The triad of severe abdominal pain, hypotension, and a tender abdominal mass characterizes rupture of an AAA. The pain is acute in onset, constant, and severe, most commonly located in the lumbar area or diffusely throughout the abdomen, with radiation into the flanks, genitals, or legs. The abdominal aorta is usually tender, and there may be peritoneal signs if free rupture into the peritoneal cavity has occurred. Less common presentations of AAA include obstructive uropathy due to ureteral compression, gastrointestinal hemorrhage when the aneurysm ruptures into the intestinal tract, high-output congestive heart failure due to an aortocaval fistula, and disseminated intravascular coagulation.

AAA can be diagnosed reliably with ultrasonography, CT, or MRI (Fig. 23-4). Angiography is not required unless the renal or peripheral arterial circulation needs to be visualized to plan treatment.

Medical management of AAA includes control of systemic hypertension (preferably with a β-adrenergic blocking agent), discontinuation of tobacco use, treatment of associated coronary and carotid artery disease, and serial noninvasive imaging tests. Noninvasive imaging should be used to assess both absolute aneurysm size and growth rate. The frequency of surveillance is based on aneurysm size at initial detection (Table 23-1).

In a good-risk patient, *selective* surgical treatment of AAA should be considered for aneurysms more than 5.0 cm in diameter. Elective surgical repair is definitely indicated when the aneurysm diameter is between 5.0 and 5.5 cm in good-risk patients. When the patient has considerable comorbid conditions (pulmonary, cardiac, renal, or liver disease), surgical therapy is individualized. Endovascular repair of AAA with stent grafts that are delivered intraluminally by catheters is an alternative to open surgical repair, and early results are comparable to those of open repair. At tertiary care centers, more than

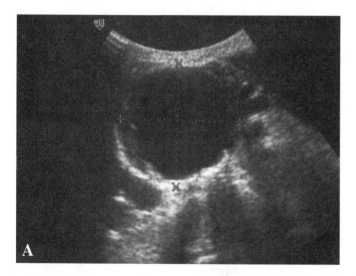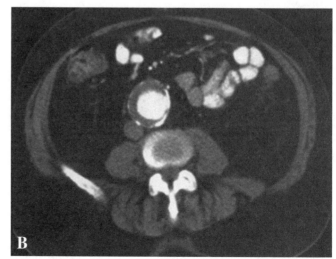

Fig. 23-4. *A*, Ultrasonogram (transverse view) shows a 4.7-cm abdominal aortic aneurysm. *B*, Computed tomogram (contrast-enhanced) shows an abdominal aortic aneurysm with moderate mural thrombus.

Table 23-1 Surveillance of Abdominal Aortic Aneurysm

Size at initial detection, cm	Surveillance interval
3.0-3.4	3 y
3.5-3.9	1 y
4.0-4.9	6 mo
≥5.0	3 mo*

*If surveillance is ongoing (vs. surgery).
Data from McCarthy RJ, Shaw E, Whyman MR, et al: Recommendations for screening intervals for small aortic aneurysms. Br J Surg 2003;90:821-826.

30% of AAA repairs are accomplished with an endovascular approach. With extended follow-up, however, postoperative complications and graft failures have been reported in some patients, resulting in reintervention, conversion to open repair, or death. The high incidence of secondary interventions brings into question the durability of endograft repair and emphasizes the need for detailed long-term follow-up care.

Inflammatory AAA accounts for approximately 2% to 4% of all AAAs. An inflammatory AAA is suggested by the triad of abdominal or back pain, weight loss, and increased erythrocyte sedimentation rate. Obstructive uropathy may occur with ureteral involvement. The findings on CT are diagnostic. The treatment is surgical resection regardless of aneurysm size. The role of corticosteroids is not well defined.

Operation is also indicated for AAAs that are symptomatic, traumatic, infectious in origin, or rapidly expanding (>0.5 cm/year).

- Elective surgical repair is definitely indicated when the AAA diameter is more than 5.0 cm in good-risk patients.
- Surgical treatment is also indicated for AAAs that are symptomatic, traumatic, infectious in origin, or are rapidly expanding (>0.5 cm/year).
- The triad of back pain, weight loss, and increased erythrocyte sedimentation rate suggests an inflammatory AAA. The findings on CT are diagnostic. Treatment is surgical resection regardless of aneurysm size.

Aortic Dissection

Etiology

The most common predisposing factors for aortic dissection are advanced age, male sex, hypertension, Marfan syndrome, and congenital abnormalities of the aortic valve (bicuspid or unicuspid valve). When aortic dissection complicates pregnancy, it usually occurs in the third trimester. Iatrogenic aortic dissection, as a result of cardiac operation or invasive angiographic procedures, also can occur.

Classification

Aortic dissection involving the ascending aorta is designated as type I or II (proximal, type A) and dissection confined to the descending thoracic aorta is designated as type III (distal, type B) (Fig. 23-5).

Clinical Features

The acute onset of severe pain (often migratory) in the anterior aspect of the chest, back, or abdomen occurs in 70% to 80% of patients, and hypertension is present in 60% to 80%. Additional findings include aortic diastolic murmur (15%-20%), pulse deficits (10%-40%), and neurologic changes (10%-30%). Syncope in association with aortic dissection occurs when there is rupture into the pericardial space, producing cardiac tamponade. Congestive heart failure is most commonly due to severe aortic regurgitation. Acute myocardial infarction (most commonly inferior infarction due to right coronary artery ostial involvement), pericarditis, and complete heart block are additional cardiac presentations.

Clues to type I aortic dissection include substernal pain, aortic valve incompetence, decreased pulse or blood pressure in the right arm, decreased right carotid pulse, pericardial friction rub, syncope, ischemic electrocardiographic changes, and Marfan syndrome.

Clues to type III aortic dissection include interscapular pain, hypertension, and left pleural effusion.

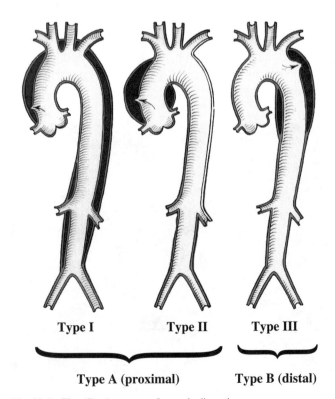

Type I   **Type II**   **Type III**

Type A (proximal)   **Type B (distal)**

Fig. 23-5. Classification system for aortic dissection.

- In a patient with a catastrophic presentation, systemic hypertension, and unexplained physical findings of vascular origin, especially in the presence of chest pain and an aortic murmur, aortic dissection should always be included in the differential diagnosis and an appropriate screening test performed on an emergency basis.

Laboratory Tests

Chest radiography may show widening of the mediastinum and supracardiac aortic shadow, deviation of the trachea to the right, a discrepancy in diameter between the ascending and descending aorta, and pleural effusion (Fig. 23-6). Normal findings on chest radiography do not exclude aortic dissection.

Electrocardiography most commonly reveals left ventricular hypertrophy, but ST-segment depression, ST-segment elevation, T-wave changes, and the changes of acute pericarditis and complete heart block can occur.

Diagnosis

Aortic dissection can be definitively diagnosed with any of the following imaging methods: echocardiography, CT, MRI, and aortography (Fig. 23-7).

Combined transthoracic and transesophageal echocardiography (TTE/TEE) can be used to identify an intimal flap, communication between the true and false lumina, a dilated aortic root (>4 cm), thrombus formation, widening of the aortic walls, aortic regurgitation, pericardial effusion or tamponade, pleural effusion, and proximal abdominal aorta involvement. Multiplane transducers have markedly improved the accuracy of TEE. Advantages of TEE include portability, safety, accuracy, rapid diagnosis, use in patients with hemodynamic instability, and intraoperative applications.

CT can accurately detect the intimal flap, identify two lumina, and demonstrate displaced intimal calcification, a disparate size between the ascending and descending aortic

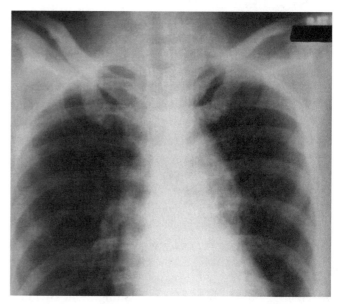

Fig. 23-6. Chest radiograph in a patient with aortic dissection shows widening of the superior mediastinum.

lumina, hemopericardium, pleural effusion, and abdominal aorta involvement. The disadvantages include nonportability (limiting use in patients with hemodynamic instability) and the need for intravenous contrast agents.

MRI is highly accurate for the diagnosis of aortic dissection. Demonstration of the intimal flap, entry or exit sites, thrombus formation, aortic regurgitation, pericardial effusion, pleural effusion, and abdominal aorta involvement is possible. MRI is also able to delineate involvement of aortic arch vessels. Disadvantages of MRI include cost and nonportability.

Aortography can accurately diagnose aortic dissection by showing the intimal flap, opacification of the false lumen, and deformity of the true lumen. Also, associated aortic regurgitation and coronary artery anatomy can be visualized. The

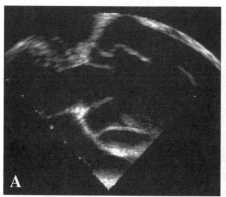
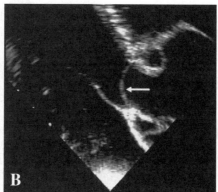
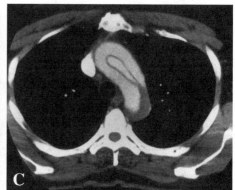

Fig. 23-7. A, Multiplane transesophageal echocardiogram (longitudinal view) shows an intimal flap in the ascending aorta. B, In diastole, the intimal flap prolapses through the aortic valve (arrow). C, Computed tomogram (contrast-enhanced) shows a spiraling intimal flap in the transverse aortic arch.

disadvantages include invasive risks, exposure to intravenous contrast agents, and nonportability.

The choice of test (TTE, TEE, CT, MRI, or aortography) in a patient with suspected acute aortic dissection depends on which is most readily available and the hemodynamic stability of the patient. Currently, one test of choice in suspected acute aortic dissection is the combination of TTE and TEE.

The initial management of suspected acute aortic dissection is shown in Figure 23-8.

The most common cause of death is rupture into the pericardial space, with cardiac tamponade. Echocardiographically guided pericardiocentesis in a patient with cardiac tamponade complicating aortic dissection is associated with an increased risk of aortic rupture and death. Cardiac tamponade due to aortic dissection is a surgical emergency, and pericardial fluid should be removed only in the operating room after cardiopulmonary bypass has been instituted. Other causes of death in aortic dissection include acute congestive heart failure due to severe aortic regurgitation, rupture through the aortic adventitia, rupture into the left pleural space, and occlusion of vital arteries.

● Aortic dissection can be diagnosed with TEE, CT, or MRI.

Treatment

Pharmacologic therapy should be instituted as soon as the diagnosis of aortic dissection is suspected (Table 23-2). Emergency operation is indicated in types I and II (proximal, type A) aortic dissection. Continued pharmacologic therapy in the coronary care unit is the preferred initial management in type III (distal, type B) aortic dissection, and surgical therapy is delayed (2-3 weeks) for selected patients whose general medical condition permits operation. When long-term pharmacologic therapy for type III aortic dissection is used, indications for operation include development of saccular aneurysm, increasing aortic diameter, or symptoms related to chronic dissection.

● Emergency operation is indicated in types I and II aortic dissection.
● Pharmacologic treatment is the preferred initial management in type III aortic dissection.

Penetrating Aortic Ulcer

Penetrating aortic ulcer occurs when an atherosclerotic plaque undergoes ulceration and penetrates the internal elastic lamina. It results in one of four possible consequences: 1) formation of an intramural hematoma, 2) formation of a saccular aneurysm, 3) formation of a pseudoaneurysm, or 4) transmural aortic rupture. Penetrating aortic ulcer most commonly involves the mid or distal descending thoracic aorta, less often the ascending or abdominal aorta. The clinical features of penetrating aortic ulcer are similar to those of aortic dissection and include acute onset of pain in the anterior or posterior chest (or both) and hypertension. Pulse deficits, neurologic signs, and acute cardiac disease (aortic regurgitation, myocardial infarction, pericardial effusion) do not occur in penetrating aortic ulcer, as they do in classic aortic dissection.

The treatment of penetrating aortic ulcer is usually nonoperative if only an intramural hematoma is present. With control of hypertension, the intramural hematoma tends to resolve spontaneously over time. Surgical therapy is indicated for patients who have ascending aortic involvement, patients in whom a saccular aneurysm or pseudoaneurysm develops, or patients with intramural hematoma who have persistent symptoms, increasing aortic diameter, or poorly controlled hypertension. The most common serious complication of surgical therapy for penetrating aortic ulcer is paraplegia.

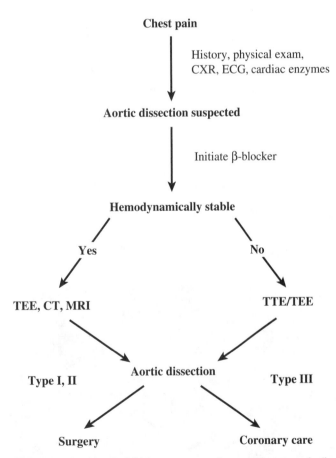

Fig. 23-8. Algorithm for initial management of suspected acute aortic dissection. CT, computed tomography; CXR, chest radiography; ECG, electrocardiography; MRI, magnetic resonance imaging; TEE, transesophageal echocardiography; TTE, transthoracic echocardiography.

Table 23-2   Initial Pharmacologic Therapy for Acute Aortic Dissection

Hypertensive patients

 Sodium nitroprusside intravenously (2.5-5.0 µg/kg per minute)

  with

 Propranolol intravenously (1 mg every 4-6 h)

  • Goal: Systolic blood pressure in the range of 110 mm Hg (or the lowest level maintaining a urine output of 25-30 mL/h) until oral medication is started

 Or Esmolol, metoprolol, or atenolol intravenously (in place of propranolol)

 Or Labetolol intravenously (in place of sodium nitroprusside and a β-blocker)

Normotensive patients

 Propranolol 1 mg intravenously every 4-6 h or 20-40 mg orally every 6 h (metoprolol, atenolol, esmolol, or labetolol may be used in place of propranolol)

Aortic Intramural Hematoma

Aortic intramural hematoma is also associated with cystic medial necrosis that occurs in the absence of an intimal tear. Aortic intramural hematoma is increasingly recognized, largely due to advances in noninvasive imaging techniques. The exact cause of aortic intramural hematoma is not well defined. Aortic intramural hematoma is diagnosed in the same manner as aortic dissection. The classification schemes are also identical, and traditionally the management has been similar—operation for type A intramural hematoma and medical treatment for type B lesions.

Incomplete Aortic Rupture

Incomplete rupture of the thoracic aorta (in the region of the aortic isthmus) results from a sudden deceleration injury. It occurs most often in victims of motor vehicle accidents and should be suspected when there is evidence of chest wall trauma, decreased or absent leg pulses, left-sided hemothorax, or widening of the superior mediastinum on chest radiography. Affected patients are usually hypertensive at initial presentation. TEE, CT, MRI, or angiography can confirm the diagnosis (Fig. 23-9). Treatment is emergency surgical repair in patients who are suitable surgical candidates. At initial presentation, the condition of 40% to 50% of patients is unstable. No clinical or imaging criteria accurately predict future complete rupture, so even if a patient presents with a chronic incomplete rupture, operation is still indicated. Most patients are young, and the risk of elective surgical repair is low, with an otherwise good prognosis for long-term survival if aortic repair is successful.

• Incomplete rupture of the thoracic aorta (in the region of the aortic isthmus) results from a sudden deceleration injury, frequently a motor vehicle accident.

Thoracic Aortic Atherosclerosis

Atherosclerosis of the thoracic aorta usually involves the origin of the brachiocephalic arteries, principally the left subclavian and occasionally the innominate artery. Although atherosclerotic disease of the aortic arch branches is usually asymptomatic, stenosis of the origin of the left or right subclavian artery may cause intermittent claudication of the arm

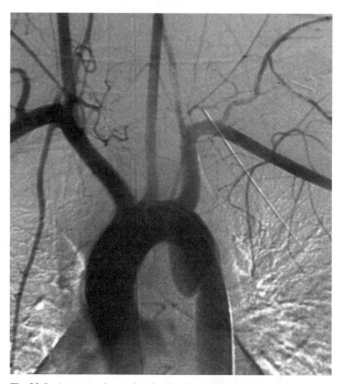

Fig. 23-9. Aortogram in a patient involved in a severe motor vehicle accident shows a contained rupture of the proximal descending thoracic aorta just distal to the origin of the left subclavian artery.

of sufficient degree to warrant surgical treatment. With complete occlusion of the origin of either subclavian artery, collateral blood flow to the arm may be derived principally from the cerebral circulation via reversed flow through the ipsilateral vertebral artery, so-called subclavian steal. This may result in episodes of transient cerebral ischemia, especially when the ipsilateral arm is exercised. A similar situation may occur on the right side if the obstruction occurs at the origin of the innominate artery, in which case flow in the right vertebral artery can "reverse" to enter the right subclavian artery. In addition to the symptoms of transient cerebral ischemia, physical signs of this condition include reduced arm and wrist pulses and reduced blood pressure on the affected side.

Furthermore, a coronary-subclavian steal phenomenon may occur in patients who have undergone prior coronary artery bypass grafting in which the internal mammary artery is used. When a hemodynamically significant subclavian artery stenosis is present ipsilateral to the internal mammary artery graft, flow through the internal mammary artery may reverse or "steal" during upper extremity exercise. The astute examiner, when palpating both radial pulses simultaneously, may also detect a delay in pulsation on the affected side.

Acquired coarctation of the thoracic aorta due to focally obstructive calcific atherosclerotic disease is rare. Symptomatic patients present with upper extremity hypertension and reduced blood pressure in the lower extremities, with or without intermittent claudication.

Microemboli or macroemboli from atherosclerotic plaque and thrombus in the thoracic aorta are important causes of cerebral and systemic embolization. Aortic atheroma occurs in approximately 27% of patients with previous embolic events and is also a strong predictor of coronary artery disease. Thoracic aortic atherosclerotic plaque is most accurately assessed with TEE. Plaque thickness more than 4 mm or mobile thrombus (of any size) is associated with an increased risk of embolism. Embolism can occur spontaneously, in relation to invasive angiographic procedures, as a result of warfarin or thrombolytic therapy, and from cardiac surgical procedures requiring cardiopulmonary bypass. Treatment is surgical resection if a focal source of embolism is present and the patient's general medical condition permits. Antiplatelet agents and a statin medication should be used for the management of all patients unless an absolute contraindication is present. Warfarin therapy may be beneficial for reducing subsequent embolic events, but further randomized trials are required.

- Emboli from atherosclerotic plaque and thrombus in the thoracic aorta are important causes of cerebral and systemic embolization.

PERIPHERAL ARTERIAL OCCLUSIVE DISEASE

Intermittent Claudication

Clinical Features

Patients with significant lower extremity arterial occlusive disease usually present with intermittent claudication. The discomfort of intermittent claudication (aching, cramping, or tightness) is always exercise-induced and may involve one or both legs, and symptoms occur at a fairly constant walking distance. Relief is obtained by standing still. Supine ankle:brachial systolic pressure indices before and after exercise testing (treadmill walking or active pedal plantar flexion) can confirm the diagnosis (Table 23-3). Furthermore, a low ankle:brachial systolic pressure index (<0.9) is associated with an increased risk of stroke, cardiovascular death, and all-cause mortality.

Pseudoclaudication

Pseudoclaudication, due to lumbar spinal stenosis, is the condition most commonly confused with intermittent claudication. Pseudoclaudication is usually described as a "paresthetic" discomfort that occurs with standing *and* walking (variable distances). Symptoms are almost always bilateral and are relieved by sitting or leaning forward. The patient often has a prior history of chronic back pain or lumbosacral spinal operation. The diagnosis of lumbar spinal stenosis can be confirmed with normal or minimally abnormal ankle:brachial systolic pressure indices before and after exercise, in combination with characteristic findings on electromyography and CT or MRI of the lumbar spine (Table 23-4).

- The discomfort of intermittent claudication is always exercise-induced; standing still provides relief.
- Pseudoclaudication occurs with standing *and* walking.

Table 23-3   Grading System for Lower Extremity Arterial Occlusive Disease*

Grade	ABI	
	Supine resting	Post-exercise
Normal	≥1.0	No change or increase
Mild disease	0.8-0.9	>0.5
Moderate disease	0.5-0.8	>0.2
Severe disease	<0.5	<0.2

ABI, ankle:brachial systolic pressure index.
*After treadmill exercise, 1-2 mph, 10% grade, 5 minutes or symptom-limited or active pedal plantar flexion, 50 repetitions or symptom-limited.

Table 23-4   Differential Diagnosis of True Claudication and Pseudoclaudication

	Claudication	Pseudoclaudication
Onset	Walking	Standing and walking
Character	Cramp, ache	"Paresthetic"
Bilateral	+/−	+
Walking distance	Fairly constant	More variable
Cause	Atherosclerosis	Spinal stenosis
Relief	Standing still	Sitting down, leaning forward

Natural History

Peripheral arterial occlusive disease is associated with considerable mortality because of its association with coronary and carotid atherosclerosis. The 5-year mortality rate in patients with intermittent claudication is 29%, and the overall amputation rate over 5 years is 4%. More than half of patients have stable or improved symptoms over this same period. Continued use of tobacco results in a 10-fold increase in the risk for major amputation and a more than 2-fold increase in mortality. The effect of diabetes mellitus on patients with intermittent claudication deserves special mention because it accounts for 60% of amputations in a community (12-fold increased risk of below-knee amputation and a cumulative risk of major amputation exceeding 11% over 25 years). Other clinical features that predict an increased risk of limb loss include ischemic rest pain, ischemic ulceration, and gangrene.

- The 5-year mortality rate in patients with intermittent claudication is 29%, predominantly due to associated coronary atherosclerosis.
- Diabetes mellitus, ischemic rest pain, ulceration, and gangrene are associated with an increased risk of limb loss in patients with intermittent claudication.

Diagnosis

Peripheral angiography is rarely needed to diagnose intermittent claudication. The diagnosis is made clinically. Further quantification of disease severity can readily be obtained by noninvasive testing (determination of ankle:brachial systolic pressure indices before and after exercise or duplex ultrasonography). Angiography is indicated for 1) defining arterial anatomy preoperatively, 2) evaluating therapy, or 3) documenting disease (medicolegal issue). Angiography also is indicated when an "uncommon" type of arterial disease is suspected. Magnetic resonance angiography is an accurate alternative to standard angiography; it is also useful for preoperative planning in patients with contraindications to invasive angiography (i.e., renal insufficiency or allergy to contrast media).

- Peripheral angiography is rarely needed to diagnose intermittent claudication.

Treatment

Medical management of intermittent claudication is effective and includes discontinuation of tobacco use (all forms), weight reduction (if obese), lipid reduction, glucose management in patients with diabetes mellitus, foot care and protection, a walking program, pharmacologic therapy, and avoidance of vasoconstrictive drugs.

A regular walking program, performed on level ground 4 or more days a week, can result in a significant increase in initial claudication distance over 2 to 3 months. This is a useful initial approach to patients with intermittent claudication.

Antiplatelet agents (aspirin, clopidogrel) reduce both the risk of limb loss and the need for surgical revascularization in patients with intermittent claudication. All patients with intermittent claudication should be managed with one of these agents, unless an absolute contraindication exists.

Pentoxifylline, a methylxanthine, has vasoactive properties, including vasodilation, inhibition of cyclic adenosine monophosphate phosphodiesterase, stimulation of prostacyclin formation, and increased erythrocyte and leukocyte deformability. These properties result in relaxation of vascular smooth muscle, inhibition of platelet aggregation, and decreased blood viscosity. A "target population" of patients with intermittent claudication most likely to benefit from pentoxifylline are those with symptoms present for more than 1 year and an ankle:brachial index less than 0.8. Only one dosing regimen (400 mg 3 times daily) is used clinically.

Cilostazol, a phosphodiesterase inhibitor, is also useful in patients with intermittent claudication, substantially improving both walking distance and quality of life. Cilostazol seems to be more effective than pentoxifylline, but it is contraindicated in patients with congestive heart failure of any severity. The dose is 100 mg orally daily (50 mg orally twice daily in patients taking diltiazem, ketoconazole, or other inhibitors of cytochrome P-450 3A4).

Propionyl-L-carnitine appears to improve alterations in carnitine metabolism in patients with a severe functional impairment from intermittent claudication, resulting in improvement in maximal walking distance and quality of life. The dose is 1 gram orally twice daily.

In hypercholesterolemic patients with symptomatic peripheral arterial occlusive disease, simvastatin in high doses (40 mg/day) may improve walking performance and the symptoms of intermittent claudication.

Indications for endovascular or surgical revascularization in a patient with peripheral arterial occlusive disease are "disabling" (lifestyle-limiting) symptoms despite optimal medical therapy, diabetes mellitus with symptoms, or critical limb ischemia (ischemic rest pain, ischemic ulceration, or gangrene).

Revascularization is *elective* in nondiabetic patients with intermittent claudication because 1) it does not improve coronary or cerebrovascular disease, the major cause of mortality, and consequently does not affect overall long-term survival, 2) the incidence of severe limb-threatening ischemia is relatively low because runoff is usually adequate, 3) perioperative complications of peripheral vascular operation, although infrequent, do occur, and 4) reocclusion may occur.

Revascularization in patients with ischemic rest pain or ischemic ulceration or in those with diabetes mellitus with intermittent claudication is *indicated* because 1) the incidence of limb loss is increased without revascularization, 2) operation may permit a lower anatomical level of amputation, and 3) the risks of the procedure are generally less than the risk of amputation.

Percutaneous transluminal angioplasty is an effective alternative to surgical therapy in patients with proximal disease, short, partial occlusions, and good distal runoff. The ideal lesion for angioplasty is an iliac stenosis less than 5 cm. Advantages of angioplasty over operation include less morbidity, shorter convalescence, lower cost, and preservation of the saphenous vein for future use. Percutaneous transluminal angioplasty in aortic or iliac disease also may allow for an infrainguinal surgical procedure to be performed at reduced perioperative risk (compared with intra-abdominal aortic operation).

- For intermittent claudication, medical management is important as initial therapy, including antiplatelet agents, cessation of tobacco use, lipid reduction, foot care and protection, a walking program, and, in selected cases, pentoxifylline or cilostazol.
- Diabetes mellitus with symptoms and critical limb ischemia (ischemic rest pain, ischemic ulceration, and gangrene) are associated with an increased risk of limb loss in patients with lower extremity arterial occlusive disease. The presence of these features warrants an invasive approach (angiography followed by endovascular or surgical revascularization).

Cardiac Risk and Vascular Surgery

Patients with peripheral arterial disease (AAA, lower extremity arterial occlusive disease, and cerebrovascular disease) have a 60% incidence of significant coronary artery disease (>70% stenosis of one or more epicardial coronary arteries). Up to 30% of patients have severe correctable three-vessel coronary artery disease with reduced left ventricular function, the group

most likely to benefit from coronary artery bypass grafting. Clinical markers that identify patients who are at increased risk for a perioperative "cardiac event" when undergoing vascular operation include age older than 70 years, angina, diabetes mellitus, ventricular ectopy, Q waves on electrocardiography, and a carotid bruit. If the preoperative clinical evaluation indicates that further noninvasive cardiac testing is indicated, pharmacologic stress (i.e., dobutamine, dipyridamole, or adenosine) is usually performed because patients with intermittent claudication often cannot achieve an adequate double product during standard treadmill exercise. The presence of reversible defects (thallium-201 or sestamibi scintigraphy) or new regional wall motion abnormalities on stress echocardiography predicts an increased perioperative cardiac risk (30% and 53%, respectively). In contrast, the absence of perfusion abnormalities or stress-induced regional wall motion abnormalities predicts a perioperative cardiac risk of 3% and less than 1%, respectively. An assessment of resting left ventricular function alone, by either radionuclide angiography or echocardiography, is not predictive of perioperative cardiac risk during vascular operation.

- Clinical markers that identify patients who are at increased risk for a perioperative cardiac event when undergoing vascular operation include age older than 70 years, angina, diabetes mellitus, ventricular ectopy, pathologic Q waves on electrocardiography, and carotid bruit.
- An assessment of resting left ventricular function alone is not predictive of perioperative cardiac risk during vascular operation.

Acute Arterial Occlusion

The symptoms of acute arterial occlusion are sudden in onset (<5 hours) and include the "5 Ps": pain, pallor, paresthesia (numbness), poikilothermy (coldness), and pulselessness (absence of peripheral pulses).

Features that suggest a *thrombotic* cause of acute arterial occlusion include previous occlusive disease in the involved limb, occlusive disease involving other extremities, acute aortic dissection, hematologic disease, arteritis, inflammatory bowel disease, neoplasm, and ergotism.

An *embolic* cause of acute arterial occlusion is suggested by the presence of cardiac disease, atrial fibrillation, proximal aneurysm, or proximal atherosclerotic disease.

After confirmation by angiography, the initial therapeutic options for acute arterial occlusion include intra-arterial thrombolysis and surgical therapy (thromboembolectomy). If thrombolytic therapy is the initial treatment, percutaneous transluminal angioplasty or surgical therapy is usually indicated to treat the underlying stenosis (if present) to improve long-term patency rates.

- The "5 Ps" suggestive of acute arterial occlusion include pain, pallor, paresthesia, poikilothermy (coldness), and pulselessness.

Peripheral Arterial Aneurysms

Because aneurysms are most commonly caused by atherosclerosis, they are more common in men 60 years or older. Coronary and carotid occlusive disease are frequent comorbid conditions. Other predisposing factors for aneurysmal disease include hypertension, familial tendency, connective tissue disease, trauma, infection, and inflammatory disease.

Most aneurysms are asymptomatic. Complications of aneurysms include embolization, pressure on surrounding structures, infection, and rupture. Aneurysms of certain arteries develop specific complications more often than other complications. For example, the most common complication of aortic aneurysms is rupture, whereas embolism is a more common complication of femoral and popliteal artery aneurysms.

An iliac artery aneurysm usually occurs in association with an AAA, but it may occur as an isolated finding. Iliac artery aneurysms may cause atheroembolism, obstructive urologic symptoms, unexplained groin or perineal pain, or iliac vein obstruction. Ultrasonography, CT with intravenous contrast agent, and MRI are the preferred diagnostic procedures. Surgical resection is indicated when the aneurysm is symptomatic or larger than 3 cm in diameter.

Thrombosis, venous obstruction, embolization, popliteal neuropathy, popliteal thrombophlebitis, rupture, and infection can complicate popliteal artery aneurysm. Popliteal artery aneurysms are bilateral in 50% of patients, and 40% of patients will have one or more aneurysms at other sites, usually the abdominal aorta. The diagnosis is readily made with ultrasonography, but angiography is necessary before surgical treatment to evaluate the proximal and distal arterial circulation. When a popliteal aneurysm is diagnosed, surgical therapy is the treatment of choice to prevent serious thromboembolic complications.

- An iliac artery aneurysm usually occurs in association with an AAA, but it may occur as an isolated finding.
- Popliteal artery aneurysms are bilateral in 50% of patients, and 40% of patients will have one or more aneurysms at other sites.

UNCOMMON TYPES OF ARTERIAL OCCLUSIVE DISEASE

The clinical features that suggest an uncommon type of peripheral arterial occlusive disease include young age, acute ischemia without a history of arterial occlusive disease, and involvement of only the upper extremity or digits (Fig. 23-10).

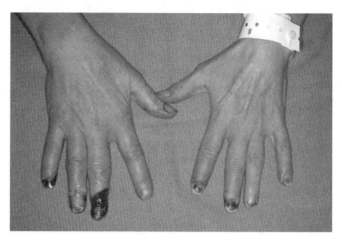

Fig. 23-10. Patient with thromboangiitis obliterans has gangrene of the tips of multiple upper extremity digits.

Uncommon types of arterial occlusive disease include thromboangiitis obliterans, arteritis associated with connective tissue disease, giant cell arteritis (cranial and Takayasu disease), and arterial occlusive disease due to blunt trauma or arterial entrapment.

Thromboangiitis Obliterans (Buerger Disease)

The diagnostic clinical criteria for thromboangiitis obliterans (Buerger disease) are listed in Table 23-5. More definitive diagnosis of thromboangiitis obliterans requires angiography, which usually reveals multiple, bilateral focal segments of stenosis or occlusion with normal proximal vessels. Treatment of thromboangiitis obliterans is the same as for other types of occlusive peripheral arterial disease, but particular emphasis

Table 23-5 Clinical Criteria for Thromboangiitis Obliterans

Age	<40 years (often <30 years)
Sex	Males most often
Habits	Tobacco, cannabis use
History	Superficial phlebitis
	Claudication, arch or calf
	Raynaud phenomenon
	Absence of atherosclerotic risk factors other than smoking
Examination	Small arteries involved
	Upper extremity involved (positive Allen test)
	Infrapopliteal artery disease
Laboratory	Normal glucose, blood counts, sedimentation rate, lipids, and screening tests for connective tissue disease and hypercoagulable disorders
Radiography	No arterial calcification

is placed on the need for permanent abstinence from all forms of tobacco. Smoking cessation ameliorates the course of the disease but does not invariably stop further exacerbations. Abstinence from tobacco also substantially reduces the risk of ulcer formation and amputation, thus improving quality of life in patients with thromboangiitis obliterans. Because the arteries involved are small, arterial reconstruction for ischemia in patients with Buerger disease is technically challenging. Distal arterial reconstruction, if necessary, is indicated to prevent ischemic limb loss. Collateral artery bypass is an option when the main arteries are affected by the disease. A patent but diseased artery should be avoided as a target for reconstruction. Sympathectomy may be useful in severe digital ischemia with ulceration to control pain and to improve cutaneous blood flow. Therapeutic angiogenesis with phVEGF165 gene transfer may be beneficial in patients with advanced Buerger disease that is unresponsive to standard medical or surgical treatment methods.

- Treatment of thromboangiitis obliterans is the same as for other types of occlusive peripheral arterial disease, but particular emphasis is placed on the need for permanent abstinence from all forms of tobacco.

Popliteal Artery Entrapment

Popliteal artery entrapment (PAE) is an uncommon congenital abnormality that is often overlooked clinically. PAE is important because repeated compression of the popliteal artery can lead to localized atherosclerosis, poststenotic dilation, or thrombosis resulting in serious ischemia in the distal leg or foot. PAE occurs most often in young men, who may present with a complaint of intermittent claudication in the arch of the foot or calf. If the popliteal artery is not already occluded, the finding of reduced pedal pulses with sustained active plantar flexion should increase suspicion of the disorder.

PAE can occur by several mechanisms. The artery can be compressed because of its anomalous relationship to the medial head of the gastrocnemius (looping around and under or through the gastrocnemius), by its displacement by an anomalous insertion of the plantaris muscle, or by passing beneath rather than behind the popliteal muscle.

The diagnosis of PAE can be made noninvasively with duplex ultrasonography, CT, and MRI. MRI is superior to ultrasonography and CT for defining the exact abnormality in PAE, with results similar to those with digital subtraction angiography. The combined morphologic and functional evaluation of the popliteal fossa makes MRI the investigation of choice in the management of young adults with intermittent claudication. MRI is particularly useful when the popliteal artery is occluded, in which situation ultrasonography and angiography are of limited value.

Angiographic findings in PAE include irregularity of the wall of the popliteal artery in an otherwise normal arterial tree, often associated with prestenotic or poststenotic dilatation. If the artery is still patent, medial displacement of the popliteal artery from its normal position in the popliteal space and popliteal artery compression with extension of the knee and dorsiflexion of the foot are diagnostic angiographic findings. If the mechanism of compression is by the plantaris or popliteal muscle, the position of the artery may appear normal on angiography. If PAE has been diagnosed in one limb, the contralateral limb should be screened because bilateral disease occurs in more than 25% of patients.

The management of PAE depends on the clinical presentation and anatomical findings. Although the natural history of PAE is not well defined, surgery has been advocated to prevent progression of the disease from repetitive arterial trauma. Detection and treatment of PAE at an early stage appear to permit better long-term results.

Thoracic Outlet Compression Syndrome

Compression of the subclavian artery in the thoracic outlet (thoracic outlet compression syndrome) can occur at several points, but the most common site of compression is in the costoclavicular space between the uppermost rib (cervical rib, or first rib) and the clavicle. If the patient is symptomatic, the presentation may be any one of the following: Raynaud phenomenon in one or more fingers of the ipsilateral hand, digital cyanosis or ulceration, and "claudication" of the arm or forearm. Occlusive arterial disease in the affected arm or hand is readily detected on examination of the arterial pulses and with the Allen test. Compression of the subclavian artery in the thoracic outlet can be determined by noting a decreased or absent pulse in the ipsilateral radial artery during performance of thoracic outlet maneuvers. The diagnosis is confirmed with duplex ultrasonography, magnetic resonance angiography, or angiography, with the involved arm in the neutral and hyperabducted position.

The optimal therapy for thoracic outlet compression is controversial. In general, treatment depends on the severity of symptoms. In minimally symptomatic patients, physical therapy and education regarding the relationship of arm and body position to arterial compression may be sufficient treatment. In patients who have more severe symptoms, aneurysm formation, distal embolization, or digital ischemia, surgical treatment is indicated. Surgical resection of the first thoracic or cervical rib is the most effective way to relieve the arterial compression. In some cases, thrombectomy and reconstruction of the subclavian artery in patients with subclavian artery stenosis, thrombosis, or occlusion are also indicated. Sympathectomy may be used as an adjunctive surgical procedure when there is extensive digital or hand ischemia. Stent placement in residual subclavian artery stenoses has been successful but needs to be performed after surgical decompression of the costoclavicular space to decrease the likelihood of recurrence or stent damage.

It is important to remember that all of the connective tissue disorders and giant cell arteritides can involve peripheral arteries and that symptoms of peripheral arterial involvement may dominate the clinical picture. Other than the conservative measures already discussed for ischemic limbs, therapy is directed mainly at the underlying disease. Only after the inflammatory process is controlled should surgical revascularization of chronically ischemic extremities be performed.

Heparin-Induced Thrombocytopenia

Heparin-induced thrombocytopenia (HIT) affects between 5% and 10% of patients who receive heparin therapy, but the incidence of arterial or venous thrombosis is less than 1% to 2%. HIT (type II) typically occurs 5 to 14 days after heparin exposure and is associated with arterial thrombosis (arterial occlusion, ischemic strokes, myocardial infarction) and venous thrombosis (pulmonary embolism, phlegmasia cerulea dolens [venous gangrene], and sagittal sinus thrombosis) (Fig. 23-11). The diagnosis of HIT is primarily clinical (occurrence of thrombocytopenia during heparin therapy, resolution of thrombocytopenia when heparin therapy is discontinued, and exclusion of other causes of thrombocytopenia) and can be confirmed by demonstration in vitro of a heparin-dependent platelet antibody. Treatment of HIT includes discontinuation of all forms of heparin exposure (subcutaneous, intravenous, or heparin flushes and heparin-coated catheters), including low-molecular-weight heparins. The current anticoagulant of choice for HIT is a direct thrombin inhibitor, that is, lepirudin or argatroban. Other therapeutic options that may be effective for patients with HIT include dextran, plasmapheresis, intravenous

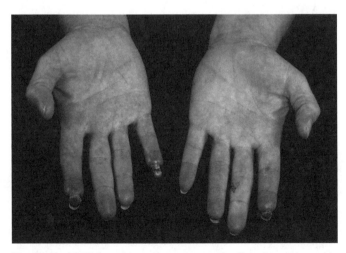

Fig. 23-11. Multiple gangrenous upper extremity digits in a patient with heparin-induced thrombocytopenia.

gamma globulin, and aspirin (acetylsalicylic acid), but these approaches have not been tested in rigorous clinical trials.

VASOSPASTIC DISORDERS

Vasospastic disorders are characterized by episodic color changes of the skin resulting from intermittent spasm of the small arteries and arterioles of the skin and digits. Vasospastic disorders are important because they frequently are a clue to another underlying disorder such as arterial occlusive disease, connective tissue disorders, neurologic disorders, or endocrine disease. Vasospastic disorders also can appear as side effects of drug therapy, specifically of ergot preparations, estrogen replacement therapy, and certain β-blockers.

Raynaud Phenomenon

When Raynaud phenomenon is present, several clinical features can help to differentiate primary Raynaud disease from secondary Raynaud phenomenon (Table 23-6).

Primary Raynaud disease is more common in women than men and usually has its onset before age 40 years. Episodes are characterized by triphasic color changes (white, blue, then red). Symptoms are usually bilateral and often symmetric and precipitated by cold exposure or emotion. Ischemic or gangrenous changes are not present. The absence of any causal condition and the presence of symptoms for at least 2 years are also required for diagnosis. Raynaud disease is generally a benign condition; treatment emphasizes protection from cold exposure and other vasoconstrictive influences. Patients with severe symptoms not controlled by local measures may benefit from a trial of a calcium-channel blocker or an α_1-adrenergic receptor antagonist.

Secondary Raynaud phenomenon affects men more often than women, and in most patients the onset is after age 40 years. It is usually unilateral or asymmetric at onset. Associated pulse deficits, ischemic changes, and systemic signs and symptoms are often present. Identification of the underlying

Table 23-6 Characteristic Clinical Features of Primary and Secondary Raynaud Phenomenon

	Primary	Secondary
Age at onset, y	<40	>40
Sex	Women	Men
?Bilateral	+	+/−
?Symmetric	+	+/−
?Toes involved	+	−
Ischemic changes	−	+
Systemic manifestations	−	+

cause is basic to appropriate treatment for secondary Raynaud phenomenon.

The initial laboratory evaluation in a patient with Raynaud phenomenon includes a complete blood count, test for erythrocyte sedimentation rate, urinalysis, serum protein electrophoresis, antinuclear antibody test, tests for cryoglobulin, cryofibrinogen, and cold agglutinins, and chest radiography to detect disorders not identified by the medical history and physical examination.

- Primary Raynaud disease is a benign condition more common in women than men, and its onset is usually before age 40 years.
- Secondary Raynaud phenomenon affects men more often than women, and in most patients the onset is after age 40 years.

Livedo Reticularis

Spasm or occlusion of dermal arterioles causes livedo reticularis, the bluish mottling of the skin in a lacy, reticular pattern. Primary livedo reticularis is idiopathic and not associated with an identifiable underlying disorder. Secondary livedo reticularis is suggested by an abrupt, severe onset of symptoms, ischemic changes, and systemic symptoms. Most commonly, it is the result of embolism of atheromatous debris from thrombus within a proximal aneurysm or from proximal atheromatous plaques. The appearance of livedo reticularis in a patient older than 50 years should suggest the possibility of atheroembolism. Other causes of secondary livedo reticularis include connective tissue disease, vasculitis, myeloproliferative disorders, dysproteinemias, reflex sympathetic dystrophy, cold injury, and as a side effect of amantadine hydrochloride (Symmetrel) therapy.

- The appearance of livedo reticularis in a patient older than 50 years should suggest the possibility of atheroembolism.

Chronic Pernio

Chronic pernio is a vasospastic disorder characterized by sensitivity to cold in patients (usually women) with a past history of cold injury. Chronic pernio presents with symmetric blueness of the toes in the autumn and resolution of the discoloration in the spring (Fig. 23-12). Without treatment, the cyanosis may be accompanied by blistering of the skin of the affected toes. The cyanosis can often be relieved in a few days after instituting treatment with an α_1-adrenergic receptor antagonist, which can then be used to prevent recurrence.

ERYTHROMELALGIA

Erythromelalgia is the occurrence of red, hot, painful, burning extremity digits on exposure to warm temperatures or after

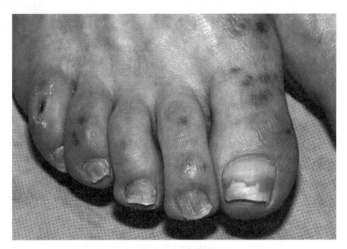

Fig. 23-12. Characteristic lesions of chronic pernio.

exercise. It is not a vasospastic disorder but is associated with color change of the skin. It may be primary (idiopathic) or be due to an underlying disorder, most commonly myeloproliferative disorders (polycythemia rubra vera), diabetes mellitus, or small fiber neuropathy. Treatment of the primary form includes avoidance of exposure to warm temperatures, aspirin, and a nonselective β-blocker, which is helpful in some patients. In persons with secondary erythromelalgia, treatment of the underlying disorder usually relieves the symptoms.

EDEMA

Lower extremity edema is commonly encountered in clinical practice. Aside from edema due to underlying cardiac disease, other causes of regional edema can usually be identified from characteristic clinical features (Table 23-7).

LYMPHEDEMA

Lymphedema can be primary (idiopathic) or due to an underlying disorder. Primary lymphedema (lymphedema praecox) usually affects young women (nine times more frequently than

Table 23-7 Differential Diagnosis of Regional Types of Edema

Feature	Venous	Lymphedema	Lipedema
Bilateral	Occasional	+/−	Always
Foot involved	+	+	0
Toes involved	0	+	0
Thickened skin	0	+	0
Stasis changes	+	0	0

men) and begins before the age of 40 years (often before age 20 years). In women, the symptoms often first appear at the time of menarche or with the first pregnancy. Edema is bilateral in about half the cases. The initial evaluation in a young woman with lymphedema should include a complete history and physical examination (including pelvic examination and Papanicolaou smear) and CT of the pelvis to exclude a neoplastic cause of lymphatic obstruction.

● In a healthy young woman with painless progressive swelling of one or both lower extremities in a pattern consistent with lymphedema, lymphedema praecox is the most likely diagnosis.

Secondary lymphedema is broadly classified into obstructive (postsurgical, postradiation, neoplastic) and inflammatory (infectious) types. Obstructive lymphedema due to neoplasm typically begins after the age of 40 years and is due to pelvic neoplasm or non-Hodgkin lymphoma. The most frequent cause in men is prostate cancer.

● In a man older than 60 years with painless progressive swelling of one leg, the diagnosis is prostate cancer until proved otherwise.

Inflammatory (infectious) lymphedema occurs as a result of chronic or recurring lymphangitis (or both) or cellulitis. The portal of entry for infection is usually dermatophytosis (tinea pedis), which is often overlooked. The diagnosis of lymphedema can be confirmed noninvasively with lymphoscintigraphy.

Medical management of lymphedema includes edema reduction therapy, followed by daily use of custom-fitted graduated compression (usually 40-50 mm Hg compression) elastic support. Manual lymphatic drainage is a type of massage used in combination with skin care, support and compression therapy, and exercise in the management of lymphedema. A combined multimodality approach may substantially reduce excess limb volume and improve quality of life. Antifungal treatment is essential if dermatophytosis is present. Weight reduction in obese patients is also beneficial. Surgical treatment of lymphedema (lymphaticovenous anastomosis, lymphedema reduction) is indicated in highly selected patients.

VENOUS DISEASE

Deep venous thrombosis (DVT) is the third most common cardiovascular disease, after acute coronary syndromes and stroke. Approximately 1 in 1,000 individuals is affected by venous thromboembolism each year, and more than 200,000 new cases occur in the United States annually. Of these, 30%

of patients die within 30 days; one-fifth suffer sudden death due to pulmonary embolism. The Virchow triad of stasis, hypercoagulability, and vascular endothelial damage contributes in varying degrees to the development of DVT. Independent risk factors for venous thromboembolism include increasing age, male sex, surgery, trauma, hospital or nursing home confinement, malignancy, neurologic disease with extremity paresis, central venous catheter or transvenous pacemaker, prior superficial vein thrombosis, varicose veins, and liver disease; among women, additional risk factors include pregnancy, oral contraceptive use, and hormone replacement therapy. A major clinical risk factor (immobility, trauma, or recent operation) is present in approximately half of patients with confirmed DVT. A family history of thrombophilia is important, because there are several identifiable and treatable inherited disorders of coagulation.

Causes of recurrent DVT are listed in Table 23-8.

Protein C Deficiency

Protein C deficiency is characterized by recurrent venous thrombosis and is inherited in an autosomal dominant fashion. Episodes of thrombosis are generally spontaneous and usually begin before the age of 30 years. Protein C levels are about 50% of normal. Treatment is lifelong oral anticoagulation, and there is a potential risk of warfarin necrosis. Acquired protein C deficiency can develop in patients with liver disease or disseminated intravascular coagulation, or it can occur postoperatively. Purpura fulminans occurs in persons homozygous for this condition.

Table 23-8 Causes of Recurrent Deep Venous Thrombosis

Primary
    Idiopathic
Secondary
    Neoplasm
    Connective tissue disease
    Inflammatory bowel disease
    Myeloproliferative disorder
    Thromboangiitis obliterans
    Oral contraceptives
Coagulation disorders
    Antithrombin III deficiency
    Protein C deficiency
    Protein S deficiency
    Activated protein C resistance
    Prothrombin 20210 G-A mutation
    Antiphospholipid antibody syndrome
    Hyperhomocystinemia

Protein S Deficiency

Protein S deficiency also causes recurrent venous thrombosis and is inherited as an autosomal dominant trait. Onset of episodes usually begins before the age of 35 years, and the episodes are generally spontaneous. Protein S levels are about 50% of normal. Treatment is lifelong oral anticoagulation, and there is no risk of warfarin necrosis. Acquired protein S deficiency can occur in association with the nephrotic syndrome, warfarin therapy, pregnancy, antiphospholipid antibody syndrome, and disseminated intravascular coagulation.

Antithrombin III Deficiency

Antithrombin III deficiency, characterized by recurrent venous and arterial thrombosis, is also inherited in an autosomal dominant fashion. The first thrombotic episode is usually after age 20 years and is usually provoked by infection, trauma, operation, or pregnancy. Antithrombin III levels are usually 40% to 60% of normal. Treatment is lifelong oral anticoagulation. An acquired form of antithrombin III deficiency can occur in patients with nephrotic syndrome or severe liver disease and in those receiving estrogen therapy.

Factor V (Leiden) Mutation

Factor V Leiden mutation, the genetic defect underlying resistance to activated protein C, is the most common risk factor for venous thrombosis. Heterozygous carriers of a mutation in factor V (factor V Leiden) are at increased risk for venous thrombosis (i.e., activated protein C resistance). This mutation may occur in 5% to 10% of the general population and may account for as many as 50% of patients with recurrent venous thromboembolism. Heterozygous carriers of factor V mutation have an 8-fold increased risk of venous thromboembolism, whereas homozygous carriers have an 80-fold increased risk. Of interest, in patients who have had myocardial infarction without significant coronary artery stenosis, the prevalence of factor V Leiden is considerably higher than in controls, suggesting that factor V Leiden mutation is an independent risk factor for myocardial infarction. Factor V Leiden mutation also increases the risk of cerebrovascular accident and paradoxic embolism (in patients with a patent foramen ovale).

Prothrombin 20210 G-A Mutation

Recently, a mutation in the prothrombin gene has been identified in some patients with venous thromboembolism. The mechanism whereby this abnormality might cause thrombosis has been assumed to be an increase in prothrombin levels. Available data indicate that this mutation may be associated with an increased risk of venous thrombosis but not arterial thrombosis (with a possible exception for myocardial infarction).

Hyperhomocysteinemia

Hyperhomocysteinemia, a disorder of methionine metabolism, is a risk factor for premature atherosclerosis and recurrent DVT. Inherited forms (disorders of transsulfuration and remethylation) and acquired forms (chronic renal failure, organ transplantation, acute lymphoblastic leukemia, psoriasis, vitamin deficiencies [vitamins B_6 and B_{12} and folate], and medications [phenytoin, carbamazepine, theophylline]) occur. Hyperhomocysteinemia is an independent risk factor for stroke, coronary artery disease, peripheral arterial disease, and DVT. A normal plasma homocysteine level is 5 to 15 μmol/L. Folic acid at a dosage of 0.4 mg per day reduces homocysteine levels, but higher doses of folate are required in patients with chronic renal failure. Screening for hyperhomocysteinemia should be considered in patients with premature atherosclerotic disease, a strong family history of premature atherosclerosis, idiopathic DVT, chronic renal failure, systemic lupus erythematosus, or severe psoriasis and in organ transplant recipients.

Clinical Evaluation of DVT

Symptoms of DVT include extremity pain, redness, and swelling, although many patients may be asymptomatic. Signs of DVT include pitting edema, warmth, erythema, tenderness, and a dilated superficial venous pattern in the involved extremity. Although leg veins are the most common location of DVT, upper extremity DVT may occur, especially in patients with a central venous line or transvenous permanent pacemaker. Extensive DVT involving an entire extremity may lead to venous gangrene (phlegmasia cerulea dolens), most commonly in association with an underlying malignancy. The clinical diagnosis of DVT is neither sensitive (60%-80%) nor specific (30%-72%), and three-fourths of patients who present with suspected acute DVT have other causes of leg pain such as cellulitis, leg trauma, muscular tear or rupture, postphlebitic syndrome, or Baker cysts. Therefore, objective noninvasive tests are required to establish a diagnosis of DVT.

Important historical features in a patient with DVT which should increase suspicion of a hypercoagulable disorder include spontaneous event, unusual site (mesenteric or cerebral), young age, positive family history, and recurrent events.

Although venography is the reference standard for the diagnosis of DVT and is highly accurate for both proximal and calf DVT, it is invasive, expensive, and technically inadequate in about 10% of patients, and it may precipitate a DVT in approximately 3% of patients. Noninvasive tests for diagnosing DVT are accurate for diagnosing proximal DVT but not calf vein thrombosis. If the results of noninvasive testing are nondiagnostic or are discordant with the clinical assessment, venography is indicated.

- Noninvasive tests for diagnosing DVT are accurate for diagnosing proximal DVT but not calf vein thrombosis.

- If the results of noninvasive testing are nondiagnostic or are discordant with the clinical assessment, venography is indicated.

Continuous-Wave Doppler

Doppler assessment at the bedside, which evaluates each limb systematically for spontaneous venous flow, phasic flow with respiration, augmentation with distal compression, and venous competence with the Valsalva maneuver and proximal compression, is useful in the diagnosis of proximal DVT. Continuous-wave Doppler is relatively insensitive to calf vein thrombosis.

Impedance Plethysmography and Strain-Gauge Outflow Plethysmography

Impedance plethysmography and strain-gauge outflow plethysmography both reliably detect occlusive thrombi in the proximal veins (popliteal, femoral, and iliac veins) but are less reliable for detecting nonocclusive thrombi and are insensitive for calf DVT. False-positive results do occur (extrinsic venous obstruction, increased central venous pressure). The reported sensitivity of impedance plethysmography for proximal DVT ranges from 70% to 90%.

Compression Ultrasonography

Compression ultrasonography (venous noncompressibility is diagnostic of DVT; venous compressibility excludes DVT) is highly sensitive and specific for detecting proximal DVT. It is currently the most accurate noninvasive test for the diagnosis of a first symptomatic proximal DVT. Compression ultrasonography is less accurate for symptomatic patients with isolated calf vein thrombosis. It should be noted that both impedance plethysmography and compression ultrasonography have decreased sensitivity when used to evaluate asymptomatic patients (22% and 58%, respectively). Withholding anticoagulant therapy in symptomatic patients with suspected DVT who have normal results on serial compression ultrasonography or impedance plethysmography is safe.

D-Dimer

Plasma levels of D-dimer, a product of fibrin degradation, are increased in patients with acute DVT. D-Dimer functions as an exclusionary test in patients with suspected DVT. For example, in a patient with both a negative objective test (compression ultrasonography or impedance plethysmography) and normal results of D-dimer test, a diagnosis of DVT becomes highly unlikely.

Evaluation of Idiopathic DVT

In a patient with idiopathic DVT, a clinical evaluation that includes a complete history and physical examination, routine laboratory testing (hematology group with differential count, chemistry profile, urinalysis, fecal hemoglobin test), and chest radiography appears to be appropriate for detecting cancer.

Mammography, pelvic examination, and Papanicolaou smear should be included in a woman with idiopathic DVT. Additional testing should be guided by any abnormalities detected by the initial clinical evaluation.

Treatment of DVT

Treatment options for acute DVT include anticoagulant therapy (heparin, warfarin), thrombolytic therapy, vena caval filter, and surgical thrombectomy.

Anticoagulant therapy is initiated with intravenous heparin, followed within 24 hours by institution of warfarin therapy. The optimal duration of warfarin anticoagulation for a first episode of DVT is controversial. Available data suggest that it is necessary to tailor the duration of anticoagulation individually according to the topography of DVT and the presence of continuing risk factors. For proximal DVT, a short course seems sufficient in patients with temporary risk factors (3 to 6 months), and a longer course (6 months at least) is recommended for patients with continuing risk factors or idiopathic DVT. The inherited or acquired hypercoagulable states can be divided into those that are common and associated with a modest risk of recurrence (i.e., isolated factor V Leiden or 20210 G-A prothrombin gene mutation) and those that are uncommon but associated with a high risk of recurrence (i.e., antithrombin III, protein C or S deficiencies, and antiphospholipid antibodies). The presence of one of the latter abnormalities favors more prolonged anticoagulant therapy. For patients with a high risk of recurrence, there is a paucity of evidence-based medicine, particularly for patients with biological thrombophilia, and randomized controlled trials in this population are required. An assessment of low- or fixed-dose oral anticoagulation is also needed to reduce hemorrhagic complications.

When problems with anticoagulation (i.e., contraindications, complications, failed effect, or unacceptable risk) are present, insertion of a vena cava filter may be indicated. Vena cava filters are also indicated for prophylactic use in patients at high risk of pulmonary embolism and as an adjunct to an urgent surgical procedure in the patient with acute DVT. Complications of vena cava filters include pulmonary embolism (1%-4%), caval thrombus (19%-24%), penetration of the cava (9%), filter migration (6%), fracture (2%), and lower extremity edema (25%).

Thrombolytic therapy may be indicated when DVT is extensive, with thrombosis extending into the iliac veins or inferior vena cava, or in upper extremity DVT. Thrombolytic therapy has the best results when initiated less than 7 days after the onset of DVT, and it may decrease the incidence of the postphlebitic syndrome by salvaging venous valve function. Systemic infusion or catheter-directed delivery of the thrombolytic agent directly into the thrombus is used. Surgical thrombectomy is reserved for patients with limb-threatening DVT (i.e., phlegmasia cerulea dolens).

Reduction of limb edema, initially by leg elevation and woven elastic (Ace) wrapping, is an integral part of the initial therapy of acute DVT. When edema has been reduced, a graduated compression elastic support stocking is required to both control edema and prevent development of the postphlebitic (postthrombotic) syndrome with venous ulceration. A 30- to 40-mm Hg graduated elastic support garment is usually sufficient. Customized, graduated compression stockings significantly reduce the occurrence of the postphlebitic syndrome in patients with a first episode of proximal DVT.

Postphlebitic Syndrome

Chronic venous insufficiency (postphlebitic syndrome) is a common disorder that results in significant morbidity. In approximately 30% of patients with DVT, postphlebitic syndrome develops within 20 years after the initial DVT. Chronic venous insufficiency most commonly results in swelling, pain, fatigue, and heaviness in the involved extremity. Secondary varicose vein formation, venous stasis changes, and cutaneous ulceration can occur in untreated chronic venous insufficiency (Fig. 23-13). Venous claudication in the setting of prior iliofemoral or vena cava thrombosis causes discomfort, fullness, tiredness, and aching of the extremity during exercise. In contrast to patients with intermittent claudication, patients with venous claudication must sit down and elevate the extremity for relief. Postphlebitic syndrome due to chronic deep venous incompetence is frequently misdiagnosed as recurrent DVT. The correct diagnosis is suggested by the clinical findings of chronic venous insufficiency (edema, venous stasis changes, secondary varicose vein formation) and confirmed by exclusion of new thrombus formation by objective testing (e.g., compression ultrasonography). "Side-by-side" comparison of current ultrasonographic studies with previous ultrasonographic or venographic studies is invaluable for documenting new venous thrombosis. Treatment of postphlebitic syndrome includes initial aggressive efforts at edema reduction with woven elastic (Ace) wrapping and pumping devices until edema is reduced, followed by fitting with a graduated compression elastic support stocking (30-40

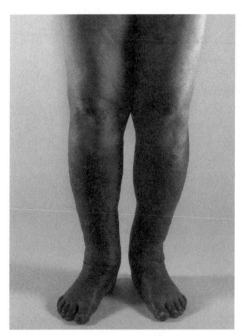

Fig. 23-13. A patient with severe deep venous incompetence and perforator vein incompetence with severe venous stasis changes and indurated cellulitis.

mm Hg). Periodic leg elevation during the day and weight reduction in obese patients are also beneficial.

- The treatment of postphlebitic syndrome includes initial aggressive efforts at edema reduction with woven elastic (Ace) wrapping and pumping devices until edema is reduced, followed by fitting with a graduated compression elastic support stocking (30-40 mm Hg).
- Periodic leg elevation during the day and weight reduction in obese patients are also beneficial.

Leg Ulcer

The cause of lower extremity ulceration usually can be determined with clinical examination. Clinical features of the four most common types of leg ulcer are summarized in Table 23-9.

Table 23-9 Clinical Features of the Four Most Common Types of Leg Ulcer

Feature	Type of ulcer			
	Venous	Arterial	Arteriolar	Neurotrophic
Onset	Trauma +/−	Trauma	Spontaneous	Trauma
Course	Chronic	Progressive	Progressive	Progressive
Pain	No (unless infected)	Yes	Yes	No
Location	Medial aspect of leg	Toe, heel, foot	Lateral, posterior aspect of leg	Plantar
Surrounding skin	Stasis changes	Atrophic	Normal	Callous
Ulcer edges	Shaggy	Discrete	Serpiginous	Discrete
Ulcer base	Healthy	Eschar, pale	Eschar, pale	Healthy or pale

Vascular Diseases Pharmacy Review
Laura J. Odell, PharmD, Kevin W. Odell, PharmD

Drug (trade name)	Dosing	Toxic/adverse effects	Comments
Warfarin (Coumadin)	Patient specific, adjusted to maintain INR in target range	Bleeding, skin necrosis in patients with protein C deficiency, purple toe syndrome, osteoporosis, alopecia, rash	Anticoagulant effect reversible with vitamin K 2.5-5 mg PO or fresh frozen plasma Lab monitor: PT and INR Pregnancy category X
Aspirin	81-325 mg once daily	Bleeding, hypoglycemia (high doses), dyspepsia, gastric ulcers, dysgeusia, hepatotoxicity (rare), urticaria, rash	Use with caution in children and teens with viral infections (risk of Reye syndrome), use with caution in patients with asthma (risk of bronchospasm) Lab monitor: bleeding time
Clopidogrel (Plavix)	75 mg once daily	Bleeding, rash, urticaria, edema, hypertension, gastrointestinal upset, increased liver function tests, rare decrease in platelets, leukocytes and hemoglobin	Rare cases of thrombotic thrombocytopenic purpura have been reported with use Lab monitor: platelet aggregation if suspected adverse effects
Pentoxyfylline (Trental)	400 mg three times daily with meals	Bleeding, dizziness, headache, dyspepsia, GI bleed, nausea and vomiting, rash, brittle fingernails, leukopenia (rare)	Decrease dose to twice daily if GI or CNS side effects. Consider discontinuing if GI or CNS side effects persist
Cilostazol (Pletal)	100 mg twice daily	Palpitations, tachycardia, dizziness, vertigo, headache, diarrhea, rash	No effect on PT and INR or bleeding time
Heparin	Dose usually based on weight	Bleeding, thrombocytopenia, skin necrosis, disseminated intravascular coagulation, erythematous plaques, alopecia, osteoporosis	Anticoagulant effect reversible with protamine Lab monitor: aPTT, platelet counts

Low-molecular-weight heparins
  Dalteparin (Fragmin)
  Enoxaparin (Lovenox)
  Tinzaparin (Innohep)
	Once or twice daily subcutaneously based on weight or condition	Bleeding, pain or bruising at injection site, osteoporosis, rash	Anticoagulant effect partially reversible with protamine, use with caution in patient with history of heparin-induced thrombocytopenia
			Lab monitor: antifactor Xa activity

aPTT, activated partial thromboplastin time; CNS, central nervous system; GI, gastrointestinal; INR, international normalized ratio; PT, prothrombin time.

QUESTIONS

Multiple Choice (choose the one best answer)

1. A 75-year-old man presents to the emergency department with sudden onset of severe chest pain radiating to the interscapular area. The initial blood pressure is 190/95 mm Hg, there is a grade 2/6 diastolic murmur, and the left femoral pulse is reduced. All of the following statements are true about this patient's condition *except*:
   a. Type A aortic dissection is a surgical emergency
   b. Bicuspid aortic valve is a risk factor for aortic dissection
   c. The electrocardiographic changes may mimic acute myocardial infarction
   d. Intravenous sodium nitroprusside is the initial treatment of choice
   e. Mortality in untreated patients is 1% per hour in the first 48 hours

2. A 65-year-old woman with diabetes mellitus complains of left lower extremity discomfort when she walks one block. The ankle:brachial systolic pressure index (ABI) is determined in the office. All of the following statements regarding the ABI are true *except*:
   a. An ABI <0.5 is consistent with severe arterial occlusive disease
   b. The resting ABI may be normal in patients with isolated iliac arterial occlusive disease
   c. ABI measurements are performed with a patient's feet in a dependent position
   d. A reduced ABI predicts an increased risk of future cardiovascular events
   e. Medial calcinosis in patients with diabetes may invalidate the ABI

3. A 56-year-old man in the hospital complains of pain and swelling of his left leg. The limb is swollen and erythematous. Duplex ultrasonography shows thrombosis of the left superficial femoral and popliteal veins. True statements regarding low-molecular-weight heparin (LMWH) therapy include all of the following *except*:
   a. It is effective for inpatient treatment of deep venous thrombosis (DVT)
   b. Heparin-induced thrombocytopenia is a potential complication
   c. It is approved for outpatient treatment of uncomplicated DVT
   d. It is approved for outpatient management of uncomplicated pulmonary embolism
   e. It has greater bioavailability than unfractionated heparin

4. A 32-year-old man presents with cold-induced color changes of two fingers on his left hand, and he is also complaining of right foot and calf discomfort when he walks. He smokes two packs of cigarettes per day and is otherwise healthy. Clinical features of thromboangiitis obliterans include all of the following *except*:
   a. Arch and calf claudication
   b. An increased erythrocyte sedimentation rate
   c. Involvement of medium-sized and small arteries
   d. Episodes of migratory superficial thrombophlebitis
   e. Recurrent DVT

5. A 68-year-old man with chronic systemic hypertension is noted to have a pulsatile abdominal mass during a routine physical examination. All of the following statements regarding this physical examination finding are true *except*:
   a. Familial clustering of cases occurs in 15%
   b. A diameter more than 5.0 cm is an indication for surgical resection
   c. CT is diagnostic
   d. The majority of patients are asymptomatic
   e. The average rate of expansion is 0.5 cm/year

6. A 75-year-old woman with acute anterior myocardial infarction underwent emergency percutaneous transluminal coronary angioplasty. Later, in the evening, she is noted to have hypertension, multiple cyanotic toes on each foot, and an increasing total leukocyte count. Other clinical features suggestive of this condition include all of the following *except*:
   a. Subacute onset
   b. Renal insufficiency
   c. Transient eosinophilia
   d. Increased erythrocyte sedimentation rate
   e. Recurrent episodes

7. A 48-year-old woman presents with episodic color changes of two fingers on the right hand and three fingers on the left hand. The episodes are induced by anxiety and also cold weather. The patient could be expected to have any of the following conditions *except*:
   a. Dermatomyositis
   b. Pheochromocytoma
   c. Scleroderma
   d. Paroxysmal nocturnal hemoglobinuria
   e. Pseudoxanthoma elasticum

8. A 72-year-old man complains of sudden severe pain in his left foot and calf. On examination, the lower calf and foot are pale and cold, and the posterior tibial and dorsalis pedis pulses are absent. He has chronic obstructive

pulmonary disease and a history of left carotid endarterectomy. All of the following are potential causes of this condition *except*:

a. Acute aortic dissection

b. Inflammatory bowel disease

c. Polycythemia vera

d. Chronic renal failure

e. Ergotism

ANSWERS

1. Answer d.

Acute aortic dissection is one of the most common fatal aortic conditions in clinical practice. When dissection involves the ascending aorta (type I and type II, type A, proximal), mortality is high without emergency surgical repair. Systemic hypertension, bicuspid and unicuspid aortic valve, and the Marfan syndrome are major risk factors for acute aortic dissection. Electrocardiography in patients with acute dissection may show left ventricular hypertrophy (with or without strain), ST-segment depression or elevation, and T-wave changes, as well as the changes of acute pericarditis. The initial treatment of choice in hypertensive patients is β-adrenergic blockade, often in combination with intravenous sodium nitroprusside. Sodium nitroprusside without concomitant β-adrenergic blockade results in an increase in left ventricular ejection velocity and promotes propagation of the dissecting process.

2. Answer c.

The ABI is a simple bedside test used to diagnose lower extremity arterial occlusive disease. ABI measurements are performed in the supine position. A normal ABI is 0.9-1.0; values of 0.8-0.9 indicate mild, 0.5-0.8 moderate, and <0.5 severe arterial occlusive disease. In patients with isolated iliac artery stenosis, the resting ABI may be normal but will decrease considerably after treadmill exercise. A reduced ABI (<0.8) is a strong independent predictor of future cardiac events. In patients with diabetes, elderly patients, and patients with chronic renal insufficiency, medial calcinosis of the lower extremity arteries may preclude determination of the ABI because of arterial noncompressibility.

3. Answer d.

LMWH has greater bioavailability and a longer anticoagulant effect than unfractionated heparin. It is given subcutaneously twice daily in a fixed dosage based on a patient's body weight, and it does not require monitoring of the activated partial thromboplastin time. Although less common than with unfractionated heparin, heparin-induced thrombocytopenia can occur. LMWH is approved for use in the prophylaxis of patients at increased risk of DVT, for the inpatient treatment of DVT and outpatient management of uncomplicated DVT, and for hospitalized patients with DVT complicated by pulmonary embolism. LMWH is not approved for outpatient management of pulmonary embolism.

4. Answer b.

Thromboangiitis obliterans (Buerger disease) is an inflammatory arteriopathy associated with tobacco exposure. Male sex, onset at less than 30 years of age, a history of migratory superficial thrombophlebitis, intermittent claudication involving the arch of the foot and calf, involvement of medium-sized and small arteries, and involvement of the wrist or hand are diagnostic clinical criteria. Results of tests for other disorders are negative or normal, including fasting glucose, lipids, erythrocyte sedimentation rate, connective tissue disease screening tests, and special coagulation tests (as indicated). Diagnosis requires angiography. Recurrent DVT is associated with Buerger disease.

5. Answer e.

An abdominal aortic aneurysm is defined as a focal dilatation of the abdominal aorta to a diameter more than 3.0 cm. Abdominal aortic aneurysm is usually an acquired condition, but 15% of patients have a familial tendency toward aneurysm development. The majority of patients are asymptomatic, and the aneurysm is discovered by clinical examination or incidentally during abdominal ultrasonography or CT performed for another purpose. The average annual expansion rate for an abdominal aortic aneurysm is 0.25 cm/year, rapid expansion being defined as >0.5 cm/year. Surgical resection is indicated when the aneurysm diameter exceeds 5.0 cm in patients whose general medical condition permits operation.

6. Answer a.

Clinical features of atheroembolism include livedo reticularis, multiple blue toes, systemic hypertension, renal insufficiency, leukocytosis, transient eosinophilia, and an increased erythrocyte sedimentation rate. Proximal atherosclerosis and aneurysmal disease are the source of embolic material. The episodes are acute in onset, are frequently recurrent, and can mimic multisystem disease when multiple territories are involved by the embolic event. Atheroembolism can occur spontaneously or after trauma, can be due to invasive angiographic procedures and cardiac surgery, and can occur with warfarin and thrombolytic therapy. Medical treatment includes antiplatelet agents, statins, vasodilator therapy, protection of the ischemic limb(s), and identification of the source of embolism. Definitive treatment requires surgical resection or revascularization if a focal source of embolism is diagnosed.

7. Answer e.

Features suggestive of secondary Raynaud phenomenon include male sex, onset after 40 years of age, asymmetric symptoms, pulse deficits, ischemic changes, and systemic symptoms. The differential diagnosis of secondary Raynaud phenomenon is extensive and includes occupation-related injury (pneumatic hammer disease, occupational arterial occlusive disease of the hand, occupational acro-osteolysis, vasospasm of typists and pianists), neurologic conditions (thoracic outlet syndrome, carpal tunnel syndrome), occlusive arterial disease (arteriosclerosis obliterans, thromboangiitis obliterans, postembolic or thrombotic arterial occlusion), and miscellaneous conditions (scleroderma, systemic lupus erythematosus, rheumatoid arthritis, dermatomyositis, Fabry disease, paroxysmal nocturnal hemoglobinuria, cold agglutinins or cryoglobulinemia, primary pulmonary hypertension, myxedema, certain neoplasms and after combination chemotherapy for testicular cancer, hepatitis B antigenemia, pheochromocytoma, and ergotism). Pseudoxanthoma elasticum is not known to be a cause of secondary Raynaud phenomenon.

8. Answer d.

The symptoms of acute arterial occlusion are sudden in onset (<5 hours) and include the "5 Ps": pain, pallor, paresthesia (numbness), poikilothermy (coldness), and pulselessness (absence of peripheral pulses). An embolic acute arterial occlusion is suggested when there is a history of cardiac disease, atrial fibrillation, a proximal aneurysm, and proximal atherosclerosis. A thrombotic cause of acute arterial occlusion is suggested by a prior history of occlusive disease, occlusive disease of other extremities, acute aortic dissection, hematologic disease, inflammatory bowel disease, and ergotism. Chronic renal failure is not a cause of acute arterial occlusion.

INDEX

Note: Page numbers in *italics* indicate figures. Page numbers followed by "t" indicate tables.

A

Abacavir, 491, 606
Abattoir worker, disease etiology, 8t
Abciximab, 907
Abdominal aortic aneurysm, 1014–1016, *1015*, 1016t
  surveillance, 1016t
Acanthamoeba, 184
Acanthocytes, 476
Acanthosis nigricans, 176, *194*
ACAS. *See* Asymptomatic Carotid Atherosclerosis Study
Accutane, 172
ACE inhibitors. *See* Acetylcholinesterase inhibitors
Acebutolol, 992
ACEIs. *See* Angiotensin-converting enzyme inhibitors
Acetaminophen, 532, 734
Acetazolamide, 700, 705
Acetylcholine, 839
Acetylcholinesterase inhibitors, 116, 392
Acetylcysteine, 682
Achondrogenesis type II, 955
Achondroplasia, 365, 955
Acid-base balance, 148–152
  metabolic acidosis, 150–151
  metabolic alkalosis, 151
  mixed acid-base disorders, 151–152
  patterns, 150t, 150–152
  respiratory acidosis, 150
  respiratory alkalosis, 150
Acid-base disorders, 150t, 691, 695–701
  delta gap, 700–701
  metabolic acidosis, 695–698t
  metabolic alkalosis, 698–699, *699*
  mixed acid-base disorders, 700
  respiratory acidosis, 699–700
  respiratory alkalosis, 700, 700t
  steps for interpreting, 697t
Acidosis
  metabolic, 150–151
  respiratory, 150
Acitretin, 172
Acne vulgaris, treatment, 172t
Acquired immunodeficiency syndrome, 59, 465
  dementia, 393, 486
  with diarrhea, diagnostic evaluation, 279

gastrointestinal manifestations, 278–279
  adenovirus, 278
  bacteria, 278
    Mycobacterium avium-intracellulare, 278
  fungi, 278
    Candida albicans, 278
    Histoplasma capsulatum, 279
  protozoa, 279
    Cryptosporidium, 279
    Isospora belli, 279
    Microsporida, 279
  viral, 278
    cytomegalovirus, 278
    herpes simplex virus, 278
hematology, 465
malignancies, 488–489
  Kaposi sarcoma, 488
  non-Hodgkin lymphoma, 488–489
  primary central nervous system lymphoma, 489
psychologic aspects, 832
Acrodermatitis enteropathica, 178
Acromegaly, 203–204
  biochemical diagnosis, 203
  clinical features, 203
  diagnosis, 203
  radiologic diagnosis, 203
  therapy, 203–204
ACTH, 3, 514
  deficiency, 200
ACTH-adrenocortical axis, 200
ACTH-producing tumors, 204
Actinomycosis, 560, 916
Acute alcoholic myopathy, 746
Acute arterial occlusion, 1022–1023
Acute bacterial arthritis, 600
Acute cerebral infarction, management, 748–749
Acute confusional state, 725, 726
Acute coronary syndromes, 101–109, *102*
  acute mechanical complications, myocardial infarction, 107t, 107–108
  prehospital dismissal evaluation, 108–109
  presentation, 103
  reperfusion therapy, 105–107
  ST-segment elevation myocardial infarction, 103
  treatments, 103–105

unstable angina, non–ST-segment elevation myocardial infarction, 102–103
Acute eosinophilic pneumonia, 878
Acute febrile neutrophilic dermatosis, 177
Acute hemolytic transfusion reaction, 459
Acute intermittent porphyria, 232
Acute interstitial nephritis, 677–678t
Acute interstitial pneumonitis, 891
Acute leukemias, 436–438
  acute lymphoblastic leukemia, 437–438
  acute nonlymphocytic leukemia, 436–437
Acute lymphoblastic leukemia, 437–438
Acute motor neuropathy, 742
Acute myelogenous leukemia, 436–437
Acute nonlymphocytic leukemia, 436–437
Acute renal failure, 681–687
  diagnosis, 685t, 685–686
  dialysis, 686–687
  intrinsic acute renal failure, 683t, 683–684
  management, 686–687
  postrenal failure, 684–685
  in pregnancy, 707
  prerenal failure, 681–683
    due to liver disease, 682–683
Acute respiratory distress syndrome, 154–157
  criteria for diagnosis, 155
  disorders associated with, 155t
  etiology, 155, 155t
  therapy for, 155–157
Acute respiratory syndrome. *See* Severe acute respiratory syndrome (SARS)
Acute tubular necrosis, urinary indices in, 685t
Acyclovir, 259, 606, 628–631, 705
  amantadine, 630–631
  cidofovir, 630
  famciclovir, 629
  foscarnet, 630
  ganciclovir, 629
  oseltamivir, 631
  rimantadine, 630–631
  valacyclovir, 629
  valganciclovir, 629–630
  zanamivir, 631
Adefovir, 298
Adenocarcinoma, 896

Adenosine triphosphatase, 695
Adjustment disorder with anxious mood, 829
Adjustment disorder with depressed mood, 825
Adjuvant therapy, 872–873
Adolescent medicine, percentage of board examination devoted to, 2
Adrenal failure, 219–220
    acute adrenocortical failure or adrenal crisis, 220
    clinical features, 220
    diagnosis, 220
    endocrine diagnosis, 220
    etiology, 219–220
    primary adrenal failure, 219
    secondary adrenal failure, 219–220
    therapy, 220
Adrenal gland disorders, 219–225
    adrenal failure, 219–220
        acute adrenocortical failure, 220
        clinical features, 220
        diagnosis, 220
        endocrine diagnosis, 220
        etiology, 219–220
        primary adrenal failure, 219
        secondary adrenal failure, 219–220
        therapy, 220
    adrenal incidentaloma, 224–225
        evaluation, 224
        therapy, 224–225
    Cushing syndrome, 220–222
        cause, 221–222
        clinical features, 221
        confirmation, 221
        diagnosis, 221
        etiology, 220–221
        therapy, 222
    etiology, 224
    pheochromocytoma, 223–224
        clinical features, 223
        diagnosis, 223–224
        etiology, 223
        therapy, 224
    primary aldosteronism, 222–223
        clinical features, 222
        diagnosis, 222–223
        etiology, 222
        therapy, 223
Adrenal incidentaloma, 224–225
    evaluation, 224
    therapy, 224–225
Adrenergic agonists, 870
Adrenergic inhibitors, with hypertension, 518–520
Adrenoleukodystrophy, 372
    X-linked, 372
Adult respiratory distress syndrome, 891
Adult-onset Still disease, 950–951
Advance directive, 650–652
Afibrinogenemia, 450

Afterdepolarization
    delayed, 65
    early, 65
Afterload, 113
Agglutination, *476*
Agnogenic myeloid metaplasia, *478*
AIDS. *See* Acquired immunodeficiency syndrome
Airway management, 152–153
Albumin, 682
Albuterol, 16, 869, 870
    pirbuterol, for asthma, 16t
Alcohol, 232, 514, 833
    abuse, dependency, 334
Alcoholic liver disease, 301–302
    alcoholic cirrhosis, 302
    alcoholic hepatitis, 301–302
Alcoholism, 726, 833–834
Aldosterone, 695
    antagonist, 223
Alendronate, 217, 259
Alkalosis
    compensation, 698t
    metabolic, 151
    respiratory, 150
Alkaptonuria, 954
Allergic alveolitis, 890–891
    extrinsic, 890–891
Allergic bronchopulmonary aspergillosis, 20, 20t, 877, 879
    as cause of eosinophilia, 31
    diagnostic features, 20t
Allergic fungal sinusitis, 24
Allergic granulomatosis, 178
Allergic rhinitis, 21
    as cause of eosinophilia, 31
    methacholine challenge, 15
Allergy, 11–38
    allergic bronchopulmonary aspergillosis, 20, 20t
    allergy testing, 11–12
        patch tests, 11
        in vitro allergy testing, 11–12
    asthma, 12t, 12–20
        pathology, 12
        pathophysiology, 12–13t
    drug allergy, 29–32
    food allergy, 27
    percentage of board examination devoted to, 2
    rhinitis, chronic, 20–24
    stinging insect allergy, 27–29
    urticaria, 24–26
Allergy medications, 514
    use, 514
Allergy skin testing in food allergy, 27
Allergy testing, 11–12, 28
    cutaneous tests, 11
    in vitro allergy testing, 11–12
    patch tests, 11

Allopurinol, 388, 678, 704, 705, 871
Almotriptan, 732
Alopecia, 481
Alpha$_1$-alkaptonuria, 369
Alpha$_1$-antiprotease deficiency, in diagnosis of wheezing, 16t
Alpha$_1$-antitrypsin deficiency, 868–869
Alpha$_1$-receptor blockers, 518
Alpha-adrenergic blockade, 224, 404
Alpha-thalassemia, 369
Alport syndrome, 676–677
Alveolar damage, 891
Alveolar hemorrhage syndromes, 907
Alveolar microlithiasis, 892
Alzheimer disease, 391–392, 726
Amantadine, 606, 630–631, 752, 753, 754, 817
Amaurosis fugax, 747
Ambulatory monitoring, 66
Amenorrhea, 227–228
    clinical features, 227
    diagnosis, 227–228
    disorders associated with, 228
        anorexia nervosa, 228
        Turner 45/XO gonadal dysgenesis, 228
    estrogen replacement therapy, 228
    etiology, 227
    ovulation induction, 228
    primary amenorrhea, 227, 228
    secondary amenorrhea, 227–228
    therapy, 228
American Heart Association
    prophylactic regimens, 588t
    step I diet, 232
American Rheumatism Association, diagnosis of rheumatoid arthritis, 949t
American Society of Anesthesiologists, classification of anesthetic mortality, 337t
Amikacin, 484, 623, 923
Amiloride, 223, 518
Aminoglycoside, 272, 554, 590, 606, 607, 608, 613–614, 744
    renal toxicity, 684
Aminopenicillins, 605–606
Aminosalicylate, 276, 880
Aminosalicylic acid, 923
Amiodarone, 69, 70, 71, 72, 83, 115, 175, 751
Amitriptyline, 707, 733, 834
Amlodipine, 110, 522
Amoxicillin, 556, 583, 588, 605
Amoxicillin-clavulanate, 556
Amphetamines, 532, 833
Amphotericin, 607
Amphotericin B, 484, 487, 684
    products, 627
Ampicillin, 551, 588, 590, 605, 608, 757
    plus chloramphenicol, 590

plus gentamicin, 588
Ampicillin sodium, 587
Ampicillin-mononucleosis rash, 30
Ampicillin-sulbactam, 555
Amprenavir, 492, 493
Amrinone, 115
Amyl nitrite, 118
Amylase, 883
Amyloidosis, 56–57, *194, 195,* 256,
        273–274, 365, 435–436, 675
    clinical features, 56–57
    diagnosis, 57
Amyotrophic lateral sclerosis, 256
Anabolic steroids, 232
Anaerobic bacteria, 558–560, 913–914
    Bacteroides, 558–559
    Clostridia, 559–560
        Clostridium botulium, 559
        Clostridium tetani, 559
    Peptococcus, 559
Analgesic chronic interstitial nephritis,
        678–679
Anaphylaxis, 28–29
    food allergy, 27
    stinging insect allergy, 28–29
Anaplastic carcinoma, 212
ANCA vasculitis, signs, symptoms, 669t
Androgen replacement, 225
Androgens in normal females, 228–229
Anemia, 411–421
    of chronic disease, 412
    cold agglutinin syndrome, 418
        immunology, 418
    Coombs-negative hemolytic anemias, 419
    enzymopathies, 420
    erythropoietin, 415–416
    evaluation, *411,* 411t, 411–415, *413, 414*
    glucose-6-phosphate dehydrogenase
        deficiency, 419–420
    hemolytic anemia, *416,* 416–418
        Coombs-positive hemolytic anemia,
            417
        drug-induced hemolytic anemia,
            417–418
            autoantibody mechanism, 417
            drug adsorption mechanisms, 417
            immune-complex mechanism,
                417–418
        inheritance patterns, 416
        intravascular hemolysis, differential
            diagnosis, 417
        laboratory findings, 416
        peripheral smear, differential diagnosis,
            417
    hereditary spherocytosis, 421
    Mycoplasma pneumoniae, 418–419
        infectious mononucleosis, 419
    paroxysmal cold hemoglobinuria, 419
    paroxysmal nocturnal hemoglobinuria,
        420

Anesthesia, risks, 336–338t
Aneurysmal disease, 1013–1016
    abdominal aortic aneurysm, 1014–1016,
        1015, 1016t
    thoracic aortic aneurysm, *1013,*
        1013–1014, *1014*
Angioedema, 24–26
    urticaria, relation between, 25
Angiotensin II, 700
    receptor blockers, with hypertension,
        522–523
Angiotensin receptor blockers, 672, 674,
        688
Angiotensin-converting enzyme inhibitors,
        14, 53, 94, 99, 109, 110, 113, 115,
        528, 667, 672, 674, 682, 688, 696,
        974
    adverse response, 14
    with hypertension, 521–522
Animal dander, 14, 23
    environmental modification, 23
    rhinitis, 23
Anisoylated plasminogen streptokinase
        activator complex, 106
Ankylosing spondylitis, 59, 880, 984–986
    differential diagnosis, 986
    disease etiology, 8t
    extraskeletal involvement, 985–986
    extraspinal involvement, 985
    features, 984–986t
    findings in, 985t
    gender, 986
    laboratory findings, 985
    results of testing in, 986t
    treatment, 986
Anorexia, 481
Anorexia nervosa, 231, 832
Anthrax, 604
    in disease etiology, 8t
Anti-allergic compounds, for asthma, 16t
Antianxiety medications, 837
Antiarrhythmic drugs
    properties, 69t
    relative effectiveness, 70t
    toxicity, side effects, 71t
Antibacterial agents, 605–625
    aminoglycosides, 613–614
    anti-tuberculosis agents, 621–625
    aztreonam, 613
    carbapenems, 612–613
        imipenem, 612–613
    cephalosporins, 609–612
        adverse reactions to cephalosporins,
            612
        first-generation cephalosporins,
            609–610
        fourth-generation cephalosporins,
            612
        second-generation cephalosporins,
            610–611

third-generation cephalosporins,
            611–612
    chloramphenicol, 615–616
    clindamycin, 616
    cotrimoxazole, 619
    fluoroquinolones, 620–621
    macrolides, 616–617
        azithromycin, 617
        clarithromycin, 617
        erythromycin, 616–617
    metronidazole, 616
    other antibacterial agents, 621
    penicillins, 606–609
        adverse reactions to penicillins, 609
        aminopenicillins, 605–606
        beta-lactam/beta-lactamase inhibitors,
            607–609
        carboxypenicillins, 607
        natural penicillins, 605
        penicillinase-resistant penicillins,
            606–607
        ureidopenicillins, 607
    tetracyclines, 614–615
    vancomycin, 617–619
Antibiotic prophylaxis, perioperative,
        343–345
Antibiotics, 172, 678, 871
Anticholinergic agents, 394, 753, 870
Anticholinergic drugs, 827
    for asthma, 16t
Anticoagulant therapy, 346–348
    bioprosthetic heart valves, 347
        anticoagulation, 347
    hemorrhagic complications, 347–348
    hemorrhagic disorders, test results in,
        450t
    mechanical prosthetic heart valves,
        346–347
        anticoagulation, 346–347
    oral anticoagulant therapy, INR
        therapeutic ranges for, 346, 346t
    prosthetic heart valve, systemic
        embolism, 347
    prosthetic heart valves, 346–347
        anticoagulation in, 346–347
    venous thromboembolic disease,
        antithrombotic therapy for, 346, 347t
    warfarin
        anticoagulant effect of, reversal,
            347–348
        reversal, 347–348
Anticoagulants, 452
Anticoagulation, in adults with venous
        thromboembolic disease, guidelines,
        347t
Anticoagulation issues, perioperative,
        monitoring for, 341–342
Anticonvulsant blood levels, 730–731
Anticonvulsant therapy, 728–730t
Anticytokine therapy, 950, 978

Antidepressants, 514, 834–835t
    side effects, 835t
Antidiuretic hormone, 695
Antiepileptic drugs, 728
    guidance for use, 729t
    side effects, 730t
    systemic side effects, 730t
    use, 729t
Antifungal therapy, 625–628
    azole antifungal agents, 625–627
        fluconazole, 625–626
        itraconazole, 626
        ketoconazole, 627
        voriconazole, 626–627
    flucytosine, 628
    glucan synthesis inhibitors, 627–628
        caspofungin, 627–628
    polyenes, 627
        amphotericin B products, 627
Anti-GBM antibody-mediated
        glomerulonephritis, 670
Antihistamines, 15, 22, 872
    rhinitis, 22
Antihypertensive therapy, 514t
Antileukotrienes, 871–872
    for asthma, 16t
Antimalarials, 175, 975
Antimicrobials, 605, 606t, 607t, 608t, 610t,
        615t, 618t, 619t, 622t, 623t, 624t,
        625t
    mechanisms of action, 607t
Antimony, 880
    in disease etiology, 8t
Antinuclear antibody patterns, 990t
Antiparkinsonian medications, 274
Antiphospholipid antibody syndrome, 993t,
        993–994
    clinical features, 994
    treatment, 994
Antiplatelet drugs, 690, 748
Antipsychotic agents, 394, 753, 835–837
    side effects, 836, 837t
Antiretroviral agents, 489–495
    classes, 489
    drug resistance testing, 494
    fusion inhibitors, 493
    guidelines for use, 493–495
    nonnucleoside reverse transcriptase
        inhibitors, 490–492t
    nucleoside/nucleotide analogue reverse
        transcriptase inhibitors, 489–490
    postexposure prophylaxis, 495
    in pregnant women, 494–495
    protease inhibitors, 491–493
        dual protease-inhibitor regimens,
            492–493
    replication cycle of human
        immunodeficiency virus, 489
Antirheumatic drug therapies, 972–978
    anti-cytokine therapies, 978

disease-modifying antirheumatic drugs,
        975–976
    antimalarial compounds, 975
    azathioprine, 976–977
    cyclophosphamide, 977
    leflunomide, 976
    methotrexate, 976
    sulfasalazine, 975–976
glucocorticosteroids, 977–978
nonacetylated salicylates, 975
nonsteroidal anti-inflammatory drugs,
        972–975
    gastrointestinal side effects of NSAIDs,
        974–975
    mechanisms of action of NSAIDs,
        972–973
    mechanisms of toxicity of NSAIDs,
        973–974t
    other toxic effects of NSAIDs, 975
Antithrombin III deficiency, 1028
Antitrypsin deficiency, 369
Antituberculosis medications, 621–625
    dosages, 923t
    first-line, 622t
    second-line, 623t
Anti-tubular basement membrane
        antibodies, 678
Antitumor cell activity, in asthma, 13t
Anti-tumor necrosis factor, 950
Antiviral activity, in asthma, 13t
Antiviral agents, 628–631, 637–638t
    acyclovir, 628–631
    amantadine, 630–631
    cidofovir, 630
    famciclovir, 629
    foscarnet, 630
    ganciclovir, 629
    oseltamivir, 631
    valacyclovir, 629
    valganciclovir, 629–630
Anxiety disorders, 828–829
    adjustment disorder with anxious mood,
        829
    generalized anxiety disorder, 828
    obsessive-compulsive disorder, 829
    panic disorders with or without
        agoraphobia, 828
    post-traumatic stress disorder, 828
Aorta, disease, 1013–1020
    aneurysmal disease, 1013–1016
        abdominal aortic aneurysm,
            1014–1016, 1015, 1016t
        thoracic aortic aneurysm, 1013,
            1013–1014, 1014
    aortic dissection, 1016–1018
        classification, 1016, 1016
        clinical features, 1016–1017
        diagnosis, 1017, 1017–1018, 1018
        etiology, 1016
        laboratory tests, 1017, 1017

    treatment, 1018, 1019t
    aortic intramural hematoma, 1019
    incomplete aortic rupture, 1019
    penetrating aortic ulcer, 1018–1019
    thoracic aortic atherosclerosis,
        1019–1020
Aortic aneurysm, 1014
Aortic dissection, 1016–1018, 1017
    classification, 1016, 1016
    clinical features, 1016–1017
    diagnosis, 1017, 1017–1018, 1018
    etiology, 1016
    laboratory tests, 1017, 1017
    pharmacologic therapy for, 1019t
    treatment, 1018, 1019t
Aortic intramural hematoma, 1019
Apatite microcrystals, 956
Aphthous ulceration, 179
Apical impulse, 40
Aplastic anemia, 454–456
APSAC. See Anisoylated plasminogen
        streptokinase activator complex
Ardeparin, 452
Aredia, 779
Argatroban, 452
Aripiprazole, 835
Arrhythmias, 65–66, 78–93
    acute cardioversion to normal sinus
        rhythm, 84–85
    acute myocardial infarction, role of
        pacing in, 91–92
    atrial fibrillation, 82–85
        nonpharmacologic AV node rate
            control, 84
        rate control, 83–84
        rhythm control, 84
        therapy for atrial fibrillation, 83, 83t
    atrial flutter, 81–82, 82, 83
    automaticity, 65–66, 66, 66t
    carotid sinus syndrome, 80–81, 81
    conduction system disorders, 78–80, 79,
        80, 81
    pacemakers, summary of indications for,
        81
    parasystole, 66
    reentry, 65, 65
    sinus node dysfunction, 78, 78
    stroke prevention, 84–85t
    supraventricular tachycardia, 85–87, 86,
        87, 88
    tachycardia-mediated cardiomyopathy,
        89–90
    torsades de pointes, 91
    triggered activity, 65
    ventricular arrhythmias, during acute
        myocardial infarction, 91
    ventricular ectopy, nonsustained
        ventricular tachycardia, 90
    ventricular tachycardia, fibrillation,
        90–91

Wolff-Parkinson-White syndrome, 87–89, *89, 90*
  atrial fibrillation in, 89
Arsenic, 827, 880
  in disease etiology, 8t
Arterial blood gases, 148–152
  clinical approach to, 152–154
Arterial occlusive disease, lower extremity, grading system for, 1020t
Arterial pulse, 39–40
Arteritis, temporal, 389, 668, 905
Arthralgias, 669
Arthritis
  associated with inflammatory bowel disease, 987
  in chronic renal failure, 958
  rheumatoid, criteria for diagnosis, 949t
Arthroplasty, total joint, indications for, 958t
Asbestos, 880, 891
  in disease etiology, 8t
Asbestosis, 880, 948
  disease etiology, 8t
Ascariasis infection, 579
Ascites, 334
  protein, to determine cause of ascites, 307t
Ascorbic acid, 259
Aseptic meningitis, 589, 756
Aseptic necrosis, of bone, 956
  causes of, mnemonic device for, 956t
Aspergillus, 20, 569–570, 928
  with sinusitis, 23
Aspergillus fumigatus, 20, 632
Aspiration, in diagnosis of wheezing, 16t
Aspiration pneumonia, 916
Aspirin, 85, 99, 101, 104, 107, 109, 116, 175, 176, 690, 734, 880, 974
  ingestion, asthma from, 14
Aspirin-sensitive asthma, 14
Astemizole, 872
Asthma, 12t, 12–20, 869
  acute, management, 17–20, *19*
  assessment of severity, 15
  asthma-provoking drugs, 14–15
  bronchial, chronic bronchitis, emphysema, differential features, 866t
  as cause of eosinophilia, 31
  chronic, management, 17, *18*
  cigarette smoking, 15
  corticosteroid therapy, 16–17
  differential diagnosis, 16, 16t
  fumes producing, 8t
  gastroesophageal reflux, 14
  genetics, 13
  goals of management, 17, 17t
  histologic hallmarks, 12t
  management, 17t, 17–20, *19*
  medical history, 15

  medications for, 16, 16t
  metals, fumes producing, 8t
  methacholine challenge, 15t, 15–16
  occupational, 13–14t, 880
  pathology, 12
  pathophysiology, 12–13t
  severity, assessment, 15
Asymptomatic Carotid Atherosclerosis Study, 748
Ataxia-telangiectasia, 179
Atenolol, 83, 519, 733, 1019
Atheroembolism, *1015*
Atherosclerosis
  mechanism, *95*, 95–96
  pathophysiology, 96
Atherosclerotic renal vascular disease, *524*
Atomoxetine, 834
Atopic dermatitis, as cause of eosinophilia, 31
Atovaquone, 482, 486
Atrial fibrillation
  nonrheumatic, management, 85t
  pharmacologic therapy for, 83t
Atrial rhythm, 79
Atrioventricular canal, partial, 48
Atrioventricular conduction defect, 730
Atypical antipsychotics, 753
Autoimmune bullous diseases, 177
Autoimmune hepatitis, 301
Autoimmune mechanism, in disease etiology, 8t
Automaticity, factors enhancing, 66t
Autonomic neuropathy, 743–744
Autosomal dominant inheritance, 364–368
  diseases with, 365t
    Ehlers-Danlos syndrome, 365
    hypertrophic cardiomyopathy, 365–366
    Marfan syndrome, 366–367
    myotonic dystrophy, 367
    neurofibromatosis, 367–368
      type 1, 367
      type 2, 367–368
    osteogenesis imperfecta, 368
    tuberous sclerosis, 368
    von Hippel-Lindau disease, 368
Autosomal dominant polycystic kidney disease, 680
Autosomal recessive inheritance, 368–371
  diseases with, 369t
    Friedreich ataxia, 369
    Gaucher disease, 369–370
    glycogen storage diseases, 370
    homocystinuria, 370–371
    pseudoxanthoma elasticum, 371
    Refsum disease, 371
    Tay-Sachs disease, 371
Autosome, 379
Azathioprine, 277, 301, 624, 744, 746, 950, 966, 976–977
Azithromycin, 484, 557, 588, 591, 606, 617

Azole antifungal agents, 607, 624–627
  fluconazole, 625–626
  itraconazole, 626
  ketoconazole, 627
  pharmacologic properties, 625t
  voriconazole, 626–627
AZT. *See* Zidovudine
Aztreonam, 606, 607, 613

B

Bacillary angiomatosis, 184
  with human immunodeficiency virus, 488
Bacillus species, 558
Bacillus subtilis, 14
  as cause of asthma, 14
Bacitracin, 690
Back pain, 351–352
Back symptoms, nonspecific, 352
Baclofen, 735, 754
Bacteremia, 598
Bacteria, 678
  in acute, chronic sinusitis, 911t
Bacterial abscess, 601
Bacterial arthritis, 998–999
Bacterial diarrhea, 270–272, 594–597
  causes, 270t, 271t
Bacterial infections, 459, 911–916
  aspiration pneumonia, 916
  community-acquired pneumonia, 914–916
    actinomycosis, 916
    Burkholderia pseudomallei, 915
    Chlamydia pneumoniae, 914
    Chlamydia psittaci, 914–915
    Coxiella burnetti, 915
    Francisella tularensis, 915
    Mycoplasma, 914
    Nocardia pneumonia, 915–916
    Yersinia pestis, 915
  nosocomial hospital-acquired pneumonia, 916
  otitis media, 911–912
  pharyngitis, 912
  pneumonia, 912–914
    anaerobic bacteria, 913–914
    Haemophilus influenzae, 913
    Klebsiella pneumoniae, 913
    Legionella pneumophila, 913
    Moraxella catarrhalis, 913
    Pseudomonas aeruginosa, 912–913
    Staphylococcus aureus, 912
    Streptococcus pneumoniae, 912
  sinusitis, 911, 911t
Bacterial meningitis, 583–587, 589t, 590t
  causes, management, 757t
  empiric therapy for, 590t
  organisms involved, 589t
Bacterial peritonitis, spontaneous, variants, 308t
Bacterial vaginosis, 594

Bacteroides, 558–559
Bactrim, 272
Bagassosis, 880
  disease etiology, 8t
Bakers' asthma, 881
  disease etiology, 8t
Ball valve, 60
Barbiturates, 183, 730, 734, 833
Baritosis, 880
  disease etiology, 8t
Barium, 880
  in disease etiology, 8t
Bauxite, in disease etiology, 8t
Bauxite lung, 880
  disease etiology, 8t
B-cell activation, 13t
Beau lines, 184
Becker muscular dystrophy, 372
Beclomethasone, for asthma, 16t
Bee allergy, 28
Behçet disease, 906, 987
Beneficence, 655
  vs. nonmaleficence, in principle of double
    effect, 656
Benzathine penicillin, 605
Benzodiazepines, 532, 686, 690, 727, 730,
    752, 833, 837
  long-acting, 22
  sedative-hypnotics, 834
Benzoyl peroxide, 172
Bernard-Soulier syndrome, 446
Berylliosis, 880
  disease etiology, 8t
Beta₂-agonist drugs, 16t, 869–871
Beta-blockers, 14, 16, 17, 53, 83, 84, 94, 96,
    99, 104, 105, 109, 110, 115, 116,
    208, 209, 210, 224, 232, 237, 341,
    386, 394, 518–519, 528, 532, 686,
    688, 733, 734, 735, 752, 869, 871,
    974
  renal-excreted, 690
Beta-hemolytic streptococcus, chaining in
    blood culture, *631*
Beta-hydroxylase, 230
Beta-hydroxysteroid dehydrogenase, 230
Beta-lactamases, 272
Beta-lactam/beta-lactamase inhibitors,
    607–609
Beta-thalassemia, 369
Betaxolol, 519
Bethanechol, 258, 265
Bicap heater probe, 263
Bile acid sequestrants, 349
Biliary cirrhosis, primary, 302–303
Biliary tract disease, 309
  bile duct stones, 310
  gallbladder carcinoma, 310
  gallstones, 309–310
  malignant biliary obstruction, 310
  sphincter of Oddi dysfunction, 310

Bilirubin, 707
Biologic enzymes, as cause of asthma, 14
Bioprosthetic heart valves, anticoagulation,
    347
Biopsy urease tests, 261
Bioterrorism, 602, 604t
  infections, treatment for, 604t
Bipolar disorder, 826
Bird fancier's lung disease, 890–891
Birds, in disease etiology, 8t
Bisoprolol, 110
Bisphosphonates, 218, 259, 978
Bivalirudin, 452
Blastomyces dermatitidis, *632*
Blastomycosis, 568, 927
  disease etiology, 8t
Bleomycin, 880, 995
Blood gases, 866
Blood pool RNA, 61
Blood pressure
  classification, 511t
  drugs increasing, 514t
Blood products, 175
Board examination, 1–9
  aim of examination, 1
  clinical skills self-evaluation module, 7
  connections between etiologic factors,
    disease, 7, 8t
  content, 2, 2t
  contents of, by subject area, 2
  day of examination, 6–7
  examples, 3–5
  format, 1–2
  medical knowledge self-evaluation
    module, 7
  one best answer, 3
  patient feedback module, 7–9
  peer feedback module, 7–9
  practice improvement module, 9
  preparation for test, 5–6
  question format, 2–3
  recertification, 7–9
  scoring, 2
  security of examination, 9
  single-best answer on examination, 3
Bone, aseptic necrosis of, causes of,
    mnemonic device for, 956t
Bone marrow suppression, 730
Bone metabolism, disorders, 213–219
Bone/joint infections, 600–601
  acute bacterial arthritis, 600
  chronic monarticular arthritis, 600
  osteomyelitis, 600–601
  vertebral osteomyelitis, 601
  viral arthritis, 600
BOOP, 891
Bordetella pertussis, 555–556
Borrelia burgdorferi, 180, 1000
Botulin, 271
Botulinum toxin, 752, 753

Botulism, 559, 604, 744–745
Bowel bypass syndrome, 179
Brain death, 725
Branhamella catarrhalis, 23
Breast cancer, 775–779
  clinical scenarios, 779
  magnitude of problem, 775
  mortality, 808
  natural history, 776–777
    grade, 777
    hormone receptor status, 777
    nodal status, 776, *777*
    tumor size, 776–777t
  node-negative
    adjuvant therapy, 778t
    treated surgically, 777t
  node-positive, adjuvant therapy, 778t
  pathology, 776, *776*
  risk factors, 775, 775t
  screening, 775, 809–810
  staging, 776, 776t
  treatment, 777–779
    adjuvant treatment, 778, 778t
    chemotherapy, 778
    herceptin, 779
    hormonal agents, 778
    primary or local-regional therapy,
      777
    treatment of advanced disease, 778
    zoledronic acid, 779
Bromide, 827
Bromocriptine, 201, 202, 228, 752, 753
Bronchial asthma, chronic bronchitis,
    emphysema, differential features,
    866t
Bronchial gland tumors, 897
Bronchiectasis, 875–878
  causes, associations, 876–878
    allergic bronchopulmonary
      aspergillosis, 877
    ciliary dyskinesia syndrome, 876–877
    hypogammaglobulinemia, 877
    infections, 876
    obstructive azoospermia, 877
    right middle lobe syndrome, 877
    unilateral hyperlucent lung syndrome,
      877–878
    yellow nail syndrome, 877
  complications, 878
  in diagnosis of wheezing, 16t
  treatment, 878
Bronchiolitis, in diagnosis of wheezing, 16t
Bronchiolitis obliterans, 16
  croup, in diagnosis of wheezing, 16
Bronchitis, 880
  chronic, 868
  disease etiology, 8t
Bronchoalveolar cell carcinoma, 896
Bronchoalveolar lavage, 866–867
Bronchodilator compounds, for asthma, 16t

Bronchodilators, 869
Bronchogenic cancer, 880
disease etiology, 8t
Bronchopulmonary aspergillosis
allergic, 20, 20t
diagnostic features, 20t
Bronchopulmonary dysplasia, in diagnosis
of wheezing, 16t
Bronchoscopy, 866
Bronchus cancer, mortality, 808
Brown syndrome, 947
Brucella, 556
Brucellosis, 948
disease etiology, 8t
Budesonide, for asthma, 16t
Bulimia, 832
Bullous emphysema, 880
disease etiology, 8t
Bullous eruption, of systemic lupus
erythematosus, 174
Bullous lung disease, 868
Bullous pemphigoid, 193
Bull's-eye calcification, *861*
Bumetanide, 517
Bupropion, 834, 835, 873
Burger disease. *See* Thromboangiitis
obliterans
Burkholderia pseudomallei, 915
Bursitis, 960
Buspirone, 532, 837
Bypass arthritis, 987–988
Byssinosis, 880
disease etiology, 8t

C

C1 esterase inhibitor, 25–26
Cabergoline, 201, 202, 228
Cadmium, 8t, 880
Caffeine, use, 532, 833, 871
Calcitonin, 215, 218, 269, 397
Calcitriol, 216
Calcium, 216, 218, 695, 978
disorders, 213–219
Calcium carbonate, 705
Calcium channel blockers, 83, 105, 258,
624, 733, 734, 735, 744
with hypertension, 522
Calcium gluconate, 216, 536
Calcium oxalate arthropathy, 983
Calcium oxalate stone, 703–704, *704*
risk factors for, 704t
Calcium phosphate disease, 983
Calcium phosphate stone, 704, 705
Calcium pyrophosphate deposition disease,
983
etiologic classification, 983
pseudogout, 983
treatment of pseudogout, 983
cAMP. *See* Cyclic adenosine
monophosphate

Campylobacter jejuni, 278, 279
Cancer. *See also* Oncology
mortality from, 808t
Cancer screening, 809–813
breast cancer, 809–810
cervical cancer, 812
colorectal cancer, 810–811
lung cancer, 809
ovarian cancer, 812–813
prostate cancer, 811–812
Candesartan, 522
Candida, 183, 258, 278
Candida albicans, with human
immunodeficiency virus, 487
Candidiasis, 481, 570–571, 928
Canine saliva, as cause of asthma, 14
Cannabis, 833
Capastat, 923
Capnocytophaga, 557
Capreomycin, 623, 923
Capsaicin, 734
Captopril, radionuclide renal scan, with
renovascular hypertension, 525–526
Captopril test, 53
with renovascular hypertension, 527
Carbamazepine, 727, 729, 735, 754, 871,
992
Carbapenems, 606, 607, 612–613
ertapenem, 612–613
imipenem, 612–613
meropenem, 612–613
Carbidopa, 752
Carboxypenicillins, 607
Carcinoid heart disease, 57–58
Carcinoid syndrome, 788–789
in diagnosis of wheezing, 16t
Carcinoma, increased incidence, 8t
Cardiac death, sudden, pharmacologic
prevention, 72t
Cardiac failure, in diagnosis of wheezing,
16t
Cardiac imaging methods, 61t
Cardiac palpation, 40
Cardiac risk stratification, noncardiac
surgical procedures, 338t
Cardiac risks, anesthesia, management,
337–340, *340*
Cardiac trauma, 59
Cardiogenic shock, diagnosis of cause, 107t
Cardiology, 39–146
acquired immunodeficiency syndrome,
59
acute coronary syndromes, 101–109, *102*
acute mechanical complications,
myocardial infarction, 107t,
107–108
prehospital dismissal evaluation,
108–109
presentation, 103
reperfusion therapy, 105–107

ST-segment elevation myocardial
infarction, 103
treatments, 103–105
unstable angina, non–ST-segment
elevation myocardial infarction,
102–103
amyloidosis, 56–57
clinical features, 56–57
diagnosis, 57
angina, chronic, 96–101
ankylosing spondylitis, 59
apical impulse, 40
arrhythmias, 65–66, 78–93
acute cardioversion to normal sinus
rhythm, 84–85
acute myocardial infarction, role of
pacing in, 91–92
atrial fibrillation, 82–85
nonpharmacologic AV node rate
control, 84
rate control, 83–84
rhythm control, 84
therapy for atrial fibrillation, 83, 83t
atrial flutter, 81–82, *82, 83*
automaticity, 65–66, *66*, 66t
carotid sinus syndrome, 80–81, *81*
conduction system disorders, 78–80,
79, 80, 81
pacemakers, summary of indications
for, 81
parasystole, 66
reentry, 65, *65*
sinus node dysfunction, 78, *78*
stroke prevention, 84–85t
supraventricular tachycardia, 85–87,
86, 87
with aberrancy, ventricular
tachycardia, differentiating, 87,
87t, *88*
tachycardia-mediated cardiomyopathy,
89–90
torsades de pointes, 91
triggered activity, 65
ventricular arrhythmias, during acute
myocardial infarction, 91
ventricular ectopy, nonsustained
ventricular tachycardia, 90
ventricular tachycardia, fibrillation,
90–91
Wolff-Parkinson-White syndrome,
87–89, *89, 90*
atrial fibrillation in, 89
arterial pulse, 39–40
atherosclerosis, *95*, 95–96
mechanism, *95*, 95–96
pathophysiology, 96
carcinoid heart disease, 57–58
cardiac murmurs, maneuvers altering,
41–47
cardiac palpation, 40

Cardiology *(contd.)*
  cardiac trauma, 59
  cardiomyopathies, 111t, 111–127
    dilated cardiomyopathy, 111–116
      clinical presentation, 112
      etiology, 111–112
      evaluation, 112
      pathophysiology, 112–113, *113, 114*
      recapitulation of drug therapy for
          heart failure, 116
      treatment, 113–116, *114*
    hypertrophic cardiomyopathy, 116–121
      diagnostic testing, 118–120, *119*
      etiology, 116–117
      examination, 118, 118t
      pathophysiology, 117–118
      symptoms, 117
      treatment, 120–121
        asymptomatic patients, 120–121,
            121
        symptomatic patients, 120, *120*
    restrictive cardiomyopathy, 121–122
      definition, 121
      diagnosis, 122
      signs, symptoms, 121
      treatment, 122
  congenital heart disease, 47–52
    atrial septal defect, 47–48
      diagnosis, 48, *48*
      physical examination, 48
      primum atrial septal defect, 48
      secundum atrial septal defect, 47–48
      sinus venosus atrial septal defect, 48
    coarctation of aorta, 50–51
      diagnosis, 51
      physical examination, 51
      treatment, 51
    Ebstein anomaly, 51–52
      diagnosis, 52
      physical examination, 51–52
    Eisenmenger syndrome, 49
    patent ductus arteriosus, 49
    pulmonary stenosis, 49–50
      diagnosis, 50, *50*
      physical examination, 49–50
    ventricular septal defect, 49
  contrast angiography, 61
  coronary angiography, 98
  coronary artery disease, symptomatic
      chronic, 96
  coronary artery spasm, 101
  coronary heart disease, 94–95
    prevention, 94–95
  diabetes mellitus, 56
  echocardiography, 61–62
    contrast echocardiography, 62
    Doppler-color Doppler
        echocardiography, 62
    M-mode echocardiography, 62
    two-dimensional echocardiography, 62

electron beam computed tomography, 64
Friedreich ataxia, 59
heart failure, 109–111
  acute heart failure syndromes, 111
  etiology, 110, 110t
  precipitating factors, 110–111t
heart sounds, 40–41
  first, 40
  fourth, 41
  opening snap, 41
  second, 40–41
  third, 41
hemochromatosis, 57
hypereosinophilic syndrome, 58
  clinical features, 58
  effects, 58
hyperthyroidism, 55
  effects, 55
  physical examination, 55
hypothyroidism, 55–56
  effects, 55–56
  physical examination, 56
imaging, 61t, 61–64
jugular venous pressure, 39
Lyme disease, 59
magnetic resonance imaging, 64
Marfan syndrome, 59
murmurs, 41
  maneuvers altering, 41–47
osteogenesis imperfecta, 59
pericardial disease, 53–55
  constrictive pericarditis, 54–55
    diagnosis, 55
    physical examination, 55
    symptoms, 54–55
  inflammatory pericarditis, 54
    causes, 54
    diagnosis, 54
    presenting symptoms, 54
  pericardial effusion, 54
    clinical features, 54
    treatment, 54
physical examination, 39–41
positron emission tomography, 64
postcardiotomy syndrome, 101
pregnancy, 52–53
  cardiac disease, 52–53
    delivery, 53
    drugs, 53
    hypertension, 53
    physiologic changes of pregnancy,
        52–53
    prosthetic valves, 53
prosthetic valves, 59–60
  bioprostheses, 59–60
  mechanical valves, 60
radionuclide imaging, 62–64
  first-pass radionuclide angiography,
      63
  gated sestamibi imaging, 64

myocardial perfusion imaging, *63,*
    63–64
radionuclide angiography, 62
rheumatoid arthritis, 59
  effects, 59
rhythm disorders, 65–93
  ambulatory electrocardiographic
      monitoring, 66–67
  antiarrhythmic drugs, 69t, 69–74, *70,*
      70t, 71t, *72,* 72t
    adenosine, 73
    amiodarone, 73
    class I antiarrhythmic drugs, 70
    electrophysiology-guided serial drug
        testing, 73
  antitachycardia surgery, 74–75t
  device therapy, 75
  electrocardiography, 66
  electrophysiologic study, *68,* 68–69
  exercise testing, 67–68
  implantable cardioverter-defibrillators
    complications of permanent pacing,
        75–76, *76*
      implantable cardioverter-
          defibrillators, 76–77
      indications for permanent pacemaker
          implantation, 76, 77t
  permanent cardiac pacemaker
      implantation, 75–76t
  signal-averaged ECG, 68
    heart rate variability, 68
  transcatheter radiofrequency ablation,
      74, 74t
scleroderma, 58
  effects, 58
silent ischemia, 96–97
stable angina, chronic, 96–101
syncope, 92t, 92–93t
systemic disease, 55–59
systemic lupus erythematosus, 58
  effects, 58
thrills, 40
tumors of heart, 60–61
  embolization, 60–61
  primary cardiac neoplasm, 61
valvular heart disease, 41–47
  aortic regurgitation, 43–45
    etiology, 43–44
      aortic root dilatation, 44
      diagnosis, 44
      physical examination, 44
      symptoms, 44
      valvular, 43–44
      timing of surgery, 44–45
  aortic stenosis, 41–43
    subvalvular, 42
      diagnosis, 42
      physical examination, 42
    supravalvular, 41–42
      physical examination, 42

valvular, 42–43
 diagnosis, 43
 physical examination, 43
 symptoms, 43
 types, 42–43
 mitral regurgitation, 46–47
 diagnosis, 47
 etiology, 46
 pathophysiology, 47
 physical examination, 46–47
 symptoms, 46
 timing of surgery, 47
 mitral stenosis, 45–46
 diagnosis, 45–46, *46*, 46t
 indications for surgery, 46
 physical examination, 45
 tricuspid regurgitation, 47
 physical examination, 47
 surgical therapy, 47
 tricuspid stenosis, 47
 tricuspid valve prolapse, 47
Cardiomyopathies, 111t, 111–127
 anatomical, pathophysiologic processes
  for, 111t
 dilated, 111–116
 clinical presentation, 112
 drug therapy for heart failure, 116
 etiology, 111–112
 evaluation, 112
 pathophysiology, 112–113, *113, 114*
 treatment, 113–116, *114*
 hypertrophic, 116–121, 365
 diagnostic testing, 118–120, *119*
 etiology, 116–117
 examination, 118, 118t
 pathophysiology, 117–118
 symptoms, 117
 treatment, 120–121
  asymptomatic patients, 120–121, *121*
  symptomatic patients, 120, *120*
 restrictive, 121–122
 definition, 121
 diagnosis, 122
 signs, symptoms, 121
 treatment, 122
Cardiopulmonary resuscitation, 157–158
 airway control, 157–158
 electrical therapy, 158
 legal rulings, 659t
 unlikely to prolong life, situations, 658t
Cardiovascular disease
 percentage of board examination devoted
  to, 2
 preventive geriatrics, 395
Carotid endarterectomy, 748
Carpal tunnel syndrome, 946
Carteolol, 519
Carvedilol, 83, 110, 519, 520
Caspofungin, 606, 607, 627–628
Castor bean, as cause of asthma, 14

Catechol *O*-methyltransferase, 752
Catecholamines, 224, 532, 695, 700, 827
 measurement of, drugs interfering with,
  532t
Cats, in disease etiology, 8t
Cat-scratch disease, 557
Cattle, in disease etiology, 8t
Cavernous sinus thrombosis, with sinusitis, 23
Caves, in disease etiology, 8t
Cefaclor, 610
Cefadroxil, 588, 610
Cefamandole, 610
Cefazolin, 584, 588, 610
Cefdinir, 610
Cefepime, 554, 610
Cefixime, 610
Cefmetazole, 610
Cefonicid, 610
Cefoperazone, 610
Cefotaxime, 554, 555, 590, 610
Cefotetan, 610
Cefoxitin, 610
Cefpodoxime, 610
Cefprozil, 610
Ceftazidime, 554, 557, 590, 610
Ceftibuten, 610
Ceftizoxime, 610
Ceftriaxone, 555, 590, 591, 610, 757
Cefuroxime, 610
Celiprolol, 519
Cell counts, 883
Cell-mediated immunity, 603
Cellulitis, with sinusitis, 23
Central airway tumors, in diagnosis of
  wheezing, 16t
Central diabetes insipidus, 693–694
Central nervous system
 depressants, 827
 infectious syndromes in, 756t
Central venous catheterization, 158
Centrilobar emphysema, 8t, 880
Cephalexin, 557, 588, 610
Cephalosporins, 555, 557, 584, 586, 587,
  599, 606, 607, 609–612
 adverse reactions to, 612
 first-generation cephalosporins, 609–610
 fourth-generation cephalosporins, 612
 with methylthiotetrazole side group, 610t
 second-generation cephalosporins,
  610–611
 third-generation cephalosporins, 611–612
Cephalothin, 610
Cephradine, 610
Cerebrospinal fluid analysis, 74–725
Cerebrovascular accident, 256
Cerebrovascular disease, 746–749
 hemorrhagic, differential diagnosis, 750t
 ischemic cerebrovascular disease,
  746–749
 antiplatelet agents, 748

 carotid endarterectomy, 748
 management of acute cerebral
  infarction, 748–749
 pathophysiologic mechanisms,
  746–747
 risk factors, 747
 stroke risks with nonvalvular atrial
  fibrillation, 749
 transient ischemic attacks, 747–748
Cervical cancer, 779
 background, 779
 screening, 812
 treatment, 779
Cervical cord, 723
Cervical osteophytes, 256
Cervical spondylosis, 739
Cervicitis, 591
Charcot joint, 956
Cheeses, tyramine in, 514
Chemoprophylaxis, 604, 814–819
Chemotherapy, 255, 604, 705, 789–790
 with advanced solid tumors, 790
 applications, 789
 basic concepts, 789, *789*
 cardiac toxicity, 461–462
 colony-stimulating factors, 790
 mechanisms of tumor cell drug
  resistance, 790
 side effects, 790
 solid tumors sensitive to, 789
Chest pain, 848
Chewing tobacco, use, 514
Chicken coops, in disease etiology, 8t
Chipmunks, in disease etiology, 8t
Chlamydia, 95, 396
Chlamydia pneumoniae, 567, 914
Chlamydia psittaci, 914–915
Chlorambucil, 746, 966
Chloramphenicol, 272, 590, 604, 606, 607,
  615–616
Chloroquine, 388
Chlorpromazine, 175, 880, 992
Chlorpropamide, 404
Cholestasis, 293, 294t
 causes, 294t
Cholestatic liver disease, chronic, 302–303
Cholestyramine, 17, 212, 233, 302, 706
Choline salicylate, 14
Chondromalacia, in diagnosis of wheezing,
  16t
Christmas disease, 448
Chromate, 880
 in disease etiology, 8t
Chrome, as cause of asthma, 14t
Chromosome abnormalities, 361–364, *363*
 Down syndrome, 361, *362*
 fragile X-linked mental retardation,
  363–364, *364*
 sex chromosome aneuploidy syndromes,
  361–363, *362*

Chromosomes, 379
  rearrangement, oncogenes, 445t
Chronic active hepatitis, 948
Chronic bronchitis, 868
  bronchial asthma, emphysema,
    differential features, 866t
Chronic eosinophilic pneumonia, 878–879
Chronic leukemias, 438–440
  myelodysplastic syndromes, 438
  myelogenous leukemia, 438–440
Chronic monarticular arthritis, 600
Chronic obstructive lung disease
  complications, causes for exacerbation,
    873
  treatment, 869
    adjuvant therapy, 872–873
    adrenergic agonists, 870
    anticholinergic agents, 870
    antihistamines, 872
    antileukotrienes, 871–872
    bronchodilators, 869
    corticosteroids, 872
    long-acting beta-adrenergic agonists,
      870
    mast cell inhibitors, 871
    nonsteroidal anti-inflammatory agents,
      872
    oxygen, 873
    phosphodiesterase inhibitors, 870–871
    reducing risk factors, 869
    short-acting beta-adrenergic agonists,
      869–870
Chronic obstructive pulmonary disease
  managing, 867t
  methacholine challenge, 15
Chronic pain disorder, 830
Chronic pernio, 1026
Chronic predominantly motor neuropathies,
    743
Chronic rejection, graft failure, 706
Chronic renal failure, 687t, 687–690
  complications of dialysis, 689–690t
  dialysis, 689
  uremia, 688–689
Churg-Strauss granulomatosis, 178
Churg-Strauss syndrome, 668, 669–670,
    879, 905–906
Churg-Strauss vasculitis, 967
  as cause of eosinophilia, 31
  clinical features, 967
  treatment, 967
Chylous effusion, 883
Chylous fistula, 707
Cicatricial pemphigoid, 173
Cidofovir, 604, 606, 630
Cigarette cutters' asthma, 880
  disease etiology, 8t
Cigarette smoking, 232
  asthma, 15
Ciliary dyskinesia, 24, 876–877

Cimetidine, 16, 678, 706, 827, 871
Ciprofloxacin, 271, 484, 487, 589, 604, 623,
    871, 923
Circulatory overload, 459
Cirrhosis, 871
Cisplatin, 684
Citalopram, 834
Clarithromycin, 484, 588, 606, 617
Classic hemophilia A, 450
Claudication, pseudoclaudication,
    differential diagnosis, 1021t
Clindamycin, 550, 588, 606, 616, 756
Clinical epidemiology, percentage of board
    examination devoted to, 2
Clinical features of rheumatoid arthritis,
    944, *944*
Clinical skills self-evaluation module, 7
Clinical syndromes, 581
Clofibrate, 690, 880
Clomiphene citrate, 228
Clonazepam, 729, 735, 752
Clonidine, 274, 520, 734
  withdrawal from, 532
Clopidogrel, 748
Clostridia, 559–560
  botulism, 559
  Clostridium tetani, 559
Clostridium botulinum, 744
Clostridium difficile, 271, 279
Clostridium perfringens, 271
Clostridium tetani, 559
Clotrimazole, 259, 487
Cloxacillin, 606
Clozapine, 752, 753, 835, 837
Clubbing, 849
Cluster headache, 733–734
Coagulase-negative staphylococci, 553–554
  clinical syndromes, 553
  treatment, 553–554
Coagulation, 444–464
  anticoagulants, 452
  aplastic anemia, 454–456
  Bernard-Soulier syndrome, 446
  chemotherapeutic agents, cardiac toxicity,
    461–462
  direct thrombin inhibitors, 453–454
  disseminated intravascular coagulopathy,
    446–447
  factor-deficiency states, 447–449
    factor V deficiency, 449
    factor VII deficiency, 449
    factor VIII deficiency, 448–449t
    factor IX deficiency, 448
    factor X deficiency, 449
    factor XI deficiency, 448
    factor XII deficiency, 448
    factor XIII deficiency, 447
    treatment, 449–450
  Gaucher disease, 461
  Glanzmann thrombasthenia, 446

  hypercalcemia, 463–464
  liver disease, 447, 448t
  low-molecular-weight heparin, 453
  neutropenia, 456
  porphyria, 461, 462t
  postsplenectomy state, 459
  post-transfusion purpura, 459
  prolonged bleeding time, 444
  spontaneous splenic ruptures, 459
  storage pool disease, 446
  superior vena cava syndrome, 462–463
  thrombocytopenia, 456–459
  thrombocytopenia in pregnancy, 459
  thrombolytic therapy, 454
  thrombophilia, 450–451
  thrombopoietin, 461
  transfusion reactions, 459t, 459–461
  unfractionated heparin, 453
  von Willebrand disease, 444–445
  warfarin, 452–453
Coagulation tests, characterizing lupus
    anticoagulant, 993t
Coal, 880
  in disease etiology, 8t
Coarctation of aorta, *532,* 532–533
Coarctation with tortuous aorta, *856*
Cocaine, 514, 833, 880
Coccidioidomycosis, 567, 927
  disease etiology, 8t
Codeine, 734
Coffee, use, 532
Cognitive disturbances, 730
Cognitive impairment, 481
Colchicine, 388, 389, 675
Cold agglutinin disease, 418
Cold agglutinin syndrome, 418
  immunology, 418
Cold formulas, use, 514
Colesevelam, 233
Collagenopathies, type II, 955
Collapsed left lower lung lobe, *852*
Collapsed left upper lung lobe, *852*
Collapsed right lower lung lobe, *853*
Collapsed right upper lung lobe, *853*
Colon, 279–287
  amebic colitis, 281
  angiodysplasia, 283
  antibiotic colitis, 280
  colon polyps, 283–284
    familial polyposis, 284
    Gardner syndrome, 284
    hereditary polyposis syndromes,
      284
    Turcot-Despres syndrome, 284
  colorectal cancer, 284–287
    diagnosis, 286
    epidemiology, 284–285
    etiology, 285
    genetic factors, 285
    pathology, 285–286

postoperative management, no apparent metastases, 286
prevention of colorectal carcinoma, 286–287
risk factors for colorectal cancer, 285
treatment, 286
congenital megacolon, 282
diverticular disease of colon, 282–283
definitions, 282, 283t
diverticulitis, 282–283
irritable bowel syndrome, 281
ischemia, 280–281
acute ischemia, 280–281
ischemic colitis, chronic, 281
review of vascular anatomy, 280
lower gastrointestinal tract bleeding, 282
nontoxic megacolon, 281–282
polyposis syndromes, not associated with risk of cancer, 284
juvenile polyposis, 284
Peutz-Jeghers syndrome, 284
pseudomembranous enterocolitis, 279
radiation colitis, 280
tuberculosis, 281
Streptococcus bovis endocarditis, 281
Colon cancer, mortality, 808
Colony-stimulating factors, 790
Color blindness, 372
Colorectal cancer, 779–781
background, 779
carcinoembryonic antigen, 780
clinical scenarios, 781
risk factors, 779–780
screening, 810–811
staging, 780t
treatment, 780
adjuvant therapy, 780
metastatic disease, 780
surgery, 780, 780t
Coma, 725–726
Combination DMARD therapy, 950
Common variable immunodeficiency, 32
Complications of dialysis, 689–690t
Compression ultrasonography, 1029
Computed tomography
magnetic resonance imaging, comparison, 722t
pulmonary disease, 862
COMT inhibitors, 753
Confidentiality, 654
Conflict of interest, 656
Congenital bicuspid stenosis, 42
Congenital heart disease, 47–52
atrial septal defect, 47–48
diagnosis, 48, *48*
physical examination, 48
primum atrial septal defect, 48
secundum atrial septal defect, 47–48
sinus venosus atrial septal defect, 48
coarctation of aorta, 50–51

diagnosis, 51
physical examination, 51
treatment, 51
Ebstein anomaly, 51–52
diagnosis, 52
physical examination, 51–52
Eisenmenger syndrome, 49
patent ductus arteriosus, 49
pulmonary stenosis, 49–50
diagnosis, 50, *50*
physical examination, 49–50
ventricular septal defect, 49
Congestive heart failure, 687, 871
perioperative, monitoring for, 342
Connections between etiologic factors, diseases, example, 7, 8t
Connective tissue, inherited disorders, 955t
Connective tissue disease
undifferentiated, 993
vasculitis associated with, 971
large vessel vasculitis, 971
obliterative endarteropathy, 971
small, medium-sized vessel vasculitis, 971
Contact dermatitis, 30
Continuous-wave Doppler, 1029
Contraceptives, oral, 175, 514, 624, 871
Contrast angiography, 61
Contrast media reactions, 31
Conversion disorder, 829–830
Coombs-negative hemolytic anemias, 419
Cooperative Study of Sickle Cell Disease, 423, 424
COPD. *See* Chronic obstructive pulmonary disease
Coronary, 110
Coronary angiography, 98
Coronary artery disease, symptomatic chronic, 96
Coronary artery spasm, 101
Coronary heart disease, prevention, 94–95
Coronary revascularization, 110
Cortical lesions, 736
Corticosteroid therapy, 21–22, 209, 302, 754, 755
in diagnosis of wheezing, 16–17
rhinitis, 21–22
Corticosteroids, 17, 21, 158, 230, 273, 276, 277, 301, 388, 389, 514, 624, 667, 670, 672, 732, 734, 758, 872, 905, 918, 963, 964
Corynebacterium diphtheriae, 557–558
Cotrimoxazole, 555, 556, 606, 619
Cotton, as cause of asthma, 14
Cottonseed, as cause of asthma, 14
Cough, 847
methacholine challenge, 15
Coumadin, 450
Courvoisier sign, 290
COX–2 inhibitors. *See* Cyclooxygenase

Coxiella burnetii, 915
Cranial arteritis, 735
Craniopharyngioma, 204
Crescentic glomerulonephritis, 668–670, *669*
CREST syndrome, *196*, 996–997t
Creutzfeldt-Jakob disease, 393, 577, 726
Cricopharyngeal dysfunction, 256
Critical care medicine, 147–167
acid-base balance, 148–152
acute respiratory distress syndrome, 154–157
arterial blood gases, 148–154
cardiopulmonary resuscitation, 157–158
disease severity scoring systems, 160–161
ethics in ICU, 161, 161t
hemodynamic monitoring, 158–159
percentage of board examination devoted to, 2
respiratory failure, 147–149
shock states, 159–160
vascular access, 158–159
Crohn disease, cutaneous, 179
Cromolyn, 16, 880
for asthma, 16t
Croup, 16
in diagnosis of wheezing, 16
Cryoglobulinemia, 970–971
laboratory studies, 971
outcome, 971
Cryoglobulinemia infection, 676
Cryoglobulinemic glomerulonephritis, 675–676t
Cryoglobulinemic vasculitis, 668
Cryoglobulins, 676, 676t
type I, 970
type II, 970
type III, 970
Cryptococcosis, 570, 927–928
Cryptococcus, 184
Cryptococcus neoformans, 632
Cryptococcus neoformans, with human immunodeficiency virus, 484
Cryptosporidiosis, with human immunodeficiency virus, 487
Cryptosporidium, 279
Crystalline arthropathy, 388–389, 979–984
calcium oxalate arthropathy, 983
calcium pyrophosphate deposition disease, 983
etiologic classification, 983
pseudogout, 983
treatment of pseudogout, 983
hydroxyapatite deposition disease, 983
diagnosis, 983, 984t
presentation, 983
hyperuricemia, 979–983
causes, 979
causes of secondary hyperuricemia, 979, 981t

Crystalline arthropathy, hyperuricemia
    (contd.)
  clinical manifestations of acute gout,
    980–981
  enzyme abnormalities in uric acid
    pathway, 979, *980*
  factors predisposing to gout, 980
  points of importance, 982–983
  renal disease, 982
  treatment during intercritical period,
    981–982
  treatment of acute gouty arthritis,
    981
  hypouricemia, 979–980
  other crystals implicated in joint disease,
    983–984
Crystalluria, 707
CT. *See* Computed tomography
Cushing syndrome, 220–222
  cause, 221–222
  clinical features, 221
  confirmation, 221
  diagnosis, 221
  etiology, 220–221
  therapy, 222
Cutaneous amyloidosis, 177
Cutaneous leukocytoclastic vasculitis,
  668
Cutaneous metastasis, 176
Cutaneous purpura, 669
Cutaneous reactions to drugs, 175t
Cutaneous vasculitis, 969–970t
Cyanosis, 848–849
Cyclic adenosine monophosphate, 869
Cyclobenzaprine, 532
Cyclooxygenase, 261
Cyclooxygenase–2 inhibitors, 261
Cyclophosphamide, 670, 674, 744, 746,
  905, 966, 992
Cycloserine, 623, 923
Cyclospora, with human immunodeficiency
  virus, 488
Cyclosporine, 514, 624, 672, 674, 678, 681,
  696, 706, 744, 746, 758, 950
Cystic fibrosis, 369, *857*, 874–875
  in diagnosis of wheezing, 16t
Cystic renal disease, 680–681
  acquired renal cystic disease, 680–681
  autosomal dominant polycystic kidney
    disease, 680
  medullary sponge kidney, 680–681
Cystine stones, 705
Cytokines, characteristics, 13t
Cytomegalovirus, 573–574
  with human immunodeficiency virus,
    484–485t
Cytomegalovirus agents, 606
Cytomegalovirus retinitis, induction
  treatment, 485t
Cytotoxic agents, 676, 992

D

Dalfopristin, 606, 607
Dalteparin, 452
Danaparoid, 452
Danazol, 25
Dander, rhinitis, 23
Dapsone, 482, 624
D-dimer, 1029
de Quervain thyroiditis, 209
Dead space ventilation, 148
Death, 656–657
  definition, 660
Decaffeinated coffee, use, 532
Decongestants, use, 532
Decubitus CXR, *854*
Deep venous thrombosis, 1027
  coagulation disorders predisposing to
    development, 899t
  incidence, 900t
  recurrent, causes, 1027t
Defective chemotaxis, 603t
Defective neutrophilic killing, 603t
Degenerative aortic valve disease, 43
Dehydroepiandrosterone, produced by
  adrenals, 228
Delavirdine, 606
Delayed afterdepolarization, 65
Delayed hemolytic transfusion reaction,
  459
Deletion, 379
Delirium, 393–394t, 831
  causes, 394, 394t
Delta gap, 700–701
Demeclocycline, 206
Dementia, 723, 725, 831–832
  causes, 728
  as complication of Lyme disease, 393
  differential diagnosis, 726t
  in elderly, 391–394
    Alzheimer disease, 391–392
    Creutzfeldt-Jakob disease, 393
    delirium, 393–394t
    frontotemporal dementia, 393
    with Lewy bodies, 393
    with Parkinson disease, 393
    vascular dementia, 393
Demerol, 289, 835
Dental procedures, American Heart
    Association prophylactic regimens,
    588t
Depression, treatment, 825
Dermatitis herpetiformis, 173, 179, *193*
Dermatology, 169–196
  acne vulgaris, 172, 172t
    systemic retinoids, 172
  allergic contact dermatitis, 171–172
  atopic dermatitis, 171
  autoimmune bullous diseases, 172–175
  cardiovascular, 178

  cutaneous T-cell lymphoma, 170
  drug reactions, 175t, 175–176
  endocrine, 182–183
    diabetes mellitus, 182–183
    thyroid, 183
  erythema multiforme, 175
  erythema nodosum, 175
  gastrointestinal, 178–179
  hematologic, 182
  human immunodeficiency virus infection,
    cutaneous manifestations, 184
  internist's perspective, 177–183
  malignancy, cutaneous signs, 176–177
  melanoma, 169t, 169–170
    prevention, 170
  metabolic, 183
  nail clues, to systemic disease, 183–184
  nephrology, 179
  neurocutaneous, 179–180
  nonmelanoma skin cancer, 170
    prevention, 170
  percentage of board examination devoted
    to, 2
  psoriasis, 170–171
    narrow-band UVB, 171
    PUVA, 171
    targeted therapy in psoriasis, 171
    ultraviolet light, 171
  respiratory, 177–178
  rheumatology, 180–182
  skin cancer, 169
Dermatomyositis, 177, *194*, 256, 789
Desipramine, 834, 880
Desmopressin, 205
Desquamation, 481
Desquamative interstitial pneumonia,
  889–890
Dexamethasone, 734
Diabetes Control and Complications Trial,
  235
Diabetes insipidus, 204–205, 693–694
  clinical features, 205
  diagnosis, 205
  endocrine diagnosis, 205
  etiology, 204–205
  polyuria, 693–694
    central diabetes insipidus, 693–694
    nephrogenic diabetes insipidus, 694,
      694t
  primary polydipsia, comparison, 694t
  therapy, 205
Diabetes mellitus, 56, 232, 233–239, 687
  chronic complications, 238
  clinical features, 234
  complications, 237–238
  diabetic ketoacidosis, 237
    prognosis, 237
    treatment, 237
  diagnosis, 234
  etiology, 233–234

hyperglycemic hyperosmolar nonketotic
    coma, 237–238
  diagnosis, 238
  therapy, 238
  hyperlipidemia in, 238
  hypoglycemia in, 236–237
  infections, 238
  ischemic heart disease in, 238
  microvascular disease in, 238
  oral glucose tolerance test, 234
  pregnancy, 239
    treatment, 239
  therapy, 235–236
    combination therapy, 236
    drug therapy for T2D, 236
    exercise, 235
    glycemic goals of optimal therapy, 235
    insulin therapy, 235
    monitoring, 235
    nutrition, 235
Diabetic ketoacidosis, 237
  prognosis, 237
  treatment, 237
Diabetic nephropathy, 673t, 673–674
  stages, 673t
Diabetic neuropathy, 744
*Diagnostic and Statistical Manual of the
    American Psychiatric Association,*
    823
Diagnostic tests, 331t, 331–336, 897
  absolute risk reduction, 335
  number needed to harm, 336
  number needed to treat, 335
  odds, likelihood ratios, 333–334
  relative risk reduction, 335
  therapeutic results, 334–335
  two by two table, 332–333t
Dialysis, 686–687, 689
  complications, 689–690t
  drugs not removed with, 690
  drugs removed with, 690
  medications to avoid with, 690
Dialysis and overdoses, 690t
Diaphragmatic calcification, 880
  disease etiology, 8t
Diarrhea, 265t, 266t, 265–268, 481
  acute diarrhea, 266
  anatomy of nutrient absorption, 266–269t
  bacterial, 595t
  bacterial overgrowth, 270
  chronic, 266, 267t
  clinical approach, 266, 266t
  functional, organic diarrhea,
    differentiating, 267t
  infectious diarrheas, 270, 270t, 271t
  mechanisms of diarrhea, 265–266
  noninvasive bacterial diarrhea, 270–272
    Clostridium perfringens, 270
    Escherichia coli, 270
    Staphylococcus aureus, 270

  osmotic, secretory diarrhea, features
    differentiating, 267t
  systemic illnesses causing, 269t
  watery diarrhea, chronic, 266, 267t
Diazepam, 624, 731
Diazoxide, 240, 538
Dibenzyline, 532
Dicloxacillin, 606
Didanosine, 489, 491, 606
Diet pills, use, 514
Diffuse idiopathic skeletal hyperostosis, 953
Diffuse lung disease, 878–881, *885,*
    885–888, *888*
  abbreviations for, types of, 886t
  causes, 878–880
    acute eosinophilic pneumonia, 878
    allergic bronchopulmonary
      aspergillosis, 879
    chronic eosinophilic pneumonia,
      878–879
    Churg-Strauss syndrome, 879
    drug reactions, 880
    hypereosinophilic syndrome, 880
    neoplasms, 880
    parasitic infections, 879
    tropical eosinophilia, 880
  clinicopathologic classification, 887t
  diagnosis, 888–892
    IPF/UIP, 888–889
  epidemiology, 886t
  hypersensitivity pneumonitis, 880–881t
  idiopathic, 886t
Diffuse urticaria, 481
Digital venous subtraction angiography, with
    renovascular hypertension, 526–527
Digitalis, 827
Digoxin, 53, 83, 110, 115, 116, 122, 624,
    686, 690
Dihydroergotamine, 732, 734
Dihydropyridines, 522
Dilantin, 690, 871
Diltiazem, 83, 84, 522, 686, 706
Diphenhydramine, 404
Diphtheria, 256
Diphtheria vaccine, 814
Direct thrombin inhibitors, 453–454
Dirithromycin, 606t
Disclosure, 653
Discoid lupus erythematosus, *196*
Discontinued feedings, right to, 659
Disease severity scoring systems, 160–161
Diseases causing diarrhea, 268–272
    Aeromonas hydrophila, 272
    Bacillus cereus, 271
    bile acid malabsorption, 269–270
    Campylobacter jejuni, 272
    carcinoid syndrome, 269
    Escherichia coli, 271
    invasive bacterial diarrhea, 271
    laxative abuse, 269

    osmotic diarrhea, 268
    Salmonella, 271
    secretory diarrhea, 268
    Shigella, 271
    Vibrio cholerae, 271
    Yersinia enterocolitica, 272
Disequilibrium, 737, 738
Disk disease, 723
Disopyramide, 69, 70, 71, 83, 110
    procainamide, 83
Disseminated intravascular coagulopathy,
    446–447
Disulfiram, 827
Diuretics, 110, 115, 122, 678, 753, 974
    loop, with hypertension, 517
    potassium-sparing, with hypertension,
      517–518
    thiazide, with hypertension, 516–517
Diverticular disease, complications, 283t
Dizziness, types, 737t
DNA analysis, diagnosis of genetic disease
    by, 374–379
  diseases amenable to DNA diagnosis, 377
  family history, 374–375, *375*
  fluorescent in situ hybridization, 377–379
  linkage analysis, 375–376, *376*
  multifactorial causation, 373–374t
  polymerase chain reaction, 377, *378*
  Southern blot procedure, 376–377, *377,
    378*
DNR. *See* "Do Not Resuscitate" order
"Do Not Resuscitate" order, 658, 658t
Dobutamine, 116
Dofetilide, 69, 70, 71, 72
Dogs, in disease etiology, 8t
Domperidone, 265
Donepezil, 727
Dopamine, 839
Dopamine agonists, 201
Dopaminergic agonists, 752, 753
Double effect, principle, 656
Down syndrome, 361, *362*
Doxepin, 834
Doxycycline, 259, 488, 556, 591, 604, 606
Drug allergy, 29–32
  ampicillin-mononucleosis rash, 30
  classes, 29–30
  common variable immunodeficiency, 32
  contact dermatitis, 30
  eosinophilia, 31t, 31–32
  erythema nodosum, 30
  fixed drug eruptions, 30
  IgE, 29–32
  immediate-type reactions, 29–32
  involving IgE, immediate-type reactions,
    30–32
  macular "drug red" syndrome, 29–30
  mastocytosis, 31
  not involving IgE, immediate-type
    reactions, 29–30

Drug allergy *(contd.)*
  penicillin allergy, 30–31
  radiographic contrast media reactions, 31
  terminal complement component deficiencies, 32
  toxic epidermal necrolysis syndrome, 29
Drug eruptions, fixed, 30
Drug hypersensitivity, as cause of eosinophilia, 31
Drug reactions, 175t, 175–176
Drug-induced liver disease, 306
Drug-induced lupus, 991–993
  agents in, 992t
  clinical features, 991–992
  implicated agents, 992t
  laboratory abnormalities, 992–993
  metabolism, 993
  treatment, 993
Drug-induced myopathies, 998
  muscle disease, 998
Drug-induced stone disease, 705, 705t
DSM. *See Diagnostic and Statistical Manual of the American Psychiatric Association*
d-sotalol, 72
Dual-chamber pacing, 110
Duchenne muscular dystrophy, 372, *375, 377, 378*
Duffy antibody, undetected before transfusion, 49–50
Duke criteria, for diagnosis of infective endocarditis, 582t
Duodenal ulcer, 260
Duodenum, 259–265
  biopsy urease tests, 261
  breath test, 261
  culture, 261
  duodenal ulcer, 260
  gastric tumors, 260
  gastric ulcer, 260
  gastritis, active, chronic, 260
  Helicobacter pylori, 259–260
    diagnostic tests for, 260
    epidemiology, 260
    organism, 259–260
    histology, 261
    nonulcer dyspepsia, 260
    serology, 260–261
    stool antigen test, 261
    treatment, 261
Duplex ultrasonography, with renovascular hypertension, 526
Durable power of attorney for health care, 651
Dust mite control, 23t
DVT. *See* Deep venous thrombosis
Dysfibrinogenemia, 450
Dysgammaglobulinemia, 603
Dysglobulinemia, 232

Dysplasia
  spondyloepimetaphyseal, 955
  spondyloepiphyseal, 955
Dyspnea, 848
Dysthymia, 825

E

Early afterdepolarization, 65
Eating disorders, 832
  anorexia nervosa, 832
  bulimia, 832
Echocardiography, 61–62
  contrast echocardiography, 62
  Doppler-color Doppler echocardiography, 62
  M-mode echocardiography, 62
  two-dimensional echocardiography, 62
Edema, 1026, 1026t
  regional types of, differential diagnosis, 1026t
Efavirenz, 606
Egg protein, as cause of asthma, 14
Eggs, as cause of food allergy, 27
Eggshell calcification, 880
  disease etiology, 8t
Ehlers-Danlos syndrome, 178, 365, 955
Elderly, preoperative assessment, 394
Electrocautery, 263
Electroconvulsive therapy, 839
Electroencephalogram, 724
Electrolyte disorders, 691
Electrolyte imbalance, 746
Electrolyte replacement, 238
Electrolyte-induced interstitial nephritis, 679–680
Electromyographic nerve conduction velocity studies, 723–724
Electron beam computed tomography, 61, 64
Eletriptan, 732
Embolism, prepulmonary, *854*
Emery, 880
  in disease etiology, 8t
Emphysema, 868, 880
  centrilobar, 8t
  chronic bronchitis, bronchial asthma, differential features, 866t
  disease etiology, 8t
  generalized, 8t
Emtricitabine, 491
Enalaprilat, 538
Encainide, 72
Encephalitis, 756
Encephalomyelitis, postinfectious, 756
Endocarditis
  Duke criteria for diagnosis, 582t
  infective
    native valve, treatment, 584–585t
    prophylactic regimens to prevent, American Heart Association, 588t

prosthetic valve, treatment, 586–587t
  prosthetic valve, organisms causing, 586t
Endocrine disease, 182–183, 746
  diabetes mellitus, 182–183
  thyroid, 183
Endocrine neoplasia type IIB
  marfanoid appearance, 539
  oral neurinomas associated with, *539*
Endocrinologic risks, management, 343
Endocrinology, 197–252
  adrenal gland disorders, 219–225
    adrenal failure, 219–220
      acute adrenocortical failure or adrenal crisis, 220
      clinical features, 220
      diagnosis, 220
      endocrine diagnosis, 220
      etiology, 219–220
      primary adrenal failure, 219
      secondary adrenal failure, 219–220
      therapy, 220
    adrenal incidentaloma, 224–225
      evaluation, 224
      therapy, 224–225
    Cushing syndrome, 220–222
      cause of, 221–222
      clinical features, 221
      confirmation of, 221
      diagnosis, 221
      etiology, 220–221
      therapy, 222
    etiology, 224
    pheochromocytoma, 223–224
      clinical features, 223
      diagnosis, 223–224
      etiology, 223
      therapy, 224
    primary aldosteronism, 222–223
      clinical features, 222
      diagnosis, 222–223
      etiology, 222
      therapy, 223
  basic principles, 197
  bone metabolism, disorders, 213–219
  calcium, disorders, 213–219
  diabetes mellitus, 233–239
    chronic complications, 238
    clinical features, 234
    complications, 237–238
    diabetic ketoacidosis, 237
      prognosis, 237
      treatment, 237
    diagnosis, 234
    etiology, 233–234
    hyperglycemia, 237–238
      diagnosis, 238
      therapy, 238
    hyperlipidemia in diabetes, 238
    hypoglycemia, 236–237
    infections, 238

ischemic heart disease in diabetes, 238
microvascular disease in diabetes, 238
oral glucose tolerance test, 234
pregnancy, 239
    treatment, 239
therapy, 235–236
    combination therapy, 236
    drug therapy for T2D, 236
    exercise, 235
    glycemic goals of optimal therapy, 235
    insulin therapy, 235
    monitoring, 235
    nutrition, 235
esophagus, 253–330
hypercalcemia, 213–215
    clinical features, 213–214
    etiology, 213
    familial hypocalciuric hypercalcemia, 214
    hypercalcemia of malignancy, 214–215
    laboratory features, 214
    lithium, 214
    management, 215
    parathyroid-dependent hypercalcemia, 213–214
    parathyroid-independent hypercalcemia, 214–215
    primary hyperparathyroidism, 213–214
    radiographic features, 214
    sarcoidosis, 215
    therapy, 214
    thiazide-induced hypercalcemia, 214
    vitamin D intoxication, 215
hyperlipidemias, 230–233
    clinical features, 230–232
    diagnosis, 232
    etiology, 230–233
    therapy, 232
        behavior modification, 232
        diet therapy, 232
        drug therapy, 232–233
        HDL, low, treatment of, 233
        hypertriglyceridemia, treatment of, 233
        increased LDL, treatment of, 233
        lipoprotein, increased, treatment of, 233
hypoglycemia, in nondiabetic patients, 239–240
    clinical features, 239
    diagnosis, 239–240
        insulinoma, 240
        postprandial hypoglycemia, 240
    etiology, 239
    therapy, 240
hypoparathyroidism, 215–216
    clinical features, 216
    diagnosis, 216
    diagnostic approach, 216

differential diagnosis, 216
    etiology, 215–216
    therapy, 216
hypothalamic-pituitary disorders, 197–206
    acromegaly, 203–204
        biochemical diagnosis, 203
        clinical features, 203
        diagnosis, 203
        radiologic diagnosis, 203
        therapy, 203–204
    ACTH-producing tumors, 204
    craniopharyngioma, 204
    diabetes insipidus, 204–205
        clinical features, 205
        diagnosis, 205
        endocrine diagnosis, 205
        etiology, 204–205
        therapy, 205
    gonadotropin-producing tumors, 204
    hypopituitarism, 198–200
        ACTH deficiency, 198
        clinical presentation in adults, 198, 199t
        diagnosis, 198–200
        endocrine evaluation, 200
        etiology, 198
        gonadotropin deficiency, 198
        growth hormone deficiency, 198
        prolactin deficiency, 198
        structural evaluation, 200
        therapy in adults, 200
        TSH deficiency, 198
    lymphocytic hypophysitis, 204
    pituitary apoplexy, 204
    pituitary incidentaloma, 204
    pituitary tumors, 200–201
        drug therapy, 201
        follow-up, 201
        radiotherapy, 201
        surgery, 201
        treatment, 201
    prolactinoma, 201–203
        clinical features, 202
        diagnosis, 202
        differential diagnosis, 202
        dopamine agonists, 202–203
        surgical treatment for prolactinomas, 203
        therapy, 202–203
    syndrome of inappropriate ADH secretion, 205–206
        clinical features, 206
        diagnosis, 206
        etiology, 205–206
        pathophysiology, 206
        therapy, 206
    TSH-producing tumors, 204
multiple endocrine neoplasia, 241
    MEN I, 241

islet cell neoplasia, 241
        pituitary tumors, 241
        primary hyperparathyroidism, 241
        screening for, 241
    MEN II, 241
        genetics of, 241
    MEN IIA, 241
    MEN IIB, 241
osteomalacia, 218–219
    clinical features, 218
    therapy, 218–219
osteoporosis, 216–218
    clinical features, 217
    diagnosis, 217
    etiology, 217
    prevention, 217–218
ovary, 227–230
    amenorrhea, 227–228
        clinical features, 227
        diagnosis, 227–228
        disorders associated with, 228
            anorexia nervosa, 228
            Turner 45/XO gonadal dysgenesis, 228
        estrogen replacement therapy, 228
        etiology, 227
        ovulation induction, 228
        primary amenorrhea, 227, 228
        secondary amenorrhea, 227–228
        therapy, 228
    androgens in normal females, 228–229
    hirsutism, 229–230
        clinical features, 229
        diagnosis, 229
        etiology, 229
        idiopathic hirsutism, 229
        late-onset congenital adrenal hyperplasia, 230
        polycystic ovarian syndrome, 229–230
        selected hyperandrogenic states, 229–230
        therapy of hirsutism, 230
        virilizing tumors of ovary, adrenal gland, 230
Paget disease, 219
    clinical features, 219
    diagnosis, 219
    therapy, 219
percentage of board examination devoted to, 2
testis, 225–226
    gynecomastia, 226
        clinical features, 226
        diagnosis, 226
        etiology, 226
    male hypogonadism, 225–226
        androgen therapy, 225
        clinical features, 225
        diagnosis, 225

Endocrinology, testis *(contd.)*
  etiology, 225
    Kallmann syndrome, 226
    Klinefelter syndrome, 226
    selected disorders of male
      hypogonadism, 226
    therapy, 225
  thyroid gland disorders, 206–213
    hyperthyroidism, 207–210
      clinical features, 207–208
      diagnosis of hyperthyroidism,
        208–209
      etiology, 207, 208, 208t
      exogenous hyperthyroidism, 209
      Graves disease, 208
      multinodular goiter, 209
      painless lymphocytic thyroiditis,
        208–209
      radioactive iodine, 209–210
      subacute painful thyroiditis, 209
      supportive therapy, 210
      surgery, 210
      therapy, 209–210
      thionamides, 209
      thyroid storm, 210
      thyrotoxicosis in pregnancy, 210
      toxic adenoma, 209
    hypothyroidism, 210–213
      amiodarone, 213
      circumstances, 211–212
      clinical features, 210–211
      diagnosis, 211
      differentiated thyroid cancer,
        212–213
      Hashimoto thyroiditis, 210
      lithium, 213
      myxedema coma, 211–212
      sick euthyroid syndrome, 213
      subclinical hypothyroidism, 211
      therapy, 211
      thyroxine replacement therapy
        in patients with angina, 211
        in pregnancy, 211
    laboratory assessment of thyroid
      function, 206–207
    thyroid nodules, 212
End-of-life care, percentage of board
  examination devoted to, 2
Endothelial cells, in asthma, 13t
End-stage liver disease
  ascites, 306–307t
  complications, 306–309
  hepatorenal syndrome, 308, 308t
  portal systemic encephalopathy, 308–309t
  spontaneous bacterial peritonitis,
    307–308t
  variceal hemorrhage, 309
Enfuvirtide, 493
Enoxaparin, 452
Entacapone, 753

Entamoeba histolytica, 281
Enteric infections, with human
  immunodeficiency virus, 487
Enterobacter, 554–555, 704
Enterococci, 551–552
Enterocytozoon bieneusi, 279
Environmental medicine, percentage of
  board examination devoted to, 2
Enzymopathies, 420
Eosinophil proliferation, differentiation, in
  asthma, 13t
Eosinophilia, 31t, 31–32
  common causes, 31t
Eosinophilia-myalgia syndrome, 906, 997
  as cause of eosinophilia, 31
Eosinophilic fasciitis, 181
  as cause of eosinophilia, 31
Eosinophilic gastroenteritis, as cause of
  eosinophilia, 31
Eosinophilic leukemia, as cause of
  eosinophilia, 31
Eosinophilic pneumonia, 891–892
  as cause of eosinophilia, 31
Ephedra, 705
Epidemiology, 479
Epidermal necrolysis syndrome, 29
Epidermolysis bullosa acquisita, 173
Epididymitis, 594
Epigenetic, 379
Epilepsy, surgery for, 731
Epinephrine injection, 263
Eplerenone, 517
Eprosartan, 522
Epstein-Barr virus, 572–573t, 678
Ergocalciferol, 216
Ergotamine tartrate, 734
Erosive osteoarthritis, 953
Ertapenem, 606, 612–613
Erythema chronicum migrans, 180
Erythema marginatum, 178
Erythema multiforme, *193*
Erythema nodosum, 30, 175, 178, *195*
Erythrocytosis, 442, 443t
  differential diagnosis, 443t
Erythromelalgia, 1026
Erythromycin, 16, 265, 271, 488, 558, 606,
  616–617, 706
Erythropoietin, 415–416, 514
Escherichia coli, 271, 273, 419, 554
Escitalopram, 834
Esmolol, 519, 538, 1019
Esophageal procedures, American Heart
  Association prophylactic regimens,
  588t
Esophagitis, evaluation, 257t
Esophagus, 253–330
  dysphagia, 253–256, *254*
    achalasia, 255
    Barrett esophagus, 254
    benign tumor, 254

    diffuse esophageal spasm, 255–256
    functional cause, 255–256
    malignant tumor, 254–255
    mechanical cause, 253–255
    mechanical obstruction, 253–254
    oropharyngeal dysphagia, 256, 256t
    peptic stricture, 254
    ring, 255
    scleroderma, 256
    web, 255
  esophageal function, 253
  esophageal perforation, 259
  gastroesophageal reflux disease, 256–258
    reflux, 256–257t
    tests for reflux, 257–258
    treatment of reflux, 258
  infections of esophagus, 258–259
  Mallory-Weiss syndrome, 259
  medication-induced esophagitis, 259
  noncardiac chest pain, 258
  normal motility, 253
Esophagus, cancer of, mortality, 808t
Essential cryoglobulinemia, 676
Essential hypertension, factors inconsistent
  with, 513t
Essential thrombocythemia, 441
Essential tremor, 751–752
Estrogen replacement, 217, 218, 228, 233
Estrogens, 232
Ethacrynic acid, 517
Ethambutol, 484, 561, 622, 706, 919–922,
  923t, 926
  toxicity, 926
Ethanol, 532, 692, 706
Ethical issues. *See* Medical ethics
Ethionamide, 623, 923t
Ethosuximide, 727, 729, 992
Ethylene glycol, 690
Ethylenediamine, as cause of asthma, 14
Etiologic factors, diseases, connections
  between, example, 8t
Euthanasia, 657–659
Euvolemic hyponatremia, 692
Evoked potentials, 724
Examination, format, 1–2
Exercise testing, 866
Exogenous dexamethasone, 228
Exogenous gonadotropin, 228
Extradural abscess, with sinusitis, 23
Extragonadal germ cell tumor, 787
Extramammary Paget disease, 176
Extrapulmonary tuberculosis, 561
Extrinsic allergic alveolitis, 890–891
Eyedrops, 14

F

Fabry disease, 179, 372, 373
Factitious disorders, 830
Factor-deficiency states, 447–449
  factor V deficiency, 449

factor V (Leiden) mutation, 1029
factor VII deficiency, 449
factor VIII deficiency, 448–449t
factor IX deficiency, 448
factor X deficiency, 449
factor XI deficiency, 448
factor XII deficiency, 448
factor XIII deficiency, 447, 450
Falls in elderly, 384–385
   evaluation, 385
   prevention, treatment, 385
Famciclovir, 606, 629
Familial Mediterranean fever, 369
Familial precocious osteoarthropathy, 955
Farmer's lung disease, 8t, 880, 890–891
Fat malabsorption, mechanisms, 268t
Febrile, nonhemolytic, reaction to
   transfusion, 459t
Febrile neutropenia, 791
Febrile neutrophilic dermatosis, 177
Felbamate, 727, 729, 730
Feline saliva, as cause of asthma, 14t
Felodipine, 522
Felty syndrome, 951, 951t
   features, 951t
Fenofibrate, 233
Fenoldopam, 538
Ferrous sulfate, 211, 259
Fetal anticonvulsant syndrome, 729
Fever, 13t
Fibrates, 350
Fibroblast
   activation, 13t
   in asthma, 13t
Fibromuscular dysplasia, *524*
Fibromuscular renal vascular disease, *524*
Fibromyalgia, 958–959
   diagnosis, 958–959
   natural history, 959
Fibrosis, progressive, massive, disease
   etiology, 8t
Filariasis, 948
First heart sound, 40
First-generation cephalosporins, 609–610
First-pass RNA, 61
Fistula, chylous, 707
Fixed drug eruptions, 30
Flecainide, 69, 70, 71, 72, 83
Flies, in disease etiology, 8t
Florists, disease etiology in, 8t
Flour, as cause of asthma, 14
Floxin, 923
Fluconazole, 259, 484, 487, 606, 625–626,
   755
Flucytosine, 484, 606, 607, 628, 755
Fludrocortisone, 695, 753
Flunisolide, for asthma, 16t
Fluorescent in situ hybridization, 377–379
Fluoroquinolones, 555, 556, 557, 599, 606,
   607, 620–621

Fluoroscopy, pulmonary disease, 851–861
Fluorouracil, 286
Fluoxetine, 834
Fluvoxamine, 834
Focal segmental glomerulosclerosis,
   671–672
Follicular carcinoma, 212
Fondaparinux, 452
Food allergy, 27
   anaphylaxis, 27
   causes, 27, 27t
   in chronic urticaria, 26
   clinical history, 27
   common causes, 27, 27t
   food-related anaphylaxis, 27
   skin testing in, 27
Food industry agents, as cause of asthma,
   14
Foreign body, in diagnosis of wheezing, 16t
Formoterol, 16
   for asthma, 16t
Fortovase, 492
Foscarnet, 485, 574, 606, 630
Fosphenytoin, 731
Fourth heart sounds, 41
Fourth-generation cephalosporins, 612
Fragile X syndrome, *364*
Fragile X-linked mental retardation,
   363–364, *364*
Francisella tularensis, 915
Friedreich ataxia, 59, 369
Frontotemporal dementia, 393, 726
Frovatriptan, 732
Fulminant hepatic failure, 305t, 305–306
   causes, 305t
Functional diarrhea, organic diarrhea,
   differentiating, 267t
Fungal diseases of lung, 927–929
   aspergillosis, 928
   blastomycosis, 927
   candidiasis, 928
   coccidioidomycosis, 927
   cryptococcosis, 927–928
   histoplasmosis, 927
   Pneumocystis carinii, 929
   sporotrichosis, 928–929
   zygomycosis, 928
Fungal infections, 567–571
   aspergillosis, 569–570
   blastomycosis, 568
   candidiasis, 570–571
   coccidioidomycosis, 567
   cryptococcosis, 570
   histoplasmosis, 568
   mucormycosis, 571
   sporotrichosis, 568–569
Fungus, 678
Furosemide, 517, 692, 871
Fusion inhibitors, 489
Futility, 654–655

G

Gabapentin, 727, 729, 733, 735
Gaisböck syndrome, 443
Galantamine, 727
Ganciclovir, 485, 574, 606, 629, 755
Ganglionic blockers, 274
Gardeners, disease etiology in, 8t
Gardner syndrome, 176, 179
Gardnerella vaginalis, 594
Gastric cancer, 263–264
   clinical aspects, 264
   precancerous lesions, 264
   treatment, 264
Gastric polyps, 264
Gastric tumors, 260
Gastric ulcer, 260
Gastritis
   active, chronic, 260
   chronic, nonerosive nonspecific, 263
Gastroduodenal dysmotility syndromes,
   264t, 264–265
   treatment, 264–265
Gastroenterology, 253–330
   acquired immunodeficiency syndrome
     with diarrhea, diagnostic evaluation,
     279
     gastrointestinal manifestations,
     278–279
   colon, 279–287
   duodenum, 259–265
   esophagus, 253–330
   pancreas, 287–291
   percentage of board examination devoted
     to, 2
   small intestine, 265–268
   stomach, 259–265
Gastroesophageal reflux, asthma and, 14
Gastrointestinal cancer, disease etiology, 8t
Gastrointestinal disorders, 178–179, 921
Gastrointestinal infection, 594–597
   bacterial diarrhea, 594–597
   viral diarrhea, 597
Gastrointestinal procedures, American Heart
     Association, prophylactic regimens,
     588t
Gastrointestinal tract cancer, 880
Gastroparesis, conditions causing, 264t
Gaucher cells, *478*
Gaucher disease, 369–370, 461
GBM abnormalities, diseases with, 676–677
   Alport syndrome, 676–677
   thin GBM disease, 677
Gemfibrozil, 233
General internal medicine, 331–360
   anticoagulant therapy, current concepts
     in, 346–348
   clinical problems in, 348–352
   diagnostic tests, interpretation, 331t,
     331–336

General internal medicine (contd.)
preoperative medical evaluation, 336–346
Generalized anxiety disorder, 828
Generalized emphysema, 880
Generalized pruritus, 177
Genetic linkage, 379
Genetics, 361–382
chromosome abnormalities, 361–364
Down syndrome, 361, 362
fragile X-linked mental retardation,
363–364, 364
other chromosome abnormalities, 363,
363
sex chromosome aneuploidy
syndromes, 361–363, 362
DNA analysis, diagnosis of genetic
disease by, 374–379
diseases amenable to DNA diagnosis,
377
family history, 374–375, 375
fluorescent in situ hybridization,
377–379
linkage analysis, 375–376, 376
multifactorial causation, 373–374t
polymerase chain reaction, 377, 378
Southern blot procedure, 376–377,
377, 378
mitochondrial mutations, 373
patterns of inheritance, 364–373
autosomal dominant, 364–368
Ehlers-Danlos syndromes, 365
hypertrophic cardiomyopathy,
365–366
Marfan syndrome, 366–367
myotonic dystrophy, 367
neurofibromatosis, 367–368
type 1, 367
type 2, 367–368
osteogenesis imperfecta, 368
tuberous sclerosis, 368
von Hippel-Lindau disease, 368
autosomal recessive, 368–371
Friedreich ataxia, 369
Gaucher disease, 369–370
glycogen storage diseases, 370
homocystinuria, 370–371
pseudoxanthoma elasticum, 371
Refsum disease, 371
Tay-Sachs disease, 371
X-linked recessive, 371–373
Duchenne, Becker muscular
dystrophies, 372
Fabry disease, 373
Genitourinary procedures, American Heart
Association, prophylactic regimens,
588t
Gentamicin, 551, 556, 584, 587, 588, 604,
757
Gentamicin sulfate, 586, 587
Geriatric medicine, 383–410

assessment, 383–384
dementia, 391–394
Alzheimer disease, 391–392
Creutzfeldt-Jakob disease, 393
delirium, 393–394t
frontotemporal dementia, 393
with Lewy bodies, 393
with Parkinson disease, 393
vascular dementia, 393
falls, 384–385
evaluation, 385
prevention, treatment, 385
hearing changes, 387
immunizations, 396–397
medications, use of, in elderly, 402–404
osteomalacia, 398
osteoporosis, 397–398
percentage of board examination devoted
to, 2
preoperative assessment of elderly, 394
pressure ulcers, 398–399
preventive geriatrics, 394–395
cardiovascular disease, 395
malignancy, 395
pulmonary changes, 395
respiratory disease, 395–396
rheumatologic problems, 387–389
crystalline arthropathy, 388–389
osteoarthritis, 387–388
polymyalgia rheumatica, temporal
arteritis, 389
rheumatoid arthritis, 388
sexual function, 390–391
syncope, 385–386
thyroid disease, 389–390
urinary incontinence, 399–402
anatomy, 399
effects of age, 399
established incontinence, 400
evaluation of incontinence, 400–401
medications affecting urination,
continence, 399–400
treatment of incontinence, 401
urologic consultation, 402
use of urinary catheters, 402
urinary tract infection, 402
vision changes, 386–387
Geriatric surgical patients, 345–346
perioperative medication management,
346
Geriatrics patients, perioperative medication
management, 346
Giant cell arteritis, 735, 905, 962–964
clinical features, 963, 963t
diagnosis, 963, 963t
diagnostic criteria for, 963t
outcome, 964
pathology, 962–963
relationship to, 961
treatment, 963–964

Giant cell pneumonitis, 892
Glanzmann thrombasthenia, 446
Glargine insulin, 235
Glaucoma, 386
Glomerular disorders, 673–675
with nephritic syndrome, 666–668
Henoch-Schönlein purpura, 667
IgA nephropathy, 666–667
membranoproliferative
glomerulonephritis, 667–668
poststreptococcal glomerulonephritis,
666
with nephrotic syndrome, 670–673
focal segmental glomerulosclerosis,
671–672
human immunodeficiency virus-
associated nephropathy, 672–673
minimal change nephropathy, 670–671
Glomerular injury, clinical manifestations,
665–666
nephritic syndrome, 666
nephrotic syndrome, 665–666
Glomerulonephritis, 687, 908
with hepatitis C virus infection, 675–676
cryoglobulinemic glomerulonephritis,
675–676t
Glossopharyngeal neuralgia, 735
Glucagonoma syndrome, 176, 179, 194
Glucan synthesis inhibitors, 607, 627–628
caspofungin, 627–628
Glucocorticoids, 16, 212, 215, 220, 222,
232, 827
for asthma, 16t
Glucocorticosteroid psychosis, 978
Glucocorticosteroids, 960, 977–978
Glucose, 240, 692
Glucose-6-phosphate dehydrogenase
deficiency, 372, 419–420
Glycerol, 692
Glyceryl trinitrate, 538
Glycine, 692
Glycogen storage disease, 369, 370
Glycoprotein IIb/IIIa inhibitors, 105
Glycyrrhizinic acid, 514
Goats, in disease etiology, 8t
Goiter, 256
Gold salts, 872
Goldman Cardiac Risk Index, 339t
Gonadotropin, 225, 226
Gonadotropin axis, 200
Gonadotropin deficiency, 200
Gonadotropin-producing tumors, 204
Gonococcal arthritis, 999–1000
Goodpasture syndrome, 668, 907–908
Gottron papules, 194
Gout, 180, 979–983
Graft failure, 706
Graft-versus-host disease, 182, 459, 997
Grain, as cause of asthma, 14
Gram-negative bacilli, 554–557

Bordetella pertussis, 555–556
Brucella, 556
Capnocytophaga, 557
cat-scratch disease, 557
Escherichia coli infections, 554
Haemophilus influenzae, 555
Klebsiella, Enterobacter, Serratia
        infections, 554–555
Legionella, 556
Pasteurella multocida, 556–557
plague, 556–557
Pseudomonas aeruginosa, 554–555
Salmonella, 555
Stenotrophomonas maltophilia, 555
tularemia, 556
Vibrio species, 557
Gram-negative cocci, 558
    Moraxella, 558
    Neisseria, 558
Gram-positive bacilli, 557–558
    Bacillus species, 558
    Corynebacterium diphtheriae, 557–558
    Listeria, 557
Gram-positive cocci, 549–552
    enterococci, 551–552
    group A beta-hemolytic streptococci,
        549
    group B streptococci, 551
    group D streptococci, 551
    invasive group A streptococcal infection,
        549–551
        nonsuppurative complications, 550,
            550t
    Streptococcus agalactiae, 551
    Streptococcus pneumoniae, 551–552
    Streptococcus pyogenes, 549
    Viridans streptococci, 552
Granulocytes, macrophages, stimulation, 13
Granulocytic leukemia, chronic, 438–440
Granuloma, *861*
Granuloma annulare, 182, *196*
Granulomatosis, Wegener, 668
Granulomatous disease, chronic, 372
Graphite, 880
    in disease etiology, 8t
Green coffee, as cause of asthma, 14
Griseofulvin, 175
Guaifenesin, 705
Guanabenz, 520
Guanethidine, 518
Guanfacine, 520
Guillain-Barré syndrome, 481t
Gum, hypertrophy, 730
Gums, as cause of asthma, 14
Gynecology, percentage of board
        examination devoted to, 2
Gynecomastia, 226
    clinical features, 226
    diagnosis, 226
    etiology, 226

H

Haemophilus influenzae, 23, 395, 555, 757,
    913
Hairy cell leukemia, 427–428, *477*
"Half-and-half" nails, 184
Hallucinogens, 827, 833
Haloperidol, 624
Hamartoma, popcorn calcification,
    861
Handgrip, 41
Hantavirus, 576, 678
Hantavirus pulmonary syndrome, 576,
    910–911
Hashimoto encephalopathy, 726
Hashimoto thyroiditis, 390
HDL. *See* High-density lipoprotein
Headache, 481, 730, 733t
Health food products, use, 514
Hearing changes, in elderly, 387
Heart failure, 109–111
    acute heart failure syndromes, 111
    causes, 110t
    etiology, 110, 110t
    precipitating factors, 110–111t
Heart rhythms, amenable to catheter
        ablation, 74t
Heart sounds, 40–41
    first, 40
    fourth, 41
    opening snap, 41
    second, 40–41
    third, 41
Heavy metals, 827
Helicobacter, 95
Helicobacter pylori, 259–264
    diagnostic tests for, 260
    epidemiology, 260
Heliotrope discoloration, *194*
HELLP syndrome, 459
Helminth, 578–579
    as cause of eosinophilia, 31
Hematite, 880
    in disease etiology, 8t
Hematite lung, 880
    disease etiology, 8t
Hematology, 411–478
    acquired immunodeficiency, 465
    anemias, 411–421
        cold agglutinin syndrome, 418
            immunology of, 418
        Coombs-negative hemolytic anemias,
            419
        enzymopathies, 420
        erythropoietin, 415–416
        evaluation, *411,* 411t, 411–415, *413,*
            414
        glucose-6-phosphate dehydrogenase
            deficiency, 419–420
        hemolytic anemia, *416,* 416–418

Coombs-positive hemolytic anemia,
    417
        drug-induced hemolytic anemia,
            417–418
            autoantibody mechanism, 417
            drug adsorption mechanisms, 417
            immune-complex mechanism,
                417–418
        inheritance patterns, 416
        intravascular hemolysis, differential
            diagnosis of, 417
        laboratory findings, 416
        peripheral smear, differential
            diagnosis, 417
    hereditary spherocytosis, 421
    Mycoplasma pneumoniae, 418–419
        infectious mononucleosis, 419
        paroxysmal cold hemoglobinuria, 419
        paroxysmal nocturnal hemoglobinuria,
            420
    coagulation, 444–464
        anticoagulants, 452
        aplastic anemia, 454–456
        Bernard-Soulier syndrome, 446
        chemotherapeutic agents, cardiac
            toxicity, 461–462
        direct thrombin inhibitors, 453–454
        disseminated intravascular
            coagulopathy, 446–447
        factor-deficiency states, 447–449
            factor V deficiency, 449
            factor VII deficiency, 449
            factor VIII deficiency, 448–449t
            factor IX deficiency, 448
            factor X deficiency, 449
            factor XI deficiency, 448
            factor XII deficiency, 448
            factor XIII deficiency, 447
            treatment of, 449–450
        Gaucher disease, 461
        Glanzmann thrombasthenia, 446
        hypercalcemia, 463–464
        liver disease, 447, 448t
        low-molecular-weight heparin, 453
        neutropenia, 456
        porphyria, 461, 462t
        postsplenectomy state, 459
        post-transfusion purpura, 459
        prolonged bleeding time, 444
        spontaneous splenic ruptures, 459
        storage pool disease, 446
        superior vena cava syndrome, 462–463
        thrombocytopenia, 456–459
        thrombocytopenia in pregnancy, 459
        thrombolytic therapy, 454
        thrombophilia, 450–451
        thrombopoietin, 461
        transfusion reactions, 459t, 459–461
        unfractionated heparin, 453
        von Willebrand disease, 444–445

Hematology, coagulation (contd.)
    warfarin, 452–453
  hemochromatosis, 464–465
  malignancies, 425–444
    acute leukemias, 436–438
      acute lymphoblastic leukemia,
        437–438
      acute nonlymphocytic leukemia,
        436–437
    chronic leukemias, 438–440
      myelodysplastic syndromes, 438
      myelogenous leukemia, 438–440
    hairy cell leukemia, 427–428
    Hodgkin lymphoma, 428–431t
    infectious mononucleosis, 428
    lymphocytic leukemia, chronic,
      425–427
    monoclonal gammopathies, 433–436
      amyloidosis, 435–436
      monoclonal gammopathies of
        undetermined significance, 434
      multiple myeloma, 434–435
      solitary plasmacytomas, 435
      Waldenström macroglobulinemia,
        435
    myeloproliferative disorders, 440–442
      erythrocytosis, 442, 443t
      essential thrombocythemia, 441
      myelofibrosis, 440–441
    non-Hodgkin lymphoma, 430–433t
    oncogenesis, 444, 445t
    polycythemia rubra vera, 442–444
  parapoxvirus infection, 465
  percentage of board examination devoted
    to, 2
  sickle cell disorders, 422–425
  thrombotic microangiopathies, 421–422
    hemolytic uremic syndrome, 422
    thrombotic thrombocytopenic purpura,
      421–422
Hematopoietic tissues, tumors of,
    classification, 432t
Hematuria, 669
Heme pigments, comparison, 683t
Hemizygote, 379
Hemochromatosis, 57, 369, 464–465, 954
Hemoglobinuria, 707
Hemolytic anemia, 416, 416–418
  Coombs-positive hemolytic anemia, 417
  drug-induced hemolytic anemia, 417–418
    autoantibody mechanism, 417
    drug adsorption mechanisms, 417
    immune-complex mechanism, 417–418
  inheritance patterns, 416
  intravascular hemolysis, differential
    diagnosis, 417
  laboratory findings, 416
  peripheral smear, differential diagnosis,
    417
Hemolytic transfusion reaction

acute, 459
delayed, 459
Hemolytic uremic syndrome, 422, 676
Hemophilia A, 448–449t
  von Willebrand disease, differences
    between, 449t
Hemophilia B, 448
Hemophilia C, 448
Hemophilic arthropathy, 956
Hemoptysis, 669, 848
Hemorrhagic cerebrovascular disease,
    749–750
  cerebellar hemorrhage, 749–750
  differential diagnosis, 750t
  intracerebral hemorrhage, 749
  subarachnoid hemorrhage, 750, 750t
Hemorrhagic complications, anticoagulant
    therapy, 347–348
Hemorrhagic disorders, anticoagulant
    therapy, test results in, 450t
Hemorrhagic fevers, viral, 604
Hemorrhagic sinusitis, 669
Hemorrhagic telangiectasia, hereditary, 178,
    365
Henoch-Schönlein purpura, 667, 668
Heparin, 104, 107, 342, 347, 450, 696
  thrombocytopenia, 1025, 1025
Hepatic abscess, 601
Hepatitis, causes, 293t
Hepatitis A, vaccine, 817
Hepatitis B, 459
  serologic markers, 297t
  serologic patterns, interpretation, 298t
  vaccine, 817–818
Hepatitis C, 459
Hepatocellular disorders, 293, 293t
Hepatology, 253–330
  abnormal liver tests, interpretation, 292
  cholestatic disorders, 293, 294t
  hepatocellular disorders, 293, 293t
  jaundice, 293–295, 294
  liver disease, 295–310
  liver tests
    abnormal, algorithms for patients with,
      295, 295, 296
    commonly used, 292–293
Hepatorenal syndrome, differential
    diagnosis, 308t
Herceptin, 779
Hereditary hemorrhagic telangiectasia, 178,
    365
Hereditary liver diseases, 303–305
  alpha$_1$-antitrypsin deficiency, 305
  genetic hemochromatosis, 303–304
  Wilson disease, 304–305
Hereditary spherocytosis, 365, 421
Heroin, 880
Herpes genitalis, 591
Herpes gestationis, 173
Herpes simplex virus, 572

Herpesviruses, 571–575
  cytomegalovirus, 573–574
  Epstein-Barr virus, 572–573t
  herpes simplex virus, 572
  human herpesvirus 6, 575
  human herpesvirus 8, 575
  varicella-zoster virus, 574–575
Heterozygote, 379
HFE gene, 303
High-density lipoprotein, HDL, decrease in,
    232
Hirsutism, 177, 229–230, 730
  clinical features, 229
  diagnosis, 229
  etiology, 229
  idiopathic hirsutism, 229
  late-onset congenital adrenal hyperplasia,
    230
  polycystic ovarian syndrome, 229–230
  selected hyperandrogenic states, 229–230
  therapy of hirsutism, 230
  virilizing tumors of ovary, adrenal gland,
    230
Hirudin, 105, 452
Histamine, 29
Histamine receptor antagonists, 258
Histiocytosis X, 856
Histoplasma, 678t
Histoplasma capsulatum, 279
Histoplasmosis, 568, 927
  disease etiology, 8t
HIV. See Human immunodeficiency virus
HMG-CoA reductase inhibitors, 349
Hodgkin disease, 477
  Cotswolds staging classification, 429t
  staging procedures for, 430t
  suggested initial therapy, 431t
Hodgkin lymphoma, 428–431t
Holter monitoring, 66
Homocystinuria, 369, 370–371
Homogentisic acid, 707
Homozygote, 379
Hookworm, 579
Horner syndrome, 849
Horse dander, as cause of asthma, 14
Hospital-acquired pneumonia, 916
Hot-tub lung, 890–891
House dust mites, 22–23t
HPV infection. See Human papillomavirus
  infection
HTLV. See Human T-cell lymphotropic
  viruses
Human herpesvirus 6, 575
Human herpesvirus 8, 575
Human immunodeficiency virus, 459,
    479–509
  acquired immunodeficiency syndrome-
    associated malignancies, 488–489
    Kaposi sarcoma, 488
    non-Hodgkin lymphoma, 488–489

primary central nervous system
lymphoma, 489
antiretroviral agents, 489–495
drug resistance testing, 494
fusion inhibitors, 493
guidelines for use, 493–495
nonnucleoside reverse transcriptase
inhibitors, 490–492t
nucleoside/nucleotide analogue reverse
transcriptase inhibitors, 489–490
postexposure prophylaxis, 495
in pregnant women, 494–495
protease inhibitors, 491–493
dual protease-inhibitor regimens,
492–493
replication cycle of human
immunodeficiency virus, 489
clinical manifestations, 481, 481t
cutaneous manifestations, 184
dementia, 726
epidemiology, 479
infections associated with, 481–488
acquired immunodeficiency syndrome
dementia complex, 486
bacillary angiomatosis, 488
Candida albicans, 487
Cryptococcus neoformans, 484
cryptosporidiosis, 487
Cyclospora, 488
cytomegalovirus, 484–485t
enteric infections, 487
isosporiasis, 487
microsporidiosis, 487–488
Mycobacterium avium complex,
483–484
Pneumocystis pneumonia, 481–482t
progressive multifocal leukoencephalopathy, 486–487
Salmonella infections, 487
syphilis, 485
toxoplasmosis, 485–486t
tuberculosis, 482–483t
laboratory diagnosis, 480, 480–481
life cycle, 496
nephropathy, 672–673
pathogenesis, 481
primary human immunodeficiency
virus infection, 481, 481t
rheumatologic manifestations, 1002t,
1002–1003
human immunodeficiency virus-
associated vasculitis, 1003
lupus-like illnesses in human
immunodeficiency virus infection,
1003
other human immunodeficiency virus-
associated rheumatic syndromes,
1003
reactive arthritis, undifferentiated
spondyloarthropathy, 1003

toxoplasmosis, 486t
transmission, 479–480
Human papillomavirus infection, 812
Human T-cell lymphotropic viruses, 459, 578
Huntington disease, 256, 365, 393, 726
Hyaluronic acid, 388
Hydralazine, 110, 115, 520, 536, 538, 992
Hydrocephalus, 736
Hydrochloric acid, 700
Hydrochloride, phenazopyridine, 707
Hydrocortisone, 220
Hydroxocobalamin, 537
Hydroxyapatite deposition disease, 983
diagnosis, 983, 984t
presentation, 983
Hydroxychloroquine, 949, 975, 992
Hypercalcemia, 213–215, 463–464,
790–791
clinical features, 213–214
etiology, 213
familial hypocalciuric hypercalcemia, 214
hypercalcemia of malignancy, 214–215
laboratory features, 214
lithium, 214
management, 215
parathyroid-dependent hypercalcemia,
213–214
parathyroid-independent hypercalcemia,
214–215
primary hyperparathyroidism, 213–214
radiographic features, 214
sarcoidosis, 215
therapy, 214
thiazide-induced hypercalcemia, 214
vitamin D intoxication, 215
Hypercalciuria, 705
Hypercholesterolemia, 365
Hypereosinophilic syndrome, 58, 880
clinical features, 58
effects, 58
Hypergammaglobulinemic purpura, 948
Hyperglycemic hyperosmolar nonketotic
coma, 237–238
diagnosis, 238
therapy, 238
Hyperhomocysteinemia, 1028
Hyperkalemia, 695, 695t, 696
diagnosis, 695t
Hyperlipidemia, 230–233
case, 348
clinical features, 230–232
diagnosis, 232
etiology, 230–233
overview of therapy for, 233t
primary, features, 231t
secondary, causes, 232, 232t
therapy, 232
behavior modification, 232
diet therapy, 232
drug therapy, 232–233

HDL, low, treatment, 233
hypertriglyceridemia, treatment, 233
increased LDL, treatment, 233
lipoprotein, increased, treatment, 233
treatment, 348–349
Hypersensitivity pneumonitis, 880–881t,
890–891
Hypertension, 511–547, 687
causes, 523–539
coarctation of aorta, 532, 532–533
definition, 511, 511t
diagnosis, 512–513
epidemiology, 511–512
evaluation, 513t, 513–515
drugs, 514, 514t
laboratory studies, 515
factors inconsistent with, 513t
hypertensive emergencies, urgencies,
536–539
avoidance of drugs, conditions
requiring, 538–539
causes, 537
definitions, 536–537
evaluation, management, 537–538
hypertensive emergency, 536–537
hypertensive urgency, 537
perioperative, monitoring for, 342
pheochromocytoma, 530–532
diagnosis, treatment, 531–532
screening, 531, 532t
symptoms, 531
pregnancy, hypertension in, 533–536
chronic hypertension in pregnancy,
535
definition, 534–535
hypertensive crisis, 536
preeclampsia-eclampsia, 535–536
primary aldosteronism, 529–530
clinical features, 529
diagnosis, 529–530
laboratory features, 529
renal parenchymal disease, 528
renovascular hypertension, 523–528, 524
screening tests, 525–527
captopril radionuclide renal scan,
525–526
captopril test, 527
digital venous subtraction
angiography, 526–527
duplex ultrasonography, 526
intravenous pyelography, 525
magnetic resonance angiography,
526
renal arteriography, 526
renal vein renins, 527
spiral computed tomography
angiography, 526
therapy for, 527–528
treatment, 515–523
adrenergic inhibitors, 518–520

Hypertension, treatment *(contd.)*
  angiotensin II receptor blockers, 522–523
  angiotensin-converting enzyme inhibitors, 521–522
  calcium channel blockers, 522
  lifestyle modifications, 515
  loop diuretics, 517
  pharmacologic therapy, 515–516
  potassium-sparing diuretics, 517–518
  thiazide diuretics, 516–517
  traditional vasodilators, 521
Hypertensive emergency, 536–539
  avoidance of drugs, conditions requiring, 538–539
  causes, 537
  definitions, 536–537
  evaluation, management, 537–538
Hypertensive urgency, 536–539
Hyperthyroidism, 55, 207–210, 256, 871
  clinical features, 207–208
  diagnosis of hyperthyroidism, 208–209
  effects, 55
  etiology, 207, 208, 208t
  exogenous hyperthyroidism, 209
  Graves disease, 208
  multinodular goiter, 209
  painless lymphocytic thyroiditis, 208–209
  physical examination, 55
  radioactive iodine, 209–210
  subacute painful thyroiditis, 209
  supportive therapy, 210
  surgery, 210
  therapy, 209–210
  thionamides, 209
  thyroid storm, 210
  thyrotoxicosis in pregnancy, 210
  toxic adenoma, 209
Hypertrichosis, 177
Hypertriglyceridemia, 232
Hypertrophic cardiomyopathy, 365–366
Hypertrophic osteoarthropathy, 849, 956
Hyperuricemia, 979–983
  causes of, 979–981t
  clinical manifestations of acute gout, 980–981
  enzyme abnormalities in uric acid pathway, 979, *980*
  factors predisposing to gout, pseudogout, 980
  points of importance, 982–983
  renal disease, uric acid, 982
  secondary, causes, 981t
  treatment during intercritical period, 981–982
  treatment of acute gouty arthritis, 981
Hyperventilation syndrome, in diagnosis of wheezing, 16t
Hypervolemic hyponatremia, 692
Hypnotics, 394, 833

Hypochondriasis, 830
Hypochondrogenesis, 955
Hypochromic microcytic anemias, *476*
  comparison, 412t
Hypofibrinogenemia, 450
Hypogammaglobulinemia, 24, 603, 877
Hypoglycemia in nondiabetic patients, 239–240
  clinical features, 239
  diagnosis, 239–240
   insulinoma, 240
   postprandial hypoglycemia, 240
  etiology, 239
  therapy, 240
Hypoglycemic agents, oral, 624, 690
Hypogonadism, male, 225–226
  androgen therapy, 225
  clinical features, 225
  diagnosis, 225
  etiology, 225
  Kallmann syndrome, 226
  Klinefelter syndrome, 226
  selected disorders of male hypogonadism, 226
  therapy, 225
Hypokalemia, 695, 695t, *696*
  diagnosis, 695t
Hyponatremia, 730
Hypoparathyroidism, 215–216
  clinical features, 216
  diagnosis, 216
  differential diagnosis, 216
  etiology, 215–216
  therapy, 216
Hypopituitarism, 198–201
  ACTH deficiency, 198
  clinical presentation in adults, 198, 199t
  diagnosis, 198–200
  endocrine evaluation, 200
  etiology, 198
  gonadotropin deficiency, 198
  growth hormone deficiency, 198
  prolactin deficiency, 198
  structural evaluation, 200
  therapy in adults, 200
  TSH deficiency, 198
Hyposplenism, 603
Hypothalamic-pituitary disorders, 197–206
  acromegaly, 203–204
   biochemical diagnosis, 203
   clinical features, 203
   diagnosis, 203
   radiologic diagnosis, 203
   therapy, 203–204
  ACTH-producing tumors, 204
  craniopharyngioma, 204
  diabetes insipidus, 204–205
   clinical features, 205
   diagnosis, 205

   endocrine diagnosis, 205
   etiology, 204–205
   therapy, 205
  gonadotropin-producing tumors, 204
  hypopituitarism, 198–200
   ACTH deficiency, 198
   clinical presentation in adults, 198, 199t
   diagnosis, 198–200
   endocrine evaluation, 200
   etiology, 198
   gonadotropin deficiency, 198
   growth hormone deficiency, 198
   prolactin deficiency, 198
   structural evaluation, 200
   therapy in adults, 200
   TSH deficiency, 198
  lymphocytic hypophysitis, 204
  pituitary apoplexy, 204
  pituitary incidentaloma, 204
  pituitary tumors, 200–201
   drug therapy, 201
   follow-up, 201
   radiotherapy, 201
   surgery, 201
   treatment, 201
  prolactinoma, 201–203
   clinical features, 202
   diagnosis, 202
   differential diagnosis, 202
   dopamine agonists, 202–203
   surgical treatment for prolactinomas, 203
   therapy, 202–203
  syndrome of inappropriate ADH secretion, 205–206
   clinical features, 206
   diagnosis, 206
   etiology, 205–206
   pathophysiology, 206
   therapy, 206
  TSH-producing tumors, 204
Hypothalamic-pituitary hormones
  clinical syndromes, 199t
  functions, 199t
Hypothyroidism, 55–56, 210–213, 232, 256, 687, 726
  amiodarone, 213
  circumstances, 211–212
  clinical features, 210–211
  diagnosis, 211
  differentiated thyroid cancer, 212–213
  effects, 55–56
  Hashimoto thyroiditis, 210
  lithium, 213
  myxedema coma, 211–212
  physical examination, 56
  sick euthyroid syndrome, 213
  subclinical hypothyroidism, 211
  therapy, 211

thyroxine replacement therapy
  in patients with angina, 211
  in pregnancy, 211
Hypovolemic hyponatremia, 691–692
Hypoxia, 147–149
  dead space ventilation, 148
  mixed venous oxygen saturation, 148
  oxygen delivery, 148
  PAO2, calculation, 148
  shunt fraction, 148–149

I

Ibuprofen, 880, 992
Ibutilide, 69, 70, 71
Ichthyosis, acquired, 177
Idiopathic diffuse lung disease, 886t
Idiopathic hypereosinophilic syndrome, as
    cause of eosinophilia, 31
Idiopathic pulmonary fibrosis, 948
Idiopathic pulmonary hemosiderosis, 909
IgA
  anaphylaxis, 459
  nephropathy, 666–667
IgE, 30–32
  synthesis, in asthma, 13t
IgG, synthesis, in asthma, 13t
Imidazoles, 624
Imipenem, 555, 606, 612–613
Imipramine, 834
Immotile cilia syndrome, 876–877
  in diagnosis of wheezing, 16t
Immune disorders, 753–755
Immunizations, 814–819, 815
  chemoprophylaxis, 814–819
  in elderly, 396–397
  vaccines, 814–819
    diphtheria, 814
    hepatitis A, 817
    hepatitis B, 817–818
    influenza, 816–817
    measles, 816
    mumps, 816
    pneumococcal disease, 818
    polio, 819
    rabies, 819
    rubella, 816
    smallpox, 818–819
    tetanus, 814–816
    varicella, 819
Immunodeficiency
  infections in, 602, 602t, 603t
  pathogens associated with, 603t
Immunology, percentage of board
    examination devoted to, 2
Immunosuppression, 459, 706, 706
Immunotherapy, 22
Impaired physician, 656
Impedance plethysmography, 1029
Implied consent, 653
Inclusion body encephalitis, 577

Incomplete aortic rupture, 1019
Incontinence, urinary, in elderly, 399–402
  anatomy, 399
  effects of age, 399
  established, 400
  evaluation, 400–401
  medications affecting, 399–400
  treatment, 401
  urinary catheters, use, 402
  urologic consultation, 402
Incurable disease, 656–657
Indinavir, 492, 705
Indinavir nelfinavir combination, 493
Indomethacin, 707, 733
Industrial agents, as cause of asthma, 14t
Infected joint prostheses, 1000
Infections, as cause of eosinophilia, 31
Infections associated with human
    immunodeficiency virus, 481–488
  acquired immunodeficiency syndrome
    dementia complex, 486
  bacillary angiomatosis, 488
  Candida albicans, 487
  Cryptococcus neoformans, 484
  cryptosporidiosis, 487
  Cyclospora, 488
  cytomegalovirus, 484–485t
  enteric infections, 487
  isosporiasis, 487
  microsporidiosis, 487–488
  Mycobacterium avium complex, 483–484
  Pneumocystis pneumonia, 481–482
  progressive multifocal leukoencephalopa-
    thy, 486–487
  Salmonella infections, 487
  syphilis, 485
  toxoplasmosis, 485–486t
  tuberculosis, 482–483t
Infections in solid organ transplantation,
    immunodeficiency states, 602, 602t,
    603t
Infectious arthritis, 998–1000
  bacterial arthritis, 998–999
  gonococcal arthritis, 999–1000
  infected joint prostheses, 1000
  mycobacterial, fungal joint infections,
    1000
  spinal septic arthritis, 1000
Infectious disease
  actinomycosis, 560
  anaerobic bacteria, 558–560
  antibacterial agents, 605–625
  antifungal therapy, 625–628
  antimicrobials, 605, 606t, 607t, 608t,
    610t, 615t, 618t, 619t, 622t, 623t,
    624t, 625t
  antiviral agents, 628–631
  bacteremia, 598
  bioterrorism, 602, 604t
  bone infections, 600–601

Chlamydia pneumoniae, 567
clinical syndromes, 581
fungal infections, 567–571
gastrointestinal infection, 594–597
gram-negative bacilli, 554–557
gram-negative cocci, 558
gram-positive bacilli, 557–558
gram-positive cocci, 549–552
hepatic abscess, 601
in immunodeficiency states, 602, 602t,
    603t
infective endocarditis, 581–583
joint infections, 600–601
meningitis, 583–589
mycobacterial diseases, 560–563
Mycoplasma pneumoniae, 566–567
neutropenia, 598
nocardiosis, 565–566
parasitic diseases, 578–580
percentage of board examination devoted
    to, 2
rickettsial infections, 566
sepsis, 598
septic shock, 598
severe acute respiratory syndrome,
    602–605
sexually transmitted diseases, 589–595
sinusitis in adults, 601
soft tissue infection, 599–600
in solid organ transplantation, 602, 602t,
    603t
spirochetes, 563–565
staphylococci, 552–554
streptococcal toxic shock syndrome, 602
toxic shock syndrome, 601
urinary tract infection, 598–599
viral diseases, 571–578
Infectious mononucleosis, 428, 477, 948
Infectious mononucleosis-like syndromes,
    573t
Infective endocarditis, 581–583
  additional information about infective
    endocarditis, 581–583
  Duke criteria for diagnosis, 582t
  native valve infective endocarditis, 581,
    582t, 584–585t
  prevention, 583, 588t
  prophylactic regimens to prevent,
    American Heart Association, 588t
  prosthetic valve, infective endocarditis,
    581, 586t, 586–587t
  prosthetic valve, treatment, 586–587t
  surgical therapy, 583
Inferior vena cava interruption, 903
Inflammatory bowel disease, 275–278
  Crohn disease, 277–278
    corticosteroids, 277
    nutrition, 277–278
  extraintestinal manifestations of
    inflammatory bowel disease, 275

Inflammatory bowel disease *(contd.)*
 indications for colonoscopy, 275–276
 toxic megacolon, 276
 ulcerative colitis, 276–277
  corticosteroids, 276–277
  surgical, 277
Inflammatory disorders, 753–755
 demyelinating diseases, 753–754
 paraneoplastic disorders, 754–755
Inflammatory myopathies, 745–746,
  997–998
 inclusion body myositis, 998
Infliximab, 277
Influenza, 575–576, 910, 948
Influenza vaccine, 816–817
Informed consent, 652–653, 659
INH. *See* Isoniazid
Inhalants, 833
Inhaled pentamidine, 880
Inheritance patterns, 364–373
 autosomal dominant, 364–368
  Ehlers-Danlos syndromes, 365
  hypertrophic cardiomyopathy,
   365–366
  Marfan syndrome, 366–367
  myotonic dystrophy, 367
  neurofibromatosis, 367–368
   type 1, 367
   type 2, 367–368
  osteogenesis imperfecta, 368
  tuberous sclerosis, 368
  von Hippel-Lindau disease, 368
 autosomal recessive, 368–371
  Friedreich ataxia, 369
  Gaucher disease, 369–370
  glycogen storage diseases, 370
  homocystinuria, 370–371
  pseudoxanthoma elasticum, 371
  Refsum disease, 371
  Tay-Sachs disease, 371
 X-linked recessive, 371–373
  Duchenne, Becker muscular
   dystrophies, 372
  Fabry disease, 373
Inhibitors of crystallization, 705
Insect allergy, 27–29
Insect stings, hypersensitivity to, 29t
Insomnia, 730
Inspiration, 41
Insulin, 236, 237, 238, 695
 short-acting, 235
Insulin pump, 235
Insulin replacement therapy, 235
Intensive care unit
 ethics in, 161, 161t
  withholding life support, *versus*
   withdrawal of existing support,
   161
Interferon alfa
 in combination with ribavirin, 300

ribavirin, combination treatment with,
  676
Interleukin 2, 880
Interleukin-1 inhibitors, 950
Intermittent claudication, 1020–1022
 cardiac risk, vascular surgery, 1022
 clinical features, 1020, 1020t
 diagnosis, 1021
 natural history, 1021
 pseudoclaudication, 1020–1021t
 treatment, 1021–1022
Internal medicine, 331–360
 anticoagulant therapy, current concepts
  in, 346–348
 clinical problems in, 348–352
 preoperative medical evaluation, 336–346
Interstitial nephritis
 common causes, 678t
 with nephrotic syndrome, renal
  insufficiency, 678
Intestinal angina, 281
Intestinal pseudo-obstruction, chronic,
  274–275
 approach to patient with, 274–275
Intimal flap
 in ascending aorta, *1017*
 in transverse aortic arch, *1017*
Intracranial tumors, 723
Intravascular coagulopathy, laboratory
  findings, 448t
Intravenous pyelography, with renovascular
  hypertension, 525
Intrinsic acute renal failure, 683t, 683–684
Iodinated contrast, 532, 880
Iodinated radio-contrast agents, 744
Ipratropium bromide, 16
 for asthma, 16t
Irbesartan, 522
Iritis, 987
 rheumatologic diseases, 987
Iron deficiency anemia, 412
Ischemia, silent, 96–97
Isolated angiitis of central nervous system,
  967–968
 clinical features, 967–968
 diagnosis, 968
 treatment, 968
Isoniazid, 483, 561, 563, 622, 814, 871,
  919–923, 992
 toxicity, 926
Isosporiasis, with human immunodeficiency
  virus, 487
Isotretinoin, 172
Isradipine, 522
Itraconazole, 484, 487, 606, 625, 626
Ixodes dammini, 180

J

Jaundice, 293–295, *294*
Joints, congenital malformations, 954

Jones criteria, for diagnosis of initial attack
  of rheumatic fever, 550t
Jugular venous pressure, 39
Justice, 657
Justifiable parentalism, 653–654

K

Kala-azar, 948
Kaletra, 493
Kanamycin, 623, 923
Kantrex, 923
Kaolin, 880
 in disease etiology, 8t
Kaposi sarcoma, 488
 epidemic, 184
Karyotype, 379
Kartagener syndrome, 876
Kawasaki disease, 668
Kayser-Fleischer ring, 304, 305
Kearns-Sayre syndrome, 373
Kell antibody, undetected before
  transfusion, 49–50
Kerley B lines, *858*
Ketoconazole, 606, 625, 627, 706, 871
Kidd antibody, undetected before
  transfusion, 49–50
Kidney function, evaluation, 707–708
 renal imaging, 708
 urinalysis, 707t, 707–708
Kidney stones, 730
 activity, 704t
 characteristics, 703t
 formation, medications increasing
  tendency for, 705t
Kinetic tremor, 751
Klebsiella, 273, 554–555, 704
Klebsiella pneumoniae, 913
Kniest dysplasia, 955
Koilonychia, 184

L

Labetalol, 532, 536, 538, 1019
Laboratory animal workers, epidemiologic
  factors affecting. *See* Rodent urine
Lambert-Eaton syndrome. *See* Myasthenic
  syndrome
Lamivudine, 491, 606
Lamotrigine, 727, 729, 730, 733
Langerhans cell histiocytosis, 890
Large cell carcinoma, 896
Large-vessel vasculitis, 971
Laryngeal edema, in diagnosis of wheezing,
  16t
Laser photocoagulation, 263
Latent tuberculosis infection, treatment, 563
Laundry detergent workers. *See Bacillus
  subtilis*
LDL. *See* Low-density lipoprotein
L-dopa, 274
 as antiparkinsonian medication, 274

LDUH. *See* Low-dose unfractionated
     heparin
Lead, 827
Leflunomide, 949, 976
Left ventricular aneurysmectomy, 110
Left ventricular outflow tract obstruction,
     118t
Leg ulcer, 1030, 1030t
     clinical features, 1030t
Legionella, 396, 556, 678
Legionella pneumophila, 913
Legionellosis, disease etiology, 8t
Leiden mutation, 1029
Leopard syndrome, 365
Lepirudin, 452
Leprosy, 948
Leptomeningeal lesions, 735
Leptospirosis, disease etiology, 8t
Lethargy, 481
Leukemia
     acute lymphoblastic, 437–438
     acute nonlymphocytic, 436–437
     myelogenous, 438–440
Leukemic infiltration, 678
Leukocytes, in asthma, 13t
Leukoplakia, oral hairy, 184
Leukotriene modifiers, in aspirin-sensitive
     asthma, 14
Leukotriene receptor antagonists, for
     asthma, 16t
Levalbuterol, 869
Levamisole, 286
Levetiracetam, 727, 729
Levocabastine, 36
Levodopa, 532, 707, 752
Levodopa-carbidopa, 753
Levofloxacin, 604, 623
Lewy bodies, dementia with, 393
Lewy body disease, diffuse, 726
Lidocaine, 69, 70, 71, 734
Life support, withholding, *versus*
     withdrawal of existing support, 161
Lifestyle modifications, with hypertension,
     515
Light chain deposition disease, 675
Light-headedness, presyncopal, 737
Limbic encephalitis, 726
Lindsay nails, 184
Linear IgA bullous dermatosis, 173
Linezolid, 606, 607
Linkage analysis, DNA analysis, 375–376,
     376
Lipodystrophy, partial, 179
Lipoxygenase inhibitors, for asthma, 16t
Lispro, 235
Listeria, 557, 757
Lithium, 690, 734, 751, 837–839, 974
     levels, conditions increasing, 838t
     toxicity, signs, symptoms, 838t
Lithium carbonate, 992

Livedo reticularis, 1026
Liver disease, 295–310
     cancer, mortality, 808
     coagulation, 447, 448t
     laboratory findings, 448t
     viral hepatitis, 295–301
         hepatitis A, 295–296
         hepatitis B, 296–298, *297*, 297t, 298t
         hepatitis C, 298–301, *299*, 299t, *300*
         hepatitis D, 298
         hepatitis E, 301
Liver failure, 730
Liver risks, management, 343
Liver tests
     abnormal
         algorithms for patients with, 295, *295,
             296*
         interpretation, 292
     alkaline phosphatase, 292
     aminotransferases, 292
     bilirubin, 292
     commonly used, 292–293
     prothrombin time, albumin, 292–293
Liver tumors, 306
     adenoma, 306
     cavernous hemangioma, 306
     cholangiocarcinoma, 306
     hepatocellular carcinoma, 306
     metastases, 306
Living will, 651
LMWH. *See* Low-molecular-weight heparin
Locked-in syndrome, 725
Loffler syndrome
     as cause of eosinophilia, 31
     in diagnosis of wheezing, 16t
Long-acting insulin, 235
Loop diuretics, 215
     with hypertension, 517
Lopinavir-ritonavir, 492
Loracarbef, 610
Lorazepam, 731, 752
Losartan, 522
Lovastatin, 690, 992
Low back pain, 351–352, 959–960
     diagnosis, 959, 960t
     spinal radiography, indications, 960t
     treatment, 959–960
Low-density lipoprotein cholesterol
     goals, therapeutic lifestyle changes, 349t
     increase in, 232
     receptor deficiency, 365
Low-dose unfractionated heparin, 344
Low-molecular-weight heparin, 342, 452,
     453
Lumbar puncture
     cerebrospinal fluid analysis, 724–725
     contraindications for, 725
     indications for, 724–725
Lumbar spine disease, 739–740
Lung abscess, 916

Lung biopsy, 866
Lung cancer, 781–783
     clinical scenarios, 783
     histologic types, characteristics, 781
     magnitude of problem, 781
     mortality, 808
     natural history, 781, *782*
     primary, 893–898
         adenocarcinoma, 896
         bronchial gland tumors, 897
         bronchoalveolar cell carcinoma, 896
         carcinoid, 897
         cell types, 894
         clinical features, 894–896
         diagnostic tests, 897
         endocrine, 898
         large cell carcinoma, 896
         lymphoma, 897
         mesenchymal tumors, 897
         nervous system, 898
         overall survival, 894
         paraneoplastic syndromes, 897
         skeletal, 898
         small cell carcinoma, 896–897
         squamous cell carcinoma, 896
     risk factors, 781
     screening, 781, 809
     staging, 781, 782t, 895t
     treatment, 781–782
         chemotherapy for NSCLC, 782
         non–small-cell lung cancer, 781–782
         small-cell lung cancer, 782
Lung disease, diffuse
     abbreviations for, 886t
     clinicopathologic classification, 887t
     epidemiology, 886t
     idiopathic, 886t
Lung functions, preoperative evaluation,
     866
Lung volumes, 147
Lungs, disease etiology, pathology in, 8t
Lunula, blue-colored, 184
Lupus erythematosus, 180
     subacute, cutaneous, *196*
Lyme disease, 59, 393, 564–565,
     1000–1001
     clinical stages, 1001
         stage I, 1001
         stage II, 1001
         stage III, 1001
     clinical syndromes, 564
     diagnosis, 564–565, 1001
     epidemiology, 564
     prevention, 565
     spirochete, 1000–1001
     treatment, 565, 1001
Lymphadenopathy, 256, 481
Lymphangioleiomyomatosis, 890
Lymphangitic carcinoma, *855*
Lymphedema, 1026–1027

Lymphoblastic leukemia, acute, *478*
Lymphocyte activation, 13t
  in asthma, 13, 13t
Lymphocytes, in asthma, 13t
Lymphocytic hypophysitis, 204
Lymphocytic interstitial pneumonitis, 892
Lymphocytic leukemia
  chronic, 425–427, *477*
  classification, 426t
Lymphoid tissues, tumors of, classification, 432t
Lymphoma, 676, 678, 897

M

Macleod syndrome, 877–878
Macroglobulinemia, Waldenström, 435
Macroglossia, *194*
Macrolides, 556, 607, 616–617, 871
  azithromycin, 617
  clarithromycin, 617
  erythromycin, 616–617
Macrophages
  in asthma, 13t
  maturation, 13
  stimulation, 13
Macular degeneration, 387
Macular "drug red" syndrome, 29–30
Maculopapular rash, 481
Magnesium, 690
Magnesium sulfate, 536
Magnetic resonance angiography, with renovascular hypertension, 526
Magnetic resonance imaging, 61, 64
  computed tomography, comparison, 722t
  pulmonary disease, 862
Mahogany, as cause of asthma, 14
Major depression, 824–826
  adjustment disorder with depressed mood, 825
  dysthymia, 825
  pharmacotherapy, 826
  psychotherapy, 825–826
  seasonal affective disorder, 824–825
  treatment of depression, 825
Malabsorption
  due to disease of small intestine, 272–273
    celiac sprue, 272–273
    eosinophilia gastroenteritis, 273
    intestinal lymphangiectasia, 273
    systemic mastocytosis, 273
    tropical sprue, 273
    Whipple disease, 273
  symptoms, 268t
Malaria, 948
Malignancy, 425–444, 948
  cutaneous signs, 176–177
  preventive geriatrics, 395
Malignant melanoma, survival in, by tumor thickness, 169t
Malingering, 830–831

Manganese, 827
Mania, 826
Mannitol, 690, 692
MAO-B inhibitors, 753
Marfan syndrome, 59, 365, 366–367, 955
Marijuana, 871
  use, 514, 871
Mast cells
  in asthma, 13t
  inhibitors, 871
  proliferation, in asthma, 13t
  stimulation, in asthma, 13t
Mastocytosis, 31, 182
Measles, 577
Measles vaccine, 816
Meat wrappers' asthma, 880
  disease etiology, 8t
Mechanical prosthetic heart valves, anticoagulation, 346–347
Mechanical ventilation, 153t, 153–154
  complications, 153t, 153–154
  modes, 154
  PEEP in mechanical ventilation, 154
Meclizine, 737
Medial fibromuscular dysplasia, *524*
Medical consultation, art, 336
Medical ethics, 649–663
  autonomy of patient, 649–655
    advance directive, 650–651
    advance medical care directive, 652
    confidentiality, 654
    conflicts, 652
    disclosure, 653
    durable power of attorney for health care, 651
    futility, 654–655
    implied consent, 653
    informed consent, 652–653
    justifiable parentalism, 653–654
    living will, 651
    Patient Self-Determination Act of 1990, 652
    preservation, 650
    principles, 649–657
    surrogate, 651–652
  beneficence, 655
  death, definition, 660
  "Do Not Resuscitate," 658, 658t
  ethical dilemmas, 649
  in intensive care units, 161t
  justice, 657
  nonmaleficence, 655–657
    conflict of interest, 656
    double effect, principle, 656
    impaired physician, 656
    incurable disease, death, 656–657
    nonabandonment, 655–656
  percentage of board examination devoted to, 2
  persistent vegetative state, 658–660

  physician-assisted suicide, euthanasia, 657–658
  principles of medical ethics, 649–657
  withholding, withdrawing life support, 658, 659t
Medical knowledge self-evaluation module, 7
Medical oncology, percentage of board examination devoted to, 2
Medication-overuse headache, 734–735
Medications, use of, in elderly, 402–404
Mediterranean fever, 675
Medullary sponge kidney, 680–681
Mees lines, 184
Melanin, 707
Melanoma, 783
  background, 783
  clinical scenarios, 783
  diagnosis, prognosis, 783, 783t
  management, 783
  ten-year survival in, 783t
Melioidosis, disease etiology, 8t
Melphalan, 675
Membranoproliferative glomerulonephritis, 667–668
Meniere syndrome, 737
Meningitis, 583–589
  aseptic meningitis, 589
  bacterial meningitis, 583–587, 589t, 590t
  chronic, 726, 756
  meningococcal meningitis, 587–589
  recurrent, 756
  with sinusitis, 23
Meningococcal meningitis, 587–589
Meningoencephalitis, 481
Meperidine, 289, 404, 835
Mercaptopurine, 277
Mercury, 827
Meropenem, 555, 606, 612–613
Mesalamine, 276, 880
Mesenchymal tumors, 897
Mesothelioma, 880
  disease etiology, 8t
Metabolic, 183
Metabolic acidosis, 150–151, 695–698t
  compensation, 698t
Metabolic alkalosis, 151, 698–699, *699*
Metabolic-toxic disorders, 726
Metabolism, percentage of board examination devoted to, 2
Metabolites, measurement of, drugs interfering with, 532t
Metal fume fever, 880
  disease etiology, 8t
Metals, as cause of asthma, 13
Metaproterenol, 869
Metformin, 230, 236
Methacholine challenge, 15t, 15–16
  positive findings, 15t
Methadone, 624
Methanol, 690

Methazolamide, 752
Methenamine, 690
Methicillin, 606
Methimazole, 209
Methotrexate, 388, 746, 872, 880, 949, 966, 974, 976
Methyldopa, 520, 532, 707, 992
Methylglucamine, 532
Methylprednisolone, for asthma, 16t
Methylxanthines, 751, 869
   for asthma, 16t
Methysergide, 734
Metoclopramide, 258, 264
Metoprolol, 83, 110, 519, 733, 1019
Metronidazole, 277, 606, 607, 616, 707
Metyrosine, 532
Mexiletine, 69, 70, 71, 871
Microangiopathies, thrombotic, 421–422
Micropolyspora, 880
   in disease etiology, 8t
Microscopic polyangiitis, 668, 669, 908
Microsporidiosis, with human immunodeficiency virus, 487–488
Midodrine, 753
Migraine, 732–733
Military camps, in disease etiology, 8t
Military tuberculosis, *857*
Milk, as cause of food allergy, 27
Milrinone, 115, 116
Mineralocorticoid replacement, 220, 222
Minimal change nephropathy, 670–671
Minocycline, 880, 949, 992
Minor allergic reaction, 459
Minoxidil, 520
Misoprostol, 682
Mississippi River valley, in disease etiology, 8t
Mitochondrial mutations, 373
Mitomycin, 907, 909
Mitral stenosis, severity of, by valve area, 46t
Mitral valve disease, 908–909
Mixed acid-base disorders, 151–152, 700
Mixed connective tissue disease, 993
Mixed cryoglobulinemia, 906–907, 948
Mixed venous oxygen saturation, 148
Molluscum contagiosum, 184
Monday morning sickness, 880
   etiologic factor, 8t
Monoamine oxidase inhibitors, 404, 514, 752, 834, 835
Monoclonal gammopathies, 433–436, 675
   amyloidosis, 435–436, 675
   light chain deposition disease, 675
   multiple myeloma, 434–435, 675
   solitary plasmacytomas, 435
   of undetermined significance, 434
   Waldenström macroglobulinemia, 435
Monocytes, in asthma, 13t
Mononeuritis multiplex, 669

Mononeuropathy multiplex, 742
Mononucleosis-like syndromes, 573t
Montelukast, 16, 16t
Mood disorders, 824–827
   adjustment disorder with depressed mood, 825
   caused by general medical condition, 826–827
   dysthymia, 825
   major depression, 824–826
   mania, bipolar disorder, 826
   pharmacotherapy, 826
   psychotherapy, 825–826
   seasonal affective disorder, 824–825
   substance-induced mood disorders, 827
   treatment of depression, 825
Moraxella, 558
Moraxella catarrhalis, 396, 913
Moricizine, 72
Morphea, 181
Mortality
   in United States, causes, 808t
Motility patterns, 255
Movement disorders, 751–753
   botulinum toxin therapy, 753
   tremor, 751–753
      essential tremor, 751–752
      Parkinson disease, 752–753t
Moxalactam, 610
Moxifloxacin, 623
MRI. *See* Magnetic resonance imaging
Mucocutaneous ulceration, 481
Mucormycosis, 24, 571, 928
Muehrcke lines, 184
Multifactorial causation
   conditions, 374t
   DNA analysis, 373–374t
Multiple endocrine neoplasia, 241, 365
   islet cell neoplasia, 241
   marfanoid appearance, *539*
   MEN II, 241
      genetics, 241
   oral neurinomas associated with, *539*
   pituitary tumors, 241
   primary hyperparathyroidism, 241
   screening for, 241
Multiple myeloma, 434–435, 675
Multiple sclerosis, 256, 726
Multisensory dizziness, 737, 738
Mumps, 578
Mumps vaccine, 816
Murmurs, 41
   maneuvers altering, 41–47
Muscle weakness, causes, 747t
Muscles, reflexes and, 792t
Myalgia, 481
Myalgias, 669
Myambutol, 923
Myasthenia gravis, 256, 744
Myasthenic syndrome, 744, 789

Mycobacterial, fungal joint infections, 1000
Mycobacterial diseases, 560–563, 916–927
   Mycobacterium tuberculosis, 560–563, 916–922, 919–920t, 921t, 922t, 923t, 924t
      clinical disease, 560
      extrapulmonary tuberculosis, 561
      screening for tuberculosis, 561–563
      treatment of latent tuberculosis infection, 563
      treatment of pulmonary tuberculosis, 560–562t
   nontuberculous mycobacteria, 922–926
   toxicity from antituberculous drugs, 926–927
      ethambutol, 926
      isoniazid, 926
      pyrazinamide, 926
      rifampin, 926
      streptomycin, 926–927
Mycobacterium avium complex, 3
   with human immunodeficiency virus, 483–484
      Cryptococcus neoformans, 484
Mycobacterium tuberculosis, 560–563, 813, 916–922, 919–920t, 921t, 922t, 923t, 924t
   clinical disease, 560
   extrapulmonary tuberculosis, 561
   latent tuberculosis infection, treatment, 563
   pulmonary tuberculosis, treatment, 560–562t
   screening for, 561–563
   treatment, 560–562t, 563
Mycophenolate mofetil, 672, 674, 744, 746
Mycoplasma infection, 5, 914
Mycoplasma pneumonia, 5, 418–419, 566–567
   infectious mononucleosis, 419
Mycoplasmosis, disease etiology, 8t
Myectomy, 110
Myelodysplastic syndromes, 438
Myelofibrosis, 440–441
Myelogenous leukemia, 436–440
   acute, 436–437
   chronic, *478*
Myeloma, 676
Myeloproliferative disorders, 440–442
   erythrocytosis, 442, 443t
   essential thrombocythemia, 441
   features, 441t
   myelofibrosis, 440–441
Myocardial disease, abnormal diastolic function in, 110t
Myocardial ischemia, perioperative, monitoring for, 341
Myoglobinuria, 707
Myopathies, classification, 745t
Myotonic dystrophy, 256, 365, 367
Myxedema, 274

N

Nadolol, 519
Nafcillin, 606, 608
Nail clues, to systemic disease, 183–184
Nalidixic acid, 607, 690
Naproxen, 733
Naratriptan, 732
Narcotics, 274, 734
Nasal polyposis, 21, 24
Nasal septal deviation, 21
Nasogastric tube, removal, 659
Nateglinide, 236
National Childhood Vaccine Act, 814
National Cholesterol Education Program
        Guidelines, 232
Native valve infective endocarditis, 581,
        582t, 584–585t
    treatment, 584–585t
Natural penicillins, 605
Nausea, vomiting, 481
Necrobiosis lipoidica diabeticorum, 182,
        196
Necrobiotic xanthogranuloma, 182
Necrolytic migratory erythema, 176, 194
Necrotizing sinusitis, 669
Nedocromil, 16
    for asthma, 16t
Nefazodone, 834
Neisseria, 558, 589–591
Neisseria meningitidis, 757
Nelfinavir, 492
Nelfinavir-saquinavir combination, 493
Neomycin, 690
Neoplasia, 676, 726
Neoplastic disease, 750–751
    as cause of eosinophilia, 31
Nephritic syndrome, 666
Nephritis
    interstitial, common causes, 678t
    renal insufficiency, 678
Nephrogenic diabetes insipidus, 694, 694t
Nephrology, 179, 665–719
    acid-base disorders, 695–701
        delta gap, 700–701
        metabolic acidosis, 695–698t
        metabolic alkalosis, 698–699, 699
        mixed acid-base disorders, 700
        respiratory acidosis, 699–700
        respiratory alkalosis, 700, 700t
    acute interstitial nephritis, 677–678t
    acute renal failure, 681–687
        diagnosis of, 685t, 685–686
        dialysis, 686–687
        intrinsic acute renal failure, 683t,
            683–684
        management of, 686–687
        postrenal failure, 684–685
        prerenal failure, 681–683
            due to liver disease, 682–683

analgesic chronic interstitial nephritis,
        678–679
    chronic renal failure, 687t, 687–690
        complications of dialysis, 689–690t
        dialysis, 689
        uremia, 688–689
    cystic renal disease, 680–681
        autosomal dominant polycystic kidney
            disease, 680
        medullary sponge kidney, 680–681
    diabetes insipidus, 693–694
        polyuria, 693–694
            central diabetes insipidus, 693–694
            nephrogenic diabetes insipidus, 694,
                694t
    diabetic nephropathy, 673t, 673–674
    electrolyte disorders, 691
    electrolyte-induced interstitial nephritis,
        679–680
    GBM abnormalities, diseases with,
        676–677
        Alport syndrome, 676–677
        thin GBM disease, 677
    glomerular disease with nephritic
        syndrome, 666–668
        Henoch-Schönlein purpura, 667
        IgA nephropathy, 666–667
        membranoproliferative
            glomerulonephritis, 667–668
        poststreptococcal glomerulonephritis,
            666
    glomerular disease with nephrotic
        syndrome, 670–673
        focal segmental glomerulosclerosis,
            671–672
        human immunodeficiency virus-
            associated nephropathy, 672–673
        minimal change nephropathy, 670–671
    glomerular disorders, 673–675
    glomerular injury, clinical manifestations,
        665–666
        nephritic syndrome, 666
        nephrotic syndrome, 665–666
    glomerulonephritis with hepatitis C virus
        infection, 675–676
        cryoglobulinemic glomerulonephritis,
            675–676t
    hemolytic uremic syndrome,
        thrombocytopenic purpura, 676
    kidney function, evaluation, 707–708
        renal imaging, 708
        urinalysis, 707t, 707–708
    monoclonal gammopathies, 675
        amyloidosis, 675
        light chain deposition disease, 675
        multiple myeloma, 675
    percentage of board examination devoted
        to, 2
    potassium balance disorders, 695
        hyperkalemia, 695, 695t, 696

hypokalemia, 695, 695t, 696
    pregnancy, kidney in, 706–707
        acute renal failure in pregnancy, 707
        parenchymal renal disease in
            pregnancy, 707
        urinary tract infections, 707
    rapidly progressive glomerulonephritis,
        668–670, 669
        ANCA vasculitides, 668t, 668–670
            Churg-Strauss syndrome, 669–670
            microscopic polyangiitis, 669
            myalgias, arthralgias, 669
            polyarteritis nodosa, 670
            Wegener granulomatosis, 669
        Goodpasture disease, 670
    sodium balance, disorders, 694
    systemic lupus erythematosus nephritis,
        674t, 674–675
    transplantation, 705–706
        graft failure, 706
        immunosuppression, 706, 706
        recurrent allograft renal disease, 706
    tubulointerstitial renal disease, clinical
        manifestations, 677
    urolithiasis, 702–705
        calcium oxalate stones, 703–704, 704
        calcium phosphate stones, 704
        cystine stones, 705
        drug-induced stone disease, 705, 705t
        epidemiology, 702, 702, 703
        inhibitors of crystallization, 705
        metabolic activity, 703, 704t
        risk factors, 702–703t
        struvite stones, 704–705
        uric acid stones, 704
        urolithiasis, bowel disease, 705
    water balance, disorders, 691–693
        hypernatremia, 692–693, 693
        hyponatremia, 691–692, 692
            diagnosis, 691
            euvolemic hyponatremia, 692
            hypervolemic hyponatremia, 692
            hypovolemic hyponatremia, 691–692
            therapy for hyponatremia, 691
Nephropathy, diabetic, stages, 673t
Nephrotic syndrome, 232, 665–666
Neural tube defect, 730
Neuroarthropathy, 956
Neurocutaneous, 179–180
Neurofibromatosis, 180, 195, 365,
        367–368
    type 1, 367
    type 2, 367–368
Neurologic infectious diseases, 755–758
    acquired immunodeficiency syndrome,
        neurologic complications, 755–757
    Lyme disease, 755
    organ transplantation, neurologic
        complications, 758
        CNS infections, 758

lymphoproliferative diseases, de novo, CNS involvement by, 758
sepsis, neurology, 757–758
  critical illness polyneuropathy, 757–758
  septic encephalopathy, 757
Neurologic signs, symptoms, 721–722
  diffuse cerebral symptoms, 721
  findings in elderly, 722
  ill-defined symptoms, 721
  localization, 722
  negative phenomena, 722
  positive phenomena, 721–722
Neurology, 721–774
  cerebrovascular disease, 746–749
    ischemic cerebrovascular disease, 746–749
      antiplatelet agents, 748
      carotid endarterectomy, 748
      management of acute cerebral infarction, 748–749
      pathophysiologic mechanisms, 746–747
      risk factors, 747
      stroke risks with nonvalvular atrial fibrillation, 749
      transient ischemic attacks, 747–748
  cervical cord, 723
  dementia, 723
  disk disease, 723
  EEG, 724
  electromyographic nerve conduction velocity studies, 723–724
  evoked potentials, 724
  hemorrhagic cerebrovascular disease, 749–750
    cerebellar hemorrhage, 749–750
    intracerebral hemorrhage, 749
    subarachnoid hemorrhage, 750, 750t
  inflammatory, immune disorders, 753–755
    demyelinating diseases, 753–754
    paraneoplastic disorders, 754–755
  intracranial tumors, 723
  lumbar puncture
    cerebrospinal fluid analysis, 724–725
    contraindications for, 725
    indications for, 724–725
  movement disorders, 751–753
    botulinum toxin therapy, 753
    tremor, 751–753
      essential tremor, 751–752
      Parkinson disease, 752–753t
  neoplastic disease, 750–751
  neurologic infectious diseases, 755–758
    acquired immunodeficiency syndrome, neurologic complications, 755–757
    Lyme disease, 755

organ transplantation, neurologic complications, 758
  CNS infections, 758
  lymphoproliferative diseases, de novo, CNS involvement by, 758
sepsis, neurology, 757–758
  critical illness polyneuropathy, 757–758
  septic encephalopathy, 757
neurologic signs, symptoms, 721–722
  diffuse cerebral symptoms, 721
  findings in elderly, 722
  ill-defined symptoms, 721
  localization, 722
  negative phenomena, 722
  positive phenomena, 721–722
percentage of board examination devoted to, 2
peripheral level, symptoms, clinical correlations, 740–746
  acute muscle weakness, 746, 747t
  muscle disease, 745t, 745–746
    acute alcoholic myopathy, 746
    electrolyte imbalance, 746
    endocrine diseases, 746
    inflammatory myopathy, 745–746
    toxic myopathies, 746
  neuropathy, 740–741t, 740–745
    acute motor neuropathy, 742
    autonomic neuropathy, 743–744
    botulism, 744–745
    chronic predominantly motor neuropathies, 743
    clinical scenarios, 742–743
    diabetic neuropathy, 744
    mononeuropathy, 742
    mononeuropathy multiplex, 742
    myasthenia gravis, 744
    myasthenic syndrome, 744
    neuromuscular transmission disorders, 744
    organophosphate toxicity, 745
    painful neuropathy, 743
    sensory ataxic neuropathy, 743
posterior fossa level, symptoms, clinical correlations, 736–738
  brainstem lesions, 736
  cerebellar lesions, 736
  dizziness, 736–738
  vertigo, 736–738
    disequilibrium, 738
    multisensory dizziness, 738
    physiologic dizziness, 737
    presyncopal light-headedness, 737–738
    psychophysiologic dizziness, 738
spinal level, symptoms, clinical correlations, 738–740
  anterior horn cell disease, 739
  degenerative disease of spine, 739–740

  cervical spondylosis, 739
  lumbar spine disease, 739–740
  radiculopathy, 739
  spinal cord disease-related weakness, 738–739
supratentorial level, symptoms, clinical correlations, 725–736
  anticonvulsant therapy, 729
    anticonvulsant blood levels, 730–731
    status epilepticus, 731, 732
    surgery for epilepsy, 731
  consciousness, disorders, 725–726
    acute confusional states, 726
    stupor, coma, 725–726
  dementia, 726t, 726–727
    anticonvulsant therapy, 728–730t
    causes, 728
    clinical scenarios, 727
    seizure disorders, 728t, 728–729
  headache, facial pain, 731–735
    clinical scenarios, 734
    cluster headache, 733–734
    glossopharyngeal neuralgia, 735
    medication-overuse headache, 734–735
    migraine and tension headache, 732–733
    temporal arteritis, 735
    trigeminal neuralgia, 735
  intracranial lesions, 735–736
    cortical lesions, 736
    leptomeningeal lesions, 735
    parasagittal lesions, 735–736
  ventricular system, 736
    hydrocephalus, 736
trauma, 723
vascular diseases, 722t, 722–723
white matter lesions, 723
Neuromuscular transmission disorders, 744
Neuropathy, peripheral, 669
Neurosyphilis, 726
Neutropenia, 456, 598, 603
  febrile, 791
Neutrophil chemotaxis, in asthma, 13t
Neutrophil maturation, in asthma, 13t
Nevirapine, 606
NHL. See Non-Hodgkin lymphoma
Niacin, 233, 349
Nicardipine, 522, 538
Nickel, 880
  chrome, as cause of asthma, 14t
  in disease etiology, 8t
Nicotine, 532, 833
Nicotinic acid, 349
Nifedipine, 105, 522
Nisoldipine, 522
Nitrates, 110, 115, 116, 118
Nitrofurantoin, 690, 880
Nitrogen dioxide, 880
  in disease etiology, 8t

Nitroglycerin, 104, 258, 538
Nitroprusside, sodium, 1019
NNRTIs. *See* Nonnucleoside reverse
    transcriptase inhibitors
Nocardia asteroides, 632
Nocardia pneumonia, 915–916
Nocardiosis, 565–566
Nonabandonment, 655–656
Nonacetylated salicylates, 14, 975
Nonalcoholic fatty liver disease, 302
Nonarticular rheumatism, 958–961
    bursitis, 960
    features, 961, 961t
    fibromyalgia, 958
        diagnosis, 958–959
        natural history, 959
    giant cell arteritis, relationship to, 961
    low back pain, 959–960
        diagnosis, 959, 960t
        treatment, 959–960
    nonarticular rheumatism, fibromyalgia,
        958–959
    polymyalgia rheumatica, 960–961
    treatment, 961
Nondihydropyridines, 522
Nonfibrogenic pneumoconioses, 880
    disease etiology, 8t
Nongonococcal acute bacterial arthritis,
    600
Nongonococcal urethritis, 591
Non-Hodgkin lymphoma, 430–433t,
    488–489
    treatment strategies for, 433t
Noninfectious pulmonary complications in
    acquired immunodeficiency
    syndrome, 930
Nonlymphocytic leukemia, acute, *478*
Nonmaleficence, 655–657
    conflict of interest, 656
    double effect, principle, 656
    impaired physician, 656
    incurable disease, death, 656–657
    nonabandonment, 655–656
    vs. beneficence, in principle of double
        effect, 656
Nonnucleoside reverse transcriptase
    inhibitors, 489, 490–492t, 606, 922
    general characteristics, 492t
Nonrheumatic atrial fibrillation
    management, 85t
    thromboembolism, risk factors for, 85t
Non–small-cell lung cancer, 781–782
Nonspecific back symptoms, 352
Nonspecific interstitial pneumonia, 889
Nonsteroidal anti-inflammatory drugs, 14,
    101, 209, 388, 389, 394, 514, 671,
    678, 681, 684, 686, 688, 696, 734,
    735, 872, 972–975, 992
    gastrointestinal side effects of NSAIDs,
        974–975

mechanisms of action of NSAIDs,
    972–973
mechanisms of toxicity of NSAIDs,
    973–974t
other toxic effects of NSAIDs, 975
side effects, 974t
ulcers induced by, 261–262
    duodenal ulcer, 262
    gastric ulcer, 262
Nonthiazide diuretics, 705
Nontuberculous mycobacteria, 922–926
    classification, 925t
Nonulcer dyspepsia, 260
Nonvalvular atrial fibrillation, stroke risks
    with, 749
Noonan syndrome, 365
Norepinephrine, 839
Norepinephrine reuptake inhibitors, 834
Norfloxacin, 271, 871
Normal-pressure hydrocephalus, 726
Nosocomial pneumonia, 916
NSAIDs. *See* Nonsteroidal anti-
    inflammatory drugs
NSCLC. *See* Non–small-cell lung cancer
n-TPA, 106
Nucleotide analogue reverse transcriptase
    inhibitors, 489–490, 491t
Nutrition, 343
Nutrition, percentage of board examination
    devoted to, 2
Nuts, as cause of food allergy, 27
Nystatin, 259, 487

O

Oak, as cause of asthma, 14
Obesity, 232
Obliterative endarteropathy, 971
Obsessive-compulsive disorder, 829
Obstetrics, percentage of board examination
    devoted to, 2
Obstruction, 687
Obstructive azoospermia, 877
Obstructive liver disease, 232
Obstructive lung diseases, 866t, 866–868
    etiology, 867
    pathology, 867–868
    physiology, 868
Occupational asthma, 13–14t, 880
Occupational health, percentage of board
    examination devoted to, 2
Ochronosis, 707, 954
Octreotide, 201, 203, 204, 269
Ocular albinism, 372
Ocular dizziness, 737
Oculocutaneous albinism, 369
Oculopharyngeal myopathy, 256
Ofloxacin, 923
Ohio River valley, in disease etiology, 8t
Olanzapine, 752, 753, 835, 837
Olmesartan, 522

Olsalazine, 276
Omega–3 fatty acids, 667
Oncogenesis, 444, 445t
Oncologic complications, emergencies,
    790–792
    febrile neutropenia, 791
    hypercalcemia, 790–791
    spinal cord compression, 791–792t
    tumor lysis syndrome, 791
Oncology, 775–806
    breast cancer, 775–779
        clinical scenarios, 779
        magnitude of problem, 775
        natural history, 776–777
            grade, 777
            hormone receptor status, 777
            nodal status, 776, 777
            tumor size, 776–777t
        pathology, 776, *776*
        risk factors, 775, 775t
        screening, 775
        staging, 776, 776t
        treatment, 777–779
            adjuvant treatment, 778, 778t
            chemotherapy, 778
            herceptin, 779
            hormonal agents, 778
            primary or local-regional therapy,
                777
            treatment of advanced disease, 778
            zoledronic acid, pamidronate, 779
    cervical cancer, 779
        background, 779
        treatment, 779
    chemotherapy, 789–790
        applications, 789
        basic concepts, 789, *789*
        colony-stimulating factors, 790
        mechanisms of tumor cell drug
            resistance, 790
        side effects, 790
        solid tumors sensitive to chemotherapy,
            789
        why chemotherapy fails to cure most
            advanced solid tumors, 790
    colorectal cancer, 779–781
        background, 779
        carcinoembryonic antigen, 780
        clinical scenarios, 781
        risk factors, 779–780
        treatment, 780
            adjuvant therapy, 780
            metastatic disease, 780
            surgery, 780, 780t
    lung cancer, 781–783
        clinical scenarios, 783
        histologic types, 781
        magnitude of problem, 781
        natural history, 781, *782*
        risk factors, 781

screening, 781
staging, 781, 782t
treatment, 781–782
chemotherapy for NSCLC, 782
non–small-cell lung cancer, 781–782
small-cell lung cancer, 782
melanoma, 783
background, 783
clinical scenarios, 783
diagnosis, prognosis, 783, 783t
management, 783
oncologic complications, emergencies, 790–792
febrile neutropenia, 791
hypercalcemia, 790–791
spinal cord compression, 791–792t
tumor lysis syndrome, 791
ovarian cancer, 783–784
CA 125, 784
clinical scenario, 784
outcome, 784
screening, 784
staging, 784
treatment, 784
palliative care, 792
background, 792
evaluation, 792
treatment, 792
general principles, 792
three-tiered approach, 792
paraneoplastic syndromes, 788–789
carcinoid syndrome, 788–789
dermatomyositis, 789
general, 788, 788t
Lambert-Eaton syndrome, 789
prostate cancer, 784–786
background, 784
clinical scenarios, 786
management, 785–786
androgen deprivation, 786
bisphosphonates, 786
chemotherapy, 786
management of stages, 785
prostatectomy, 785
radiation therapy, 785–786
prostate-specific antigen, 784–785t
testicular cancer, 786–787
background, 786–787
extragonadal germ cell tumor, 787
management, 787, 787t
staging, 787
unknown primary lesion, 787–788
background, 787–788
treatment, 788
Onycholysis, 183
Opening snap, heart sounds, 41
Ophthalmology, percentage of board examination devoted to, 2
Opioids, 624, 833
Opisthorchis infection, 306

Oral procedures, American Heart Association prophylactic regimens, 588t
Orbital infection, with sinusitis, 23
Organ transplantation, neurologic complications
CNS infections, 758
lymphoproliferative diseases, de novo, CNS involvement by, 758
Organophosphate toxicity, 745
Oropharyngeal dysphagia, causes, 256, 256t
Orthopedics, percentage of board examination devoted to, 2
Oseltamivir, 606, 631
Osler-Weber-Rendu disease, 365
Osler-Weber-Rendu syndrome, 178
Osmotic diarrhea, secretory diarrhea, features differentiating, 267t
Osteoarthritis, 387–388, 952–958, 957
clinical features, 952–953
clinical subsets, 953–954
primary, 953–954
diffuse idiopathic skeletal hyperostosis, 953
erosive, 953
generalized, 953
isolated hip, 953
isolated nodal, 953
pathogenesis of, 952
radiographic features of, 957, 957
secondary, 954–957
therapy for, 957–958t
Osteogenesis imperfecta, 59, 365, 368, 955
Osteoid osteoma, 987
Osteomalacia, 218–219
clinical features, 218
in elderly, 398
therapy, 218–219
Osteomyelitis, 600–601
with sinusitis, 23
Osteophytes, cervical, 256
Osteoporosis, 216–218
clinical features, 217
diagnosis, 217
in elderly, 397–398
etiology, 217
prevention, treatment, 217–218
Otitis media, 911–912
Ovarian cancer, 783–784
CA 125, 784
clinical scenario, 784
mortality, 808
outcome, 784
screening, 784, 812–813
staging, 784
treatment, 784
Ovary, 227–230. See also Ovarian cancer
amenorrhea, 227–228
clinical features, 227
diagnosis, 227–228

disorders associated with, 228
anorexia nervosa, 228
Turner 45/XO gonadal dysgenesis, 228
estrogen replacement therapy, 228
etiology, 227
ovulation induction, 228
primary amenorrhea, 227, 228
secondary amenorrhea, 227–228
therapy, 228
androgens in normal females, 228–229
hirsutism, 229–230
clinical features, 229
diagnosis, 229
etiology, 229
idiopathic hirsutism, 229
late-onset congenital adrenal hyperplasia, 230
polycystic ovarian syndrome, 229–230
selected hyperandrogenic states, 229–230
therapy, 230
virilizing tumors of ovary, adrenal gland, 230
virilization, 229–230
Overdoses, dialysis, 690t
Overlap syndromes, 993
mixed connective tissue disease, 993
undifferentiated connective tissue disease, 993
Oxacillin, 606, 608
Oxalate, 705
Oxcarbazepine, 727, 729, 730
Oxygen, 873
Oxypurinol stones, 705

P

Pacemaker implantation, indications for, 77t
Pacemaker syndrome, 75
Pacemaker-mediated tachycardia, 76
Pacing, code, 76t
Paget disease, 176, 219
clinical features, 219
diagnosis, 219
extramammary, 176
therapy, 219
Painful neuropathy, 743
Palliative care, 255, 792
background, 792
evaluation, 792
percentage of board examination devoted to, 2
treatment, 792
general principles, 792
three-tiered approach, 792
Palpable purpura, differential diagnosis, 972t
Pamidronate, 215, 779
Pancoast tumor, 859
Pancreas, 287–291

Pancreas *(contd.)*
  acute, 287
    assessment of severity, 289, 289t
    clinical presentation, 287–288
    complications, 289
    diagnosis of acute pancreatitis, 288
    etiologic factors, 287
    treatment, 288–289
  chronic, 289–290
    cystic fibrosis, 291
    laboratory diagnosis, 290
    malabsorption, 290
    pain, 290
    pancreatic carcinoma, 290–291
    pancreatic endocrine tumors, 291
    triad, 290
  classification, 287
  embryology, 287
Pancreatic cancer, 290
  mortality, 808
Pancreatic enzymes
  in blood, 669
  as cause of asthma, 14
Panic disorders, with or without
      agoraphobia, 828
Panlobular emphysema, *855*
PaO2, calculation, 148
Papillary thyroid carcinoma, 212
Para-aminosalicylic acid, 880
Paraneoplastic syndromes, 788–789, 897
  carcinoid syndrome, 788–789
  classification, 788t
  dermatomyositis, 789
  general, 788, 788t
  Lambert-Eaton syndrome, 789
Parasagittal lesions, 735–736
Parasites, 678
Parasitic diseases, 578–580, 879, 929
  helminths, 578–579
  protozoan parasites, 579–580
Parapoxvirus infection, 465
Parenchymal renal disease in pregnancy,
      707
Pargyline, 834
Parkinson disease, 256, 274, 385, 752–753t
  dementia with, 393
  treatment, 753t
Paromomycin, 487
Paroxetine, 834
Paroxysmal cold hemoglobinuria, 419
Paroxysmal nocturnal dyspnea, 848
Paroxysmal nocturnal hemoglobinuria, 420
Parvovirus B19, 578
Pasteurella multocida, 556–557
Pathophysiologic mechanisms, 746–747
Patient autonomy, 649–655
  advance directive, 650–652
  confidentiality, 654
  conflicts, 652
  disclosure, 653

    durable power of attorney for health care,
        651
    futility, 654–655
    implied consent, 653
    informed consent, 652–653
    justifiable parentalism, 653–654
    living will, 651
    Patient Self-Determination Act of 1990,
        652
    preservation, 650
    right to, 659
    surrogate, 651–652
Patient feedback module, 7–9
Patient Self-Determination Act of 1990,
      652
Patterns of inheritance, 364–373
  autosomal dominant, 364–368
    Ehlers-Danlos syndrome, 365
    hypertrophic cardiomyopathy, 365–366
    Marfan syndrome, 366–367
    myotonic dystrophy, 367
    neurofibromatosis, 367–368
      type 1, 367
      type 2, 367–368
    osteogenesis imperfecta, 368
    tuberous sclerosis, 368
    von Hippel-Lindau disease, 368
  autosomal recessive, 368–371
    Friedreich ataxia, 369
    Gaucher disease, 369–370
    glycogen storage diseases, 370
    homocystinuria, 370–371
    pseudoxanthoma elasticum, 371
    Refsum disease, 371
    Tay-Sachs disease, 371
  X-linked recessive, 371–373
    Duchenne, Becker muscular
        dystrophies, 372
    Fabry disease, 373
PCP. *See* Phencyclidine
Peanuts, as cause of food allergy, 27
PEEP in mechanical ventilation, 154
Pegvisomant, 204
Pelvic inflammatory disease, 593–594
  Trichomonas vaginalis, 593–594
Pemphigus, 174
Pemphigus foliaceus, *193*
Penbutolol, 519
Penetrating aortic ulcer, 1018–1019
Penicillamine, 907, 992
Penicillin, 30, 175, 176, 551, 554, 556, 557,
      583, 585, 604, 606–609, 678, 880
  adverse reactions to, 609
  allergy, 30–31
  aminopenicillins, 605–606
  beta-lactam/beta-lactamase inhibitors,
      607–609
  carboxypenicillins, 607
  as cause of asthma, 14
  microorganisms, 608t

    microorganisms for which penicillin is
        drug of choice, 608t
    natural penicillins, 605
    penicillinase-resistant penicillins,
        606–607
    ureidopenicillins, 607
Penicillin G, 553, 558, 564, 605, 608
Penicillin V, 605, 608
Penicillinase-resistant penicillins,
      606–607
Pentamidine, 482
Pentazocine, 404
Peptococcus, 559
Peptostreptococcus, 559
Pergolide, 753
Pericardial disease, 53–55
  constrictive pericarditis, 54–55
    diagnosis, 55
    physical examination, 55
    symptoms, 54–55
  inflammatory pericarditis, 54
    causes, 54
    diagnosis, 54
    presenting symptoms, 54
  pericardial effusion, 54
    clinical features, 54
    treatment, 54
Perioperative antibiotic prophylaxis,
      343–345
Perioperative medical therapy, 341
  geriatrics patients, 346
Peripheral arterial aneurysms, 1023
Peripheral arterial occlusive disease,
      1020–1023
  acute arterial occlusion, 1022–1023
  intermittent claudication, 1020–1022
    cardiac risk, vascular surgery, 1022
    clinical features, 1020, 1020t
    diagnosis, 1021
    natural history, 1021
    pseudoclaudication, 1020–1021t
    treatment, 1021–1022
  peripheral arterial aneurysms, 1023
Peripheral level, symptoms, clinical
      correlations, 740–746
  acute muscle weakness, 746, 747t
  muscle disease, 745t, 745–746
    acute alcoholic myopathy, 746
    electrolyte imbalance, 746
    endocrine diseases, 746
    inflammatory myopathy, 745–746
    toxic myopathies, 746
  neuropathy, 740–741t, 740–745
    acute motor neuropathy, 742
    autonomic neuropathy, 743–744
    botulism, 744–745
    chronic predominantly motor
        neuropathies, 743
    clinical scenarios, 742–743
    diabetic neuropathy, 744

mononeuropathy, 742
mononeuropathy multiplex, 742
myasthenia gravis, 744
myasthenic syndrome, 744
neuromuscular transmission disorders, 744
organophosphate toxicity, 745
painful neuropathy, 743
sensory ataxic neuropathy, 743
Peripheral neuropathy, 481
clinical features, differential diagnosis, 740t
evaluation, 742t
Permanent pacing, code, 76t
Pernio, chronic, lesions, *1026*
Persistent vegetative state, 658–660, 725
Peutz-Jeghers syndrome, 179
Pharyngitis, 481, 912
Phenacetin, 679
Phencyclidine, 827, 833
Phenelzine, 834
Phenobarbital, 706, 727, 729, 871
Phenothiazine, 532, 690, 707
Phenothiazines, 175, 176, 274
Phenotype, 379
Phenoxybenzamine, 224, 532
Phentolamine, 538
Phenylglycine acid chloride, as cause of asthma, 14
Phenylketonuria, 369
Phenytoin, 53, 69, 211, 624, 678, 690, 706, 727, 729, 730, 731, 735, 880, 992
Pheochromocytoma, 223–224, 530–532
clinical features, 223
diagnosis, 223–224
treatment, 531–532
etiology, 223
screening, 531, 532t
symptoms, 531
therapy, 224
Phosphodiesterase inhibitors, 115, 116, 870–871
Phthalic anhydrides, as cause of asthma, 14
Physical urticaria, 26
Physician-assisted suicide, 659
euthanasia, 657–658
Pick disease, 393, 726
PIE syndrome, drugs causing, 880
Pilocarpine, 386
Piperacillin, 554
Pirbuterol, 16, 869
for asthma, 16t
Pitting, 183
Pituitary apoplexy, 204
Pituitary incidentaloma, 204
Pituitary tumors, 200–201
drug therapy, 201
follow-up, 201
radiotherapy, 201
surgery, 201

treatment, 201
Plague, 556–557, 604
disease etiology, 8t
Pasteurella multocida, 556–557
Plain chest radiography, pulmonary disease, 849–851, *852–861*
Plants, in disease etiology, 8t
Plaquenil, 992
Plasma cell, *477*
Plasmacytomas, solitary, 435
Plasmapheresis, 676
Plasmodium falciparum, *632*, 678
Plastics, as cause of asthma, 14t
Platinum, 880
in disease etiology, 8t
Pleural biopsy, 884
Pleural effusion, 881–884
amylase, 883
causes, 882t
cell counts, 883
chylous effusion, 883
complement, 883
complications, 884
cultures, 883–884
cytology, 883
glucose, pH, 882
pleural biopsy, 884
transudate *versus* exudate, 882, 882t
Plexiform neurofibroma, *195*
Plicatic acid. *See* Western red cedar
PML. *See* Progressive multifocal leukoencephalopathy
Pneumococcal disease vaccine, 818
Pneumocystis, 481, 482
Pneumocystis carinii, 929
Pneumocystis pneumonia
drugs used for treatment, 482t
with human immunodeficiency virus, 481–482t
prophylaxis of, drugs used for, 482t
Polio, 256
Polio vaccine, 819
Poliovirus, 576
Pollen, 23
rhinitis, 23
Polyarteritis, 964–967
clinical features, 965, 965t
diagnosis, 966, *966*
outcome, 966–967
pathology, 964–965
treatment, 966
Polyarteritis nodosa, 668, 670, 907, *966*
Polychondritis
in diagnosis of wheezing, 16
relapsing, 178
Polycystic kidney disease, 365, 687
Polycythemia rubra vera, 442–444
Polyenes, 627
amphotericin B products, 627
Polymerase chain reaction, 377, *378*

Polymyalgia rheumatica, 389, 960–961
Polymyalgia-like syndrome, systemic illnesses presenting with, 961t
Polyuria, 693–694
central diabetes insipidus, 693–694
nephrogenic diabetes insipidus, 694, 694t
Polyvinyl chloride, as cause of asthma, 14
Popcorn calcification, of hamartoma, *861*
Popliteal artery entrapment, 1024
Porphyria, 183, 365, 461, 462t, 707
acute, intermittent, 462
comparison, 462t
Porphyria cutanea tarda, *196*, 462
Porphyria variegata, 462
Portal systemic encephalopathy, grading system for, 309t
Positron emission tomography, 64
Postcardiotomy syndrome, 101
Posterior fossa level, symptoms, clinical correlations, 736–738
brainstem lesions, 736
cerebellar lesions, 736
vertigo, dizziness, 736–738
disequilibrium, 738
multisensory dizziness, 738
physiologic dizziness, 737
presyncopal light-headedness, 737–738
psychophysiologic dizziness, 738
vertigo, 736–737
Postexposure prophylaxis, human immunodeficiency virus, antiretroviral agents, 495
Postinfectious encephalomyelitis, 756
Postpartum thyroiditis, 208–209
Postphlebitic syndrome, 1030, *1030*
Postproctoscopic purpura, *195*
Postrenal failure, 684–685
Postsplenectomy state, 459
Poststreptococcal glomerulonephritis, 666
Post-transfusion purpura, 459t
Post-traumatic stress disorder, 828
Postural tremor, 751
Posture, 41
Potassium, 237, 695
balance disorders, 695
hyperkalemia, 695, 695t, *696*
hypokalemia, 695, 695t, *696*
supplements, 259
Potassium chloride, 237, 695
Potassium-sparing diuretics, 688
with hypertension, 517–518
Pramipexole, 753
Prednisone, 16t, 21, 220, 389, 674, 675, 676, 734, 735, 744, 746
Preeclampsia-eclampsia, 535–536
Pregnancy
antiretroviral agents, 494–495
cardiac disease, 52–53
delivery, 53
drugs, 53

Pregnancy, cardiac disease *(contd.)*
  hypertension, 53
  physiologic changes of pregnancy, 52–53
  prosthetic valves, 53
  hypertension in, 533–536
    chronic hypertension in pregnancy, 535
    definition, 534–535
    hypertensive crisis, 536
    preeclampsia-eclampsia, 535–536
  kidney in, 706–707
    acute renal failure in pregnancy, 707
    parenchymal renal disease in pregnancy, 707
    urinary tract infections, 707
Preload, 113
Preoperative laboratory tests, 345, 345t
Preoperative medical evaluation, 336–346
  anesthesia, risks, 336–338t
  anticoagulation issues, 341–342
  cardiac risks, management, 337–340, *340*
  congestive heart failure, 342
  endocrinologic risks, management, 343
  geriatric surgical patients, 345–346
    perioperative medication management, 346
  hematologic risks, management, 342–343
  hypertension, 342
  liver risks, management, 343
  medical consultation, art, 336
  myocardial ischemia, perioperative, monitoring for, 341
  nutrition, 343
  perioperative antibiotic prophylaxis, 343–345
  perioperative medical therapy, 341
  preoperative laboratory tests, 345, 345t
  pulmonary risks, management, 337
  thromboembolism, prophylaxis, 343, 344t
  valvular heart disease, 341
Prepulmonary embolism, *854*
Prerenal failure, 681–683
  due to liver disease, 682–683
  urinary indices in, 685t
Presbyopia, 386
Preservation of autonomy of patient, 650
Pressure ulcers, in elderly, 398–399
Presyncopal light-headedness, 737–738
Preventive geriatrics, 394–395
  cardiovascular disease, 395
  malignancy, 395
Preventive medicine, 583, 588t, 807–822
  cancer screening, 809–813
    breast cancer, 809–810
    cervical cancer, 812
    colorectal cancer, 810–811
    lung cancer, 809
    ovarian cancer, 812–813
    prostate cancer, 811–812
  immunizations, 814–819, *815*

chemoprophylaxis, 814–819
  vaccines, 814–819
    diphtheria, 814
    hepatitis A, 817
    hepatitis B, 817–818
    influenza, 816–817
    measles, 816
    mumps, 816
    pneumococcal disease, 818
    polio, 819
    rabies, 819
    rubella, 816
    smallpox, 818–819
    tetanus, 814–816
    varicella, 819
  percentage of board examination devoted to, 2
  screening characteristics, 808
  screening for disease, principles, 807–814
  tuberculosis prevention, 813–814
Prevotella, 558–559
Primary aldosteronism, 222–223, 529–530
  clinical features, 222, 529
  diagnosis, 222–223, 529–530
  etiology, 222
  laboratory features, 529
  therapy, 223
Primary central nervous system lymphoma, 489
Primary osteoarthritis, 953–954
Primary polydipsia, diabetes insipidus, comparison, 694t
Primary sclerosing cholangitis, 303
Primary thrombocythemia, 441
Primidone, 729, 752
Principle of double effect, 656
Printers' asthma, 8t
Prion-associated central nervous system diseases, 576–577
Privacy, right to, 659
Proband, 379
Probenecid, 388, 690
Procainamide, 53, 69, 70, 71, 83, 744, 992
Procaine penicillin, 605
Prochlorperazine, 734
Progesterone, 228, 700
Progestins, 232
Progressive multifocal leukoencephalopathy, 576
  with human immunodeficiency virus, 486–487
  Candida albicans, 487
Progressive supranuclear palsy, 726
Prokinetic drugs, 264
Prolactin, 200
Prolactinoma, 201–203
  clinical features, 202
  diagnosis, 202
  differential diagnosis, 202
  dopamine agonists, 202–203

surgical treatment for prolactinomas, 203
  therapy, 202–203
Proliferative/neoplastic disease, as cause of eosinophilia, 31
Promethazine, 737
Promyelocytic leukemia, acute, *478*
Propafenone, 69, 70, 71, 83
Prophylactic regimens, to prevent infective endocarditis, American Heart Association, 588t
Propranolol, 83, 519, 624, 733, 744, 752, 871, 1019
Propylthiouracil, 209, 992
Prostaglandins, 29, 269
Prostate cancer, 784–786
  background, 784
  clinical scenarios, 786
  management, 785–786
    androgen deprivation, 786
    bisphosphonates, 786
    chemotherapy, 786
    management of stages, 785
    prostatectomy, 785
    radiation therapy, 785–786
  prostate-specific antigen, 784–785t
  screening, 811–812
  staging, 785t
Prostate-specific antigen, 225, 784–785t
Prosthetic heart valve, 59–60
  anticoagulation in, 346–347
  bioprostheses, 59–60
  endocarditis, 581, 586t, 586–587t
    organisms causing, 586t
    treatment, 586–587t
  mechanical valves, 60
  systemic embolism, 347
Protease inhibitors, 489, 491–493, 606, 624
  dual protease-inhibitor regimens, 492–493
  general characteristics, 492t
Protein C deficiency, 1027
Protein S deficiency, 1028
Protein synthesis, 607
Proteinuria, 669t
Proteus, 704
Prothrombin 20210 G-A mutation, 1029
Proton pump inhibitors, 258
Protozoan parasites, 579–580
Protriptyline, 834
"Prudent patient test," 659
PSA. *See* Prostate-specific antigen
Pseudoachondroplasia, 955
Pseudoclaudication, 1020–1021t
  claudication, differential diagnosis, 1021t
Pseudoephedrine, 22
Pseudomonas, 183, 238, 704
Pseudomonas aeruginosa, 554–555, 912–913
Pseudo-obstruction, megacolon, 281–282

Pseudoxanthoma elasticum, 178, 365, 369, 371
Psittacosis, disease etiology, 8t
Psoriatic arthritis, 180, 987
Psychiatry, 823–845
    acquired immunodeficiency syndrome, psychologic aspects, 832
    alcoholism, 833–834
    anxiety disorders, 828–829
        adjustment disorder with anxious mood, 829
        generalized anxiety disorder, 828
        obsessive-compulsive disorder, 829
        panic disorder with or without agoraphobia, 828
        post-traumatic stress disorder, 828
    benzodiazepines, sedative-hypnotics and anxiolytics, 834
    delirium, 831
    dementia, 831–832
    eating disorders, 832
        anorexia nervosa, 832
        bulimia, 832
    electroconvulsive therapy, 839
    factitious disorders, 830
    lithium, 837–839
    malingering, 830–831
    mood disorders, 824–827
        major depression, 824–826
            adjustment disorder with depressed mood, 825
            dysthymia, 825
            pharmacotherapy, 826
            psychotherapy, 825–826
            seasonal affective disorder, 824–825
            treatment of depression, 825
        mania, bipolar disorder, 826
        mood disorders caused by general medical condition, 826–827
        substance-induced mood disorders, 827
    percentage of board examination devoted to, 2
    psychopharmacology, 834–837
        antianxiety medications, 837
        antidepressants, 834–835t
        antipsychotic agents, 835–836
            side effects, 836, 837t
        monoamine oxidase inhibitors, 835
        newer antipsychotic agents, 836–837
    psychotic disorders, 827t, 827–828
    somatoform disorders, 829–830
        chronic pain disorder, 830
        conversion disorder, 829–830
        hypochondriasis, 830
        somatization disorder, 829
    substance abuse disorders, 833t, 833–834
    suicidal patient, 823–824
Psychopharmacology, 834–837
    antianxiety medications, 837
    antidepressants, 834–835t

antipsychotic agents, 835–836
    extrapyramidal reactions, 836, 837t
    side effects, 836, 837t
    monoamine oxidase inhibitors, 835
    newer antipsychotic agents, 836–837
Psychophysiologic dizziness, 737, 738
Psychophysiologic vocal cord adduction, 16, 16t
    in diagnosis of wheezing, 16
Psychotherapy, 825–826
Psychotic disorders, 827t, 827–828
Psychotic symptoms, drugs producing, 827t
Pulmonary alveolar proteinosis, 892
Pulmonary angiography, pulmonary disease, 862
Pulmonary artery catheterization, 158, 159t
    hemodynamic data obtained with, 159t
Pulmonary changes in elderly, 395
Pulmonary disease, 847–941
    alpha$_1$-antitrypsin deficiency, 868–869
    alveolar microlithiasis, 892
    asbestos-related lung disease, 891
    asthma, 869
    BOOP, 891
    bronchiectasis, 875–878
        causes, associations, 876–878
            allergic bronchopulmonary aspergillosis, 877
            ciliary dyskinesia, 876–877
            hypogammaglobulinemia, 877
            infections, 876
            obstructive azoospermia, 877
            right middle lobe syndrome, 877
            unilateral hyperlucent lung syndrome, 877–878
            yellow nail syndrome, 877
        complications, 878
        treatment, 878
    bullous lung disease, 868
    causes, associations, 881t
    chest pain, 848
    chronic bronchitis, 868
    chronic obstructive pulmonary disease
        complications, causes for exacerbation, 873
        treatment, 869
            adjuvant therapy, 872–873
            adrenergic agonists, 870
            anticholinergic agents, 870
            antihistamines, 872
            antileukotrienes, 871–872
            bronchodilators, 869
            corticosteroids, 872
            long-acting beta-adrenergic agonists, 870
            mast cell inhibitors, 871
            nonsteroidal anti-inflammatory agents, 872
            oxygen, 873

phosphodiesterase inhibitors, 870–871
            reducing risk factors, 869
            short-acting beta-adrenergic agonists, 869–870
    clubbing, 849
    cough, 847
    cyanosis, 848–849
    cystic fibrosis, 874–875
    desquamative interstitial pneumonia, 889–890
    diagnostic tests, 849–866
        blood gases, oximetry, 866
        bronchoalveolar lavage, 866–867
        bronchoscopy, 866
        exercise testing, 866
        lung biopsy, 866
        preoperative evaluation of lung functions, 866
        pulmonary function tests, 863–864
            interpretation of pulmonary function tests, 863–864
            provocation inhalational challenge, 863
        radiology, 849–861
            computed tomography, 862
            fluoroscopy, 851–861
            magnetic resonance imaging, 862
            plain chest radiography, 849–851, *852–861*
            pulmonary angiography, 862
        radionuclide lung scans, 862
        sputum microscopy, 863
    diffuse alveolar damage, adult respiratory distress syndrome, 891
    diffuse lung disease, 878–881, *885,* 885–888, *888*
        causes, 878–880
            acute eosinophilic pneumonia, 878
            allergic bronchopulmonary aspergillosis, 879
            chronic eosinophilic pneumonia, 878–879
            Churg-Strauss syndrome, 879
            drug reactions, 880
            hypereosinophilic syndrome, 880
            neoplasms, 880
            parasitic infections, 879
            tropical eosinophilia, 880
        diagnosis, 888–892
        IPF/UIP, 888–889
        hypersensitivity pneumonitis, 880–881t
    dyspnea, 848
    emphysema, 868
    eosinophilic pneumonia, 891–892
    examination, 849, 850t
    giant cell pneumonitis, 892
    hemoptysis, 848
    history, physical examination, 850t
    Horner syndrome, 849

Pulmonary disease *(contd.)*
  hypersensitivity pneumonitis, 890–891
    extrinsic allergic alveolitis, 890–891
  hypertrophic pulmonary osteoarthropathy,
    849
  Langerhans cell histiocytosis, 890
  lymphangioleiomyomatosis, 890
  lymphocytic interstitial pneumonitis, 892
  nonspecific interstitial pneumonia, 889
  obstructive lung diseases, 866t, 866–868
    etiology, 867
    pathology, 867–868
    physiology, 868
  percentage of board examination devoted
    to, 2
  pleural effusion, 881–884
    amylase, 883
    cell counts, 883
    chylous effusion, 883
    complement, 883
    complications, 884
    cultures, 883–884
    cytology, 883
    glucose, pH, 882
    pleural biopsy, 884
    transudate *versus* exudate, 882, 882t
  pulmonary alveolar proteinosis, 892
  pulmonary infections, 910–930
    bacterial infections, 911–916
      aspiration pneumonia, 916
      community-acquired pneumonia,
        914–916
        actinomycosis, 916
        Burkholderia pseudomallei, 915
        Chlamydia pneumoniae, 914
        Chlamydia psittaci, 914–915
        Coxiella burnetti, 915
        Francisella tularensis, 915
        Mycoplasma, 914
        Nocardia pneumonia, 915–916
        Yersinia pestis, 915
      hospital-acquired pneumonia, 916
      otitis media, 911–912
      pharyngitis, 912
      pneumonia, 912–914
        anaerobic bacteria, 913–914
        Haemophilus influenzae, 913
        Klebsiella pneumoniae, 913
        Legionella pneumophila, 913
        Moraxella catarrhalis, 913
        Pseudomonas aeruginosa,
          912–913
        Staphylococcus aureus, 912
        Streptococcus pneumoniae, 912
      sinusitis, 911, 911t
    fungal diseases of lung, 927–929
      aspergillosis, 928
      blastomycosis, 927
      candidiasis, 928
      coccidioidomycosis, 927

        cryptococcosis, 927–928
        histoplasmosis, 927
        Pneumocystis carinii, 929
        sporotrichosis, 928–929
        zygomycosis, 928
      lung abscess, 916
      mycobacterial diseases, 916–927
        Mycobacterium tuberculosis,
          916–924t
        nontuberculous mycobacteria,
          922–926
        toxicity from antituberculous drugs,
          926–927
          ethambutol, 926
          isoniazid, 926
          pyrazinamide, 926
          rifampin, 926
          streptomycin, 926–927
      noninfectious pulmonary complications
        in acquired immunodeficiency
        syndrome, 930
      parasitic diseases, 929
      viral infections, 910–911
        Hantavirus pulmonary syndrome,
          910–911
        influenza, 910
        severe acute respiratory syndrome,
          911
        viral pneumonia, 910
  pulmonary neoplasms, 893–898
    primary lung cancer, 893–898
      adenocarcinoma, 896
      bronchial gland tumors, 897
      bronchoalveolar cell carcinoma, 896
      carcinoid, 897
      cell types, 894
      clinical features, 894–896
      diagnostic tests, 897
      endocrine, 898
      large cell carcinoma, 896
      lymphoma, 897
      mesenchymal tumors, 897
      nervous system, 898
      overall survival, 894
      paraneoplastic syndromes, 897
      skeletal, 898
      small cell carcinoma, 896–897
      squamous cell carcinoma, 896
    pulmonary metastases, 898
    solitary pulmonary nodule, 893
      clinical evaluation, 893
      decision making, 893, 894t
      diagnosis, 893
  respiratory bronchiolitis, 889–890
  sarcoidosis, 889
  silicosis, 891
  sputum, 847–848
  symptoms, 847–849
  vascular diseases, 898–909
    pulmonary embolism, 898–904

      clinical features, 900
      complications of PE, 903–904
      diagnostic tests, 900–902, *901*
      etiology, 899t, 899–900t
      inferior vena cava interruption, 903
      prophylaxis, 903
      treatment, 902t, 902–903
    pulmonary vasculitides, 904–909
      alveolar hemorrhage syndromes, 907
      Behçet disease, 906
      Churg-Strauss syndrome, 905–906
      eosinophilia-myalgia syndrome, 906
      giant cell arteritis, 905
      glomerulonephritis, 908
      Goodpasture syndrome, 907–908
      idiopathic pulmonary hemosiderosis,
        909
      microscopic polyangiitis, 908
      mitral valve disease, 908–909
      mixed cryoglobulinemia, 906–907
      polyarteritis nodosa, 907
      secondary vasculitis, 907
      Takayasu arteritis, 906
      toxic alveolar hemorrhage, 909
      urticarial vasculitis, 906
      vasculitides, 908
      Wegener granulomatosis, 904–905
Pulmonary edema, 880
  disease etiology, 8t
Pulmonary embolism, 898–904
  clinical features, 900
  coagulation disorders predisposing to
    development, 899t
  complications of PE, 903–904
  in diagnosis of wheezing, 16t
  diagnostic tests, 900–902, *901*
  etiology, 899t, 899–900t
  inferior vena cava interruption, 903
  prophylaxis, 903
  treatment, 902t, 902–903
Pulmonary function tests, pulmonary
  disease, 863–864
  interpretation of pulmonary function
    tests, 863–864
  provocation inhalational challenge, 863
Pulmonary infections, 910–930
  bacterial infections, 911–916
    aspiration pneumonia, 916
    community-acquired pneumonia,
      914–916
      actinomycosis, 916
      Burkholderia pseudomallei, 915
      Chlamydia pneumoniae, 914
      Chlamydia psittaci, 914–915
      Coxiella burnetti, 915
      Francisella tularensis, 915
      mycoplasma, 914
      Nocardia pneumonia, 915–916
      Yersinia pestis, 915
    hospital-acquired pneumonia, 916

otitis media, 911–912
pharyngitis, 912
pneumonia, 912–914
    anaerobic bacteria, 913–914
    Haemophilus influenzae, 913
    Klebsiella pneumoniae, 913
    Legionella pneumophila, 913
    Moraxella catarrhalis, 913
    Pseudomonas aeruginosa, 912–913
    Staphylococcus aureus, 912
    Streptococcus pneumoniae, 912
sinusitis, 911, 911t
fungal diseases of lung, 927–929
    aspergillosis, 928
    blastomycosis, 927
    candidiasis, 928
    coccidioidomycosis, 927
    cryptococcosis, 927–928
    histoplasmosis, 927
    Pneumocystis carinii, 929
    sporotrichosis, 928–929
    zygomycosis, 928
lung abscess, 916
mycobacterial diseases, 916–927
    Mycobacterium tuberculosis, 916–924t
    nontuberculous mycobacteria, 922–926
    toxicity from antituberculous drugs,
        926–927
        ethambutol, 926
        isoniazid, 926
        pyrazinamide, 926
        rifampin, 926
        streptomycin, 926–927
noninfectious pulmonary complications
    in acquired immunodeficiency
    syndrome, 930
parasitic diseases, 929
viral infections, 910–911
    Hantavirus pulmonary syndrome,
        910–911
    influenza, 910
    severe acute respiratory syndrome, 911
    viral pneumonia, 910
Pulmonary infiltrates, 669
Pulmonary metastases, 898
Pulmonary neoplasms, 893–898
    primary lung cancer, 893–898
        adenocarcinoma, 896
        bronchial gland tumors, 897
        bronchoalveolar cell carcinoma, 896
        carcinoid, 897
        cell types, 894
        clinical features, 894–896
        diagnostic tests, 897
        endocrine, 898
        large cell carcinoma, 896
        lymphoma, 897
        mesenchymal tumors, 897
        nervous system, 898
        overall survival, 894

paraneoplastic syndromes, 897
skeletal, 898
small cell carcinoma, 896–897
squamous cell carcinoma, 896
pulmonary metastases, 898
solitary pulmonary nodule, 893
    clinical evaluation, 893
    decision making, 893, 894t
    diagnosis, 893
    World Health Organization classification,
        894t
Pulmonary-renal syndrome, differential
    diagnosis, 972t
Pulmonary risks, anesthesia, management,
    337
Pulmonary tuberculosis, treatment,
    560–562t
Pulmonary vasculitides, 904–909
    alveolar hemorrhage syndromes, 907
    Behçet disease, 906
    Churg-Strauss syndrome, 905–906
    eosinophilia-myalgia syndrome, 906
    giant cell arteritis, 905
    glomerulonephritis, 908
    Goodpasture syndrome, 907–908
    idiopathic pulmonary hemosiderosis, 909
    microscopic polyangiitis, 908
    mitral valve disease, 908–909
    mixed cryoglobulinemia, 906–907
    polyarteritis nodosa, 907
    secondary vasculitis, 907
    Takayasu arteritis, 906
    toxic alveolar hemorrhage, 909
    urticarial vasculitis, 906
    vasculitides, 908
    Wegener granulomatosis, 904–905
Pyoderma gangrenosum, 176, 179, *194*
Pyrazinamide, 561, 622, 919–923, 926
    toxicity, 926
Pyridium, 707
Pyridoxine, 704
Pyrimethamine, 486, 756
Pyuria, 707

Q

Q fever, disease etiology, 8t
Question format, 2–3
Quetiapine, 752, 753, 835
Quinidine, 53, 69, 70, 71, 83, 115, 259, 624,
    744, 992
Quinine, 744
Quinolone antibiotics, 16
Quinupristin, 606, 607

R

Rabbits, in disease etiology, 8t
Rabies, 576
Rabies vaccine, 819
Racing workers, epidemiologic factors
    affecting. *See* Horse dander

Radiculopathy, 481
Radioactive iodine uptake, 208t
Radiographic contrast media reactions, 31
Radionuclide imaging, 62–64
    first-pass radionuclide angiography, 63
    gated sestamibi imaging, 64
    myocardial perfusion imaging, *63*, 63–64
    radionuclide angiography, 62
Radionuclide lung scans, pulmonary
    disease, 862
Rai classification, staging, 426t
RAIU. *See* Radioactive iodine uptake
Raloxifene, 397
Ranitidine, 706
Ranson criteria, 289t
Rapidly progressive glomerulonephritis,
    668–670, *669*
    ANCA vasculitides, 668t, 668–670
        Churg-Strauss syndrome, 669–670
        microscopic polyangiitis, 669
        myalgias, arthralgias, 669
        polyarteritis nodosa, 670
        Wegener granulomatosis, 669
    Goodpasture disease, 670
Rats, in disease etiology, 8t
Raynaud phenomenon, 994–995t, 1025t,
    1025–1026
    characteristic clinical features, 1025t
    secondary, causes, 995t
Reactive arthritis, 986–987
Recombinant PTH, 218
Rectum cancer, mortality, 808
Recurrent allograft renal disease, 706
Red wine, tyramine in, 514
Redwood, as cause of asthma, 14
Reflexes, 792t
Refsum disease, 369, 371
Reiter syndrome, 180
Rejection, chronic, graft failure, 706
Relapsing polychondritis, 178
Relative risk reduction, 335
Remicade, 277
Renal arteriography, with renovascular
    hypertension, 526
Renal disease, causes, 687t
Renal imaging, 708
Renal insufficiency, 232
    reversible causes, 687t
Renal parenchymal disease, 528
Renal transplant rejection, 678
Renal vein renins, with renovascular
    hypertension, 527
Renal-excreted beta-blockers, 690
Renovascular hypertension, 523–528, *524*
    screening tests, 525–527
        captopril radionuclide renal scan,
            525–526
        captopril test, 527
        digital venous subtraction angiography,
            526–527

Renovascular hypertension, screening tests
(contd.)
    duplex ultrasonography, 526
    intravenous pyelography, 525
    magnetic resonance angiography, 526
    renal arteriography, 526
    renal vein renins, 527
    spiral computed tomography
        angiography, 526
    therapy for, 527–528
Repaglinide, 236
Replication cycle of human
        immunodeficiency virus, 489
Reserpine, 518
Respiratory acidosis, 150, 699–700
    alkalosis, compensation, 698t
Respiratory alkalosis, 150, 700, 700t
    disorders causing, 700, 700t
Respiratory bronchiolitis-associated
        interstitial lung disease, 889–890
Respiratory disease, in elderly, 395–396
Respiratory failure, 147–149
    hypoxia, 147–149
        A-a gradient, 148
        dead space ventilation, 148
        Fick equation, 148–149
        mixed venous oxygen saturation, 148
        oxygen delivery, 148
        P_{AO_2}, calculation, 148
        shunt fraction, 148–149
    physiologic definitions, 147
        compliance, 147
        lung volumes, 147
        resistance, 147
        relationships, 147
Respiratory infection, methacholine
        challenge, 15
Respiratory tract procedures, American
        Heart Association prophylactic
        regimens, 588t
Rest tremor, 751
Resuscitation
    legal rulings, 659t
    unlikely to prolong life, situations, 658t
Retin A, 172
Retro-orbital pain, 481
Retrovir, 489
Rheumatic diseases, 43
    autoantibodies in, 991t
Rheumatic fever
    initial attack of, Jones diagnosis criteria,
        550t
    poststreptococcal reactive arthritis, 1002
Rheumatoid arthritis, 59, 180, 388, 943–950
    adult-onset Still disease, 950–951
    clinical features of rheumatoid arthritis,
        944, *944*
    conditions related to, 950–952
    constitutional features of rheumatoid
        arthritis, 944–945t

criteria for diagnosis, 949t
diagnosis, 948, 949t
effects, 59
extra-articular complications, 946–947
    cardiac complications, 947
    liver abnormalities, 947
    neurologic manifestations, 946
    ophthalmic abnormalities, 947
    pulmonary manifestations, 946–947
    rheumatoid nodules, 946
    rheumatoid vasculitis, 946
Felty syndrome, 951, 951t
laboratory findings, 947–948t
musculoskeletal complications, 945t,
        945–946
    carpal tunnel syndrome, 946
    cervical spine, 945
    popliteal cyst, 945
    tenosynovitis, 945–946
natural history, 948–949, *949*
pathogenesis of rheumatoid arthritis,
        943–944
radiographic findings, 948
seronegative rheumatoid arthritis, 950
Sjögren syndrome, 951–952t
treatment, 949–950
    surgery, 950
Rheumatoid factor, diseases with, 948t
Rheumatoid nodules, 946
Rheumatoid vasculitis, 946
Rheumatologic disease, 987
Rheumatologic manifestations of human
        immunodeficiency virus infection,
        1002t, 1002–1003
    human immunodeficiency virus-
        associated rheumatic syndromes,
        1003
    human immunodeficiency virus-
        associated vasculitis, 1003
    lupus-like illnesses in human
        immunodeficiency virus infection,
        1003
    reactive arthritis, undifferentiated
        spondyloarthropathy, 1003
Rheumatologic problems, in elderly,
        387–389
    crystalline arthropathy, 388–389
    osteoarthritis, 387–388
    polymyalgia rheumatica, temporal
        arteritis, 389
    rheumatoid arthritis, 388
Rheumatology, 180–182, 943–1011
    antiphospholipid antibody syndrome,
        993t, 993–994
        clinical features, 994
        treatment, 994
    antirheumatic drug therapies, 972–978
        anti-cytokine therapies, 978
        disease-modifying antirheumatic drugs,
        975–976

        antimalarial compounds, 975
        azathioprine, 976–977
        cyclophosphamide, 977
        leflunomide, 976
        methotrexate, 976
        sulfasalazine, 975–976
    glucocorticosteroids, 977–978
    nonacetylated salicylates, 975
    nonsteroidal anti-inflammatory drugs,
        972–975
        gastrointestinal side effects of
            NSAIDs, 974–975
        mechanisms of action of NSAIDs,
            972–973
        mechanisms of toxicity of NSAIDs,
            973–974t
        other toxic effects of NSAIDs, 975
    arthritis in chronic renal failure, 958
    Behçet syndrome, 987
    Buerger disease, 967
    bypass arthritis, 987–988
    Churg-Strauss vasculitis, 967
        clinical features, 967
        treatment, 967
    cryoglobulinemia, 970–971
        laboratory studies, 971
        outcome, 971
    crystalline arthropathies, 979–984
        calcium oxalate arthropathy, 983
        calcium pyrophosphate deposition
            disease, 983
            etiologic classification, 983
            pseudogout, 983
            treatment of pseudogout, 983
        hydroxyapatite deposition disease, 983
            diagnosis, treatment, 983, 984t
            presentation, 983
        hyperuricemia, gout, 979–983
            causes of hypouricemia, 979–980
            causes of secondary hyperuricemia,
                979, 981t
            clinical manifestations of acute gout,
                980–981
            enzyme abnormalities in uric acid
                pathway, 979, *980*
            factors predisposing to gout and
                pseudogout, 980
            points of importance, 982–983
            renal disease, uric acid, 982
            treatment during intercritical period,
                981–982
            treatment of acute gouty arthritis,
                981
        other crystals implicated in joint
            disease, 983–984
    drug-induced lupus, 991–993
        clinical features, 991–992
        laboratory abnormalities, 992–993
        metabolism, 993
        treatment, 993

drug-induced myopathies, 998
  muscle disease, 998
giant cell arteritis, 962–964
  clinical features, 963, 963t
  diagnosis, 963, 963t
  outcome, 964
  pathology, 962–963
  treatment, 963–964
infectious arthritis, 998–1000
  bacterial arthritis, 998–999
  gonococcal arthritis, 999–1000
  infected joint prostheses, 1000
  mycobacterial, fungal joint infections,
    1000
  spinal septic arthritis, 1000
inflammatory myopathies, 997–998
  inclusion body myositis, 998
iritis, rheumatologic diseases, 987
isolated angiitis of central nervous
    system, 967–968
  clinical features, 967–968
  diagnosis, 968
  treatment, 968
Lyme disease, 1000–1001
  clinical stages, 1001
    stage I, 1001
    stage II, 1001
    stage III, 1001
  diagnosis, 1001
  spirochete, 1000–1001
  tick, 1000
  treatment, 1001
nonarticular rheumatism, 958–961
  bursitis, 960
  features, 961, 961t
  fibromyalgia, 958
    diagnosis, 958–959
    natural history, 959
  giant cell arteritis, relationship to,
    961
  low back pain, 959–960
    diagnosis, 959, 960t
    treatment, 959–960
  nonarticular rheumatism, fibromyalgia,
    958–959
  polymyalgia rheumatica, 960–961
  treatment, 961
osteoarthritis, 952–958
  clinical features of osteoarthritis,
    952–953
  clinical subsets of osteoarthritis,
    953–954
    primary osteoarthritis, 953–954
  diffuse idiopathic skeletal hyperostosis,
    953
  erosive osteoarthritis, 953
  generalized osteoarthritis, 953
  isolated hip osteoarthritis, 953
  isolated nodal osteoarthritis, 953
  pathogenesis of osteoarthritis, 952

radiographic features of osteoarthritis,
    957, 957
  secondary osteoarthritis, 954–957
  therapy for osteoarthritis, 957–958t
osteoid osteoma, 987
overlap syndromes, 993
  mixed connective tissue disease, 993
  undifferentiated connective tissue
    disease, 993
percentage of board examination devoted
    to, 2
polyarteritis, 964–967
  clinical features, 965, 965t
  diagnosis, 966, 966
  outcome, 966–967
  pathology, 964–965
  treatment, 966
Raynaud phenomenon, 994–995t
rheumatic fever, poststreptococcal
    reactive arthritis, 1002
rheumatoid arthritis, 943–950
  adult-onset Still disease, 950–951
  clinical features of rheumatoid arthritis,
    944, 944
  conditions related to, 950–952
  constitutional features of rheumatoid
    arthritis, 944–945t
  diagnosis, 948, 949t
  extra-articular complications, 946–947
    cardiac complications, 947
    liver abnormalities, 947
    neurologic manifestations, 946
    ophthalmic abnormalities, 947
    pulmonary manifestations, 946–947
    rheumatoid nodules, 946
    rheumatoid vasculitis, 946
  Felty syndrome, 951, 951t
  laboratory findings, 947–948t
  musculoskeletal complications,
    945–946
    carpal tunnel syndrome, 946
    cervical spine, 945
    popliteal cyst, 945
    tenosynovitis, 945–946
  natural history, 948–949, 949
  pathogenesis of rheumatoid arthritis,
    943–944
  radiographic findings, 948
  seronegative rheumatoid arthritis,
    950
  seronegative rheumatoid arthritis of
    elderly, 950
  Sjögren syndrome, 951–952t
  treatment, 949–950
  surgery, 950
rheumatologic manifestations of human
    immunodeficiency virus infection,
    1002t, 1002–1003
  human immunodeficiency virus-
    associated vasculitis, 1003

lupus-like illnesses in human
    immunodeficiency virus infection,
    1003
  other human immunodeficiency virus-
    associated rheumatic syndromes,
    1003
  reactive arthritis, undifferentiated
    spondyloarthropathy, 1003
scleroderma-like syndromes, 997
  disorders associated with occupation or
    environment, 997
  eosinophilic fasciitis, 997
  metabolic causes of scleroderma-like
    syndrome, 997
sinusitis, vasculitis, 972
small vessel vasculitis/cutaneous
    vasculitis, 969–970t
  clinical features, 969
  diagnosis, 969–970
  histopathology, 969
  treatment, outcome, 970
spondyloarthropathies, 984–987, 985
  ankylosing spondylitis, 984–986
    differential diagnosis, 986
    extraskeletal involvement, 985–986
    extraspinal involvement, 985
    features, 984–986t
    laboratory findings, 985
    in men, women, 986
    treatment, 986
  arthritis associated with inflammatory
    bowel disease, 987
  psoriatic arthritis, 987
  reactive arthritis, 986–987
systemic lupus erythematosus, 988–991
  clinical manifestations, 989
    articular, 989
    cardiopulmonary, 989
    dermatologic, 989
    neuropsychiatric, 989
  diagnosis, 988
  epidemiology, 988
  etiology, 988
  genetics, 988
  laboratory findings, 990, 990t, 991t
  outcome, 991
  pathogenesis, 988–989
  pregnancy, 989
  renal involvement, 989–990
  treatment, 990–992t
systemic sclerosis, 995
  clinical manifestations, 995–996
    articular, 995–996
    cardiac, 996
    gastrointestinal, 996
    pulmonary, 996
    Raynaud phenomenon, 995
    renal, 996
    skin, 995
  laboratory findings, 996

Rheumatology, systemic sclerosis *(contd.)*
treatment, 996
Takayasu arteritis, 964
clinical, laboratory features, 964
treatment, outcome, 964
vasculitic syndromes, 961, 962t,
962–971, *963*
differential diagnosis, 971–972t, *973*
vasculitis
associated with connective tissue
diseases, 971
large vessel vasculitis, 971
obliterative endarteropathy, 971
small, medium-sized vessel
vasculitis, 971
skin lesions associated with, 971–972
viral arthritis, 1002
Wegener granulomatosis, 968–969
ANCA, 969
clinical features, 968–969
pathologic diagnosis, 969
treatment, outcome, 969
Rhinitis
allergy skin tests, 21
antihistamines, 22
chronic, 20–24
allergy skin tests in allergic rhinitis, 21
antihistamines, decongestants, 22
corticosteroid therapy for rhinitis,
21–22
environmental modification, 22–23
immunotherapy for allergic rhinitis,
22
medical history, 20–21t
corticosteroid therapy, 21–22
decongestants, 22
differential diagnosis, 21t
environmental modification, 22–23
animal dander, 23
house dust mites, 22–23t
pollen, 23
immunotherapy, 22
medical history, 20–21t
Rhinitis medicamentosus, 21
Rhizopus species, 571
Rhythm disorders, 66–77
ambulatory electrocardiographic
monitoring, 66–67
antiarrhythmic drugs, 69t, 69–74, *70*, 70t,
71t, *72*, 72t
adenosine, 73
amiodarone, 73
class I antiarrhythmic drugs, 70
electrophysiology-guided serial drug
testing, 73
antitachycardia surgery, 74–75t
device therapy, 75
electrocardiography, 66
electrophysiologic study, *68*, 68–69
exercise testing, 67–68

implantable cardioverter-defibrillators
complications of permanent pacing,
75–76, *76*
implantable cardioverter-defibrillators,
76–77
indications for permanent pacemaker
implantation, 76, 77t
permanent cardiac pacemaker
implantation, 75–76t
signal-averaged ECG, 68
heart rate variability, 68
transcatheter radiofrequency ablation, 74,
74t
transtelephonic event recording, 66–67
Ribavirin, 604
interferon alfa, combination treatment
with, 676
interferon alfa in combination with, 300
Rickets, hypophosphatemic, 372
Rickettsial infections, 419, 566
Rifabutin, 483, 484, 606, 607
Rifadin, 923
Rifamate, 923
Rifampin, 211, 302, 483, 554, 556, 561,
586, 589, 606, 607, 622, 624t, 707,
871, 919–923, 926
drugs with reduced serum concentrations
in presence, 624t
toxicity, 926
Rifamycins, 483, 606
Rifapentine, 483, 606, 607
Rifater, 923
Right middle lobe syndrome, 877
Right-sided diarrhea, left-sided, clinical
presentation, 266t
Rimactane, 923
Rimantadine, 606, 630–631, 817
Risedronate, 217, 259
Risk factors, 747
Risperidone, 835, 837
Ritonavir, 492
Ritonavir-indinavir combination, 493
Ritonavir-nelfinavir combination, 493
Ritonavir-saquinavir combination, 493
Rivastigmine, 727
Rizatriptan, 732
RNA synthesis, 607
Rochalimaea quintana, 184
Rodent urine, as cause of asthma, 14
Roots, reflexes and, 792t
Ropinirole, 753
Roseola-like rash, 481
Rouleaux, *476*
Rubella, 577
Rubella vaccine, 816
Rubeola, 577

S

SAAG. *See* Serum-ascites albumin gradient
Salicylates, 700

Salmeterol, 16, 870
formoterol, for asthma, 16t
Salmonella, 265, 279, 419, 555
with human immunodeficiency virus, 487
Salmonella enteritidis, 278
Salmonella typhimurium, 271
Salmonellosis, 948
Salts of platinum, as cause of asthma, 14
Saquinavir, 492
Sarcoid, 880
in disease etiology, 8t
Sarcoid-like disease, 880
disease etiology, 8t
Sarcoidosis, 177, 678, *856, 857*, 889, 948
SARS. *See* Severe acute respiratory
syndrome (SARS)
Schistocytes, *477*
Schistosomiasis, 579, 948
Sciatica, 351
Scleroderma, 58, *196*, 948, 995
clinical findings in, 997t
clinical manifestations, 995–996
skin, 995
effects, 58
laboratory findings, 996
systemic, 181
treatment, 996
Scleroderma-like syndromes, 997
disorders associated with occupation or
environment, 997
eosinophilic fasciitis, 997
metabolic causes of scleroderma-like
syndrome, 997
Scleromyxedema, 997
Screening for disease, principles, 807–814
Seasonal affective disorder, 824–825
Second heart sounds, 40–41
Secondary osteoarthritis, 954–957
Secondary urticaria, 24
Secondary vasculitis, 907
Second-generation cephalosporins, 610–611
Secretin, 269
Sedatives, 833
Sedentary life, 232
Seizures, classification, 728t
Selegiline, 752, 753
Sensory ataxic neuropathy, 743
Sepsis, neurology
critical illness polyneuropathy, 757–758
septic encephalopathy, 757
Septic meningitis, 756
Seromycin, 923
Seronegative rheumatoid arthritis, 950
Serotonin, 514, 732, 839
Serratia infections, 554–555
Sertraline, 834
Serum-ascites albumin gradient, ascites
protein, 307t
Severe acute respiratory syndrome (SARS),
602–605, 911

Sex chromosome aneuploidy syndromes, 361–363, *362*

Sexual function, in elderly, 390–391

Sexually transmitted diseases, 589–595
  epididymitis, 594
  Gardnerella vaginalis, 594
  Herpes genitalis, 591
  Neisseria gonorrhoeae, 589–591
  nongonococcal urethritis, cervicitis, 591
  pelvic inflammatory disease, 593–594
    Trichomonas vaginalis, 593–594
  syphilis, 592t, 592–593
  vulvovaginal candidiasis, 594

Shellfish, as cause of food allergy, 27

Shigella, 265, 271

Shigella flexneri, 278, 279

Shock states, 159–160

Short-acting insulin, 235

Shy-Drager syndrome, 385

Sickle cell disorders, 369, 422–425

Side effects of chemotherapy, 790

Siderosis, 880
  disease etiology, 8t

Silent ischemia, 96–97

Silicosis, 880, 891
  disease etiology, 8t

Silo filler's lung, 880
  disease etiology, 8t

Sinemet, 752, 753

Sinusitis, 21, 23t, 23–24, *24*, 24t, 334, 601, 911, 911t
  bacteria in, 911t
  complications, 23t
  persistent, causes, 24t
  recurrent, causes, 24t
  vasculitis, 972

Sjögren syndrome, 676, 678, 948, 951–952t
  features, 952t

Skin rash, 730

Slow viruses, 576–577
  Creutzfeldt-Jakob disease, 577
  inclusion body encephalitis, 577
  prion-associated central nervous system diseases, 576–577
    Creutzfeldt-Jakob disease, 577
    progressive multifocal leukoencephalopathy, 576
    subacute sclerosing panencephalitis, 577
  progressive multifocal leukoencephalopathy, 576
  subacute sclerosing panencephalitis, 577

Small cell carcinoma, 896–897

Small cell lung cancer, 782

Small intestine, 265–268

Small-bowel disorders, 274
  aortoenteric fistula, 274
  Meckel diverticulum, 274

Smallpox, 604

Smallpox vaccine, 818–819

Small-vessel vasculitis, 668, 969–970t
  clinical features, 969
  conditions with, 970t
  diagnosis, 969–970
  histopathology, 969
  treatment, outcome, 970

Smoking, methacholine challenge, 15

Sodium, 690, 695

Sodium balance, disorders, 694

Sodium bicarbonate, 695

Sodium nitrite, 537

Sodium nitroprusside, 536, 537, 1019

Soft tissue infection, 599–600

Soil, in disease etiology, 8t

Solid organ transplantation
  immunodeficiency states, infections in, 602, 602t, 603t
  infections in, 602, 602t, 603t
  opportunistic infections in, 602t

Solitary pulmonary nodule, 893
  clinical evaluation, 893
  decision making, 893, 894t
  diagnosis, 893

Somatization disorder, 829

Somatoform disorders, 829–830
  chronic pain disorder, 830
  conversion disorder, 829–830
  hypochondriasis, 830
  somatization disorder, 829

Sorbitol, 692

Sotalol, 69, 70, 71, 72, 83, 532

South America, travel to, in disease etiology, 8t

Southeast Asia, travel to, in disease etiology, 8t

Southern blot procedure, 376–377, *377, 378*

Southwestern United States, travel in, disease etiology, 8t

Soybean, as cause of food allergy, 27

Spherocytes, *476*

Spherocytosis, hereditary, 365

Spinal conditions, potentially serious, 351

Spinal cord compression, 791–792t
  outcome of patients with, 792t

Spinal level, symptoms, clinical correlations, 738–740
  anterior horn cell disease, 739
  degenerative disease of spine, 739–740
    cervical spondylosis, 739
    lumbar spine disease, 739–740
  radiculopathy, 739
  spinal cord disease-related weakness, 738–739

Spinal septic arthritis, 1000

Spiral computed tomography angiography, with renovascular hypertension, 526

Spiramycin, as cause of asthma, 14

Spirochetes, 563–565
  leptospirosis, 563–564
  Lyme disease, 564–565

clinical syndromes, 564
  diagnosis, 564–565
  epidemiology, 564
  prevention, 565
  treatment, 565

Spironolactone, 223, 230, 517, 682, 696

Spondyloarthropathies, 984–987, *985*
  ankylosing spondylitis, 984–986
    differential diagnosis, 986
    extraskeletal involvement, 985–986
    extraspinal involvement, 985
    features, 984–986t
    laboratory findings, 985
    in men, women, 986
    treatment, 986
  arthritis associated with inflammatory bowel disease, 987
  psoriatic arthritis, 987
  reactive arthritis, 986–987

Spondyloepimetaphyseal dysplasia, 955

Spondyloepiphyseal dysplasia, 955

Spontaneous splenic ruptures, 459

Spoon nails, 184

Sporotrichosis, 568–569, 928–929
  disease etiology, 8t

Spur cells, *476*

Sputum, 847–848
  microscopy, pulmonary disease, 863

Squamous cell carcinoma, 896

Squirrels, in disease etiology, 8t

Stable angina, chronic, 96–101

Standard preoperative tests, in nonemergency situations, indications for, 345t

Stannosis, 880
  disease etiology, 8t

Stanozolol, 25

Staphylococci, 552–554, 704
  coagulase-negative staphylococci, 553–554
  clinical syndromes, 553
  treatment, 553–554

Staphylococcus aureus, 171, 271, 552–553, 670, 912
  clinical syndromes, 552–553
  mechanisms of resistance, 553
  toxins, 552
  treatment, 553

Starling roosts, in disease etiology, 8t

Statins, 109, 233, 349

Status epilepticus, 731, *732*

Stavudine, 489, 491, 606

Stenotrophomonas maltophilia, 555

Steroids, 705, 992

Steroid-sparing agents, 872

Stevens-Johnson syndrome, 730

Stickler syndrome, 955

Stiff hand syndrome, 182

Stimulants, use, 827

Stinging insect allergy, 27–29

Stinging insect allergy *(contd.)*
  allergy testing, 28
  anaphylaxis, 28–29
  avoidance, 28, 29t
  bee allergy, 28
  venom immunotherapy, 28, 28t
  vespid allergy, 28
Stomach, 259–265
  biopsy urease tests, 261
  breath test, 261
  culture, 261
  duodenal ulcer, 260
  gastric tumors, 260
  gastric ulcer, 260
  gastritis, active, chronic, 260
  Helicobacter pylori, 259–260
    epidemiology, 260
    organism, 259–260
  histology, 261
  nonulcer dyspepsia, 260
  serology, 260–261
  stool antigen test, 261
  treatment, 261
Stone formation, medications increasing
    tendency for, 705
Stool antigen test, 261
Stool composition, normal, 265t
Storage pool disease, 446
Strain-gauge outflow plethysmography,
    1029
Straw, in disease etiology, 8t
Streptococcal toxic shock syndrome, 602
Streptococcus agalactiae, 551
Streptococcus pneumoniae, 23, 395, 396,
    551–552, 757, 912
  in sputum, 631
Streptococcus pyogenes, 549
  infections, 549
Streptokinase, 107
Streptomycin, 551, 556, 561, 604, 622,
    919–923
  toxicity, 926–927
Stress ulcers, 263
Structural lesions, 726
Struvite stones, 704–705
Stupor, 725–726
Sturge-Weber-Dimitri syndrome, 180
Subacute bacterial endocarditis, 948
Subacute cutaneous lupus erythematosus,
    196
Subacute sclerosing panencephalitis, 577
Subdural abscess, with sinusitis, 23
Subdural hematoma, 726
Subepidermal blisters, 182
Substance abuse, 833t, 833–834
  percentage of board examination devoted
      to, 2
Substance-induced mood disorders, 827
Substituted judgment, 659
Sucralfate, 211

Sudden cardiac death, trials on
    pharmacologic prevention, 72t
Suicidal patient, 823–824
Suicide, physician-assisted, 659
Sulfa derivatives, 678
Sulfa drugs, 707
  allergy to, 730
Sulfadiazine, 756
Sulfamethoxazole, 482, 486, 619, 706
Sulfamethoxazole-trimethoprim, 606
Sulfasalazine, 276, 277, 880, 949, 975–976,
    992
Sulfonamides, 175, 176, 183, 705
Sulfonylurea, 236, 240
Sulindac, 880
Sumatriptan, 732, 734
Superior vena cava syndrome, 462–463
Supratentorial level, symptoms, clinical
    correlations, 725–736
  anticonvulsant therapy, 729
    anticonvulsant blood levels, 730–731
    status epilepticus, 731, *732*
    surgery for epilepsy, 731
  consciousness, disorders, 725–726
    acute confusional states, 726
    stupor, coma, 725–726
  dementia, 726t, 726–727
    anticonvulsant therapy, 728–730t
    causes, 728
    clinical scenarios, 727
    seizure disorders, 728t, 728–729
  headache, facial pain, 731–735
    clinical scenarios, 734
    cluster headache, 733–734
    glossopharyngeal neuralgia, 735
    medication-overuse headache,
        734–735
    migraine and tension headache,
        732–733
    temporal arteritis, 735
    trigeminal neuralgia, 735
  intracranial lesions, 735–736
    cortical lesions, 736
    leptomeningeal lesions, 735
    parasagittal lesions, 735–736
  ventricular system, 736
    hydrocephalus, 736
Surgical myectomy, 110
Surgical therapy, 583
Surrogate, 651–652
  right to refuse treatment by, 659
Sweet syndrome, 177
Swine, in disease etiology, 8t
Swyer-James syndrome, 877–878
Sympathomimetics, 514, 870
Syncope, 92t, 92–93t
  in elderly, 385–386
  major causes, 92t
  unexplained, risk stratification in patients
      with, 93t

Syndrome of inappropriate ADH secretion,
    205–206
  clinical features, 206
  diagnosis, 206
  etiology, 205–206
  pathophysiology, 206
  therapy, 206
Synercid, 606
Synovial fluid analysis, 984t
Syphilis, 592t, 592–593, 948
  with human immunodeficiency virus, 485
  laboratory diagnosis, 592t
Systemic lupus erythematosus, 58, 232,
    678, 948, 988–991
  clinical manifestations, 989
    articular, 989
    cardiopulmonary, 989
    dermatologic, 989
    neuropsychiatric, 989
  complications of treatment, 992t
  diagnosis, 988
  effects, 58
  epidemiology, 988
  etiology, 988
  genetics, 988
  laboratory findings, 990, 990t, 991t
  nephritis, 674t, 674–675
  outcome, 991
  pathogenesis, 988–989
  pregnancy, 989
  renal involvement, 989–990
  treatment, 990–992t
  WHO classes of renal diseases in, 674t
Systemic sclerosis, 995
  clinical manifestations, 995–996
    articular, 995–996
    cardiac, 996
    gastrointestinal, 996
    pulmonary, 996
    Raynaud phenomenon, 995
    renal, 996
    skin, 995
  laboratory findings, 996
  treatment, 996

T

T cells, in asthma, 13t
Tabes dorsalis, 256
Tachyarrhythmia therapy, summary, 75t
Tacrolimus, 514, 827
Takayasu, 964
  arteritis, 668, 906
  clinical, laboratory features, 964
  treatment, outcome, 964
Tamoxifen, 880
Target cells, *476*
Tay-Sachs disease, 369, 371
TB. *See* Tuberculosis
T-cell activation, in asthma, 13t
Telmisartan, 522

Temporal arteritis, 668, 735, 905
Tenofovir, 491
Tension headache, 732–733
Terbutaline, 869
Teriparatide, 397
Terlipressin, 682
Terminal complement component
    deficiencies, 32
Terry nails, 183
Testicular cancer, 786–787
    background, 786–787
    extragonadal germ cell tumor, 787
    management, 787, 787t
    staging, 787
Testicular feminization, 372
Testis, 225–226
    gynecomastia, 226
        clinical features, 226
        diagnosis, 226
        etiology, 226
    male hypogonadism, 225–226
        androgen therapy, 225
        clinical features, 225
        diagnosis, 225
        etiology, 225
        Kallmann syndrome, 226
        Klinefelter syndrome, 226
        selected disorders of male
            hypogonadism, 226
        therapy, 225
Testosterone, 25, 225, 226
Testosterone enanthate, 225
Tetanus, 256, 559, 814–816
Tetracyclines, 53, 175, 176, 259, 271, 272,
    273, 556, 557, 604, 606, 607,
    614–615, 690, 707, 880
    clinical indications for, 615t
TH1. See T cells
TH2. See T cells
Thalassemia minor, 412
Thallium, 827
Theophylline, 16, 624, 690, 869
    for asthma, 16t
    clearance, 871t
Thermoactinomyces, 880
    disease etiology, 8t
Thiamine, 731
Thiazides, 175, 176, 205, 215, 216, 678
    with hypertension, 516–517
    steroids, 232
Thiazolidinediones, 236
Thin GBM disease, 676–677
Thionamides, 209
Third heart sound, 41
Third-generation cephalosporins, 611–612
Thoracic aorta, rupture, *1019*
Thoracic aortic aneurysm, *1013*,
    1013–1014, *1014*
Thoracic aortic atherosclerosis,
    1019–1020

Thoracic outlet compression syndrome,
    1024–1025
Thrills, 40
Thrombasthenia, Glanzmann, 446
Thromboangiitis obliterans, 967, *1023*,
    1023t, 1023–1024
    clinical criteria for, 1023t
Thrombocythemia
    essential, 441
    primary, 441
Thrombocytopenia, 456–459
    in pregnancy, 459
Thrombocytopenic purpura, 676
    idiopathic, 457t
Thromboembolism, prophylaxis, 343, 344t
Thrombolytic therapy, 454
Thrombopoietin, 461
Thrombotic microangiopathies, 421–422
    hemolytic uremic syndrome, 422
    thrombotic thrombocytopenic purpura,
        421–422
Thrombotic thrombocytopenic purpura,
    421–422
Thyroid disease, in elderly, 389–390
Thyroid function, laboratory assessment,
    206–207
Thyroid gland disorders, 206–213
    hyperthyroidism, 207–210
        clinical features, 207–208
        diagnosis, 208–209
        etiology, 207, 208, 208t
        exogenous hyperthyroidism, 209
        Graves disease, 208
        multinodular goiter, 209
        painless lymphocytic thyroiditis,
            208–209
        radioactive iodine, 209–210
        subacute painful thyroiditis, 209
        supportive therapy, 210
        surgery, 210
        therapy, 209–210
        thionamides, 209
        thyroid storm, 210
        thyrotoxicosis in pregnancy, 210
        toxic adenoma, 209
    hypothyroidism, 210–213
        amiodarone, 213
        circumstances, 211–212
        clinical features, 210–211
        diagnosis, 211
        differentiated thyroid cancer, 212–213
        Hashimoto thyroiditis, 210
        lithium, 213
        myxedema coma, 211–212
        sick euthyroid syndrome, 213
        subclinical hypothyroidism, 211
        therapy, 211
        thyroxine replacement therapy
            in patients with angina, 211
            in pregnancy, 211

laboratory assessment of thyroid function,
    206–207
thyroid nodules, 212
Thyroid hormone replacement therapy, 211
Thyroid nodules, 212
Thyroid stimulating hormone, 211
    deficiency, 200
    thyroid axis, 200
    tumors producing, 204
Thyroiditis
    de Quervain, 209
    postpartum, 208–209
Tiagabine, 727, 729
Ticarcillin, 554
Ticks. See also Lyme disease
    in disease etiology, 8t
Ticlopidine, 748
Tilting disc, 60
Timolol, 519, 733
Tin, 880
    in disease etiology, 8t
Tinzaparin, 452
TIPS. See Transjugular intrahepatic
    portosystemic shunt
Tissue plasminogen activator, 106, 107, 749
Titanium, 880
    in disease etiology, 8t
Tizanidine, 754
TNK-TPA, 106
Tobacco, use, 350–351, 514, 871
Tolbutamide, 624
Toluene diisocyanate, 880
    as cause of asthma, 14
    in disease etiology, 8t
Topiramate, 705, 727, 729, 730, 733
Torsemide, 517
Total joint arthroplasty, indications for, 958t
Toxic alveolar hemorrhage, 909
Toxic epidermal necrolysis syndrome, 29
Toxic myopathies, 746
Toxic oil syndrome, as cause of
    eosinophilia, 31
Toxic shock syndrome, 601
Toxin-induced interstitial nephritis, 679–680
Toxoplasma, 486
Toxoplasmosis, with human
    immunodeficiency virus, 485–486t
    drugs used for treatment, 486t
TPA. See Tissue plasminogen activator
Traditional vasodilators, with hypertension,
    521
TRALI. See Transfusion-related acute lung
    injury
Transfusion, reactions to, 459t, 459–461
Transfusion-related acute lung injury, 459
Transfusions, risks of complications from,
    459t
Transient ischemic attacks, 747–748
Transjugular intrahepatic portosystemic
    shunt, 307

Translocation, 379
Transplantation, 110, 705–706
    graft failure, 706
    immunosuppression, 706, *706*
    opportunistic infections in, 602t
    recurrent allograft renal disease, 706
Transtelephonic event recording, 67
Tranylcypromine, 834
Trauma, 723, 954
Trazodone, 834, 880
Trecator-SC, 923
Tretinoin, 172
Triamcinolone acetonide, for asthma, 16t
Triamterene, 223, 518, 705
Trichinosis, 579
Trichomonas vaginalis, 593–594
Tricyclic antidepressants, 274, 404, 514,
    532, 734, 735, 834
Trigeminal neuralgia, 735
Triglycerides, 273
    increase in, 232
Trihexyphenidyl, 753
Trimellitic anhydrides, 909
    as cause of asthma, 14t
Trimethoprim, 606
Trimethoprim-sulfamethoxazole, 271, 272,
    273, 482, 486, 487, 488, 599, 619,
    905
Trimipramine, 834
Tropheryma whippelii, 1003
Tropical eosinophilia, 880
    in diagnosis of wheezing, 16t
Trousseau sign, 290
Trypanosoma cruzi, 255
Trypanosomiasis, 948
TSH. *See* Thyroid stimulating hormone
Tuberculin testing, 562t
    for latent tuberculous infection, 924t
Tuberculosis, 948
    according to human immunodeficiency
        virus status, 922t
    first-line drugs for, 921t
    with human immunodeficiency virus,
        482–483t
    increased incidence, 8t
    prevention, 813–814
    prophylaxis of, drugs used for, 483t
    pulmonary, treatment, 561t
    treatment, 562t, 919–920t
Tuberous sclerosis, 179, *195*, 365, 368
Tubulointerstitial renal disease, clinical
    manifestations, 677
Tularemia, 556, 604
    disease etiology, 8t
Tumor cell drug resistance, mechanisms,
    790
Tumor lysis syndrome, 791
Tumors of heart, 60–61
    embolization, 60–61
    primary cardiac neoplasm, 61

Turner syndrome, *362*
TWAR strain, *Chlamydia pneumoniae*, 914
Two-dimensional echocardiography, 61
Tylosis, 177
Typhimurium, 278
Tyramine, 835

U

Ulcers, pressure, in elderly, 398–399
Ultralente, 235
Uncommon types of arterial occlusive
    disease, *1023*, 1023–1025
    heparin-induced thrombocytopenia, 1025,
        1025
    popliteal artery entrapment, 1024
    thoracic outlet compression syndrome,
        1024–1025
    thromboangiitis obliterans, 1023t,
        1023–1024
Unfractionated heparin, 452, 453
Unilateral hyperlucent lung syndrome,
    877–878
United States, causes of death in, 808t
Unknown primary lesion, 787–788
    background, 787–788
    treatment, 788
Uranium, 880
    in disease etiology, 8t
Urapidil, 532
Urates, 707
Ureidopenicillins, 607, 608
Uremia, 688–689
Uremic pruritus, 179
Uric acid stones, 704
Urinalysis, 707t, 707–708
Urinary incontinence, in elderly, 399–402
    anatomy, 399
    effects of age, 399
    established, 400
    evaluation, 400–401
    medications affecting, 399–400
    treatment, 401
    urinary catheters, use, 402
    urologic consultation, 402
Urinary tract infection, 598–599, 707
    in elderly, 402
    in females, 598–599
    in males, 599
Urine discoloration, causes, 707t
Urolithiasis, 702–705
    bowel disease, 705
    calcium oxalate stones, 703–704, *704*
    calcium phosphate stones, 704
    cystine stones, 705
    drug-induced stone disease, 705, 705t
    epidemiology, 702, *702, 703*
    inhibitors of crystallization, 705
    metabolic activity, 703, 704t
    risk factors, 702–703t
    struvite stones, 704–705

uric acid stones, 704
Urology, percentage of board examination
    devoted to, 2
Urticaria, 24–26
    angioedema, relation between, 25
    chronic
        food allergy in, 26
        histopathology, 26
    histopathology, 26
    management, 26
    secondary, 24
Urticarial vasculitis, 906

V

Vaccine Adverse Event Reporting System,
    814
Vaccines, 814–819, 948
    diphtheria, 814
    hepatitis A, 817
    hepatitis B, 817–818
    influenza, 816–817
    measles, 816
    mumps, 816
    pneumococcal disease, 818
    polio, 819
    rabies, 819
    rubella, 816
    smallpox, 818–819
    tetanus, 814–816
    varicella, 819
Vaccinia, 818–819
VAERS. *See* Vaccine Adverse Event
    Reporting System
Vaginosis, 594
Valacyclovir, 606, 629
Valganciclovir, 606, 629–630
Valproic acid, 727, 729, 733, 734, 839
Valsalva maneuver, 41
Valsartan, 522
Valvular diseases, effects of physical
    maneuvers, 42t
Valvular heart disease, 41–47
    aortic regurgitation, 43–45
        etiology, 43–44
            aortic root dilatation, 44
            diagnosis, 44
            physical examination, 44
            symptoms, 44
            valvular, 43–44
        timing of surgery, 44–45
    aortic stenosis, 41–43
        subvalvular, 42
            diagnosis, 42
            physical examination, 42
        supravalvular, 41–42
            physical examination, 42
        valvular, 42–43
            diagnosis, 43
            physical examination, 43
            symptoms, 43

types, 42–43
mitral regurgitation, 46–47
  diagnosis, 47
  etiology, 46
  pathophysiology, 47
  physical examination, 46–47
  symptoms, 46
  timing of surgery, 47
mitral stenosis, 45–46
  diagnosis, 45–46, *46*, 46t
  indications for surgery, 46
  physical examination, 45
perioperative, monitoring for, 341
tricuspid regurgitation, 47
  physical examination, 47
  surgical therapy, 47
  tricuspid valve prolapse, 47
tricuspid stenosis, 47
Vancomycin, 553, 554, 584, 586, 587, 588,
    590, 606, 607, 617–619, 757
  plus gentamicin, 588
  situations in which use discouraged, 618t
  therapeutic indications for, 619t
Varicella vaccine, 819
Varicella-zoster virus, 574–575
Vascular access, hemodynamic monitoring,
    158–159
  central venous catheterization, 158
  pulmonary artery catheterization, 158,
    159t
Vascular dementia, 393, 726
Vascular diseases, 722t, 722–723, 898–909,
    1013–1034
  aorta, disease, 1013–1020
    aneurysmal disease, 1013–1016
      abdominal aortic aneurysm,
        1014–1016, *1015*, 1016t
      thoracic aortic aneurysm, *1013*,
        1013–1014, *1014*
    aortic dissection, 1016–1018
      classification, 1016, *1016*
      clinical features, 1016–1017
      diagnosis, *1017*, 1017–1018, *1018*
      etiology, 1016
      laboratory tests, 1017, *1017*
      treatment, 1018, 1019t
    aortic intramural hematoma, 1019
    incomplete aortic rupture, 1019
    penetrating aortic ulcer, 1018–1019
    thoracic aortic atherosclerosis,
      1019–1020
  edema, 1026, 1026t
  erythromelalgia, 1026
  lymphedema, 1026–1027
  peripheral arterial occlusive disease,
    1020–1023
    acute arterial occlusion, 1022–1023
    intermittent claudication, 1020–1022
      cardiac risk, 1022
      clinical features, 1020, 1020t

diagnosis, 1021
natural history, 1021
pseudoclaudication, 1020–1021t
treatment, 1021–1022
vascular surgery, 1022
peripheral arterial aneurysms, 1023
pulmonary embolism, 898–904
  clinical features, 900
  complications, 903–904
  diagnostic tests, 900–902, *901*
  etiology, 899t, 899–900t
  inferior vena cava interruption, 903
  prophylaxis, 903
  treatment, 902t, 902–903
pulmonary vasculitides, 904–909
  alveolar hemorrhage syndromes, 907
  Behçet disease, 906
  Churg-Strauss syndrome, 905–906
  eosinophilia-myalgia syndrome, 906
  giant cell arteritis, 905
  glomerulonephritis, 908
  Goodpasture syndrome, 907–908
  idiopathic pulmonary hemosiderosis,
    909
  microscopic polyangiitis, 908
  mitral valve disease, 908–909
  mixed cryoglobulinemia, 906–907
  polyarteritis nodosa, 907
  secondary vasculitis, 907
  Takayasu arteritis, 906
  toxic alveolar hemorrhage, 909
  urticarial vasculitis, 906
  vasculitides, 908
  Wegener granulomatosis, 904–905
uncommon types of, arterial occlusive
    disease, *1023*, 1023–1025
  heparin-induced thrombocytopenia,
    1025, *1025*
  popliteal artery entrapment, 1024
  thoracic outlet compression syndrome,
    1024–1025
  thromboangiitis obliterans, 1023t,
    1023–1024
vasospastic disorders, 1025–1026
  chronic pernio, 1026
  livedo reticularis, 1026
  Raynaud phenomenon, 1025t,
    1025–1026
venous disease, 1027t, 1027–1030
  antithrombin III deficiency, 1028
  clinical evaluation of DVT, 1029–1029
  compression ultrasonography, 1029
  continuous-wave Doppler, 1029
  D-dimer, 1029
  evaluation of idiopathic DVT, 1029
  factor V mutation, 1029
  hyperhomocysteinemia, 1028
  impedance plethysmography, 1029
  leg ulcer, 1030, 1030t
  postphlebitic syndrome, 1030, *1030*

protein C deficiency, 1027
protein S deficiency, 1028
prothrombin 20210 G-A mutation,
    1029
strain-gauge outflow plethysmography,
    1029
treatment of DVT, 1029–1030
Vascular ring affecting trachea, in diagnosis
    of wheezing, 16t
Vasculitic syndromes, 961, 962t, 962–971,
    963
  differential diagnosis, 971–972t, *973*
Vasculitides, 908
Vasculitis, 676, 726
  ANCA, signs, symptoms, 669t
  clinical features, 962t
  connective tissue, as cause of
    eosinophilia, 31
  with connective tissue diseases, 971
    large vessel vasculitis, 971
    obliterative endarteropathy, 971
    small, medium-sized vessel vasculitis,
      971
  cutaneous, 969–970t
    clinical features, 969
    diagnosis, 969–970
    histopathology, 969
    treatment, outcome, 970
  diagnostic approach to, 962t
  large-vessel, 668
  medium-sized vessel, 668
  skin lesions associated with, 971–972
  syndromes mimicking, 962t
  systemic, Chapel Hill consensus on
    nomenclature, 668t
Vasoactive intestinal peptide, 269
Vasoconstrictors, 753
Vasodilators, 118, 753
  traditional, with hypertension, 521
Vasomotor rhinitis, 21
Vasopressin, 259
Vasospastic disorders, 1025–1026
  chronic pernio, 1026
  livedo reticularis, 1026
  Raynaud phenomenon, 1025t, 1025–1026
Vegetable dusts, as cause of asthma, 14
Venlafaxine, 834, 835
Venom immunotherapy, 28, 28t
  indications for, 28t
Venous disease, 1027t, 1027–1030
  antithrombin III deficiency, 1028
  clinical evaluation of DVT, 1029–1029
  compression ultrasonography, 1029
  continuous-wave Doppler, 1029
  D-dimer, 1029
  evaluation of idiopathic DVT, 1029
  factor V mutation, 1029
  hyperhomocysteinemia, 1028
  impedance plethysmography, strain-gauge
    outflow plethysmography, 1029

Venous disease *(contd.)*
    leg ulcer, 1030, 1030t
    postphlebitic syndrome, 1030, *1030*
    protein C deficiency, 1027
    protein S deficiency, 1028
    prothrombin 20210 G-A mutation, 1029
    treatment of DVT, 1029–1030
Venous thromboembolic disease
    antithrombotic therapy for, 346, 347t
    duration of treatment for, 902t
Venous thromboembolism, prevention, 344t
Ventilator support, criteria for, 153t
Ventricular escape rhythm, 79
Ventricular tachycardia, identification, 87t
Verapamil, 53, 83, 84, 105, 110, 115, 120, 522, 706, 734
Vertebral osteomyelitis, 601
Vertigo, 736–737
Vespid allergy, 28
Veterinarians, disease etiology in, 8t
Vibrio species, 557
Videx, 489
Vinblastine, 995
Vincristine, 465
Viral arthritis, 600, 1002
Viral diarrhea, 597
Viral diseases, 571–578
    Hantavirus infection, Hantavirus pulmonary syndrome, 576
    herpesviruses, 571–575
        cytomegalovirus, 573–574
        Epstein-Barr virus, 572–573t
        herpes simplex virus, 572
        human herpesvirus 6, 575
        human herpesvirus 8, 575
        varicella-zoster virus, 574–575
    human T-cell lymphotropic viruses, 578
    influenza, 575–576
    measles, 577
    mumps, 578
    parvovirus B19, 578
    poliovirus, 576
    rabies, 576
    rubella, 577
    slow viruses, prion-associated central nervous system diseases, 576–577
        Creutzfeldt-Jakob disease, 577
        progressive multifocal leukoencephalopathy, 576
        subacute sclerosing panencephalitis, 577
    viral meningoencephalitis, 578

Viral hemorrhagic fevers, 604
Viral infection, 871, 910–911. *See also under specific infection*
    Hantavirus pulmonary syndrome, 910–911
    influenza, 910
    severe acute respiratory syndrome, 911
    viral pneumonia, 910
Viral meningoencephalitis, 578
Viral pneumonia, 910
Viridans streptococci, 552
Visceral larva migrans, as cause of eosinophilia, 31
Vision changes, in elderly, 386–387
Vitamin B$_{12}$, deficiency in, 726
Vitamin C, 705
Vitamin D, 216, 217, 218, 705, 978
    supplementation, 218
Vitamin E, 727
Vitamin K, 729
    deficiency in, laboratory findings, 448t
Vocal cord adduction, psychophysiologic, 16
    in diagnosis of wheezing, 16
von Hippel-Lindau disease, 365, 368
von Willebrand disease, 365, 444–445, 450
    hemophilia A, differences between, 449t
Voriconazole, 606, 625, 626–627
Vulvovaginal candidiasis, 594

W

Waldenström macroglobulinemia, 435, 676
Warfarin, 53, 85, 109, 116, 342, 344, 347, 450, 452–453, 624, 749
    anticoagulant effect of, reversal, 347–348
Water balance, disorders, 691–693
    hypernatremia, 692–693, *693*
    hyponatremia, 691–692, *692*
        diagnosis, 691
        euvolemic hyponatremia, 692
        hypervolemic hyponatremia, 692
        hypovolemic hyponatremia, 691–692
        therapy for hyponatremia, 691
Water-cooling tower, in disease etiology, 8t
Weakness, muscle, causes, 747t
Weevil, as cause of asthma, 14
Wegener granulomatosis, 24, 178, 668, 669, 904–905, 968–969
    ANCA, 969
    clinical features, 968–969
    pathologic diagnosis, 969
    treatment and outcome, 969

Weight loss, 481
Welder's lung, 880
Welding, in disease etiology, 8t
Western red cedar, as cause of asthma, 14
Wheat, as cause of food allergy, 27
Wheezing, differential diagnosis, 16t
Whipple disease, 726
White matter lesions, 723
Wilson disease, 369, 955
Wines, red, tyramine in, 514
Withholding, withdrawing life support, 161, 658, 659t
Women's health, percentage of board examination devoted to, 2
Wood, decaying, in disease etiology, 8t
Wood dusts, as cause of asthma, 14
World Health Organization, classification of pulmonary neoplasms, 894t

X

Xanthine stones, 705
Xanthines, 700
Xanthogranuloma, necrobiotic, 182
Xanthomonas maltophilia, 555
X-linked adrenoleukodystrophy, 372
X-linked recessive conditions, 371–373
    Duchenne, Becker muscular dystrophies, 372
    Fabry disease, 373

Y

Yellow nail syndrome, 184, 877
Yersinia pestis, 556–557, 915
Young syndrome, 877

Z

Zafirlukast, 16, 16t
Zalcitabine, 489, 491, 606
Zanamivir, 631
ZDV, 489
Zenker diverticulum, 256
Zerit, 489
Zidovudine, 489, 490, 491, 494, 522, 606, 755, 756, 992
Zileuton, 16, 16t
Ziprasidone, 835
Zoledronic acid, 779
Zollinger-Ellison syndrome, 262–263
Zolmitriptan, 732
Zometa, 779
Zonisamide, 727, 729, 730
Zygomycetes, 571
Zygomycosis, 928